Fundamentals of
Sleep Medicine

Fundamentals of

Sleep Medicine

SECOND EDITION

Richard B. Berry, MD, FAASM
Professor of Medicine
University of Florida
Gainesville, Florida

Mary H. Wagner, MD, FAASM
Professor of Pediatrics
University of Florida
Gainesville, Florida

Scott M. Ryals, MD, FAASM
Sleep Physician
Atrium Health Sleep Medicine
Charlotte, North Carolina

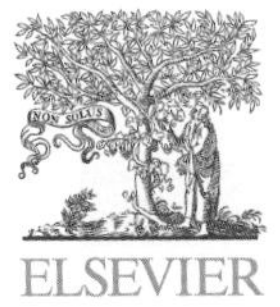

ELSEVIER

Elsevier
1600 John F. Kennedy Blvd.
Ste 1800
Philadelphia, PA 19103-2899

FUNDAMENTALS OF SLEEP MEDICINE, SECOND EDITION ISBN: 978-0-323-81081-4

Previous edition 2012

Videos 15.1, 15.2, 15.5, 18.1, 36.1, 36.2, 36.3 and 36.7 are borrowed from: Berry RB, Wagner MH. *Sleep Medicine Pearls*, 3rd ed, Philadelphia: Elsevier, 2015.

Senior Content Strategist: Melanie Tucker
Content Strategist: Mary Hegeler
Senior Content Development Specialists: Jinia Dasgupta, Priyadarshini Pandey
Publishing Services Manager: Shereen Jameel
Project Manager: Gayathri S
Design Direction: Christian Bilbow

Printed in India

Last digit is the print number: 9 8 7 6 5 4 3 2 1

This book is dedicated to our families:
David, Sarah, and Catherine Berry
Daniel, Analiese, and Barry Wagner
Will, Luke, Rosemary, and Sara Ryals
They are our greatest joy!

Preface

The goal of this book is to provide the reader with a core of fundamental knowledge regarding sleep medicine and polysomnography in a concise format with numerous figures and tables summarizing the important points. Since the first edition of *Fundamentals of Sleep Medicine* was published in 2012, there has been an explosion of information about sleep physiology and sleep disorders. A text revision of the third edition of the International Classification of Sleep Disorders (ICSD-3-TR) was published as well as Version 3.0 of the American Academy of Sleep Medicine Scoring Manual. Numerous clinical practice guidelines have been published and revised. The field of sleep medicine is changing so rapidly that any text is "out of date" before it is even published. Thus, the task of writing a second edition is one we have found quite challenging. However, our inspiration for writing the second edition is feedback from numerous readers that the first edition was valuable to them in the daily practice of sleep medicine. We have tried to cover aspects of sleep-monitoring technology and sleep study interpretation that many who are new to the field of sleep medicine find difficult.

A single text cannot hope to cover all aspects of sleep medicine and sleep physiology. Therefore, we have focused on information we feel is the most clinically useful. The goal of this book is not to be a comprehensive text of sleep physiology and sleep disorders; other excellent and much larger texts address this need. The science of sleep medicine is extremely complex and, in many areas there are many (and sometimes conflicting) models to explain fundamental processes. This book attempts to summarize relevant physiology in a manner that that is useful to the practicing clinician. However, some degree of simplification was unavoidable. The reader should supplement the information provided in this text with published updates in the literature. In summary, although this task has been challenging, we hope the second edition will serve as a useful introduction to those entering the field of sleep medicine and as a source of information for physicians actively caring for patients with sleep disorders.

Acknowledgments

We would like to express our gratitude for the support and encouragement of the University of Florida sleep physicians, including Dr. Stephan Eisenschenk, Dr. Michael Jaffee, Dr. Emily Beck, Dr. Susheela Hadigal, and Dr. Semiramis Carbajal Mamani, as well as physicians in clinical practice, including Dr. Michael Johnson, Dr. Holly Skinner, and Dr. Craig Foster. It is a pleasure to work with such a dedicated and talented group of individuals.

The patience and assistance of the Elsevier editorial staff is also greatly appreciated. Melanie Tucker, Senior Content Strategist, was instrumental in developing the concept for the book and provided critical support in the planning stages. Mary Hegeler, Content Strategist, provided encouragement during the final stages of book preparation. Priyadarshini Pandey, Senior Content Development Specialist, helped assemble the chapters and many figures. We are also grateful for the patience and diligence of Gayathri S, Project Manager, during the production process.

Contents

Video Table of Contents

36.8: Kicking during rapid eye movement (REM) sleep during continuous positive airway pressure (CPAP) titration. The patient is wearing a chin strap.

36.9: Rapid eye movement (REM) sleep behavior disorder—falling out of bed. This patient experiences an episode of activity occurring out of REM sleep. He sits up, moves his arms, and wakes up as he begins for fall out of bed. His eyes are closed during this episode.

36.10: Talking and violent movements during rapid eye movement (REM) sleep (REM sleep behavior disorder). The patient is dreaming about snakes and hitting them (she talks about big snakes).

36.11: Rapid eye movement (REM) sleep behavior disorder. This is an episode of violent movements (trying to hit snakes) during REM sleep. At the end of the episode, the patient says, "Go away from me." The snoring and coughing are from the patient's daughter, who slept in the monitoring room. In the unblurred version of the video, one can see that the patient's eyes are closed during the event.

36.12: An example of catathrenia in a 24-year-old woman wearing a sleep mask. A very short episode is followed by an arousal, then a longer episode of expiratory groaning. The events appear to be central apneas but occur during exhalation. (Note: increase the volume to hear the groaning.) Here, catathrenia is noted out of non–rapid eye movement (NREM) sleep.

Sleep Stages and Basic Sleep Monitoring

Chapter 1

SLEEP STAGE NOMENCLATURE

Sleep is divided into non–rapid eye movement (NREM) and rapid eye movement (REM) sleep. Sleep staging is based on electroencephalographic (EEG), electrooculographic (EOG), and submental (chin) electromyographic (EMG) criteria. EOG (eye movement recording) and chin EMG are used to detect REM sleep, which is characterized by REMs and reduced muscle tone. From 1968 to 2007 sleep was staged according to *A Manual of Standardized Terminology, Techniques and Scoring System for Sleep Stages of Human Subjects,* edited by Rechtschaffen and Kales (R&K).[1] In the R&K scoring manual, NREM sleep was divided into sleep stages 1, 2, 3, and 4. REM sleep was referred to as stage REM. Sleep stage nomenclature changed after the publication of the American Academy of Sleep Medicine (AASM) *Manual for the Scoring of Sleep and Associated Events: Rules, Terminology and Technical Specifications* (hereinafter the AASM scoring manual) in 2007.[2,3] The new nomenclature was introduced to denote sleep stages defined by new criteria. The old and new nomenclatures are shown in Table 1–1. Stages 3 and 4 are combined into stage N3. Stage W refers to Wakefulness in both the R&K and AASM scoring manual nomenclature. Revisions of the AASM scoring manual are published as needed to update and clarify scoring rules, and the reader should consult the latest version.[4]

Today, digital polysomnography (PSG) (complex sleep recording) has replaced recording on paper. However, previously sleep recording was performed with polygraphs using ink writing pens with a paper speed of 10 mm/second. At this paper speed, a 30-cm page of paper contained 30 seconds of recording. A sleep stage was identified for each page (30 seconds), termed an *epoch*. The tradition of staging sleep in 30-second epochs has been retained in the AASM scoring manual. The sleep stage assigned to each epoch is the stage occupying the majority of time within that epoch. Digital recording allows display of data in one of several time windows (typically 5, 10, 30, 60, 90, 120, and 240 seconds). The 10-second window corresponds to a paper speed of 30 mm/second and is used for clinical EEG monitoring; it also approximates the appearance of electrocardiographic (ECG) recording that was typically performed using a paper speed of 25 mm/second before the current use of digital ECG recording.

EEG MONITORING DURING SLEEP

Understanding EEG monitoring during PSG requires knowledge of EEG electrode placement, EEG derivations, and important EEG patterns. These topics will be discussed in the following sections.

EEG Electrode Placement

The nomenclature for the EEG electrodes follows the International 10–20 system.[5] The "10–20" refers to the fact that the electrodes are positioned at either 10% or 20% of the distance between landmarks. The major landmarks include the nasion (where the top of the bridge of the nose meets the forehead), inion (prominence at base of the occiput), and preauricular points (Figs. 1–1 and 1–2). In the 10–20 system, even-numbered subscripts refer to the right side of the head and odd-numbered subscripts to the left. The nomenclature of EEG electrodes used for sleep monitoring is listed in Table 1–2. Electrodes are named for the part of the brain they are over. For example, **Fp1** and **Fp2** are the left and right **frontal pole** electrodes, **F3** and **F4** are the left and right **frontal** electrodes, **C3** and **C4** are the left and right **central** electrodes, and **O1** and **O2** are the left and right **occipital** electrodes. Electrodes in the midline in the frontopolar, frontal, central, and occipital regions are named Fpz, Fz, Cz, and Oz, respectively. The position of the electrode Cz is at the top of the head and is called the **vertex.** In EEG monitoring electrodes are placed on the ear lobes and are denoted as A1 (left) and A2 (right). However, in sleep monitoring electrodes are placed on the left and right mastoid areas and in the AASM scoring manual nomenclature are named **M1** (left) and **M2** (right).

EEG Derivations

EEG signals are displayed as voltage differences between two electrodes. The term **derivation** refers to a set of two electrodes (and the voltage difference between the electrodes). The term **montage** refers to a set of derivations. The AASM scoring manual[4] recommends that the following EEG electrodes be placed for sleep monitoring (F3, F4, C3, C4, O1, O2, M1, and M2). In sleep monitoring, electrodes in the frontal, central, and occipital electrodes are referenced against the contralateral **mastoid electrode. The EEG derivations recommended for staging sleep by the AASM scoring manual are F4-M1, C4-M1, and O2-M1 (standard derivations in** Table 1-3**).** The AASM scoring manual also lists backup derivations (F3-M2, C3-M2, and O1-M2) that are displayed if one of the electrodes in the recommended derivations malfunctions during the study (additional derivations in Table 1-3). For example, if electrode F4 or M1 malfunction during the study, the derivations **F3-M2,** C4-M1, and O2-M1 are used (not F3-M1). That is, if F3 must be used instead of F4 it is referenced against M2 not M1. Note that derivations C4-M1 and O2-M1 can still be used. If M1 fails, then the backup derivations using M2 are displayed. In digital recording, one can easily display all six derivations (F4-M1, F3-M2, C4-M1, C3-M2, O2-M1, O1-M2) if desired at the same time. Of note, in the original R&K scoring manual, only central derivations were used to stage sleep. Although the recommended derivations are the most widely used, the AASM scoring manual lists alternative **acceptable** derivations (Fz-Cz, Cz-Oz, C4-M1). The acceptable derivations use the electrodes Fz, Cz, Oz, C4, and M1 with the backup electrodes Fpz (to replace Fz), C3 (to replace Cz or C4),

Table 1–1 Sleep Stage Nomenclature

	R&K	AASM
Wake	Stage W	Stage W
NREM	Stage 1 Stage 2 Stage 3 Stage 4	Stage N1 Stage N2 Stage N3
REM	Stage REM	Stage R

Stages 3 and 4 are combined into stage N3, Stage W (Wakefulness).
AASM, American Academy of Sleep Medicine; *NREM,* non–rapid eye movement; *R&K,* Rechtschaffen and Kales; *REM,* rapid eye movement.

O1 (to replace Oz), and M2 (to replace M1) if electrodes in the acceptable derivations malfunction during the study.

Commonly used additional electrodes beyond those discussed in the AASM scoring manual include a ground electrode and a common reference electrode(s). In sleep monitoring, a ground electrode is usually placed at or near Fpz and connected to the isolated ground (or iso-ground) input on the electrode box. As discussed in Chapter 2, the ground is used to balance the individual AC differential amplifiers giving them a common reference. One electrode (or two linked electrodes) is also placed to serve as a reference for referential recording (see Chapter 2). The reference electrode(s) are commonly placed at or near Cz depending on which EEG electrodes are to be

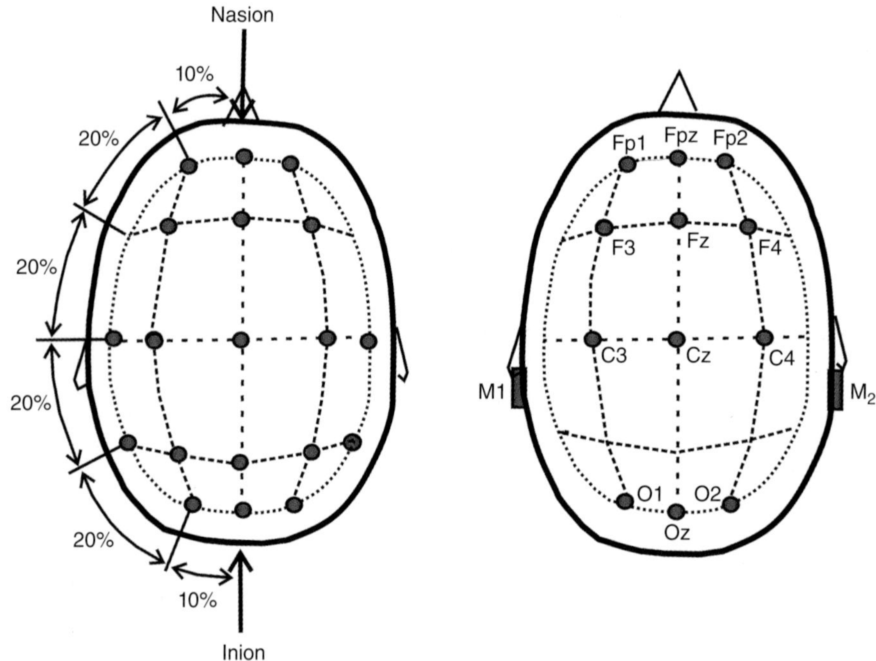

Figure 1–1 Top view of electrode positions using the 10–20 system. (Adapted from Berry RB. *Fundamentals of Sleep Medicine.* Saunders; 2012:2.)

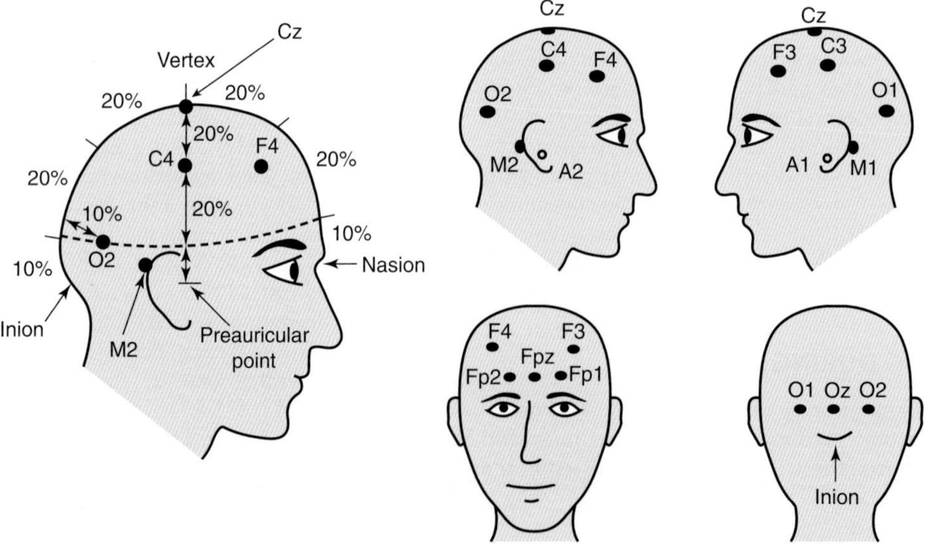

Figure 1–2 Electrode positions using the 10-20 system. A1 and A2 are earlobe (auricular) electrodes described in the electroencephalographic literature. However, the left and right mastoid electrodes (M1 and M2) are used in sleep monitoring. (Adapted from Berry RB. *Fundamentals of Sleep Medicine.* Saunders; 2012:3.)

Table 1–2 Electroencephalographic Electrode Nomenclature

	Left	Right	Midline
Frontopolar	Fp1	Fp2	Fpz
Frontal	F3	F4	Fz
Central	C3	C4	Cz
Occipital	O1	O2	Oz
Mastoid	M1	M2	

Table 1–3 Electroencephalographic Derivations Used to Stage Sleep

Standard	Additional
F4-M1	F3-M2
C4-M1	C3-M2
O2-M1	O2-M2

recorded for sleep monitoring. Some digital PSG systems do not use a dedicated reference electrode(s) and instead use linked standard electrodes as the reference (e.g., C3-C4).

EEG Waveform Patterns

Recognition of certain characteristic EEG waveform patterns is essential for sleep staging.[1-4] EEG activity is recorded using a differential AC amplifier such that the signal recorded is the **difference in voltage** between two inputs (G1 and G2). By EEG convention, if input G1 is **negative** with respect to G2, this results in an **upward** deflection (negative up polarity). As noted previously, the term *derivation* is used to describe the differential signal between two inputs. For example, in the derivation C4-M1, a change in the voltage between these electrodes results in an upward deflection if C4 is negative with respect to M1. EEG activity is described by frequency in cycles per second (hertz [Hz]), amplitude (microvolts [μV]), and shape. The classically described EEG frequency ranges are delta (0 to 3.99 Hz), theta (4 to 7.99 Hz), alpha (8–13 Hz), and beta (>13 Hz).[4] Activity that is faster results in narrower deflections and slower frequency results in wider deflections. **Sharp waves** are narrow waves of 70 to 200 msec duration, and **spikes** have an even shorter duration of 20 to 70 msec.

Some of the EEG waveforms important for sleep staging are illustrated in Figure 1–3 with their major characteristics detailed in Figures 1–4 and 1–5. In addition to frequency, the region of highest activity (amplitude) and the effects of maneuvers on the EEG activity are also important for waveform identification. The term *alpha activity* is used to describe any EEG activity with a frequency in the alpha range (8–13 Hz). However, **posterior dominant rhythm** (PDR, also known as alpha rhythm in adults) consists of alpha activity most prominent in occipital derivations that is attenuated by eye opening and increased by eye closure. The term *posterior dominant rhythm* instead of *alpha rhythm* is preferred as the frequency of occipital activity attenuated by eye opening and increased by eye closure has a frequency lower than 8 Hz in infants and young children (see Chapter 5). An important part of biocalibrations (see Chapter 2) at the start of sleep recording is to ask patients to close and then open their eyes to document if they produce alpha rhythm (PDR) with eye closure. About 10% of normal individuals do not demonstrate PDR with eye closure and an additional 10% generate limited alpha rhythm.[2,3] As discussed in Chapter 3, scoring sleep onset is different if an individual does not generate alpha rhythm with eye closure. Bursts of alpha waves often occur during stage R typically at a frequency 1 to 2 Hz slower than during wakefulness.[3,6] Prominent alpha activity in frontal and central derivations during NREM sleep is also noted in individuals with

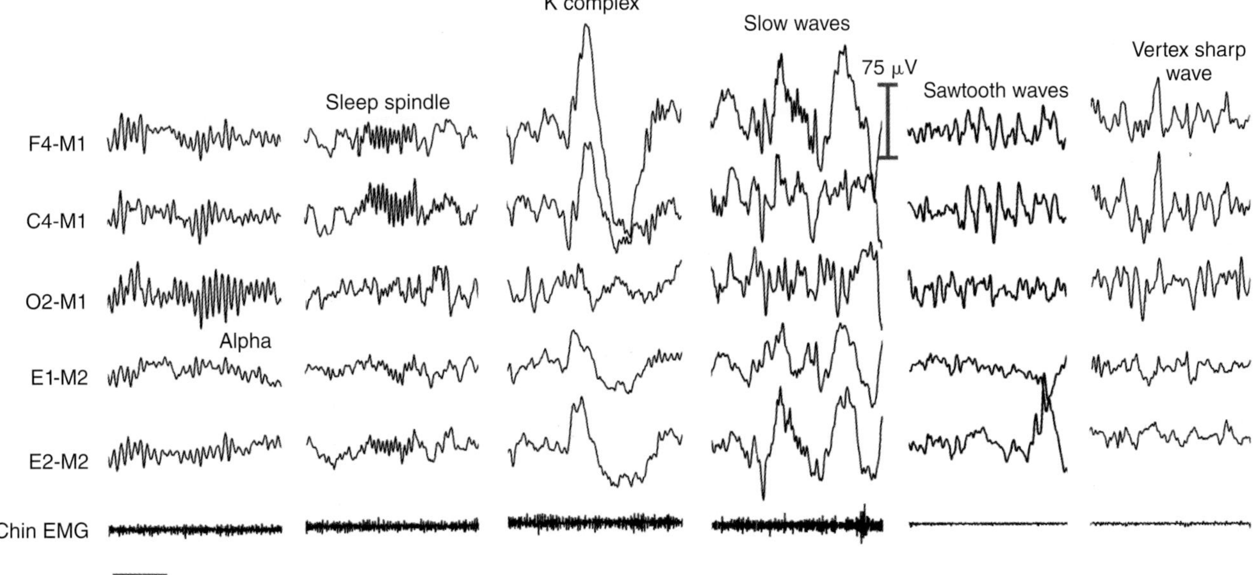

Figure 1–3 Common electroencephalographic waveforms useful for staging sleep. (Adapted from Berry RB, Wagner MH. *Sleep Medicine Pearls*. 3rd ed. Elsevier; 2015:11.)

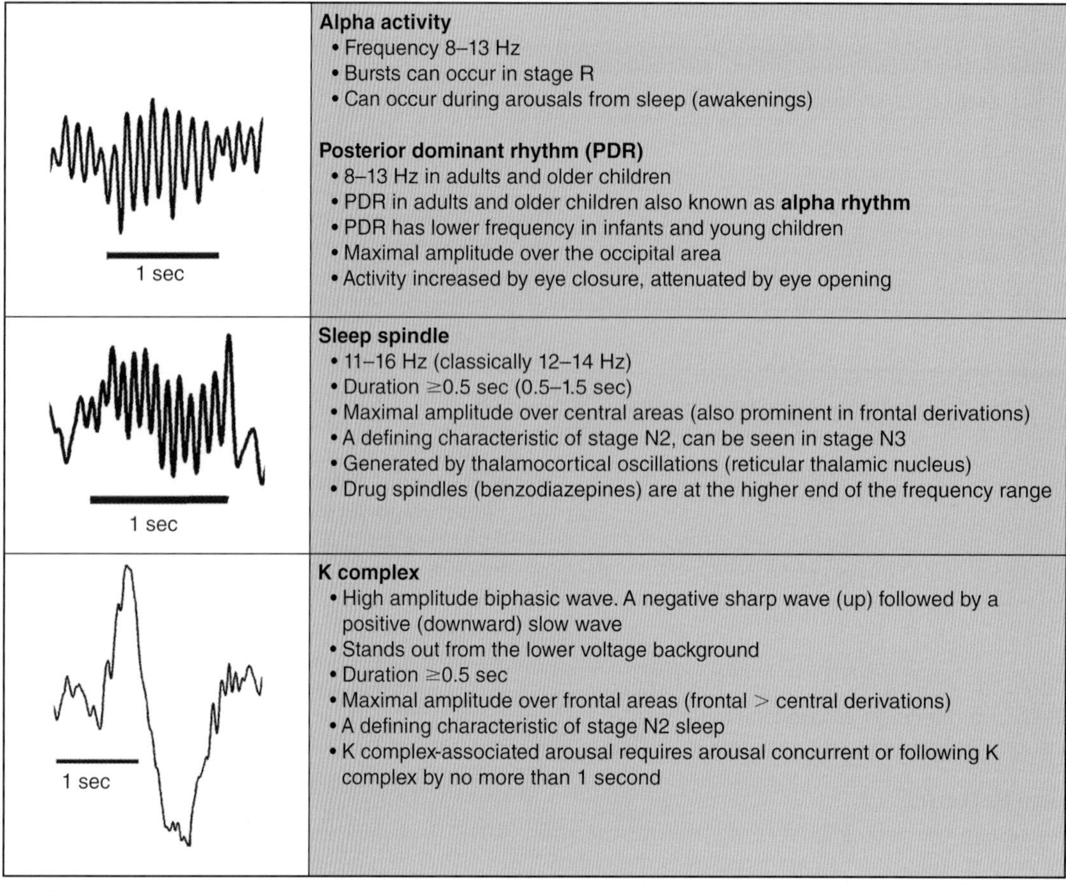

1 sec
Alpha activity
• Frequency 8–13 Hz
• Bursts can occur in stage R
• Can occur during arousals from sleep (awakenings)
Posterior dominant rhythm (PDR)
• 8–13 Hz in adults and older children
• PDR in adults and older children also known as alpha rhythm
• PDR has lower frequency in infants and young children
• Maximal amplitude over the occipital area
• Activity increased by eye closure, attenuated by eye opening
1 sec
Sleep spindle
• 11–16 Hz (classically 12–14 Hz)
• Duration ≥0.5 sec (0.5–1.5 sec)
• Maximal amplitude over central areas (also prominent in frontal derivations)
• A defining characteristic of stage N2, can be seen in stage N3
• Generated by thalamocortical oscillations (reticular thalamic nucleus)
• Drug spindles (benzodiazepines) are at the higher end of the frequency range
1 sec
K complex
• High amplitude biphasic wave. A negative sharp wave (up) followed by a positive (downward) slow wave
• Stands out from the lower voltage background
• Duration ≥0.5 sec
• Maximal amplitude over frontal areas (frontal > central derivations)
• A defining characteristic of stage N2 sleep
• K complex-associated arousal requires arousal concurrent or following K complex by no more than 1 second

Figure 1–4 Properties of some important electroencephalographic waveforms used for staging sleep. Here alpha activity, posterior dominant rhythm, a sleep spindle, and a K complex are illustrated. (Adapted from Berry RB, Wagner MH. *Sleep Medicine Pearls*. 3rd ed. Elsevier; 2015:11.)

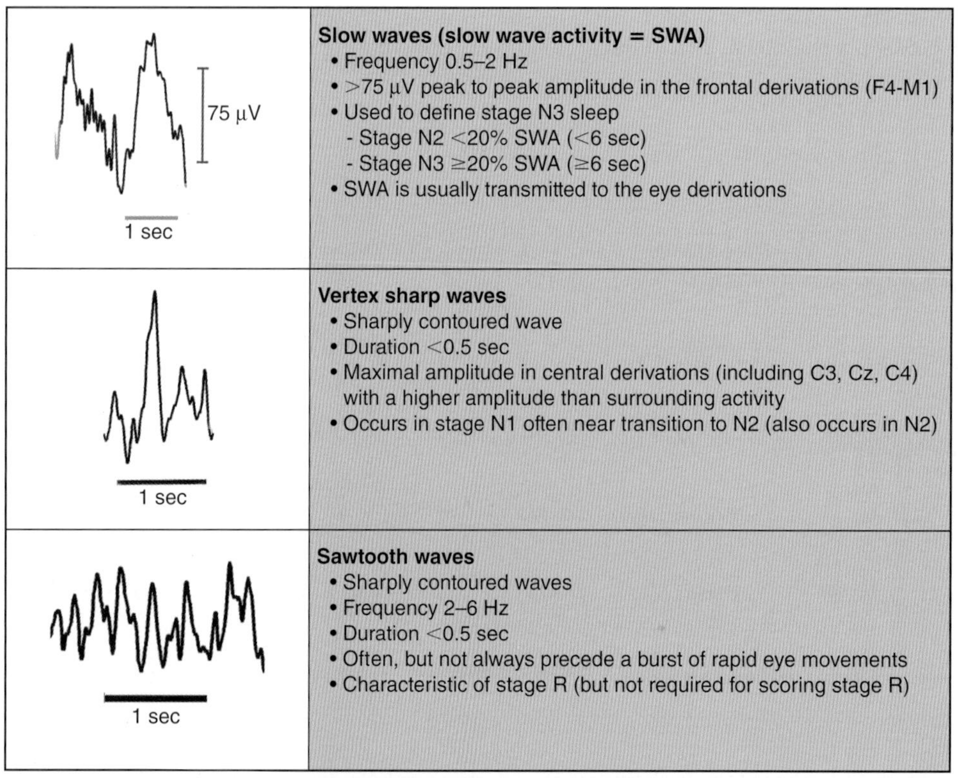

75 μV
1 sec
Slow waves (slow wave activity = SWA)
• Frequency 0.5–2 Hz
• >75 μV peak to peak amplitude in the frontal derivations (F4-M1)
• Used to define stage N3 sleep
- Stage N2 <20% SWA (<6 sec)
- Stage N3 ≥20% SWA (≥6 sec)
• SWA is usually transmitted to the eye derivations
1 sec
Vertex sharp waves
• Sharply contoured wave
• Duration <0.5 sec
• Maximal amplitude in central derivations (including C3, Cz, C4) with a higher amplitude than surrounding activity
• Occurs in stage N1 often near transition to N2 (also occurs in N2)
1 sec
Sawtooth waves
• Sharply contoured waves
• Frequency 2–6 Hz
• Duration <0.5 sec
• Often, but not always precede a burst of rapid eye movements
• Characteristic of stage R (but not required for scoring stage R)

Figure 1–5 Waveforms used for staging sleep. Here slow waves, a vertex sharp wave, and sawtooth waves are illustrated. Although the presence or absence of sawtooth waves does not define stage R, this waveform is characteristic of that sleep stage and may assist in recognition of stage R. Frontal derivations are C4-M1 or C3-M2. (Adapted from Berry RB, Wagner MH. *Sleep Medicine Pearls*. 3rd ed. Elsevier; 2015:11.)

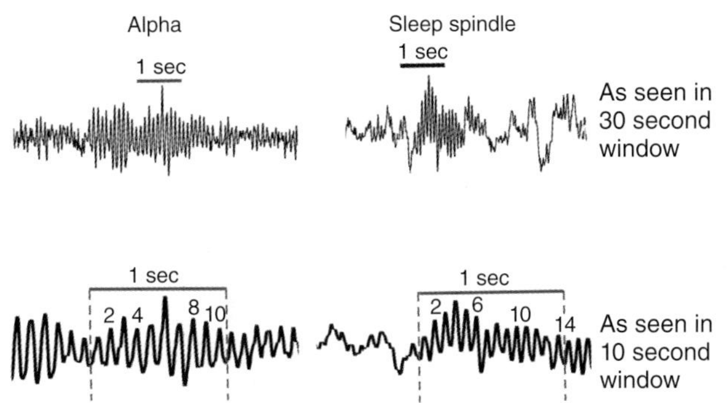

Figure 1–6 Alpha activity and a sleep spindle are shown as seen in a 30-second window and a 10-second window. Counting the number of waves in 1 second can help differentiate alpha activity (8–13 Hz) and sleep spindles (11–16 Hz), although there is some overlap in frequency. Posterior dominant rhythm (alpha rhythm in adults and older children) is most prominent in occipital derivations.

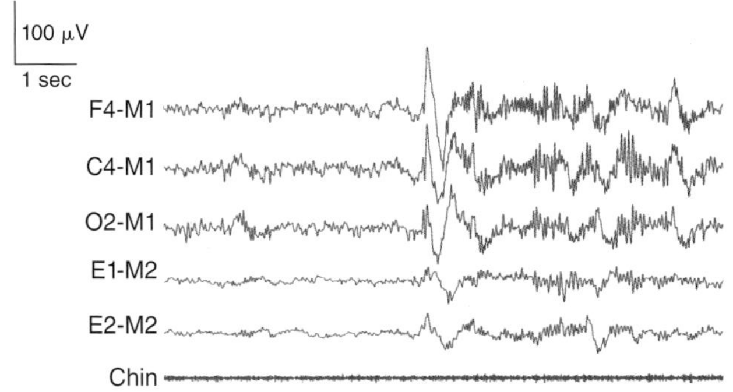

Figure 1–7 A 20-second tracing showing a K complex associated with an arousal. (Adapted from Berry RB, Wagner MH. *Sleep Medicine Pearls.* 3rd ed. Elsevier; 2015:21.)

alpha sleep anomaly (sometimes referred to as alpha intrusion) (see Chapter 4).

Sleep spindles[1-4,7,8] are bursts of activity with a frequency range of 11 to 16 Hz (usually 12–14) with a duration of 0.5 second or greater (usually 0.5–1.5 seconds). The term *spindle* is used because the shape of sleep spindle bursts sometimes resembles a yarn spindle (larger in the middle and smaller on both ends). If there is uncertainty about whether activity is a burst of alpha activity or a sleep spindle, one can display a 10-second window (see Fig. 1–6) and count the deflections (waves) per second. Sleep spindles are usually maximal in amplitude in central derivations but can occasionally be more prominent in frontal derivations. Some studies have suggested that spindles of a slower frequency (≈12 Hz) are more prominent over frontal brain areas, whereas faster spindles (≈14 Hz) are more prominent over central-parietal areas.[7-9] In contrast, alpha rhythm is maximal in amplitude in occipital derivations. Sleep spindles arise from thalamocortical oscillations. The **reticular nucleus** of the thalamus is responsible for generating sleep spindles.

A **K complex**[1-4,8] is a high-amplitude biphasic wave composed of an initial negative sharp wave (deflection up) followed by a slow wave (Figs. 1–3 and 1–4). A burst of spindle activity is often superimposed on a K complex. A K complex stands out from the lower voltage background. K complex amplitude is greatest in frontal derivations (also central > occipital). A K complex is said to be associated with an arousal if the arousal is either concurrent with the K complex or if the arousal commences no more than 1 second after the termination of the K complex.[4] An arousal during sleep stages N1, N2, and N3 is scored if there is an abrupt shift of EEG frequency including alpha, theta, and/or frequencies greater than 16 Hz (but not spindles) that lasts at least 3 seconds, with at least 10 seconds of stable sleep preceding the change.[2,4] Scoring arousals during stage R also requires 1 second or more of an increase in the chin EMG concurrent with the arousal. Arousals are discussed in more detail in Chapter 3. An example of a K complex associated with an arousal is shown in Figure 1–7. Also note that the K complex activity is visualized in the EOG derivations E1-M1 and E2-M2 as in-phase deflections. Eye movements and EOG electrodes are discussed later.

As noted previously, the frequency of delta activity is less than 4 Hz. EEG activity in this range produces relatively wide duration deflections, often called *delta* or *slow waves* (see Figs. 1–3 and 1–5). However, for sleep staging, the designation **slow wave activity (SWA)**[2-4] specifically refers to waves with a frequency range of 0.5 to 2 Hz (2 to 0.5 seconds duration) and peak-to-peak amplitude of **greater** than 75 μV in the **frontal derivations** (F4-M1,F3-M2). Slow waves have the greatest amplitude over the frontal areas. K complexes that meet SWA criteria can be considered slow waves and included in the determination of the duration of SWA. Of note, sleep staging according to the R&K manual used only central derivations. Because slow wave amplitude is higher over the frontal areas, a given epoch of EEG activity would be expected to have greater SWA (greater duration meeting amplitude criteria) using the AASM scoring manual definition[2,4] (frontal derivations) compared with the R&K manual (using central derivations) in some patients. The recommended derivation for determining SWA is F4-M1 (or F3-M2 if necessary). If using the acceptable EEG derivations, Fz-Cz is not appropriate for determination of slow wave activity. Using a differential AC amplifier, the activity common to both electrodes is rejected, and because Fz and Cz are close together, this reduces the amplitude of slow wave activity. If using acceptable EEG derivations and acceptable EOG derivations (as discussed in the next section), E1-Fpz is used to determine slow wave activity. Used in this way, Fpz will be the active electrode recording frontal activity and E1 the reference electrode. If using the acceptable EEG derivations and recommended EOG derivations, C4-M1 (or C3-M2 if either the C4 or M1 electrodes malfuntion) is used to determine slow wave activity.

Vertex sharp waves (see Figs. 1–3 and 1–5) are narrow-duration waves (<500 msec measured at the base of the wave according to the AASM scoring manual[2,4]) prominent in derivations containing electrodes near the vertex (Cz, C3, C4). They are often seen near the transition between stage N1 and stage N2 sleep but can occur in either sleep stage. **Sawtooth waves** (see Figs. 1–3 and 1–5) occur during REM sleep, although they are not always present during this sleep stage. They are triangular waves of 2 to 6 Hz of highest amplitude in the central derivations. The presence of sawtooth waves is not required to score stage R. However, the presence of sawtooth waves is very helpful for stage R recognition when they are noted.

EOG MONITORING FOR SLEEP

Recording of eye movements is possible because a potential difference exists across the eyeball with the front/cornea

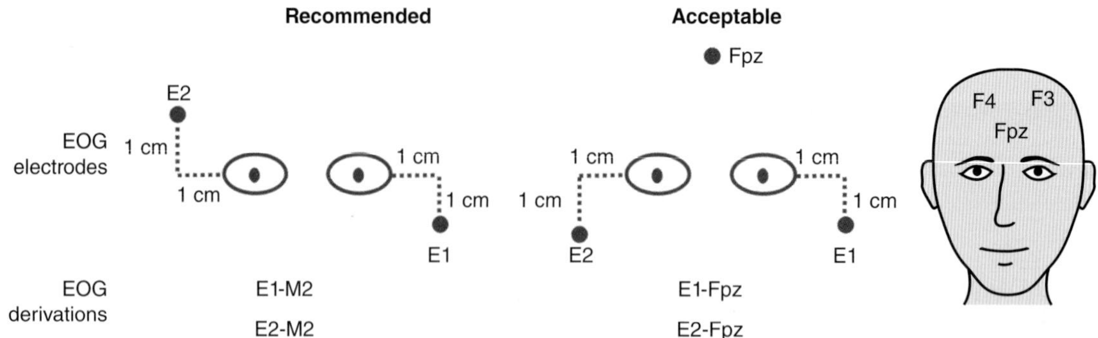

Figure 1–8 Electrooculographic electrode positions and derivations (recommended and acceptable) as specified in the *AASM Manual for the Scoring of Sleep and Associated Events: Rules, Terminology and Technical Specifications.*

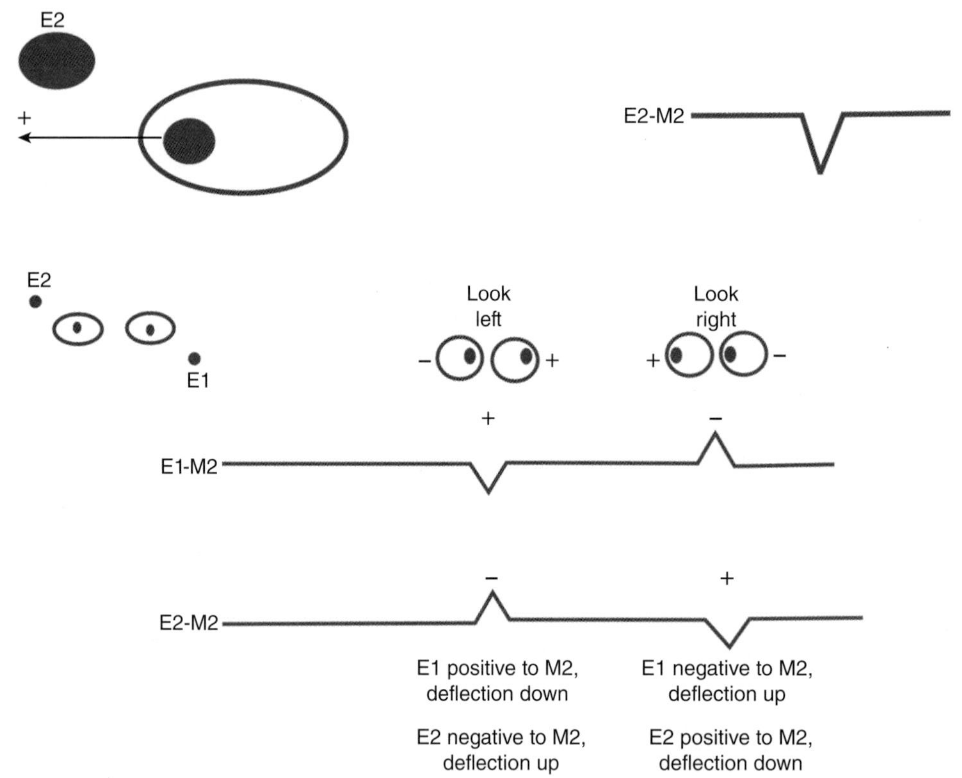

Figure 1–9 Schematic showing the effect of lateral eye movements on deflections in the electrooculographic derivations. Remember the front of the eye is positive and when moving toward E1 or E2 causes a downward deflection in E1-M2 or E2-M2. (Adapted from Berry RB. *Fundamentals of Sleep Medicine*. Saunders Elsevier; 2012:7.)

positive (+) and back/retina negative (−). Eye movements are detected by EOG electrodes (near the eyes) recording voltage changes associated with eye movement.

EOG Electrode Placement and EOG Derivations

The **recommended** EOG electrodes in the AASM scoring manual[2,4] are illustrated in Figure 1–8. E1 and E2 refer to the left and right eye electrodes, respectively. Previously EOG electrodes were named *right outer canthus (ROC)* and *left outer canthus (LOC)*. Electrode E1 is placed 1 cm below and 1 cm lateral to the LOC, and E2 is located 1 cm above and 1 cm lateral to the ROC. Because E1 is below and E2 above the eyes, both vertical and horizontal eye movement can be detected. The **recommended EOG derivations** are E1-M2 and E2-M2. Note that M2 is used in both derivations. If electrode M2 fails, then electrode M1 is used for EOG monitoring.

The AASM scoring manual also specifies **acceptable** (alternative) EOG electrodes and EOG derivations. Electrode E1 is located 1 cm below and 1 cm lateral to the LOC, and E2 is located 1 cm below and E2 is located 1 cm below and 1 cm lateral to the ROC (Fig. 1–8). The E1 placement is the same as the recommended E1 electrode but the location of the acceptable E2 electrode is different (below rather than above the ROC). The **acceptable** EOG derivations are E1-Fpz and E2-Fpz using the central frontopolar electrode (Fpz) as the reference electrode for both E1 and E2 (see Fig. 1–8).

When the eyes move toward an electrode, a positive voltage is recorded (Fig. 1–9). EOG recording follows the same polarity convention used in EEG recording. That is, if an eye electrode is negative compared with the reference electrode (M2), the signal has an upward deflection. Thus, eye movement (cornea +) **toward an electrode** referenced to another electrode further away from the eyes results in a **downward** deflection. In the recommended EOG derivations, eye movements result in **out-of-phase deflections.** This is because eye movements are conjugate (both eyes move laterally or vertically in the same direction). That is, they both move toward one EOG electrode and away from the other EOG electrode. The polarity of the eye electrodes determines the net voltage difference of the EOG derivations because the electrodes are much closer to the eyes than M2. The schematic in Figure 1–9 illustrates eye movements and the resulting deflections (this assumes that both eye derivation tracings have the standard negative polarity upward). Note that when the **acceptable** EOG derivations E1-Fpz and E2-Fpz are used, both E1 and E2 are 1 cm *below* and 1 cm lateral to the LOC and ROC, respectively. In this scheme, **vertical** eye movements result in **in-phase deflections** and **lateral** eye movements result in **out-of-phase deflections.** Upward movement results in an upward deflection (E1 and E2 more negative than Fpz) and downward movement results in a downward defection (both E1 and E2 more positive than Fpz). The advantages of the **acceptable** EOG derivations are that vertical eye movements tend to produce larger deflections (e.g., vertical REMs and blinks are more prominent), and one can also distinguish vertical (in-phase) from horizontal (out-of-phase) eye movements. In addition, it is easy to remember that downward eye movements result in downward deflections in the eye derivations, and upward eye movements result in upward deflections. Alternatively, the **recommended** eye derivations make it easier to recognize EEG activity transmitted to the eye derivations (e.g., activity associated with a K complex), which results in in-phase deflections, whereas eye movements cause out-of-phase deflections (Fig. 1–10).

Eye Movement Patterns

Typical eye movement patterns include blinks, slow eye movements, REMs, and reading eye movements (Fig. 1–11). Slow eye movements consist of fairly sinusoidal conjugate movements with an initial deflection greater than 0.5 seconds and are typically noted during drowsy wakefulness with the eyes closed and stage N1 sleep. Rapid eye movements (REMs) are conjugate, irregular, sharply peaked eye movements with an initial deflection of less than 0.5 seconds and are seen in eyes open wakefulness or stage R sleep. During wakefulness the chin EMG activity is high, and during stage R the activity is low. Slow eye movements typically disappear with the onset of stage N2 sleep. However, patients taking selective serotonin reuptake inhibitors (SSRIs) can have eye movements that are a mixture of slow and more rapid activity that persist into stage N2.[10,11] This pattern is called "Prozac eyes," which can occur with patients taking fluoxetine but can also occur with any SSRI (see Chapter 4).

Blinks are vertical eye movements (fast eyelid closure and then opening) that usually occur during wakefulness but also may occur during sleep. They are typically short in duration, less than 0.5 seconds. Knowledge about the Bell phenomenon is helpful for understanding the EOG pattern of blinks or changes in the EOG derivations with the eyes opening or closing. The Bell phenomenon consists of a reflex upward movement of the eye globe with eyelid closure. With eye opening, the globe returns to a neutral position (Fig. 1–12). A blink consists of fast eye movement upward with a return to neutral. The movement away from E1 results in an initial upward deflection in E1-M2 and toward E2 results in a downward deflection in E2-M2 (Fig. 1–12).

The EOG pattern of reading eye movements (Fig. 1–13) occurs because of a slow gaze to the right (reading from left to right) followed by fast eye movement to the left (to begin reading the next line of print). The slow gaze to the right results in a slowly increasing upward deflection in E1-M2 and downward deflection in E2-M2 (Fig. 1–13). The quick eye movement to the left results in a sharp downward deflection in E1-M2 and an upward deflection in E2-M2. Observation of the patient reading on the synchronized video recorded with the sleep study can confirm that reading did produce the observed EOG pattern.

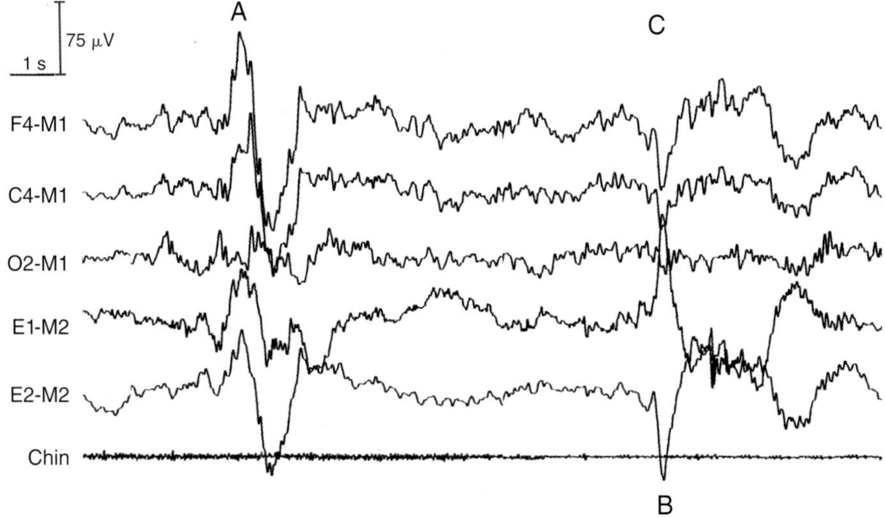

Figure 1–10 A 15-second tracing of a K complex associated with in-phase deflections in the electrooculographic derivations (A), whereas rapid eye movements (REMs) result in out-of-phase deflections (B). Also note that the REM (at B) results in a deflection in F4-M1 (C) as F4 is relatively close to the right eye. Deflections in F4-M1 and E2-M2 from eye movements are in the same direction as both F4 and E2 are on the right side and positioned above the eyes.

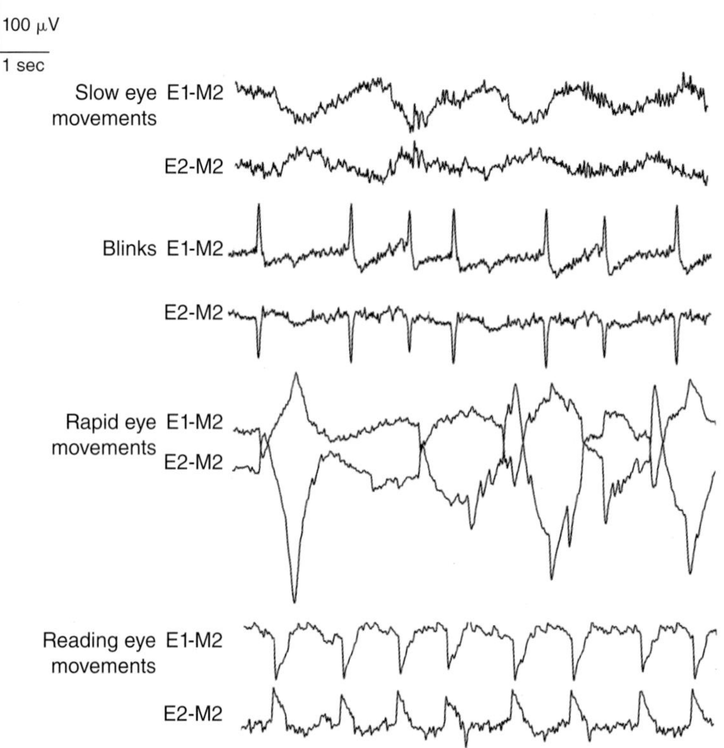

Figure 1–11 Common eye movement patterns during sleep. (Adapted from Berry RB. *Fundamentals of Sleep Medicine*. Saunders Elsevier; 2012:9.)

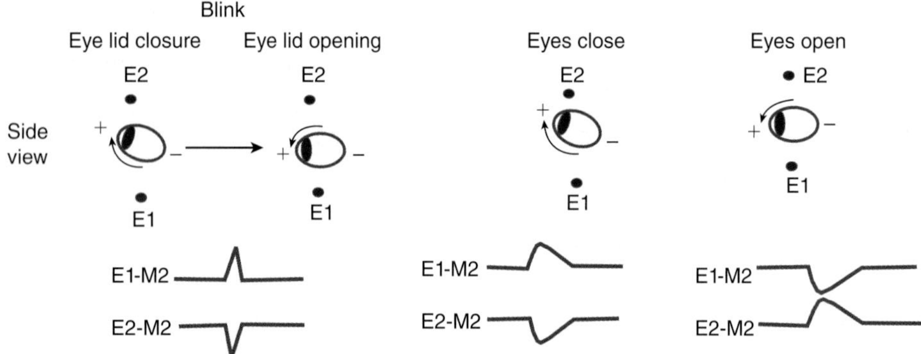

Figure 1–12 Effects of blinks, eye closure, and eye opening on electrooculographic derivations. Closure of the eyelid results in upward rotation of the eye and eyelid opening results in a return to a neutral position. (Adapted from Berry RB, Wagner MH. *Sleep Medicine Pearls*. 3rd ed. Elsevier; 2015:13.)

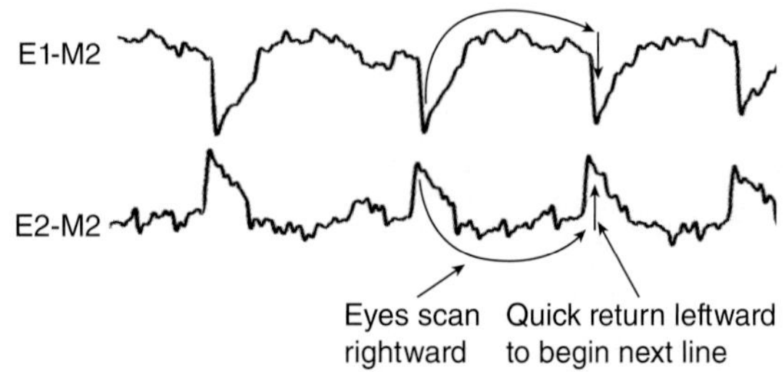

Figure 1–13 Etiology of electrooculographic activity during reading (reading eye movements). When reading, the eyes scan slowly to the right and then quickly return to the left to read the next line. (Adapted from Berry RB, Wagner MH. *Sleep Medicine Pearls*. 3rd ed. Elsevier; 2015:13.)

It is also worth noting that vertical eye movements including REMs (stage W and stage R) or those associated with opening and closing of the eyelids may result in deflections in frontal derivations as F3 and F4 are relatively close to the eyes (Fig. 1–10). With eyelid closure the eyes move upward (downward deflection in F3-M2 and F4-M1), and with opening and eye movement downward there is an upward deflection in the frontal derivations.

CHIN (SUBMENTAL) EMG MONITORING

The AASM scoring manual defines the position and nomenclature of the chin electrodes (Fig. 1–14). ChinZ

Three electrodes are recommended to record the chin EMG

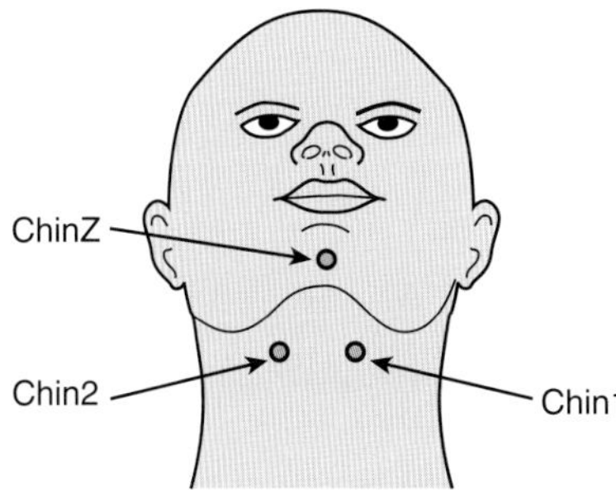

ChinZ electrode	Midline 1 cm above inferior edge of mandible
Chin2 electrode	2 cm below inferior edge of the mandible and 2 cm to the right of the midline
Chin1 electrode	2 cm below inferior edge of mandible and 2 cm to the left of the midline

Recommended Chin EMG derivations: Chin1 - ChinZ or Chin2 - ChinZ

Figure 1–14 Positions of the chin electrodes and recommended chin electromyographic derivations as specified in the *American Academy of Sleep Medicine Manual for the Scoring of Sleep and Associated Events.* The recommended derivations are to use either electrode below the mandible referred to the midline electrode above the mandible. (Adapted from Berry RB. *Fundamentals of Sleep Medicine.* Saunders; 2012:9.)

refers to the midline electrode above the mandible and Chin1 and Chin2 refer to the electrodes below the mandible on the patient's left (Chin1) and right (Chin2). The recommended derivations are either Chin1-ChinZ or Chin2-ChinZ. The electrode not used in the displayed derivation is placed as a backup. For example, if the Chin1 electrode is faulty the derivation Chin2-ChinZ is used for staging sleep. If ChinZ is faulty, ideally it should be replaced. If this is not feasible, the derivation Chin1-Chin2 can be used.[4] The monitoring of chin EMG activity is *an essential element only for identifying stage R (REM sleep) and arousals from stage R.* In stage R, the chin EMG is relatively reduced, that is, the amplitude is equal to or lower than the lowest chin EMG amplitude during NREM sleep. Chin activity during stage R is the lowest during recording. Chin EMG amplitude during other sleep stages is variable. Depending on the EMG channel sensitivity (gain), a reduction in EMG amplitude from wakefulness to sleep and often a further reduction on transition from stage N1 to stage N2 to stage N3 may be seen. A further drop may be seen on transition from NREM to REM sleep. However, the chin EMG activity may drop to the stage R level several epochs before the onset of REM sleep. In Figure 1–10, a subtle fall in chin EMG amplitude is noted at the transition to Stage R just before REMs occur. Of note, the reduction in chin EMG amplitude during REM sleep reflects the generalized skeletal muscle hypotonia present in this sleep stage. In sleep tracings in this book "chin EMG" is used for brevity to identify the chin activity channel with the understanding that the actual EMG derivation is either Chin1-ChinZ or Chin2-ChinZ.

SUMMARY OF KEY POINTS

1. In the EEG or EOG derivation G1-G2, an upward deflection in the tracing is noted if input to the G1 electrode becomes negative with respect to input to the G2 electrode (conventional negative upward polarity).
2. The recommended EEG derivations are F4-M1, C4-M1, and O2-M1.
3. The recommended EOG derivations are E1-M2 and E2-M2. Both eye electrodes are referred to a common mastoid electrode M2.
4. Sleep is staged in 30-second epochs using a 30-second window view.
5. To differentiate whether alpha waves (8–13 Hz) or sleep spindles (11–16 Hz) are present, change to a 10-second window and count the individual deflections in one second (see Fig. 1–6). Posterior dominant rhythm (alpha rhythm) is more prominent (greater amplitude) in occipital derivations and sleep spindles in central and frontal derivations.
6. K complexes and slow waves have the greatest amplitude in frontal derivations. Sleep spindles and sawtooth waves have the greatest amplitude in central derivations. Slow wave activity has a frequency of 0.5 Hz to 2 Hz with a peak to peak amplitude > 75 μV measured over the frontal regions referenced to the contralateral mastoid (F4-M1, F3-M2).
7. **Alpha activity** is any waveform with a frequency of 8 to 13 Hz. **Posterior dominant rhythm** (PDR) in adults and older children has a frequency of 8 to 13 Hz, is most prominent in the occipital derivations, and is enhanced by eye closure and attenuated by eye opening. The term *alpha rhythm* is often used to describe the PDR in adults and older children. In young children the PDR has a frequency lower than 8 Hz.
8. The front of the eye (cornea) is positive with respect to the back of the eye (retina). If the eyes move toward E1 and away from E2, this causes a downward deflection in E1-M2 and an upward deflection in E2-M2 (assuming standard negative polarity upward).
9. In the recommended EOG derivations, eye movements result in out-of-phase deflections and K complexes and slow waves result in in-phase deflections.
10. In stage R, the chin EMG amplitude is equal to or lower than the lowest level in NREM sleep. The chin EMG activity can reach the REM level during NREM sleep. Transitions from NREM to stage R are not always associated with a decrease in chin activity. Chin EMG activity is useful in differentiating stage R from stage W with the eyes open (REMs present).

CLINICAL REVIEW QUESTIONS

1. The standard electroencephalographic (EEG) montage for sleep recording is F4-M1, C4-M1, and O2-M1. If electrode C4 fails, which of the following montages should be used?
   A. F4-M1, C3-M2, O2-M1
   B. F4-M1, C3-M1, O2-M2
   C. F3-M2, C3-M2, O1-M2
   D. F4-M2, C3-M2, O2-M2
2. **Posterior dominant rhythm** in adults and older children is characterized by which of the following?
   A. 8–13 Hz, attenuated by eye opening, most prominent in occipital derivations
   B. 8–13 Hz, attenuated by eye closure, most prominent in occipital derivations
   C. 8–13 Hz, attenuated by eye opening, most prominent in frontal derivations
   D. 8–13 Hz, attenuated by eye closure, most prominent in central derivations

3. Sleep spindles are characterized by which of the following?
   A. 12–14 Hz activity, most prominent in the occipital areas
   B. 8–13 Hz, thalamocortical oscillations
   C. 11–16 Hz, most prominent in frontal derivations
   D. 11–16 Hz, generated by the reticular nucleus of the thalamus
4. **Slow wave activity** for sleep staging is characterized by which of the following?
   A. Minimum EEG amplitude peak to peak >75 μV in C4-M1, frequency 0.5–2 Hz
   B. Minimum EEG amplitude peak to peak >75 μV in F4-M1, frequency 0.5–2 Hz
   C. Minimum EEG amplitude peak to peak ≥75 μV in F4-M1, frequency <4 Hz
   D. Minimum EEG amplitude peak to peak >75 μV in F4-M1, frequency <4 Hz
5. On right lateral gaze, which of the following deflections are noted in the recommended EOG derivations?
   A. E1-M2 Deflection **up;** E2-M2 Deflection **down**
   B. E1-M2 Deflection **down;** E2-M2 Deflection **up**
   C. E1-M2 Deflection **up;** E2-M2 Deflection **up**
   D. E1-M2 Deflection **down;** E2-M2 Deflection **down**
6. Which of the following is true about slow eye movements (using the **recommended** eye derivations)?
   A. Can occur during stage W or N1, are sinusoidal out-of-phase eye movements
   B. Can occur during stage W only, are sinusoidal out-of-phase eye movements
   C. Can occur during stage W or N1, are sinusoidal in-phase movements
   D. Can occur during stage W only, are sinusoidal out-of-phase movements
7. In Figure 1–10, what is causing the deflection at C?
   A. Upward eye movement
   B. Downward eye movement
8. What are the waveforms at A and B in Figure 1–15?

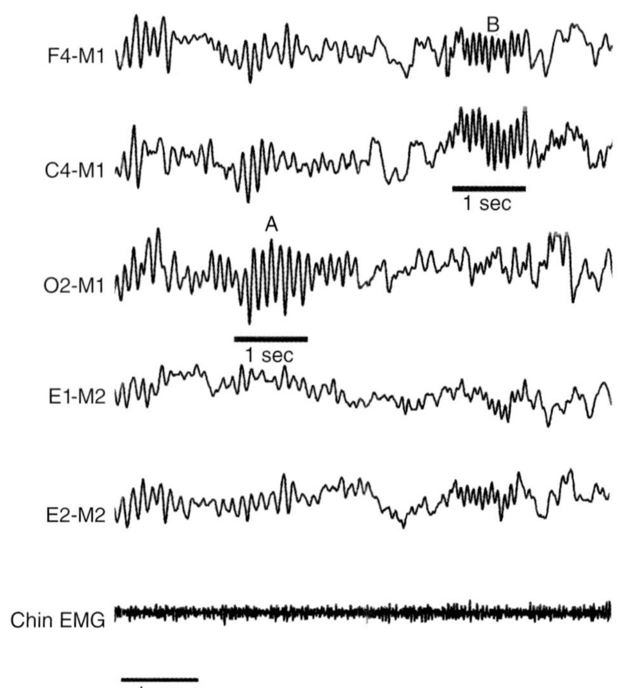

Figure 1–15 This figure is used in question 8. What are the waveforms at A and B?

ANSWERS

1. **A.** The alternate derivation for C4-M1 is C3-M2. It is not necessary to change the other derivations.
2. **A.** Posterior dominant rhythm is 8–13 Hz in adults and older children, attenuated by eye opening, most prominent in occipital derivations.
3. **D.** Sleep spindles have a frequency of 11–16 Hz and represent thalamocortical oscillations generated by the reticular nucleus of the thalamus. Sleep spindles are usually most prominent in central derivations.
4. **B.** Slow wave activity is characterized by a minimum amplitude peak to peak of > (not ≥) 75 μV in the **frontal** derivations (F4-M1) with a frequency of 0.5 to 2 Hz.
5. **A.** In the recommended derivations, eye movements cause out-of-phase deflections. Because the cornea is positive with respect to the retina, a rightward gaze results in E2 being positive with respect to M2 (E2 is closer to the cornea), and this results in a downward deflection. With a rightward gaze, E1 is negative with respect to M2 (upward deflection).
6. **A.** Slow eye movements can occur during wake (eyes closed drowsy wake) or stage N1 and are sinusoidal out-of-phase movements.
7. **A.** Upward eye movement. Movement upward toward F4 (+) is causing a downward deflection in the derivation F4-M1. Remember with eye closure the globe turns upward and with eye opening downward.
8. **A.** alpha (more prominent in occipital derivation, and you can count oscillations in 1 second = 8) **B.** sleep spindle (more prominent in central and frontal derivations, and you can count oscillations in 1 second ≈ 12 or 13 Hz)

ABBREVIATIONS

AASM, American Academy of Sleep Medicine; EEG, electroencephalographic; EMG, electromyographic; EOG, electrooculographic (eye movement recording); LOC, left outer canthus; NREM, non–rapid eye movement; PDR, posterior dominant rhythm; PSG, polysomnography; REM, rapid eye movement; REMs, rapid eye movements; ROC, right outer canthus; SEM, slow eye movement.

SUGGESTED READING

McCormick L, Nielsen T, Nicolas A, Ptito M, Montplaisir J. Topographical distribution of spindles and K complexes in normal subjects. *Sleep.* 1997;20(11):939-941.

Silber MH, Ancoli-Israel S, Bonnet MH, et al. The visual scoring of sleep in adults. *J Clin Sleep Med.* 2007;3(2):121-131. Erratum in: *J Clin Sleep Med.* 2007;3(5):table of contents.

Troester MM, Quan SF, Berry RB, et al; for the American Academy of Sleep Medicine. *The AASM Manual for the Scoring of Sleep and Associated Events: Rules, Terminology and Technical Specifications. Version 3.* American Academy of Sleep Medicine; 2023.

REFERENCES

1. Rechtschaffen A, Kales A, eds. *A Manual of Standardized Terminology, Techniques and Scoring System for Sleep Stages of Human Sleep.* Brain Information Service/Brain Research Institute, UCLA; 1968.

2. Iber C, Ancoli-Israel S, Chesson A, Quan SF for the American Academy of Sleep Medicine. *The AASM Manual for the Scoring of Sleep and Associated Events, Rules, Terminology and Technical Specifications*. American Academy of Sleep Medicine; 2007.
3. Silber MH, Ancoli-Israel S, Bonnet MH, et al. The visual scoring of sleep in adults. *J Clin Sleep Med*. 2007;3(2):121-131. Erratum in: *J Clin Sleep Med*. 2007;3(5):table of contents.
4. Troester MM, Quan SF, Berry RB, et al; for the American Academy of Sleep Medicine. *The AASM Manual for the Scoring of Sleep and Associated Events: Rules, Terminology and Technical Specifications. Version 3*. American Academy of Sleep Medicine; 2023.
5. Jasper HH. The ten-twenty electrode system of the International Federation of Societies for Electroencephalography and Clinical Neurophysiology: Report of the committee on methods of clinical examination in electroencephalography: Ten twenty electrode system. *EEG Clin Neurophysiol*. 1958;10:371-375.
6. Cantero JL, Atienza M, Salas RM. Human alpha oscillations in wakefulness, drowsiness period, and REM sleep: different electroencephalographic phenomena within the alpha band. *Neurophysiol Clin*. 2002;32(1): 54-71.
7. De Gennaro L, Ferrara M. Sleep spindles: an overview. *Sleep Med Rev*. 2003;7(5):423-440.
8. McCormick L, Nielsen T, Nicolas A, et al. Topographical distribution of spindles and K-complexes in normal subjects. *Sleep*. 1997;20(11):939-941.
9. Alfonsi V, D'Atri A, Gorgoni M, et al. Spatiotemporal dynamics of sleep spindle sources across NREM sleep cycles. *Front Neurosci*. 2019;13:727.
10. Schenck CH, Mahowald MW, Kim SW, et al. Prominent eye movements during NREM sleep and REM sleep behavior disorder associated with fluoxetine treatment of depression and obsessive-compulsive disorder. *Sleep*. 1992;15(3):226-235.
11. Armitage R, Trivedi M, Rush AJ. Fluoxetine and oculomotor activity during sleep in depressed patients. *Neuropsychopharmacology*. 1995;12(2): 159-165.

Chapter 2

The Technology and Methods of Sleep Monitoring (Differential Amplifiers, Digital Polysomnography, and Biocalibration)

DIGITAL POLYSOMNOGRAPHY OVERVIEW

Polysomnography (PSG) is the detailed monitoring of sleep. Digital PSG systems provide the ability to record many more channels than during the era of paper recording. In Table 2–1 the commonly recorded parameters and purposes are displayed. These include electroencephalographic (EEG), electrooculographic (EOG), and electromyographic (EMG) signals to detect and stage sleep; airflow sensors to detect apnea and hypopnea; respiratory effort sensors to classify apnea (obstructive, central, and mixed); pulse oximetry to measure the arterial oxygen saturation; and bilateral anterior tibial EMG electrodes to detect leg movements. During positive airway pressure (PAP) titration PSG signals from the laboratory PAP device including PAP flow, delivered PAP pressure, and PAP leak are usually recorded and can be viewed. There are three main versions of PSG: diagnostic PSG, PAP titration PSG, and split PSG (initial portion diagnostic, second portion PAP titration). In clinical EEG the term *montage* refers to the derivations being recorded and how the signals are arranged. In PSG a montage can refer to the set of EEG and EOG derivations, respiratory signals, and leg movement channels to be viewed. In some PSG systems the term used is *display view* or *workspace*. Different

Table 2–1 Polysomnography—Channels Recorded

Parameter	Electrodes/Sensor	Purpose
EEG derivations	F4-M1, C4-M1, O2-M1 (frontal, central, occipital)	Staging of sleep
EOG derivations	E1-M2, E2-M2	Staging of sleep
Chin EMG	Chin1, Chin2, ChinZ	Staging of sleep
ECG	Electrocardiogram	Cardiac rate and rhythm
Airflow (diagnostic study)	Nasal pressure	Detection of hypopnea
	Oronasal thermal flow	Detection of apnea
Airflow (PAP titration)	PAP device flow	Detection of apnea and hypopnea
Snoring	Microphone, piezoelectric sensor	Detection of snoring
Respiratory effort	Chest and abdominal RIP belts	Classify apnea (central, mixed or obstructive)
Arterial oxygen saturation (SpO_2)	Pulse oximetry	Detect desaturation
Left anterior tibial (LAT) EMG	Surface EMG electrodes	Detect PLMS
Right anterior tibial (RAT) EMG	Surface EMG electrodes	Detect PLMS
End-tidal PCO_2	Diagnostic study—recommended in children, optional in adults	Detect hypoventilation Detect apnea or RERAs in children
Optional		
Pulse rate	Oximeter output (pulse rate)	Moving time average of pulse rate
Estimate of tidal volume	RIPsum	Alternate sensor for apnea and hypopnea
Estimate of airflow	RIPflow	Alternate sensor for apnea and hypopnea
Intercostal EMG	Right costal EMG electrodes	Detect inspiratory effort
Transcutaneous PCO_2	Diagnostic and PAP titrations	Detect hypoventilation
PAP pressure, leak	PAP device pressure and leak	Monitor delivered pressure, leak

ECG, Electrocardiogram; *EEG*, electroencephalographic; *EMG*, electromyogram; *EOG*, electrooculographic; *LAT*, left anterior tibial; *PAP*, positive airway pressure; *PCO_2*, partial pressure of carbon dioxide; *PLMS*, periodic limb movements in sleep; *RAT*, right anterior tibial; *RERA*, respiratory effort arousal; *RIP*, respiratory inductance plethysmography; *RIPflow*, time derivative of RIPsum; *RIPsum*, sum of signals of chest and abdomen RIP belts.

Table 2–2 Sample Polysomnographic Display Views (Montages)

Channel	Diagnostic 1	Diagnostic 2	PAP Titration
1	F4-M1	E1-M2	F4-M1
2	C4-M1	E2-M2	C4-M1
3	O2-M1	F4-M1	O2-M1
4	E1-M2	F3-M2	E1-M2
5	E2-M2	C4-M1	E2-M2
6	Chin EMG	C3-M2	Chin EMG
7	ECG	O2-M1	ECG
8	Pulse rate	O1-M2	Pulse rate
9	Snoring	Chin EMG	Snoring
10	Nasal pressure	ECG	PAP flow
11	Oronasal thermal flow	Pulse rate	Chest
12	Chest	Snoring	Abdomen
13	Abdomen	Nasal pressure	SpO_2
14	SpO_2	ON therm	LAT
15	LAT	Chest	RAT
16	RAT	Abdomen	PAP leak
17	Exhaled PCO_2	SpO_2	PAP pressure
18	End-tidal PCO_2	LAT	PAP tidal volume
19		RAT	$PtcCO_2$

ECG, Electrocardiogram; *EEG*, electroencephalography; *EMG*, electromyogram; *LAT*, left anterior tibial; *ON therm*, Oronasal thermal flow; *PAP*, positive airway pressure device; *$PtcCO_2$*, transcutaneous Pco_2; *RAT*, right anterior tibial; *SpO_2*, arterial oxygen saturation by pulse oximetry. Pulse rate by oximetry a surrogate of heart rate, Chest and Abdomen are RIP effort belts around the chest and abdomen.

default display views for each of the three types of PSG studies can be customized for different viewers (Table 2–2). In some sleep centers a body position sensor is used, whereas in most PSG systems body position is entered by the monitoring technologist along with the current treatment PAP pressure and oxygen flow (if indicated). Digital PSG systems allow one to view all or a portion of the parameters recorded. A channel is a horizontal display of a recorded parameter versus time. The number of channels displayed can be customized. Display windows of 5, 10, 15, 30, 60, 90, 180, and 240 seconds are typically available. The current epoch number, body position, and PAP level (if applicable) are displayed along with the selected tracings. This information can also be displayed as a watermark in some PSG systems. In addition, an all-night summary is available (Figure 2–1) and can be displayed (or toggled on and off) below the main window containing the viewed channels. A typical all-night summary view would include a hypnogram (graphical representation of sleep stages) and vertical lines to indicate the timing of respiratory events, arterial oxygen desaturations, and leg movements, as well as a condensed tracing of the arterial oxygen saturation by pulse oximetry, PAP level, and body position. A line showing the current position of the main window in the all-night summary is provided. Double-clicking on a point in the summary window will move the main tracings window to that time. The contents of the all-night summary view can be edited and a default view saved. For example, one might display the individual respiratory event types. In Figure 2–2 an all-night summary of a split sleep study (initial portion diagnostic, second portion PAP titration) is shown. The dramatic reduction in respiratory events as the continuous PAP (CPAP) increases is illustrated. In subsequent chapters the monitoring of respiration, the electrocardiogram (ECG), leg movements, and the recording and use of PAP device signals will be discussed in detail. This chapter discusses the technology of monitoring sleep, although some aspects are relevant to the other parameters being recorded.

RECORDING SLEEP

In sleep monitoring EEG, EOG, and EMG signals are recorded by differential alternating current (AC) amplifiers that amplify the difference in voltage between two inputs[1-5] (Figures 2–3 and 2–4). Each differential amplifier has two

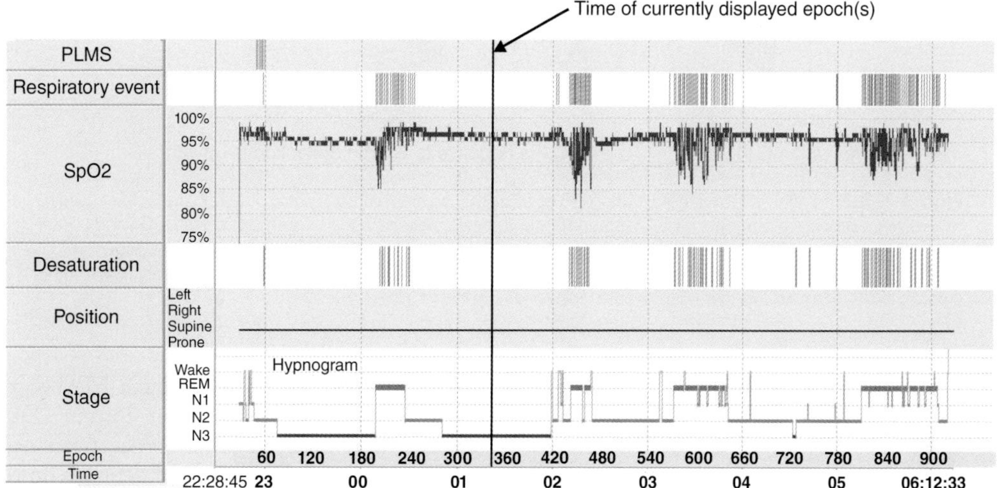

Figure 2–1 The vertical line shows the position of the currently displayed detailed tracings in the main window in the all night summary. The reviewer can choose additional parameters to be displayed (e.g., the level of positive airway pressure). *PLMS*, Periodic limb movements in sleep; *SpO_2*, arterial oxygen saturation by pulse oximetry. (Adapted from Berry RB, Wagner MH. *Sleep Medicine Pearls*. 3rd ed. Elsevier; 2015:81.)

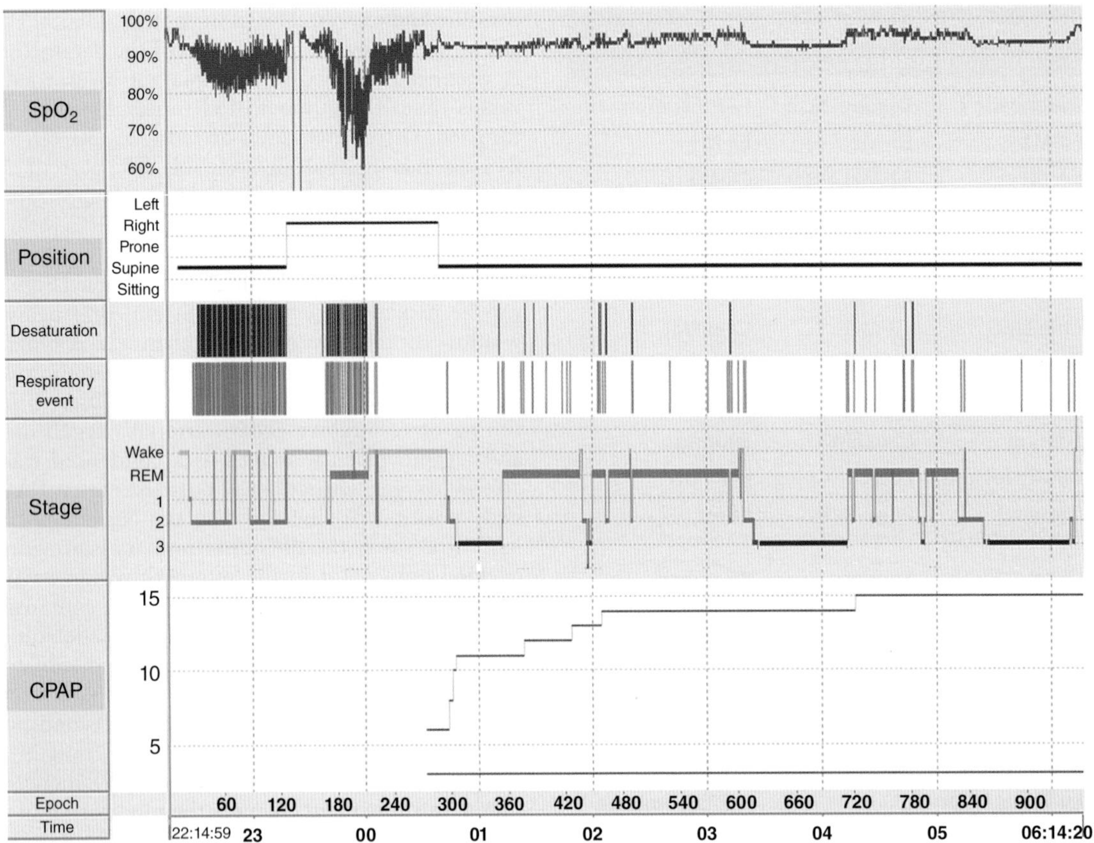

Figure 2–2 An all-night summary of a split sleep study. One can see frequent respiratory events and desaturations in the first part of the study with a significant decrease in these events as the level of continuous positive airway pressure *(CPAP)* is increased. This patient had large amounts of stage R and stage N3 on CPAP (N3 and rapid eye movement *[REM]* sleep rebound). *SpO$_2$* arterial oxygen saturation using pulse oximetry.

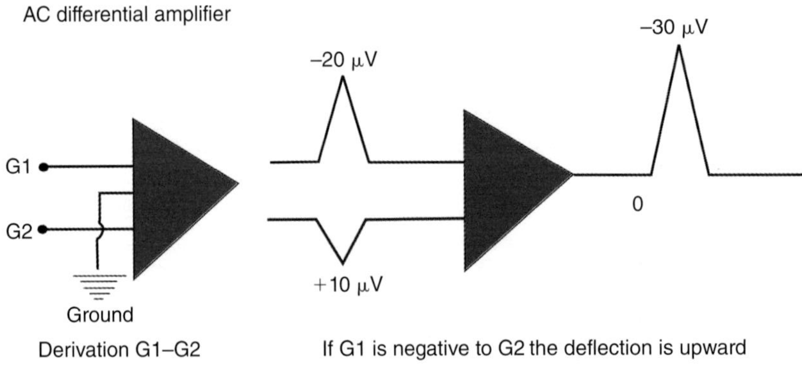

Figure 2–3 Simplified schematic illustration of the output of an alternating current differential amplifier used to record electroencephalographic (EEG) and electrooculographic signals. Signals common to inputs G1 and G2 are rejected, and only the difference is amplified. Here the gain is 1. Note that when G1 is negative with respect to G2, the deflection is upward. This is the negative polarity upward convention used for EEG recording. *AC,* alternating current. (From Berry RB, Wagner MH. *Sleep Medicine Pearls.* 3rd ed. Elsevier; 2015:3.)

inputs and a ground. By convention, in EEG recording, if input-1 (G1) is negative relative to input-2 (G2), the deflection is upward (negative up polarity). Signals common to both inputs are not amplified (common mode rejection). Each of the inputs is recorded against the common ground and input 2 is inverted (Figure 2–4). This allows common signals to cancel each other but differences between input-1 and input-2 to be amplified. Use of differential amplifiers permits the recording of very-low-voltage EEG signals that are superimposed upon larger direct current (DC) scalp voltage changes and 60-cycle interference from nearby AC power lines. Common mode rejection depends on the impedance at input-1 and input-2 being relatively equal. Otherwise, common signals will produce unequal voltages at the two inputs. Making the intrinsic impedance of the inputs much higher than the impedance of the electrodes minimizes the effect of

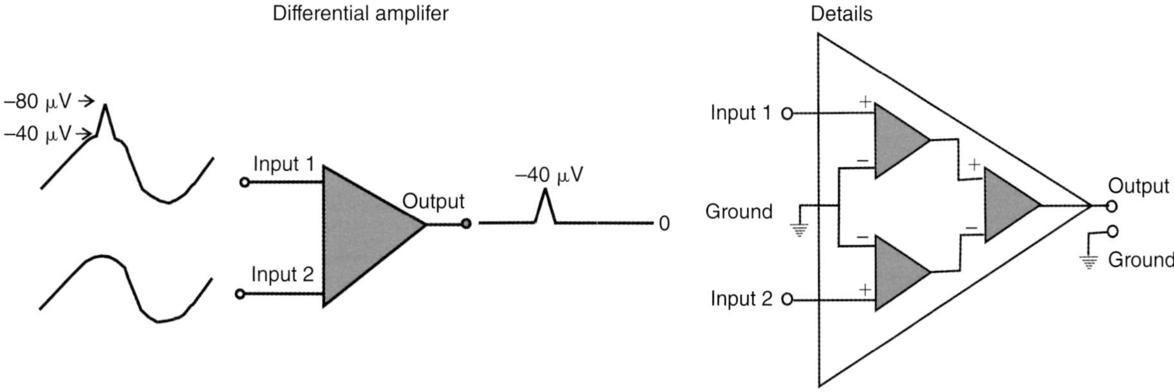

Figure 2–4 Simplified schematic illustrating common mode rejection *(left panel)*. The portion of the signal common to both inputs cancels, and only what is different is amplified. Here a gain of 1 is chosen for simplicity. The *right panel* shows that there are two components to the differential amplifier, and one portion is inverted so that common signals are rejected. The schematic is for illustration of the concept of common mode rejection. Actual differential amplifers are more complex.

unequal electrode impedances. However, a poorly conducting electrode (high impedance) will typically result in a large amount of 60-Hz artifact (signal contamination). The ground of each differential AC amplifier is connected to the common patient ground (commonly, an electrode placed on the forehead). This common ground helps balance the inputs to all the differential amplifiers, thereby improving common mode rejection. The patient ground is isolated from instrument ground for patient safety. The use of grounds in EEG recording is discussed at the end of the chapter. It should be noted that a localized short-duration wave (such as a sharp wave) that is located midway between two electrodes will produce an equal signal at both inputs of the differential AC amplifier that will cancel out (output approximately zero). This cancellation effect will reduce the overall EEG signal amplitude less if electrodes are further apart. Thus a greater distance between two electrode inputs will increase the amplitude of the recorded signal (less cancellation). This is one reason the recommended EEG derivations use *contralateral* mastoid references (C4-M1, not C4-M2).

Referential and Bipolar Recording

Most digital recording systems use a combination of referential, true bipolar, and DC recording (Table 2–3). In true bipolar recording, each amplifier records the difference between two electrodes of interest (A–B, C–D). However, changing the derivation once the signal is recorded (changing from A–B to A–D) is not possible. True bipolar recording (two inputs to one differential amplifier) is still used for inputs that one would not desire to change in review—for example, the two inputs of the thermal flow sensor, respiratory effort bands (thorax and abdomen), leg EMG inputs, and ECG inputs. In referential recording, multiple electrodes are recorded against a common electrical reference (often a single or two linked electrodes placed near the vertex). In some PSG systems a virtual reference is used composed of linked electrodes (e.g., C3-C4) rather than a separate reference electrode. A **display** of any derivation using two referentially recorded electrodes is then obtained by digital subtraction [(electrode A − reference) − (electrode B − reference) = electrode A − electrode B] either during live recording or during review (see Figure 2–5). The digital subtraction for display does *not* change the recorded data. For example, if the sleep technologist failed to observe that the electrode M2 was not functioning properly during the a portion of the recording, the reviewer can change the viewed eye derivations to E1-M1 and E2-M1. For this reason, EEG, EOG, M1, M2, and chin EMG electrodes for both the recommended and backup derivations are referentially recorded (each against the reference electrode), even though only the recommended derivation may be displayed in the default montage (set of derivations automatically displayed). Of note, if the reference electrode is faulty, all referential signals are affected (Figure 2–6). Note that the true bipolar channels are not affected by a faulty reference electrode. In summary, the EEG, EOG, mastoid, and chin EMG electrodes are recorded referentially in nearly all PSG systems (see Table 2–3). The ECG can be recorded as a bipolar input, or multiple ECG electrodes can be recorded referentially. One may then choose the pair of ECG electrodes with the best signal. DC recording is used for nasal pressure, pulse oximetry, and other DC signals such as those from the PAP device (flow, leak, tidal volume, delivered pressure), and signals from partial pressure of carbon dioxide (Pco_2) monitoring devices (end-tidal PCO_2 value, exhaled PCO_2 waveform, or transcutaneous PCO_2 value).

Table 2–3 Types of Recording

Referential recording	EEG: F4, F3, C4, C3, O2, O1, M1, M2 EOG: E_1, E_2, M_1, M_2 Chin1, Chin2, ChinZ Reference (a single electrode, or linked electrodes near the location of Cz), isolated ground electrode
True bipolar (two inputs each)	• ECG • Oronasal thermal airflow • Thorax and abdominal effort sensors • LAT and RAT EMG • Snoring sensor
DC	• Nasal pressure • SpO_2 • PAP device signals (flow, leak, pressure) • End-tidal PCO_2, transcutaneous PCO_2

DC, Direct current; *ECG,* electrocardiography; *EEG,* electroencephalography; *EMG,* electromyography; *EOG,* electrooculography; *LAT,* left anterior tibial; *PAP,* positive airway pressure; *PCO_2,* partial pressure of carbon dioxide; *RAT,* right anterior tibial; *SpO_2,* pulse oximetry.

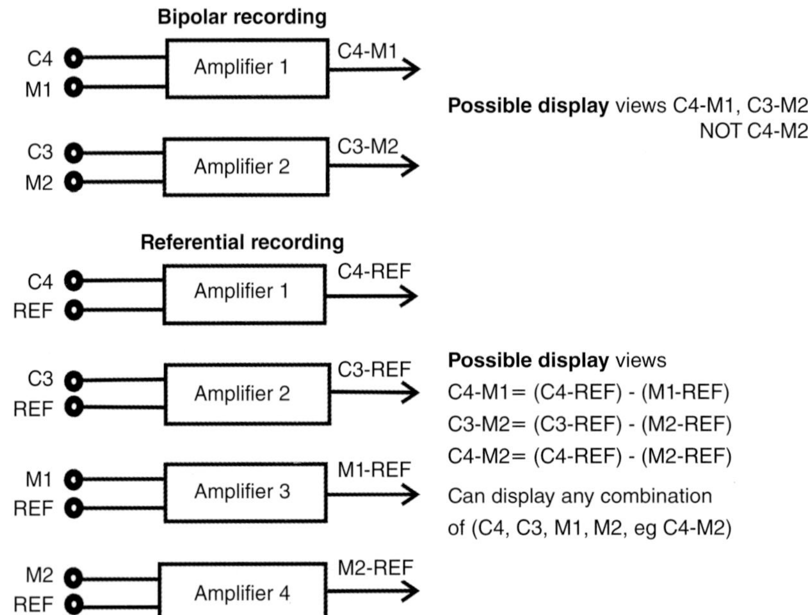

Figure 2–5 Difference between bipolar and referential recording. In referential recording all electrodes are recorded relative to the reference electrode. Then, using digital subtraction, any combination of the referentially recorded electrodes can be displayed. (Adapted from Berry RB, Wagner MH. *Sleep Medicine Pearls.* 3rd ed. Elsevier; 2015:82.)

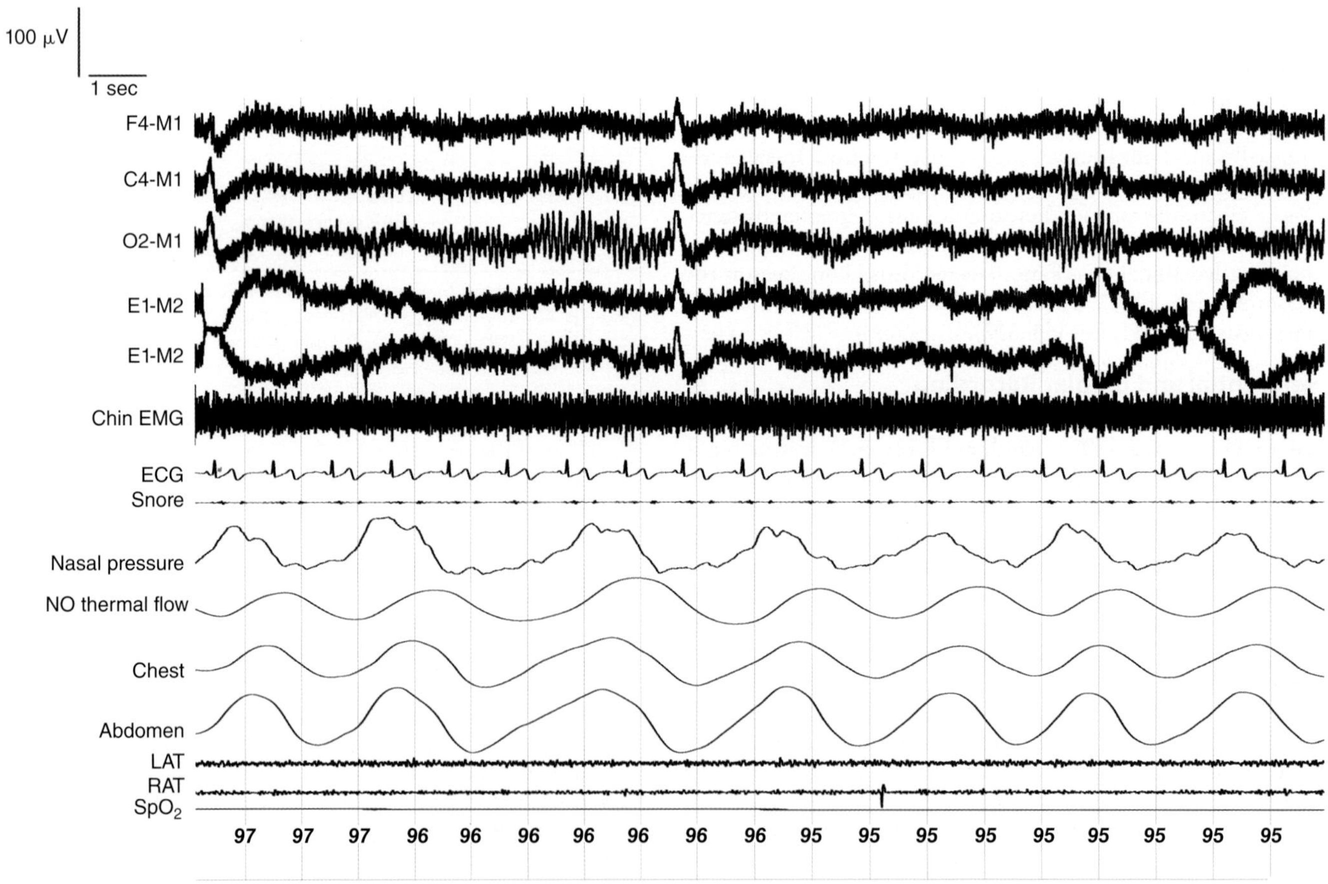

Figure 2–6 A 20-second tracing showing the results when the reference electrode is faulty. A 60-Hz artifact is visible in all channels using referential recording but not in channels with bipolar recording. *ECG,* Electrocardiogram; *EMG,* electromyogram; *LAT,* left anterior tibial electromyogram; *NO,* nasal oral; *RAT,* right anterior tibial electromyogram; *SpO_2,* arterial oxygen saturation by pulse oximetry. (From Berry RB, Wagner MH. *Sleep Medicine Pearls.* 3rd ed. Elsevier; 2015:88.)

Time Window for Staging Sleep

During traditional paper-ink recording for sleep, the paper speed was 10 mm/sec, which produced 30-second pages (30-cm-wide paper). Each 30-second page was an epoch of sleep. A faster speed was used for clinical EEG (30 mm/sec, 10 seconds per page). However, such a fast paper speed would have produced a very large amount of paper for each sleep study, and therefore a slower speed was used. In digital recording, one can choose various time windows during either acquisition or review. A 30-second window is used for sleep staging and for scoring arousals. Time windows of 60 to 240 seconds may be used to view and score respiratory events and leg movements. Alternatively, viewing tracings in a 10-second window (equivalent to 30 mm/sec) is the usual time window for clinical EEG viewing. This allows better visualization of very brief events (sharp waves and spikes) used to identify interictal or ictal (seizure) activity. The 10-second window can also be useful for measuring the frequency of a group of oscillations or viewing the ECG tracing. The traditional ECG speed is 25 mm/sec, which is quite close to 30 mm/sec. Some systems allow split screens with different time windows in each screen. There is usually an option to synchronize or not to synchronize the two windows. For example, the top window shows a 30-second view with signals used to stage sleep and the bottom window a 90- to 120-second window to visualize respiratory and leg movement events.

Sampling Rate

Most digital recording systems use analog amplifiers that produce a continuous signal output. The signal is then sampled by an analog-to-digital (A/D) conversion board that converts the signal to a digital form that can be manipulated by a computer and stored in memory. The sampling rate must be more than twice the frequencies being recorded to reduce aliasing signal distortion **(Nyquist theorem).**[1-7] If lower sampling rates are used, the recorded digital signal can be distorted with the addition of frequencies lower than the original analog signal sampled (Figure 2–7). Here "alias" means an assumed or additional frequency. For example a 4 Hz analog signal is sampled at 3 Hz and the stored digital signal is 1 Hz. The digital 1 Hz signal is an alias for the 3 Hz analog signal (Figure 2–7). It is not possible to remove the distorted component of the signal (the 1 Hz signal) once the A/D converter outputs the signal in digital form to the computer for storage. For this reason, signals with a frequency higher than half the sampling rate must be filtered out (significantly attenuated) before being sent to the A/D converter because they can cause aliasing distortion.[1-7] For example, if the sampling rate is 200 samples/sec, the amplified signal must be processed by a high-frequency filter with a cutoff frequency of 100 Hz or lower before being sampled (A/D converter). The aliasing frequency (1 Hz in the above example) is equal to the absolute value of [(N × the sampling rate) minus the signal frequency] where N is the integer bringing the product of N and the sampling rate closest to the signal frequency.[8] For the example of a sampling rate of 3 Hz for a 4 Hz signal the aliasing frequency is the absolute value of [(1 × 3) - 4] which equals 1 Hz. The required sampling rate depends on the frequency of the signal to be recorded. Slower varying signals require a lower sampling rate. Of note, accurate representation of a signal requires a sampling rate much higher than twice the frequency of a signal. In Table 2–4 the sampling rates recommended by the American Academy of Sleep Medicine (AASM) scoring manual[9-11] are illustrated. Some digital PSG systems can record different signals at different sampling rates. Using only the minimum acceptable sampling rate reduces the size of the data file. However, today storage capacity is not an issue, and often the same sampling rate is used for all signals being sent to the A/D converter. However, some lower frequency PSG signals may be downsampled by the PSG software (additional digital filtering as indicated followed by digital sampling at a lower than the original sampling rate) before being stored in computer memory. Most computer systems record synchronized video and even when compressed, the video data can easily exceed PSG data in file size. Ultimately, the computer program uses only a small portion of the signal data for the display because monitor resolution (in pixels per displayed time duration) is usually much less than the sampling rate.[7]

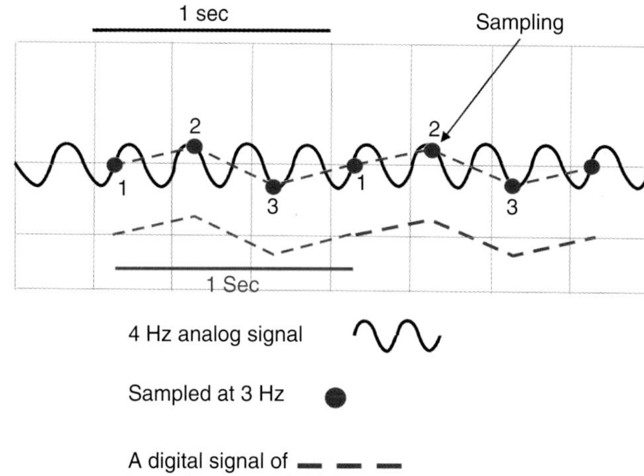

Figure 2–7 Undersampling a signal (sampling at <2X the frequency to be recorded) can result in the introduction of a signal of lower frequency than the original signal. Here, sampling a 4-Hz signal at 3 Hz results in introduction of a 1-Hz signal. A 4-Hz signal should be sampled at 8 Hz or greater (Nyquist theorem). However, accurate representation of a signal requires a sampling rate much higher than twice the frequency of the signal being recorded. For a 4 Hz signal a sampling rate of 40 Hz or higher would provide a more accurate representation of the signal.

Table 2-4 Standard Sampling Rates for Various Polysomnographic Signals

Minimal (Hz)	Desirable (Hz)	Signal Type
≥200	500 or greater	EEG, EOG, EMG, ECG, snoring
≥25	100 or greater	Nasal pressure Thermal airflow PAP device flow End-tidal PCO_2 waveform Chest and abdominal effort belt signals
≥10	25	Oximetry Transcutaneous PCO_2
>1 Hz	≥1 Hz	Body position

The sampling rates are consistent with the recommendations in the AASM scoring manual.

ECG, Electrocardiography; *EEG*, electroencephalography; *EMG*, electromyography; *EOG*, electrooculography.

Adapted from Troester MM, Quan SF, Berry RB, et al; for the American Academy of Sleep Medicine. *The AASM Manual for the Scoring of Sleep and Associated Events: Rules, Terminology and Technical Specifications. Version 3.*

This can produce "monitor aliasing," in which the signal visualized on the monitor is distorted because of the low number of pixels per inch compared with the frequency of the signal (discussed below)[1,2]. The high resolution of current monitors diminishes this issue. A/D conversion is also characterized by the dynamic range (the range of voltages accepted by the A/D converter) and the resolution. The dynamic range may be expressed as the amplified or unamplified signal range. The resolution depends on the A/D converter, as well as the dynamic range. A 12-bit DC converter produces $2^{12} = 4096$ digital values (bits) across the dynamic range. A typical A/D converter might have a dynamic range for the amplified signal of 5 V (± 2.5 V). Commonly, a set amplification is applied to all AC signals before A/D conversion (e.g., a gain of 1250). If one assumes an amplification of 1250, then the dynamic range (peak to peak) of an A/D converter with an amplified voltage range of 5 V expressed as the unamplified signal would be approximately 4000 μV (−2000 to +2000 μV) as (4000 μV × 1250 = 5,000,000 μV = 5.0 V). If a 12-bit A/D converter is used, this would result in a resolution of 0.97 μV/ bit (4000 μV/4096 digital values) (Figure 2–8).

Ultimately, the signal resolution that matters is the accuracy of the visual representation of the signal on the computer monitor. Lower resolution monitors may suffer from monitor aliasing.[6,7]. For example, if there are 1600 horizonal pixels and a 30-second window is displayed, the maximum pixel sampling rate is 53/sec (ignoring pixels needed for channel labels and so on). A sampling rate of 53/sec means that signals over about 26 Hz would be affected by monitor aliasing. Most sleep EEG waveforms of interest have a frequency rate lower than 26 Hz. However higher frequency components of the signal could result in aliasing if not attenuated. This issue is less of a concern as the EEG signal is processed by a high frequency filter of 35 Hz before being displayed. However, when using a 60-second window the pixel sampling rate falls to about 27 pixels per second. Thus, the effective monitor "sampling rate or pixels/second" depends on both the monitor resolution and the duration (seconds) to be displayed. Undersampling a signal by the monitor display can result in the addition of a waveform of lower frequency than the signal (Figure 2–7) as well as providing a less acccurate representation of the signal. If the EEG signal contains a significant amplitude of 60 Hz artifact after filtering, a 53 pixel per second representation (30 second window) would add a 7 Hz waveform to the display (aliasing frequency). In addition, although a monitor "sampling rate" of 53 pixels/second is more than twice 12 Hz, this would not be expected to provide a smooth representation of a 12 Hz signal and monitor undersampling is associated with a jagged appearance of waveforms. A number of computational techniques are available to minimize the effects of monitor aliasing/undersampling, but discussion of these is beyond the scope of this chapter). Fortunately, technological advances have made large higher resolution monitors more affordable, and this provides a more accurate visual representation of waveforms.

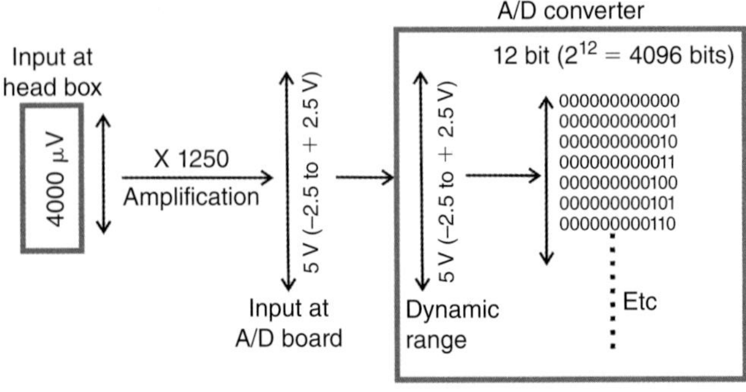

Figure 2–8 Conversion of an analog signal to a digital signal. The resolution depends on the dynamic range and the digital resolution ($2^{\text{no. of bits}}$). *A/D*, Analog to digital. (From Berry RB, *Fundamentals of Sleep Medicine*, Elsevier Saunders; 2012:16)

Filters (Low Frequency, High Frequency, and Notch)

Any signal of interest can be contaminated by unwanted low- or high-frequency signals or 50- to 60-Hz artifact (from nearby AC power lines). Filters allow these components to be diminished. For example, a low-frequency filter (high-pass filter) attenuates the amplitude of low-frequency signals. A high-frequency filter (low-pass filter) attenuates the amplitude of high-frequency signals (Figure 2–9).[1-4,12-14] Another way of visualizing the effect of a filter is to plot attenuation versus signal frequency (Figure 2–10). The amount of signal reduction due to a given analog or digital filter is given in decibels (dB) (Equation 2–1). Here voltage-in and voltage-out are the amplitudes of the signal entering and leaving the filter, respectively.

$$\text{dB} = 20 \log (\text{Voltage-out/Voltage-in}) \qquad \text{Equation 2–1}$$

$$-3\ \text{dB} = 20 \log (0.707) \text{ or } -6\text{dB} = 20 \log (0.501)$$

A signal reduction of ≈30% and ≈50% (voltage-out/voltage-in ratios of ≈0.707 and ≈0.5, respectively) corresponds to −3 dB and −6 dB amplitude reductions, respectively. Filter settings (e.g., 0.3, 1 Hz) are named by the "cutoff frequency," which is the frequency of the signal that is reduced by 3 or

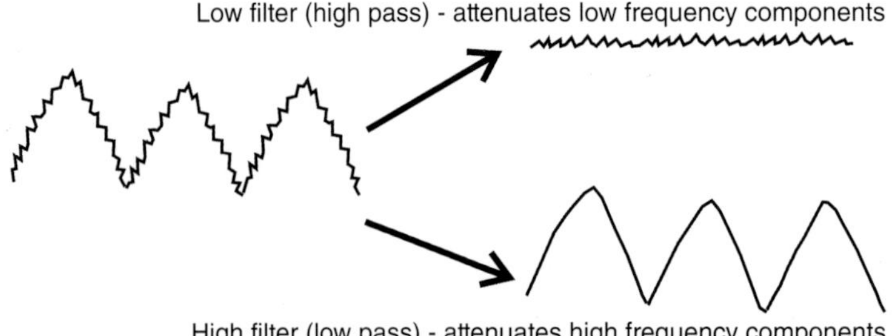

Figure 2–9 Schematic examples of the effects of a low-frequency filter (high pass) and a high-frequency filter (low pass). (From Berry RB, Wagner MH. *Sleep Medicine Pearls.* 3rd ed. Elsevier; 2015:86.)

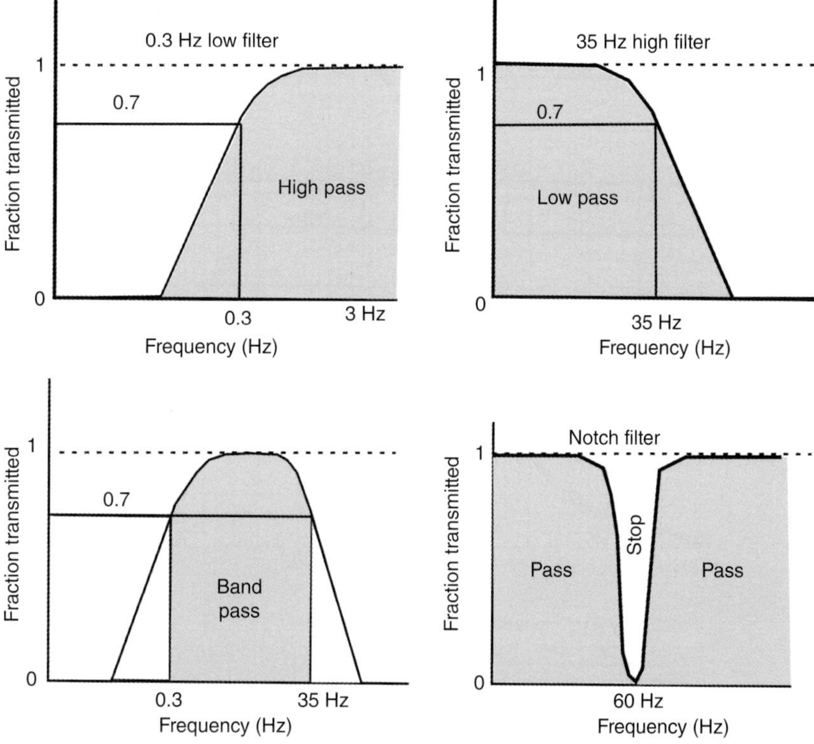

Figure 2–10 Schematic illustration of filter types. A low-frequency filter is also known as a high pass filter and a high-frequency filter is known as a low pass filter. A band pass filter "passes" (does not significantly attenuate) signals with a frequency above and below certain frequencies (the bandwidth). A notch filter attenuates signals in a narrow range of frequencies. A 0.3 Hz low frequency filter attenuates a 0.3 Hz signal to approximately 0.7 of the incoming signal amplitude (assuming a -3 dB filter, see Equation 2-1). A 35 Hz high frequency filter attenuates a 35 Hz signal to approximately 0.7 of the incoming amplitude.

6 dB depending on the terminology and the type of filter the manufacturer of the PSG equipment uses. Therefore, a filter setting of "X Hz" means that the amplitude of a signal with a frequency of X is diminished by approximately 30% or 50% depending on whether the −3 dB or −6 dB cutoff frequency is used to name the filter. The following discussion assumes use of a −3 dB filter (commonly used in PSG recording). It should also be noted that the figures in this section are based on a simple resistance-capacitance (RC) circuit for filters with voltage across the resistance equivalent to the output of a low-frequency filter and across the capacitor for a high-frequency filter. The figures represent the effect of a first-order Butterworth filter. More complex filter systems using arrangements of multiple RC circuits may produce different results. Although digital filters attempt to mimic analog filters, the effect of digital filters from different computer software may vary and may not exactly reproduce the behavior represented by the figures in this chapter.

Low-Frequency Filter

A 0.3 Hz low-frequency filter (−3 dB) attenuates a 0.3 Hz signal by approximately 30% (or to ≈70% of the original signal). The signal strength of frequencies below 0.3 Hz would be attenuated even more. Signals with a frequency slightly above 0.3 Hz are slightly attenuated, and frequencies above 3 Hz are not attenuated at all (Figure 2–11). This is an example of a Bode plot that is often used to illustrate the effect of a filter on signals of different frequency. This is usually a semilogarithmic plot with a logarithmic scale on the X-axis (frequency) and a linear scale on the Y-axis (attenuation). This allows frequencies of very different amplitudes to be displayed (Figure 2–11). In Figure 2–12 an example of the effects of a 0.3 Hz low-frequency filter on signals of different frequencies is illustrated. It is important to realize that frequencies **slightly above** the low-frequency filter setting of 0.3 Hz will also be attenuated by a 0.3 Hz low-frequency filter, although to a lesser degree. An example of the effect of different filters on a 1-Hz signal is shown in Figure 2–13. This figure also illustrates the fact that filters not only affect the amplitude of a signal, but they also change the phase (signal vs. time characteristics). In this figure the 1-Hz peak is shifted to the left. A range of possible low-frequency filter settings (off, 0.01, 0.03, 0.1, 0.3, 1, 3, and 10) is commonly provided. Sometimes low-frequency filter settings are specified as a time constant (T_C) rather than as a cutoff frequency (Figure 2–14). The lower the low-frequency filter setting, the longer the time constant (Equation 2–2).

$$\text{Time Constant } Tc = \frac{1}{2\pi fc} \quad (fc = \text{low-frequency filter cutoff value}) \qquad \text{Equation 2–2}$$

Traditional analog filters used RC circuits.[1,12,13] In RC circuits, an increase in step voltage produces an abrupt increase in voltage across the resistor and then an exponential fall in voltage to 1/e (0.37) of the maximum voltage in one time constant. In a simple, low-frequency filter RC circuit, the frequency (fc) at which the output voltage across the resistor is attenuated to 0.37 of the input voltage is related to the T_C by the formula

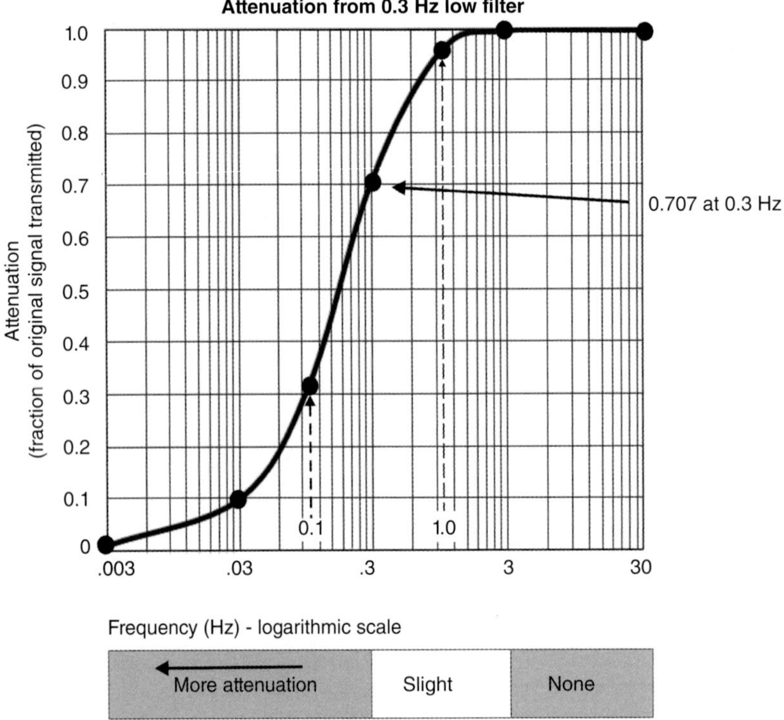

Figure 2–11 Plot displaying the attenuation of different frequency signals by a −3 dB 0.3-Hz low-frequency filter. A signal with a frequency of 0.3 Hz is attenuated to 0.707 of the original signal. Higher-frequency signals are attenuated less, and lower-frequency signals are attenuated more. Note that some attenuation of signals with frequencies slightly greater than 0.3 Hz occurs, but signals greater than 1 Hz undergo minimal or 3 Hz no attenuation. The Y-axis is linear, and the X-axis is logarithmic. This allows a wide range of frequencies to be displayed. This is an example of a Bode plot. The data is for a simple first-order Butterworth filter. The precise attenuation varies with the type of digital filter.

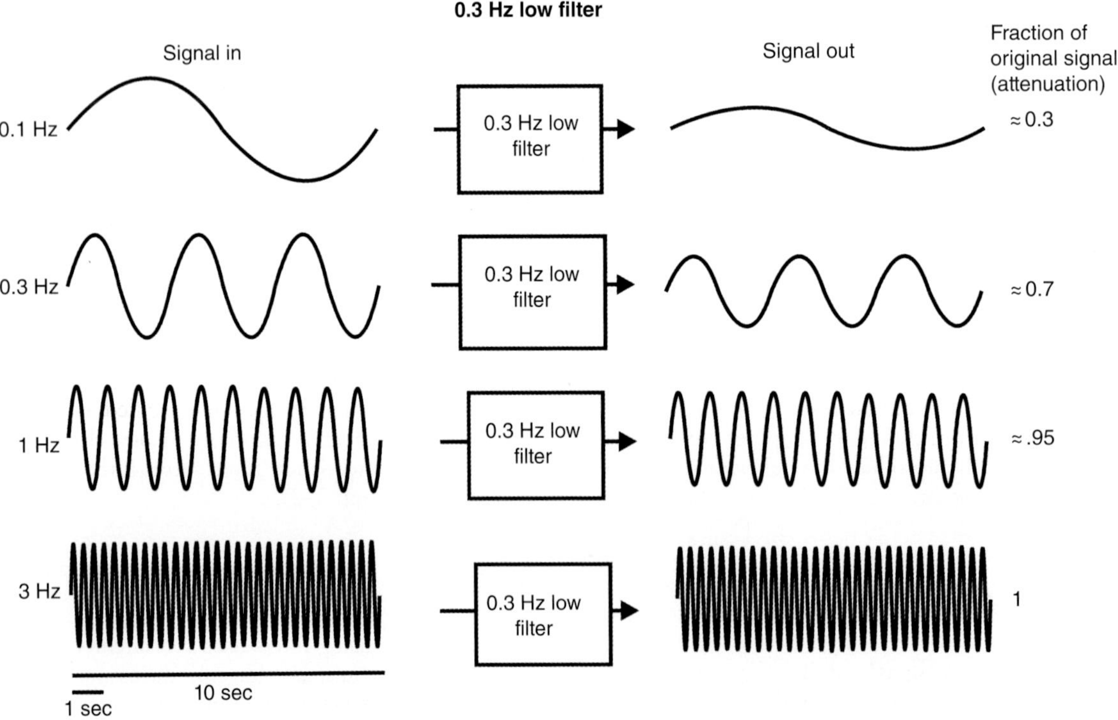

Figure 2–12 Illustration of the effect of a −3 dB 0.3-Hz filter on different frequency signals. A 0.3-Hz signal is attenuated to approximately 0.707 of the original signal amplitude. For frequencies less than 0.3 Hz, greater attenuation is noted. For a signal with a slightly higher frequency than 0.3 Hz (1 Hz), the attenuation is less, and by 3 Hz the signal undergoes no attenuation.

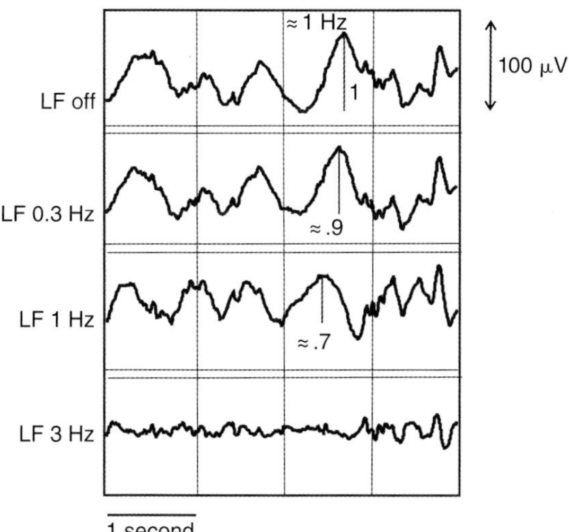

Figure 2–13 Effects of different low-frequency filters on a typical tracing showing frequencies close to 1 Hz. A 1-Hz low-frequency filter attenuates a 1-Hz signal to about 0.7 of the unfiltered amplitude. The 0.3-Hz filter attenuates the signal only slightly. A 3-Hz low-frequency filter dramatically attenuates all activity near or below 1 Hz. *LF,* Low filter setting.

$fc = 1/(2\pi/T_C)$. In RC circuits, the $T_C = RC$, where R is the resistance and C the capacitance of the circuit. Even if digital filters are used, the relationship between the T_C and the −3 dB frequency is given by Equation 2–2. For example, a 0.3-Hz low-frequency filter has a TC of approximately 0.53 seconds. Of note, the actual T_C after a step increase in voltage may vary depending on the high-frequency filter setting as well. As the high-frequency filter is decreased, the amplitude of the signal after a step increase in voltage input is also decreased. The lower the cutoff frequency, the longer the time constant (see Figure 2–14). If a step calibration signal (square wave) voltage change is recorded, the T_C can be determined from the time it takes for the deflection to return to 0.37 of the maximum deflection. Step calibration voltages can be applied at the start of recording. Of note, the measured time constant on the display may not be equal to one calculated using from Equation 2–2 using the digital filter setting in Hz. As discussed below, the amplified signal (including the calibration signal) is processed by one or more low-frequency filters before being digitized so the filtered signal that is viewed has been processed by two or more low-frequency filters in series.

High-Frequency Filters

A 35-Hz high-frequency filter attenuates a signal of 35 Hz by about 30% (−3 dB filter), and frequencies above 35 Hz would be attenuated more. In addition, frequencies slightly below the high-frequency filter setting will also be slightly attenuated. Figure 2–15 illustrates the effects of a −3 dB 30-Hz filter. A range of high-frequency filter settings is typically provided (off, 3, 15, 35, 70, and 100 Hz). Note that using a 30-Hz high-frequency filter (see Figure 2–15) significantly attenuates 60-Hz signals (although less than a 60-Hz notch filter). Therefore, the addition of a 60-Hz notch filter adds less attenuation if a 35-Hz high-frequency filter is already being used. Using the combination of a low-frequency and a high-frequency filter, a range of frequencies is visualized with little or no attentuation (the bandwidth).

Band Pass Filter

The combination of a low and a high filter applied to a signal is called a band pass filter. The frequency range of signals that are minimally or not attenuated by the filter is called the bandwidth (Figure 2–16). Amplified signals are band pass filtered before being converted to digital data. The high filter setting is chosen based on the sampling rate, and the low filter setting is chosen to allow visualization of slowly varying

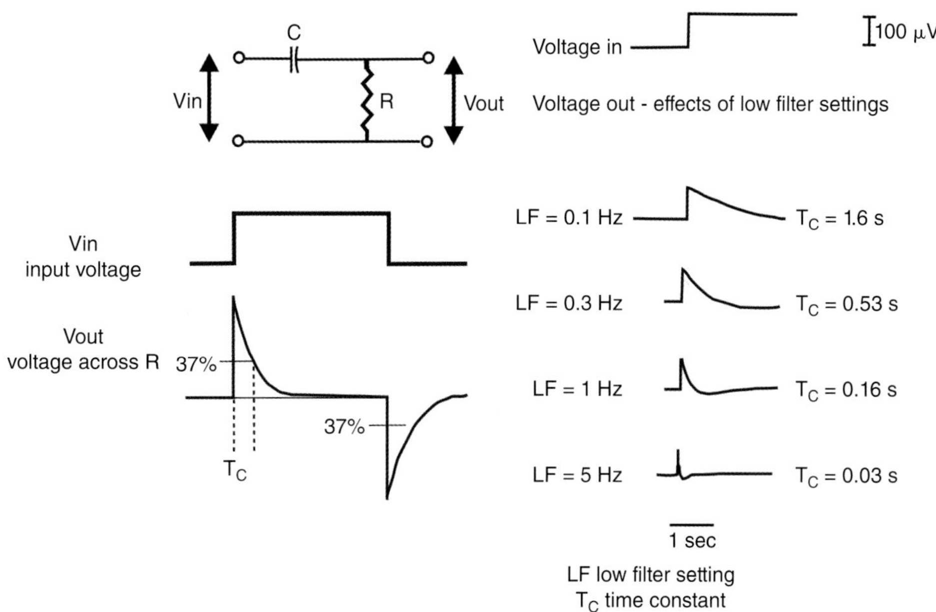

Figure 2–14 Effect of a square wave voltage across a resistance-capacitance circuit acting as a low-frequency filter. After an initial sharp increase in voltage, the amplitude decreases to 37% of the original in one time constant *(TC)*. The *right side* of the figure shows the effects of various low-frequency filters and the associated time constants. The lower the cutoff filter frequency, the longer the T_C. *LF,* Low filter setting.

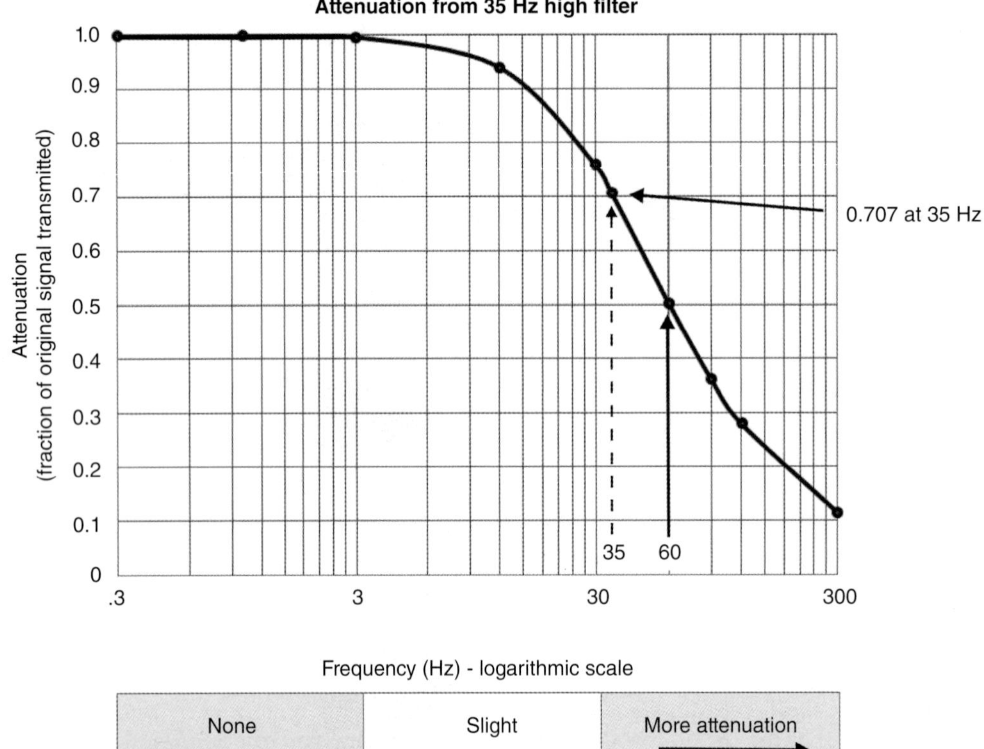

Figure 2–15 The effect of a 35-Hz high-frequency filter (−3 dB) on signals of various frequencies. The Y-axis is linear and the X-axis logarithmic. A 35-Hz signal is attenuated to about 0.7 of the original amplitude. Higher frequencies are attenuated more. Frequencies slightly lower than 35 Hz are attenuated slightly. At 12 Hz there is minimal attenuation, and below 3 Hz there is no attenuation at all. Also note the 60-Hz frequencies are attenuated to about 50% of the original amplitude. The result shown here is for a simple first-order filter. The effects of digital filters used in various polysomnography software may be different.

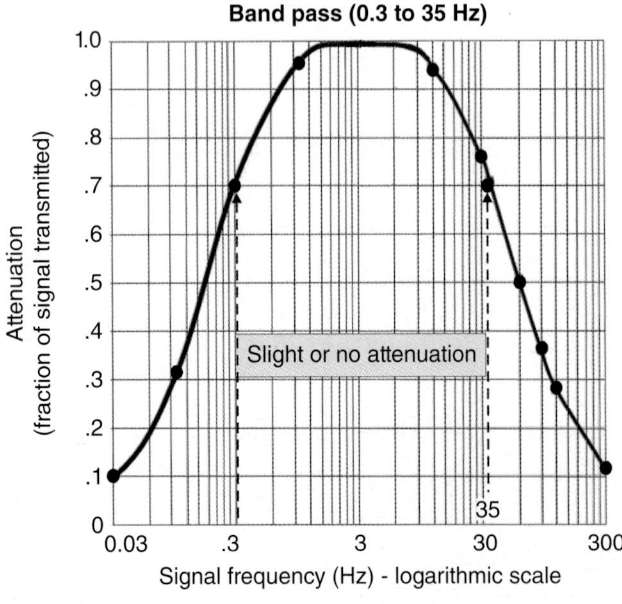

Figure 2–16 The effects of a band pass filter using a combination of a 0.3-Hz low-frequency filter and 35-Hz high-frequency filter. Frequencies between 0.3 and 35 Hz undergo slight or no attenuation. Signals with frequencies outside the 0.3- to 35-Hz bandwidth are attenuated more with greater attenuation of signals much lower than 0.3 Hz or higher than 35 Hz. The results shown here are for a simple first-order filter. Various digital filters may produce different results.

signals while still rejecting unwanted very slowly varying signals due to changes in skin/electrode impedance. Typical band pass settings for a 200 Hz sampling rate might be 0.1 to 100 Hz or 0.08 to 100 Hz.

60-Hz or Notch Filters

Digital PSG systems provide notch filters to significantly attenuate a narrow range of frequency associated with power line signal contamination (e.g., 50 or 60 Hz). The notch filter can be turned on or off. If the notch filter is turned on, it is applied to the signal in addition to the low-frequency and high-frequency filters. The routine use of a notch filter is not recommended. *The appearance of increased 60-Hz activity in a derivation is a clue that one or more electrodes is faulty.* Routine use of notch filters may prevent identification of a problem electrode. Turning on and off the 60-Hz (notch) filter can be useful in determining the degree of signal contamination by 60-Hz interference. If turning off the notch filter dramatically increases signal amplitude, this suggests considerable 60-Hz signal contamination (Figure 2–17). However, as previously mentioned, use of a high-frequency filter of 35 Hz (commonly used for EEG and EOG derivations) already substantially attenuates a 60-Hz signal (but not as much as turning on the 60-Hz filter). Turning on the notch filter will have more effect if a high-frequency filter of 100 Hz is used (commonly used for EMG derivations) compared with a high-frequency filter of 35 Hz (EEG and EOG derivations). For this reason, 60-Hz contamination is most

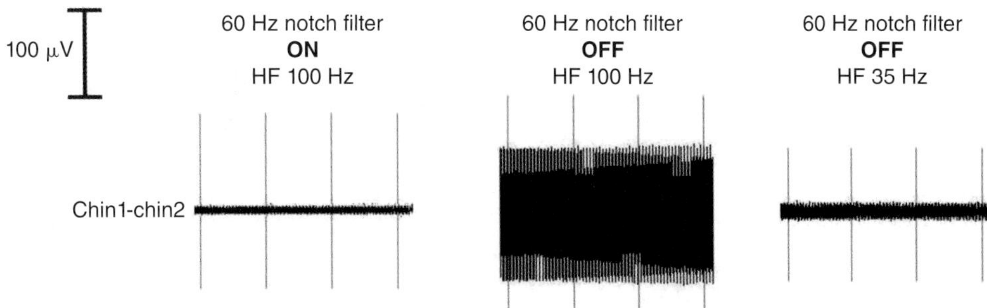

Figure 2–17 The effect of a 60-Hz notch filter on a chin derivation containing a significant amount of 60-Hz signal contamination. Due to use of a notch filter, the contamination may not be detected (left panel). The severity of the 60 Hz contamination can be appreciated by the dramatic increase in signal amplitude when the 60-Hz filter is turned off *(center panel).* However, when a 35-Hz high-frequency filter is used, the 60-Hz activity is also attenuated (even if the notch filter is turned off) but not as much as when the notch filter is used *(right panel).* A 60-Hz artifact is more prominent in derivations using a 100-Hz high-frequency filter compared with those using a 35-Hz filter. *HF,* high filter setting.

frequently visualized in the chin and leg EMG derivations (if the notch filter is off). Artifacts including 60-Hz artifact are discussed in more detail in Chapter 4.

Amplifier (Channel) Filter Setting for Digital Polysomnography

As noted, most PSG amplifiers used for digital recording (referential and true bipolar) output a signal for A/D conversion with a wide band pass using a low-frequency filter (0.03–0.1) and a high-frequency filter setting usually at or less than half the sampling rate (e.g., 100 Hz for a sampling rate of 200/sec). Thus "raw" signals are actually recorded over a wide frequency range or bandwidth (between default low and high frequencies) but are viewed (displayed) after application of selected digital low-frequency and high-frequency filters. The digital filters alter the *displayed* signal but *not* the recorded data. This allows a choice of multiple filter settings if desired by the technologist or reviewer. In Table 2-5 typical combinations of low and high filter settings are shown and the signal type(s) usually recorded using these settings. The low/high filter setting combinations recommended by the AASM scoring manual[9-11] are as follows: EEG and EOG (0.3, 35 Hz); ECG (0.3, 100 Hz); EMG (10, 100 Hz); and airflow/respiratory effort belts (0.1, 15 Hz). The recent edition of the scoring manual changed the high filter setting of the ECG from 70 to 100 Hz to improve visualization of pacer spikes. For nasal pressure the filter combination is (DC or <0.03 Hz, 100 Hz) and PAP device flow, oximetry, the end-tidal Pco_2 waveform, and the transcutaneous PCO_2 are recorded as DC signals. The importance of the nasal pressure filter settings is discussed later. The filter settings for a given signal are selected to include the frequencies of interest in sleep monitoring. For example, to detect slow waves and eye movements but avoid the effect of scalp DC voltage changes (very low frequency), a low-frequency filter of 0.3 Hz is selected. This filter only slightly attenuates 0.5 to 2 Hz signals but effectively reduces unwanted slower frequencies. Setting the low-frequency filter of the EEG or EOG channels higher would reduce slow wave and eye movement amplitude. For EEG and EOG monitoring, selection of a 35-Hz high-frequency filter allows visualization of sleep spindles (11–16 Hz) but removes unwanted higher frequencies. For EMG channels, a low-frequency filter of 10-Hz is used, because the relevant activity is of a much higher frequency. The typical high-frequency filter is 100 Hz. Most systems allow recording of DC signal directly (or with a low-frequency filter of ≤0.08), and a high-frequency filter can be applied for visualization of the waveform if desired in some PSG systems.

Table 2–5 Standard Filter Settings

Low Frequency	High frequency	Signal type
0.3 Hz	35 Hz	EEG, EOG
0.3 Hz	100 Hz	ECG
10 Hz	100 Hz	EMG Snoring sensor
0.1 Hz	15 Hz	Oronasal thermal flow Chest and abdominal effort belts
DC or <0.03 Hz	100 Hz	Nasal pressure
DC	DC	PAP device flow Oximetry End-tidal Pco_2 waveform and value Transcutaneous PCO_2 value

The filter settings are consistent with the recommendations in the AASM scoring manual.

DC, direct current; ECG, Electrocardiography; *EEG,* electroencephalography; *EMG,* electromyography; *EOG,* electrooculography.

Adapted from Troester MM, Quan SF, Berry RB, et al; for the American Academy of Sleep Medicine. *The AASM Manual for the Scoring of Sleep and Associated Events: Rules, Terminology and Technical Specifications. Version 3.*

Clinical Example of the Effects of Filter Settings

As discussed in Chapter 10, monitoring nasal pressure provides a more accurate estimate of airflow than thermal sensors. During upper airway narrowing, the nasal pressure signal shows a flattening (flow plateau) during inspiration. Some sleep centers record nasal pressure with an AC amplifier instead of acquiring the signal in the DC mode. However, a low-frequency filter setting of 0.03 or less (or a long T_C) is ideal to allow visualization of a flow plateau in the nasal pressure signal (Figure 2–18). To accurately record or display a very slowly varying signal, a sufficiently low cutoff frequency must be used for the low

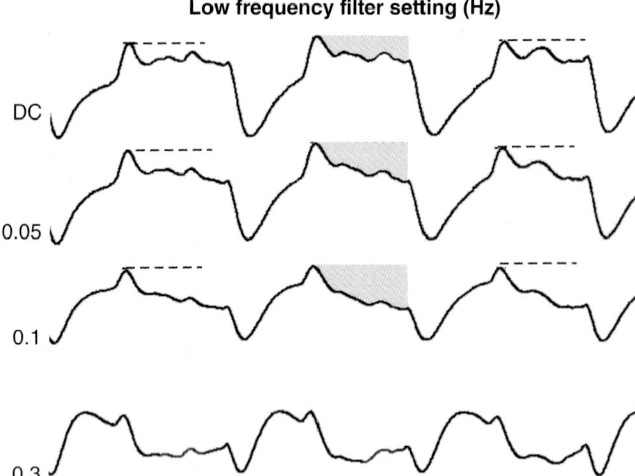

Figure 2–18 Effects of various low-frequency filters on a nasal pressure signal showing flattening (inspiration upward). The plateau is seen best when acquired as a direct current *(DC)* signal or when a low-frequency filter with a very low cutoff frequency is used (0.05). Even using a low-frequency filter of 0.1 Hz, some flattening can be noted, but a 0.3 filter dramatically alters the waveform shape.

filter. If the nasal pressure signal is unfiltered, high-frequency vibration in the signal (airflow) during snoring is often visible. However, the ability to see snoring (high-frequency vibration) depends on the appropriate high-frequency filter settings. Using a low setting for the high-frequency filter will reduce high-frequency signals such as noted in the nasal pressure tracing during snoring (Figure 2–19). Ideally, one would use a high-frequency filter setting of 70 to 100 Hz. However, as previously mentioned the maximum high-frequency filter setting would be one-half the sampling rate. Digital PSG systems will provide only appropriate filter setting choices based on the sampling rate. Many PSG systems record all signals using the same sampling rate, but downsample some signals with additional filtering if appropriate before the data is stored in a digital format.

DIGITAL SYSTEM OVERVIEW

The typical PSG system uses a headbox for connection of the individual electrodes to the PSG amplifier.[14,15] This includes the EEG, the EOG, chin EMG electrodes for referential recording, and inputs from the bipolar signals. The head box may also contain an integrated pressure transducer (nasal pressure monitoring) and input for the pulse oximeter probe (arterial oxygen saturation). An accessory box for DC channel inputs or dedicated input jacks on the amplifier is also usually available. The amplifier is then connected to the A/D converter. The A/D converter transforms the analog signals into digital data. Today, the A/D converter is usually contained within the amplifier case that is located at the patient's bedside. The digitized signal can then be sent over ethernet cables to the computer or sent in wireless mode to a computer, which then records the digital data. This arrangement avoids the difficulties that occur when an analog signal is sent over a long distance (60-Hz contamination or loss of signal strength). In some systems digital data is also stored on a device in the patient room to avoid interruptions, especially if connection with the computer in the monitoring room is over a network rather than a dedicated ethernet cable. Storage in the patient room also prevents loss of data if the computer in the monitoring room crashes. A schematic of a typical system is shown in Figure 2–20. A typical PSG amplifier often has a fixed gain and default low- and high-frequency filter settings (e.g., 0.08 and 100 Hz). As discussed in the section on sampling rate, the high-frequency filter is chosen to avoid aliasing distortion. As previously discussed, for a sampling rate of 200 Hz the value is 100 Hz. AC signals are recorded over a wide frequency range (bandwidth). The A/D converter samples the signal, and raw digital data are stored in the computer. After the raw data are digitized and stored, extensive manipulation is possible to produce the desired signal display. During acquisition and review, the computer program performs digital subtraction of referentially recorded signals to display the desired derivations and processes the data with the selected digital low-frequency and high-frequency filters. A display sensitivity is also chosen to determine the upper and lower limits of data

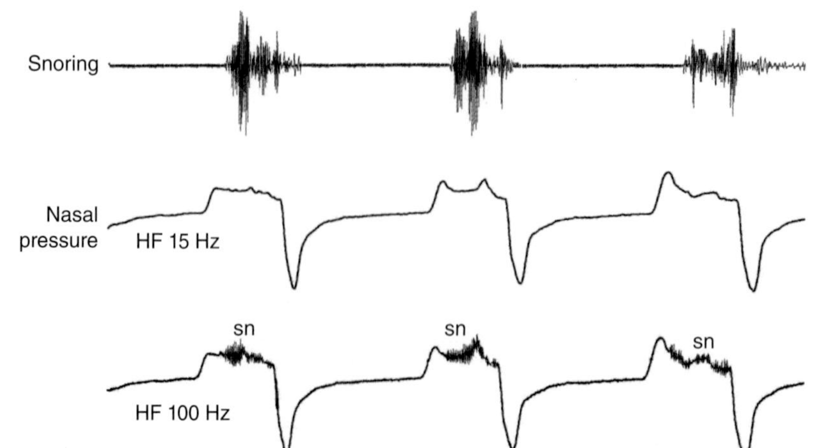

Figure 2–19 Using a high-frequency filter setting *(HF)* of 100 Hz for visualization of the nasal pressure signal allows visualization of high-frequency pressure vibration associated with snoring (sn). This activity is removed if a high-frequency filter of 15 Hz is used.

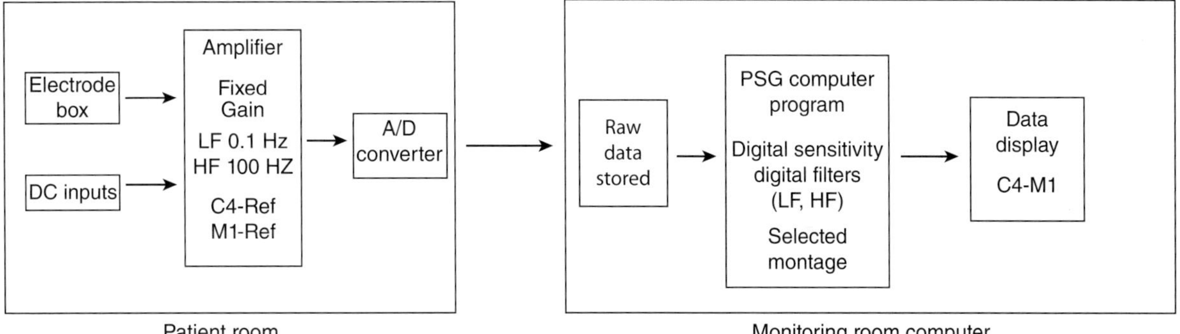

Figure 2–20 A simplified schematic of data flow during polysomnography. Data is acquired and amplified with a default gain and band pass filtered before being converted to digital data. Digital data is then transmitted to the monitoring room where it is stored. In some systems additional appropriate digital filtering is performed before storage in cases where all the digital data for a given channel is not stored (reduced effective sampling rate). The raw data is manipulated by the computer program to produce the display view using the selected montage (including filter settings). The raw stored data (acquired with a wide band pass) is not changed by the program. This allows display of the data using multiple montages and channel settings. Converting data to digital form before transfer to the monitoring room prevents corruption of the analog data by long cables and exposure to sources of signal contamination. In many systems the data is also stored in the patient room as a backup to prevent loss of data due to malfunction of the computer in the control room. Data is also often transferred from the patient room to the monitoring room over a network, and issues with the network can cause problems with data transmission. Saving the data in the patient room prevents loss of data due to network issues. *A/D*, Analog-to-digital; *DC*, direct current; *HF*, high filter setting; *LF*, low filter setting; *PSG*, polysomnography.

to be displayed in the channel width (sensitivity). The changes in the display view (specific derivations, digital filters, display sensitivity) do not change the raw data that are recorded and stored on the computer.

Channel Settings/Montages

Each channel (tracing) display can be changed by the viewer with respect to the inputs, sensitivity (sometimes called gain), low-frequency and high-frequency filters, channel width, tracing color, and inversion of signal. Montages (collection of signals to be displayed) can be defined (Table 2–2) and stored in the PSG program. Most systems have a montage editor where one can specify standard sensitivity, color, and digital filter settings for each channel for each montage (or workplace view) and store them with the montage information (Table 2–6), so they do not have to be individually set for each recording (or each time a recording is viewed). Figure 2–21 illustrates typical channel controls. As previously mentioned, changes in channel settings do not change the recorded (and digitally stored) data. In sleep recording using paper, the EEG was usually recorded at a sensitivity of 50 to 70 μV/cm in adults. In children, a lower sensitivity (100 μV/cm) was used because of the very high amplitude EEG activity. The term *gain* rather than *sensitivity* was also used. However, this implies an amplification of signal. In digital recording, amplification occurs before the signal is digitized. The size of the display of a given signal is varied by the computer program that scales the display based on the available channel width and the voltage limits or sensitivity. For example, if a channel width of 100 pixels represents 100 μV peak to peak, a signal of 50-μV peak to peak would vary between the 25th and the 75th pixel. If the channel is 50 μV peak to peak, the signal would occupy the entire channel width of 100 pixels. The default digital displays for EEG often use 100 or 150 μV peak to peak per channel width (200 μV for children). Some PSG systems also scale EEG signals with a goal of a displaying a desired size on the monitor screen. A 50-μV deflection at 5 μV/mm would occupy 1 cm on the monitor screen. This method requires knowledge of the monitor resolution and mimics visualization of the signal as if printed on paper. Figure 2–22 shows the same EEG derivation displayed at different sensitivity settings using two formats. A range of sensitivity options is usually available; for example, 25, 50, 100, 150, or 300 μV peak to peak (or using the μV/mm format, 3 μV/mm, 5 μV/mm, 7 μV/mm, 10 μV/mm). In either approach it is confusing that a lower number corresponds to a bigger signal. In some systems if the signal voltage exceeds the voltage limits of the channel, the signal is truncated (clipped). In other systems the signal simply overlaps onto the adjacent channel tracings.

Impedance Checking and Referential Display View

Traditionally, after electrodes were applied to the patient's head, the impedance of each electrode was checked by plugging the electrodes into an impedance box that allowed comparison of any electrode referred to the ground electrode or a combination of all the other electrodes. However, most digital systems can measure impedance online during recording using a signal from the amplifier often sent to the ground electrode or reference electrode. Then the results of the signal are recorded at each electrode. Knowing the frequency and voltage of the signal sent and the measured value at each electrode, the impedance of each electrode is calculated. The values can then be stored with other digital data for later review. The AASM scoring manual[9,10] recommends a maximum EEG, EOG, and chin EMG electrode impedance of 5 KΩ (kiloohms) (impedance ≤5 kiloohms). Leg EMG recording is more challenging, thus impedance of ≤10 KΩ is acceptable. The AASM scoring manual does not currently specify and impedance of ECG electrodes, but a low impedance will reduce the noise in the baseline signal. Another useful method of looking at the quality of each individual electrode is to display all of the unfiltered (except for bandpass filter before digitizing), referentially recorded electrodes

Table 2–6 Sample Settings for Each Channel in a Diagnostic Montage

Channel	Diagnostic 1	Low-Frequency Filter(Hz)	High-Frequency Filter(Hz)	Sensitivity (μV p-p)	NotchFilter	Channel Size	Color
1	F4-M1	0.3	35	150	OFF	100	Black
2	C4-M1	0.3	35	150	OFF	100	Black
3	O2-M1	0.3	35	150	OFF	100	Black
4	E1-M2	0.3	35	150	OFF	100	Black
5	E2-M2	0.3	35	150	OFF	100	Blue
6	Chin EMG	10	100	150	OFF	100	Blue
7	ECG	0.3	70	150	OFF	100	Black
8	Pulse rate	DC	DC	150	OFF	100	Black
9	Snoring	10	100	150	OFF	100	Black
10	Nasal Pressure	DC	100	150	OFF	100	Black
11	Oronasal thermal flow	0.1	15	150	OFF	100	Black
12	Chest	0.1	15	150	OFF	100	Black
13	Abdomen	0.1	15	150	OFF	100	Black
14	SpO_2	DC	DC	150	OFF	100	Black
15	LAT	10	100	150	OFF	100	Black
16	RAT	10	100	150	OFF	100	Black
17	Exhaled PCO_2	DC	DC	150	OFF	100	Black
18	End-tidal PCO_2	DC	DC	150	OFF	100	Black

Channel size is relative (four channels 100, 100, 100, 200 means the first three channels each occupy one-fifth of the viewing area, and the last channel occupies two-fifths of the viewing area). Exhaled PCO_2 is the capnography waveform, End-tidal PCO_2 is the reading (value).

DC, Direct current; *ECG,* electrocardiography; *EMG,* electromyography; *LAT,* left anterior tibial; *PCO_2,* partial pressure of carbon dioxide; *RAT,* right anterior tibial; *SpO_2,* pulse oximetry; *μV p-p,* peak-to-peak channel voltage.

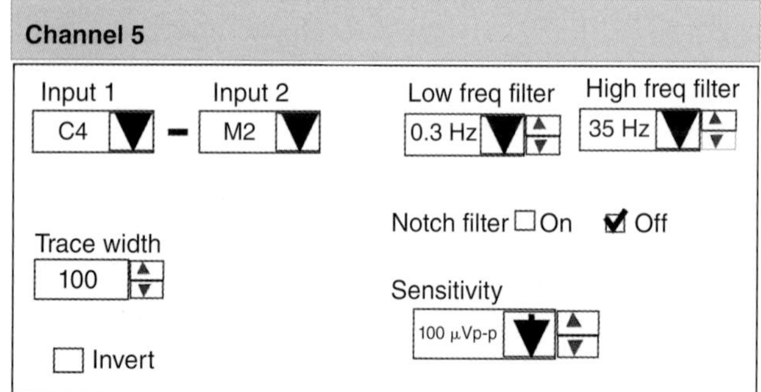

Figure 2–21 Example of a typical referential channel control. The two inputs can be specified, as well as the low- and high-frequency filter settings chosen; the notch filter can be turned on or off; the signal can be inverted; the sensitivity can be specified; and the channel width specified. Typically, the channel trace color can also be chosen (not shown). All of these parameters can be specified for each channel in a saved montage. Multiple montages can be saved specifying the channels viewed and the order on the screen, as well as the chosen settings for each channel.

against the common reference (rather than the digital subtraction of two referentially recorded electrodes). Figure 2–23 displays a referential view with all high-frequency filters set to 100 Hz. Electrode impedance is also displayed. One can tell that O2 and Chin2 are faulty and should be changed or fixed. The figure also shows the electrode impedance, which was very high for the two faulty electrodes. As previously noted, if all tracings on the referential view are bad, this suggests a problem with the reference electrode. However, a faulty reference electrode does not affect the true bipolar channels (see Figure 2–6).

Calibration

Calibration was critical during paper recording to document the individual amplifier sensitivity, polarity, and filter settings because these could not be changed once data were recorded on paper. Calibration was usually performed by sending a square wave voltage pulse (typically 50 μV). The sensitivity control was adjusted until a 50-μV signal produced a 10-mm pen deflection (others used 75 μV for 10 mm). In the digital era, EEG, EOG, and EMG data are acquired using a default amplifier gain and filtered with a wide bandpass (e.g., 0.03 and 100 Hz) before conversion to digital data. Different digital filters may be applied to the stored signal data for display, but this does not change the stored data. Recording of calibration signals is usually still performed, but the goal is to display that the system is working correctly and that sensitivity and filter settings are appropriate and not for adjustment of amplifier gain. Modern solid-state amplifiers are adjusted at the factory and remain very stable over time. The appearance of a calibration signal is affected by both low- and high-frequency filter settings. Even if there is an error in default display filter settings, this can be corrected for an individual channel during review by application of the appropriate filter. Figure 2–24 shows an example of recording during calibration mode. One can see that the tracing in F4-M1 has a slightly different shape than the other EEG/EOG derivations. Here the

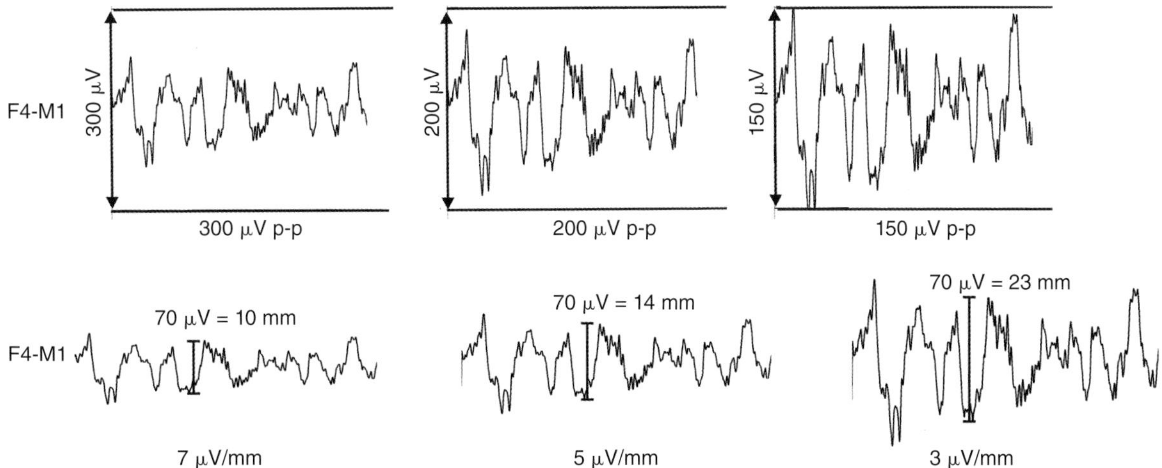

Figure 2–22 Two methods of specifying gain or sensitivity for data display. Although the terms *sensitivity* and *gain* are used, the original raw data is not changed. The data is scaled by the computer program based on the monitor resolution, screen size, and the number of channels displayed. The *top row* shows data display by specifying channel peak-to-peak voltage. The *bottom row* shows specification as voltage to waveform size. This method attempts to mimic paper recording and depends on the monitor resolution. In both cases a lower number is actually more sensitive (moving from left to right).

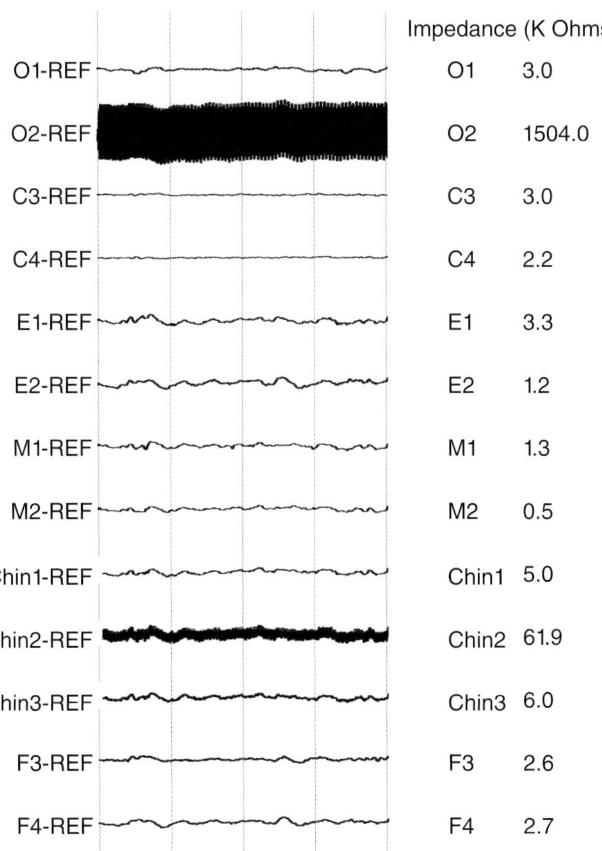

Figure 2–23 An example of a referential montage and the corresponding impedance values for the different electrodes. One can see that there is an issue with electrodes O2 and Chin2. The very dark, rope-like waveform is due to 60-Hz artifact. Note that the impedance values for these electrodes are high. The recommended electrode impedance is 5 KΩ or less. (From Berry RB, Wagner MH. *Sleep Medicine Pearls.* 3rd ed. Elsevier; 2015:89.)

low filter setting LF has been turned off. The signal still decreases while the calibration voltage is constant, showing that a low filter was already applied before the analog signal was converted to digital form. Compare this to the square shape of DC signals (SpO_2 and CPAP leak tracings).

Calibration of DC signals (Figure 2–25) is usually performed using a two-point calibration method. This is performed by knowing what the reading on the device supplying the signal input corresponds to a given voltage (V). For example, a PAP device and analog module outputs 0 V for 0 cm H_2O pressure and 1 V for 30 cm H_2O pressure. The voltage input and corresponding digital value are specified and the calibration factor (30 cm H_2O/1 volt) is stored in the software. In Figure 2–25, digital values 0 and 30 cm H_2O are specified to correspond to 0 and 1 V, respectively. In Figure 2–24 the SpO_2 tracing uses 0 to 1 V for 0 to 100% and the CPAP leak signal uses 0 to 1 V for 0 to 120 L/min. The calibration tracing verifies that the calibration factors have been correctly set in the software.

Physiological Calibration (Biocalibration)

Biocalibration (Figure 2–26) is an important part of every PSG recording, but the value of the procedure is often unrecognized. The AASM scoring manual[10] contains a recommended biocalibration procedure, as follows:

1. Perform/document an impedance check of the EEG, EOG, and EMG electrodes
2. Record at least 30 seconds of EEG with patient awake lying quietly with **eyes open**
3. Record at least 30 seconds of EEG with patient lying quietly with **eyes closed**
4. **Look up and down** without moving the head (×5)
5. **Look left and right** without moving the head (×5)
6. Blink (×5)
7. Grit teeth and/or chew (5 seconds)
8. Simulate a snore or hum (5 seconds)

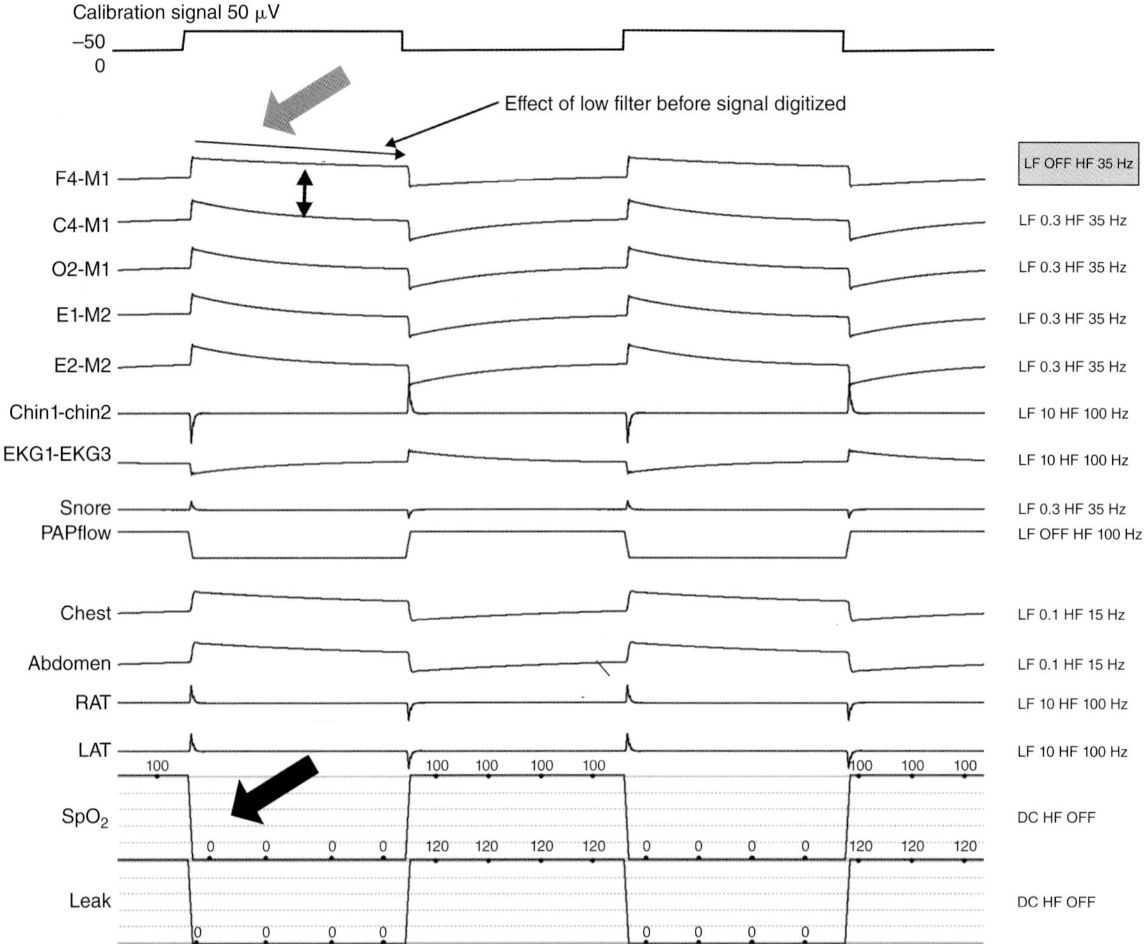

Figure 2–24 A recording of a typical calibration signals using a step voltage (square wave voltage) calibration signal. In the alternating current (AC) channels there is an initial sharp deflection followed by a slow decrease in the signal amplitude that depends on the low-frequency filter setting (time constant). Recall that a steady constant input to an AC amplifier results in zero deflection. An AC amplifier responds to changes in the signal. The low-frequency filter is turned off in F4-M1 *(gray arrow)*, but the signal still has a slow decrease consistent with the fact that the signal has been changed by one or more low-frequency filters before the signal is converted to digital form. In contrast, direct current *(DC)* signals *(large dark arrow)* remain constant as long as the input voltage is constant. *HF*, High filter setting; *LAT*, left anterior tibial electromyogram; *LF*, low filter setting; *RAT*, right anterior tibial electromyogram; *SpO*$_2$, arterial oxygen saturation by pulse oximetry; *Leak*, PAP device leak signal.

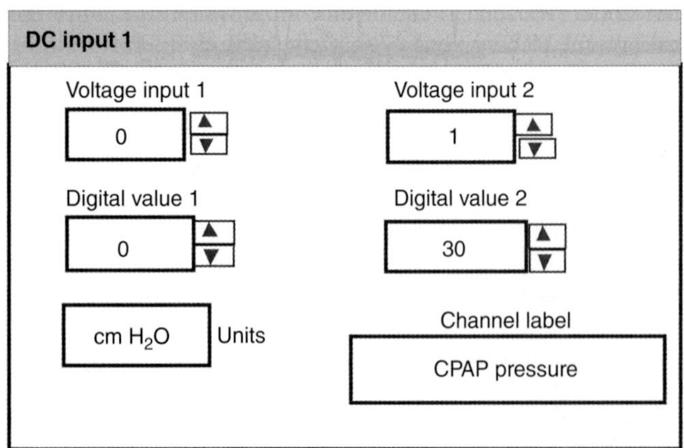

Figure 2–25 An example of direct current *(DC)* calibration. Values of 0 and 1 V correspond to 0 and 30 cm H_2O pressure. The proper calibration factors are supplied by the manufacturer of the laboratory positive airway pressure device or other instruments such as the capnography or transcutaneous partial pressure of carbon dioxide (PCO_2) device (e.g., a PCO_2 value of 0–100 mm Hg corresponding to 0–1 V). *CPAP*, Continuous positive airway pressure.

9. **Breathe normally;** verify that the polarity of airflow and effort channels is synchronized
10. **Breath hold** (10 seconds); simulates apnea
11. Ask the patient to breathe normally and, upon instruction, to take a breath in and out; check polarity and mark the record with the timing of the commands IN and OUT accordingly
12. Breathe through the **nose only** (10 seconds); documents that nasal breathing is detected
13. Breathe through the **mouth only** (10 seconds); documents that oral breathing is detected
14. Deep breath and exhale slowly (prolonged expiration: 10 seconds)
15. Flex the left foot/raise the toes on the **left foot** (×5)
16. Flex the right foot/raise the toes on the **right foot** (×5)
17. Flex/extend the fingers on the left hand, as appropriate, if upper extremity EMG is recorded
18. Flex/extend the fingers on the right left hand, as appropriate, if upper extremity EMG is recorded
19. Adjust the ECG signal to provide a clear waveform (R wave should deflect upward)

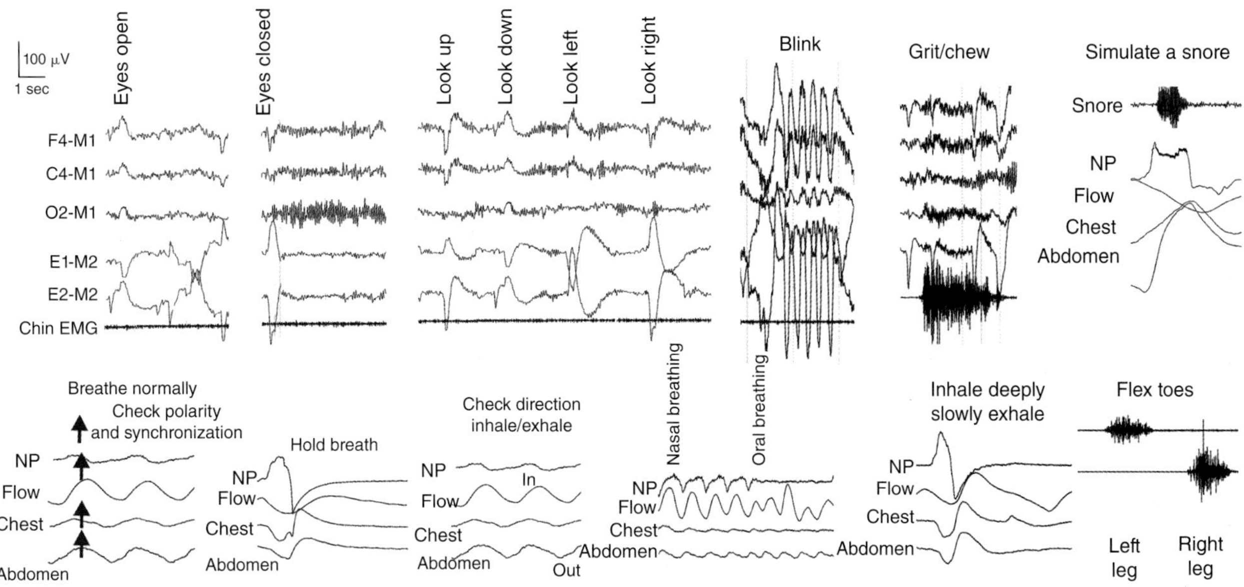

Figure 2–26 Selected portions of a biocalibration procedure. Biocalibration procedures move from left to right on the top line then left to right on the bottom line. For simplicity, only one or a small number of repetitions for each maneuver are illustrated. Note that the eyes closed command produced posterior dominant rhythm in the occipital derivation (O2-M1). (Adapted from Berry RB, Wagner MH. *Sleep Medicine Pearls.* 3rd ed. Elsevier; 2015:84.)

20. Perform and document a repeat impedance check of the EEG, EOG, and EMG electrodes at the end of the PSG recording
21. Repeat physiological calibrations at the end of the PSG recording

During the biocalibration procedure, signals are recorded while the patient performs maneuvers that verify the monitoring equipment, electrodes, and sensors are working properly. The impedance of all EEG, EOG, and EMG electrodes should also be checked. The AASM scoring manual recommends that biocalibration be performed at the beginning and end of the night's recording. Some useful information that can be determined from biocalibration is summarized in Table 2–7. For the reviewer, noting the patient's EEG, EOG, and EMG pattern of eyes-open and eyes-closed stage W can help with recognition of this sleep stage during the recording and during scoring of sleep. It is especially important to know whether the person being recorded generates posterior dominant (alpha) rhythm with eye closure because this affects the scoring criteria for stage W and stage N1 (see Chapter 3). It is important that signals from all the respiratory sensors be both functional and synchronized. Most sleep centers use the convention of inspiratory upward. All flow signals and effort belt signals should have a polarity consistent with the convention used in the sleep center.

Table 2–7 Information Provided by Biocalibration

Procedure	Information Provided
Eyes open	• Attenuation of alpha • EEG of wakefulness • Pattern of eyes-open stage W • REMs during wake
Eyes closed	• Quality of alpha production • Slow eye movements
Eye movements up-down-left-right Blink eyes	• Integrity of eye electrodes • Pattern of the patient's REMs and blinks • Ability to detect horizontal and vertical eye movements
Grit teeth	• Function of chin EMG • Sensitivity should be adjusted so that some activity is present during relaxed wake
Hold your breath and quiet breathing maneuvers	• Airflow sensors show airflow working properly, adjust sensitivity • Proper polarity for all respiratory sensors including oronasal airflow, nasal pressure, and chest and abdominal effort belts (i.e., during inspiration, all deflections are upward or downward, depending on sleep center protocol) • Adjust sensitivity of chest and abdomen tracings • Ability to detect apnea
Nasal-only then oral-only breathing	• Ability to detect nasal and oral breathing
Extremity maneuvers	• Ability to detect leg movements • Adjust leg derivation sensitivity so movements can be easily seen in both legs

EEG, Electroencephalogram; *EMG,* electromyogram; *REMs,* rapid eye movements.

Video-Audio Polysomnography

Today most digital systems allow for the simultaneous recording of video and audio signals. Ideally the video should be synchronized with the recorded EEG and other signals. This will allow the reviewer to see patient movement corresponding exactly to a given time point in the recorded PSG signals. For example, one could note facial twitching during a particular EEG pattern. The AASM scoring manual requires that recorded video data must be synchronized with PSG data within one second and have an accuracy of at least one video frame per second (higher when monitoring for a parasomnia).

Video PSG is an important development and allows the reviewer to confirm the position of the patient (supine, lateral) and document unusual behavior (e.g., parasomnias) during the night. Simultaneous audio is also usually available, which is very useful for documenting teeth grinding (bruxism), talking during parasomnias, snoring, and other behaviors during the recording. A definitive diagnosis of bruxism requires a typical EEG/EMG pattern associated with audible teeth grinding. Video files are often quite large and are usually compressed (e.g., MPEG4). The size of the file will depend on the quality of the video (10 or 25 frames/sec). Review of the video can elucidate the reason for the sudden appearance of artifact in the tracings (patient scratching the head).

GROUNDS AND ELECTRICAL SAFETY

The terminology is confusing with three different grounds being used in modern PSG recording.[16] These include:

1. *Patient ground* (isoground input on the electrode box). This neutral electrode is usually connected to the forehead. It is used to balance the inputs of all the differential amplifiers (essential for common mode rejection). This ground should be isolated from other grounds to avoid current entering the body via this electrode.
2. *Chassis ground* (container ground). Because a metal chassis is rarely used today, this would be the amplifier circuit ground (or the ground of the nonisolated portion of the amplifier).
3. *Earth ground.* In the three-wire power line (three-prong plug) AC input, the three wires are designated "hot" (H), "neutral" (N), and "earth ground."

Essentially all PSG systems use an isolated medical-grade power supply that outputs low-level DC voltage to power the amplifiers. The power supplies have a circuit to smooth the output voltage (regulated). The low-voltage DC portions of the power supply are isolated from the high-voltage AC portions. This is another safeguard to improve electrical safety.

In modern systems, the patient ground is never directly connected to the amplifier circuit or earth ground. A current-limiting device or isolation device is always placed between the patient ground and the earth ground. A common method is to use optical isolation in which the signal is transmitted by light within a small element of the circuit. That is, the amplifier consists of an isolated portion (connected to patient ground) and a nonisolated portion connected to circuit/chassis ground.

Routine testing of equipment used for human monitoring is essential for electrical safety. Table 2–8 shows the effects of various 60 Hz AC currents applied to the chest.[17] Of note, **100 milliamperes (mA)** is the ventricular fibrillation threshold. Note also that the same voltage applied to wet skin (a skin electrode) or internal monitoring devices results in much greater current (less resistance) than when applied to dry skin. Therefore, the safety standards require very low leakage current for medical devices. Testing of monitoring equipment is essential to assure proper grounding and measurement of leakage current (must be <100 μA for PSG and <10 μA for high-risk areas). All equipment should be connected to the same power strip or ground to avoid ground loops. These occur due to voltage differences between different grounds. Using a single ground minimizes the chances of failure of the grounding wiring (ground fault) when multiple grounds are used. Turning equipment on before attaching the patient and disconnecting the patient before turning the equipment off can avoid exposure to power surges.

Table 2–8 Estimated Effects of 60-Hz Alternating Currents

1 mA	Barely perceptible
16 mA	Maximum grasp and let go
20 mA	Paralysis of respiratory muscles
100 mA	Ventricular fibrillation threshold
2 Amps	Cardiac standstill, organ damage
15/20 Amps	Common fuse breaker opens

This is for currents applied to the chest. The same applied voltage to wet skin results in much greater current.
mA, Milliampere.
From NIOSH: The National Institute for Occupational Safety and Health. *Worker Deaths by Electrocution.* NIOSH Publication No. 98-131. https://stacks.cdc.gov/view/cdc/6385

SUMMARY OF KEY POINTS

1. PSG uses three types of recording: referential, true bipolar, and DC. In referential recording each electrode is recorded compared with a reference electrode. Any combination of referentially recorded electrodes can be displayed.
2. The recommended EEG, EOG, and chin EMG electrode impedance is 5 KΩ or less (≤5 kiloohms).
3. A signal of X frequency must be sampled at a frequency greater than 2X to avoid aliasing distortion. A more accurate representation is obtained by an even higher sampling rate (10X or greater).
4. A high-frequency filter of one-half the sampling rate must be applied before signals are digitized to avoid distortion. For example, for a sampling rate of 200 Hz, the high filter setting should be 100 Hz.
5. A filter setting of X Hz means a X-Hz signal will be reduced to about 0.7 of the original amplitude (−3 dB filter).
6. A low-frequency filter of 0.3 Hz attenuates signals less than 0.3 Hz (the lower the frequency below 0.3 Hz, the greater the attenuation), slightly attenuates signals with a frequency slightly above 0.3 Hz, and has minimal or no effect on signals with a frequency of 1 Hz or greater.
7. A high-frequency filter of 35 Hz attenuates signals higher than 35 Hz (the higher the frequency is above 35 Hz, the greater the attenuation), slightly attenuates signals with a frequency slightly below 35 Hz, and has no or minimal attenuation of signals lower than approximately 12 Hz.
8. The recommended band pass of 0.3 to 35 Hz allows visualization of slow wave activity and sleep spindles with minimal attenuation while reducing unwanted lower and higher frequencies.
9. Routine use of the 60-Hz notch filter is not recommended. The presence of 60-Hz contamination alerts the technologist that an electrode has a high impedance.
10. Biocalibration should be performed at the start and end of each sleep study. It is important to note if the individual monitored generates posterior dominant rhythm (alpha rhythm) with the eyes closed. All respiratory signals should have inspiration in the same direction (usually up).
11. Once signals are recorded and stored in the computer, they can be modified for appropriate viewing (application of digital filters), but the original data is not changed.

CLINICAL REVIEW QUESTIONS

1. What (low, high) filter settings are recommended for PSG recording (display) of EEG and EOG derivations?
   A. 0.5, 70 Hz
   B. 0.3, 35 Hz
   C. 0.5, 70 Hz
   D. 0.5, 35 Hz
2. What are the recommended (low, high) filter settings for display of EMG?
   A. 1 Hz, 70 Hz
   B. 0.3 Hz, 35 Hz
   C. 10 Hz, 100 Hz
   D. 10 Hz, 70 Hz
3. What is the minimum recommended sampling rate for recording EEG, EOG, EMG, and ECG signals?
   A. 100 samples/sec
   B. 200 samples/sec
   C. 400 samples/sec
   D. 500 samples/sec
4. Which of the following is true about the effect of a low filter setting of 0.3 Hz?
   A. It has minimal effect on a 10-Hz signal.
   B. It does not affect the amplitude of slow wave activity (0.5–2 Hz).
   C. It decreases the amplitude of a 0.1-Hz signal more than a 0.3-Hz signal.
   D. A and B
   E. A and C
5. If a sampling rate of 400 samples/sec is used, what is the highest-frequency cutoff for the high filter that can be used and still avoid significant aliasing distortion?
   A. 400 Hz
   B. 200 Hz
   C. 100 Hz
   D. 50 Hz
6. Signals X, Y, and Z are recorded against a reference (referential) and W1 and W2 are acquired by bipolar recording (W1-W2) using digital PSG. Which of the following is **NOT** true?
   A. The derivation X-Y can be displayed.
   B. The derivation W1-X can be displayed.
   C. If all derivations containing X, Y, and Z show artifact, the reference electrode is probably faulty.
   D. The filter settings of the displayed derivation W1-W2 can be changed.
7. What is the recommended EEG, EOG, and chin EMG electrode impedance?
   A. ≤10 KΩ
   B. ≤5 KΩ
   C. ≤20 KΩ
   D. ≤1 KΩ
8. What high-frequency filter setting for ECG will best allow visualization of pacer spikes?
   A. 100 Hz
   B. 35 Hz
   C. 70 Hz
   D. 10 Hz
9. Using a high filter of 35 Hz for the EEG and EOG display (recording) reduces 60-Hz activity in the displayed signal.
   A. True
   B. False
10. What are the recommended (low, high) filter settings for display of the thermal airflow or chest and abdominal respiratory inductance plethysmography signals?
    A. 0.3, 35 Hz
    B. 0.1, 15 Hz
    C. 0.3, 15 Hz
    D. 0.1, 35 Hz
11. A 100-μV signal with a frequency of 1 Hz is processed by a 1 Hz (−3 dB) low-frequency filter. What is the approximate resulting amplitude?
    A. 30 μV
    B. 50 μV
    C. 70 μV
    D. 90 μV
12. What is the minimum sampling rate recommended by the AASM for recording the oximetry signal?
    A. Minimal 10 Hz, optimal 25 Hz
    B. Minimal 5 Hz, optimal 20 Hz
    C. Minimal 20 Hz, optimal 50 Hz
    D. Minimal 5 Hz, optimal 15 Hz

ANSWERS

1. **B**
2. **C**
3. **B**
4. **E.** A low filter of X Hz has some effect on signals with a slightly higher frequency than X. Therefore, a 0.3-Hz filter does slightly attenuate signals in the lower part of the 0.5- to 2-Hz frequency range. The lower a frequency signal is compared with X Hz, the larger the decrement in amplitude. A 0.3-Hz filter decreases the amplitude of a 0.1-Hz signal more than a 0.3-Hz signal.
5. **B.** 200 Hz. The Nyquist theorem states that the minimum sampling frequency to record a signal of X Hz is 2X Hz. Conversely, all frequencies greater than X Hz are undersampled if a sampling rate of 2X Hz is used and this can result in aliasing signal distortion. For this reason, a high frequency filter of X Hz must be applied to a signal sampled at 2X Hz before the signal reaches the A/D converter and is converted to digital data.
6. **B.** True bipolar recording does not allow one part of the derivation (W1, W2) to be displayed against another electrode.
7. **B.** ≤5 KΩ is recommended, but ≤10 KΩ is acceptable for limb EMG.
8. **A.** For rapidly changing waveforms, a higher setting of the high-frequency filter will allow better visualization.
9. **A. True.** A high filter with a cutoff setting of 35 Hz reduces the activity of frequency of signals higher than 35 Hz. Therefore a 35-Hz high filter does reduce 60-Hz contamination but not as much as the 60-Hz notch filter.
10. **B.** Using a low filter of 0.1 instead of 0.3 allows more accurate visualization of a slowly varying signal. A high-frequency filter of 15 Hz is recommended to minimize unwanted artifact.
11. **C.** A −3 dB 1-Hz low filter will attenuate the signal to approximately 0.707 of the original amplitude.
12. **A.** The AASM scoring manual states that using 25 Hz is desirable to assist with artifact evaluation. Oximeters display a moving average of several beats to avoid artifactual changes due to inaccuracy in a single reading due to movement. Averaging a large number of beats reduces artifact

(inaccurate value due to movement), but too long an average time reduces the ability to detect transient desaturations. The AASM scoring manual specified an averaging time ≤3 seconds at a heart rate of 80 beats per minute. This is equivalent to a moving time average of 4 beats.

ABBREVIATIONS

AASM, American Academy of Sleep Medicine; *AC,* alternating current; *CPAP,* continuous positive airway pressure; *DC,* direct current; *ECG,* electrocardiographic; *EEG,* electroencephalography; *EMG,* electromyography; *EOG,* electrooculography; *HF,* high frequency; *Hz,* hertz, *LAT,* left anterior tibial; *NREM,* non–rapid eye movement; *PAP,* positive airway pressure; *PSG,* polysomnography; *RC,* resistance-capacitance; *REM,* rapid eye movement; *Tc,* time constant; *RAT,* right anterior tibial.

SUGGESTED READING

Libenson MH. *Practical Approach to Electroencephalography.* Saunders Elsevier; 2010:146-170.

Patil SP. What every clinician should know about polysomnography. *Respir Care.* 2010;55(9):1179-1195.

Silber MH, Ancoli-Israel S, Bonnet MH, et al. The visual scoring of sleep in adults. *J Clin Sleep Med.* 2007;15:121-131.

Troester MM, Quan SF, Berry RB, et al; for the American Academy of Sleep Medicine. *The AASM Manual for the Scoring of Sleep and Associated Events: Rules, Terminology and Technical Specifications. Version 3.* American Academy of Sleep Medicine; 2023.

REFERENCES

1. Tyner FS, Knott JR, Brem Mayer W. *Fundamentals of EEG Technology.* Raven; 1983.
2. Fisch BJ. *Spehlman's EEG Primer.* Elsevier; 1991:39-65.
3. Berry RB, Wagner MH. *Sleep Medicine Pearls.* 3rd ed. Elsevier; 2015: 80-90.
4. Patil SP. What every clinician should know about polysomnography. *Respir Care.* 2010;55(9):1179-1195.
5. Beniczky S, Schomer DL. Electroencephalography: basic biophysical and technological aspects important for clinical applications. *Epileptic Disord.* 2020;22(6):697-715.
6. Epstein C. Digital EEG. Trouble in paradise? *J Clin Neurophysiol.* 2006;23:190-193.
7. Epstein CM. Aliasing in the visual EEG: a potential pitfall of video display technology. *Clin Neurophysiol.* 2003;114:1974-1976.
8. Lockhart R, DATAQ Instruments. What You Really Need to Know About Sampling Rate. https://www.dataq.com/resources/pdfs/article_pdfs/sample-rate.pdf, 2023. [Accessed 01 October 2023].
9. Iber C, Ancoli-Israel S, Chesson A, Quan SF, for the American Academy of Sleep Medicine. *The AASM Manual for the Scoring of Sleep and Associated Events: Rules, Terminology and Technical Specifications.* American Academy of Sleep Medicine; 2007.
10. Troester MM, Quan SF, Berry RB, et al., for the American Academy of Sleep Medicine. *The AASM Manual for the Scoring of Sleep and Associated Events: Rules, Terminology and Technical Specifications.* Darien, IL: American Academy of Sleep Medicine; 2023.
11. Silber MH, Ancoli-Israel S, Bonnet MH, et al. The visual scoring of sleep in adults. *J Clin Sleep Med.* 2007;3(2):121-131. Erratum in: *J Clin Sleep Med.* 2007;15;3(5):table of contents.
12. Shrivastava D, Kalra M. Understanding digital filters in polysomnography for clinicians. *Indian J Sleep Med.* 2013;8(3):111-115.
13. Sinclair CM, Gasper MC, Blum AS. Basic electronics in clinical neurophysiology. In: Blum AS, Rutkove SB, eds. *The Clinical Neurophysiology Primer.* Humana Press; 2007:3-18.
14. Libenson MH. *Practical Approach to Electroencephalography.* Saunders Elsevier; 2010:146-170.
15. Penzel T, Conradt R. Computer based sleep recording and analysis. *Sleep Med Rev.* 2000;4(2):131-148.
16. Burgess RC. Electrical safety. *Handb Clin Neurol.* 2019;160:67-81.
17. Fish RM, Geddes LA. Conduction of electrical current to and through the human body: a review. *Eplasty.* 2009;9:e44.

Chapter 3

Staging Sleep in Adults

INTRODUCTION

The American Academy of Sleep Medicine (AASM) *Manual for the Scoring of Sleep and Associated Events: Rules, Terminology, and Technical Specification* was published in 2007 (hereinafter the AASM scoring manual).[1-3] The manual changed the rules of staging sleep and made recommendations about the methods used to monitor sleep. Previously, sleep was staged according to the manual edited by Rechtschaffen and Kales (R&K).[4] Non–rapid eye movement (NREM) sleep now consists of stages N1, N2, and N3 rather than 1, 2, 3, and 4 in the R&K system. The R&K manual stages 3 and 4 are combined into stage N3 in the AASM scoring manual. Frontal, central, and occipital derivations are now used to stage sleep (see Chapter 1). In the R&K manual, only central derivations are used. The AASM scoring manual also contains rules for scoring arousals.[1,2,5,6] The AASM scoring manual is periodically updated to clarify and edit the rules based on questions submitted by the sleep community, recent published evidence, or technological advances. The reader is referred to the most updated version. The definitions of the electroencephalography (EEG) and eye movement (electrooculography [EOG]) patterns used for staging sleep are discussed in Chapter 1.

OVERVIEW OF STAGING SLEEP IN ADULTS

In staging sleep, it is important to keep in mind that sleep occurs in cycles of NREM followed by rapid eye movement (REM) sleep (Fig. 3–1). Usually there are three to six NREM/REM cycles per night. In adults the first cycle lasts about 70 to 100 minutes and later cycles approximately 90 to 120 minutes. Overall, the average length of each sleep cycle is about 90 minutes. The first epoch of sleep in adults is typically stage N1. The initial brief period of stage N1 is usually followed by a longer period of stage N2, then stage N3, and finally the first episode of REM sleep, which is typically brief. As the night progresses, fewer stage N3 episodes occur, and the duration of stage R episodes increases. The number of REMs per epoch of stage R (REM density) also increases in the second part of the night. Brief episodes of wakefulness occur during the night. The hypnogram shown in Figure 3–1 is a graphical representation of sleep with different sleep stages represented by different levels on the Y-axis and time on the X-axis. Note that stage N3 episodes decrease in length as the night progresses, whereas the length of stage R episodes increases. The pattern of sleep known as "sleep architecture" changes with age, medications, and disease and will be discussed in Chapters 6, 7, and 9.

The rules of scoring sleep are detailed, and a brief overview is helpful. The characteristics of **stage W** (Wakefulness) depend on whether an individual has their eyes open or closed. During eyes open wakefulness, the EEG consists of a low-amplitude mixture of alpha (8–13 Hz) and beta (>13 Hz) frequencies. The EOG derivations may demonstrate blinks, voluntary REMs, or reading eye **movements** (Figs. 3-2 and 3-3). See Chapter 1 for an example of reading eye movements. Chin electromyography (EMG) activity is usually relatively high compared with the activity during sleep. In this chapter Chin EMG in the figures refers to the Chin1-ChinZ or Chin2-ChinZ derivation. As individuals become drowsy, the blink frequency decreases and the eyes close. Following eye closure, **posterior dominant rhythm** (PDR) (in adults also known as alpha rhythm) is the predominant pattern (>50% of the epoch), and **slow eye movements** (SEMs) may be present (Fig. 3–4). As discussed in Chapter 1, PDR is characterized by 8- to 13-Hz sinusoidal waves most prominent in the occipital derivations with the amplitude attenuated by eye opening and increased with eye closure. SEMs are sinusoidal, conjugate EOG waves (out of phase in E1-M2 and E2-M2) that may be seen in stages W or N1. Epochs of stage W may also contain a mixture of portions with PDR activity and portions with the pattern of eyes open stage W (Fig. 3–5). About 10% of individuals do *not* generate alpha rhythm on eye closure, and a further 10% may generate limited alpha rhythm.[1-3] The eyes open and eyes closed EEG patterns during stage W are similar in these individuals. In both alpha generators and non–alpha generators, stage W is scored if *majority of the epoch* contains (1) PDR; (2) the eye movements associated with wake (blinks, REMs with normal or high EMG tone, or reading eye movements); or (3) a combination of (1) and (2). Epochs of wake vary in appearance as individuals open and close their eyes as they become drowsy.

On transition to stage N1, **low-amplitude mixed-frequency (LAMF)** EEG activity replaces alpha rhythm for the majority of the epoch (Fig. 3–6). The LAMF EEG is characterized by predominantly 4- to 7-Hz activity. SEMs often persist into stage N1. The chin EMG in stage N1 is variable but usually lower than stage W (Fig. 3–6). Stage N1 is usually brief, as the transition from stage N1 to stage N2 occurs quickly after sleep onset unless sleep is disturbed by frequent brief awakenings (arousals). Episodes of stage N1 may also occur following periods of wakefulness during the night (see the hypnogram in Fig. 3–1). In *individuals who do not generate PDR with eye closure,* stage N1 is scored at the first appearance of SEMs or vertex sharp waves, or when there is a perceptible slowing of the EEG (EEG of 4 to 7 Hz and at least 1 Hz slower than wake) (Fig. 3–7).

The onset of **stage N2** is characterized by the presence of sleep spindles (SS, 11- to 16-Hz bursts), K-complexes (KC, large biphasic deflections), or both (Fig. 3–8) in the

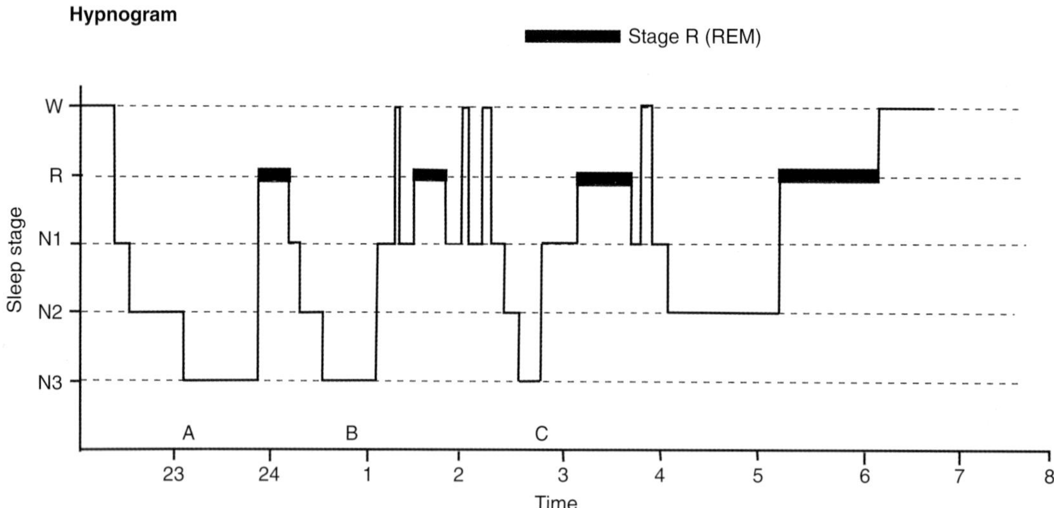

Figure 3–1 A hypnogram showing the progression of sleep stages through the night. Note that the length of episodes of stage N3 (A, B, C) decreases during the night, and the length of stage R episodes increases. Periods of stage W followed briefly by stage N1 also occur during the night.

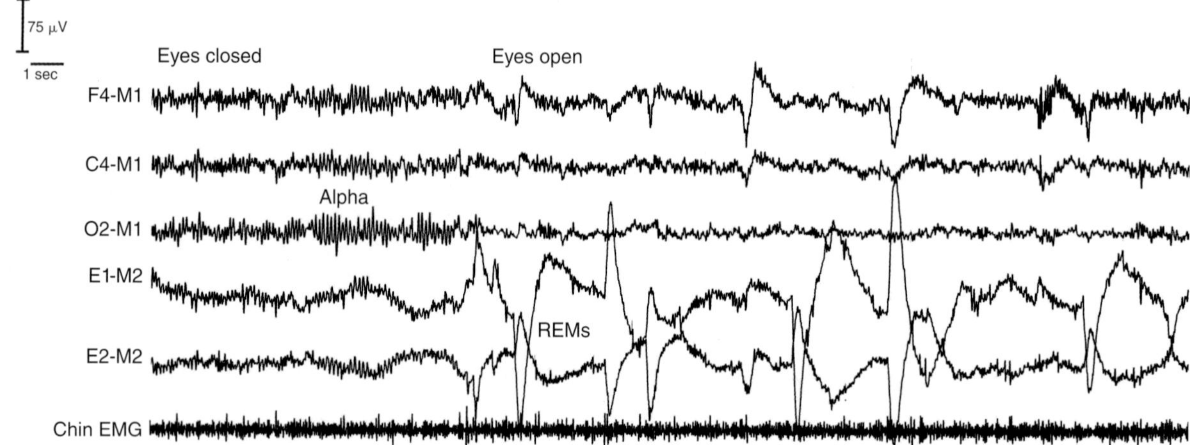

Figure 3–2 A 30-second tracing of stage W. In the first part of the epoch, eyes are closed and posterior dominant rhythm (alpha rhythm) is observed. With the eyes open, posterior dominant rhythm is attenuated and the electroencephalogram shows a low-amplitude pattern with a mixture of alpha and beta activity associated with rapid eye movements *(REMs)* concurrent with chin electromyogram *(EMG)* activity that is normal or increased.

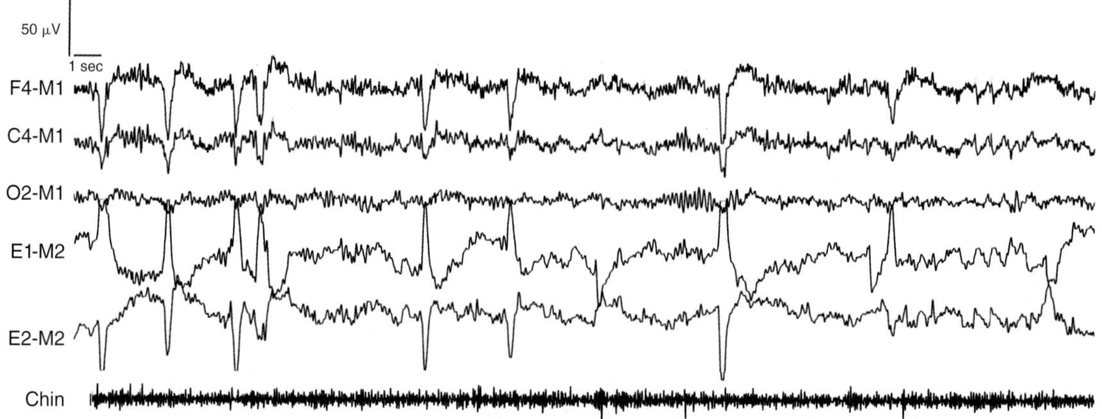

Figure 3–3 A 30-second epoch of eyes-open stage W is shown containing blinks and low-amplitude high-frequency electroencephalographic activity. Blinks have a characteristic appearance different from most rapid eye movements (REMs). The eye quickly looks up (upward deflection in E1-M2 and downward deflection in E2-M2) with eye lid closure, and the deflection is narrow and usually high amplitude (see Chapter 1). REMs with an upward deflection in E1-M2 and a downward deflection in E2-M2 can have the same pattern but usually the duration is wider. Blinks all have the same morphology in a given individual, whereas REMs have variable appearance. Blinks occur during stage W with the eyes open or closed.

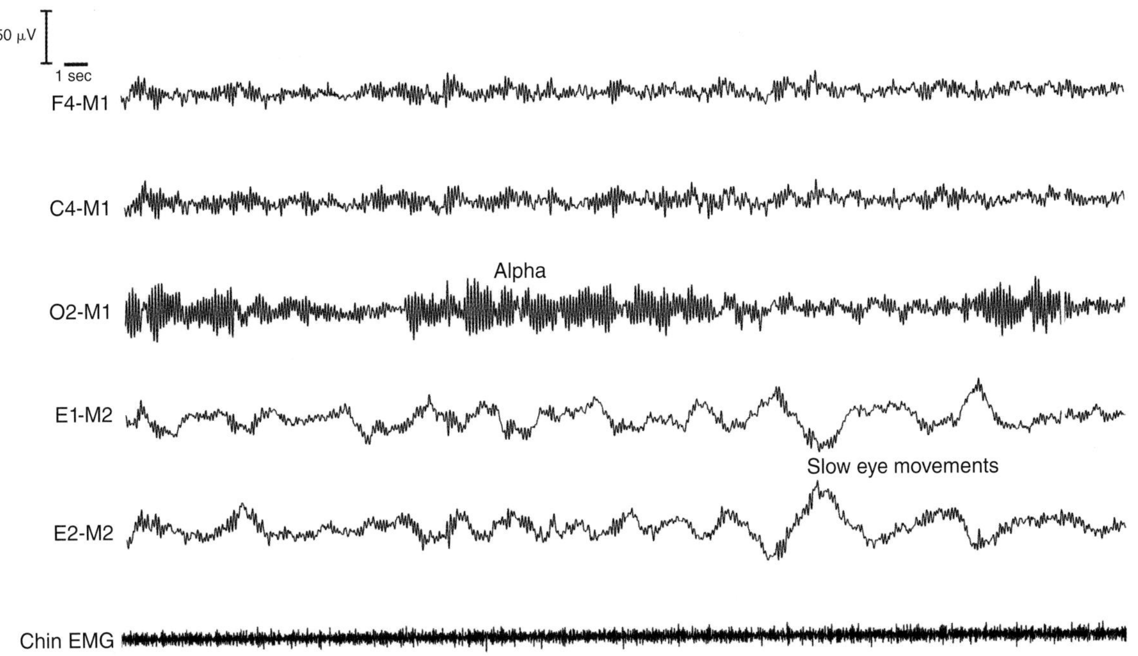

Figure 3–4 A 30-second epoch of eyes-closed stage W with posterior dominant rhythm, also known as alpha rhythm in adults, is present in more than 50% of the epoch. Slow eye movements (SEMs) are also noted. SEMs can occur in stage W or stage N1. *EMG*, Electromyogram.

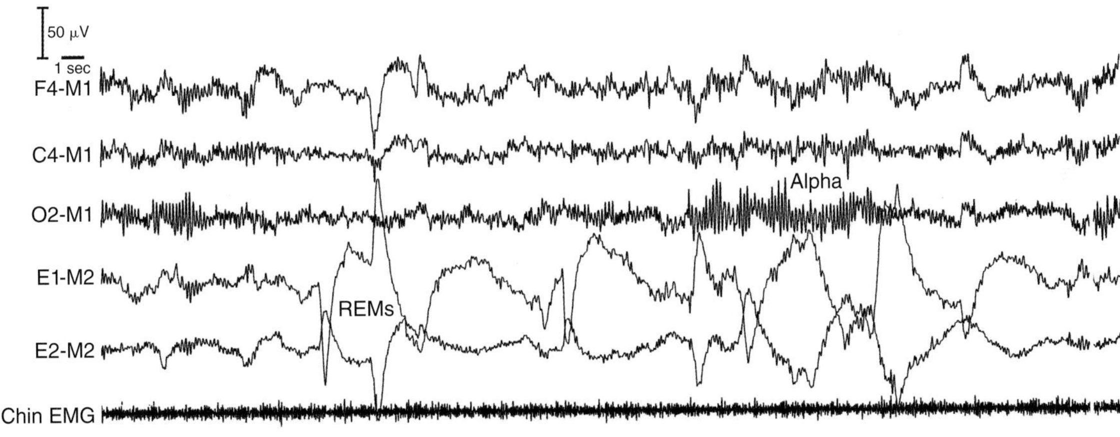

Figure 3–5 A 30-second epoch of eyes-open stage W. Note the mixture of rapid eye movements *(REMs)* with a variable electroencephalogram showing periods of low-amplitude high-frequency activity mixed with periods of alpha activity (posterior dominant rhythm). The chin electromyogram *(EMG)* of stage W is usually higher than during sleep.

EEG. However, these waveforms may not be present in every epoch of stage N2. As noted in the scoring rules, once an epoch of stage 2 is scored, this sleep stage is considered to continue until evidence of a transition to another stage of sleep or a brief awakening (arousal) is noted. As stage N2 continues, an increasing amount of slow wave activity (SWA) is usually noted (0.5- to 2-Hz activity with a peak-to-peak amplitude >75 μV **in F4-M1 or F3-M2**) but occupies less than 20% of the epoch (<6 seconds). Eye movement activity has usually ceased during stage N2, and chin EMG is variable in amplitude. Stage N3 is scored when SWA activity (waves with 0.5 to 2 Hz activity **>75μV** in F4-M1 or F3-M2) occupies 20% or more of an epoch **(≥6 seconds)** (Fig. 3–9). SWA is also noted in the EOG derivations, and sleep spindles may be superimposed on the slow waves. An abrupt transition from stage N3 to stage R may occur, or the SWA (and EEG amplitude) may decrease sufficiently so that stage N3 transitions briefly into stage N2 before the onset of stage R. A reduction in SWA, chin EMG activity, or both is a clue that stage R may soon occur. Epochs of **definite stage R** (Fig. 3–10) are characterized by the absence of sleep spindles or K complexes in the EEG and the concurrent presence of REMs and low chin EMG activity. **Low chin activity** is defined as baseline EMG activity in the chin derivations that is no higher than that associated with any other sleep stage and usually the lowest of the night. However, REMs do not occur in every epoch of

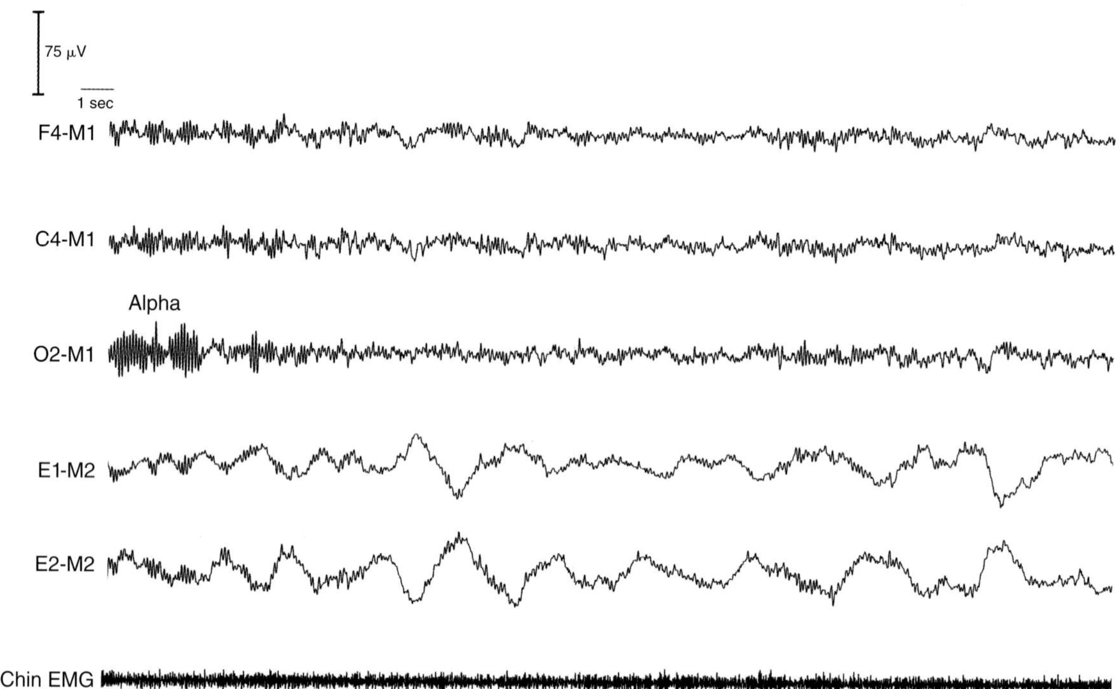

Figure 3–6 A 30-second epoch showing the transition from wake with posterior dominant rhythm (alpha rhythm) to stage N1 sleep. Posterior dominant rhythm is attenuated for the majority of the epoch and is replaced by a low-amplitude mixed-frequency electroencephalographic pattern. Slow eye movements are present but are not required to score stage N1. *EMG,* Electromyogram.

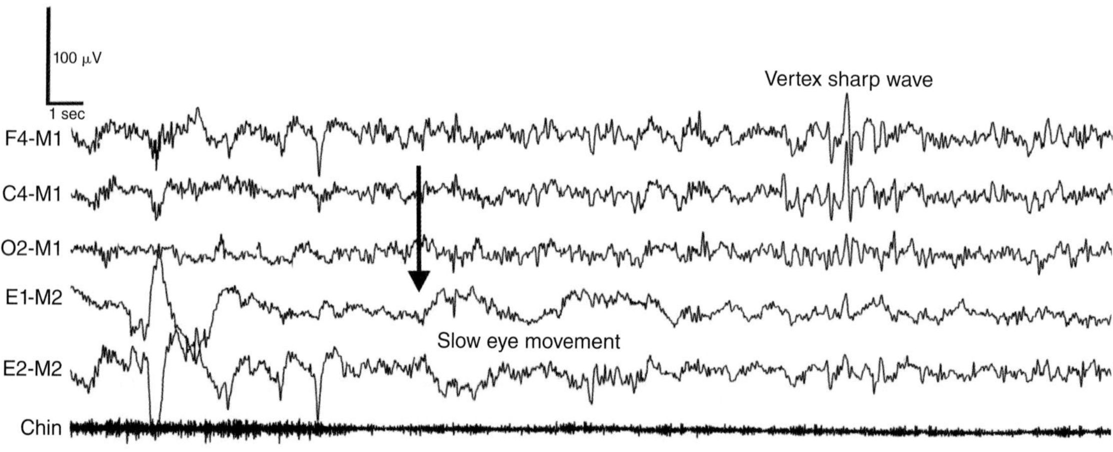

Figure 3–7 A 30-second epoch from a patient who did not generate alpha with eye closure. **The previous epoch was scored as wake.** Sleep onset starts when the first slow eye movement *(arrow)* or vertex sharp wave appears, or the electroencephalographic frequency is 4–7 Hz and at least 1 Hz lower than stage W.

stage R, and the chin EMG may reach the REM level during NREM sleep before REMs appear. Detailed scoring rules exist for the start, continuation, and end of stage R and will be discussed in detail in later sections of this chapter. The LAMF activity in stage R resembles that in stage N1 sleep. Of interest, prominent alpha activity can be seen during stage R with a frequency typically 1 to 2 Hz slower than stage W (Fig. 3–10). In fact, some individuals have a greater amount of alpha activity in stage R than stage N1. Sawtooth waves (see Fig 3-10 and Chapter 1) are characteristic of stage R but are not required to score an epoch of definite stage R.

SCORING BY EPOCHS

The AASM scoring manual continues the convention of staging sleep in sequential 30-second epochs. Each epoch is assigned a sleep stage. If an epoch contains EEG/EOG/EMG activity consistent with two stages, the stage occupying the majority of the epoch is assigned the sleep stage for the epoch. If three segments of an epoch meet criteria for different sleep stages, first *score the epoch as sleep* if the majority of the epoch contains stage N1, N2, N3, or R. Second, assign the epoch the stage that occupies the *majority of sleep within the epoch*. For

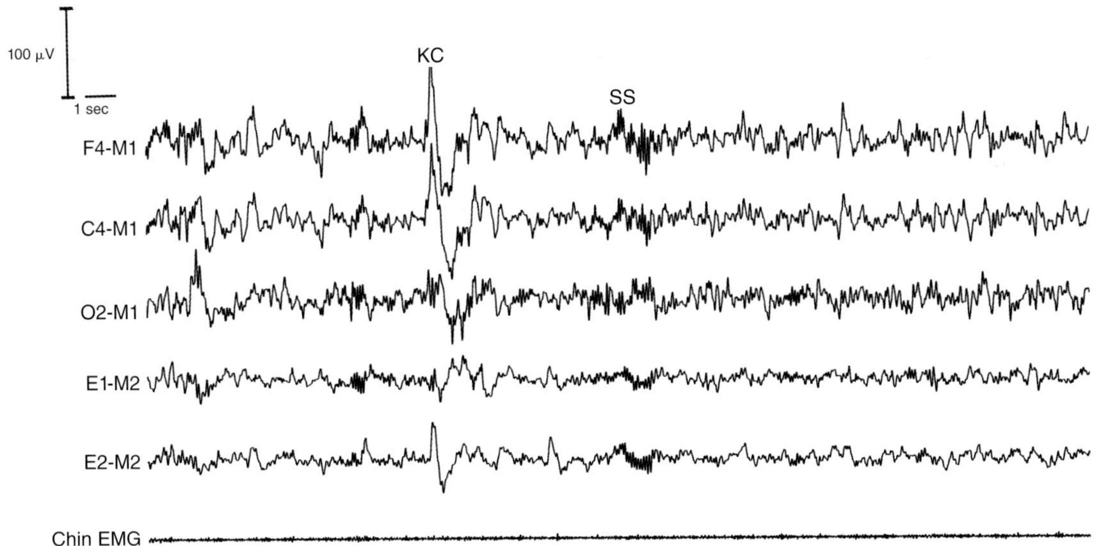

Figure 3–8 A 30-second epoch of the start of stage N2 with both a K complex *(KC)* not associated with an arousal and a sleep spindle *(SS)*. The KC is clearly in the first half of the epoch, so the epoch is stage N2. *EMG*, Electromyogram.

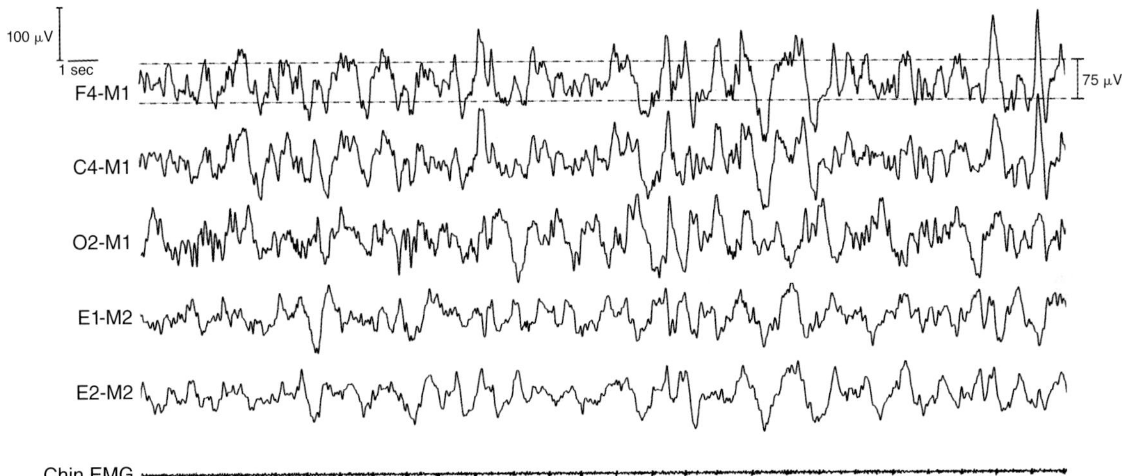

Figure 3–9 A 30-second epoch of unequivocal stage N3 with ≥6 seconds of slow wave activity meeting amplitude and frequency criteria (>75 μV peak to peak in F4-M1 and frequency 0.5–2 Hz). Amplitude grid lines separated by 75 μV are shown in F4-M1. Note that the amplitude criterion is >75 μV, not ≥75 μV. *EMG*, Electromyogram.

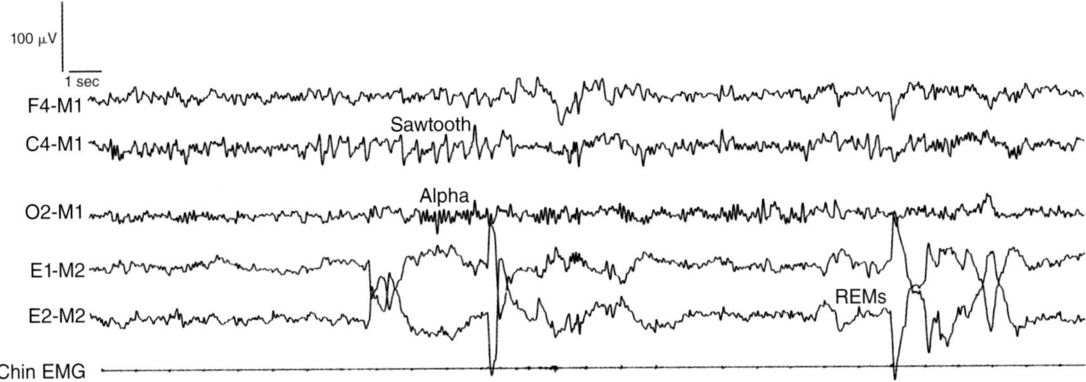

Figure 3–10 A 30-second epoch of definite stage R with low chin electromyogram *(EMG)* concurrent with rapid eye movements *(REMs)* and an electroencephalogram showing a low-amplitude mixed-frequency pattern with an absence of K complexes or sleep spindles. Bursts of alpha are common in stage R. Sawtooth waves are characteristic of stage R but are not required to score stage R.

example, an epoch containing 20% stage W, 60% stage N1, and 20% stage N2 would be assigned sleep stage N1.

SCORING STAGE W (WAKE FULNESS)

As noted previously, the EEG of eyes open stage W consists of low amplitude activity, typically a mixture of alpha (8–13 Hz) and beta activity (>13 Hz) without rhythmicity, and is associated with REMs, blinks, or reading eye movements and relatively high chin EMG activity. See Chapter 1 for examples of reading eye movements. The differentiation between eyes open stage W and eyes closed stage R (both have REMs) when the chin EMG in stage W happens to be low can be difficult. Time synchronized video showing open eyes helps identify the epoch as stage W with REMs. The EEG of drowsy eyes closed stage W consists of PDR often with SEMs. Epochs of stage W typically contain a mixture of these patterns as the individual opens and closes their eyes on transition to sleep. As noted previously, about 10% of individuals do not generate alpha with eye closure, whereas another 10% exhibit limited/equivocal alpha activity. The EEG of wake in these individuals is similar with eyes open or closed (mixture of alpha and beta activity). In those individuals generating alpha activity with eye closure, stage W is scored when more than 50% of an epoch contains PDR (Fig. 3–4). In all individuals stage W is scored when EOG findings consistent with stage W are noted including eye blinks, REMs with normal or high chin muscle tone, or reading eye movements for the majority of the epoch. Finally, if the majority of the epoch contains segments with alpha rhythm, eye movements consistent with wake, or both, the epoch is scored as stage W (Figs. 3-2 to 3-5).

Summary of Scoring Stage W[2]:

- Greater than 50% of the epoch contains PDR, eye movements associated with stage W (EMW), or a combination of PDR and EMW.
- EMW includes blinks, reading eye movements, and REMs (with normal or high chin EMG activity).
- SEMs may or may not be present.
- Chin EMG is variable but usually high.

SCORING STAGE N1

Sleep onset is defined as the first epoch of stage of sleep (N1, N2, N3, R). Stage N1 is usually the first epoch of sleep in adults and is usually of short duration. The predominant EEG activity during stage N1 is LAMF EEG activity defined as low amplitude, predominantly 4- to 7-Hz EEG activity. This EEG activity is in the theta range of EEG frequency. Vertex sharp waves (see Chapter 1 and Fig. 3–7) are also common in stage N1, often near the transition to stage N2. *SEMs are characteristic of stage W but commonly persist into stage N1.* In individuals generating alpha rhythm with eye closure, stage N1 is scored when alpha rhythm is replaced by LAMF for more than 50% of the epoch (Fig. 3–6)[2]. In individuals who do not generate alpha rhythm, score stage N1 at the first instance of an EEG with 4- to 7-Hz activity and a slowing of at least 1 Hz compared with stage W, SEMs, or a vertex sharp wave (Fig. 3–7). *Note that neither SEMs nor vertex sharp waves are required to score stage N1 when other defining characteristics are present.* However, in non–alpha generators the presence of these waveforms is used to score the onset of stage N1. An epoch is scored as stage N1 if the majority of the epoch meets criteria for stage N1 (EEG showing LAMF EEG activity) in the absence of evidence for another sleep stage. Subsequent epochs with an EEG showing LAMF EEG activity are scored as stage N1 until there is evidence for another sleep stage (usually stage W, stage N2, or stage R).

An arousal (brief awakening) is characterized by an abrupt shift of EEG frequency including alpha, theta, and/or frequencies greater than 16 Hz (but not spindles) that lasts **at least 3 seconds,** with at least 10 seconds of stable sleep preceding the change.[2] Scoring of arousals during REM requires a concurrent increase in submental EMG lasting **at least 1 second** (concurrent with EEG changes meeting criteria for an arousal). Scoring arousals is discussed at the end of this chapter. Stage N1 is scored following an arousal that occurs in stage N2 or N3 if the EEG following the arousal shows LAMF without K complexes or sleep spindles (Fig. 3–11, right panel) unless there is evidence for another sleep stage. Stage N1 continues until there is evidence for another sleep stage (usually N2 or R). However, if an arousal interrupts stage R and the following EEG pattern continues to show LAMF activity without PDR and low chin EMG activity (at the REM level), stage N1 is scored only if SEMs (not associated with PDR) are present providing evidence of a shift in sleep stage. If SEMs are not present, stage R continues until there is evidence for another sleep stage. Note that the presence of SEMs with PDR would be suggestive of a transition to stage W. Scoring sleep after arousals in stage N2 and stage R will be discussed (with examples) in detail in later sections of this chapter.

Summary of Scoring Stage N1:

1. Transition from stage W to stage N1 (PDR generators)
   - PDR for less than 50% of the epoch
2. Transition from stage W to stage N1 (PDR not generated with eye closure)
   - First instance of one of the following:
     - SEMs
     - Vertex sharp waves
     - EEG 4 to 7 Hz with slowing of background frequencies ≥ 1 Hz from those of stage W
3. Stage N1 in all individuals
   - SEMs may be present.
   - Chin is EMG variable but often lower than stage W.
   - An epoch containing a majority of LAMF EEG(without K Complexes or sleep spindles is scored as stage N1 unless the epoch meets criteria for another sleep stage (usually based on surrounding epochs). Subsequent epochs continue to be scored as stage N1 unless there is evidence for transition to another sleep stage.
   - Stage N1 following an arousal.
     - Score stage N1 following an arousal from NREM sleep if the following segment contains LAMF with or without SEMs (chin EMG activity is variable) and criteria for other sleep stages are not met. Stage N1 continues until there is evidence for another sleep stage.
     - Score stage N1 following an arousal from stage R if the segment following the arousal contains LAMF EEG activity and **SEMs (not associated with PDR)** even if the chin EMG activity remains low. Stage N1

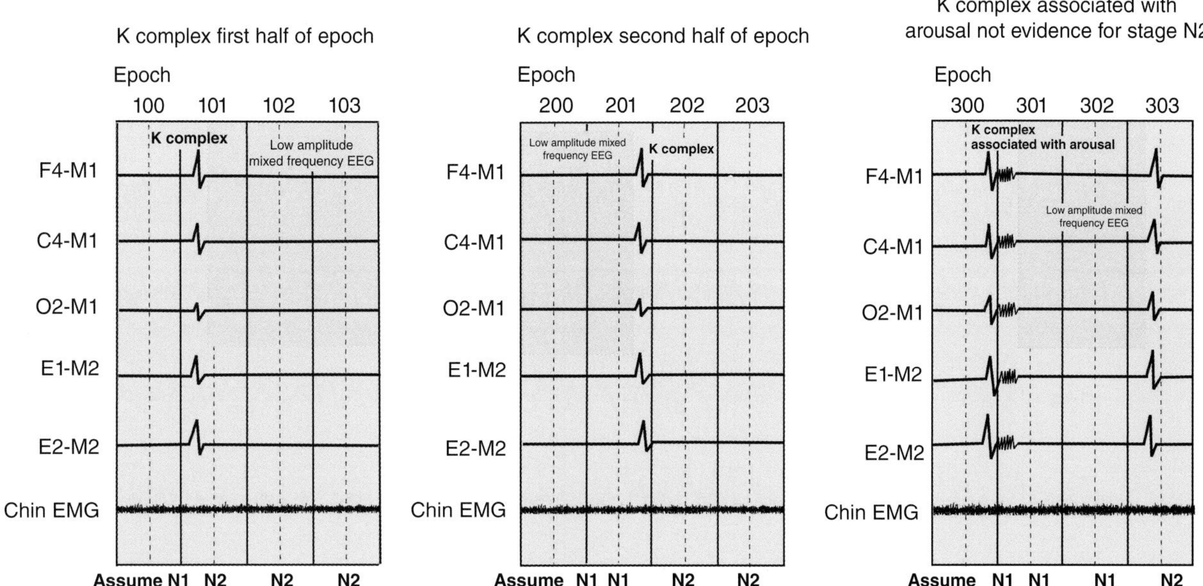

Figure 3–11 Schematics illustrating the start of stage N2. The electroencephalogram *(EEG)* is assumed to contain low-amplitude mixed-frequency activity without K complexes or sleep spindles *(gray area)* unless otherwise labeled. An epoch is scored as stage N2 if a K complex unassociated with an arousal, sleep spindle, or both occurs in the first half of the current epoch (epoch 101) or last half of the previous epoch (epoch 202). Stage N2 continues to be scored in the following epochs even if sleep spindles or K complexes are absent as long as there is no intervening arousal (epochs 102, 103, 203). A K complex associated with an arousal occurs in the beginning of epoch 301 and does not provide evidence for stage N2. Epoch 301 is scored as stage N1 as an arousal occurs in the first half of the epoch and continues until there is evidence for stage N2 (epoch 303). *EMG,* Electromyogram.

continues until there is evidence of another sleep stage.

- Score stage N1 following an arousal from stage R if the following segment following the arousal has LAMF EEG activity **and the chin EMG is above the REM level.** Stage N1 continues until there is evidence of another sleep stage.

SCORING STAGE N2

Start of Stage N2

Stage N2 usually occupies the greatest percentage of total sleep time. Begin scoring stage N2 if one or more K complexes **unassociated** with an arousal and/or one or more sleep spindles occur in the first half of the current epoch or the last half of the previous epoch[2]. (Figs. 3-8 and 3-11). This assumes the epoch does not meet criteria for another sleep stage (N3 or R). The chin tone in stage N2, though variable, is usually less than stage W and sometime less than stage N1. SEMs typically cease in stage N2. Note that a K complex **associated** with an arousal (arousal concurrent with K complex or following by no more than 1 second) does **not provide** evidence for the start or continuation of stage N2 (Fig. 3–11, right panel).

Stage N2 After Stage N3

As noted later, to score stage N3 an epoch must have 6 seconds or greater of SWA meeting amplitude and frequency requirements. In some individuals an epoch meeting stage N3 criteria is followed by an epoch of lower-amplitude slow waves not meeting criteria for stage N3 but without discrete K complexes or sleep spindles in the first half of the epoch. In this case the epoch is considered stage N2. This assumes that there is no intervening arousal and that the epoch following the stage N3 epoch does not meet criteria for stage R. Stage N2 continues until there is evidence for another sleep stage (Fig. 3–12).

Summary of the Start of Stage N2:

- KC, SS, or both in the first half of current epoch or in the last half of the previous epoch.
- If an arousal interrupts a period of stage N2, stage N2 is considered to be present until the arousal. If the majority of the epoch containing the arousal is considered stage N2, the epoch is scored as stage N2.
- Epochs following an epoch of stage N3 without an intervening arousal are scored as stage N2 unless there is evidence for another sleep stage.

Continuation of Stage N2

Once an epoch of stage N2 is scored, the following epochs are considered stage N2 even in the absence of a K complex or sleep spindle until there is an arousal or transition to a different sleep stage (Fig. 3–11). In the case of the arousal, all segments preceding the arousal are considered stage N2. If stage N2 constitutes the majority of any epoch, the epoch is scored as stage N2. A major body movement (MBM) is an event consisting of movement and muscle artifact obscuring the EEG for **more than half an epoch** to the extent that the sleep stage cannot be determined. When an MBM interrupts stage N2, the MBM epoch is followed by an EEG with LAMF without K complexes or sleep spindles, and the EOG

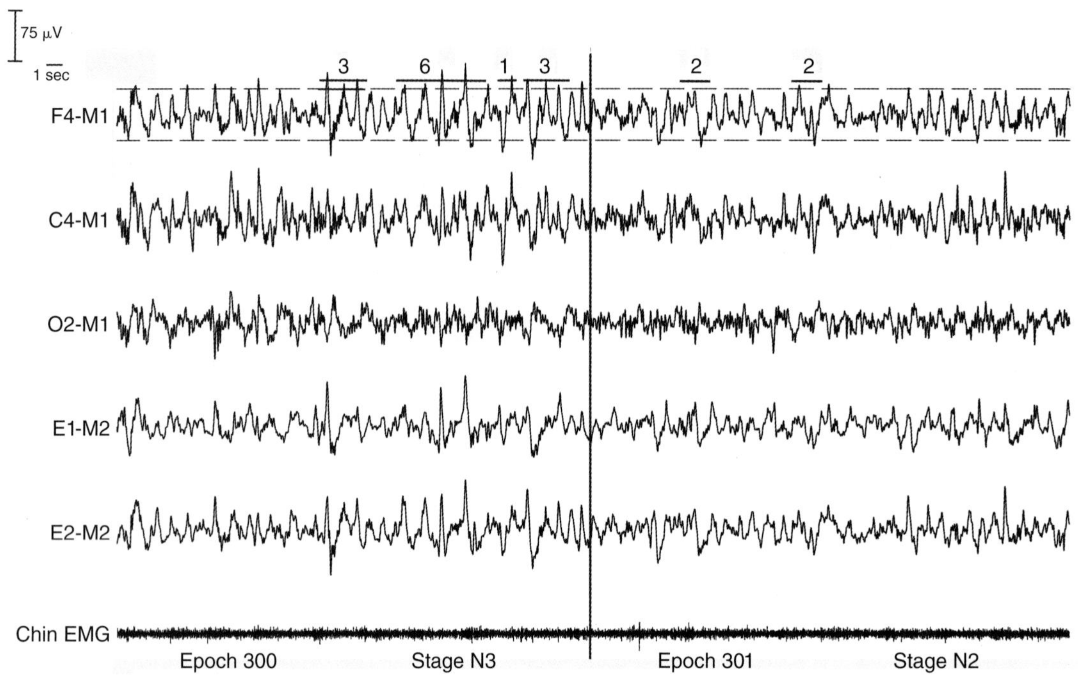

Figure 3–12 Two 30-second epochs are shown. Epoch 300 meets criteria for stage N3. Epoch 301 is scored as stage N2 as it does not have sufficient slow wave activity (SWA) to meet criteria for stage N3 even in the absence of a sleep spindle or K complex. Portions of both epochs meeting SWA criteria are shown by lines above the F4-M1 derivation with the duration in seconds. *EMG,* Electromyogram.

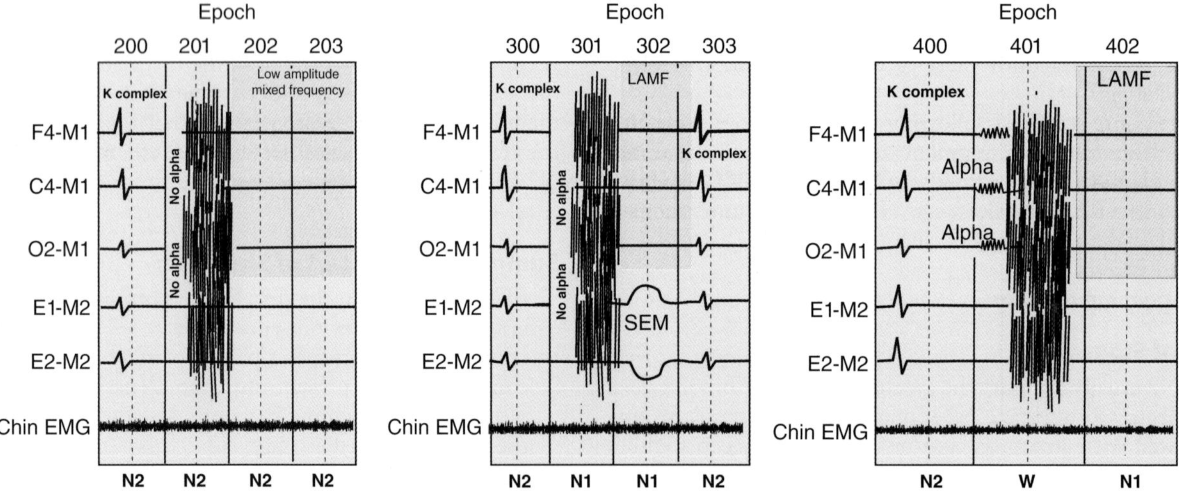

Figure 3–13 A major body movement (MBM) interrupts stage N2 sleep. In the *left panel,* low-amplitude mixed-frequency (LAMF) electroencephalogram *(gray area)* without slow eye movements *(SEMs)* occurs in epoch 202 and stage N2 continues. The MBM epoch is scored as stage N2 (see MBM rules). In the *middle panel,* an MBM epoch is followed by an epoch with both LAMF activity and SEMs. A transition to stage N1 is scored. In the *right panel,* alpha activity is noted in the MBM epoch, which is scored as stage W. Stage N2 ends, and the following epoch is scored as stage N1 based on LAMF activity and no evidence for other sleep stages.

does *not show SEMs, stage N2 continues until there is evidence* for another sleep stage (Fig. 3–13, left panel). The MBM epoch is scored according to the MBM rules. *Note that if the MBM epoch is scored as wake, then stage N2 ends* (see MBM rules, later). If SEMs are present after the MBM epoch (not scored as wake) and the EEG shows LAMF activity, stage N1 is scored (Fig. 3–13, middle panel). If the MBM epoch is scored as wake (alpha activity is present, see MBM rules), then stage N2 ends (Fig. 3–13, right panel).

Summary of Continuation of Stage N2:

- Stage N2 continues following epochs containing a defining KC (not associated with an arousal) or SS until there is evidence for another sleep stage, or an arousal.
- When stage N2 is interrupted by an MBM (MBM epoch not scored as stage W), stage N2 continues (Fig. 3–13, left panel) unless SEMs are present following the MBM (evidence for stage N1) (Fig. 3–13, middle panel) unless there is evidence for another sleep stage.

End of Stage N2

Stage N2 ends if there is a transition to wake, an arousal in the first half of an epoch otherwise meeting criteria for stage N2 up until the arousal, an MBM (not scored as wake) followed by SEMs and an EEG that meets criteria for stage N1, or a transition to stage N3 or R. As previously noted, when an arousal interrupts stage N2, *sleep up to the arousal is considered stage N2* (and if the majority of the epoch is considered stage N2, stage N2 is scored). However, after the arousal sleep is scored as stage N1 if the EEG contains LAMF EEG activity without K complexes or sleep spindles until there is evidence for another sleep stage (Fig. 3–14). This assumes there is no evidence of a transition to wake or stage R. If an MBM interrupts stage N2 and the MBM epoch contains any amount of alpha activity, the MBM epoch is scored as stage W and stage N2 ends (Fig. 3–13, right panel). If the MBM epoch does not contain alpha activity and the MBM epoch is followed by LAMF activity **and SEMs,** stage N2 ends, and stage N1 is scored unless there is evidence of another sleep stage (Fig. 3–13, middle panel). The presence of SEMs is considered evidence of a transition to stage N1. Stage N1 will continue to be scored until there is evidence for another sleep stage. As will be discussed later, there are situations in which stage N2 and stage R rules are in conflict. In such cases *stage R rules are predominant.* Transitions to stage R are discussed in a later section.

Summary of End of Stage N2:

- Arousal (segments up until arousal considered N2). Segments following the arousal with LAMF activity and no KC or SS are scored as stage N1 unless (until) there is evidence for another sleep stage (Fig. 3–14).
- Transition to stage W, N3, or R.
- MBM interrupts stage N2 followed by SEMs and LAMF without SS or KC.
- An epoch scored as N2 by N2 rules and R by REM rules is scored as stage R (REM rules are predominant).

SCORING STAGE N3

An epoch is scored as stage N3 if **at least 6 seconds** of SWA is present (Figs. 3-9 and 3-15). *Sleep spindles may also occur.* Eye movements are not typically seen. The chin EMG amplitude is variable but may be lower than in stage N2 sleep and can be as low as the chin EMG during stage R. SWA is transmitted to the EOG derivations (in-phase deflections). Using

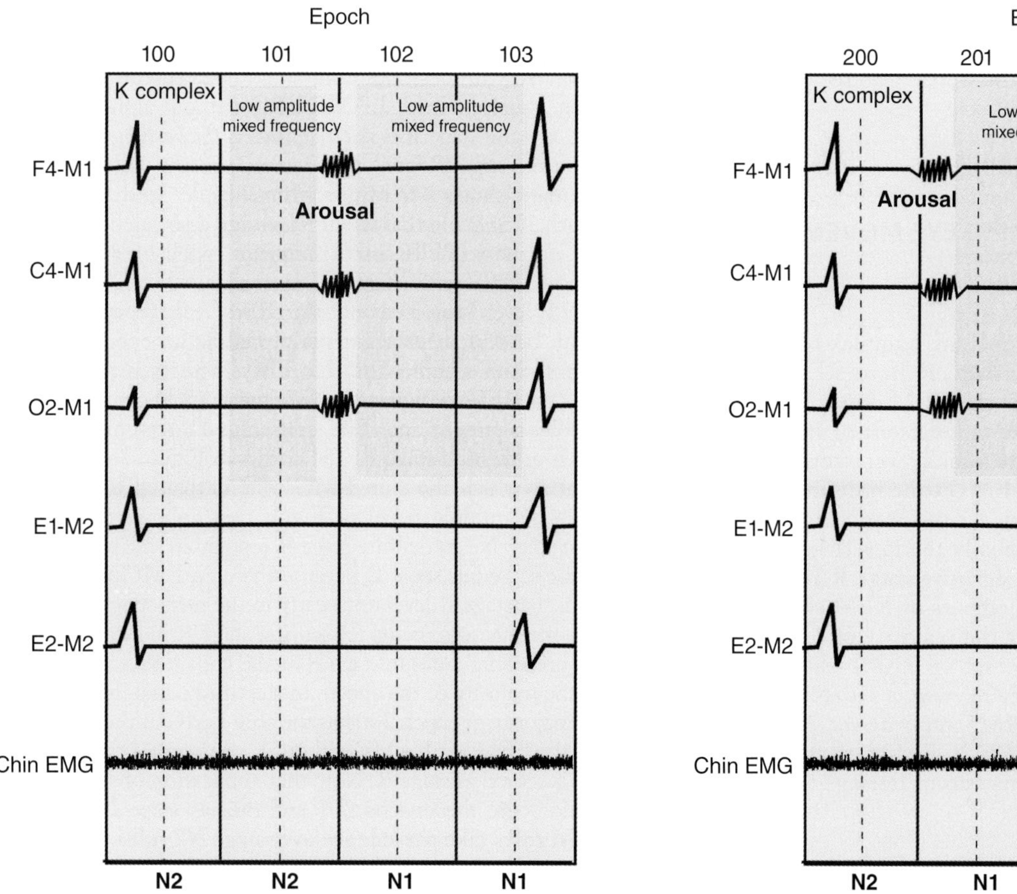

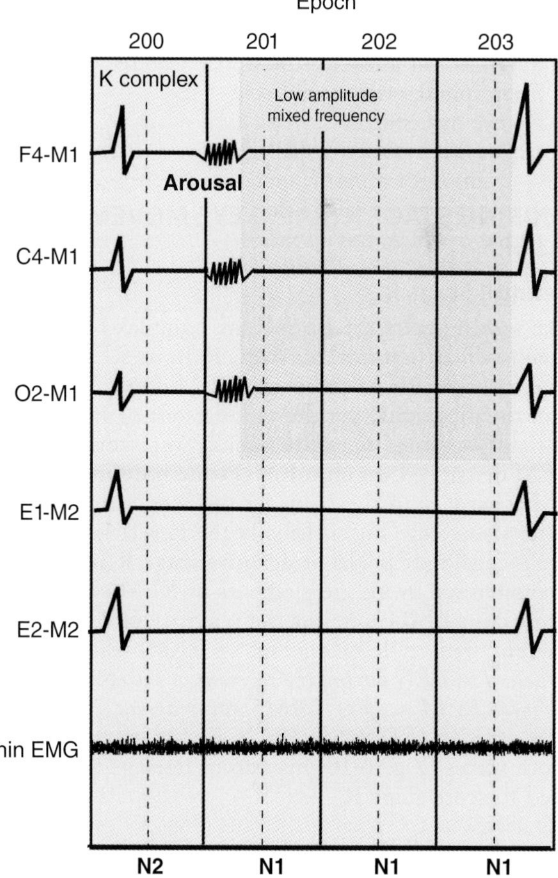

Figure 3–14 An arousal interrupts stage N2 sleep. Epoch 102 is scored as stage N1 as the electroencephalogram after the arousal contains low-amplitude mixed-frequency activity without K complexes or sleep spindles *(gray area).* Stage N2 is scored up until the occurrence of the arousal at the end of epoch 101. Stage N1 continues in epochs 102 and 103. Epoch 103 is scored as stage N1 as the K complex occurs in the last half of the epoch. In the *right panel,* stage N2 ends at the start of epoch 201. Stage N1 continues until there is evidence of another sleep stage. Epoch 203 is scored as stage N1 as the K complex does not occur until the second half of the epoch. *EMG,* Electromyogram.

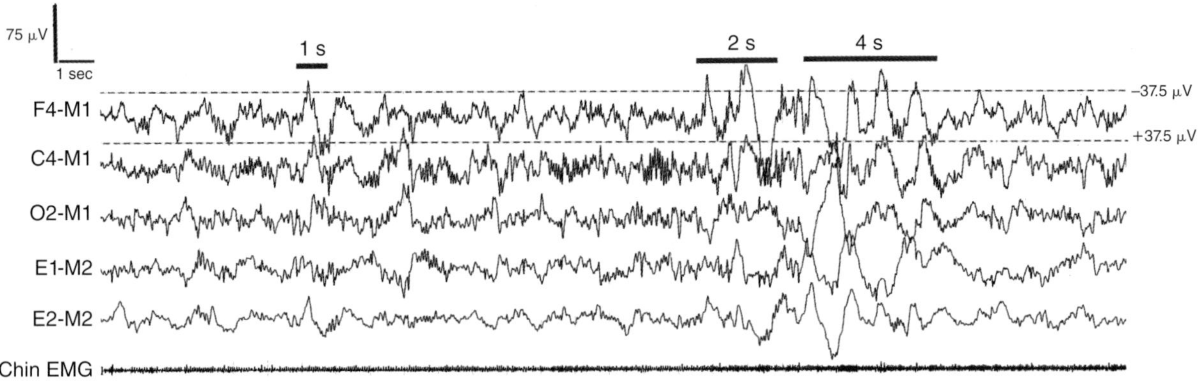

Figure 3–15 A 30-second epoch barely meets criteria for stage N3. Slow wave activity is marked with duration in seconds. There is only about 50% agreement between different individuals staging sleep for borderline epochs at the transition between stage N2 and N3. Sleep spindles are also visible in this epoch. *EMG*, Electromyogram.

the frontal derivations, more stage N3 will be scored in some patients compared with scoring using central derivations. Slow waves have higher amplitude in frontal than central derivations. Epochs at the transition from stage N2 to N3 have a low degree of agreement between scorers as it is often difficult to determine the duration of SWA (meeting amplitude and frequency criteria).[7] In Figure 3–15, an epoch barely meeting criteria for stage N3 is shown.

Summary of Scoring Stage N3:

- SWA 20% or greater of the epoch (≥6 seconds)
- Sleep spindles may occur
- No eye movements
- Chin EMG variable usually low

SCORING STAGE R (RAPID EYE MOVEMENT SLEEP)

Definite Stage R

The scoring rules for stage R are complex because not all epochs of an episode of stage R have REMs. The frequency of REMs is called the *REM density* and increases over the night. Scoring the first episode of stage R is more difficult because there are usually very few REMs (low REM density). **Low chin EMG tone** is defined as baseline EMG activity in the chin derivation no higher than any other sleep stage and is usually the lowest level of the entire recording. Epochs of **definite stage R** (Fig. 3–10) are characterized by all the elements of REM sleep including a low chin EMG tone for the majority of the epoch **concurrent** with at least one set of REMs anywhere in the epoch. *The EEG during the segment of the epoch used to score definite REM sleep is LAMF with absent K complexes or sleep spindles (REM-like EEG).* Bursts of alpha and sawtooth waves (Fig. 3–10) may occur during stage R but not used to score stage R.

Summary of Criteria for Scoring Definite Stage R:

- No KC or SS, and EEG is LAMF.
- REMs occur in any part of the epoch.
- Chin EMG at REM level for majority of the epoch and concurrent with REMs.
- Bursts of alpha and sawtooth waves may occur but are not required to score stage R.

Epochs Preceding Definite Stage R

One or more epochs contiguous and *preceding an epoch of definite stage R* are scored as stage R (even in the absence of REMs) if the chin EMG remains at the stage R level, the EEG contains LAMF activity with no K complexes or sleep spindles, there is no intervening arousal, and SEMs following an arousal or stage W are not present (Figs. 3-16 and 3-17). There are additional rules discussed below for intervening arousals. Although SEMs can occur during episodes of stage R, the presence of SEMs *after a period of wake or an arousal* are typical of stage W when associated with posterior dominant (alpha rhythm) or stage N1 when associated with LAMF EEG without alpha rhythm. Of note, scoring stage **R is *not an option if the baseline chin EMG is not at the stage R level.*** In Figure 3–16 the left panel of the schematic shows a transition from stage W to definite stage R (epoch 103). Note that when SEMs are associated with LAMF EEG activity (PDR absent) after an epoch of stage W or an arousal, they signify stage N1 even if the chin EMG is at the stage R level. However, once the SEMs cease (epoch 102), stage R can be scored for segments preceding an epoch of definite stage R. This assumes the chin EMG activity is at the stage R level, an EEG exhibiting LAMF without K complex or sleep spindles is present, and there is no arousal intervening before the epoch of definite stage R. The arrows in Figure 3–16 shows the point at which the chin EMG tone decreased to the stage R level. The middle panel of Figure 3–16 shows the transition from stage N2 to definite stage R (epoch 203). Epoch 200 cannot be scored as stage R because the chin EMG tone does not reach the stage R level until early in the next epoch. Epoch 201 does meet requirements for scoring stage R in a contiguous epoch preceding definite stage R as the chin EMG activity is low for the majority of the epoch. In the third panel in Figure 3–16, the majority of epoch 300 has the chin EMG at the stage R level and the EEG has LAMF without K complexes or sleep spindles and is scored as stage R. Note that application of stage N2 rules would score the epochs 301 and 302 as stage N2. However, **REM rules take precedence over stage N2 rules.**

Summary for Scoring Epochs Preceding Definite Stage R:

- Segments preceding an epoch of definite R can be scored as stage R even if REMs are not present if:
    - EEG contains no KC or SS.
    - No SEMs following wake or an arousal are present.

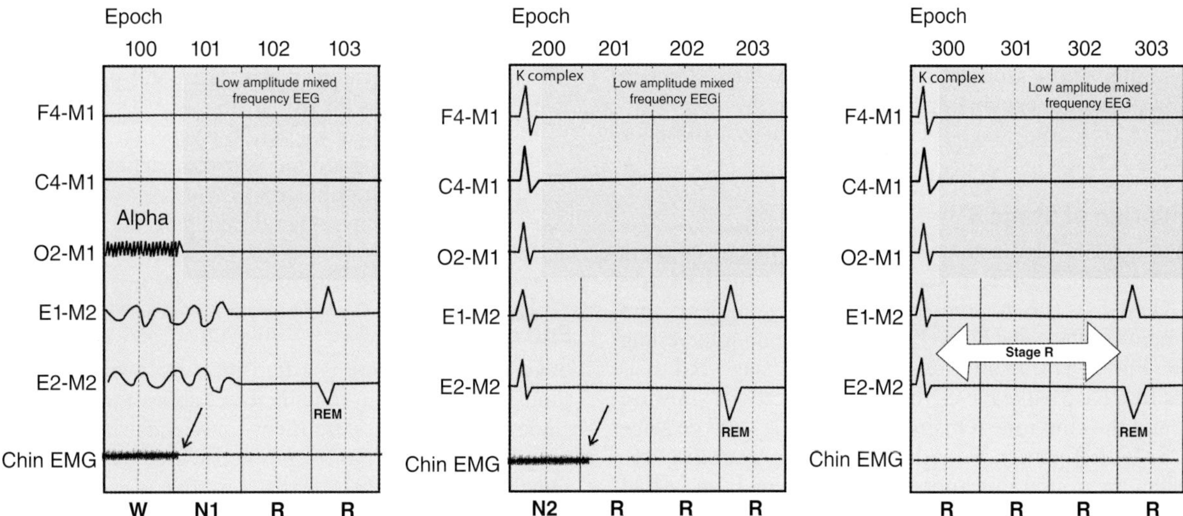

Figure 3–16 Schematics illustrating the start of stage R. Epoch 103 is definite stage R. Epoch 102 is scored as stage R as the electroencephalogram *(EEG)* shows low-amplitude mixed-frequency activity (LAMF) without K complexes or sleep spindles, the chin electromyogram *(EMG)* is at the rapid eye movement *(REM)* level, and there is no intervening arousal between epoch 102 and 103. Epoch 101 has the chin EMG at the REM level but is not scored as stage R as SEMs occupy the majority of the epoch and follow an epoch of stage W. In the *middle panel,* epochs preceding definite stage R in epoch 203 can be scored as stage R as the chin EMG is at the REM level, the EEG has LAMF activity, and there is no intervening arousal. In the *right panel,* the segments following the K complex at the start of epoch 300 all meet criteria for stage R preceding an epoch of definite stage R in epoch 303. The *gray area* means LAMF EEG is present without K complexes or sleep spindles.

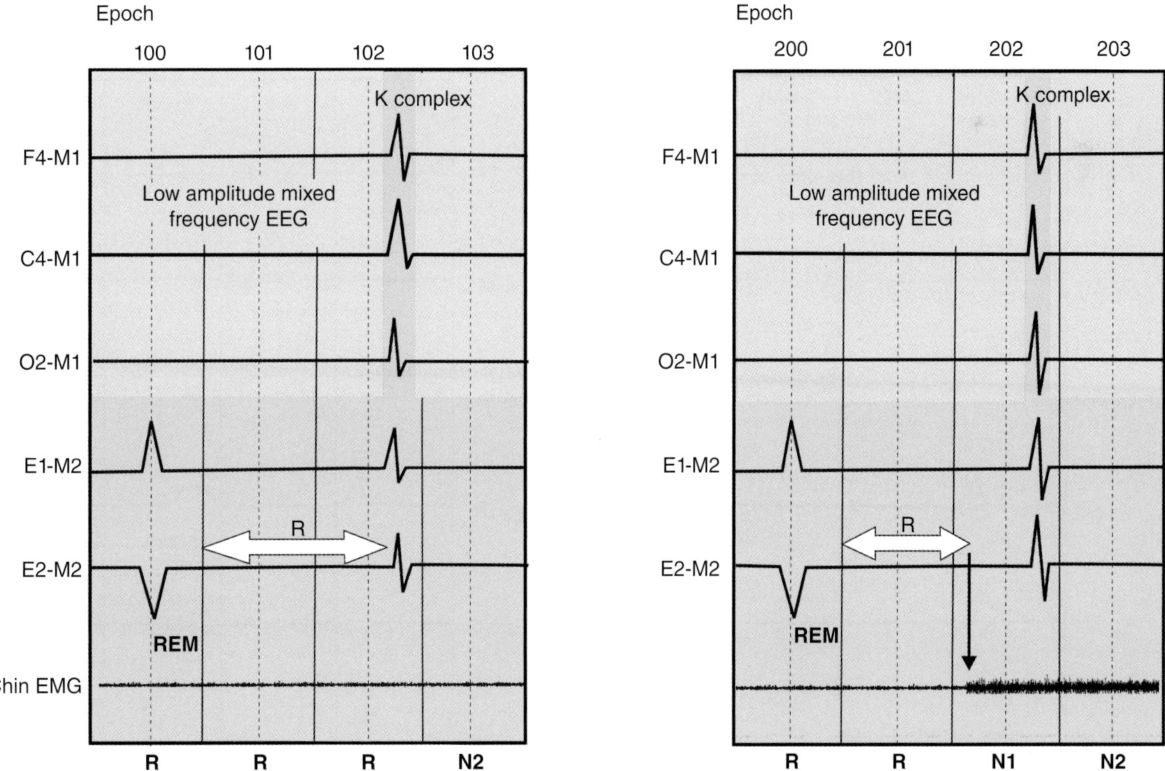

Figure 3–17 Schematic illustrating the continuation of stage R following an epoch of definite stage R. Stage R continues to be scored (even in the absence of rapid eye movements *[REMs]*) as long as the electroencephalogram *(EEG)* shows low-amplitude mixed-frequency (LAMF) activity, the chin electromyogram *(EMG)* remains at the REM level, and there is no intervening arousal. Stage R ends with the appearance of a K complex. However, because the K complex does not occur until the second half of epoch 102, the epoch is scored as stage R. Stage R can no longer be scored in epoch 202 as the chin EMG activity has increased above the REM level. Stage N1 is scored, as the EEG shows LAMF and there is no evidence of another sleep stage.

- Chin EMG is at the REM level for the majority of the epoch.
- No intervening arousal (between definite stage R epoch and preceding epochs).
- Rules for scoring stage R take precedence over those for stage N2.

Continuation of Stage R

Continue to score segments of sleep that follow one or more epochs of definite stage R as stage R as long as the EEG remains REM-like (no K complexes or sleep spindles), chin tone remains at the stage R level, and there are no intervening arousals (Fig. 3–17). If an arousal interrupts stage R but is followed by a REM-like EEG, the EOG derivations **show no SEMs,** and the chin tone remains low, continue to score stage R (Fig. 3–18, left panel). Note that this differs from the situation when an arousal interrupts stage N2 sleep. If an MBM epoch (without alpha activity) interrupts stage R and is followed by a REM-like EEG, the EOG derivations contain no SEMs, and the chin activity remains at the REM level, continue to score stage R (Fig. 3–19, left panel). This assumes that the MBM epoch is not scored as stage W (contains any amount of alpha activity; see MBM rules, later). If the MBM epoch is scored as stage W, stage R ends. If there are SEMs after the MBM epoch, see the following section for the scoring rule for this circumstance.

Summary of Continuation of Stage R:

- Segments following an epoch of definite R continue to be scored as stage R even if REMs are not present if:
  - EEG contains no KC or SS
  - Chin EMG is at the REM level
  - No intervening arousal (between definite stage R epoch and subsequent epochs)
  - Rules for scoring stage R take precedence over those for stage N2
  - Criteria for the end of stage R are not met

End of Stage R

Stage R ends if there is a transition to stage W or stage N3 (unlikely). If the chin tone increases above the REM level (excludes brief increases, transient muscle activity), the segments with higher chin tone are not considered stage R (Fig. 3–17, right panel, epoch 202). If the chin tone is at the stage R level for the majority of the epoch, the epoch can still be scored as stage R (Fig. 3–17, epoch 201). If stage R is interrupted by an arousal and the chin tone after the arousal is higher than the stage R level, then stage R ends. However, what if the chin tone remains at the stage R level after the arousal and the EEG remains REM-like? As noted, stage R continues until there is evidence for another sleep stage. An exception is when the EEG shows LAMF activity *without PDR and the EOG shows SEMs after the arousal* (Fig. 3–18, right panel). This suggests a

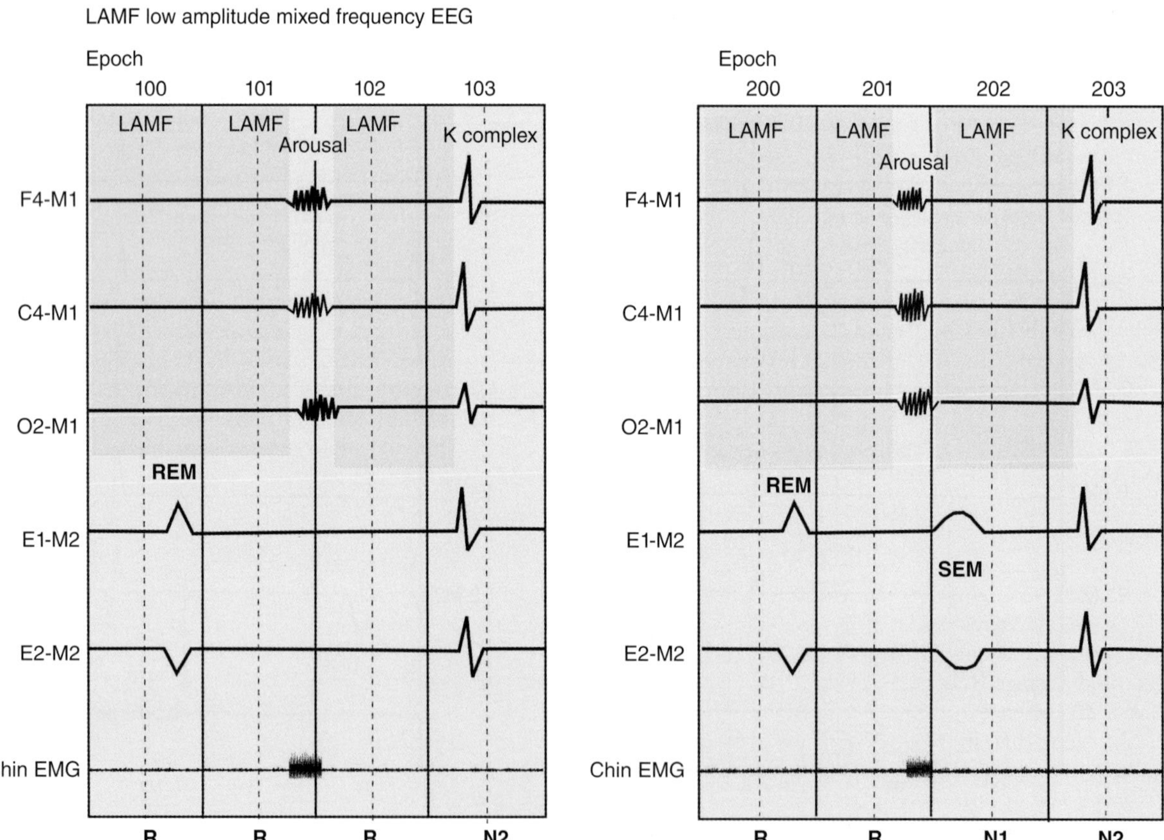

Figure 3–18 Schematics illustrating the interruption of stage R by an arousal. In the *left panel,* stage R continues to be scored in epoch 102 following an arousal as the electroencephalogram *(EEG)* shows low-amplitude mixed-frequency *(LAMF)* activity and the chin electromyogram *(EMG)* remains at the rapid eye movement *(REM)* level. No slow eye movements *(SEMs)* follow the arousal. In the *right panel,* a SEM follows the arousal, and stage N1 is scored until there is evidence of another sleep stage (stage N2 in epoch 203).

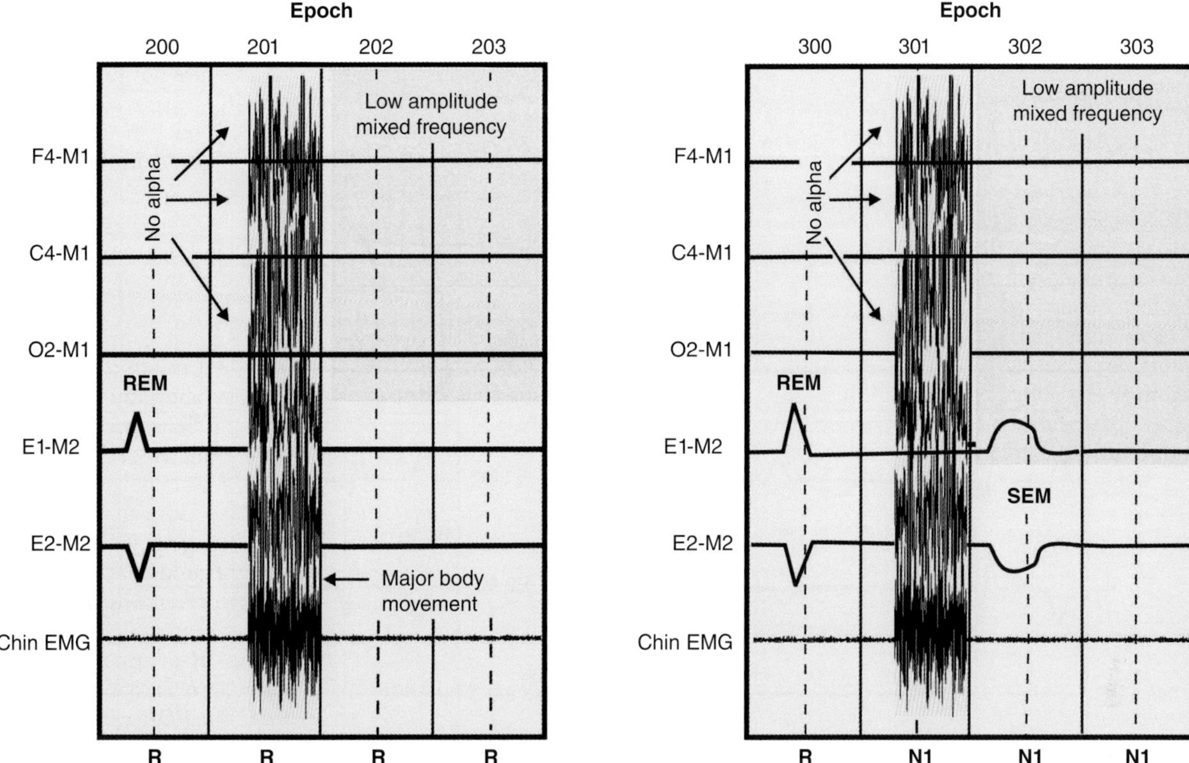

Figure 3–19 A major body movement (MBM) interrupts stage R. As no slow eye movements *(SEMs)* are present after the MBM, the chin activity remains low, and the electroencephalogram (EEG) shows low-amplitude mixed-frequency (LAMF) activity with no K complexes or sleep spindles, epoch 202 remains stage R. By the MBM rules, if the MBM epoch is not scored as stage W, it is scored the same as the epoch that follows. Therefore 201 is stage R. In the *right panel,* a SEM follows the MBM epoch, the chin activity remains low, and the EEG is LAMF. The appearance of the SEM is evidence of a stage shift in this circumstance, epoch 302 is scored as N1, and stage N1 continues unless there is evidence for another sleep stage. The MBM epoch is scored as stage N1 based on the scoring of the epoch that follows the MBM epoch. See the section on MBM scoring. The absence of alpha in epoch 201 is important because an MBM epoch containing alpha is scored as stage W.

transition to stage N1 even if the chin activity remains low (stage N1 scored). If PDR is noted along with the SEMs, this suggests a transition to stage W. If an MBM interrupts stage R and the MBM epoch is scored as stage W, stage R ends (unless the next epoch after the MBM meets criteria for stage R). If the MBM epoch is not scored as stage W, and the epoch afterward has LAMF EEG with SEMs, the epoch is scored as stage N1 even if the chin EMG tone remains low (Fig. 3–19, right panel). The presence of SEMs suggest a sleep stage transition. If a K complex (not associated with an arousal) or sleep spindle interrupts stage R, score stage R up until the K complex of sleep spindle (Fig. 3–17, epoch 102). If the K complex or sleep spindle does not occur until the second half of the epoch, the epoch is scored as stage R, but the following epoch is stage N2 unless there is evidence for another sleep stage (Fig. 3–17, epoch 103). Note that in Figure 3–17 had the K complex occurred in the first half of epoch 102, the epoch would be scored as stage N2. It is important to remember that epochs 101 and 102 in Figure 3–17 would not be scored as stage R if the chin activity did not remain low (at the stage R level).

Summary for end of stage R:

- K complex, sleep spindle in first half of epoch (even if chin EMG remains low)
- Chin EMG increases above REM level
- Note that stage R continues up until the KC, SS, or increase in chin EMG
- Arousal **followed by SEMs** without PDR (even if chin EMG remains low, EEG LAMF)
- MBM **followed by SEMs** (even if chin EMG remains low, EEG LAMF)
- Transition to another sleep stage (W, N2)

Scoring Epochs With a Mixture of K Complexes, Sleep Spindles, and Rapid Eye Movements

Segments of sleep ***with low chin EMG activity*** can contain a mixture of K complexes, sleep spindles, and REMs (Fig. 3–20). This is especially common during the first REM period of the night. First, any segment of the record between two K complexes, two sleep spindles, or a K complex and a sleep spindle without intervening REMs is considered to be stage N2. Second, any segment between two sets of REMs without intervening K complexes or sleep spindles is considered stage R (assumes chin EMG activity is at the REM level). Each epoch is scored based on whether stage N2 or stage R segments predominate in a given epoch. The above rules assume that the chin EMG stays at the REM sleep level.

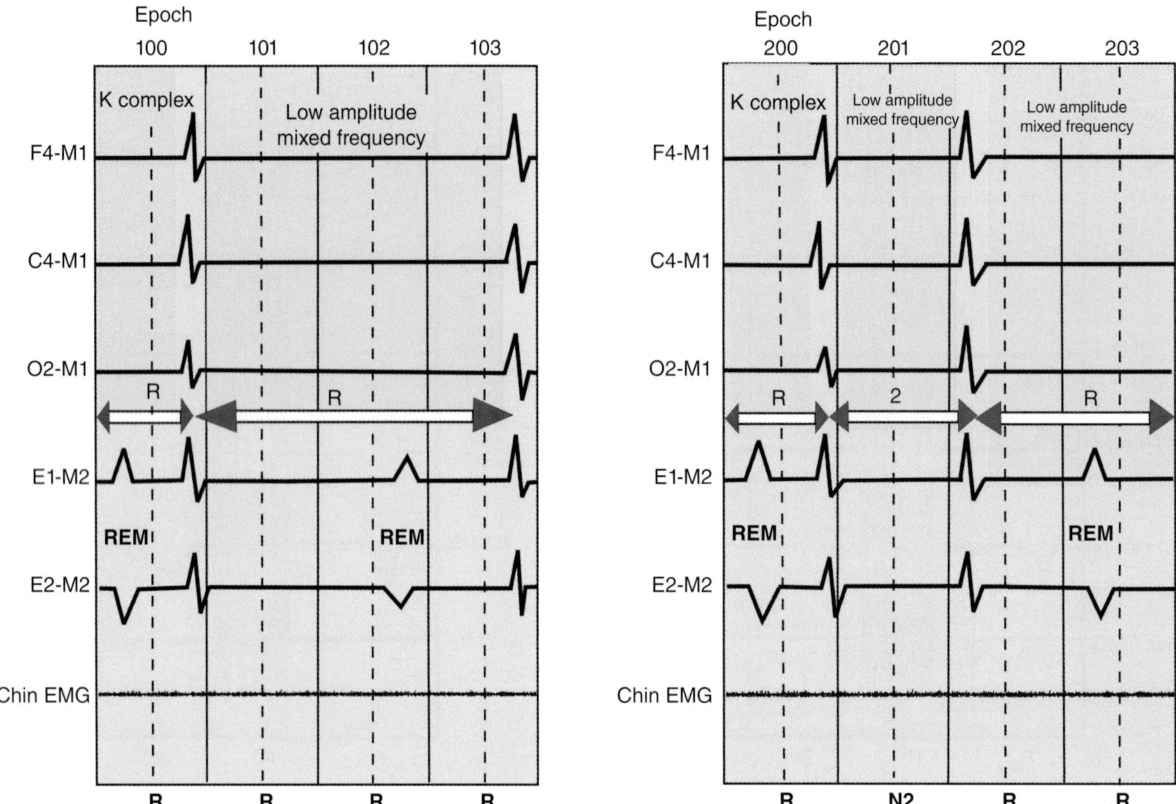

Figure 3–20 Schematics illustrate the scoring of epochs that contain a mixture of rapid eye movements *(REMs)*, K complexes, and sleep spindles **when the chin electromyogram (EMG) is at the REM level.** Segments containing REMs without a K complex or sleep spindle are considered stage R. Segments between two K complexes or two sleep spindles (or a K complex and a sleep spindle) without REM are considered stage N2. Each epoch is scored based on the sleep stage occupying the majority of the epoch.

Summary for Scoring Mixture of K Complexes, Sleep Spindles, REMs:

- Chin EMG must be at REM level to score stage R.
- Segments between two KCs, two SSs, or a KC and SS without REMs are considered stage N2.
- Segments without KC or SS that contains REMs and low chin activity are considered stage R.
- Score each epoch based on the majority of segments (N2 or R).

MAJOR BODY MOVEMENTS

An **MBM** is an event consisting of movement and muscle artifact obscuring the EEG for **more than half an epoch** to the extent that the sleep stage cannot be determined.

The three rules that apply to MBM epochs are illustrated in Figure 3–21.

1. If alpha rhythm is present in the epoch with a MBM (even <15 seconds duration), score the epoch as stage W.
2. If no alpha rhythm is discernible in the epoch containing an MBM, but an epoch scoreable as stage W either precedes or follows the epoch with an MBM, score the MBM epoch as stage W.
3. If no alpha rhythm occurs in an MBM epoch and neither the preceding nor following epoch is stage W, score the MBM epoch as the same stage as the epoch that follows it.

The situations in which an MBM interrupts stage N2 or stage R have already been discussed.

SCORING AROUSALS

The rule for scoring arousals specify different requirements for NREM and REM sleep. This is necessary because bursts of alpha activity are common during stage R.

An arousal is scored during sleep stages N1, N2, N3 if there is an abrupt shift of EEG frequency including alpha, theta, and/or frequencies greater than 16 Hz (but not spindles) that lasts ***at least 3 seconds,*** *with at least 10 seconds of stable sleep preceding the change* (Fig. 3–22)[2].

At sleep onset there are often periods of LAMF EEG alternating with periods of alpha activity. A period of 3 seconds or more of alpha activity would not be scored as an arousal unless the EEG activity meeting criteria for an arousal is preceded by at least 10 seconds of sleep. Of note, scoring arousals during NREM sleep does not include a chin EMG criterion. An increase in chin EMG activity in the absence of EEG changes meeting arousal criteria is not scored as an arousal.

Score an arousal during sleep stage R if there is an abrupt shift of EEG frequency including alpha, theta, and/or frequencies greater than 16 Hz (but not spindles) that lasts ***at least 3 seconds,*** *with at least 10 seconds of stable sleep preceding the change. In addition, an increase in the chin EMG lasting* ***at least 1 second***

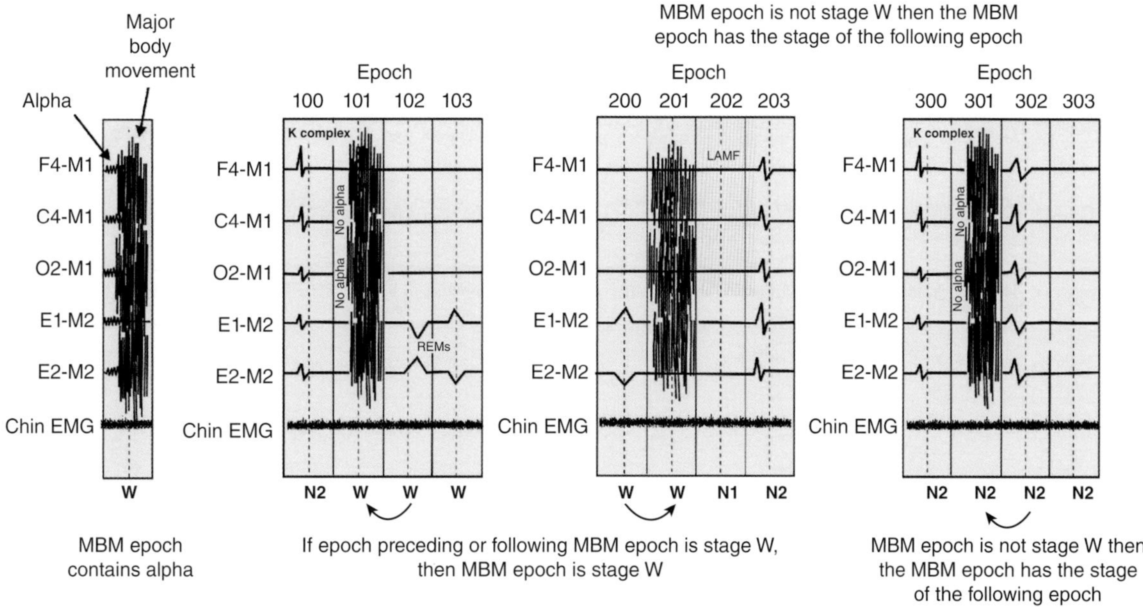

Figure 3–21 Schematics illustrate the major body movement *(MBM)* rules. If the MBM epoch contains any alpha activity, it is scored as stage W *(left panel)*. If an epoch preceding or following the MBM epochs is scored as stage W, then the MBM epoch is stage W *(middle two panels)*. If the MBM epoch is not scored as stage W, it is scored the same as the following epoch *(right panel)*. Epochs 102 and 103 are scored as stage W and not stage R even though REMs are present, as **the chin electromyogram (*EMG*) activity is *not* low** (assumed to be above the stage R level).

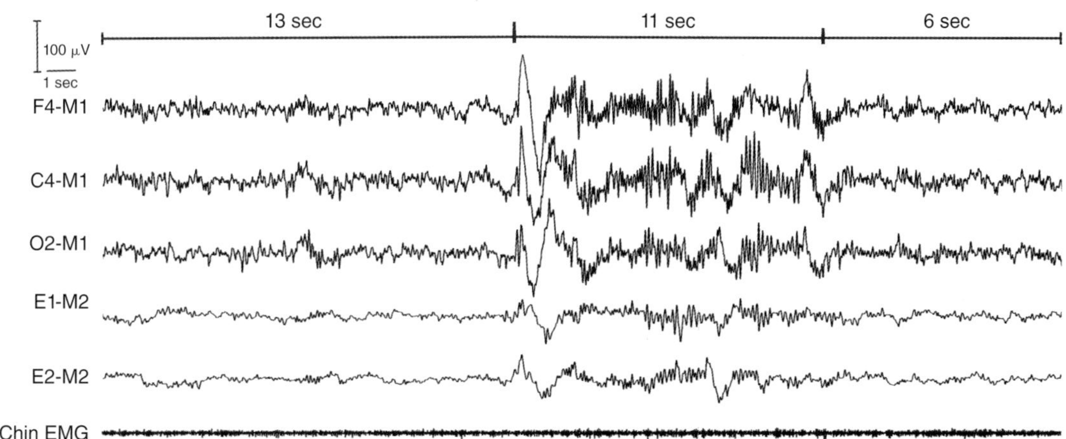

Figure 3–22 A 30-second epoch of non–rapid eye movement (NREM) sleep containing an arousal. Here the previous epoch is assumed to be stage N2. The portion of the epoch preceding the arousal is considered a continuation of stage N2 (there is also an equivocal sleep spindle in the middle of the tracing before the arousal). Note that there is no change in the chin electromyogram *(EMG)* (not required for an arousal for NREM sleep). There is a K complex followed by an abrupt shift in the electroencephalogram (EEG) meeting criteria for an arousal (≥3 seconds in duration). The EEG shift cannot be sleep spindle activity, which can also be associated with K complexes. In this tracing the fast EEG activity is in the alpha frequency range. **K complexes and bursts of slow waves can be associated with arousals but neither qualifies as evidence of an arousal using the American Academy of Sleep Medicine scoring manual rules in absence of qualifying EEG activity.** How should this epoch be scored? The first and third segments are sleep (13 + 6 = 19), whereas 11 seconds would qualify as wake. Therefore the epoch is sleep. Then what sleep stage predominates? The longest segment of 13 seconds would be stage N2 based on the preceding epoch assumed to be stage N2. The 6 seconds would be scored as stage N1 (recall an arousal ends stage N2). Therefore, as the majority of sleep is stage N2, the epoch is scored as stage N2. However, the following epoch would be scored as stage N1 until there was evidence of another sleep stage.

must be present *(concurrent with EEG changes meeting criteria for an arousal).*[2]

As noted above, this extra requirement of an increase in chin EMG activity to score an arousal from stage R is necessary as bursts of alpha activity are common during stage R and do not necessarily mean an arousal (sleep stage change) has occurred. An example of arousal scoring during stage R is shown in Figure 3–23. At A there is an abrupt change in the EEG (burst of alpha activity) meeting criteria for an arousal. However, there is no concurrent increase in chin EMG activity. At B there is an increase in chin EMG activity but no associated EEG change meeting arousal criteria. At C there is

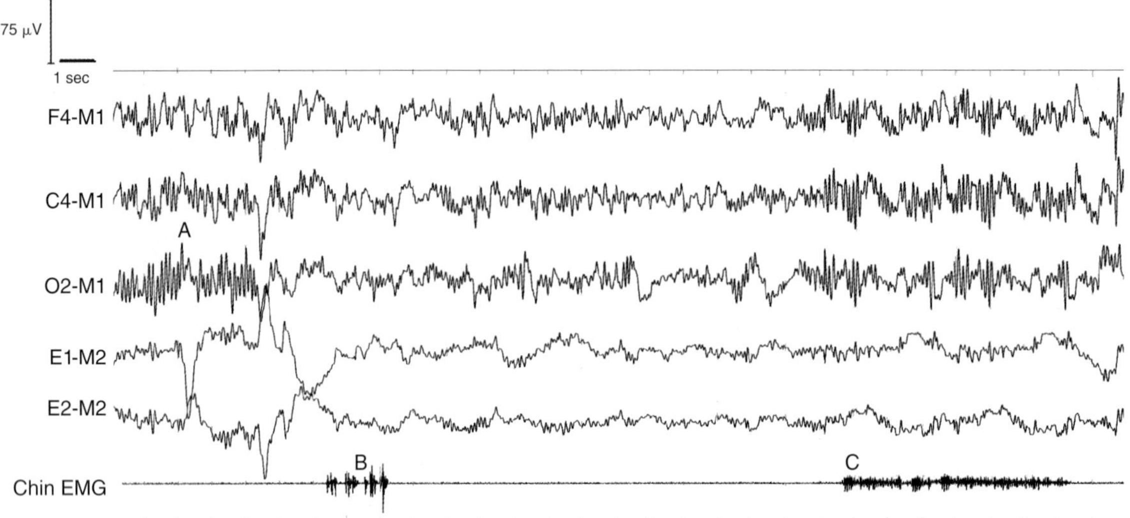

Figure 3–23 A 30-second epoch of definite stage R. The electroencephalogram (EEG) shows an abrupt alpha burst at A that would meet EEG criteria for arousal, but there is no associated increase in chin EMG (must be at least 1 second in duration). The burst of chin electromyogram *(EMG)* activity at B is not associated with an EEG change meeting arousal criteria. At C there is a greater than 3-second change in the EEG meeting arousal criterion (preceded by 10 seconds of sleep). There is a concurrent increase in chin EMG. Therefore an arousal can be scored at C.

both a qualifying EEG change for an arousal and a concurrent increase in chin EMG of at least 1 second. Note that up to C, the epoch meets criteria for definite stage R (the majority of the epoch meets criteria for stage R).

Arousals immediately preceding an epoch of stage W are still scored (both an arousal and stage W can be scored). Arousal scoring should use information from the frontal, central, and occipital derivations.

The sudden appearance of a K complex or slow waves is not evidence for an arousal even if associated with an increase in the chin *EMG unless there is a change in the EEG that meets the arousal rule criteria.* In Figure 3–22, a K complex followed by EEG activity meeting criteria for arousal is noted. The K complex is associated with the arousal, but the K complex alone does not qualify the event as an arousal. Transitions between sleep stages are not scored as arousals unless arousal EEG criteria are met. Note that it is possible that an arousal could be scored in the middle of an epoch scored as stage W, assuming 10 seconds of sleep preceded the EEG changes meeting criteria for an arousal.

SUMMARY OF KEY POINTS

1. The AASM scoring manual uses updated nomenclature for wake fullness and sleep (stages W, N1, N2, N3, and R). Stage N3 replaces stages 3 and 4 and stage R replaces stage REM.
2. Sleep is scored in sequential 30-second epochs. If more than one sleep stage occurs in an epoch, the epoch is scored based on the sleep stage occupying the majority of the epoch.
3. In individuals who do generate PDR (alpha) on eye closure, when the PDR is replaced by LAMF activity for more than 50% of the epoch, stage N1 is scored.
4. In individuals who do not generate posterior dominant (alpha) rhythm on eye closure, the onset of stage N1 is based on the earliest occurrence of SEMs, EEG activity in the 4- to 7-Hz range with slowing of the background frequency by 1 Hz or greater compared with wake, or vertex sharp waves.
5. Begin scoring stage N2 when one or more sleep spindles or K complexes (not associated with an arousal) occur in the first half of the current epoch or last half of the previous epoch. This assumes criteria for stages W, N3, or R are not met.
6. Epochs following an epoch of stage N2 continue to be scored as stage N2 (even in the absence of a sleep spindle or K complex) until there is a reason to change to another sleep stage (arousal, stage W, stage N3, stage R). If the majority of an epoch is considered N2 then the epoch is scored as N2.
7. The scoring of stage N3 is based on SWA in the frontal derivations (≥6 seconds of SWA, not >6 seconds). SWA is defined as an EEG showing 0.5- to 2-Hz activity with an amplitude greater than 75 μV (not ≥) peak to peak in F4-M1 or F3-M2.
8. An epoch of definite stage R is characterized by all of the following:
   - REMs in any part of the epoch
   - LAMF EEG activity without K complexes or sleep spindles
   - Low chin EMG tone for the **majority of the epoch and concurrent with REMs**
9. Epochs immediately preceding or following an epoch of definite stage R can be scored as stage R in the absence of REMs if the EEG has a LAMF pattern without K complexes or sleep spindles and the chin EMG is at the REM level as long as there are no intervening arousals.
10. Scoring sleep when an arousal interrupts stage N2 is different than when an arousal interrupts stage R. When an arousal interrupts stage N2 the stage ends until there is new evidence for sleep stage N2. The following epoch is usually stage N1 or stage W. When an arousal interrupts stage R, the stage continues until there is evidence for a different sleep stage.
11. When an arousal interrupts stage N2 and the EEG following the arousal is LAMF without K complexes or sleep spindles, a transition to stage N1 has occurred. When an arousal interrupts stage R and the chin EMG activity following the arousal remains low, the EEG shows a LAMF pattern without K complexes or sleep spindles, and no SEMs are present, stage R continues. If SEMs are present (not associated with

PDR in the EEG), stage N1 is scored until there is evidence for another sleep stage.

12. Score arousals during sleep stages N1, N2, N3, or R if there is an abrupt shift of EEG frequency including alpha, theta, and/or frequencies greater than 16 Hz (but not spindles) that lasts at least 3 seconds, with at least 10 seconds of stable sleep preceding the change. Scoring of arousals during REM requires an increase in the submental EMG lasting at least 1 second (concurrent with EEG changes meeting criteria for an arousal).

CLINICAL REVIEW QUESTIONS

1. Which of the following criteria describe SWA?
   A. Frequency 0.5–2 Hz and amplitude $\geq 75\ \mu V$ in F4-M1 or F3-M2
   B. Frequency 0.5–2 Hz and amplitude $> 75\ \mu V$ in F4-M1 or F3-M2
   C. Frequency 0.5–2 Hz and amplitude $\geq 75\ \mu V$ in F4-M2 or F3-M1
   D. Frequency 0.5–2 Hz and amplitude $> 75\ \mu V$ in F4-M2 or F3-M1
2. Which of the following describes an epoch of stage N3 (SWA meets amplitude criteria)?
   A. SWA > 6 seconds
   B. SWA ≥ 6 seconds
   C. SWA > 15 seconds
   D. SWA ≥ 15 seconds
3. Which of the following describes an arousal from sleep?
   A. Preceded by at least 5 seconds of sleep
   B. A burst of slow waves with a brief increase in chin EMG activity
   C. An abrupt shift in EEG frequency for at least 3 seconds
   D. A sudden burst of 3 seconds of alpha activity during REM sleep but no change in the chin EMG
4. An MBM epoch is preceded by an epoch of stage W and followed by an epoch of stage N2. What is the sleep stage of the MBM epoch?
   A. Stage W
   B. Stage N1
   C. Determined by presence or absence of alpha activity in the MBM
   D. Determined by the level of chin activity in the MBM
5. Which of the following statements about stage N1 is true?
   A. Must contain SEMs
   B. PDR < 50% of the epoch (PDR/alpha generator)
   C. Must contain vertex sharp waves
   D. Chin EMG activity must be lower than stage W
6. In Figure 3–24, what is the sleep stage of epochs 301, 302, and 303?

Epoch	301	302	303
A	N2	N1	N2
B	N2	N2	N2
C	N1	N1	N2
D	N2	W	N2

7. In Figure 3–25, what is the sleep stage of epochs 101, 102, and 103?

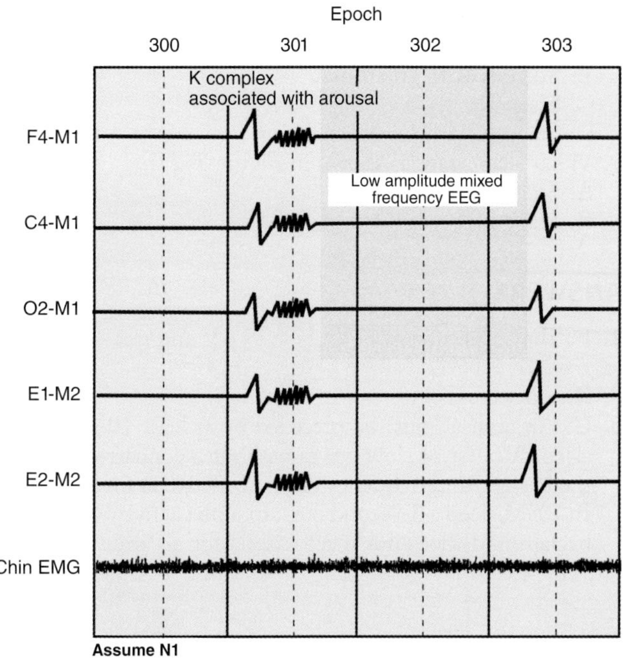

Figure 3–24 This figure is for review question 6. What is the sleep stage for epochs 301, 302, and 303?

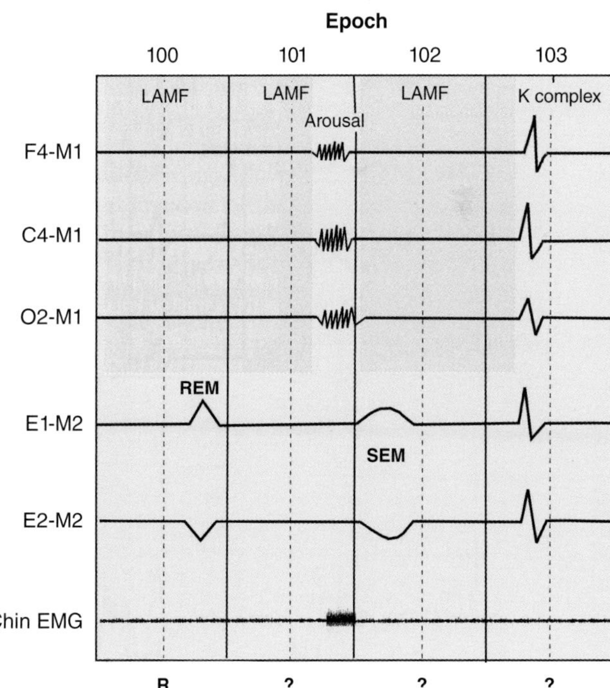

Figure 3–25 This figure is for review question 7. What is the sleep stage for epochs 101, 102, and 103?

Epoch	101	102	103
A	R	R	N2
B	R	N1	N2
C	N1	N1	N2
D	N1	W	N2

8. What sleep stage is shown in Figure 3–26?
   A. Stage W
   B. Stage R with an arousal
   C. Stage R
   D. Stage R with sawtooth waves
9. What sleep stage is shown in Figure 3–27?
   A. Stage N2
   B. Stage N1

ANSWERS

1. **B.** The amplitude of SWA is >75 μV and not ≥75 μV in F4-M1, F3-M2.
2. **B.** ≥6 seconds.
3. **C.** An arousal must be preceded by at least 10 seconds of sleep. A burst of slow waves without a concurrent shift in the background frequency does meet criteria for an arousal. In REM sleep a 3-second burst of alpha activity (shift from background) does not meet criteria for an arousal in stage R unless accompanied by at least a 1-second increase in chin EMG activity concurrent with the EEG evidence of an arousal.
4. **A.** Stage W. If an MBM is preceded or followed by an epoch of stage W, the MBM epoch is scored as stage W.
5. **B.** In a patient generating PDR, an epoch of stage N1 must have <50% PDR activity. Although SEMs and vertex sharp waves may be present in stage N1, they are not required if the epoch otherwise meets qualifying criteria. The magnitude of chin EMG activity is not a criterion for staging N1, N2, or N3. The amplitude is usually less than stage W.
6. **C.** Stages N1, N1, N2. In epoch 301 there is a K complex associated with an arousal. This does *not* provide evidence for stage N2, so stage N1 continues until epoch 303, which has a K complex not associated with an arousal in the first part of the epoch.
7. **B.** Stages R, N1, and N2. As the arousal in epoch 101 occurs in the last half of epoch 101, stage R is considered to be present in the majority of the epoch.

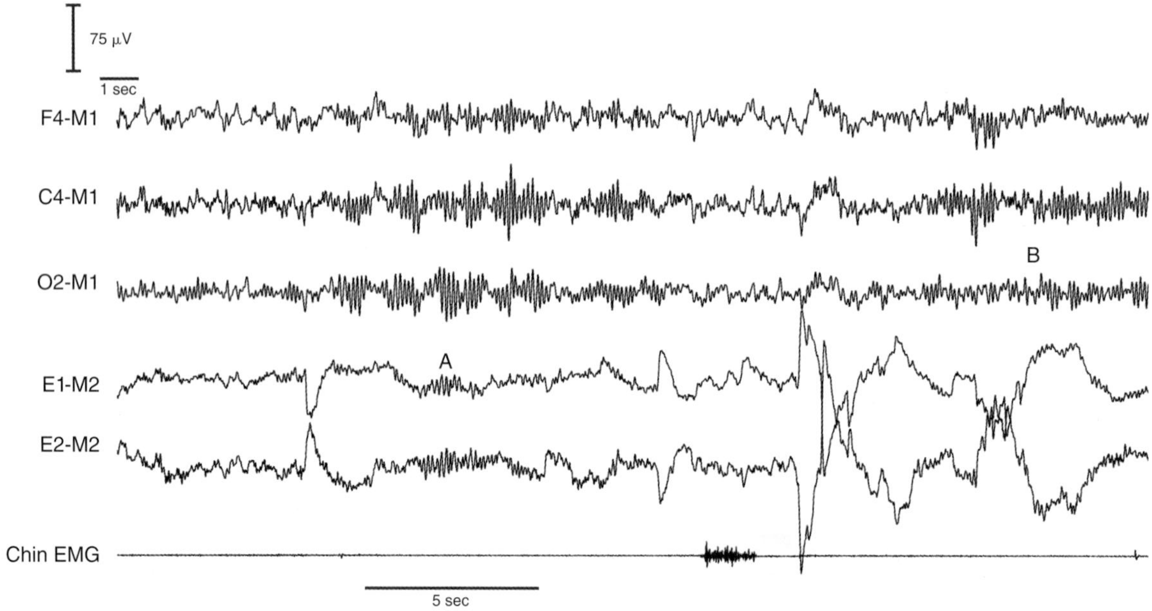

Figure 3–26 This figure is for review question 8. What sleep stage is shown in this figure?

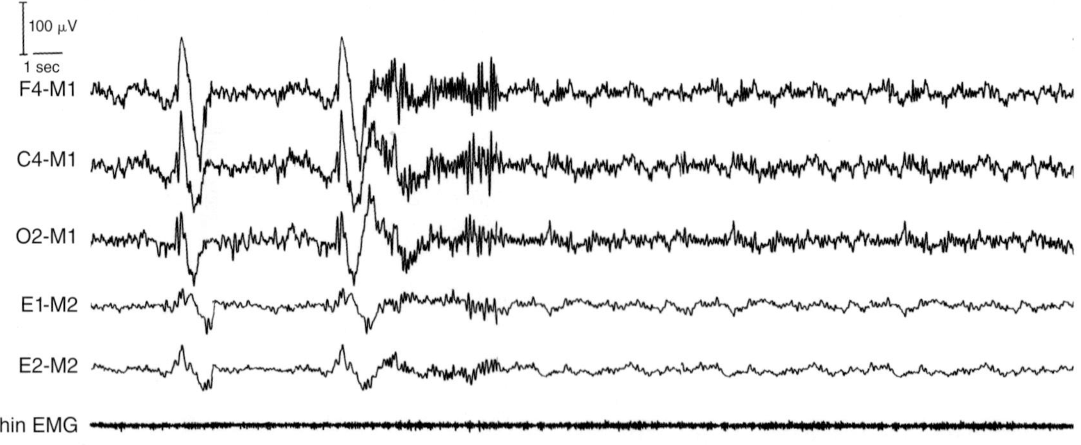

Figure 3–27 This figure is for review question 9. What sleep stage is shown?

The arousal-interrupting stage R is followed by a SEM, and epoch 102 is considered to be a transition to N1 even if the EEG has LAMF activity without K complexes or sleep spindles and the chin EMG remains at the REM level. The K complex in the first half of epoch 103 indicates the start of stage N2.

8. **C.** An epoch of stage R is shown with bursts of alpha activity (A, B), REMs, and low chin EMG activity for the majority of the epoch. An arousal is not present as the increase in chin activity is not concurrent with the alpha bursts. If the chin EMG was higher than the REM level for the majority of the epoch, the epoch would be scored as stage W. Sawtooth waves can occur in stage R but are not required for the diagnosis.
9. **B.** Stage N1. Stage N2 is scored up until the K complex associated with an arousal. Stage N2 ends. The sleep after the arousal has LAMF activity and is scored as stage N1. As the majority of the epoch meets criteria for stage N1, the epoch is stage N1. This assumes that the following epoch does not provide evidence that a different sleep stage should be scored in this epoch. For example, if the chin EMG was considered to be at the REM level and the next epoch was definite stage R then the epoch would be scored as stage R if there was no intervening arousal.

SUGGESTED READING

Silber MH, Ancoli-Israel S, Bonnet MH, et al. The visual scoring of sleep in adults. *J Clin Sleep Med.* 2007;15:121-131.

Troester MM, Quan SF, Berry RB, et al. *The AASM Manual for the Scoring of Sleep and Associated Events: Rules, Terminology and Technical Specifications. Version 3.* American Academy of Sleep Medicine; 2023.

REFERENCES

1. Iber C, Ancoli-Israel S, Chesson A, Quan SF. *The AASM Manual for Scoring of Sleep and Associated Events: Rules, Terminology and Technical Specifications.* American Academy of Sleep Medicine; 2007.
2. Troester MM, Quan SF, Berry RB, et al. *The AASM Manual for the Scoring of Sleep and Associated Events: Rules, Terminology and Technical Specifications. Version 3.* American Academy of Sleep Medicine; 2023.
3. Silber MH, Ancoli-Israel S, Bonnet MH, et al. The visual scoring of sleep in adults. *J Clin Sleep Med.* 2007;15:121-131.
4. Rechtschaffen A, Kales A, eds. *A Manual of Standardized Terminology Techniques and Scoring System for Sleep Stages of Human Sleep.* Brain Information Service/Brain Research Institute, UCLA; 1968.
5. Bonnet MH, Doghramji K, Roehrs T, et al. The scoring of arousal in sleep: reliability, validity, and alternatives. *J Clin Sleep Med.* 2007; 3(2):133-145.
6. EEG arousals: scoring rules and examples: a preliminary report from the Sleep Disorders Atlas Task Force of the American Sleep Disorders Association. *Sleep.* 1992;15(2):173-184.
7. Rosenberg RS, Van Hout S. The American Academy of Sleep Medicine inter-scorer reliability program: sleep stage scoring. *J Clin Sleep Med.* 2013;9(1):81-87.

Chapter 4

Artifacts and Common Variants of Sleep

ARTIFACTS

Artifacts in electroencephalographic (EEG), electrooculographic (EOG), and electromyographic (EMG) derivations that are caused by inadequate electrode application, the effects of patient movement (with respiration, awakening, changing sleep position), and the environment (warm room) are common in polysomnography (PSG).[1-6] It is essential that they be recognized during recording to allow for intervention by the sleep technologist. Postrecording interventions can minimize the effects of most of the artifacts on the ability to accurately stage sleep. For example, the application of backup electrodes allows a change in derivation to one not using a faulty electrode.

Electrode Popping

Electrode popping is a common and significant artifact that makes the staging of sleep difficult[2] (Table 4–1). It is characterized by a sudden high-amplitude deflection secondary to movement of an electrode pulling away from the skin (sudden loss of signal) (Figure 4–1). The temporary loss of the electrical connection to the skin can occur with either direct pressure on the electrode or pulling on the electrode wire. If the electrode gel/paste dries out, this makes an electrode more susceptible to popping. The high amplitude of the artifact may be clipped (not displayed beyond a certain positive and negative amplitude) in some PSG programs to avoid overlap into the next channel. The deflection can be of a short duration (very sharp) or longer depending on the cause of the popping. The deflections often tend to be regular and correspond to body movement during breathing. Electrode popping may also be caused by the patient lying on one mastoid electrode or pulling on the wire connecting the electrode with the electrode box during respiration. For example, if the wire runs under the patient's body or through chest or abdominal respiratory effort bands, patient movement or respiration can pull on the electrode wire. At the time of recording, adding electrode gel or reapplication of the problem electrode may eliminate the problem. After recording, the artifact can frequently be handled by switching to an alternative derivation that does not use the problem electrode. For example, if O2 is the problem, the exploring occipital electrode is switched to O1 (derivation O1-M2). This is one reason that redundant electrodes are routinely placed. In Figure 4–1, regular high-voltage deflections are noted in all derivations containing M1. Therefore, the problem is most likely in electrode M1. Video monitoring confirmed that the patient was sleeping on the left side. After changing the reference electrode to M2 (using derivations F3-M2, C3-M2, O1-M2, E1-M2, and E2-M2), the problem was eliminated. During testing, adding gel to the electrode, replacing the electrode, or rerouting the electrode wire are interventions that might resolve this issue. Displaying O2-M2 would also eliminate the artifact. However, the alternate derivations recommended by the American Academy of Sleep Medicine (AASM) scoring manual[1] use a reference electrode on the opposite side of the exploring electrode. For example, if electrode O2 fails, use F4-M1, C4-M1, O1-M2 (see Chapter 1).

Finding the Problem Electrode

Interventions for many artifacts at the time of reading of a sleep study require determination of the problem electrode and changing derivations to minimize the problem. First, determine if the artifact is present in more than one channel containing a common electrode but not in channels not using this electrode. The common electrode is the faulty electrode (e.g., M1 in Figure 4–1). Second, if the artifact is present in only one derivation, the electrode unique to that derivation is likely the issue. If changing the channel derivation to one not using the suspected electrode eliminates the issue, this confirms that this is the problem electrode. One must also not be confused if M1 and M2 are linked (or averaged) to reduce electrocardiographic (ECG) artifact. Then, changing M1 or M2 may not have the desired effect. For troubleshooting, use derivations that do not link or average M1 and M2.

60-Hz Artifact

A 60-cycle artifact in EEG, EOG, or EMG tracings is a common problem in sleep study recording (Table 4–2). It is caused by 60-Hz electrical activity from power lines contaminating the recorded signal. A 60-Hz artifact can be minimized by correct application of electrodes and proper design of the sleep laboratory. All power lines should be as far from the PSG amplifier and headbox as possible. EEG signals are recorded using differential alternating current (AC) amplifiers, which allows them to record low-voltage EEG activity while

Table 4–1 Electrode Popping Artifact
• Electrode popping artifact is a sudden, high-voltage deflection occurring at regular intervals, usually coincident with respiration.
• Electrode popping artifact is due to an electrode pulling away from the skin or the drying of electrode gel or paste.
• Noting the affected derivations can identify the problem electrode: • Several derivations with a common electrode • One derivation with a unique electrode
• Reapplication of the problem electrode, the addition of electrode paste, or change in the position of the electrode wire is indicated during recording.
• Review using a derivation not including the problem electrode will usually allow staging of sleep.

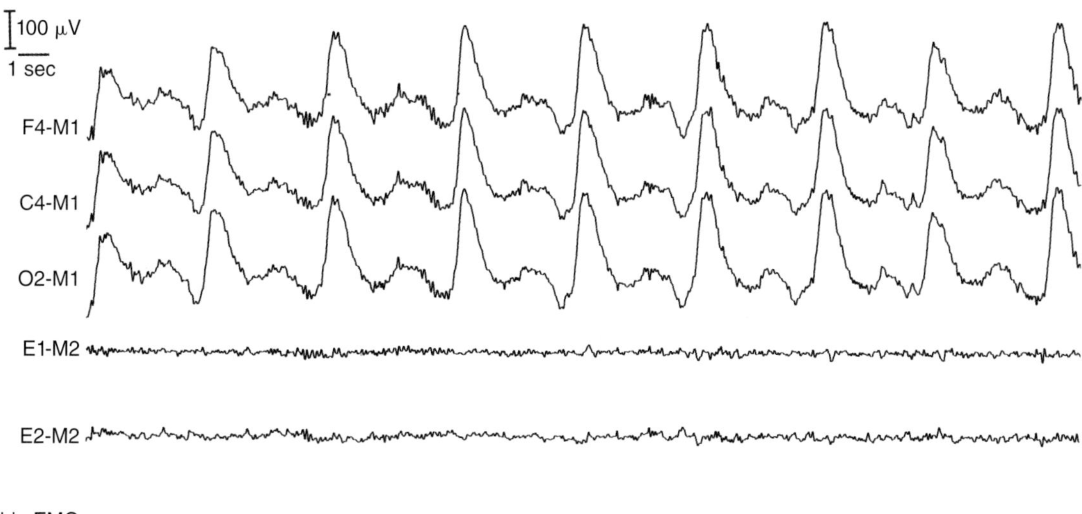

Figure 4–1 A 30-second tracing showing popping artifact. The artifact is noted in all derivations containing M1 and none using electrode M2. Therefore M1 is the problem electrode. Changing the display to F3-M2, C3-M2, and O2-M2 eliminated the problem. During recording repair of electrode M1 (adding electrode gel or reapplication) or rerouting the electrode wire would have been the ideal solution. *EMG,* Electromyogram. (From Berry RB, Wagner MH. *Sleep Medicine Pearls.* 3rd ed., Philadelphia, Elsevier; 2015:102.)

Table 4–2 60-Hz Artifact
• A 60-Hz artifact often produces a thick band or rope-like appearance in the tracing.
• A 60-Hz contamination of the recorded signal may not be recognized if both a 35-Hz high-frequency filter and a 60-Hz notch filter are used for display.
• Recording with **60-Hz filter off** will increase the ability to recognize the presence of 60-Hz signal contamination (usually a clue that an electrode needs replacement).
• A 60-Hz artifact is more apparent in channels using a 100-Hz high-frequency filter setting (especially when the 60-Hz notch filter is turned off).
• If turning on and off the 60-Hz notch filter significantly reduces (filter on) or increases (filter off) the signal/artifact amplitude, this is another clue that 60-Hz contamination is present in a given derivation.

rejecting unwanted and sometimes higher-voltage AC or direct current (DC) activity. Differential amplifiers can record low-voltage physiologic signals by amplifying the difference in voltage between two electrodes while rejecting the common-mode signal consisting of higher-voltage, 60-Hz, background activity. When recording the voltage difference between two electrodes, the background AC activity is rejected only if the electrode impedances are relatively equal. While EEG channels have an option to use a 60-Hz notch filter to minimize 60-Hz signal contamination, use of the notch filter may not prevent prominent 60-Hz activity when electrode impedances are very different (usually one defective electrode has a very high impedance). The **maximum** electrode impedance recommended by the AASM scoring manual for EEG, EOG and chin EMG electrodes is 5 KΩ (impedance ≤5 kiloohms). A maximum impedance for ECG electrodes has not been specified (it should be adjusted to minimize noise in the baseline signal amplitude). The ideal leg EMG impedance is 5KΩ or less. However, an impedance less than 10 KΩ is acceptable. Electrode impedance should be checked by the sleep technician after electrode application before recording starts and then periodically during recording. Post PSG systems allow recording of the electrode impedances when they are checked during recording. An impedance is calculated for each electrode by having the amplifier send a very low amperage oscillating signal to the patient (usually through the ground or reference electrode) and recording the voltage at each electrode. Knowing the input signal and the signal recorded at each electrode, an impedance can be calculated. Routine use of 60-Hz notch filters is not recommended as this makes recognition of a faulty electrode more difficult because it masks 60-Hz contamination. *However, it should be appreciated that use of a 35-Hz high- frequency filter for EEG and EOG derivations significantly attenuates 60-Hz activity.* The effect of adding or removing the notch filter is more prominent in chin and leg EMG derivations that use a high-frequency filter of 100 Hz. The sudden appearance of 60-Hz artifact usually means one electrode is faulty (disconnected or high impedance). In the days of paper PSG recording with ink pens, the 60 Hz artifact caused a characteristic humming of the pens as they oscillated at 60 cycles/sec. If 60-Hz contamination of a derivation is significant, turning off the 60 Hz notch filter will **significantly increase** the amplitude of the artifact (especially if a high filter of 100 Hz is used for the derivation). A 60-Hz artifact can also be recognized on the usual 30-second view by a very dense, uniform, squared-off or "rope-like" tracing that does not vary (Figure 4–2). If 60-Hz artifact is due to a single electrode, it should be replaced or repaired during recording. Using a different display derivation during postrecording viewing may solve the problem. In Figure 4–3 (left panel), prominent 60-Hz artifact is noted in the chin derivation and produces a band or rope-like tracing. In Figure 4–3 (center panel), application of the 60-Hz filter dramatically reduced the amplitude consistent with a significant amount of 60-Hz artifact. When the derivation was

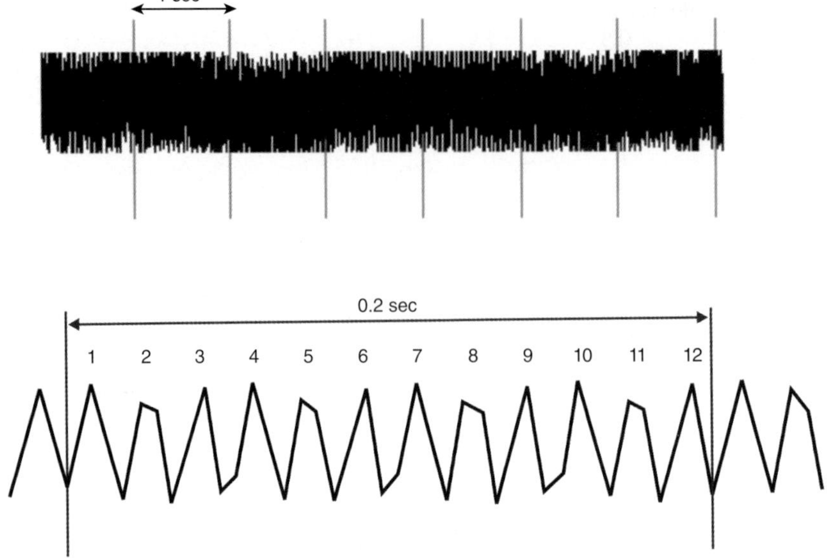

Figure 4–2 The top line shows a 60-Hz artifact as it appears in a 30-second window (7 seconds shown). The bottom tracing shows a blowup of an actual tracing with 60-Hz artifact allowing counting of the frequency with 60 oscillations (5 × 12) in 1 second (60 Hz). (From Berry RB, Wagner MH. *Sleep Medicine Pearls.* 3rd ed., Philadelphia, Elsevier; 2015:103.)

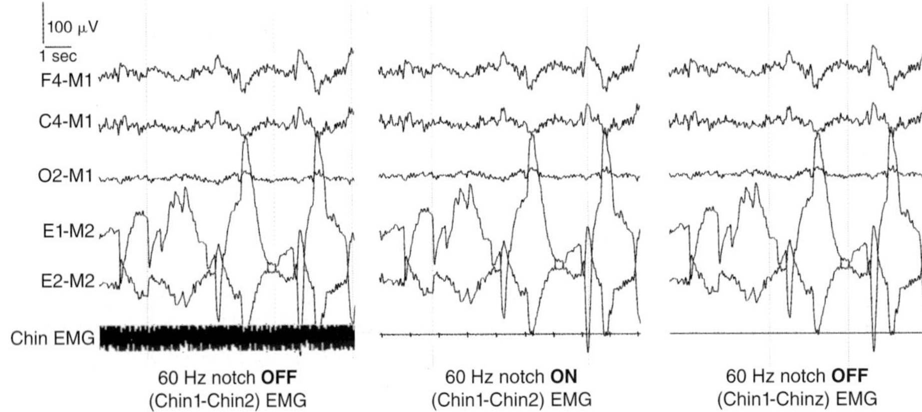

Figure 4–3 The *left panel* shows stage R with significant 60-Hz artifact in the chin electromyogram *(EMG)*. The *middle panel* shows the effect of turning on the 60-Hz notch filter. This demonstrates that this artifact is from 60-Hz contamination of the chin signal. One could assume that either Chin1 or Chin2 is the faulty electrode. Eliminating Chin2 from the derivation *(right panel)* using Chin1-ChinZ eliminated the artifact without the need to turn the 60 Hz notch filter on. (From Berry RB, Wagner MH. *Sleep Medicine Pearls.* 3rd ed., Philadelphia, Elsevier; 2015:104.)

changed to one not including Chin2 (Figure 4–3, right panel), the artifact was eliminated without the use of a 60-Hz filter. The ideal intervention would have been replacement of the Chin2 electrode during recording by the technologist. The problem was the Chin2 electrode.

Slow-Frequency (Sweat and Respiratory) Artifact

Slow-frequency artifact is characterized by a slowly undulating movement (sway or oscillation) of the baseline of affected channels (Table 4–3; Figures 4–4, 4–5, and 4–6). The movement may or may not be synchronous with the patient's respiration. When not in phase with respiration, slow-frequency artifact is often called "sweat artifact" (Figure 4–4), and typically has a slower frequency than the patient's respiration and involves all the EEG and EOG electrodes. When in phase with the patient's respiration, the artifact is called

Table 4–3 Slow Frequency (Sweat or Respiratory Artifact)
• A slowly undulating signal (sway) is typical of sweat artifact.
• If the undulations are in phase with respiration (same frequency) respiratory artifact is said to be present.
• If sweat artifact is present in all derivations and the room or patient is warm, cooling of the patient should be attempted.
• If sway is present only in derivations using a given mastoid electrode, the artifact may be due to movement of the mastoid electrode during respiration or perspiration surrounding the mastoid electrode.
• Slow-frequency artifact may make scoring stage N3 very difficult.

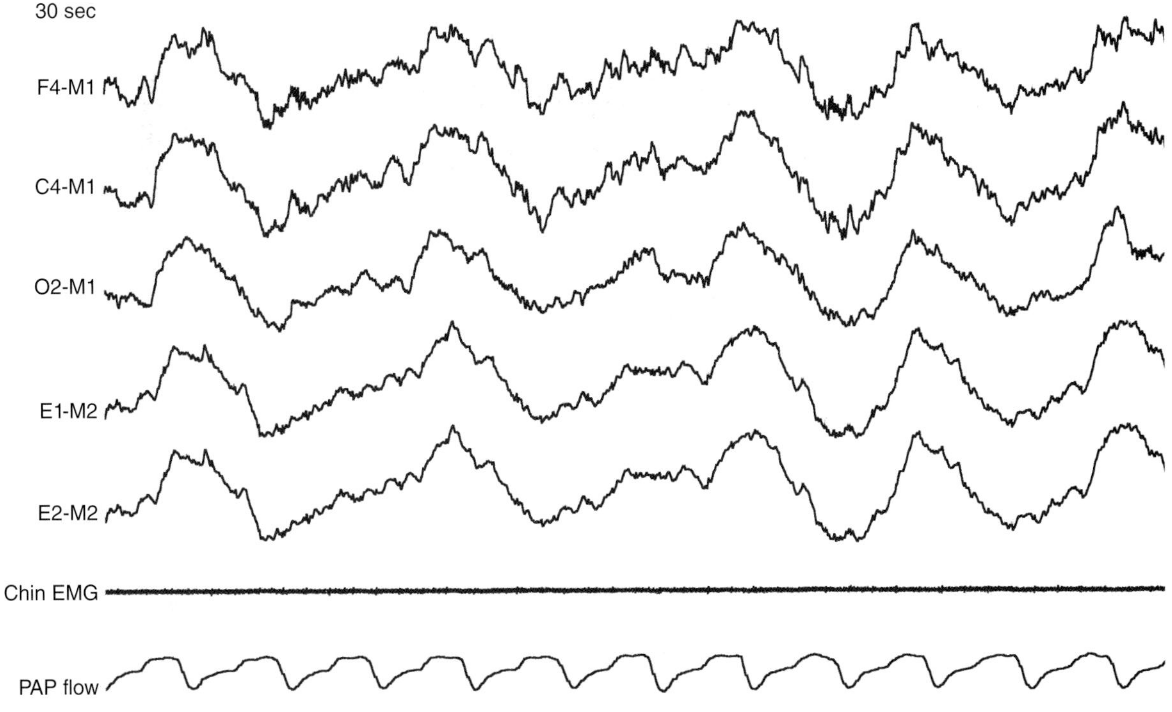

Figure 4–4 A 30-second tracing of slow-frequency artifact. The frequency of the large undulations is much lower than the respiratory frequency as noted in the positive airway pressure *(PAP)* device flow signal. The artifact is also present in derivations using both M1 and M2, therefore the issue is generalized and likely due to "sweat artifact." Reduction in room temperature and removing some blankets resolved the issue. *EMG,* Electromyogram.

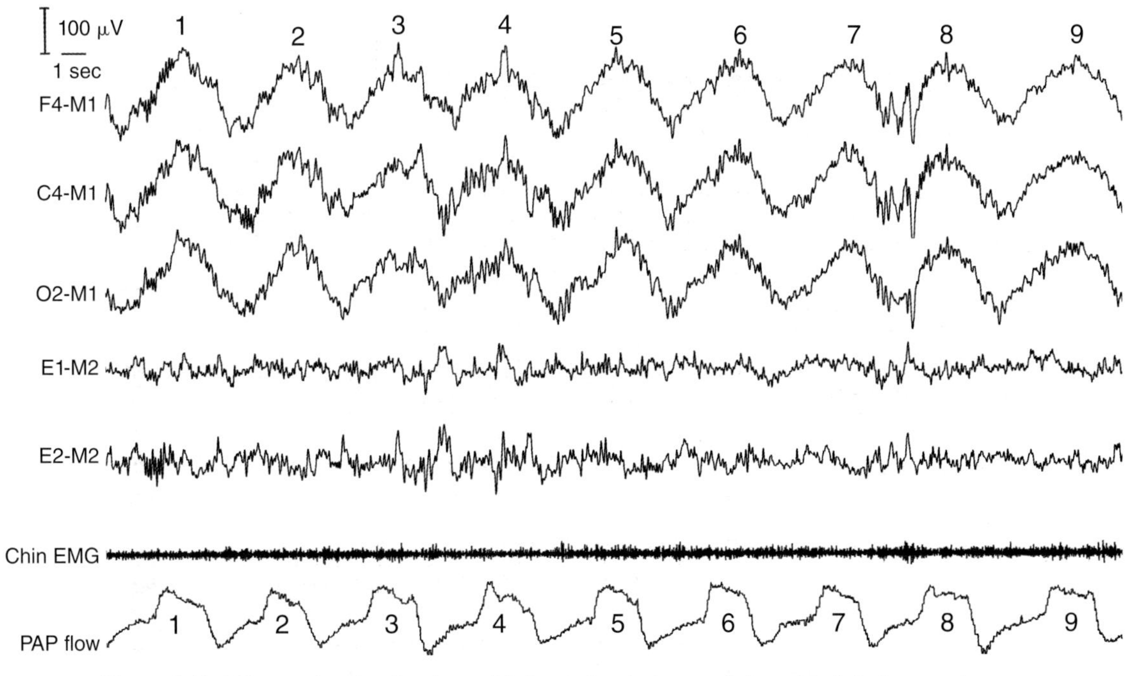

Figure 4–5 A 30-second tracing showing undulations in the electroencephalographic derivations synchronous with positive airway pressure *(PAP)* airflow. This is an example of respiratory artifact. *EMG,* Electromyogram. (Adapted from Berry RB, Wagner MH. *Sleep Medicine Pearls.* 3rd ed., Philadelphia, Elsevier; 2014:112.)

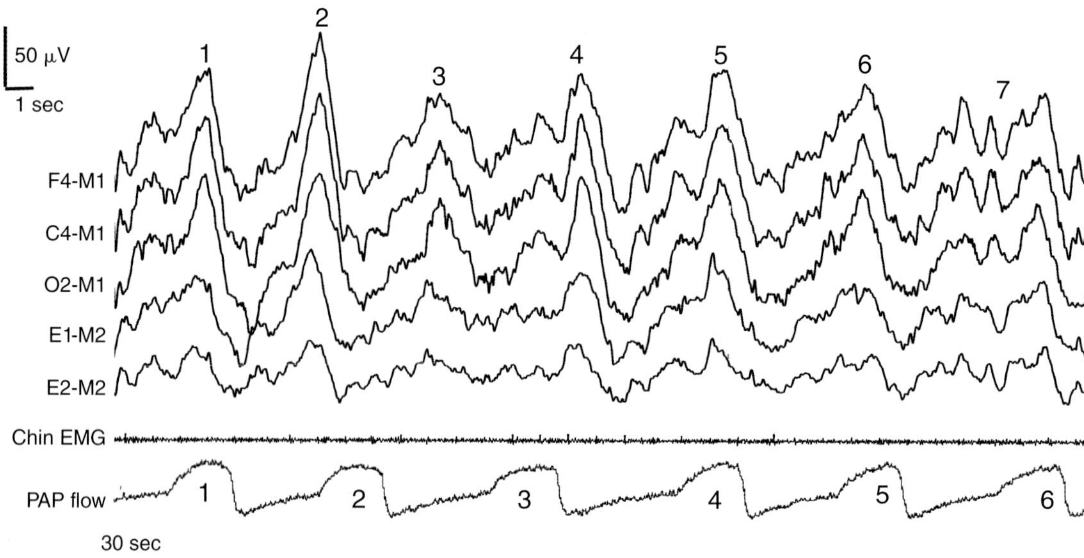

Figure 4–6 A 30-second tracing of sweat artifact with a frequency slightly higher than respiration (positive airway pressure *[PAP]* flow). Also note that the artifact is present in derivations containing both M1 and M2 in contrast to the situation in Figure 4–5.

respiratory artifact (Figure 4–5). However, a given patient can have both sweat and respiratory artifact during a given night.[6] In Figure 4–6 the frequency of the artifact is slightly faster than respiration and involves derivations using both M1 and M2, so this is an example of sweat artifact. Slow-frequency artifact is believed to be secondary to the effects of perspiration. Sweat alters the electrode potential, thereby producing a high amplitude artifact that mimics delta waves and results in overscoring of stage N3. When the artifact is *not* present in all channels, the artifact may be secondary to pressure on an electrode (or pulling on the electrode) with respiration or due to perspiration surrounding selected electrodes (e.g., an electrode between the head and a pillow). In this case, the artifact is usually coming from one or more electrodes on the side on which the patient is lying. For example, if the patient is sleeping with the left side down, derivations containing M1 would be affected, but not those containing M2. In Figure 4–5 only derivations containing the M1 electrode are affected. If a single electrode is the problem, changing derivations to one that does not use the faulty electrode may be a solution. If "sweat artifact" is believed to be present during recording, options include reducing the room temperature, uncovering the patient, and/or using a fan. As a last-ditch alternative, the setting of the low-frequency filter setting may be increased (e.g., from 0.3 to 0.5 or 1 Hz). Unfortunately, this maneuver decreases the amount of slow wave activity (SWA) that is displayed, but still may be preferable to a totally unscorable record. Sweat artifact can be prevented by maintaining a low room temperature, especially when very obese or heavily perspiring patients are studied. One can quickly add a blanket, but cooling down a sleep room takes more time.

Electrocardiographic and Pulse Artifact

ECG artifact is one of the most common and easily recognizable recording artifacts (Table 4–4; Figure 4–7). It can be identified by sharp deflections in the signals of affected channels corresponding exactly in time with the QRS complex of the ECG tracing. Fortunately, this artifact does not usually interfere with visual sleep staging because the artifact does not mimic the usual sleep EEG waveforms of interest. It can mimic spike activity. The artifact can be minimized by placing the mastoid electrodes sufficiently high (behind the ear) so that they are over bone instead of neck tissue (fat). As M1 is on the same side of the body as the heart, derivations involving M1 are commonly involved. Either linking the two mastoid electrodes physically by a jumper cable at the electrode box or using derivations in which the reference electrode is an average of M1 and M2 can minimize ECG artifact. This intervention is also called *double referencing*. These techniques work because if the ECG voltage vector is toward one mastoid, it is away from the other. Hence, the ECG components of the two signals tend to cancel each other out. In Figure 4–7, the right panel shows that ECG artifact is prominent in all derivations except one using an average of M1 and M2 (F4-AVG). Three ellipses mark the artifact in F4-M1 and F4-AVG. In the tracing shown, ECG artifact is larger than desirable, but the record still can be scored. Today many PSG programs have a feature to allow removal of the "R wave" from all channels including leg EMG channels without the need for averaging M1 and M2.

A pulse artifact is similar to an ECG artifact except that rather than electrical interference, the artifact is caused by movement of an electrode resulting from the pulsation of an underlying artery. As the arterial pulse occurs after the QRS complex, the

Table 4–4 Electrocardiogram Artifact

- ECG artifact can be easily recognized as sharp deflections in the affected leads corresponding to the QRS complex in the ECG lead.
- Proper application of the mastoid electrodes and double referencing (using an average of M1 and M2) can prevent or minimize this artifact.

ECG, Electrocardiogram.

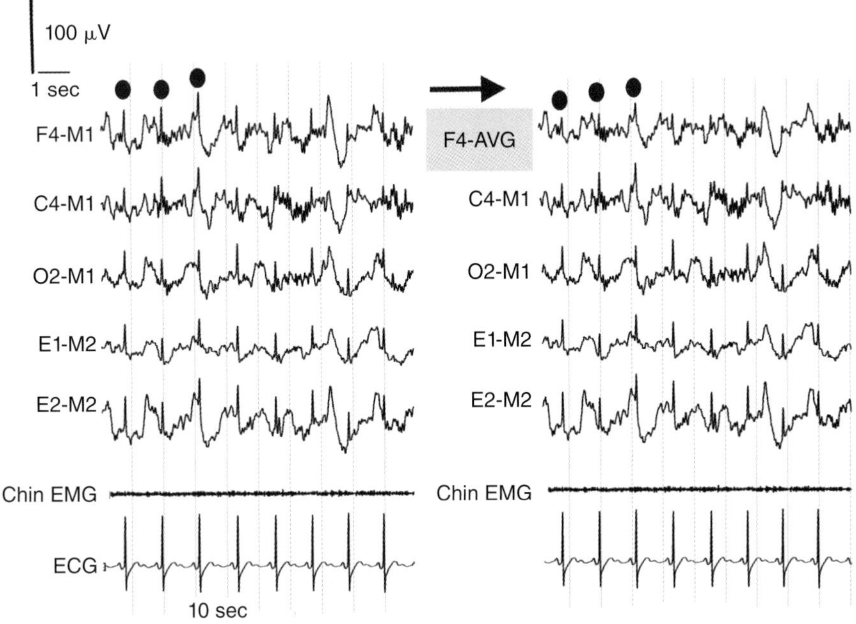

Figure 4–7 The *left panel* shows electrocardiographic *(ECG)* artifact in all electroencephalographic and electro-oculographic derivations. The *dark circles* mark three sharp deflections in the F4-M1 derivation. Using the average of M1 and M2 (linked mastoids) results in reduction (but not elimination) of the artifact *(three dark circles in the right panel). EMG,* Electromyogram. (From Berry RB, Wagner MH. *Sleep Medicine Pearls.* 3rd ed., Philadelphia, Elsevier; 2015:111.)

timing of the artifact is delayed (after) each QRS complex. In Figure 4–8, a patient with both ECG and pulse artifact is shown.

Muscle Artifact and Suck Artifact

Muscle artifact in the EEG and EOG is caused by increased muscle tone in the muscles underlying the EEG and EOG electrodes (Figure 4–9). This can occur during patient movement and sometimes at the beginning of a sleep study if the patient is anxious. Often, this issue will resolve as the patient relaxes and falls asleep. Reducing the high-frequency filter setting can also reduce muscle artifact but will also decrease the amplitude of EEG waveforms used to stage sleep. Prominent EMG activity in the EEG and EOG electrodes can also be seen during episodes of bruxism (tooth grinding) and may actually be more prominent than changes in the chin EMG. An example of a tracing of bruxism is shown in Chapter 15. In Figure 4–10 an example of chin EMG artifact due to an infant sucking on a pacifier is illustrated ("suck artifact"). A similar pattern can be seen with chewing. *It is very useful to observe the video when an unusual EEG/EOG/EMG pattern is noted.* Often the etiology of the artifact is immediately obvious from observing the video.

Snoring/Respiratory Artifact

An increase in chin EMG amplitude can sometimes be seen with each inspiration (Figure 4–11). This is especially common when the upper airway resistance is high (e.g., during snoring). The genioglossus (tongue protrusion) has inspiratory EMG activity (phasic activity) that increases with more negative upper airway pressure.[7] The muscle attaches to the mandible in the midline. EMG electrodes below the mandible may pick up the increased inspiratory activity of the genioglossus or other nearby neck muscles associated with increased inspiratory effort induced by a high upper airway resistance. As discussed in the chapter on respiratory monitoring (chapter 10), nasal pressure is used to score hypopneas. If the signal is visualized using an appropriate high-frequency filter setting (100 Hz), rapid oscillations in the signal can be seen during airway vibration/airflow fluctuations associated with snoring (Figure 4–11).

Eye Movement Artifact/Effect of Prosthetic Eye

Eye movements often cause deflection in the signals of the frontal EEG derivations because F3 and F4 are close to the eyes. This is really not an artifact but simply the recording of relatively high-voltage changes due to the eye movements in an EEG electrode close to the eyes. These can be recognized when signal deflections in the frontal derivations are synchronous with eye movements. Sometimes the same deflection can also be seen in central derivations but only smaller in amplitude. As might be expected, vertical eye movements are more likely to be associated with frontal EEG deflections than horizontal movements. Figure 4–12 shows a 30-second tracing of stage R in a patient with a prosthetic left eye. This explains the lack of deflections in E1-M2. One can also see deflections in F4-M1 (less in C4-M1) synchronous with the eye movement deflections. Selected portions of the biocalibration in the patient with the prosthetic left eye are shown in Figure 4–13. Recall that when the eyes move toward electrode F4, this results in a downward deflection in F4-M1 as the cornea is positive with respect to the retina. In general, E2-M2 and F4-M1 will have deflections in the same direction (upward or downward) as both F4 and E2 are above the eyes and F4 is also on the right side of the head, so lateral eye movements result in deflections in the same direction in F4 and E2. Deflections in the frontal derivations with eye movements can be seen with eye opening and closing and with blinks. The direction of the deflections in F4-M1 and F3-M2 with eye

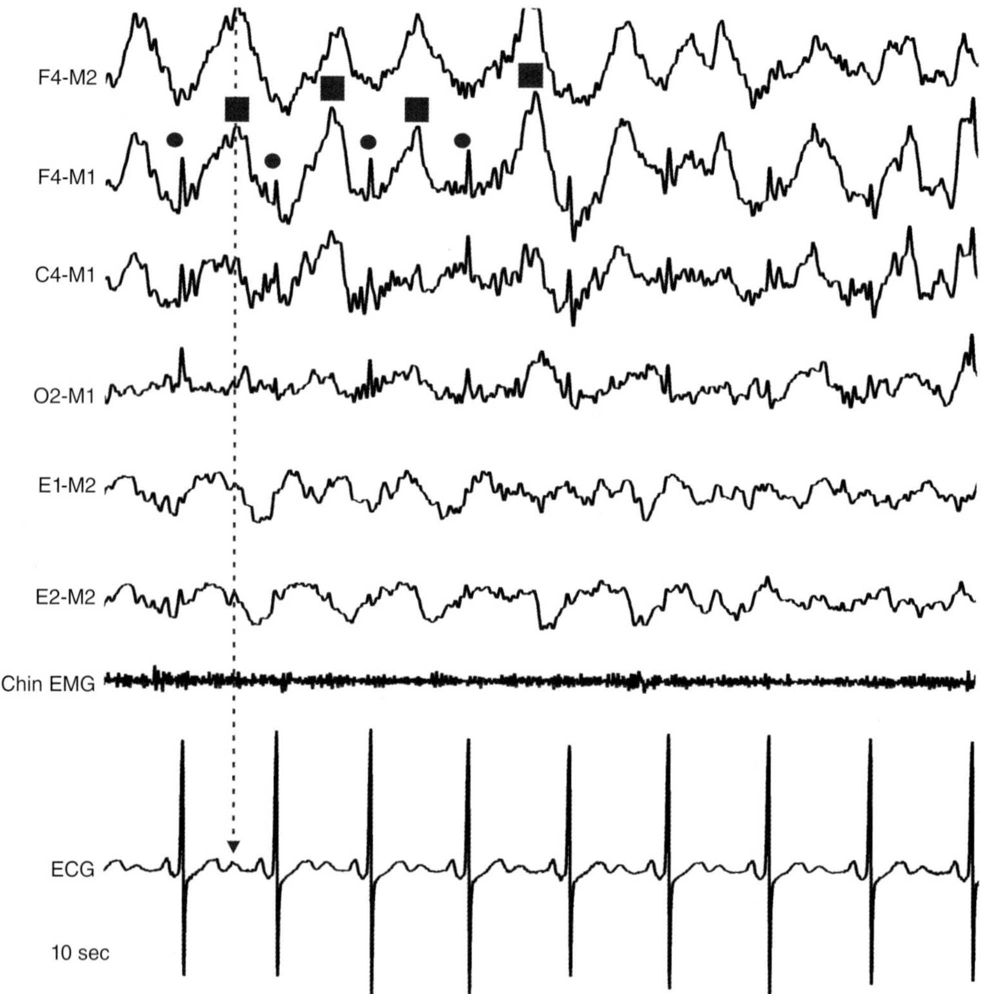

Figure 4–8 A 10-second tracing showing pulse artifact. The undulations occur about the time of the electrocardiographic *(ECG)* T wave and are delayed from the time of the ECG QRS complex. This is due to the timing of the pulse of blood compared with the ECG waveform. In F4-M1 you can see the *round dot* over the deflection due to the ECG and *squares* marking deflections due to the pulse. Note that the ECG artifact is noted in all derivations containing M1 but that the pulse artifact is best localized to the area of F4 and C4. Note that the ECG artifact is present in F4-M1 but not F4-M2 documenting that the artifact is associated with electrode M1. *EMG*, Electromyogram.

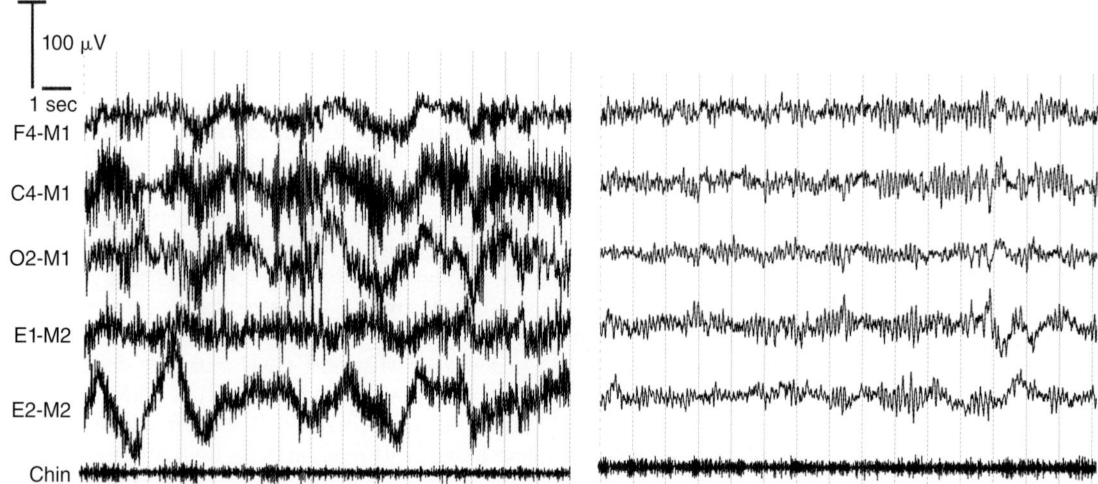

Figure 4–9 The tracing on the *left* was recorded just after the start of a sleep study showing electromyographic artifact in all channels. As the patient relaxed and became drowsy the tracing on the *right* shows posterior dominant rhythm (alpha rhythm) as the patient closed their eyes and started to transition to sleep.

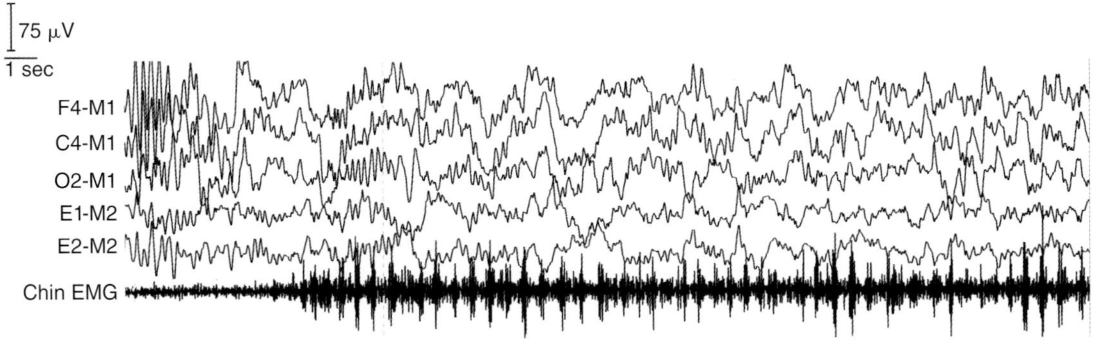

Figure 4–10 A 30-second epoch of artifact in the chin electromyogram *(EMG)* due to an infant sucking on a pacifier ("suck artifact"). A similar pattern can be seen with chewing or bruxism. When evaluating unusual patterns in the electroencephalogram or chin EMG, it is essential to look at the associated video (which often reveals an obvious cause).

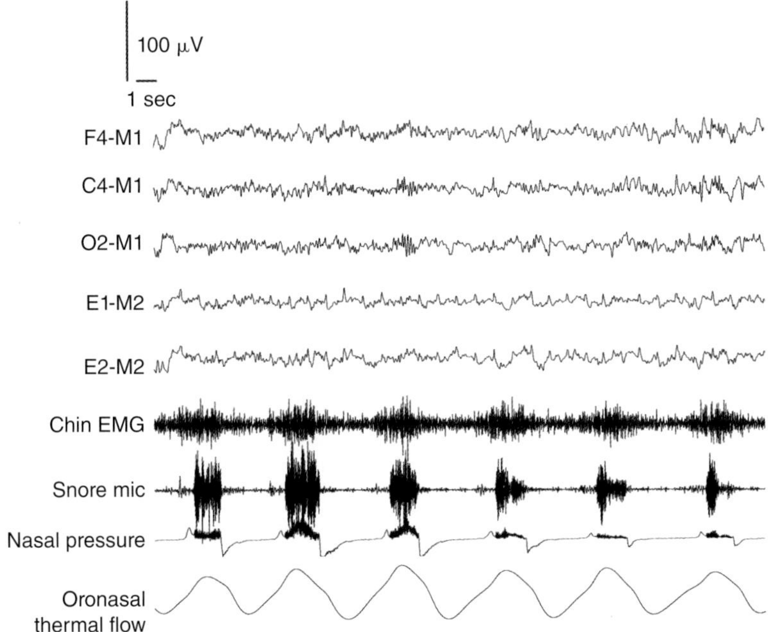

Figure 4–11 Snoring artifact is seen in the chin electromyogram *(EMG)* tracing synchronous with snoring in the snore microphone tracing *(Snore mic)* and rapid oscillations in the nasal pressure signal. The high filter setting for the nasal pressure was 100 Hz. (From Berry RB, Wagner MH. *Sleep Medicine Pearls.* 3rd ed., Philadelphia, Elsevier; 2015:106.)

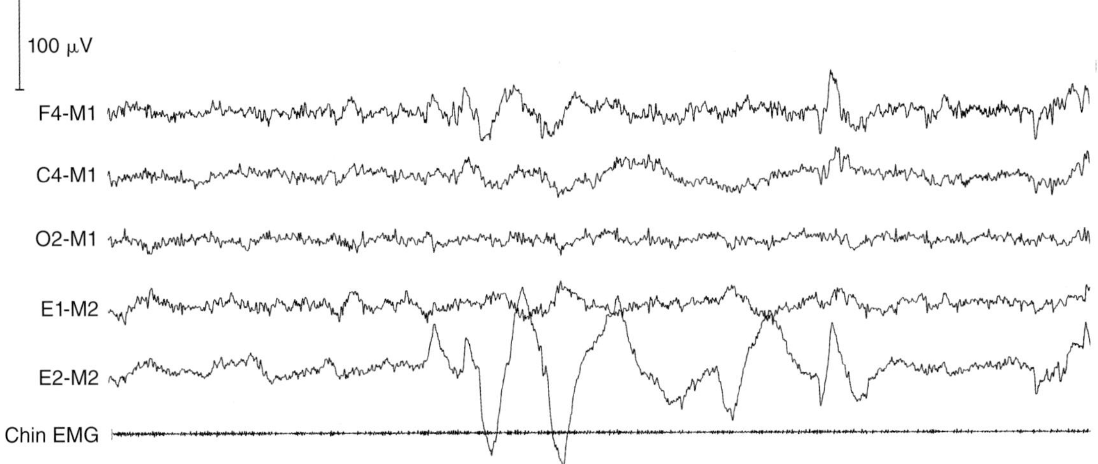

Figure 4–12 A 30-second tracing of a patient with unusual eye movements. *EMG,* Electromyogram. (From Berry RB, Wagner MH. *Sleep Medicine Pearls.* 3rd ed., Philadelphia, Elsevier; 2015:108.)

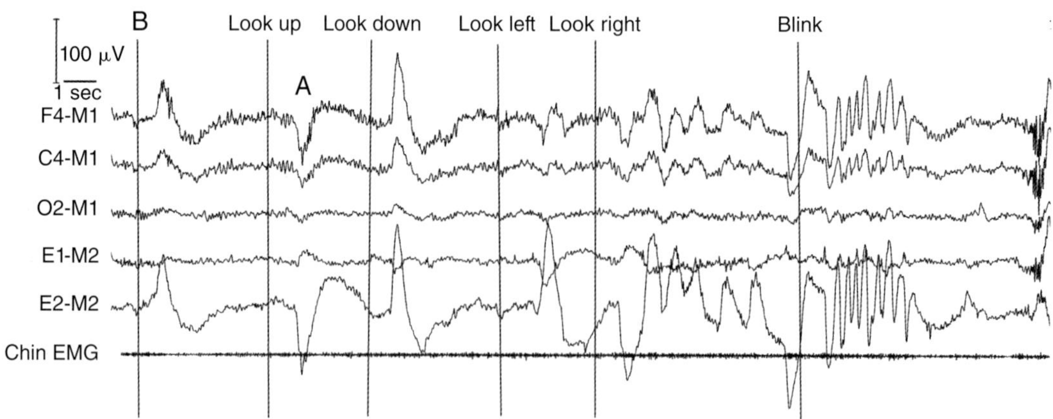

Figure 4–13 Biocalibration tracings for a patient with a prosthetic left eye. As expected, there are minimal deflections in E1-M2 due to the absence of the left eye. It is also instructive that the eye movement deflections in F4-M1 have the same direction as E2-M2 as both electrodes are on the right side and both are above the eyes. The command at B was "Open your eyes," as eyes were previously closed. The command at A was "Look up." See the text and Chapter 1 for a discussion of changes in the electroencephalographic and electrooculographic derivations due to eye movements. For simplicity, a single eye movement in each direction is depicted. *EMG,* Electromyogram. (From Berry RB, Wagner MH. *Sleep Medicine Pearls.* 3rd ed., Philadelphia, Elsevier; 2015:109.)

opening and closure can be deduced by remembering that the cornea is positive with respect to the retina and that eye closure results in an upward movement of the eye, whereas eye opening results in a downward movement of the eye (Bell phenomenon, see Chapter 1). With eye opening the globe moves downward resulting in an upward deflection in F4-M1 (F4 negative compared with M1). With eye closure the upward rotation of the eyeball results in a downward deflection in F4-M1 (F4 positive compared with M1). In the biocalibration tracing of a patient (Figure 4–13), the command at B (after a period of eye closure) was "Open the eyes." With eye opening the eye globe moves downward (away from F4 and E2), which results in an upward deflection in F4-M1 and E2-M2. The command at A was "Look up"; eye movement upward caused a downward deflection in F4-M1 and E2-M2.

Ground Artifact/Reference Artifact

If one of the two inputs to a differential amplifier (say, G1 in the derivation G1-G2) is disconnected (electrode unattached), the amplifier actually records the difference between G2 and the ground electrode. Because the *ground electrode is typically attached to the forehead near the eyes,* one can see deflections associated with eye movements in channels in which they are usually not visible (say, O2-M1). Usually, considerable 60-Hz artifact would also be seen. However, if the display of the derivation uses a 35-Hz high frequency and 60-Hz filter, which attenuate a great deal of the 60-Hz signal contamination, this might be missed. Therefore the appearance of eye movements in unusual channels should trigger the technologist or reviewer to consider whether "ground artifact" is present. Recall if there is an issue with the reference electrode, all signals recorded referentially may show 60-Hz artifact. Bipolar channels such as the left and right leg EMG would not show the artifact as bipolar recording does not depend on the reference electrode (see Chapter 2).

Channel Clipping, Channel Saturation Artifact, and Polarity Issues

The issue of a tracing exceeding channel display width is handled differently in different PSG computer programs (e.g., if the channel displays ±100 μV and the value at a given point is −200 μV). In some PSG programs, signal deflections can cross channel borders and be superimposed on the adjacent channel tracings. In other programs channels are clipped, meaning the deflections cannot exceed the channel voltage limits. See an example of channel clipping in Figure 4–14.

Signal saturation is a different issue than clipping and occurs when a signal (usually DC) input exceeds the dynamic range of the analog-to-digital (A/D) converter. This issue commonly occurs when a separate nasal pressure transducer system supplies a voltage that exceeds the dynamic range due to an excessive increase in gain set on the separate device. For example, if +3 V is sent to the A/D converter and the dynamic range is ±2.5 V, the highest signal that can be visualized corresponds to +2.5 V. This gives a truncated waveform (Figure 4–15). Decreasing the gain using the computer program will make the waveform smaller, but it will still be truncated. When the nasal pressure cannula amplification is adjusted at the start of the study, the gain should be able to accommodate larger than tidal breaths. If adjusted so that small breaths are full scale on the PSG tracing, large breaths will result in signal saturation. Today the majority of PSG systems have a pressure transducer integrated into the PSG amplifier and the default gain is set at a value to avoid this problem.

In most sleep centers the polarity used for respiratory signals is inspiration upward. Part of biocalibration is to ensure that the polarity of flow and effort sensors is consistent. It is especially important to determine if the polarity of the nasal pressure signal is as expected. Polarity can be opposite the expected direction due to montage defaults or placement of the end of the nasal cannula on the wrong side of a pressure transducer with two pressure inlets. If the nasal pressure signal is displayed with inspiration down in a sleep center with the inspiration upward convention, it has an unusual pattern; flow plateaus during airflow limitation are on the bottom of the signal, and the upward deflection in the nasal pressure signal is not in phase with the respiratory effort (chest and abdomen) signals (Figure 4–16). This assumes the inspiration upward convention is used. When the nasal pressure signal is inverted,

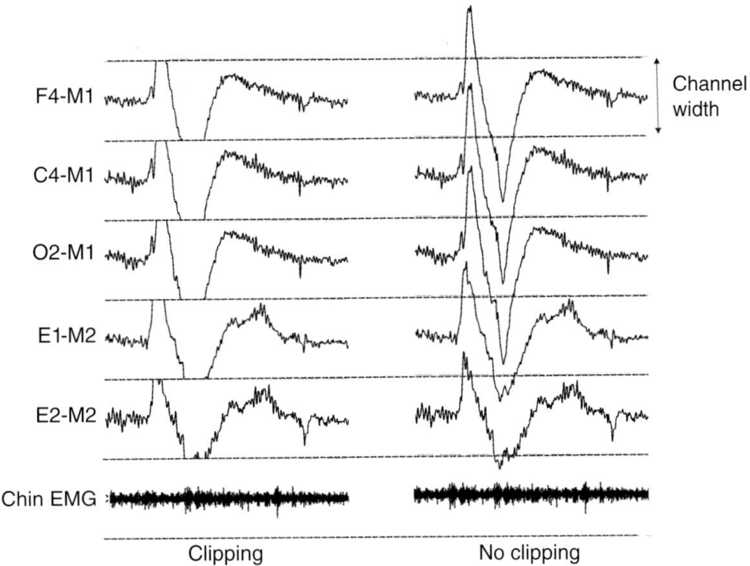

Figure 4–14 Tracings showing a high-amplitude K complex displayed with channel clipping *(left panel)* and without channel clipping *(right panel)*. An option for channel clipping is offered by many brands of polysomnographic software.

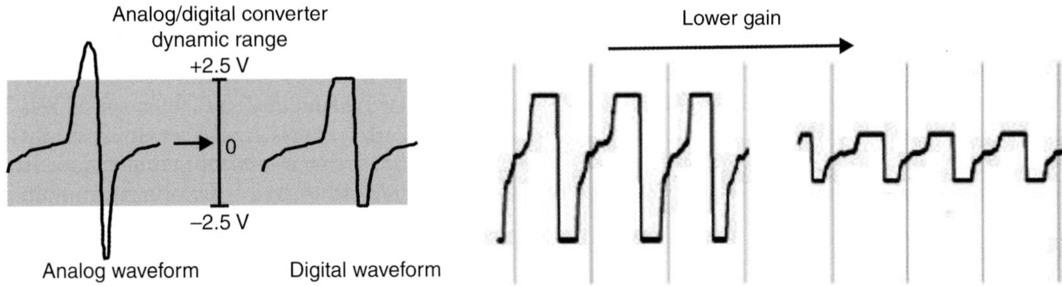

Figure 4–15 An example of channel saturation. An analog signal exceeds the dynamic range of the analog to digital converter and results in a truncated signal. Note that a change in gain (sensitivity) reduces the size of the displayed signal compared with the channel width but does not change the shape.

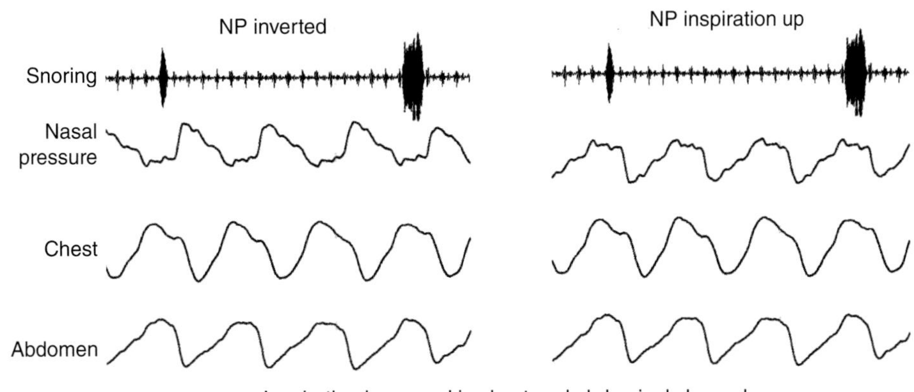

Figure 4–16 An example of inadvertent "flipped" polarity in the nasal pressure channel in the left panel. The chest and abdomen have inspiration-up polarity, whereas the nasal pressure *(NP)* has inspiration-down polarity. This can be recognized as the flat portion of the nasal pressure signal (airflow limitation during inspiration) is downward in the *left panel* and is associated with snoring. Snoring can occur in expiration but is usually present during inspiration. In the right panel the NP channel control option to invert the signal is selected and direction of the NP is signal is corrected.

the normal relationship between snoring, nasal pressure flattening, and inspiratory effort is restored.

Cardioballistic and Inaccurate Oximetry Artifacts

Small deflections in the chest or abdominal effort belts due to transmission of pulsation of the heart may sometimes be noted (at the same frequency as the heart rate). If the heart rate is slow, they can rarely be misinterpreted as respiratory effort during a central apnea. However, even with a slow heart rate the respiratory rate is much lower (and time between respiratory deflections in the effort belts is greater). A central apnea with cardioballistic artifact is noted in Figure 4–17.

When reviewing sleep studies an unexpectedly low arterial oxygen saturation by pulse oximetry can be encountered (e.g., a period of low SpO_2 without apparent cause [no associated respiratory events]). In these situations, looking at the oximetry plethysmography signal can be very helpful. Most PSG systems today provide several oximetry signals including the oxygen saturation (SpO_2), pulse rate (based on oximetry) and a plethysmography signal reflecting the increased light absorption (increase in blood volume in the finger) associated with each pulse.[8] A reduction in the signal implies poor perfusion of the digit either due to pressure (laying on a hand), a digit with poor perfusion, or displacement of the oximetry probe. In Figure 4–18, the left panel shows a low SpO_2 associated with movement and a very low amplitude plethysmography signal. Later, after readjustment of the oximetry probe, the expected normal SpO_2 associated with a good plethysmography signal is noted. There can be other causes of an unexpectedly low SpO_2 signal, but checking the oximetry plethysmography signal can help identify oximetry artifact. Fingernail polish, acrylic nails, and poor perfusion to the digit attached to the oximetry probe can all impair oximetry accuracy. A change in the position of the oximetry electrode or using an earlobe sensor may improve the signal. More information on pulse oximetry is provided in Chapter 10. It is also worth noting that the oximetry pulse rate and actual pulse rate can be very different if small pulsations (as with premature ventricular contractions) are not counted by the oximetry software.

Artifacts due to Implanted Devices

Artifacts associated with implanted devices are common and include artifact from pacemakers, hypoglossal nerve stimulation, phrenic nerve stimulation, deep brain stimulation, and vagal nerve stimulation. These can be challenging if the history supplied with the sleep study is not comprehensive. Examples of pacemaker artifact in the ECG signal are presented in Chapter 14, hypoglossal nerve stimulation artifact in the chin EMG in Chapter 26, and phrenic nerve pacing artifact in the ECG in Chapter 30. Vagal nerve stimulation (VNS) is used for intractable epilepsy and has been used for depression.[9-11] Stimulation occurs for 30 seconds every 3 to 5 minutes and can often be seen as an increase in the chin EMG activity (Figure 4–19). VNS can cause respiratory events (obstructive apneas, hypopneas, and central apneas), and if a periodicity of events every 3 to 5 minutes is noted, then VNS could be suspected.

COMMON VARIANTS SEEN DURING SLEEP MONITORING

Alpha Non–Rapid Eye Movement Sleep Anomaly

The finding of prominent alpha activity (8–13 Hz) during non–rapid eye movement (NREM) sleep is often called *alpha sleep, alpha intrusion,* or *alpha-delta* sleep (if noted in association with stage N3).[12-15] It makes sleep staging more challenging

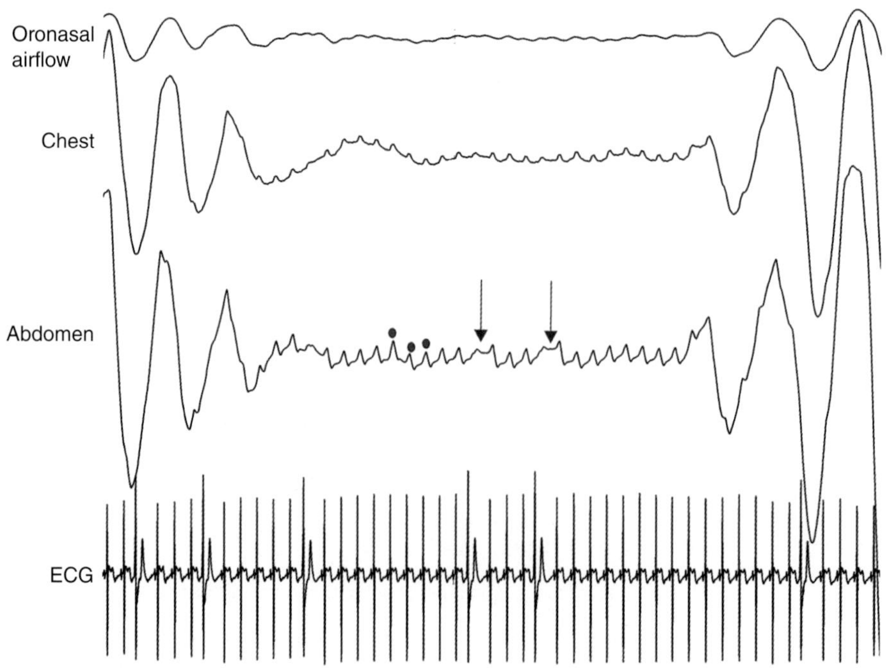

Figure 4–17 An example of cardioballistic artifact *(dark circles)* noted in the chest and abdomen respiratory inductance plethysmography effort belt channel during a central apnea. Note the pause in cardioballistic artifact *(arrows)* during premature beats associated with decreased stroke volume and chest wall movement. *ECG,* Electrocardiogram.

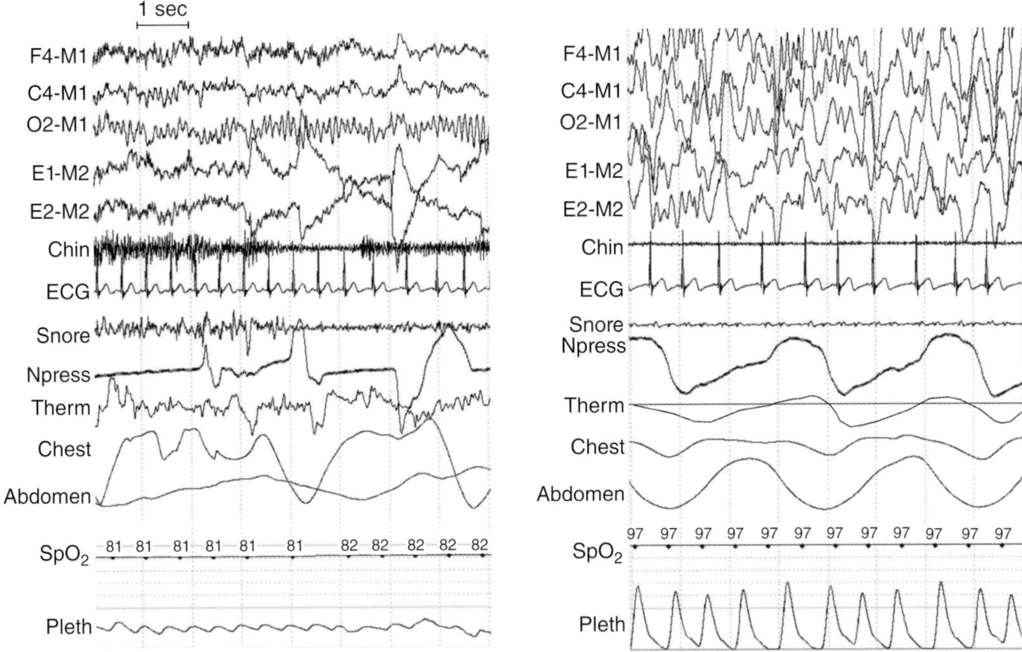

Figure 4–18 Tracings illustrating an inaccurate arterial oxygen saturation by oximetry *(SpO_2)* reading *(left panel)* with poor oximetry plethysmography signal *(Pleth)* compared with accurate readings *(right panel)* with a good plethysmography signal. *ECG,* Electrocardiogram.

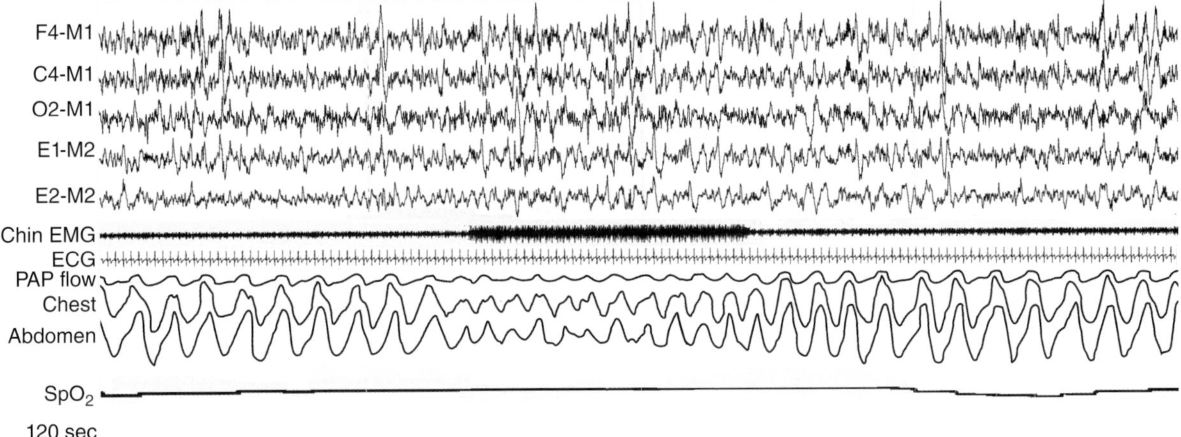

Figure 4–19 A 120-second tracing during a continuous positive airway pressure *(PAP)* titration. This is an example of vagal nerve stimulation with artifact seen in the chin electromyogram *(EMG).* In this patient, stimulation lasted 30 seconds every 5 minutes. Stimulation was associated with a hypopnea with arterial oxygen desaturation *(SpO_2)* and an increase in respiratory rate. *ECG,* Electrocardiogram.

(Table 4–5 and Figure 4–20). The alpha activity may be more prominent in frontal than occipital regions in contrast to the typical alpha (posterior dominant) rhythm. When viewing a tracing of alpha-delta sleep in a 30-second window, there is the impression of a background of diffuse higher-frequency activity. By changing to a 10-second window (Figure 4–21), one can count the smaller wave form oscillations in 1 second that are superimposed on slower activity (alpha, 8–13 Hz). First described in 1973 by Hauri and Hawkins,[12] alpha-delta sleep was once thought to be a characteristic finding associated with fibromyalgia (FM).[13] However, alpha sleep is not seen in all patients with FM and can occur in patients with other psychiatric and chronic pain disorders. Mahowald and Mahowald[14] concluded

Table 4–5 Alpha Sleep Anomaly
• Alpha sleep anomaly is characterized by the persistence of prominent alpha activity during NREM sleep (especially stage N3 sleep).
• The pattern has been associated with chronic pain syndromes or psychiatric disorders but can occur in normal individuals.
• Alpha anomaly makes scoring stage N1 and sometimes stage N2 sleep difficult.
• Scoring stage N3 is less problematic (the amplitude of slow waves is not affected).

NREM, Non–rapid eye movement.

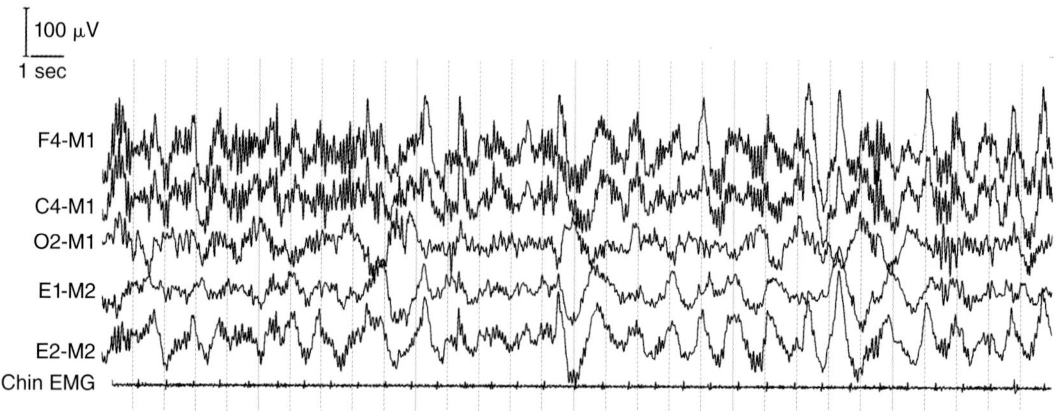

Figure 4–20 A 30-second tracing showing prominent alpha activity during stage N3 sleep. This is an example of alpha sleep (or alpha-delta sleep). Note that the alpha activity is more prominent in the frontal and central derivations than in the occipital derivation. In posterior dominant (alpha) rhythm the highest amplitude is in occipital derivations. The patient was being treated for a chronic pain syndrome. *EMG*, Electromyogram. (Adapted from Berry RB, Wagner MH. *Sleep Medicine Pearls.* 3rd ed., Philadelphia, Elsevier; 2015:34.)

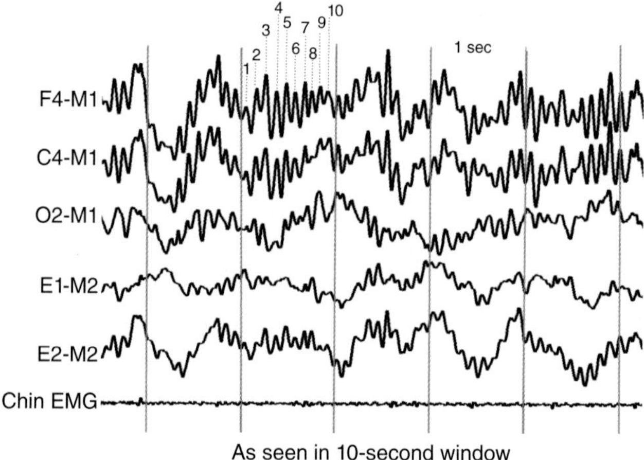

Figure 4–21 An enlargement of a portion of the tracing shown in Figure 4–20. The presence of alpha activity (about 10 Hz) is demonstrated. Such activity is superimposed on underlying slow wave activity as seen in Figure 4-20. *EMG*, Electromyogram. (From Berry RB, Wagner MH. *Sleep Medicine Pearls.* 3rd ed., Philadelphia, Elsevier; 2015:34.)

that alpha sleep was not specific for FM and was not necessarily associated with symptoms of myalgia. It was present in 15% of normal subjects in undisturbed sleep in some studies.

Roizenblatt and coworkers[15] also studied patients with FM off medications that could interfere with sleep and normal controls. Prominent alpha rhythm was noted during sleep in 70% of FM patients and 16% of normal individuals. Three distinct patterns were noted: a phasic alpha pattern consisting of episodic alpha occurring simultaneously with delta activity (70% FM, 7% controls); tonic alpha continuously present throughout NREM sleep independent of delta activity (20% of FM and 9% of controls); and a low alpha pattern, seen in 30% of FM patients and 84% of controls. The phasic pattern was associated with lower sleep efficiency, decreased slow wave (stage N3) sleep, longer morning pain, and subjective feeling of superficial sleep. Further research is needed to confirm the findings.

Drug Spindles

Patients who are taking benzodiazepine receptor agonists (BZRAs) often have increased sleep spindle activity (Table 4–6; Figure 4–22).[16-18] Sleep spindle activity has a frequency of 11 to 16 Hz. Drug spindles often have a frequency in the higher end of the range. Benzodiazepines are associated with a decrease in slow wave amplitude (less stage N3 sleep) and an increase in higher EEG frequencies.[17,18] The nonbenzodiazepine BZRAs (zolpidem, zaleplon, eszopiclone) tend to have less effect on the amplitude of slow waves and, therefore, do not usually decrease the amount of stage N3 sleep. However, they do increase EEG frequencies during sleep, including sleep spindle activity. One might ask, what is the maximum number of sleep spindle bursts per epoch (spindle density) that could be considered normal? A

Table 4–6 Drug Spindles
• Frequent and prominent sleep spindle activity is often noted in patients taking BZRAs.
• The frequency of medication associated sleep spindles is often at the higher end of the sleep spindle range (12–14 Hz).
• The pattern may be a useful clue that a hypnotic medication was taken before the sleep study.

BZRAs, Benzodiazepine receptor agonists.

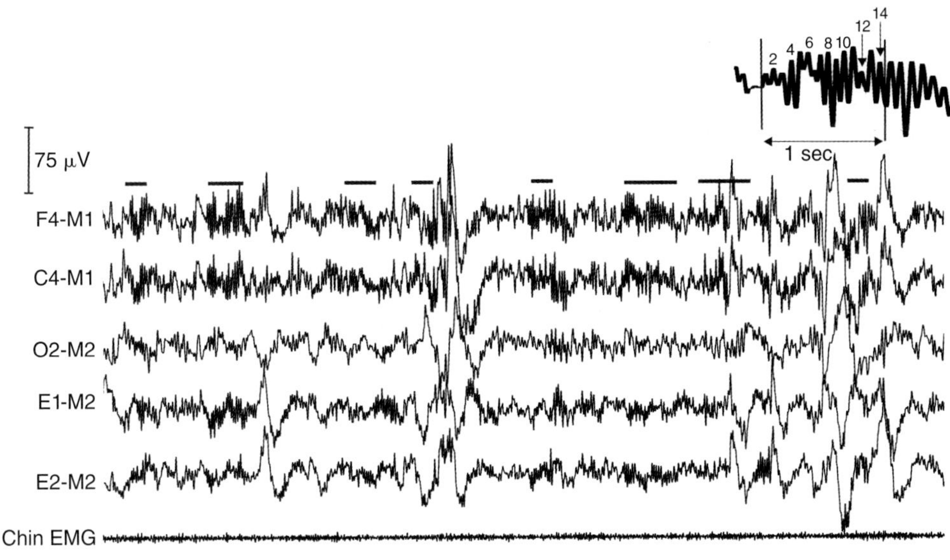

Figure 4–22 A 30-second tracing of a patient taking clonazepam for anxiety. Very frequent sleep spindles (horizontal bars) are shown (frequency about 14 Hz). *EMG*, Electromyogram.

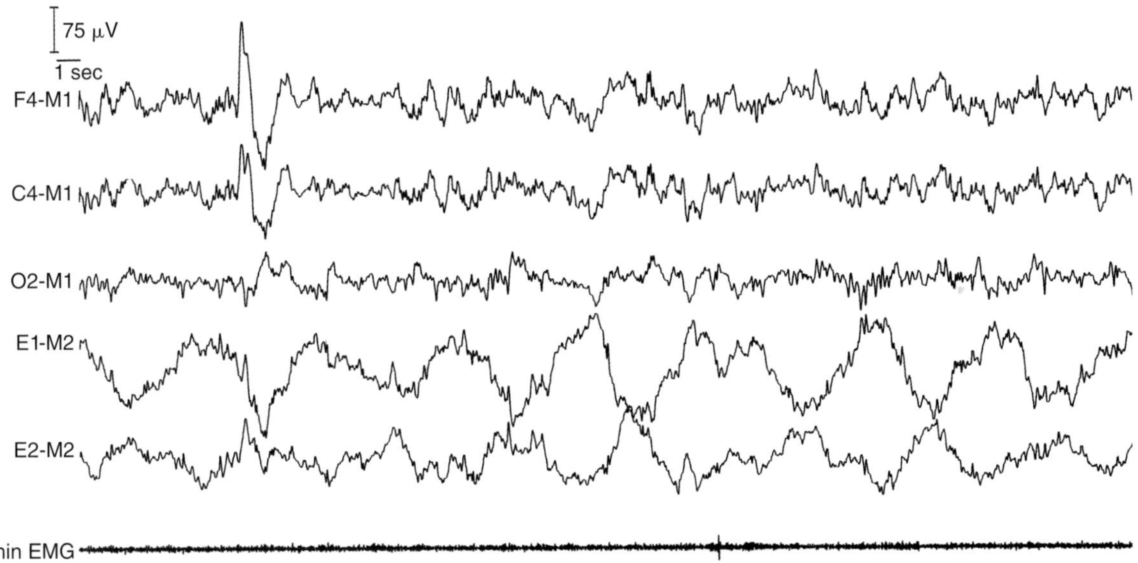

Figure 4–23 A 30-second tracing of stage N2 sleep with persistent slow eye movements. The patient was taking fluoxetine for depression. *EMG*, Electromyogram.

large study of the sleep health cohort found that the maximum spindle density was around four per minute (mean, ~2/min) for the entire group.[19] Based on this data, two to three spindle bursts per epoch would be a reasonable upper limit of normal. In the example in Figure 4–22 there are at least eight spindle bursts per epoch (indicated by dark lines above F4-M1.

Eye Movements Associated With Selective Serotonin Reuptake Inhibitor Medications

Slow eye movements are typically present during stage W with the eyes closed and during stage N1. They typically vanish with the onset of stage N2. However, in patients taking selective serotonin reuptake inhibitors (SSRIs), a mixture of slow and more rapid eye movements may persist into stage N2 or stage N3.[20,21] Because this phenomenon was first described with patients taking fluoxetine, such eye movements are often called "Prozac eyes." Figure 4–23 shows a tracing from a patient taking fluoxetine (Table 4–7).

Table 4–7 Eye Movements Associated With Selective Serotonin Reuptake Inhibitor Medications
• Prominent slow and rapid eye movement activity may be seen in stage N2 (and less commonly in stage N3) in patients taking SSRI antidepressants.
• The SSRI eye movements can be a mixture of slow and more rapid eye movements.
• Although called "Prozac eyes", the eye movements can occur with all SSRI medications.

SSRI, Selective serotonin reuptake inhibitor.

Transient Muscle Activity During Rapid Eye Movement Sleep

Stage R (REM [rapid eye movement] sleep) is characterized by low chin EMG tone; that is, the baseline chin EMG activity in the chin derivation is no higher than in any other sleep stage and usually at the lowest level of the entire recording. However, transient bursts of EMG activity termed *transient muscle activity* (TMA; formerly called "phasic activity"), consisting of short irregular bursts of EMG activity (usually <0.25 second), may be seen in the chin or anterior tibial EMG derivations during stage R.[1,22] This activity is often seen in association with bursts of REMs (Figure 4–24). The AASM scoring manual[1] defines TMA as chin or leg EMG activity of 0.1 to 5 seconds in duration and at least two times as high in amplitude as the stage R atonia level or lowest amplitude in NREM, if no stage R atonia is present. There is a characteristic spiky pattern. In normal individuals, twitching in muscles may occur but usually no gross motor movements. The scoring of epochs exhibiting REM sleep without atonia (RWA) based on *excessive* tonic or phasic (TMA) chin EMG activity and/or *excessive* TMA in leg or arm EMG will be discussed in Chapter 15.[1] However, even if TMA is prominent, it is important to note that demonstration of RWA alone does not confirm a diagnosis of the REM sleep behavior disorder. It would be appropriate to review the sleep history of a patient with TMA to determine if a history of dream enactment was reported. Patients taking SSRIs often show some TMA, although they usually do not meet criteria for excessive TMA. Winkelman and James[23] determined the number of 2-second bins during REM sleep that contained phasic chin (defined as EMG activity lasting 0.1–5 seconds with an amplitude four times the background EMG activity). The mean percentages of 2-second REM sleep bins containing phasic activity in the control group and SSRI groups were 2.36% and 9.54%, respectively ($P = .07$). Antidepressants can increase TMA in patients with and without the REM sleep behavior disorder (RBD).[24] A modest amount of TMA might be considered a normal variant in the absence of a history or video evidence consistent with the RBD, especially if the patient is taking an SSRI. On the other hand, it is possible that the patient might develop RBD manifestations at a later time. See Chapter 15 for information on scoring the EMG activity associated with the REM sleep behavior disorder.

SUMMARY OF KEY POINTS

1. If an artifact occurs in all derivations containing a given electrode and none of the derivations not containing the given electrode, this electrode is likely the cause of the artifact. Note that if M1 and M2 are linked or averaged, this makes electrode troubleshooting difficult (unable to identify M1 or M2 as a problem electrode).
2. If an electrode is suspected to be causing an artifact, try using an alternative derivation not containing the electrode to see if this resolves the issue. For example, change from Chin1-ChinZ to **Chin2**-ChinZ.
3. The recommended electrode impedance for EEG, EOG, and chin EMG electrodes is 5 KΩ or less (≤ 5 kiloohms).
4. A 60-Hz artifact can be recognized as dense and rope-like pattern. If turning on (or off) the 60-Hz notch filter changes the amplitude substantially, this documents that a 60-Hz artifact is present. A 60-Hz artifact is most obvious in derivations using a high-frequency filter of 100 Hz (e.g., leg EMG) rather than 35 Hz, which does attenuate 60-Hz activity.
5. Slow-frequency artifact can be due to "sweat" or pulling/pressure on an electrode during respiration. If the slow undulations are synchronous with respiration, the pattern is called respiratory artifact. Sweat artifact is characterized by slow undulations not synchronous with respiratory and often affecting all EEG derivations. If sweat artifact is present, try cooling the room or using a fan. If respiratory artifact is noted, try to identify the problem electrode (often M1 or M2) by using an alternative derivation.

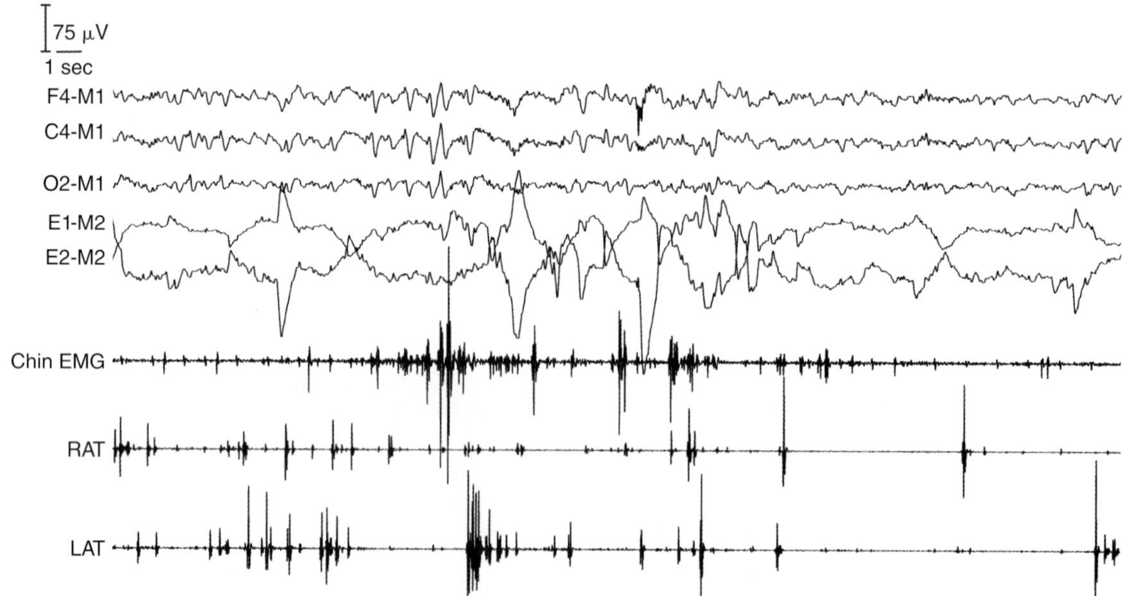

Figure 4–24 A 30-second tracing of a patient with transient muscle activity in the chin electromyogram *(EMG)* and in the left *(LAT)* and right anterior tibial *(RAT)* EMG tracings during stage R. Excessive transient muscle activity is present as there is activity in at least 50% of 10 three-second mini-epochs. The activity is more than twice the rapid eye movement atonia level, which in this case is the lowest activity between bursts.

6. Electrode popping can have a variable appearance but tends to be repetitive and often has a high-voltage amplitude. This artifact occurs when an electrode intermittently pulls away from the skin. If the problem electrode is identified, it should be repaired (with more gel) or replaced. The electrode wire could also be rerouted to avoid pulling on the electrode during each breath.
7. ECG artifact is easy to recognize by a repetitive narrow deflection synchronous with the ECG. It is often noted in derivations using M1 (on the same side as the heart). Using an average of M1 and M2 as the reference electrode will often reduce the artifact.
8. It is important to know the direction of inspiration used in a sleep recording. If inspiration is upward, it is important to note if the nasal pressure waveform has a polarity consistent with this convention. Otherwise, periods of inspiratory flattening may be missed.
9. If oximetry readings are of questionable accuracy, observe the plethysmography signal available in most PSG systems. A reduction in signal suggests that the signal is likely not accurate. Try switching the oximetry sensor to another finger or ask the patient not to lie on the hand with an oximetry sensor attached.
10. Alpha sleep anomaly is characterized by persistent prominent alpha activity (often in the frontal and central derivations) during NREM sleep. The pattern is thought to be nonspecific but is often seen in patients with chronic pain disorders or psychiatric disorders.
11. Slow eye movement typically cease during stage N2 sleep but can be present in patients taking an SSRI.
12. An increased number of sleep spindle bursts per epoch can be seen in patients taking a BZRA (more than 2 or 3 sleep spindle bursts per epoch).

CLINICAL REVIEW QUESTIONS

1. During review of a sleep study an abnormality in F4-M1 was noted (Figure 4–25). What type of artifact is present, and what could you do to resolve the issue?
2. A tracing from a patient with depression and anxiety is shown in Figure 4–26. What are the medications the patient is likely taking?
3. What are the artifacts at A and B of Figure 4–27? Which is the problem electrode in A? Is the artifact in B respiratory artifact or sweat artifact?
4. What is the recommended impedance for EEG, EOG, and chin EMG electrodes?
   A. ≤1 KΩ
   B. ≤5 KΩ
   C. ≤10 KΩ
   D. ≤15 KΩ
5. ECG artifact is noted in EEG and EOG derivations. Which of the following may reduce the artifact?
   A. Place M1 and M2 in the proper position.
   B. Use the PSG program ECG filter if available.
   C. Link M1 and M2 electrically (jumper cable) or computationally (PSG program).
   D. All of the above.

ANSWERS

1. A 60-Hz artifact is present in F4-M1. As the artifact is not present in other derivations containing M1, the problem electrode is F4. Removing the 60-Hz filter (if turned on) and/or changing the high-frequency filter to 100 Hz should cause a worsening of the problem. Changing to the derivation F3-M2 would eliminate the problem.
2. The patient is taking fluoxetine (an SSRI), and this explains the presence of eye movements in stage N2. The frequent spindles are from clonazepam, a BZRA used for anxiety.
3. **A.** Popping artifact due to faulty signal from electrode M1. **B.** Slow-frequency ("sweat") artifact. The undulations are less frequent than the breathing frequency (respiratory rate), and unlike the example in A, all electrodes are affected.
4. EEG, EOG, and chin EMG electrode impedance should be ≤5 KΩ.
5. **D.** If M1 or M2 are placed too low at the mastoid/neck junction, this predisposes to ECG artifact as obtaining a good electrode impedance is easier to accomplish higher over the mastoid bone. Many PSG programs offer an ECG filter that can be applied to each derivation that reduces the artifact. Physically or computationally (software option) linking M1 and M2 also reduces the artifact.

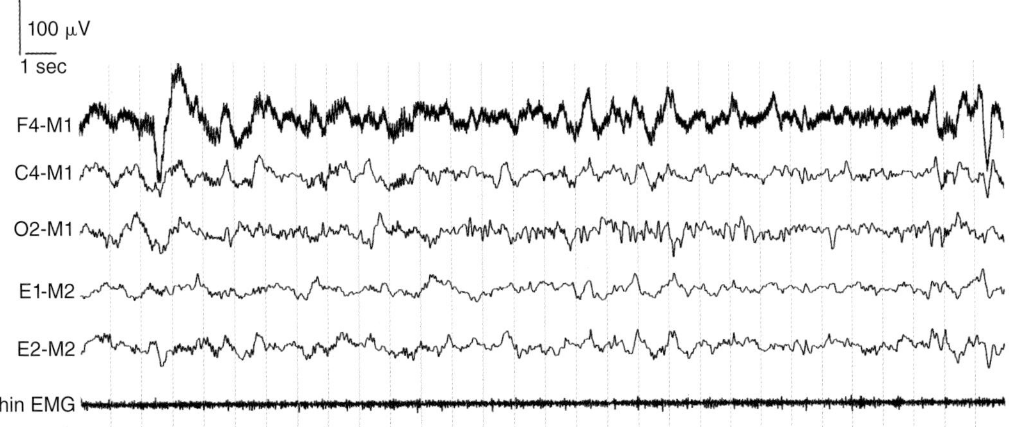

Figure 4–25 A 30-second tracing of a patient with an artifact in F4-M1. What is the artifact, and which electrode is the problem? This figure is associated with review question 1. *EMG,* Electromyogram. (From Berry RB, Wagner MH. *Sleep Medicine Pearls.* 3rd ed. Philadelphia, Elsevier; 2015:26.)

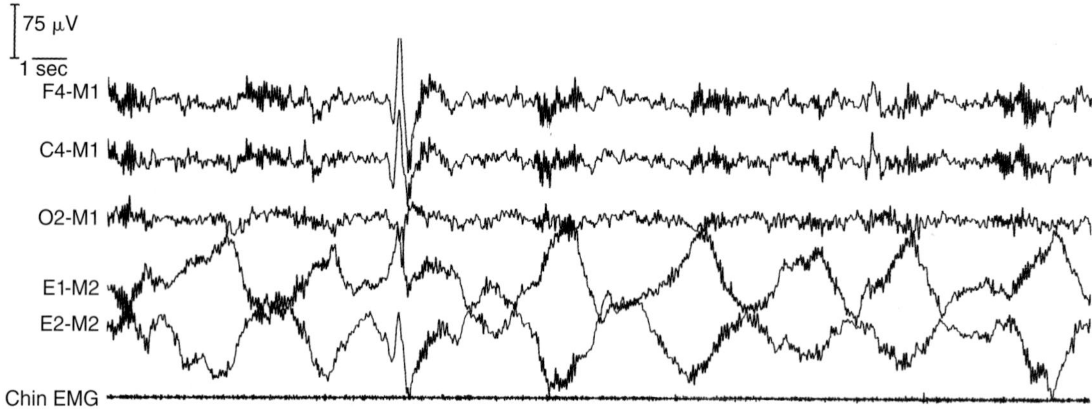

Figure 4–26 A 30-second tracing associated with review question 2. *EMG*, Electromyogram.

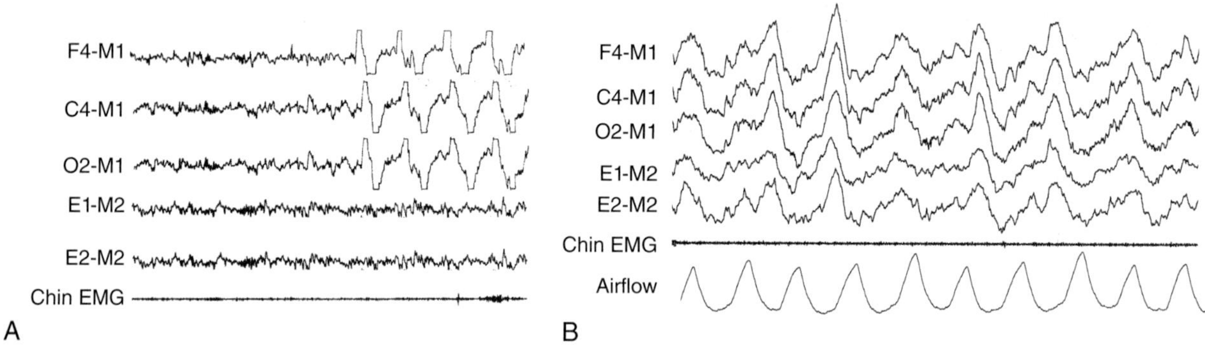

Figure 4–27 This figure shows two types of artifacts and is associated with review question 3. *EMG*, Electromyogram.

ABBREVIATIONS

AASM, American Academy of Sleep Medicine; *AC,* alternating current; *BZRA,* benzodiazepine receptor agonist; *DC,* direct current; *ECG,* electrocardiography; *EEG,* electroencephalography; *EMG,* electromyography; *EOG,* electrooculography; *FM,* fibromyalgia; *LAT,* left anterior tibial; *NP,* nasal pressure; *NREM,* non–rapid eye movement; *PAP,* positive airway pressure; *PSG,* polysomnography; *RAT,* right anterior tibial; *RBD,* rapid eye movement sleep behavior disorder; *REM,* rapid eye movement; *SSRI,* selective serotonin reuptake inhibitor; *SWA,* slow wave activity; *TMA,* transient muscle activity; *VNS,* vagal nerve stimulation.

SUGGESTED READING

Berry RB, Wagner MH. *Sleep Medicine Pearls.* 3rd ed. Elsevier; 2015:102-107.

Geyer JD, Carney PD. Chapter 45. In: Avidan A, Barkoukis TJ, eds. *Review of Sleep Medicine.* 4th ed. Elsevier Saunders; 2018:695-745.

Grigg-Damberger M. Polysomnographic artifacts. In: Tatum WO, eds. *Atlas of Clinical Neurophysiology.* Springer; 2018.

Libenson MH. *Practical Approach to Electroencephalography.* Elsevier; 2010:124-145.

Siddiqui F, Osuna E, Walters AS, et al. Sweat artifact and respiratory artifact occurring simultaneously in polysomnogram. *Sleep Med.* 2006;7(2):197-199.

Troester MM, Quan SF, Berry RB, et al. *The AASM Manual for the Scoring of Sleep and Associated Events: Rules, Terminology and Technical Specifications. Version 3.* American Academy of Sleep Medicine; 2023.

REFERENCES

1. Troester MM, Quan SF, Berry RB, et al. *The AASM Manual for the Scoring of Sleep and Associated Events: Rules, Terminology and Technical Specifications. Version 3.* American Academy of Sleep Medicine; 2023.
2. Berry RB, Wagner MH. *Sleep Medicine Pearls.* 3rd ed. Elsevier; 2014:102-107.
3. Libenson MH. *Practical Approach to Electroencephalography.* Elsevier; 2010:124-145.
4. Grigg-Damberger M. Polysomnographic artifacts. In: Tatum WO, ed. *Atlas of Clinical Neurophysiology.* Springer; 2018.
5. Geyer JD, Carney PD. Artifacts. In: Avidan A, Barkoukis TJ, eds. *Review of Sleep Medicine.* 4th ed. Elsevier Saunders; 2018:695-745.
6. Siddiqui F, Osuna E, Walters AS, Chokroverty S. Sweat artifact and respiratory artifact occurring simultaneously in polysomnogram. *Sleep Med.* 2006;7(2):197-199.
7. White DP. Pathogenesis of obstructive and central sleep apnea. *Am J Respir Crit Care Med.* 2005;172:1363-1370.
8. Chan ED, Chan MM, Chan MM. Pulse oximetry: understanding its basic principles facilitates appreciation of its limitations. *Respir Med.* 2013;107(6):789-799.
9. Parhizgar F, Nugent K, Raj R. Obstructive sleep apnea and respiratory complications associated with vagus nerve stimulators. *J Clin Sleep Med.* 2011;7(4):401-407.
10. Ebben MR, Sethi NK, Conte M, et al. Vagus nerve stimulation, sleep apnea, and CPAP titration. *J Clin Sleep Med.* 2008;4(5):471-473.
11. Upadhyay H, Bhat S, Gupta D, et al. The therapeutic dilemma of vagus nerve stimulator-induced sleep disordered breathing. *Ann Thorac Med.* 2016;11(2):151-154.
12. Hauri P, Hawkins DR. Alpha-delta sleep. *Electroencephalogr Clin Neurophysiol.* 1973;34:233-237.
13. Moldofsky H, Scarisbrick P, England R, Smythe H. Musculoskeletal symptoms and non-REM sleep disturbance in patients with "fibrositis syndrome" and healthy subjects. *Psychosom Med.* 1975;37:341-351.
14. Mahowald ML, Mahowald MW. Nighttime sleep and daytime functioning (sleepiness and fatigue) in less well defined chronic rheumatic disease with particular reference to "alpha-delta NREM sleep anomaly". *Sleep Med.* 2000;1:195-207.
15. Roizenblatt S, Moldofsky H, Benedito-Silva AA, Tufik S. Alpha sleep characteristics in fibromyalgia. *Arthritis Rheum.* 2001;44:222-230.

16. Johnson LC, Hanson K, Bickford RG. Effect of flurazepam on sleep spindles and K complexes. *Electroencephalogr Clin Neurophysiol.* 1976;40:67-77.
17. Johnson LC, Spinweber CL, Seidel WF, et al. Sleep spindle and delta changes during chronic use of a short acting and a long acting benzodiazepine hypnotic. *Electroencephalogr Clin Neurophysiol.* 1983;55: 662-667.
18. Leong CWY, Leow JWS, Grunstein RR, et al. A systematic scoping review of the effects of central nervous system active drugs on sleep spindles and sleep-dependent memory consolidation. *Sleep Med Rev.* 2022;62:101605.
19. Purcell SM, Manoach DS, Demanuele C, et al. Characterizing sleep spindles in 11,630 individuals from the National Sleep Research Resource. *Nat Commun.* 2017;8:15930.
20. Schenck CH, Mahowald MW, Kim SW, et al. Prominent eye movements during NREM sleep and REM sleep behavior disorder associated with fluoxetine treatment of obsessive compulsive disorder. *Sleep.* 1992; 15:226-235.
21. Armitage R, Trivedi M, Rush AJ. Fluoxetine and oculomotor activity during sleep in depressed patients. *Neuropsychopharmacology.* 1995;12:159-165.
22. Silber MH, Ancoli-Israel S, Bonnet MH, et al. The visual scoring of sleep in adults. *J Clin Sleep Med.* 2007;15:121-131.
23. Winkelman JW, James L. Serotonergic antidepressants are associated with REM sleep without atonia. *Sleep.* 2004;15:317-321.
24. McCarter SJ, St Louis EK, Sandness DJ, et al. Antidepressants increase REM sleep muscle tone in patients with and without REM sleep behavior disorder. *Sleep.* 2015;38(6):907-917.

Chapter 5

Sleep Staging in Infants and Children

AGE RANGE AT WHICH SCORING RULES APPLY

The current version of the American Academy of Sleep Medicine (AASM) scoring manual[1-3] now provides scoring rules for infants (0–2 months post-term or more precisely 37–48 weeks postmenstrual age), older infants, and children. The age terminology[4] used for infants is shown in Table 5–1 and Figure 5–1. The term conceptual age has been replaced by postmenstrual age (PMA). The gestational age is the time from the first day of the last menstrual period until birth in completed weeks. The PMA is gestational age + time in weeks since birth (chronological age). For an infant born at less than 37 weeks PMA (premature infants), no AASM scoring rules are provided. The AASM scoring manual refers the reader to discussion in the AASM Pediatric Scoring Task Force review and a recent review of infant sleep.[5,6] Other references also provide a useful discussion of the electroencephalogram (EEG) in premature infants.[7] A very brief discussion of premature infant sleep will be provided for information. Of note, the traditional sleep stage nomenclature for infants 0 to 2 months post-term has been changed from Quiet sleep and Active sleep[8] to Non–Rapid Eye Movement (NREM) sleep (stage N) and Rapid Eye Movement (REM) sleep (stage R), respectively.

SLEEP IN PREMATURE INFANTS

The sleep of premature infants differs from that of term infants (PMA 37–48 weeks) and changes substantially with increasing age. The timing of the appearance of different EEG patterns characteristic of different sleep stages is illustrated in Figure 5–2. The trace discontinue (TD) pattern (Fig. 5–3) is a discontinuous EEG pattern occurring in premature infants with 10 to 20 seconds or longer of very diminished EEG activity separated by short bursts of high-voltage activity. Before 30 weeks gestational age, TD is the EEG pattern associated with Wake, Stage N, and REM sleep. Thus before 30 weeks the infant's clinical appearance is used to differentiate wake and sleep. The TD pattern is gradually replaced by more mature EEG patterns as shown in Figure 5–2. The EEG patterns of term infants will be discussed in detail later. Even in term infants, behavioral observations are essential for sleep staging because a given EEG pattern may be associated with more than one sleep stage. In addition, all the usual waveforms for scoring sleep (sleep spindles, K complexes, and slow waves) may not be present until 6 months of age. The time of appearance of several waveforms used to stage sleep is displayed in Table 5–2.

Table 5–1 Age Nomenclature for Infants

Gestational age (GA) = time from the first day of LMP until delivery (in completed weeks)
At birth, classification based on GA • Premature (<37 weeks) • Full term (37 to 42 weeks) • Post-term (>42 weeks)
Postmenstrual age = gestational age at birth + weeks post-partum (chronological age)
Chronological age (postnatal or legal age) − time since birth (in weeks, months, years) • Neonate: 0 to 28 days after birth • Infant: 1 to 12 months of age (after birth)

LMP, Last menstrual period.

AASM SCORING RULES FOR TERM INFANTS POSTMENSTRUAL AGE 37-48 WEEKS

As noted above, infant scoring rules for scoring sleep and wake are used for infants 0 to 2 months post-term (37– 48 weeks PMA). Before the publication of infant scoring rules in the AASM scoring manual, sleep was scored according to the recommendations of Anders, Emde, and Parmelee.[8] The AASM term infant scoring rules are based on the former recommendations with some modifications including different terminology for sleep stages.[5,6] The new rules still adhere to the general concept of sleep staging based on behavioral and respiratory patterns as well as the EEG.

Technical Differences From Adults

Electrode distances are smaller because of a smaller head size. Sleep spindles are often *asynchronous* in children until 2 years of age (Fig. 5–4) and may be more prominent in the midline central derivations (C4-Cz, C3-Cz), where Cz is a central electrode in the midline (at the vertex). Use of a derivation to provide optimal visualization of sleep spindles could be considered (e.g., F4-M1, C4-M1, O2-M1, F3-M2, C3-M2, O1-M2, C4-Cz, C3-Cz). EEG electrode positions are discussed in Chapter 1. Sleep spindles are typically 12 to 14 Hz in this age group and often low voltage. Because behavioral patterns are so important to stage sleep, recording of synchronized audio and video is recommended.

General Scoring Rules for Term Infants (PMA 37 to 48 weeks)

- Sleep stages include:
  - Stage W (Wakefulness)
  - Stage N (NREM): formerly Quiet sleep
  - Stage R (REM): formerly Active sleep
  - Stage T (Transitional): formerly Indeterminant sleep

The nomenclature of Quiet sleep, Active sleep, and Indeterminant sleep has been replaced by stage N, stage R, and stage T, respectively. Sleep is staged in sequential 30-second

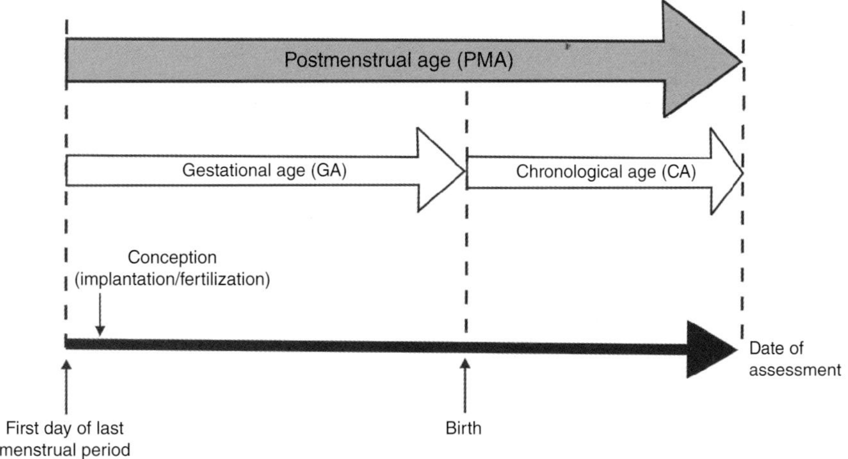

Figure 5–1 Schematic of the various age definitions for the newborn.

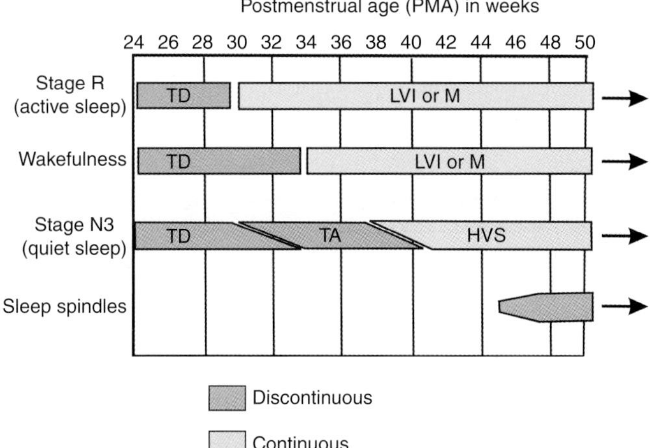

Figure 5–2 Appearance of different electroencephalogram patterns by postmenstrual age (PMA) in weeks. Note that the trace discontinue pattern is seen in all sleep stages before 30 weeks MA. Before this time, differentiation between wakefulness and sleep can only be made on the basis of the baby's clinical appearance, and specific sleep stages are hard to differentiate. The continuous background pattern is highlighted in a light color to emphasize the stages during which continuous activity is seen. *HVS,* High-voltage sleep; *LVI,* low-voltage irregular; *M,* mixed pattern; *TA,* trace alternant; *TD,* trace discontinue. (Adapted from Libenson MH. *Practical Approach to Electroencephalography.* Elsevier Saunders; 2010:321.)

epochs with a stage assigned to each epoch. If two stages coexist in an epoch, the epoch is scored based on the stage occupying the majority of the epoch. Sleep staging is based on the following five characteristics: *behavioral observation, respiration pattern, EEG pattern, electrooculogram (EOG) pattern, and chin electromyogram (EMG) pattern. If two or more polysomnographic (PSG) characteristics are discordant for stage N or stage R, the epoch is scored as stage T.* However, stage T is not scored if there is unequivocal evidence for stage W (eyes are wide open for most of the epoch) or vocalization (e.g., whimpering, crying), or if the infant is actively feeding.

Behavioral Characteristics

During wake the eyes are open, scanning eye movements are present (analogous to reading eye movements in adults), although brief eye closure may occur with crying. *If an infant maintains eye closure for 3 minutes or longer, they are considered to be asleep.* During stage N, the eyes are closed; few movements are noted but sucking can occur. During stage R the eyes are closed but REMs may be seen under the eyelids. Motor activity, including squirming, sucking, and small movements of the face or limbs, may be seen during stage R.

Summary of Behavioral Characteristics:

- Stage W: Eyes open (calm or active), scanning eye movements, brief eye closure with crying
- Stage N: Eyes closed, few body movements, sucking can occur
- Stage R: Eyes closed, REMs under eyelids, squirming, sucking, grimacing, small facial/limb movements
- If an infant maintains eye closure for 3 minutes of longer, they are considered to be asleep

Respiration Characteristics

During wake the pattern of respiration is irregular, rapid, and shallow. During stage N respiration is regular, but brief postsigh pauses can be noted. During stage R respiration is irregular and some central pauses may be noted (they may or may not meet criteria for central apnea). *The regularity or irregularity of respiration is the most reliable characteristic for differentiating stage N (regular) versus stage R (irregular).*

Summary of Respiration Characteristics:

- Stage W: Irregular, rapid, shallow breaths
- Stage N: Regular with occasional postsigh pauses
- Stage R: Irregular, central pauses (may or may not meet criteria for scoring apnea)

EEG Patterns

The EEG patterns in term infants aged 0 to 2 months are classified as discontinuous or continuous based on the presence or absence of periods of very reduced EEG activity (discontinuous). Of note, *some of the EEG patterns can be associated with more than one sleep stage.*[1,6]

The trace alternant (TA) pattern is discontinuous (Fig. 5–5) and characterized by *three or more periods* of high-voltage activity (3–8 seconds each) alternating with periods of low-voltage activity (4–12 seconds each). The TA high-voltage EEG activity consists of bilaterally symmetrical and synchronous slow waves (1–3 Hz), and the low voltage activity is in the theta

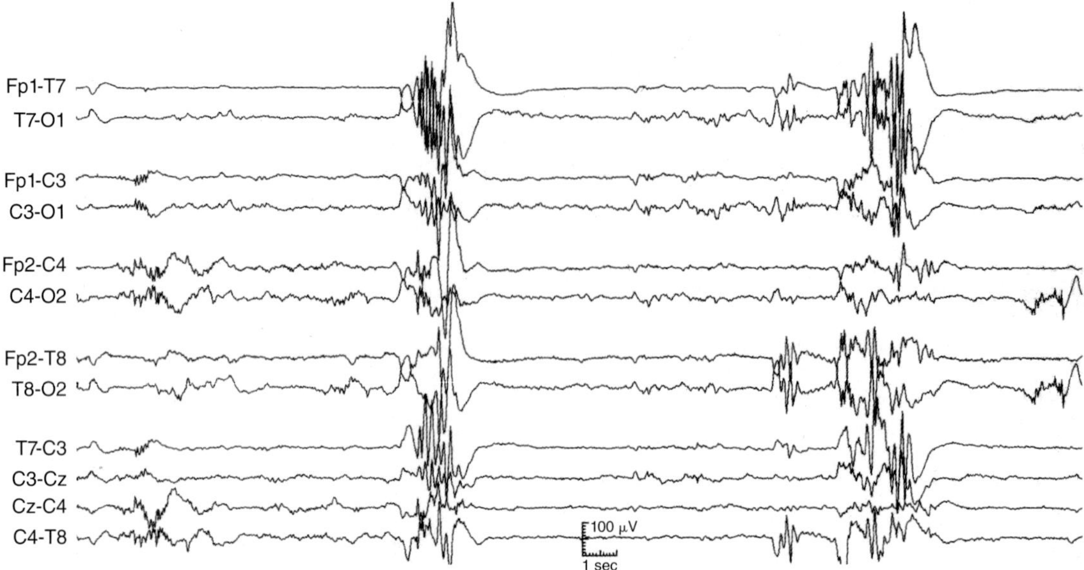

Figure 5–3 Trace discontinue (TD). Bursts of high-voltage activity alternate with long periods of flat electroencephalogram (EEG) activity. Electrode nomenclature is as follows: Fp1 is the left frontopolar, T7 left temporal, C3 left central, Fp2 right frontopolar, T8 right temporal, Cz vertex, and C4 right central. More details on electrode position are provided in Chapters 1 and 35. In premature infants before 30 weeks postmenstrual age, trace discontinue is noted in wake, stage N, and stage R sleep. (From Libenson MH. *Practical Approach to Electroencephalography.* Elsevier Saunders; 2010:320.)

Table 5–2 Age of Waveform Appearance

Waveform	Age of Initial Appearance	
Sleep spindles	6 weeks to 3 months post-term	(usually present by 2–3 months)
Slow wave activity	2–5 months post-term	(usually present by 4–5 months)
K complexes	3–6 months post-term	(usually present by 5–6 months)
Vertex sharp waves	4–6 months post-term	
Hypnagogic hypersynchrony	3–6 months post-term	
Posterior Dominant Rhythm		
Frequency 3.5–4.5 Hz	3–4 months post-term	
Frequency 5–6 Hz	5–6 months post-term	
Frequency 7.5–9 Hz	3 years post-term	
Mean frequency of 9 Hz	9 years (63%)	
Mean frequency of 10 Hz	15 years (65%)	

Adapted from Grigg-Damberger MM. The visual scoring of sleep in infants 0 to 2 months of age. *J Clin Sleep Med.* 2016;12(3):429-445.

range (4–7 Hz). TA differs from the TD pattern in premature infants as TD is characterized by *longer periods* of electrical quiescence rather than the shorter periods of reduced (but not absent) EEG activity in TA. The TA pattern is *only associated with the EEG pattern of stage N* but can be present in epochs scored as stage T (the TA EEG pattern is consistent with stage N, but the stage of the epoch depends on the other four characteristics). Low-voltage irregular (LVI) (Fig. 5–5) is characterized by continuous low-voltage mixed-frequency (delta and predominantly theta) EEG activity and is associated with stage R and wake. When LVI is present, sleep staging depends on chin activity as both wake and stage R can be associated with irregular respiration and REMs. In stage W chin EMG activity is present, whereas in stage R the chin EMG activity is absent or the lowest of the night. The high-voltage slow (HVS) pattern is analogous to stage N3 in adults and is characterized by continuous high-voltage 1- to 3-Hz activity (Fig. 5–5). The HVS pattern is associated with stage N (rarely R). The mixed (M) pattern is also continuous and composed of both high amplitude slow activity (similar to that seen in HVS but lower in amplitude) intermingled with low-voltage polyrhythmic activity with minimal periodicity (Fig. 5–5). The mixed EEG pattern can be associated with sleep stages W, R, and rarely N.

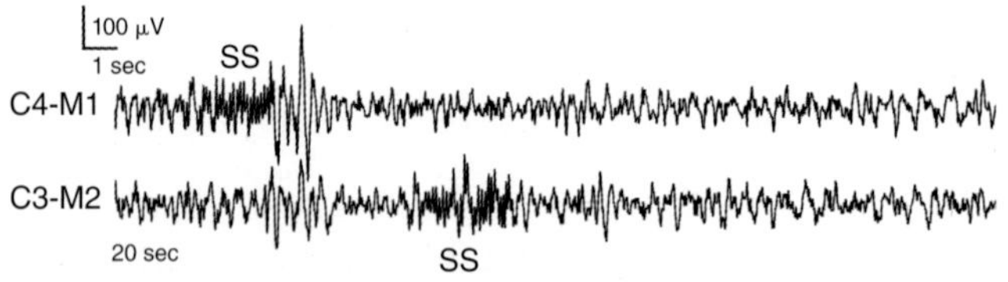

Figure 5–4 An example of asymmetric and asynchronous sleep spindles in a 5-month-old child. A sleep spindle in C4-M1 occurs without corresponding activity in C3-M2. Then a sleep spindle occurs in C3-M2 but not C4-M1.

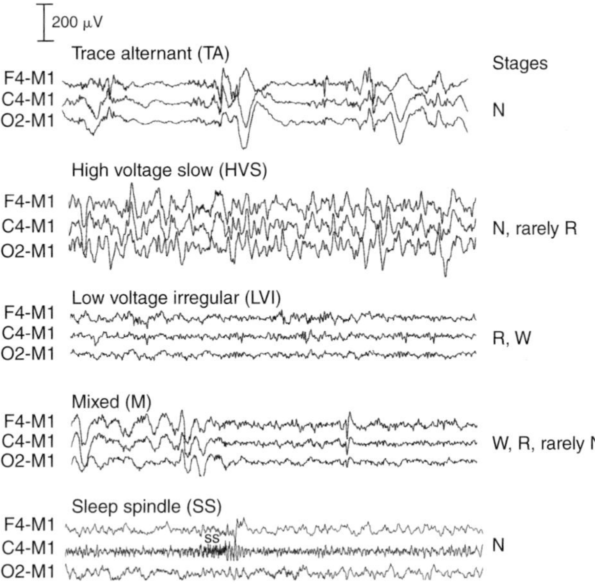

Figure 5–5 Samples of the electroencephalogram patterns that are used to stage sleep in post-term infants younger than 2 months of age (postmenstrual age 37 to 48 weeks). The corresponding sleep stages in which the patterns can appear are shown at the right border. Note that all patterns can occur in stage T sleep.

In summary, TA is consistent with stage N; HVS is consistent with stage N and rarely R; LVI is consistent with stage W or R; and the M pattern can be seen in W, N, or R. In addition, if a sleep spindle is present, the EEG pattern is consistent with stage N. However, the *ultimate sleep stage assigned an epoch depends on all five of the defining characteristics.*

From the sleep stage point of view, stage W can be associated with LVI and M; stage N can be associated with TA, HVS, and rarely M; and stage R is associated with LVI, M, and rarely HVS. *If sleep spindles are present, this is unequivocal evidence for the presence of a stage N* EEG pattern similar to the TA pattern. However, the final stage assigned to an epoch with an EEG pattern consistent with stage N (TA, sleep spindles) depends on the other scoring criteria, and such an epoch could be staged as stage T if the characteristic patterns are discordant. For this reason, stage T can be associated with any of the EEG patterns (TA, LVI, HVS, and M).

Summary of Sleeping EEG Patterns in Term Infants:

A. Discontinuous pattern:
- Trace alternant (TA): Three or more periods (3–8 seconds) of high-voltage activity alternating with periods (4–12 seconds) of low-voltage activity, consistent with stage N

B. Continuous patterns:
- High-voltage slow (HVS): Continuous high-voltage activity (1 to 3 Hz), consistent with stage N (rarely R)
- Low-voltage irregular (LVI): Continuous low-voltage mixed-frequency activity (delta and predominantly theta activity) consistent with stages R and W (wakefulness)
- Mixed: A combination of high high amplitude slow activity (similar to HVS but lower in amplitude) intermingled with low-voltage polyrhythmic activity and minimal periodicity, consistent with stages W, R, and rarely N

C. Sleep spindles: 12-14 Hz, consistent with stage N

D. By sleep stage:
- Stage W: LVI, M
- Stage N: TA, HVS, rarely M, sleep spindles
- Stage R: LVI, M, rarely HVS
- Stage T: any EEG pattern

EOG Patterns

During stage W, REMs, blinks, and scanning eye movements may be present. REMs and blinks are similar to those in adults. Scanning eye movements are similar to reading eye movements in adults (see Chapter 1), with conjugate eye movements displaying a slow phase followed by a rapid phase opposite the direction of the slow phase as the infant scans the environment or follows objects. Transient eye closure can be seen with crying. In stage N the eyes are closed and not moving; in stage R the eyes are closed with either no eye movements or REMs. As in adults, REMs may not be seen in all epochs scored as stage R.

Summary of Eye Movement Patterns:
- Stage W: REMs, blinks, scanning eye movements
- Stage N: Eyes closed, no eye movements
- Stage R: Eyes closed with REMs or no eye movements

Chin EMG Patterns

In stage W the chin EMG activity is present and often high, sometimes with movement artifact. During stage N the chin EMG activity is present (variable but often lower than stage W). During stage R the chin EMG activity is low, but transient muscle activity can be present. **Low chin EMG activity** is defined as no higher than any other sleep stage and usually at the lowest level of the recording. Transient muscle activity consists of short, irregular bursts of EMG activity, usually with a duration less than 0.25 seconds superimposed on low chin muscle tone.

Summary of Chin EMG Patterns:
- Stage W: EMG activity present and variable
- Stage N: EMG activity present and often lower than stage W
- Stage R: EMG activity is low (lowest of the night), transient muscle activity may be present

SCORING THE SLEEP STAGES IN TERM INFANTS WITH A PMA 37 TO 48 WEEKS

As noted above, sleep stage scoring is based on the five characteristics: behavioral, respiration, EEG pattern, eye movement pattern, and chin EMG pattern. Stage W is also scored when there is obvious behavioral evidence of wakefulness, as noted below. As in adults, sleep is staged in 30 second epochs and if more than one sleep stage is present in a given epoch, the epoch is scored as the sleep stage occupying the greatest portion of the epoch.

Rules for Scoring Stage W: PMA Age 37 to 48 Weeks[1,2]

Score stage W if either 1, 2, or 3 is present for the majority of the epoch:

1. Eyes are wide open (for the majority of the epoch)
2. Vocalization (e.g., whimpering, crying) or actively feeding
3. **All of the following are met:**
   - Eyes are open intermittently
   - REMs or scanning eye movements
   - Sustained chin EMG tone with bursts of muscle activity
   - Irregular respiration
   - EEG: LVI or M (may have superimposed movement artifacts)

Wake is most reliably scored by behavioral observation as many of the EEG waveforms used to stage sleep are not present until after 2 months post-term. A tracing of stage W in an infant is displayed in Figure 5–6. This stage is characterized by an infant with eyes open (often crying), irregular respiration, an EEG of the LVI or M pattern, REMs, blinks, or scanning eye movements with present EMG tone of variable magnitude. *Note that in the absence of meeting criteria "1" or "2" in the scoring rules for stage W, all five characteristics listed in criteria "3" must be present.*

Rules for Scoring Stage N: PMA Age 37 to 48 Weeks[1,2]

Score stage N if **four or more** of the following are present for the majority of the epoch:

- Eyes closed, no eye movements
- Chin EMG activity present
- Regular respiration (postsigh pauses may occur)
- EEG: TA, HVS, or sleep spindles
- Reduced movement compared with wake

Two examples of stage N are shown in Figures 5-7 and 5-8. A TA EEG pattern is shown in Figure 5–7 and HVS in Figure 5–8. Note that the TA EEG pattern is only associated with the EEG of stage N (or stage T if characteristics are discordant). Stage N is characterized by regular respiration and an EEG with a TA, HVS, or M pattern **or the presence of sleep spindles.** The eyes are closed, no eye movements are noted, and chin EMG activity is present but often lower than stage W. Sleep spindles are associated with the EEG of stage N (or stage T if the other characteristics are discordant). *If an infant's eyes are closed for more than 3 minutes, the infant is considered asleep.*

Rules for Scoring Stage R: PMA Age 37 to 48 Weeks[1,2]

- Score stage R (definite R) in epochs with **four or more** of the following criteria present, **including irregular respiration *and* REMs:**
  - Low chin EMG (for the majority of the epoch)
  - Eyes closed with at least one REM (concurrent with low chin tone)
  - Irregular respiration
  - Mouthing, sucking, twitches, or brief head movements
  - EEG exhibits a continuous pattern (usually LVI or M, rarely HVS) **without sleep spindles**
- Score segments of sleep contiguous with and **after** an epoch of definite R as defined above in the absence of REMs, as stage R if *all of the following are present:*
  - The EEG shows low- or medium-amplitude mixed-frequency activity (LVI or M) without TA activity or sleep spindles
  - The chin muscle tone is low for the majority of the epoch
  - There is no intervening arousal (defined by the same arousal rule as for children and adults)

Note that both irregular respiration and at least one REM concurrent with low EMG activity must be present to score an

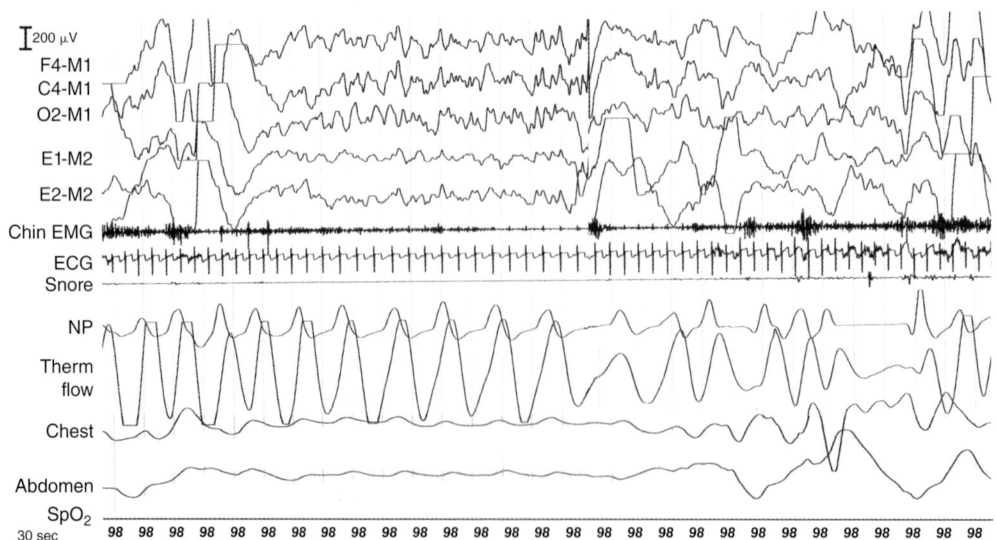

Figure 5–6 Stage W. A 30-second tracing from a 1-month-old infant shows an EEG M pattern; behavior: movement artifact noted (*video shows eyes open and head movement*); respiration: irregular; electrooculogram derivations shows rapid eye movements present; chin electromyogram activity present with bursts of activity. However, the most definitive evidence is the video. NP nasal pressure, Therm flow using an oronasal thermal sensor, Chin Chin EMG (Chin1-ChinZ or Chin2-ChinZ).

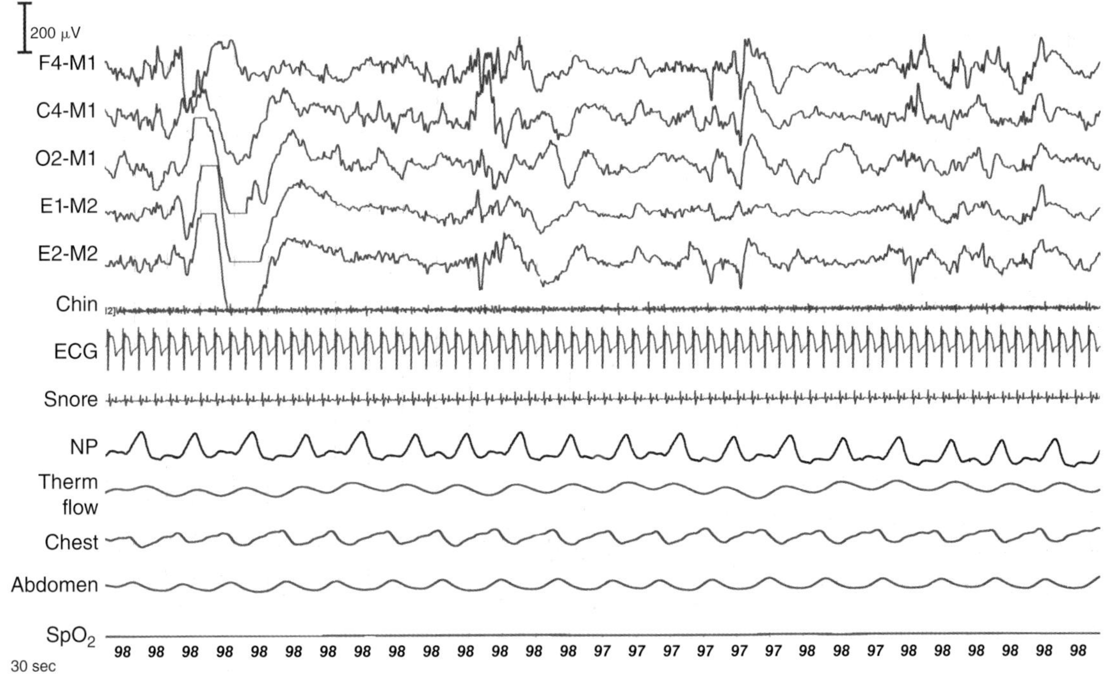

Figure 5–7 Stage N. A 30-second epoch in a 1-month-old infant of stage N showing an EEG pattern: trace alternant; EOG: absent eye movements; chin EMG: chin tone is present; and respiration: regular. *The video showed no infant movement, and the eyes were closed.* NP nasal pressure, Chin is Chin EMG (Chin1-ChinZ or Chin2-ChinZ).

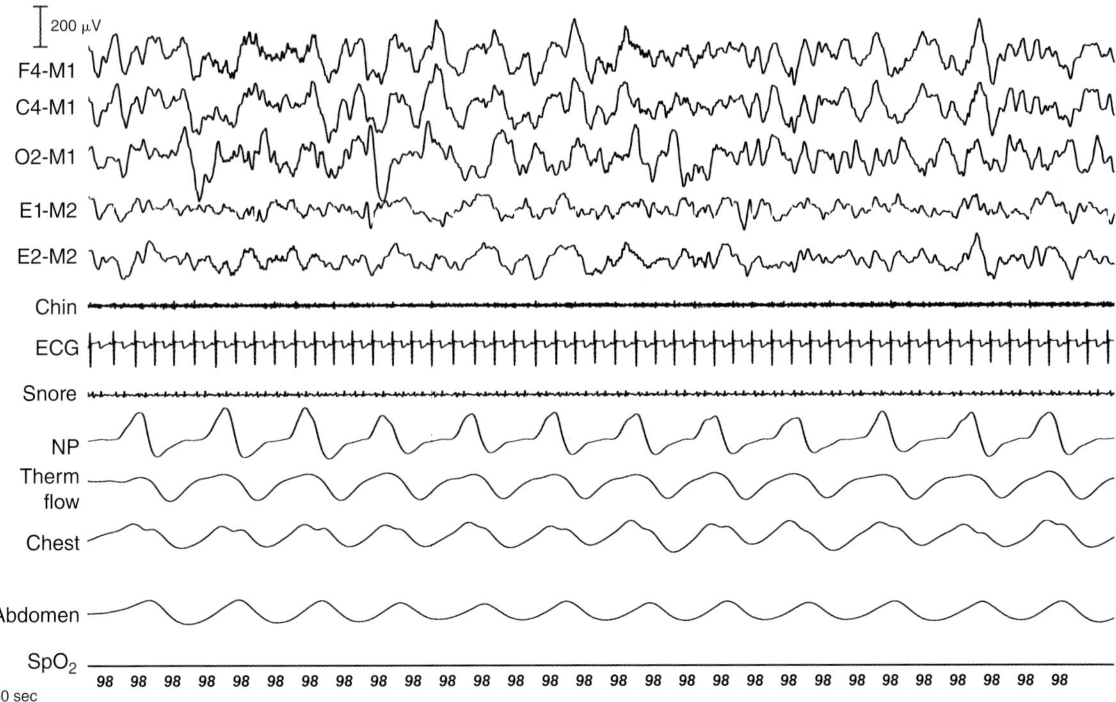

Figure 5–8 A 30-second epoch of stage N in a 1-month-old infant. The electroencephalogram shows a high-voltage slow (HVS) activity, there are no eye movements, respiration is regular, and chin EMG activity is present. *The video showed the infant not moving with the eyes closed.* NP nasal pressure, inspiration is upward. Chin is Chin EMG (Chin1-ChinZ or Chin2-ChinZ).

epoch as *definite stage R*. In infants up to 2 to 3 months, the first epoch of sleep is most commonly stage R. Given the difficulty in determining sleep onset, **an epoch of definite stage R is required to begin scoring this sleep stage in infants with a PMA of 37 to 48 weeks.** Note that this scoring of stage R onset differs from scoring stage R in children and adults as the first epoch(s) of an episode of stage R may not have REMs, although contiguous and preceding an epoch of definite stage R. Here the start of stage R must be an epoch of definite stage R. Stage R is characterized by eyes closed, irregular respirations, an EEG of LVI or M (rarely HVS), REMs, closed eyes, and low chin EMG activity (Fig. 5–9). Irregular respiration is the most reliable sign of stage R. Readers most familiar with adult tracings can be confused by the relatively high-voltage EEG present in this sleep stage (if an M pattern is noted) in many infants as well as the presence of stage R at sleep onset.

Rules for Scoring Stage T (Transitional Sleep): PMA Age 37 to 48 Weeks

- Score an epoch as stage N, stage W, or stage R if only one PSG characteristic is discordant for this sleep stage.
- Score an epoch as stage T (transitional) if it contains three NREM and two REM characteristics or two NREM and three REM characteristics.

Stage T usually represents a transition from one sleep stage to another; for example, from stage R to stage N or from stage N to stage R. An example of an epoch of stage T is illustrated in Figure 5–10. The rules for scoring stage T assume that an epoch does not follow an epoch of definite stage R. In that case if REMs were not be present the epoch could be scored as stage R rather than stage T if other criteria for stage R were met. For example in Figure 5–10 if the epoch followed an epoch of definite stage R wihout an intervening arousal it would be scored as stage R rather than stage T even though REMs are not present.

SLEEP ARCHITECTURE IN TERM INFANTS AND CHILDREN

Some information about the differences in sleep architecture in newborn infants compared with children and adults is useful in scoring sleep.[9-12] For a more detailed discussion of sleep architecture in children see Chapter 7. Newborn infants typically have periods of sleep lasting 3 to 4 hours interrupted by feeding, and the total sleep duration in 24 hours is usually 16 to 18 hours. They have cycles of sleep with a *45- to 60-minute periodicity* with about 50% REM sleep. In newborns the *presence of REM at sleep onset is the norm.* In contrast, the adult sleep cycle is 90 to 100 minutes, REM occupies about 20% to 25% of sleep, and NREM sleep is noted at sleep onset.

After about age 3 months, the percentage of REM sleep starts to diminish and the intensity of body movements during REM begins to decrease. The pattern of NREM at sleep onset begins to emerge. However, the sleep cycle period does not reach the adult value of 90 to 100 minutes until adolescence.[9-12]

Sleep Scoring In Children 2 Months Post-term or Older

Ages for Which AASM Pediatric Sleep Scoring Rules Apply

Pediatric sleep scoring rules can be used to score sleep and wakefulness in children 2 months post-term or older (PMA of 48 weeks or older). The AASM scoring manual does not define a precise upper limit for using pediatric sleep scoring rules.[1,2] Note that rarely there is some overlap in the age ranges for using infant versus pediatric sleep staging rules. If an infant born at 38 weeks PMA is aged 2 months (PMA 46 weeks) the age criteria for infant rules is satisfied (37-48 weeks PMA) as well as pediatric scoring rules (2 months post-term or older). One has the option of using the scoring rules that best describe the sleep of the infant.

Terminology of Sleep Stages

The following terminology should be used when scoring sleep in children age 2 months post-term or older:

- Stage W (wakefulness)
- Stage N1 (NREM 1)
- Stage N2 (NREM 2)

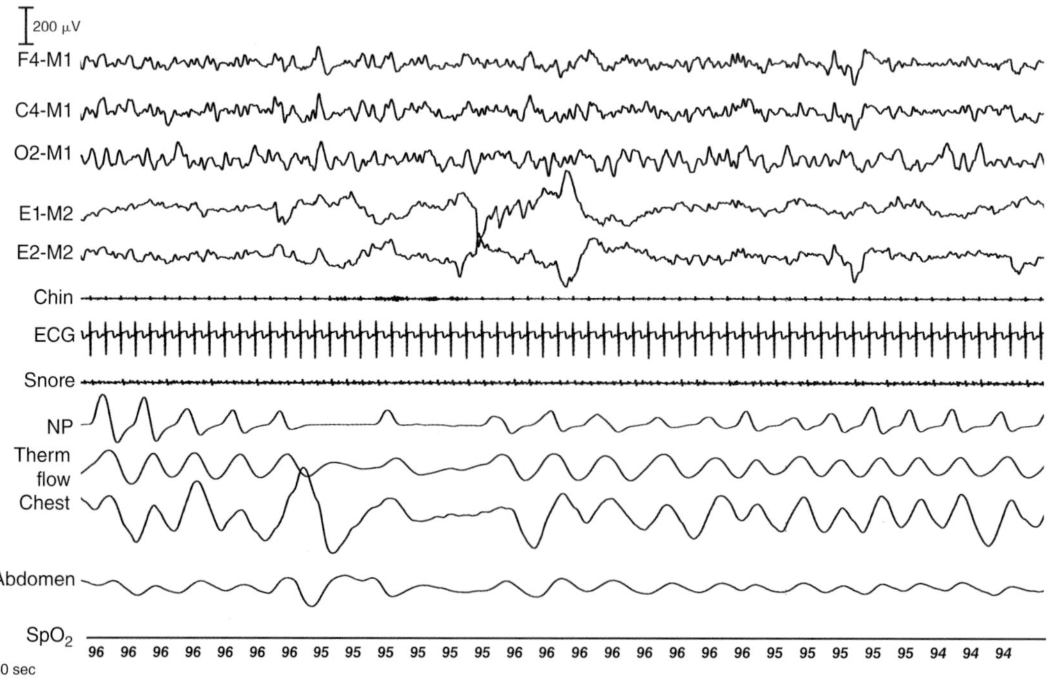

Figure 5–9 A 30-second epoch of stage R in a 1-month-old infant. The electroencephalographic pattern is low-voltage irregular (LVI), rapid eye movements are present, the chin electromyogram shows low tone, and respiration is irregular. The video showed eyes closed and small twitches of the corners of the mouth. NP nasal pressure,Chin is Chin EMG (Chin1-ChinZ or Chin2-ChinZ).

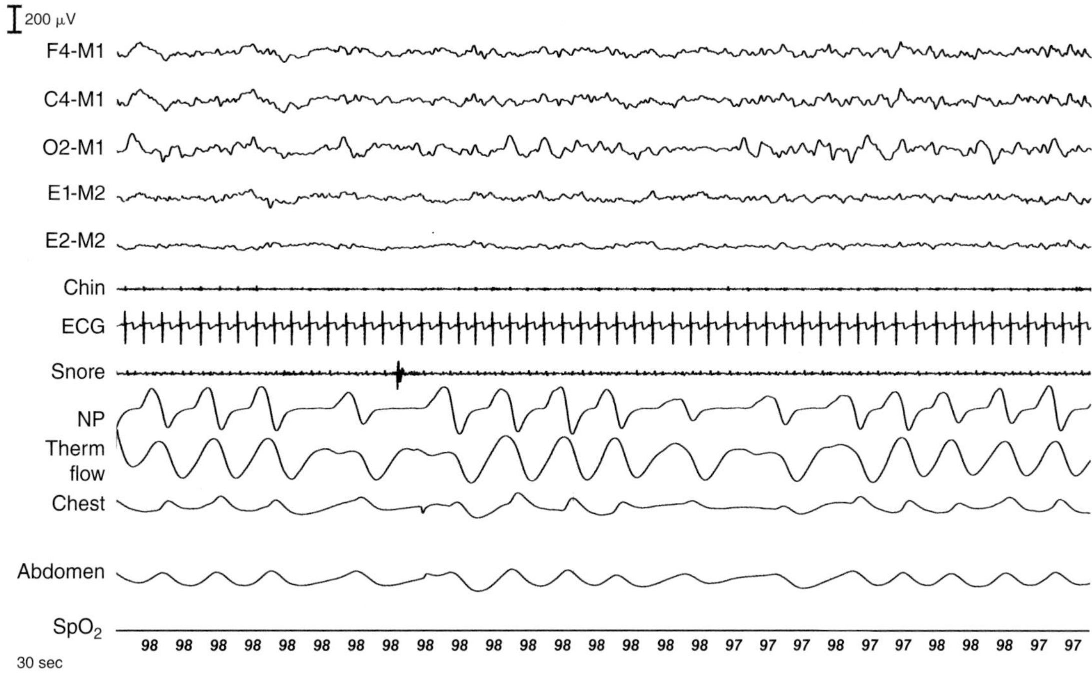

Figure 5–10 Stage T. A 30-second epoch in a 1-month-old infant with three N features and two R features. For N (no eye movements; behavioral, no movement), for R (EEG pattern: low-voltage irregular; respiration: irregular; EMG low/absent). NP nasal pressure,Chin is Chin EMG (Chin1-ChinZ or Chin2-ChinZ).

- Stage N3 (NREM 3)
- Stage N (NREM)
- Stage R (REM)

The sleep stage terminology differs from adults to account for the fact that not all features of sleep may be present in infants 2 to 6 months post-term. By 6 months sleep spindles, K complexes and slow waves should be present and stages N1, N2, and N3 can usually be scored (and sometimes younger). In the scoring of infant sleep, four possible scenarios are described.

A. If all epochs of NREM sleep contain no recognizable sleep spindles, K complexes, or high-amplitude 0.5- to 2-Hz slow wave activity, score all epochs as stage N (NREM).
B. If some epochs of NREM sleep contain sleep spindles or K complexes, score those as stage N2 (NREM 2). If the remaining NREM epoch contains no slow wave activity constituting more than 20% of the duration of epochs, score as stage N (NREM).
C. If some epochs of NREM sleep contain greater than 20% slow wave activity, score these as stage N3 (NREM 3). If the remaining NREM epochs contain no K complexes or spindles, score as stage N (NREM).
D. If NREM is sufficiently developed that some epochs contain sleep spindles and K complexes and other epochs contain sufficient amounts of slow wave activity, score NREM sleep in this infant as either stage N1, N2, or N3 as in an older child or adult.

Scenarios A, B, and C are uncommonly noted unless a sleep center studies a large number of very young infants. *An infant is defined as a child 1 to 12 months of age.* An example of scenario C is shown in Figure 5–11. Here the infant has developed slow waves but not K complexes or sleep spindles.

Rules for Scoring Sleep Stages in Children 2 Months Post-term or Older (Pediatric Sleep Staging Rules)

Scoring Stage W

Scoring stage W in children 2 months post-term or older uses both familiar waveforms used for sleep staging in adults and some waveforms not seen in adults. These will be discussed followed by the stage W rules.

Waveforms Used to Score Wake

A. Posterior Dominant Rhythm (PDR)
- PDR in both adults and children is defined as the predominant rhythm seen over occipital derivations during eyes closed wakefulness that is reactive (reactive = activity blocks or attenuates with eye opening and appears with passive eye closure). PDR in adults is often called "alpha rhythm" in older children and adults and consists of activity most prominent over occipital derivations with an amplitude of less than 50 μV and a frequency of 8 to 13 Hz; it is reactive to eye opening (decreased amplitude). Of note, 10% to 25% of adults have no or poorly defined alpha rhythm. PDR frequency in infants and children changes with age. Table 5–3 shows the characteristic changes. A simple rule to remember is "at least three at 3 months, at least four at 4 months, nine by age 9," meaning that in normal awake children older than age 9, PDR is usually greater than 9 Hz (8–13 Hz). In Figure 5–12 a tracing of PDR in a 3-month-old infant is shown with a frequency of 4 to 5 Hz.

B. Additional Waveforms of Wakefulness
- Posterior slow waves (PSWs) of youth: This waveform occurs in children 8 to 14 years of age and has a frequency of 2.5 to 4.5 Hz *during wake*. PSW usually occurs at the same time as PDR with eyes closed wake and disappears with

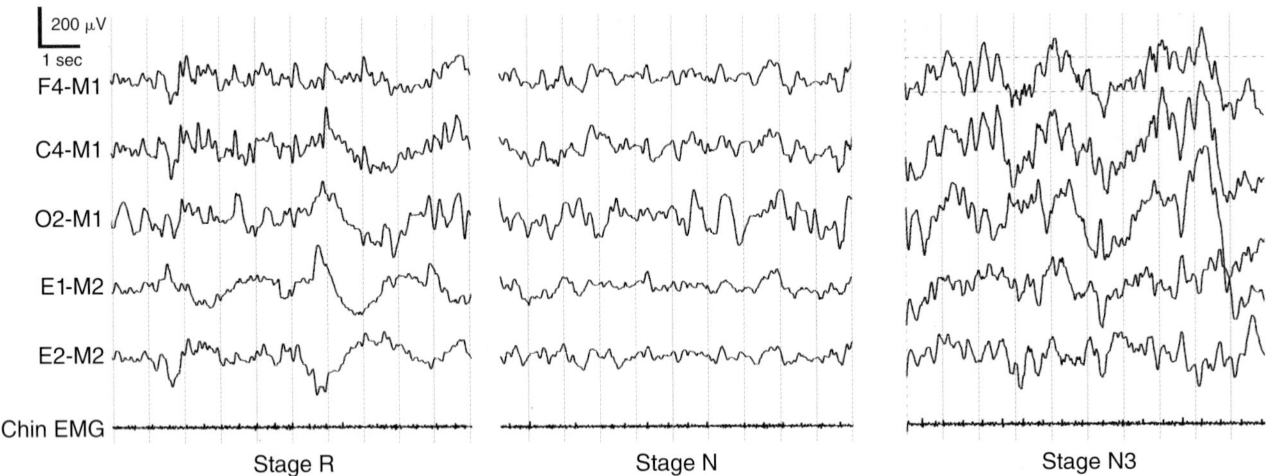

Figure 5–11 Three 10-second segments of different stages in a 3-month-old infant. No sleep spindles or K complexes were present. However, slow wave activity was present allowing the scoring of stage N3 sleep. The epochs of sleep that were not stage N3 or stage R were scored as stage N. (From Berry RB, Wagner MH. *Sleep Medicine Pearls.* 3rd ed. Elsevier; 2015:56.)

Table 5–3 Waveforms for Scoring Stage W and N1 in Children

PDR	• Dominant reactive rhythm over the occipital region in relaxed wakefulness (eyes closed) and attenuates with eye opening. The frequency is 8–13 Hz in adults and older children but slower in infants and young children (see below).	
PDR changes with age	Frequency 3.5–4.5 Hz Frequency 5–6 Hz Frequency 7.5–9 Hz Mean frequency of 9 Hz Mean frequency of 10 Hz	3–4 months post-term 5–6 months post-term 3 years 9 years 15 years
LAMF	• Low amplitude predominantly 4–7 Hz	
Vertex sharp waves	• Less than 0.5 seconds (as measured at the base of the wave) • Maximal over the central region • Often at transition from N1 to N2 but can occur in N1 and N2.	
HH	• Stage N1, stage N2 • High-amplitude (75–350 μV) sinusoidal shape • Rhythmic 3- to 4.5-Hz activity • Widely distributed (central, frontal, front-central) • 95% of normal children 6–8 years • 10% of healthy 11-year-old children • Rare after age 12 years	

HH, Hypnagogic hypersynchrony; *LAMF*, low-amplitude mixed-frequency; *PDR*, posterior dominant rhythm.
Adapted from Grigg-Damberger MM, Gozal D, Marcus CL, et al. The visual scoring of sleep and arousal in infants and Children. *J Clin Sleep Med.* 2007;3(2):201-240.

drowsiness or transition to stage N1 sleep. Maximal incidence is 8 to 14 years of age and is rare in children younger than 2 years or adults older than 21 years[1,5] (Fig. 5–13).

- Blinks: Conjugate vertical eye movements at a frequency of 0.5 to 2 Hz in wakefulness with eyes open or closed. Eye blinks in children, as in adults, are associated with the eyeball turning upward (Bell phenomenon). In children, they cause occipital sharp waves that are monophasic or biphasic (200–400 msec) and less than 200 μV that follow eye blinks.[5]
- Slow eye movements (SEMs) or REMs are defined the same as in adults. See Chapter 1 for examples.

Pediatric Stage W Rules.[1,2] Score stage W when more than 50% of the epoch contains either or both of the following:

- Age-appropriate PDR occupies more than 50% of the epoch over the occipital region (individuals generating PDR with eye closure)
- Other findings consistent with stage W (all individuals)
  - Eye blinks at a frequency of 0.5 to 2 Hz
  - REMs associated with normal or high chin muscle tone
  - Reading eye movements

An example of stage W exhibiting PDR for nearly all of the epoch is shown in Figure 5–12.

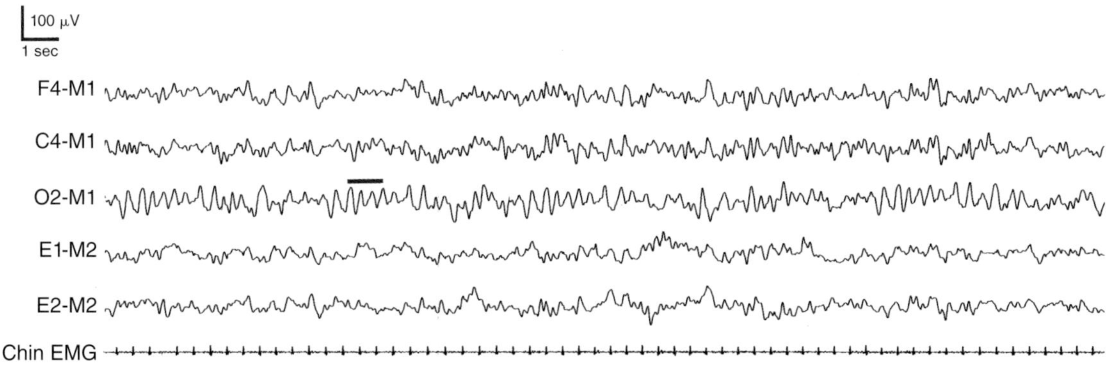

Figure 5–12 A 30-second epoch of stage W in a 3-month-old infant showing a posterior dominant rhythm of 4 Hz that is normal for this age group.

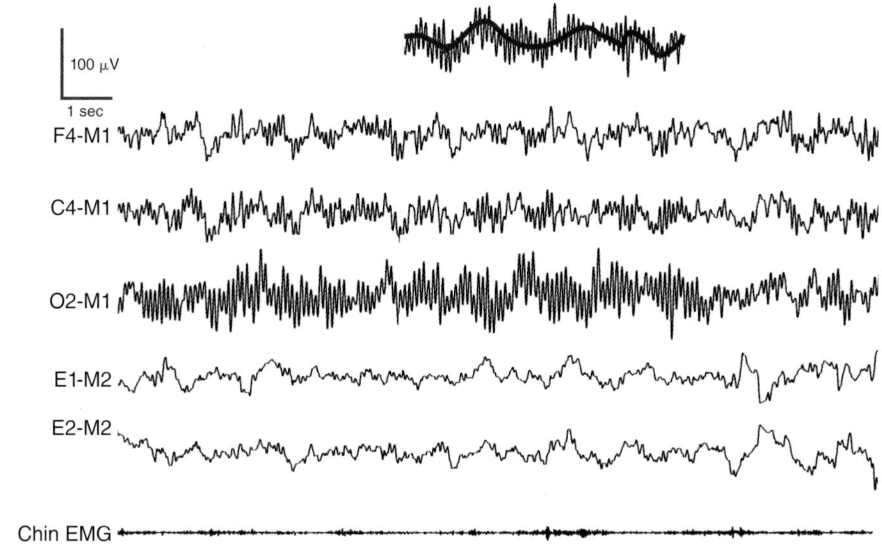

Figure 5–13 An example of posterior slow waves (PSW) of youth during stage W (30-second epoch) in an 8-year-old child. This pattern is seen during **relaxed wakefulness** and disappears with sleep onset. The usual posterior dominant rhythm is superimposed on underlying slow waves activity. PSW occurs only with the eyes closed during wake and disappears as the individual becomes drowsy and transitions to sleep. The pattern is most common in children aged 8 to 14 years. (From Berry RB, Wagner MH. *Sleep Medicine Pearls.* 3rd ed. Elsevier; 2015:57.)

Scoring Stage N1

Scoring stage N1 in children 2 months post-term or older (PMA 48 weeks or older) both familiar waveforms used in adult sleep staging and some unique to children. After discussion of the important waveforms, pediatric scoring rules for stage N1 will be discussed.

Waveforms for Scoring Pediatric Stage N1. In staging N1, the presence or absence of certain waveforms is important (Table 5–3).

A. Hypnagogic hypersynchrony (HH) is characterized by bursts of *very high amplitude* 3 to 4.5 Hz sinusoidal waves maximal in frontal and central derivations and smallest in the occipital derivation (widely distributed) (see Fig. 5–14). HH can occur in stages N1 or N2.
B. Low-amplitude mixed-frequency (LAMF): Low amplitude, predominantly 4- to 7-Hz activity.
C. Vertex sharp waves are sharply contoured waves with duration less than 0.5 second maximal over the central region and distinguishable from background activity (see Chapter 1).
D. Slow eye movements (SEMs): Conjugate, reasonably regular, sinusoidal eye movements with initial deflection that last longer than 500 msec (see Chapter 1).

Pediatric Stage N1 Rules[1,2]

- In individuals generating age appropriate PDR with eye closure, score stage N1 if PDR is attenuated or replaced by LAMF activity for more than 50% of the epoch (Fig. 5–15).
- In individuals not generating PDR with eye closure, score stage N1 commencing with the earliest of any of the following phenomena:
    - Activity in range 4 to 7 Hz with slowing of background frequencies by 1 to 2 Hz from those of stage W (e.g., 5 Hz activity is noted and stage W activity was 7 Hz)
    - SEMs
    - Vertex sharp waves

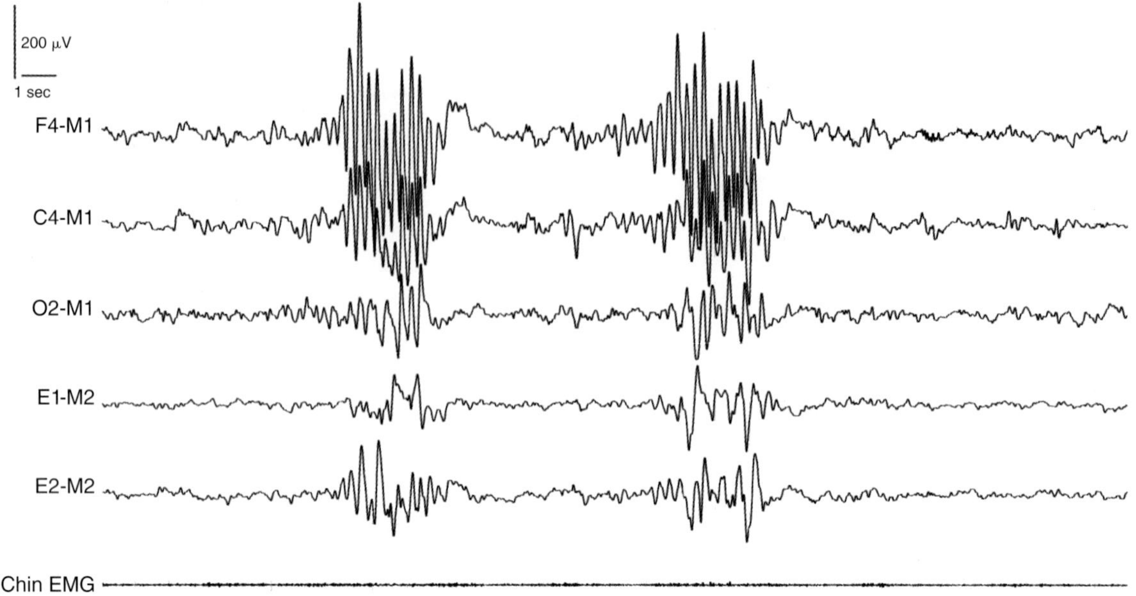

Figure 5–14 A 30-second epoch of stage N1 in a 5-year-old child with two bursts of hypnogogic hypersynchrony. (From Berry RB, Wagner MH. *Sleep Medicine Pearls.* 3rd ed. Elsevier; 2015:62.)

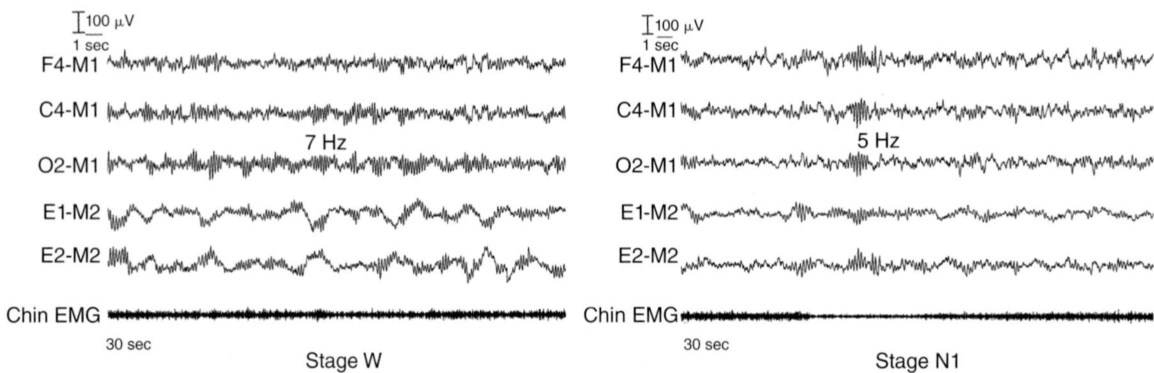

Figure 5–15 Two 30-second epochs of stage W and stage N1 in a 3-year-old child. The entire epoch of stage W exhibits posterior dominant rhythm at 7 Hz. Slow eye movements are also noted. In stage N1 the posterior dominant rhythm has been attenuated and replaced by slower activity.

- Hypnagogic Hypersynchrony (HH)
- Diffuse or occipital predominant high-amplitude, rhythmic 3- to 5-Hz EEG activity

The stage N1 rules of children differ from adults based on the addition of HH or diffuse/occipital high-amplitude, rhythmic 3-to-5 Hz activity to determine the onset of stage N1 in individuals that do not generate PDR with eye closure. HH is a distinctive EEG pattern of **drowsiness and stage N1**[1,5] that often disappears with deeper stages of NREM sleep (but can occur in stage N2). HH is seen in approximately 30% of infants at 3 months post-term, in *95% of all normal children aged 6 to 8 months,* and is less prevalent after 4 to 5 years of age. The waveform is seen in only 10% of healthy children by age 11 and is rarely seen after 12 years of age. Of note, HH can also be seen in children who generate PDR activity with eye closure, but in these PDR-generating individuals stage N1 can usually be scored before the appearance of HH based on the decrease in PDR. Figure 5–14 shows an example of stage N1 with two bursts of HH. However, HH can occur in stage N2 (Figure 5–16). In Figure 5–17 stage N1 can be scored based on the presence of high-voltage, fairly diffuse 4-Hz activity in an individual not generating PDR. In earlier versions of the AASM scoring manual, rhythmic anterior theta (RAT) was specified as a waveform enabling scoring of age N1 in individuals not generating PDR with eye closures. RAT is characterized by 5-to-7 Hz activity seen in the frontal regions that is first noted around age 5 years and is common in children and adolescents. Although the pattern is no longer separately delineated in the current version of the AASM scoring manual or used to score N1, the pattern is common during transition from stage W to N1.

Pediatric Stage N2 Rules. Score stage N2 as per adult rules[1,2] (see Chapter 3).

Sleep spindles in young children differ somewhat from those in adults. In infants, sleep spindles are often asynchronous until age 1 to 2 years (Fig. 5–4). Sleep spindles occur independently at two different locations and frequencies in

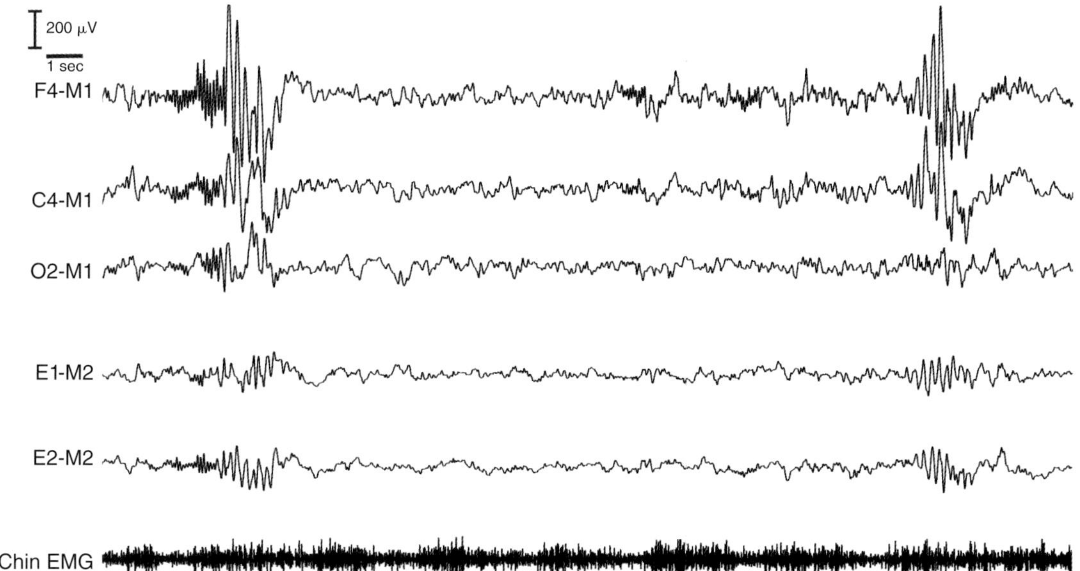

Figure 5–16 A 30-second epoch of stage N2 in a 5-year-old child. A sleep spindle occurs just before a burst of hypnogogic hypersynchrony (HH). Of note, HH is characteristic of stage N1 but can persist into stage N2. Another burst of HH is noted at the end of the epoch.

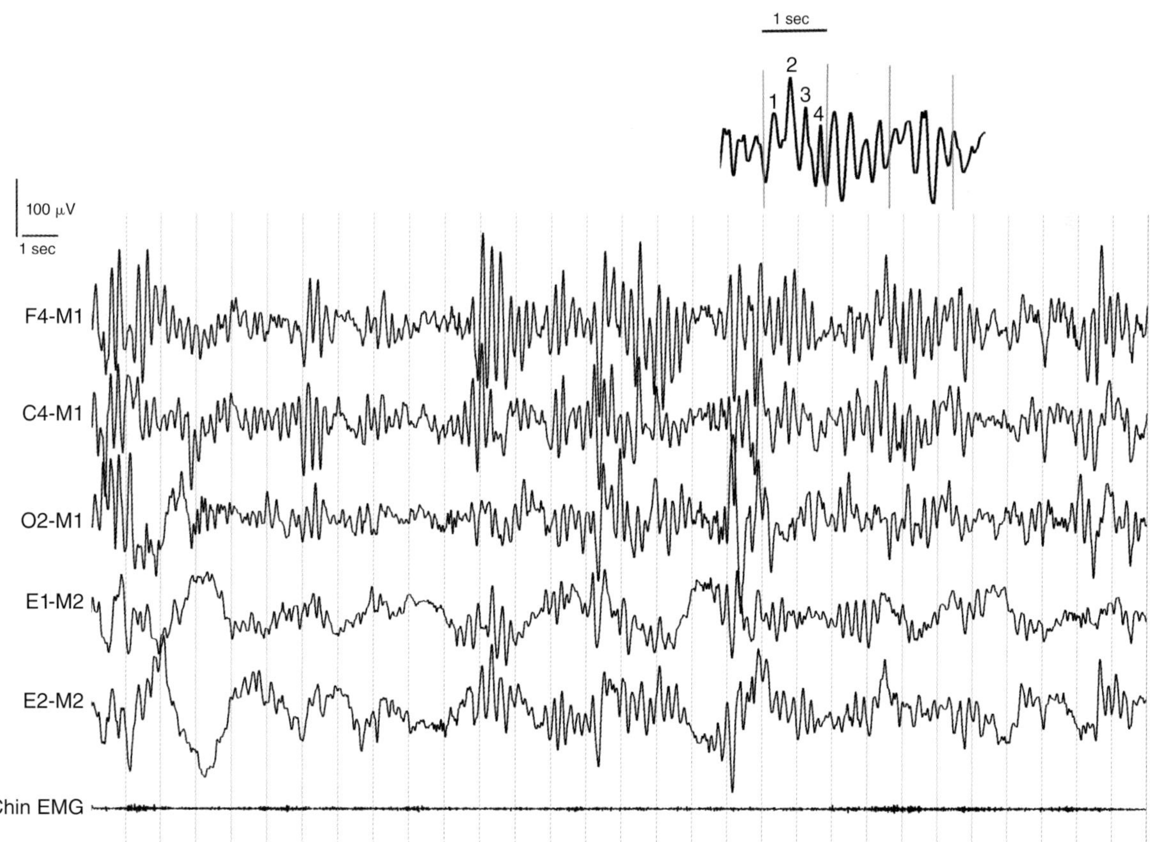

Figure 5–17 A 30-second epoch of stage N1. The tracing exhibits diffuse electroencephalogram activity of 4 Hz. The epoch immediately followed an epoch of stage W in an individual who did not generate PDR. Neither sleep spindles nor hypnogogic hypersynchrony is present. (From Berry RB, Wagner MH. *Sleep Medicine Pearls*. 3rd ed. Elsevier; 2015:62.)

children and adolescents. Frontal spindles typically are 11 to 12.5 Hz compared with 12.5 to 14.5 Hz in centroparietal regions. Centroparietal spindles show little change between ages 4 and 24 years, whereas frontal spindles decrease dramatically in power and become stable at about age 13 years.[9]

Pediatric Stage N3 Rules. Score stage N3 as per adult rules[1,2] (see Chapter 3).

Slow-wave activity for sleep staging is defined as greater than 75 μV peak to peak in the frontal derivation (F3-M2 or F4-M1) with a frequency of 0.5 to 2 Hz (corresponding to 2- to 0.5-second width, respectively). Slow waves in children are often much larger than in adults (100 to 400 μV) in amplitude. Slow waves appear as early as 3 months but more often about 3 to 4.5 months post-term. In scoring adult sleep, the major question for epochs containing slow-frequency activity is "Is the amplitude criteria met for at least 6 seconds?" In children, the major decision is what constitutes slow activity based on frequency because nearly all activity exceeds 75 μV peak to peak. A 30-second epoch of stage N3 sleep is shown in Figure 5–18.

Pediatric Stage R Rules. Stage R is scored as per adult rules (see Chapter 3).

Stage R of pediatric sleep differs from adults in that the background activity may not show a familiar pattern until after age 5 to 10 years (LAMF). In infants and younger children, the activity is slower and often with higher amplitude.[5] The background activity may be 4 to 5 Hz at age 5 months, 5 to 6 Hz at age 9 months, and 5 to 7 Hz at ages 1 to 5 years. An example of stage R in a child is shown in Figure 5–19. Note the relatively high background activity.

Pediatric Arousal Rules

Score arousals in children using adult rules (see Chapter 3).

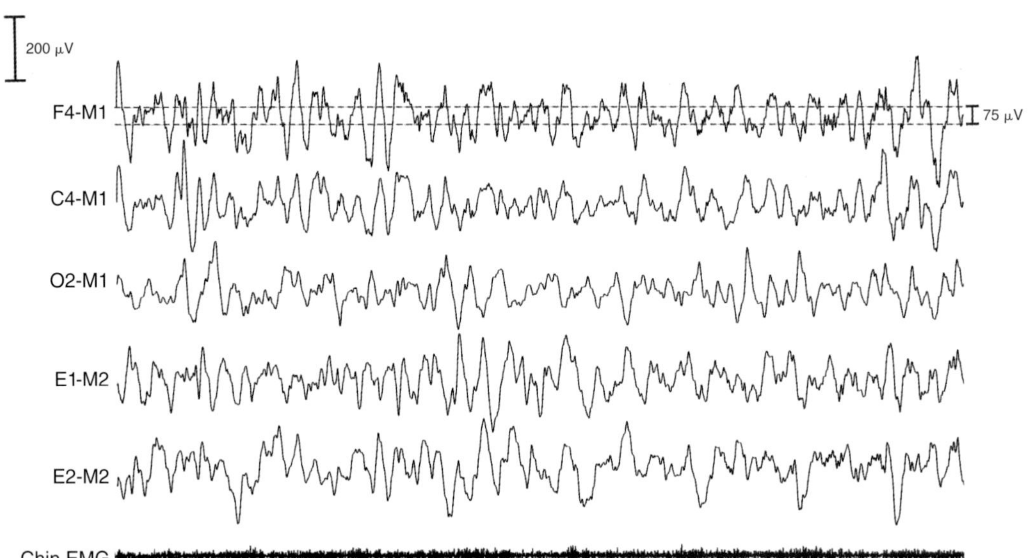

Figure 5–18 A 30-second epoch of stage N3 in a 3-year-old child. Nearly all of the electroencephalogram activity in F4-M1 meets criteria for slow wave activity (amplitude greater than 75 μV peak to peak, 0.5 to 2 Hz). (From Berry RB, Wagner MH. *Sleep Medicine Pearls.* 3rd ed. Elsevier; 2015:62.)

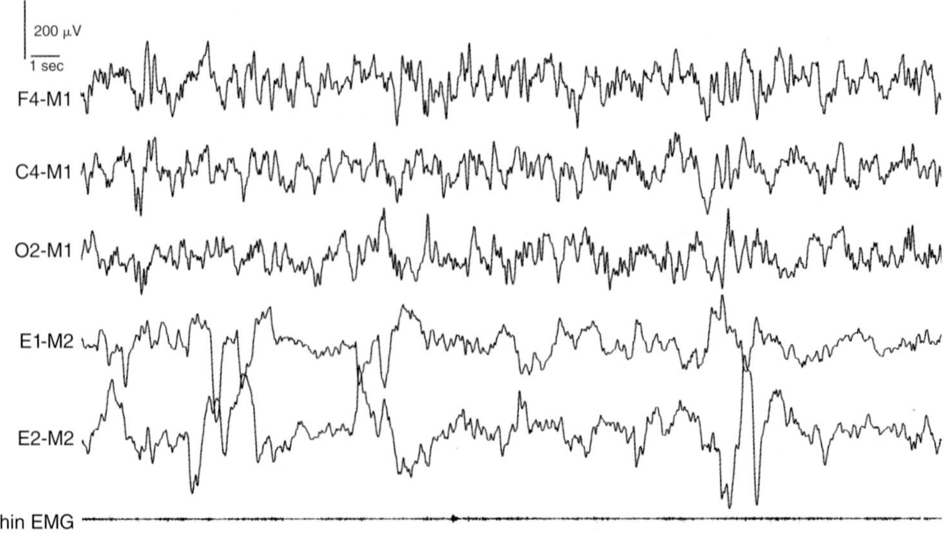

Figure 5–19 A 30-second epoch of stage R in a 5-year-old child. In children the electroencephalogram background activity during stage R often has a higher amplitude than that which is typical of stage R in adults.

SUMMARY OF KEY POINTS

1. For full-term infants aged 0 to 2 months (37–48 weeks PMA), sleep is staged using the AASM scoring rules for infants. The terms Quiet Sleep, Active Sleep, and Indeterminate Sleep used in the scoring rules of Anders, Emde, and Parmelee have been changed to stage N (NREM), stage R (REM), and transitional (stage T) sleep, respectively.
2. Scoring of sleep in infants is based on five characteristics: behavioral observation, respiration pattern, EEG pattern, EOG pattern, and chin EMG pattern.
3. Sleep spindles and the TA EEG pattern are found only in stage N (can be found in stage T if characteristics are discordant). The TA pattern evolves into HVS soon after birth in term infants.
4. Eye closure for more than 3 minutes in an infant is evidence of sleep.
5. The most important characteristic differentiating stage N and stage R in infants is respiration. Respiration is regular in stage N and irregular in stage R.
6. Pediatric sleep staging rules can be used to score sleep in children 2 month post-term and older.
7. Timing of appearance of characteristic EEG patterns of sleep (age post-term):
   - Sleep spindles (6 weeks to 3 months post-term)
   - Slow wave activity (2–5 months post-term)
   - K complex (3–6 months post-term; usually present at 5–6 months)
8. By age 6 months, stages N1, N2, and N3 can usually be scored (sometimes younger).
9. PDR is the dominant rhythm over the occipital regions in relaxed wakefulness with eyes closed. PDR is attenuated by eye opening.
10. The frequency of PDR increases with age, from around 4 Hz at 4 months to a mean of 9 Hz by age 9 years.
11. HH is high-voltage 3- to 4.5-Hz activity maximal in frontal and central derivations and is *used to identify the onset of stage N1 sleep in children who do not generate PDR with eye closure* (along with SEMs, vertex sharp waves, slowing of the EEG, and the presence of diffuse or occipital theta activity). HH is also present in children who generate PDR with eye closure, but in these children stage N1 is identified by PDR being replaced by LAMF EEG for most of the epoch. HH is most common in stage N1 but can occur in stage N2 sleep.
12. In children aged 2 months post-term or older stage W is scored when more that 50% of an epoch contains contains either or both of the following: age appropriate PDR (in individuals generating PDR with eye closure) or other findings consistent with stage W (all individuals) including eye blinks, reading eye movements, and REMs associated with high or normal chin msucle tone.
13. In children aged 2 month post-term or older stage N1 is scored if PDR is attenuated or replaced by LAMF activity for more than 50% of the epoch (individuals generating PDR with eye closure) or in individuals not generating PDR commencing with the earliest of the following: EEG activity 4 to 7 Hz (and 1 to 2 Hz slower than wake), slow eye movements, vertex sharp waves, hypnogogic hypersynchrony, or diffuse or occipital-predominant high amplitude 3 to 5 Hz EEG activity.
14. The rules for staging N2, N3, and R in childrens aged 2 months post-term or older are the same as for adults. However, the voltage of the EEG is much higher than in adults (even during stage R).

CLINICAL REVIEW QUESTIONS

1. Which of the following is true about stage R in a term infant age 1 month?
   A. Commonly the first epoch of sleep
   B. Respiration is regular
   C. Small jerks and facial twitches are **never** seen given atonia of REM sleep
   D. The first epoch of an episode of stage R may not contain REMs

2. Which of the following is true of HH?
   A. Required to score N1 in children generating PDR with eye closure
   B. A key feature for scoring N2
   C. Very high amplitude, stands out from EEG background
   D. Frequency usually 5 to 8 Hz

3. Which of the following EEG patterns is never found in an epoch of stage R?
   A. TA
   B. LVI
   C. M
   D. HVS

4. What is the typical sleep duration and duration of sleep cycles in a term infant age 1 month?
   A. Sleep duration 20 hours, duration of sleep cycles 60 minutes
   B. Sleep duration 16 hours, duration of sleep cycles 90 minutes
   C. Sleep duration 16 hours, duration of sleep cycles 45 minutes
   D. Sleep duration 20 hours, duration of sleep cycles 30 minutes

5. PSWs of youth occur in what sleep stage?
   A. Stage W
   B. Stage N1
   C. Stage N2
   D. Stage R

6. At what age post-term do sleep spindles appear?
   A. 6 weeks to 3 months
   B. 2 weeks to 4 months
   C. 3 to 4 months
   D. 4 to 5 months

7. In an infant 1 month of age, the following data are noted:

Characteristic	Pattern
EEG	LVI
Respiration	Irregular
Behavior	Eyes closed, small jerks
Chin EMG	Present, but less than stage W
Eyes	No REMs

What is the sleep stage?

8. Which of the following EEG patterns is not seen in a term infant of 1 month of age?
   A. TD
   B. TA
   C. LVI
   D. M

ANSWERS

1. **A.** In infants aged 0 to 2 months, post-term entry into sleep via stage R is the expected pattern. In stage R, respiration is irregular, small jerks and facial twitches are common, *and* the first epoch of a group of epochs scored as stage R must be definite stage R (contain REMs). Later epochs of definite stage R epochs can be scored as stage R without REMs as long as they meet the criteria in the stage R rule.
2. **C.** Stage N1 can be scored when PDR occupies less than 50% of an epoch and is replaced by LAMF activity (individuals generating PDR with eye closure). HH can be used to score the onset of N1 in individuals that do not generate PDR with eye closure. HH is high-amplitude activity with a frequency of 3.5 to 4.5 (5 Hz) and is characteristic of stage N1 but can occur in N2.
3. **A.** TA is present in stage N but never stage R. TA can also occur in stage T if the five characteristics are discordant (three N; two R or two N; three R). The typical EEG pattern of stage R is LVI, but M and rarely HVS can be seen.
4. **C.** The sleep duration in 24 hours is 16 to 18 hours, and the cycle time is about 45 minutes.
5. **A.** (stage W).
6. **A.** (6 weeks to 3 months).
7. Stage T. The EEG, respiration, and behavior are consistent with stage R, and the chin EMG and lack of REMs is consistent with stage N. Therefore, the properties are discordant.
8. **A.** TD is a pattern seen in premature infants. TA is seen in term infants and gradually converts to HVS as the infant matures.

SUGGESTED READING

Grigg-Damberger MM. The visual scoring of sleep in infants 0 to 2 months of age. *J Clin Sleep Med.* 2016;12(3):429-445.

Grigg-Damberger M, Gozal D, Marcus CL, et al. The visual scoring of sleep and arousal in infants and children. *J Clin Sleep Med.* 2007;3:201-240.

Troester MM, Quan SF, Berry RB, et al. *The AASM Manual for the Scoring of Sleep and Associated Events: Rules, Terminology and Technical Specifications. Version 3.* American Academy of Sleep Medicine; 2023.

REFERENCES

1. Troester MM, Quan SF, Berry RB, et al. *The AASM Manual for the Scoring of Sleep and Associated Events: Rules, Terminology and Technical Specifications. Version 3.* American Academy of Sleep Medicine; 2023.
2. Berry RB, Quan SF, Abreu AR, et al. *The AASM Manual for the Scoring of Sleep and Associated Events: Rules, Terminology and Technical Specifications. Version 2.6.* American Academy of Sleep Medicine; 2020.
3. Iber C, Ancoli-Israel S, Chesson AJ, Quan S. *The AASM Manual for the Scoring of Sleep and Associated Events: Rules, Terminology and Technical Specification.* American Academy of Sleep Medicine; 2007.
4. Engle WA, American Academy of Pediatrics Committee on Fetus and Newborn. Age terminology during the perinatal period. *Pediatrics.* 2004;114(5):1362-1364.
5. Grigg-Damberger M, Gozal D, Marcus CL, et al. The visual scoring of sleep and arousal in infants and children. *J Clin Sleep Med.* 2007;3:201-240.
6. Grigg-Damberger MM. The visual scoring of sleep in infants 0 to 2 months of age. *J Clin Sleep Med.* 2016;12(3):429-445.
7. Libenson MH. *Practical Approach to Electroencephalography.* Elsevier Saunders; 2010:321.
8. Anders T, Emde R, Parmelee A. *A Manual of Standardized Terminology, Techniques and Criteria for Scoring of Stages of Sleep and Wakefulness in Newborn Infants.* Brain Information Service, UCLA; 1971.
9. Sheldon S. Polysomnography in infants and children. In: Sheldon SH, Ferber R, Kryger MH, eds. *Principles and Practice of Pediatric Sleep Medicine.* Elsevier Saunders; 2005:49-71.
10. Kahn A, Dan B, Grosswasser J, et al. Normal sleep architecture in infants and children. *J Clin Neurophysiol.* 1996;13:184-297.
11. Iglowstein I, Jenni OG, Molinari L, Largo RH. Sleep duration from infancy to adolescence: reference values and generational trends. *Pediatrics.* 2003;111:302-307.
12. Montgomery-Downs HE, O'Brien LM, Gulliver TE, et al. Polysomnographic characteristics in normal preschool children. *Pediatrics.* 2006;117:741-753.

Normal Sleep Architecture in Adults

Chapter 6

SLEEP ARCHITECTURE TERMINOLOGY

A number of parameters concerning the quantity and quality of sleep are usually included in polysomnography (PSG) reports[1,2] (Table 6–1; Figure 6–1). Typically, PSG data recording starts before lights out to verify that the electrodes and monitoring equipment are providing adequate signals. In addition, calibrations and biocalibrations are recorded as described in Chapter 2. **Lights out time** is the time at which the patient is allowed to fall asleep and marks the start of the data that will be staged and analyzed. **Lights on time** is the time that analysis of the recording of sleep is terminated. However, most sleep centers continue actual recording until the electrodes and monitoring equipment are removed (including a biocalibration at the end of the study). **Total recording time** (TRT) is the time from lights out to lights on. The TRT is sometimes called the time in bed (TIB). The **sleep latency** is the time from lights out to the start of the first epoch of sleep. **Wake after sleep onset** (WASO) as defined by the *AASM Manual for the Scoring of Sleep and Associated Events: Rules, Terminology and Technical Specifications* (hereafter referred to as the AASM Scoring manual) includes all stage W after sleep onset (from the *start of the first epoch of sleep*) until lights on. The WASO also includes out-of-bed wake time during the period from sleep onset until lights on. The total amount of stage W (during TRT) = sleep latency + WASO. That is, TRT = sleep latency + WASO + TST. The rapid eye movement **(REM) latency** is the time from sleep onset until the *start of the first epoch of stage R*. The **total sleep time** (TST) is the total minutes spent in stages of sleep (N1, N2, N3, R). **Sleep efficiency** (SE, in %) is the (TST in minutes/TRT in minutes) × 100. The AASM scoring manual also recommends presentation of the durations of the sleep stages both as an absolute duration and as a percentage of TST. The terminology for sleep stages changed from 1, 2, 3, 4, and REM in the manual of Rechtschaffen and Kales (R&K)[3] to N1, N2, N3, and R in the AASM scoring manual.[1] Stages 3 and 4 are combined into N3. Stages N1, N2, and N3 compose non–rapid eye movement (NREM) sleep and, for staging, REM sleep is referred to as stage R. Although the sleep architecture parameters listed in Table 6–1 are useful, they obviously do not convey details about the pattern of sleep over the night. Hypnograms can be very informative, and many sleep centers include a hypnogram in their sleep report. The hypnogram is a graphical representation stage of sleep versus clock time. Stage W and each stage of sleep are assigned levels (Figure 6–1). In this figure the sleep latency, REM latency, and TRT are depicted. The hypnogram in Figure 6–1 illustrates normal sleep and shows that sleep occurs in cycles of NREM-REM sleep with most stage N3 in the first cycles of sleep. As the night progresses the amount of stage N3 decreases and stage R increases.

Previously, some clinicians used the term "sleep period time" (SPT) (Figure 6–1), defined as the time from sleep onset to the final awakening.[4-7] That is, the SPT is the number of minutes from the first to the last epoch scored as stage N1, N2, N3, or R. WASO was then defined as the duration of wake during the sleep period time ($WASO_{SPT}$). That is, $WASO_{SPT}$ = SPT − TST, where TST = total sleep time. This allowed WASO to be expressed as a percentage of SPT. The AASM scoring manual uses a different definition of WASO and does not use the SPT as a standard parameter. However, a considerable number of publications previously used SPT and $WASO_{SPT}$ (formerly identified as WASO), so the reader should be familiar with this terminology.[4-7] Some authors previously presented the sleep stages as a percentage of SPT. The arousal index (ArI) is the number of arousals × 60/TST

Table 6–1 Sleep Architecture Parameters

Parameter	Clinical Example 1		Clinical Example 2	
	Male Age 25 Years		**Male Age 65 Years**	
Lights out time	10:30 PM		10:30 PM	
Lights on time	6:00 AM		6:00 AM	
Total recording time (TRT) (min)	450		450	
Total sleep time (TST) (min)	430		390	
Sleep latency (min)	5		20	
REM latency (min)	90		75	
Sleep efficiency (%)	95		87	
Stage W (min)	20		60	
Wake after sleep onset (WASO) (min)	15		40	
Sleep Stages	(min)	%TST	(min)	%TST
Stage N1	10	2.3	30	7.7
Stage N2	240	55.8	265	68
Stage N3	80	18.6	15	3.8
Stage R	100	23.2	80	20.5
Arousal Index (#/hour)	5		15	

Arousal index = number of arousals/hour of sleep, see text for parameter definitions

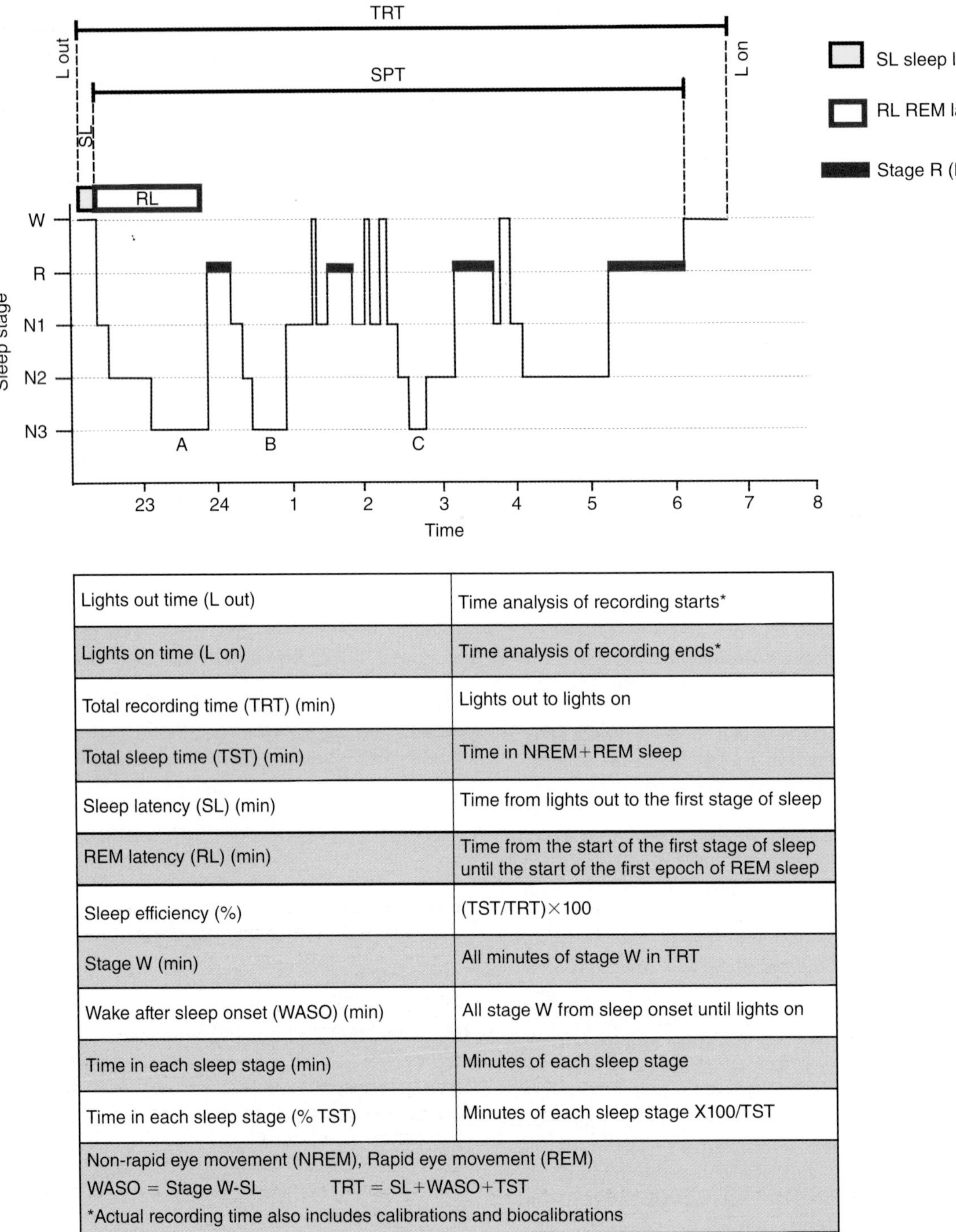

Lights out time (L out)	Time analysis of recording starts*
Lights on time (L on)	Time analysis of recording ends*
Total recording time (TRT) (min)	Lights out to lights on
Total sleep time (TST) (min)	Time in NREM+REM sleep
Sleep latency (SL) (min)	Time from lights out to the first stage of sleep
REM latency (RL) (min)	Time from the start of the first stage of sleep until the start of the first epoch of REM sleep
Sleep efficiency (%)	(TST/TRT)×100
Stage W (min)	All minutes of stage W in TRT
Wake after sleep onset (WASO) (min)	All stage W from sleep onset until lights on
Time in each sleep stage (min)	Minutes of each sleep stage
Time in each sleep stage (% TST)	Minutes of each sleep stage X100/TST
Non-rapid eye movement (NREM), Rapid eye movement (REM) WASO = Stage W-SL TRT = SL+WASO+TST *Actual recording time also includes calibrations and biocalibrations	

Figure 6–1 A hypnogram showing a normal sleep pattern in a young adult. Time from Lights out (L out) to Lights on (L on) is the period of time sleep is staged and analyzed TRT (total recording time). The sleep latency *(SL)* and REM latency *(RL)* are depicted. There are four NREM/REM cycles. Stage N3 is confined to the first part of the night and (A > B > C) showing the longest episode of stage N3 is in the first cycle. The episodes of REM sleep increase in duration over the night with the longest period usually in the early morning. The sleep period time *(SPT)* is the time from the first sleep until the final awakening. The definitions of sleep architecture parameters are listed below the hypnogram.

in minutes. The total number of arousals and ArI are included in PSG reports. Other parameters not routinely used include the number of sleep stage shifts, the latency to persistent sleep (time from lights out to the first 10-minute period containing less than 2 minutes of wakefulness or stage N1 sleep) and the latency to unequivocal sleep (time from lights out to three consecutive epochs of N1 or an epoch of stage N2, N3, or R).

NORMAL SLEEP IN ADULTS

Sleep occurs in cycles, each usually composed of a period of NREM sleep followed by a period of REM sleep. In adults the first sleep NREM/REM cycle lasts from 70 to 100 minutes, whereas later sleep cycles are 90 to 120 minutes in duration.[8] For the entire night, the average NREM/REM cycle is

Box 6–1 SLEEP ARCHITECTURE FACTS

- Three to five sleep (NREM-REM) cycles during the night
- First sleep cycle ≈70 to 100 minutes in duration
- Later sleep cycles ≈90 to 120 minutes in duration
- Stage N3
  - Most stage N3 is during the first half of the night
  - Delta power usually decreases with each NREM cycle
- Stage R
  - Episodes of stage R are longer in the second part of the night
  - REM density (number of eye movements per time during REM sleep) is higher in the later episodes of REM sleep

NREM, Non–rapid eye movement; *REM,* rapid eye movement.

about 90 to 110 minutes. There are usually three to five NREM-REM cycles per night (Box 6–1). In contrast to the hypnogram in Figure 6–1, a less ideal night of sleep is illustrated in Figure 6–2. The sleep latency is prolonged, there is no REM sleep in the first sleep cycle, the amount of stage N3 is decreased, and stage W is increased with nine brief awakenings during the night.

Sleep architecture is a term used to denote the structure of sleep. In young adults, stage N1 usually occupies approximately 5% to 10% of the TST.[8] It is a transitional state between wake and the other stages of sleep. Stage N2 occupies the greatest proportion of the TST and accounts for approximately 50% to 60% of sleep. Stage N3 occupies approximately 15% to 20% of the TST in young adults and stage R occupies approximately 20% to 25% of the TST. The amplitude of the slow waves (0.5 to 2 Hz) and amount of stage N3 is greatest in the first sleep cycle (A in Figure 6–1). Recall slow wave activity (SWA) for sleep staging is EEG activity in F4-M1 that has a peak to peak amplitude > 75 μV and a frequency of 0.5 to 2 Hz. Stage N3 has SWA ≥ 6 seconds (20%) in each epoch. Using power spectral analysis, one can compute the delta power (usually defined as the power in the 0.5 to 4 Hz range of electroencephalographic [EEG] activity) (Figure 6–3A). The delta power (an estimate of the contribution of this frequency range to the power of the total EEG signal in units of μV^2) is usually the highest during the initial cycle of NREM sleep. Higher delta power is associated with a greater duration of slow wave activity (SWA) (see Figure 6–3B). For example, 15 to 30 seconds of SWA in typical epochs of stage N3 in the first NREM cycle but 6 to 15 seconds in typical epochs of stage N3 later in the night. The episodes of stage R occur about every 90 to 120 minutes, and they are usually of longer duration as the night progresses (Figure 6–1). The **REM density** is the number of eye movements per time. The REM density tends to be highest in the later REM periods.[9] In fact, the initial REM period of the night is often difficult to score owing to infrequent REMs. The first REM period may have K complexes or sleep spindles with low chin electromyogram (EMG) mixed with one or more REMs. The AASM scoring manual[1] provides detailed rules for scoring such epochs (see Chapter 3). In general, an isolated K complex or sleep spindle during a segment that otherwise meets criteria for stage R is scored as stage R. During the last half of the night, most sleep is composed of stage N2 and stage R with intervening W and stage N1 (Figures 6-1 and 6-2). Although more than 50% of total sleep time is composed of stage N2, stage N2 epochs can be very different with one epoch having a SWA duration of 0 seconds and another 5 seconds (just shy of qualifying for stage N3).

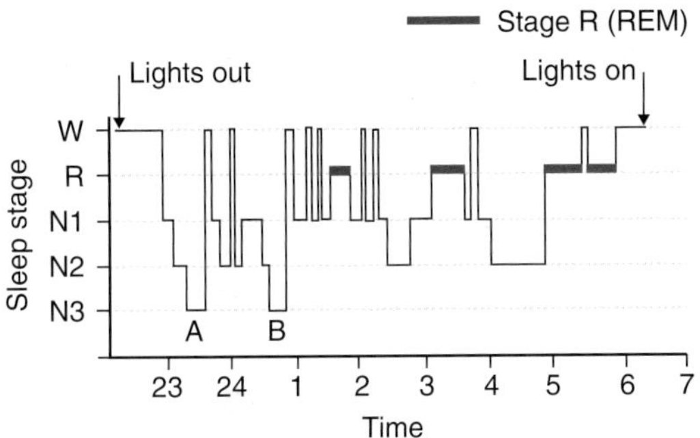

Figure 6–2 This is a hypnogram of a patient with fragmented sleep. The sleep latency is increased (compare with Figure 6–1). The first NREM cycle is not followed by an episode of stage R. Therefore, there is a long REM latency. Multiple periods of awakening (stage W episodes are noted). The amount of stage N1 is increased. Only two episodes of stage N3 are noted (A, B).

Changes in Sleep Architecture With Aging in Adults

Many studies have analyzed sleep architecture in normal populations with variable results (Tables 6-2 and 6-3).[4-7,10-15] Some expressed the sleep stage duration as a percentage of sleep period time.[4-7] Some of the studies combined men and women for the primary analysis but then analyzed differences between the sexes.[11] In most analyses there were relatively few individuals in the older age groups. The studies published before 2007[11,12] scored sleep using the Rechtschaffen and Kales criteria.[3] Some of the new studies[6,13,14] used the AASM scoring manual rules.[1]

There is a consistent decrease in the sleep efficiency over the entire age range up to and beyond age 90 years.[11] Most other age-dependent changes in sleep architecture occur before the age of 60 years, with relatively minor changes in stage N3, REM sleep, and stage N1 percentage after that age. A summary of changes in overall sleep architecture based on two large studies is given in Table 6–2[1,2] and a summary of findings from multiple studies in Table 6–3.[8-14] A summary of changes can be visualized looking at a figure from the study by Ohayon et al.[11] (Figure 6–4). Of note, this analysis comprised studies in which sleep was staged using the scoring rules of Rechtschaffen and Kales[3] rather than the AASM scoring manual. The study of sleep architecture in older adults is complicated by inclusion of individuals with medical or mental disorders in some studies of the effect of aging on sleep architecture. Many studies did not include a sufficient number of women or older individuals. This is important as the data at the lower and upper limits of the age spectrum can influence the regression line or analysis of the effect of age on a given sleep architecture parameter. Ohayon et al.[11] performed a large meta-analysis of sleep architecture and attempted to determine the effect of age on different sleep parameters with and without exclusion of patients with mental diseases that could alter sleep architecture. Data were fit to an exponential line reflecting the changes in a given parameter versus age. Redline et al.[12] published another analysis of the effects of age on sleep architecture in a large group of individuals in the Sleep Heart Health Study (ages 37–92).

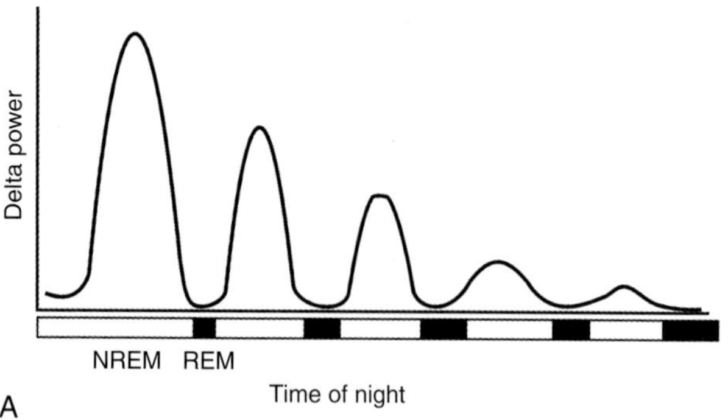

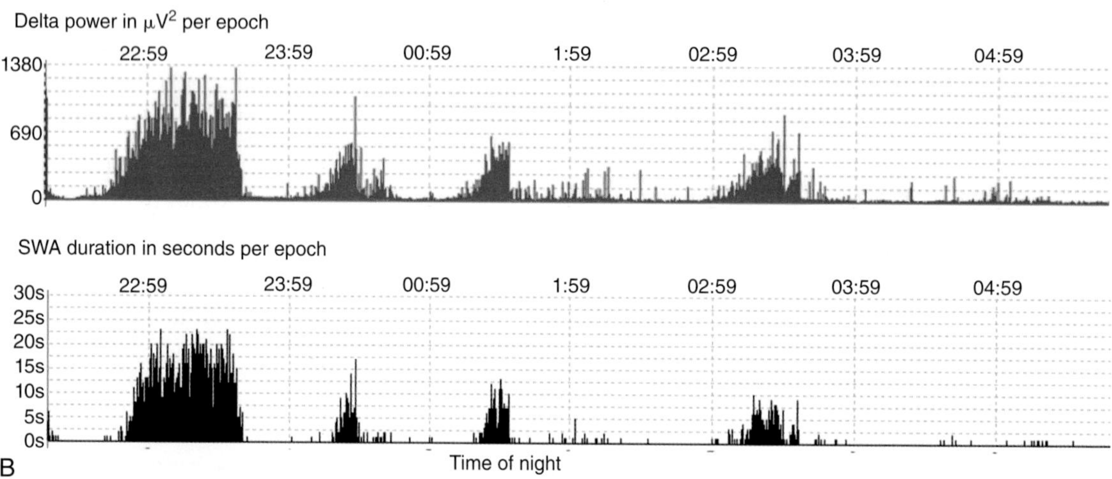

Figure 6–3 (A) An idealized schematic illustrating decreasing delta power during the five sleep cycles across the night. Higher delta power is associated with increased amplitude and duration of slow wave activity (SWA) in the electroencephalogram (EEG). The delta power is derived using fast Fourier analysis of the EEG from the derivation F4-M1. Note that the delta power is low during stage R (REM), which is characterized by low-amplitude mixed-frequency EEG activity with minimal SWA. (B) Actual delta power for each epoch in μV^2 for the first four NREM cycles in the top tracings and SWA duration (seconds) for each epoch in the lower tracing. Higher delta power is associated with a greater duration SWA. The delta power is much higher in the first cycle in this patient but similar in the next 3 cycles. In other individuals, there is a progressive decrease in delta power over the night in periods of NREM sleep as illustrated in the idealized schematic (A).

Table 6–2 Changes in Sleep Architecture With Age

Increase With Age	Decrease With Age
Sleep latency*	Sleep efficiency*
WASO (most change after 40 yr)*	TST*
Stage N1 (%TST)*	Stage N3 (%TST)*
Stage N1 (%TST), men only†	Stage N3 (%TST), men only†
Stage N2 (%TST)*	Stage R (%TST)*,†
Stage N2 (%TST), men only†	REM latency*

REM, Rapid-eye movement; *TST*, total sleep time; *WASO*, wake after sleep onset.
*Ohayon MM, Carskadon MA, Guillemenault C, Vitiello MV. Meta-analysis of quantitative sleep parameters from childhood to old age in healthy individuals: developing normative sleep values across the human lifespan. *Sleep*. 2004;27(7):1255-1273.
†Redline S, Kirchner L, Quan S, et al. The effects of age, sex, ethnicity, and sleep-disordered breathing on sleep architecture. *Arch Intern Med*. 2004;164:406-418.

Participants were excluded from the analysis if there was a history of sleep-altering medications, heavy alcohol use, or other disorders known to disrupt sleep. In this analysis separate findings were presented for men and women. PSG was performed at home and central and occipital derivations were used to score sleep. Van Cauter et al.[5] also published findings concerning the age-related changes in slow wave and REM sleep in healthy men. Moraes et al.[13] analyzed 1024 normal individuals ages 20 to 80 years from a population in Brazil. Boulos et al.[14] performed a meta-analysis of studies determining sleep architecture using 5273 participants. The results for some sleep architecture parameters differ between the studies. Some had relatively few individuals in the older age groups. Results are often presented as the mean ± 1 standard deviation (SD) for different age ranges or give the results of regression analysis. It is difficult to establish a normal range for a given age range for a given parameter as the data is often not normally distributed, and if the lower limit is defined as the mean minus 2 SDs, the lower limit would be a negative number. A few studies[6,7] analyzed cohorts of normal individuals and derived percentile curves for standard sleep stage parameters to help define an expected range of values for a given age group. A normal range might be defined as values between the 10th and 90th percentiles. In the following sections, the changes in specific sleep parameters with age will be discussed. A previously noted, the findings are summarized in Tables 6-2 and 6-3.

Table 6–3 Summary of Changes in Sleep Architecture With Age From Different Studies

Study	Ohayon[11]	Redline[12]	Moraes[13]	Boulos[14]	Mitterling[6*]
N	3577	2683	1024	5273	100
Publication Year	2004	2004	2014	2019	2015
TST	Decrease	–	Decrease (M, F)	Decrease	Decrease
Sleep efficiency	Decrease	Decrease	Decrease (M, F)	Decrease	Decrease
REM latency	**Decrease**	**–**	**Increase (F)**	**No change**	**Trend for decrease until age 60 then increase for age > 60 years (*P* = .098)**
Sleep latency (min)	Increase	–	Increase (M, F)	Increase (small)	No change
WASO (min)	Increase	–	Increase (M, F)	Increase	Increase
Arousal index	–	Increase	Increase (M, F)	Increase	No change
Stage N1(%TST)	Increase	Increase (M)	Increase (M, F)	Increase	No change*
Stage N2 (%TST)	Increase	Increase (M)	Increase (M)	No change	No change*
Stage N3 (%TST)	Decrease	Decrease (M)	Decrease (M)	No change	Decrease*
Stage R (%TST)	Decrease	Decrease	Decrease (F)	No change	Decrease*

*Analysis as %SPT; M, male; F, female.
F, female; *M*, male; *REM*, Rapid eye movement; *SPT*, sleep period time; *TST*, total sleep time; *WASO*, wake after sleep onset; – not analyzed, if M/ F not specified analysis combined men and women

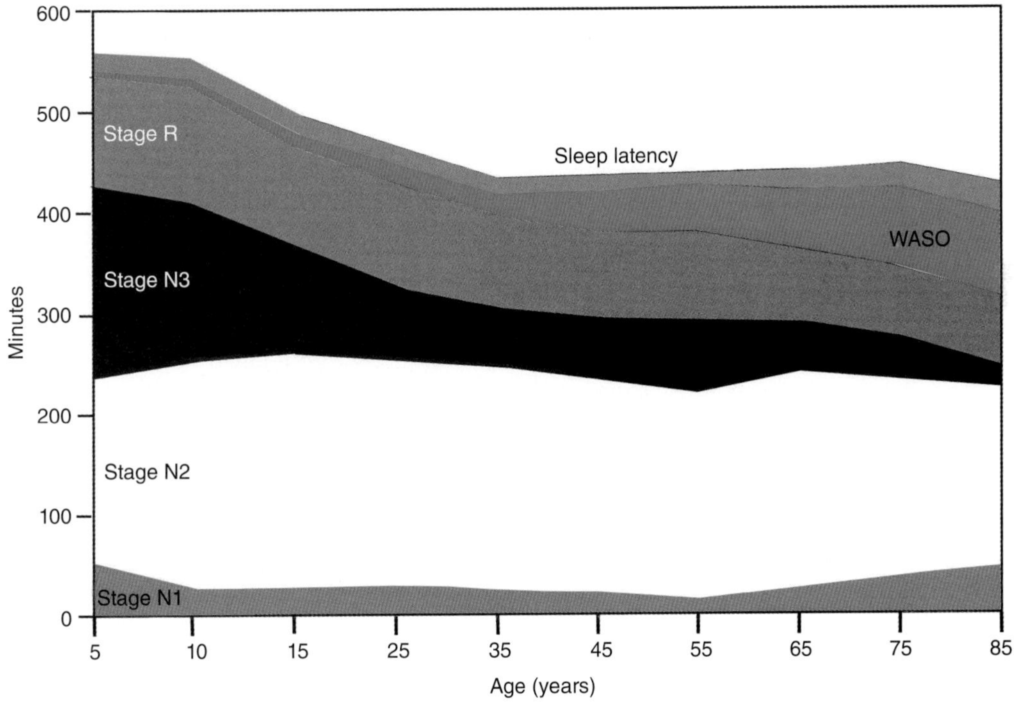

Figure 6–4 Age related trends for stages N1, N3, N3, R as well as sleep latency and wake after sleep onset (WASO) in minutes. The major changes are an increase in WASO and decrease in stage N3 with increasing age. More recent studies suggest that the decrease in stage N3 occurs in men but not women. There is a slight decrease in the amount of REM sleep, whereas the sleep latency changes very little until it increases slightly in the older age groups. (From Ohayon MM, Carskadon MA, Guilleminault C, Vitiello MV. Meta-analysis of quantitative sleep parameters from childhood to old age in healthy individuals: developing normative sleep values across the lifespan. *Sleep.* 2004;27(7):1255-1273.)

Sleep Latency and REM Latency

In the meta-analysis by Ohayon et al.,[11] when studies that included individuals with sleep and medical disorders were excluded, *sleep latency increased only minimally* from ages 20 to 80 (~10 minutes) (Figure 6–5A). If those patients with sleep and medical disorders were included, there was not a significant change in sleep latency with age. This is consistent with more reports of early morning awakening rather than sleep onset problems in the healthy elderly. In general, a sleep latency of 30 minutes or more is considered abnormal. In the same meta-analysis, Ohayon et al. found *REM latency decreased with* age (Figure 6–5B). However, the largest

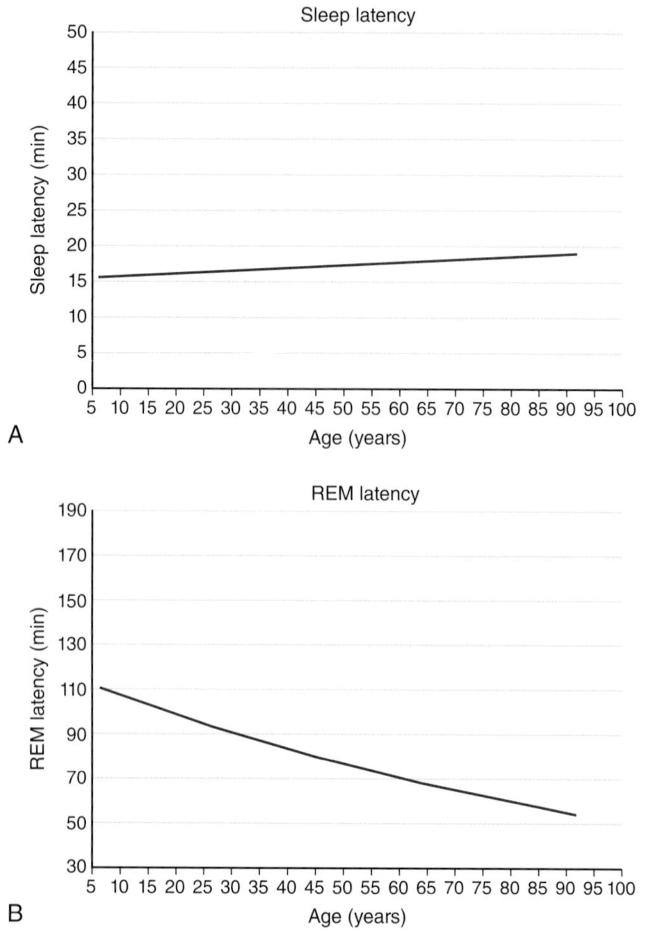

Figure 6–5 (A) The sleep latency across age groups. The sleep latency shows a very slight increase in age. In general, a sleep latency greater than 30 minutes is considered abnormal in any age group. (B) The REM latency decreases with age. In older individuals, values in the 50- to 70-minute range may be normal. The lines in A and B represent an exponential equation fit of the data. (Graphs A and B plotted from data from Ohayon MM, Carskadon MA, Guillemenault C, Vitiello MBV. Meta-analysis of quantitative sleep parameters from childhood to old age in healthy individuals: developing normative sleep values across the human lifespan. *Sleep.* 2004;27(7):1255-1273.)

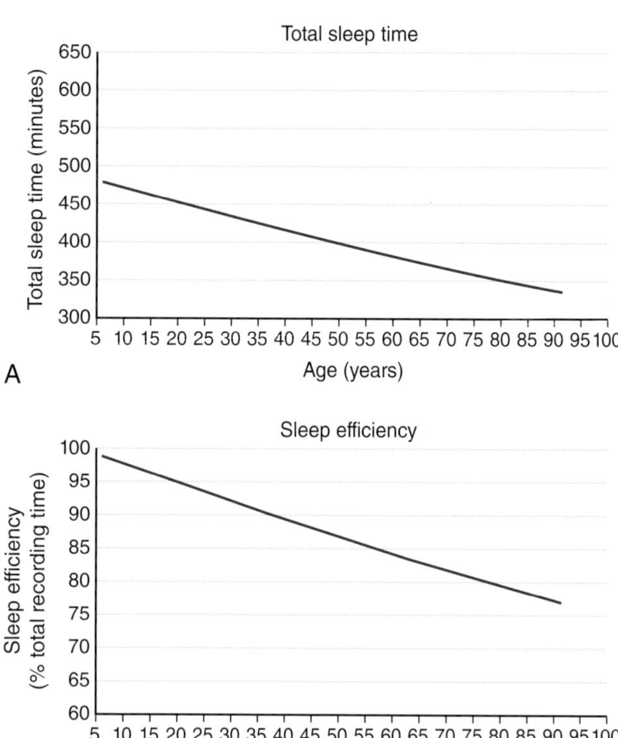

Figure 6–6 (A) The total sleep time decreases with age with the biggest decrease from childhood to adolescence. There was no change between the 60- to 70-year age group and older patients (age > 70). (B) Sleep efficiency decreases with age showing a progressive significant decrease across all age groups. The lines represent the exponential equations fitted to the data. (Graphs A and B were plotted using data from Ohayon MM, Carskadon MA, Guillemenault C, Vitiello MV. Meta-analysis of quantitative sleep parameters from childhood to old age in healthy individuals: developing normative sleep values across the human lifespan. *Sleep.* 2004;27(7):1255-1273.)

decrease was from childhood to adolescence. Boulos et al. did not find a decrease in the REM latency with age.[14] In contrast, the study of Moraes et al. found the REM latency to change with age only in women (an increase).[13] In summary, the REM latency likely decreases slightly with age, but the magnitude of the effect is relatively small in the older age groups.

TST and Sleep Efficiency

TST decreases with age as does the sleep efficiency [(TST/TRT) × 100][10-14] (Figure 6–6). There tends to be a more rapid decrease in TST from childhood to adolescence and then a slower decrease from age 20 to 80 years. Sleep efficiency decreases most rapidly after age 50.[11] Of interest, Ohayon et al.[11] found no change in TST between the elderly (60 to 70 years) compared with old elderly (>70 years) individuals. However, there was a significant decrease in sleep efficiency from elderly to old elderly. As previously noted, *sleep efficiency shows a consistent decrease with age in adults over the entire life span.*

Wake After Sleep Onset (WASO)

In the meta-analysis by Ohayon et al.,[11] WASO (minutes) increased from ages 20 to 60 years (Figure 6–7). The largest increase is in the older age groups. The meta-analysis by Boulos also found an increase in the WASO for men and women.[14]

Stage N1 (as a Percentage of TST)

In the meta-analysis by Ohayon et al.,[11] stage N1 (as %TST) increased from ages 20 to 60 years (Figure 6–8A). In the analysis by Redline et al.,[12] the amount of stage N1 (%TST) increased with age in men but not women (Figure 6–9A). In the study of Moraes et al., stage N1 (%TST) increased with age in both men and women.[13] The meta-analysis by Boulos also found an increase stage N1 as a percentage of TST with increasing age (men and women combined).[14]

Stage N2 (as a Percentage of TST)

In the meta-analysis by Ohayon et al.,[11] the amount of stage N2 as a percentage of TST increased with age (combined men and women) (Figure 6–8B). Redline et al.[12] found stage N2 as a percentage of TST to increase with age in men but not women (Figure 6–9B). This is consistent with the findings of a decrease in stage N3 (%TST) with age in men but not women in their study, as discussed in the next section. The amount of stage N2 (%TST) was higher in men than in

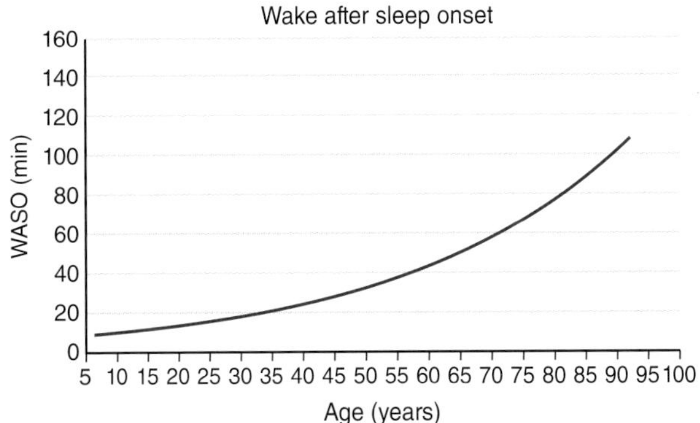

Figure 6–7 The change with wake after sleep onset (WASO) with age is depicted. WASO increased with age especially after 60 years. The line represents the exponential equation fitted to the data. (Plotted from data from Ohayon MM, Carskadon MA, Guillemenault C, Vitiello MV. Meta-analysis of quantitative sleep parameters from childhood to old age in healthy individuals: developing normative sleep values across the human lifespan. *Sleep.* 2004;27(7):1255-1273.)

women when all age groups were considered. Moraes et al. found an increase in stage N2 (%TST) with age only in men.[13] In general, if stage N2 (%TST) increases with age, it is associated with a decrease in stage N3 (%TST).

Stage N3 (as a Percentage of TST)

In the large meta-analysis by Ohayon et al.[11] the amount of stage N3 decreased with age (men and women combined) (Figure 6–8C). The effect size was greater in men than in women. In the study by Redline et al.,[12] the amount of stage N3 (%TST) decreased with age only in men (Figure 6–9C). The decrease in stage N3 in men was associated with increases in stage N1 and N2 as a percentage of total sleep time. For the entire group of women (all ages) the amount of stage N3 (%TST) was higher in women compared with men. The values for stage N3 (%TST) in the older age groups were higher than noted in the study of Ohayon et al.[11] Van Cauter also found a decrease in stage N3 in men (as %SPT).[5]

Stage R (as a Percentage of TST)

Ohayon et al.[11] found a decrease in stage R with age (men and women combined) (Figure 6–8D). Most of the decrease in REM as a percentage of TST was noted between 10 and 35 years of age. In the data from Redline et al.,[12] there was a small but statistically significant decrease in stage R with age for both men and women (Figure 6–9D). Men and women did not differ in the rate of decrease. Moraes et al.[13] found a decrease in stage R (%TST) with age only in women but Boulos et al. found no change in either sex.[14] Van Cauter et al. found a decrease in stage R (%SPT) in men but only after age 50.[5] Floyd et al.[15] found a linear decrease in REM (%TST) with age until the mid-70s, after which there was a small increase in REM (%TST) due to increased minutes of stage R and a decrease in TST.

Sleep Architecture (as a Percentage of SPT)

Van Cauter et al.[5] published information on sleep architecture in normal men. They found an increase in stage W but minimal change in combined Stage N1 and N2 with age. The sleep stage data were expressed as a percentage of sleep period time.

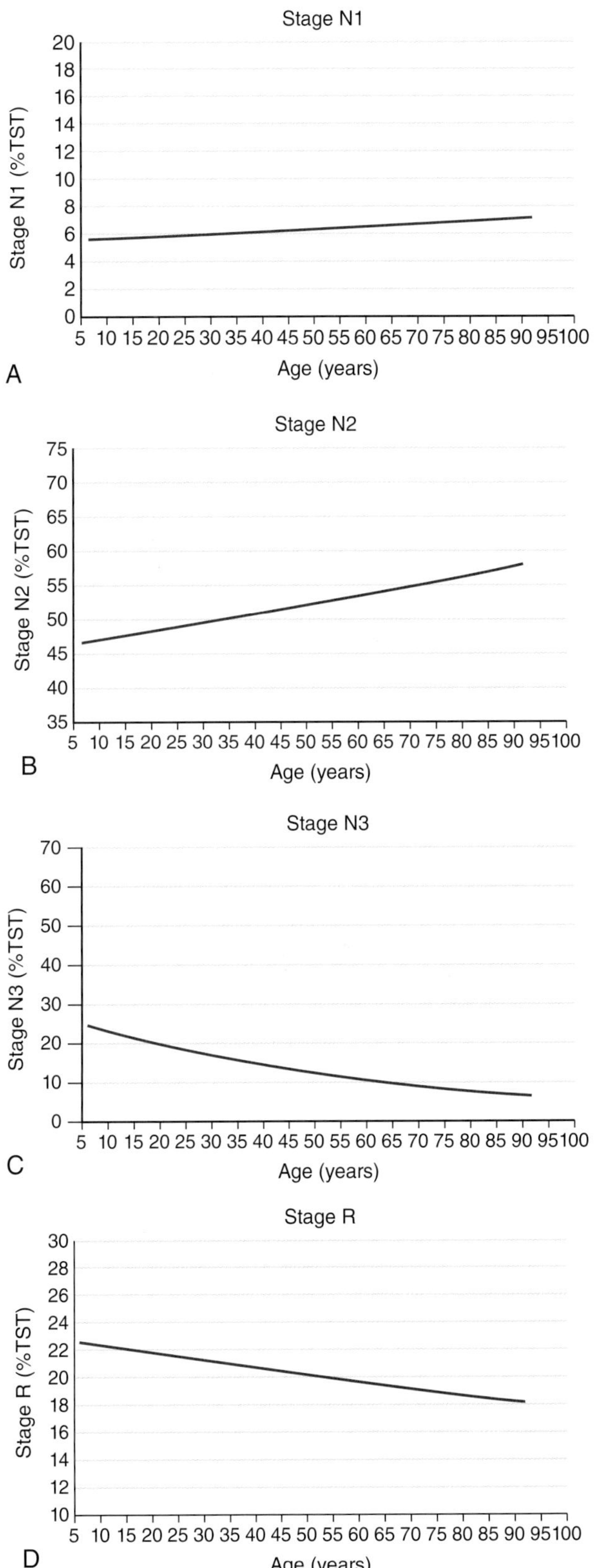

Figure 6–8 (A) Stage N1 (%TST) increases slightly with age (data from men and women combined). (B) Stage N2 (%TST) shows an increase with age. (C) Stage N3 (%TST) decreases with age. (D) Stage R (%TST) decreases with age. In A–D, data from men and women are combined. The lines represent the exponential equations fitted to the data. (A–D drawn from data from Ohayon MM, Carskadon MA, Guillemenault C, Vitiello MV. Meta-analysis of quantitative sleep parameters from childhood to old age in healthy individuals: developing normative sleep values across the human lifespan. *Sleep.* 2004;27(7):1255-1273.)

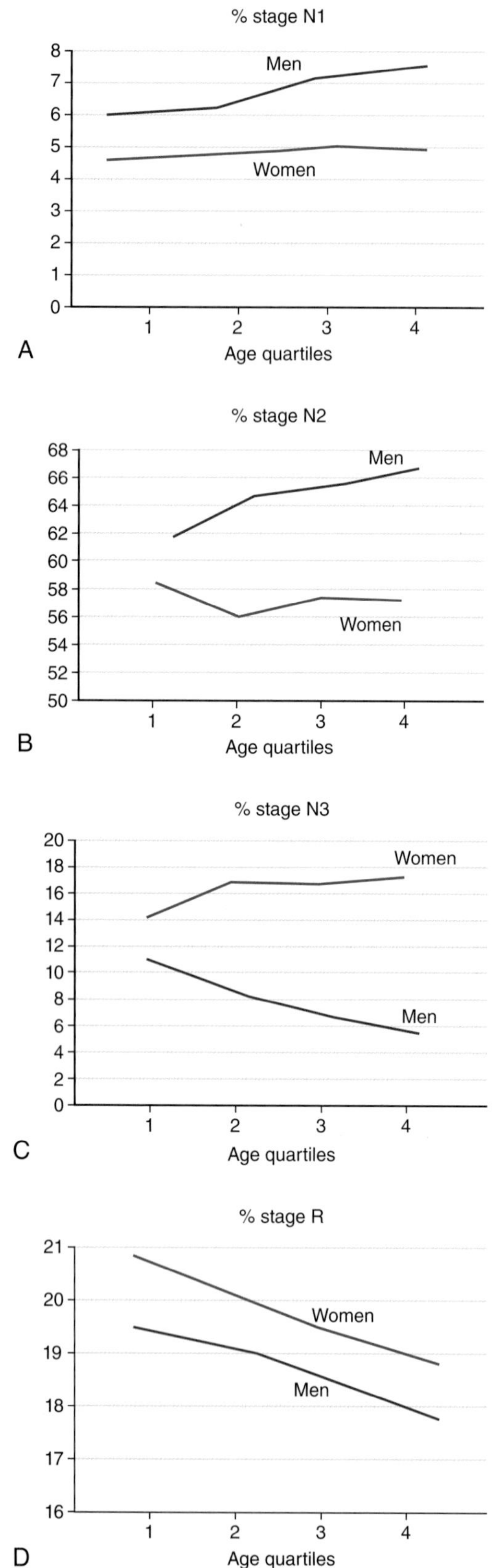

Figure 6–9 Changes in stage N1 (A), stage N2 (B), stage N3 (C), and stage R (D) as a percentage of total sleep time across age quartiles. Stages N1 and N2 increase and stage N3 decreases in men but not women. Stage R decreases slightly with age, but the change is similar in men and women. The lines represent plots of least square means for age quartiles (Q1 ≤ 54 years, Q2 > 54 to ≤ 61 years, Q3 > 61 to ≤ 70 years, Q4 > 70 years). (Drawn from data from Redline S, Kirchner L, Quan S, et al. The effects of age, sex, ethnicity, and sleep-disordered breathing on sleep architecture. *Arch Intern Med.* 2004;164:406-418.)

They also found a decrease in stage N3 with age and a decrease in stage R (%SPT) most prominent after age 50.

GENDER DIFFERENCES IN SLEEP ARCHITECTURE

The large meta-analysis by Ohayon et al. found that men had higher mean values of TST, sleep latency, stage N3 (%TST), REM (%TST), and the REM latency.[11] The finding for stage N3 is not consistent with most other studies and is likely due to the composition of the studies analyzed or the methods. Stage N2 (%TST) and WASO were higher in women. In contrast, the analysis of Redline et al.[12] found men to have higher stage N1 (%TST) and stage N2 (%TST) and lower stage N3 (%TST) in the older age quartiles. Men but not women had a significant decrease in stage N3 (%TST) with increasing age. Both men and women had a small decrease in stage R (%TST) with age, but the values did not differ between men and women. This study had the advantage of directly comparing men and women recruited for a single study.[12] Boulos et al.[14] found an increase in sleep latency with older age in women but not men. In summary, there is conflicting evidence concerning the effect of gender on sleep architecture. However, it appears that stage N3 decreases in men more than women with age, and this is associated with larger amounts of stage N1 (%TST) and N2 (%TST) in some studies. There appears to be no clinically significant difference in men and women with respect to REM sleep.

FIRST-NIGHT EFFECT

The first-night effect was described by Agnew et al.[16] from analysis of individuals undergoing multiple sleep studies. The phenomenon consists of lower sleep efficiency (more wakefulness), lower amount of REM sleep, and longer REM latency on the first night in the sleep center. Patients may also miss the first episodes of REM sleep (an initial NREM cycle without stage R) (Figure 6–2). A meta-analysis of subjects used as controls in several studies found a first-night effect with lower stage 4 (used older classification in which N3 divided into stage 3 and 4), lower stage N2, and a lower sleep efficiency on the first night of multiple-night studies.[17]

COMPARISON OF SLEEP STAGING BETWEEN THE AASM SCORING MANUAL AND RECHTSCHAFFEN AND KALES

Given that most previous work on sleep architecture was based on the scoring manual of R&K,[3] normative values could be altered by the new AASM scoring manual scoring rules. Sleep staging by R&K used only central derivations, and scoring rules differed. Therefore, studies comparing sleep architecture between R&K and the AASM scoring manual were needed. Moser et al.[18] found that sleep latency, REM latency, TST, and sleep efficiency were not affected (similar in AASM and R&K). The amounts of stage N1 and N3 increased in absolute duration and as a percentage of TST using AASM scoring criteria compared with those of R&K. The amount of stage N2 increased in absolute duration and as a percentage of TST using AASM scoring criteria. WASO also increased slightly with AASM versus R&K rules (mean increase of 4 minutes). Stage R differed but was age dependent being slightly higher in absolute duration and as a percentage of TST using AASM scoring rules only in older individuals. The higher amount of stage N3 using AASM scoring rules would be expected with the use of frontal derivations to assess SWA (slow waves have higher amplitude in frontal compared to central derivations). Danker-Hopfe et al.[19] compared interscorer reliability between the AASM and the R&K criteria and found slightly better agreement with the AASM criteria, although the difference was small.

AROUSAL INDEX

The AASM scoring manual[1] recommends reporting of the total of arousals and ArI in sleep reports. Many sleep centers also report arousals associated with respiratory events, periodic limb movements in sleep, snoring or respiratory effort–related arousals, and spontaneous arousals. Arousals can result in nonrestorative sleep even in the absence of a decrement in TST. The ArI (number of arousals/hour of sleep) in normal individuals increases with age (Figure 6–10).[20-23] Bonnet and Arand[20] found the ArI in 61- to 70-year-old individuals to be 21.9 ± 6.8/hr (mean ± SD). Therefore, the 95% confidence limits may slightly exceed 30/hr in older age groups Conversely, an ArI of 25/hr would be high for a young adult (Figure 6-10).

DEFINING A NORMAL RANGE

When reading a sleep study, some guidance on whether or not a sleep architecture parameter is within a normal range for a given age group could be helpful, but establishing a normal range is challenging. Most sleep reports do not provide a normal range, and some physicians would object to the idea of defining a normal range for individuals being studied for suspected sleep pathology. Individual sleep centers have different schedules for typical lights out and lights on. In addition, one would **not** expect overall sleep architecture to be similar for diagnostic, positive airway pressure titrations and split-night studies. There is also a first-night effect for many patients. Published studies of normative sleep architecture targeted nonclinical populations, and the results may not be relevant to the populations being studied in sleep centers. Even using the data from large studies is challenging as the data for a given parameter (e.g., total sleep time for men aged 40–50 years) may not be normally distributed, and using the mean ± 2 SDs for some sleep architecture parameters may result in a number less than zero. One option for defining a normal range would be to use percentile values and define normal as between the 10th and 90th percentile values. However, outliers are still a problem and may result in a lower or higher limit of normal for a parameter that does not seem to correspond to clinical experience. Mitterling et al.[6] presented data from their study of sleep in 100 normal individuals (AASM scoring manual criteria) using the 10th- and 90th-percentile approach; examples for total sleep time and the ArI are given in Figure 6–11. The plot of the ArI shows the 90th-percentile values suddenly decreasing at the highest age group. This does not seem consistent with data from other studies and could be due to the existence of few individuals in the higher age range. One can also appreciate that the width of the ranges of values at different age points can vary.

With all these limitations in mind, Tables 6-4 and 6-5 provide an estimate of "normal ranges" for common sleep architecture parameters but should be considered only an approximation of the range of values commonly encountered in sleep centers for different age groups in adult men and women. No effort is made to define different values based on the type of sleep study (diagnostic vs. split). However, several sleep centers have found similar tables useful. The values in Table 6-4 and Table 6-5 are adapted from work of Williams et al.[4] using normal as the mean ± 1 SD for different age groups of men and women with adjustment for the fact that their data were

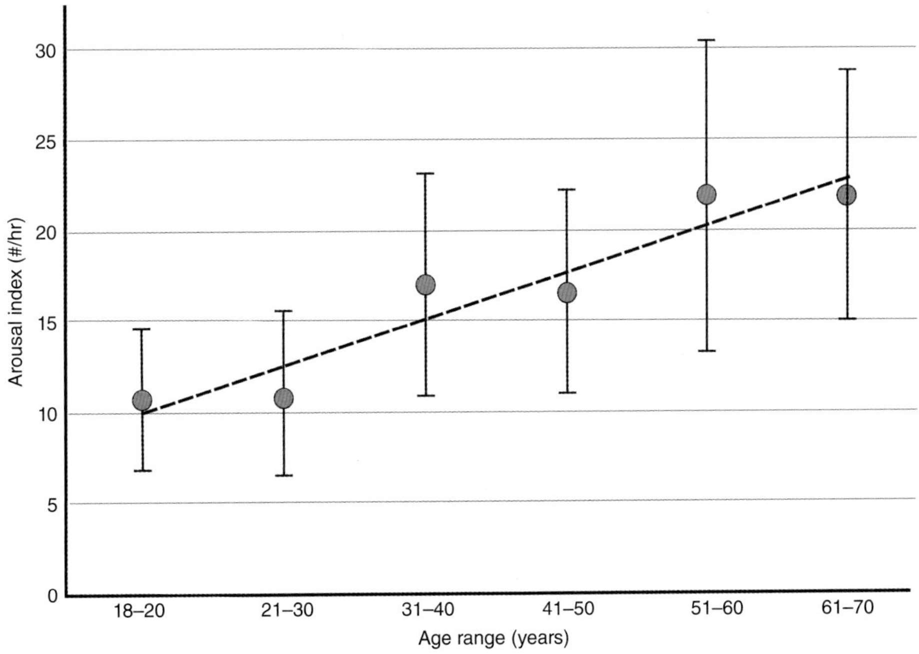

Figure 6–10 The arousal index (ArI) increases with age. The means and standard deviations are plotted. In older individuals the ArI can be in the high 20s to low 30s. (Drawn from Bonnet M, Arand D. EEG arousal norms by age. *J Clin Sleep Med.* 2007;3(3):271-274.)

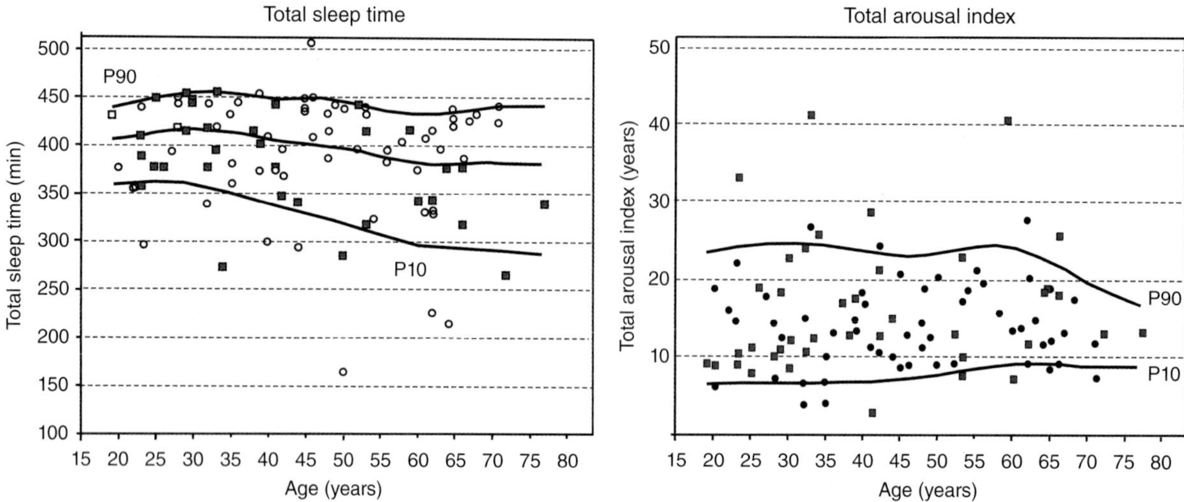

Figure 6–11 The 10th and 90th percentile curves for total sleep time (TST) *(left)* and the total arousal index (ArI) *(right)*. The individual values for TST are shown (circles women, red rectangles men). The 90th percentile line for total sleep time has minimal variation with age, whereas the 10th percentile line shows a decrease with age. Note the relatively few subjects with age range 65 to 75 years. The individual values for the ArI are shown (*circles* women, *rectangles* men). In the ArI plot note that outliers can alter the curves and that relatively few values in the >65-year age range were included. This may explain why the 90th percentile ArI curve decreased in the oldest age ranges. (Drawn from Mitterling T, Högl B, Schönwald SV, et al. Sleep and respiration in 100 healthy Caucasian sleepers—a polysomnographic study according to American Academy of Sleep Medicine standards. *Sleep.* 2015;38(6):867-875.)

Table 6–4 Sleep Architecture—Estimate of Normal Ranges (Men)

Age (yr)	20–29	30–39	40–49	50–59	60–69	70–79
TRT (min)	430–454	414–455	390–468	378–468	414–489	444–543
TST (min)	405–465	390–450	365–436	345–430	330–420	310–410
SE (%)	90–98	85–95	83–93	80–90	78–88	75–85
SL (min)	3–25	6–25	8–28	8–28	8–28	8–30
RL (min)	75–115	70–108	65–100	60–93	55–85	50–80
WASO (min)	5–25	8–35	12–45	15–55	20–75	35–100
Stage N1 (%TST)	3–8	4–9	4–9	4–10	4–10	4–11
Stage N2 (%TST)	40–59	45–63	48–68	52–70	53–73	55–75
Stage N3 (%TST)	11–25	8–20	6–16	4–14	3–13	2–12
Stage R (%TST)	18–25	18–24	17–23	17–22.5	16–22	16–22

SE = TST × 100/TRT.
RL, REM latency; *SE,* sleep efficiency; *SL,* sleep latency; *TRT,* total recording time; *TST,* total sleep time; *WASO,* wake after sleep onset.
Adapted from Williams RL, Karacan I, Hursch CJ. *Electroencephalography (EEG) of Human Sleep: Clinical Applications.* Wiley & Sons; 1974. The original formulation analyzed sleep stages as a percentage of sleep period time. Limits were also adjusted to be more consistent with reference 11.

Table 6–5 Sleep Architecture—Estimates of Normal Range (Women)

Age (yr)	20–29	30–39	40–49	50–59	60–69	70–79
TRT (min)	410–454	425–462	419–464	420–514	420–511	451–563
TST (min)	408–460	394–450	375–440	355–430	330–420	310–410
SE (%)	90–98	87–95	84–93	80–90	77–88	74–85
SL (min)	3–25	6–25	8–28	8–28	8–28	8–30
RL (min)	75–115	70–110	65–105	60–98	55–90	50–85
WASO (min)	5–25	8–35	12–45	15–55	20–75	30–100
Stage N1 (%TST)	2–8	3–9	4–9	4–10	4–10	4–11
Stage N2 (%TST)	40–57	42–58	44–59	46–61	48–63	50–65
Stage N3 (%TST)	15–28	13–25	11–24	10–23	9–22	8–22
Stage R (%TST)	18–25	18–24	17–23	17–23	16–22	16–22

SE = TST × 100/TRT.
RL, REM latency; *SE,* sleep efficiency; *SL,* sleep latency; *TRT,* total recording time; *TST,* total sleep time; *WASO,* wake after sleep onset.
Adapted from Williams RL, Karacan I, Hursch CJ. *Electroencephalography (EEG) of Human Sleep: Clinical Applications.* Wiley & Sons; 1974. The original formulation analyzed sleep stages as a percentage of sleep period time. Limits were also adjusted to be more consistent with reference 11.

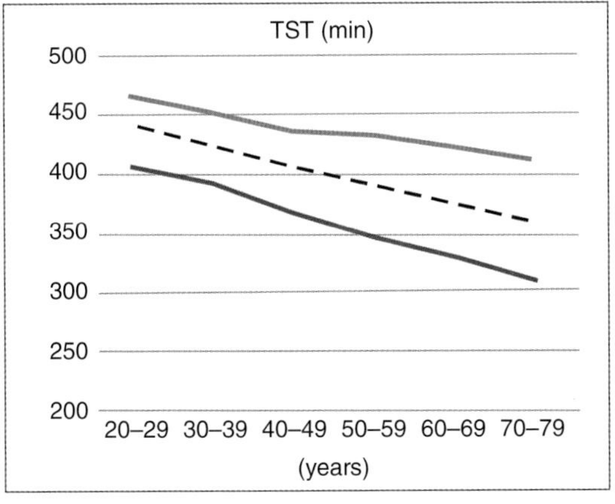

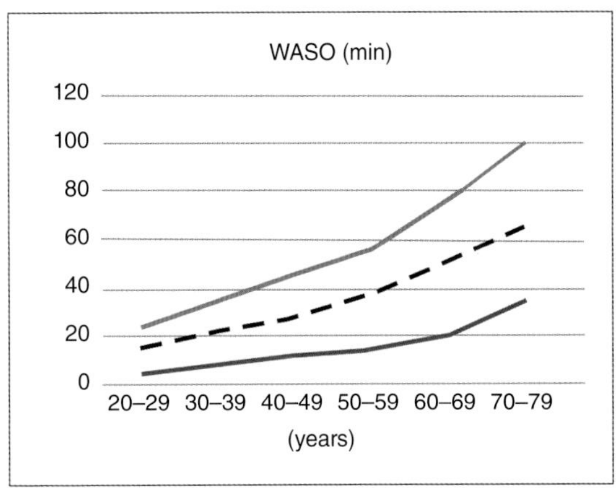

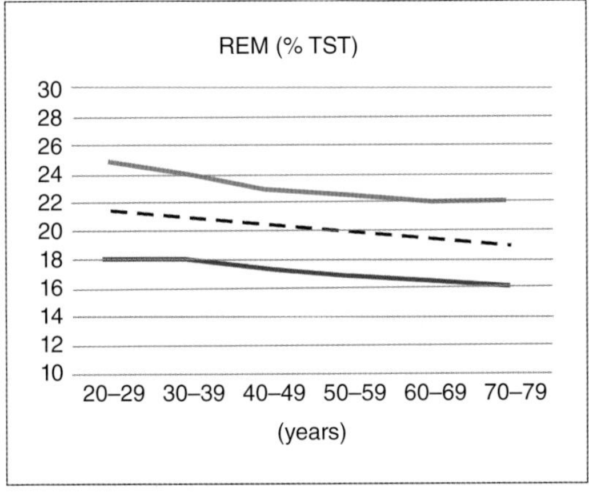

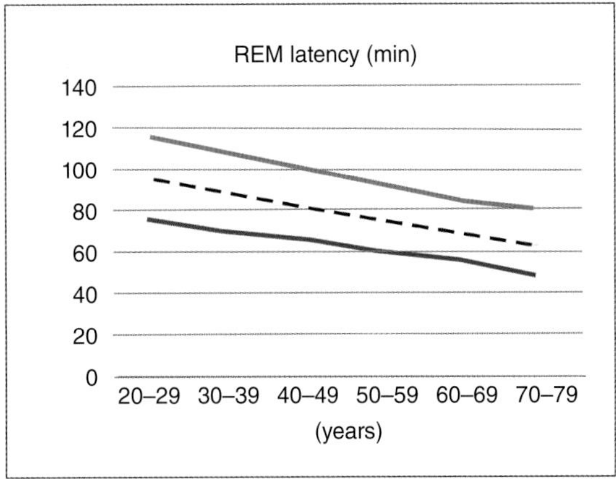

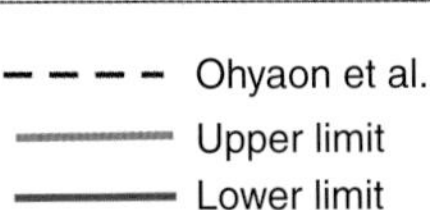

Figure 6–12 Plots of the upper and lower limits of the ranges for men (Table 6–4) for total sleep time, wake after sleep onset *(WASO)*, REM (%TST), and the REM latency. The dotted line is plotted from data obtained in the middle of an age ranges from the exponential line fitted to the data for the corresponding sleep parameter in the study by Ohayon et al.[11] (Adapted from Ohayon M, Carskadon M, Guillemenault C, Vitiello M: Meta-analysis of quantitative sleep parameters from childhood to old age in healthy individuals: developing normative sleep values across the human lifespan. SLEEP 2004;27(7):1255-1273.)

given as a percentage of sleep period time. Values just outside the limits should be considered normal. For example, for men the range of REM sleep as a percentage of total sleep time for ages 70 to 79 years is 16% to 22%. A value of 24% might be considered normal, but 30% likely reflects an increase in REM sleep. Figure 6-12 displays plots of the upper and lower limits of the "normal range" for men for several sleep parameters. For comparison, an additional plot is displayed using values in the middle of the age range for the parameter obtained from the lines determined by exponential data fitting in the study by Ohayon et al.[11] Of note, data in this article was from studies scoring sleep using the Rechtschaffen and Kales manual.[3] In general, the "normal ranges" encompass the line based on an exponential fit of the data fairly well. An example of a sleep report using "normal range" values is shown in Table 6–6. The REM latency is slightly above the upper limit of the normal range but could be considered normal. However, the striking finding is the large increase in the amount of stage R, which is much greater than the upper limit of the normal range. The sleep architecture is from a patient undergoing a continuous positive airway pressure titration and exhibiting a large increase in stage R (REM rebound).

Table 6–6 Sleep Architecture—45-Year-Old Female Continuous Positive Airway Pressure Titration

Sleep Parameter			Normal range
TRT (min)	480		(419–464)
TST (min)	427		(375–440)
SE (%)	88.9		(84–93)
SL (min)	23		(8–28)
RL (min)	113		(65–105)
Sleep stages			
WASO (min)	30		(12–45)
		(%TST)	
Stage N1 (min)	15.0	3.5	(4–9)
Stage N2 (min)	213.0	49.8	(44–59)
Stage N3 (min)	25.0	5.8	(11–24)
Stage R (min)	**174.0**	**40.7**	(17–23)

RL, REM latency; *SE*, sleep efficiency; *SL*, sleep latency; *TRT*, total recording time; *TST*, total sleep time; *WASO*, wake after sleep onset.

LIMITATIONS OF THE CURRENT SLEEP ARCHITECTURE ANALYSIS

A detailed discussion of the controversies regarding sleep architecture analysis in clinical sleep studies is beyond the scope of this chapter. However, two points are worth discussing. The first is the lack of agreement between human gold standard scorers unless an effort is made to find consensus for each epoch, which is time-consuming. Rosenberg and Van Hout[24] analyzed the scoring of 1800 epochs by more than 2500 scorers, most with 3 or more years of experience scoring. The analysis determined agreement with the score chosen by the majority of scorers. Sleep stage agreement averaged 82.6%. Agreement was highest for stage R sleep with stages N2 and W approaching the same level. Scoring agreement for stage N3 sleep was 67.4% and was lowest for stage N1 at 63.0%. Therefore comparing parameters such as stage N3 as a percentage of TST between two individuals is problematic unless the same scorer evaluates both of the sleep studies being compared, and even then, there is within scorer variability (repeat scoring by the same individual) varies. Other analysis of the reliability of scoring using AASM scoring rules has shown similar results.[25] Advanced computer techniques of EEG analysis can improve interscorer reliability for such parameters as stage N3 (%TST) using computer-derived features.[26] The second issue is that stage N2, which constitutes about 50% of sleep, varies tremendously in the EEG pattern from low-amplitude EEG with a few sleep spindles to an epoch almost qualifying for stage N3. Methods to estimate sleep depth have been developed. The odds ratio product (ORP) is a parameter estimating the probability of a given 3-second EEG segment with a given EEG pattern (relative amount of alpha/sigma, theta, delta, and beta frequency bands) for occurring in an epoch of wake or during an arousal.[27] The values range from 0 (no chance of being in a wake epoch) to 2.5 (high chance of being in a wake epoch, full wake). The average ORP can provide an estimate of sleep depth. Two individuals with nearly identical sleep architecture using conventional parameters can have very different estimates of sleep depth. If the ORP range is divided into deciles (0–0.25, 0.25–0.50, 0.50–0.75, etc.) and the percentage of total epochs in each decile is plotted in graphical form, patterns of sleep can be determined.[28] In Figure 6–13

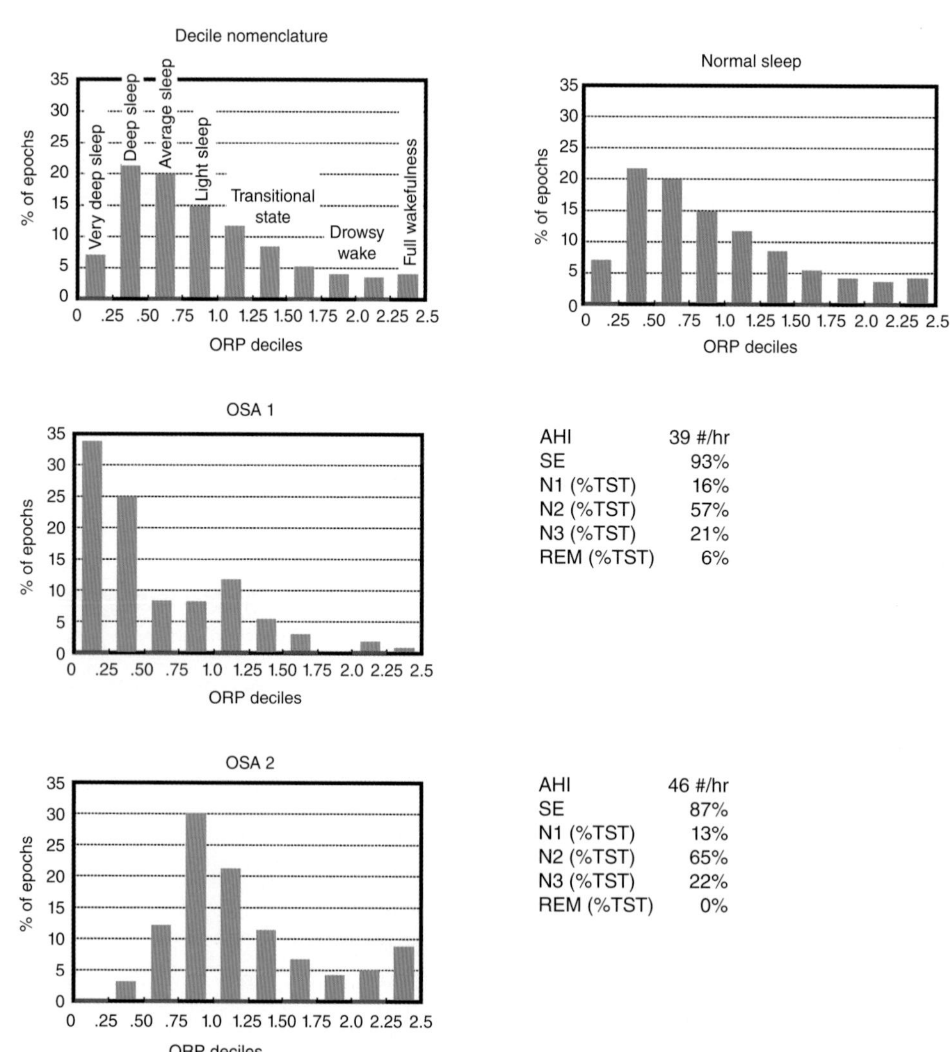

Figure 6–13 The analysis of sleep architecture using deciles of the odds ratio product (ORP), a measure of sleep depth. On the top row nomenclature of the deciles is shown with the pattern seen in a normal individual. The second and third rows show results of an ORP decile analysis showing very different patterns for two patients with obstructive sleep apnea (OSA 1, OSA 2) who have similar patterns using conventional sleep architecture. The OSA 1 patient has preserved amounts of deeper sleep (lower ORP deciles) compared with the OSA 2 patient. *SE*, Sleep efficiency. AHI apnea hypopnea index (#/hour) (Courtesy of Magdy Younes, MD.)

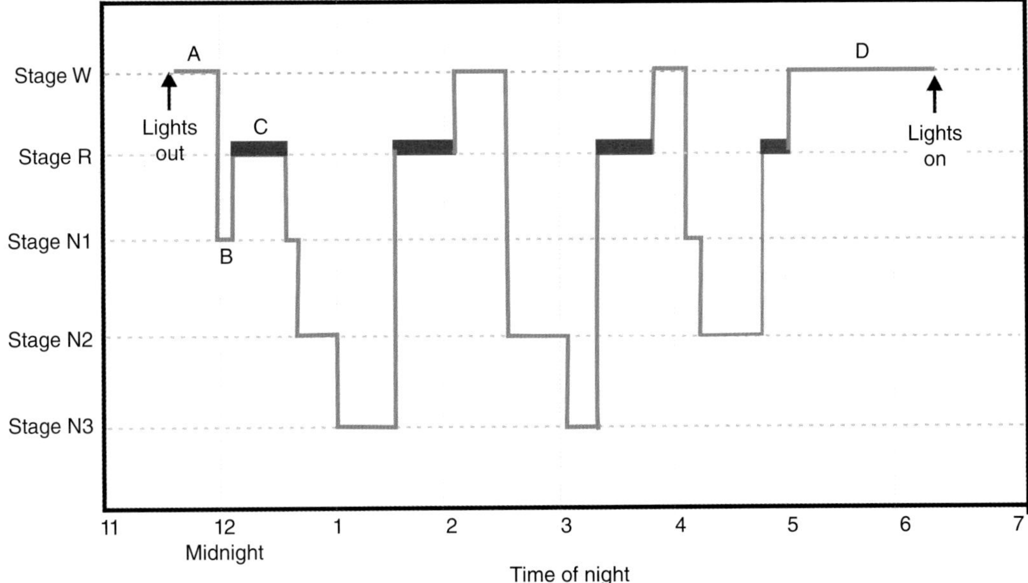

Figure 6–14 Hypnogram for review question 4.

a decile plot of a normal sleeper and definitions of the ranges are shown in the top row. In the second and third rows the analysis of two patients with obstructive sleep apnea and similar sleep architecture by conventional analysis is shown. One can see the ORP decile patterns are quite different. This type of analysis has the potential to improve the analysis of sleep architecture to better understand the changes with age or disease. The reader can consult the references for a more detailed discussion.[25-28]

SUMMARY OF KEY POINTS

1. Sleep in adults is characterized by three to five NREM-REM cycles, each lasting about 90 to 120 minutes. The initial NREM-REM cycle can be shorter (70–100 minutes).
2. The duration of stage R in each cycle is typically longer in the second part of the night. The individual episodes of REM are also increasingly longer. The REM density (eye movements/time) is greater in the second part of the night. The first episode of stage R is typically of a short duration with few REMs.
3. Most stage N3 occurs in the first part of the night and stage R in the second part of the night.
4. Most of the changes in sleep architecture occur by age 60, but sleep efficiency continues to decrease across the entire age spectrum.
5. In adults the TST and sleep efficiency decrease with age, and the amount of WASO increases with age.
6. The amounts of stage N1 (%TST) and stage N2 (%TST) increase with age. However, some studies found an increase only in men.
7. The amount of stage N3 (%TST) decreases with increasing age, but some studies have found that stage N3 (%TST) decreases with age only in men.
8. There is also a modest **increase** in the sleep latency and a **decrease** in REM (%TST) and the REM latency with increasing age in some but not all studies.
9. The normal ArI increases with age.
10. Careful review of the hypnogram provides useful information not provided in the numerical results. Overnight trends and the distribution of wake periods over the night can be appreciated (see review question 4).
11. Traditional determination of sleep architecture does not provide information about the average depth of sleep. Two patients with the same amount of stage N2 and N3 as a percentage of total sleep time can have very different average sleep depth. New methodology is being developed to better assess sleep depth.

CLINICAL REVIEW QUESTIONS

1. Which of the following decreases with age?
   A. Sleep latency
   B. WASO
   C. Arousal Index
   D. Sleep efficiency
2. Which of the following does NOT *decrease* with age?
   A. TST
   B. Stage N1 (men)
   C. Stage N3 (men)
   D. Stage R
   E. REM latency
3. The REM density shows which pattern?
   A. Increase over the night
   B. No change over the night
   C. Decrease over the night
4. In the hypnogram in Figure 6–14, all of the following are true *except*
   A. Short sleep latency
   B. Short REM latency
   C. Relatively long initial REM period
   D. Early morning awakening
5. Which of the following is the largest and most consistent change over the entire age span?
   A. Decrease in total sleep time
   B. Decrease in stage R (%TST)
   C. Decrease in REM latency
   D. Decrease in sleep efficiency

6. What percentage of the total sleep does stage N3 occupy in a normal, healthy 25-year-old individual?
   A. ≈5%
   B. ≈10%
   C. ≈20%
   D. ≈30%
7. First-night effect in the sleep center is characterized by all of the following *except*
   A. Lower sleep efficiency
   B. Lower amount of REM sleep
   C. Longer REM latency
   D. Shorter sleep latency
8. Which of the following is true?
   A. There is a large increase in stage N1 as a percentage of total sleep time with age.
   B. If stage N1 as a percentage of TST is 15%, this would be abnormal in all age groups.
   C. Stage N1 as a percentage of TST is 10% in normal young individuals.
   D. Some studies have shown stage N1 as a percentage of TST increases with age only in women.
9. A patient is being evaluated for abnormal nocturnal behavior. Assuming NREM parasomnias are more common in stage N3, and REM parasomnias are obviously associated with REM sleep, which of the following is true?
   A. REM parasomnias tend to occur in the first part of the night.
   B. NREM parasomnias tend to occur in the second part of the night.
   C. REM parasomnias tend to occur in the second part of the night.
   D. REM parasomnias are equally likely to happen in the first and second parts of the night.

ANSWERS

1. **D.** Sleep efficiency decreases with age.
2. **B.** Stage N1 increases (men only in one study) or stays the same (women in one study).
3. **A.** The REM density increases over the night (very low in initial REM period).
4. **A.** The hypnogram shows a patient with untreated depression. The sleep latency (A) is not short, but there is a very short REM latency (B), a relatively long initial REM period (C), and early morning awakening (D).
5. **D.** A decrease in sleep efficiency is the most consistent and robust across the entire life span.
6. **C.** 20% (15%–25% is commonly quoted, see Figure 6–8C).
7. **D.** Shorter sleep latency. A longer sleep latency is part of the first night effect.
8. **B.** Stage N1 as a percentage of TST is around 5% or less in healthy young adults, stage N1 as a percentage of TST increases slightly with age (some studies found the increase only in men). However, a value of 15% would be high in all age groups (see Figure 6-8A).
9. **C.** Most REM sleep occurs in the second part of the night. REM parasomnias tend to occur in the second part of the night and NREM parasomnias in the first part of the night. In children NREM parasomnias occur out of stage N3 but can also occur out of stage N2 in adults. However, even in adults an event in the second part of the night would favor a REM parasomnia.

SUGGESTED READING

Ohayon M, Carskadon M, Guilleminault C, Vitiello M. Meta-analysis of quantitative sleep parameters from childhood to old age in healthy individuals: developing normative sleep values across the human lifespan. *Sleep*. 2004;27(7):1255-1273.

Redline S, Kirchner HL, Quan SF, et al. The effects of age, sex, ethnicity, and sleep-disordered breathing on sleep architecture. *Arch Intern Med.* 2004;164:406-418.

Troester MM, Quan SF, Berry RB, et al. *The AASM Manual for the Scoring of Sleep and Associated Events: Rules, Terminology and Technical Specifications. Version 3.* American Academy of Sleep Medicine; 2023.

REFERENCES

1. Troester MM, Quan SF, Berry RB, et al. *The AASM Manual for the Scoring of Sleep and Associated Events: Rules, Terminology and Technical Specifications. Version 3.* American Academy of Sleep Medicine; 2023.
2. Kushida CA, Littner MR, Morgenthaler T, et al. Practice parameters for the indications for polysomnography and related procedures: an update for 2005. *Sleep*. 2005;28:499-521.
3. Rechtschaffen A, Kales A, eds. *A Manual of Standardized Terminology Techniques and Scoring System for Sleep Stages of Human Subjects.* Brain Information Service/Brain Research Institute, UCLA; 1968.
4. Williams RL, Karacan I, Hursch CJ. *Electroencephalography (EEG) of Human Sleep: Clinical Applications.* Wiley & Sons; 1974.
5. Van Cauter E, Leproult R, Plat L. Age-related changes in slow wave sleep and REM sleep and relationship with growth hormone and cortisol levels in healthy men. *JAMA*. 2000;284:861-868.
6. Mitterling T, Högl B, Schönwald SV, et al. Sleep and respiration in 100 healthy Caucasian sleepers: a polysomnographic study according to American Academy of Sleep Medicine standards. *Sleep*. 2015;38(6):867-875.
7. Danker-Hopfe H, Schafer M, Dorn H, et al. Percentile reference charts for selected sleep parameters for 20- to 80-year-old healthy subjects from the SIESTA database. *Somnologie*. 2005;9:3-14.
8. Carskadon MA, Dement WC. Normal human sleep: an overview. In: Kryger MH, Roth T, Dement WC, eds. *Principles and Practice of Sleep Medicine.* 6th ed. Elsevier; 2017:15-24.
9. Khalsa SB, Conroy DA, Duffy JF, et al. Sleep- and circadian-dependent modulation of REM density. *J Sleep Res*. 2002;11(1):53-59.
10. Bliwise DL, Scullin MK. Normal aging. In: Kryger MH, Roth T, Dement WC, eds. *Principles and Practice of Sleep Medicine.* 6th ed. Elsevier; 2017:25-38.
11. Ohayon MM, Carskadon MA, Guillemenault C, Vitiello MV. Meta-analysis of quantitative sleep parameters from childhood to old age in healthy individuals: developing normative sleep values across the human lifespan. *Sleep*. 2004;27(7):1255-1273.
12. Redline S, Kirchner L, Quan S, et al. The effects of age, sex, ethnicity, and sleep-disordered breathing on sleep architecture. *Arch Intern Med.* 2004;164:406-418.
13. Moraes W, Piovezan R, Poyares D, et al. Effects of aging on sleep structure throughout adulthood: a population-based study. *Sleep Med.* 2014;15(4):401-409.
14. Boulos MI, Jairam T, Kendzerska T, et al. Normal polysomnography parameters in healthy adults: a systematic review and meta-analysis. *Lancet Respir Med.* 2019;7(6):533-543.
15. Floyd JA, Janisse JJ, Jenuwine ES, Ager JW. Changes in REM-sleep percentage over the adult lifespan. *Sleep*. 2007;30(7):829-836.
16. Agnew Jr HS, Webb WB, Williams RL. The first night effect: an EEG study of sleep. *Psychophysiology*. 1966;2:263-266.
17. Hein H, Magnussin H. Literature-based values of control subjects in sleep medicine. *Somnologie*. 2003;7:28-34.
18. Moser D, Anderer P, Gruber G, et al. Sleep classification according to AASM and Rechtschaffen & Kales: effects of sleep scoring parameters. *Sleep*. 2009;32:139-149.
19. Danker-Hopfe H, Anderer P, Zeitlhofer J, et al. Interrater reliability for sleep scoring according to the Rechtschaffen & Kales and the new AASM standard. *J Sleep Res*. 2009;18(1):74-84.
20. Bonnet MH, Arand DL. EEG arousal norms by age. *J Clin Sleep Med.* 2007;3(3):271-274.
21. Mathur R, Douglas NJ. Frequency of EEG arousals from nocturnal sleep in normal subjects. *Sleep*. 1995;18(5):330-333.
22. Gosselin N, Michaud M, Carrier J, et al. Age difference in heart rate changes associated with micro-arousals in humans. *Clin Neurophysiol.* 2002;113(9):1517-1522.
23. Boselli M, Parrino L, Smerieri A, Terzano MG. Effect of age on EEG arousals in normal sleep. *Sleep*. 1998;21(4):351-357.

24. Rosenberg RS, Van Hout S. The American Academy of Sleep Medicine inter-scorer reliability program: sleep stage scoring. *J Clin Sleep Med.* 2013;9(1):81-87.
25. Younes M, Kuna ST, Pack AI, et al. Reliability of the American Academy of Sleep Medicine rules for assessing sleep depth in clinical practice. *J Clin Sleep Med.* 2018;14(2):205-213.
26. Younes M, Hanly PJ. Minimizing interrater variability in staging sleep by use of computer-derived features. *J Clin Sleep Med.* 2016;12(10):1347-1356.
27. Younes M, Ostrowski M, Soiferman M, et al. Odds ratio product of sleep EEG as a continuous measure of sleep state. *Sleep.* 2015;38(4): 641-654.
28. Younes M, Gerardy B, Pack AI, et al. Sleep architecture based on sleep depth and propensity: patterns in different demographics and sleep disorders and association with health outcomes. *Sleep.* 2022;45(6):zsac059.

Chapter 7

Normal Sleep in Children and Infants

NORMAL SLEEP IN INFANTS AND CHILDREN

The major points regarding normal sleep in infants and children are listed in Tables 7-1 and 7-2. When discussing sleep architecture, findings are usually divided into infants, children, and adolescents.[1-11] Typical sleep architecture values for pediatric polysomnography are shown in Table 7–3.

Normal Sleep in Infants

For infants younger than 2 months, staging rules are different than older infants and children (see Chapter 5 for details).

Table 7–1 Normal Sleep in Infants and Children

Infants <3 months
- Stage R (REM sleep, active sleep) at sleep onset is common
- Total sleep time 16–18 hr
- Sleep episodes of 3–4 hr duration interrupted by feeding
- Sleep cycles 45–60 min (90–100 min in adults)
- Stage R about 50% of sleep

Infants >3 months
- Percentage of REM sleep starts to decrease
- Entering sleep through NREM sleep instead of stage R
- Sleep consolidates into major episodes at night with daytime naps

Children
- NREM sleep at sleep onset
- Sleep cycle period does not reach adult values until adolescence
- Sleep cycles increase in length (40 min at 2 yr, 60 min at 5 yr), at age 5 typically 7–10 sleep cycles per night depending on sleep duration
- REM %TST 50% early infancy, 30% age 1 yr, 20%–25% at 3 to 5 yr
- REM latency
  - 3–5 yr ≈ 90 min
  - 6–7 yr ≈ 132 min

NREM, Non–rapid eye movement; *REM,* rapid eye movement; *TST,* total sleep time.

Table 7–2 Changes in Sleep Childhood to Adolescence

No Change	Decrease	Increase
• Sleep efficiency • Sleep latency	• TST (recording on non–school days) • Stage N3 as %TST • REM sleep as %TST • TST (recording on school days)	• Stage N2

REM, Rapid eye movement; *TST,* total sleep time.

Sleep is divided into wakefulness (stage W), non–rapid eye movement (NREM) (stage N) sleep, rapid eye movement (REM) (stage R) sleep, and transitional (stage T) sleep.[12] Stage R was formerly called Active sleep; stage N, Quiet sleep; and stage T, Indeterminate sleep. Infants normally enter sleep via stage R (Active sleep) and spend approximately 50% of the total sleep time (TST) in this sleep stage. Infants have shorter sleep cycles of approximately 45 to 60 minutes (in contrast to adult cycles of 90–100 minutes).[2-5] Infants have cycles of sleep interrupted by episodes of feeding around the clock. A hypnogram of a 2-month-old infant undergoing sleep monitoring is shown in Figure 7–1. Entry into sleep via stage R, frequent short sleep cycles, and episodes of wake for feeding are shown. At 3 months of age, the amount of REM sleep starts to decrease. Sleep begins to consolidate into longer nocturnal sleep periods with shorter naps during the day after 3 to 4 months of age.[2-4] By age 5 to 6 months the infant electroencephalogram (EEG) has typically matured enough for scoring stages N1, N2, N3, and R sleep.

Iglowstein et al.[3] determined sleep duration in infants and children using structured interviews. This study was before the age of widespread personal electronics. Data from this paper is plotted in Figure 7–2. One can see that total sleep duration decreased, whereas nighttime sleep increases over the first year.

Normal Sleep in Children

Total 24-hour sleep duration decreases from about 14 hours at age 1 to 11 hours at age 5. As seen in Figure 7–2, the amount of sleep during naps (total 24-hour sleep − nighttime

Table 7–3 Typical Sleep Architecture Values for Normal Children Aged 1–18

Parameter	Usual Values
Sleep efficiency (%)	89%, large variability
Sleep latency (min)	23 min, large variability
REM latency (min)	85–155 (<10 yr) 136–156 (>10 yr), large variability
Arousal index (#/hr)	9–16
Stage N1 (%TST)	4–5
Stage N2 (%TST)	44–56
Stage N3 (%TST)	29–32 (<10 yr) 20–32 (>10 yr)
Stage R (%TST)	17–21 (can be higher in younger children)

REM, Rapid eye movement; *TST,* total sleep time.
Adapted from Beck SE, Marcus CL. Pediatric polysomnography. *Sleep Med Clin.* 2009;4:393-406.

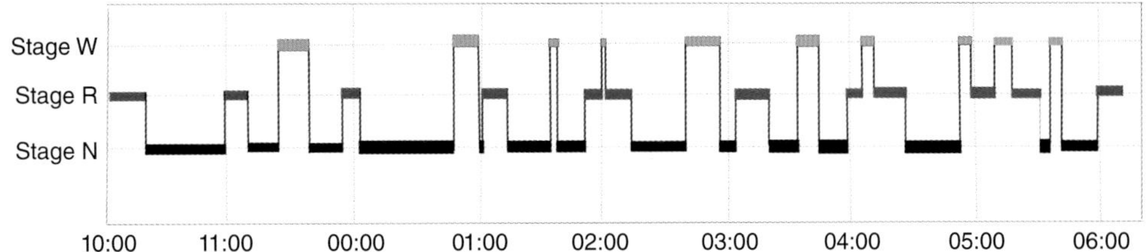

Figure 7–1 A hypnogram from a 2-month-old infant undergoing sleep monitoring. Note the short sleep cycle time, the large number of sleep cycles, and entry into sleep via stage R. In this infant waveforms to allow differentiation of stages N1, N2, and N3 were not yet present; therefore non–rapid eye movement sleep is called stage N.

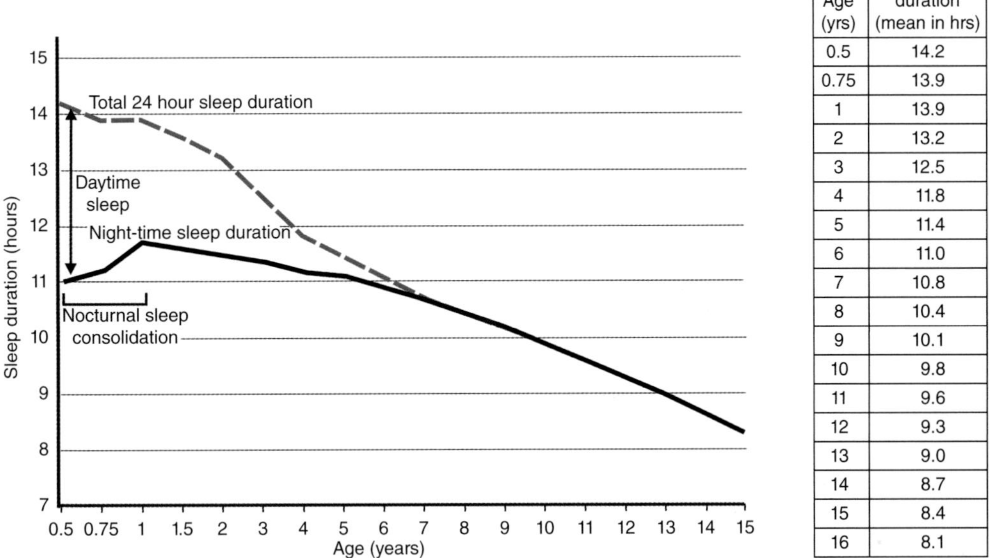

Age (yrs)	Sleep duration (mean in hrs)
0.5	14.2
0.75	13.9
1	13.9
2	13.2
3	12.5
4	11.8
5	11.4
6	11.0
7	10.8
8	10.4
9	10.1
10	9.8
11	9.6
12	9.3
13	9.0
14	8.7
15	8.4
16	8.1

Figure 7–2 Reported sleep duration in infants and children. The difference between total 24-hour sleep duration and nighttime sleep duration is the amount of sleep during naps. This progressively decreases from ages 1 to 5 years. (The figure is a plot of data from Iglowstein I, Jenni OG, Molinari L, Largo RH. Sleep duration from infancy to adolescence: reference values and generational trends. *Pediatrics.* 2003;111(2):302-307.)

sleep) decreases from age 1 to 5. Studies of normal sleep duration in children before the age of widespread use of personal electronics by children found the mean sleep duration for children ages 5, 10, and 15 years to be 11.4, 9.2, and 8.4 hours, respectively.[3] The mean nighttime sleep in each age by year is shown in the figure. Mindell et al.[5] attempted to determine sleep patterns under real world conditions in infants and toddlers. One of their findings was that bedtime was much more variable than wake times. This could be due to parental obligations. However, bedtime seemed to be variable, and total sleep duration was very dependent on the bedtime. Iglowstein et al.[3] found that **daily** napping was uncommon at 5 years of age (8% of children napping), and only 1% were napping at age 7 (Figure 7–3).[3] Napping after age 7 or a return to napping should be a clue that excessive daytime sleepiness is present.

In children the percentage of REM sleep decreases from approximately 30% at age 1 to 2 years to 20% to 25% at 3 to 5 years of age. As in adults, the duration of REM periods increases across the night (longer in the second part of the night). Montgomery-Downs et al.[6] found an increase in the REM latency in 6- to 7-year-olds to 132 minutes compared

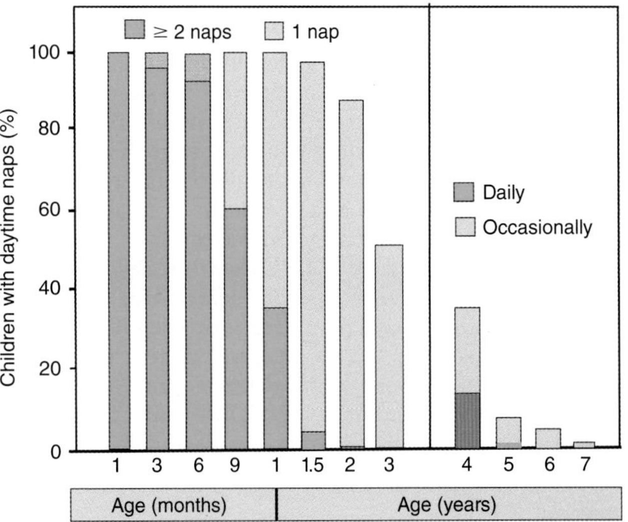

Figure 7–3 Napping at different ages is shown. Napping is uncommon after age 5 years and rare after age 7 years. (The figure is a plot of data from Iglowstein I, Jenni OG, Molinari L, Largo RH. Sleep duration from infancy to adolescence: reference values and generational trends. *Pediatrics.* 2003;111:302-307.)

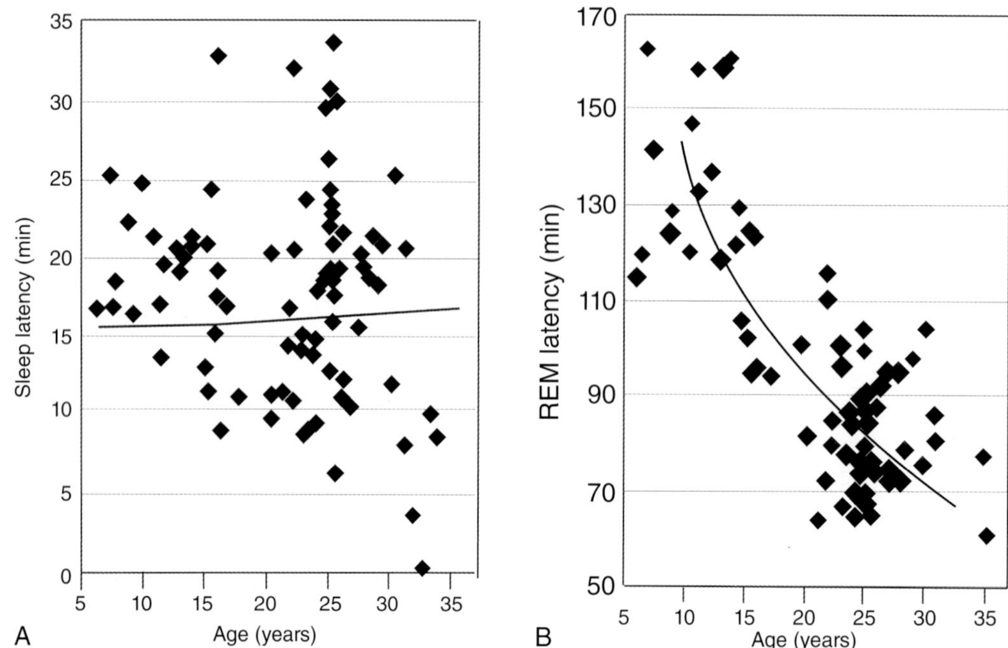

Figure 7–4 Changes in sleep latency and rapid eye movement latency with age. The lines are an exponential fit of the data. (Adapted from Ohayon MM, Carskadon MA, Guilleminault C, Vitiello MV. Meta-analysis of quantitative sleep parameters from childhood to old age in healthy individuals: developing normative sleep values across the human lifespan. ***Sleep.*** 2004;27:1255-1273.)

with 87.8 minutes in 3- to 5-year-olds but there was a large degree of variability. Others have found a decrease in REM latency with age. A plot of sleep latency and REM latency from the data of Ohayon et al. is shown in Figure 7–4. As children move toward adolescence, there tends to be a decrease in stage N3 sleep and stage R with an increase in stage N2. Total sleep duration decreases from about 11 hours in early childhood to 9 hours in early adolescence.[3] Mean sleep duration for ages from 1 to 16 is shown in Figure 7–2.

Sleep in Adolescents

Changes from childhood to adolescence are associated with no change in either the sleep latency or sleep efficiency (Table 7–2). Total sleep time decreases both on school and non–school days as does the amounts of stage N3 and REM sleep as a percentage of total sleep time.[2,3] The reduction in stage N3 and REM sleep as a percentage of total sleep time means that the amount of stage N2 increases.

One of the major findings in adolescence is the delay in bedtime and spontaneous wake time associated with a delay in circadian rhythms.[8,9] During school days sleep is of short duration due to a forced wake time. On the weekend longer sleep periods are noted with an even greater delay in sleep onset and a significant delay in rise times, especially in older adolescents. Shorter sleep duration appears to be associated with worse mood.[13] Adolescents were significantly less happy and energetic during sleep restricted to 5 hours and significantly less energetic during sleep restricted to 7.5 hours. When adolescents had 10 hour sleep opportunities their happiness significantly increased. Baker et al.[10] analyzed EEG in 141 healthy adolescents aged 12 to 21. Older age was associated with a lower percentage of N3 sleep, accompanied by higher percentages of N2, N1, and REM sleep (Figure 7–5; Table 7–4). The decrease in stage N3 with age tended to be greater in males. The slight increase in REM sleep over adolescence was also found by Feinberg et al.[11] and Ohayon et al.[1] This is somewhat surprising as the amount of REM sleep decreases from infancy to childhood. In adults there is slight decrease in REM sleep with age. Baker et al. also found that older boys compared with younger boys had more frequent awakenings and wakefulness after sleep onset, effects that were absent in girls.

RECOMMENDED SLEEP DURATION

A consensus panel of the American Academy of Sleep Medicine[14] has listed recommended minimum sleep duration for infants and children (Table 7–5). Unless there is a sufficiently early bedtime, an adequate sleep duration is difficult as today more families have both parents working on daily schedules requiring them to start work at 8 AM.

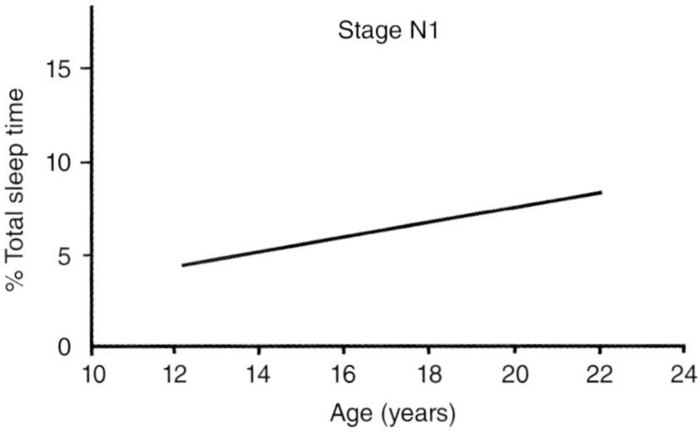

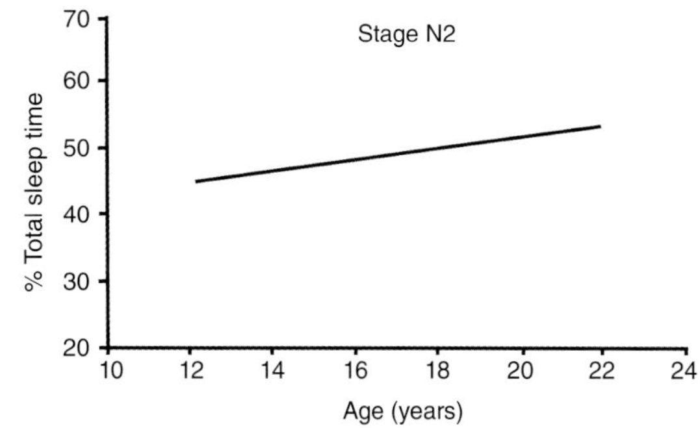

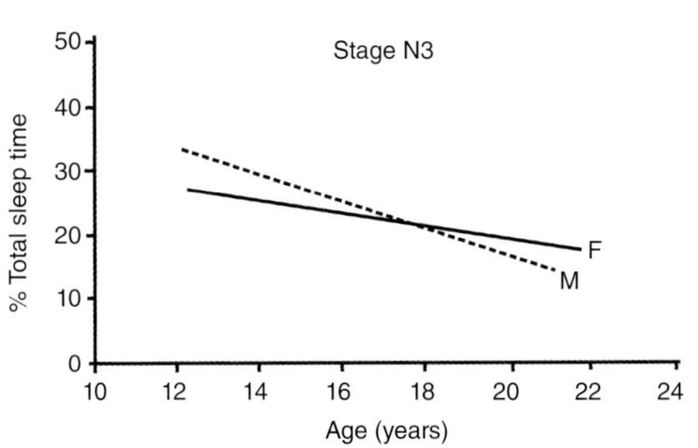

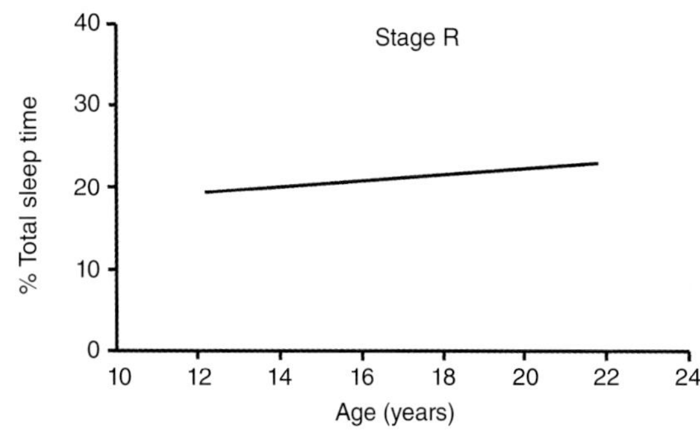

Figure 7–5 Changes in stages N1, N2, N3, and R as a function of age in older children and adolescents. The regression lines are shown. Although a decrease in stage N3 is expected, the modest increase in rapid eye movement (REM) sleep (early to late adolescence) is unanticipated but has been found in several studies. *F*, female; *M*, male. (Adapted from Baker FC, Willoughby AR, de Zambotti M, et al. Age-related differences in sleep architecture and electroencephalogram in adolescents in the National Consortium on Alcohol and Neurodevelopment in Adolescence sample. *Sleep.* 2016;39(7):1429-1439.)

Table 7–4 Changes in Sleep From Early to Late Adolescence

Stage N1	Increase
Stage N2	Increase
Stage N3	Decrease
Stage R (%TST)	Increase

Data from Feinberg I, Davis NM, de Bie E, et al. The maturational trajectories of NREM and REM sleep durations differ across adolescence on both school-night and extended sleep. *Am J Physiol Regul Integr Comp Physiol.* 2012;302(5):R533-R540.

Table 7–5 Recommended Sleep Duration in Infants and Children

Age	Recommended Sleep Duration
Infants 4–12 months	12–16 hr per 24 hr (including naps)
Children 1–2 yr	11–14 hr per 24 hr (including naps)
Children 3–5 yr	10–13 hr per 24 hr (including naps)
Children 6–12 yr	9–12 hr per 24 hr
Adolescents 13–18 yr	8–10 hr per 24 hr

Paruthi S, Brooks LJ, D'Ambrosio C, et al. Consensus statement of the American Academy of Sleep Medicine on the recommended amount of sleep for healthy children: methodology and discussion. *J Clin Sleep Med.* 2016;12(11):1549-1561.

SUMMARY OF KEY POINTS

1. In infants entry into sleep via REM sleep (formerly known as Active sleep) is common. Infants have an increased amount of REM sleep (≈50%), which decreases throughout the first year of life.
2. Sleep is consolidated with lengthening periods of nocturnal sleep at age 3 to 4 months.
3. In children sleep cycle duration is 45 to 60 minutes with seven or more sleep cycles per night.
4. The amount of stage R in each cycle is longer in the second part of the night. The REM density (number of eye movements/time) is greater in the second part of the night.
5. Most stage N3 occurs in the first part of the night. The greatest slow wave activity is typically in the first episode of stage N3 sleep.
6. TST decreases with age from infancy to adolescence. Sleep architecture also changes with a decrease in stage N3 and REM and increase in stage N2 from early childhood to adolescence to mimic adult patterns.
7. Adolescence is associated with a delay in circadian phase, a delayed bedtime but unchanged rise times (school days). The mandated earlier rise time on school days results in a decrease in TST. Over adolescence there is a decrease in stage N3 and a modest increase in REM sleep.
8. Napping is uncommon in children of age 5 years and older. By age 7 napping is rare. A return to napping is a sign of excessive sleepiness in children.

CLINICAL REVIEW QUESTIONS

1. Which statement is true about sleep in a 2-month-old infant?
   A. Stage N was formerly referred to as active sleep.
   B. In infants, entry to sleep through stage R is normal.
   C. The typical sleep cycle duration in infants is 90 to 110 minutes.
   D. Typical total sleep time in 24 hours is 12 hours.
2. A 7-year-old male is evaluated for problems with attention at school. Which of the following is true?
   A. He should be getting 8 hours of sleep at night.
   B. Taking naps during the day on weekends is normal.
   C. A REM latency of 130 minutes would be abnormal.
   D. A REM latency on polysomnography less than 15 minutes would be abnormal.
3. Which of the following is true about adolescent sleep?
   A. There is a delay in the phase of circadian rhythm.
   B. REM sleep as a percentage of TST decreases over adolescence.
   C. Stage N3 (%TST) increases over adolescence.
   D. Both bedtime and rise time are later.

ANSWERS

1. **B.** In infants entry into sleep via stage R is normal. Stage N was formerly called Quiet sleep and stage R was called Active sleep. Therefore answer A is incorrect. The typical sleep cycle in infants is 40 to 60 minutes, therefore answer C is incorrect. The typical sleep duration in infants is around 14 hours with periods of sleep alternating with periods of wakefulness for feeding. Therefore, answer D is incorrect. As infants mature the sleep episodes consolidate into a longer period at night with shorter naps during the day.
2. **D.** Entry into sleep via stage R in an infant would be normal (very short REM latency). However, by age 6 years such a short REM latency would be abnormal. A REM latency of 130 minutes would not be abnormal (wide of variability, see Table 7–3 and Figure 7–4). A child 7 years of age should be getting at least 10 hours of sleep at night. Therefore answer A is not correct. If the family wakes up at 6 AM, this would mean a bedtime around 8 PM. In the digital entertainment age, enforcing an adequate bedtime is essential. Taking a nap would be atypical at age 7 and a resumption of napping is an indication of excessive sleepiness. The amount of stage R as a percentage of TST decreases with age and would be greater in a 7-year-old than an adult.
3. **A.** There is a circadian delay during adolescence. Bedtimes are later but rise times are unchanged resulting in a decrease in TST over adolescence. REM sleep as a percentage of TST increases slightly over adolescence, and stage N3 decreases. REM latency from 130–146 min with large variability has been reported in some publications (Table 7–3).

SUGGESTED READING

Beck SE, Marcus CL. Pediatric polysomnography. *Sleep Med Clin.* 2009;4: 393-406.

Troester MM, Quan SF, Berry RB, et al; for the American Academy of Sleep Medicine. *The AASM Manual for the Scoring of Sleep and Associated Events: Rules, Terminology and Technical Specifications. Version 3.* Darien, IL: American Academy of Sleep Medicine; 2023.

Iglowstein I, Jenni OG, Molinari L, Largo RH. Sleep duration from infancy to adolescence: reference values and generational trends. *Pediatrics.* 2003;111(2):302-307.

Paruthi S, Brooks LJ, D'Ambrosio C, et al. Consensus statement of the American Academy of Sleep Medicine on the recommended amount of sleep for healthy children: methodology and discussion. *J Clin Sleep Med.* 2016;12(11):1549-1561.

REFERENCES

1. Ohayon MM, Carskadon MA, Guilleminault C, Vitiello MV. Meta-analysis of quantitative sleep parameters from childhood to old age in healthy individuals: developing normative sleep values across the human lifespan. *Sleep.* 2004;27:1255-1273.
2. Kahn A, Dan B, Groswasser J, et al. Normal sleep architecture in infants and children. *J Clin Neurophysiol.* 1996;13:184-197.
3. Iglowstein I, Jenni OG, Molinari L, Largo RH. Sleep duration from infancy to adolescence: reference values and generational trends. *Pediatrics.* 2003;111:302-307.
4. Paavonen EJ, Saarenpää-Heikkilä O, Morales-Munoz I, et al. Normal sleep development in infants: findings from two large birth cohorts. *Sleep Med.* 2020;69:145-154.
5. Mindell JA, Leichman ES, Composto J, et al. Development of infant and toddler sleep patterns: real-world data from a mobile application. *J Sleep Res.* 2016;25(5):508-516.
6. Montgomery-Downs HE, O'Brien LM, Gulliver TE, et al. Polysomnographic characteristics in normal preschool children. *Pediatrics.* 2006; 117:741-753.
7. Beck SE, Marcus CL. Pediatric polysomnography. *Sleep Med Clin.* 2009;4:393-406.
8. Carskadon MA, Wolfson AR, Acebo C, et al. Adolescent sleep patterns, circadian timing, and sleepiness at a transition to early school days. *Sleep.* 1998;21(8):871-881.
9. Crowley SJ, Acebo C, Carskadon MA. Sleep, circadian rhythms, and delayed phase in adolescence. *Sleep Med.* 2007;8(6):602-612.
10. Baker FC, Willoughby AR, de Zambotti M, et al. Age-related differences in sleep architecture and electroencephalogram in adolescents in the National Consortium on Alcohol and Neurodevelopment in Adolescence sample. *Sleep.* 2016;39(7):1429-1439.
11. Feinberg I, Davis NM, de Bie E, et al. The maturational trajectories of NREM and REM sleep durations differ across adolescence on both school-night and extended sleep. *Am J Physiol Regul Integr Comp Physiol.* 2012;302(5):R533-R540.
12. Troester MM, Quan SF, Berry RB, et al; for the American Academy of Sleep Medicine. *The AASM Manual for the Scoring of Sleep and Associated Events: Rules, Terminology and Technical Specifications. Version 3.* Darien, IL: American Academy of Sleep Medicine; 2023.
13. Booth SA, Carskadon MA, Young R, Short MA. Sleep duration and mood in adolescents: an experimental study. *Sleep.* 2021;44(5):zsaa253.
14. Paruthi S, Brooks LJ, D'Ambrosio C, et al. Consensus statement of the American Academy of Sleep Medicine on the recommended amount of sleep for healthy children: methodology and discussion. *J Clin Sleep Med.* 2016;12(11):1549-1561.

Neurobiology of Sleep and Wakefulness

Chapter 8

INTRODUCTION

In 1930 Constantin von-Economo published findings of an autopsy study of the brains of patients dying from encephalitis lethargica, a disorder sometimes manifested by sleep for more than 20 hours per day for months.[1-3] He found that patients with damage to the posterior hypothalamus (PH) and rostral midbrain often had excessive sleepiness, whereas those with injury to the anterior hypothalamus had unrelenting insomnia. Based on these observations, he hypothesized that the anterior hypothalamus contained neurons that promoted sleep, whereas neurons near the hypothalamus-midbrain junction helped promote wakefulness. Decades later, the importance of those areas of the brain for sleep and wakefulness is increasingly understood. The major brain areas involved in control of sleep and wakefulness, their abbreviations, and major neurotransmitters (neuromodulators) are listed in Table 8–1.[4-9]

The term *neurotransmitter* is currently applied to situations in which one presynaptic neuron directly influences another postsynaptic neuron. In **neuromodulation,** a given neurotransmitter regulates the activity of diverse populations of neurons in the central nervous system (CNS). Examples of neurotransmitters that are also neuromodulators include acetylcholine (ACh), serotonin (5HT), dopamine (DA), norepinephrine (NE), and histamine (HA). For simplicity this chapter will use the term neurotransmitter for all the manifestations of these neurotransmitters/neuromodulators. Neurons are often characterized with respect to sleep by the sleep stage(s) when they are most active.[4-7] Some neurons are active during wakefulness, during rapid eye movement (REM) sleep only (REM-on), during REM and wakefulness (wakefulness/REM-on), during non-rapid eye movement (NREM) sleep only (NREM-on), or during NREM and REM sleep (NREM/REM-on). Table 8–2 lists important brain areas/neurotransmitters for the control of wakefulness and sleep and their activity in wakefulness, NREM, and REM sleep. It is important to realize that a given brain area may have *more than one group of neurons* (with different neurotransmitters) important for sleep. Some of the major brain areas important for wakefulness and sleep are illustrated in Figures 8-1 to 8–3. Figure 8–1 is an overview some of the major locations. Figure 8–2 shows details of the hypothalamic area,[10] and Figure 8–3 is a schematic showing the locations of some important areas in cross section of the midbrain and pons. A brief summary of the neurotransmitters important for sleep will be followed by a discussion of the major important brain areas for sleep.

Table 8–1 Brain Areas Important for Wakefulness and Sleep

Area	Abbreviation	Major Neurotransmitter/ Neuromodulator	Abbreviation
Basal forebrain	BF	Acetylcholine, Gamma-aminobutyric acid, glutamate	Ach, GABA, Glu
Dorsal raphe nucleus	DRN	Serotonin	5HT
Lateral dorsal tegmentum	LDT	Acetylcholine	ACh
Lateral hypothalamus	LH	Hypocretin 1 and 2, Melanin Concentrating Hormone	Hcrt , MCH
Lateral pontine tegmentum	LPT	Gamma-aminobutyric acid	GABA
Locus coeruleus	LC	Norepinephrine	NE
Parabrachial area	PB	Glutamate	Glu
Parafacial zone	PFZ	Gamma-aminobutyric acid	GABA
Pedunculopontine tegmentum	PPT	Acetylcholine	ACh
Precoeruleus Area	PC	Glutamate	Glu
Reticular activating system	RAS	Glutamate	Glu
Sublaterodorsal nucleus	SLD	Glutamate	Glu
Supramammillary nucleus	SMN	Glutamate	Glu
Tuberomammillary nucleus	TMN	Histamine	HA
Ventral periaqueductal gray	vPAG	Dopamine	DA
Ventral tegmental area	VTA	Dopamine	DA
Ventrolateral preoptic area/ median preoptic area	VLPO/MnPO	Gamma-aminobutyric acid, galanin	GABA, Gal
Ventrolateral periaqueductal gray	vlPAG	Gamma-aminobutyric acid	GABA

Table 8–2 Activity of Brain Areas Important for Wakefulness and Sleep

	Wakefulness	NREM	REM
EEG	Fast, low voltage	Slow, high voltage	Fast, low voltage
PPT/LDT (ACh)			
• Wake-on/REM-on	↑↑↑	↑	↑↑↑
• REM-on	↑	↑	↑↑↑
TMN (HA)	↑↑↑	↑	↔
DRN (5HT)	↑↑↑	↑	↔
LC (NE)	↑↑↑	↑	↔
VLPO (GABA, Gal)			
• NREM-REM-on	↑	↑↑↑	↑↑↑
• NREM-on	↑	↑↑↑	↑
Parafacial Zone (GABA)	↑	↑↑↑	?
Lateral posterior hypothalamus			
• Hypocretin	↑↑↑	↔	↔
• Melanin concentrating hormone (MCH)	↔	↔	↑↑↑
VTA, vPAG (dopamine)	↑↑↑	↑	?
Parabrachial (PB) nucleus (Glutamate)	↑↑↑	?	↑↑↑
• PB Wake-on	↑↑↑	↔	↔
• PG RFM-on	↔	↔	↑↑↑
Basal Forebrain			
• Cholinergic neurons-active during wakefulness, stimulate the cortex • GABA neurons - active during wakefulness, inhibit neurons inhibiting the cortex (disinhibition) • Glutamatergic neurons - increase wakefulness, mechanisms unknown			
Other Glutamatergic neuronal Areas			
• Present in multiple brain areas including midbrain and pontine reticular formation, PB nucleus, supramaxillary area, basal forebrain, and hypothalamus • REM-on areas of pons important for the REM switch, REM atonia including the sublaterodorsal (SLD) nucleus and other components of REM sleep including the precoeruleus and parabrachial areas)			
REM-off/REM switch GABA neurons			
• Ventrolateral periaqueductal gray (vlPAG) and lateral tegmentum (LPT)			

DRN, Dorsal raphe nucleus; *EEG,* electroencephalogram; *LC,* locus coeruleus; *LDT,* lateral dorsal tegmentum; *MCH,* melanin-concentrating hormone; *NREM,* non-rapid eye movement; *PPT,* pedunculopontine tegmentum; *REM,* rapid eye movement; *TMN,* tuberomammillary nucleus; *VLPO,* ventrolateral preoptic area; *vlPAG,* ventrolateral periaqueductal gray.

Adapted from Saper CB, Chou TC, Scammell TE. The sleep switch: hypothalamic control of sleep and wakefulness. *Trends Neurosci.* 2001;24:726-731, and Lim MM, Szymusiak R. Neurobiology of arousal and sleep: updates and insights. *Curr Sleep Medicine Resp.* 2015:1:91-100.

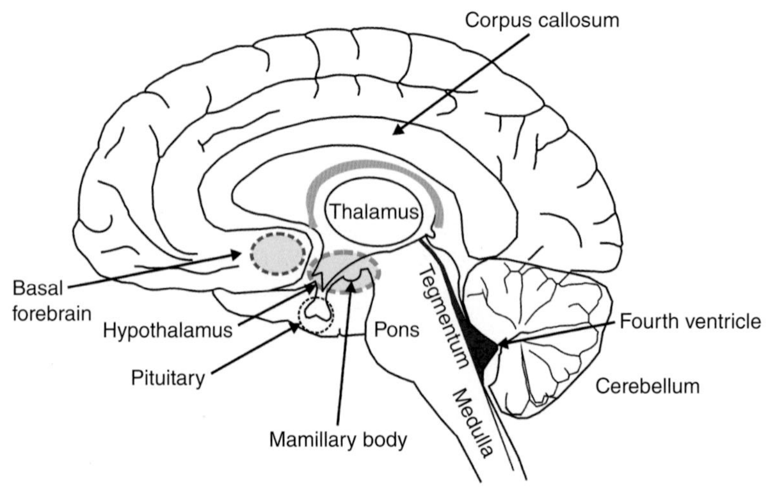

Figure 8–1 Major brain areas important for wakefulness and sleep.

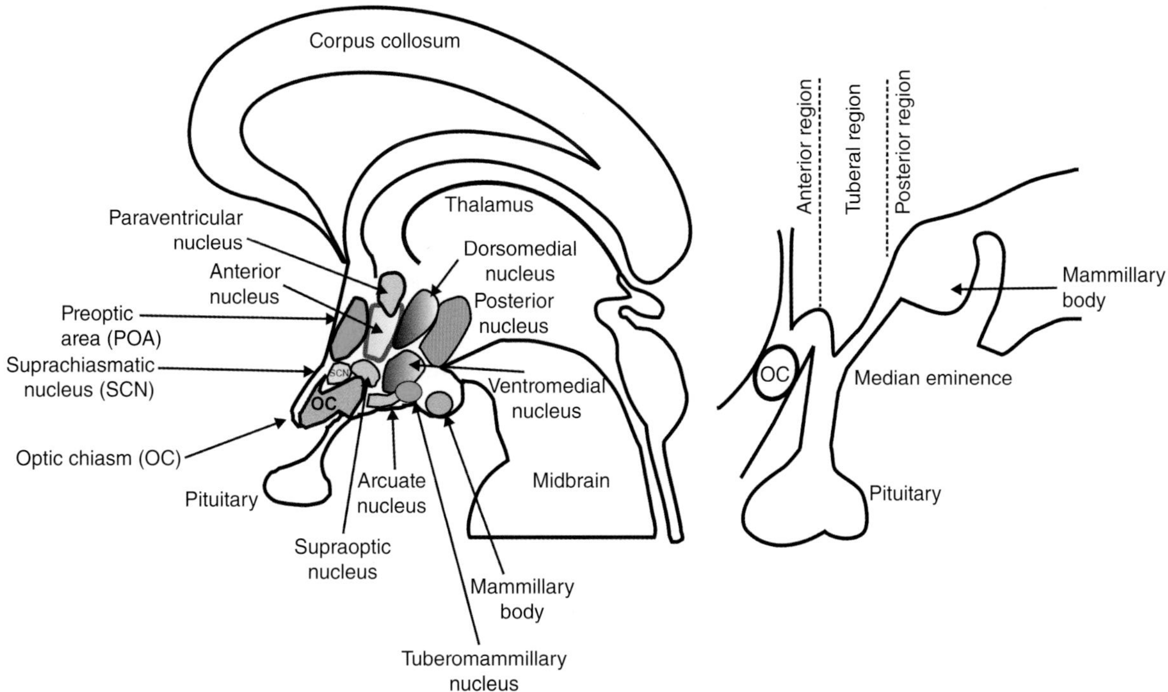

Figure 8–2 Schematic of the major nuclei in the hypothalamus. The preoptic area is also shown in the figure, as many nuclei important for wakefulness and sleep are located there. OC optic chiasm.

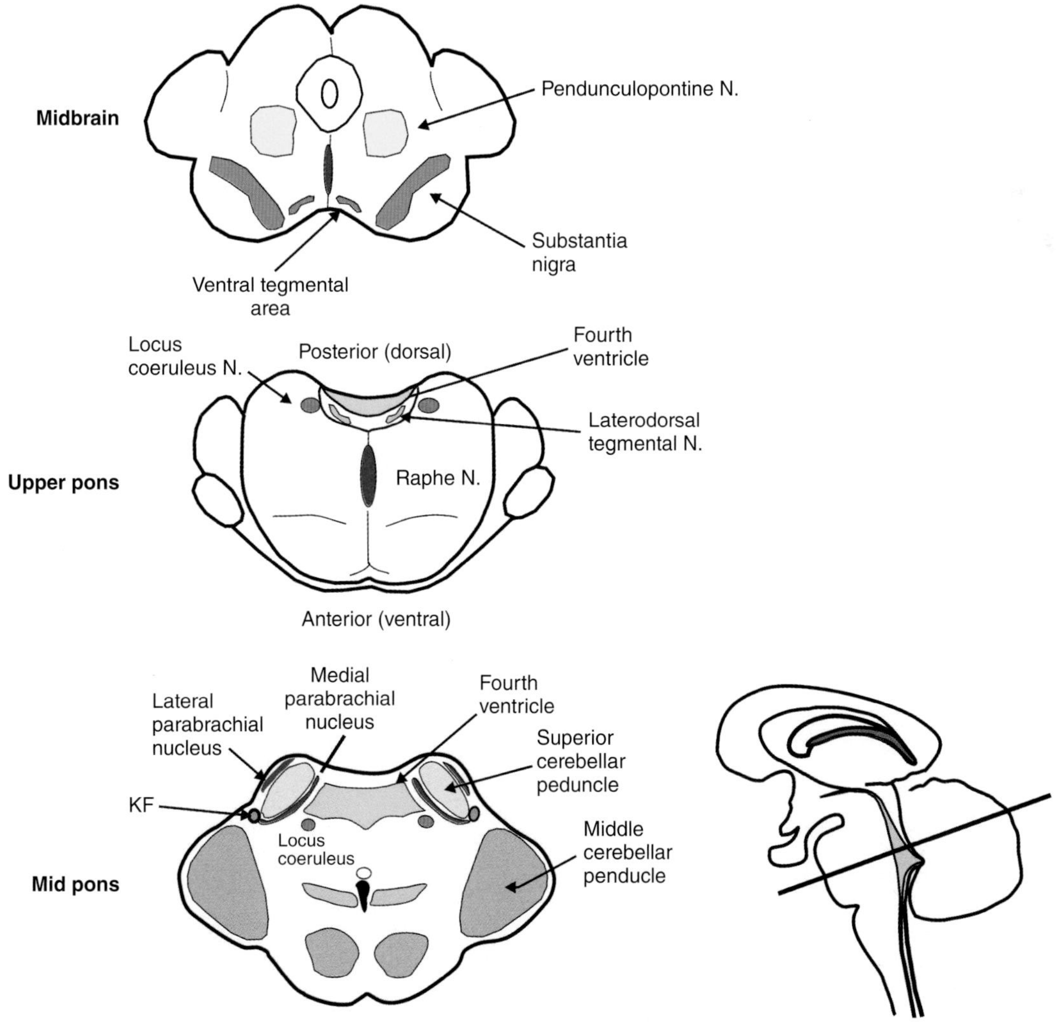

Midbrain
Pendunculopontine N.
Substantia nigra
Ventral tegmental area
Locus coeruleus N.
Posterior (dorsal)
Fourth ventricle
Laterodorsal tegmental N.
Upper pons
Raphe N.
Anterior (ventral)
Lateral parabrachial nucleus
Medial parabrachial nucleus
Fourth ventricle
Superior cerebellar peduncle
KF
Locus coeruleus
Middle cerebellar penducle
Mid pons

Figure 8–3 Schematics of brain stem sections at the midbrain, upper pons, and middle pons levels. The location of some nuclei/brain areas important for wake and sleep are illustrated. *KF,* Kölliker-Fuse nucleus.

Then the control of wakefulness, NREM sleep, and REM sleep will be discussed. It should be appreciated that the field of neurobiology is rapidly evolving, and there are several models proposed (sometimes overlapping) to explain the control of sleep and wakefulness.

NEUROTRANSMITTERS/NEUROMODULATORS

Monoamines

Cell groups producing NE, 5HT, or HA drive wakefulness and arousal and innervate the cerebral cortex, basal forebrain (BF), lateral hypothalamus (LH), and other areas important for wakefulness (Boxes 8-1 to 8-3). It is useful to remember that these cell groups share some common properties. They have higher firing rates during wakefulness (especially active wakefulness), slow firing during NREM sleep, and virtual cessation of firing during REM sleep. That is, they are **wake-on neurons.** After being released into the synaptic cleft 5HT and NE are transported back into the secreting neuron by reuptake (serotonin transporter [SERT], norepinephrine transporter [NET]. There is no reuptake of HA. The monoamines are then metabolized by monoamine oxidases or repackaged into membrane vesicles (the vesicular monoamine transporters VMAT1 and VMAT2).

The locus coeruleus (LC) is the brain area containing NE neurons and the dorsal raphe serotonergic neurons. Histaminergic neurons are confined to the posterior caudal hypothalamus in the area (Fig. 8–2) called the *tuberomammillary nucleus (TMN).* TMN neurons project to the cerebral cortex, amygdala, substantia nigra (SN), dorsal raphe nucleus (DRN), LC, and nucleus of the solitary tract. HA acting at H1 receptors is *associated with wakefulness.* More discussion of the role of HA in sleep and wakefulness is included in the section on the TMN. Although HA is not essential for maintenance of wakefulness, it is likely important for maintaining long periods of wakefulness. Antihistamines (especially first generation) cause sedation.

Box 8–1 NOREPINEPHRINE AND WAKEFULNESS/SLEEP

Brain areas: NE neurons in several areas, LC primary area
Activity/Function:
- Active in wakefulness, less active NREM, inactive REM
- Important for arousal when high attention needed
- LC projections:
  - Thalamus, hypothalamus
  - Inhibitory to VLPO

Important drug effects: Central α-2 agonists (reduce NE) associated with sleepiness (clonidine)

LC, Locus coeruleus; *NE,* norepinephrine; *NREM,* non-rapid eye movement; *REM,* rapid eye movement; *VLPO,* ventrolateral preoptic area.

Box 8–2 SEROTONIN AND WAKEFULNESS/SLEEP

Brain areas: neurons in dorsal and median raphe nuclei
Activity/Function:
- Active in wakefulness, less active NREM, very decreased activity in REM
- 14 types of 5HT receptors and effects vary depending on receptor type
- Usually wakefulness-promoting
- Low 5HT signaling may be associated with hypersomnia in some depressed patients

Important drug effects: SSRIs decrease REM sleep

5HT, Serotonin; *NREM,* non-rapid eye movement; *REM,* rapid eye movement; *SSRI,* selective serotonin reuptake inhibitors.

Box 8–3 HISTAMINE AND WAKEFULNESS/SLEEP

Brain area: TMN—posterior hypothalamus
- Only brain source of HA

Activity/Function
- Active wake, lower activity NREM, very low activity REM
- Promotes wakefulness, promote motivated behaviors, increased attention
- Widespread innervation, Inhibits VLPO (NREM)
- Lesions of TMN have little effect on wakefulness

Important drug effects:
- Antihistamines (H1 receptor)—increased sleepiness (diphenhydramine)
- Sedating antidepressants—trazodone, mirtazapine, doxepin have antihistamine activity
- H3 receptor antagonist/inverse agonist—increase HA levels and wakefulness (pitolisant)

HA, histamine; *NREM,* non-rapid eye movement; *REM,* rapid eye movement; *TMN,* tuberomammillary nucleus; *VLPO,* ventrolateral preoptic area.

Dopamine

Increased DA levels are found in multiple sites during wakefulness. It was once thought that the firing rates of DA neurons did not vary with sleep state (Box 8–4). However, more recently investigators have demonstrated that concentrations of the monoamine DA are higher during wakefulness and lower during NREM sleep in the ventral tegmental area (VTA) and ventral periaqueductal gray (vPAG).[11-13] Variations in firing (burst firing) or variable activity of the DA transporter (DAT) might also explain higher DA levels during wakefulness. After being released into the synaptic cleft DA molecules are transported back into the secreting neuron by reuptake (DAT). DA molecules are then metabolized by monoamine oxidase or repackaged into membrane vesicles (VMAT1, VMAT2). Alerting medications (modafinil, amphetamines, solriamfetol) all increase DA signaling[6,14] (Box 8–5). More discussion on DA and alerting medications follows in later sections.

Box 8–4 DOPAMINE AND WAKEFULNESS/SLEEP

Brain areas:
- VTA, vPAG, SN

Activity/Function:
- Previous findings: DA neuron firing rate does not change across sleep states
- However, high levels of extracellular DA during wakefulness in many brain areas
- Recent findings: DA neurons in VTA, vPAG active in wakefulness

DA neurons innervate:
- Frontal cortex, limbic areas, thalamus

Diseases:
- Decreased DA signaling in Parkinson disease promotes sleepiness

Important drug effects:
- Alerting medications increase DA signaling (see Box 8–5)
- D1, D2 receptor blockade (traditional antipsychotics such as chlorpromazine)—promote sleep
- D2 agonists (pramipexole, ropinirole) inhibit DA neurons (via activity at DA autoreceptors), can be sedating especially in patients with low DA (Parkinson Disease)

DA, Dopamine; *SN,* substantia nigra; *vPAG,* ventral periaqueductal gray; *VTA,* ventral tegmental area.

Box 8–5 IMPORTANT DOPAMINE MEDICATIONS FOR SLEEP

Alerting Agents (Increased Wakefulness)

- Modafinil, armodafinil
  - Decrease activity of dopamine transporter (DAT)
  - Modest increase DA and wakefulness, less abuse potential than amphetamines
- Solriamfetol—DA, NE reuptake inhibitor increased DA, NE—wakefulness-promoting

Traditional Stimulants

- Amphetamines
  - Block DA reuptake, induce reverse DAT transport (out of neuron)
  - Block NE reuptake, increase NE levels (more at higher doses)
  - Associated with motor tics (increased DA in motor pathways)
  - Abuse potential linked to increased DA in reward pathways
- Methylphenidate (Blocks DA, NE reuptake, increased DA, NE)

DA, Dopamine; *DAT*, dopamine transporter; *NE*, norepinephrine.

Acetylcholine

Important brain areas with cholinergic neurons are the lateral dorsal tegmental (LDT)/pedunculopontine tegmental (PPT) in the upper pons and in the basal forebrain (BF) (Box 8–6). Some cholinergic neurons in the LDT/PPT are **wake-on** and others are **wake-on/REM-on.** Cholinergic neurons in the BF activate the cortex and seem to inhibit cortical synchronization. Contrary to previous thinking, this activity does not appear necessary for wakefulness.[15,16]

Glutamate

Glutamate (Glu) is the major stimulating (excitatory) neurotransmitter/neuromodulator in the brain. Glutamatergic neurons are present in many **portions of the reticular activating system (RAS),** which promotes wakefulness and arousal (Table 8–2, Box 8–7). Newer models of sleep and wakefulness have emphasized their role compared with the monoamine brain regions.[7,8] Wake-on glutamatergic neurons that are present in the **parabrachial (PB) nucleus,** a brain structure located in the dorsolateral pons that surrounds the superior cerebellar peduncle (Fig. 8–3), are felt to be very important for control of wakefulness and arousal.[6,7,9] Other glutamate neurons in the **supramammillary area** (above the mamillary body in the caudal hypothalamus) and **precoeruleus** are also important wake-on neurons.[17] **REM-on glutamatergic neurons** in the brainstem (parabrachial area, precoeruleus area, sublaterodorsal nucleus) are believed to be part of the REM-off/REM-on switch to be discussed in a later section. Glutamatergic neurons in the sublateral dorsal (SLD), precoeruleus (PC) and medial parabrachial (PB) areas of the pons are active during REM sleep. Glu itself serves as metabolic precursor for the neurotransmitter gamma-aminobutyric acid (GABA), via the action of the enzyme glutamate decarboxylase.

Box 8–7 GLUTAMATE AND WAKEFULNESS/SLEEP

- Major excitatory neurotransmitter in the CNS
  - Present in many brain regions associated with wakefulness
  - PB—important for wakefulness
  - Supramammillary area—wakefulness active
  - Diffusely located neurons of RAS
  - REM-on neurons: SLD—part of REM switch, precoereleus and parabrachial areas mediate some aspects of REM sleep
  - BF—may increase wakefulness, mechanism unknown
- Precursor of GABA

BF, Basal forebrain; *CNS*, central nervous system; *GABA*, gamma-aminobutyric acid; *PB*, parabrachial nucleus; *RAS*, reticular activating system; *REM*, rapid eye movement; *SLD*, sublaterodorsal nucleus.

Gamma-aminobutyric Acid

GABA is the major inhibitory neurotransmitter of the brain (Box 8–8) but can have a stimulatory effect when GABAergic neurons inhibit other inhibitory neurons (disinhibition). For example, GABA neurons in the BF activate the cortex by inhibiting cortical interneurons that inhibit cortical neurons and promote cortical desynchronization and wakefulness.[15] Recent studies have identified GABAergic neurons in the PH that are active during sleep.[16,18] GABAergic neurons in the parafacial zone in the medulla (PZ-GABA) are both necessary and sufficient to induce deep NREM sleep, also called slow wave sleep (SWS) or stage N3, which is characterized by high-amplitude cortical delta activity, a marker of cortical synchronization and sleep depth.[16,19,20] Mutually inhibitory GABA neurons in REM-off ventrolateral periaqueductal gray (vlPAG) and REM-on sublaterodorsal (SLD) tegmental areas of the brainstem are important components of the REM

Box 8–6 CHOLINERGIC NEURONS AND SLEEP

- **Important brain areas with cholinergic neurons:** LDT/PPT and BF
- **PPT/LDT**
  - Active in wake and REM (lowest in NREM)
  - Project to thalamus, lateral hypothalamus, BF, brainstem REM-on areas
  - Activation of thalamocortical signaling—fast cortical rhythms
- **BF**
  - Active in wake, REM (lowest in NREM)
  - Project to cortex, hippocampus, amygdala
- **Important drug effects:**
  - ACh agonists (donepezil), nicotinic agonists—improve cognition
  - ACh antagonists—decrease cognition

ACh, Acetylcholine; *BF*, basal forebrain; *LDT*, lateral dorsal tegmentum; *NREM*, non-rapid eye movement; *PPT*, pedunculopontine tegmentum; *REM*, rapid eye movement.

Box 8–8 GAMMA-AMINOBUTYRIC ACID

- **Major inhibitory neurotransmitter in the brain**
  - Can have stimulatory effects if it inhibits other inhibitory neurons (disfacilitation)
- **Important brain areas:**
  - VLPO—active during NREM and REM sleep
  - BF—GABA neurons indirectly activate cortex
  - Important in mutually inhibitory REM-on and REM-off areas of pons (REM switch)
  - **Parafacial neurons** (GABA, glycine) promoted sleep by inhibiting Parabrachial nucleus
- **Precursor of GHB**
- **Important drug effects:**
  - Benzodiazepine receptor agonists increase binding of GABA to GABA-A receptors
  - Sodium oxybate binds to GABA-B receptors

BF, Basal forebrain; *CNS*, central nervous system; *GABA*, gamma-aminobutyric acid; *GHB*, gamma-hydroxybutyrate; *NREM*, non-rapid eye movement; *PB*, parabrachial nucleus; *REM*, rapid eye movement; *VLPO*, ventrolateral preoptic area.

switch.[6] In summary, the role of GABA in the control of wakefulness and sleep is complex. Whereas GABA neurons in some areas promote sleep, others (e.g., in the BF) promote wakefulness.

MAJOR BRAIN AREAS IMPORTANT FOR SLEEP AND WAKEFULNESS

Hypothalamic Areas

Lateral Hypothalamus

Neurons in the LH are the sole source of the wakefulness-promoting neuropeptides hypocretin 1 (Hcrt1) and Hcrt2, also known as orexin A and orexin B, respectively.[21,22] Neurons producing melanin-concentrating hormone (MCH) are also mixed with orexin neurons (Box 8–9). Hcrt1 can attach to both Hcrt1 and Hcrt2 receptors whereas Hcrt2 attaches only to Hcrt2 receptors. Patients with narcolepsy with cataplexy have loss of 90% or more of Hcrt-producing neurons and have low to undetectable cerebrospinal fluid (CSF) levels of Hcrt1.[23-25] Canine narcolepsy is due to a mutation in the gene for the Hcrt2 receptor.

Hcrt neurons send abundant excitatory projections to the **dorsal raphe** (Hrct1 and Hcrt2 receptors) nucleus, the **LC** (Hcrt 1 receptors), and the TMN (Hcrt2 receptors) (Fig. 8–4). These areas in turn send inhibitory projections to Hcrt neurons. Hcrt neurons also have a strong excitatory effect on **cholinergic neurons** of the BF that contribute to cortical arousal. In addition, orexin neurons stimulate areas in the SN and VTAs. As will be discussed later, Hcrt appears to stabilize transitions between wakefulness and sleep. Hcrt neurons are active during wakefulness (especially active wakefulness) and inactive during NREM and REM sleep. Of note, Hcrt activity is especially important for supporting long periods of wakefulness. Although loss of orexin is associated with sleepiness, it does not increase 24-hour total sleep time. Patients with narcolepsy with cataplexy have normal 24-hour total sleep time. On the other hand, diffuse injury to the LH and PH may cause sleep for over 15 hours per day. Orexin neurons do not have a direct effect on sleep active neurons in the ventrolateral preoptic area (VLPO) but have an indirect effect via stimulation of monoamine nuclei that inhibit neurons in the VLPO.

Mixed in with the orexin neurons of the LH are a large number of **REM sleep-active neurons** that produce both MCH and GABA.[18,26] These cells innervate nearly all the same target regions as the orexin neurons including the dorsal raphe and LC. However, both MCH and GABA are inhibitory, whereas orexin is excitatory. MCH neurons fire at a *high rate during REM sleep*, with much less firing during NREM sleep and complete inactivity during wakefulness. It is believed that the MCH neurons promote REM sleep by inhibiting the arousal regions.

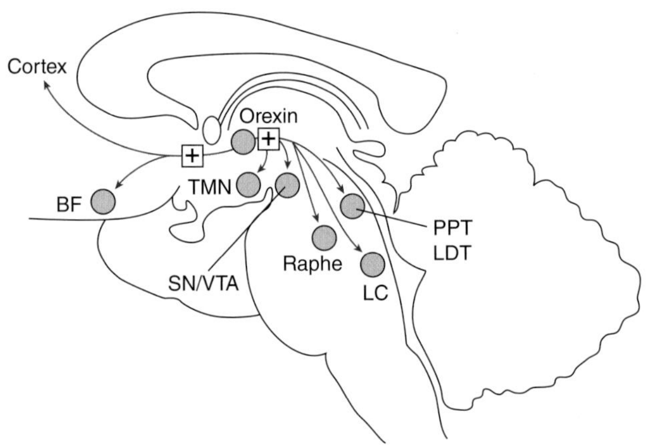

Figure 8–4 Orexin neurons in the lateral posterior hypothalamus excite multiple wakefulness-promoting brain areas. These include the pedunculopontine tegmentum *(PPT)*, lateral dorsal tegmentum *(LDT)*, substantia nigra *(SN)*, ventral tegmental area *(VTA)*, locus coeruleus *(LC)*, basal forebrain *(BF)*, and tuberomammillary nucleus *(TMN)*. Orexin neurons stabilize both wake and sleep. (Adapted from España RA, Scammell TE. Sleep neurobiology from a clinical perspective. *Sleep.* 2011;34(7):845-858.)

Box 8–9 LATERAL HYPOTHALAMUS

Hypocretins

- Neurons sole sources of wakefulness-promoting peptides:
  - Hypocretin-1 (Hcrt1, Orexin A)
  - Hypocretin-2 (Hcrt2, Orexin B)
- Stabilize wakefulness and sleep
- Hcrt neurons active during **wakefulness**
- Excitatory projections to multiple sites including TMN, DR, LC, BF
- Narcolepsy Type 1 (with cataplexy)—hypocretin deficient

Melanin-Concentrating Hormone

- Neurons secreting MCH
  - Active during **REM sleep**
  - Inhibitory actions

BF, Basal forebrain; *DR,* dorsal raphe; *LC,* locus coeruleus; *REM,* rapid eye movement; *TMN,* tuberomammillary nucleus.

Ventrolateral Preoptic Nucleus

The location of the preoptic area in the hypothalamus is shown in Figure 8–2. The VLPO is an area containing neurons active during sleep (Box 8–10, Fig. 8-5). Most sleep-active neurons in the VLPO are believed to be active *during both NREM and REM sleep*.[6,7] Many of the VLPO neurons are activated by sleep-inducing factors (somnogens) including **adenosine (AD)** and **prostaglandin D2**.[27] These neurons are *sensitive to warmth and heating this area of the brain increases their activity and decreases wakefulness (increasing sleep) [the mnemonic HOTS,*

Box 8–10 VENTROLATERAL PREOPTIC AND MEDIAN PREOPTIC AREAS

Ventrolateral Preoptic Area

- Neurons active during NREM and REM sleep
- GABA and galanin
- Inhibitory projections to multiple areas (DRN, LC, TMN, PB, BF, orexin neurons)
- Receives inhibitor projections from DRN, LC, TMN
- Essential part of wake-sleep flip-flop switch
- Neurons activated by adenosine (accumulates during wakefulness)
- Warm sensitive (active increasing sleep)
- eVLPO
  - Subset active during REM sleep
  - Inhibitory projections to DR, LC, PPT/LDP

Median Preoptic Area

- Neurons active during NREM and REM sleep
- GABA and galanin

BF, Basal forebrain; *DRN,* dorsal raphe nucleus; *eVLPO,* extended ventrolateral preoptic area; *GABA,* gamma-aminobutyric acid; *LC,* locus coeruleus; *LDT,* lateral dorsal tegmentum; *NREM,* non-rapid eye movement; *PPT,* pedunculopontine tegmentum; *REM,* rapid eye movement; *TMN,* tuberomammillary nucleus.

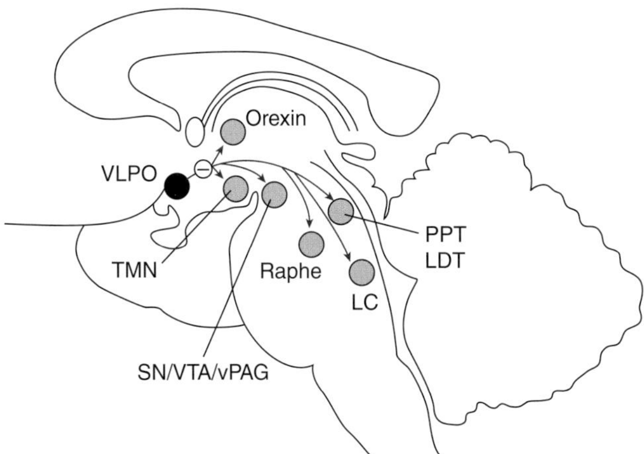

Figure 8–5 Inhibitory projections of the ventrolateral preoptic *(VLPO)* neurons to the areas important for maintaining wake are shown. VLPO neuronal activity promotes sleep. The neurotransmitters are gamma-aminobutyric acid and galanin. VLPO neurons are active during non-rapid eye movement and rapid eye movement sleep. *LC,* Locus coeruleus; *LDT,* lateral dorsal tegmentum; *PPT,* pedunculopontine; *SN/VTA,* substantia nigra/ventral tegmental areas; *TMN,* tuberomammillary nucleus; *vPAG,* ventral periaqueductal gray. (Adapted from España RA, Scammell TE. Sleep neurobiology from a clinical perspective. *Sleep.* 2011;34(7):845-858.)

for heating increases sleep]. The VLPO has inhibitory neuronal projections to the DRN, LC, TMN, PB, BF, and orexin-producing neurons[27-29] (Fig. 8-5). The neurons in the VLPO receive inhibitory projections from the DRN, LC, and TMN. A compact group of VLPO neurons (VLPO cluster) projects to the TMN and inhibits the neuronal activity of that area. A second group of VLPO neurons is located dorsal and medial to the VLPO cluster neurons, and the group is called the *extended VLPO (eVLPO)* by some authors. The eVLPO neurons make up most of the projections to the DRN and LC, as well as to the interneurons of the LDT/PPT region.[27] One study showed a subset of neurons in the eVLPO were *more active during REM than NREM.*[28] However, most VLPO neurons appear to be active during both NREM and REM. The neurons in the VLPO contain the neurotransmitters GABA and *galanin*. Injections of ACh into the VLPO also reduce neuronal activity. Destruction of the VLPO impairs sleep. A second group of sleep-active neurons in the median preoptic nucleus (MnPO) was described after the identification of the VLPO.[30] The VLPO and MnPO neurons may help mediate the homeostatic response to sleep deprivation.[6,31] Increased sleep pressure causes the neurons in the areas to fire faster during sleep deprivation and during the subsequent sleep. AD stimulates firing of these neurons. There may be two populations of sleep active neurons, one stimulated by AD and one group inhibited by NE, 5HT, and ACh.[6]

Tuberomammillary Nucleus

Histaminergic neurons are confined to the posterior caudal hypothalamus in the area (Box 8–11, Fig. 8-2) called the TMN. The TMN is so named because it sits between the tuberal hypothalamus and the mammillary body. TMN neurons project to the cerebral cortex, amygdala, SN, DRN, LC, and nucleus of the solitary tract. HA acting at H1 receptors is *associated with wakefulness*, and antihistamines (H1 receptor blockers) cause drowsiness or sleep.[32] First generation antihistamines are more lipophilic and enter the brain easily and cause prominent sedation. Nonsedating antihistamines such as loratadine or fexofenadine do not cross the blood brain barrier as easily and cause less sedation. HA is synthesized from the amino acid histidine by the enzyme histidine decarboxylase. Histaminergic neurons contain H3 autoreceptors (Fig. 8-6). When brain HA is high, binding of HA to the H3 receptors reduces HA synthesis and release. Therefore, *H3 autoreceptor agonists* could cause sleepiness possibly by stimulating autoregulatory receptors that decrease HA release. H3 receptor **antagonists** reduce the inhibitory feedback increasing HA release. H3 receptor blockers/inverse agonists not only block the H3 receptor (HA cannot bind a blocked receptor) but also increase HA synthesis and release. The difference between an antagonist and inverse agonist can be confusing, but in pharmacology, an **inverse agonist** is a drug that binds to the same receptor as an agonist but induces a pharmacological response opposite to that of the agonist. A neutral antagonist has no activity in the absence of an agonist or inverse agonist but can block the activity of either. Pitolisant (Wakix)[32,33] is an H3 receptor antagonist/inverse agonist that is approved by the U.S. Food and Drug Administration for treatment of excessive sleepiness and cataplexy in patients with narcolepsy. Pitolisant binds to the H3 autoreceptors with high affinity and selectivity, with no appreciable binding to other HA receptors. When the medication binds H3 receptors on histaminergic neurons, the synthesis and release of HA are increased. Increased HA is believed to mediate the reduction in excessive sleepiness. HA binding on H3 **heteroreceptors** on neurons in other brain areas secreting NE, 5HT, and ACh increases reuptake of those mediators, but when pitolisant binds the H3 heteroreceptors, concentration of these mediators increases in the synaptic cleft. Some H3R heteroreceptors may display constitutive activity (receptor active in the absence of an agonist). Thus H3R inverse agonists might increase neurotransmission in the absence of HA. An increase in ACh and DA may increase wakefulness, and the increase in NE may mediate the anticataplexy action of pitolisant.

The TMN receives stimulatory input from the LH (Hcrt). *The TMN firing rate is high during wakefulness, lower during NREM, and absent during REM.* Lesions of the TMN have *minimal effect on wakefulness.* However, this may simply mean that HA is not essential for wakefulness in general and that there is compensation for lack of HA. HA may be important for maintaining wakefulness during periods of high arousal.

Box 8–11 TUBEROMAMMILLARY NUCLEUS AND SUPRAMAMILLARY NUCLEUS

Tuberomammillary Nucleus

- Neurons active during wakefulness, less active NREM, nearly silent REM
- Secrete HA
- Stimulated by Hcrt neurons
- Inhibited by VLPO neurons
- Not essential for wakefulness, maybe help prolonged wakefulness
- Active during episodes of cataplexy (unlike during REM sleep)

Supramammillary Nucleus

- Neurons active during wakefulness
- Secrete glutamate
- Inhibition of glutamate releasing neurons increased NREM sleep
- Involved in production of theta activity during REM sleep

HA, Histamine; *Hcrt,* hypocretin; *NREM,* non-rapid eye movement; *REM,* rapid eye movement; *VLPO,* ventrolateral preoptic area.

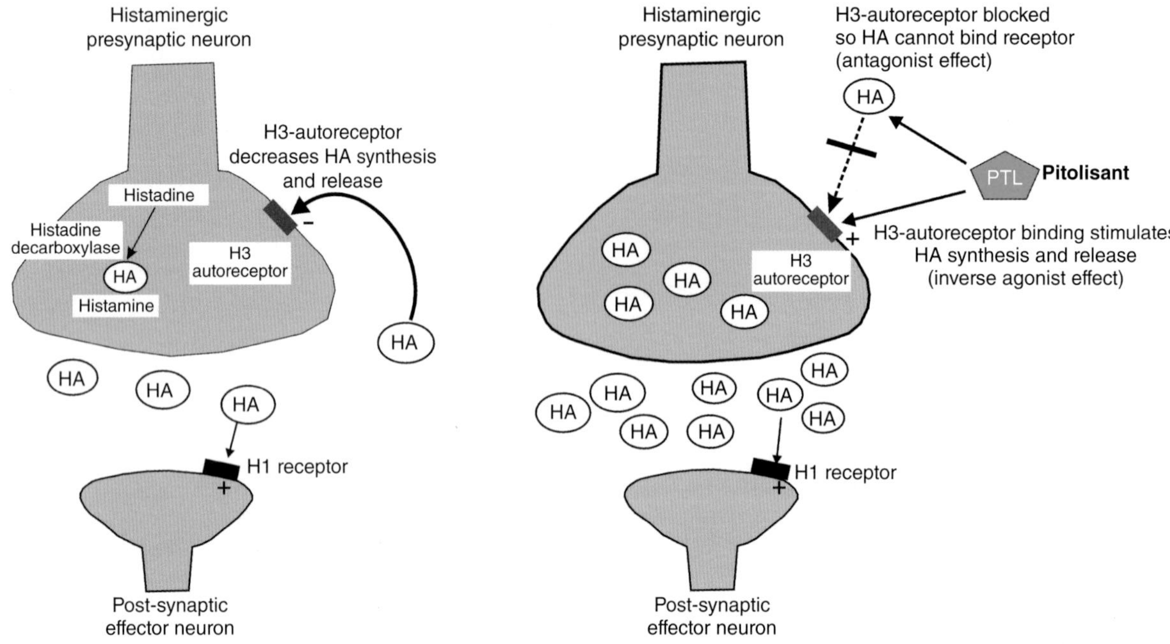

Figure 8–6 *Histamine activity* at H3 autoreceptors decreases histamine release, and at H3 heteroreceptors on norepinephrine and dopamine neurons decreases release of norepinephrine and dopamine. Pitolisant binds these receptors as an inverse agonist, both blocking the receptor preventing histamine binding and stimulating histamine or other neurotransmitter release. This action promotes wakefulness.

The number of HA-secreting neurons may be increased in narcolepsy with cataplexy (type 1),[34] but CNS levels of HA in patients with narcolepsy[32] appear to be normal. Initial studies found CSF HA to be low in narcolepsy patients and others with hypersomnia,[35] but this was *not* confirmed by later studies of large groups with a sensitive assay.[36] *In contrast to REM sleep, during attacks of cataplexy, TMN neurons have a high firing rate associated with preservation of consciousness.*[37]

Supramammillary Nucleus

The supramammillary nucleus is a thin layer of cells in the brain that lies above the mammillary body. Some neurons release glutamate and others glutamate and GABA.[17] The glutamate release is thought to be important for *maintenance of wakefulness* (Box 8–11). *The area may also be important for production of theta activity during REM sleep.* Acute inhibition of glutamate-releasing supramammillary neurons results in an increase in NREM sleep and fragmentation of wakefulness. Ascending connections from neurons in the supramammillary nucleus to GABAergic and cholinergic neurons in the BF have been demonstrated. These cell groups appear to mediate arousal and suppress cortical slowing, respectively.

Brainstem Regions

Dopamine Regions

Neurons producing DA are abundant in the SN and VTA (Box 8–4). Early studies found that DA neurons in these regions do *not* have a "wake-on" firing pattern, and it was thought that DA neurons do not change their firing rates substantially across sleep stages.[5] However, extracellular DA levels are increased in several brain regions during wakefulness. A group of DA neurons in the vPAG are active during wakefulness.[11,12] DA neurons in the vPAG project to and receive input from cholinergic neurons in the LDT area, orexin neurons, VLPO, and prefrontal cortex. Loss of vPAG DA neurons promotes sleep. DA neurons are also mixed with 5HT neurons in the dorsal raphe. One explanation of the lack of change in DA neuron firing rates with sleep is that whereas the average rate of firing of the VTA neurons does not change across states, some studies suggest that they have burst firing during wakefulness that releases more DA. Another explanation is that there is a change in DAT activity. However, Eban-Rothschild and coworkers using newer techniques have demonstrated that DA neurons in the VTA reduce their activity in NREM sleep compared with wakefulness and REM sleep.[13] DA neurons are now thought to important promoters of wakefulness, especially under conditions of motivation. Of note, the VTA also contains GABAergic and glutamatergic neurons.

DA agonists acting at D1, D2, and D3 receptors increase wakefulness and decrease NREM and REM sleep. Exactly which DA neurons are important for maintenance of wakefulness is not clear. DA blockers of D1 and D2 receptors can promote sleep (antipsychotics). In patients with low DA activity, such as those with Parkinson disease, low doses of DA agonists (pramipexole, ropinirole) that bind D2/D3 autoreceptors on DA neurons can cause sleepiness by reducing DA signaling. The effect is believed to be most significant when the overall amount of DA is reduced, as in Parkinson disease.[6] Amphetamines, modafinil, armodafinil, and solriamfetol promote wakefulness by increasing DA signaling (brain concentrations of DA). The DAT takes up DA from the synaptic cleft reducing DA signaling. Modafinil and armodafinil are weak DAT blockers. Amphetamines not only reduce DA uptake but also stimulate release of DA and NE.[5,6,14]

Dorsal Raphe Nucleus

Most serotonergic activity arises from the DRN and median raphe nuclei (MRNs). DRN serotonergic neurons are active during wakefulness, less active during NREM, and minimally

Box 8–12 DORSAL RAPHE NUCLEUS AND LOCUS COERULEUS

Dorsal Raphe Nucleus

- Active wakefulness, less active NREM, minimally active REM
- Serotonergic neurons (5HT)
- Inhibitory projections to VLPO

Locus Coeruleus

- Active wakefulness, less active NREM, silent during REM
- Noradrenergic neurons (NE)
- Inhibitory projections to VLPO

5HT, Serotonin; *NE,* norepinephrine; *NREM,* non-rapid eye movement; *REM,* rapid eye movement; *VLPO,* ventrolateral preoptic area.

active during REM sleep (Box 8–12).[5] The influences of DRN neurons are mainly stimulatory. They are part of the RAS network. DRN nuclei innervate many brain areas and also receive reciprocal innervation from multiple many brain regions. Some dopaminergic neurons also are located in the dorsal raphe area and are wakefulness active.

Locus Coeruleus

Neurons in the LC use NE as the neurotransmitter and innervate wide areas of the brain with chiefly stimulatory effects and receive reciprocal inputs from multiple areas (Box 8–12). As noted previously, LC firing rates are high during wakefulness, lower during NREM, and **absent** during REM sleep[5,6] (see Table 8–2 and Box 8–12). NE agonists increase wakefulness, and central alpha-2 agonists (clonidine), which reduce NE, are associated with sedation.

Lateral Dorsal Tegmentum/Pedunculopontine Tegmentum

The PPT and LDT are clusters of cholinergic clusters at the junction of the pons and midbrain (Fig. 8-3, Box 8–13). One group of cholinergic neurons in the LDT and PPT areas are active during REM sleep (REM-on), and another group are active during wake and REM (wake/REM-on).[38] The activity of these neurons is low during NREM sleep. These nuclei also contain populations of GABAergic and glutaminergic neurons. *Cholinergic activity induces fast electroencephalographic (EEG) activity via stimulation of thalamocortical neurons.* Glutaminergic neurons of the PPT/LDT are also thought to increase wakefulness.

Parabrachial Nucleus

The PB relays signals to the BF. Glutaminergic neurons of the *medial* PB nucleus innervate the BF and are essential for wakefulness promotion.[39] Of interest, **glutaminergic neurons** from the lateral PB are activated by hypercarbia and are likely

Box 8–13 LATERAL DORSAL TEGMENTUM/PEDUNCULOPONTINE TEGMENTUM

- Cholinergic neurons (ACh)
- Wake/REM-on neurons
- REM-on neurons
- During REM excitatory to thalamus—allowing fast EEG of REM
- Area also contains GABA and glutamate neurons

ACh, Acetylcholine; *EEG,* electroencephalogram; *GABA,* gamma-aminobutyric acid; *REM,* rapid eye movement.

Box 8–14 PARABRACHIAL AND PARAFACIAL ZONE AREAS

Parabrachial Area

- Located in the dorsolateral pons that surrounds the superior cerebellar peduncle
- Subdivided into the medial and lateral parabrachial nuclei and the Kölliker-Fuse nucleus
- Area relays sensory information (visceral malaise, taste, temperature, pain, itch) to forebrain structures including the thalamus, hypothalamus, and extended amygdala
- Glutamate secreting neurons important for **wake** (wake active)
- Lateral PB neurons—mediate arousal from hypercapnia

Parafacial Zone

- Located in medulla at the level of CN VII (facial nerve)
- GABA neurons
- **NREM on neurons**, inhibit PB nuclei promoting sleep
- Essential for slow wave sleep

GABA, Gamma-aminobutyric acid; *NREM,* non-rapid eye movement; *PB,* parabrachial area.

important for arousal due to hypercapnia (Box 8–14).[40] There are also REM-on neurons in the PB that mediate some effects of REM sleep.

Parafacial Zone

GABA-secreting neurons are present in the medulla at the level of CN VII (facial nerve) in an area called the parafacial zone (PFZ or PZ) (Box 8–14). The neurons are active during sleep (especially NREM) and inhibit wakefulness-promoting PB neurons, thus promoting sleep. PZ neurons are thought to be essential for stage N3 sleep.[6-9,19,20]

Basal Forebrain

BF neurons promote wakefulness and are necessary for cortical activation and arousal (Box 8–15). The BF contains *cholinergic neurons,* as well as neurons producing *GABA and glutamate.* As previously mentioned, the cholinergic neurons in the BF excite cortical pyramidal cells producing fast cortical activity (reducing slow wave activity), but it appears that this activity is not essential for wakefulness.[15,16] BF GABA neurons promote wakefulness likely by disinhibiting cortical neurons, that is, by inhibiting interneurons that inhibit cortical neurons. Lesions that destroy ACh and GABA neurons in the BF increase delta power. Cholinergic neurons in the caudal BF also project to the amygdala, and those in the medial septum innervate the dorsal hippocampus and drive theta activity. *The cholinergic*

Box 8–15 BASAL FOREBRAIN

Promotes Wakefulness and Electroencephalogram Activation

- Cholinergic BF neurons excite cortical pyramidal cells, active during wake and REM sleep resulting in increased fast EEG frequencies and decreased slow waves during sleep
- GABA BF neurons disinhibit cortical neurons
- (activating GABA BF neurons increases wakefulness)
- Glutamate BF neurons may also promote wakefulness
- Glutamate levels higher in cortex during wake and REM sleep compared to NREM sleep

BC, Basal forebrain; *EEG,* electroencephalogram; *GABA,* gamma-aminobutyric acid; *REM,* rapid eye movement.

neurons of the BF are active during wakefulness and REM sleep (associated with fast EEG activity) but much less so during NREM sleep. The BF glutamatergic neurons are also believed to increase wakefulness, although the mechanisms are currently not known.

Thalamus

The thalamus serves as a bilobed complex relay center (>30 nuclei) between many brain areas including the cortex and brain stem with many afferent and efferent connections. The thalamus serves as a sleep gate allowing sleep to proceed without interruptions from sensory inputs. The thalamic *reticular nucleus* (TRN) is involved in producing the thalamocortical oscillations that produce sleep spindles.[41-43] The TRN forms a thin envelope around most of the principal thalamic nuclei and covers these like an umbrella along their frontal-caudal extent (Fig. 8-7). **Sleep spindles** are bursts of neural oscillation that are generated by interplay of the TRN and other thalamic nuclei during NREM sleep in a frequency range of about 11 to 16 Hz (usually 12-14 Hz) with a duration of 0.5 seconds or greater (usually 0.5-1.5 seconds). After generation in the TRN, spindles are sustained and relayed to the cortex by thalamocortical neuronal loops.

Reticular Formation

Before identification of a number of discrete nuclei important for wakefulness and arousal, the concept of the RAS received more attention. However, the concept emphasizes that neurons scattered throughout the brain stem have important functions in maintaining wakefulness. Rather than a discrete location, the reticular formation is a loose collection of neurons extending from the caudal medulla to the core of the midbrain.[44] **Sections above the mid pons produce coma or hypersomnolence.** Wakefulness depends on the activity of the ascending RAS. This system projects to higher brain centers. One pathway ascends dorsally to the thalamus, and the second ascends ventrally through the LH and forebrain (Fig. 8-8).

Dorsal Reticular Activating System

Neurons in the LDT and PPT areas that are in the dorsal midbrain and pons make up most of the dorsal RAS pathway through the pons and are cholinergic. Some of the neurons are active during wake and REM sleep (wake/REM-on), whereas others are active mainly during REM sleep (REM-on). Acetylcholine (ACh) release in the thalamus is high during wakefulness and REM sleep. The cholinergic neurons from these areas densely innervate the thalamus (especially the medial and intralaminar thalamic nuclei), LH, and midbrain. During wakefulness and REM sleep, these cholinergic neurons depolarize thalamic relay neurons thereby activating thalamocortical signaling and produce fast cortical rhythms. During NREM sleep, these neurons are inactive. *Glutamatergic* neurons throughout the RAS are essential for wakefulness and project to the thalamus (reticular and intralaminar nuclei) and throughout the cortex.

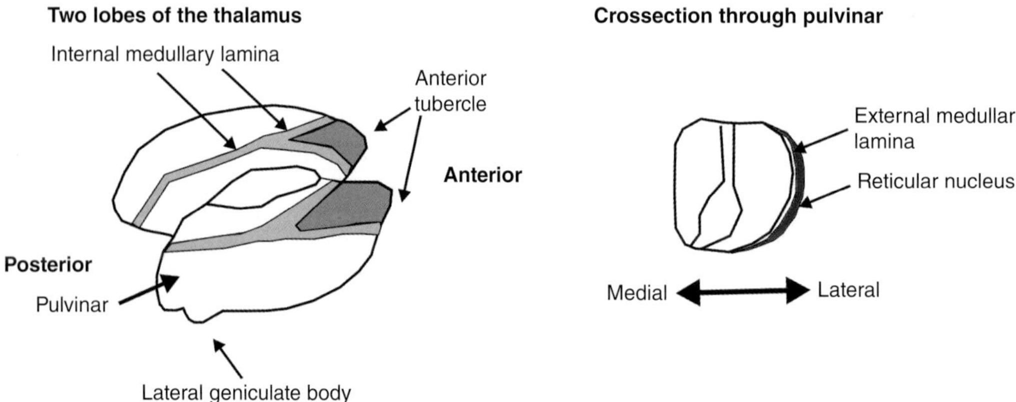

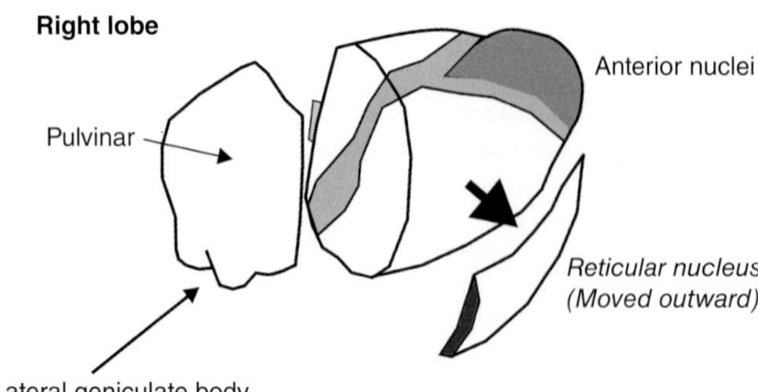

Figure 8–7 Schematic of the thalamus showing the location of the thalamic reticular nucleus (TRN). The thalamus is a bilobed group of nuclei serving as a relay station between the brain stem and the cortex. The TRN generates sleep spindles via cortical connections (spindles are the result of thalamocortical oscillations).

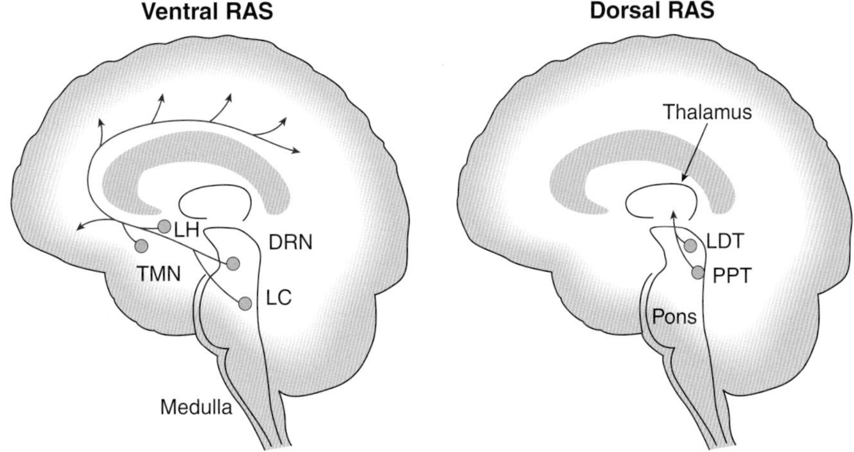

Figure 8–8 Schematic illustration of components of the reticular activating system *(RAS)*. Although not shown, glutaminergic neurons diffusely scattered throughout the brain stem also contribute to activation of the brain maintaining wakefulness and arousal. *DRN,* Dorsal raphe nucleus; *LC,* locus coeruleus; *LDT,* lateral dorsal tegmentum; *LH,* lateral hypothalamus; *PPT,* pedunculopontine nucleus; *TMN,* tuberomammillary nucleus.

Ventral Reticular Activating System

The ventral RAS projects through the LH terminating on magnocellular neurons in the substantia innominata, medial septum, and diagonal band. These regions contain neurons that project to the cortex. The ascending projections of this branch are joined by input from the TMN and LH. The ventral RAS is composed of projections from the DRN (5HT) and LC (NE).

CONTROL OF WAKEFULNESS

Areas of the brain important for wakefulness contain neurons using 5HT, NE, DA, Glu, and ACh as neurotransmitters/modulators (Fig. 8–9, Box 8–16). A network of multiple areas of the brain is believed to be important for wakefulness. Monoaminergic neurons (LC, DRN, TMN) innervate the cortex, hypothalamus, and thalamus, thus promoting wakefulness. Hcrt neurons are active during wakefulness and believed to be needed to stabilize long periods of wakefulness. During wakefulness centers triggering NREM and REM sleep are inhibited. Hcrt neurons do not innervate the VLPO directly but stimulate the TMN, DRN, or LC during wakefulness but not during NREM sleep. Then, during wakefulness, the TMN, DRN, and LC inhibit the VLPO. The activity of dopaminergic VTA and vPAG neurons is high during wakefulness, but the mechanisms by which increased DA helps maintain wakefulness are still uncertain. As noted earlier, the wakefulness-promoting medications modafinil, armodafinil,

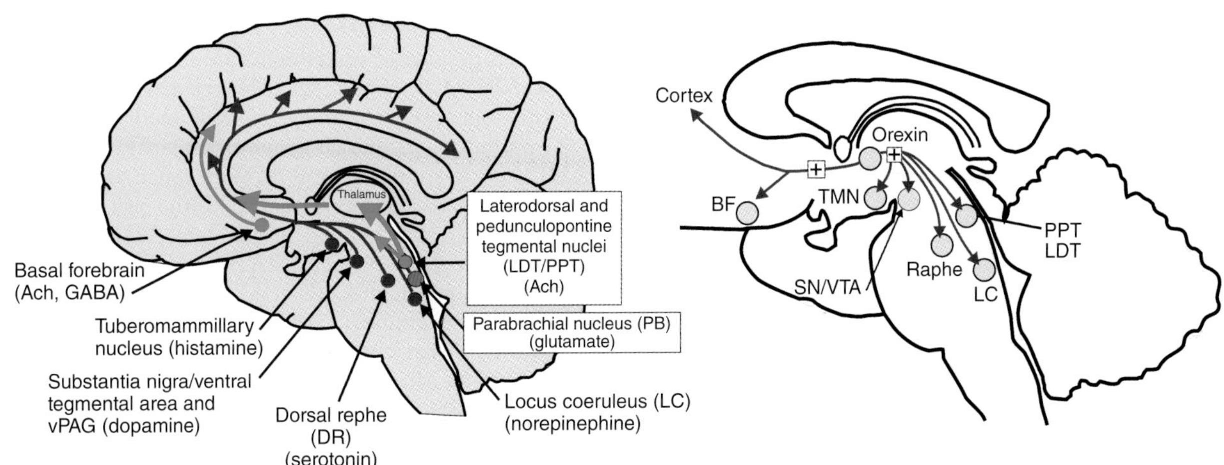

Figure 8–9 Brainstem areas involved with promoting wake and arousal. On the *left*, stimulation from monoamines (serotonin, norepinephrine, histamine), glutamate, and acetylcholine from nuclei in the brainstem and acetylcholine and gamma-aminobutyric acid *(GABA)* from the basal forebrain stimulate the cortex. The lateral dorsal tegmentum/pedunculopontine *(LDT/PPT)* also stimulates areas in the thalamus. On the *right*, orexin neurons provide excitatory innervation to the monoamine neurons, dopamine neurons, the basal forebrain, and the cortex. *Ach,* Acetylcholine; *BF,* basal forebrain; *LC,* locus coeruleus; *LDT,* lateral dorsal tegmentum; *PPT,* pedunculopontine; *SN/VTA,* substantia nigra/ventral tegmental areas; *TMN,* tuberomammillary nucleus; *vPAG,* ventral periaqueductal gray. (Adapted from España RA, Scammell TE. Sleep neurobiology from a clinical perspective. *Sleep.* 2011;34(7):845-858.)

Box 8–16 BRAIN AREAS AND NEUROTRANSMITTERS IMPORTANT FOR WAKEFULNESS

Parabrachial nucleus (PB) and Supramammillary area	Glutamate
Reticular Activating System	Glutamate
Basal Forebrain (BF)	ACh, GABA*
Locus Coeruleus	Norepinephrine
Dorsal Raphe	Serotonin
LDT/PPT	Acetylcholine
TMN	Histamine
Lateral Hypothalamus	Hypocretin (Orexin)
VTA/vPAG	Dopamine

VTA, ventral tegmental area; *vPAG*, ventral periaqueductal gray.
*BP GABA neurons may inhibit cortical inhibitory interneurons

and amphetamines all increase DA signaling. Cholinergic neurons in the LDT/PPT (innervate thalamus and hypothalamus) and BF also promote wakefulness. Cholinergic neurons in the BF directly and indirectly excite cortical pyramidal neurons promoting fast cortical activity, but it is unclear whether the neurons are needed for wakefulness itself. A subset of GABAergic BF GABAergic BF neurons likely promote wakefulness/cortical activation by reducing the activity of inhibitory cortical interneurons. Chemogenetic activation of GABAergic BF neurons dramatically increases wakefulness and fast EEG activity. Recently the importance of glutamatergic neurons in the PB and supramammillary areas for promoting wakefulness has been recogni zed.[7-9,17,39]

CONTROL OF NREM SLEEP

Flip-Flop Switch of NREM Sleep

During NREM sleep, the VLPO neurons are active and inhibit the firing of neurons in the TMN, DRN, PPT/LDT, and LC, as well as orexin neurons in the LH (Fig. 8–10). Neurons in the PZ (GABA) (Box 8–14) inhibit neurons in the PB region that promote wakefulness. Other neurons in the BF and neuronal nitric acid synthetase neurons in the cortex also promote sleep. During wakefulness the TMN, DRN, and LC inhibit the VLPO. The orexin neurons do not innervate the VLPO directley but stimulate the TMN, DRN, or LC during wakefulness (which inhibit the VLPO neurons) but not during NREM sleep. This mutually inhibitory system functions as a flip-flop switch transitioning between the two states[5,6,45] (Fig. 8–11). Although this model is useful, it does not explain the cycles of NREM (followed by REM) that occur during the night or the increase stage N3 that occurs after sleep deprivation. Two other factors influencing the flip-flop are the homeostatic sleep drive (accumulated wakefulness), which favors NREM sleep, and the circadian alerting signals, which favor wakefulness. As will be discussed later, **AD** is believed to play an important role in the increase in the homeostatic drive during wakefulness, as well as the quality of NREM sleep. There are also NREM-promoting neurons in the BF. Most neurons in the *BF are wakefulness active,* but a few are active during NREM sleep and are GABAergic. Some of these neurons innervate the cortex, so they may promote NREM sleep via direct inhibition of cortical neurons. Others may have effects within the BF (e.g., inhibiting wakefulness-promoting neurons). Neurons in the

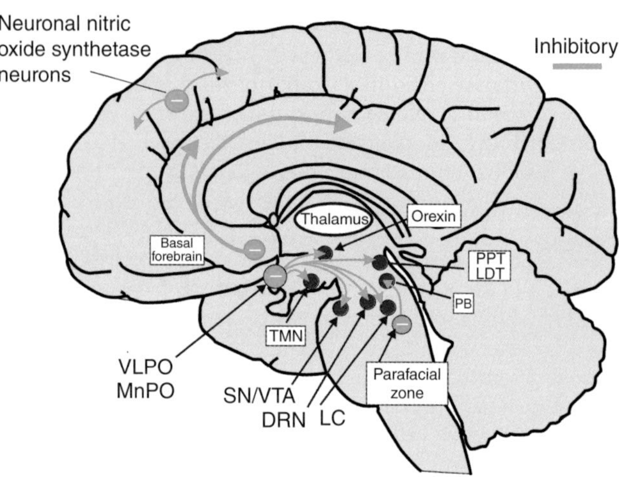

Figure 8–10 Generation of non-rapid eye movement sleep. Neurons in the ventrolateral preoptic area *(VLPO)*, median preoptic nucleus *(MnPO)*, parafacial zone, and basal forebrain inhibit wake centers. The parafacial zone neurons inhibit neurons in the parabrachial nucleus, which are wakefulness-promoting. The neurons in the VLPO/MnPO are gamma-aminobutyric acid (GABA) and galanin secreting and send inhibitory projections as shown to multiple areas. The inhibitory neurons in the basal forebrain are likely GABA type. Cortical neurons that produce nitric oxide are also believed to have inhibitory actions. *DRN*, Dorsal raphe nucleus; *LC*, locus coeruleus; *LDT*, lateral dorsal tegmentum; *PB*, parabrachial nucleus; *PPT*, pedunculopontine; *SN*, substantia nigra, *TMN*, tuberomammillary nucleus; *VTA*, ventral tegmental area. (Adapted from España RA; Scammell TE. Sleep neurobiology from a clinical perspective. *Sleep.* 2011;34(7):845-858.)

parafacial zone (PZ) located within the medulla oblongata, lateral and dorsal to the facial nerve are GABAergic/glycinergic and are active during NREM sleep. They promote sleep by inhibiting wakefulness-promoting glutamatergic neurons in the PB (thus promoting NREM sleep).[9,19,20] The cortex contains scattered NREM sleep-active neurons that contain both GABA and neuronal nitric oxide synthase.

NREM Sleep Homeostasis, Somnogens, and Caffeine

Prolonged periods of wakefulness are followed by long periods of NREM sleep with an increased amount of stage N3, and this homeostatic response is likely mediated by NREM sleep-promoting substances (somnogens) including adenosine (AD), prostaglandin D2, and cytokines such as interleukin-1 and tumor necrosis factor-alpha. AD is the best understood of these somnogens (Box 8–17). The two AD receptor types relevant to sleep are A1 and A2A. In the BF, cortex, and hippocampus extracellular levels of AD increase across prolonged periods of wakefulness and decline during sleep. It was hypothesized that the accumulation of AD might be the mechanism of sleep homeostatic drive build-up. However, AD knock-out mice still exhibit the effects of sleep restriction on stage N3 sleep (increased slow wave activity). Therefore AD is likely not the **only** substance mediating the build-up of pressure for sleep during prolonged wakefulness. AD receptor antagonists (e.g., caffeine) have potent effects on maintaining wakefulness. AD binds to A1 receptors on BF cholinergic neurons (wakefulness-promoting) decreasing the firing of these neurons.[6,31] This causes a reduction in cortical arousal. AD also may disinhibit some cells in the VLPO promoting NREM sleep. The AD-mediated reduction in activity of inhibitory BF GABAergic neuronal activity targeting galaninergic VLPO neurons (disinhibition) increases the activity of these sleep-promoting neurons. AD may also directly excite a

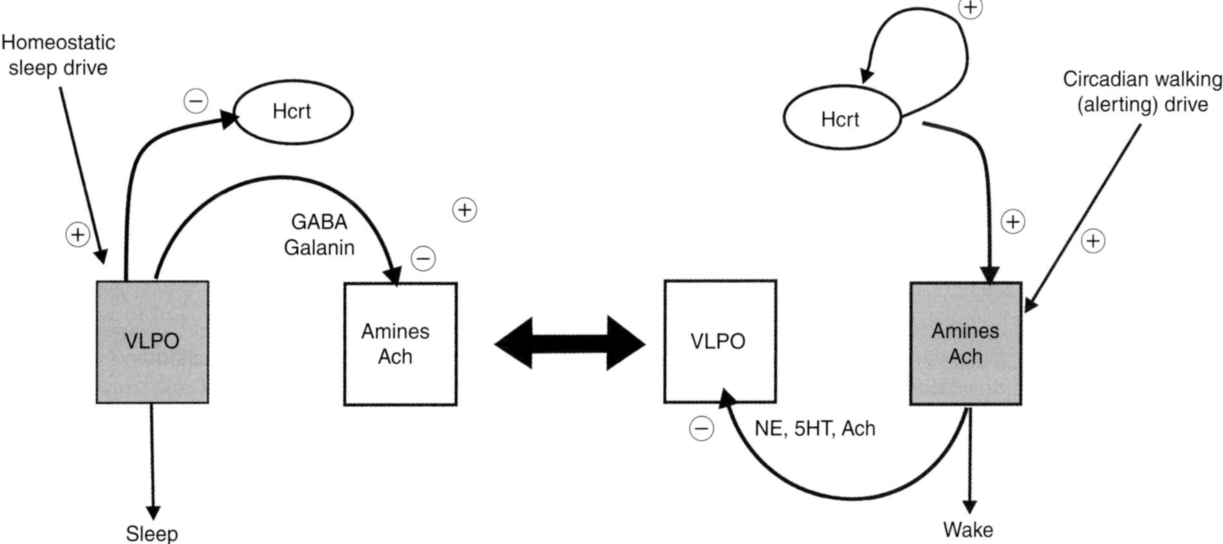

Figure 8–11 Flip-flop transition between states. When neurons in the ventrolateral preoptic area *(VLPO)* are active, they inhibit monoamine and acetylcholine *(Ach)* neurons and orexin-secreting neurons. The homeostatic sleep drive helps activate the VLPO, but this decreases during sleep. When brainstem monoamine nuclei are active, stimulated by the circadian waking (alerting) signal and hypocretin (*Hcrt;* orexin) from the lateral hypothalamus, they inhibit the VLPO favoring wakefulness. *5HT,* Serotonin; *GABA,* gamma-aminobutyric acid; *NE,* norepinephrine. (Adapted from Saper CB, Chou TC, Scammell TE. The sleep switch: hypothalamic control of sleep and wakefulness. *Trends Neurosci.* 2001;24:726-731.)

Box 8–17 ADENOSINE AND SLEEP

Adenosine Levels in Basal Forebrain

- Increase with prolonged wakefulness
- (correlated with amount of SWA during recovery sleep)
- AD levels decrease during recovery sleep

Adenosine Receptors: A1 and A2A

- AD at A1 receptors—mediates response to sleep deprivation and increased sleep need both by promoting sleep and inhibiting some arousal pathways
- AD at A2A receptors—promotes sleep mainly by decreasing arousal.
- Selective and non-selective AD agonists increase sleep and SWA

A1 Receptors (A1Rs)

- Facilitate sleep through AD inhibition of wake-active neurons in several brain areas, including both the BF and brainstem regions (LDT) of the cholinergic arousal system
- Decreased HA release at TMN
- Disinhibits some cells in VLPO (promotes NREM)
- (decreased GABAergic neuron inhibition of galaninergic VLPO neurons)
- The buildup of adenosine in the cortex and thalamus increases slow wave activity through the activation of A1Rs.

A2A Receptors

- AD action at A2A receptors in NAc an area associated with arousal induces slow wave sleep
- Caffeine (A1 and A2A antagonist)—alerting effects mediated by blocking A2A receptors in the NAc outer shell. (Mice lacking A2A receptors—no caffeine response)
- AD action at A2A receptors in TMN inhibit HA release.
- AD at A2A excites subpopulation of VLPO cells.

Nucleus Accumbens (NAc)—part of BF near preoptic area contains outer area (shell) and inner area (core) involved with arousal and dopamine reward pathways
AD, Adenosine; *BF,* basal forebrain; *GABA,* gamma-aminobutyric acid; *HA,* histamine; *NAc,* nucleus accumbens; *SWA,* slow wave activity; *TMN,* tuberomammillary nucleus; *VLPO,* ventrolateral preoptic area; *A1Rs,* adenosine 1 receptors.

subpopulation of VLPO neurons (A2A receptors). In addition, AD also decreases HA release from TMN neurons (A1, A2A receptors) favoring sleep. The effect of AD inhibition on wakefulness-promoting neurons in the nucleus accumbens (NAc) (located in the BF near the preoptic area) by binding A2A receptors is thought to be important for decreasing arousal (thereby promoting sleep).[46] Caffeine blocks both AD A1 and A2A receptors (nonselective), but blockade of A2A receptors in the outer portion (shell) of the NAc in the BF near the preoptic area is thought to be essential for caffeine's wakefulness-promoting effects. Caffeine has no alerting effect on mice lacking A2A receptors.

CONTROL AND MANIFESTATIONS OF REM SLEEP

Manifestations of REM Sleep

The major tonic and phasic features of REM sleep are listed in Box 8–18. The tonic features include EEG desynchronization (reduction in cortical EEG amplitude), theta rhythm generation by the hippocampus (sawtooth wave in the EEG), suppression of muscle tone (atonia), absent thermoregulation, penile erection, and constriction of the pupils. The phasic features of REM sleep include *ponto-geniculo-occipital* (PGO) waves that precede and occur in association with REMs during stage R, irregular respiration, an irregular heart rate (sympathetic bursts), and REMs. The PGO waves start in the pons transit to the lateral geniculate nucleus (LGN) of the thalamus and from there to the occipital area. PGO waves are an integral part of REM sleep. The density of the PGO waves coincides with the amount of eye movements measured during REM sleep.

Box 8–18 CHARACTERISTICS OF RAPID EYE MOVEMENT SLEEP

Tonic Features

1. EEG desynchronization (reduction in cortical EEG amplitude).
2. Theta rhythm generated in hippocampus (sawtooth waves in EEG).
3. Suppression of muscle tone (atonia).
4. Absent thermoregulation (no shivering).
5. Penile erections.
6. Pupils constrict (parasympathetic dominance).

Phasic Features

1. PGO waves: Precede and occur during REM sleep. PGO waves arrive in bursts in association with eye movements. PGO waves originate in pons, travel to LGN of the thalamus and then to the occipital cortex.
2. Contraction of middle ear muscles.
3. Irregular respiration and heart rate.
4. REMs.

EEG, electroencephalogram; *LGN*, lateral geniculate nucleus; *PGO*, ponticulo-occipital; *REM*, rapid eye movements

Models of Control of REM Sleep

Several models have been proposed for the control of REM sleep.[5,6,47,48] Schematic illustration of some of the important areas for the control of REM sleep is shown in Figure 8–12. In the traditional model(s), when the activity of cholinergic REM-on neurons in the LDT and PPT nuclei is high and that in the monoaminergic centers (TMN,DRN, and LC) is low, REM sleep occurs and vice versa (Fig. 8–13). TMN, DRN, and LC neurons are inhibited by REM-on neurons, and these neurons mutually inhibit the REM-on neurons. For simplicity, not all interactions are shown. The REM-on neurons stimulate the thalamus, which results in the low amplitude desynchronized EEG of REM sleep. In some early models the cholinergic REM-on LPT/PPT neurons directly stimulated neurons in the middle medulla that inhibit motor neurons (REM atonia) using the neurotransmitters GABA and galanin. Different populations of REM-on cells in the LPT and PPT stimulate effector cells in the medial pontine reticular formation (mPRF). The neurons in

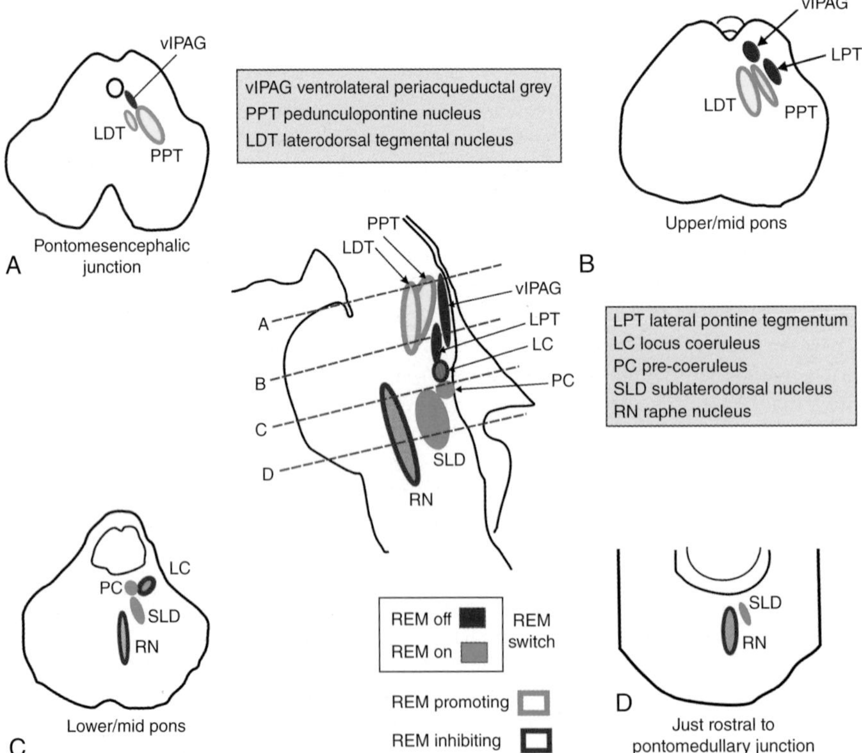

Figure 8–12 Schematic showing some of the brain areas involved in the rapid eye movement *(REM)* switch (controlling REM sleep) are shown. A, B, C, and D are cross sections at the levels shown in the lateral view of the brainstem. The REM-on areas are in *green*, including the pericoeruleus *(PC)* area and the sublaterodorsal nucleus *(SLD)*. The REM-off areas are in *red*, including the reticular nucleus *(RN)*, ventrolateral periaqueductal gray *(vlPAG)*, and the lateral pontine tegmentum *(LPT)*. The pedunculopontine *(PPN)* and lateral dorsal tegmentum *(LDT)* are also REM-on but are not part of the basic REM switch. The RN and LC are REM-inhibiting but not part of the basic REM switch. (Adapted from Boeve BF, Silber MH, Saper CB, et al. Pathophysiology of REM sleep behaviour disorder and relevance to neurodegenerative disease. *Brain*. 2007;130(Pt 11):2770-2788.)

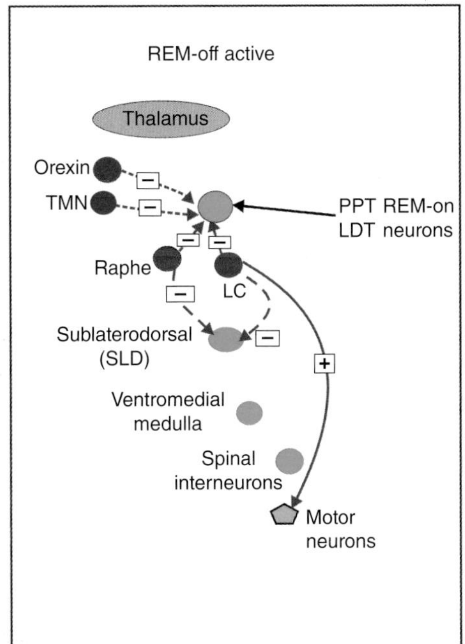

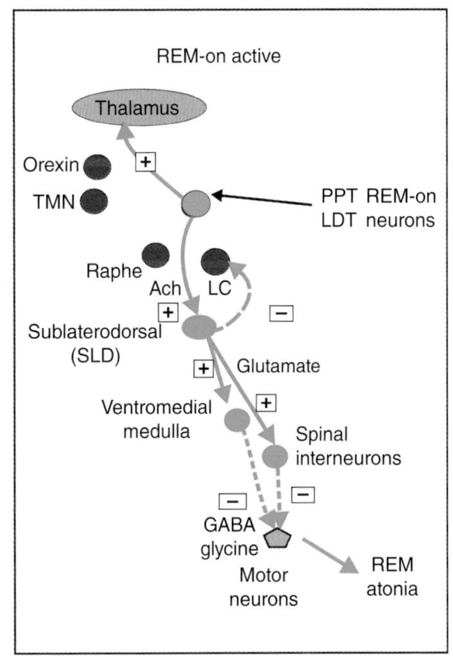

REM-off — Stimulatory
REM-on - - - Inhibitory

Figure 8–13 "Traditional" rapid eye movement *(REM)* sleep model. In this model REM-on neurons in the pedunculopontine *(PPT)* and lateral dorsal tegmentum *(LDT)* inhibit REM-off areas including the dorsal raphe nucleus and locus coeruleus *(LC)* and stimulate REM-on areas including the sublaterodorsal nucleus *(SLD)*. SLD neurons (glutamate) mediate REM atonia by exciting inhibitory neurons in the medulla, which inhibit motor neurons by secreting gamma-aminobutyric acid *(GABA)* and glycine. The SLD may also stimulate spinal interneurons that also inhibit spinal motor neurons. The PPT/LDT also excite the thalamus allowing the fast electroencephalogram of REM sleep. The REM-off neurons inhibit the PPT/LDT. Note that LC provides stimulatory input to motor neurons, which is diminished by activity in the SLD and other REM-on neurons. *TMN*, Tuberomammillary nucleus.

the mPRF are cholinoceptive. Infusion of cholinergic agonists into this area results in many of the manifestations of REM sleep. Specific areas in the mPRF provide ascending projections resulting in PGO waves and REMs. In later models the cholinergic REM-on neurons stimulate the SLD nucleus, which then stimulates the inhibitory neurons in the middle medulla (as shown in Fig. 8–13). The REM-on neurons in the SLD are glutamatergic.

Whereas some of the original models of control of REM sleep emphasized inhibition by the REM off neurons in the LC and DRN, the pons contains other REM-suppressing neurons than those found in the LC and DRN. GABAergic neurons in the vlPAG and the adjacent **lateral pontine tegmentum** (LPT), a region also known as the deep mesencephalic reticular nucleus, suppress the REM-on neurons in the pontine SLD tegmental area located below the LC. The vlPAG/LPT area is silent during REM sleep but active during wakefulness. The SLD area (also known as the pericoeruleus or subcoeruleus area) contains *REM-on glutamatergic neurons* in the sublateral dorsal (SLD) nucleus and the precoeruleus (PC) nucleus important for some manifestations of REM sleep, as well as REM-on GABAergic neurons. One should avoid confusing the lateral dorsal tegmentum (LDT) and lateral pontine tegmentum (LPT) as well as the pericoeruleus and precoeruleus areas given the similarity in nomenclature.

In a newer model of REM sleep, the vlPAG/LPT REM-off area in the pons interacts with the SLD nuclei, a REM-on area. The two areas form the two reciprocally inhibiting REM-off and REM-on areas in the model of REM sleep generation proposed by Lu and colleagues (Fig. 8–14).[47,48] GABAergic neurons in the

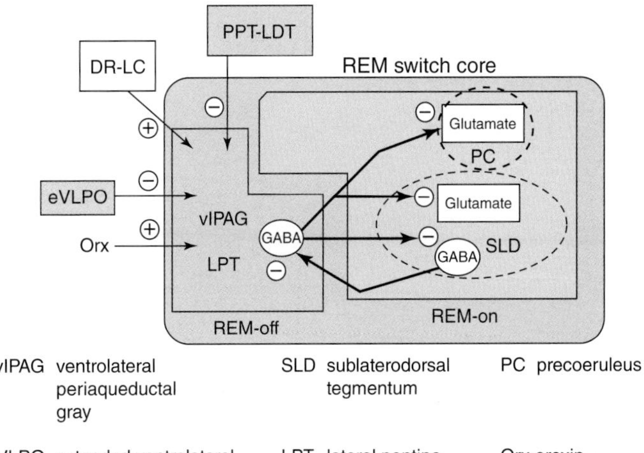

vlPAG ventrolateral periaqueductal gray
SLD sublaterodorsal tegmentum
PC precoeruleus
eVLPO extended ventrolateral preoptic neurons
LPT lateral pontine tegmentum
Orx orexin

Figure 8–14 A model of the rapid eye movement *(REM)* sleep switch in which REM-off and REM-on areas in the pons are mutually inhibitory. The core of the switch includes REM-off neurons in the ventrolateral periaqueductal gray *(vlPAG)* and Lateral pontine tegmentum and REM-on neurons in the sublaterodorsal nucleus *(SLD)* and precoeruleus area *(PC)*. Gamma-aminobutyric acid *(GABA)* neurons in each area mutually inhibit each other, as well as the opposing REM-on or REM-off neurons. REM-on neurons in the pedunculopontine *(PPT)* and lateral dorsal tegmentum *(LDT)* and extended ventrolateral preoptic area *(VLPO)* provide inhibitory input to REM-off areas and excitatory input to the REM-on areas (not shown in figure for simplicity). Orexin neurons and neurons in the dorsal raphe and locus coeruleus *(DR-LC)* stimulate the REM-off areas. (Adapted from Lu J, Sherman D, Devor M, Saper CB. A putative flip-flop switch for control of REM sleep. *Nature*. 2006;441:589-594.)

REM-off and REM-on areas mutually inhibit each other. In this REM sleep flip-flop circuit model, the REM-on GABAergic neurons in the LDT/PPT and eVLPO (high activity during REM) provide inhibitory input to the REM-off neurons (favoring the REM-on state). Orexin neurons provide stimulatory input to the REM-off neurons. REM-on glutamatergic neurons in the precoeruleus (PC) and medial parabrachial (PG) areas project to the medial septum-BF and activate the hippocampus and neocortex, mediating some of REM sleep effects on the EEG. REM-on glutamatergic neurons in the SLD produce the atonia of REM sleep as discussed later. In summary, in this model cholinergic and monoaminergic systems may modulate REM sleep by acting on either the REM-off or the REM-on groups or on both simultaneously (not shown), but the cholinergic and monoaminergic systems are located external to the REM switch. However, cholinergic neurons in the PPT/LDT may still help drive the fast EEG activity of REM sleep (via thalamic projections), as well as other REM manifestations. Another group of REM sleep-promoting neurons is scattered across the *LH and PH* and produces the neuropeptide *MCH*. These cells innervate the SLD and many other regions, and they *fire maximally during REM* sleep. Studies show that photoactivation or chemoactivation of the MCH neurons increases REM sleep.[6,16,18]

REM Atonia

The SLD area is now believed to be responsible for the manifestation of REM atonia. Different models are proposed to explain how the SLD generates the atonia (Fig. 8–15). In one model the SLD excites GABA/glycinergic neurons in the ventromedial medulla that then inhibit spinal motor neurons.[5,49] Another model proposes that the SLD glutamatergic neurons bypass the medulla and directly excite spinal interneurons that use glycine and/or GABA to inhibit spinal motor neurons.[50-52] These models are not mutually exclusive, and both mechanisms may be present. REM-on neurons are also believed to inhibit the LC. The atonia of skeletal muscles during REM sleep results not only from the inhibition by GABA and glycine at the alpha motor neurons but also from disfacilitation, or the loss of NE stimulation of spinal motor neurons (Fig. 8–13). The breakdown of REM atonia mechanisms underlies the REM sleep behavior disorder.[53,54] Some of the same circuits are involved in cataplexy in narcolepsy, which is mediated by emotional stimuli and occurs due to lack of orexin inhibition on the SLD.[55] The mechanisms promoting cataplexy are discussed in more detail in Chapter 32. Maintenance of consciousness during cataplexy is due in part to persistent activity of the TMN (HA).[37] In contrast, during REM sleep TMN activity is very reduced.

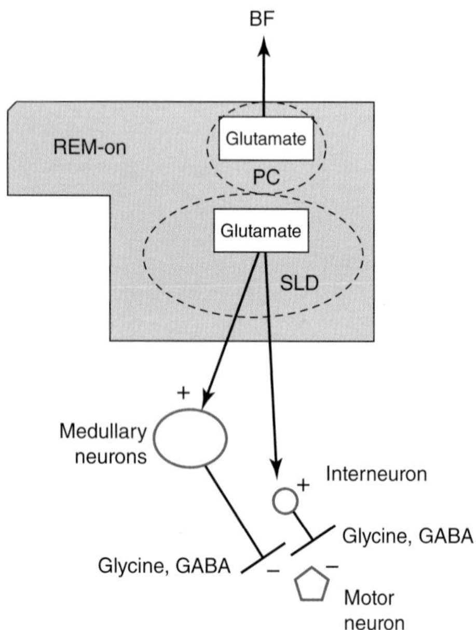

Figure 8–15 Schematic of postulated rapid eye movement *(REM)* atonia mechanisms. REM-on neurons in the precoeruleus *(PC)* area are glutaminergic and have projections to the basal forebrain *(BF)*. The glutaminergic neurons in the sublaterodorsal *(SLD)* nucleus have excitatory projections to areas in the ventral medial medulla, which have inhibitory action on motor neuron nuclei (neurotransmitters gamma-aminobutyric acid *[GABA]* and glycine) and/or stimulate interneurons that they have inhibitory innervation of motor neurons (also GABA and glycine).

MEDICATIONS AND NEUROBIOLOGY

Although discussed in individual sections, a brief summary of neurobiology and medications may highlight some important mechanisms (Table 8-3). Further information on the effects of medications on wakefulness and sleep is presented in Chapter 9. Medications that increase DA signaling increase wakefulness, including modafinil, armodafinil, solriamfetol (dual DA and NE reuptake blocker), methylphenidate, and amphetamines.[5,6,14,56] Modafinil and armodafinil are inhibitors of DAT.[57] Amphetamines increase the synaptic concentration of DA by decreasing the reuptake of DA by DAT and disrupting vesicular packaging of DA, which increases cytosolic levels of DA that can the leak out via DAT reverse transport. At high concentrations amphetamines also block the reuptake of NE and 5-HT, which can cause tachycardia, arrhythmia, and even psychosis.[14]

Medications that increase HA signaling (pitolisant) increase wakefulness, whereas antihistamines increase sedation.[32,33] Atypical antipsychotic medications that are sedating do so via antihistamine activity (quetiapine, olanzapine, clozapine).[58] Sedating antidepressants act in part due to antihistamine activity (e.g., sedating tricyclic antidepressants [doxepin], trazodone, mirtazapine). Although 5HT has multiple effects via the many receptor types, 5HT in general is wakefulness-promoting, as is NE. Selective serotonin reuptake inhibitors and serotonin-norepinephrine reuptake inhibitors inhibit REM sleep. Cholinergic agonists tend to promote wakefulness or REM sleep, and anticholinergics are sedating. For example, taking donepezil (a cholinesterase inhibitor decreasing the metabolism of acetylcholine) in the evening may promote insomnia and less commonly nightmares.

HOMEOSTATIC DRIVE AND CIRCADIAN CONTROL OF SLEEP

The timing of sleep depends on the homeostatic sleep drive (increases with the cumulative wake time since the last sleep episode) known as process S and circadian factors (process C) controlled by the suprachiasmatic nucleus (SCN). This interaction is described by the two-process model and illustrated in Figure 8–16.[59] During wakefulness there is a progressive increase in process S, which can be assessed by the amount of EEG theta activity during wakefulness. Process S increases in amplitude until the onset of sleep and then falls during sleep (the fall is assessed by the decrease in frontal slow wave activity). Process C depends on the internal circadian clock controlled by the SCN

Table 8-3 Effects of Medications/Substances on Sleep

Drug Class	Examples	Pharmacology	Neurologic Mechanism	
Selective serotonin reuptake inhibitors (SSRIs)	Fluoxetine Citalopram	Increase extracellular Levels of 5HT	5HT inhibits REM sleep producing neurons	Decreased REM sleep
Tricyclic antidepressants	Amitriptyline Nortriptyline	Increased extracellular Levels of 5HT and NE	Increased 5HT	Decreased REM sleep
Central nervous system stimulants	Amphetamine Methylphenidate	Increased extracellular levels of DA and NE	Increased DA and NE signaling	Increased wakefulness
Alerting Agents (DA)	Modafinil, armodafinil	Increased extracellular levels of DA	Increased DA signaling	Increased wakefulness
Alerting Agents (DA, NE)	Solriamfetol	Increased extracellular levels of DA	Increased DA, NE signaling	Increased wakefulness
Benzodiazepines	Diazepam Clonazepam	Enhance GABA signaling via GABA-A receptors	GABA inhibits the Arousal systems	Increased sleep
Typical antipsychotics	Haldol, Chlorpromazine	Block DA receptors	Reduced DA signaling	Increased sleep
Antihistamines (First generation)	Diphenhydramine	Block HA H1 receptors	Reduced HA signaling	Increased sleep
HA Modifiers	Pitolisant	H3 receptor antagonist/ inverse agonist	Increased HA signaling	Increased wakefulness
Adenosine receptor blocker	Caffeine	Adenosine receptor blocker	Decrease adenosine signaling	Increased wakefulness

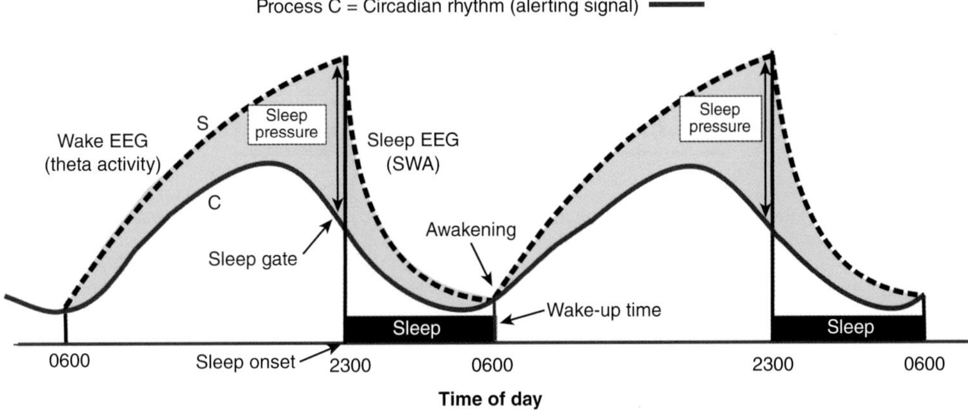

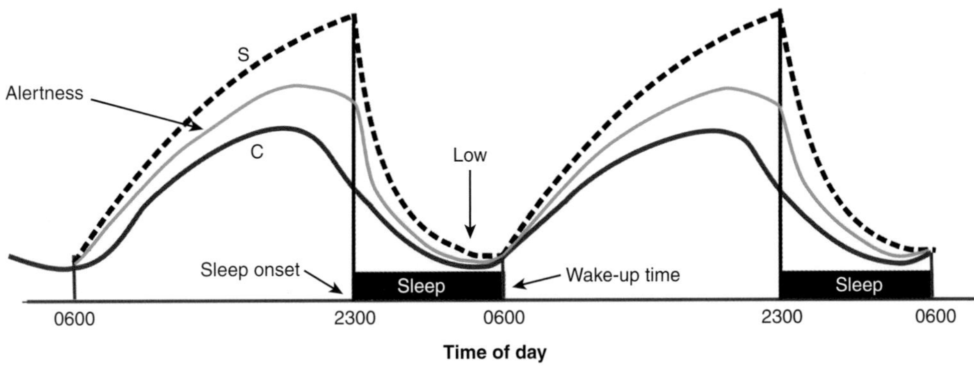

Figure 8–16 The interaction of the homeostatic sleep drive (process S) and circadian rhythm (process C) to determine the pattern of wake and sleep is shown. As the S process increases with cumulative wakefulness, the C signal increases to minimize sleep tendency but falls near bedtime. During sleep the S decreases; by morning sleep is maintained only by a decrease in circadian alerting signal. During the day the circadian alerting signal increases to maintain wake as the homeostatic sleep drive increases.

(entrained by light and other zeitgebers). The magnitude of process C reflects the amplitude of alerting signal from the SCN and can be represented by core body temperature. Process C peaks during the late evening to offset the high amplitude of process S and then starts to decrease before sleep onset (to allow sleep) with a nadir in the early morning hours (about 2 to 3 hours before awakening). In the early morning after awakening both processes S and C increase. Signals from the SCN affect sleep, and sleep state also affects SCN activity. Even during the day, during REM sleep SCN signaling is relatively higher but decreased during NREM sleep. Another method of visualizing the interaction between sleep load and the circadian alerting signal is the "opposition model" shown in Figure 8–17.

The schematic in Figure 8–18 represents the pathways by which the SCN affects sleep.[6,60] The rhythms generated by the SCN are entrained to the light/dark cycle by nonvisual information from retinal ganglion cells via the retinohypothalamic tract to the SCN. The SCN has projections to hypothalamic nuclei including the paraventricular nucleus, dorsomedial hypothalamic nucleus (DMH), ventromedial nucleus, and LH and to the preoptic area. SCN signals flow via the ventral subparaventricular zone (a region just above the SCN) to the dorsomedial hypothalamus. The DMH regulates timing of wakefulness via excitatory projections to orexin neurons (LH) and DRN and inhibitory projections to the preoptic area. The DMH also provides excitation (glutamatergic neurons) that innervate wakefulness-promoting areas including orexin neurons, TMN, LC, VTA, DR, and LDT. However, GABAergic neurons (inhibitory) from the DMH innervate sleep-promoting areas including the VLPO and MnPO (median preoptic area). Therefore, wakefulness can be promoted and sleep inhibited at appropriate times based on information from the SCN.

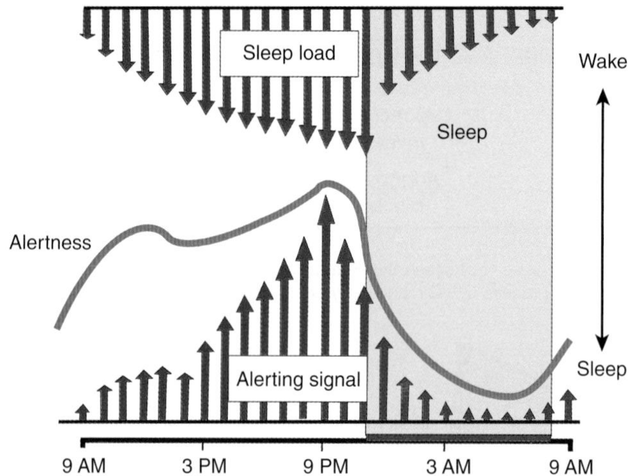

Figure 8–17 Opposition model of sleep. The alerting signal increases to compensate for the increasing sleep load (sleep pressure) until a few hours before habitual sleep and begins falling to allow for sleep onset. During sleep the alerting signal falls as the sleep load falls to allow continued sleep with a minimum a few hours before habitual wake time. Then the alerting signals rises to allow awakening and increases during the day as the sleep load increases.

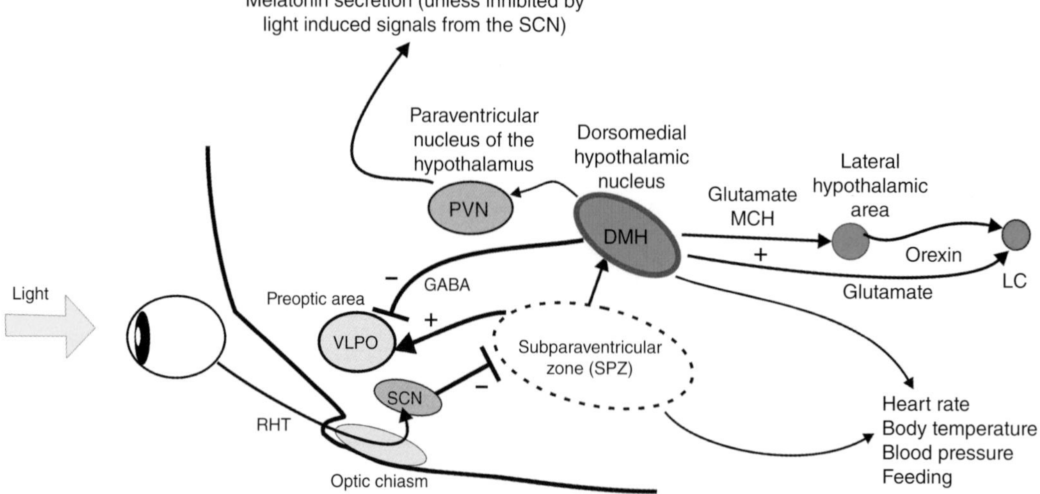

Figure 8–18 Schematic of circadian control of wake and sleep. Light information reaches the suprachiasmatic nucleus *(SCN)* via the retinohypothalamic tract *(RHT)*. Output from the SCN traverses the subparaventricular zone *(SPZ)* to the dorsal medial hypothalamic nucleus *(DMH)*. The DMH sends excitatory input to orexin other wake active neurons to facilitate wake and inhibitory neurons to sleep centers to suppress sleep. The opposite pattern occurs when the alerting signal decreases before sleep. *GABA,* Gamma-aminobutyric acid; *LC,* locus coeruleus; *MCH,* melanin-concentrating hormone; *PVN,* paraventricular nucleus of the hypothalamus; *VLPO,* ventrolateral preoptic area. (Adapted from Saper CB, Cano G, Scammell TE. Homeostatic, circadian, and emotional regulation of sleep. *J Comp Neurol.* 2005;493(1):92-98.)

SUMMARY OF KEY POINTS

1. Activity profiles of neurotransmitter systems across wakefulness and sleep:

	Wakefulness	NREM	REM
Ach	↑↑	-	↑↑
Monoamines*	↑↑	↑	↔
VLPO/MnPO†	–	↑↑	↑↑
Orexin (Hcrt)	↑↑	–	–
Glu	↑↑	–	↑
DA‡	↑↑	–	–

*Monoamines: 5HT, NE, HA.
†GABA, galanin.
‡vPAG.
Ach, Acetylcholine; *DA,* dopamine; *5HT,* serotonin; *GABA,* gamma-aminobutyric acid; *Glu,* glutamate; *HA,* histamine; *Hcrt,* hypocretin; *MnPO,* median preoptic nucleus; *NE,* norepinephrine; *VLPO,* ventrolateral preoptic area; *vPAG,* ventral periaqueductal gray.
– Little or no firing, ↑ lower activity, ↑↑ high activity.

2. Neurons producing monoamines (5HT, HA, NE), Ach, DA, and Glu promote wakefulness.
3. GABA is the major inhibitory transmitter in the CNS (but can be excitatory if it inhibits inhibitory neurons). The neurons in the VLPO that promote sleep secrete GABA and galanin.
4. Glu is the major excitatory neurotransmitter in the CNS. The PB nucleus (Glu) that surrounds the superior cerebellar peduncle is important for wakefulness. The lateral PB nucleus mediates the arousal response to hypercapnia.
5. The TMN (HA) has high activity during wakefulness, lower activity during NREM, and very low activity during REM sleep. Antihistamines cause sedation, but pitolisant (an antagonist/inverse agonist at H3 autoreceptors) increases HA release by action on HA secreting neurons and binding of H3 heteroreceptors on NE, and DA secreting neurons increases NE and DA. These actions of pitolisant increasing HA, NE, and DA increase wakefulness.
6. Although DA concentration is high during wakefulness in several brain areas, in the past DA neurons were thought *not* to have a wake-sleep-related change in firing rate. However, new techniques have shown that DA neurons in vPAG and VTA are more active during wakefulness.
7. Alerting medications including modafinil, armodafinil, and amphetamines/methylphenidate increase wakefulness by increasing DA activity.
8. Orexin (Hcrt) neurons in the lateral hypothalamus are active during wakefulness but stabilize both wakefulness and sleep. Patients with narcolepsy type I are Hcrt deficient.
9. BF cholinergic neurons (directly) and BF GABA secreting neurons (indirectly) stimulate the cortex enhancing wakefulness.
10. AD concentrations increase (accumulate) during wakefulness in the VLPO area and likely contribute to the increase in homeostatic sleep drive. Caffeine promotes wakefulness by blocking AD receptors.
11. The SLD nucleus glutamatergic neurons mediate the atonia of REM sleep by one or more pathways resulting in inhibition of spinal motor neurons with glycine and galanin.
12. Sleep spindles are generated by thalamocortical oscillations involving the reticular thalamic nucleus.
13. During REM sleep, cholinergic activity of the LPT/PPT stimulates the thalamus resulting in the desynchronized EEG pattern. However, the REM switch is mediated by mutually inhibitory areas REM-off (vlPAG, LPT) and REM-on (subdorsolateral nucleusand precoeruleus areas) via mutually inhibitory GABA neurons.
14. The cholinergic cells of the PPT/LDT regions are active during wake and REM sleep. Some are wake-on, whereas others are wake-on/REM-on.

CLINICAL REVIEW QUESTIONS

1. Which of the following brain areas is active during both NREM and REM sleep?
   A. TMN
   B. LC
   C. DRN
   D. VLPO
2. Which of the following brain areas is/are active during REM sleep?
   A. LDT/PPT
   B. LC
   C. DRN
   D. TMN
3. Which of the following areas is/are active during cataplexy but not REM sleep?
   A. LDT/PPT
   B. LC
   C. DRN
   D. TMN
4. What is/are the neurotransmitter(s) of VLPO neurons promoting sleep?
   A. GABA, galanin
   B. 5HT
   C. HA
   D. NE
5. Which of the following neurotransmitters/modulators is primarily responsible for the alerting effects of amphetamine?
   A. 5HT
   B. DA
   C. NE
   D. HA
6. Which of the following is *not* true about Hcrt neurons?
   A. Stabilize wakefulness-sleep transitions
   B. Are active during wakefulness
   C. Are located in the lateral hypothalamus
   D. Provide inhibitory input to the LC and DRN
7. What is the major transmitter of neurons in the DRN?
   A. 5HT
   B. DA
   C. NE
   D. HA
8. During REM sleep, neurons in what area(s) are responsible for hypotonia?
   A. LDT/PPT
   B. Sublaterodorsal tegmentum
   C. LC
   D. DRN
   E. TMN
9. What neurotransmitter is believed to mediate the inhibition of spinal motor neurons (by interneurons)?
   A. NE
   B. Glu
   C. 5HT
   D. GABA/glycine
10. Which of the following brain areas *do (does) not* have glutaminergic neurons important for wakefulness?
    A. Supramammillary neurons
    B. Parabrachial neurons
    C. Parafacial zone neurons
    D. Reticular activating system

11. What accumulates in the VLPO regions during periods of prolonged wakefulness?
A. GABA
B. Adenosine
C. Ach
D. Galanin

12. In the two-process model of wakefulness and sleep, which of the following is **NOT** true?
A. Homeostatic sleep drive falls during sleep or naps.
B. The circadian alerting signal is highest in the midafternoon.
C. The circadian alerting signal begins to drop before the normal sleep period.
D. The low point of the circadian alerting signal is in the early morning about 2 to 3 hours before habitual wake time.

13. Sleep spindles are generated by neurons in which brain area?
A. Supramammillary neurons
B. Reticular nucleus of the thalamus
C. VLPO
D. Ventral tegmental area

14. The alerting effects of pitolisant depends primarily on:
A. Increased DA
B. Decreased GABA
C. Increased HA
D. Increased NE

15. Which brain area(s) has/have neurons active during both wakefulness and REM sleep?
A. TMN
B. DRN
C. LC
D. LDT/PPT

16. Which hypothalamic nucleus is responsible for transmitting the circadian alerting signal to sleep/wake neurons?
A. Arcuate nucleus
B. Subparaventricular zone neurons
C. Paraventricular nucleus
D. Dorsal medial nucleus

ANSWERS

1. D.
2. A.
3. D.
4. A.
5. B.
6. D. Excitatory input to wakefulness centers.
7. A.
8. B. Although some neurons in the LD/PPT are active during REM sleep, they are not directly responsible for hypotonia.
9. D.
10. C. Parafacial zone neurons have GABA as the main neurotransmitter/modulator and promote sleep.
11. B.
12. B. The alerting signal is highest in the evening a few hours before habitual bedtime to counteract the very high homeostatic sleep drive.
13. B. Thalamic reticular nucleus (thalamocortical oscillations).
14. C. Increased histamine via drug actions on the histamine H3 auto-receptor.
15. D.
16. D.

ABBREVIATIONS

AD, Adenosine; *CSF,* cerebrospinal fluid; *DMH,* dorsomedial hypothalamic nucleus; *5HT,* serotonin; *HA,* histamine; *LDT,* lateral dorsal tegmental; *LH,* lateral hypothalamus; *LPT,* lateral pontine tegmentum; *MCH,* melanin-concentrating hormone; *MRN,* median raphe nucleus; *NAc,* nucleus accumbens; *PPT,* pedunculopontine tegmental; *PZ-GABA,* parafacial zone gamma-aminobutyric acid; *SLD,* sublaterodorsal; *SN,* serotonin; *SWS,* slow wave sleep; *TRN,* thalamic reticular nucleus; *vlPAG,* ventrolateral periaqueductal gray; *VLPO,* ventrolateral preoptic area; *VTA,* ventral tegmental area.

SUGGESTED READING

España RA, Scammell TE. Sleep neurobiology from a clinical perspective. *Sleep*. 2011;34(7):845-858.
Scammell TE, Arrigoni E, Lipton JO. Neural circuitry of wakefulness and sleep. *Neuron*. 2017;93(4):747-765.
Schneider L. Neurobiology and neuroprotective benefits of sleep. *Continuum (Minneap Minn)*. 2020;26(4):848-870.
Saper CB, Chou TC, Scammell TE. The sleep switch: hypothalamic control of sleep and wakefulness. *Trends Neurosci*. 2001;24:726-731.

REFERENCES

1. Von Economo C. Sleep as a problem of localization. *J Nerv Ment Dis*. 1930;71:249-259.
2. Reid A, McCall S, Henry JM, Taubenberger K. Experimenting on the past: the enigma of von Economo's encephalitis lethargica. *J Neuropathol Exp Neurol*. 2001;60:663-670.
3. Hoffman LA, Vilensky JA. Encephalitis lethargica: 100 years after the epidemic. *Brain*. 2017;140(8):2246-2251.
4. España RA, Scammell TE. Sleep neurobiology for the clinician. *Sleep*. 2004;27(4):811-820.
5. España RA, Scammell TE. Sleep neurobiology from a clinical perspective. *Sleep*. 2011;34(7):845-858.
6. Scammell TE, Arrigoni E, Lipton JO. Neural circuitry of wakefulness and sleep. *Neuron*. 2017;93(4):747-765.
7. Schneider L. Neurobiology and neuroprotective benefits of sleep. *Continuum (Minneap Minn)*. 2020;26(4):848-870.
8. Falup-Pecurariu C, Diaconu Ş, Ţînţ D, Falup-Pecurariu O. Neurobiology of sleep (review). *Exp Ther Med*. 2021;21(3):272.
9. Venner A, Todd WD, Fraigne J, et al. Newly identified sleep-wake and circadian circuits as potential therapeutic targets. *Sleep*. 2019;42(5):zsz023.
10. Neudorfer C, Germann J, Elias GJB, et al. A high-resolution in vivo magnetic resonance imaging atlas of the human hypothalamic region. *Sci Data*. 2020;7(1):305.
11. Lu J, Jhou TC, Saper CB. Identification of wake-active dopaminergic neurons in the ventral periaqueductal gray matter. *J Neurosci*. 2006;26(1):193-202.
12. Benarroch EE. Periaqueductal gray: an interface for behavioral control. *Neurology*. 2012;78(3):210-217.
13. Eban-Rothschild A, Rothschild G, Giardino WJ, et al. VTA dopaminergic neurons regulate ethologically relevant sleep-wake behaviors. *Nat Neurosci*. 2016;19(10):1356-1366.
14. Faraone SV. The pharmacology of amphetamine and methylphenidate: relevance to the neurobiology of attention-deficit/hyperactivity disorder and other psychiatric comorbidities. *Neurosci Biobehav Rev*. 2018;87:255-270.
15. Anaclet C, Pedersen NP, Ferrari LL, et al. Basal forebrain control of wakefulness and cortical rhythms. *Nat Commun*. 2015;6:8744.
16. Gompf HS, Anaclet C. The neuroanatomy and neurochemistry of sleep-wake control. *Curr Opin Physiol*. 2020;15:143-151.
17. Pedersen NP, Ferrari L, Venner A, et al. Supramammillary glutamate neurons are a key node of the arousal system. *Nat Commun*. 2017;8(1):1405.
18. Hassani OK, Henny P, Lee MG, Jones BE. GABAergic neurons intermingled with orexin and MCH neurons in the lateral hypothalamus discharge maximally during sleep. *Eur J Neurosci*. 2010;32(3):448-457.
19. Alam MA, Kostin A, Siegel J, et al. Characteristics of sleep-active neurons in the medullary parafacial zone in rats. *Sleep*. 2018;41(10):zsy130.
20. Anaclet C, Lin JS, Vetrivelan R, et al. Identification and characterization of a sleep-active cell group in the rostral medullary brainstem. *J Neurosci*. 2012;32(50):17,970-17,976.

21. De Lecca L, Kilduff TS, Peyron C, et al. The hypocretins: hypothalamic specific peptides with neuroexcitatory activity. *Proc Natl Acad Sci U S A*. 1998;95:322-327.
22. Sakurai T, Amemiya A, Ishii M, et al. Orexins and orexin receptors: a family of hypothalamic neuropeptides and G protein-coupled receptors that regulate feeding behavior. *Cell*. 1998;92(4):573-585.
23. Thannickal T, Moore RY, Nienbus R, et al. Reduced number of hypocretin neurons in human narcolepsy. *Neuron*. 2000;27:469-474.
24. Nishino S, Ripley B, Overeem S, et al. Hypocretin (orexin) deficiency in human narcolepsy. *Lancet*. 2003;355:39-40.
25. Inutsuka A, Yamanaka A. The physiological role of orexin/hypocretin neurons in the regulation of sleep/wakefulness and neuroendocrine functions. *Front Endocrinol (Lausanne)*. 2013;4:18.
26. Hassani OK, Lee MG, Jones BE. Melanin-concentrating hormone neurons discharge in a reciprocal manner to orexin neurons across the sleep-wake cycle. *Proc Natl Acad Sci U S A*. 2009;106(7): 2418-2422.
27. McGinty D, Szymusiak R. Brain structures and mechanisms involved in the generation of NREM sleep: focus on the preoptic hypothalamus. *Sleep Med Rev*. 2001;5(4):323-342.
28. Lu J, Bjorkum AA, Xu M, et al. Selective activation of the extended ventrolateral preoptic nucleus during rapid eye movement sleep. *J Neurosci*. 2002;2:4568-4576.
29. Saito YC, Tsujino N, Hasegawa E, et al. GABAergic neurons in the preoptic area send direct inhibitory projections to orexin neurons. *Front Neural Circuits*. 2013;7:192.
30. McGinty D, Gong H, Suntsova N, et al. Sleep-promoting functions of the hypothalamic median preoptic nucleus: inhibition of arousal systems. *Arch Ital Biol*. 2004;142(4):501-509.
31. Lazarus M, Oishi Y, Bjorness TE, Greene RW. Gating and the need for sleep: dissociable effects of adenosine A1 and A2A receptors. *Front Neurosci*. 2019;13:740.
32. Scammell TE, Jackson AC, Franks NP, et al. Histamine: neural circuits and new medications. *Sleep*. 2019;42(1):zsy183.
33. Guevarra JT, Hiensch R, Varga AW, Rapoport DM. Pitolisant to treat excessive daytime sleepiness and cataplexy in adults with narcolepsy: rationale and clinical utility. *Nat Sci Sleep*. 2020;12:709-719.
34. Valko PO, Gavrilov YV, Yamamoto M, et al. Increase of histaminergic tuberomammillary neurons in narcolepsy. *Ann Neurol*. 2013;74(6): 794-804.
35. Nishino S, Sakurai E, Nevsimalova S, et al. Decreased CSF histamine in narcolepsy with and without low CSF hypocretin-1 in comparison to healthy controls. *Sleep*. 2009;32(2):175-180.
36. Dauvilliers Y, Delallée N, Jaussent I, et al. Normal cerebrospinal fluid histamine and tele-methylhistamine levels in hypersomnia conditions. *Sleep*. 2012;35(10):1359-1366.
37. John J, Wu MF, Boehmer LN, Siegel JM. Cataplexy-active neurons in the hypothalamus: implications for the role of histamine in sleep and waking behavior. *Neuron*. 2004;42(4):619-634.
38. Thakkar MM, Strecker RE, McCarley RW. Behavioral state control through differential serotonergic inhibition in the mesopontine cholinergic nuclei: a simultaneous unit recording and microdialysis study. *J Neurosci*. 1998;18:5490-5497.
39. Xu Q, Wang DR, Dong H, et al. Medial parabrachial nucleus is essential in controlling wakefulness in rats. *Front Neurosci*. 2021;15:645877.
40. Kaur S, Saper CB. Neural circuitry underlying waking up to hypercapnia. *Front Neurosci*. 2019;13:401.
41. Lüthi A. Sleep spindles: where they come from, what they do. *Neuroscientist*. 2014;20(3):243-256.
42. Fernandez LMJ, Lüthi A. Sleep spindles: mechanisms and functions. *Physiol Rev*. 2020;100(2):805-868.
43. Dimitrov T, He M, Stickgold R, Prerau MJ. Sleep spindles comprise a subset of a broader class of electroencephalogram events. *Sleep*. 2021;44(9):zsab099.
44. Jones BE. Arousal and sleep circuits. *Neuropsychopharmacology*. 2020; 45(1):6-20.
45. Saper CB, Chou TC, Scammell TE. The sleep switch: hypothalamic control of sleep and wakefulness. *Trends Neurosci*. 2001;24(12): 726-731.
46. Quarta D, Ferré S, Solinas M, et al. Opposite modulatory roles for adenosine A1 and A2A receptors on glutamate and dopamine release in the shell of the nucleus accumbens. Effects of chronic caffeine exposure. *J Neurochem*. 2004;88(5):1151-1158.
47. Lu J, Sherman D, Devor M, Saper CB. A putative flip-flop switch for control of REM sleep. *Nature*. 2006;441:589-594.
48. Fuller PM, Saper CB, Lu J. The pontine REM switch: past and present. *J Physiol*. 2007;584:735-741.
49. Vetrivelan R, Fuller PM, Tong QA, Lu J. Medullary circuitry regulating rapid eye movement sleep and motor atonia. *J Neurosci*. 2009;29: 9361-9369.
50. Torontali ZA, Fraigne JJ, Sanghera P, et al. The sublaterodorsal tegmental nucleus functions to couple brain state and motor activity during REM Sleep and wakefulness. *Curr Biol*. 2019;29(22):3803-3813.e5.
51. Fraigne JJ, Torontali ZA, Snow MB, Peever JH. REM sleep at its core—circuits, neurotransmitters, and pathophysiology. *Front Neurol*. 2015;6:123.
52. Peever J, Fuller PM. The biology of REM sleep. *Curr Biol*. 2017; 27(22):R1237-R1248.
53. Boeve BF, Silber MH, Saper CB, et al. Pathophysiology of REM sleep behaviour disorder and relevance to neurodegenerative disease. *Brain*. 2007;130(Pt 11):2770-2788.
54. Peever J, Luppi PH, Montplaisir J. Breakdown in REM sleep circuitry underlies REM sleep behavior disorder. *Trends Neurosci*. 2014;37(5): 279-288.
55. Pintwala S, Peever J. Circuit mechanisms of sleepiness and cataplexy in narcolepsy. *Curr Opin Neurobiol*. 2017;44:50-58.
56. Boutrel B, Koob GF. What keeps us awake: the neuropharmacology of stimulants and wakefulness-promoting medications. *Sleep*. 2004; 27(6):1181-1194.
57. Wisor J. Modafinil as a catecholaminergic agent: empirical evidence and unanswered questions. *Front Neurol*. 2013;4:139.
58. Miller DD. Atypical antipsychotics: sleep, sedation, and efficacy. *Prim Care Companion J Clin Psychiatry*. 2004;6(suppl 2):3-7.
59. Borbély AA, Daan S, Wirz-Justice A, Deboer T. The two-process model of sleep regulation: a reappraisal. *J Sleep Res*. 2016;25(2):131-143.
60. Saper CB, Cano G, Scammell TE. Homeostatic, circadian, and emotional regulation of sleep. *J Comp Neurol*. 2005;493(1):92-98.

Chapter 9

Sleep Loss and Effects of Sleep Disorders and Medications on Sleep

EFFECTS OF SLEEP LOSS ON SLEEP ARCHITECTURE

Sleep loss occurs in two ways. The first is sleep fragmentation, which occurs via arousals or frequent periods of wakefulness; these cause symptoms via disrupted, noncontinuous sleep. The second way is via sleep restriction or sleep debt. This chapter details sleep loss and its effects on sleep architecture and physiology.

Sleep Fragmentation

Sleep fragmentation refers to the occurrence of arousals and brief awakenings during the night. Chapter 3 presents the scoring criteria for arousals.[1] Scoring of arousals is important because frequent arousals result in nonrestorative sleep even in the absence of a decrement of total sleep time (TST).[2] As discussed in Chapter 6, the arousal index (ArI, or number of arousals per hour of sleep) in normal individuals increases with age.[3-6] Bonnet and Arand[3] found the ArI in 61- to 70-year-old individuals to be 21.9 ± 6.8/hr (mean ± standard deviation). Therefore, the upper 95% confidence limit may approach 35/hr in older age groups. Conversely, an ArI of 25/hr would be high for a young adult. Although in clinical practice sleep fragmentation and chronic partial sleep deprivation (chronically decreased TST) commonly occur together, studies have shown that frequent arousals alone can cause decrements in performance and mood as well as increases in subjective and objective sleepiness. *Consolidated episodes of sleep in excess of 10 minutes* are needed for restorative sleep.[7] When experimental sleep disturbance occurs more frequently than every 3 minutes (<3-minute episodes of consolidated sleep, or an ArI of 20/hour), there is a sharp decrease in the sleep latency (increased daytime sleepiness) on the multiple sleep latency test (MSLT)[8] (Figure 9–1). However, a significant decrease in the sleep latency begins to occur with sleep fragmentation every 10 minutes. Several sleep fragmentation studies have carefully controlled TST to show that the effects of sleep fragmentation are not produced entirely by the reduction in total sleep time due to fragmentation.[8] Depending on the distribution of arousals over the entire night, two patients with the same ArI may differ in the amount of consolidated sleep (Figure 9–2). Sleep continuity can be measured by survival analysis, which looks at the propensity for different durations of periods (runs) of consolidated sleep to occur in an individual.[9] Better sleep quality is associated with more long runs of consolidated sleep. One can look at the hypnogram (Chapter 6) to assess the continuity of sleep. Many short segments of sleep between awakenings is evidence of poor sleep continuity. The intensity of arousals can vary between individuals,[10] as well as the rapidity of return to sleep after an arousal (Figure 9–3). Younes and coworkers developed the odds ratio product (ORP) as an index of sleep depth, with 2.5 being fully awake and 0 the deepest sleep.[11] Using the ORP, Younes and Hanly[12] found that a quick return to sleep (lower ORP in the 9 seconds after arousal) was associated with increased overall sleep depth during non–rapid eye movement (NREM) sleep (lower NREM average ORP), as well as a reduced probability of subsequent arousal. A rapid return to sleep may explain why some patients with severe obstructive sleep apnea (OSA) do not report daytime sleepiness. Box 9–1 lists the common clinical symptoms of significant sleep fragmentation.[8,13] Similar findings can occur with sleep deprivation as noted below.

Total and Partial Sleep Deprivation

Some of the effects of very severe sleep fragmentation and total and partial sleep deprivation are listed on Box 9–1 and shown in Figure 9–4. In general, the sleep latency (nocturnal and MSLT) decreases after total and partial sleep deprivation and after severe sleep fragmentation. Very severe sleep fragmentation results in essentially equivalent sleepiness as total sleep deprivation (Figures 9–4 and 9–5).[8] In partial sleep deprivation, the effects will increase with repeated nights of partial sleep deprivation and depending on the degree of sleep restriction can have neurobehavioral deficits equivalent to those after 1 to 3 nights of total sleep loss.[14] Another term used for this pattern is *chronic sleep restriction.* The adverse effects of chronic sleep restriction on daytime performance do not plateau and continue to increase over at least 14 days.[14,15] Of interest, *subjective feelings of sleepiness tend to plateau,* whereas manifestations of impaired performance continue to increase.[14,15] Individuals with chronic sleep restriction may not recognize their impairment.

Selective Sleep Deprivation

If rapid eye movement (REM) sleep is selectively impaired by induced arousals, the REM latency decreases, and the amount of REM increases on recovery nights. In some patients with OSA on the first night of continuous positive airway pressure (CPAP) treatment, there may be a large increase in the amount of stage R (REM rebound).[16] Withdrawal of REM-suppressant medications can also result in similar findings. Of note, other patients with OSA have a large increase in stage N3 on the first CPAP night.[16]

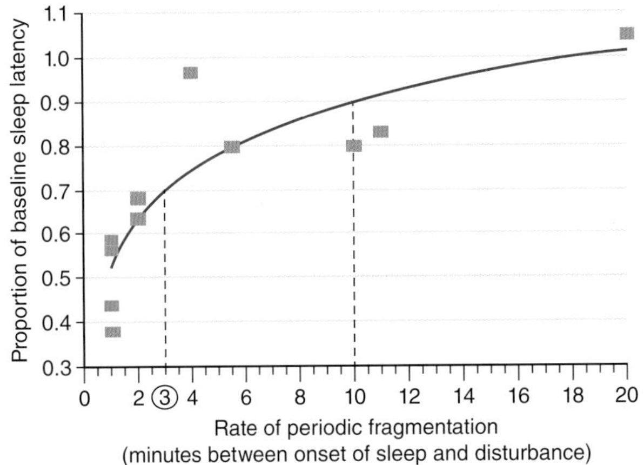

Figure 9–1 Increase in sleepiness (decrease in sleep latency) on the multiple sleep latency as the length of periods of undisturbed sleep is reduced. Sleep disturbance after every 3 minutes of sleep (3 within the ellipse) would be equivalent to an arousal index of about 20/hour. (From Bonnet MH, Arand DL. Clinical effects of sleep fragmentation versus sleep deprivation. *Sleep Med Rev.* 2003;7:297-310.)

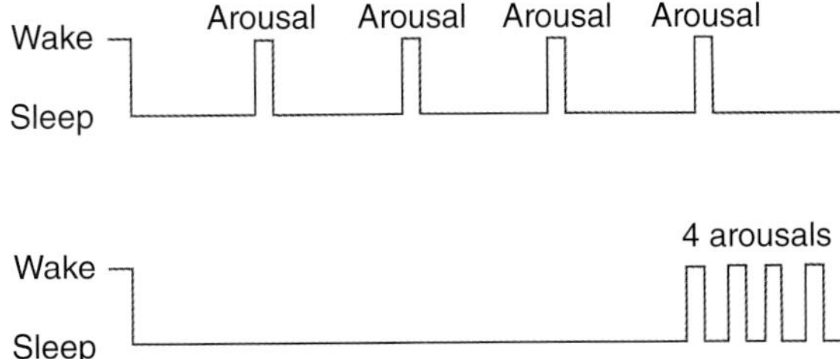

Figure 9–2 Schematic illustrating that a different patterns of consolidated sleep segments can occur with the same arousal index. (Adapted from Norman RG, Scott MA, Ayappa I, et al. Sleep continuity measured by survival curve analysis. *Sleep.* 2006;29(12):1625-1631.)

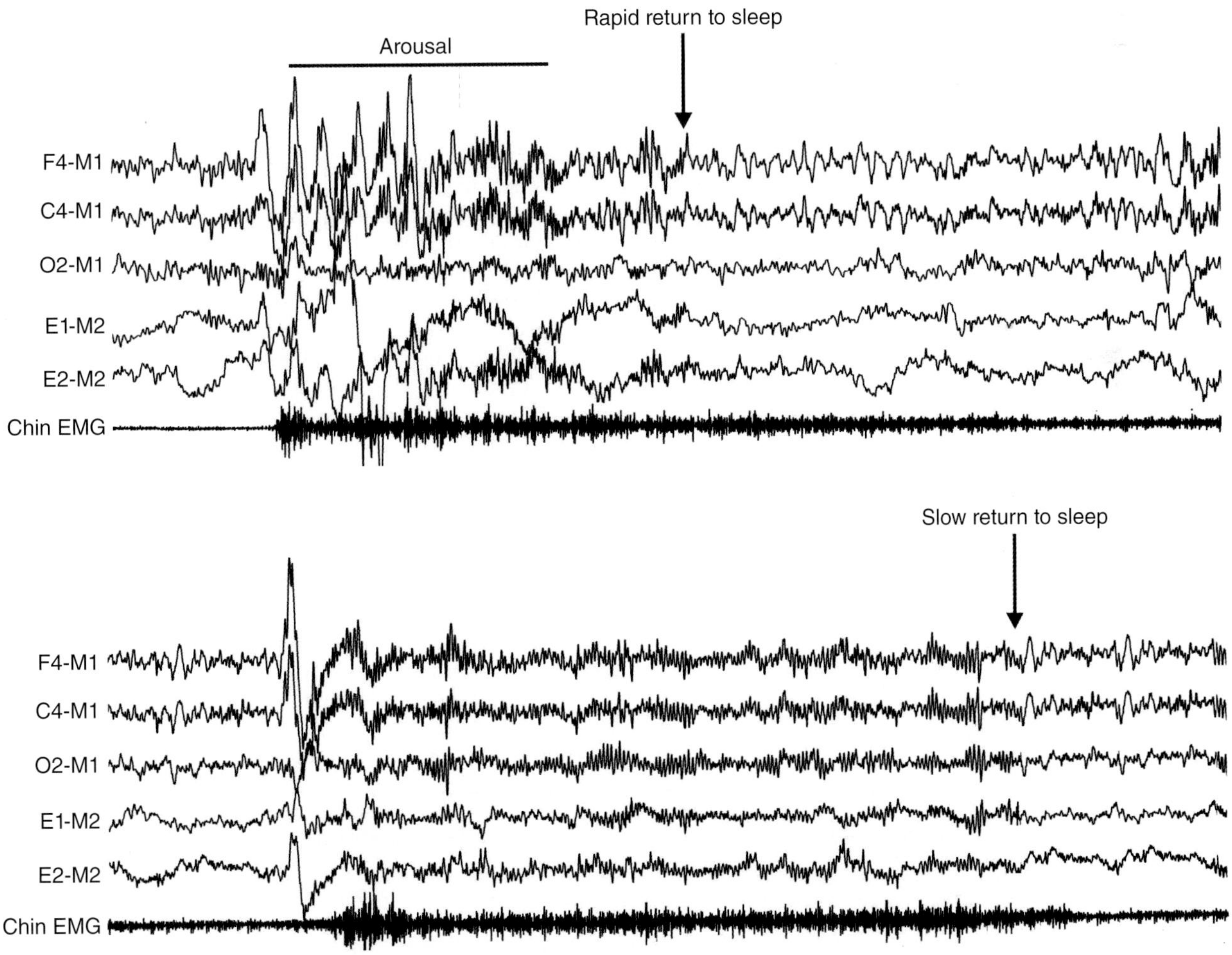

Rapid return to sleep
Arousal
F4-M1
C4-M1
O2-M1
E1-M2
E2-M2
Chin EMG

Slow return to sleep
F4-M1
C4-M1
O2-M1
E1-M2
E2-M2
Chin EMG

Figure 9–3 Two 30-second epochs of polysomnography. In the *top* tracing, following arousal there is a quick return to sleep with stage N2 beginning in the next epoch. In the *bottom* tracing the arousal is followed by long period of posterior dominant rhythm and a transition to sleep occur only near the end of the epoch. The patient remained in stage N1 sleep during the next two epochs.

Box 9–1 CLINICAL MANIFESTATIONS OF SLEEP FRAGMENTATION AND SLEEP DEPRIVATION (RESTRICTION)

- Longer reaction time
- Lapses in attention
- Lost information
- Poor short-term memory
- Poor mood
- Reduced motivation
- Sleepiness
- Poor performance
  - Worse at circadian low points
  - Worse when sedentary
  - Worse with no feedback
  - Worse with reduced light or sound
  - Worse with low motivation, interest, or novelty

From Bonnet MH, Arand DL. Clinical effects of sleep fragmentation versus sleep deprivation. *Sleep Med Rev.* 2003;7:297-310.

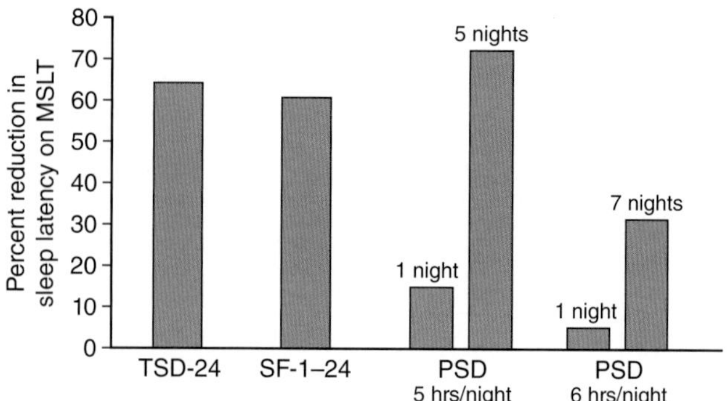

Figure 9–4 Total sleep deprivation (TSD), frequent sleep fragmentation, and chronic sleep restriction all cause significant objective sleepiness (significant reduction in the mean sleep latency). Very frequent sleep fragmentation produced a similar increase in objective sleepiness as 24 hours of TSD. The effects of five nights of sleep restriction to 5 hours are similar to 24 hours of TSD. In partial sleep deprivation (restriction) the effect increased with repeated nights of short sleep duration. (Data redrawn from Bonnet MH, Arand DL. Clinical effects of sleep fragmentation versus sleep deprivation. *Sleep Med Rev.* 2003;7:297-310.)

Recovery from Sleep Loss

The findings during recovery sleep after sleep deprivation in normal individuals are shown in Table 9–1. On the first night, there is an increase in stage N3 at the expense of the other sleep stages. On the second night, there may be an increase in REM sleep.[8,13] Therefore, at least in most patients, stage N3 rebound wins out over stage R rebound, at least during initial recovery sleep. Older patients who have less stage N3 at baseline may be more likely to exhibit an increase in REM sleep on the first recovery night than stage N3.[13,17,18] Studies of patients after abdominal surgery have shown disturbed sleep on the first and sometimes second night after surgery (reduced stage N3 and stage R). This is followed by a rebound in stage N3 and stage R on nights 2 and 3 (or nights 3 and 4). At least in one study a rebound in stage R on on the second and third nights following abdominal surgery was associated with worse desaturation on the second and third night after surgery compared with pre-surgery values.[17] Williamson and Feyer[19] found moderate sleep deprivation to produce impairment in cognitive and motor performance similar to those slightly below or at the legal alcohol level for driving. Another study found that even low-dose alcohol combined with moderate sleep deprivation worsened performance in a driving simulator after sleep deprivation.[20] Therefore the combination is especially problematic. Of interest, there is wide individual variability in the ability to tolerate sleep deprivation. In addi-

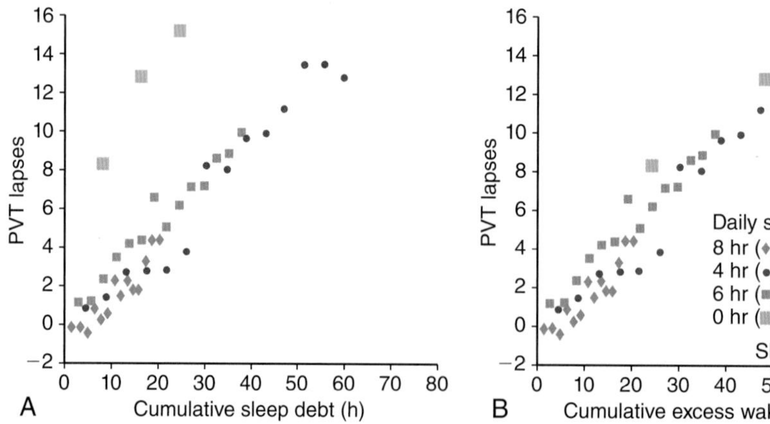

Figure 9–5 Behavioral alertness as a function of cumulative sleep debt versus cumulative wakefulness. The panels show behavioral alertness as measured by psychomotor vigilance test (PVT) performance lapses (relative to baseline), plotted as a function of cumulative sleep debt (A) or cumulative excess wakefulness (B). The PVT presents a randomly timed stimulus, and the subject presses a button in response. Lapses are stimuli that were missed (no response within 500 ms). Cumulative hour of sleep debt was calculated based on estimated daily sleep need of 8.16 hours. Each point represents the average for a day. In (B), excess wakefulness was calculated based on daily wakefulness exceeding 15.84 hours. In (B) the sleep deprivation and restriction values all lie along the same line. This illustrates a monotonic relationship between cumulative excess wakefulness and performance impairment irrespective of the daily sleep ration. (From Van Dongen HPA, Maislin G, Mullington JM, Dinges DF. The cumulative cost of additional wakefulness: dose-response effects on neurobehavioral functions and sleep physiology from chronic sleep restriction and total sleep deprivation. *Sleep.* 2003;2:117-126.)

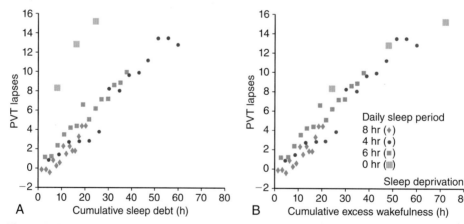

Table 9–1 Recovery From Acute Sleep Deprivation (Recovery Sleep)

First Recovery Night • Shorter sleep latency • Less stage W, stage N1, stage N2 • Longer TST (but ≤12–15 hours; if initial recovery sleep curtailed, longer TST on two or three recovery nights) • Higher % stage N3 • Lower % stage R (older individuals may experience increased % stage R) • REM latency (unchanged younger, shorter in older adults)
Second Recovery Night • Increased stage R (REM rebound) most prominent in younger sleepers • TST increased • Stage N3 normal % TST
Third Recovery Night • Sleep variables approach normal

REM, Rapid eye movement; *TST,* total sleep time.

From Bonnet MH. Acute sleep deprivation. In: Kryger MH, Roth T, Dement WC, eds. *Principles and Practice of Sleep Medicine.* 5th ed. Elsevier; 2011:54-65.

tion, other factors such as motivation, amount of ambient light, activity, and circadian timing are important. The low point of circadian alertness is around 4 to 6 AM (associated with core body temperature minimum),[21] and driving home after a night shift is especially problematic. An on-call resident with minimal sleep during the preceding night often functions well on rounds when presenting but falls asleep in a dark room during a lecture. On the other hand, the circadian alerting signal is high in the evening to maintain wakefulness despite high homeostatic sleep drive (wake maintenance zone [WMZ]). Studies have shown that after sleep deprivation, better performance is seen in the WMZ.[22]

Chronic Partial Sleep Deprivation (Restriction)

Whereas some members of society suffer from periodic sleep restriction for one or two nights, a larger segment likely suffers from chronic partial sleep deprivation. There is large *interindividual variability in the tolerance to chronic partial sleep deprivation.* Healthy humans appear to require 7 to 8 hours of sleep. A large-scale dose-response study on chronic sleep restriction estimated the daily sleep need to average 8.16 hours per night to avoid detrimental effects on waking functions.[14] The study used the psychomotor vigilance test (PVT), in which subjects respond to a randomly timed target. The time between the stimulus and the response as well as the frequency of lapses (missed target due to inattention) were determined. The study documented that the frequency of lapses on the PVT increased in proportion to total sleep debt or total accumulated **excess** wake time (Figure 9–5A and B). The sleep deprivation and partial sleep loss conditions fit the same graph when expressed as PVT lapses versus **total excess accumulated wake** (Figure 9–5B). This study also found that the *subjective feeling of sleepiness or impairment* did not continue to worsen beyond a certain point. *Therefore, the chronically sleep-deprived individual does not recognize the degree of impairment.* The results from this and other studies have demonstrated that chronic sleep restriction to less than 7 hours per night can have significant effects on cognitive functioning.[15]

Table 9–2 Effects of Chronic Partial Sleep Restriction (Deprivation)

Increase with sleep loss	**Decrease** with sleep loss
• Sleepiness (subjective and objective) • Attention lapses • Norepinephrine • Cortisol and adrenocorticotropic hormone • Ghrelin (hunger) • Insulin resistance • Medical errors • Motor vehicle accidents	• Vigilance • Pain tolerance • Cognition and attention • Seizure threshold • Leptin (increase satiety) • Acute antibody response to influenza and hepatitis A vaccine • Cognitive processing (addition/subtraction)

Data from references 23–26. Sleep loss includes sleep fragmentation, sleep restriction/deprivation, or a combination.

Consequences of Sleep Loss

Sleep loss has many additional consequences beyond daytime sleepiness, decreased attention, and cognitive dysfunction. Some of the many effects of chronic partial sleep loss are listed in Table 9–2. These include **decreased** performance, decreased serum leptin (increased leptin causes satiety), and an impaired response to immunization.[23-26] Conversely, chronic sleep loss is associated with **increased** cortisol, increased ghrelin (which causes hunger), and insulin resistance. Some have hypothesized that chronic partial sleep deprivation may contribute to the current obesity epidemic via decreased leptin and increased ghrelin. Many individuals pursue a pattern of decreased sleep during the week and increased sleep duration on the weekends to "catch up." However, depending on the severity of sleep restriction, 2 days of recovery sleep is not sufficient to reverse the effects of 5 days of sleep restriction with respect to daytime function or metabolism.[27] Sleep restriction can also reduce the morning metabolic rate, which could be a risk factor for development of obesity.[28] Indeed, studies have shown that sleep restriction is a risk factor for obesity.[29]

A review of current data concerning sleep duration and health was published as a joint venture of the American Academy of Sleep Medicine (AASM) and Sleep Research Society (SRS).[29,30] A joint consensus statement of the AASM and the SRS recommends that adults should sleep 7 or more hours per night on a regular basis to promote optimal health.[29,30] The group of experts concluded that sleeping less than 7 hours is associated with adverse health outcomes including weight gain and obesity, diabetes, hypertension, heart disease and stroke, depression, and increased risk of death. In addition, impaired immune function, increased pain, impaired performance, increased errors, and a greater risk of accidents are associated with sleeping less than 7 hours (Box 9–2). The consensus statement also said that sleeping more than 9 hours per night on a regular basis may be appropriate for young adults, individuals recovering from sleep debt, and individuals with illnesses. Although some previous studies have found sleeping more than 9 hours is associated with adverse outcomes, the consensus statement stated that it is uncertain if sleeping more than 9 hours on a regular basis is associated with health risk.

Sleep, Performance, and Learning (Memory)

Prior sleep loss results in decreased attention (vigilance), working memory (short-term memory), and cognitive throughput (addition/subtraction). As noted previously,

Box 9–2 JOINT CONSENSUS STATEMENT OF THE AMERICAN ACADEMY OF SLEEP MEDICINE AND SLEEP RESEARCH SOCIETY CONCERNING SLEEP DURATION

Sleep 7 or more hours per night on a regular basis to promote optimal health. Sleeping less than 7 hours per night is associated with:

- Weight gain and obesity
- Diabetes
- Hypertension
- Heart disease
- Stroke
- Depression
- Increased risk of death
- Impaired immune function
- Increased pain
- Impaired performance/increased errors
- Greater risk of accidents

From Watson NF, Badr MS, Belenky G, et al. Recommended amount of sleep for a healthy adult: a joint consensus statement of the American Academy of Sleep Medicine and Sleep Research Society. *J Clin Sleep Med*. 2015;11(6):591-592.

there is *considerable variability in the impact of sleep loss on individuals, and this also applies to performance after sleep loss*. Some individuals show minimal effects, others have significant impairment with some recovery during the day, and some have significant impairment during both day and night. As noted above, circadian factors also affect performance after sleep loss. Sleep is required to process the prior days' experiences and encode them into memory. Selective deprivation of either early sleep (dominated by stage N3) or late-night sleep (stage N2 and stage R) impairs overnight memory consolidation.[31] Memories (information) from the prior day are "pruned" with some less important events discarded and processed. *A period of sleep on the night after learning improves retention of information*. Some studies suggest at least 6 hours of post-training sleep is needed to enhance retesting performance (improvement proportional to the amount of sleep over 6 hours). Sleep has been shown to enhance prior learning of perceptional and motor skills, paired word associations, emotionally charged memories, and enhanced mathematical insight. In general, stages N2, N3, and REM are all important, but types of learning may depend differentially on different sleep stages. In addition, learning can also affect sleep on the night after learning. In some studies, the amount of REM sleep increases on nights after learning. Learning is also impaired *if wakefulness and sleep periods are not aligned with circadian rhythms*.

EFFECTS OF SLEEP DISORDERS AND MEDICATIONS ON SLEEP ARCHITECTURE

Both sleep disorders and medications may alter sleep architecture by influencing the amount of sleep, the latency to sleep, and the amount of specific sleep stages.[32-34] Alterations in nocturnal sleep architecture frequently occur and can include increases or decreases in the sleep latency, the REM latency, the amount of wakefulness after sleep onset (WASO, in minutes), or the amounts of stages N1, N2, N3, and R (as a percentage of TST). Some common abnormalities of sleep architecture are shown in Table 9–3.

Table 9–3 Common Abnormalities of Sleep Architecture

Sleep Latency/Early Awakening

- Increased sleep latency
  - Chronic insomnia disorder, depression, medications, medical disorders associated with pain
  - Delayed sleep-wake phase disorder, restless legs syndrome
  - Age (small effect)
  - Withdrawal from sedatives
- Decreased sleep latency
  - Hypersomnia disorders, prior sleep loss, sedating medications
- Early morning awakening—depression, advanced sleep-wake phase disorder

REM Latency

- Increased and decreased (see Table 9–4, Table 9–5, Table 9–6 and Box 9–3)

Total Sleep Time

- Decreased total sleep time—depression, pain, chronic insomnia disorder, lung disease, alerting medications near bedtime
- Increased total sleep time—recovery from sleep loss, sedating medications, hypersomnia disorders

Sleep Efficiency

- Decreased sleep efficiency—age, any cause of frequent awakenings, difficulty returning to sleep (chronic insomnia disorder, depression)
- Increased sleep efficiency—prior sleep restriction, sedating medications

Change in Stages N1, N2, N3, and R as % TST

- **Increased stage N1**—any disorder associated with frequent arousals
- **Increased stage N3**
  - First night of recovery sleep from sleep loss, rebound with initial CPAP treatment of OSA
  - Medications (gabapentin, trazodone)
- **Increased stage R (% TST)**
  - Depression, second night of recovery from sleep loss
  - Rebound with initial CPAP treatment
  - Withdrawal of REM-suppressing medications or substances (alcohol, marijuana)
- **Decreased stage R (% TST)**
  - REM-suppressing medications, untreated OSA

CPAP, Continuous positive airway pressure; *OSA*, obstructive sleep apnea; *REM*, rapid eye movement; *TST*, total sleep time.

Effects of Sleep Disorders on Sleep Architecture

Most sleep disorders can be associated with changes in sleep architecture (Table 9–3). Insomnia from any cause, including chronic insomnia disorder, depressive and bipolar disorders, chronic pain disorders, and leg movement disorders, can increase the sleep latency and decrease the TST. Increased sleep latency can occur with delayed sleep-wake phase disorder or restless legs syndrome. Early-morning awakening can be seen with depression and the advanced sleep-wake phase disorder. A decreased sleep latency is a common manifestation of hypersomnia disorders or sedating medications. Patents with idiopathic hypersomnia or hypersomnia associated with a mental disorder can have a long TST or time in bed (some types of depression). In contrast, patients with narcolepsy have a

Box 9–3 CHANGES IN SLEEP ARCHITECTURE WITH DEPRESSION

- Decreased REM latency
- Long initial REM period
- High REM density in first REM period
- Increased REM (% TST)
- Findings may differ if the patients are taking medications that affect REM sleep
- Changes in sleep architecture can persist after improvement in mood with antidepressant medication

REM, Rapid eye movement; *TST,* total sleep time.

ntormal 24-hour total sleep duration but abnormal occurrence of sleep periods over the 24-hour period. Decreased sleep efficiency can occur with disorders causing sleep fragmentation, such as sleep apnea syndromes or depression. Patients requiring a long time to return to sleep (chronic insomnia disorder) also exhibit decreased sleep efficiency. Sedating medications and prior sleep restriction can result in a decreased sleep latency. Increased stage N1 is a common manifestation of any disorder causing frequent arousals, including severe sleep apnea. An increase in stage N3 can occur on the first recovery night after sleep loss or on the first night of CPAP initiation. As will be discussed later, some medications can also increase stage N3. A very short REM latency (sleep onset REM sleep) is characteristic of narcolepsy but can occur with depression. Changes in sleep architecture associated with depression are listed in Box 9–3 and will be discussed later in more detail. In the following sections, which will describe alterations in individual sleep parameters associated with certain medications, some additional information on the effect of sleep disorders on certain parameters will also be provided.

Sleep Architecture Changes Associated With Depression

As noted above depression is often associated with changes in sleep architecture (Box 9-3). However, there are certain alterations in REM sleep that are characteristic of patients with depression.[35-37] The findings in a given patient may vary depending on whether or not they are taking antidepressant medications that can both improve depression and change the REM latency. In depression, REM latencies on the order of 40 to 60 minutes are typical (Figure 9–6) but can be as short as those seen in patients with narcolepsy. In depression, the first episode of REM sleep is often prolonged with a higher REM density (REMs per epoch) than usual.[35-37] In normal individuals relatively few eye movements are seen in the first REM period, which is typically short. There may also be an increase in the amount of REM sleep as a percentage of TST. On the other hand, some patients with depression and severe insomnia may have a decrease in TST and the amount of REM sleep. Depression can be associated with complaints of hypersomnia as well as insomnia.

Medications and Sleep

Many medications and substances may affect sleep (Tables 9–4 to 9–10).[32-34,38-40] A patient history documenting the *onset of a sleep complaint coinciding with starting a particular medication* or increase in the dose of a medication can be very helpful when identifying a medication as a cause of sleep disturbance. The medication may not be suspected by the patient as the culprit in causing their sleep problem (e.g., a medication for blood pressure causing insomnia). In some patients, withdrawing the

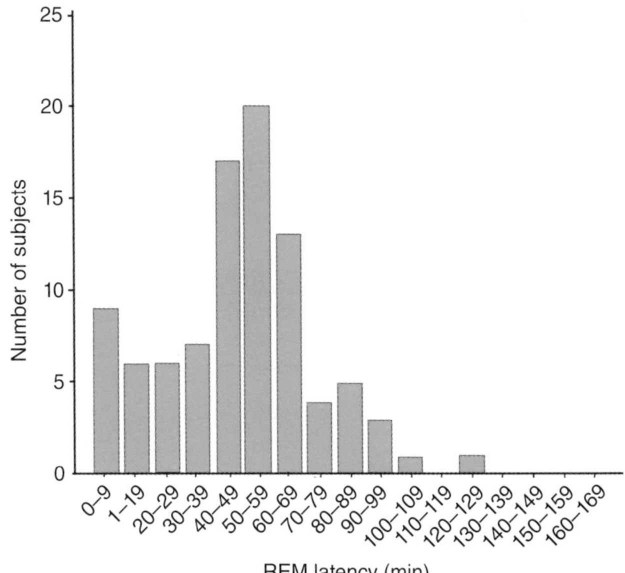

Figure 9–6 Distribution of REM latency values in a group of patients with depression. Although the majority of patients have a REM latency over 40 minutes, values can be much shorter. (From Ansseau M, Kupfer DJ, Reynolds CF 3rd, McEachran AB. REM latency distribution in major depression: clinical characteristics associated with sleep onset REM periods. *Biol Psychiatry.* 1984;19(12):1651-1666.)

suspected offending medication is indicated. In patients where continued use of a medication known to cause sleep problems is essential, addressing the sleep complaint or finding an alternative medication is appropriate. For example, after trial of many antidepressants, an effective medication is finally found. If this medication causes insomnia, one option might be the addition of a low dose of a sedating antidepressant at night. It is important to note that a different medication from the same drug class **may not necessarily** cause the same complaint. For example, nightmares that occur with one dopamine agonist (pramipexole) may not occur with another (ropinirole). One should ensure proper timing of a medication, and potentially changing the timing of a medication may be necessary. If a once-a-day medication that is often taken at bedtime (e.g., donepezil [Aricept]) causes insomnia, it should be taken in the morning. Furthermore, some medications should be taken in the morning due to their side effects; for example, long-acting bupropion (Wellbutrin XL) can be alerting and may cause sleep onset insomnia if improperly taken at night instead of in the morning.

Antidepressants and Sleep

Given the high prevalence of mental health disorders, information on the effects of different antidepressants on sleep is useful for the sleep clinician (Table 9–5). Sedating tricyclic antidepressants (TCAs: amitriptyline and doxepin), trazodone, and mirtazapine decrease sleep latency and improve sleep continuity.[38-40] The sedating antidepressants are often used at low doses for insomnia. However, low-dose doxepin (Silenor) is the only antidepressant medication approved by the U.S. Food and Drug Administration (FDA) for treatment of insomnia (difficulty with sleep maintenance). When antidepressants are used for insomnia, using a lower than antidepressant dose may prevent unwanted side effects. For example, using a low dose of doxepin avoids anticholinergic side effects,

Table 9–4 Causes of Changes in the REM Latency

Short REM Latency	Long REM Latency	No or Small Change
• Narcolepsy (≤15 min) • Depression (typically 40–60 min) • Withdrawal of REM-suppressing medications • Untreated sleep apnea (uncommon) • Previous REM sleep deprivation	• Untreated sleep apnea • SSRIs, SNRIs • TCAs • MAOIs? (Minimal data) • Ethanol • Lithium • First-night effect	• Mirtazapine • Trazodone • Bupropion*

*Bupropion associated with conflicting and limited data (see text) may increase or decrease the REM latency depending on population studied but the changes are relatively small.
MAIO, Monoamine oxidase inhibitors; *REM*, rapid eye movement; *SNRI*, selective serotonin and norepinephrine uptake inhibitor; *SSRI*, selective serotonin reuptake inhibitor; *TCA*, tricyclic antidepressant.
From Berry R, Wagner M. Effects of sleep disorders and medications on sleep architecture. In: Berry R, Wagner M, eds. *Sleep Medicine Pearls*. 3rd ed. Elsevier Saunders; 2014:75.

which can be problematic for men with urinary retention issues. Trazodone has no significant anticholinergic activity, but lower doses minimize daytime sedation. Doxepin, trazodone, mirtazapine, and quetiapine (a sedating atypical antipsychotic) have significant antagonist activity at H1 histamine receptors at relatively low doses, which results in sedation. Trazodone and mirtazapine have antagonist activity at 5HT2 receptors, which is also believed to enhance sedation. Most of the other *nonsedating* antidepressants tend to increase sleep latency and decrease sleep continuity. Nonsedating TCAs, selective serotonin reuptake inhibitors (SSRIs), selective serotonin and norepinephrine reuptake inhibitors (SNRIs), and norepinephrine reuptake inhibitors all increase the REM latency (Table 9–4) and decrease the amount of REM sleep. In contrast, mirtazapine has little impact on REM sleep, trazodone may slightly decrease REM sleep, and there is limited information about the effects of bupropion on REM sleep.[41-43] In a study by Nofzinger et al.,[41] a small group ($N = 7$) of depressed patients received bupropion and the REM latency decreased (≈11 minutes) and the minutes of REM sleep and REM sleep as %TST increased. However, as there was no placebo comparison some of the effects could be due to the first night effect (increased REM latency, decreased REM sleep in the initial sleep study). Ott and coworkers studied the effects of one dose of bupropion SR using a randomized crossover design in 20 depressed patients. Overall, bupropion had no effect on REM sleep measures. There was a subgroup with an increase in the REM latency and this was predictive of a clinical response to bupropion. In a study of a single patient with narcolepsy with short nocturnal REM latency, bupropion increased this parameter (21 to 52 minutes).[43] In summary, based on limited data bupropion likely has small effects on REM sleep but may increase the REM latency in some patients with depression or narcolepsy. Monoamine oxidase inhibitors (MAOIs) are rarely used but effective antidepressants. They increase sleep latency and REM latency but decrease sleep continuity and are potent inhibitors of REM sleep. Clozapine, a TCA used for obsessive-compulsive disorder, is also a very potent REM sleep suppressor.

Information about atypical antipsychotic medications, mood stabilizers, and antiepileptic medications is presented in Table 9–6. Of special interest is that olanzapine and quetiapine are the most sedating of the atypical antipsychotics.[44,45] Lithium increases slow wave sleep (SWS, stage N3) and decreases REM sleep.[46,47] Gabapentin is included here as it can be used as a mood stabilizer and less commonly as a sleep aid. It is known to increase TST, SWS, and REM sleep.[48]

Changes in Sleep Latency with Medications

Sleep latency may be prolonged because of the first-night effect (sleep in a novel setting), chronic insomnia disorder (sleep onset insomnia), comorbid insomnia (depression), stimulant medications, nonsedating antidepressants, and bronchodilators (see Table 9–7). βeta (β)-blockers can cause insomnia, with propranolol carrying the highest risk (Table 9–8). Those β-blockers with higher lipophilicity (propranolol, metoprolol, carvedilol, labetalol) are associated with a greater incidence of insomnia compared with those that are less lipophilic (atenolol, bisoprolol).[33,49,50] It also appears that the relative affinity of these medications for 5-HT receptors also affects the risk for insomnia (Table 9–8).[33] For example, sotalol has low lipid solubility and high affinity for serotonin receptors and is believed to have a moderate risk of sleep disruption. Propranolol has high lipid solubility and affinity for serotonin receptors and has the *highest risk of sleep disturbance*. β-Blockers are also associated *with fatigue, vivid dreams,* and *nightmares*. There have been case reports of lipophilic β-blockers associated with the REM sleep behavior disorder. Sedating antidepressants may shorten sleep latency when compared with the untreated state. Depression and medical disorders associated with pain can increase sleep latency and WASO. Statin medications are often listed as medications associated with insomnia, but the supporting evidence is limited. Data mining of side effect databases did find an association, but small trials in normal individuals have failed to clearly show an effect.[33] Lipophilic statins (atorvastatin [Lipitor], simvastatin [Zocor], lovastatin [Altoprev]) are thought to be more likely to cause sleep disturbance that hydrophilic statins (rosuvastatin [Crestor], pravastatin [Pravachol]).

Changes in the REM Latency

Circumstances that prolong or shorten the REM latency are listed in Table 9–4.[32,33] A sleep onset REM period (REM latency < 15 minutes) on an overnight PSG may rarely be associated with untreated OSA (≈1%)[51] and is present in 25% to 40% of patients with narcolepsy. A short REM latency can also be seen with withdrawal of a REM-suppressing medication. As mentioned earlier, a short REM latency is often noted with untreated depression,[35-37] REM latencies on the order of 40 minutes are typical but may be as short as those in patients with narcolepsy (Figure 9–6). Other

Table 9–5 Effects of Antidepressants on Sleep

Drug Class	Medications	Sleep Latency	Sleep Continuity	N3	REM Latency	REM Sleep	Mechanism of Action
Sedating TCA	Amitriptyline, doxepin, trimipramine	↓	↑	↔	↑	↓	Antihistamine Inhibition of 5HT and NE uptake
Activating TCA	Imipramine, nortriptyline	↑	↓	↓	↑	↓	Inhibition of 5HT and NE uptake
MAOI	Phenelzine (Nardil) Selegiline (Emsam) Tranylcypromine (Parnate)	↔	↔	?*	?*	↓	Prevent breakdown of DA, 5HT, NE Inhibition MAO
SSRI	Fluoxetine, citalopram, escitalopram, sertraline, paroxetine	↑	↔↑	↔	↑	↓	Inhibit 5HT reuptake Fluoxetine also NE reuptake
SNRI	Venlafaxine, duloxetine	↑	↓	↔	↑	↓	Inhibit NE, 5HT reuptake
NRI	Strattera	↑	↓	↔	↑	↓	Inhibit NE reuptake
Non-sedating "atypical anti-depressant"	Bupropion (Wellbutrin)	↔	↔↓	↔	↔↓↑**	↔↑↓**	Inhibit NE, DA reuptake
Sedating "atypical" Antidepressants	Trazodone	↓	↑	↑	↔↑	↔ or small ↓	Antihistamine, antagonism 5HT2A receptors, weak serotonin reuptake inhibitor
	Mirtazapine (Remeron)	↓	↑	↔	↔↑	↔↓	Antihistamine (HA1 receptor antagonism) central presynaptic alpha-2 receptors (increases NE,5HT), blocks 5HT2A, 5HT3 receptors
Serotonin Modulators	Vortioxetine (Trintellix)	?	↔↓	?	?	?	Inhibits 5HT reuptake, modulation of the activity of multiple serotonergic receptors*
	Vilazodone (Viibryd)	?	?	?	?	↓	5HT1A partial agonist and serotonin reuptake inhibitor

*Very limited data.
**conflicting results.
DA, Dopamine; *5HT*, serotonin; *MAOI*, monoamine oxidase inhibitor; *NE*, norepinephrine; *NRI*, norepinephrine reuptake inhibitor; *SSRI*, selective serotonin reuptake inhibitor; *SNRI*, serotonin norepinephrine reuptake inhibitor; *TCA*, tricyclic antidepressant, *HA*, histamine.
↑ increased, ↓ decreased, ↔ no or minimal change.
Data from references 38–43.

Table 9–6 Effects on Atypical Antipsychotic, Mood Stabilizer, and Anti-epilepsy Medications

Generic Medication	Brand Name	Sedation	Weight Gain	Sleep Latency	REM Latency	TST	SWS	REM
Olanzapine	Zyprexa	+++	+++	↓	↑	↑	↑↑	↓
Quetiapine	Seroquel	++	++	↓	↔	↑		↓
Aripiprazole	Abilify	+	0					
Risperidone	Risperdal	+	++	↓	↔	↑	↑	
Ziprasidone	Geodon	+	0	↓	↑	↑	↑	↓
Lithium	Eskalith, Lithobid	+			↑	↔	↑	↓
Lamotrigine	Lamictal	+ /insomnia	–			–	↓	↑
Gabapentin	Neurontin	+	+	⟷	–	↑	↑	⟷
Phenytoin	Dilantin	++					↓	
Valproic acid	Depakote and others	+				↑		
Carbamazepine	Tegretol	++		?↓		↑	↑	↓
Levetiracetam	Keppra	++				↑	↑	

REM, Rapid eye movement; *SWS*, slow wave sleep; *TST*, total sleep time, Blank cells no data.
Data from references 44, 45.

Table 9–7 Medications Commonly Associated With Insomnia and Long Sleep Latency

Class	Examples	Comments
Stimulants	Methylphenidate Dextroamphetamine Atomoxetine (adults > children)	Especially sustained release medications if taken too late
Xanthines	Caffeine; theophylline	
Anticholinergic medications	Donepezil (Aricept)	2% to 14% incidence of insomnia; if so, take in the morning
β-Blockers	Propranolol, metoprolol	Atenolol lower risk—can be associated with nightmares
Ethanol	Ethanol	May shorten sleep latency but fragments sleep
Drugs for hyperlipidemia	Atorvastatin	? Lipophilic statins more likely Evidence not convincing
Selective serotonin reuptake inhibitors	Fluoxetine, sertraline, paroxetine, citalopram, escitalopram	Take in the morning (unless sedating)
Nonsedating tricyclic antidepressants	Nortriptyline	Amitriptyline and doxepin are sedating
Other antidepressants	Bupropion, venlafaxine, duloxetine	Mirtazapine is sedating
Angiotensin-converting enzyme inhibitors	Enalapril	Rare nightmares and insomnia

From Berry RB, Wagner MH. Effects of sleep disorders and medications on sleep architecture. In: Berry R, Wagner M, eds. *Sleep Medicine Pearls*. 3rd ed. Philadelphia, Elsevier Saunders; 2014:74.

Table 9–8 Risk of Insomnia With Commonly Used β-Blocker Medications

Drug	Lipid Solubility	β Selectivity	Relative Affinity for HT Receptors	Risk for Insomnia
Atenolol	Low	β-1	Low	Low
Sotalol	Low	Nonselective	High	? Moderate
Carvedilol	Moderate	Nonselective α-1 antagonism	High	Moderate
Metoprolol	Moderate	β-1	Low	High
Propranolol	High	Nonselective	High	Highest

Adapted from Schweitzer PK, Randazzo AC. Drugs that disturb sleep and wakefulness. In: Kryger M, Roth T, Dement WD, eds. *Principles and Practice of Sleep Medicine*. 6th ed. Elsevier; 2017:480-498.

REM findings in patients with depression were previously discussed.

A number of medications may prolong REM latency (see Table 9–4). As discussed previously, medications known to prolong REM latency include TCAs, SSRIs, MAOIs, and lithium. MAOIs are said to be the most potent suppressors of REM sleep. Some substances such as alcohol may also increase REM latency. Mirtazapine, trazodone,[38] and bupropion appear to have minimal if any effects on the REM latency. As mentioned previously, there is conflicting information about bupropion, but the changes in the REM latency were relatively small (10–20 minutes) in the studies documenting a change in the REM latency.[41,42] Due to the effects of medications on the REM latency, careful consideration of current medications is necessary when considering evaluation of a patient with a MSLT (see Chapter 17).

Changes in the Amount of REM Sleep

The amount of REM sleep may increase after prior REM sleep deprivation, during the first night of treatment of OSA (REM rebound), and after withdrawal of REM-suppressing medications (Table 9–9).[32,33] Factors that shorten REM latency also typically increase the duration of REM sleep. However, a number of exceptions exist. For example, patients with narcolepsy may exhibit a very short nocturnal REM latency (about 20%–50% of patients) but have a normal amount of REM sleep. As noted above, the first night of recovery after sleep loss is often characterized by a rebound in stage N3 but can be associated with REM rebound in older patients. REM rebound in OSA patients on the first night of CPAP treatment is a fairly common finding, especially in patients with very severe sleep apnea. Most antidepressants tend to decrease the amount of REM sleep. Bupropion may increase the amount of REM sleep in depressed patients, and mirtazapine and trazodone have minimal effects on the amount of REM sleep. In the case of trazodone, studies have shown increases and decreases in REM as a percentage of TST but no change in the absolute amount.[38]

Changes in Stage N3

Several medications may decrease or increase stage N3 (Table 9–10). Patients with a very high apnea-hypopnea index

Table 9–9 Factors Affecting the Duration of REM Sleep

Decreased REM Sleep	Increased REM Sleep	Minimal Change or Increase/Decrease in REM Sleep
• SSRIs • TCAs • MAOIs • Morphine • Lithium • Benzodiazepines (slight) • First-night effect	• Withdrawal of REM suppressant medication • Prior REM sleep deprivation • REM rebound on first night of PAP treatment • Nefazodone* • Withdrawal from cannabis	• Mirtazapine • Bupropion (or increase/decrease in different studies) • Trazodone

*No longer available in the United States (hepatic toxicity).
MAIO, monoamine oxidase inhibitor; *PAP*, positive airway pressure; *REM*, rapid eye movement; *SSRI*, selective serotonin reuptake inhibitor; *TCA*, tricyclic antidepressant.
From Berry R, Wagner M. Effects of sleep disorders and medications on sleep architecture. In: Berry R, Wagner M, eds. *Sleep Medicine Pearls*. 3rd ed. Elsevier Saunders; 2014:76.

Table 9–10 Medications Affecting the Duration of Stage N3 Sleep

Increased	Decreased
• Trazodone • Mirtazapine • Lithium • Pregabalin • Gabapentin • Carbamazepine • Sodium oxybate • Levetiracetam • Sedating tricyclic antidepressants	• Benzodiazepines* • Phenytoin • Caffeine • Theophylline • Stimulants (amphetamines)

*Benzodiazepine receptor agonist hypnotics that are not benzodiazepines (zolpidem, zaleplon, eszopiclone) do not decrease stage N3 sleep.
From Berry R, Wagner M. Effects of sleep disorders and medications on sleep architecture. In: Berry R, Wagner M, eds. *Sleep Medicine Pearls*. 3rd ed. Elsevier Saunders; 2014:76.

often have little or no stage N3 due to the repetitive arousals. Benzodiazepines tend to decrease stage N3 because of a decrease in the amplitude of sleep waves.[32,33] Nonbenzodiazepine receptor agonist hypnotics (zaleplon, zolpidem, eszopiclone) do not decrease stage N3 (no change in amplitude but do increase higher electroencephalographic [EEG] frequencies). Caffeine and theophylline may decrease stage N3.[33,1] Medications that may increase stage N3 include trazodone, gabapentin, pregabalin, lithium, levetiracetam, carbamazepine, and some sedating antidepressants. Sodium oxybate increases stage N3 (duration and delta power) in patients with narcolepsy,[53,54] and this may be one mode of its beneficial action.

Medications and Nightmares

Nightmares are unpleasant dreams that occur predominantly in REM sleep. A number of medications have been reported to cause nightmares (Table 9–11).[33,55] Medications such as varenicline (Chantix), pramipexole, and efavirenz are notorious for causing vivid or unpleasant dreams in some people. The treatment of nightmare disorder will be discussed in Chapter 36. However, a trial of discontinuation (if possible) of a medication possibly inducing nightmares should be the first approach.

Over-the-Counter Medications Used as Hypnotics

An extensive discussion of the effects of over-the-counter (OTC) medications on sleep is beyond the scope of this chapter. The hypnotic effects of melatonin will be discussed in Chapter 33. The antihistamines diphenhydramine and doxylamine are the active ingredients in many OTC sleeping pills. They are often used in "PM" medications in combination with ibuprofen or acetaminophen. They provide a subjective feeling of sedation and for this reason are popular OTC hypnotics. The half-life of diphenhydramine is 9 to 10 hours, and that of doxylamine is 10 to 12 hours. Therefore, morning sedation is an issue. Valerian root is an extract of a tall grassy plant with variable components depending on the preparation. Valerian root is also used in many OTC sleeping pills. A placebo-controlled study[56] compared a combination of the herbal medications valerian and hops (valerian-hops), 50 mg of diphenhydramine, and placebo taken over 6 weeks. At 2 weeks there was no difference in the three groups in polysomnography variables. TST increased by 40 minutes with the valerian combination and 35 minutes with placebo and diphenhydramine. Diphenhydramine produced a trend for increased subjective TST relative to placebo during the first 14 days of treatment. Valerian produced a significant reduction in subjective sleep latency at week 6 but the absolute reduction in time was only a few minutes greater than placebo. An AASM clinical practice guideline for pharmacological treatment of insomnia[57] did not recommend use of diphenhydramine or valerian root as hypnotics. In one meta-analysis diphenhydramine reduced sleep latency by only 8 minutes greater than placebo and increased TST by 12 minutes compared with placebo. Valerian root decreased sleep latency by 9 minutes greater than placebo. Neither result is clinically significant. Thus, although diphenhydramine is symptomatically sedating, the objective effects on sleep (at least with use for 14 days) are minimal. The first generation antihistamines can significantly worsen the restless legs syndrome. Urinary retention can worsen due to the anticholinergic activity of diphenhydramine and doxylamine. This issue can be more significant in men with benign prostatic hypertrophy.

CAFFEINE, CANNABIS, ALCOHOL, AND SLEEP

The effects of caffeine, cannabis, and alcohol on sleep are of interest given the widespread use of these substances. A brief discussion of important points about each of these follows. The reader is referred to the references for more detailed information.

Caffeine

Caffeine's alerting effects are believed to be due to antagonism of adenosine receptors in the central nervous system.[58,59] It is

Table 9–11 Medications Commonly Associated With Nightmares

Class of Agent	Examples	Comments
Amphetamines/amphetamine-like agents	Dextroamphetamine	Chronic use
Cholinergic medications	Donepezil (Aricept)	Chronic use
Benzodiazepines, BZRAs	Alprazolam, zolpidem	Chronic use and withdrawal
Melatonin	Melatonin	Chronic use
Ethanol	Ethanol	REM rebound on withdrawal
TCAs	Amitriptyline, doxepin, imipramine, nortriptyline	Chronic use
SSRIs	Fluoxetine, sertraline, paroxetine, citalopram, escitalopram	Insomnia, nightmares
Other antidepressants	Bupropion, venlafaxine, duloxetine	Insomnia, nightmares
Antiviral	Amantadine, oseltamivir	Chronic, Aute use
Antiretroviral medications	Efavirenz (Sustiva), tenofovir	Chronic use
β-Blockers	Propranolol, metoprolol, carvedilol > atenolol	Chronic use
β-Agonists	Albuterol	Chronic use
α-Agonists	Methyldopa, clonidine	Chronic use
Dopaminergic agents	Levodopa, pramipexole (up to 11%), ropinirole	Acute or chronic use
Agents for smoking cessation	Varenicline (Chantix)	10%–13%
Calcium channel blockers	Verapamil, amlodipine	Chronic use
Antibiotics	Erythromycin, levofloxacin, ciprofloxacin	Acute use
Angiotensin-converting enzyme	Enalapril	Rare nightmares and insomnia
Agents for hyperlipidemia	Atorvastatin?	Limited data

BZRA, Benzodiazepine receptor agonist; *REM,* rapid eye movement; *SSRI,* selective serotonin reuptake inhibitor; *TCA,* tricyclic antidepressant.
From Berry R, Wagner M. Effects of sleep disorders and medications on sleep architecture. In: Berry R, Wagner M, eds. *Sleep Medicine Pearls.* 3rd ed. Elsevier Saunders; 2014:77.

known that endogenous adenosine levels rise with continued wakefulness and may be a fundamental part of the homeostatic sleep drive. The cause of the rise in adenosine is unknown. Actions of adenosine on neurons in the ventral lateral preoptic nucleus of the hypothalamus are believed to mediate some of the effect, but other areas are important. Whereas caffeine blocks both adenosine A1 and A2A receptors, blockade of the A2A receptors in the shell region of the nucleus accumbens is believed to be responsible for the effect of caffeine on wakefulness.[59] Caffeine in doses ranging from 200 to 400 mg helps maintain alertness and performance in the context of sleep deprivation, sedation, and sleep restriction. Caffeine consumption is increasing (large servings of brewed coffee can have up to 500 mg of caffeine), and use of energy drinks with high caffeine is also increasing. A short half-life is one limitation on the effectiveness of caffeine, although sustained release preparations have been used. The duration of caffeine's effect on alertness appears to be dose dependent, with 75 to 150 mg of caffeine (one cup of coffee) lasting up to 90 minutes after administration, 200 mg (approximately two cups of coffee) improving performance up to 4 hours after administration, and 300 to 400 mg (three to four cups of coffee) sustaining alertness for up to 5.5 to 7.5 hours.[52] One of the few head-to-head studies comparing the effects of caffeine (600 mg), dextroamphetamine (20 mg), and modafinil (400 mg) on psychomotor vigilance after 44 hours of wakefulness found similar improvements in performance with all three stimulants, although caffeine had a shorter duration of action.[60] High doses of caffeine (200 to 600 mg) may approximate the efficacy of standard doses of modafinil (200 to 400 mg) in maintaining alertness and performance during long-term sleep deprivation.[63]

The effects of caffeine on sleep depend on individual susceptibility, metabolism, time of administration and dose, and chronicity of use.[61] After oral ingestion, caffeine reaches peak plasma levels within 30 to 120 minutes. Caffeine then undergoes hepatic metabolism, with metabolites excreted in the urine. The half-life of caffeine varies, ranging between 4 and 6 hours (3.5 to 5 hours in some references). Its effects may also depend on polymorphisms of the adenosine A2A receptor gene.[62] Caffeine is metabolized in the liver to active metabolites including paraxanthine, theobromine, and theophylline. There is interest in the potential use of paraxanthine because its wakefulness-promoting activity is higher than caffeine but produces less anxiety. The half-life of caffeine is reduced (metabolism increased) in smokers, but metabolism is reduced in women on oral contraceptives or during pregnancy (hormonal and CYP1A interactions). Older adults also have reduced metabolism.

Because of the high variability in the elimination half-life of caffeine administered to healthy adults, specific recommendations on what time of day to discontinue caffeine use to optimize sleep vary widely, from 4 to 11 hours before bedtime. Drake et al.[64] found that 400 mg of caffeine taken 0, 3, and 6 hours before habitual bedtime all affected self-reported sleep quality compared with placebo in a group in normal individuals with normal sleep. TST was reduced by 1 hour. Individuals consuming more than five caffeinated beverages daily were excluded. In most studies consumption of caffeine within a few hours of bedtime postpones sleep onset and reduces TST, sleep efficiency, the amount of SWS (stage N3), and the amount of EEG delta activity. The effectiveness of caffeine as a stimulant is reduced by the development of tolerance. Multiple sleep latency testing after repeated caffeine doses shows the wakefulness-promoting effects (increase in sleep latency) decreases with the continued dosing. However, the alerting effects of caffeine were higher than placebo suggesting persistent benefit despite some possible development of tolerance.[65,66] Caffeine in even moderate doses can produce a withdrawal syndrome with symptoms including headache, increased sleepiness, fogginess, and depressed mood with symptoms emerging 12 to 24 hours after caffeine cessation and lasting 20 to 51 hours.[67] In summary, caffeine can be a useful stimulant in some situations. The adverse effects of caffeine on sleep occur with administration as much as 6 hours before bedtime and vary between individuals. In patients with insomnia, cessation of caffeine after 12:00 PM is a reasonable recommendation. A large dose of caffeine administered 3 hours before habitual bedtime induced a 40-minute delay in circadian rhythms.[68] However, chronic caffeine exposure in the morning and early afternoon does not appear to alter the circadian rhythm of melatonin secretion.[69] In moderate doses caffeine appears to be safe and has some potential health benefits.[70]

Cannabis

Cannabis use is prevalent in the U.S. population[71,72] and can complicate treatment of sleep disorders and multiple sleep latency testing. Dzodzomenyo et al.[73] performed a retrospective review of 383 urine drug screens in patients less than 21 years of age having an MSLT. They found 14 individuals with a positive drug screen for tetrahydrocannabinol (THC), and 45% had a result meeting diagnostic criteria for narcolepsy or having multiple sleep-onset REM periods (a higher percentage than those without a positive drug screen). Of interest, 10% of the urine drug screens were positive for some substance. The cannabis plant, also known as marijuana, contains over 500 different compounds, but the main psychoactive drug is THC (also known as delta-9 THC). The plant contains many other cannabinoids including cannabidiol (CBD).[71,72,74] Approved cannabinoid products include dronabinol (delta-9–THC, synthetic THC), nabilone (a THC analogue), and CBD, which differ in their pharmacology and may thus have different effects on sleep. Dronabinol (Marinol) is used to treat loss of appetite and associated weight loss with AIDS and to treat severe nausea and vomiting caused by chemotherapy. Dronabinol is usually given after antiemetic medicines have been tried without success. Nabilone is also used to treat chemotherapy-induced nausea (usually after other medications have failed) and severe weight loss. The FDA has approved only one CBD-based drug (Epidolex), used to treat two rare types of epilepsy (Lennox-Gastaut syndrome and Dravet syndrome) and seizures caused by tuberous sclerosis complex. The medication is approved for adults and children over 1 year old. The FDA has not approved CBD for any other use at this time. In a review of the effects of illicit recreational drugs on sleep Schierenbeck et al.[72] found that smoked marijuana and oral delta-9 THC reduced REM sleep (Table 9–12). Moreover, acute administration of cannabis appears to facilitate falling asleep and to increase stage N3 sleep.[75] Difficulty sleeping and strange dreams are among the most consistently reported symptoms of acute and subacute cannabis withdrawal. Longer sleep onset latency, reduced SWS, and a REM rebound can be observed.[76] Prospective studies are needed in order to verify whether sleep disturbances during cannabis withdrawal predict treatment outcome. However, sleep disturbances are a major cause of difficulties in withdrawing from cannabis.[76] In patients chronically using cannabis, acute withdrawal at the time of an MSLT could cause longer sleep latency but of greater importance REM rebound and the appearance of sleep onset REM periods. Spanagel and Bilbao[74] reviewed cannabinoids approved as therapeutics and found that pharmaceutical THC (nabilone, dronabinol) does not affect sleep or appetite. In addition, there was no evidence that CBD had a significant effect on sleep. Another review also found no conclusive evidence of an effect of CBD on sleep[75] (although the quality of published evidence was low).

Because drug screen urine tests are used with MSLT, it is important to understand that these tests usually detect the major metabolite of THC, which is 11-Nor-9-carboxy-THC, also known as THC-COOH. Most cannabis drug tests yield a positive result when the concentration of THC-COOH in urine exceeds 50 ng/mL.[77] THC itself has a short

Table 9–12 Effects of Cannabis on Sleep

	Acute Use	Chronic Use	Withdrawal
Sleep latency	Decrease	Increase	Increase
Total sleep time	Increase	Decrease	Decrease
Stage N3	Increase	Decrease	Decrease
Stage R	Decrease	Not consistent (decreased in one study)	Increase stage R (%TST), vivid dreams Acute withdrawal REM rebound
WASO	Decrease	Increase	Increase
REM latency	?	Increased	Decreased
Comments	Could vary with dose and timing	Varies with dose and frequency of use	Vivid dreams, worse in heavy users Onset 24–72 hours, persists for 6–7 weeks

REM, Rapid eye movement; *WASO*, wake after sleep onset.

Based on Kaul M, Zee PC, Sahni AS. Effects of cannabinoids on sleep and their therapeutic potential for sleep disorders. *Neurotherapeutics.* 2021;18(1):217-227.

Table 9–13 Effects of Alcohol on Sleep

Acute*	Sleep Latency	NREM	REM%	Wakefulness	REM Latency
First half of night	Decreased	Increased SWS	Decreased	Decreased	Increased
Second half of night	N/A	Decreased More N1	Increased	Very increased	–

Withdrawal	Sleep Latency	TST	SWS	REM%	REM Latency
	Increased	Decreased	Decreased	Increased	Unchanged

Abstinence†	Sleep Latency	Sleep Quality	Wakefulness	Slow Wave Sleep	Melatonin Release
	Increased	Poor and fragmented	Frequent arousals	Reduced or increased	Decreased

*With chronic alcohol use, tolerance develops to the sleep-inducing effects of alcohol but not to other negative effects of alcohol on sleep quality and duration of uninterrupted sleep. In acute low dose can be stimulatory in some indviduals and increase the sleep latency.
†Can persist for months and years after abstinence.
NREM, Non–rapid eye movement; *REM*, rapid eye movement; *SWS*, slow wave sleep; *TST*, total sleep time. Withdrawal means recently sober (usually within 30 days of stopping alcohol consumption).
Adapted from references 78–82.

half-life and may only be detectable in saliva and oral fluid for 2 to 24 hours in most cases. Urine tests are usually positive up to 3 days following THC exposure in on and off users and up to 7 days with chronic use. However, testing can be positive for up to 6 weeks in heavy users. False positive results can occur with pantoprazole and hemp-containing foods.

Alcohol

Alcohol can have significant effects on sleep (Table 9–13) including an increase in the REM latency.[78,79] Alcohol may aid sleep onset but tends to cause frequent awakenings in the second part of the night. A study by Landholt et al.[80] of middle aged men found alcohol consumption 6 hours before bedtime (alcohol level at bedtime = 0) still caused sleep disturbance. Sleep efficiency, TST, stage 1, and REM sleep were reduced. In the second half of the sleep episode, wakefulness exhibited a twofold increase. A study using actigraphy found low doses of alcohol in normal subjects to be more disruptive with decreased TST due to increase wakefulness in the second part of the night.[81] Of note, not all studies have shown dramatic effects on alcohol on sleep, but this may be due to the age of subjects and the amount of alcohol consumption. Younger individuals may be less affected by alcohol.

A number of studies of sleep during abstinence of alcohol-dependent patients have been performed. Common findings are prolonged sleep latency, decreased sleep efficiency, shorter sleep duration, and reduced amounts of SWS (stage N3) when compared with healthy controls. The sleep patterns of the abstinent patients are fragmented, and the typical time course of EEG delta wave activity is severely disrupted. The amount of REM sleep may be reduced or increased. Sleep changes can persist during months or years of abstinence, and studies indicate that certain alterations in sleep architecture, as well as subjective sleep complaints, predict relapse to alcoholism.[82]

SUMMARY OF KEY POINTS

1. Sleep loss occurs in two ways: sleep fragmentation and sleep restriction.
2. Frequent arousals result in nonrestorative sleep even in the absence of a decrement in TST. Consolidated episodes of sleep in excess of 10 minutes are needed for restorative sleep.
3. For the same arousal index the impact can vary depending on the clustering of arousals and the ability to return to sleep quickly.
4. After sleep deprivation, recovery sleep is usually characterized by an increase in stage N3 on the first recovery night with an increase in REM sleep on subsequent nights.
5. Chronic sleep restriction can have a number of adverse health consequences. These include a reduction in leptin, an increase in ghrelin, and impaired glucose metabolism. Sleep loss may reduce the response to immunization.
6. Performance on the PVT decreases proportional to the amount of sleep debt, whereas subjective feelings of sleepiness do not continue to worsen beyond a certain point. Therefore, the chronically sleep-deprived individual does not recognize the degree of impairment.
7. Both sleep disorders and medications may alter sleep architecture by influencing the total amount of sleep, sleep efficiency, sleep latency, REM latency, and the amounts of specific sleep stages.
8. Medical conditions (narcolepsy, depression) are associated with short REM latency, as is the withdrawal of REM-suppressing medications or previous sleep/REM restriction.
9. Antidepressants in general (except mirtazapine and perhaps bupropion) are REM suppressing and prolong REM latency. Trazodone has less effect on the REM latency or amount of REM sleep than MAOIs, TCAs, SSRIs, and SNRIs.
10. A number of medications are associated with nightmares or vivid dreams including levodopa, pramipexole (up to 11%), ropinirole, efavirenz (Sustiva), varenicline (Chantix), donepezil (Aricept), amantadine, oseltamivir (Tamiflu), β-blockers (propranolol, metoprolol, carvedilol > atenolol), antidepressants (especially during withdrawal including SSRIs, SNRIs, TCAs, bupropion), hypnotics (eszopiclone,

zaleplon, zolpidem), statins (rare), semaglutide, calcium channel blockers, diphenhydramine, steroids, and exogenous melatonin.

11. The effect of depression on sleep includes a short REM latency, a long first REM period, an increased REM density (eye movements per time) in the initial REM period and an increased total duration of REM sleep. Depression can be associated with either insomnia or hypersomnia.
12. Alcohol consumption can decrease sleep latency (depending on timing of consumption) but increases the REM latency and causes sleep fragmentation during the second part of the night. Even alcohol consumption confined to "happy hour" can have an effect on sleep in some individuals. Alterations in sleep architecture during abstinence in treated alcoholic patients may persist, and some studies suggest continued poor sleep can be a risk factor for relapse. A decrease in stage N3 sleep is a common finding.
13. Cannabis withdrawal after chronic use is associated with significant sleep disturbance. Acute withdrawal (as before sleep testing) can cause REM rebound and affect the accuracy of the multiple sleep latency test.
14. Caffeine metabolism decreases with age, pregnancy, and oral contraceptive medication but increases with cigarette smoking. The recommended time for caffeine consumption to stop to improve sleep quality depends on the individual, amount of consumption, and tolerance to caffeine.

CLINICAL REVIEW QUESTIONS

1. Sleep deprivation results in which of the following?
   A. Increased leptin
   B. Increased ghrelin
   C. Augmented response to immunization
   D. Stage R rebound before stage N3 rebound during the first night of recovery sleep
2. Which of the following increases the REM latency?
   A. Depression
   B. Narcolepsy
   C. Withdrawal of Tricyclic antidepressants
   D. Lithium
3. Which β-blocker has the highest likelihood of causing insomnia?
   A. Atenolol
   B. Carvedilol
   C. Nadolol
   D. Propranolol
4. Which of the following is ***not*** associated with nightmares/vivid dreams?
   A. Varenicline (Chantix)
   B. Pramipexole
   C. Efavirenz
   D. Prazosin
5. Which of the following medications is ***not*** associated with insomnia?
   A. Donepezil (Aricept)
   B. Fluoxetine
   C. Amitriptyline
   D. Methylphenidate
6. Which of the following is true about chronic sleep restriction?
   A. Sleep duration of 5 hours or less is needed for impairment.
   B. Individuals with sleep restriction may not feel progressively impaired.
   C. Performance deficits plateau after 5 days.
   D. Sleeping longer on the weekend can reverse 5 days of sleep restriction.
7. Which of the following is true about *withdrawal* of cannabis?
   A. Decreased REM latency, increased amount of REM sleep (%TST)
   B. Increased REM latency, decreased amount of REM sleep (%TST)
   C. Decreased REM latency, increased total sleep time
   D. Increased REM latency, decreased total sleep time
8. Which of the following statements is ***not*** true?
   A. Donepezil can cause insomnia and nightmares.
   B. If pramipexole causes nightmares, so will ropinirole.
   C. Gabapentin, trazodone, and mirtazapine may increase stage N3 sleep.
   D. A common mechanism by which trazodone, doxepin, mirtazapine, and quetiapine improve sleep is antagonism of H1 receptors (antihistamine).
9. Which of the following does not exhibit significant anticholinergic side effects?
   A. Diphenhydramine
   B. Trazodone
   C. Amitriptyline
   D. Paroxetine

ANSWERS

1. B. Sleep deprivation increases ghrelin but decreases leptin and the response to immunization. In recovery sleep, an increase in stage N3 occurs on the initial recovery night and increased REM on subsequent nights. In older individuals with little stage N3 sleep at baseline, an increase in REM sleep can be more prominent on the first recovery night.
2. D. Lithium increases the REM latency (decreases the amount of REM sleep but increases stage N3). Withdrawal of TCAs decreases the REM latency.
3. D. Propranolol is the most lipophilic β-blocker, and those with more lipophilicity (propranolol, metoprolol, carvedilol, labetalol) are more likely to cause insomnia than those that are less lipophilic (nadolol, atenolol). However, the affinity for serotonin receptors may also play a role. Of the β-blocker medications, atenolol may be the best for sleep.
4. D. Prazosin may reduce nightmares (especially associated with PTSD). The other medications are associated with disturbed dreaming.
5. C. Amitriptyline is a sedating antidepressant.
6. B. Individuals with chronic sleep restriction may not recognize an impairment. Sleep restriction to 6 hours will result in deficits. Deficits with chronic sleep restriction do not plateau (at least up to 2 weeks), and two nights of recovery sleep do not recover deficits from 5 nights of sleep restriction.
7. A. Withdrawal of cannabis can result in a decreased REM latency and an increase in the relative amount of REM sleep, although the total sleep time is usually reduced. Acute withdrawal of cannabis can affect the accuracy of an MSLT.

8. B. Dopamine agonists are associated with nightmares. However, sometimes a patient will tolerate a different dopamine agonist. Doxepin, trazodone, mirtazapine, and quetiapine all have potent antihistamine activity at low doses. Doxepin and amitriptyline have anticholinergic activity, whereas trazodone does not. Very low-dose doxepin is sedating without significant anticholinergic effects. Trazodone and mirtazapine block 5HT2A receptors that may also promote sleep. However, at low doses the antihistamine effect is predominant.

9. B. Trazodone. The other medications have significant anticholinergic side effects including dry mouth, dry eyes, blurred vision, and in susceptible men a risk of urinary retention. Paroxetine has the most anticholinergic activity of all the SSRIs. The medication has a relatively high affinity for M1 muscarinic receptors.

SUGGESTED READING

Berry R, Wagner M. Effects of sleep disorders and medications on sleep architecture. In: Berry R, Wagner M, eds. *Sleep Medicine Pearls.* 3rd ed. Elsevier Saunders; 2014:74-77.

Bonnet MH. Acute sleep deprivation. In: Kryger MH, Roth T, Dement WC, eds. *Principles and Practice of Sleep Medicine.* 5th ed. Elsevier; 2011:54-65.

Buysse DJ, Tyagi S. Clinical pharmacology of other drugs used as hypnotics. In: Kryger M, Roth T, Dement WC, eds. *Principles and Practice of Sleep Medicine.* 5th ed. Elsevier; 2017:432-445.

Schweitzer PK, Randazzo AC. Drugs that disturb sleep and wakefulness. In: Kryger M, Roth T, Dement WC, eds. *Principles and Practice of Sleep Medicine.* 5th ed. Philadelphia: Elsevier; 2017:480-498.

Van Dongen HPA, Maislin G, Mullington JM, et al. The cumulative cost of additional wakefulness: dose-response effects of neurobehavioral function and sleep physiology from chronic sleep restriction and total sleep deprivation. *Sleep.* 2003;26:117-126.

REFERENCES

1. Troester MM, Quan SF, Berry RB, et al. *The AASM Manual for the Scoring of Sleep and Associated Events: Rules, Terminology and Technical Specifications. Version 3.* Darien, IL: American Academy of Sleep Medicine; 2023:12.
2. Bonnet MH, Doghramji K, Roehrs T, et al. The scoring of arousal in sleep; reliability, validity, and alternatives. *J Clin Sleep Med.* 2007;3:133-145.
3. Bonnet M, Arand DL. EEG arousal norms by age. *J Clin Sleep Med.* 2007;3:271-274.
4. Mathur R, Douglas NJ. Frequency of EEG arousals from nocturnal sleep in normal subjects. *Sleep.* 1995;18:330-333.
5. Gosselin N, Michaud M, Carrier J, et al. Age difference in heart rate changes associated with micro-arousals in humans. *Clin Neurophysiol.* 2002;113:1517.
6. Boselli M, Parrino L, Smerieri A, et al. Effect of age on EEG arousals in normal sleep. *Sleep.* 1998;21:351-357.
7. Bonnet MH. Performance and sleepiness as a function of frequency and placement of sleep disruption. *Psychophysiology.* 1986;23:263-271.
8. Bonnet MH, Arand DL. Clinical effects of sleep fragmentation versus sleep deprivation. *Sleep Med Rev.* 2003;7(4):297-310.
9. Norman RG, Scott MA, Ayappa I, et al. Sleep continuity measured by survival curve analysis. *Sleep.* 2006;29(12):1625-1631.
10. Azarbarzin A, Ostrowski M, Hanly P, Younes M. Relationship between arousal intensity and heart rate response to arousal. *Sleep.* 2014;37(4): 645-653.
11. Younes M, Ostrowski M, Soiferman M, et al. Odds ratio product of sleep EEG as a continuous measure of sleep state. *Sleep.* 2015;38(4): 641-654.
12. Younes M, Hanly PJ. Immediate postarousal sleep dynamics: an important determinant of sleep stability in obstructive sleep apnea. *J Appl Physiol (1985).* 2016;120(7):801-808.
13. Bonnet MH. Acute sleep deprivation. In: Kryger MH, Roth T, Dement WC, eds. *Principles and Practice of Sleep Medicine.* 5th ed. St. Louis, MO: Elsevier; 2011:54-65.
14. Van Dongen HP, Maislin G, Mullington JM, Dinges DF. The cumulative cost of additional wakefulness: dose-response effects on neurobehavioral functions and sleep physiology from chronic sleep restriction and total sleep deprivation. *Sleep.* 2003;26(2):117-126.
15. Banks S, Dinges DF. Behavioral and physiological consequences of sleep restriction. *J Clin Sleep Med.* 2007;3(5):519-528.
16. Verma A, Radtke RA, VanLandingham KE, et al. Slow wave sleep rebound and REM rebound following the first night of treatment with CPAP for sleep apnea: correlation with subjective improvement in sleep quality. *Sleep Med.* 2001;2(3):215-223.
17. Rosenberg J, Wildschiødtz G, Pedersen MH, et al. Late postoperative nocturnal episodic hypoxaemia and associated sleep pattern. *Br J Anaesth.* 1994;72(2):145-150.
18. Rosenberg J. Sleep disturbances after non-cardiac surgery. *Sleep Med Rev.* 2001;5(2):129-137.
19. Williamson AM, Feyer AM. Moderate sleep deprivation produces impairments in cognitive and motor performance equivalent to legally prescribed levels of alcohol intoxication. *Occup Environ Med.* 2000;57(10): 649-655.
20. Vakulin A, Baulk SD, Catcheside PG, et al. Effects of moderate sleep deprivation and low-dose alcohol on driving simulator performance and perception in young men. *Sleep.* 2007;30(10):1327-1333.
21. Dijk DJ, Duffy JF, Czeisler CA. Circadian and sleep/wake dependent aspects of subjective alertness and cognitive performance. *J Sleep Res.* 1992;1(2):112-117.
22. Zeeuw J, Wisniewski S, Papakonstantinou A, et al. The alerting effect of the wake maintenance zone during 40 hours of sleep deprivation. *Sci Rep.* 2018;8(1):11,012.
23. Van Cauter E, Spiegel K, Leproult R. Metabolic consequences of sleep and sleep loss. *Sleep Med.* 2008;9(suppl 1):S23-S28.
24. Spiegel K, Tasali E, Penev P, Van Cauter E. Sleep curtailment in healthy young men is associated with decreased leptin levels, elevated ghrelin levels, and increase hunger and appetite. *Ann Intern Med.* 2004;141:846-850.
25. Donga E, van Dijk M, van Dijk JG, et al. A single night of partial sleep deprivation induces insulin resistance in multiple metabolic pathways in healthy subjects. *J Clin Endocrinol Metab.* 2010;95(6):2963-2968.
26. Spiegel K, Sheridan JF, Van Cauter E. Effect of sleep deprivation on response to immunization. *JAMA.* 2002;288:1471-1472.
27. Depner CM, Melanson EL, Eckel RH, et al. Ad libitum weekend recovery sleep fails to prevent metabolic dysregulation during a repeating pattern of insufficient sleep and weekend recovery sleep. *Curr Biol.* 2019;29(6):957-967.
28. Spaeth AM, Dinges DF, Goel N. Resting metabolic rate varies by race and by sleep duration. *Obesity (Silver Spring).* 2015;23(12):2349-2356.
29. Watson NF, Badr MS, Belenky G, et al. Joint consensus statement of the American Academy of Sleep Medicine and Sleep Research Society on the recommended amount of sleep for a healthy adult: methodology and discussion. *Sleep.* 2015;38(8):1161-1183.
30. Watson NF, Badr MS, Belenky G, et al. Recommended amount of sleep for a healthy adult: a joint consensus statement of the American Academy of Sleep Medicine and Sleep Research Society. *Sleep.* 2015;38(6):843-844.
31. Walker MP, Stickgold R. Sleep-dependent learning and memory consolidation. *Neuron.* 2004;44(1):121-133.
32. Berry R, Wagner M. Effects of sleep disorders and medications on sleep architecture. In: Berry R, Wagner M, eds. *Sleep Medicine Pearls.* 3rd ed. Philadelphia: Elsevier Saunders; 2014:74.
33. Schweitzer PK, Randazzo AC. Drugs that Disturb Sleep and Wakefulness. In: Kryger M, Roth T, Dement WD, eds. *Principles and Practice of Sleep Medicine.* 6th ed. Philadelphia: Elsevier; 2017:480-498.
34. Schutte-Rodin S, Broch L, Buysse D, et al. Clinical guideline for the evaluation and management of chronic insomnia in adults. *J Clin Sleep Med.* 2008;4(5):487-504.
35. Ansseau M, Kupfer DJ, Reynolds CF III, McEachran AB. REM latency distribution in major depression: clinical characteristics associated with sleep onset REM periods. *Biol Psychiatry.* 1984;19(12):1651-1666.
36. Palagini L, Baglioni C, Ciapparelli A, et al. REM sleep dysregulation in depression: state of the art. *Sleep Med Rev.* 2013;17(5):377-390.
37. Wang YQ, Li R, Zhang MQ, et al. The neurobiological mechanisms and treatments of REM sleep disturbances in depression. *Curr Neuropharmacol.* 2015;13(4):543-553.
38. Buysse DJ, Tyagi S. Clinical pharmacology of other drugs used as hypnotics. In: Kryger M, Roth T, Dement WC, eds. *Principles and Practice of Sleep Medicine.* 6th ed. Philadelphia: Elsevier; 2017:432-445.
39. Wichniak A, Wierzbicka A, Walęcka M, Jernajczyk W. Effects of antidepressants on sleep. *Curr Psychiatry Rep.* 2017;19(9):63.
40. Gursky JT, Krahn LE. The effects of antidepressants on sleep: a review. *Harv Rev Psychiatry.* 2000;8(6):298-306.

41. Nofzinger EA, Reynolds CF III, Thase ME, et al. REM sleep enhancement by bupropion in depressed men. *Am J Psychiatry*. 1995;152(2):274-276.
42. Ott GE, Rao U, Lin KM, et al. Effect of treatment with bupropion on EEG sleep: relationship to antidepressant response. *Int J Neuropsychopharmacol*. 2004;7(3):275-281.
43. Rye DB, Dihenia B, Bliwise DL. Reversal of atypical depression, sleepiness, and REM-sleep propensity in narcolepsy with bupropion. *Depress Anxiety*. 1998;7:92-95.
44. Monti JM, Torterolo P, Pandi Perumal SR. The effects of second generation antipsychotic drugs on sleep variables in healthy subjects and patients with schizophrenia. *Sleep Med Rev*. 2017;33:51-57.
45. Muench J, Hamer AM. Adverse effects of antipsychotic medications. *Am Fam Physician*. 2010;81(5):617-622.
46. Kupfer DJ, Wyatt RJ, Greenspan K, et al. Lithium carbonate and sleep in affective illness. *Arch Gen Psychiatry*. 1970;23(1):35-40.
47. Billiard M. Lithium carbonate: effects on sleep patterns of normal and depressed subjects and its use in sleep-wake pathology. *Pharmacopsychiatry*. 1987;20(5):195-196.
48. Liguori C, Toledo M, Kothare S. Effects of anti-seizure medications on sleep architecture and daytime sleepiness in patients with epilepsy: a literature review. *Sleep Med Rev*. 2021;60:101559.
49. Yamada Y, Shibuya F, Hamada J, et al. Prediction of sleep disorders induced by beta-adrenergic receptor blocking agents based on receptor occupancy. *J Pharmacokinet Biopharm*. 1995;23:131-145.
50. Chang CH, Yang YH, Lin SJ, et al. Risk of insomnia attributable to β-blockers in elderly patients with newly diagnosed hypertension. *Drug Metab Pharmacokinet*. 2013;28(1):53-58.
51. Aldrich MS, Chervin RD, Malow BA. Value of the multiple sleep latency test (MSLT) for the diagnosis of narcolepsy. *Sleep*. 1997;20(8):620-629.
52. Bazalakova M, Benca RM. Wake-Promoting Medication. In: Kryger MH, Dement WC, Roth T, eds. *Principles and Practice of Sleep Medicine*. 6th ed. Philadelphia: Elsevier; 2017:462-479.
53. Pardi D, Black J. Gamma-hydroxybutyrate/sodium oxybate: neurobiology, and impact on sleep and wakefulness. *CNS Drugs*. 2006;20(12):993-1018.
54. Mamelak M, Black J, Montplaisir J, Ristanovic R. A pilot study on the effects of sodium oxybate on sleep architecture and daytime alertness in narcolepsy. *Sleep*. 2004;27:1327-1334.
55. Pagel JF, Helfter P. Drug induced nightmares—an etiology based review. *Hum Psychopharmacol*. 2003;18(1):59-67.
56. Morin CM, Koetter U, Bastien C, et al. Valerian-hops combination and diphenhydramine for treating insomnia: a randomized placebo-controlled clinical trial. *Sleep*. 2005;28(11):1465-1471.
57. Sateia MJ, Buysse DJ, Krystal AD, et al. Clinical Practice Guideline for the Pharmacologic Treatment of Chronic Insomnia in Adults: an American Academy of Sleep Medicine Clinical Practice Guideline. *J Clin Sleep Med*. 2017;13(2):307-349.
58. Drake CL, Jefferson C, Roehrs T, Roth T. Stress-related sleep disturbance and polysomnographic response to caffeine. *Sleep Med*. 2006;7(7):567-572.
59. Lazarus M, Shen HY, Cherasse Y, Qu WM, et al. Arousal effect of caffeine depends on adenosine A2A receptors in the shell of the nucleus accumbens. *J Neurosci*. 2011;31(27):10,067-10,075.
60. Killgore WD, Rupp TL, Grugle NL, et al. Effects of dextroamphetamine, caffeine and modafinil on psychomotor vigilance test performance after 44 hours of continuous wakefulness. *J Sleep Res*. 2008;17(3):309-321.
61. Clark I, Landolt HP. Coffee, caffeine, and sleep: a systematic review of epidemiological studies and randomized controlled trials. *Sleep Med Rev*. 2017;31:70-78.
62. Landolt HP. "No thanks, coffee keeps me awake": individual caffeine sensitivity depends on ADORA2A genotype. *Sleep*. 2012;35(7):899-900.
63. Wesensten NJ, Belenky G, Kautz MA, et al. Maintaining alertness and performance during sleep deprivation: modafinil versus caffeine. *Psychopharmacology (Berl)*. 2002;159(3):238-247.
64. Drake C, Roehrs T, Shambroom J, Roth T. Caffeine effects on sleep taken 0, 3, or 6 hours before going to bed. *J Clin Sleep Med*. 2013;9:1195-1200.
65. Bonnet MH, Arand DL. Caffeine use as a model of acute and chronic insomnia. *Sleep*. 1992;15(6):526-536.
66. Gyllenhaal C, Merritt SL, Peterson SD, et al. Efficacy and safety of herbal stimulants and sedatives in sleep disorders. *Sleep Med Rev*. 2000;4(3):229-251.
67. Silverman K, Evans SM, Strain EC, Griffiths RR. Withdrawal syndrome after the double-blind cessation of caffeine consumption. *N Engl J Med*. 1992;327:1109-1114.
68. Burke TM, Markwald RR, McHill AW, et al. Effects of caffeine on the human circadian clock in vivo and in vitro. *Sci Transl Med*. 2015;7(305):305ra146.
69. Weibel J, Lin YS, Landolt HP, et al. Caffeine-dependent changes of sleep-wake regulation: Evidence for adaptation after repeated intake. *Prog Neuropsychopharmacol Biol Psychiatry*. 2020;99:109851.
70. O'Keefe JH, Bhatti SK, Patil HR, et al. Effects of habitual coffee consumption on cardiometabolic disease, cardiovascular health, and all-cause mortality. *J Am Coll Cardiol*. 2013;62(12):1043-1051.
71. Kaul M, Zee PC, Sahni AS. Effects of cannabinoids on sleep and their therapeutic potential for sleep disorders. *Neurotherapeutics*. 2021;18(1):217-227.
72. Schierenbeck T, Riemann D, Berger M, Hornyak M. Effect of illicit recreational drugs upon sleep: cocaine, ecstasy and marijuana. *Sleep Med Rev*. 2008;12(5):381-389.
73. Dzodzomenyo S, Stolfi A, Splaingard D, et al. Urine toxicology screen in multiple sleep latency test: the correlation of positive tetrahydrocannabinol, drug negative patients, and narcolepsy. *J Clin Sleep Med*. 2015;11(2):93-99.
74. Spanagel R, Bilbao A. Approved cannabinoids for medical purposes—comparative systematic review and meta-analysis for sleep and appetite. *Neuropharmacology*. 2021;196:108680.
75. Gates PJ, Albertella L, Copeland J. The effects of cannabinoid administration on sleep: a systematic review of human studies. *Sleep Med Rev*. 2014;18(6):477-487.
76. Gates P, Albertella L, Copeland J. Cannabis withdrawal and sleep: a systematic review of human studies. *Subst Abus*. 2016;37(1):255-269.
77. Hoffman RJ. Testing for drugs of abuse (DOAs). In: Ganetsky M, Traub SJ, eds. UptoDate; September 21, 2022. Accessed April 3, 2022.
78. Colrain IM, Nicholas CL, Baker FC. Alcohol and the sleeping brain. *Handb Clin Neurol*. 2014;125:415-431.
79. Koob GF, Colrain IM. Alcohol use disorder and sleep disturbances: a feed-forward allostatic framework. *Neuropsychopharmacology*. 2020;45(1):141-165.
80. Landolt HP, Roth C, Dijk DJ, Borbély AA. Late-afternoon ethanol intake affects nocturnal sleep and the sleep EEG in middle-aged men. *J Clin Psychopharmacol*. 1996;16(6):428-436.
81. Geoghegan P, O'Donovan MT, Lawlor BA. Investigation of the effects of alcohol on sleep using actigraphy. *Alcohol Alcohol*. 2012;47(5):538-544.
82. Landolt HP, Gillin JC. Sleep abnormalities during abstinence in alcohol-dependent patients. Aetiology and management. *CNS Drugs*. 2001;15(5):413-425.

Chapter 10

Monitoring Respiration—Technology and Techniques

INTRODUCTION

The three major components of respiratory monitoring during polysomnography (PSG) include measurement (or detection) of airflow (or tidal volume), detection of respiratory effort, and measurement of the arterial oxygen saturation (SaO_2). These parameters allow detection of apnea (cessation of airflow), hypopnea (reduction in airflow), and arterial oxygen desaturation. Apneas can be classified as obstructive, mixed, or central (see Chapters 11 and 12). Signals from respiratory inductive plethysmography (RIP) thoracoabdominal effort belts can be used to detect respiratory effort and signals derived from them used to detect apnea and hypopnea. Ancillary monitoring may include detection of snoring and recording surrogates of the arterial partial pressure of carbon dioxide ($PaCO_2$) including end-tidal PCO_2 ($P_{ET}CO_2$) and transcutaneous PCO_2 ($TcPCO_2$). These surrogates of the $PaCO_2$ are used to detect hypoventilation. The American Academy of Sleep Medicine (AASM) *Manual for the Scoring of Sleep and Associated Events* (hereinafter "AASM scoring manual")[1,2] specifies sensors recommended for detection of respiratory events and rules for scoring respiratory events. The reader should consult the most current version of the manual. The background and rationale for the recommendations concerning respiratory sensors and respiratory event definitions has also been published.[3-5] For different respiratory event types, recommended and alternative sensors are specified. Alternative sensors are used if the recommended sensor is not functioning or providing reliable information. There are two levels of recommendation: "recommended" and "acceptable." The techniques employed for respiratory monitoring for both adults and pediatric individuals are discussed in detail in this chapter. Criteria for scoring respiratory events for adults are discussed in Chapter 11 and for pediatric patients in Chapter 12. The convention used in this book is for inspiratory signals to be upward and expiratory signals downward. Home sleep apnea testing (HSAT) is increasingly used as an alternative to PSG for the diagnosis of obstructive sleep apnea in adult patients. Sensors recommended for HSAT using airflow monitoring are discussed at the end of this chapter.

MEASURING AIRFLOW OR TIDAL VOLUME

The techniques used to detect (measure) airflow during PSG are listed in Table 10–1. Advantages and disadvantages of the methods are also listed and will be discussed in the following sections. Standard and other apnea and hypopnea sensors are shown in Tables 10–2 and 10–3.

Pneumotachograph

The pneumotachograph (PNT) is the most accurate method to measure airflow during sleep studies (Figure 10–1).[3,5,6] This device quantifies airflow by measurement of the pressure drop across a linear (constant) resistance (usually a wire screen). The relationship between the pressure change, flow rate, and resistance is given by the following equation:

$$\text{Pressure change} = \text{Flow} \times \text{Resistance} \qquad \text{Equation 10–1}$$

The PNT is worn in a mask covering the nose and mouth. Although a PNT is commonly used to measure airflow during sleep research, this device is rarely used during clinical sleep studies.

Oronasal Thermal Sensors

Thermal devices were the first to be used to monitor airflow during clinical sleep studies.[5-9] These devices detect changes in temperature induced by airflow (cooler inspired air, warmer exhaled air). The changes in device temperature result in changes in voltage output (thermocouples) or resistance (thermistors). Thermal sensors are generally adequate to detect an absence of airflow (apnea), but their signal does not vary in proportion to airflow.[7,8] Therefore, thermal sensors are not an ideal means of detecting a reduction in airflow (hypopnea). Results of a study comparing thermistor and thermocouple signals in a nose model with a PNT as the gold standard (accurate measure of flow) are shown in Figure 10–2.[8] Note that thermal signals and PNT flow are equal at 1 L/sec (by design). However, as airflow decreases, the thermal signals overestimate flow. This figure illustrates that thermal sensors are not ideal sensors to detect hypopneas (reductions in flow). The same study demonstrated that the thermal sensor signal decreases when the nostrils are large, or the thermal sensor is further from the nares. Of note, thermal devices composed of polyvinylidene fluoride (PVDF) film may offer a better estimate of the amplitude flow[9] (Figure 10–3). PVDF sensors respond to changes in pressure as well as temperature. Oronasal thermal sensors usually have a portion of the device placed within or just outside the nostrils with another portion over the mouth (detection of oral flow) (Figure 10–4). A major advantage of thermal sensors is that they can detect both nasal and oral airflow without the need for a cumbersome mask covering the face. An oronasal thermal airflow sensor is recommended by the American Academy of Sleep Medicine (AASM) scoring manual for **detection of apnea** in both adult and pediatric patients during diagnostic studies.[1]

Nasal Pressure

Nasal pressure (NP) is measured using a nasal cannula (inserted into the nares) connected to an accurate pressure transducer. Because the cannula tips are inside the nares and the other side of the pressure transducer is open to the atmosphere, the pressure being measured is the pressure change across the resistance of the nasal inlet associated with nasal airflow. Measurement of NP provides an estimate of nasal

Table 10–1 Methods to Monitor Airflow or Tidal Volume

Device	Physiology
Pneumotachograph (PNT)	• Pressure drop across PNT = Flow × Resistance • Flow = Pressure difference/Resistance • PNT usually placed in a mask covering the nose and mouth • Used for research studies

Oronasal thermal sensor	• Changes in temperature induced by airflow result in changes in resistance (thermistor) or voltage output (thermocouple)
	  • Accurate for the presence or absence of airflow
	  • Can detect nasal and oral airflow
	  • Signal not proportional to flow
	• Polyvinylidene fluoride devices respond to both temperature and pressure changes
	  • Accurate for the presence or absence of airflow
	  • Can detect nasal and oral airflow
	  • Signal more proportional to flow than other thermal sensors

Nasal Pressure (NP)	• Measures pressure difference across the nares • $NP = K1 \times (Flow)^2$ K1 = constant • $FLOW = K2 \times \sqrt{NP}$ K2 = constant • Flattening of the inspiratory flow contour detects airflow limitation • Oral breathing not well detected

RIP	• RIPsum = (K1 × RIPchest + K2 × RIPabdomen)
	  • Changes in RIPsum are an estimate of tidal volume
	  • Most accurate if calibrated (determine K1 and K2)
	• RIPflow is the time derivative of the RIPsum and RIPflow is an estimate of airflow

PAP device flow	• Accurate flow sensor in the laboratory positive airway pressure (PAP) device. A DC signal is output that can be recorded • Flattening of inspiratory flow contour indicates airflow limitation • Signal quality not sufficient to demonstrate snoring

NP, Nasal pressure; *PNT,* pneumotachograph; *RIP,* respiratory inductance plethysmography.

Table 10–2 Apnea Sensors

Standard Apnea Sensors

- Diagnostic study: oronasal thermal airflow sensor (thermistor, thermocouple, or PVDF)
- PAP titration study—PAP device flow

Other Apnea Sensors (Diagnostic Study)

- Nasal pressure transducer (with or without square root transformation)
- RIPsum (calibrated or uncalibrated)—deflections an estimate of tidal volume
- RIPflow (calibrated or uncalibrated)—deflections in the signal an estimate of airflow
- Polyvinylidene fluoride (PVDF) sum = sum of chest and abdominal PVDF belt signals . Signal is a surrogate of airflow used to detect apnea and hypopnea.
- Exhaled PCO_2 waveform (used in children)

RIP, respiratory inductance plethysmography; *PAP,* positive airway pressure

Table 10–3 Standard and Other Hypopnea Sensors

Adults and Children

Standard Hypopnea Sensors

Diagnostic study
- NP (with or without square root transformation)

PAP titration study
- PAP flow

Other Hypopnea Sensors (Diagnostic Study)

- Oronasal thermal airflow sensor
- RIPsum (calibrated or uncalibrated)—deflections estimate of tidal volume
- RIPflow (calibrated or uncalibrated)—estimate of airflow
- Dual thoracoabdominal RIP belts
- PVDFsum

NP, Nasal pressure; *PAP,* positive airway pressure; *PVDF,* polyvinylidene fluoride; *RIP,* respiratory inductance plethysmography; *RIPflow,* time derivative of RIPsum; *RIPsum* and *PVDFsum,* sum of chest and abdominal belt signals.

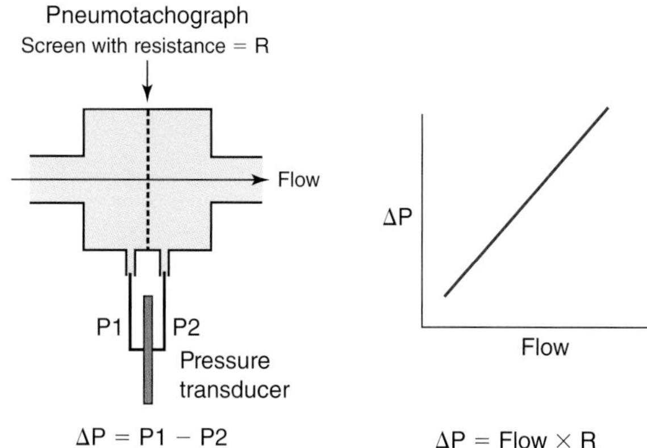

Figure 10–1 The pneumotachograph (PNT) measures airflow by determining the pressure drop across a linear (constant) resistance, which is usually some type of screen. The PNT is usually inserted in the entrance of a mask covering the nose and mouth.

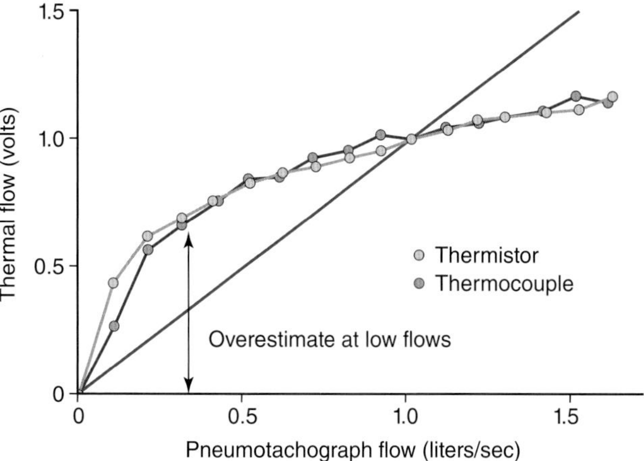

Figure 10–2 Comparison of signals from a thermistor and thermocouple with the gold-standard pneumotachograph using a nose model of simulated breathing. The signals were normalized to be equal at a flow rate of 1 L/min. Thermal devices overestimate the actual flow (underestimate the drop in flow) as flow decreases. The *straight line* is the line of identity. (Reproduced with permission of the © ERS 2023: European Respiratory Journal 11 (1) 179-182; DOI: 10.1183/09031936.98.11010179 Published 1 January 1998.)

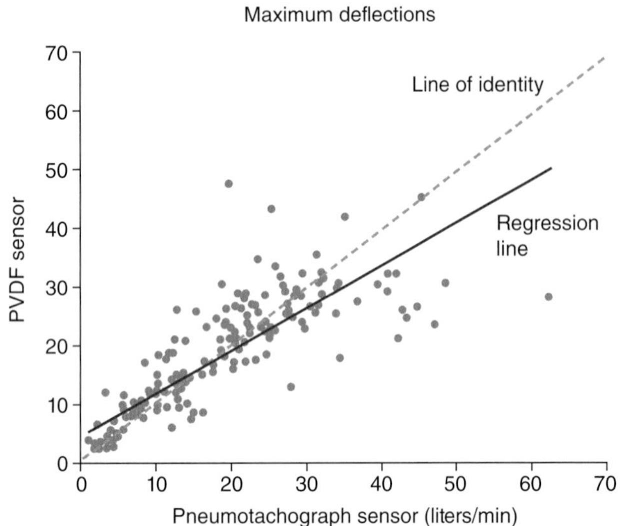

Figure 10–3 Comparison of the flow signal from a polyvinylidene fluoride (PVDF) oronasal airflow sensor with that of a pneumotachograph. The results are the maximum deflections in each signal during breathing. PVDF sensor signals appear to provide a fairly accurate estimate of airflow. (Reproduced from Berry RB, Koch GL, Trautz S, Wagner MH. Comparison of respiratory event detection by a polyvinylidene fluoride film airflow sensor and a pneumotachograph in sleep apnea patients. *Chest.* 2005;128:1331-1338.)

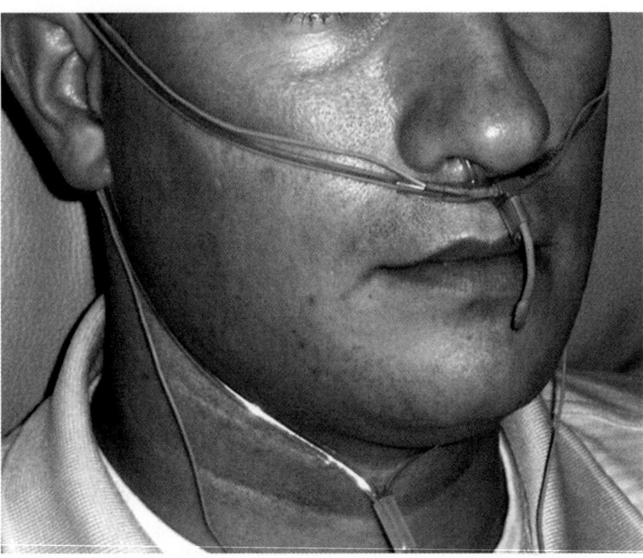

Figure 10–4 The photograph shows the simultaneous use of a nasal pressure cannula and an oronasal thermal device. The sensors provide complementary information. The nasal pressure signal is recommended for detection of hypopnea and the oronasal thermal sensor for detection of apnea. If one sensor is not working, the other can be used as a backup (alternative) sensor.

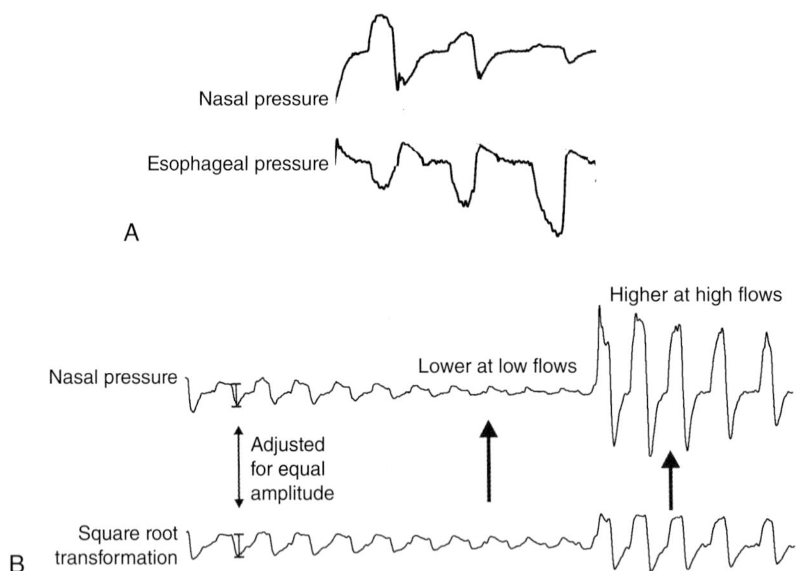

Figure 10–5 (A) The nasal pressure signal and esophageal pressure at the start of an obstructive respiratory event. The inspiratory waveform is round on the first breath with a small esophageal pressure deflection. The second and third breaths show a decrease in nasal pressure amplitude, and the third breath shows inspiratory flattening (airflow limitation). Esophageal pressure deflections increase progressively from the first breath to the third. On the third breath, lower flow associated with greater driving pressure means the upper airway resistance is increased. The third breath exhibits airflow limitation (defined as constant flow [flat profile] with increasing effort). (B) The nasal pressure signal *(top)* and the signal with a square root transformation *(bottom)*. Assuming the transformed signal is the better estimate of airflow, the nasal pressure signal *(top)* underestimates airflow at low flow rates and overestimates flow at high flow rates. However, this makes reductions in airflow easier to detect visually.

airflow that is more accurate than one obtained with most thermal sensors.[10-15] However, the resistance of the nasal inlet is not a constant (nonlinear). The relationship of NP and flow is given by the following equations.[8,13]

$$\text{NP} \approx \text{K1} \times (\text{Flow})^2 \quad \text{K1} = \text{constant} \qquad \text{Equation 10–2}$$

$$\text{Flow} = \text{K2} \times \sqrt{NP} \quad \text{K2} = \text{constant} \qquad \text{Equation 10–3}$$

Because NP varies with the square of flow, the NP signal tends to underestimate airflow at low flow rates and overestimate flow at high flows (Figure 10–5). This makes reductions in airflow more visually apparent. As noted in Equation 10–3, nasal airflow is proportional to the square root of the NP signal. A square root transformation of the NP signal ("linearized") is a more accurate estimate of nasal airflow.

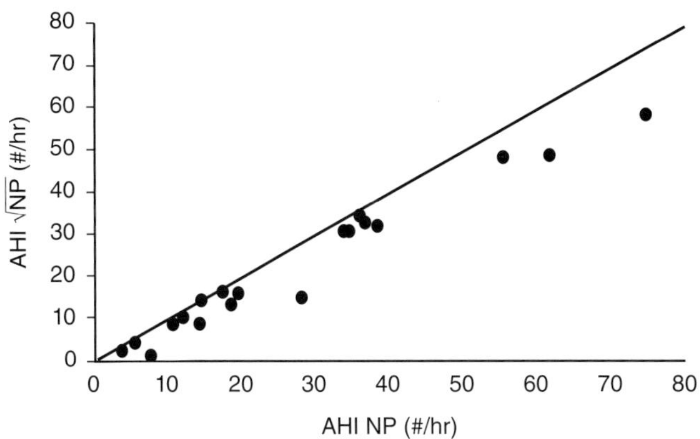

Figure 10–6 The average AHI values were determined using the nasal pressure signal NP and the transformed NP signal ($\sqrt{NP}$). The NP values tended to be slightly higher. (Plotted from data from Thurnheer R, Xie X, Bloch KE. Accuracy of nasal cannula pressure recordings for assessment of ventilation during sleep. *Am J Respir Crit Care Med.* 2001;146: 1914-1919.)

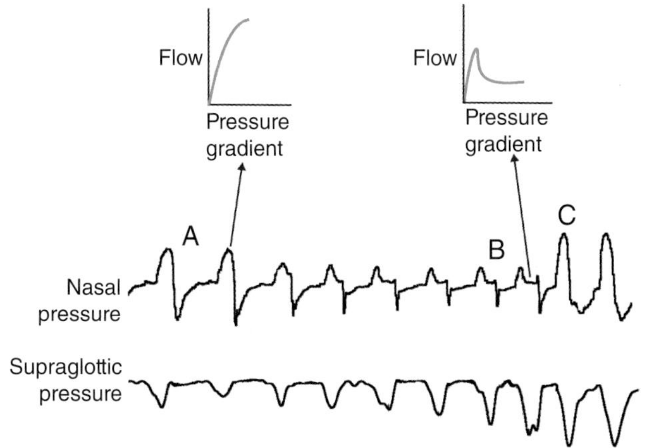

Figure 10–7 Changes in nasal pressure and supraglottic pressure recorded below the site of upper airway narrowing during a hypopnea (reduction in airflow). Inspiration is upward. At (A) the flow is rounded, whereas at (B) the flattened airflow contour is associated with an increase in pressure drop across the upper airway and airflow limitation (unchanged or decreased flow associated with an increased pressure gradient across the upper airway). Finally, at (C) the upper airway is open associated with rounded inspiratory airflow.

However, even with a square root transformation, the NP signal may not provide an exact estimate of total airflow over the entire night. Changes in cannula position, periods of partial or total oral airflow, and obstruction of the cannula by nasal secretions make the linearized NP signal a less accurate measure of airflow over the entire night. Thurnheer and coworkers[14] compared the NP and the square root transformed NP signals with the PNT (flowmeter = pneumotachograph) for detection of respiratory events. The number of apneas and hypopneas per hour of sleep (apnea-hypopnea index [AHI]) was determined using each of the three signals. Hypopnea was defined as a reduction in signal to 50% or less of the baseline. The AHI values by PNT and NP with and without a square root transformation were highly correlated. The mean difference ± 2 standard deviations in the AHI values between NP and PNT was 3.9/hr with limits of agreement (± 2 SD) of ± 4.6/hr. The mean difference in AHI values between the $\sqrt{NP}$ and the PNT was 0.9/hr ± 9.0/hr. The AHI values detected by the untransformed NP signal tended to be slightly higher than the $\sqrt{NP}$ signal, but the differences were usually small (Figure 10–6). Other investigations have also documented the utility of the NP signal for detection of apneas and hypopneas.[15]

In addition to the signal amplitude, the shape (contour) of both the PNT and the NP signals during inspiration provides additional useful information.[5,10,11,13] During normal unobstructed flow, the inspiratory shape (contour) of the NP signal is round (see Figures 10–5 and 10–7), whereas during airflow limitation (a constant or decreased airflow associated with an increasing driving pressure) the inspiratory shape of the PNT and NP signals is flattened. Of note, airflow limitation is characteristically present during obstructive reductions in airflow (hypopnea) or snoring. In contrast, when reductions in airflow are simply due to a fall in inspiratory effort, the NP signal amplitude is reduced but the shape is round. Airflow limitation is usually associated with an increased pressure drop across the upper airway (more negative inspiratory pressure below the site of upper airway narrowing) and increased inspiratory effort as reflected by more negative pressure as measured by a supraglottic pressure-sensing catheter (Figure 10–7) or esophageal manometry (Figure 10–8).

The NP signal can show vibration in airflow associated with snoring as well as airflow limitation if appropriate high filter and low filter settings are used (Figure 10–9).

The most important limitation of the NP technique is that approximately 10% of patients are "mouth breathers" and the NP signal may be misleading.[12] Even if a patient breathes mainly through the nasal route, intermittent mouth breathing can result in a NP signal showing minimal deflections (apparent apnea), whereas the oronasal thermal sensor continues to show airflow (Figure 10–10). Because of this phenomenon, an event that is actually a hypopnea may be misclassified as apnea if only the NP signal is used to detect airflow. For this reason, the AASM scoring manual recommends an oronasal thermal sensor for scoring apnea and the NP signal (with or without square root transformation of the signal) for detection of hypopnea during diagnostic PSG.[1] Simultaneous use of both NP and oronasal thermal sensors is recommended during PSG for optimal scoring of both apnea and hypopnea events. Using both sensors has the additional advantage of having a backup sensor if one of the airflow sensors fails to function appropriately during the study (see Figure 10–4).

Respiratory Inductance Plethysmography

RIP uses changes in the inductance of thoracic and abdominal effort belts with respiration to detect respiratory effort, and derived signals also provide estimates of tidal volume and airflow. The inductance of wires in bands around the entire circumference of the thorax and abdomen changes during respiration as the thoracic and abdominal belts expand or contract.[5,16-24] Each RIP band consists of a wire attached to a cloth band in a zigzag pattern. This produces a larger change in inductance of the band for a given change in band circumference. The band inductance varies proportionately with the cross-sectional area the band encircles. An oscillator produces an AC signal that is applied to each belt circuit, and changes in inductance are converted into a voltage output that is usually recorded as a bipolar AC signal. As the sensing element covers the entire circumference,

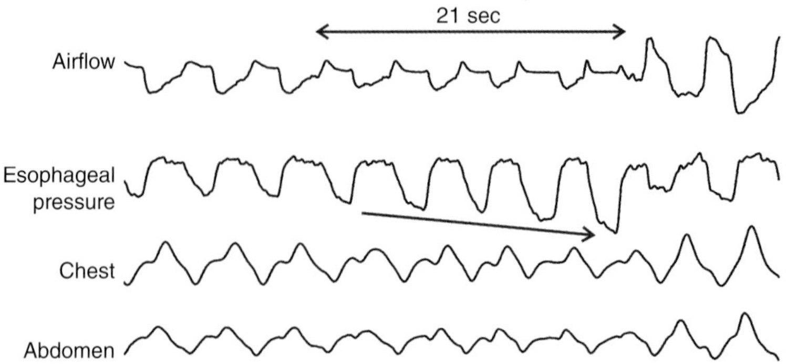

Figure 10–8 This figure shows a progressive drop in airflow and flattening of the inspiratory waveform using the nasal pressure signal associated with increasingly negative esophageal pressure deflections. There are more subtle changes in the chest and abdominal respiratory inductive plethysmography (RIP) signals (decrease in amplitude associated with decreased tidal volume), but they do not clearly reflect the increase in respiratory effort. Depending on the manufacturer of the RIP belts and the presence or absence of calibration, RIP belts may or may not exhibit paradox (paradoxical motion) during obstructive events.

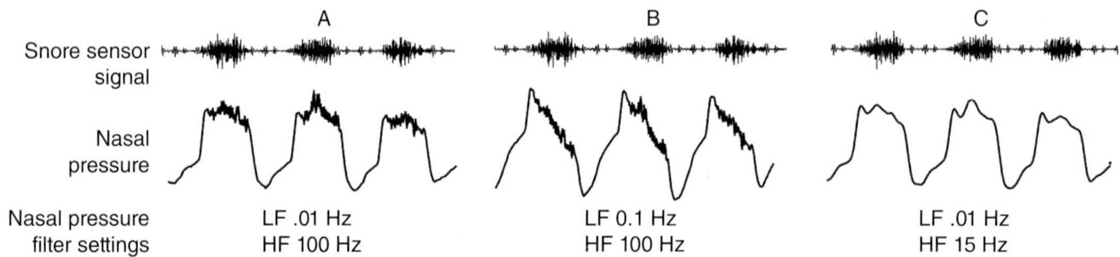

Figure 10–9 The nasal pressure signal can reveal evidence of snoring (high-frequency vibration in airflow) if the high filter setting is appropriate (A and B). The nasal pressure can also show inspiratory flattening if the signal is acquired and visualized either as a DC signal or as an AC signal with a sufficiently reduced low frequency filter setting (0.01 Hz) (A and C). Recording in the DC mode or with an appropriate low-frequency filter setting allows one to visualize a flow plateau. The snoring sensor signal is from a piezoelectric sensor placed on the upper neck near the trachea that responds to vibration. *LF*, low frequency filter setting; *HF*, high frequency filter setting. (Adapted from Berry RB, Wagner MH. *Sleep Medicine Pearls*. 3rd ed. Elsevier; 2015:120.)

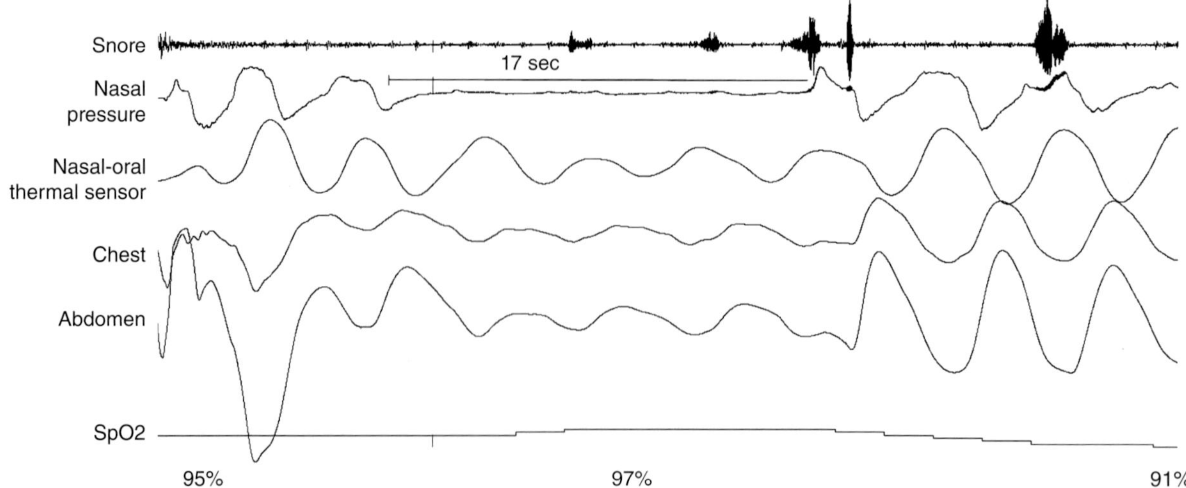

Figure 10–10 An example of a hypopnea with absent nasal pressure deflections. The oronasal thermal sensor deflections are not consistent with apnea. The is an example of oral breathing with absent NP defections. Note some evidence of snoring is also present consistent with persistent airflow (apnea not present). Inspiration is in the upward direction.

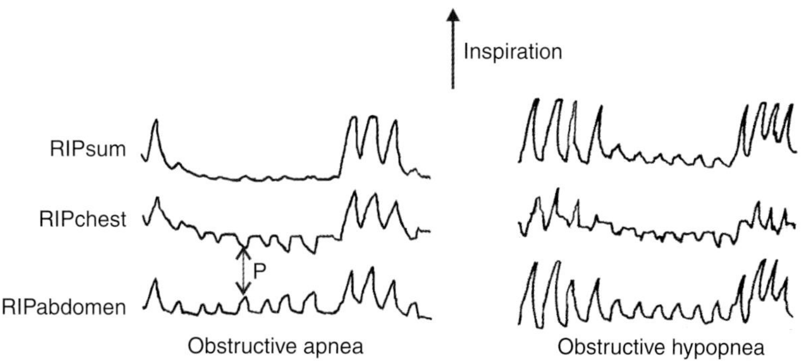

Figure 10–11 Examples of respiratory inductance plethysmography (RIP) tracings during obstructive apnea and hypopnea. During obstructive apnea the RIPchest and RIPabdomen signals show a paradoxical pattern (P), and the deflections cancel with the RIPsum deflections being near zero. The cancellation is more accurate (RIPsum closer to zero) when the RIP belts are calibrated. During obstructive hypopnea the deflections of the RIPchest and RIPabdomen also show paradoxical breathing, and the RIPsum signal shows reduced deflections consistent with reduced tidal volume. (From Berry RB, Wagner MH. *Sleep Medicine Pearls*. 3rd ed. Elsevier; 2015:133.)

changes in breathing can be detected in any body position. In contrast, effort belts using a single sensor (piezoelectric [PE] belts) have the sensing element on a small portion of the belt length. When a patient is lying on top of the PE sensor, the effort signal can be dampened or not detected, producing erroneous readings or unexplained changes in polarity that look like paradoxical movement. In general, RIP belts provide a more accurate method of detecting changes in thoracic and abdominal motion during respiration than belts using a single sensor. Of course, this assumes the RIP belts are located properly and sized (tightened) appropriately. The signals from the thoracic (RIPchest) and abdominal band (RIPabdomen) sensors can be summed (RIPsum = K1 × RIPchest + K2 × RIPabdomen), where K1 and K2 are calibration constants. If one takes the time derivative of the RIPsum signal, the result is an estimate of airflow (RIPflow). Several brands of PSG software automatically calibrate the RIP signals in real time based on the patient's pattern of breathing or the ability of RIPflow to mimic the transformed NP flow. A number of different techniques have been used to calibrate the RIP belts.[18-24] The belts can also be used in an uncalibrated manner (typically K1 and K2 = 0.5). The deflections in the RIPsum provides an estimate of tidal volume, which is more accurate if the RIPs are calibrated. Even if uncalibrated, changes in the deflections in the RIPsum signal reflect changes in tidal volume. In the case of an obstructive apnea (see Figure 10–11), the RIPchest and RIPabdomen signal deflections cancel each other (paradox) so that the RIPsum shows minimal deflections (apnea). The RIPflow shows the same pattern during apnea. In the case of hypopnea, there is a reduction in the deflections in the RIPsum signal (low tidal volume) and the deflections in both the RIPchest and RIPabdomen signal deflections, and the RIPflow signal. In the case of obstructive hypopnea, there may also be paradox with chest and abdomen signals moving in opposite directions (see Figure 10–11). If a RIPsum signal is not available, one can detect hypopnea by a reduction in both the thoracic and abdominal RIP signals. In the study of Thurnheer and coworkers discussed earlier,[14] detection of apnea and hypopnea by the calibrated RIPsum and RIPflow signals was compared with the PNT (flowmeter) signal. The AHI values obtained from the RIPsum and RIPflow showed good agreement with AHI values from the PNT signal. In Figure 10–12 an obstructive apnea is shown with associated changes in the oronasal thermal signal and the RIPsum and RIPflow. Of note, it is possible that the oronasal thermal sensor signal is flat consistent with an apnea while the RIPsum signal has continued deflections (deflections in the two bands are opposite in directions but the sum is not zero) (Figure 10–13). This scenario is more likely with uncalibrated RIP signals. In fact, one method of calibration of RIP signals is to have the patient simulate apnea (the isovolume maneuver) and adjust the K1 and K2 constants such that the sum is as close to zero as possible. The accuracy of the RIPsum signal to estimate tidal volume can deteriorate if body position changes or the positions of the bands change during sleep. The RIPsum and RIPflow signals provide useful alternative signals for detection of apnea and hypopnea. If the oronasal thermal sensor should fail, using the

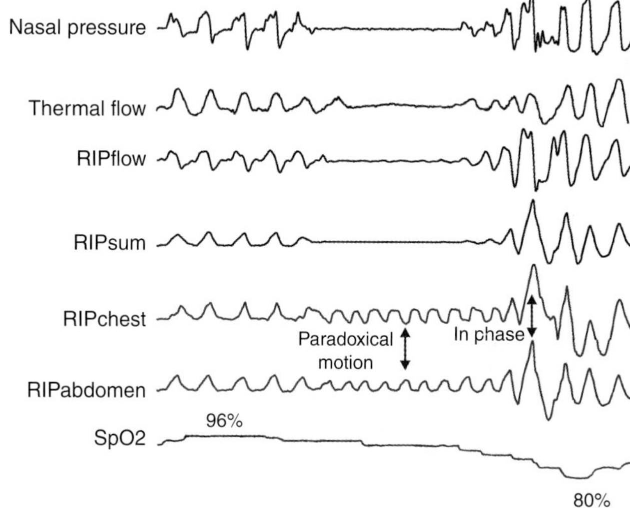

Figure 10–12 A tracing showing an obstructive apnea with absent airflow (or tidal volume) as shown by absent deflections in the RIPsum, RIPflow, and oronasal thermal sensor (thermal flow) signals. If the thermal flow is not functioning, one can use the nasal pressure or the RIPsum and RIPflow to identify apneas (recommended alternative apnea sensors/signals). If the nasal pressure signal is used to score apneas as noted in Figure 10-10, oral breathing may result in an event being classified as an apnea when it is actually a hypopnea. However, the RIPsum and RIPflow do not depend on the route of breathing. If the RIPchest and RIPabdomen signals are calibrated the RIPsum and RIPflow deflections will be near zero during an apnea. Note the paradoxical movement of the chest and abdomen during the apnea but not following apnea (in phase). *RIP,* Respiratory inductance plethysmography.

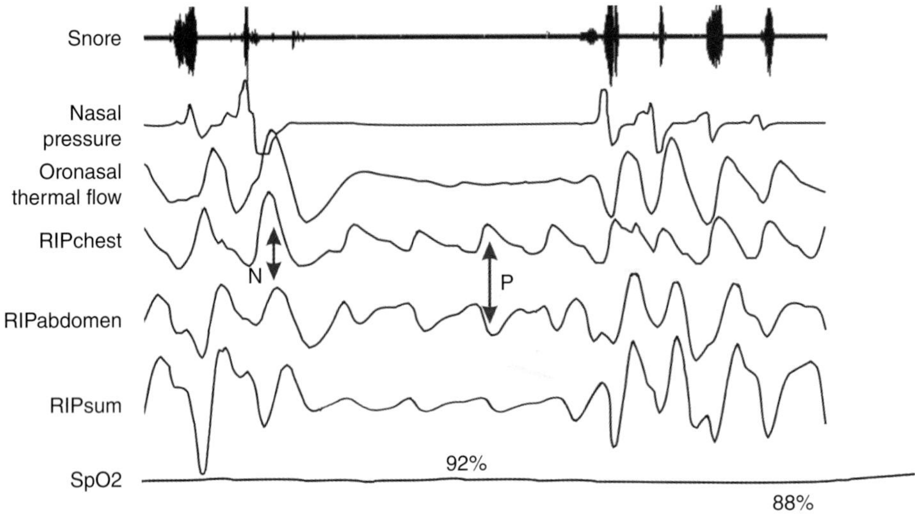

Figure 10–13 This tracing shows an obstructive apnea based on absent deflections in the oronasal thermal flow sensor. Paradoxical breathing is noted during the event (P) but before the event chest and abdominal signals were in nearly in phase (N). The chest and abdominal signals are from uncalibrated RIP belts, and the chest and abdominal deflections do not quite cancel. The RIPsum is quite reduced although showing some small deflections (signal reduced to about 80% of baseline). The RIPsum is a useful alternative signal for scoring apnea and hypopnea. However, depending on effort belt placement and the presence or absence of calibration, some events that are actually apneas may appear to be hypopneas using the RIP signal.

NP alone might falsely classify an event as an apnea during mouth breathing. However, the deflections in the RIPsum and RIPflow signals are not affected by mouth breathing and, in this scenario, should be near zero if an apnea is truly present (Figure 10–12). Small deflections in the RIPsum and RIPflow signals can be present during apnea if the RIPchest and RIPabdomen signals are not calibrated. Of note, different brands of RIP belt vary considerably in the ability to accurately reflect changes in tidal volume or airflow.[21]

Polyvinylidene Fluoride Belt Sum

Effort bands using PVDF sensors are also available. The ability to detect respiratory effort has been validated by a few studies, but generally there is less evidence than for RIP bands (in addition, the RIP signals can be calibrated). The PVDF effort belts typically consist of a single sensor per band. The sum of output from PVDF thoracic and abdominal bands is called PDVF-sum.[25,26] The sum can be used as a surrogate of airflow to score apnea and hypopnea. The AASM scoring manual lists PVDF effort belts[1] as **acceptable** for detecting respiratory effort and the PVDFsum signal an ***acceptable*** *alternative* sensor for scoring apnea and hypopnea in adults and children.

Positive Airway Pressure Device Flow

The positive airway pressure (PAP) devices used for PAP titration PSG provide several signals that can be recorded (flow, leak, and pressure). The signals are discussed in detail in Chapters 23 and 24. The airflow signal (PAP flow) uses an accurate flow sensor in the device. Like the NP signal, flattening of the PAP flow signal can be used to detect airflow limitation. However, due to the sampling rate or filtering the signal output from the PAP device does not exhibit vibrations during snoring (unlike NP with appropriate high filter settings). The AASM scoring manual recommends PAP device flow for scoring apnea and hypopnea during PAP titrations. No alternate sensor is available for use during PAP titrations.

End-Tidal PCO_2 Waveform

Use of end-tidal PCO_2 is listed as an acceptable alternative apnea sensor in children.[1] The waveform of exhaled PCO_2 versus time is what is actually used (capnogram). Exhaled PCO_2 measuring devices typically output both a capnography wave form (PCO_2 versus time) and a running estimate of end-tidal values derived from the waveform.[5] These two signals can be recorded during PSG. In the side stream method, air is continually sampled via a nasal cannula with constant suction from a measurement device usually at bedside. The alternative is direct sampling with the measuring device below the nostrils. Split nasal cannulas are available allowing both exhaled PCO_2 and NP to be sampled. Children have small nares, and separate cannulas would be not practical. Apnea, which is associated with absent airflow, results in only room air being suctioned (no exhaled PCO_2 sampled) and a value of zero during the event. There is a time delay between a change in the PCO_2 at the nostril and the associated change measured by the capnography device at bedside due to the time for the suctioned sample to reach the bedside device. This results in a delay between the onset of an apnea in the flow signals and the time the exhaled PCO_2 reaches zero (Figure 10–14). Obstruction of the cannula with nasal secretions or mouth breathing are limitations of this method to detect apnea. More discussion of the use of the end-tidal PCO_2 signal is provided in the section on monitoring hypoventilation.

RECOMMENDED AND ALTERNATIVE SENSORS FOR SCORING APNEA AND HYPOPNEA DURING POLYSOMNOGRAPHY

During diagnostic PSG in adults and children an oronasal thermal sensor is recommended for detecting apnea, and the NP (with or without square root transformation) is recommended for scoring hypopnea. During PAP titrations, as noted, the PAP flow is recommended for scoring of both apnea

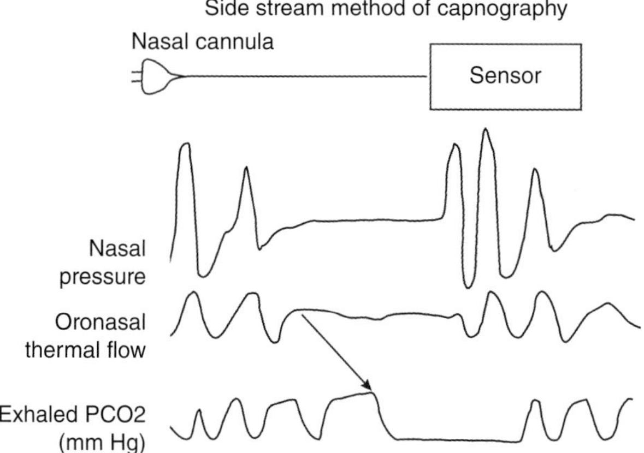

Figure 10–14 Use of the exhaled partial pressure of carbon dioxide *(PCO_2)* signal to detect apnea. A nasal cannula was connected to a bedside capnograph (side stream method). Absent deflections in the exhaled PCO_2 waveform are consistent with no exhaled PCO_2 (no flow = apnea). Note the delay in the start of the apnea by PCO_2 waveform compared with the flow signals *(arrow)*. The delay is due to the time it takes for increased PCO_2 in an exhaled breath sampled by the nasal cannula to reach the bedside sensor (side stream method). It is important to note that the amplitude of the exhaled PCO_2 deflections represents the value of the PCO_2 being exhaled and *not* the flow. Small breaths with a high PCO_2 will cause a large deflection. Limitations of this method for detecting apnea include mouth breathing and obstruction of the nasal cannula by secretions. The waveform of the exhaled PCO_2 signal (end-tidal PCO_2 monitoring) is an acceptable alternative apnea sensor in pediatric patients.

and hypopnea. The AASM scoring manual[1] notes that if the recommended sensor signal is not functioning or the signal is not reliable, an alternative sensor can be used. In adults, the **recommended** alternative airflow sensors for apnea detection include the NP signal (transformed or untransformed), RIPsum and RIPflow signals, and an **acceptable** alternative apnea sensor the PVDFsum signal. The RIP signals can be calibrated or uncalibrated. The recommended alternative sensors for hypopnea detection include an oronasal thermal flow sensor, calibrated or uncalibrated RIP signals (RIPsum, RIPflow), and the dual thoracoabdominal RIP effort belt signals. The PVDFsum is also listed as an acceptable alternative signal for scoring hypopnea. In children the recommended and alternative apnea and hypopnea sensors are the same as for adults with the exception that the end tidal PCO_2 signal (exhaled PCO_2 versus time) is an acceptable alternative sensor for scoring apnea.

Summary:

- Apnea (diagnostic study)
  - Recommended: oronasal thermal sensor
  - Alternative sensors (**recommended**): nasal pressure, RIPsum, RIPflow. The NP signal is with or without a square root transformation. The RIP signals can be calibrated or uncalibrated.
  - Alternative sensors (**acceptable**): PVDFsum, end-tidal PCO_2 (children only)
- Hypopnea (diagnostic study)
  - Recommended: nasal pressure (with or without square root transformation)
  - Alternative sensors (recommended): oronasal thermal sensor, RIPsum, RIPflow, dual thoracoabdominal RIP signals. The RIP signals can be calibrated or uncalibrated.
  - Alternative sensor (acceptable): PVDFsum
- Apnea and hypopnea (PAP titration study)
  - Recommended: PAP device flow signal

MONITORING RESPIRATORY EFFORT

Determination of respiratory effort is essential to classify apneas as obstructive (continued respiratory effort), central (absent effort), or mixed (a central portion followed by an obstructive portion in adults or in either order in children)[1]. Paradoxical motion in the thoracic and abdominal RIP bands is also a criterion for classifying a hypopnea as obstructive. Some available respiratory effort sensors are listed in Table 10–4. The AASM scoring manual lists recommended methods to detect respiratory effort (esophageal manometry, dual thoracoabdominal RIP effort belts) and an acceptable method (dual thoracoabdominal PVDF belts) in both adults and children. The most sensitive and accurate method of detecting respiratory effort is by measurement of esophageal pressure[5,16,17,27] (Figure 10–8). Changes in esophageal pressure are estimates of changes in pleural pressure that occur during respiration (negative intrathoracic pressure during inspiration). Esophageal pressure monitoring can detect rather feeble respiratory efforts even when thoracic and abdominal movements are small. In addition, the size of the pressure deflections provides an estimate of the magnitude of respiratory effort. Measurement of supraglottic pressure is another option for assessing respiratory effort. Esophageal pressure may be measured with air-filled balloons, fluid-filled catheters, or catheters with a small pressure sensor on the tip.[16,27] The technique does require special equipment and expertise and is performed mainly during research sleep studies. Some research sleep studies measure supraglottic pressure instead of esophageal pressure using a transducer tip placed just below the tongue base in a supraglottic location. This allows direct measurement of the pressure drop across the upper airway. However, due to the invasive nature of the technique, esophageal manometry is not suitable for clinical studies. Staats and colleagues[17] compared calibrated RIP belts and esophageal pressure monitoring (the gold standard) for accurate detection of respiratory effort. The RIP belts correctly identified the central versus obstructive nature of over 90% of the events. A few events were misclassified as central by RIP associated with "feeble" inspiratory effort detected by esophageal monitoring. Obstructive events were associated with paradoxical motion of the chest and abdomen. Thus, RIP belts are adequate for classification of central versus obstructive events for clinical studies with the understanding that a few events may be incorrectly classified as central.

In addition to classification of apneas, demonstration of increased respiratory effort is needed to detect respiratory effort–related arousals (RERAs) (see Chapters 11 and 12). The definition of a RERA is an event characterized by increased respiratory effort or a flattened inspiratory NP waveform for 10 seconds or more leading to an arousal when the event does not qualify for scoring as a hypopnea. As discussed

Table 10–4 Available Respiratory Effort Sensors
Adults and Children
• Esophageal manometry • Dual thoracoabdominal RIP belts (calibrated or uncalibrated) • Dual thoracoabdominal PVDF belts • Dual piezoelectric effort belts

PVDF, Polyvinylidene fluoride; *RIP*, respiratory inductance plethysmography.

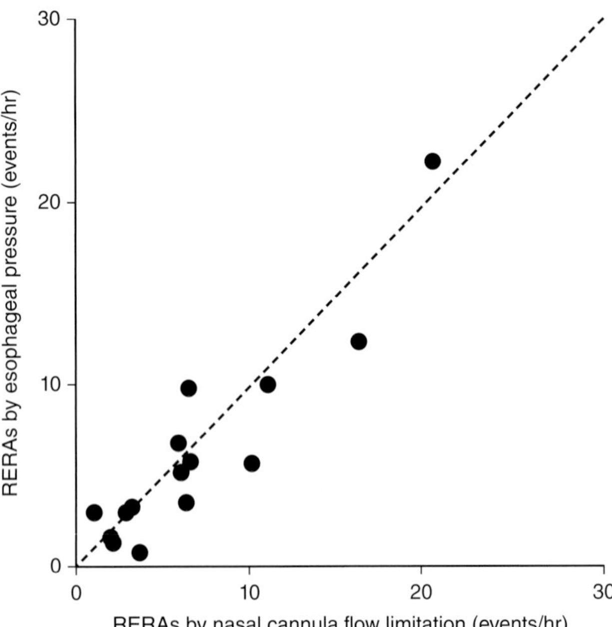

Figure 10–15 This figure shows respiratory effort related arousals *(RERAs)* identified by nasal pressure (inspiratory flattening) preceding an arousal versus identification using esophageal pressure (showing an increase in negative pressure deflections preceding an arousal). Each point represents the number of RERAs per hour for each subject using the two methods. The line of identity is shown. This study showed that nasal pressure inspiratory flattening is fairly accurate in determining periods of increased inspiratory effort before an arousal. However, there are airflow limitation events that are not associated with an increase in pressure deflections (below the line of identity) as well as increases in respiratory effort by esophageal pressure monitoring without evidence of airflow limitation (above the line of identity). (From Ayappa I, Norman RG, Krieger AC, Rosen A, O'Malley RL, Rapoport DM. Non-invasive detection of respiratory effort-related arousals (RERAs) by a nasal cannula/pressure transducer system. *Sleep.* 2000;23(6):763-771.)

earlier, the NP signal shows flattening of the inspiratory waveform during airflow limitation, which is usually associated with increased respiratory effort. Ayappa and coworkers[28] compared RERA detection using NP and esophageal manometry (Figure 10–15). The two methods provided very similar results. A few airflow limitation events were not associated with increased respiratory effort, and a few events with increased respiratory effort did not have an easily recognizable NP flattening. Therefore, detection of airflow limitation using NP is a suitable method to identify RERAs, but NP flattening (airflow limitation) can rarely occur without increased respiratory effort.

In summary, dual RIP effort belts (chest and abdominal) are the recommended respiratory effort sensors that are used in most sleep centers for PSG. As noted earlier, dual RIP belts are not 100% sensitive for detection of respiratory effort, but if positioned and tensioned (appropriately sized), they will accurately detect respiratory effort (if present) during the study in most patients.

Paradoxical Motion

Staats and colleagues[17] found obstructive events to be associated with paradoxical motion of the chest and abdomen as reflected in the RIP effort belts being out of phase. In Figures 10–11 to 10–13, note the paradox in the chest and abdominal belt signals during obstructive apnea and hypopnea. In Figure 10–13, before the event the two signals are slightly out of phase (maximal excursions do not occur precisely at the same time), but the lack of asynchrony increases during the event to become frank paradoxical motion (P). After event termination the chest and abdomen signals are nearly in phase. Paradoxical movement of the chest and abdomen is often noted during obstructive apnea or hypopnea. However, although thoracoabdominal paradox during respiratory events is consistent with upper airway narrowing or closure, this finding is not always present even if RIP effort belts are used to detect respiratory effort. In Figure 10–8 only subtle changes in the chest and abdominal RIP signals are seen during an obstructive hypopnea. In this case the NP signal is much more sensitive for detecting increased respiratory effort. The ability to see paradox depends on optimal placement of the effort belts, may differ between different brands of RIP belts and may be influenced by how negative the intrathoracic pressure swings are during an obstructive event (level of respiratory effort). Most RIP effort belt manufacturers recommend that effort bands should be placed at the point of maximum thoracic and abdominal contraction, respectively. Another option is placement of the chest belt at the level of the upper axilla to minimize movement during sleep. Using *calibrated* RIP may also improve the ability to see paradox and/or detect when the chest and abdominal movements are out of phase.

During normal inspiration both the chest and abdomen expand as intrathoracic pressure becomes more negative. Paradoxical motion is characterized by chest compartment expansion and abdominal compartment contraction or vice versa (Figure 10–16). Paradox in the chest and abdominal band signals occurs during episodes of high upper airway resistance, with chest wall muscle weakness (worse during rapid eye movement [REM] sleep), with diaphragmatic weakness (also worse during REM sleep), or with an immature flexible chest wall. During episodes of high upper airway resistance, the intrathoracic pressure swings may become very negative, and this can pull a weak or paralyzed diaphragm upward (abdomen sucked inward). On the other hand, with a weak or unstable chest wall the chest may be sucked inward during inspiration while the abdomen expands (contraction of the diaphragm pushes abdominal contents downward). Staats and colleagues[17] found that abdominal paradox was typical in their patients with obstructive apnea monitored with both dual thoracoabdominal RIP belts and esophageal manometry. In patients with diaphragmatic weakness, abdominal paradox (inward motion during inspiration) can be seen, especially during REM sleep when inspiration depends on this respiratory muscle. Such events are sometimes called "pseudo-obstruction," that is, the upper airway is not the problem. However, in fact, there is usually evidence of airflow limitation, so some degree of increased upper airway resistance is also present. The take-home message is that interventions to prevent upper airway narrowing and provide pressure support to augment ventilation (assist the weak diaphragm) are both needed in this setting.

If respiratory inductance bands are calibrated, during an obstructive apnea the chest and abdominal band excursions are exactly equal but opposite in direction and the RIPsum (RIPchest + RIPabdomen) is zero. Use of RIP effort belts may also detect more subtle alterations of chest and abdominal synchrony as seen when movements are slightly out of phase (peak chest deflection is earlier than peak abdominal belt deflection or vice versa). Obstructive events may result in out-of-phase motion of the chest and abdomen even if paradox is absent. In the AASM scoring manual classification of a hypopnea as central requires absence of airflow flattening in the NP signal, chest/abdominal paradox, and snoring during the event.

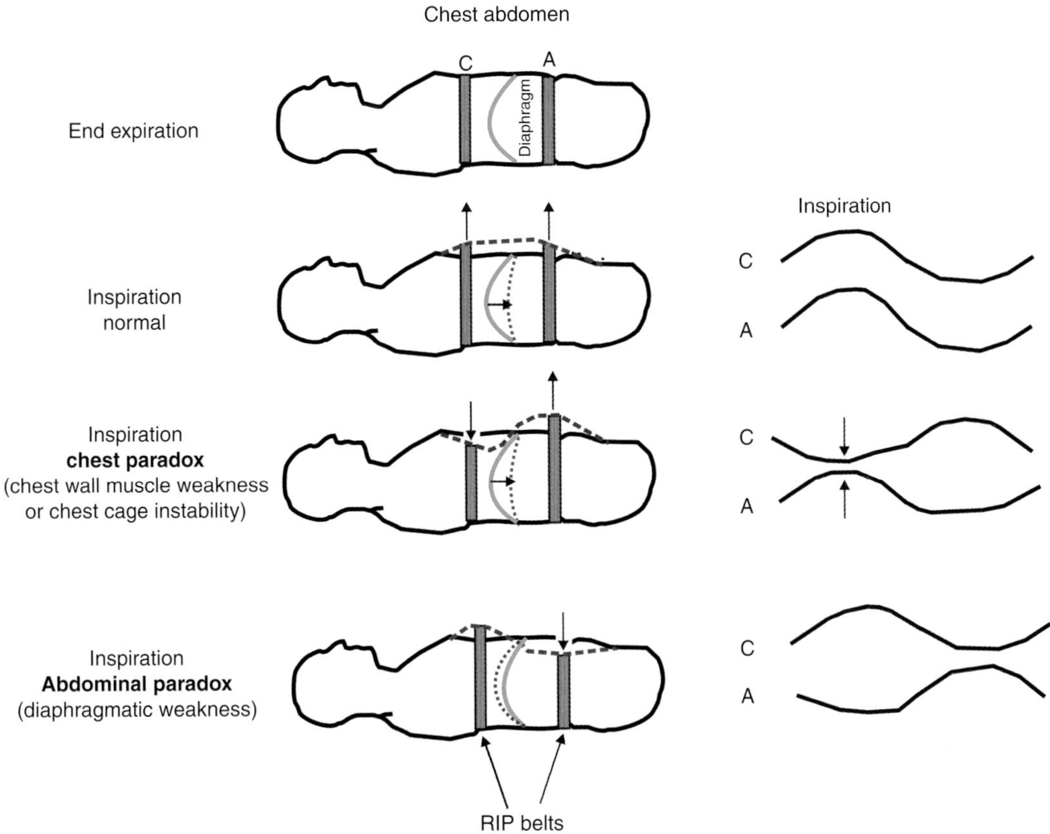

Figure 10–16 This figure shows examples of paradoxical chest and abdominal movement. During normal inspiration the chest and abdominal respiratory inductance plethysmography *(RIP)* band signals increase (inspiration upward). During normal inspiration the chest volume increases, and the diaphragm moves downward causing the abdomen to expand. The RIP signal reflects the area encircled by the band, and both will increase during normal inspiration. During chest wall paradox the chest band shows a decreasing signal (smaller chest area) and the abdominal band an increasing signal with downward movement of the diaphragm, as the chest is "sucked" inward. An example of abdominal paradox is shown at the bottom. The chest moves outward (chest wall muscles), but the abdomen moves inward due to a weak diaphragm, which moves upward due to the negative intrathoracic pressure. Paradoxical motion of the chest and abdomen can occur in patients with a normal chest wall and diaphragm during periods of high upper airway resistance.

Dual thoracic and abdominal PVDF effort belts are listed as acceptable in the AASM scoring manual for detecting respiratory effort. There is more evidence for use of RIP effort belts than PVDF belts, but all brands of RIP belts may not be equal in the ability to record respiratory effort or thoracic abdominal paradox. Another method for detecting respiratory effort in clinical sleep studies uses piezoelectric (PE) sensors connected to bands around the chest and abdomen. Changes in the tension on the PE transducer as the chest and abdomen expand and contract produce a voltage that can be measured. The signal from these devices depends on the degree of tension on the transducer. The PE belts are adequate for detection of respiratory effort in most patients but do not really quantify the changes in thoracic or abdominal size. Although relatively inexpensive compared with RIP effort belts, the PE effort belts may provide misleading information (false absence of respiratory effort), especially if not properly positioned and tensioned. They are not listed as recommended or acceptable respiratory effort sensors for PSG in the AASM scoring manual *but are listed as acceptable effort sensors for HSAT. Of note, during polysomnography for titration of hypoglossal nerve stimulation, PE effort belts are currently recommended. RIP belts can interfere with communication between the tablet used remotely by the sleep technologist to change the stimulation voltage and the implanted device. An external wand is placed over the implanted pulse generator and allows communication between the tablet and the pulse generator.*

Respiratory effort can also be detected by recording a chest wall respiratory muscle electromyogram (EMG) activity using bipolar surface electrodes[16,29] (Figures 10–17 and 10–18). The presence of inspiratory bursts documents respiratory effort. Surface diaphragm EMG recording uses two electrodes, but the optimal electrode placement varies between patients. One common method is to place electrodes about 2 cm apart horizontally in the seventh and eighth intercostal spaces in the right anterior or midaxillary line. Other electrode placement is used in some sleep centers (Figure 10–17), and several positions must often be tried to obtain a good signal. Depending on electrode placement, activity from other chest wall muscles and the diaphragm is recorded. The right side of the body is used to reduce electrocardiogram (ECG) artifact. Many PSG computer programs have an option to remove or reduce ECG artifact in EMG signals. Typical low and high filter settings for recording the surface EMG are 10 and 100 Hz, respectively. Using a low filter setting of 25 or 40 Hz can reduce ECG artifact but also reduces the amplitude of the signal. Intercostal EMG recording often uses the right parasternal area (second and third intercostal spaces in the midaxillary

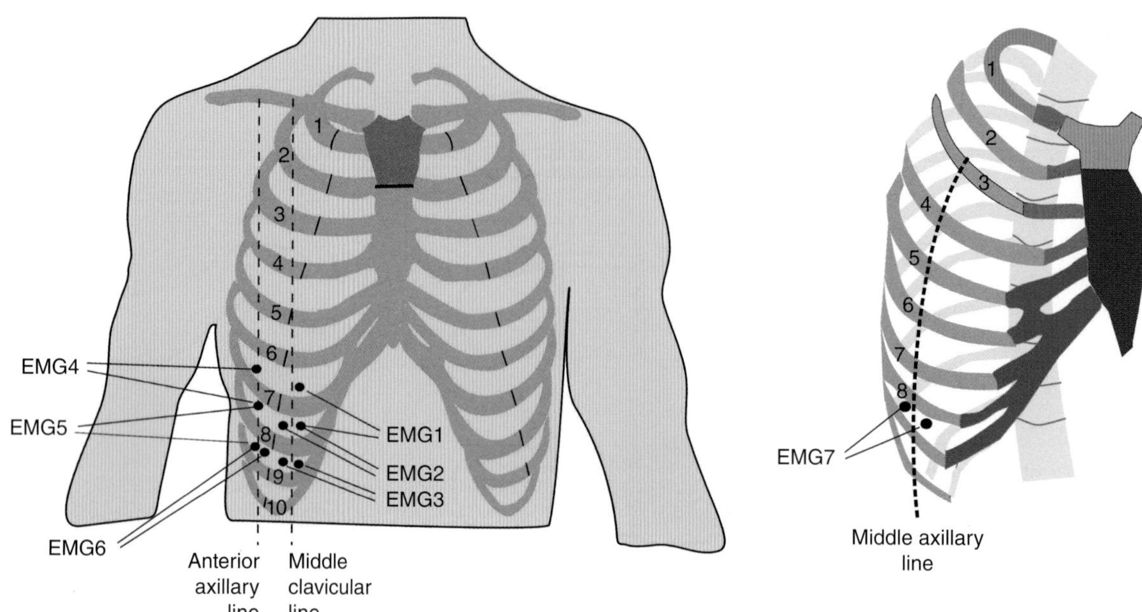

Figure 10–17 Possible locations for placement of surface electrodes to record electromyographic (EMG) signals from the diaphragm and chest wall muscles. The right side is used to minimize electrocardiogram artifact. Depending on the location of electrode placement, activity from both the diaphragm and chest wall muscles may contribute to the signal. However, the signal is often called the diaphragmatic EMG. More anterior electrode locations record primarily diaphragmatic activity. At times, multiple electrode positions must be tried before a good signal can be recorded. Sometimes recording a useful signal is not possible. Other surface EMG options include recording the surface EMG of the intercostal muscles (parasternal location) or neck muscle EMG (scalene).

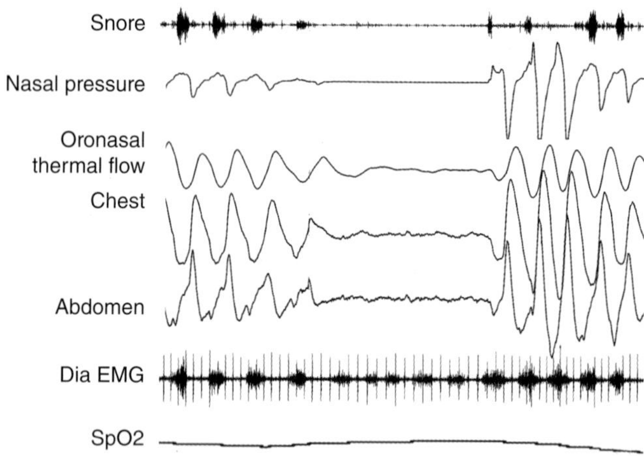

Figure 10–18 A tracing showing an event that might be scored as a central apnea based on the chest and abdominal signals but is obviously an obstructive apnea based on the surface electromyographic *(EMG)* signal showing inspiratory bursts. Electrocardiogram artifact in the signal is common but can be removed by some polysomnography programs.

line), or the activity of neck muscles (scalene) is recorded. Inspiratory EMG activity is noted in the intercostal muscles and the diaphragm during non–rapid eye movement (NREM) sleep. During REM sleep, the intercostal activity is inhibited but diaphragmatic activity persists, although often diminished in amplitude during bursts of eye movements. The current version of the AASM scoring manual states that "a surface diaphragmatic/intercostal EMG signal may be used for detection of respiratory effort during apnea, hypopnea, or RERA to complement effort belt signals when unambiguous EMG bursts are present during normal breathing." An example of an apnea that would likely be classified as central but is clearly shown to be obstructive by a surface EMG signal is shown in Figure 10–18. If the diaphragmatic EMG is rectified and integrated, it can be used to assess the magnitude of respiratory effort similar to esophageal pressure monitoring.[30]

MEASURING THE ARTERIAL OXYGEN SATURATION

Continuous measurement of the arterial partial pressure of oxygen (PaO_2) during sleep studies is not feasible. Spot checks of arterial blood gases (ABGs) are only rarely performed during sleep studies, and many facilities do not have the capability to process arterial blood samples. Instead of PaO_2, measurement of the arterial oxygen saturation (SaO_2) by continuous recording of pulse oximetry (SpO_2), typically with finger or ear probes, is recorded during PSG. An understanding of the utility and limitations of pulse oximetry is important for the sleep physician.[31,32] The SaO_2 is defined as the ratio of oxygenated hemoglobin (O_2Hb) to the total amount of hemoglobin (Hb) *that can bind oxygen* (Equation 10–4). The amount of Hb that can bind oxygen is the sum of the O_2Hb and deoxygenated (reduced) hemoglobin (RHb).

$$SaO_2 = 100 \times \frac{[O_2Hb]}{([O_2Hb] + [RHb])} \text{ (as \%)} \qquad \text{Equation 10–4}$$

This assumes that all the Hb is available to bind oxygen. The SaO_2 value for a given PaO_2 depends on the position of the

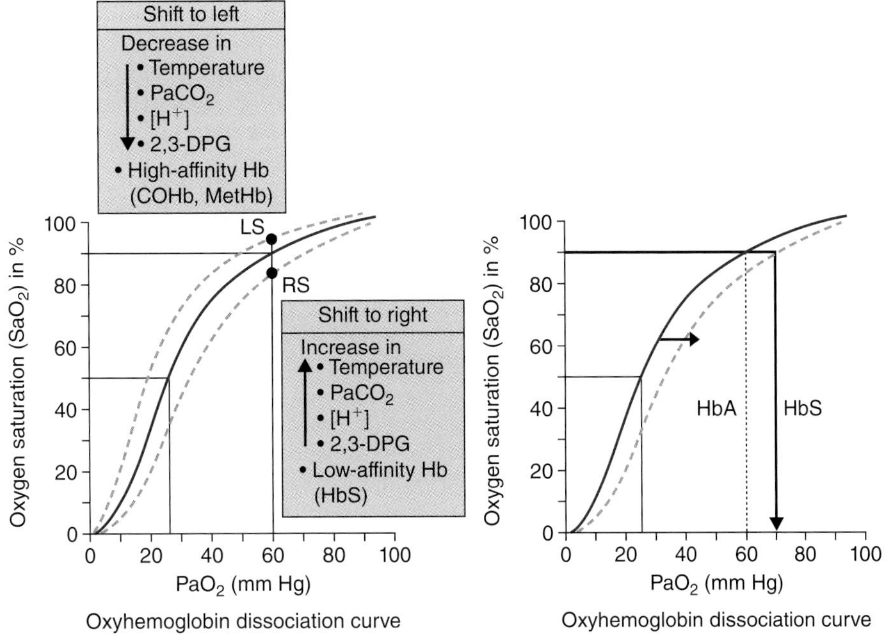

Figure 10–19 In the *left panel*, changes in the position of the oxyhemoglobin dissociation curve with changes in temperature, partial pressure of carbon dioxide *($PaCO_2$)*, hydrogen ion concentration *($[H^+]$)*, and the amount of 2,3-diphosphoglycerate *(2,3-DPG)* are shown. High-affinity hemoglobin (carboxyhemoglobin, methemoglobin), and decreased temperature, $PaCO_2$, $[H^+]$, and 2,3-DPG concentration are associated with a left shift. Low affinity means for a given partial pressure of oxygen *(PaO_2)* there is a higher arterial oxygen saturation *(SaO_2)*. Another description of a left shift is that for a given SaO_2, the PaO_2 is lower. Low-affinity hemoglobin and increased temperature, $PaCO_2$, hydrogen ion concentration, and 2,3-DPG concentration are associated with a right shift. The *right panel* illustrates a right shift as seen in sickle hemoglobin (HbS). Low affinity means for a given partial pressure of oxygen *(PaO_2)* there is a lower arterial oxygen saturation *(SaO_2)*. Another description of a right shift is that for a given SaO_2, the PaO_2 is higher.

oxygen-hemoglobin saturation curve (also called the oxygen-hemoglobin dissociation curve)[33,34] (Figure 10–19). At the usual body temperature and pH, a PaO_2 of 60 mm Hg corresponds to an SaO_2 of approximately 90%. A left shift of the oxygen saturation curve results in a given PaO_2 being associated with a higher SaO_2 (higher affinity). A shift to the left can occur with decreasing temperature, hydrogen ion concentration $[H^+]$, $PaCO_2$, or level of 2,3-diphosphoglycerate (2,3-DPG). An abnormal high oxygen affinity Hb, elevated carboxyhemoglobin (COHb)[35,36] or methemoglobin (MetHb)[37] can also cause a left shift. COHb is produced when carbon monoxide binds to Hb and the amount of COHb is commonly increased in smokers. Hb binds carbon monoxide (CO) 200 to 300 times more than with oxygen, resulting in the formation of COHb and preventing the binding of oxygen to Hb due to competition for the same binding sites. The binding of one CO molecule to Hb increases the affinity of the other binding spots for oxygen, leading to a left shift in the dissociation curve.[37] MetHb occurs when the normal ferrous state (Fe^{2+}) of the iron moiety in Hb is oxidized to the ferric stage (Fe^{3+}). Significant methemoglobinemia can occur after exposure to certain medications[38] (e.g., dapsone, topical sprays containing benzocaine) but is uncommon in the sleep center. Neither COHb nor MetHb can bind oxygen. A shift to the right means that a given PaO_2 is associated with a lower SaO_2 (low affinity for oxygen). A shift to the right can occur with increasing temperature, hydrogen ion concentration $[H^+]$, $PaCO_2$, or level of 2,3-DPG. Abnormal Hbs with lower or higher than normal affinity for oxygen binding can also result in a different relationship between the SaO_2 and the PaO_2. For example, in patients with sickle cell disease (SCD), the PaO_2 for a given SaO_2 is higher due to the rightward shift of the O_2Hb saturation curve for hemoglobin S (HbS) compared with hemoglobin A (HbA) (Figure 10–19).[39,40] The position of the O_2Hb dissociation curve is often defined by the P50, which is the PaO_2 corresponding to an SaO_2 of 50%. For HbA, the P50 is 26 mm Hg but for SCD patients is 42 to 56 mm Hg.[39] This is consistent with a rightward shift in the O_2Hb dissociation curve for HbS. This means that for a given SaO_2, the PaO_2 is higher in SCD patients than would be expected based on the normal O_2Hb dissociation curve. The amount of right shift varies considerably between SCD patients and can be influenced by transfusion with blood (HbA). It is useful to remember that for PaO_2 values of 30, 40, and 60 mm Hg, the corresponding SaO_2 values are approximately 60%, 75%, and 90% values, respectively.

The SaO_2 is measured noninvasively during sleep studies by pulse oximetry (SpO_2) to detect arterial oxygen desaturation and hypoxemia. The majority of the oxygen-carrying capacity of the blood is due to oxygen bound to Hb with a small fraction of dissolved oxygen (Equation 10–5) where the oxygen content of the blood is abbreviated as CaO_2 with units (mL O_2/100 mg of blood).[33,34] When fully saturated, a gram of Hb carries about 1.34 mL/dL of oxygen (1 dL = 100 mL). The PaO_2 in Equation 10-5 is the partial pressure of oxygen in mm Hg.

$$(CaO_2\ [\text{mL } O_2/100\text{ mL}]) = 1.34\ (\text{mL/g}) \times \text{Hb}\ (\text{g}/100\text{ mL}) \times SaO_2 + 0.003\ PaO_2$$

Equation 10–5

However, determining the oxygen-carrying capacity of Hb is complicated by the fact that both COHb and MetHb are forms of circulating Hb that do not bind oxygen. The sum of the concentrations of RHb, O_2HB, COHb, and MetHb represented by the symbols [RHb], [O_2Hb], [COHb], [MetHb] equals the total Hb concentration [Hb-total] (Equation 10–6).[34] The fractional concentration of O_2Hb (FO_2Hb in %) is equal to ([O_2Hb] × 100/[Hb-total]), where [O_2Hb] and [Hb-total] are the concentrations of O_2Hb and total Hb, respectively (Equation 10–7). Similar equations define the fractional concentration of the other Hb moieties. The sum of the fractional concentrations of O_2Hb, RHb, COHb, and MetHb equal 100% (Equation 10–8). The true fraction of Hb bound to oxygen (FO_2Hb) is given by Equation 10–9 and depends on the concentrations of COHb, MetHb, RHb, and O_2Hb.[34,40]

$$[\text{Hb-total}] = [O_2\text{Hb}] + [\text{RHb}] + [\text{COHb}] + [\text{MetHb}] \quad \text{Equation 10–6}$$

$$FO_2\text{Hb} = \frac{[O_2\text{Hb}] \times 100}{[\text{Hb- total}]} \text{ fractional concentration as \%} \quad \text{Equation 10–7}$$

$$100\% = FO_2\text{Hb} + \text{FRHb} + \text{FCOHb} + \text{FMetHb} \quad \text{Equation 10–8}$$

$$\text{or} \quad FO_2\text{Hb} + \text{FRHb} = 100 - \text{FCOHb} - \text{FMetHb}$$

$$FO_2\text{Hb} = \frac{[O_2\text{Hb}] \times 100}{[\text{Hb} - \text{total}]} = \frac{[O_2\text{Hb}] \times 100}{([O_2\text{Hb}] + [\text{RHb}] + [\text{COHb}] + [\text{MetHb}])} \text{ as \%} \quad \text{Equation 10–9}$$

In Equation 10-9 [O_2Hb], [RHb], [COHb], and [MetHb] are the concentrations of the types of Hb and equal the total Hb concentration [Hb-total]. Note that the *SaO_2* depends on [RHb] and [O_2Hb] and is the fraction of *Hb capable of binding oxygen* that is bound to oxygen. In contrast, the *FO_2Hb* is the *fraction of the total Hb* that is bound to oxygen. One can express the SaO_2 using fractional concentrations (Equation 10–10).

$$SaO_2 = \frac{FO_2\text{Hb} \times 100}{(FO_2\text{Hb} + \text{FRHb})} = \frac{FO_2\text{Hb} \times 100}{(100 - \text{FCOHb} - \text{FMetHb})} \text{ all values in \%} \quad \text{Equation 10–10}$$

$$\text{Or} \quad FO_2\text{Hb} = SaO_2(\text{in \%}) \times [(100 - \text{FCOHb} - \text{FMetHb})/100] \quad \text{Equation 10–11}$$

For example, if the FO_2Hb = 85%, FCOHb = 8%, and FMetHb = 1%, then the FRHb is 6%. Using these numbers and Equation 10–10, the SaO_2 equals [(85 × 100)]/[100 – 9] or 93.41%, which is considerably higher than an FO_2Hb of 85%. Conversely using Equation 10-11 if the SaO_2 = 93.41%, FCOHb = 8%, and FMetHb=1%, the FO_2Hb is [93.41 × (100-8-1)/100)] or 85%. The FO_2Hb and the amount of Hb are the main determinants of the blood's oxygen-carrying capacity. When significant COHb or MetHb is present, Equation 10–5 should have SaO_2 replaced by FO_2Hb. The difference between the SaO_2 and the FO_2Hb (in %) at normal PO_2 values is approximately equal to the sum of FCOHb and FMetHb. The FO_2Hb is sometimes called the fractional saturation and the SaO_2 the functional or effective saturation. Of note, the oxyhemoglobin dissociation curve associates a given PaO_2 with the SaO_2 and NOT the FO_2Hb. That is, the oxyhemoglobin saturation curve expresses the ratio of oxygenated Hb to the total Hb *available for oxygen binding*. Neither COHb nor MetHb binds oxygen. However, as noted above, the position of the oxyhemoglobin saturation curve is shifted to the left by the presence of COHb or MetHb.[35-37] An example of the effect of the presence of COHb is shown in Figure 10–20. What is most important during sleep studies is knowing the approximate value of the PaO_2, which depends on the SaO_2 and not the FO_2Hb.

The four fractions of Hb ([O_2Hb], [RHb], [COHb], and [MetHb]) can be accurately measured by co-oximeters that measure the absorption of four or more wavelengths of electromagnetic radiation by blood.[34,41,42] This is possible because the four forms of Hb differ in their absorption for the different wavelengths of radiation. In contrast, routine pulse oximetry[31,32] uses only two wavelengths—660 nm (red) and 940 nm (infrared)—to measure the O_2Hb and RHb. The absorption of radiation at 660 nm is much greater with RHb than O_2Hb, whereas O_2Hb absorbs more radiation at 940 nm (Figure 10–21A). The SpO_2 (not the SaO_2), which depends on measured relative absorptions of two wavelengths of radiation, is based on the empirical observation that the ratio (R) of absorbance at the two wavelengths is related to the oxygen saturation (see Figure 10–21B). This relationship (calibration curve) is calculated experimentally by determining R at varying oxygen saturations. To specifically determine the absorbance of arterial blood, the AC (pulse added absorbance) at each wavelength is divided by the DC (background absorbance) to account for the effect of the absorption of the radiation by venous blood and tissue.

$$R = (AC_{660}/DC_{660})/AC_{940}/DC_{940} \quad \text{higher R associated with lower } SpO_2 \quad \text{Equation 10–12}$$

AC is the pulse added absorption and DC the steady-state absorption at the indicated wavelength of light (660 nm or 940 nm). Figure 10–21 shows that O_2Hb and RHb have about the same absorption at 940 nm, but RHb has greater absorption at 660 nm. The relative amounts of O_2Hb and RHb determine the value of R and the SpO_2. Higher O_2Hb lowers the relative absorption at 660 nm, decreasing R and increasing the SpO_2. However, when forms of Hb that cannot bind oxygen are present, R does not depend only on the concentrations of O_2Hb and RHb. COHb has about the same absorbance at 660 nm as O_2Hb but very low absorbance at 940 nm and decreases the relative absorbance at 660 nm, so R decreases and the measured SpO_2 increases (Figure 10–22). An easy way to think about this is that the COHb mimics the effect of O_2Hb. In normal individuals, FCOHb is 2% or less but can be 8% or more in cigarette smokers. Patients with Sickle Cell Disease (SCD) often have FCOHb values of 4% or more due to production of CO from chronic hemolysis. Based on a canine experiment,[32,43] it has been estimated that the pulse oximeter reading (SpO_2) can be estimated by FO_2Hb + 0.9 FCOHb. For example, from the values FO_2Hb = 85%, COHb = 4%, MetHb = 0%, RHb = 11%, one can estimate the SpO_2 as 88.6% (85 + 0.9 × 4). This is essentially the same as the SaO_2 computed from Equation 10–10 (85×100)/(85+11) which equals 88%. Thus, the SpO_2 is a much better estimate of the SaO_2 than the FO_2Hb is in this situation. In patients who are heavy smokers, it is important to remember that the SpO_2 overestimates the FO_2Hb. In the case of MetHb, the absorption is similar at 660 nm and 940 nm (R ≈ 1). As the amount of MetHb increases, the R moves toward 1 and the SpO_2 moves toward 85%.[31,32,42,44] As noted earlier, dapsone and topical anesthetic sprays containing benzocaine (Cetacaine and others) are the most common causes of acquired methemoglobinemia and give blood a chocolate color.[38] Mild to moderate levels of MetHb cause cyanosis, but increased COHb does not. In summary, both COHb and MetHb cause a divergence between the SaO_2 (and SpO_2) and

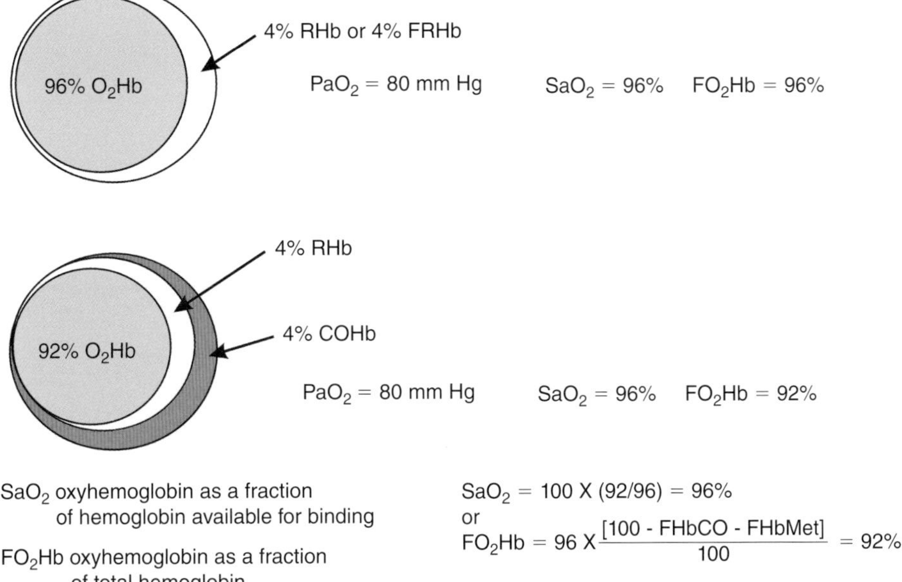

Figure 10–20 Schematic illustration of the difference between the arterial oxygen saturation *(SaO_2)* and the fraction of hemoglobin bound to oxygen *(FO_2Hb)*. The *top circle* illustrates the circumstance in which all of the hemoglobin is available to bind oxygen. The partial pressure of oxygen *(PaO_2)* is 80 mm Hg and the *SaO_2* is approximately 96%. The SaO_2 and FO_2Hb as a percentage are identical. In the *bottom circle* 4% of the hemoglobin is bound to carbon monoxide and not available for binding of oxygen. If the PaO_2 is 80 mm, the corresponding SaO_2 is still approximately 96% based on the hemoglobin available for oxygen binding. This assumes the relationship between the PaO_2 and SaO_2 has not changed. However, the FO_2Hb is based on the total hemoglobin ($FO_2Hb = 96 \times [(100 - 4)/100]$ or $96 \times 0.96 = 92\%$ using Equation 10-11). For simplicity, this analysis assumes that the carboxyhemoglobin (COHb) affects the total Hb available for binding but not the relationship of SaO_2 and PaO_2 (position of the oxygen hemoglobin saturation curve). However, COHb does cause a leftward shift of the oxygen hemoglobin dissociation curve[35] (higher SaO_2 for a given PaO_2; for example, for $PO_2 = 80$ mm Hg, $SaO_2 > 96\%$). The effect is small at low levels of COHb. (Adapted from Berry RB, Wagner MH. *Sleep Medicine Pearls*. 3rd ed. Elsevier; 2015:146.)

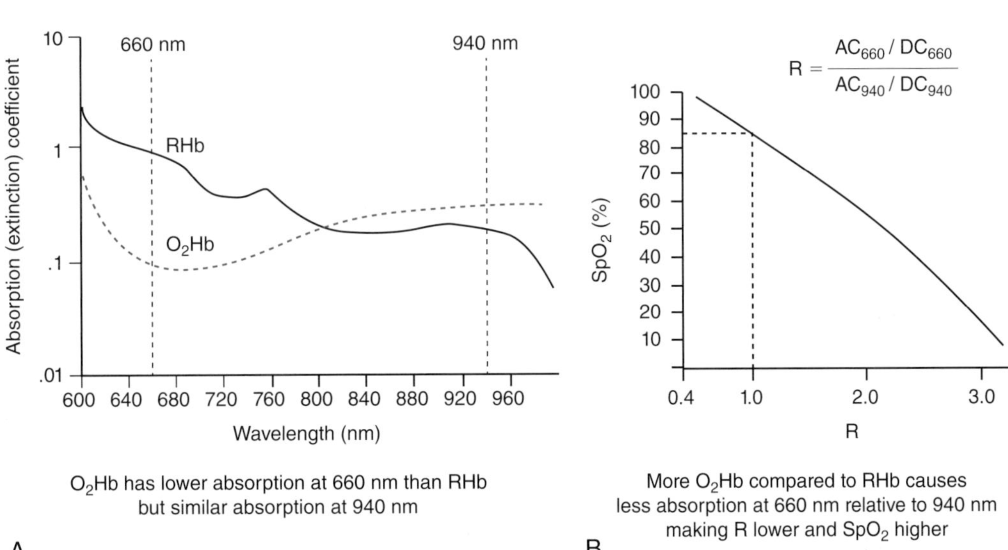

Figure 10–21 The *left panel* illustrates the absorption of two wavelengths of light by oxyhemoglobin (O_2Hb) and reduced hemoglobin (RHb). Oxyhemoglobin absorbs much less light at 660 nm than reduced hemoglobin (RHb). These two wavelengths of light are used in routine oximetry. It was discovered empirically that a ratio of absorption of light at 660 nm and 940 nm was related to the oxygen saturation by Equation 10-12 as illustrated in the right panel. A lower R is associated with a higher SpO_2. At R = 1 the SaO_2 is 85%. In the equation shown, AC (the pulse added absorption representing the absorption during an arterial pulse), is divided by the DC steady state or background absorbance. This allows correction for light absorption by veins and other surrounding structures. In summary, the ratio of absorption of the two wavelengths of light allows measurement of the SpO_2. (A, From Barker SJ and Tremper KK: Pulse Oximetry: Applications and limitations, International Anesthesiology Clinics, 25(3):p 155-175, Fall 1987; B, From JA Pologe: Pulse Oximetry: Technical aspects of machine design, International Anesthesiology Clinics, 25(3):p 137-153, Fall 1987.

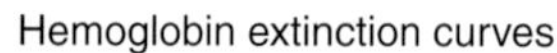

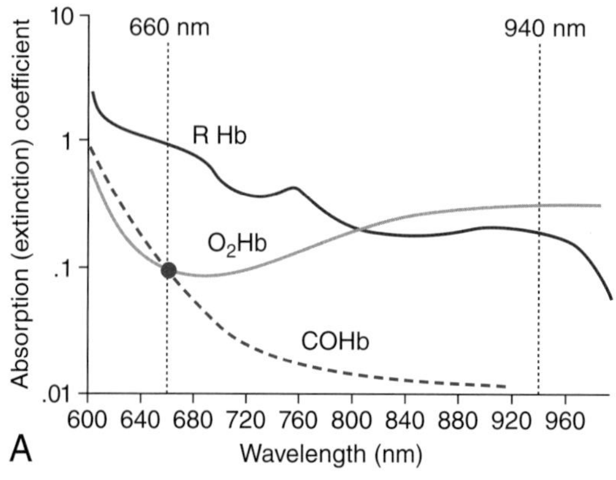

COHb similar absorption at 660 nm at O_2Hb measured SpO_2 is higher

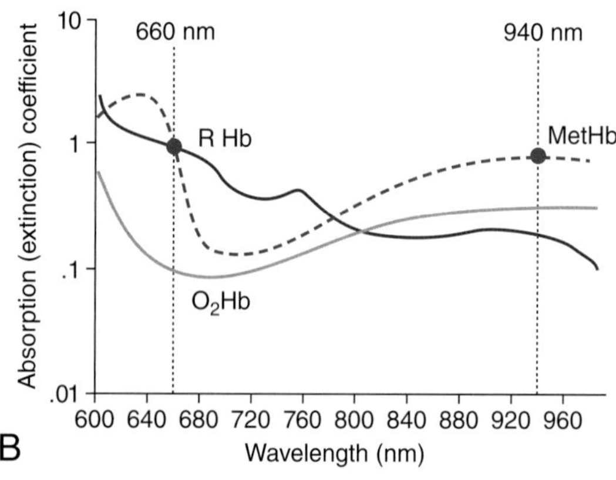

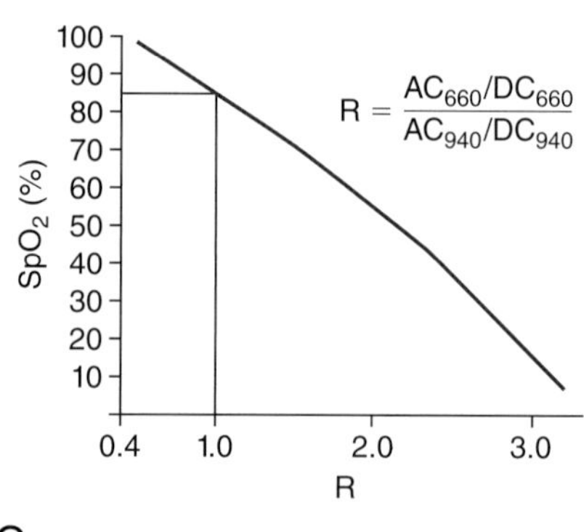

MetHb has similar absorption at 660 nm and 940 nm—as the amount of Met Hb increases—which makes R approach 1 and the SpO_2 approach 85%

Figure 10–22 The absorption curves for (A) carboxyhemoglobin and (B) methemoglobin are illustrated. The absorption curves for O_2Hb and RHb (deoxyhemoglobin) are also shown. At 660 nm the absorption of COHb is similar to O_2Hb, whereas there is minimal absorption by CO at 940 nm. COHb "mimics" the presence of O_2Hb lowering the overall absorption at 660 nm, which lowers R and increases the measured SpO_2. For methemoglobin the absorption at 660 nm and 940 nm is similar, and the higher the methemoglobin concentration, the closer R is to 1 and the SpO_2 to 85%. As shown in (C), R = 1 corresponds to a SpO_2 of 85%. Therefore, at normal PO_2 and SaO_2 the SpO_2 will be falsely lower than the true value if methemoglobin is present.

FO_2Hb. COHb at the low values likely to be encountered in the sleep center has relatively little effect on the SpO_2 in comparison to the SaO_2 (SpO_2 slightly higher) but a greater effect on the FO_2Hb. There is also a shift to the left in the Hb oxygen saturation curve, meaning a given SpO_2 is associated with a lower PaO_2. However, MetHb impairs the accuracy of the oximetry (the SpO_2), which underestimates the SaO_2 at values over 85% and overestimates the SaO_2 at values below 85% as the measured SpO_2 converges to 85%. Thus, methemoglobinemia is one cause of a lower than expected SpO_2 in a patient with a normal PaO_2.

If a patient has a lower than expected SpO_2 (no history of lung disease or hypoventilation) while awake in the sleep center, a number of possibilities should be considered, including a faulty oximetry probe, poor signal quality due to poor perfusion, artificial fingernails/dark polish, a shift in the O_2Hb saturation curve due to the factors illustrated in Figure 10–19, or an abnormal Hb.[31,32] For example, a patient with Sickle cell disease could have a reduced SaO_2 but normal PaO_2. If oximetry issues are ruled out, an ABG is needed to determine whether hypoxemia is really present. In this situation, co-oximetry analysis could also determine whether significant COHb or MetHb is present and determine the true FO_2Hb (fraction of Hb that is oxygenated). Note that not all laboratories use a co-oximeter, and the SaO_2 is often reported based on the PaO_2 using a nomogram. That is, the FO_2Hb is not directly measured (this assumes no COHb or MetHb). It is important in this situation to perform co-oximetry.

Most oximeters provide a plethysmography signal reflecting the perfusion of fingertip (or earlobe) in the oximetry probe. If the signal shows low and erratic amplitude, the SpO_2 reading is likely not accurate. An example of this situation is provided in Figure 10–23. Recently, it has been noted some oximeters may overestimate the SaO_2 in some dark-skinned individuals.[45]

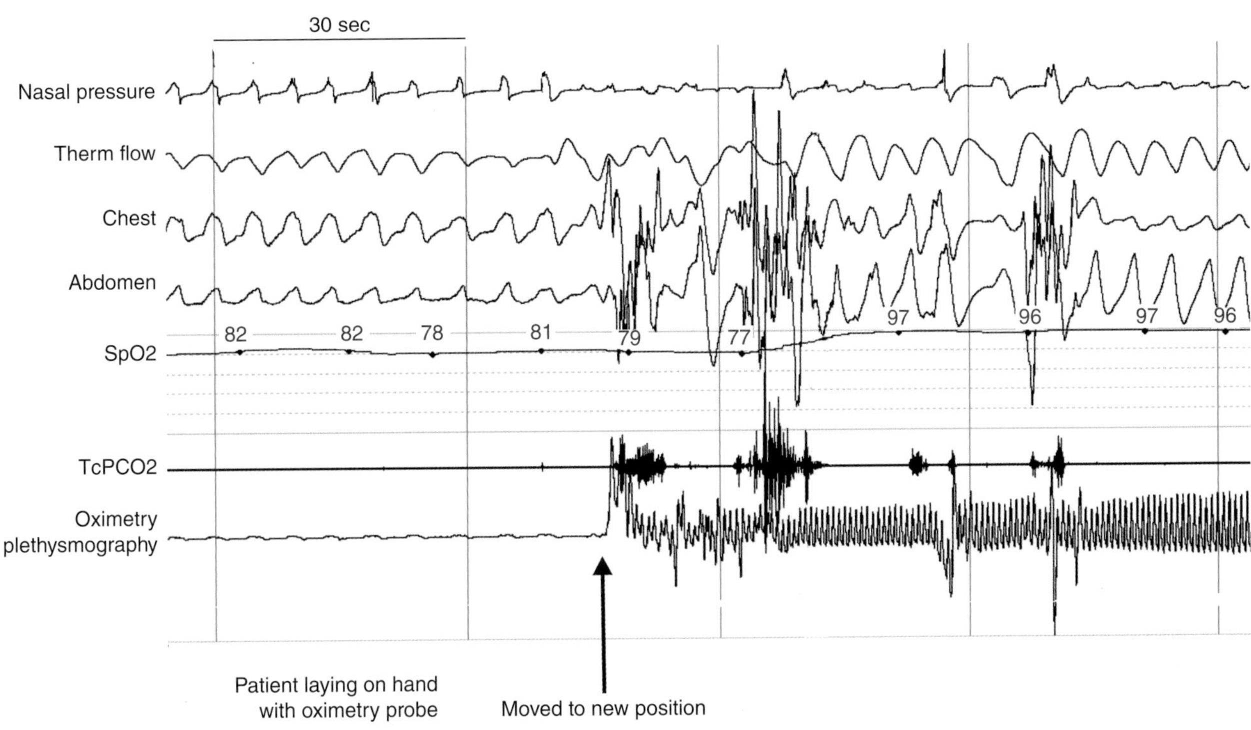

Figure 10–23 This tracing illustrates the utility of recording the plethysmography ("pleth") signal from the oximeter. A dampened (reduced amplitude) pleth signal is often associated with erroneous reading in the SpO_2. This can occur with poor oximetry probe position or any factor decreasing perfusion to the area where the oximetry probe is attached. Changing the oximetry probe to another digit or hand or moving the patient (as illustrated) to improve perfusion to the oximetry probe will improve the pleth signal and the SpO_2 accuracy.

As noted earlier, it is important to realize that the SaO_2 often reported with an ABG is simply determined from the measured PaO_2 and a nomogram. If clinically indicated, analysis with a co-oximeter will provide more accurate information.

In sleep monitoring, an *arterial oxygen desaturation* is usually defined as a decrease in the SpO_2 of 3% or 4% or more from baseline. Note that the nadir in SaO_2 commonly follows apnea (hypopnea) termination by approximately 6 to 8 seconds (longer in severe desaturations) (Figure 10–24). This delay is secondary to circulation time and instrumental delay (the oximeter averages over several pulses to determine a moving time average). The AASM scoring manual states "the maximum acceptable averaging time for a pulse oximeter is 3 seconds. Longer averaging times increase the likelihood of not detecting transient desaturations from baseline." At a heart rate of 80 bpm, this corresponds to averaging 4 pulses.

SEVERITY OF ARTERIAL OXYGEN DESATURATION

Several apneas of variable length and the associated arterial oxygen desaturation are shown in Figure 10–24. Typically the number of desaturations (drops in the $SaO_2 \geq 3$ or 4% from baseline) is determined. Various measures have been used to assess the severity of desaturation, including computing the number of desaturations, the average minimum SpO_2 during desaturations, the time below 80%, 85%, 90%, as well as the mean SpO_2 and the minimum saturation during NREM and REM sleep. The time with an SpO_2 of 88% or less is also commonly determined. The AASM scoring manual[1] recommends reporting of the lowest SpO_2 during sleep, the time below a specified threshold (often ≤88%), and the average SpO_2. Reporting the number of desaturations (drop in the $SpO_2 \geq 3\%$ or 4%) or an oxygen desaturation index (ODI = desaturations × 60/TST in minutes) are optional, but these values are usually reported. The hypoxic burden specific to sleep apnea is a new parameter computed as the sum of the areas between the baseline SpO_2 and the arterial oxygen desaturation divided by the total sleep time in hours (% min/hour) (Figure 10–24).[46] The hypoxic burden may be a better predictor of cardiovascular morbidity than the AHI.

Factors Determining the Severity of Desaturation

A number of factors can worsen the severity of arterial oxygen desaturation in patients with obstructive sleep apnea (Box 10–1).[47-52] Patients with a higher body mass index desaturate more severely, and the effect of obesity is accentuated during REM sleep, in the supine position, and in men more than women.[49] A low baseline SpO_2 (PaO_2) also worsens desaturation because for a given fall in the PaO_2, the fall in the SaO_2 (desaturation) is greater if the baseline PaO_2 values is on the steep part of the oxygen hemoglobin desaturation curve (Figure 10–25). The baseline awake supine SpO_2 values should be included in the sleep report. Long respiratory events with only a few breaths between back-to-back apneas or hypopnea also worsen desaturation. The expiratory reserve volume is the difference between the functional residual capacity (FRC) (end expiratory lung volume) and the residual volume (RV) (lung volume at maximum exhalation). A low FRC means that oxygen stores are lower at the time of breath hold.[50] In addition, breathing at low lung volumes causes increased ventilation perfusion mismatch as some airways are closed during tidal volume breathing at low lung volumes.

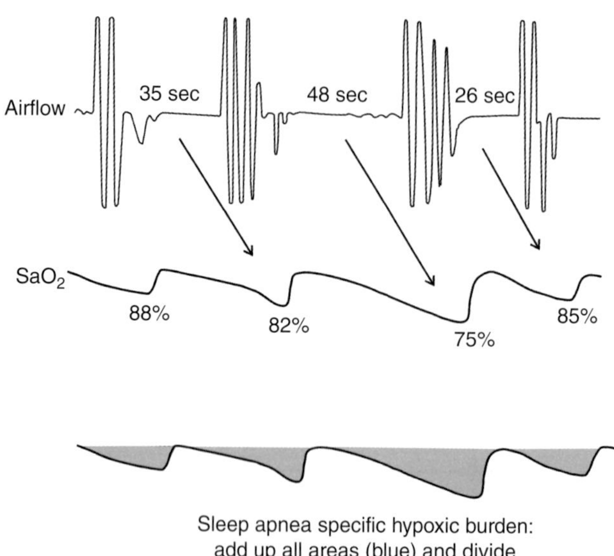

Figure 10–24 The *top* portion of the figure illustrates the relationship between apnea events of various lengths and the associated arterial oxygen desaturations. Longer events are associated with more severe desaturations and a longer delay in the SpO_2 nadir after event termination. In patients with a decreased cardiac output (long circulation time) the nadir can be very delayed. The *bottom* portion of the figure shows an example of the method for computing the sleep apnea specific hypoxic burden (see reference 46). See the reference for more details. (Reproduced from Berry RB: Sleep medicine pearls , ed 2, Philadelphia, 2003, Saunders, p 86.)

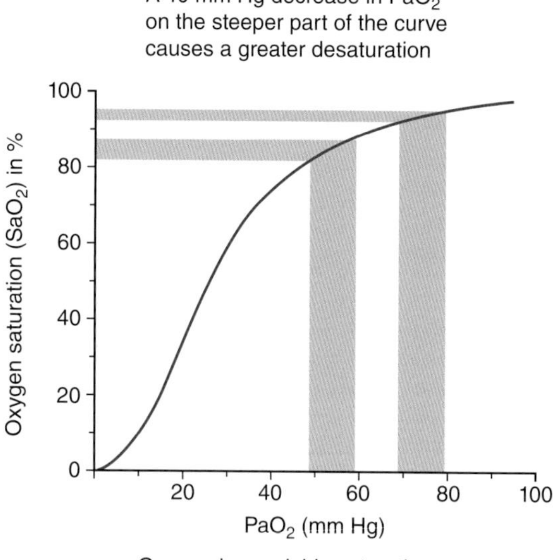

Figure 10–25 The amount of arterial oxygen desaturation for a given decrease in the PaO_2 depends on the starting point (baseline SaO_2) on the oxygen hemoglobin association curve. At normal PO_2 values the curve is flat, and a drop in the PaO_2 of 10 mm Hg is associated with a minimal drop in the arterial oxygen saturation. However, if the baseline PaO_2 is low (e.g., due to lung disease) and the position is on the steeper part of the curve, a fall in PaO_2 of 10 mm Hg is associated with a much greater desaturation.

Box 10–1 FACTORS WORSENING ARTERIAL OXYGEN DESATURATION

- Higher BMI
  - More effect REM > NREM sleep
  - More effect supine > lateral sleep
  - More effect men > women
- Lower baseline awake supine PaO_2 or SaO_2
- Lower ERV = FRC − RV
  - Low FRC—obesity
  - High RV—obstructive airway disease (COPD)
- Longer event duration
- Greater decrease in tidal volume (hypopnea)
- Short ventilatory period between apneas or hypopneas
- REM sleep versus NREM sleep (REM events are also longer)
- Supine versus lateral position

BMI, body mass index; *COPD,* chronic obstructive pulmonary disease; *ERV,* expiratory reserve volume; *FRC,* functional residual capacity; *NREM,* non-rapid eye movement; *PaO_2,* arterial partial pressure of oxygen; *REM,* rapid eye movement; *RV,* residual volume; *SaO_2,* arterial oxygen saturation; *VT,* tidal volume.

Obesity tends to lower the FRC (especially compared with the RV). In pulmonary function testing the most common finding in obesity is a low ERV (FRC-RV) mainly due to a fall in the FRC. A high RV can occur with airtrapping due to chronic lung disease. Patients with both obstructive sleep apnea and chronic obstructive pulmonary disease tend to have severe desaturation, especially if they have a low awake SpO_2.

REM sleep has several important consequences in patients with obstructive sleep apnea. First, the AHI is usually higher during REM sleep. The respiratory events tend to be longer and the arterial oxygen desaturation more severe.[52] An exception is when patients have most REM sleep in the lateral position. There is an interaction between body position and REM sleep as far as the severity of arterial oxygen desaturation.[52] The circumstance most likely to be associated with worsened desaturation is supine REM sleep.

Oximeters may vary considerably in the number of desaturations they detect and their ability to discard movement artifact. Using long averaging times may dramatically decrease the detection of desaturations.[53] As most PSG monitoring equipment has integrated oximeters with the amplifier, the oximetry settings are optimized for sleep.

MEASUREMENT OF $PACO_2$ DURING SLEEP

Documentation of hypoventilation during sleep requires measurement (or estimate) of the $PaCO_2$. The gold standard for measurement of $PaCO_2$ is an ABG. However, continuous ABG monitoring during PSG to determine the $PaCO_2$ is not practical. Instead, the end-tidal PCO_2 ($P_{ET}CO_2$) or transcutaneous PCO_2 ($TcPCO_2$) is used as a surrogate for the $PaCO_2$ determined with an ABG. However, the AASM scoring manual recommendations for measuring the $PaCO_2$ can be confusing. The first issue is that monitoring for hypoventilation is recommended for pediatric diagnostic studies but optional in adult diagnostic studies and optional in both adult and pediatric PAP titration studies. **If monitoring for hypoventilation**, end-tidal PCO_2 or $TcPCO_2$ is recommended for diagnostic studies, but only $TcPCO_2$ is recommended for PAP titration studies.[1] The advantage of measurement of the $P_{ET}CO_2$ is the ability to determine an estimate of the $PaCO_2$ on a breath by breath basis. However, this measurement is not recommended during PAP titration studies due to potential dilution of the end tidal PCO_2 sample by PAP airflow. The $TcPCO_2$ measurements do not have this issue but have a slow response rate often laging changes in the $PaCO_2$ by several minutes depending on the device being used.[5] The AASM scoring manual[1] defines sleep-related hypoventilation in **adults** as an increase in the $PaCO_2$ during sleep greater than 55 mm Hg for ≥10 minutes or an increase in the $PaCO_2$ of ≥10 mm Hg compared with an awake supine value to greater than 50 mm Hg for ≥10 minutes. An ABG performed at the start or at the end of the study could be used to validate a surrogate measure of $PaCO_2$. If an ABG sample is taken just at awakening, it may be used to infer hypoventilation during sleep. However, ABG sampling requires special expertise and can be difficult and painful. Instead, an arterialized capillary blood gas is often performed rather than an arterial sample. A small incision 1 to 2 mm deep on a fingertip or ear lobe with lancet is performed, and the blood sample is obtained by placing a capillary tube where blood exits the skin, and the sample is drawn into the tube by capillary action. Before sampling, heat or a vasodilatory substance is applied to the skin. Studies have shown that capillary ABGs provide an accurate estimate of the arterial PCO_2; the capillary gas PCO_2 is usually within a few mm Hg of the $PaCO_2$.[54-58] The capillary ABG is more commonly used in pediatric medicine, but it could be potentially useful in adult patients. In particular, a capillary ABG PCO_2 value can be used with simultaneous measurement of $TcPCO_2$ to determine the accuracy of the $TcPCO_2$ measurement. Due to the slow response time of $TcPCO_2$ to a change in the $PaCO_2$, the capillary ABG measurement of PCO_2 should be compared to the transcutaneous PCO_2 several minutes later (depending on response time of the $TcPCO_2$ device). The use of the capillary PCO_2 and venous PCO_2 to estimate the $PaCO_2$ is discussed by Huttman and colleagues.[54]

Summary of PCO_2 monitoring:

- AASM recommendations for PCO_2 monitoring
  - Recommended: pediatric diagnostic studies
  - Optional: pediatric PAP titration studies, all types of adult studies
- Arterial blood gas determination of $PaCO_2$ is the gold standard measurement
- AASM recommended surrogates of the $PaCO_2$
  - Diagnostic studies: end-tidal PCO_2 or transcutaneous PCO_2
  - PAP titration studies: transcutaneous PCO_2

End-Tidal PCO_2 ($P_{ET}CO_2$)

Capnography[54,59-61] consists of the continuous measurement of the fraction of CO_2 in exhaled gas. This is usually performed using an infrared sensor and, less commonly, a mass spectrophotometer. The PCO_2 is determined by multiplication of the fraction of CO_2 by (Patm—47 mm Hg). Here, the Patm is the atmospheric pressure (760 mm Hg at sea level), and 47 mm Hg is the partial pressure of H_2O in exhaled gas at body temperature. A schematic tracing of exhaled PCO_2 versus time is shown in Figure 10–26. During initial exhalation, the dead space (PCO_2 = 0) reaches the sensor (phase 1), then a mixture of dead space and alveolar gas (phase 2), and, finally, alveolar gas (phase 3). The alveolar plateau occurs because the PCO_2 in the exhaled air from the different alveoli differs slightly. The differences are larger (the slope of the alveolar plateau is steeper) in patients with lung disease. The $P_{ET}CO_2$ is an estimate of the mean alveolar PCO_2 (and therefore an estimate of the $PaCO_2$). Of note, there is a gradient between the $PaCO_2$ and the $P_{ET}CO_2$ ($PaCO_2 - P_{ET}CO_2$) with the $PaCO_2$ being typically 2 to 7 mm Hg higher than the $P_{ET}CO_2$ (2 to 5 mm Hg in some references).[5] The gradient is due to anatomic (PCO_2 = 0) and physiologic (high ventilation to perfusion units with low alveolar PCO_2) dead space, which dilutes the alveolar PCO_2 sample. The gradient can be larger in patients with lung disease. To be valid, a plateau should be seen in the exhaled PCO_2 waveform. Small breaths may not clear the dead space and produce a rounded pattern with a lower PCO_2. As noted earlier, the two common methods of capnography are mainstream and side stream. In the mainstream method, the sensor is located directly in the path of exhaled gas. In the side stream method, gas is continually suctioned through a tube to a more remote sensor (in the instrument at bedside).

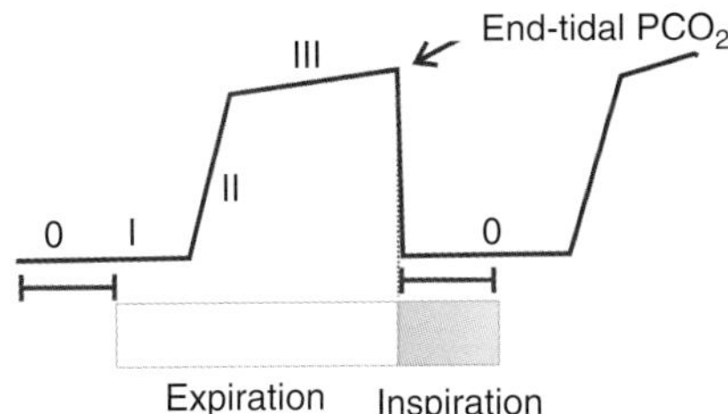

Phases of exhaled PCO_2
0 Inspiration (PCO_2 = 0, inhaled gas)
I Dead space (no CO_2 exhaled)
II Mixture of dead space and alveolar gas
III Alveolar plateau

Figure 10–26 A schematic illustrating the phases of the exhaled PCO_2 wave form (capnography). This is an idealized example with a clear plateau. The value at end-expiration (end-tidal) is an estimate of the alveolar PCO_2 and therefore the arterial PCO_2. The arterial PCO_2 usually exceeds the end-tidal PCO_2 by about 5 mm Hg (range, 2–7 mm Hg). The arterial to end-tidal PCO_2 difference is larger in patients with lung disease. In patients with lung disease the alveolar plateau is steeper due to inhomogeneity in the lung units, some with lower and some with higher alveolar PCO_2.

Exhaled PCO_2 measuring devices typically output both a capnography wave form (PCO_2 vs. time) and a running estimate of end-tidal values derived from the waveform (Figure 10–27).[1-4] The waveform assists in visualizing changes, and ideally there should be a plateau in the exhaled PCO_2 waveform for the end-tidal PCO_2 value to be considered an accurate measurement. The AASM scoring manual recommends end-tidal PCO_2 measurement to assess hypoventilation in diagnostic sleep studies, but PCO_2 **monitoring is for hypoventilation recommended** only in pediatric patients during diagnostic studies (optional in adults). Capnography is especially useful in pediatric diagnostic sleep studies as children may have long periods of obstructive hypoventilation (see Chapter 12) due to high upper airway resistance (airflow limitation without discrete apneas or hypopneas). Other than a mild decrease in the SpO_2, the significance of these events would be underestimated except for the demonstration of an increase in the $P_{ET}CO_2$. Pediatric patients with obstructive sleep apnea may have a relatively mild AHI but evidence of significant hypoventilation during sleep.[61,62] An analysis of the utility of end-tidal PCO_2 was performed by Paruthi and colleagues.[61] Valid data was found in a large proportion of patients and often contributed information for clinical decision-making that was not available with a simple AHI or

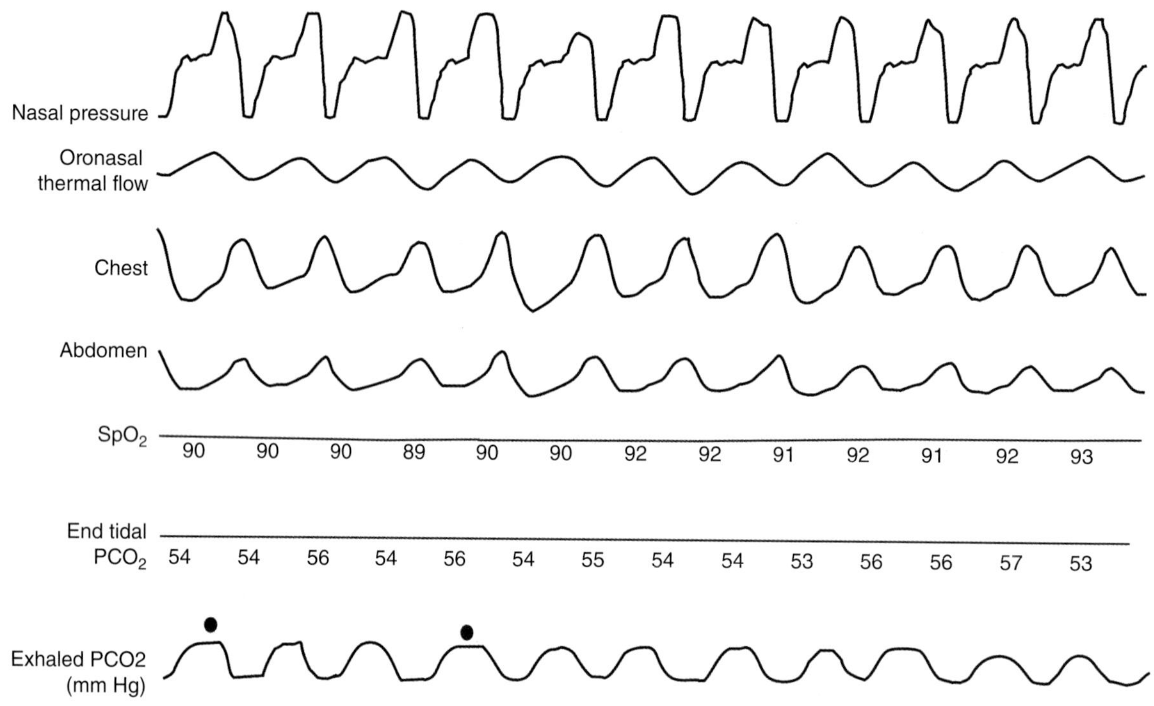

Figure 10–27 This tracing recorded both outputs of a capnography device including the recent end-tidal PCO_2 number and the exhaled PCO_2 waveform. Note the plateaus in waveforms (best seen during breaths with a circle on top). Notice that although the PCO_2 was elevated, the SaO_2 was only mildly reduced. When the exhaled PCO_2 waveform has a plateau, the end-tidal PCO_2 value is more reliable.

determination of arterial oxygen desaturation. Although capnography can be performed during a PAP titration using a nasal cannula under the mask, the sample is often diluted and can cause mask leaks. The AASM scoring manual does not recommend exhaled CO_2 monitoring during PAP titrations (although some clinicians find this measurement to be useful). $TcPCO_2$ monitoring is the method of choice in this situation. The AASM scoring manual[1] does provide guidance on assessing the accuracy of the end-tidal PCO_2 signal. The manual emphasizes that if an alveolar plateau is not present, the $P_{ET}CO_2$ value may not be an accurate estimate of $PaCO_2$. Other problems for exhaled PCO_2 monitoring include oral breathing and occlusion of the nasal cannula with secretions. In addition, if tidal volumes are very small, a true alveolar sample may never reach the sensor. If only a mixture of dead space ($PCO_2 = 0$) and alveolar gas is sampled, the $P_{ET}CO_2$ value will likely be much lower than the $PaCO_2$. Of note, an elevation in the end-tidal PCO_2 above baseline can be used to score respiratory effort related arousals in children (see Chapter 12).

Transcutaneous PCO_2 Monitoring

Measurement of $TcPCO_2$[5,54,63] depends on the fact that heating of capillaries in the skin causes increased capillary blood flow and makes the skin permeable to the diffusion of CO_2. The CO_2 in the capillaries diffuses through the skin and is measured by an electrode at the skin surface. The measured value is corrected for the fact that heat increases the skin CO_2 production as the measured value exceeds the $PaCO_2$ measured at 37°C. Typically, $TcCO_2$ electrodes are calibrated with a reference gas. A thermostat controls the heating of the membrane-skin interface. It is usually recommended that the probe of most $TcPCO_2$ monitoring devices be moved every 3 to 4 hours to avoid skin irritation/damage. New $TcPCO_2$ devices use lower probe temperature, and the probe may be changed less frequently. The response time of newer $TcPCO_2$ units has improved, but in general, the measured PCO_2 may not increase rapidly enough to correlate with short respiratory events. However, $TcPCO_2$ can be a good instrument for documenting trends in the PCO_2 during the night. In addition, $TcPCO_2$ is the recommended method to measure PCO_2 during a PAP titration, as dilution by PAP device delivered airflow makes measurement of end-tidal PCO_2 problematic. Figure 10–28 shows trends in the SpO_2 and $TcPCO_2$. Decreases in the SpO_2 occur in association with increases in the $TcPCO_2$ during episodes of REM sleep. Kirk and colleagues found reasonable agreement between the $P_{ET}CO_2$ and the $TcPCO_2$ during pediatric PSG.[63] Having two measures could potentially be useful. If there is reasonable agreement, this may increase confidence in the accuracy. Storre and colleagues[64] found reasonable agreement between $PaCO_2$ and $TcPCO_2$ values during noninvasive PAP titration. The best agreement was between a given $PaCO_2$ value and the corresponding $TcPCO_2$ value about 2 minutes later. The response time varies between $TcPCO_2$ devices. To improve the accuracy, the $TcPCO_2$ sensor should be calibrated with a reference gas according to the manufacturer's recommendations and when the accuracy of the current reading is doubtful. If there is a steady substantial trend upward in the reading over several hours, this is likely drift, and the results may not be accurate. At times, after recalibration the values may differ significantly from previous ones. Obtaining a capillary ABG with a concurrent measurement may be useful. As noted above, the $TcPCO_2$ value corresponding to the capillary ABG PCO_2 may not occur until several minutes after the capillary sample was obtained (slower response time).

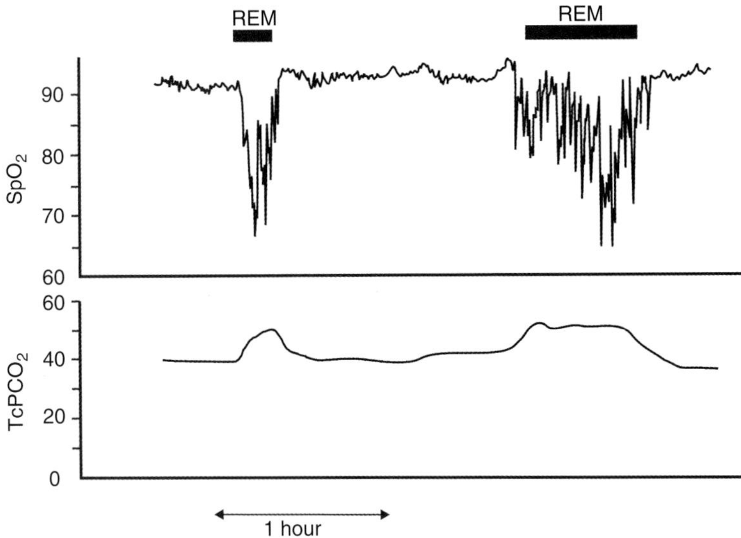

Figure 10–28 A tracing of arterial saturation by pulse oximetry and the transcutaneous PCO_2. The transcutaneous PCO_2 responds slowly to change (not breath to breath) but is useful for observing trends. Here during episodes of REM sleep significant arterial oxygen desaturation is noted along with elevations in the PCO_2. That is, hypoventilation during REM sleep.

Snoring

Snoring is a sound produced by vibration of upper airway structures. Although snoring sensors are widely used, there is little published evidence to demonstrate the utility of measurement/detection of snoring during sleep. When snoring is present, upper airway narrowing of some degree can be inferred. There is evidence that vibration of different areas of the upper airway causes different sounds. However, the utility of this information remains to be determined. Snore sensors are usually microphones or PE transducers that are commonly applied to the neck near the trachea. Microphones/sensors can also be attached to the upper chest area or the face. The ability of the sensor to detect simulated snoring is typically tested during polysomnography before lights-out as part of the biocalibration procedure. Snoring can also be seen in the NP signal as a rapid oscillation in the pressure tracing (Figure 10–9) if an appropriate high-frequency filter setting (100 Hz) is used and the transducer is sufficiently sensitive. The AASM scoring manual[1] says the monitoring snoring is optional. When monitoring snoring, an acoustic sensor (microphone), piezoelectric sensor, or nasal pressure is a recommended sensor (signal). Detection of snoring is part of the adult respiratory scoring rules only for the optional classification of hypopneas as central or obstructive. In pediatrics the presence of snoring is used to score RERAs.

Table 10–5 Sensors for Home Sleep Apnea Testing (Adults)

Monitoring Flow (or Tidal Volume)—Detecting (Apnea or Hypopnea)

At least one of the following:

Standard sensors:

- Oronasal thermal sensor (including PVDF sensors)
- Nasal Pressure (with or without square root transformation)

Alternative Sensors:

- Respiratory inductance Plethysmography sum (RIPsum) or flow (RIPflow)
- PVDF Thoracoabdominal belt Sum*

Monitoring Respiratory Effort

Use one of the following:

- Dual Thoracoabdominal RIP belts
- Single RIP thoracoabdominal RIP belt * (simple but provides less information)
- Single or dual thoracoabdominal PFDF belt*
- Single or dual thoracoabdominal piezo belts*
- Single or dual pneumatic belts*

Monitoring arterial oxygen saturation: use pulse oximetry

Monitoring snoring (optional), use an acoustic sensor (eg microphone), piezoelectric sensor, or nasal pressure

NP, Nasal pressure; *PE,* piezoelectric; *PVDF,* polyvinylidene fluoride; *RIP,* respiratory inductance plethysmography; *RIPflow,* time derivative of RIPsum; *RIPsum,* sum of chest and abdominal belt signals. * acceptable level of recommendation

MONITORING TECHNOLOGY FOR HOME SLEEP APNEA TESTING

Essentially the same respiratory monitoring sensors are used for home sleep apnea tests that monitor airflow as for PSG with a few exceptions (Table 10–5). If the patient must place the sensors on themselves, simplicity has advantages. Devices with more sensors provide more information and have backup sensors. See Chapter 16 for information of home sleep apnea testing (HSAT). The AASM scoring manual provides recommendations for sensors used in HSAT with airflow measurement.[1] Alternative sensors are used if the recommended sensor is not functioning. The levels of recommendation are "recommended" and "acceptable." The recommended airflow sensors are an oronasal thermal sensor and NP monitoring.[1] Unlike PSG, only one is required (although use of both is optimal). Most often the NP signal is used to score apneas and hypopneas. In those HSAT devices using dual RIP effort belts, RIPsum and RIPflow can be derived and used as **recommended** alternative airflow (RIPflow) or tidal volume (RIPsum) sensors. If dual PVDF effort belts are used, the PVDFsum can be used to monitor airflow as an **acceptable** alternative sensor. Home sleep apnea testing using peripheral arterial tonometry (PAT)[1] must have the ability to calculate an REI (respiratory event index = respiratory events/hour of monitoring time) as a surrogate of the apnea-hypopnea index, ability to measure oximetry, and ability to record a measure of heart rate. More information on PAT devices is available in Chapter 16.

For monitoring respiratory effort during HSAT, use of dual RIP effort belts is recommended by the AASM scoring manual[1]. Use of a single RIP effort belt, single or dual PVDF belts, or single or dual PE belts is acceptable. In addition, a single or dual pneumatic sensor belt(s) is also acceptable[1]. PE effort belts use a single sensor constructed of PE material that outputs a signal in response to belt tension. Pneumatic effort belts produce a signal by pulling on a volume sensitive sensor. For monitoring SaO_2 pulse oximetry is recommended. Of note, many HSAT devices also have a body position sensor and a sensor to detect snoring (microphone or piezoelectric sensor). Snoring can also be detected (actually airflow vibration) using NP with a high frequency filter setting of 100 Hz. Monitoring snoring is considered optional.

SUMMARY OF KEY POINTS

1. A pneumotachograph (PNT) in a mask covering the nose and mouth is the most accurate method to measure airflow but is practical only for research studies. Airflow is measured in this device by determining the pressure drop across a linear resistance.
2. Oronasal thermal airflow sensors (thermistors, thermocouples, PVDF film) are placed under the nose with a portion extending over the mouth and can detect both nasal and oral airflow. The signal from thermistors or thermocouples is based on changes in temperature associated with cooler inhaled air and warmed exhaled air. The signal of thermal sensors is not proportional to airflow and overestimates airflow at low flow rates. PVDF flow sensors respond to both pressure and temperature, and the signal deflections more accurately estimate the magnitude of changes in flow. Oronasal thermal airflow sensors are the recommended sensors to score apnea in adults and children.
3. NP monitoring detects the pressure change across the nasal inlet. The resistance is nonlinear, and the flow can be approximated by taking the square root of the signal (NP is proportional to the square of airflow). A nasal cannula in the nose is connected to a sensitive pressure transducer. The NP signal with or without a square root transformation is used to detect hypopneas (reduction in airflow). When using a square root transformation of the NP signal the determined AHI may be slightly lower than when using the untransformed NP signal as the untransformed NP signal underestimates low flow rates and overestimates high flow rates. However, the difference is not usually clinically significant. The NP signal may not detect oral breathing and can be flat when the oronasal thermal sensor shows deflections consistent with the presence of airflow. Flattening of the inspiratory waveform of the NP signal can detect airflow limitation (narrowing) of the upper airway. A NP sensor with or without square root transformation is the recommended sensor for scoring hypopneas in adults and children.
4. Use of both an oronasal thermal airflow sensor and a NP sensor is recommended for monitoring airflow during diagnostic PSG in both adults and children. If the oronasal thermal sensor is not functioning, NP is a recommended alternative sensor for detecting apnea. If the NP signal is not functioning the oronasal thermal sensor is a recommended alternative hypopnea sensor.
5. The flow signal from the laboratory PAP device (often called PAPflow or Cflow) is the recommended apnea and hypopnea sensor for use during PSG PAP titrations for adults and children. Flattening of the inspiratory portion of the signal is used to detect airflow limitation (airflow narrowing). There is no alternative flow sensor for use in PAP titration sleep studies.
6. RIP measures changes in inductance of wire coils in chest and abdominal bands that occur with chest and abdominal movement associated with respiration. Deflections in the sum of the two signals is an estimate of tidal volume (RIPsum), and deflections in the signal *derived from the first derivative of the RIPsum* (RIPflow) is an estimate of changes in airflow. When calibrated, deflections in the RIPsum and RIPflow are more accurate. That is, constants a and b are determined with RIPsum = a × RIP chest + b × RIP abdomen. RIPsum and RIPflow are alternative sensors recommended for detection of apnea and hypopnea when the oronasal thermal airflow signal (apnea) or NP signal (hypopnea) is not functioning properly in adults and children. The combination of chest and abdominal RIP signals is a recommended alternative hypopnea sensor (used if RIPsum is not available) in adults and children. The sum of signals from chest and abdominal bands using PVDF sensors (PVDFsum = PVDFchest + PVDFabdomen) is an acceptable alternative sensor for detection of apnea or hypopnea when the oronasal thermal airflow signal (apnea) or NP signal (hypopnea) is not functioning properly in adults and children.
7. In children only, the end-tidal PCO_2 signal (actually the exhaled PCO_2 waveform) is an alternative apnea sensor. During apnea the value is zero (no CO_2 is exhaled). In the AASM scoring manual the signal is considered an "acceptable" alternative apnea sensor in children.
8. Respiratory effort can be determined by esophageal manometry, RIP, or effort belts using piezoelectric (PE) or PVDF sensors. Esophageal manometry or dual thoracoabdominal RIP belts are recommended effort sensors for PSG and PVDF thoracoabdominal belts are acceptable effort sensors in children and adults. Dual RIP belts are recommended for home sleep apnea testing (HSAT). One or ideally two effort belts using PE or pneumatic sensors are acceptable for detecting effort in HSAT (not PSG).
9. Pulse oximetry is the recommended method for monitoring oxygen saturation during PSG in children and adults.
10. Recommended surrogate methods of measuring the PCO_2 during sleep studies include end-tidal PCO_2 (diagnostic studies) or $TcPCO_2$ (diagnostic and PAP titration studies), if appropriately calibrated. The exhaled PCO_2 waveform used in capnography should exhibit a plateau for the end-tidal PCO_2 values to be considered accurate. Note that in the AASM scoring manual, monitoring PCO_2 during PSG (both diagnostic and titration) is optional in adults, but in children, monitoring PCO_2 during diagnostic PSG is recommended (essential; see Chapter 12). In children, monitoring the PCO_2 during PAP titration studies is optional.
11. The SaO_2 is equal to the concentration of Hb bound to oxygen divided by the total amount of Hb available for oxygen transport.
12. The relationship between the SaO_2 and the corresponding PaO_2 depends on many factors affecting the position of the oxyhemoglobin saturation curve (including $PaCO_2$, temperature, the hydrogen ion concentration, the amount of 2,3 DPG, and abnormal Hb).
13. Carboxyhemoglobin (COHb) and methemoglobin (MetHb) are forms of Hb that are not available for oxygen transport.

The fraction of the total Hb available for oxygen transport that is bound to oxygen is often called the fractional concentration of oxyhemoglobin (FO_2Hb) (see Equation 10–10).

14. Routine pulse oximeters measure absorption of two wavelengths of light to determine the SaO_2 by oximetry (SpO_2). The accuracy can be affected by the presence of significant amounts of COHb or MetHb. Co-oximeters can detect the amounts of oxyhemoglobin, RHb, COHb, and MetHb using at least four wavelengths of light. Co-oximetry can determine the true fraction of the total Hb that is bound to oxygen (FO_2Hb) if significant amounts of COHb or MetHb are present. If a co-oximeter is NOT used the SaO_2 reported with ABG results is based on measurement of the PaO_2 and values from tables that assume COHb and MetHb are not present. The reported SaO_2 can differ from the values of the SaO_2 and the FO_2Hb measured by co-oximetry.

CLINICAL REVIEW QUESTIONS

1. Deflections in the sum of the thorax and abdominal band RIP signals (RIPsum) is an estimate of:
   A. Airflow (flow rate)
   B. Tidal volume
2. Which of the following is ***not*** true about the nasal pressure (NP) signal?
   A. It is a more accurate estimate of flow than most thermal sensors.
   B. The signal is proportional to the flow rate (Flow = K × NP signal).
   C. It measures the pressure drop across the nasal inlet.
   D. Flattening of the inspiratory NP waveform suggests airflow limitation is present.
   E. The NP signal (without square root transformation) tends to underestimate flow at low flow rates and overestimate flow at high flow rates.
3. Which of these can cause a greater than expected PaO_2 for a given SpO_2?
   A. Lower PCO_2
   B. Lower temperature
   C. Higher pH (lower hydrogen ion concentration)
   D. Higher PCO_2
4. What statement is correct?
   A. The recommended sensor to detect apnea during a diagnostic study is the nasal pressure signal.
   B. The recommended hypopnea sensor during a diagnostic study is the oronasal sensor.
   C. The RIPsum (calibrated or uncalibrated) is a recommended alternative apnea sensor.
   D. For children the exhaled PCO_2 waveform is a recommended alternative apnea sensor.
5. A patient has a significant increase in carboxyhemoglobin (fractional concentration is 10%). The fractional concentration of oxygenated blood is 80%. Which of the following is closest to the computed SaO_2?
   A. 80%
   B. 84%
   C. 90%
   D. 94%
6. Which of the following is associated with a shift of the oxyhemoglobin saturation curve to the right?
   A. Decreased $PaCO_2$
   B. Decreased pH
   C. Decreased 2,3-DPG
   D. Decreased temperature
7. What column (A, B, or C) lists the correct expected approximate PO_2 values for the SaO_2 values?

		A	B	C
SaO_2 = 60%	PaO_2	40	30	30
SaO_2 = 75%	PaO_2	60	40	40
SaO_2 = 90%	PaO_2	75	60	80

8. Which of the following is **NOT** true about methemoglobinemia?
   A. If the PaO_2 is normal, MetHb causes a falsely high SpO_2.
   B. Blood can have a chocolate color.
   C. It reduces the oxygen carrying capacity of hemoglobin.
   D. It causes a left shift of the oxyhemoglobin dissociation curve.
9. Given the capnography tracings in Figure 10–29. What is the most likely $PaCO_2$ value?
   A. 48 mm Hg
   B. 40 mm Hg
   C. 52 mm Hg
   D. 35 mm Hg

ANSWERS

1. **B.** The deflection in the RIPsum is an estimate of tidal volume. When calibrated deflections in the RIPsum signal is a more accurate estimate of tidal volume. The time derivative of the RIPsum signal is an estimate of flow (RIPflow).

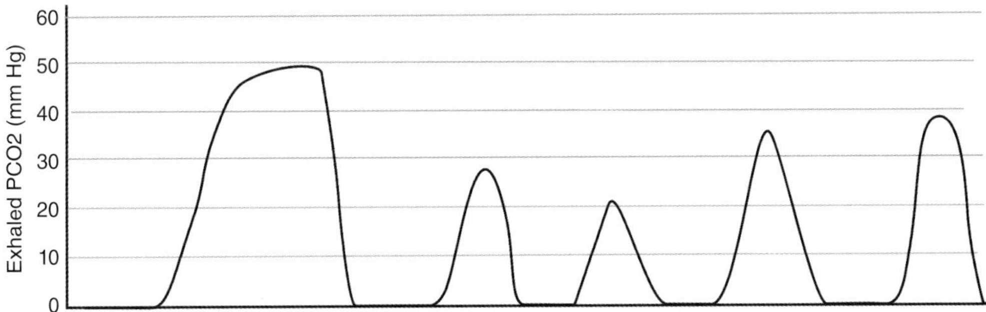

Figure 10–29 Given the capnography tracing of several breaths, what is the most likely $PaCO_2$ value?

2. **B.** The NP signal is proportional to the square of the flow rate. For this reason, a square root transformation of the NP signal is a better estimate of airflow. However, the clinical importance of using this transformation has not been demonstrated.
3. **D.** When the oxyhemoglobin saturation curve is shifted to the right, a given SaO_2 is associated with a higher PaO_2. The curve is shifted to the right by an increase in $PaCO_2$.
4. **C.** The RIPsum is a recommended alternative apnea sensor. A and B are incorrect because during a diagnostic study the recommended apnea sensor is an oronasal thermal flow sensor, and the recommended hypopnea signal is from a nasal pressure transducer. The exhaled PCO_2 wave form is an alternative apnea sensor in children, but the AASM **level** of recommendation is "**acceptable**," not "recommended."
5. **C.** 90%. The fractional concentration of reduced (deoxygenated hemoglobin) is 100 − 80 − 10 = 10%. The SaO_2 = 100 × (FO_2Hb)/(FO_2Hb + FRHb) = 80/90 = 88%.
6. **B.** A decreased pH is associated with a higher hydrogen ion concentration [H^+], which is associated with a right shift.
7. **B.**
8. **A.** Methemoglobin is a cause of a falsely low SpO_2. Methemoglobin causes the SpO_2 to move toward 85% as the levels increase. With a normal PaO_2 the SaO_2 would likely be approximately 96% and the SpO_2 be lower than 96% but above 85%. The other answers are true.
9. **C.** 52 mm Hg. The only breath with a good plateau is the breath with an end-tidal PCO_2 value just below 50 mm Hg. The $PaCO_2$ is usually 2 to 5 mm Hg above the end-tidal PCO_2 value.

SUGGESTED READING

Chan ED, Chan MM, Chan MM. Pulse oximetry: understanding its basic principles facilitates appreciation of its limitations. *Respir Med.* 2013;107(6):789-799.

Huttmann SE, Windisch W, Storre JH. Techniques for the measurement and monitoring of carbon dioxide in the blood. *Ann Am Thorac Soc.* 2014;11(4):645-652.

Paruthi S, Rosen CL, Wang R, et al. End-tidal carbon dioxide measurement during pediatric polysomnography: signal quality, association with apnea severity, and prediction of neurobehavioral outcomes. *Sleep.* 2015;38(11):1719-1726.

Troester MM, Quan SF, Berry RB, et al. *The AASM Manual for the Scoring of Sleep and Associated Events: Rules, Terminology and Technical Specifications. Version 3.* American Academy of Sleep Medicine; 2023.

REFERENCES

1. Troester MM, Quan SF, Berry RB, et al. , for the American Academy of Sleep Medicine. *The AASM Manual for the Scoring of Sleep and Associated Events: Rules, Terminology and Technical Specifications. Version 3.* Darien, IL: American Academy of Sleep Medicine; 2023.
2. Iber C, Ancoli-Israel S, Chesson A, Quan SF, American Academy of Sleep Medicine. *The AASM Manual for the Scoring of Sleep and Associated Events: Rules, Terminology and Technical Specifications.* Westchester, IL: American Academy of Sleep Medicine; 2007.
3. American Academy of Sleep Medicine Task Force. Sleep related breathing disorders in adults: recommendation for syndrome definition and measurement techniques in clinical research. *Sleep.* 1999;22:667-689.
4. Redline S, Budhiraja R, Kapur V, et al. The scoring of respiratory events in sleep: reliability and validity. *J Clin Sleep Med.* 2007;3:169-200.
5. Berry RB, Budhiraja R, Gottlieb DJ, et al. Rules for scoring respiratory events in sleep: update of the 2007 AASM Manual for the Scoring of Sleep and Associated Events. Deliberations of the Sleep Apnea Definitions Task Force of the American Academy of Sleep Medicine. *J Clin Sleep Med.* 2012;8(5):597-619.
6. Farré R, Montserrat JM, Navajas D. Noninvasive monitoring of respiratory mechanics during sleep. *Eur Respir J.* 2004;24(6):1052-1060.
7. Berg S, Haight JSJ, Yap V, et al. Comparison of direct and indirect measurement of respiratory airflow: implications for hypopneas. *Sleep.* 1997;20:60-64.
8. Farre R, Montserrat JM, Rotger M, et al. Accuracy of thermistors and thermocouples as flow-measuring devices for detecting hypopneas. *Eur Respir J.* 1998;11:179-182.
9. Berry RB, Koch GL, Trautz S, Wagner MH. Comparison of respiratory event detection by a polyvinylidene fluoride film airflow sensor and a pneumotachograph in sleep apnea patients. *Chest.* 2005;128:1331-1338.
10. Norman RG, Ahmed M, Walsben JA, Rapoport DM. Detection of respiratory events during NPSG: nasal cannula/pressure sensor versus thermistor. *Sleep.* 1997;20:1175-1184.
11. Hosselet J, Normal RG, Ayapa I, Rapoport DM. Detection of flow limitation with a nasal cannula/pressure transducer system. *Am J Respir Crit Care Med.* 1988;157:1461-1467.
12. Hernandez L, Ballester E, Farre R, et al. Performance of nasal prongs in sleep studies. *Chest.* 2001;119:442-450.
13. Farre R, Rigau J, Montserrat JM, et al. Relevance of linearizing nasal prongs for assessing hypopneas and flow limitation during sleep. *Am J Respir Crit Care Med.* 2001;163:494-497.
14. Thurnheer R, Xie X, Bloch KE. Accuracy of nasal cannula pressure recordings for assessment of ventilation during sleep. *Am J Respir Crit Care Med.* 2001;146:1914-1919.
15. Heitman SJ, Atkar RS, Hajduk EA, et al. Validation of nasal pressure for the identification of apneas/hypopneas during sleep. *Am J Respir Crit Care Med.* 2002;166:386-391.
16. Vandenbussche NL, Overeem S, van Dijk JP, Simons PJ, Pevernagie DA. Assessment of respiratory effort during sleep: esophageal pressure versus noninvasive monitoring techniques. *Sleep Med Rev.* 2015;24:28-36.
17. Staats BA, Bonekat HW, Harris CD, Offord KP. Chest wall motion in sleep apnea. *Am Rev Respir Dis.* 1984;130(1):59-63.
18. Tobin MJ, Cohen MA, Sackner MA. Breathing abnormalities during sleep. *Arch Intern Med.* 1983;143:1221-1228.
19. Kogan D, Jain A, Kimbro S, Gutierrez G, Jain V. Respiratory inductance plethysmography improved diagnostic sensitivity and specificity of obstructive sleep apnea. *Respir Care.* 2016;61(8):1033-1037.
20. Sackner MA, Watson H, Belsito AS, et al. Calibration of respiratory inductive plethysmograph during natural breathing. *J Appl Physiol (1985).* 1989;66(1):410-420.
21. Montazeri K, Jonsson SA, Agustsson JS, et al. The design of RIP belts impacts the reliability and quality of the measured respiratory signals. *Sleep Breath.* 2021;25(3):1535-1541.
22. Poole KA, Thompson JR, Hallinan HM, Beardsmore CS. Respiratory inductance plethysmography in healthy infants: a comparison of three calibration methods. *Eur Respir J.* 2000;16(6):1084-1090.
23. Stradling JR, Chadwick GA, Quirk C, Phillips T. Respiratory inductance plethysmography: calibration techniques, their validation and the effects of posture. *Bull Eur Physiopathol Respir.* 1985;21(4):317-324.
24. Strömberg NO, Dahlbäck GO, Gustafsson PM. Evaluation of various models for respiratory inductance plethysmography calibration. *J Appl Physiol (1985).* 1993;74(3):1206-1211.
25. Koo BB, Drummond C, Surovec S, Johnson N, Marvin SA, Redline S. Validation of a polyvinylidene fluoride impedance sensor for respiratory event classification during polysomnography. *J Clin Sleep Med.* 2011; 7(5):479-485.
26. Griffiths AG, Patwari PP, Loghmanee DA, Balog MJ, Trosman I, Sheldon SH. Validation of polyvinylidene fluoride impedance sensor for respiratory event classification during polysomnography in children. *J Clin Sleep Med.* 2017;13(2):259-265.
27. Berry RB. Esophageal and nasal pressure monitoring during sleep. In: Lee-Chiong TL, Sateia MJ, Caraskadon MA, eds. *Sleep Medicine.* Philadelphia: Hanley & Belfus; 2002:661-671.
28. Ayappa I, Norman RG, Krieger AC, Rosen A, O'Malley RL, Rapoport DM. Non-invasive detection of respiratory effort-related arousals (RERAs) by a nasal cannula/pressure transducer system. *Sleep.* 2000;23(6):763-771.
29. Berry RB, Ryals S, Girdhar A, Wagner MH. Use of chest wall electromyography to detect respiratory effort during polysomnography. J Clin Sleep Med. 2016;12(9):1239-1244.
30. Stoohs RA, Blum HC, Knaack L, et al. Comparison of pleural pressure and transcutaneous diaphragmatic electromyogram in obstructive sleep apnea syndrome. *Sleep.* 2005;28:321-329.
31. Chan ED, Chan MM, Chan MM. Pulse oximetry: understanding its basic principles facilitates appreciation of its limitations. *Respir Med.* 2013;107(6):789-799.
32. Tremper KK, Barker SJ. Pulse oximetry. *Anesthesiology.* 1989;70(1): 98-108.

33. West JB, Wagner P. Ventilation, blood flow, and gas exchange. In: Murray JF, Nadel JA, eds. *Textbook of Respiratory Medicine*. 3rd ed. Baltimore: WB Saunders; 2000:55-89.
34. Toffaletti J, Zijlstra WG. Misconceptions in reporting oxygen saturation. *Anesth Analg*. 2007;105(suppl 6):S5-S9.
35. Roughton FJW, Darling RC. The effect of carbon monoxide on the oxyhemoglobin dissociation curve. *Am J Physiol*. 1944;141:17-31.
36. Zwart A, Kwant G, Oeseburg B, Zijlstra WG. Human whole-blood oxygen affinity: effect of carbon monoxide. *J Appl Physiol Respir Environ Exerc Physiol*. 1984;57(1):14-20.
37. Haymond S, Cariappa R, Eby CS, Scott MG. Laboratory assessment of oxygenation in methemoglobinemia. *Clin Chem*. 2005;51(2):434-444.
38. Rehman HU. Methemoglobinemia. *West J Med*. 2001;175(3):193-196.
39. Seakins M, Gibbs WN, Milner PF, Bertles JF. Erythrocyte Hb-S concentration. An important factor in the low oxygen affinity of blood in sickle cell anemia. *J Clin Invest*. 1973;2(2):422-432.
40. Wagner MH, Berry RB. A patient with sickle cell disease and a low baseline sleeping oxygen saturation. *J Clin Sleep Med*. 2007;3(3):313-315.
41. Mack E. Focus on diagnosis: co-oximetry. *Pediatr Rev*. 2007;28(2):73-74.
42. Barker SJ, Curry J, Redford D, Morgan S. Measurement of carboxyhemoglobin and methemoglobin by pulse oximetry: a human volunteer study. *Anesthesiology*. 2006;105(5):892-897. [Erratum in: *Anesthesiology*. 2007;107(5):863].
43. Barker SJ, Tremper KK. The effect of carbon monoxide inhalation on pulse oximetry and transcutaneous PO_2. *Anesthesiology*. 1987;66(5):677-679.
44. Barker SJ, Tremper KK, Hyatt J. Effects of methemoglobinemia on pulse oximetry and mixed venous oximetry. *Anesthesiology*. 1989;70(1): 112-117.
45. Sjoding MW, Dickson RP, Iwashyna TJ, Gay SE, Valley TS. Racial bias in pulse oximetry measurement. *N Engl J Med*. 2020;383(25):2477-2478. [Erratum in: *N Engl J Med*. 2021;385(26):2496].
46. Azarbarzin A, Sands SA, Taranto-Montemurro L, et al. The sleep apnea-specific hypoxic burden predicts incident heart failure. *Chest*. 2020; 158(2):739-750.
47. Bradley TD, Martinez D, Rutherford R, et al. Physiological determinants of nocturnal arterial oxygenation in patients with obstructive sleep apnea. *J Appl Physiol*. 1985;59:1364-1368.
48. Series F, Cormier Y, La Forge J. Influence of apnea type and sleep stage on nocturnal postapneic desaturation. *Am Rev Respir Dis*. 1990;141:1522-1526.
49. Peppard PE, Ward NR, Morrell MJ. The impact of obesity on oxygen desaturation during sleep disordered breathing. *Am J Respir Crit Care Med*. 2009;180:788-793.
50. Findley LJ, Ries AL, Tisi GM, Wagner PD. Hypoxemia during apnea in normal subjects: mechanisms and impact of lung volume. *J Appl Physiol*. 1983;55:1777-1783.
51. Findley LJ, Wihoit SC, Surrat PM. Apnea duration and hypoxemia during REM sleep in patients with obstructive sleep apnea. *Chest*. 1985;87:432-436.
52. Oksenberg A, Arons E, Nasser K, Vander T, Radwan H. REM-related obstructive sleep apnea: the effect of body position. *J Clin Sleep Med*. 2010;6(4):343-348.
53. Davila DG, Richards KC, Marshall BL, et al. Oximeter performance: the influence of acquisition parameters. *Chest*. 2002;122:1654-1660.
54. Huttmann SE, Windisch W, Storre JH. Techniques for the measurement and monitoring of carbon dioxide in the blood. *Ann Am Thorac Soc*. 2014;11(4):645-652.
55. Zavorsky GS, Cao J, Mayo NE, Gabbay R, Murias JM. Arterial versus capillary blood gases: a meta-analysis. *Respir Physiol Neurobiol*. 2007;155(3):268-279.
56. Hollier CA, Maxwell LJ, Harmer AR, et al. Validity of arterialised-venous PCO_2, pH and bicarbonate in obesity hypoventilation syndrome. *Respir Physiol Neurobiol*. 2013;188(2):165-171.
57. Lambert LL, Baldwin MB, Gonzalez CV, Lowe GR, Willis JR. Accuracy of transcutaneous CO_2 values compared with arterial and capillary blood gases. *Respir Care*. 2018;63(7):907-912.
58. Yildizdaş D, Yapicioğlu H, Yilmaz HL, Sertdemir Y. Correlation of simultaneously obtained capillary, venous, and arterial blood gases of patients in a paediatric intensive care unit. *Arch Dis Child*. 2004;89(2):176-180.
59. Kodali BS. Capnography outside the operating rooms. *Anesthesiology*. 2013;118(1):192-201.
60. D'Mello J, Butani M. Capnography. *Indian J Anaesthesiol*. 2002;46: 269-278.
61. Paruthi S, Rosen CL, Wang R, et al. End-tidal carbon dioxide measurement during pediatric polysomnography: signal quality, association with apnea severity, and prediction of neurobehavioral outcomes. *Sleep*. 2015;38(11):1719-1726.
62. Amaddeo A, Fauroux B. Oxygen and carbon dioxide monitoring during sleep. *Paediatr Respir Rev*. 2016;20:42-44.
63. Kirk VG, Batuyong ED, Bohn SG. Transcutaneous carbon dioxide monitoring and capnography during pediatric polysomnography. *Sleep*. 2006;29:1601-1608.
64. Storre JH, Steurer B, Kabitz HJ, et al. Transcutaneous PCO_2 monitoring during initiation of noninvasive ventilation. *Chest*. 2007;132: 1810-1816.

Chapter 11

Respiratory Events in Adults—Event Definitions and Scoring Rules

ABBREVIATIONS

PAP positive airway pressure, $PaCO_2$ arterial partial pressure of carbon dioxide, AHI apnea hypopnea index

HISTORY OF RESPIRATORY DEFINITIONS

A historical perspective is helpful to understand the origin of the current respiratory event definitions and associated controversy. The apnea hypopnea index (AHI) is the number of apneas and hypopneas per hour of sleep. This metric is used to make the diagnosis of sleep apnea and to grade the severity. This metric is not ideal but continues to be the standard for diagnosis of obstructive sleep apnea (OSA).[1] Definitions of apnea have been relatively standard (typically absent or nearly absent airflow for ≥10 sec), but different definitions of hypopnea (reductions in airflow) have resulted in a "floating metric."[2] Major developments in definitions of apnea and hypopnea are listed in Table 11–1.

Guilleminault et al. published a summary of the Stanford sleep clinic experience with diagnosis and treatment of OSA.[3] Diagnosis of the OSA syndrome required excessive daytime sleepiness and 30 or more apneas per night over 7 hours of monitoring. An apnea was defined as absent airflow for 10 seconds or more. Later an apnea index ≥ 5/hour was used to diagnose OSA. In 1978, Block and coworkers[4] were the first to use the term *hypopnea,* defined as a reduction (rather than an absence) in airflow detected by an oronasal thermal sensor and a decrease in chest movement associated with a 4% or greater desaturation (drop in the arterial oxygen desaturation by oximetry [SpO_2]). The choice of 4% was arbitrary but chosen to exceed the variability of the signal and was the smallest change that could be reliably scored using paper recording. Of note, the thermal airflow sensors used in these studies could detect the presence or absence of airflow but were less sensitive for detection of changes in airflow. In 1987, the Centers for Medicare and Medicaid Services (CMS; then known as the Health Care Finance Administration) accepted 30 **apneas** per night as evidence of OSA qualifying a patient for treatment with continuous positive airway pressure (CPAP). In 1988, Gould and colleagues[5] published findings in a group of patients that fit the clinical picture of OSA, but the majority of their respiratory events were hypopneas rather than apneas. They defined hypopnea as a 50% reduction in respiratory inductance plethysmography (RIP) belt deflections lasting greater than 10 seconds. The term *sleep apnea hypopnea syndrome* began to be used by some clinicians rather than OSA. Using a definition of hypopnea based on a discernable drop in airflow (thermal sensor) associated with a ≥4% desaturation, Young et al. described the incidence of OSA in a middle-aged population as comprising 4% in men and 2% in women (AHI ≥ 5/hour + symptoms).[6]

Table 11-1 History of Apnea and Hypopnea Definitions

Year	Event
1976	Guilleminault describes OSA (≥30 apneas per night)[3]
1978	Block et al. describe hypopneas[4]
1980s	Use of the apnea index to diagnose OSA
1987	CMS (HCFA) accepts 30 **apneas** per night for diagnosis of OSA and payment for CPAP
1988	Gould et al. describe the sleep hypopnea syndrome[5]
1993	Wisconsin cohort study—occurrence of OSA in middle-aged adults (H4, hypopnea based on ≥ 30% drop in flow associated with a ≥ 4% desaturation)[6]
1993	Upper airway resistance syndrome described[7]
1997	Nasal pressure measurement described[8,9]
1999	Chicago Criteria for an obstructive apnea/hypopnea event published (Table 11-2)[10]
2000	Sleep Heart Health Study—association of AHI and hypertension (H4 hypopnea)[11]
2001	CMS accepts hypopneas for diagnosis of OSA (AH4I, AHI based on H4)[12]
2007	AASM scoring manual: two hypopnea definitions:[13] • Recommended: H4 (≥30% drop in airflow for ≥10 seconds + ≥4% drop in SaO_2) • Alternative: H3A-50 (≥50% drop in airflow for ≥10 seconds + ≥3% drop in SaO_2 or arousal)
2012	Sleep Apnea Definition Task Force[14] recommends: • H3A (≥30% drop in airflow for ≥10 seconds + ≥3% drop in SaO_2 or arousal)
2012	AASM scoring manual[15] recommends H3A (≥30% drop in flow + ≥ 3% desaturation or arousal)—single rule with a provision to report AH4I additionally if required by insurance
2017	AASM scoring manual: (two hypopnea definitions) • Recommended: H3A • Acceptable: H4
2018	AASM Position Paper: arousal-based scoring of respiratory events should be included in the PSG evaluation of obstructive sleep apnea[27]
2024	AASM Scoring Manual Version 3.0[30]. Recommended hypopnea definition H3A, option to report H4 in addition to H3A if needed for insurance reimbursement

AASM, American Academy of Sleep Medicine; *AHI,* apnea hypopnea index; *AH3AI,* AHI based on H3A; *AH4I,* AHI based on H4; *CMS,* Centers for Medicare and Medicaid Services; *CPAP,* continuous positive airway pressure; *H3A,* hypopnea based on ≥ 30% drop in airflow for ≥ 10 seconds + ≥3% desaturation or arousal; *H4,* hypopnea based on ≥30% drop in airflow for ≥10 seconds + ≥4% desaturation; *OSA,* obstructive sleep apnea.
Health Care Finance Administration (HCFA) renamed the **Centers for Medicare and Medicaid Services** in July, 2001.

Subsequently it was recognized that reductions in airflow from obstructive events not associated with desaturations could be associated with consequences such as arousal from sleep, sleep fragmentation, and daytime symptoms. In 1993, the *upper airway resistance syndrome* was defined in patients without significant apnea/hypopnea using thermal sensors but with evidence of high upper airway resistance associated with arousal using esophageal manometry.[7] Esophageal manometry was not widely adopted because of its invasive nature. However, measurement of airflow using a nasal cannula connected to a pressure transducer was demonstrated to be more accurate for detection of changes in airflow than thermal sensors.[8,9] A flattened nasal pressure inspiratory signal was also shown to reflect airflow limitation and upper airway narrowing. Hypopneas based on arousal as well as desaturation began to be used by some clinicians. The lack of agreement on respiratory event definitions was recognized. A consensus conference[10] published the "Chicago criteria" in 1999, which described an apnea/hypopnea respiratory event defined as a >50% drop in airflow (determined by an accurate measure of airflow) or a smaller but discernable drop in airflow associated with either a ≥3% drop in the arterial oxygen desaturation by oximetry (SpO_2) or an arousal (Table 11–2). The use of 3% versus 4% was based on reanalysis (unpublished) of the Wisconsin cohort data[6], which found that using a ≥3% drop in the SpO_2 produced similar results as a ≥4% drop.

Publications of results from the Sleep Heart Health Study,[11] a large multicenter population-based investigation, found an association between hypertension and an increased AHI based on hypopnea (H4) defined by a ≥30% decrease in airflow or thoracoabdominal excursions for 10 seconds or more accompanied by a 4% or greater decrease in oxygen saturation. Airflow was monitored with an oronasal thermal sensor and respiratory effort with RIP belts. The choice of 4% was arbitrary but based on historical precedent. In 2001, CMS accepted an AHI based on a hypopnea definition of ≥30% drop in airflow associated with a ≥4% drop in the SpO_2 (AH4I) for diagnosis of OSA.[12] In 2007, the American Academy of Sleep Medicine (AASM) published the first edition of the *AASM Manual for the Scoring of Sleep and Associated Events* manual[13] (hereinafter referred to as the AASM scoring manual) with a *recommended* hypopnea definition (≥30% drop in airflow for ≥ 10 seconds associated with a ≥4% arterial oxygen desaturation, H4) and an *alternative* hypopnea definition (**50% drop in airflow for ≥ 10 seconds and an associated** ≥3% desaturation OR arousal, H3A-50) (Table 11–2). Use of the H3A-50 definition resulted in an increased percentage of patients diagnosed with OSA in a study of a sleep clinic population.[14] The sleep apnea definition task force of the AASM developed consensus respiratory event definitions and recommended use of a hypopnea definition based on a ***≥30% drop in airflow*** for ≥ 10 seconds and an associated ≥3% arterial oxygen desaturation or arousal (H3A).[15] In 2012, a revision of the AASM scoring manual recommended *only the H3A hypopnea definition* with a provision to report AH4I if required for CPAP reimbursement for patients.[16] Because a large fraction of sleep centers used only the AH4I as required for CPAP reimbursement in their locales, the 2017 the AASM scoring manual defined hypopnea based on two definitions: H3A (recommended) and H4 (acceptable).[17] These hypopnea definitions are also present in the 2020 version of the AASM scoring manual.[18] Studies have documented the wide variation of the percentage of individuals diagnosed with OSA depending on the hypopnea definition.[19,20] Analysis of the sleep heart health cohort by Ho and coworkers[21] found the following median values of the AHI using various definitions: 5.4/hour (AH4I), 9.7/hour (AH3I), and 13.4/hour (AH3AI), where the AHI values were determined using a hypopnea definition based on a ≥4% desaturation, ≥3% desaturation, and a ≥3% desaturation or arousal, respectively. Of interest, much less divergence in the metrics is seen at the higher AHI values.

Proponents of the H4 definition contend that this metric is associated with cardiovascular morbidity[21,22] and has a better interscorer reliability[23] than a metric based on arousal. Proponents of the H3A definition contend that the H4 definition excludes individuals that would benefit from treatment of sleep apnea. Thin individuals and those with normal lungs tend to have milder drops in the SpO_2 with respiratory events. In a study by Won et al. the AH3A metric identified additional patients with OSA diagnosed with AH3AI compared with the AH4I metric (AH4I < 5/hour, AH3AI ≥ 5/hour) who were sleepy but who were not at increased risk for cardiovascular disease.[24] The *inclusion of arousal in the hypopnea diagnostic criteria* was required for 63% of the group to reach the AH3A ≥5/hour cutoff.[24] That is, most would not have been diagnosed using oxygen saturation (≥3% desaturation) alone. This has implications for home sleep apnea testing, which cannot detect EEG-based arousals. The fact that the milder group diagnosed by AH3AI but not AH4I was not at increased risk for cardiovascular disease is not surprising. In fact, an increased risk of cardiovascular disease in most studies is documented only in severe OSA (AHI ≥ 30/hour) using any definition of AHI.[11,24] Therefore, an emphasis on improving symptoms rather than cardiovascular risk is likely most

Table 11-2 Summary of Hypopnea Definitions

Chicago Criteria[10]	• Obstructive apnea/hypopnea event >50% decrease in valid measure of airflow Clear amplitude reduction in valid measure of airflow (less than 50% reduction) with ≥3% oxygen desaturation OR arousal
CMS[12]	• Hypopnea ≥30% reduction in airflow and ≥4% oxygen desaturation
AASM 2007[13]	• Recommended hypopnea definition (H4) ≥30% reduction in airflow and ≥4% oxygen desaturation • Alternative hypopnea definition ≥**50% reduction** in airflow and ≥3% oxygen desaturation OR arousal
AASM scoring manual, version 2.6[18]	• Recommended hypopnea definition (H3A) ≥30% reduction in airflow and ≥3% oxygen desaturation OR arousal • Acceptable hypopnea (H4) ≥30% reduction in airflow and ≥4% oxygen desaturation
AASM scoring manual, version 3.0[30]	Recommended hypopnea definition (H3A), AHI using H3A must be reported Optional: report number of hypopneas (H4) and related AHI

AASM, American Academy of Sleep Medicine; AHI, apnea hypopnea index; *CMS*, Centers for Medicare and Medicaid Services.
Chicago Criteria Sleep-related breathing disorders in adults: recommendations for syndrome definition and measurement techniques in clinical research. The Report of an American Academy of Sleep Medicine Task Force. *Sleep*. 1999;22(5):667-689.

relevant to the discussion of choosing a hypopnea definition in patients with mild to moderate OSA.

Proponents of the H3A definition point out that use of the *H4 definition is less likely to result in a diagnosis of OSA in women and younger individuals*.[25] In fact, **using either** definition of hypopnea (H3A or H4), the percentage of normal populations with an AHI ≥ 5/hour is quite large.[20] In the study by Hirotsu et al about 47% of a general population had an AH4I ≥ 5/hr and 72% and AH3AI ≥ 5/hr.[20] Recall that a diagnosis of the *OSA syndrome* is based on both an AHI and symptoms in the lower range of AHI values. For example, diagnosis of OSA in the third edition text revision of the *International Classification of Sleep Disorders* requires that if the AHI is ≥ 5/hour but less than 15/hour, there must be associated symptoms.[26] The hypopnea controversy continues at the time of writing of this text. CMS and most private insurers still mandate use of the H4 hypopnea definition. In 2018, the AASM issued a position statement stating that arousal-based hypopnea scoring should be included when polysomnography was performed to diagnose OSA.[27] Indeed, the intent of the AASM board of directors was to have the AASM scoring manual have a recommended hypopnea definition (H3A) that must be reported with the option of also reporting hypopneas scored based on a ≥4% desaturation (H4). It was recognized that many sleep centers would need to report an AHI based on the H3A definition as well as an AHI based on the H4 definition. A hypopnea scoring rule task force was appointed by the board of directors of the AASM with the mandate to create a strategy for adoption and implementation of the AASM-recommended adult hypopnea scoring criteria (H3A) among members, payers, and device manufacturers in advance of the planned change in the AASM scoring manual. The task force identified the group of patients diagnosed with OSA using AH3AI but not AH4I (H4NOSA)[28] as the group of interest to support use of the AH3AI. There is limited data on this group, but one study suggested that they are as sleepy as other patients with OSA and could benefit from treatment.[29] In this study the inclusion of arousals was required for diagnosis in about one-third of the H4NOSA group. In this investigation home sleep apnea testing with an artificial intelligence algorithm to detect arousal was the method to diagnose OSA. Patients were randomized to treatment with auto-adjusting positive airway pressure (autoCPAP, APAP) with Standard Care (sleep hygiene education plus a follow-up telephone call to check on progress with improvement in sleep behaviors) versus Standard Care alone. Improvement in subjective sleepiness and a vitality scale were demonstrated in the APAP group but not the Standard Care alone group. More studies of the effects of PAP treatment on the H4NOSA group are needed. The hypopnea task force conferred with polysomnography software vendors about the need of many sleep centers to report two different AHI values. It was determined that this requires minimal additional scoring time as the H4 events can be identified by software from those H3A events already scored. The newly published version 3.0 of the AASM scoring manual[30] mandates that the H3A recommended definition must be used (and the number of H3A events as well as the AH3AI reported). There is the *option* of *also* reporting the number of H4 events and the derived AH4I if required by insurance.

RESPIRATORY EVENT DEFINITIONS

This chapter discusses scoring respiratory events from signals recorded using polysomnography. The rules for scoring respiratory events in home sleep apnea testing using airflow are similar, but fewer respiratory signals are usually recorded. Home sleep apnea testing and the rules for scoring respiratory events in this type of monitoring are discussed in Chapter 16.

Apnea

The AASM scoring manual[17,30] defines apnea as a ≥90% drop in the peak signal excursion compared with pre-event baseline for ≥10 seconds using an **oronasal thermal sensor** (diagnostic study), PAP device flow (titration study), or alternative apnea sensor (diagnostic study). The recommended apnea sensor is an **oronasal thermal sensor** rather than a nasal pressure sensor (nasal cannula connected to a pressure transducer). Nasal pressure sensors may not detect oral airflow, and an event that appears to be an apnea (using nasal pressure) may be a hypopnea (reduced but not absent airflow using an oronasal thermal sensor) (Figure 11–1). If the oronasal sensor is not functioning or the signal is not reliable, alternative apnea sensors are to be used. Recommended alternative apnea sensors (diagnostic study) include the nasal pressure signal and respiratory inductance

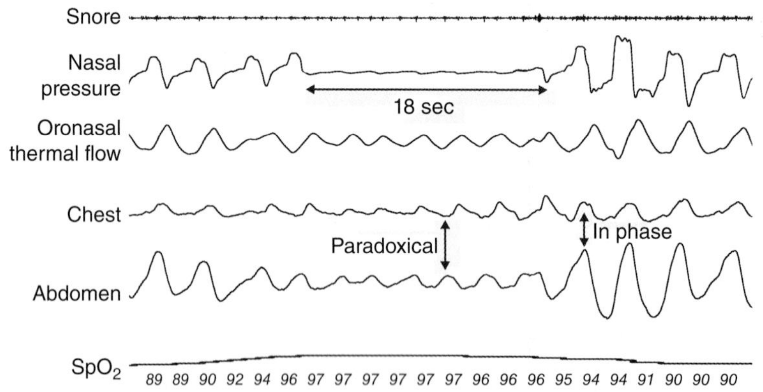

Figure 11–1 Hypopnea, not apnea. The oronasal thermal flow signal is the recommended sensor for scoring apnea, and the deflections have not decreased ≥90% (therefore insufficient to score an apnea). The nasal pressure signal has absent deflections, and a hypopnea can be scored. Note the paradoxical breathing in the chest and abdomen during the event but in phase deflections before and after the event. This is an obstructive hypopnea. Nasal pressure monitoring may not detect oral breathing and for this reason, oronasal thermal sensors are used to complement the nasal pressure signal for detection of airflow. The chest and abdomen tracings are from chest and abdominal respiratory inductance plethysmography belts. The direction of inspiration is upward.

plethysmopgraphy (RIP) sum and flow signals (RIPsum, RIPflow). RIPsum is the sum of the RIPchest and RIPabdomen effort belt signals and RIPflow is the time derivative of RIPsum. The nasal pressure signal can be used with or without a square root transformation. RIP signals can be used with or without calibration. Deflections in the RIPsum and RIPflow are estimates of tidal volume and flow, respectively. The polyvinylidene (PVDF) sum signal (PVDFsum) is the sum of the signals from chest and abdominal PVDF belts and is an acceptable alternative signal to score apneas. See Chapter 10 for a complete discussion of airflow sensors. Apneas are classified as obstructive, central, or mixed based on the associated respiratory effort. Respiratory effort sensors include esophageal manometry and dual RIP effort belts (classified as recommended by the AASM scoring manual) and PVDF effort belts (classified as acceptable). An obstructive apnea is associated with continued or increased effort during the event. A central apnea is associated with absent effort during the entire event. A mixed apnea has an initial central portion followed by an obstructive portion (once respiratory effort returns during the event). Examples of the different types of apneas are shown in Figure 11–2. Note that scoring an apnea (including a central apnea) does NOT require an associated desaturation in adults. Patients with frequent respiratory events often have epochs of wake occurring between respiratory events. A portion of a respiratory event may be present in an epoch scored as wakefulness. The AASM scoring manual states:[17,30]

> *If an apnea or hypopnea event begins or ends during an epoch that is scored as sleep, then the corresponding respiratory event can be scored and included in the computation of the AHI. In this situation a portion of the respiratory event may occur in an epoch scored as wake. However, if the apnea or hypopnea occurs entirely during an epoch scored as wake, it should not be scored or counte d toward the apnea-hypopnea index.*

Summary of Apnea Detection

Apnea Rule

- ≥90% decrease in the peak signal excursion compared to baseline breathing using an oronasal thermal sensor (diagnostic study), PAP device flow (titration study), or an alternative apnea sensor (diagnostic study)
- Duration of the ≥90% decrease in the apnea sensor signal is ≥10 seconds

Alternative Apnea Sensors

- Recommended: nasal pressure (with or without square root transformation), RIPsum and RIPflow (calibrated or non-calibrated)
- Acceptable: (sum of PVDF chest and abdominal effort belt signals)

Apnea Classification:

- Obstructive: respiratory effort present during the entire event
- Central: respiratory effort absent during the entire event
- Mixed: initial central portion followed by an obstructive portion

Hypopnea

The hypopnea definition recommended by the AASM scoring manual[17,30] is a ≥30% reduction in the peak signal excursion compared with pre-event baseline for ≥10 seconds using a nasal pressure transducer (diagnostic study), PAP device flow (titration study), or alternative hypopnea sensor (diagnostic study) associated with either a ≥3% drop in the arterial oxygen saturation or an arousal. The definition for scoring arousals is discussed in Chapter 3. Here nasal pressure can be used with or without a square root transformation. Alternative hypopnea sensors for diagnostic studies are used if the nasal pressure signal is not functioning or the signal is not reliable. The recommended alternative hypopnea sensors include an oronasal thermal sensor, the RIPsum or RIPflow signals (calibrated or uncalibrated), and dual thoracoabdominal RIP effort belts. The PVDF sum is an acceptable alternative signal to score hypopneas. There is a detailed discussion of sensors used to detect hypopneas in Chapter 10. In version 2.6 of the AASM scoring manual,[17] the ***acceptable*** hypopnea definition was a ≥30% reduction in hypopnea sensor signal for ≥10 seconds associated with a ≥4% drop in the arterial oxygen saturation. The presence or absence of an arousal was not considered. With the publication of version 3.0 of the AASM scoring manual,[30] the recommended hypopnea definition must be used and an AHI determined using this definition reported. Now the previously "acceptable" hypopnea definition is identified as *optional rather than acceptable.* That is, the number of hypopneas based on the newly defined optional hypopnea definition and an AHI based on this hypopnea definition *may also be reported.* In summary, sleep reports must list the number of hypopneas scored using the recommended definition and the derived AHI based on this definition. There is the option of also reporting the number of hypopneas using the optional hypopnea definition and the derived AHI based on this hypopnea definition. An example of a hypopnea meeting both recommended and optional (formerly acceptable) criteria is shown in Figure 11–3.

Reduction in the amplitude of the chest and abdominal RIP belt signals can be used as an alternative hypopnea sensor (Chapter 10). If RIPsum or RIPflow are available these signals rather than a reduction in the dual RIP effort belt signals is typically used as an alternative signal to score hypopneas.

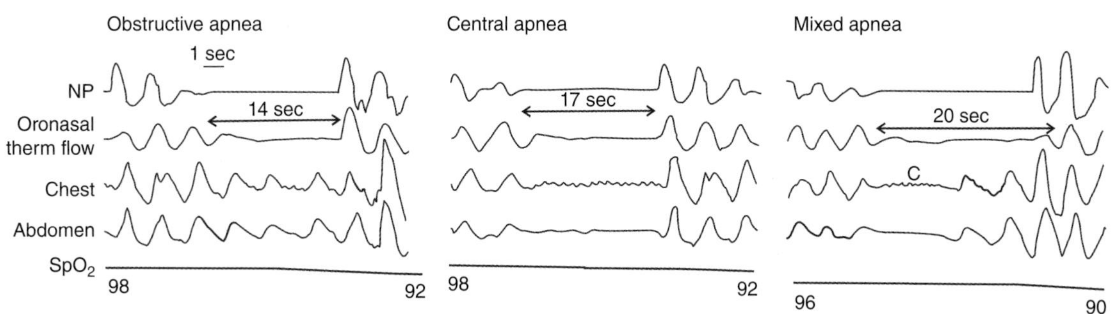

Figure 11–2 The three types of apneas are illustrated. and the direction of inspiration is upward. Although arterial oxygen desaturation is illustrated, desaturation is not required to score an apnea in adults. *C,* Central portion of the event; *NP,* nasal pressure. (Adapted from Berry RB: Fundamentals of sleep medicine, Philadelphia, 2012, Saunders, p 124.)

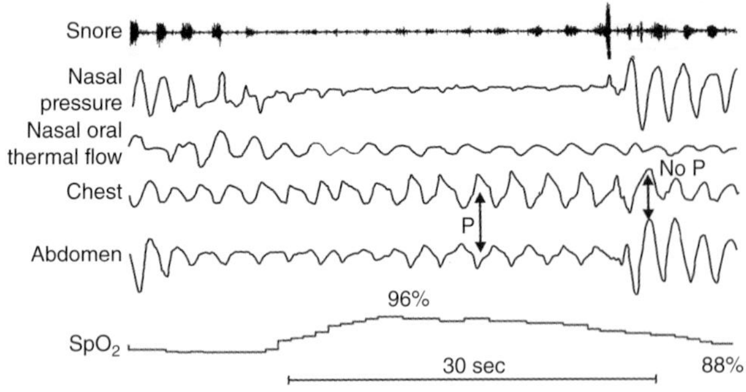

Figure 11–3 Obstructive hypopnea with snoring, flattening of the inspiratory nasal pressure waveform, and paradoxical motion of the chest and abdomen tracings (respiratory inductance plethysmography effort belts). In this tracing, inspiration is upward. (Reproduced from Berry RB: Fundamentals of sleep medicine, Philadelphia, 2012, Saunders, p 130.)

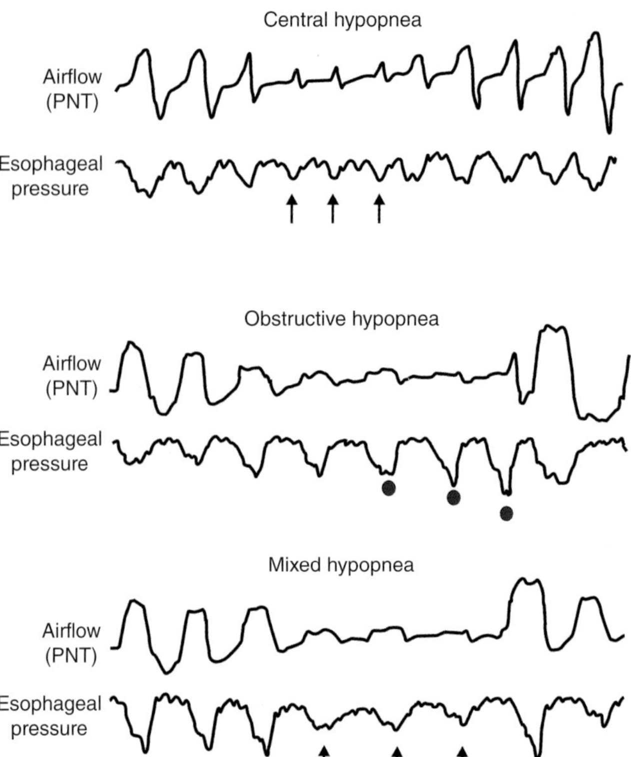

Figure 11–4 Hypopnea types as demonstrated by airflow monitoring using a pneumotachograph *(PNT)* in a mask over the nose and mouth and respiratory effort monitoring using esophageal pressure. Inspiration is upward. The central hypopnea shows the reduced effort *(small arrows)*. The airflow inspiratory profile is rounded. The obstructive hypopnea shows increasing pressure deflections (*round red dots* show increased effort) while flow is decreasing. In the "Mixed Hypopnea," there is evidence of upper airway narrowing (flattened inspiratory flow) and reduced respiratory effort. Classification of hypopneas as obstructive or central is difficult for "mixed" events with evidence of both increased upper airway resistance and reduced respiratory effort even with the use of sophisticated monitoring that is not available for clinical sleep studies (supraglottic or esophageal pressure monitoring and use of a PNT for accurate measurement of airflow). (From Berry RB. *Fundamentals of Sleep Medicine,* Elsevier; 2012:129.)

Note in Figure 11–1 the reduction in amplitude in the chest and abdominal RIP tracings during the first portion of the hypopnea as well as the paradoxical motion during the event. Depending on the type of RIP effort belts and whether or not the signals are calibrated, paradoxical movement is often noted during obstructive hypopneas (reduced airflow due to increased upper airway resistance). In Figure 11–3 the chest and abdominal RIP tracings do not decrease during the event but do show paradoxical breathing at the end of the event but not after the event. A good example of a reduction in the deflections in the chest and abdominal RIP tracings during a hypopnea can be seen in Chapter 10 (Figure 10-11).

Classification of Hypopneas

Hypopneas may be classified as obstructive (reduced airflow due to upper airway narrowing) or central (reduced airflow due to reduced respiratory effort). Definitive classification depends on an accurate measure of airflow (pneumotachograph or PAP flow sensor) and a measure of respiratory effort (or pressure drop across the upper airway). This requires esophageal manometry or a pressure sensor above the epiglottis to measure supraglottic airway pressure. Examples of obstructive and central hypopneas with accurate measures of airflow and effort are shown in Figure 11–4. An example of a "mixed" hypopnea with evidence of both increased upper airway narrowing (airflow limitation, flattening of the inspiratory airflow waveform) and reduced effort is also shown. The AASM scoring manual does not provide diagnostic criteria for mixed hypopneas. Airflow limitation is discussed in Chapter 10 and is usually associated with an increase in upper airway resistance.[9,31,32] The AASM scoring manual[17,30] provides the *option* to score hypopneas as obstructive or central. The main utility is that patients with the central sleep apnea syndrome with Cheyne-Stokes breathing (CSB) may exhibit hypopneas rather than apneas associated with the crescendo-decrescendo pattern of breathing. To characterize the severity of central sleep apnea in these patients, it is useful to provide a central apnea + central hypopnea index. This is discussed in more detail below. Because pneumotachographs (accurate airflow measurement) and esophageal pressure measurements are not used in clinical studies, the obstructive nature of the hypopnea is assumed by the presence or absence of associated snoring during the event, increased flattening of the airflow sensor signal, or thoracoabdominal paradox during the event but not pre-event. In the absence of these findings, the hypopnea is assumed to be central. Examples of obstructive hypopneas are shown in Figure 11–1 and 11-3 and a central hypopnea in Figure 11–5.

The ability to identify hypopneas as obstructive or central was evaluated by two studies[32,33] with different algorithms and found only fair interscorer reliability. Another approach to classify apneas and central or obstructive is to use the surface EMG of the chest wall to reflect inspiratory effort. The signal can be recorded with methods similar to those used to record limb EMG[34,35] and detects the inspiratory activity of the diaphragm and chest wall muscles.[34,35] Use of the surface EMG is discussed in Chapter 10. One issue with this signal is contamination of the signal with ECG artifact (although there are methods to remove artifact from the signal), and the other problem is that a good signal cannot be obtained in many patients. However, if recorded, rectified, and integrated, this signal provides a surrogate for esophageal pressure and an estimate of respiratory effort.[35] The signal is often referred to as the diaphragmatic EMG, but depending on the placement of the surface EMG electrodes the inspiratory activity of the external intercostal muscles may also contribute to the signal (hence

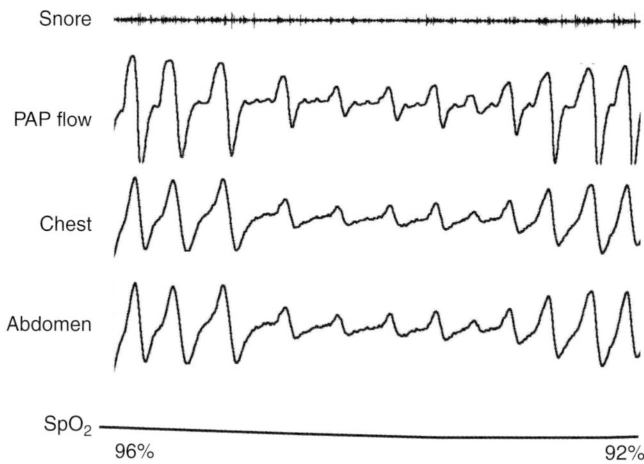

Figure 11–5 A central hypopnea is shown. Snoring, airflow flattening (PAP flow signal), and paradoxical movement of the chest and abdomen are not present. The PAP flow is the accurate airflow signal from a positive airway pressure device. Inspiration is upward. In central hypopneas there is a symmetrical decrease then increase in respiratory effort in parallel with changes in airflow.

referred to here as *chest wall EMG*). Using this signal and airflow one can compute a surrogate for airway resistance (resistance ratio or RR) for each breath as Δ *chest wall effort*/Δ flow with the value normalized to the pre-event breath.[34] The pattern of flow and effort across the event can be visualized (Figure 11–6). As one might expect, the average resistance surrogate for hypopneas meeting AASM criteria for an obstructive hypopnea is higher than that for hypopneas meeting criteria for a central hypopnea, but there is overlap (Figure 11–7). If one analyzes the average resistance surrogate (RR) over the first half (RR1) and last half of the hypopneas (RR2), a higher RR2/RR1 provides a better separation between AASM obstructive and central hypopneas (Figure 11–7). Central hypopneas have a symmetric fall and rise of effort and flow, but obstructive events show an increase in resistance over the last half of the hypopnea. As can be seen in Figure 11–7, whereas some hypopneas are obviously obstructive or central, there is a "gray" zone of intermediate RR values. Given the spectrum of the relative importance of decreased drive and increased upper airway resistance in characterizing hypopneas, efforts at characterizing the nature of all respiratory events to give an index of the degree of obstruction using complex analysis has been proposed.[36] Conductance (the inverse of resistance) is often used to analyze respiratory events because when flow is zero (apnea), resistance (pressure/flow) goes to infinity whereas the conductance is zero.

Summary of Hypopnea Detection

Hypopnea Rule (recommended)

- ≥30% decrease in the peak signal excursion compared to baseline breathing using nasal pressure (with or without square root transformation, diagnostic study), PAP device flow (titration study), or an alternative hypopnea sensor (diagnostic study)
- Duration of the ≥30% decrease in the apnea sensor signal is ≥10 seconds

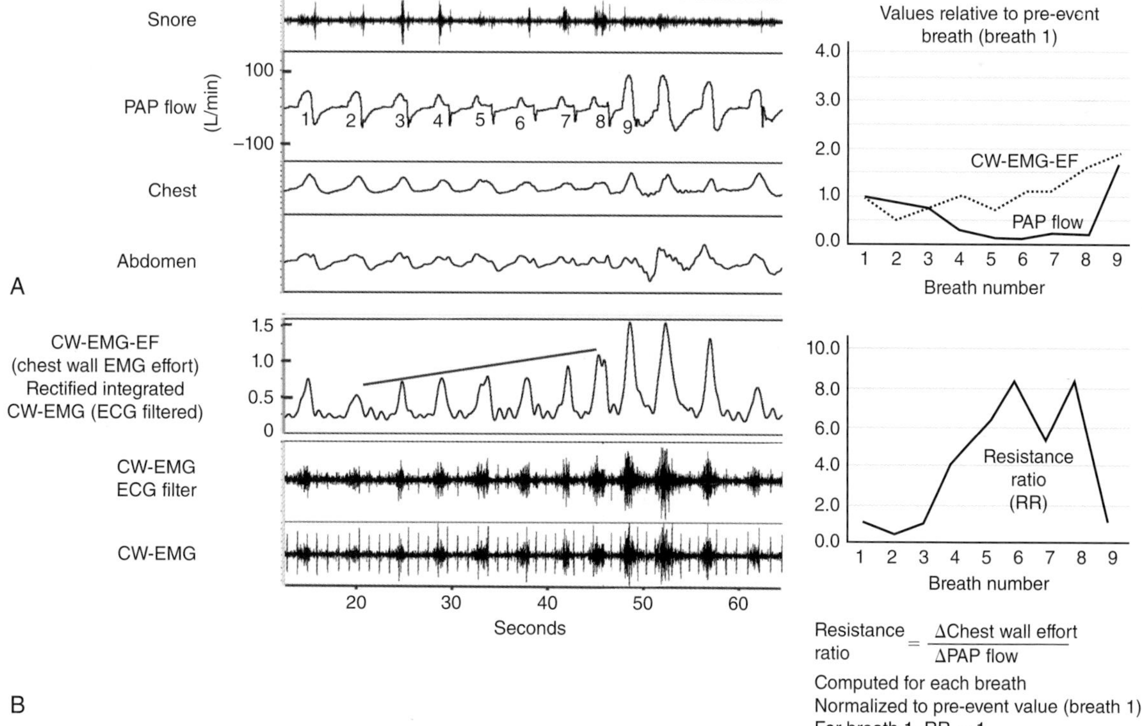

Figure 11–6 Characterization of an obstructive hypopnea using the rectified and integrated chest wall EMG signal to reflect effort *(CW-EMG-EF)* as a surrogate of the driving pressure for airflow. The resistance ratio (RR, a surrogate for airway resistance) is computed by dividing the change in effort by the change in flow for each breath and normalized to the pre-event breath (breath 1 with RR = 1 for breath 1. In this sample the airflow falls as the effort increases consistent with an increase in resistance **(A)** and the resistance ratio increases compared with pre-event values **(B)**. (Adapted from Berry RB, Ryals S, Wagner MH. Use of chest wall EMG to classify hypopneas as obstructive or central. *J Clin Sleep Med.* 2018;14(5):725-733.)

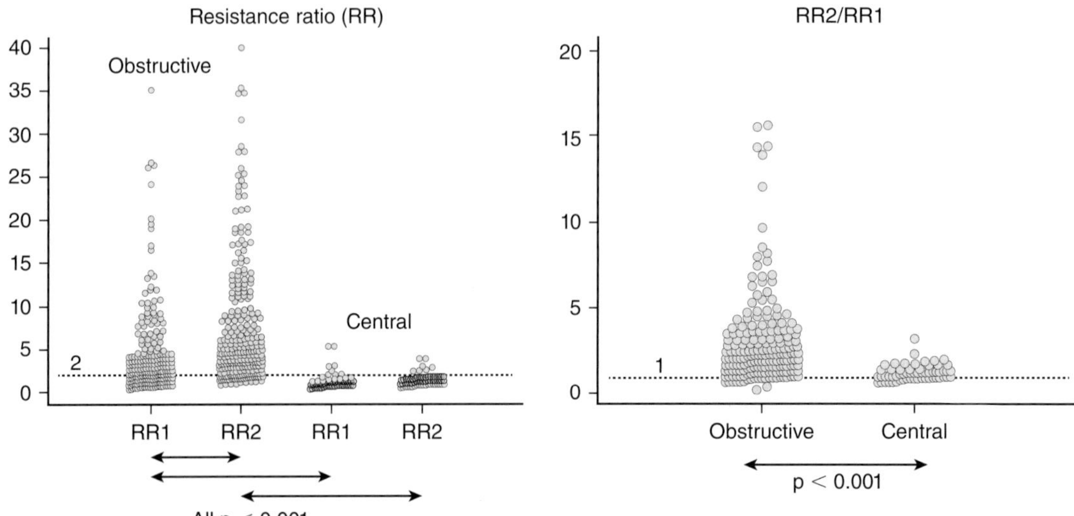

Figure 11–7 The resistance ratio (*RR*; a surrogate of upper airway resistance) for the first half *(RR1)* and second half *(RR2)* of the hypopneas is shown for hypopneas classified as obstructive and central by AASM criteria. There is overlap in the measurements. In all cases the RR values for each event are normalized based on the prehypopnea breath. In the right panel the RR2/RR1 ratio for each hypopnea is illustrated. Hypopneas are grouped by AASM classification as obstructive or central. Most obstructive hypopneas were characterized by a RR2/RR1 ratio greater than 1. That is, resistance is higher in the second half of events in obstructive hypopneas, but in central hypopneas the resistance in the first and second half of the events is similar (RR2/RR1 ≈ 1). (Adapted from Berry RB, Ryals S, Wagner MH. Use of chest wall EMG to classify hypopneas as obstructive or central. *J Clin Sleep Med.* 2018;14(5):725-733.)

- There is an associated ≥3% oxygen desaturation from pre-event baseline or an arousal

Alternative Hypopnea Sensors

- Recommended: oronasal thermal sensor, RIPsum, RIPflow, dual thoracoabdominal belts (RIP calibrated or non-calibrated)
- Acceptable: PVDF sum

Hypopnea Rule (option) - same as recommended except change in flow is associated with a ≥ 4% oxygen desaturation

Hypopnea Classification (optional)

- Obstructive: one or more of the following criteria are present
  1. Increased inspiratory flattening of nasal pressure or PAP device flow signal compared to baseline breathing
  2. Snoring
  3. Thoracoabdominal paradox that occurs during the event but not during pre-event breathing
- Central - if none of the above obstructive criteria are present

Determining Event Duration and Scoring Apnea Rather Than Hypopnea

Determining event duration is often difficult because the exact start and end of an event may be ambiguous. The AASM scoring manual[17,30] provides rules for determine event duration, but they are not always easy to apply. This is especially true when there is no stable breathing between events or when there is a gradual decrease in airflow before the event starts. The apnea or hypopnea duration is measured from the nadir preceding the first breath that is clearly reduced to the beginning of the first breath that approximates the baseline breathing amplitude. The signals used to measure the duration should use the recommended sensors (apnea or hypopnea sensors). The rules for determining event duration are illustrated in Figure 11–8 (Table 11–3). There are rare events in which a longer duration would qualify as a hypopnea, but a shorter portion qualifies as an apnea (Figure 11–9). The scoring manual states that "if a portion of a respiratory event that would otherwise meet criteria for a hypopnea meets criteria for an apnea, the event should be scored as an apnea."[17,30]

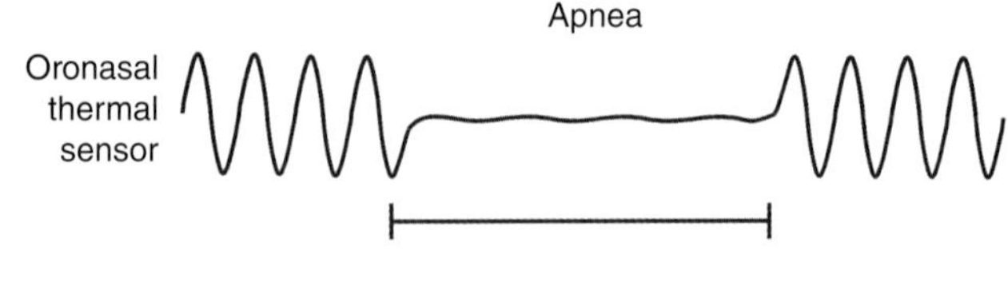

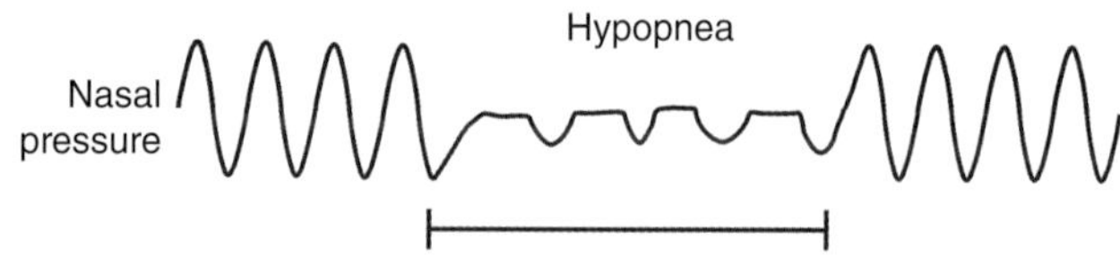

Figure 11–8 This figure shows measurement of event duration for an apnea (oronasal thermal airflow sensor) and for a hypopnea (nasal pressure sensor). During a positive airway pressure (PAP) titration study the PAP device flow is used for measurement of apnea and hypopne durations. The event starts with the nadir before the first clearly decreased breath and ends with the start of normal respiration. This is very idealized because airflow may slowly decrease before the event making identification of the starting point difficult.

Respiratory Effort–Related Arousals

Respiratory effort–related arousals (RERAs) are respiratory events characterized by increasing respiratory effort or flattening of the inspiratory portion of the nasal pressure or PAP flow signal leading to an arousal that ***do not meet* criteria for apnea or hypopnea.**[17,30] The AASM scoring manual states that scoring

Table 11-3 Measuring Respiratory Event Duration

- Apnea or hypopnea duration is measured from the nadir preceding the first breath that is clearly reduced to the beginning of the first breath that approximates the baseline breathing amplitude.
- For apnea duration, use the oronasal thermal sensor signal (diagnostic study) or PAP device flow signal (PAP titration study) to determine the event duration.
- For hypopnea event duration, use the nasal pressure signal (diagnostic study) or PAP device flow signal (PAP titration study).
- When diagnostic study sensors fail or are inaccurate, *alternative* sensors may be used.

PAP, Positive airway pressure.

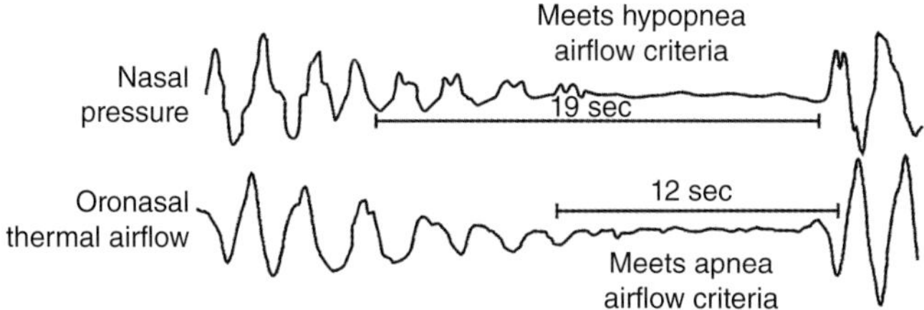

Figure 11–9 The illustrated event shows that if a portion of a respiratory event that would otherwise meet criteria for a hypopnea has a portion that would qualify as an apnea, the entire event is scored as an apnea.

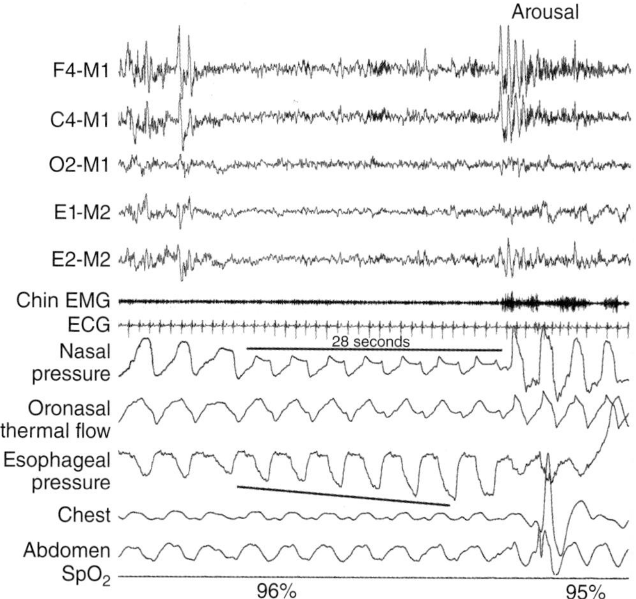

Figure 11–10 Hypopnea or respiratory effort-related arousal (RERA)? The event shown is a hypopnea using the recommended hypopnea definition (arousal present) but not using the optional (formerly named acceptable) hypopnea definition (only a 1% desaturation). If the optional definition of hypopnea (H4) is used, the event meets criteria for a RERA. Note the increasing esophageal effort (slanted line) with only subtle changes in the chest and abdominal respiratory inductance plethysmography (RIP) effort belts in this example. Now that scoring and reporting of H3A hypopneas is mandated by the American Academy of Sleep Medicine for all sleep studies, very few RERAs will be scored. Note that the scoring of RERAs is optional. (Adapted from Berry RB. *Fundamentals of Sleep Medicine.* Elsevier; 2012:127.)

RERAs is *optional.* Increasing respiratory effort can be accurately documented by esophageal pressure manometry (Figure 11–10), but this is rarely used in clinical practice. However, flattening of the inspiratory portion of the nasal pressure signal or PAP device flow signal identifies airflow limitation, a surrogate for increasing upper airway resistance, which is *usually* accompanied by increasing effort as the patient tries to maintain airflow.[9,31] As discussed in Chapter 10, flow limitation arousals (nasal pressure flattening associated with an arousal) and arousals associated with increased inspiratory effort by esophageal or supraglottic pressure monitoring are highly correlated, although not identical.[9,31] Airflow limitation (flattening of airflow signal) can occur without increased respiratory effort (Figure 11–4, bottom tracing). However, nasal pressure flattening is sufficient for identification of increased respiratory effort for most events and is used in clinical practice for detection of RERA events. Flattening of the airflow signal from positive airway pressure devices will also demonstrate flattening during events with airflow limitation. Of note, subtle changes in the chest and abdominal RIP effort belt tracings during RERAs may sometimes be noted with deflections out of phase or flattened reflecting periods of airflow limitation. The ability to detect more subtle change in effort depends on the type of RIP belt used, the placement of the belts, and whether or not the belt signals are calibrated. In Figure 11–10 there are subtle changes in the deflections of the chest and abdominal RIP signals, which are slightly out of phase and reduced in amplitude. However, these changes do not reflect the large increase in respiratory effort as noted in the esophageal pressure tracing or in the increasing amount of flattening in the nasal pressure signal. For most events, flattening of the inspiratory portion of the nasal pressure signal is a more sensitive method for detection of increased respiratory effort than changes in the effort belt signals.

A given respiratory event could be a hypopnea or a RERA depending on the hypopnea definition used. For example, a respiratory event is characterized by a ≥30% reduction in the nasal pressure signal for 15 seconds with inspiratory flattening of the nasal pressure signal, a 2% oxygen desaturation, and an associated arousal. Such an event would be a RERA if one used the optional hypopnea definition (H4) or a hypopnea using the *recommended* definition (H3A). If using the recommended hypopnea definition (H3A), there are very few RERAs.[37,38] Since publication of the new version of the scoring manual, a RERA would be scored only if it does not meet criteria for hypopnea using the H3A definition. Using the recommended hypopnea definition, an event associated with an arousal that exhibits inspiratory flattening but not a ≥30% drop in amplitude from baseline would meet criteria for a RERA but not a hypopnea (Figure 11–11). Such events are not common. If scoring RERAs, it is useful to calculate a RERA index = number of RERA/hours of sleep or number of RERAs × 60/total sleep time (min). Some patients may have an AH4I < 5 hour but an AH4I + RERA index ≥ 5/hour. RERA events are sometimes called *upper airway resistance events.* Now that reporting H3A hypopneas and an AHI based on this definition is recommended (must be included in all sleep reports), reporting RERAs has much less utility. As noted above, scoring RERAs is optional.

Summary of RERA Detection

- Scoring RERAs is optional.
- A sequence of breaths lasting ≥10 seconds characterized by increasing respiratory effort or by flattening of the inspiratory portion of the nasal pressure (diagnostic study) or PAP device flow (titration study) waveform leading to an arousal from sleep when the sequence of breaths does not meet criteria for an apnea or hypopnea.

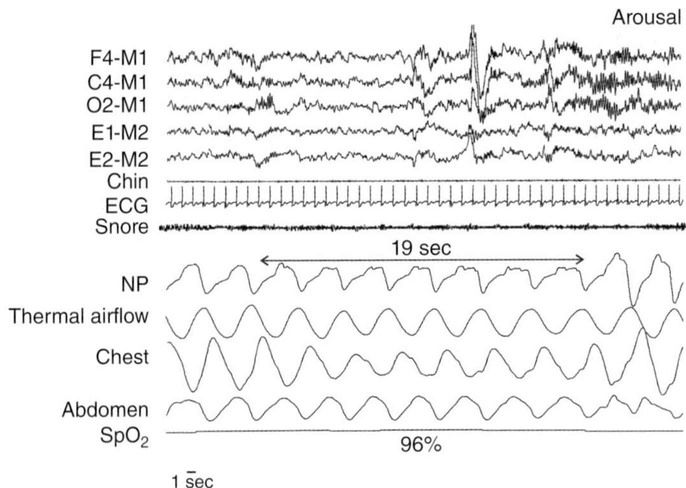

Figure 11–11 A respiratory effort–related arousal (RERA) is shown. Because the nasal pressure signal (NP) does not show a 30% decrease in amplitude from baseline, the event does not meet either the recommended or optional hypopnea definition. However, there is flattened inspiratory nasal pressure and an associated arousal. In this example, inspiration is upward. (Adapted from Berry RB. *Fundamentals of Sleep Medicine.* Elsevier; 2012:126.)

- Now that H3A hypopneas are scored as standard practice, there will be very few RERAs

AHI and RDI

The AHI is the number of apneas and hypopneas per hour of sleep. Another metric, the *respiratory disturbance index* (RDI), is often used as another designation for the AHI. However, the AASM scoring manual[17,30] recommends that the RDI be defined as the sum of the AHI and the RERA index **(RDI = AHI + RERA index),** where the RERA index is the number of RERAs per hour of sleep. To add to the RDI ambiguity, the CMS definitions use the term RDI for the number of apneas and hypopneas per hour of monitoring during home sleep testing when sleep is not recorded. The AASM scoring manual recommends use of the term *respiratory event index* (REI) for that circumstance. In any case, it is important to carefully determine the definition of RDI when reading publications or sleep study reports as well as the definition used for scoring hypopneas. Calculating an RDI is most useful if the AHI is based on hypopneas scored solely on the basis of arterial oxygen desaturation. In this case the RDI provides an estimate of the impact of respiration on sleep fragmentation not associated with desaturation. For most patients an AHI (based on a H4 definition) + RERA index is very similar to the AHI calculated with hypopneas based on both desaturation and arousals (AH3A).

Cheyne-Stokes Breathing (CSB)

CSB is a form of periodic breathing, with central apneas or central hypopneas at the nadir of effort and a crescendo-decrescendo pattern of breathing between respiratory events[17,30] (Figure 11–12). CSB is most often seen in patients with congestive heart failure (systolic and diastolic) and less commonly after a cerebrovascular accident. The cycle length is the time from the start of a central apnea to the end of the next crescendo-decrescendo respiratory phase (start of next apnea) (Figure 11–12). The longer the *ventilatory phase between central apneas,* the longer the circulation time and the lower the cardiac output and ejection fraction.[39] The cycle length is patients with congestive heart failure and a reduced ejection fraction is usually 60 to 90 seconds (see Chapter 30). Patients with congestive heart failure

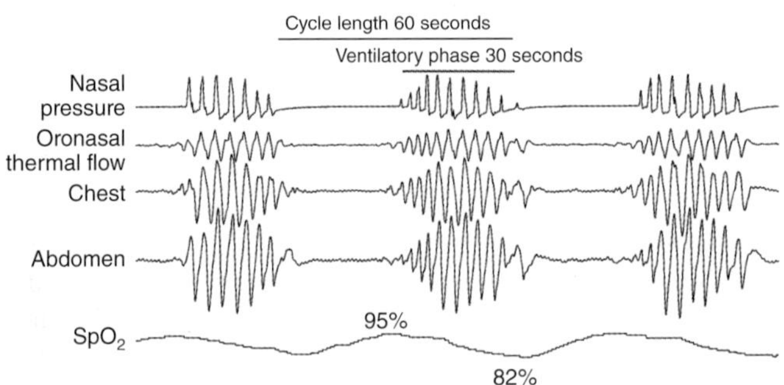

Figure 11–12 Cheyne-Stokes breathing with central apneas is shown. The cycle time is 60 seconds. The ventilatory phase between breaths is long and is suggestive of a long circulation time. In fact, the nadir in the arterial oxygen saturation by oximetry (SpO_2) is very delayed. (Reproduced from Berry RB: Fundamentals of sleep medicine, Philadelphia, 2012, Saunders, p 133.)

(CHF) and a normal (preserved) ejection fraction (HFPEF, diastolic heart failure) have a shorter cycle time than those with systolic dysfunction, but the cycle time is usually >40 seconds.[39] The crescendo decrescendo pattern of ventilation can also be see in individuals without heart failure but the cycle length is usually 40 to 50 seconds in duration. The AASM scoring manual (version 2.6) rules for scoring CSB[18] require both of the following to be present: (a) ≥3 consecutive central apneas or central hypopneas separated by a crescendo-decrescendo pattern of respiration and a *cycle length ≥40 seconds* and (b) there must be ≥ 5 central apneas and/or central hypopneas per hour of sleep associated with the crescendo-decrescendo breathing pattern recorded over ≥2 hours of monitoring. Criterion (b) is arbitrary and based on consensus[15] but is similar to CMS requirements for the minimal number of obstructive events to make a diagnosis of OSA. As mentioned previously, some patients with CSB have a significant proportion of events with central hypopneas at the nadir of breathing (Figure 11–13). Ideally, these events should be used to determine the amount of CSB. However, not every sleep center classifies hypopneas as central or obstructive (optional). Version 3.0 of the AASM scoring manual[30] has changed the scoring rule for CSB to address this issue. The revised CSB scoring rule states "there are episodes of ≥3

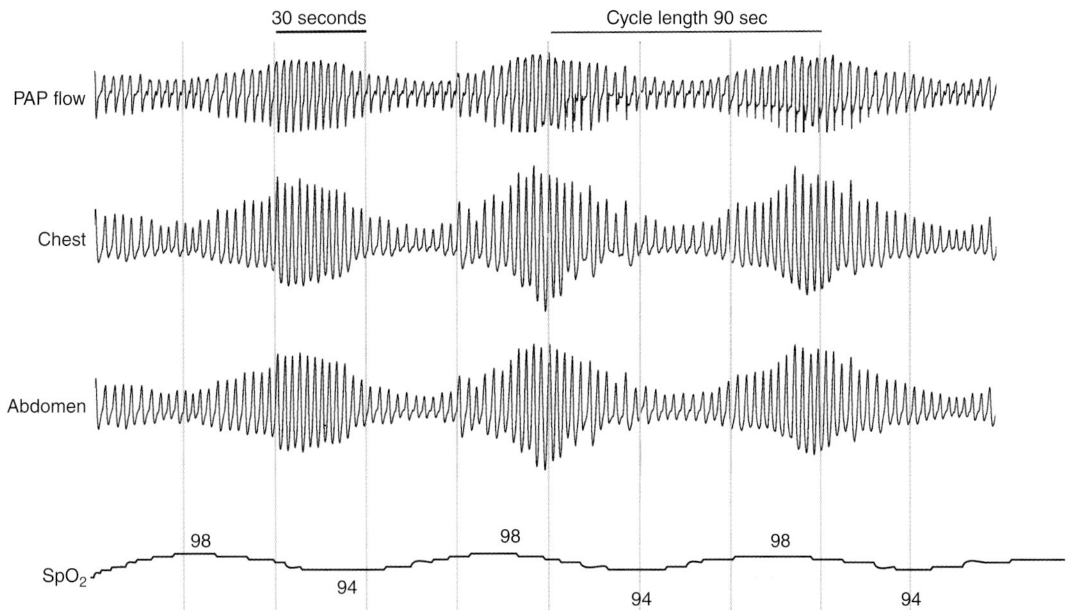

Figure 11–13 Cheyne-Stokes breathing with central hypopneas at the nadir in PAP flow and respiratory effort. In this case note the rounded inspiratory profile in the PAP flow during the hypopneas. Although not shown, snoring was absent. The hypopneas meet criteria for central hypopneas. The cycle length is measured from peak effort to peak effort. Note unlike central apneas, central hypopneas must be associated with a ≥ 3% desaturation or arousal (that is meet hypopnea criteria). Chest and Abdomen are RIP effort belts.

consecutive central apneas *and/or hypopneas* (hypopneas replaces central hypopneas) separated by a crescendo and decrescendo change in breathing amplitude with a cycle length of ≥40 seconds. To be included, the hypopneas must have a symmetrical decrescendo-crescendo pattern of tidal volume or flow." In version 3.0 of the AASM scoring manual, a note states that individual apneas and hypopneas during a run of CSB can be scored as individual apneas and hypopneas. To qualify patients with complex sleep apnea for a PAP device with a backup rate, residual central events during a PAP titration (after obstructive events are effectively reduced) must make up more than 50% of the total respiratory events (see Chapter 24), hence the desire to include the hypopneas associated with CSB as central events (central hypopnea). The hypopneas occurring during a run of CSB can be scored as central hypopneas if they meet central hypopnea criteria.

Summary of Cheyne-Stokes Breathing Detection

Both of the following are present:

- Episodes of ≥3 consecutive central apneas and/or **hypopneas** separated by a crescendo and decrescendo change in breathing amplitude (respiratory effort) with a **cycle length of ≥40 seconds.**
- To be included the hypopneas must have a symmetrical crescendo-decrescendo pattern of tidal volume or flow.
- There must be ≥5 central apneas and/or **hypopneas** per hour of sleep associated with the crescendo-decrescendo breathing pattern recorded over ≥ 2 hours of monitoring.
- Cycle length is the time from the start of a central apnea to the end of the next crescendo-decrescendo respiratory phase (start of next apnea). Individual central apneas/hypopneas within a run of CSB are also scored if they meet criteria for apnea and hypopnea. Although not stated in the AASM scoring manual, the cycle length of CSB with hypopneas can be defined as the time between two consecutive zeniths in airflow (Figure 11–13). If a hypopnea associated with CSB meets criteria it can be scored as a central hypopnea (optional).

Hypoventilation

Hypoventilation during **wakefulness** is usually defined as a partial pressure of arterial carbon dioxide ($PaCO_2$) > 45 mm Hg (some use ≥45 mm Hg). During clinical sleep monitoring, continuous monitoring of the $PaCO_2$ is not practical. According to the AASM scoring manual,[17,30] acceptable surrogates of the $PaCO_2$ include end-tidal PCO_2 (diagnostic study) or transcutaneous PCO_2 (diagnostic or PAP titration studies) (Figure 11–14). For adults, monitoring for hypoventilation is

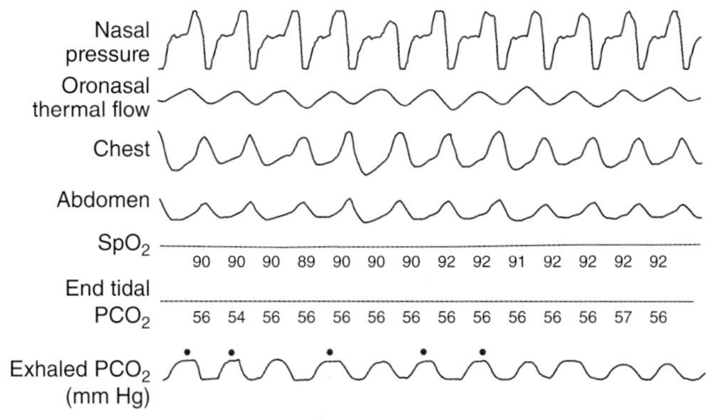

Figure 11–14 A tracing from a patient with hypoventilation. There is a mild and stable decrease in the arterial oxygen saturation by pulse oximetry (SpO_2) but end-tidal PCO_2 monitoring reveals hypoventilation. This patient had more than 10 minutes with a PCO_2 above 55 mm Hg. The end-tidal PCO_2 channel simply registers the recent value, whereas the exhaled PCO_2 waveform show the instantaneous exhaled PCO_2 value versus time tracing. A plateau in the PCO_2 waveform *(dots)* is required for an accurate estimate of the arterial PCO_2. (Adapted from Berry RB, Wagner MH. *Sleep Medicine Pearls.* 3rd ed. Elsevier; 2015:123.)

optional for both diagnostic and PAP titration studies. For children, monitoring for hypoventilation is recommended during diagnostic studies. The AASM criteria for hypoventilation include either (a) an increase in the $PaCO_2$ (or surrogate) to a value **> 55 mm** Hg (not ≥) for ≥10 minutes or (b) there is a ≥10 mm Hg increase in the $PaCO_2$ (or surrogate) during sleep (in comparison to an awake supine value) to a value **exceeding 50 mm Hg** for ≥10 minutes. Although one might infer that hypoventilation is present in the setting of a low SpO_2 without discrete respiratory events, the AASM scoring manual requires documentation of a qualifying measurement of the PCO_2 for a diagnosis of hypoventilation. Technical aspects of CO_2 monitoring are discussed in Chapter 10. It is important to note that for adults, scoring hypoventilation is **optional** but is very useful for evaluation of patients with chronic hypoventilation during diagnostic or PAP titration sleep studies. Figure 11–14 shows an example of a patient with a mild decrease in the SpO_2 without obvious change in flow signals. However, hypoventilation is documented by the measure of the end-tidal PCO_2 as the patient had more than 10 minutes with an end-tidal PCO_2 above 55 mm Hg.

Summary for Scoring Hypoventilation

- An increase in the $PaCO_2$ (or surrogate) to >55 mm Hg for ≥10 minutes

or

- An increase in the $PaCO_2$ (or surrogate) by ≥10 mm Hg (in comparison to an awake supine value) to a value **exceeding 50 mm Hg** for ≥10 minutes

ADDITIONAL CONSIDERATIONS FOR SCORING RESPIRATORY EVENTS

Positive Airway Pressure Titrations With a Backup Rate

During PAP titration sleep studies when bilevel positive airway pressure with a backup rate is being used, there are events associated with machine-triggered pressure pulses (pressure support) with the PAP flow showing a pattern consistent with an apnea (Figure 11–15). There has been controversy as to whether to score such an event as a central apnea or an obstructive apnea. Because there is no spontaneous patient effort, the AASM scoring manual[17,30] scores this event as a central apnea. This phenomenon is likely because of a closed (or nearly closed) upper airway, which can occur during central events.[40] A small amount of flow can be present and sometimes small deflections are seen in chest and abdominal tracings, but these deflections are concurrent with the machine-triggered pulses (pressure support) and are not spontaneous efforts.

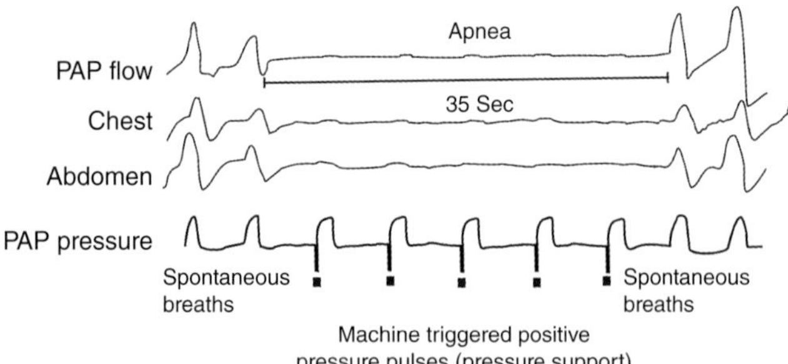

Figure 11–15 An example of an apnea during machine-triggered pressure pulses. The positive pressure pulses (pressure support) that are machine-triggered are marked by the downward artifact added to the patient pressure signal from the laboratory positive airway pressure *(PAP)* device. The small deflections in the chest and abdomen are associated with very small amounts of airflow and are not spontaneous inspiratory efforts. The PAP flow signal shows ≥ 90% reduction from baseline (meets apnea criteria). The American Academy of Sleep Medicine (AASM) scoring manual classifies such an event as a central apnea. The upper airway is closed (or very narrow), consistent with a closed airway central apnea. However, the AASM scoring manual does not use this terminology. Different laboratory PAP devices mark device-triggered events in different ways. This figure illustrates the method used by Philips-Respironics devices. See Chapter 24 for more information on this topic.

The AASM scoring manual states:

Score a respiratory event occurring during PAP device triggered breaths as central apnea if ALL of the following criteria are met:

- There is no evidence of spontaneous (patient triggered) respiratory effort during the event
- There is a decrease in the PAP flow signal meeting apnea criteria
- Device triggered pressure pulses (pressure support) occur during the event

False Classification of Apneas as Central

During obstructive respiratory events, movement in the chest and abdomen often decreases. In some circumstances minimal or ambiguous deflections in the chest and abdominal bands can result in an event being incorrectly scored as central when it is actually obstructive.[41] One approach is to increase the sensitivity of chest and abdominal tracings (Figure 11–16), although this may result in chest or abdominal effort belt signal intrusion into other adjacent traces. The second is to use surface chest wall/diaphragmatic EMG recording[42] (Figure 11–17), as discussed in Chapter 10. In Figure 11–17 inspiratory bursts of EMG activity are seen during an event that might otherwise have been scored as a central apnea.

Relationship of Arousal and Respiratory Event

The AASM scoring manual does not specify a maximum time interval from respiratory event termination until arousal initiation for the arousal to be considered respiratory. Arousals associated with respiratory event termination can occur slightly before, concurrent with, or after event termination.[43] A recent study found that 90% of hypopnea-associated arousals started

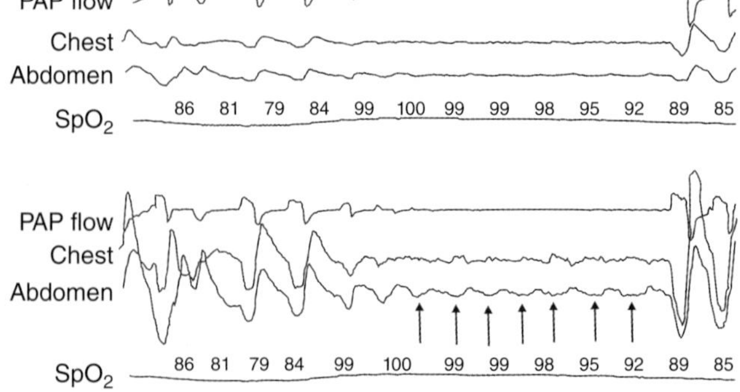

Figure 11–16 False classification of apnea as central. The *upper panel* shows minimal deflection in the chest and abdominal tracings during apnea. The *lower panel* shows definite deflections *(arrows)* after an increase in sensitivity (gain) of the chest and abdominal channels. (Adapted from Ryals et al with permission. Ryals S, McCullough L, Wagner M, Berry R, Dibra M. A case of treatment-emergent central sleep apnea? *J Clin Sleep Med.* 2020;16(2):331-334.)

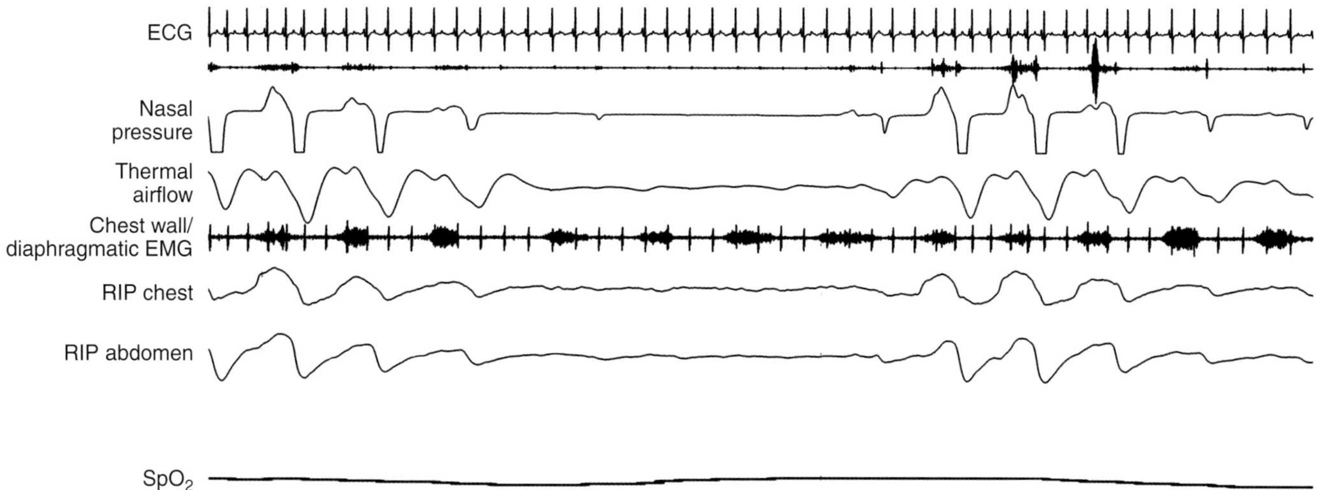

Figure 11–17 Demonstration of respiratory effort during apnea using chest wall/diaphragmatic EMG. Inspiratory bursts are noted, although there are minimal if any deflections during apnea in the chest and abdominal effort channels. The events would likely be misclassified as a central apnea based on the respiratory effort belt deflections.

no earlier than 6 seconds before and no later than 14 seconds after the end of hypopneas, with the peak of the distribution coinciding with event end time.[44] Of note, arousals associated with CSB are often noted just before or at the zenith of inspiratory effort that can follow the termination of apnea by over 10 seconds in some cases. However, the start of the arousal is usually before the zenith of inspiratory effort. Arousals associated with CSB can be grouped into early (within 3 seconds before or after apnea termination) or late arousals (starting >8 seconds after apnea termination.[45] A study[46] found that a substantial number of arousals start just before or at the start of the ventilatory phase of CSB. However, the second quarter of the ventilatory phase was found to be the most common location of the start of arousals. In the literature CSB is usually characterized as having arousals preceding the zenith of respiratory effort rather than soon after apnea termination.[39]

SUMMARY OF KEY POINTS

1. The AASM scoring manual defines apnea as a ≥90% reduction in the peak signal excursion compared with pre-event baseline for ≥10 seconds using an **oronasal thermal sensor** (diagnostic study), PAP device flow (titration study), or an alternative apnea sensor (diagnostic study). The oronasal thermal sensor can detect both nasal and oral breathing.
2. An obstructive apnea is associated with continued or increased respiratory effort during the event. A central apnea is associated with absent effort during the entire event. A mixed has an initial central portion followed by an obstructive portion (once respiratory effort returns during the event).
3. The hypopnea definition recommended by the AASM scoring manual (H3A) is a ≥30% reduction in the peak signal excursion compared with pre-event baseline for ≥10 seconds using a nasal pressure transducer (diagnostic study), PAP device flow (titration study), or an alternative hypopnea sensor (diagnostic study) associated with either a ≥3% drop in the arterial oxygen saturation or an arousal. Alternative hypopnea sensors for diagnostic studies are also recommended if the nasal pressure signal is not functioning or the signal is not reliable on the type of sensor.
4. The AASM scoring manual includes an option to **also** report hypopnea based an optional hypopnea definition (previously acceptable definition) defined as a ≥30% reduction in hypopnea sensor signal for ≥10 seconds associated with a ≥4% drop in the arterial oxygen saturation. The presence or absence of an arousal is not considered.
5. The number of hypopneas and derived AHI using the recommended hypopnea definition must be reported. There is an option of also reporting the number of hypopnea and derived AHI using the optional (previously acceptable) hypopnea definition.
6. Classifying hypopneas as obstructive or central is optional. An obstructive hypopnea is characterized by one or more of the following: (a) increased flattening of nasal pressure signal (diagnostic study) or PAP device flow (titration study) compared with baseline breathing; (b) snoring during the event; or (c) thoracoabdominal paradox during the event but not during pre-event breathing. A central hypopnea has none of these characteristics.
7. RERAs are respiratory events characterized by increasing respiratory effort or flattening of the inspiratory portion of the nasal pressure or PAP flow signal for ≥10 seconds leading to an arousal that ***do not meet*** **criteria for apnea or hypopnea. Now that scoring H3A hypopnea is mandated, there will be very few RERAs.**
8. The RDI is the sum of the AHI and the RERA index (RDI = AHI + RERA index). The RERA index is the number of RERAS per hour of sleep.
9. In adults scoring hypoventilation is *optional.* Score *hypoventilation during sleep* if EITHER of the following is present: (a) an increase in the arterial $PaCO_2$ (or surrogate) to a value >55 mm Hg for ≥10 minutes or (b) there is a ≥10 mm Hg increase in the arterial PCO_2 (or surrogate) during sleep

(in comparison to an awake supine value) to a value exceeding >50 mm Hg for ≥10 minutes. Note: >55 mm Hg and >50 mm Hg (not ≥ these values).

10. Score a respiratory event as CSB if BOTH of the following are present:
    (a) There are ≥3 consecutive central apneas or hypopneas separated by a crescendo-decrescendo change in breathing (respiratory effort) with a cycle length ≥**40 seconds**. To be included, the hypopneas must have a symmetrical decrescendo-crescendo pattern of tidal volume or flow.
    (b) There are ≥5 central apneas or hypopneas per hour of sleep associated with the crescendo-decrescendo breathing pattern over ≥2 hours of recording.
11. The cycle length of CSB is measured from the beginning of the central apnea to the end of the next crescendo-decrescendo respiratory phase (start of next central apnea). Apneas or hypopneas (meeting event criteria) that occur within a run of CSB should be scored as individual apneas or hypopneas

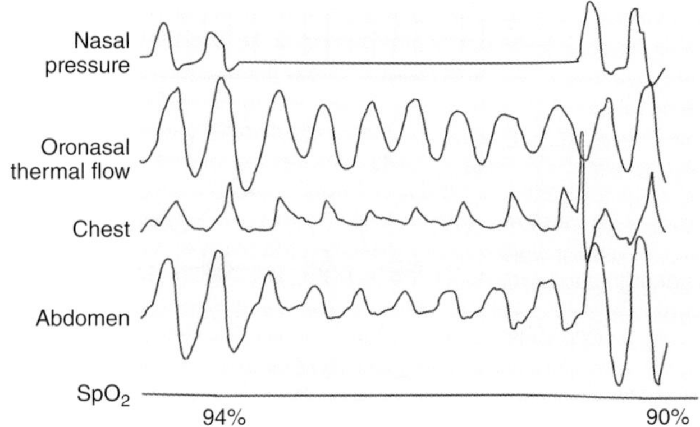

Figure 11–18 What is the respiratory event depicted in this figure? (Adapted from Berry RB, Wagner MH. *Sleep Medicine Pearls.* 3rd ed. Elsevier; 2015:131.)

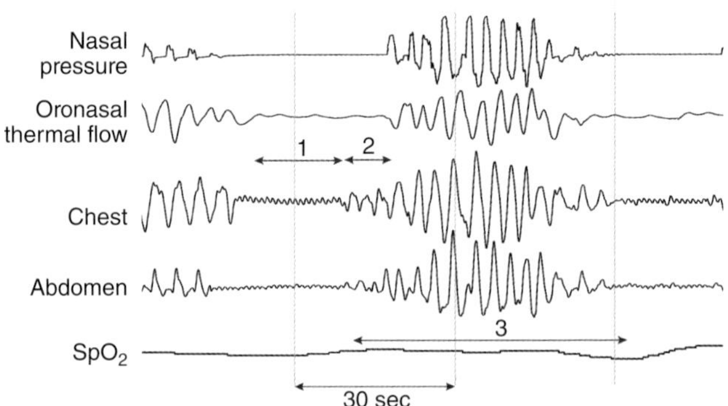

Figure 11–19 What is the respiratory event depicted in this figure? What is unusual about the position of the nadir in desaturation at 3? Inspiration is upward. (Adapted from Berry RB, Wagner MH. *Sleep Medicine Pearls.* 3rd ed. Elsevier; 2015:131.)

CLINICAL REVIEW QUESTIONS

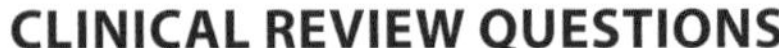

1. What is the minimum cycle length of Cheyne-Stokes breathing (CSB)?
   A. >40 seconds
   B. ≥40 seconds
   C. >50 seconds
   D. ≥50 seconds
2. What is the respiratory event shown in Figure 11–18?
3. What is the respiratory event shown in Figure 11–19?
4. What is the respiratory event shown in Figure 11–20?
5. Is CSB present in Figure 11–21?

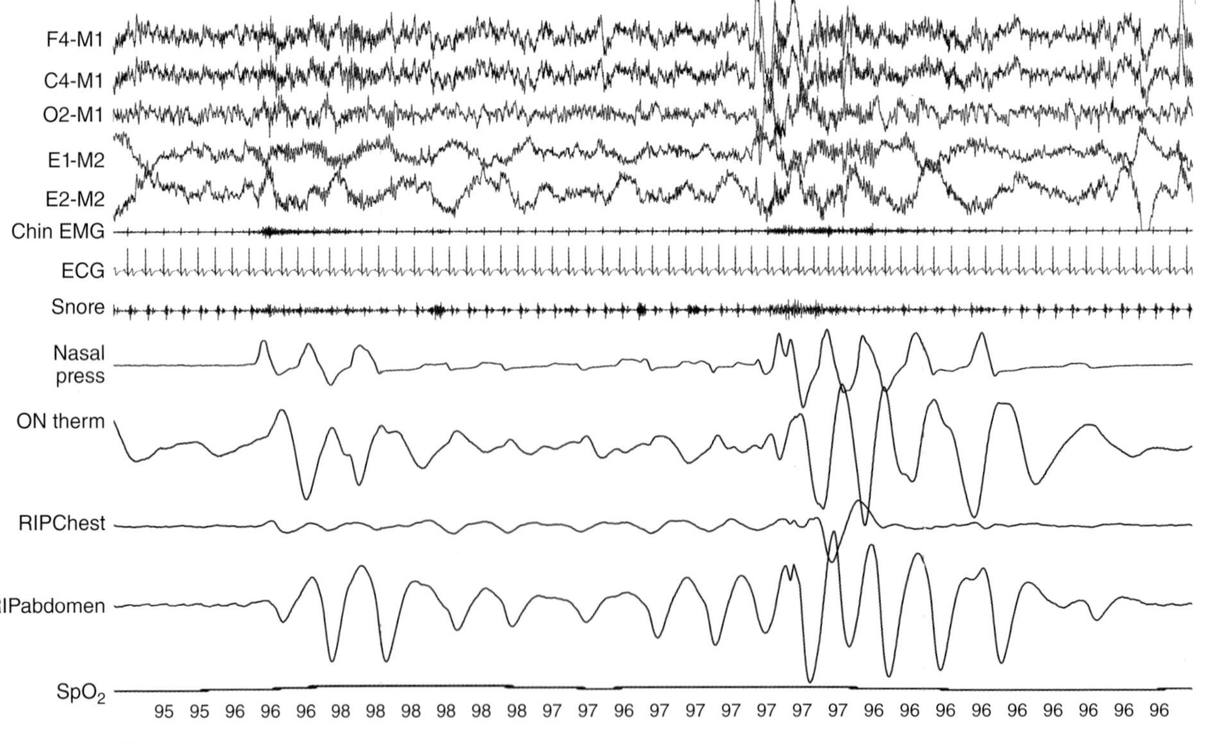

Figure 11–20 What respiratory event is depicted? Inspiration is upward. *NP,* Nasal pressure; *ON Therm,* oronasal thermal airflow signal. (Adapted from Berry RB, Wagner MH. *Sleep Medicine Pearls.* 3rd ed. Elsevier; 2015:131.)

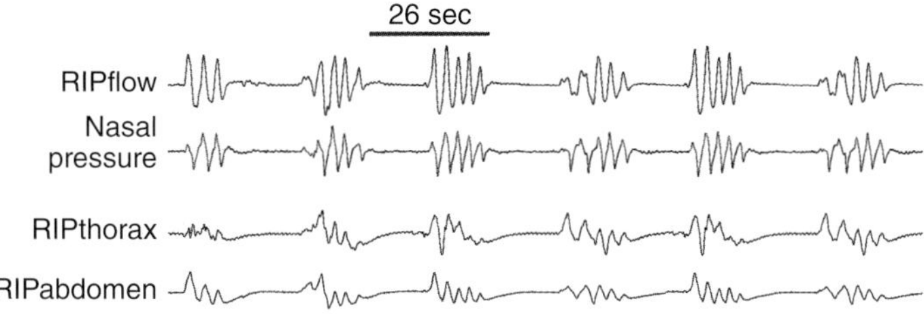

Figure 11-21 What type of respiratory events are shown in this tracing? *RIP*, respiratory inductance plethysmography), *RIPflow* is the time derivative of *RIPsum* (the sum of *RIPthorax* and *RIPabdomen*).

6. Hypoventilation requires which of the following ($PaCO_2$ or surrogate):
   A. $PaCO_2 > 45$ mm Hg for >10 minutes
   B. $PaCO_2 > 55$ mm Hg for ≥10 minutes
   C. $PaCO_2 \geq 55$ mm Hg for >10 minutes
   D. Increase in $PaCO_2$ of ≥5 mm Hg from baseline to a value >50 mm Hg for ≥10 minutes

ANSWERS

1. B.
2. Hypopnea, NOT an apnea. Apneas are scored using the oronasal thermal flow sensor, and the tracing does not meet apnea criteria. The event does meet hypopnea criteria by either recommended or the optional hypopnea definition.
3. Mixed apnea. There is a central portion (1) followed by an obstructive portion (2). The small deflections in the central portion are cardioballistic artifact. A long delay in the SaO_2 nadir after the apnea is noted (3). This is consistent with a long circulation time (reduced cardiac output). This patient has underlying CSB (note the long ventilatory phase between apneas with a crescendo-decrescendo pattern best seen in the chest and abdominal RIP tracings). When placed on positive pressure the obstructive component was eliminated and CSB with central apneas was noted.
4. Hypopnea. Using the recommended hypopnea rule (H3A) the event meets criteria for a hypopnea (associated arousal). Therefore it would not meet criteria for a RERA. Previously, if one was using the H4 hypopnea definition, the event would have been a RERA. However, currently all studies must be scored using H3A (with the option of also reporting hypopneas based on the H4A definition).
5. The tracing shows repeated central apneas. Some have a crescendo-decrescendo pattern but the cycle length is too short to score CSB (cycle length must be ≥ 40 seconds).
6. B. Hypoventilation can **also** be scored if there is ≥10 mm Hg increase in arterial PCO_2 (or surrogate) during sleep (in comparison to an awake supine value) to a *value exceeding 50 mm Hg for ≥10 minutes.*

SELECTED READINGS

Berry RB, Abreu AR, Krishnan V, Quan SF, Strollo PJ, Malhotra RK. A transition to the American Academy of Sleep Medicine-recommended hypopnea definition in adults: initiatives of the Hypopnea Scoring Rule Task Force. *J Clin Sleep Med.* 2022;18(5):1419-1425.

Berry RB, Budhiraja R, Gottlieb DJ, et al; American Academy of Sleep Medicine. Rules for scoring respiratory events in sleep: update of the 2007 AASM Manual for the Scoring of Sleep and Associated Events. Deliberations of the Sleep Apnea Definitions Task Force of the American Academy of Sleep Medicine. *J Clin Sleep Med.* 2012;8(5):597-619.

Troester, MM, Quan, SF, Berry RB, et al; for the American Academy of Sleep Medicine. *The AASM Manual for the Scoring of Sleep and Associated Events: Rules, Terminology and Technical Specifications.* Version 3. American Academy of Sleep Medicine; 2023.

Won CHJ, Qin L, Selim B, Yaggi HK. Varying hypopnea definitions affect obstructive sleep apnea severity classification and association with cardiovascular disease. *J Clin Sleep Med.* 2018;14(12):1987-1994.

REFERENCES

1. Malhotra A, Ayappa I, Ayas N, et al. Metrics of sleep apnea severity: beyond the apnea-hypopnea index. *Sleep.* 2021;44(7):zsab030.
2. Redline S, Sander M. Hypopnea, a floating metric: implications for prevalence, morbidity estimates, and case finding. *Sleep.* 1997;20:1209-1217.
3. Guilleminault C, Tilkian A, Dement WC. The sleep apnea syndromes. *Ann Rev Med.* 1976;27:465-484.
4. Block AJ, Boysen PG, Wynne JW, et al. Sleep apnea, hypopnea, and oxygen desaturation in normal subjects: a strong male predominance. *N Engl J Med.* 1979;330:513-517.
5. Gould GA, Whyte KF, Rhind GB, et al. The sleep hypopnea syndrome. *Am Rev Respir Dis.* 1988;137:895-898.
6. Young T, Palta M, Dempsey J, et al. The occurrence of sleep disorders breathing among middle-aged adults. *N Engl J Med.* 1993;28:1230-1235.
7. Guilleminault C, Stoohs R, Clerk A, et al. A cause of excessive daytime sleepiness: the upper airway resistance syndrome. *Chest.* 1993;104: 781-787.
8. Norman RG, Ahmed M, Walsben JA, Rapoport DM. Detection of respiratory events during NPSG: nasal cannula/pressure sensor versus thermistor. *Sleep.* 1997;20:1175-1184.
9. Ayappa I, Norman RG, Krieger AC, et al. Non-invasive related arousals (RERAs) by a nasal cannula/pressure transducer system. *Sleep.* 2000;23: 763-771.
10. Sleep-related breathing disorders in adults: recommendations for syndrome definition and measurement techniques in clinical research. The Report of an American Academy of Sleep Medicine Task Force. *Sleep.* 1999;22(5):667-689.
11. Nieto FJ, Young TB, Lind BK, et al. Association of sleep-disordered breathing, sleep apnea, and hypertension in a large community-based study. Sleep Heart Health Study. *JAMA.* 2000;283(14):1829-1836. Erratum in: *JAMA.* 2002;288(16):1985.
12. Centers for Medicare and Medicaid Services. *Continuous Positive Airway Pressure (CPAP) Therapy for Obstructive Sleep Apnea (OSA).* Centers for Medicare and Medicaid Services; 2001. Publication CAG-00093N. Available at: https://www.cms.gov/medicare-coverage-database/view/ncacal-decision-memo.aspx?proposed=N&NCAId=19&LCDId=38310&ver=7&NCDId=11&ncdver=1&CoverageSelection=Both&ArticleType=All&PolicyType=Final&s=All&KeyWord=sleep+apnea&KeyWordLookUp=Title&KeyWordSearchType=And&bc=gAAAAAgAAAAA&. Accessed August 23, 2023.
13. Iber C, Ancoli-Israel S, Chesson A, Quan SF, for the American Academy of Sleep Medicine. *The AASM Manual for the Scoring of Sleep and Associated Events: Rules, Terminology and Technical Specifications.* American Academy of Sleep Medicine; 2007.
14. Ruehland WR, Rochford PO, O'Donoghue FJ, et al. The new AASM criteria for scoring hypopneas: impact on the apnea hypopnea index. *Sleep.* 2009;32:150-157.

15. Berry RB, Budhiraja R, Gottlieb DJ, et al; American Academy of Sleep Medicine. Rules for scoring respiratory events in sleep: update of the 2007 AASM Manual for the Scoring of Sleep and Associated Events. Deliberations of the Sleep Apnea Definitions Task Force of the American Academy of Sleep Medicine. *J Clin Sleep Med.* 2012;8(5):597-619.
16. Berry RB, Brooks R, Gamaldo CE, et al; for the American Academy of Sleep Medicine. *The AASM Manual for the Scoring of Sleep and Associated Events: Rules, Terminology and Technical Specifications.* Version 2.0. American Academy of Sleep Medicine; 2012.
17. Berry RB, Brooks R, Gamaldo CE, et al; for the American Academy of Sleep Medicine. *The AASM Manual for the Scoring of Sleep and Associated Events: Rules, Terminology and Technical Specifications.* Version 2.4. American Academy of Sleep Medicine; 2017.
18. Berry RB, Quan SF, Abreu AR, et al; for the American Academy of Sleep Medicine. *The AASM Manual for the Scoring of Sleep and Associated Events: Rules, Terminology and Technical Specifications.* Version 2.6. American Academy of Sleep Medicine; 2020.
19. Redline S, Kapur VK, Sanders MH, et al. Effects of varying approaches for identifying respiratory disturbances on sleep apnea assessment. *Am J Respir Crit Care Med.* 2000;161(2 Pt 1):369-374.
20. Hirotsu C, Haba-Rubio J, Andries D, et al. Effect of three hypopnea scoring criteria on OSA prevalence and associated comorbidities in the general population. *J Clin Sleep Med.* 2019;15(2):183-194.
21. Ho V, Crainiceanu CM, Punjabi NM, Redline S, Gottlieb DJ. Calibration model for apnea-hypopnea indices: impact of alternative criteria for hypopneas. *Sleep.* 2015;38(12):1887-1892.
22. Punjabi NM, Newman AB, Young TB, Resnick HE, Sanders MH. Sleep-disordered breathing and cardiovascular disease: an outcome-based definition of hypopneas. *Am J Respir Crit Care Med.* 2008;177(10): 1150-1155.
23. Whitney CW, Gottlieb DJ, Redline S, et al. Reliability of scoring respiratory disturbance indices and sleep staging. *Sleep.* 1998;21(7):749-757.
24. Won CHJ, Qin L, Selim B, Yaggi HK. Varying hypopnea definitions affect obstructive sleep apnea severity classification and association with cardiovascular disease. *J Clin Sleep Med.* 2018;14(12):1987-1994.
25. Khalid F, Ayache M, Auckley D. The differential impact of respiratory event scoring criteria on CPAP eligibility in women and men. *J Clin Sleep Med.* 2021;17(12):2409-2414.
26. American Academy of Sleep Medicine. *International Classification of Sleep Disorders.* 3rd ed., text revision. American Academy of Sleep Medicine; 2023.
27. Malhotra RK, Kirsch DB, Kristo DA, et al; American Academy of Sleep Medicine Board of Directors. Polysomnography for obstructive sleep apnea should include arousal-based scoring: an American Academy of Sleep Medicine position statement. *J Clin Sleep Med.* 2018;14(7):1245-1247.
28. Berry RB, Abreu AR, Krishnan V, Quan SF, Strollo PJ, Malhotra RK. A transition to the American Academy of Sleep Medicine–recommended hypopnea definition in adults: initiatives of the Hypopnea Scoring Rule Task Force. *J Clin Sleep Med.* 2022;18(5):1419-1425.
29. Wimms AJ, Kelly JL, Turnbull CD, et al; MERGE trial investigators. Continuous positive airway pressure versus standard care for the treatment of people with mild obstructive sleep apnoea (MERGE): a multicentre, randomised controlled trial. *Lancet Respir Med.* 2020;8(4):349-358.
30. Troester, MM, Quan, SF, Berry RB, et al; for the American Academy of Sleep Medicine. *The AASM Manual for the Scoring of Sleep and Associated Events: Rules, Terminology and Technical Specifications.* Version 3. American Academy of Sleep Medicine; 2023.
31. Hosselet JJ, Norman RG, Ayappa I, Rapoport DM. Detection of flow limitation with a nasal cannula/pressure transducer system. *Am J Respir Crit Care Med.* 1998;157(5 Pt 1):1461-1467.
32. Randerath WJ, Treml M, Priegnitz C, Stieglitz S, Hagmeyer L, Morgenstern C. Evaluation of a noninvasive algorithm for differentiation of obstructive and central hypopneas. *Sleep.* 2013;36(3):363-368.
33. Dupuy-McCauley KL, Mudrakola HV, Colaco B, Arunthari V, Slota KA, Morgenthaler TI. A comparison of 2 visual methods for classifying obstructive vs central hypopneas. *J Clin Sleep Med.* 2021;17(6):1157-1165.
34. Berry RB, Ryals S, Wagner MH. Use of chest wall EMG to classify hypopneas as obstructive or central. *J Clin Sleep Med.* 2018;14(5):725-733.
35. Stoohs RA, Blum HC, Knaack L, Butsch-von-der-Heydt B, Guilleminault C. Comparison of pleural pressure and transcutaneous diaphragmatic electromyogram in obstructive sleep apnea syndrome. *Sleep.* 2005;28(3):321-329.
36. Tolbert TM, Parekh A, Sands SA, Mooney AM, Ayappa I, Rapoport DM. Quantification of airway conductance from noninvasive ventilatory drive in patients with sleep apnea. *J Appl Physiol (1985).* 2021;131(5): 1640-1652.
37. Cracowski C, Pépin JL, Wuyam B, Lévy P. Characterization of obstructive nonapneic respiratory events in moderate sleep apnea syndrome. *Am J Respir Crit Care Med.* 2001;164(6):944-948.
38. Masa JF, Corral J, Teran J, et al. Apnoeic and obstructive nonapnoeic sleep respiratory events. *Eur Respir J.* 2009;34(1):156-161.
39. Hall MJ, Xie A, Rutherford R, Ando S, Floras JS, Bradley TD. Cycle length of periodic breathing in patients with and without heart failure. *Am J Respir Crit Care Med.* 1996;154(2 Pt 1):376-381.
40. Badr MS, Toiber F, Skatrud JB, Dempsey J. Pharyngeal narrowing/occlusion during central sleep apnea. *J Appl Physiol (1985).* 1995;78(5): 1806-1815.
41. Ryals S, McCullough L, Wagner M, Berry R, Dibra M. A case of treatment-emergent central sleep apnea? *J Clin Sleep Med.* 2020;16(2): 331-334.
42. Berry RB, Ryals S, Girdhar A, Wagner MH. Use of chest wall electromyography to detect respiratory effort during polysomnography. *J Clin Sleep Med.* 2016;12(9):1239-1244.
43. Younes M. Role of arousals in the pathogenesis of obstructive sleep apnea. *Am J Respir Crit Care Med.* 2004;169(5):623-633.
44. Zitting KM, Lockyer BJ, Azarbarzin AA, et al. Association of cortical arousals with sleep-disordered breathing events. *J Clin Sleep Med.* 2023; 19(5):899-912.
45. Trinder J, Merson R, Rosenberg JI, Fitzgerald F, Kleiman J, Douglas Bradley T. Pathophysiological interactions of ventilation, arousals, and blood pressure oscillations during Cheyne-Stokes respiration in patients with heart failure. *Am J Respir Crit Care Med.* 2000;162(3 Pt 1):808-813.
46. Pinna GD, Robbi E, Terzaghi M, Corbellini D, La Rovere MT, Maestri R. Temporal relationship between arousals and Cheyne-Stokes respiration with central sleep apnea in heart failure patients. *Clin Neurophysiol.* 2018;129(9):1955-1963.

Respiratory Events in Children—Event Definitions and Scoring Rules

Chapter 12

INTRODUCTION

Current respiratory event definitions for children are based on recommendations of an American Academy of Sleep Medicine task force published in 2012[1] and are continually updated by the *AASM Manual for the Scoring of Sleep and Associated Events* (hereafter referred to as the AASM scoring manual).[2] The manual is updated periodically, and the reader is referred to the most current version for updates. The pediatric scoring rules differ from adult rules in several important aspects. If an adult is breathing at 12 breaths per minute, a minimum apnea duration of 10 seconds corresponds to two breaths (5 seconds per breath). Normal respiratory rates (breaths per minute) in children are much faster. Approximate (50th percentile) values are in the low 40s at age 3 months, mid-30s at 1 year, mid-20s at 4 years, and around 20 breaths per minute at age 10.[3] As children breathe at much faster rates than adults, event duration criteria are based on the duration of two breaths during baseline breathing rather than the absolute duration of 10 seconds. This minimum duration is used for obstructive and mixed apnea and hypopnea. As discussed below, central apneas are scored differently in children than in adults, as central apneas frequently occur after large breaths in normal children and likely have no clinical significance unless prolonged or followed by an arousal or arterial oxygen desaturation. In young children central pauses in respiration can be scored based on associated bradycardia, as discussed below.

AGES FOR WHICH PEDIATRIC RESPIRATORY SCORING RULES APPLY

The pediatric scoring rules for respiratory events should be used for children <18 years, but there is an option to use adult rules for children ≥13 years with an adult body habitus (note <18 and ≥13 years).[2] Several studies suggest that the apnea hypopnea index (AHI) will be higher in adolescent patients when using pediatric compared with the adult rules when the adult hypopnea definition requires a drop in airflow associated with a ≥4% arterial oxygen desaturation (H4) rather than a ≥3% desaturation OR an arousal (H3A).[4-6] If using the currently recommended adult hypopnea definition based on H3A, adult and pediatric hypopnea rules are similar except for the duration of the event. Therefore, there will be less difference in the AHI when using the adult rules based on the recommended hypopnea definition (H3A) versus pediatric rules in adolescent patients.

MEASURING EVENT DURATIONS

For scoring either an apnea or a hypopnea, the event duration is measured from the nadir preceding the first breath that is clearly reduced to the beginning of the first breath that approximates the baseline breathing amplitude. For apneas use the oronasal thermal sensor, and for hypopneas use the nasal pressure sensor (or alternative sensors if these sensors are not functional or accurate) (Fig. 12–1). During a positive airway pressure (PAP) titration sleep study, the PAP device flow is used to measure event duration.[2]

SCORING RESPIRATORY EVENTS IN SLEEP VERSUS WAKE

The AASM scoring manual[2] provides guidance for respiratory events occurring partially or completely within an epoch scored as wake.

> *"If the apnea or hypopnea event begins or ends during an epoch that is scored as sleep, then the corresponding respiratory event can be scored and included in the computation of the apnea-hypopnea index (AHI). This situation usually occurs when an individual has a high AHI with events occurring so frequently that sleep is severely disrupted, and epochs may end up being scored as wake even though <15 seconds of sleep is present during the epochs containing that portion of the respiratory event." However, if the apnea or hypopnea occurs entirely during an epoch scored as wake they are not included in the calculation of the AHI.*

SCORING RULES FOR RESPIRATORY EVENTS IN CHILDREN

The rules of scoring respiratory events are similar to those in adults with a few exceptions. Scoring central apneas uses different rules, there is only one hypopnea definition based on a decrease in flow associated with a ≥3% desaturation or an arousal, and periodic breathing rather than Cheyne-Stokes breathing is scored. The definition of hypoventilation is also different from the one used in adults.

Apnea Events

This apnea definition differs from the adult rule as central apneas require special considerations in pediatric patients. An arterial oxygen desaturation is not required to score an apnea if the event *otherwise meets apnea criteria*. If a portion of a respiratory event that would otherwise meet criteria for a hypopnea meets criteria for apnea (including the two-breath minimum if applicable), the entire event should be scored as an apnea.[2] In children the apnea sensors recommended by the AASM scoring manual are the same as for adults with the exception that the exhaled PCO_2 waveform can be used as an acceptable alternative apnea sensor. The recommended standard apnea sensor is an oronasal thermal flow sensor (diagnostic study) or positive airway pressure (PAP) flow signal (PAP titration sleep study).

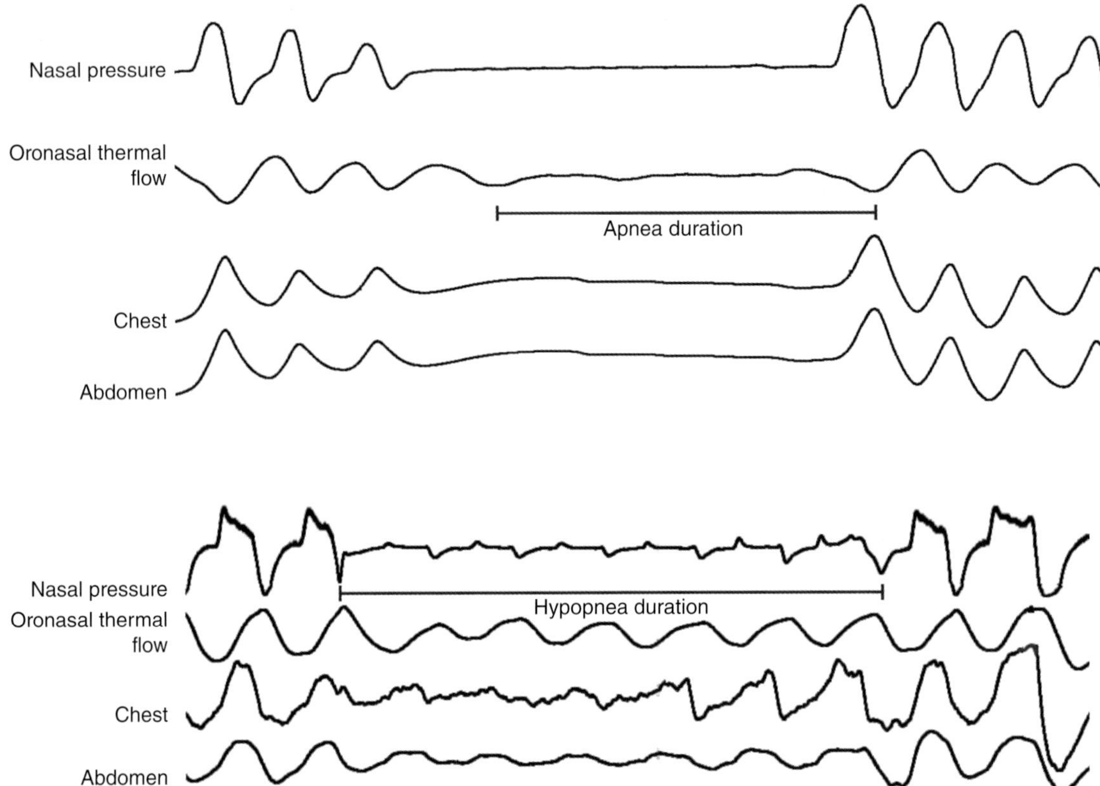

Figure 12–1 Measurement of event duration is shown for an apnea and a hypopnea. To determine the apnea duration, the oronasal thermal sensor signal is used, and for hypopnea the nasal pressure signal is used (inspiration is upward in this figure). Event duration begins with the nadir preceding the first breath that is clearly reduced until the start of the first breath that approximates baseline breathing.

Recommended alternative apnea sensors are used if the recommended sensor is not reliable and include the nasal pressure (with or without square root transformation), and respiratory inductance plethysmography (RIP) sum and flow signals (RIPsum and RIPflow). The RIP signals can be calibrated or uncalibrated. The sum signal is the sum of the signals from chest and abdominal RIP effort belts, and RIPflow is the time derivative of the RIPsum signal (see Chapter 10). Deflections in the RIPsum are estimates of tidal volume, and deflections in the RIPflow are estimates of airflow. Use of polyvinylidene fluoride (PVDF) sum and end-tidal PCO_2 signals are alternative apnea sensors specified as "acceptable" because of the lower level of evidence supporting their use. The PVDF sum is the sum of thoracic and abdominal PVDF effort belt signals, and the waveform of the exhaled PCO_2 rather than the end-tidal values is used as a signal to score apnea (see Chapter 10). During PAP titration the recommended sensor for scoring apnea and hypopnea is the PAP device flow signal (there is no alternative sensor for scoring apnea or hypopnea during a positive pressure titration). Although not required for reporting, the AASM scoring manual states, "it is valuable to describe any airway protective maneuvers, such as persistent mouth opening/mouth breathing, neck hyperextension and avoidance of sleep in the supine position, as these can be supplemental evidence of obstructive sleep apnea."

Respiratory effort is used to classify apneas as obstructive, mixed, or central. The recommended respiratory effort sensors include esophageal manometry and dual thoracoabdominal RIP effort belts. Acceptable respiratory effort sensors include dual thoracoabdominal PVDF effort belts.

Pediatric Apnea Rule

Score a respiratory event as an apnea if it meets **ALL** of the following criteria:

a. There is a drop in the peak signal excursion by ≥90% of the pre-event baseline using an oronasal thermal sensor (diagnostic study), PAP device flow (titration study), or an alternative apnea sensor (diagnostic study).
b. The duration of the ≥90% drop lasts at least the **minimum duration as specified by obstructive, mixed, or central apnea duration criteria.**
c. The event meets respiratory effort criteria for obstructive, central, or mixed apnea.

Obstructive Apnea Rule

An **obstructive apnea is scored if the event meets** apnea criteria (≥90% drop in apnea sensor signal compared with baseline) for at least the duration of two breaths during baseline breathing **AND** is associated with the presence of respiratory effort throughout the entire period of absent airflow.

In Figure 12–2 a short obstructive apnea is noted lasting only two breaths (two inspiratory efforts). Even though the duration is short, an associated arterial oxygen desaturation is noted. In Figure 12–3 an obstructive apnea is shown associated with changes in the exhaled PCO_2 waveform (can be used as an acceptable alternative apnea sensor). Apnea is associated with no exhaled CO_2 and the measured $PCO_2 = 0$. Note that there is a delay in the start of the drop in the PCO_2 waveform to zero compared with the start of the apnea in the

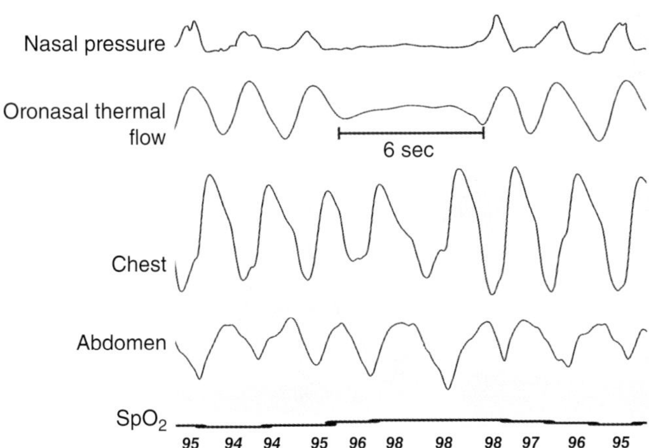

Figure 12–2 Obstructive apnea in a 4-year-old child. The oronasal airflow signal shows absent deflections for 6 seconds or the duration of two inspiratory efforts (at least the duration of two baseline breaths). Even though the event is short, a fall in arterial oxygen saturation by pulse oximetry *(SpO₂)* still occurs. Inspiration is upward. *Chest* and *Abdomen* are chest and abdominal respiratory inductance plethysmography effort belt signals, respectively.

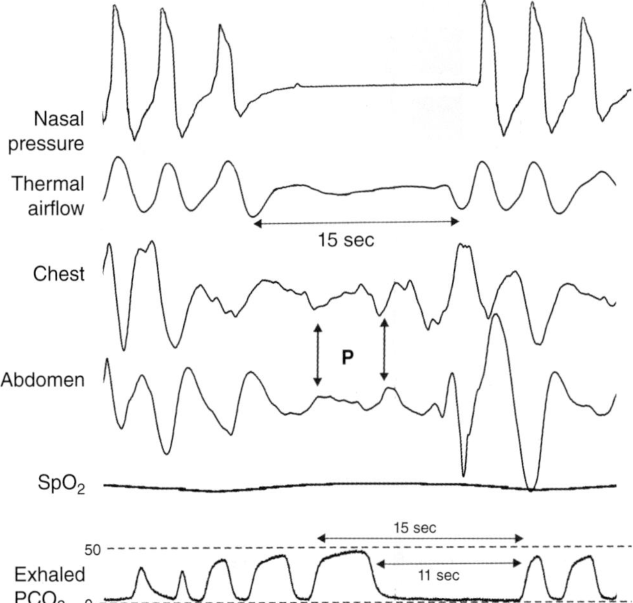

Figure 12–3 An obstructive apnea in a 4-year-old child. Note the paradoxical motion *(P)* in the chest and abdominal RIP effort belt signals. Thermal airflow is an oronasal thermal sensor signal. The oronasal thermal flow is the recommended apnea sensor for diagnostic studies; if the signal was not reliable, one could use alternative sensors including the nasal pressure signal (a recommended alternative apnea sensor) or the exhaled PCO_2 signal (acceptable alternative apnea sensor, in mm Hg). Note that evidence of the apnea in the exhaled PCO_2 signal is delayed compared with the airflow signals and that the duration of the exhaled PCO_2 = 0 mm Hg is shorter than the duration of apnea by airflow signals (the duration of exhalation during the last breath before apnea is prolonged compared with baseline breathing).

thermal flow signal. This is because of the side stream method of exhaled PCO_2 measurement (see Chapter 10).

Mixed Apnea Rule

A **mixed apnea** is scored if the event meets apnea criteria (≥90% drop in apnea sensor signal compared with baseline) for at least the **duration of two breaths** during baseline breathing AND is associated with **absent** respiratory effort during one portion of the event AND the presence of inspiratory effort in another portion, **regardless of which portion comes first.**

In Figure 12–4 a mixed apnea is shown with the obstructive portion preceding the central portion. Note that in adult rules, the central portion is specified to be first.

Central Apnea Rule

A central apnea is scored if an event *meets apnea criteria (≥90% drop in apnea sensor signal compared with baseline), is associated with absent inspiratory effort throughout the entire duration of the event,* ***AND at least one of the following is met:***

a. *The event lasts* ***≥20 seconds.***
b. *The event lasts at least the* ***duration of two breaths*** *during baseline breathing and is associated with an* ***arousal or a ≥3% arterial oxygen desaturation.***
c. The event lasts at least the duration of two breaths during baseline breathing and is associated with a decrease in heart rate to fewer than **50 beats per minute for at least 5 seconds.** *For infants* ***younger than 1 year,*** *the decrease in heart rate requirement adjusts to* ***less than 60 beats per minutes for at least 15 seconds*** *due to the higher baseline heart rates.*

An example of a central apnea in a 2-month-old child is shown in Figure 12–5. The drop in the oronasal thermal flow signal meets apnea criteria, there is absent inspiratory effort, and the event is associated with a ≥3% arterial oxygen desaturation. Note that in young children very short apneas can result in arterial oxygen desaturation. In Figure 12–6 a 4-second breathing pause in the same patient as in Figure 12–5 meets apnea **airflow** and **effort** criteria (absent inspiratory effort) to score a central apnea. However, the event is NOT scored as a central apnea as it is not associated with an arousal, a ≥3% arterial oxygen desaturation, or a qualifying drop in the heart rate. In Figure 12–7 an event can be scored as a central apnea as the duration is ≥20 seconds. The central apnea follows a large breath.

SCORING PEDIATRIC HYPOPNEAS

There is only one hypopnea scoring rule, and there is an option to score hypopneas and obstructive or central. The recommended hypopnea sensor is a nasal pressure transducer with or without a square root transformation (diagnostic study) or PAP device flow signal (PAP titration sleep study). **Alternative hypopnea sensors** are used (diagnostic study) if the nasal pressure signal is not functional or reliable. The *recommended alternative hypopnea sensors* (signals) include an oronasal thermal airflow sensor, RIPsum, and RIP flow, and dual RIP thoracoabdominal belts. The RIP signals can be calibrated or uncalibrated. *The acceptable alternative hypopnea sensor* (signal) is the PVDF sum. Obstructive hypoventilation is not given a separate scoring rule but is discussed below. Hypoventilation does have a specific scoring rule.

Pediatric Hypopnea Rule

The following is the rule for scoring hypopneas as defined by the AASM scoring manual.[2]

Score a respiratory event as a **hypopnea** if it meets **ALL** of the following criteria:

a. The peak signal excursions drop by ≥30% of pre-event baseline using nasal pressure (diagnostic study), PAP device flow (titration study), or an alternative hypopnea sensor (diagnostic study).

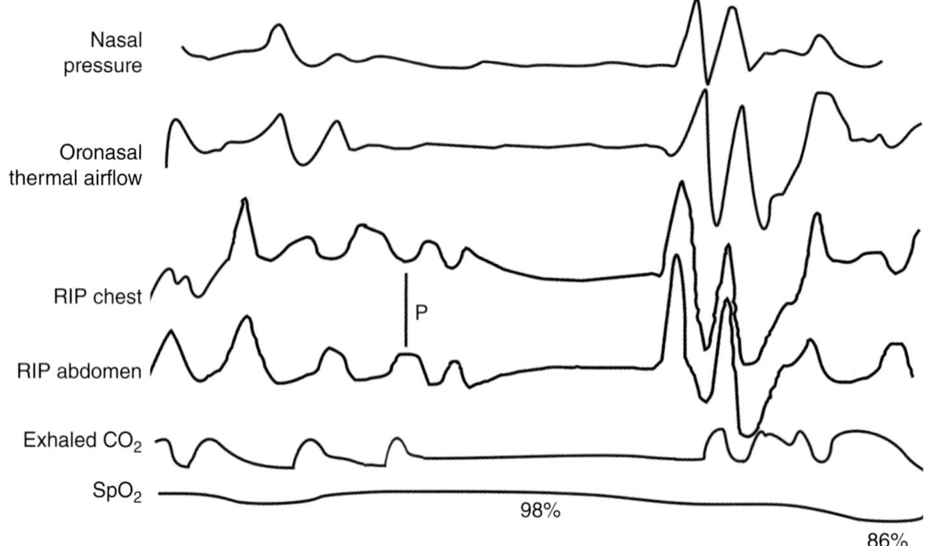

Figure 12–4 A mixed apnea with an initial obstructive portion and a terminal central portion. Paradoxical chest and abdominal RIP belt deflections are seen at P. In adults the initial portion of a mixed apnea is always central. Inspiration is upward.

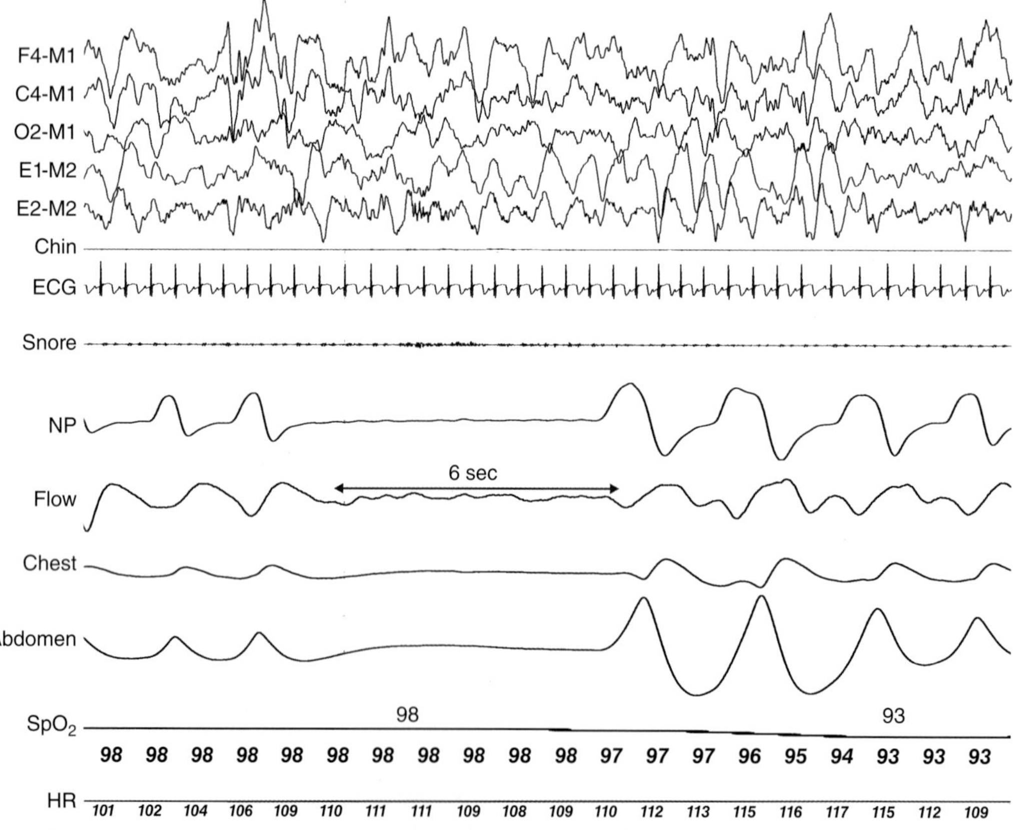

Figure 12–5 A 20-second tracing of central apnea in a 2-month-old child. The event duration exceeds the duration of two respiratory cycles with absent inspiratory effort and is associated with a ≥3% arterial oxygen desaturation. Flow is an oronasal thermal airflow sensor. There is no associated arousal. *Chest* and *Abdomen* are respiratory inductance plethysmography effort belt signals. Inspiration is upward.

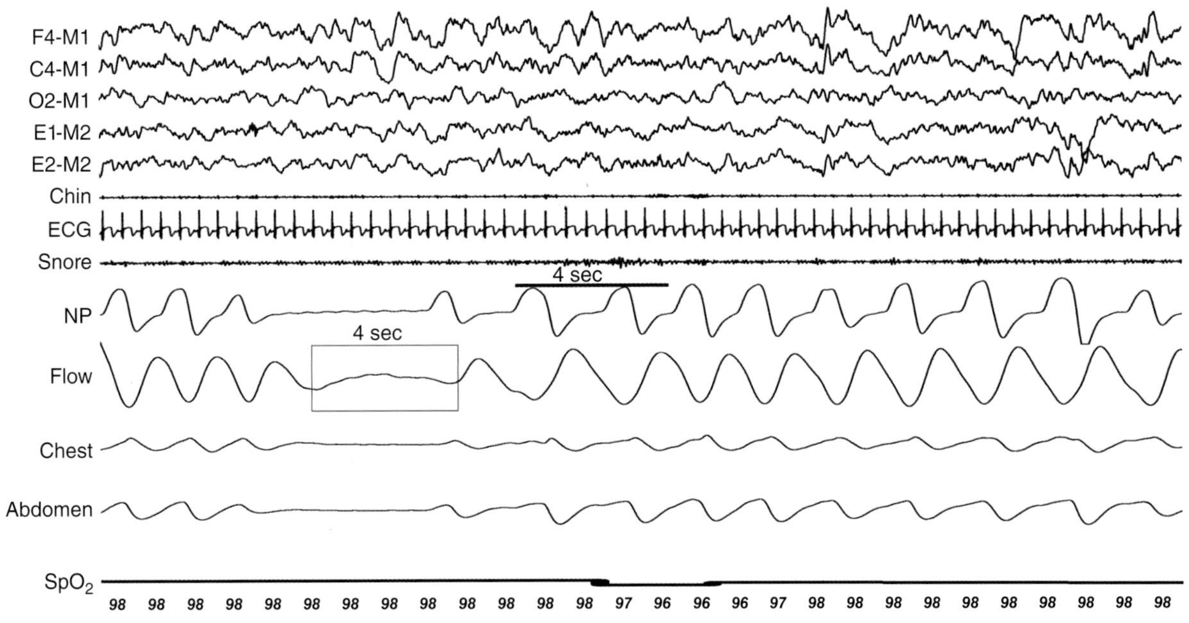

Figure 12–6 A 30-second tracing in a 2-month-old child with a 4-second breathing pause that meets apnea airflow criteria with absent inspiratory effort. However, the event is NOT scored as a central apnea as it is not >20 seconds in duration, not associated with an arousal or a ≥3% arterial oxygen desaturation, and there is no qualifying drop in heart rate. *Chest* and *Abdomen* are chest and abdominal respiratory inductance plethysmography effort belt signals, respectively. Flow is an oronasal thermal airflow sensor. Inspiration is upward.

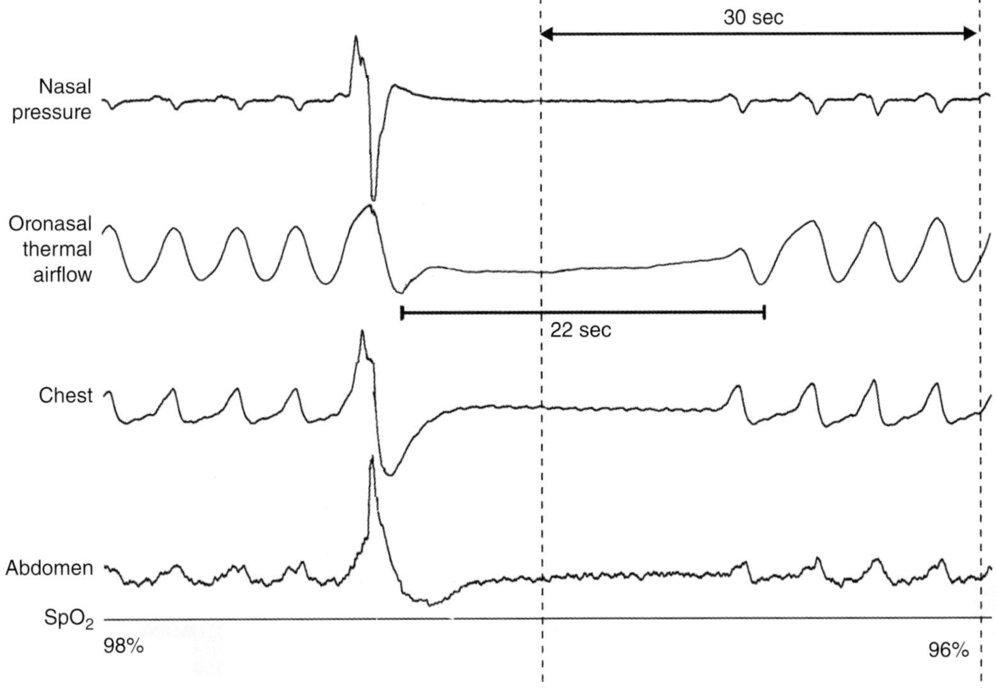

Figure 12–7 A central apnea in a 10-year-old child. There was no associated ≥3% desaturation or arousal. However, as the duration was ≥20 seconds a central apnea can be scored. Chest and Abdomen are RIP effort belt signals.

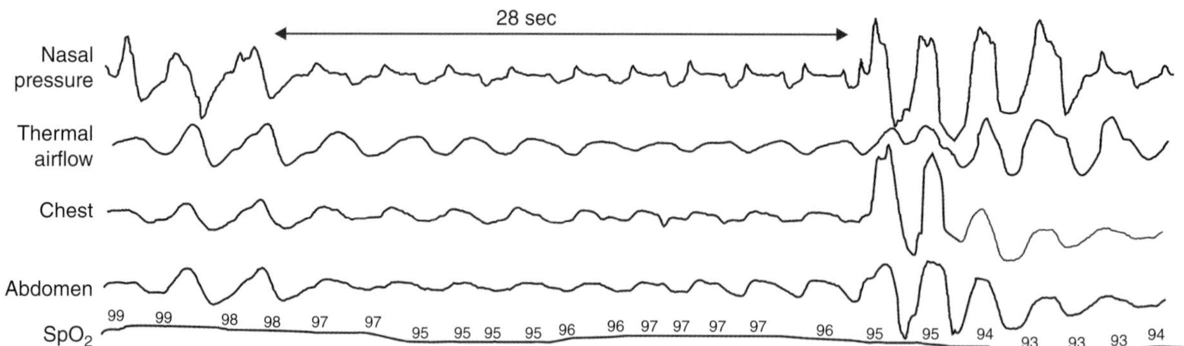

Figure 12–8 A 45-second tracing of a respiratory event in a 10-year-old child scored as a hypopnea based on the qualifying decrease in the nasal pressure signal and an associated ≥3% arterial oxygen desaturation. Thermal flow is the oronasal thermal flow signal. Inspiration is upward. Note the evidence of airflow limitation (flattened inspiratory profile). The hypopnea shown could be classified as an obstructive hypopnea if hypopneas are being classified as central or obstructive (scoring a hypopnea as obstructive or central is optional).

b. The duration of the ≥30% drop in signal excursion lasts for at least two breaths.
c. There is ≥3% oxygen desaturation from pre-event baseline or the event is associated with an arousal.

In Figure 12–8 a 28-second hypopnea is noted as the qualifying drop in the nasal pressure signal is associated with a ≥3% arterial oxygen desaturation.

Scoring Hypopneas as Obstructive or Central

The scoring of hypopneas as central or obstructive events is ***optional*** as noted in parameters to be reported in the AASM scoring manual. The following are rules for scoring hypopneas as obstructive or central.

Pediatric Obstructive Hypopnea Rule

If **electing to score obstructive hypopneas,** score a hypopnea as obstructive if **ANY** of the following criteria are met:
a. Snoring during the event
b. Increased inspiratory flattening of the nasal pressure or PAP device flow signal compared with baseline breathing
c. Associated thoracoabdominal paradox occurs during the event but not during pre-event breathing

Pediatric Central Hypopnea Rule

If **electing to score central hypopneas,** score a hypopnea as central if **NONE** of the following criteria are met:
a. Snoring during the event
b. Increased inspiratory flattening of the nasal pressure or PAP device flow signal compared with baseline breathing
c. Associated thoracoabdominal paradox occurs during the event but not during pre-event breathing

An example of an obstructive hypopnea in a 10-year-old child is shown in Figure 12–8. There is definite inspiratory flattening of the nasal pressure signal compared to baseline breathing.

PEDIATRIC RERA RULE

Scoring respiratory effort–related arousals (RERAs) is ***optional*** as noted in parameters to be reported in the AASM scoring manual. Note that when using a hypopnea definition based on arousals as well as arterial oxygen desaturation there are relatively few RERAs. If the nasal pressure signal showed flattening but NOT a ≥30% drop in flow from pre-event baseline associated with an arousal, this event would be scored as a RERA but not a hypopnea. Reporting the occurrence of snoring is optional in adults but recommended in children chiefly because it is a current criterion for scoring a RERA event.

If electing to score respiratory effort-related arousals:
Score a respiratory event as a RERA if there is a sequence of breaths lasting at least two breaths (or the duration of two breaths during baseline breathing) **that do not meet criteria for an apnea or hypopneas** and lead to an **arousal** from sleep. The breathing sequence can be characterized when **one or more** of the following is present:
a. Increasing respiratory effort
b. Flattening of the inspiratory portion of the nasal pressure (diagnostic study) or PAP device flow (titration study) waveform
c. **Snoring**
d. An elevation in the end-tidal PCO_2 above pre-event baseline

Note that the amount of elevation in the end-tidal PCO_2 above baseline is not specified. An example of a RERA event is shown in Figure 12–9. Here there is flattening of the nasal pressure signal but NOT a ≥30% reduction in deflection (so a hypopnea cannot be scored). In this example note the increase in the end-tidal PCO_2 during the event. RERAs can be scored based on flattening of the inspiratory portion of the nasal pressure flow signal (or PAP flow in a titration study), increased respiratory effort, snoring, or an elevation in the end-tidal PCO_2 from pre-event baseline.

PEDIATRIC HYPOVENTILATION

For detection of hypoventilation during a diagnostic study, monitoring of end-tidal PCO_2 or transcutaneous PCO_2 is recommended. For detection of hypoventilation during a PAP titration study, transcutaneous PCO_2 is recommended. **Monitoring hypoventilation** in children is **recommended** during a diagnostic study and **optional** during a PAP titration study. The reason is that the recommended surrogate device for monitoring hypoventilation during a PAP titration

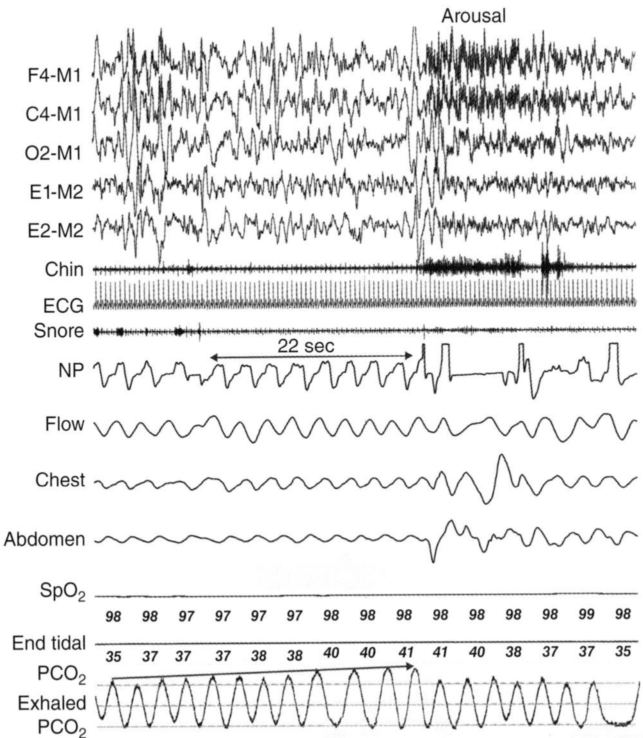

Figure 12–9 A respiratory effort–related arousal (RERA) in a 10-year-old child. The amplitude reduction in nasal pressure signal was minimal although showing a flattened profile compared with pre-event breathing. The reduction in the nasal pressure signal was NOT ≥30% of baseline. Therefore a RERA and not a hypopnea was scored. In this example one can see an increase in the end-tidal PCO_2 before the arousals. Increased inspiratory effort, flattening of the nasal pressure signal, snoring, an increase in end-tidal PCO_2, or snoring can all be used to score a RERA. NP is nasal pressure; Flow is an oronasal thermal sensor signal. Inspiration is upward.

is a transcutaneous PCO_2 device, and these are relatively expensive. In a study of normal children Montgomery-Downs et al.[7] found that 20% of all children spent ≥50% of TST with end-tidal carbon dioxide value of ≥ 45 mm Hg, whereas only 2.2% spent ≥50% TST with an end-tidal PCO_2 ≥ 50 mm Hg. Although end-tidal PCO_2 monitoring can be challenging in children, an analysis by Paruthi et al.[8] found that usable tracings were obtained in about 90% of studies. However, the tracings came from sleep centers experienced at this type of monitoring.

Pediatric Hypoventilation rule (scoring recommended during a diagnostic study)

Score hypoventilation during sleep when >25% of the total sleep time as measured by either the arterial PCO_2 or surrogate is spent with a PCO_2 > 50 mm Hg. **(Note: > not ≥ is used.)**

An example of hypoventilation is shown in Figure 12–10 in a patient with muscular dystrophy. Note that the SpO_2 is relatively well preserved as the lungs of this patient were normal.

Obstructive Hypoventilation

In children there may be episodes of prolonged loud snoring and/or airflow limitation associated with only mild drops in the SpO_2 but evidence of hypercapnia. Whereas the AASM scoring manual does not provide criteria for the scoring of obstructive hypoventilation as a discrete event, the cumulative increase in PCO_2 may qualify for a diagnosis of hypoventilation. An example of an episode of obstructive hypoventilation is illustrated in Figure 12–11.

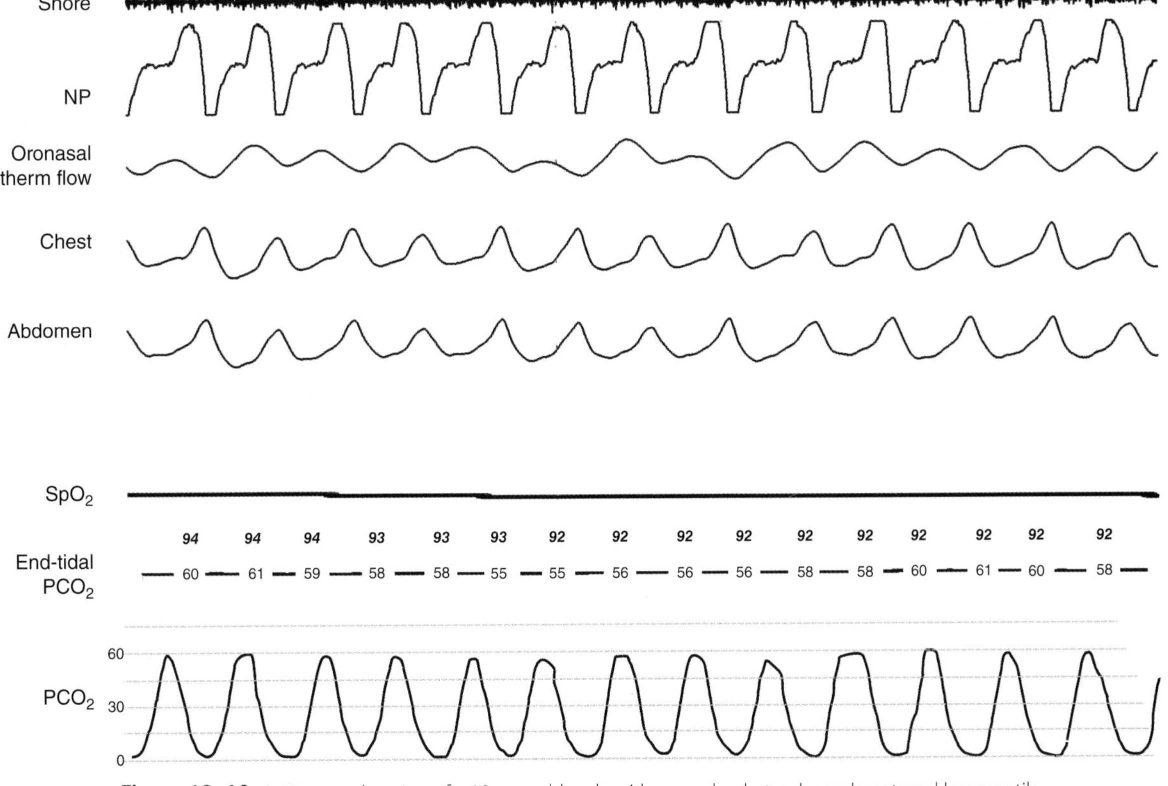

Figure 12–10 A 30-second tracing of a 10-year-old male with muscular dystrophy and nocturnal hypoventilation. The end-tidal PCO_2 was > 50 mm Hg for about 48% of total sleep time. Therefore, hypoventilation was scored.

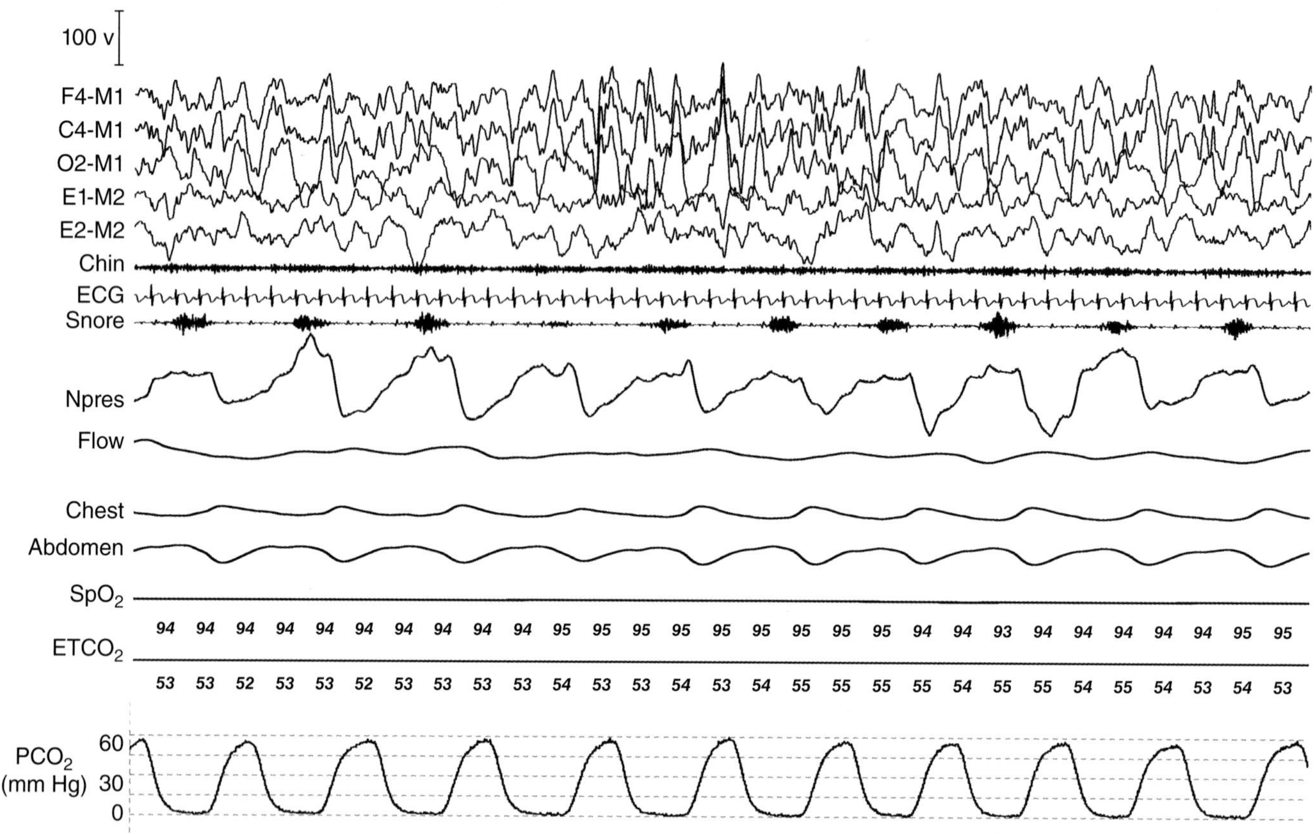

Figure 12–11 A 30-second tracing of an 8-year-old child with a body mass index of 34 kg/m². The patient had an AHI of 24/hour on the sleep study. The event shown is an example of obstructive hypoventilation with a long period of airflow limitation, snoring, and increased PCO_2 without a discrete apnea or hypopnea. Also note the paradoxical breathing pattern in the chest and abdominal effort belt signals.

Periodic Breathing

It should be noted that periodic breathing is normal in premature and young infants (see below) and is most commonly noted during stage R. Central pauses in breathing (no airflow or respiratory effort) that occur within a run of periodic breathing should be scored as central apneas if they meet central apnea criteria.

Pediatric Periodic Breathing Rule:

Score a respiratory event as periodic breathing if there are ≥3 episodes of central pauses in respiration (absent airflow and inspiratory effort) lasting >3* seconds separated by ≤20 seconds of normal breathing. (Note >3 seconds not ≥3 seconds.)

An example of periodic breathing is shown in Figure 12–12. The central pauses are scored a central apneas, as they are associated with a ≥3% desaturation.

At what age is periodic breathing normal? Kelly et al.[9] analyzed 287 pneumographic recordings from 123 full-term infants (63 males) obtained during the first 12 months of life to establish normative values for apnea, periodic breathing, and bradycardia. The results of the analysis were tabulated by sex and age. The number of infants who exhibited periodic breathing decreased significantly over time (78% at 0–2 weeks vs. 29% at 39–52 weeks; $P < 0.05$). No bradycardia was identified. Normal full-term infants occasionally had central apneas of 10, 11, or 12 seconds. Until 6 months of age, the majority of infants had a small amount of periodic breathing (<1% of sleep time) during sleep at home. It is important to note that scoring periodic breathing does NOT require that the central pauses are associated with desaturation. A ≥3% desaturation associated with each central pauses is used as one criteria to determine if the central pause can be scored as a central apnea.

Special Circumstances for Scoring Respiratory Events

During PAP titration sleep studies with a PAP device using a backup rate, there may be events that qualify as an apnea based on airflow in which the entire duration of the event is associated with machine-triggered pressure pulse (breaths) (Fig. 12–13). The following rule applies.

Score a respiratory event occurring during PAP device-triggered breaths as a central apnea if all the following criteria are met:

a. There is a decrease in the PAP flow signal meeting apnea criteria.
b. Device-triggered pressure pulses (pressure support) occur during the event.
c. There is no evidence of spontaneous (patient-triggered) respiratory effort during the event.

It is important to note that there may be small deflections in the chest and abdominal effort belt signals at the time of pressure pulses. These do NOT represent patient efforts. The method of documenting a machine triggered breath varies between laboratory PAP devices manufactured by different companies.

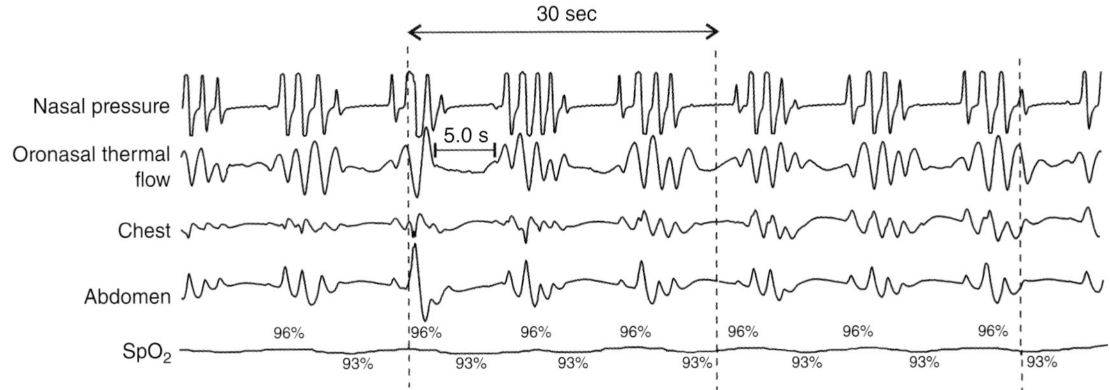

Figure 12–12 Periodic breathing is shown. There are three or more central pauses in breathing for a duration >3 seconds separated by ≤20 seconds (in this case much less) of normal breathing. All central pauses can be scored as central apneas as each is associated with a ≥3% arterial oxygen desaturation. Chest and Abdomen are RIP effort belts.

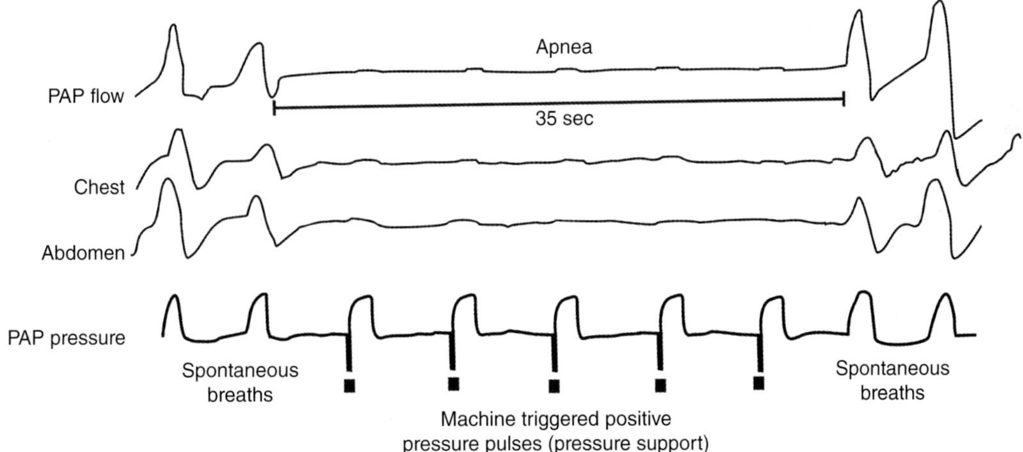

Figure 12–13 An example of an apnea during machine-triggered pressure pulses. The positive pressure pulses (pressure support) that are machine-triggered are marked by the downward artifact added to the PAP pressure signal from the laboratory positive airway pressure (PAP) device. The small deflections in the chest and abdomen are associated with very small amounts of airflow and are not spontaneous inspiratory efforts. The PAP flow signal shows ≥90% reduction from baseline for ≥20 seconds (meets apnea criteria). The AASM scoring manual classifies such an event as a central apnea. The upper airway is closed (or very narrow) consistent with a closed airway central apnea. However, the AASM scoring manual does not use this terminology.

RESPIRATORY PARAMETERS REPORTED IN PEDIATRIC POLYSOMNOGRAPHY

The AASM scoring manual[2] recommends that the following respiratory parameters be reported. Index parameters are the number of events divided by total sleep time (TST). Note that in pediatric polysomnography an *obstructive AHI* is usually specified given that infants and young children often have some central apneas. In the following list, * denoted reporting is recommended,** optional.

1. Number of obstructive, mixed, and central apneas;* number of hypopneas;* number of apneas + hypopneas (AH);* apnea hypopnea index (AHI)* = number of apneas and hypopneas per hour of sleep = (60 × AH)/TST in minutes
2. Apnea index (AI),* Hypopnea index (HI)*
3. AHI during supine and non-supine sleep—useful, not required by AASM scoring manual
4. AHI NREM and AHI REM—useful, not listed in AASM scoring manual
5. Minimum SpO_2 during sleep,* mean SpO_2,* time below a specified oxygen saturation threshold*
6. OD** = number of arterial oxygen desaturations (≥3% or 4%)
7. Oxygen desaturation index (ODI)** = (OD × 60)/TST in minutes
8. Number of RERAs**
9. RERA index* = number of RERAs × 60/TST (minutes)
10. RDI** = AHI + RERA index
11. Obstructive AHI (OAHI)** = number of *obstructive and mixed apneas* + obstructive hypopneas per hour of sleep
12. Central apnea index (CAI)**
13. Occurrence of hypoventilation if present* (recommended diagnostic study). Further details are not specified but usually one reports the maximum $P_{ET}CO_2$ and time spent with a $P_{ET}CO_2$ > 50 mm Hg (absolute time or as % TST) and similar values if using transcutaneous PCO_2.
14. Obstructive apnea hypopnea index (OAHI)** = (number of obstructive and mixed apneas + hypopneas) × 60/TST (in minutes).
15. Occurence of periodic breathing (if present).

SUMMARY OF KEY POINTS

1. Pediatric scoring rules can be used for children **less than** 18 years of age. However, for children ≥13 years with an adult body habitus, respiratory events may be scored using adult criteria.
2. Scoring of central pauses in respiration as central apneas has special requirements including a reduction in the apnea sensor signal by ≥90% of baseline breathing using a recommended or alternative apnea sensor, absent inspiratory effort during the entire event, and at least one of the following: a duration ≥20 seconds, a duration of at least two breaths during baseline breathing and an associated ≥3% desaturation or an arousal, or a duration of at least two breaths during baseline breathing, and is associated with a decrease in heart rate to fewer than 50 beats per minute for at least 5 seconds. For infants younger than 1 year of age, the decrease in heart rate requirement is adjusted to less than 60 beats per minute for at least 15 seconds on account of the higher baseline heart rates.
3. Periodic breathing is normal in premature infants and is present in about 80% of full-term infants for ages 1 to 2 months; some degree of periodic breathing is present in normal full-term infants up to about 6 months of age.
4. Central pauses in respiration occurring as part of episodes of periodic breathing can be scored as central apneas if they meet criteria for central apneas.
5. The end-tidal PCO_2 waveform can be used to score apneas in pediatric patients (acceptable alternative apnea sensor) and is used to score hypoventilation during diagnostic studies.
6. Scoring of hypoventilation during sleep in children during diagnostic studies is recommended but is optional during titration sleep studies. The difference between diagnostic and titration studies is the expense of transcutaneous PCO_2 devices. The recommended hypoventilation sensors are end-tidal PCO_2 (diagnostic study) and transcutaneous PCO_2 (diagnostic or titration study). In sleep centers monitoring pediatric patients with hypoventilation, use of a transcutaneous PCO_2 device is extremely valuable if properly calibrated.
7. Obstructive and mixed apneas have a duration ≥ the duration of two breaths during baseline breathing with a reduction in the apnea sensor signal by ≥90% of baseline breathing. In obstructive apneas inspiratory effort is present during the entire period of apnea. In mixed apneas one portion has absent respiratory effort and one portion inspiratory effort is present regardless of which comes first.
8. In children there is only one hypopnea definition. A reduction in the nasal pressure signal or an alternative hypopea sensor (diagnostic studies), PAP devide flow signal (titration studies) of ≥30% from baseline breathing for a duration ≥ the duration of two breaths during baseline breathing associated with an arousal or a ≥3% arterial oxygen desaturation.
9. RERAs are not common in children as most respiratory events associated with arousals can be scored as apnea or hypopneas. RERAs are sequences of breaths with a duration of at least two breaths during baseline breathing associated with (a) increased inspiratory effort; (b) flattening of the inspiratory waveform (nasal pressure diagnostic study, PAP device flow during PAP titration); (c) snoring; or (d) an increase in end-tidal PCO_2 above baseline.
10. Hypoventilation is defined as a $PaCO_2$ (or surrogate) > 50 mm Hg for >25% of total sleep time.

CLINICAL REVIEW QUESTIONS

1. What type of respiratory event is present in Figure 12–14?
2. In Figure 12–15, are there one or two central apneas?
3. In Figure 12–16, what is the respiratory event? What apnea sensor can be used?
4. In a 16-year-old patient with an adult body habitus, can adult scoring rules be used?
5. Which of the following is the definition of hypoventilation in children?
   A. PCO_2 > 55 mm Hg for >25% total sleep time
   B. PCO_2 ≥ 50 mm Hg for ≥25% total sleep time
   C. PCO_2 > 50 mm Hg for >25% total sleep time
   D. PCO_2 > 50 mm Hg for ≥25% total sleep time
6. What PCO_2 sensor (surrogate for $PaCO_2$) is recommended during positive airway pressure titration studies?
7. Which of the following statements is **NOT** true about periodic breathing in children?
   A. Up until 6 months of age the majority of full-term infants will have a small amount of periodic breathing.
   B. In the first 2 weeks of life about 80% of full-term infants have periodic breathing.
   C. The inspiratory pauses during periodic breathing can be scored as central apneas even if they otherwise meet criteria for central apnea.
   D. ≥20 seconds of normal breathing must separate the inspiratory pauses in breathing.

ANSWERS

1. A RERA event is shown. There is flattening of the nasal pressure signal without a ≥30% decrease in amplitude. Therefore a hypopnea is not scored.
2. Only the first central pause in breathing meets the desaturation criteria for a central apnea. Although both pauses in breathing were the same duration, the desaturation was milder after the second event for reasons that are not known.
3. A central apnea. The nasal pressure and oronasal thermal airflow signals were not functional, but the PCO_2 waveform can be used to score an apnea (acceptable alternative apnea sensor). The patient was being monitored by a divided nasal cannula that was displaced slightly outside the nares but continued to suction exhaled air and record an exhaled PCO_2 signal. The oronasal thermal sensor had been removed by the patient. A central apnea can be scored as the duration is longer at least the duration of two breaths and the event is associated with a ≥3% arterial oxygen desaturation.
4. Yes
5. C (> and >)
6. Transcutaneous PCO_2
7. D. ≤20 seconds, NOT ≥20 seconds of normal breathing between central pauses.

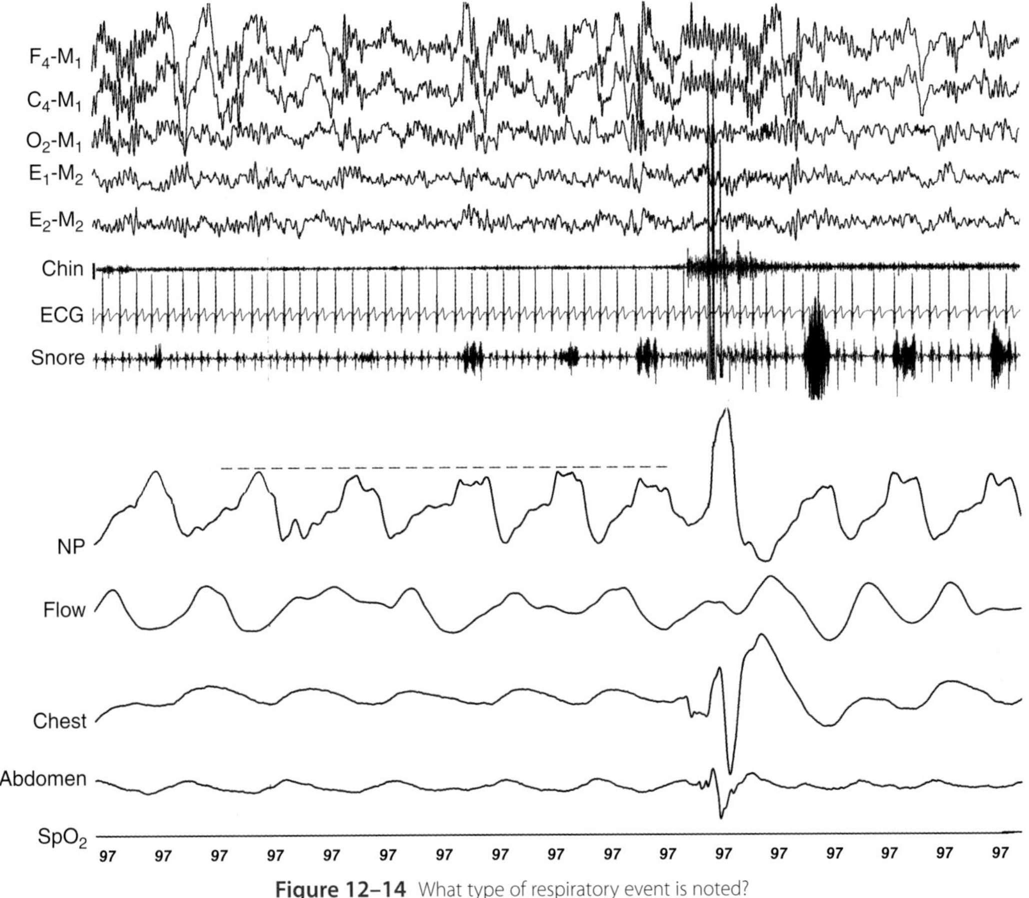

Figure 12–14 What type of respiratory event is noted?

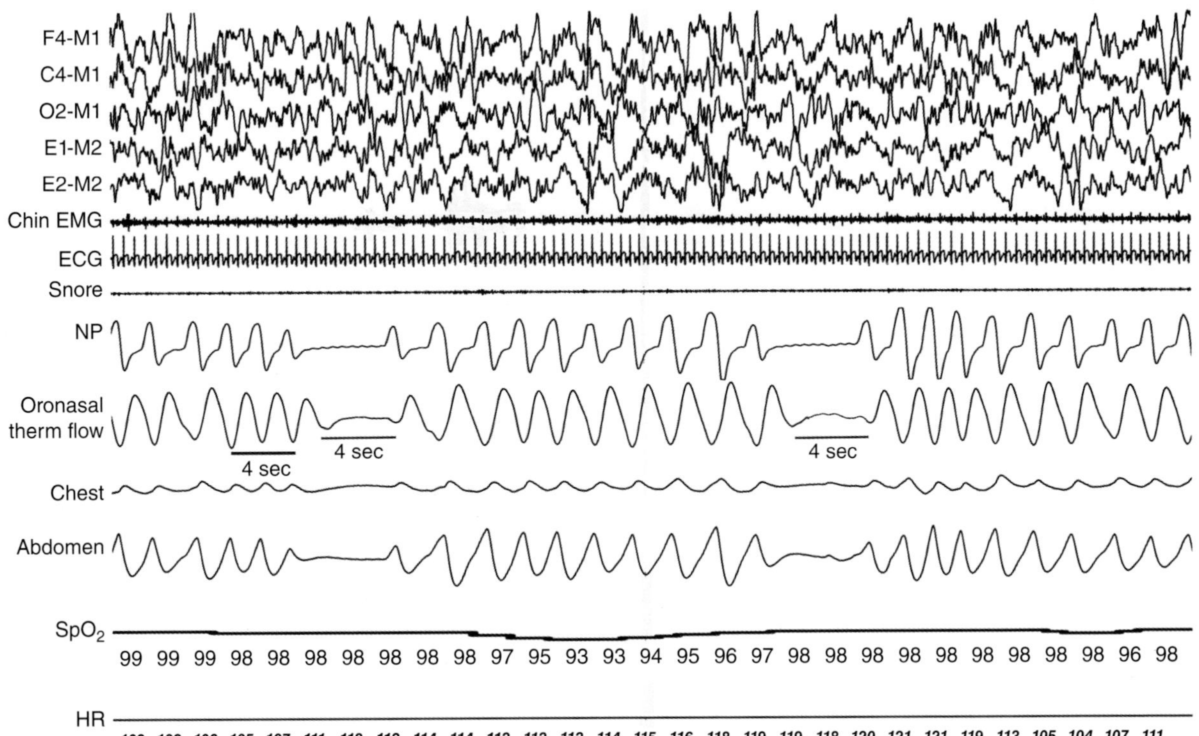

Figure 12–15 How many central apneas are present?

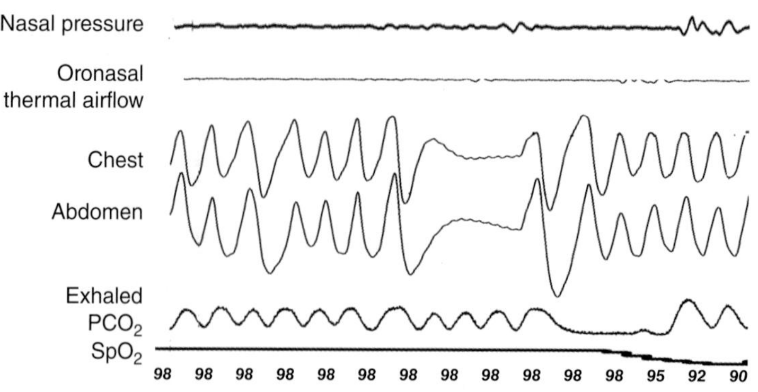

Figure 12–16 What type of respiratory event is present?

SUGGESTED READING

Berry RB, Budhiraja R, Gottlieb DJ, et al. Rules for scoring respiratory events in sleep: update of the 2007 AASM Manual for the Scoring of Sleep and Associated Events. *J Clin Sleep Med.* 2012;8(5):597-619.

Paruthi S, Rosen CL, Wang R, et al. End-tidal carbon dioxide measurement during pediatric polysomnography: signal quality, association with apnea severity, and prediction of neurobehavioral outcomes. *Sleep.* 2015;38(11): 1719-1726.

REFERENCES

1. Berry RB, Budhiraja R, Gottlieb DJ, et al. Rules for scoring respiratory events in sleep: update of the 2007 AASM Manual for the Scoring of Sleep and Associated Events. *J Clin Sleep Med.* 2012;8(5):597-619.
2. Troester MM, Quan SF, Berry RB, et al; for the American Academy of Sleep Medicine. *The AASM Manual for the Scoring of Sleep and Associated Events: Rules, Terminology and Technical Specifications.* Version 3. American Academy of Sleep Medicine; 2023.
3. Fleming S, Thompson M, Stevens R, et al. Normal ranges of heart rate and respiratory rate in children from birth to 18 years of age: a systematic review of observational studies. *Lancet.* 2011;377(9770):1011-1018.
4. Rosen C, D'Andrea L, Haddad G. Adult criteria for obstructive sleep apnea do not identify children with severe obstruction. *Am Rev Respir Dis.* 1992;146:1231-1234.
5. Tapia IE, Karamessinis L, Bandla P, et al. Polysomnographic values in children undergoing puberty: pediatric vs. adult respiratory rules in adolescents. *Sleep.* 2008;31:1737-1744.
6. Accardo JA, Shults J, Leonard MB, Traylor J, Marcus CL. Differences in overnight polysomnography scores using the adult and pediatric criteria for respiratory events in adolescents. *Sleep.* 2010;33:1333-1339.
7. Montgomery-Downs HE, O'Brien LM, Gulliver TE, Gozal D. Polysomnographic characteristics in normal preschool and early school-aged children. *Pediatrics.* 2006;117:741-753.
8. Paruthi S, Rosen CL, Wang R, et al. End-tidal carbon dioxide measurement during pediatric polysomnography: signal quality, association with apnea severity, and prediction of neurobehavioral outcomes. *Sleep.* 2015; 38(11):1719-1726.
9. Kelly DH, Stellwagen LM, Kaitz E, Shannon DC. Apnea and periodic breathing in normal full-term infants during the first twelve months. *Pediatr Pulmonol.* 1985;1(4):215-219.

Sleep and Respiratory Physiology

Chapter 13

INTRODUCTION

The goal of this chapter is to present a brief overview of aspects of respiratory physiology useful for the sleep physician. Most patients who exhibit arterial oxygen desaturation in the sleep center do so from apnea or hypopnea. However, patients with other respiratory disorders may have sleep-related arterial oxygen desaturation and/or hypoventilation without a significant number of discrete apnea or hypopnea events. These abnormalities in gas exchange can occur because the normal effects of sleep on ventilation and oxygenation are magnified by abnormal function of the lung, chest wall, respiratory muscles, or ventilatory control centers. The effects of lung disease on breathing during sleep are discussed in more detail in Chapter 29 and disorders of ventilatory control and respiratory muscle weakness in Chapter 30.

ARTERIAL BLOOD GASES

Alveolar hypoventilation during wakefulness is usually defined as an arterial partial pressure of carbon dioxide ($PaCO_2$) > 45 mm Hg (or ≥ 45 mm Hg in some references). Sleep hypoventilation is defined in the American Academy of Sleep Medicine scoring manual as a $PaCO_2$ (or surrogate) > 55 mm Hg for at least 10 minutes or an increase in $PaCO_2$ ≥ 10 mm Hg above an awake supine value with the absolute value >50 mm Hg for ≥ 10 minutes.[1,2] This is based on limited observations in normal subjects of an increase in $PaCO_2$ during sleep of 2 to 7 mm Hg (on average about 4–5 mm Hg).[2] Surrogates for the arterial PCO_2 include end-tidal PCO_2 or transcutaneous PCO_2 (appropriately calibrated). Hypoxemia is defined as a low arterial partial pressure of oxygen (PaO_2) relative to predicted values. A PaO_2 less than 55 mm Hg while awake and breathing room air is considered severe and an indication for chronic 24-hour supplemental oxygen therapy. Milder degree of hypoxemia can be identified by comparing a PaO_2 with a predicted value for age. A simple estimate of a normal predicted PaO_2 is [105 − ½ age (in years)].

The alveolar gas equation[3] (Equation 13-1) allows one to compute the alveolar (ideal) partial pressure of oxygen (**PAO_2**) from the fractional concentration of oxygen in inspired gas (FiO_2), which is 0.21 when breathing room air, and the $PaCO_2$. The respiratory exchange ratio (R) is the CO_2 elimination divided by the O_2 uptake. At steady state, R is equal to the respiratory quotient (RQ), which equals the CO_2 production/O_2 consumption $\dot{V}CO_2/\dot{V}O_2$. R is usually assumed to be 0.8.[3] In Equation 13-1, P_B is the barometric pressure (760 mm Hg at sea level) and PH_2O is the partial pressure of water vapor (47 mm Hg at 37°C). The inspired partial pressure of oxygen $PiO_2 = (P_B - 47) \times FiO_2$. The FiO_2 remains the same at increased altitude (0.21), but the P_B is decreased with ascent above sea level. Breathing room air, Equation 13-1 becomes Equation 13-2, which is used to compute the ideal (alveolar) PAO_2. The alveolar-arterial (A-a) gradient is the difference between the ideal PAO_2 and the actual (measured) PaO_2 (Equation 13-3).[3-5] Studies have determined the A-a gradient in normal individuals,[4-7] and Equation 13-4 gives several formulas for a predicted A-a gradient (usually <25 mm Hg).[7] Computing the A-a gradient allows one to identify hypoxemia solely due to hypoventilation (increased $PaCO_2$) as the A-a gradient is normal. Hypoxemia due to lung disease is associated with an increased A-a gradient.

$$PAO_2 = FiO_2 \times (P_B - PH_2O) - PaCO_2/R \qquad \text{Equation 13–1}$$

$$R = RQ = \dot{V}CO_2/\dot{V}O_2 \text{ (assumed to be 0.8)}$$

$$\dot{V}CO_2 = CO_2 \text{ elimination}$$

$$\dot{V}O_2 = O_2 \text{ uptake}$$

Breathing room air at sea level — Equation 13–2

$$PAO_2 = 0.21\,(760 - 47) - PaCO_2/0.8 = 150 - PaCO_2/0.8$$

$$\text{A-a gradient} = PAO_2 - PaO_2 \qquad \text{Equation 13–3}$$

Predicted estimates of normal A-a gradient (age in years) — Equation 13–4

$$\text{A-a gradient} = 4 + (\text{age in years})/4$$

$$\text{A-a gradient} = 2.5 + 0.21\,(\text{age})$$

$$\text{A-a gradient} = (10 + \text{age})/4$$

For example, using the second equation for a 48-year-old, the A-a gradient = 2.5 + 0.21 (48) = 12.1, and for a 60-year-old the A-a gradient would be 15.2.

The major causes of hypoxemia[3] are listed in Table 13–1. Causes of hypoxemia include a low FiO_2, a low P_B (high altitude), hypoventilation (increased $PaCO_2$), ventilation perfusion ($\dot{V}/\dot{Q}$) mismatch, shunt, and diffusion abnormality. In ($\dot{V}/\dot{Q}$) mismatch, some alveoli are underventilated for their blood flow (low ($\dot{V}/\dot{Q}$) and blood is incompletely oxygenated. This can be overcome by increasing the FiO2, thereby increasing the effective oxygen flow to underventilated alveoli. If shunt is causing hypoxemia, blood completely bypasses the alveoli. The deoxygenated blood mixes with oxygenated blood to give a lower than ideal PaO_2. Raising the FiO_2 has no effect on shunted blood. Diffusion abnormality is also frequently listed as a cause of hypoxemia due to impaired diffusion of oxygen from the alveolus to the pulmonary capillaries due to fibrosis or inflammation (thickened membrane) or interstitial

Table 13–1 Major Causes of Hypoxemia

	A-a Gradient	Responds to Supplemental Oxygen
Low FiO_2, low P_B	Normal	Yes
Hypoventilation	Normal	Yes
($\dot{V}/\dot{Q}$) mismatch	Increased	Yes
Shunt	Increased	No
Diffusion abnormality	Increased	Yes

A-a, alveolar-arterial gradient; *FiO_2,* fractional concentration of inspired oxygen; *PB,* barometric pressure; ($\dot{V}/\dot{Q}$), ventilation-perfusion ratio.

edema. This abnormality results in incomplete oxygenation of blood leaving the pulmonary capillaries but is not due to inadequate ventilation. However, diffusion impairment is usually associated with some degree of ($\dot{V}/\dot{Q}$) mismatch. Raising the FiO_2 in the alveoli increases diffusion and can overcome diffusion abnormality. Most patients with lung disease also have defects in CO_2 excretion due to high ($\dot{V}/\dot{Q}$) lung units ("wasted ventilation," high physiological dead space).[3] This may not result in alveolar hypoventilation (increased $PaCO_2$) because the patient may compensate by increasing the minute ventilation (discussed later). Hypoxemia can occur simply because of isolated hypoventilation. As noted above, a patient with normal lungs may have an increased $PaCO_2$ due to muscle weakness or abnormal ventilatory control. In this case, the measured PaO_2 is close to the ideal (PAO_2) computed from the alveolar gas equation (Equation 13-1) using the known $PaCO_2$ and the computed A-a gradient (Equation 13-3) would be normal. Lung disease severe enough to cause an increased $PaCO_2$ is always associated with an increased A-a gradient. Box 13-1 presents examples of use of the alveolar gas equation (Equation 13-1). In a patient with amyotrophic lateral sclerosis (ALS; Example 1), an arterial blood gas reveals a PaO_2 of 60 mm Hg and a $PaCO_2$ of 65 mm Hg. The computed A-a gradient is 8.7 mm Hg (normal). Hypoxemia is due to hypoventilation secondary to respiratory muscle weakness. In Example 2, a patient with chronic obstructive pulmonary disease has evidence of both hypoxemia and hypercapnia and the A-a gradient is increased. The hypoxemia is due to both ($\dot{V}/\dot{Q}$) mismatch and hypoventilation. In patients with hypoventilation of unclear etiology, calculating an A-a gradient can provide an important clue as to whether the hypoxemia is due to lung disease or due entirely to hypoventilation. *A normal A-a gradient in a patient with hypoventilation would suggest a disorder of ventilatory control or a neuromuscular disorder (muscle weakness).* The pattern can also be seen with thoracic cage disorders. However, patients with abnormalities in ventilatory control or muscle weakness can have an *increased A-a gradient if lung disease is also present.* The A-a gradient increases with the FiO_2;[5] therefore, it is most useful when patients are breathing room air.

The physiology of oxygen transport, the hemoglobin-oxygen dissociation curve, and pulse oximetry are discussed in detail in Chapter 10 and will not be repeated here. An understanding of oximetry is important as this measurement assesses oxygenation in the sleep center and determination of arterial oxygen desaturation is important for detection of respiratory events during polysomnography.

Box 13-1 EXAMPLES OF CALCULATION OF THE A-A GRADIENT

Example 1: Hypoventilation due to amyotrophic lateral sclerosis (normal A-a gradient) in a 60-year-old patient

Laboratory: PaO_2 = 60 mm Hg and $PaCO_2$ = 65 mm Hg (breathing room air)
Predicted A-a gradient = 4 + 60/4 = 19
Computation: PAO_2 = 150 − 65/0.8 = 68.8
A-a gradient = PAO_2 − PaO_2 = 68.8 − 60 = 8.8 (normal)

Example 2: Hypoventilation due to chronic obstructive pulmonary disease (increased A-a gradient) in a 60-year-old patient

Laboratory: PaO_2 = 50 mm Hg and $PaCO_2$ = 55 mm Hg (breathing room air)
PAO_2 = 150 − (55/0.8) = 81
A-a gradient = PAO_2 − PaO_2 = 81 − 50 = 31 (increased)

A-a, gradient Alveolar-arterial gradient; *$PaCO_2$,* arterial partial pressure of carbon dioxide; *PAO_2,* alveolar partial pressure of oxygen; *PaO_2,* arterial partial pressure of oxygen.

DETERMINANTS OF $PaCO_2$

The $PaCO_2$ is determined by the CO_2 production ($\dot{V}CO_2$) and the alveolar ventilation ($\dot{V}_A$) (Equation 13-5). The $PaCO_2$ is inversely related to the alveolar ventilation. For the same CO_2 production, if the alveolar ventilation doubles, the $PaCO_2$ decreases to half the original value. The $\dot{V}_A$ equals the minute ventilation ($\dot{V}_E$) minus the dead space ventilation ($\dot{V}_D$) (Equation 13-6). The $\dot{V}_D$ can be written as the product of the respiratory rate (RR) and the dead space (V_D). The dead space includes the anatomic dead space (no alveoli) and overventilated areas of the lung (high $\dot{V}/\dot{Q}$ units).[8] The $\dot{V}_D$ is "wasted ventilation." If the minute ventilation $\dot{V}_E$ is expressed as the respiratory rate (RR) × tidal volume (V_T), then the alveolar ventilation can be expressed using the dead space to tidal volume ratio (V_D/V_T as shown in Equation 13-7). The equation for $PaCO_2$ can be written so that $PaCO_2$ depends on the minute ventilation (VT × RR) and the V_D/V_T ratio (Equation 13-8).

$$PaCO_2 = K \times \frac{\dot{V}CO_2}{\dot{V}A} \quad K = \text{constant} \qquad \text{Equation 13–5}$$

$$\dot{V}_A = \dot{V}_E - \dot{V}_D \qquad \text{Equation 13–6}$$

$$\dot{V}_A = (RR \times V_T) - (RR \times V_D) \qquad \text{Equation 13–7}$$

$$= RR \times V_T\left(1 - \frac{V_D}{V_T}\right)$$

$$PaCO_2 = \frac{K \times \dot{V}CO2}{RR \times VT\left(1 - \frac{V_D}{V_T}\right)} \qquad \text{Equation 13–8}$$

Table 13–2 illustrates the effect of different patterns of breathing on the alveolar ventilation and the $PaCO_2$. For the same minute ventilation, breathing with a low V_T and high RR is associated with an increased V_D/V_T ratio, a decreased $\dot{V}_A$, and

Table 13–2 Effects of Changing Dead Space and Tidal Volume

		$\frac{V_D}{V_T}$	V_D (ml)	V_T (ml)	RR (bpm)	$\dot{V}_E$ (L/min)	$\dot{V}_D$ (L/min)	$\dot{V}_A$ (L/min)	$PaCO_2$* (mm Hg)
						$RR \times V_T$	$RR \times V_D$	$\dot{V}_E - \dot{V}_D$	
A	Normal	0.3	200	600	10	6.0	2.0	4.0	40
B	Low V_T, same $\dot{V}_E$	0.5	200	400	15	6.0	3.0	3.0	53
C	High V_D, higher $\dot{V}_E$	0.42	300	700	10	7.8	3.8	4.0	40
D	High V_D, low V_T	0.6	300	500	20	10.0	6.0	4.0	40

$\dot{V}_E$ Minute ventilation $\dot{V}_A$ Alveolar ventilation $\dot{V}_D$ Dead space ventilation

Notes

A V_T tidal volume RR respiratory rate

$*PaCO_2 = K \times \dot{V}CO_2/\dot{V}_A$ * assumes $K \times \dot{V}CO_2 = 160 \frac{ml}{min}$ V_T tidal volume RR respiratory rate

B Lower tidal volume and higher respiratory rate results in a lower alveolar ventilation for the same minute ventilation.

C Higher minute ventilation is needed to achieve a normal alveolar ventilation due to an increased V_D.

D Higher minute ventilation in needed to achieve a normal alveolar ventilation due to an increased V_D and decreased V_T.

an increased $PaCO_2$ (Table 13–2, example B). Patients with lung disease often have an increased dead space. However, the $PaCO_2$ can still be normal if there is a compensatory increase in minute ventilation (Table 13–2 example C). The combination of a high dead space and low tidal volume requires an even greater increase in minute ventilation (produced by an increased respiratory rate) to provide compensation (Table 13–2, example D). The anatomic dead space is approximately the lean body weight in pounds and is approximately one-third of the tidal volume in normal individuals. The normal V_D/V_T ratio in percent is equal to 24.6 + 0.17 × age (in years).[9] For example, a 40-year-old individual would have a V_D/V_T of about 31%, or a ratio of 0.31. Hart and coworkers developed a prediction equation for the physiological V_D based on height.[10] The physiologic V_D equals the anatomic V_D + the effect of high $\dot{V}/\dot{Q}$ lung units. In lung disease, the physiologic V_D is increased and *higher than normal minute ventilation is needed to produce the same alveolar ventilation* (and $PaCO_2$). Patients who have a rapid, shallow breathing pattern are predisposed to hypoventilation because this is an inefficient method of breathing (high V_D/V_T). However, patients with muscle weakness or a stiff chest wall (high work of breathing) may use a pattern of ventilation with a small V_T and high RR to avoid respiratory muscle fatigue.

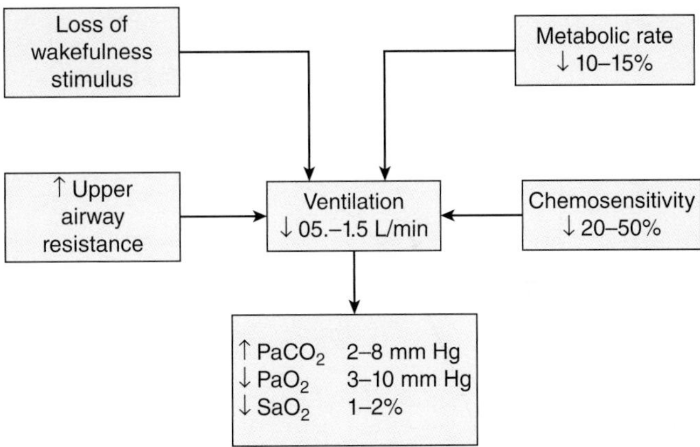

Figure 13–1 Changes in ventilation and gas exchange with normal sleep. The loss of wakefulness stimuli and reduced ventilatory drive + increased upper airway resistance result in a reduction in minute ventilation. Although the metabolic rate and CO_2 excretion are lower, the net effect is a mild increase in the arterial partial pressure of carbon dioxide ($PaCO_2$) and decrease in the arterial pressure of oxygen (PaO_2). *SaO_2*, Arterial oxygen saturation. Of note, here the increase in PaCO2 with sleep is 2 to 8 mmHg while another reference gives a range of 2 to 7 mm Hg for the increase in PaCO2 during sleep 2. (From Mohsenin V. Sleep in chronic obstructive pulmonary disease: sleep and respiration. *Semin Respir Crit Care Med.* 2005;26:109-115.)

Normal Changes in Ventilation During Sleep

The changes in respiratory physiology during normal sleep are summarized in Figure 13–1 and Table 13–3. During sleep, the metabolic rate falls (hence, decreased CO_2 production), but this is offset by a proportionately greater fall in minute ventilation (and alveolar ventilation) with the result that the $PaCO_2$ increases slightly. The fall in ventilation is due to increased upper airway resistance and decreased chemosensitivity as well as the loss of the wakefulness stimulus to breathe.[11-12] The result is that the $PaCO_2$ rises and the PaO_2 falls slightly. Because of the normal position on the flat portion of the O_2Hb dissociation curve, there is little change in the SaO_2 as a result of the fall in PO_2 associated with sleep (Figure 13–2). If the baseline awake PaO_2 is lower, the fall in SaO_2 will be greater for the same drop in PaO_2. In patients with lung disease and a lower awake PaO_2, even a normal sleep-related drop in PaO_2 will be associated with a larger decrease in the SaO_2.

The decrease in minute ventilation with sleep is due to a fall in V_T with minimal change in the respiratory rate (RR)[11-14] (Figure 13–3). Studies of changes in respiration during sleep have uniformly found a reduction in minute ventilation during sleep due to a decrease in tidal volume. Kreiger et al. found no change in respiratory rate on transition from wakefulness to NREM sleep and no change in tidal volume from NREM to REM sleep.[13] However the respiratory rate was

Table 13–3 Changes in Ventilation With Sleep (Compared With Wake)

Parameter	NREM	REM
Respiratory rate	Unchanged or increased	Variable, central apnea can occur Higher in phasic REM*
Tidal volume	Decreased	Further decreased from NREM—during phasic (REMs present) REM sleep*
Minute ventilation	Decreased (≈20% from wake)	Decreased more than NREM more in some studies Decreased in phasic REM sleep > tonic REM*
Alveolar ventilation	Decreased	Decreased more than NREM in some studies. Decreased in phasic more than tonic REM
$PaCO_2$	Slightly increased (2–8 mm Hg)	Increased slightly more
PaO_2	Decreased slightly (3–10 mm Hg)	Decreased slightly more
SaO_2	Decreased 1%–2%	Decreased slightly more
Hypercapnic ventilatory response	Decreased	Decreased more
Hypoxic ventilatory response	Decreased (NREM men), REM (men and women)	Decreased more
Upper airway resistance	Increased	Increased more during phasic REM*

Phasic REM, Rapid eye movements present.

Data from Krieger J, Maglasiu N, Sforza E, Kurtz D. Breathing during sleep in normal middle-aged subjects. *Sleep*. 1990;13(2):143-154; Douglas NJ, White DP, Pickett CK, Weil JV, Zwillich CW. Respiration during sleep in normal man. *Thorax*. 1982;37(11):840-844; and *Wiegand L, Zwillich CW, Wiegand D, White DP. Changes in upper airway muscle activation and ventilation during phasic REM sleep in normal men. *J Appl Physiol (1985)*. 1991;71(2):488-497.

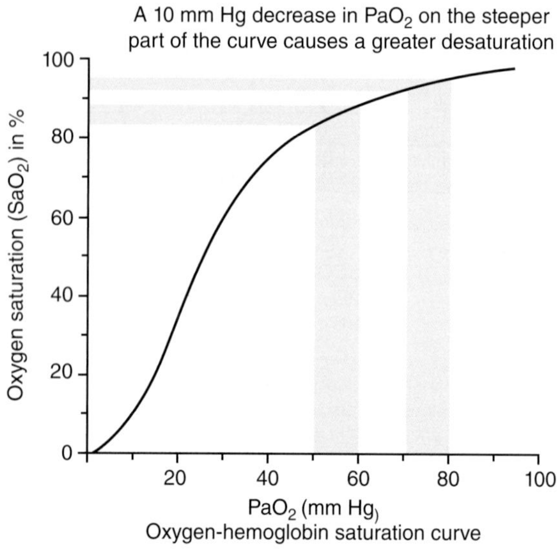

Figure 13–2 The same drop in arterial partial pressure of oxygen (PaO_2) causes a greater drop in the arterial oxygen saturation (SaO_2) if the starting point is on the steeper slope of the oxygen-hemoglobin saturation curve (dissociation curve). Patients with lung disease and a wake PaO_2 of 60 mm Hg will experience a greater drop in the SaO_2 with sleep onset. (From Berry RB. *Fundamentals of Sleep Medicine*. Elsevier; 2012:413.)

higher during REM sleep compared to both wakefulness and NREM sleep. Douglas et al.[14] found a small increase in respiratory rate from wake to sleep (both NREM and REM) and *a decrease in tidal volume from stage N2* to REM sleep without a change in respiratory rate. Other studies have found the respiratory rate during REM sleep to be slightly higher and variable. As REM sleep is not homogenous measurement of the tidal volume is influenced by the amount of rapid eye movements (REMs) present. In phasic REM sleep (REMs present) ventilation is more variable than during tonic REM sleep (no or minimal REMs). During bursts of REMs the tidal volume is often decreased as ventilation is inhibited. Some studies have found lower minute ventilation during REM sleep compared with NREM sleep[14] but others have not. **Phasic** REM sleep appears to have lower ventilation than non–rapid eye movement (NREM) and a higher and variable respiratory rate. The end-tidal PCO_2 increases 1 to 2 mm Hg from wake to NREM and another 1 to 2 mm Hg from NREM to REM sleep. The gradient from the end-tidal PCO_2 to the arterial PCO_2 is about 2 to 7 mm Hg and the $PaCO_2$ increases on average about 4 to 5 mm Hg (range 2 - 8 mm Hg) during sleep.[2] During the transition from wake to stage N1 and early stage N2, the ventilation can be slightly irregular and transitional central apneas can occur at the transition from wake to sleep. However, in stable stage N2 and stage N3, the V_T and RR are nearly constant. During REM sleep, ventilation is irregular with periods of decreased V_T associated with bursts of REMs and the respiratory rate is variable.[15,16] In Figure 13–4 note the reduction in airflow and respiratory effort (esophageal pressure deflections) associated with a burst of REMs. The moving time average of the genioglossus (GG) activity is also reduced. The functional residual capacity, which is the resting end expiratory lung volume, decreases from wake to sleep.[17] In some individuals, there may be a further decrease from NREM to REM sleep, at least during periods with a reduced tidal volume.[18] Changes in ventilatory parameters are summarized in Table 13–3.

APNEIC THRESHOLD

During NREM sleep there is an apneic threshold (AT) in $PaCO_2$ below which central apnea occurs.[19-21] This will be discussed in more detail in Chapter 30. The AT is usually near the awake eucapnic $PaCO_2$ level. For example, with sleep onset the $PaCO_2$ might increase from 40 to 45 mm Hg (Figure 13–5). In this figure an isometabolic hyperbola shows

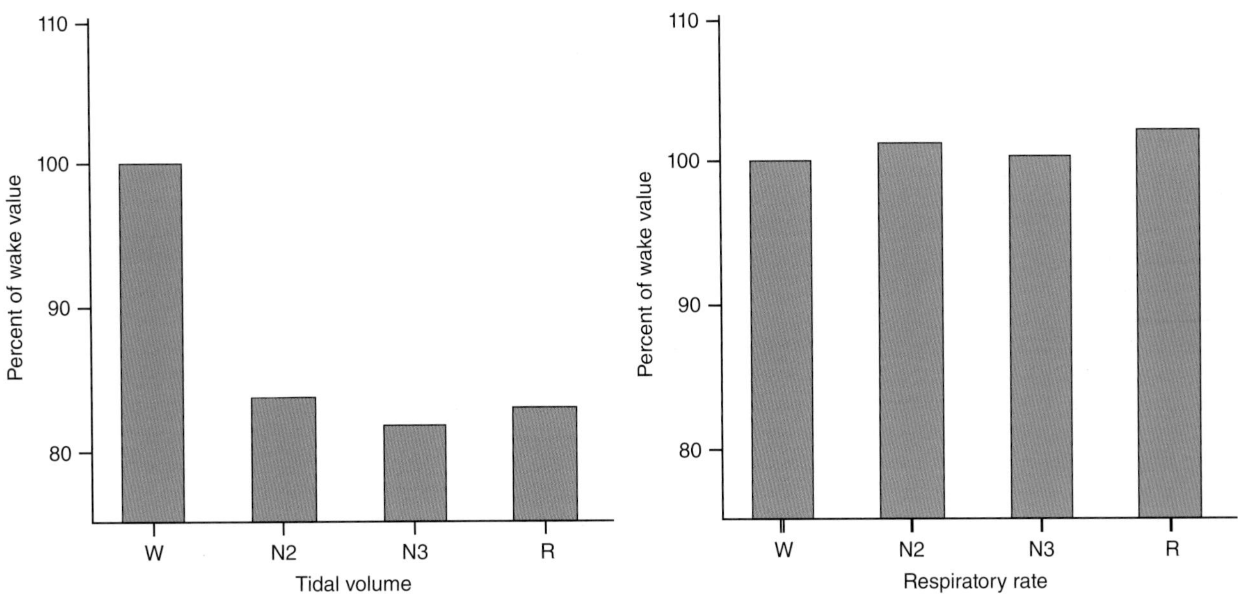

Figure 13–3 The fall in minute ventilation from wakefulness to sleep is due to a fall in tidal volume (VT) with no significant change in respiratory rate (RR). REM, Rapid eye movement; N2, stage N2; N3, stage 3–4 (stage N3); W, wakefulness. (From Krieger J. Respiratory physiology: breathing in normal subjects. In: Kryger MH, Roth T, Dement WC, eds. *Principles and Practice of Sleep Medicine*. Elsevier; 2005:232-255.)

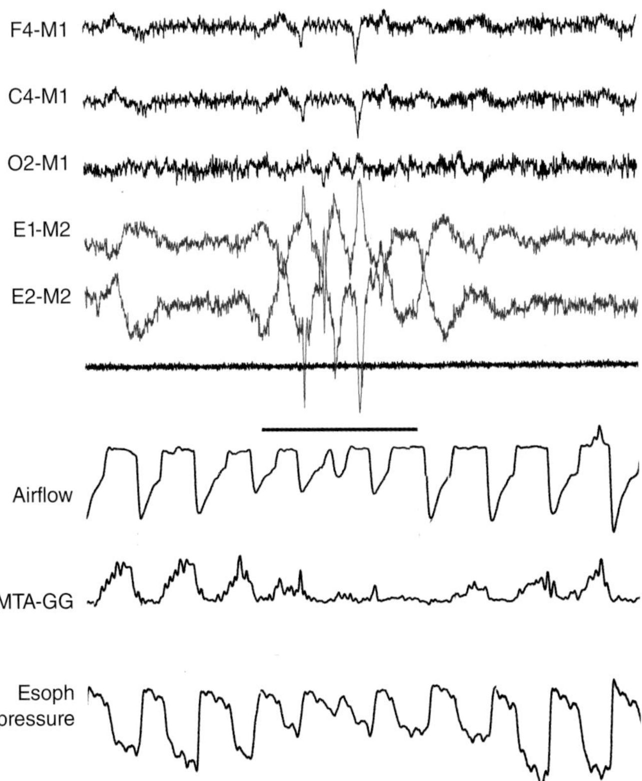

Figure 13–4 During a burst of rapid eye movements in REM sleep, a decrease in airflow, respiratory effort (esophageal pressure deflections), and moving time average of the EMG of the genioglossus muscle (MTA-GG) is noted. Phasic REM sleep is characterized by periods of inhibition of respiration and sometimes increased respiratory rate. During these periods a reduction in tidal volume and ventilation is common. Esoph is esophageal pressure.

the relationship between alveolar ventilation and the $PaCO_2$. If the CO_2 production remains constant, all possible combinations of $PaCO_2$ and alveolar ventilation fall along the line. The sleeping eucapnic $PaCO_2$ (45 mm Hg) and the line showing the relationship between $PaCO_2$ and ventilation above and below eucapnia (slope = hypercapnic ventilatory response) are illustrated. If ventilation transiently increases and the $PaCO_2$ falls to 40 mm Hg (the AT), ventilation ceases (central apnea). For example, if a patient arouses and increases ventilation so that the $PaCO_2$ decreases from 45 mm Hg to below 40 mm Hg (the AT) on return to sleep, a central apnea will occur. The change in $PaCO_2$ needed to reach the AT is the CO_2 reserve[20] – the larger the reserve, the larger the de-

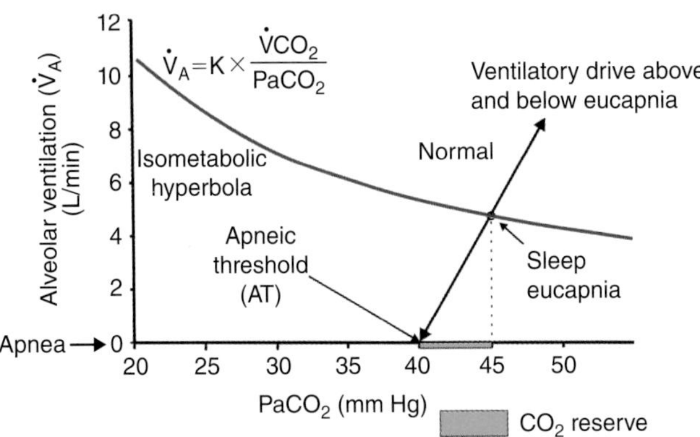

Figure 13–5 The isometabolic hyperbola is shown in *red* and represents the steady state relation between alveolar ventilation and $PaCO_2$ (arterial partial pressure of carbon dioxide). The apneic threshold (AT) is the $PaCO_2$ at which ventilation is zero. In this normal individual the eucapnic set point during sleep and the ventilatory drive above and below eucapnia are shown. The slope of the alveolar ventilation versus $PaCO_2$ line is the hypercapnic ventilatory response. If alveolar ventilation increases sufficiently to reduce the $PaCO_2$ to the AT, central apnea occurs. The drop in the $PaCO_2$ needed to reach the AT is called the CO_2 reserve. In normal individuals the AT is close to the waking $PaCO_2$ value.

crease in the $PaCO^2$ and increase in ventilation needed to reach the AT. Patients with an increased hypercapnic ventilatory drive have a lower awake and sleeping $PaCO_2$ (for example certain patients with congestive heart failure). In this case the CO_2 reserve is smaller and the change in ventilation needed to reach the AT is also smaller. This is illustrated in Figure 13–6. However, the high ventilatory drive and not the lower eucapnic sleeping (and awake) $PaCO_2$ is the cause of the low CO_2 reserve. As shown in Figure 13–7, a lower sleeping eucapnic $PaCO_2$ actually decreases plant gain (change in $PaCO_2$ for a given change in alveolar ventilation) due to the position of the $PaCO_2$ set point on the steeper part of the isometabolic hyperbola. That is, a larger increase in ventilation is needed for the same decrease in the $PaCO_2$. As Figure 13–6 shows, the effect of the increased ventilatory response to $PaCO^2$ (steeper slope) is the predominant effect and the CO_2 reserve is smaller and the increase in ventilation needed to reach the AT is also smaller. The low awake and sleeping $PaCO_2$ values are simply a marker for the high ventilatory drive. As will be discussed in Chapter 30, patients with primary central sleep apnea and central apnea associated with Cheyne-Stokes respiration have an increased ventilatory drive during wakefulness and sleep.[21]

During REM sleep it is not possible to define an AT and hypocapnic central apnea does not occur. The ventilatory drive in REM sleep is lower, making excessive ventilation effects of less likely and therefore less likely to produce hypocapnia. In addition, ventilation during REM sleep is not completely under chemoreceptor control. Not only is there a generalized decreased in tonic muscle activity (diaphragm spared), but there are periodic decreases in the inspiratory (phasic) neural drive to breathe to both the diaphragm and upper airway muscles (Figure 13–4). The chemical drive (increased $PaCO_2$, decreased PO_2) does not decease during these periods but the response of the motor neurons does. *This is believed to be due to the inhibitory influence of nonrespiratory neurons (manifesting phasic REM changes) acting on respiratory neurons (neuromodulation). More information about the effects of REM sleep on upper airway muscles and the diaphragm is provided in chapter 19.* There may also be periods of higher respiratory rate, and breathing is irregular. The clinical significance of the lack of an AT during REM sleep is that hypocapnic central sleep apnea as associated with primary central sleep apnea, treatment emergent central sleep apnea, and central sleep apnea during Cheyne-Stokes breathing is usually NOT present during REM sleep.[19-21] Central sleep apnea due to opioids is also less likely to occur during REM sleep.

BRIEF SUMMARY OF BRAINSTEM CENTERS INVOLVED IN VENTILATORY CONTROL

A detailed discussion of ventilatory control is beyond the scope of this chapter. Some major elements are summarized in Table 13–4 and illustrated in schematic form in Figures 13–8 and 13–9. The peripheral chemoreceptors include the bilateral carotid bodies (located near the bifurcation of carotid arteries) and aortic bodies (located along the aortic arch) that respond rapidly to changes in PaO_2 (NOT SaO_2), but the response depends on $PaCO_2$ and pH.[22-24] A higher $PaCO_2$ and lower pH are associated with a greater response to falls in PaO_2.

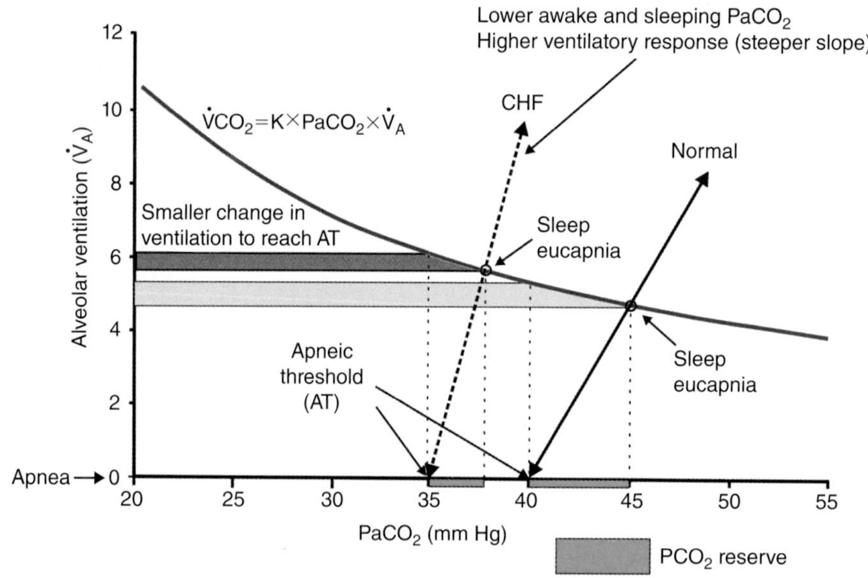

Figure 13–6 The isometabolic hyperbola is shown in *red* (the steady state relation between alveolar ventilation and $PaCO_2$ (arterial partial pressure of carbon dioxide). In some patients with congestive heart failure (CHF) the ventilatory drive to PCO_2 is increased compared with normal individuals above and below the sleeping eucapnia set point, which is at a lower than normal $PaCO_2$ during sleep. The apneic threshold (AT) is the $PaCO_2$ at which ventilation is zero. The difference in $PaCO_2$ at eucapnia and at the AT is called the CO_2 reserve and signifies the change in the $PaCO_2$ needed to reach the AT. The CO_2 reserve in the patient with heart failure who has a lower resting $PaCO_2$ and a greater ventilatory response to $PaCO_2$ (steeper slope) is smaller than normal. The change in **ventilation** corresponding to the change from eucapnia to the AT is also smaller in the patient with heart failure compared with normal. As shown in the next figure, the lower $PaCO_2$ sleeping set point is not the cause of a reduced CO_2 reserve and decreases plant gain (change in $PaCO_2$ for a given change in ventilation). However the increased ventilatory drive effect is predominant. Individuals with a low CO_2 reserve are more likely to have central sleep apnea. (Figure adapted from Dempsey JA. Central sleep apnea: misunderstood and mistreated! *F1000Res.* 2019;8:F1000 Faculty Rev-981.)

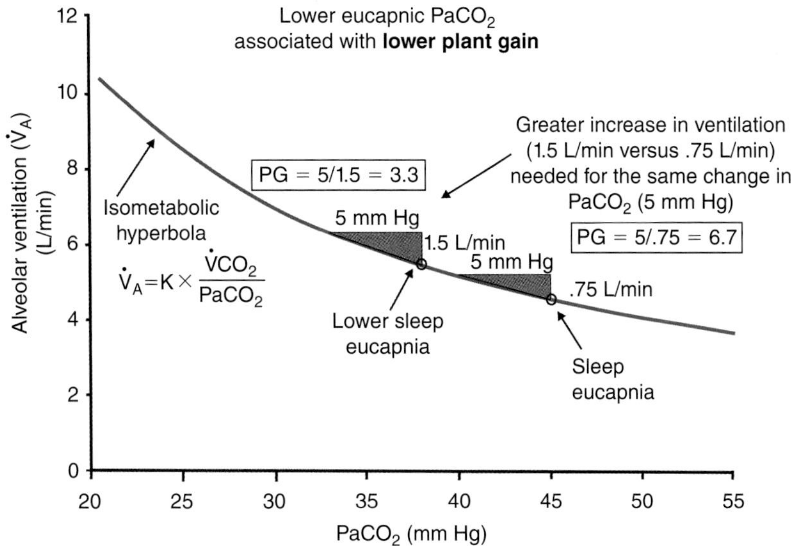

Figure 13–7 The plant gain is defined as change in PCO_2 for a given change in ventilation $(\Delta PaCO_2/\Delta\dot{V}_A)$. A lower eucapnic sleeping PCO_2 is associated with lower plant gain due to the position on the isometabolic hyperbola with a **steeper slope**. Here the same change in PCO_2 (5 mm Hg) requires a larger increase in ventilation (1.5 L/min compared with 0.75 L/min). (Figure adapted from Dempsey JA. Central sleep apnea: misunderstood and mistreated! *F1000Res.* 2019;8:F1000 Faculty Rev-981.)

Table 13–4 Elements of Ventilatory Control

Controller	Location	Afferents Stimulus	Effects
Dorsal respiratory group (DRG)	Dorsomedial medulla	Upper airway (CN 5) Arterial chemoreceptors (CN 9) Lung afferents (CN10)	Ramping pattern of firing during continued inspiration
Ventral respiratory group (VRG)	Ventrolateral medulla	Need for forced expiration	Stimulate phrenic, intercostal, abdominal motor neurons
Pre-Bötzinger area	Ventrolateral medulla	—	Pacemaker for respiration
Pneumotaxic center	Rostral pons (nucleus parabrachialis and Kölliker-Fuse nucleus	Fine adjustment of respiratory response to hypercapnia, hypoxia, and lung volume changes	Tonic input to respiratory pattern generator Control of duration of inspiration
Apneustic center	Lower pons	Pneumotaxic center and vagal input	Signals the smooth termination of inspiratory efforts
Central chemoreceptors	Medulla—ventrolateral surface	Extracellular [H+]—$PaCO_2$ diffuses into extracellular area	Responds to brain extracellular [H+]
Peripheral chemoreceptors	Carotid bodies (near bifurcation of carotid artery), aortic bodies (aortic arch)	CN 9 to medulla (carotid body), CN 10 to medulla (aortic bodies)	Respond to PaO_2, PCO_2, and pH. Increased output with low PaO_2 (increased $PaCO_2$, and decreased pH augment this effect.) Hypoxia increases sensitivity to PCO_2 and pH Quick response
Pulmonary mechanoreceptors	1. PSR in proximal airway smooth muscle 2. J-receptors lung in juxtacapillary area respond to pulmonary congestion (innervated by CN 10) 3. Bronchial C-fiber	—	1. Respond to inflation 2. Mediate dyspnea, increased repiratory rate 3. Affect bronchomotor tone and respond to pulmonary inflammation
Upper airway mechanoreceptors	Upper airway	CN 9 to NTS	Respond to negative pressure

CN 5, Cranial nerve 5 (trigeminal); *CN 9*, cranial nerve 9 (glossopharyngeal); *CN 10*, cranial nerve 10 (vagus); *DRG*, dorsal respiratory group; [*H*+], hydrogen ion concentration; *NTS*, nucleus tractus solitarius; *PSR*, pulmonary stretch receptors; *VRG*, ventral respiratory group.

Adapted from Malik V, Smith D, Lee-Chiong T. Respirator physiology during sleep. *Sleep Med Clin.* 2012;7(3):497-505.

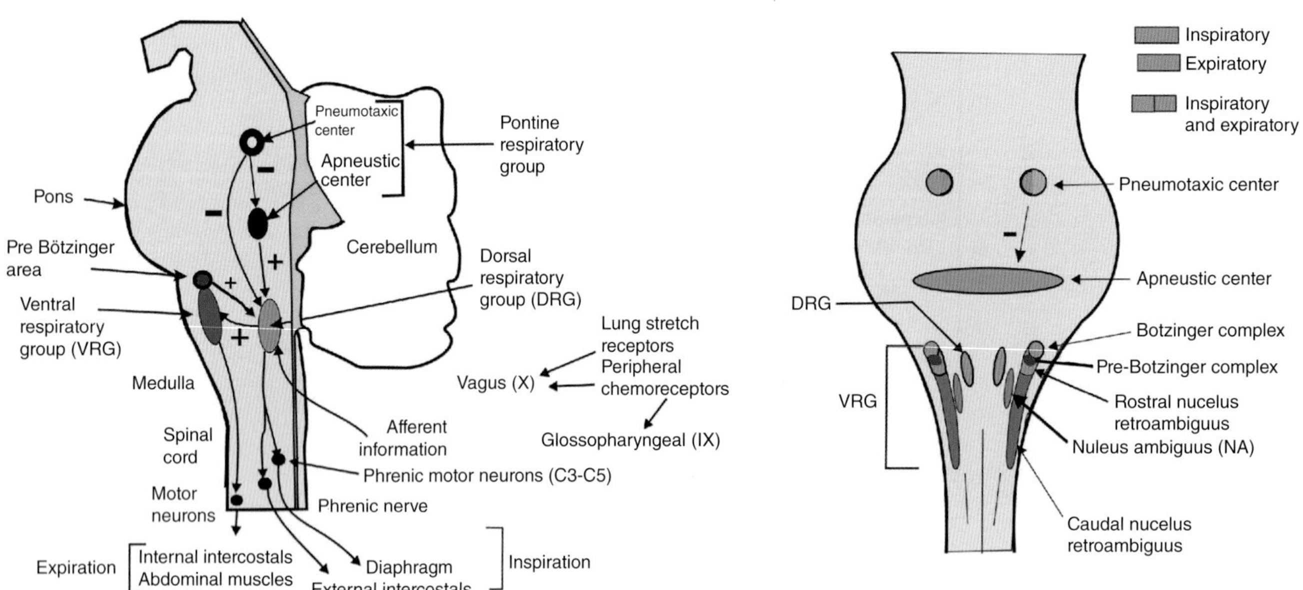

Figure 13–8 Schematic illustrating the position of important brainstem areas for the control of ventilation. The pneumotaxic center (upper pons) inhibits the apneustic center (lower pons), which together control the duration of inspiration. Without inhibition from the pneumotaxic center and vagal feedback, the apneustic center would elicit long inspiratory gasps (apneustic breathing). The dorsal respiratory group (DRG) contains inspiratory neurons and is responsible to quiet inspiration (and passive expiration). The ventral respiratory group (VRG) contains inspiratory and expiratory neurons and is responsible for forced inspiration and expiration. *The pre-Bötzinger nucleus is the respiratory pacemaker.* The DRG innervates the diaphragm and external intercostals (inspiration), whereas the VRG innervates internal intercostals and the abdominal muscles (forced expiration). *Note that while cranial nerves to not decussate (exception CN IV, Trochlear) the respiratory pre-motor neurons in the medulla innervate the* ***contralateral*** *respiratory motor neurons* (see Fig. 13–9). (Adapted from Sowho M, Amatoury J, Kirkness JP, Patil SP. Sleep and respiratory physiology in adults. *Clin Chest Med.* 2014;35(3):469-481.)

Hypoxia also increases the carotid body sensitivity to PCO_2 and pH changes. Peripheral chemoreceptor information reaches ventilatory control centers via the glossopharyngeal (carotid body) and vagal (aortic receptors) nerves. These nerves are cranial nerves IX and X, respectively. The central chemoreceptors in the medulla respond to change in brain extracellular $[H^+]$ due to changes in $PaCO_2$. The arterial $PaCO_2$ diffuses across the blood brain barrier and the enzyme carbonic anhydrase coverts $CO_2 + H_2O$ into carbonic acid (H_2CO_3), which dissociates into HCO_3^- and H^+. There is considerable interaction between the peripheral and central chemoreceptors that is still not completely understood. Pulmonary stretch receptors (PSRs in smooth muscle in proximal bronchi) relay volume information via the vagus to prevent overinflation. PSRs stimulation induces shortened inspiration and prolonged expiration. J-receptors located in the juxtacapillary area on the lungs are stimulated by pulmonary vascular congestion/pulmonary edema and communicate via the vagus nerve to the brainstem. When stimulated, they increase respiratory rate. These receptors may mediate the increase in ventilatory drive (and lower $PaCO_2$) that occurs overnight in patients with congestive heart failure as fluid is redistributed from the lower extremities to the lung.[25] Bronchial C-fibers respond to pulmonary inflammation.

There are several pontine and medullary areas that control respiration. The medullary centers include the dorsal respiratory group (DRG) and ventral respiratory group (VRG). The centers receive input from chemoreceptors, mechanoreceptors, the hypothalamus (anxiety), and cerebral cortex (conscious control of breathing, for example associated with speech). The pontine respiratory group includes the pneumotaxic (also known as the pneumatic center) and the apneustic centers. The pneumotaxic center (upper pons) controls the rate and pattern of breathing and is an antagonist to the apneustic center. Stimulation of the pneumotaxic center **shortens the inspiratory time,** which limits inspiratory volume and indirectly influences the respiratory rate. The apneustic center (lower pons) **prolongs inspiration** (smooths end of inspiration) sending signals to the DRG. Stimulation of the apneustic center results in *prolonged inspiratory gasps*. The apneustic center is inhibited by pulmonary stretch receptors and the pneumotaxic center. If there is a transection above the apneustic center (removing inhibitory input from the pneumotaxic center) and vagal input is eliminated, long inspiratory breaths are noted (apneustic breathing). The pontine pneumotaxic center also contains the **parabrachial complex** (a group of nuclei in the dorsolateral pons surrounding the superior cerebellar peduncle), which is felt to be critical in the arousal response to hypercapnia and the ventilatory response to arousal. The complex includes the Kölliker-Fuse (KF) nucleus. A hallmark respiratory response to hypercapnia and hypoxia is the emergence of active exhalation, characterized by abdominal muscle pumping during the late one-third of expiration (late-E phase). Late-E abdominal activity during hypercapnia has been attributed to the activation of expiratory neurons. The KF nucleus is believed to play a role in influencing expiratory motor neuron activity in this circumstance.

The VRG contains both inspiratory and expiratory neurons but is mainly responsible for active (forceful) inspiration and expiration. The area activates accessory respiratory muscles (inspiration and expiratory) and **internal intercostal** (expiratory) muscles. The abdominal muscles are active during forced exhalation. The pre-Bötzinger area and nucleus ambiguus are associated with the VRG. *The pre-Bötzinger area is thought to*

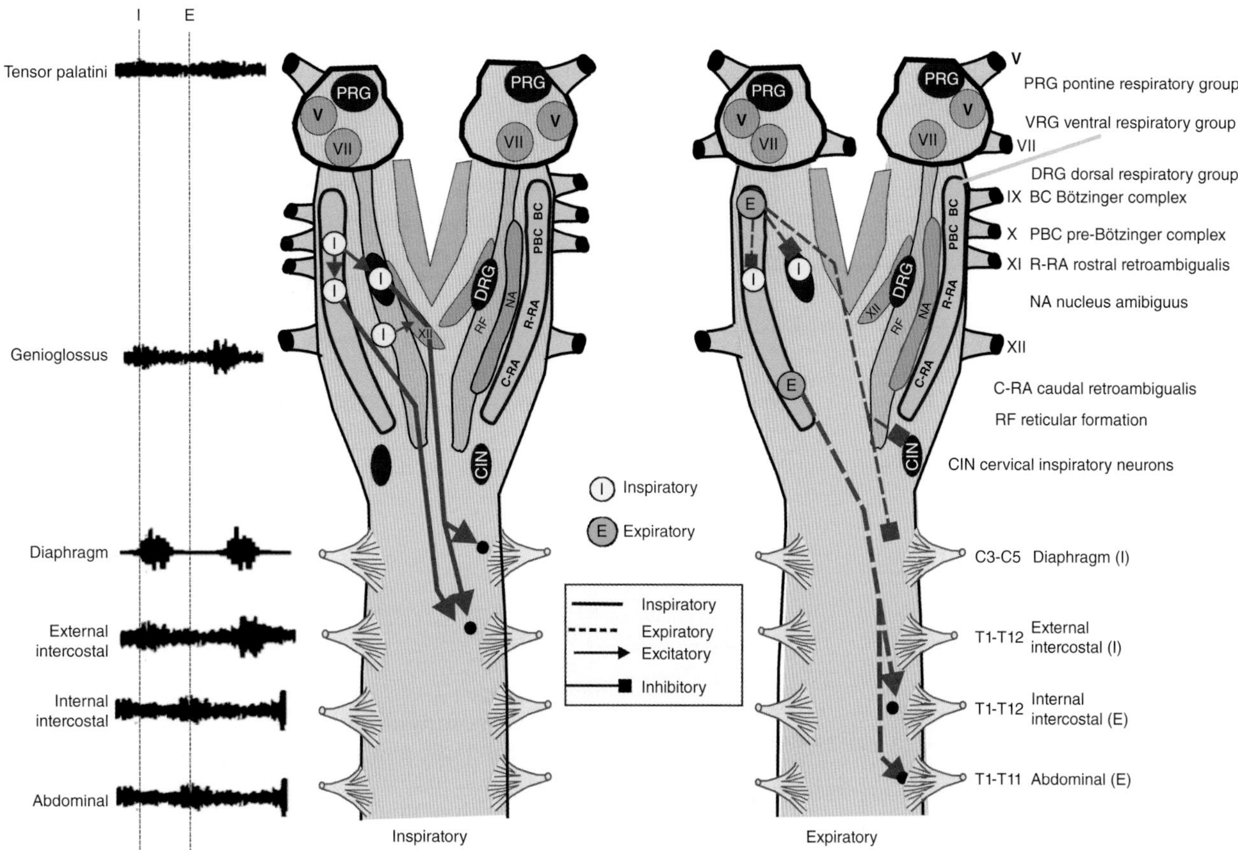

Figure 13–9 Ventral view of the brainstem (with cerebellum removed) showing the main aggregates of respiratory neurons in the dorsal and ventral respiratory groups (DRG and VRG, respectively). The VRG includes the Bötzinger complex (BC), pre-Bötzinger complex (PBC), rostral retroambigualis (R-RA), and caudal retroambigualis (C-RA). Inspiratory neurons are located in the PBC, and R-RA, and DRG. Expiratory neurons are located in the BC and C-RA. The locations of cervical inspiratory neurons (CIN) and respiratory-related neurons in the lateral reticular formation (RF) projecting to the hypoglossal motor nucleus (XII) also are shown. The projections of inspiratory and expiratory neurons are depicted as *solid and dashed lines,* respectively, whereas excitatory and inhibitory synaptic connections are depicted by *arrowheads* and *squares,* respectively. The electromyographic activities of various inspiratory-related (e.g., tongue, diaphragm, external intercostal) and expiratory (e.g., internal intercostal, abdominal) muscles are shown. Note that the level of respiratory-related and tonic activities varies for different muscles, with some muscles such as the tensor palatini expressing mainly tonic activity. The onset of muscle activity with respect to the diaphragm is shown by the dashed line. The rootlets of cranial nerves V, VII, IX, X, XI, and XII and the cervical (C) and thoracic (T) segments of the spinal cord also are shown, as are the motor nuclei of cranial nerves XII, VII, and V. The locations of the pontine respiratory group (PRG) and the nucleus ambiguus (NA) are shown, although their projections are not included for clarity. (Adapted from Horner RL. Respiratory physiology: central neural control of respirator neurons and motorneurons during sleep. In: Kryger M, Roth T, Dement WC, eds. *Principles and Practice of Sleep Medicine.* Elsevier; 2017:156.)

serve as the pattern generator (pacemaker for respiration). The center has mu opioid receptors and the depression of ventilation with opioids (decreased respiratory rate) may be mediated by a decrease in activity of this center.

The DRG contains inspiratory neurons and is the area controlling quiet breathing (depth and rate) with passive exhalation. The DRG sends activating signals to the VRG, and the DRG activates the diaphragm and external intercostal muscles (muscles of inspiration). The nucleus of the solitary tract (NTS) is part of the group and receives signals from the pontine respiratory group and the vagus (CN X) and glossopharyngeal cranial nerves (CN IX). Input includes peripheral chemoreceptors and baroreceptor input as well as lung receptors such as stretch receptors. **Phrenic motor neurons** are located in the cervical spinal cord, and axons originating from C3 to C5 (mainly C4) converge into the **phrenic** nerve innervating the diaphragm. Of note, the respiratory premotor neurons in the medulla innervate the contralateral respiratory motor neurons (Figure 13–9).

UPPER AIRWAY MUSCLES

Upper airway physiology will also be discussed in Chapter 19. The coordinated activity of multiple upper airway muscles (Table 13–5) is necessary for many functions including swallowing, speech, and breathing (Figure 13–10).[26-34] For simplicity muscles influencing the hyoid bone position and the pharyngeal constrictor muscles are not listed in Table 13–5. The reader should refer to the article by Edwards and White for more information[26]. During wakefulness the muscles maintain an open upper airway even if it is anatomically small and collapsible. During sleep there is loss of the wakefulness stimulus (tonic excitation), resulting in decreased upper airway muscle activity. In patients with unfavorable anatomy, upper airway

Table 13–5 Selected Upper Airway Muscle Properties

Tongue	Genioglossus	Phasic	Hypoglossal (medial branch)	Protrudes (and depresses) the tongue
	Styloglossus	Phasic	Hypoglossal (lateral branch)	Raises, retracts tongue
	Hyoglossus	Phasic	Hypoglossal (lateral branch)	Depresses, retracts tongue
Palate	Tensor palatini	Tonic	Trigeminal (mandibular branch)	Stiffens soft palate
	Levator palatini	Phasic	Vagus (pharyngeal branch)	Raises soft palate
	Palatoglossus	Phasic	Vagus (pharyngeal branch)	Elevates tongue and pulls palate down onto base of the tongue. The palatoglossus muscle exhibits phasic activity with inspiration and alters palatal position to facilitate the nasal route of ventilation.
	Palatopharyngeus	Phasic	Vagus (pharyngeal branch	Lifts the pharyngeal wall and may move the soft plate anteriorly

Adapted from Edwards BA, White DP. Control of the pharyngeal musculature during wakefulness and sleep: implications in normal controls and sleep apnea. *Head Neck.* 2011;33(suppl 1):S37-45.

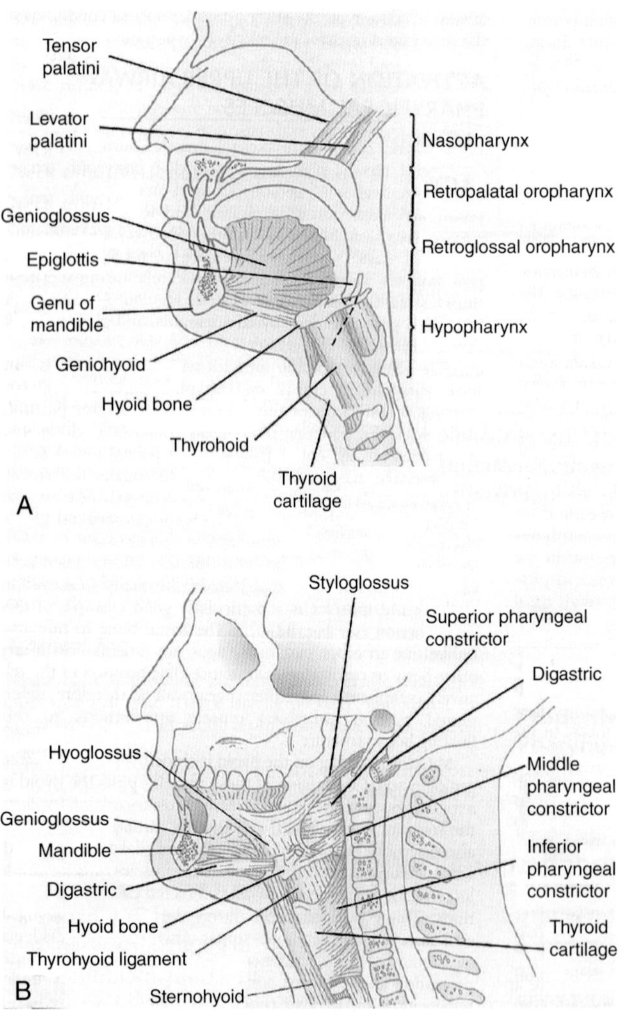

Figure 13–10 The pharyngeal airway anatomy and upper airway dilator muscles. Midsagittal (A) and parasagittal (B) representation of the pharyngeal anatomy showing tongue, soft palate, hyoid bone and pharyngeal constrictors. (Reprinted with permission from Kryger M, Roth T, Dement WC, eds. *Principles and Practice of Sleep Medicine.* Elsevier; 2005:998.)

narrowing (hypopnea or apnea) may occur with loss of the wakefulness drive. The genioglossus (GG) (tongue protruder) is innervated by the hypoglossal nerve and is the most studied upper airway muscle. Its action is to pull the posterior portion of the tongue forward away from the posterior airway wall. The muscle has tonic and phasic activity (bursts during inspiration). The GG responds to negative upper airway pressure via a reflex pathway from upper airway mechanoreceptors to the NTS and then to activation of the hypoglossal motor neurons (Figure 13–11). For example, if upper airway pressure changes from 0 to -5 cmH_2O, GG activity increases, GG activity is also increased by chemostimulation (increased $PaCO_2$ and decreased PO_2) via input from chemoreceptors to premotor neurons (central pattern generators). Reduction in several neuromodulators excitatory to hypoglossal motor neurons have been hypothesized to mediate the loss of the wakefulness stimulus and changes during REM sleep. Current understanding is that the primary effect is due to loss of noradrenergic stimulation on transition from wake to NREM (dysfacilitation) and a combination of loss of noradrenergic stimulation and cholinergic-mediated inhibition on transition from NREM to REM sleep.[26-28] During wakefulness GG activity has been shown to be elevated in patients with OSA as compared with healthy controls. This is thought to represent a neuromuscular compensation for the deficient anatomy.

GG activity and other upper airway muscle activity (tensor palatini and others) falls at sleep onset (loss of wakefulness stimuli)[29-31] (Figure 13–12). Concurrent with the reduction in GG activity is a reduction in airway caliber in healthy individuals (resulting in increased upper airway resistance and sometimes snoring). Tidal volume falls in the first few breaths after sleep onset. Airway negative pressure and chemostimulation increase after the initiation of sleep, both of which increase GG activity. After a few breaths GG activity has recovered (Figure 13–12). Tidal volume recovers but remains reduced compared with wakefulness. Studies have evaluated changes at sleep onset while individuals wear continuous positive airway pressure (CPAP) to eliminate the influences of negative upper airway (and increased upper airway resistance). A fall in GG muscle activity was documented with sleep onset. The fall in GG activity at sleep onset is believed to be due to a large effect of loss of wakefulness stimulus, mildly

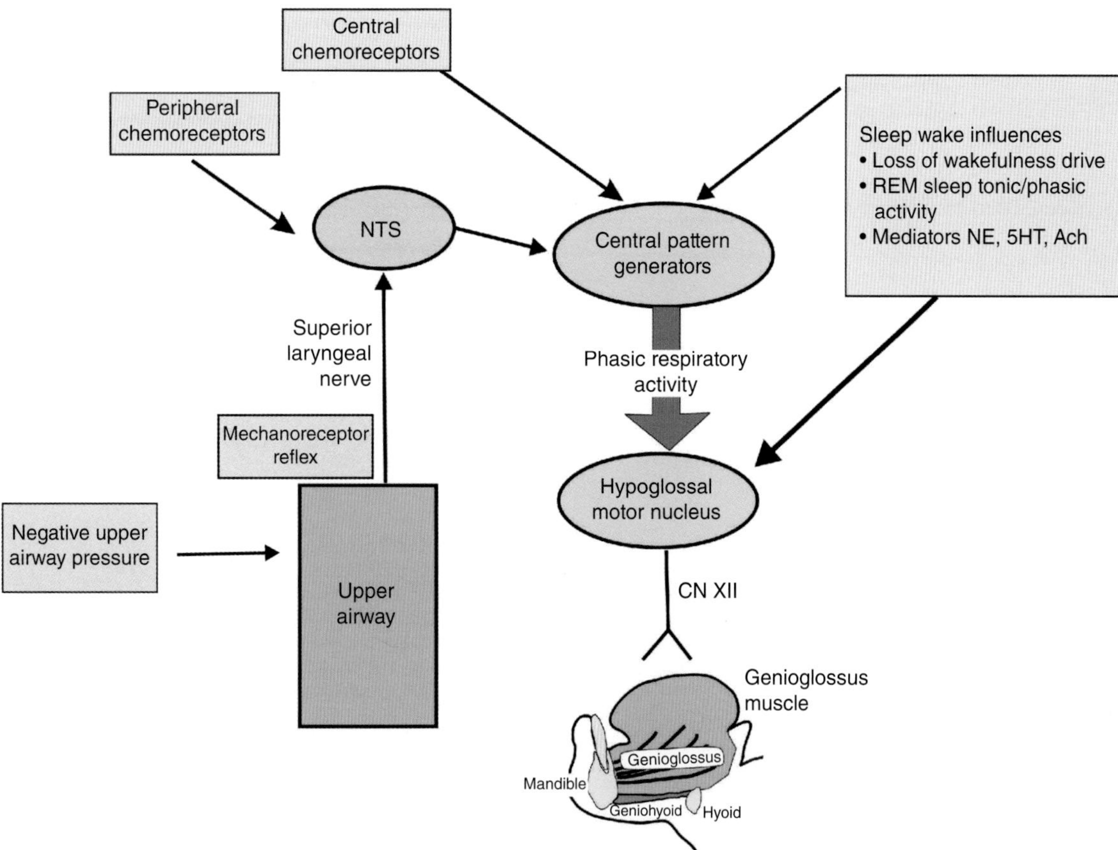

Figure 13–11 Schematic illustration of control of the genioglossus muscle (GG), an important tongue muscle for maintaining upper airway patency (protrudes the tongue). The muscle has phasic inspiratory activity generated by central pattern generators that receive input from the chemoreceptors (increased $PaCO_2$ or decreased PO_2 increase activity). Activity is also augmented by negative pressure in the upper airway through a reflex with the pathway shown in the figure. Neuromodulators facilitate hypoglossal motor neuron activity and are part of the wakefulness stimulus. With sleep onset there is loss of the wakefulness stimulus mediated in part by a decrease in norepinephrine facilitation of hypoglossal motor neuron activity resulting in decreased phasic respiratory activity. During REM sleep decreased norepinephrine facilitation and cholinergic inhibition of hypoglossal motorneurons is so believed to reduce tonic and phasic GG activity. With increased negative pressure (higher upper airway resistance due to narrowing of the airway) and chemostimulation the activity of the GG recovers during stable NREM sleep. However, in individuals with unfavorable upper airway anatomy there is significant airway narrowing or closure before there is sufficient augmentation of the GG and other upper airway muscles to maintain an open upper airway. CN XII is the hypoglossal nerve. NTS is the nucleus of the solitary tract

decreased stimulus from negative upper airway pressure and a small decrease in respiratory drive from central pattern generators.[29,30] The results of a study by Carberry et al[32] are shown in Figure 13–13. There was a fall in maximum GG EMG activity and tonic EMG activity of the tensor palatini (palatal muscle) during sleep in individuals wearing CPAP.[32] In this study there was no increase in GG activity during stable NREM sleep likely due to prevention of negative pressure influences. Of interest, the activity of the GG fell from NREM to REM, but the only change in tensor palatini tonic activity was from wake to sleep.

Note that at sleep onset ventilatory drive to the pump muscles also falls. Although negative upper airway pressure still increases in magnitude slightly, the upper airway changes are not due to the airway being narrowed due to strong negative pressure but more the occurrence of a passive collapse. In patients with obstructive sleep apnea (OSA) the fall in upper airway muscle activity is associated with partial or complete upper airway obstruction). During apnea and hypopnea ventilatory drive to respiratory pump muscles and the upper airway increases but the airway remains narrow or closed until there is sufficient augmentation of upper airway muscles to open the airway or there is an arousal (or both). Augmentation of GG (and other upper airway muscle) activity can result in periods of stable ventilation even in patients with obstructive sleep apnea (OSA). Instability in the control of breathing can result in cyclic decreases in ventilatory drive both to the pump muscles and to the GG. Upper airway narrowing or closure is more likely to occur as drive decreases. Additional discussion of the pathophysiology of OSA is presented in Chapter 19.

Upper airway patency depends on the activity of multiple muscles. Palatal muscles of interest include the palatoglossus and levator palatini, which have phasic activity, and the tensor palatini, which has mainly tonic activity. The tensor palatini **tonic** activity falls during sleep contributing to upper airway narrowing. Upper airway muscle activity is believed to be lower in NREM than wake and lower in REM than NREM (in some studies). Different studies have not always agreed with this general impression but different experimental techniques

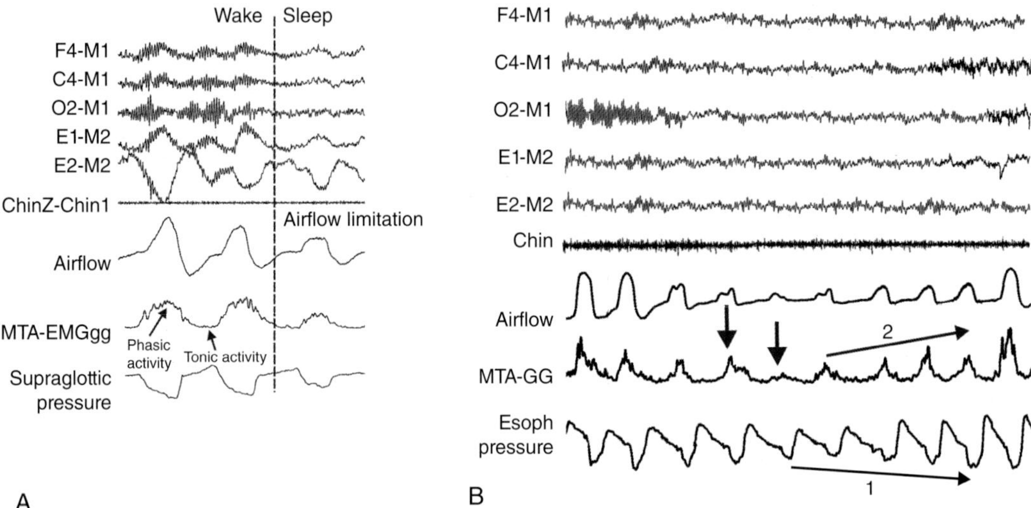

Figure 13–12 The left panel (A) shows that the transition from wake to sleep is associated with a decrease in genioglossi (GG) activity. MTA-EMGgg is the moving time average of the GG EMG. The esophageal pressure deflection falls with reduced ventilatory drive at sleep onset but due to a fall in upper airway muscle activity, upper airway resistance increases (airflow limitation is noted). (B) During sleep onset there is a fall in GG activity (down arrows) but with increased ventilatory drive and the associated more negative upper airway pressure (1) the GG activity recovers (2) and airflow recovers (at a lower level than wake). Airflow measured by a pneumotachograph in a mask over the nose and mouth. Inspiration is upward. Esoph pressure is esophageal pressure. (A, From Berry RB. *Fundamentals of Sleep Medicine*. Elsevier; 2012:265.)

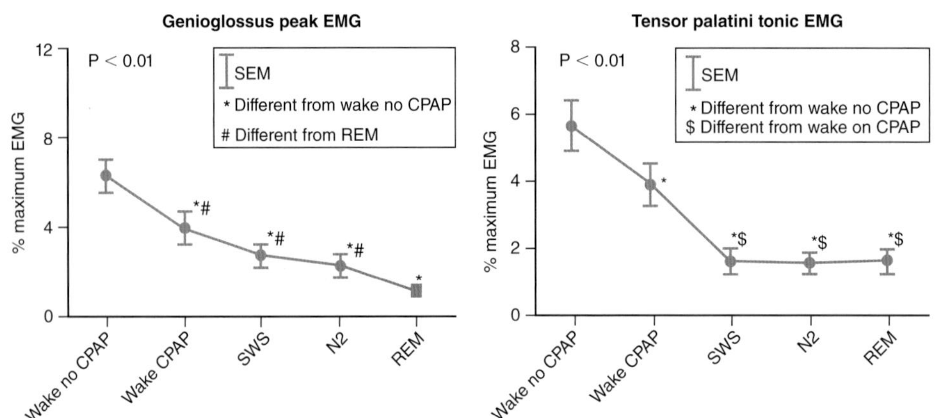

Figure 13–13 This figure shows the change in maximum EMG activity of the genioglossus muscle GG and tonic EMG activity from the tensor palatini (TP; has tonic activity) during wake with and without CPAP and the stages of sleep on CPAP. CPAP was used to stabilize the airway and minimize the influences of negative airway pressure and chemostimulation to isolate the effect of the different sleep stages. GG activity decreased from wake to sleep and from NREM to REM sleep. The TP decreased from wake to sleep but was not different between the sleep stages. SEM standard error of the mean, SWS slow wave sleep (stage N3). (From Carberry JC, Jordan AS, White DP, Wellman A, Eckert DJ. Upper airway collapsibility [Pcrit] and pharyngeal dilator muscle activity are sleep stage dependent. *Sleep.* 2016;39(3):511-521.)

or differences in the individuals may explains some differences. Using passive ventilation Lo et al.[29] documented a fall in GG and TP activity at sleep onset. During stable NREM sleep TP activity decreased and was further decreased during REM sleep. After the initial fall at sleep onset the GG activity was stable during NREM sleep but decreased on transition to REM sleep. As noted above, Carberry and coworkers[32] found a reduction from NREM to REM in the GG but not the tensor palatini (tonic EMG). The fall in GG activity noted during REM sleep is thought to be due to withdrawal of neural drive and not to impaired muscles responses during REM sleep.[33] The role of the upper airway mechanoreceptors and negative pressure has been studied using upper airway anesthesia. The importance was illustrated by a significant decrease in the augmentation of GG activity during apnea in OSA patients when mechanoreceptor contribution to GG activity was abolished by anesthesia despite large increases in ventilatory drive.[34]

TESTS OF VENTILATORY CONTROL AND CHANGES DURING SLEEP

As noted above, the major chemoreceptors are the carotid body (responding to PaO_2, $PaCO_2$, and pH) and the medullary chemoreceptors (responding to changes in the [H+] that occur with changes in $PaCO_2$).[22-24] Hypercapnic hypoxemia creates the greatest stimulus.[35] The sensitivity of the chemoreceptors and ventilatory control centers to changes in arterial blood gases can be determined by measuring the ventilatory responses to rises in $PaCO_2$ (hypercapnic ventilatory response [HCVR]) and falls in PaO_2 (hypoxic ventilatory response [HOVR]).[35] These are measured by rebreathing methods. The end-tidal partial pressure of carbon dioxide ($P_{ET}CO_2$) and end-tidal partial pressure of oxygen ($P_{ET}O_2$) are determined on a breath-by-breath basis (assumed to be alveolar values) and plotted against the ventilation at that time on a breath-by-breath basis. A line is then drawn to fit the points with the slope being the ventilatory response. The HCVR is measured under hyperoxic conditions (minimizing the effect of peripheral chemoreceptors) and the HOVR is measured under eucapnic conditions ($PaCO_2$ kept constant by removal of some of the CO_2 from the system). The slope of the HCVR is a measure of sensitivity to hypercapnia (Figure 13–14A). However, the position of the curve—that is, the set point or base point—is also important. The slope of the HOVR (see Figure 13–14B) is not constant (relationship between ventilation and the PaO^2 is not linear) and analysis is more complex. However, if expressed as ventilation versus the SaO_2 (SpO_2 is measured), the relationship between ventilation and PaO_2 is linear with a constant slope (see Figure 13–14C). However, it should be remembered that the PaO_2 and not the SaO_2 is what mediates the hypoxic ventilatory response. The ventilatory response to hypoxia is much larger below 55 mm Hg. If a person has a normal ventilatory control center but abnormal lungs, high airway resistance, or abnormal thoracic cage, the slope of the ventilatory response to CO_2 will be lower (see Figure 13–14A). Thus, measuring ventilation in a patient with a high airway resistance or low respiratory system compliance is not an ideal method to test the neural drive to breathe. The mouth occlusion pressure ($P_{0.1}$)—the mouth pressure measured 0.1 second after the start of inspiration (unexpected airway occlusion)—can be used instead of ventilation as a better index of drive. Pressures measured at 0.1 second after inspiratory occlusion occur before voluntary changes in pressure can occur. Because there is no flow during occlusion, the $P_{0.1}$ is not affected by airway resistance. Maintaining adequate ventilation with a high airway resistance requires a compensatory increase in ventilatory drive (increased $P_{0.1}$). The $P_{0.1}$ response to hypercapnia or hypoxemia is determined during rebreathing with intermittent airway occlusion (measurement of $P_{0.1}$). The $P_{0.1}$ values are plotted versus $PaCO_2$, PaO_2, or SaO_2 depending on the test. A patient with high upper airway resistance may have a reduced hypercapnic ventilatory response but a normal hypercapnic $P_{0.1}$ response. For example, in one study patients with chronic obstructive pulmonary disease (COPD) had a lower ventilatory response to hypercapnia compared with controls but had a higher $P_{0.1}$ response to hypercapnia than the control group.[36]

During sleep, the HCVR is reduced during NREM compared with wake and decreased in REM sleep compared with NREM sleep (Figure 13–15A).[37] The set point of the PCO_2 is shifted to the right. During sleep the HOVR (Figure 13–15B) is reduced in NREM sleep in men[38,39] (not pre-menopausal women) *but is reduced in both men and women during REM sleep compared to wakefulness and NREM sleep.*[38,39] Although the sleeping ventilatory response to hypoxia was similar in men and women, the men had a higher awake ventilatory drive (hence a larger change in ventilation from wake to sleep).[39] Figure 13–16 shows the breath-by-breath values of the ventilatory response to $PaCO_2$ in an OSA patient with daytime hypercapnia before (control) and after CPAP treatment.[40] The slope did not change but the set point (baseline $PaCO_2$) decreased, and the position of the curve shifted to the

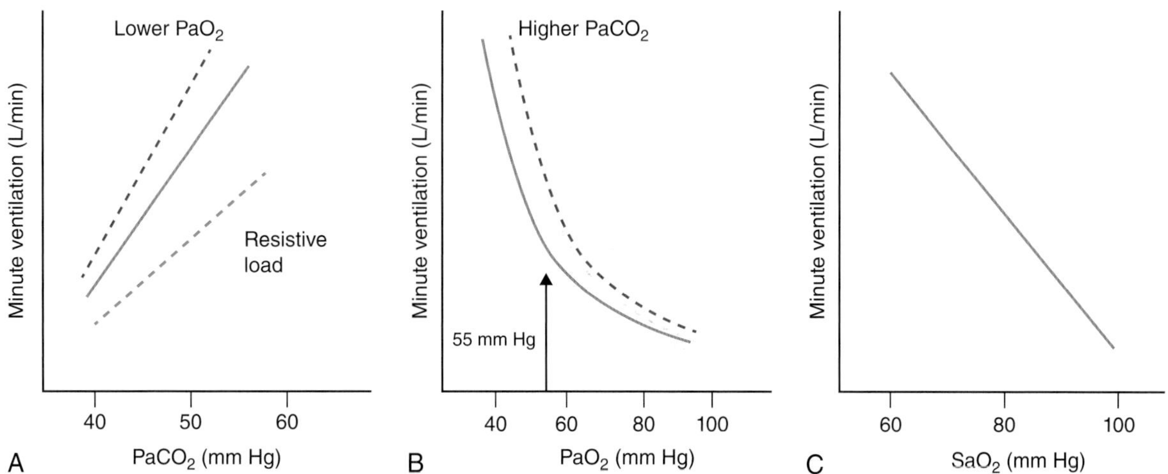

Figure 13–14 Schematic representation of the hypercapnic ventilatory response (A) and the hypoxic ventilatory response (B and C). (A) Although $PaCO_2$ is shown on the x axis the end-tidal PCO_2 is actually measured on a breath by breath basis during the rebeathing test. If the hypercapnic response (A) is tested with a resistive load, the slope is lower. This illustrates that this testing depends not simply on the ventilatory control centers (neural drive) but also on the resistance and compliance of the respiratory system. A lower PaO_2 increases the hypercapnic ventilatory response (hypoxic hypercapnia). At (B) the ventilatory response to reductions in the PaO_2 is not linear with little increase in ventilation until the PaO_2 is about 50–55 mm Hg. Athough the PaO_2 is shown on the x axis the end-tidal PO_2 is actually measured on a breath by breath basis during rebreathing as an estimate of the alveolar PO_2 (PaO_2) and the PaO2. If expressed as ventilation versus oxygen saturation (C) the hypoxic ventilatory response is linear. However, the peripheral chemoreceptors respond to PaO_2 and not the SaO_2. Note that if the $PaCO_2$ is higher, this increases the hypoxic ventilatory response. *SaO_2*, arterial oxygen saturation (actually SpO_2 from oximetry). (From Berry RB. *Fundamentals of Sleep Medicine.* Elsevier; 2012:147.)

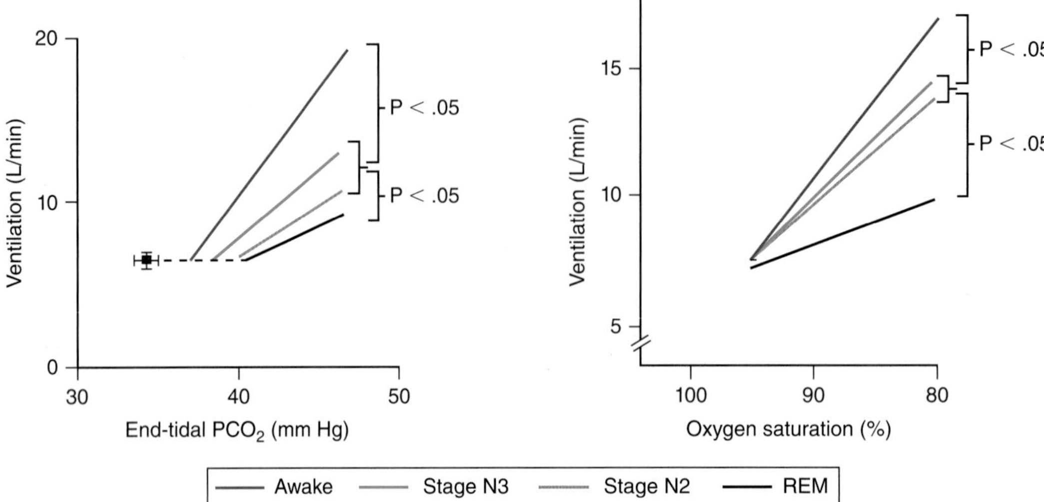

Figure 13–15 (A) The hypercapnic ventilatory response is reduced during non–rapid eye movement (NREM) sleep compared with wakefulness and decreased in rapid eye movement (REM) sleep compared with NREM sleep. (B) The hypoxic ventilatory response is also decreased during NREM compared with wakefulness and REM compared with NREM in men. *PCO_2,* partial pressure of carbon dioxide. (A and B, from Douglas NJ, White DP, Weil JV, et al. Hypercapnic ventilatory response in sleeping adults. *Am Rev Respir Dis* 1982;126:286-289.)

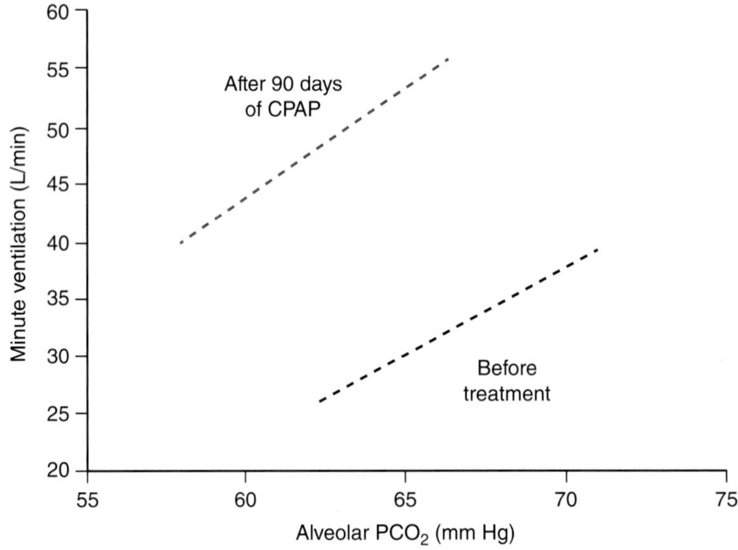

Figure 13–16 The hypercapnic ventilatory response before and after continuous positive airway pressure (CPAP) treatment. The slope did not change but the curve shifted to the left. *Alveolar CO_2,* estimated $PACO_2$ from end-tidal sample of exhaled gas during rebreathing test. (Plotted from data from Berthon-Jones M, Sullivan CE. Time course of change in ventilatory response to CO_2 with long-term CPAP therapy for obstructive sleep apnea. *Am Rev Respir Dis.* 1987;135:144-147.)

left. At any given $PaCO_2$, the ventilation is higher. Patients with *daytime hypercapnia* had a shift to the left without a change in slope of the ventilatory response to PCO_2 after CPAP treatment. Patients with OSA and a normal daytime PCO_2 exhibited no shift and no change in slope. A shift in the ventilation curve position without a change in slope can be seen with changes in HCO_3 due to chronic metabolic acidosis or alkalosis[41,42] (Figure 13–17). One explanation for the parallel shift in the hypercapnic ventilatory response curve after CPAP treatment is that the patients on CPAP with daytime hypercapnia no longer developed worsening of hypercapnia during sleep and, therefore, no longer accumulated HCO_3 at night to compensate. A fall in the serum HCO_3 due to prevention of worsening nocturnal hypercapnia with CPAP would be associated with a leftward shift in the ventilatory response (see Figure 13–17).

ACID-BASE PHYSIOLOGY

Some basic information regarding acid-base physiology can be useful in evaluating patients with sleep-related breathing disorders. The relationship of the pH ($-\log [H^+]$) to the serum HCO_3^- and $PaCO_2$ is given by the logarithmic version of the Henderson-Hasselbalch equation (Equation 13-9). Here $[H^+]$ is the hydrogen ion concentration. A nonlogarithmic form of the Henderson-Hasselbalch equation (Kassirer-Bleich) relates the $[H+]$ to the ratio of the $PaCO_2$ and HCO_3 (Equation 13-10).[43]

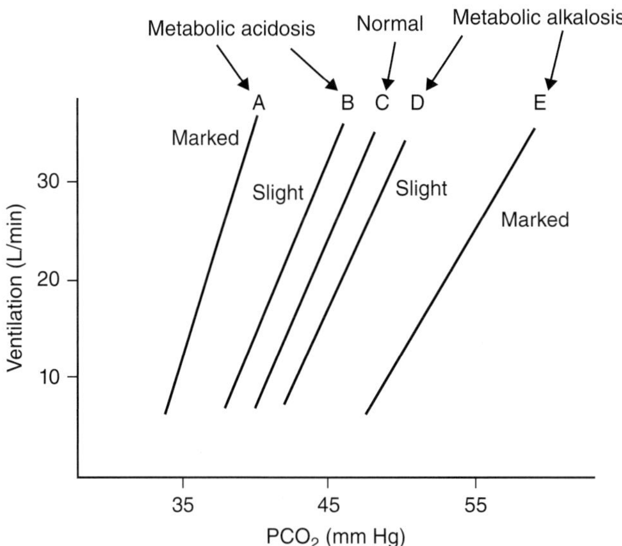

Figure 13–17 Changes in the hypercapnic ventilatory response with metabolic acidosis and alkalosis. The slope did not change but the position of the curve shifted left or right. *PCO_2*, partial pressure of carbon dioxide. (From Oren A, Whipp BJ, Wasserman K: Effects of chronic acid-base changes on the rebreathing hypercapnic ventilatory response in man. *Respiration*. 1991;58:181-185.)

$$pH = 6.10 + \log\left(HCO_3/0.03 \times PaCO_2\right) \quad \text{Equation 13–9}$$

$$\text{where } pH = -\log\left[H^+\right]$$

$$\left[H^+\right] = 24 \times PaCO_2/HCO_3 \quad \text{Equation 13–10}$$

$$\left[H^+\right] \text{ in nanomoles/L} = 10^{-9} \text{ moles/L, } HCO_3 \text{ in mEq/L}$$

For example:

$$pH = 7.40, \left[H^+\right] = 40 \text{ mEq/L, } PaCO_2 = 40 \text{ mm Hg, } HCO_3^- = 24 \text{ mEq/L} \left[40 = 24\,(40/24)\right]$$

At a pH of 7.40 the $[H^+]$ is 40 nanomoles/L and as the pH decreases the $[H^+]$ increases. At a $PaCO_2$ of 40 mm Hg, the HCO_3 is 24 mEq/L. A simplified method of using Equation 13-10 which requires conversion of pH to $[H^+]$ uses the approximation that around pH = 7.40 for every 0.01 decrease (increase) in the pH from 7.40, the $[H^+]$ increases (decreases) by 1 nanomole/L from 40 nanomoles/L (Box 13-2). Hence pH = 7.30 corresponds to an $[H^+]$ = 50 nanomoles/L and pH = 7.50 corresponds to a $[H^+]$ = 30 nanomoles/L. Examples of acute and chronic hypoventilation are shown in Box 13-2.

Equation 13-10 illustrates the useful concept that the pH or $[H^+]$ depends on the $PaCO_2/HCO_3^-$ ratio. If a change in $PaCO_2$ occurs, the body attempts to compensate by changing the HCO_3^- in the same direction, thereby minimizing the change in the $PaCO_2/HCO_3^-$ ratio (Table 13–6). However, compensation is never complete (pH remains below or above 7.40). In evaluating the acid-base status of an arterial blood gas, a few simple rules are helpful. More comprehensive rules exist, but a useful rule is that for every 10 mm Hg the $PaCO_2$ increases or decreases from 40 mm Hg, the HCO_3^- increases or decreases about 1 mEq/L acutely and 3 to 4 mEq/L chronically (metabolic compensation).[43,44] The corresponding changes in pH are 0.08 and 0.03 in the opposite direction (Table 13–6). For example, if a patient's $PaCO_2$ increased from 40 to 50 mm Hg acutely, the HCO_3^- would increase from 24 to 25 mEq/L, and after chronic renal compensation it would be expected to increase by 3 to 4 mEq/L to 27-28 mEq/L. Similarly, the pH would be expected to decrease by approximately 0.08 acutely or 0.03 to 0.04 with chronic compensation (Table 13–6). Assuming a baseline HCO_3 of 24 mEq/L, an increase in $PaCO_2$ from 40 to 50 mm Hg and chronic compensation would result in an HCO_3^- around 27 to 28 mEq/L or a pH of 7.36 to 7.37. Noting electrolyte results can be helpful when evaluating obese patients with severe sleep apnea. If such a patient has chronic respiratory acidosis (high $PaCO_2$), he or she will usually have a high HCO_3^- (or serum CO_2). An elevated HCO_3^- in the absence of a reason to have a metabolic alkalosis (e.g., diuretic) is a clue that respiratory acidosis could be present. The utility of an elevated HCO_3 (or serum CO_2) for identifying patients with the obesity hypoventilation syndrome (OHS) is discussed in Chapter 18. The serum CO_2 on routine electrolyte tests is approximately equal to the HCO_3^-. If a patient presents with significant CO_2 retention but a modest decrease in the pH, this would be consistent with chronic hypoventilation and renal compensation. A significantly decreased pH less than 7.30 would suggest an acute process. However, often hospitalized patients have acute on chronic compensation with a pH between what might be expected from an acute or chronic process. If the primary process is metabolic, rules exist to determine the expected respiratory compensation (change in the $PaCO_2$), which is fairly rapid (see Table 13–6). For a discussion of complex acid-base scenarios, the reader is referred to the practical article by Haber.[44]

Box 13-2 NONLOGARITHMIC HENDERSON-HASSELBALCH EQUATION

(approximate $[H^+]$ values near pH = 7.40)

$[H^+]$ (nanomoles/L)	pH
30	7.50
35	7.45
40	7.40
45	7.35
50	7.30

Sample calculations: $[H+] = 24 \times PaCO_2/HCO_3^-$

Normal	$40 = \frac{24(40)}{24}$	pH = 7.40 (normal)
Acute hypoventilation	$48 = \frac{24(50)}{25}$	pH = 7.32
Chronic hypoventilation	$44 = \frac{24(50)}{27}$	pH = 7.36

$[H^+]$, Hydrogen ion concentration in nanomoles/L; *HCO_3*, serum bicarbonate in mEq/L; *$PaCO_2$*, arterial partial pressure of carbon dioxide (mmHg).

PULMONARY FUNCTION TESTING

Pulmonary function testing is often needed to evaluate patients with a low awake PaO_2 (or SaO_2) or to determine the

Table 13–6 Acid-Base Changes and Compensation

Goal: Keep the PCO_2/HCO_3 ratio unchanged		
Acid-Base Change	**Primary**	**Compensation**
Respiratory acidosis	Increased $PaCO_2$	Increased HCO_3 (renal)
Respiratory alkalosis	Decreased $PaCO_2$	Decreased HCO_3 (renal)
Metabolic acidosis	Decreased HCO_3	Decreased $PaCO_2$ (increased ventilation)
Metabolic alkalosis	Increased HCO_3	Increased $PaCO_2$ (decreased ventilation)

Compensation rules[44]:
For every 10 mm Hg increase/decrease in the $PaCO_2$, the HCO_3 increases/decreases by about 1 mEq/L acutely or 3–4 mEq/L chronically (or pH changes by 0.08 acutely and 0.03 chronically in the opposite direction).
In the case of primary metabolic acidosis for every 1 mEq/L decrease in the HCO_3^- the $PaCO_2$ decreases about 1 mm Hg.
For primary metabolic alkalosis, the compensated $PaCO_2 = 0.9\ [HCO_3] + 15.6$

Sample calculations (hydrogen ion concentration in nanomoles/L):
Example: PCO_2 increases 40–50 mm Hg, assume starting $HCO_3^- = 24$ mEq/L
$[H^+] = 24 \times PaCO_2/HCO_3^-$

Acute: compensation for increase in $PaCO_2$ from 40 to 50 mmHg: HCO_3 increases 1 mEq/L
New $[H^+] = 24 \times (50/25) = 48$ or pH =7.32

Chronic compensation for increase in $PaCO_2$ from 40 50 mmHg: HCO_3 increases 4 mEq/L
New $[H^+] = 24 \times (50/28) = 43$ or pH =7.37

Adapted from Haber RJ. A practical approach to acid-base disorders. *West J Med.* 1991;155(2):146-151.

etiology of unexpected daytime hypoventilation or dyspnea on exertion. Sleep physicians may order pulmonary function testing after a sleep study reveals an unexplained low sleeping SaO_2 without discrete apneas or hypopneas. Therefore, some knowledge of pulmonary function testing can be useful for the sleep clinician. Many patients have a diagnosis of chronic obstructive pulmonary disease (COPD) that is not accurate. A fact that can be recognized with a basic knowledge of the patterns of pulmonary function abnormality. The goal of this section is to provide a basic overview of pulmonary function testing, and the reader should realize that there is considerable controversy about what is considered normal and how to define normal ranges.[45-49] Pulmonary function study results must be interpreted with the clinical picture in mind (including chest CT results) as results may be borderline or at the lower limit of normal (but showing a pattern of progression).

The patterns of impairment in lung disease include an obstructive ventilatory defect (OVD) and a restrictive ventilatory defect (RVD).[46-48] Patterns of pulmonary impairment are shown in Table 13–7. An OVD is characterized by reductions in airflow due to bronchospasm or bronchiolar narrowing due to inflammation or fibrosis. These disorders are frequently associated with changes in lung volumes due to hyperinflation and air-trapping, as described below. Disorders with an OVD pattern of impairment include asthma, chronic bronchitis, and emphysema. The term *chronic obstructive pulmonary disease* is used because patients typically have a mixture of chronic bronchitis and emphysema in variable proportions. Patients with asthma usually have a significant component of reversible airflow obstruction. Patients with COPD have a mixture of chronic bronchitis (cough and sputum production) and emphysema and may have some improvement after inhaled bronchodilator. *Chronic* bronchitis is a clinical diagnosis based on a history of sputum production, but the term is often used for COPD patients with OVD who do not have a significant component of emphysema. Emphysema is a pathological diagnosis characterized by destruction of the alveolar sacs and terminal bronchioles. A computerized axial tomography scan is a sensitive way of visualizing the changes from emphysema. Emphysema is associated with a decreased diffusing capacity for carbon monoxide (DLco).[45-47,50] An RVD is characterized by a reduction in the total lung capacity, but other lung volumes can also be decreased. The RVD disorders are divided into extrinsic RVD (involvement of the chest wall, pleura, or respiratory muscle weakness) and intrinsic RVD (lung parenchymal disorders such as interstitial lung disease) (Table 13–7). Airflow can be reduced in patients with an RVD, but the reduction is proportionate to the changes in lung volumes. Of note, patients with pulmonary vascular diseases (scleroderma and others) may have a reduced diffusing capacity with or without decreases in lung volumes. This scenario will be discussed below.

Pulmonary function testing is often ordered for patients with OSA and daytime hypercapnia and/or hypoxemia. Such patients could have the obesity hypoventilation syndrome (OHS) characterized by obesity, daytime hypercapnia, and no other reason to explain the hypercapnia. Pulmonary function testing will usually reveal an extrinsic RVD, but in some individuals lung volumes are at the lower limit of normal. An inaccurate diagnosis of COPD is sometimes made in these patients during hospitalization for acute hypercapnic respiratory failure. A diagnosis of COPD should always be confirmed by pulmonary function testing. Another group with daytime hypoxia and hypercapnia is the overlap syndrome (OSA and COPD), and these patients will display an OVD pattern on pulmonary function tests. In such patients optimal treatment of both the sleep apnea and the COPD is important.

Spirometry, lung volume determination, and measurement of the diffusing capacity for carbon monoxide (DLco) are an essential part of the evaluation of all patients with lung disease or hypoventilation. In addition, if lung function abnormalities are documented, the severity as well as response to treatment can also be assessed. Nomenclature of the lung volumes is illustrated in Figure 13–18. The total lung capacity (TLC) is the lung volume at maximal inspiration, residual volume (RV) is the lung volume at maximal expiration, and the functional residual capacity (FRC) is the end-expiratory lung volume during

Table 13–7 Disorders Associated With OVD and RVD

	Disorders	Pulmonary Function
OVD **Reduced FEV_1/FVC**	Asthma	Large BD response Increased RV, RV and FRC, RV, FRC, and TLC Normal DLco
	Chronic bronchitis	Small or no BD response Increased RV > FRC > TLC TLC, FRC may be normal Normal DLco
	Emphysema	Usually no BD response Increased RV > FRC > TLC **Decreased DLco**
	Mixed chronic brochitis and emphysema	Small BD response Increased RV> FRC > TLC (TLC may be normal), Decreased DLco
RVD **Normal FEV_1/FVC** Reduced TLC	Intrinsic RVD Pulmonary fibrosis Parenchymal disorders	Decreased TLC (FRC, RV normal or low) Reduced DLco, reduction in DLco often greater than TLC
	Extrinsic RVD Muscle weakness Chest wall disorders	Decreased TLC (FRC, RV normal or low) Normal or slightly reduced DLco FRC can be increased (ankylosing spondylitis)
Pulmonary vascular	Scleroderma Pulmonary arterial HTN Chronic PE Rheumatoid arthritis SLE Polymyositis	Normal or mild RVD on spirometry Reduced DLco
Mixed (OVD + RVD)	Mixture of Disorders Associated with OVD and RVD	Reduced FEV_1/FVC consistent with OVD and reduced TLC consistent with RVD
Special pattern	Pulmonary vascular disease, emphysema, early interstitial lung disease	Normal spirometry and reduced diffusing capacity

BD, Bronchodilator; *DLco,* diffusing capacity for carbon monoxide; *TLC,* total lung capacity; OVD, obstructive ventilatory defect; RVD, restrictive ventilatory defect.

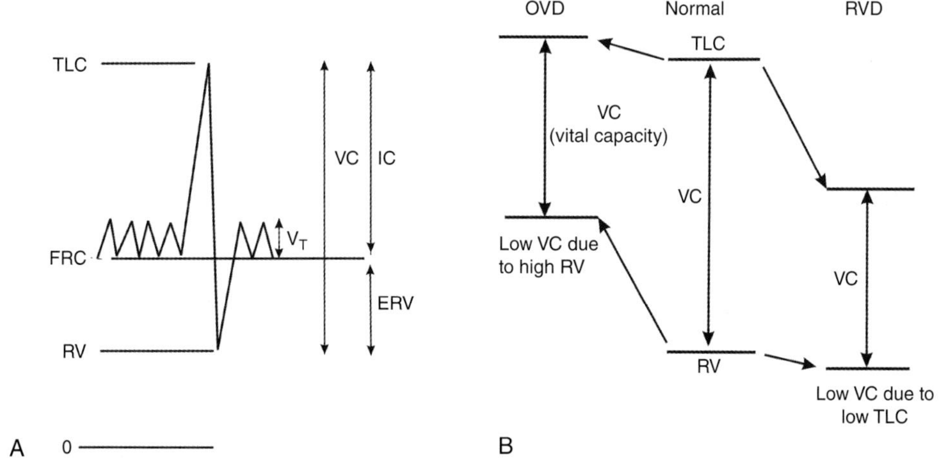

Figure 13–18 (A) Lung volume nomenclature. (B) Changes in lung volumes with disease. In an obstructive ventilatory defect (OVD), the VC can be decreased due to an increase in the RV that exceeds any increase in the TLC. In a restrictive ventilatory defect, by definition, there is a decrease in the TLC and the VC decreases due to a decrease in the total capacity that exceeds any decrease in the RV. *ERV,* Expiratory reserve volume; *FRC,* functional residual capacity; *IC,* inspiratory capacity; *RV,* residual volume; *TLC,* total lung capacity; *VC,* vital capacity; V_T, tidal volume. (From Berry RB. *Fundamentals of Sleep Medicine.* Elsevier; 2012.)

tidal breathing. The expiratory reserve volume (ERV) is the volume between FRC and RV. The inspiratory capacity (IC) is the volume between FRC and TLC. In normal individuals, the RV is about 25% of TLC, and the FRC is approximately 40% to 45% of the TLC. The ERV and IC constitute about one-third and two-thirds of the vital capacity (VC), respectively.

Spirometry is a measurement of exhaled volume versus time (Figure 13–19). Spirometry cannot measure absolute lung volumes (TLC, FRC, RV), but it is widely available as the equipment for performance of spirometry is simpler and less expensive than for complete lung function studies. Spirometry is also a convenient method to follow the course of lung disease. The most

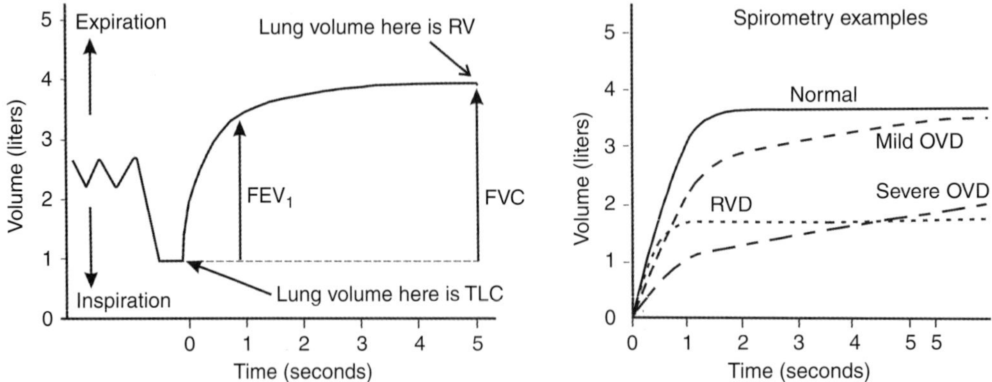

Figure 13–19 *Left,* Spirometry records exhaled volume versus time. *Right,* Typical patterns of an obstructive ventilatory defect (OVD) and a restrictive ventilatory defect (RVD) are noted. OVD is characterized by a reduced forced expiratory volume in 1 second–to–forced vital capacity (FEV_1/FVC) ratio. Either OVD or RVD can result in a reduced vital capacity—but with different alternations in the total lung capacity (TLC) and residual volume (RV) (see Fig. 13–18).

important parameters include the forced expiratory volume in 1 second (FEV_1), the forced vital capacity (FVC), and the FEV_1/FVC ratio. OVD is associated with a reduced FEV_1/FVC ratio, whereas the ratio is normal or increased in RVD (see Table 13–7).[45-48] OVD processes are associated with reductions in airflow, hence a reduced FEV_1. In very mild disease, the FEV_1 may be normal but the FEV_1/FVC reduced. In patients with OVD, the FVC may be normal but can be reduced in individuals with "air trapping," meaning air that would not come out of the lungs during the FVC maneuver, usually because of airway collapse at low lung volumes. The causes of a reduced VC differs in patients with OVD and RVD (Figure 13–18B). In RVD the TLC **decreases** more than the RV, and in OVD the RV **increases** more than the TLC. The TLC in OVD is normal or increased. The combination of a decreased FEV_1/FVC ratio and a decreased TLC can occur in a mixed defect (combined OVD and RVD).[45-48] The RVD pattern of spirometry is characterized by a normal FEV_1/FVC ratio and a reduced FVC. However, the definitive diagnosis of RVD requires demonstration of a reduced TLC (lung volume testing). The pattern of a reduced FVC, a normal FEV_1/FVC ratio, and normal TLC is present in about 10% of all lung function studies.[47] About half have evidence of OVD based on "scooping" of the expiratory flow volume curve or an increased RV. The VC is reduced due to a relative increase in the RV with normal TLC. Other patients have a FVC much less than the slow VC measure on lung volume measurements (poor performance or obstruction at low lung volumes). Still others have a clinical picture consistent with RVD including a neuromuscular disorder, obesity, or parenchymal lung disease on CT scan. Some of this discrepancy is due to the fact that prediction equations for the FVC and TLC may not be consistent with each other, for example, a reduced TLC but a FVC at the lower limit of normal. The reader is referred to the reference by Dempsey and Scanlon for a practical method of pulmonary function interpretation with discussion of "nonspecific" patterns of abnormality.[47] Although the FEV_1/FVC is pivotal in defining a normal, OVD, or RVD pattern on spirometry, there is controversy about what constitutes normal. This issue will be discussed below.

Bronchodilator testing is performed by administering inhaled bronchodilator to a patient who has not used a bronchodilator before the study. American Thoracic Society criteria[45] for a significant bronchodilator response have been an increase in the FEV1 or FVC by 12% AND an absolute increase of at least 200 mL. More recently an increase of 10% has been recommended as a significant bronchodilator response.[45-48] A large improvement of 15% to 40% is suggestive of asthma. However, patients with asthma may not have an acute bronchodilator response but may improve with chronic bronchodilator therapy (including steroids). Patients with COPD typically have no response (predominant emphysema) or a modest response of 10% to 15% (predominant chronic bronchitis). Flow volume curves are often determined during spirometry and are plots of flow versus exhaled volume.[51] Individuals inspire to TLC, then forcibly exhale until no more air comes out, and then forcibly inhale to form a flow volume loop (Figure 13–20). The expiratory flow rates over roughly the lower 70-75% of the VC are "effort independent" and determined by properties of the lung (assuming adequate expiratory effort).[3] Flow rates decrease as lung volume decreases during exhalation. The reduced flow rates are due to lower effective driving pressure (lung elastic recoil) and higher airway resistance (smaller bronchial diameter) as the lung volume decreases during exhalation. Milder forms of OVD are manifested by a normal FEV_1/FVC ratio and *scooping of the expiratory limb of the flow volume curve* (Figure 13–20B). The scooping represents lower than expected flow for a given lung volume at lower lung volumes. This is due to closure or narrowing of small airways at low lung volumes. In COPD the small airways are narrowed and there is less tethering of the airway preventing airway closure due to destruction of the surrounding parenchma. Flow volume curves are also used to diagnose reduced flows due to fixed obstruction in the lower or upper airways or a variable "central" obstruction that results in a flow pattern with a plateau. A plateau in the flow suggests something other than the lung (exhalation) or inspiratory effort (inspiration) is controlling flow. In variable central upper airway (above the sternal notch) obstruction the inspiratory limb of the flow volume curve is flat, whereas the expiratory limb is minimally affected (positive intraluminal pressure tends to expand in exhalation). In variable intrathoracic obstruction the flattening is in exhalation as inspiration tends to open the obstruction. It is also important to note that the inspiratory flow portion of the flow volume loop is effort dependent.

Lung volume testing by helium or methane dilution or body plethysmography is used to determine the FRC. The patient then performs a slow vital capacity (slow SVC) maneuver and the IC and ERV are determined (see Figure 13–21). Then the

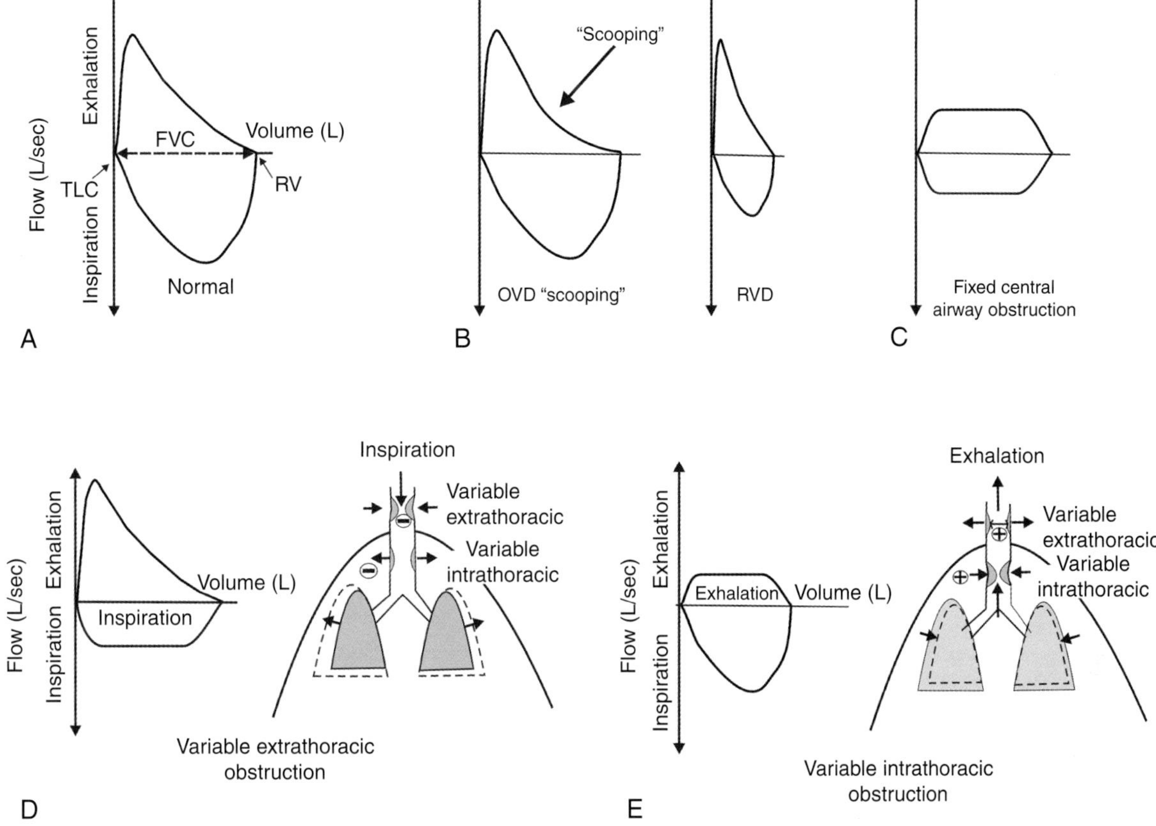

Figure 13–20 Flow volume curves. (A) The flow volume curve is a plot of flow on the *y*-axis and volume on the *x*-axis. The patient inhales to TLC and performs a forced expiration follow by a forced inspiration. (B) In an obstructive ventilatory defect (OVD) there is scooping of the expiratory curve secondary to reduced flows at low lung volumes due to airway disease and closure. In RVD the volume is reduced but flows are appropriate for the lung volume (no scooping). (C) The pattern from a fixed tracheal or upper airway obstruction showing a plateau in inspiration and expiration. (D) On the bottom left, the pattern of variable extrathoracic obstruction, which results in a plateau in the inspiratory limb as this location tends to collapse increasing the obstruction during inspiration. (E) At the bottom right, variable intrathoracic obstruction is depicted showing flattening in exhalation due to the tendency for obstruction to increase during exhalation. In fixed obstruction (flow plateau in both inspiration and exhalation) the location of the central obstruction is not known and can be in the upper airway or tracheal. Note that obstruction must be severe to give the patterns, shown in C, D, and E. Flow volume testing is not a sensitive method to detect pathology in these areas.

TLC and RV are computed (TLC = FRC + IC and RV = FRC – ERV). Note that the VC equals the difference between the TLC and the RV. *Changes in either the TLC, the RV, or both can decrease the VC.* By definition, RVD is associated with a reduced TLC. Ideally, a diagnosis of RVD based on spirometry should always be confirmed by documenting a reduced TLC. As noted previously, in OVD, the TLC is normal or increased. The RV in OVD is usually increased (air-trapping) more than the TLC, and this can result in a decrease in the VC (or FVC). In RVD, the TLC is decreased more than the RV, and this results in a decrease in the VC (see Fig. 13–18B).

Lung volume measurement is usually performed with helium or methane dilution or body plethysmography. In dilution methods the degree of dilution of a known concentration and volume of gas by the patient during tidal breathing is used to determine the FRC. In body plethysmography the patient pants against a closed airway, and change in box volume and mouth pressure are used to determine the FRC. In either case, after measurement of FRC at end expiratory lung volume the patient performs a slow VC maneuver, and all lung volumes can then be determined as illustrated in Figure 13–21. Accurate

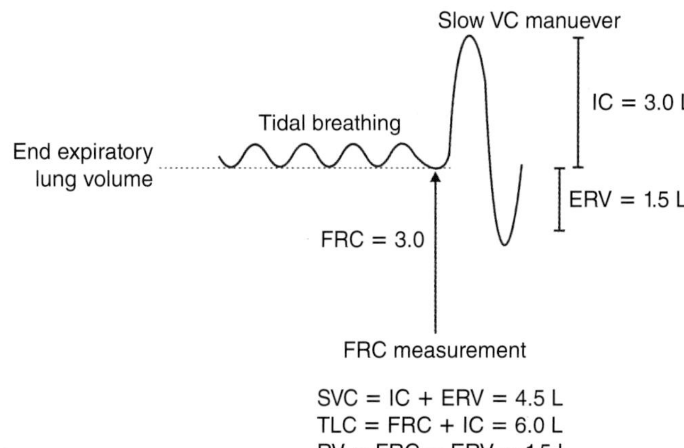

Figure 13–21 A schematic illustrating the measurement of lung volumes from the determination of FRC at end expiratory lung volume followed by performance of a slow vital capacity (SVC) maneuver. Note that the vital capacity (slow vital capacity) should be similar to the FVC for valid lung volume determination. Any error in the FRC will produce an error in the TLC and RV even if the SVC maneuver is accurate. IC, inspiratory capacity; ERV, expiratory reserve volume; FRC, functional residual capacity.

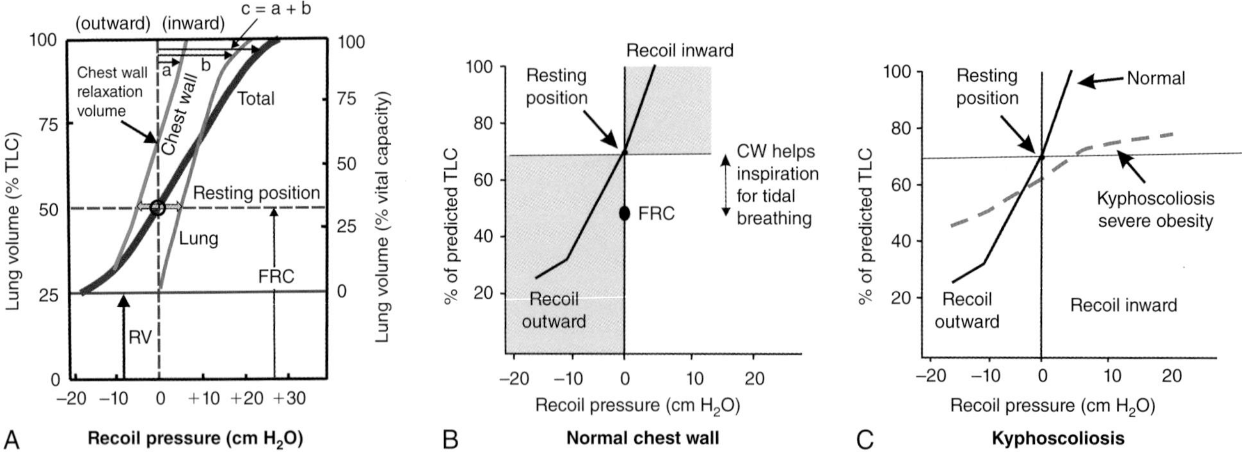

Figure 13–22 (A) Static volume versus pressure plots for the normal lung, chest wall, and respiratory system (Total). These depend entirely on the properties of the chest wall and lung (no respiratory muscle effort). The chest wall has a resting volume at about 60%–70% of TLC. Lung recoil is inward at all lung volumes. The respiratory system curve *(Total)* is plotted with the lung and chest wall curves. The resting position of the respiratory system is at FRC. Here inward lung recoil (positive) is balance by outward chest wall recoil (negative). At lung volumes greater than FRC the respiratory system has inward recoil (positive) and must be matched by outward inspiratory muscle force. Below FRC the respiratory system has outward recoil (negative) and must be balanced by inward muscle force (expiratory). In this figure RV is about 25% of TLC, FRC 50% of TLC, and the IC = TLC − FRC is twice the ERV = FRC − RV. The panels to the *right* illustrate the normal chest wall curve (B) and the difference between the chest wall curve of a normal individual and one with kyphoscoliosis (C). In kyphoscoliosis the chest has a relaxation point at a lower lung volume than normal and the curve is flat; compliance (change in volume per pressure change) is low. A larger than normal pressure change is needed to move above or below the chest wall resting point. Due to chest wall properties the TLC and FRC are reduced in kyphoscoliosis, although the RV is usually normal. (Adapted from Miller WF, Scacci R, Gast R. *Laboratory Evaluation of Pulmonary Function.* JB Lippincott; 1987:181.)

lung volume results depend on an accurate FRC and an accurate slow VC maneuver. A detailed discussion of lung volume measurement is beyond the scope of this chapter and the reader is referred to references.[9,45,47,48] Of note, lung volumes measured by dilution techniques can underestimate lung volumes in patients with OVD due to poorly ventilated lung units that do not participate in gas dilution. This is especially true if lung volumes are determined based on a single breath dilution as part of diffusing capacity testing. It is important to determine if the slow VC and the FVC are reasonably similar. If not, either poor performance on one of the tests or small airway closure at low lung volumes could have reduced the FVC.

Static pressure volume curves of the chest wall, lung, and respiratory system are illustrated in Figure 13–22. The main points to remember are (1) lung recoil is inward at all lung volumes, (2) the chest wall recoils outward at lung volumes less than about 60% to 70% of the TLC (a point between FRC and TLC) and inward above that point, and (3) the FRC is the resting end-expiratory volume and is the lung volume at which the outward recoil of the chest wall is balanced by the inward lung elastic recoil[9]. The behavior of respiratory system as a whole (lungs and chest wall) is the sum of the static behavior of lung and chest wall. Figure 13–22 shows the chest wall static behavior in a patient with kyphoscoliosis. The entire curve is displaced toward lower lung volumes and the curve is flat, showing severely reduced compliance (change in volume/change in pressure). This results in a reduced TLC and FRC with minor changes, if any, in the RV. Inspiratory activity (diaphragm, intercostals, sternocleidomastoid) is required to reach TLC and expiratory muscle activity is required (abdominal muscles) to reach RV (Figure 13–23). In OVD, the RV is the first lung volume to be significantly affected (due to air-trapping due to small airway disease). In

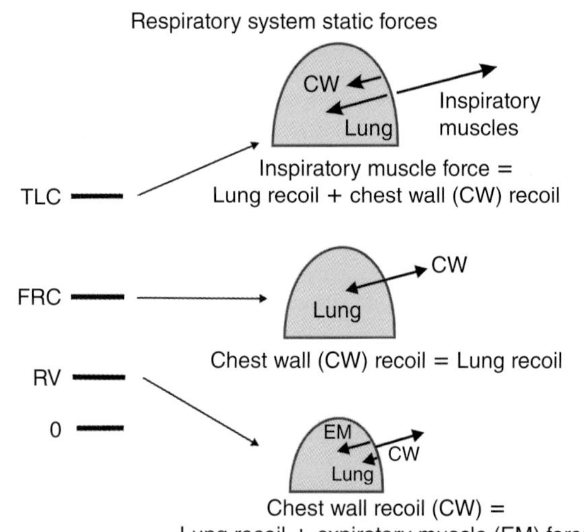

Figure 13–23 Schematic illustration of the forces at total lung capacity (TLC), functional residual capacity (FRC), and residual volume (RV). At FRC no muscle force is needed, as the outward chest recoil is balanced by inward lung recoil. At TLC both lung and chest recoil are inward, and this is balanced by outward inspiratory muscle force. At RV lung recoil is inward (small) and chest recoil is outward. Inward expiratory muscle force is needed to reach RV. From this illustration one could predict a normal FRC in a patient with muscle weakness. However, over time changes in the chest wall and lung result in a lower FRC in some individuals. *Expiratory muscle weakness would increase RV and inspiratory muscles weakness would decrease TLC.*

more advanced OVD, the RV is increased much more than the FRC and TLC, which can result in a decrease in the VC (Figure 13–18). In severe OVD, the FRC and TLC can also be increased (hyperinflation). Emphysema is characterized by loss of lung parenchymal structures (alveoli and supporting

Table 13–8 Use of the Diffusing Capacity in Pulmonary Function Testing

OVD disorders	Reduced with emphysema
Intrinsic RVD disorders	Reduced (interstitial lung disease) Reduction can occur with lung volumes still within the normal range
Extrinsic RVD disorders	Normal or mildly reduced—mild to moderate reductions in TLC Greater reduction with moderate to severe reductions in the TLC
Reduced diffusing capacity and normal spirometry	Emphysema Interstitial lung disease Pulmonary vascular disease Anemia

structures) and a reduction in elastic recoil. The result is an increase in the FRC and TLC. Hyperinflation can also occur in patients with severe asthma.

The diffusing capacity for carbon monoxide (DLco) is a noninvasive method to assess the ability of the lung to transfer gas.[45-48,50] Changes in the diffusing capacity with pulmonary disorders are summarized in Table 13–8. The DLco is usually measured with a single breath test in which the subject exhales to RV, then inhales a mixture of CO and another gas (usually helium or methane) and breath holds at TLC for 10 seconds. The individual then exhales and after discarding dead space gas and alveolar sample is collected and analyzed. The exhaled CO concentration is lower due to diffusion of CO across the alveolar membrane and the exhaled helium (or methane) concentration is lower (diluted) by diffusion into the alveolar spaces (essentially a single breath determination of the alveolar volume VA [VA = TLC − dead space]). The diffusing capacity depends on the effective surface area for gas transfer (intact membrane and lung volume), the pulmonary blood volume, and the amount of hemoglobin in the blood. If the breath hold takes place at a volume much less than TLC, the diffusing capacity can be reduced. For diffusing capacity testing to be valid, the inspired volume should exceed 80% of the VC. CO diffuses across the alveoli and binds to Hb. The diffusing capacity must be corrected for anemia if this is present. Destruction of the effective surface area for diffusion occurs with emphysema or parenchymal lung disorders associated with RVD (interstitial lung disease and others). Pulmonary vascular diseases that destroy the pulmonary arterial structures perfusing the alveoli can reduce the effective blood flow to the alveoli, thus reducing the diffusing capacity. As might be expected, obstructive diseases that affect the alveoli (emphysema) are associated with a reduced DLco. OVD due to asthma or chronic bronchitis is usually associated with a relatively normal DLco. Although $(\dot{V}/\dot{Q})$ match due to airway disease can reduce the diffusing capacity, this effect is minimized by performance of the test at TLC, which tends to open airways. Disorders causing RVD that affect the lung parenchyma (alveolar filling or interstitial lung disease) are associated with a reduced DLco. Of note, *early in these disorders, the DLco may be reduced even though the FVC and TLC are still in the normal range.* In extrinsic RVD (respiratory muscle weakness or chest wall/pleural disorders),[52] the DLco is relatively normal (normal or mildly reduced) because the structure of the alveoli is not directly affected by these disorders. However, a reduction in lung volume can reduce the surface area for gas exchange, and with severe extrinsic RVD the diffusing capacity is reduced. Table 13–7 and 13–8 presents a summary of pulmonary function findings in OVD and RVD. Of note, the pattern of near normal spirometry and a decreased diffusing capacity can occur with emphysema, interstitial lung disease, pulmonary vascular disease, or anemia. Some patients with emphysema have minimal abnormalities in airflow but a reduced diffusing capacity. As noted above, some patients with early manifestations of disorders of the lung causing RVD can have a reduction in the diffusing capacity while the FVC and TLC are still normal.[45-47] The situation is especially common in lung disease due to medications (e.g., amiodarone, chemotherapy agents). In pulmonary vascular disease (e.g., scleroderma), reduction in the diffusing capacity can occur in association with minimal changes in spirometry. A mixed pattern of OVD and RVD can occur and is characterized by a reduced FEV_1/FVC ratio in combination with a reduced TLC (should be normal or increased in OVD without a component of RVD).

Defining Normal and Severity

Prediction equations for normal values of the FEV_1, FVC, FEV_1/FVC ratio, TLC, FRC, RV, and diffusing capacity are available, and the predicted values depend on gender, age, and height.[1-4] The FEV_1, FVC, and diffusing capacity increase with height, decrease with age and are lower in female individuals at the same height and age. The RV, FRC, and TLC increase with age and are lower in women at the same height and age (TLC and FRC). A simple way of defining a normal range is shown below.[53]

Simple normal ranges include:

- FEV_1, FVC, TLC 80% to 120% of predicted
- FEV_1/FVC 90% of predicted
- Diffusing capacity: 75% to 120% of predicted
- FRC 70% to 130% of predicted
- RV: 60% to 140% of predicted

However, a more precise method is to define a lower limit of normal for the FEV_1, FVC, and FEV_1/FVC ratio and a lower and upper limit of normal (LLN, ULN) for lung volumes and diffusing capacity based on the distribution of normal values (95% confidence limits).[1-4] Of note, some pulmonary function laboratories use only a LLN for the diffusing capacity. The LLN excludes the bottom 5% and the ULN-LLN excludes 2.5% at the upper and lower bounds. The LLN = predicted − 1.64 SEE and for ULN/LLN parameters predicted ± 1.96 SEE. Here the SEE is the standard error of the estimate derived from the regression equation for the value versus age and height for a given gender. Another method is to compute the z score = (value − predicted)/SEE[48]. For values with only an LLN, the lower limit Z score is 1.64 and for ULN/LLN quantities ± 1.96 are the corresponding values. Values for the LLN for the FEV_1, FVC, and FEV1/FVC ratio and a normal range (LLN to ULN) for lung volumes and the DLco are often displayed in pulmonary function reports, as shown in Table 13–9. This table shows normal pulmonary function in an obese individual. The Global Initiative for Obstructive Lung Disease criteria define OVD based on the **post-bronchodilator** FEV_1/FVC ratio < 0.70,[54] but this value is too low for normal young individuals and possibly too high for the elderly.

Table 13–9 Pulmonary Function in an Obese Patient

Age 38	Height 63 inches	Weight 307 pounds	Gender: Female		
TEST	LLN	Pre	% predicted		
FVC (L)	2.86	4.20	117		
FEV_1 (L)	2.35	3.55	120		
FEV1/FVC	72	85	102		
	LLN	ULN	Pre	% predicted	
TLC (L)	3.78	5.76	5.47	116	
FRC (L)	1.80	3.44	1.82	69	At lower limit of normal
RV (L)	0.93	2.08	1.21	81	
ERV (L)	1.00	1.202	0.60	54	Decreased
DLco (mL/min/mm Hg)	16.5	27.9	23.3	109	

The American Thoracic Society recommends using an LLN for the FEV_1/FVC (normal is greater than the lowest 5% of values in the population). A lower limit of normal z score can also be used.[48] Pennock et al.[53] reported use of an LLN using the 90% of predicted value. The choice of what constitutes a normal FEV_1/FVC ratio is an ongoing issue. Defining a normal range is discussed in detail in references by Pennock et al.[53], Dempsey and Scanlon.[47], and Stanojevic et al.[1]

Severity criteria for OVD and RVD are somewhat arbitrary,[45-49,53,54] but some commonly used criteria are displayed in Table 13–10 for OVD and Table 13–11 for RVD and the diffusing capacity. Severity criteria can also be expressed based on the z score. For example for the FEV1: normal > −1,64, mild (−1.65 to −2.5), moderate (−2.51 to −4.0), and severe (≤ −4.1)[1]. For simplicity the z score will not be used in examples in this chapter. Examples of pulmonary function results for both OVD and RVD are displayed in Table 13–12. A useful overview of an approach to reading pulmonary function tests is contained in several references.[44,45,47,55] A simplified algorithm for pulmonary function testing is displayed in Figure 13–24. More complete and complex algorithms are supplied in the references.

Lung Volume Changes in Extrinsic Restrictive Disorders

As noted above, OVD is associated with normal or increased lung volumes (increase in RV > FRC > TLC), and RVD is associated with a reduced TLC and variable changes in the FRC and RV. In the RVD, the reduction in the TLC exceeds any reduction in the RV, and this results in a decrease in the VC. In an intrinsic RVD as disease worsens, the FRC and then RV may be reduced. In an extrinsic RVD, the pattern varies with the cause of the disorder.[56] Common patterns seen in various disorders[56-58] are shown in Figure 13–25. In simple obesity the TLC and VC are usually preserved, and the FRC may be reduced due to mass loading and a shift in the static chest wall characteristics to lower lung volumes. However, in simple obesity a reduced ERV is the most common finding as the decrease in the FRC exceeds any decrease in the RV (ERV = FRC-RV). In the OHS the TLC and

Table 13–10 Severity of Obstruction

Obstruction Grading Based on FEV_1 (%predicated)*	1986 ATS[63]	2005 ATS[46]	Gold 2018[54]
Mild	60% to LLN	>70%	≥80%
Moderate	41%–59%	60%–69%	≥50% and <80%
Moderately severe	N/A	50%–59%	N/A
Severe	31%–40%	35%–49%	≥30% and <50%
Very severe	<30%	<35%	<30%
FEV_1/FVC cutoff	Below LLN	Below LLN	<70%

*Gold criteria use post-bronchodilator FEV_1.
LLN, Lower limit of normal.

Adapted from Dempsey TM, Scanlon PD. Pulmonary function tests for the generalist: a brief review. *Mayo Clin Proc.* 2018;93(6):763-771.

Table 13–11 Restriction Grading

	Lung Volumes	Diffusing Capacity	
	TLC*	FVC	DLco†
Mild	<80%	<80%	> 60% and < LLN (or 75% of predicted)
Moderate	<60%	<60%	40%–60%
Severe	<50%	<50%	<40%
Very Severe	<35%		

Values are % predicted. FEV_1/FVC must be normal. Use FVC if prior TLC < 80% predicted. LLN lower limit of normal.
In RVD, severity depends on both lung volumes and diffusing capacity.
*Adapted from Dempsey TM, Scanlon PD. Pulmonary function tests for the generalist: a brief review. *Mayo Clin Proc.* 2018;93(6):763-771.
†Adapted from Pellegrino R, Viegi G, Brusasco V, et al. Interpretative strategies for lung function tests. *Eur Respir J.* 2005;26(5):948-968.

Table 13–12 Examples of Pulmonary Function

	Pre-BD	% Predicted	Post-BD	% Change
Asthma				
FVC (L)	3.07	67%	4.26	39
FEV_1 (L)	1.46	41%	2.21	52
FEV_1/FVC	0.48			
TLC (L)	8.35	124%		
FRC (L)	5.61	165%		
RV (L)	4.43	203%		
DLco (mL/min/mm Hg)	29.1	94%		
Reduced FEV_1/FVC, increased RV > FRC > TLC, normal DLco, large BD response				
COPD: Mixed Chronic Bronchitis/Emphysema				
FVC (L)	2.85	79	3.00	5
FEV_1 (L)	1.34	50	1.50	12
FEV_1/FVC	0.47			
TLC (L)	6.4	110		
FRC (L)	4.40	132		
RV (L)	3.55	161		
DLco(ml/min/mm Hg)	10.0	50		
Reduced FEV1/FVC, increased RV > FRC, reduced diffusing capacity, small/borderline improvement after inhaled bronchodilator				
RVD Intrinsic (Pulmonary Fibrosis)				
FVC (L)	2.45	56%		
FEV_1 (L)	1.98	61%		
FEV_1/FVC	0.81			
TLC (L)	3.61	51%		
FRC (L)	2.18	59%		
RV (L)	1.14	43%		
DLco(ml/min/mm Hg)	10.1	34%		
Normal FEV_1/FVC, reduced FVC and TLC, reduced DLco				
RVD Extrinsic (Kyphoscoliosis)				
FVC (L)	1.54	42%		
FEV_1 (L)	1.13	35%		
FEV_1/FVC	0.73			
TLC (L)	2.31	48%		
FRC (L)	1.27	50%		
RV (L)	0.74	64%		
DLco (ml/min/mm Hg)	21.0	70%		
Normal FEV_1/FVC, reduced TLC, mildly reduced diffusing capacity				

DLco diffusing capacity; L, liters

FRC are often reduced. In kyphoscoliosis the TLC and FRC are reduced. In ankylosing spondylitis the TLC is decreased but the FRC and RV can be increased due to the thoracic cage being "fixed at a high lung volume." In patients with muscle weakness, one might expect the FRC to be normal as no muscle effort is needed to reach FRC. However, chronic changes in the chest wall and/or lung result in a reduced TLC and FRC in chronic muscle weakness. In patients with primarily expiratory muscle weakness, one might expect an increase in the RV with relatively preserved TLC, such as in patients with spinal cord injury. However the pattern can vary between patients due to changes in the lung or chest wall (including obesity) with time.[58]

Maximum Inspiratory Pressure and Maximum Expiratory Pressure

The maximum inspiratory pressure (MIP) and maximum expiratory pressure (MEP) are often said to be the most sensitive tests of respiratory muscle strength. However, obtaining accurate measurement of these parameters requires patient cooperation and special expertise.[59] The apparatus to measure the MIP and MEP consists of a mouthpiece with a small orifice to provide a leak and an accurate pressure transducer. *The leak is required to prevent the patient from closing the glottis and using cheek muscles to perform the maneuvers.* The MIP is usually performed at RV, and the MEP is performed at TLC. Unfortunately, the published normal ranges are wide and vary considerably between studies. In general, the pressures decrease with age, they are higher in men than in women, and the MEP exceeds the MIP in normal individuals. For clinically significant changes in the FVC to begin to occur, the MIP is usually less than 60 cm H_2O. Of note, it has been shown that in neuromuscular disease the decrease in the FVC is greater than one might expect for a given detriment in muscle strength.[57] Therefore the FVC is actually a fairly sensitive test for following muscle strength in patients with neuromuscular disease. Note that at TLC with a normal chest wall and lungs the inward recoil of the respiratory system is about −30 cm H_2O. An MEP less than 60 cm H_2O is associated with a reduced ability to cough and clear secretions. An American College of Chest Physicians Consensus group recommended noninvasive positive-pressure ventilation for progressive neuromuscular disorders when the MIP was less than 60 cm H_2O (or FVC < 50% of predicted).[60] These MIP and FVC measurements are part of the Centers for Medicare and Medicaid criteria for paying for a bilevel PAP device with a backup rate in patients with neuromuscular disorders. Current thinking is that many individuals with neuromuscular disease would benefit from nocturnal ventilatory support at a higher FVC percent of predicted (≈70% of predicted). Of special interest is the fact that performance of FVC testing in the supine position was found to be a very sensitive test of diaphragmatic weakness.[61] In this posture the chest wall muscles are less effective, and any weakness in the diaphragm is more evident. Some patients with neuromuscular disease cannot make a good mouth seal. Nasal sniff inspiratory pressure can be performed with a soft nasal plug with a pressure-measuring catheter in the middle. The other nostril is sealed either by patient or the individual making the measurement. In one study a nasal inspiratory sniff pressure less than 40 cm H_2O predicted a high risk of death within 6 months in patients with amyotrophic lateral sclerosis.[62]

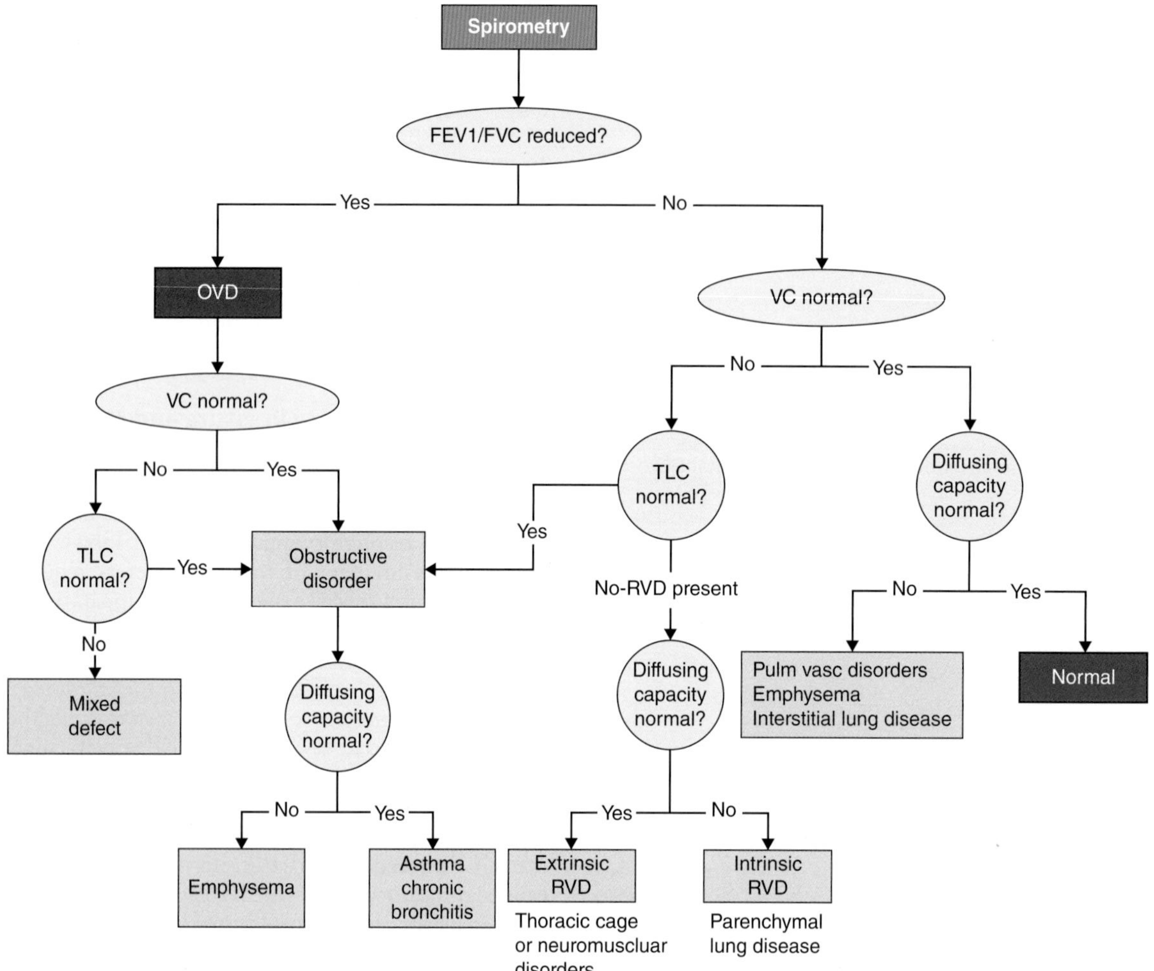

Figure 13–24 A simplified algorithm for pulmonary function test interpretation. If the FEV_1/FVC ratio is decreased, OVD is present. If the FEV1/FVC and TLC are both reduced, this suggests a mixed defect (combined OVD and RVD) is present. In OVD the TLC should be normal or increased. The presence of OVD with a reduced diffusing capacity suggests a significant component of emphysema is present. If the FEV_1/FVC ratio is normal or increased, RVD may be present, but determination of the total lung capacity is needed for a definitive diagnosis. If the TLC is normal and the diffusing capacity reduced, this pattern can be seen with pulmonary vascular disorders and the other disorders listed. If the TLC is reduced, then RVD is present and the diffusing capacity suggests if intrinsic or extrinsic RVD is present. One should keep in mind that if extrinsic RVD is associated with a severe decrease in the TLC that the diffusing capacity will be reduced. See the references by Pellegrino et al.[46] and Dempsey and Scanlon[47].

SUMMARY OF KEY POINTS

1. Mechanisms of hypoxemia include high altitude [low $FiO_2 = 0.21(P_B - 47)$ due to low barometric pressure], hypoventilation, ventilation perfusion mismatch, shunt, and diffusion defect. Supplemental oxygen (increased FiO_2) can improve the PaO_2 for all the mechanisms of hypoxemia *except for shunt.*
2. Breathing room air the predicted alveolar gas equation is $PAO_2 = 150 - PaCO_2/0.8$. The alveolar to arterial PO_2 gradient (A-a gradient) $= PAO_2 - PaO_2$.
3. If hypoxemia is due to hypoventilation alone, the A-a gradient [$PAO_2 - PaO_2$] is normal. The A-a gradient increases with age, but lung disease severe enough to cause hypercapnia is usually associated with a value $\geq$25 mm Hg.
4. Alveolar hypoventilation (increased $PaCO_2 > 45$ mm Hg) with a normal A-a gradient suggests a disorder of ventilatory control, a chest wall disorder, or muscle weakness rather than lung disease is the cause of hypoventilation.
5. Patients with alveolar hypoventilation due to parenchymal lung disease have an increased A-a gradient (usually >25 mm Hg).
6. The $PaCO_2 = \text{constant} \times \dfrac{CO_2 \text{ production}}{(\text{alveolar ventilation})}$. If the alveolar ventilation doubles, the $PaCO_2$ decreases to half the original value. The alveolar ventilation = minute ventilation − dead space ventilation. For the same minute ventilation, the alveolar ventilation will be lower with a lower tidal volume (V_T) and a higher respiratory rate as this pattern increases the V_D/V_T and the dead space **ventilation**.
7. Increases in the dead space–to–tidal volume ratio (V_D/V_T) from a high V_D and/or a low V_T reduce the alveolar ventilation for a given minute ventilation.
8. Patients with lung disease can maintain a normal $PaCO_2$ by higher than normal minute ventilation to compensate for greater physiologic dead space.

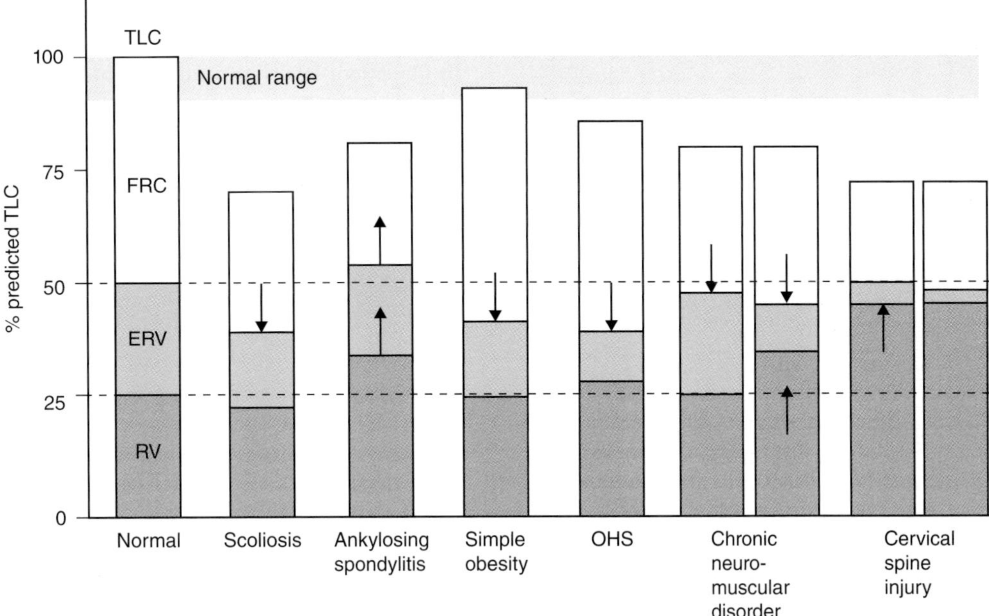

Figure 13–25 Typical alterations in lung volumes with different disorders of the chest wall or respiratory muscle weakness. *These are generalizations and the actual pattern will vary depending on the severity of the disorder and other factors such as obesity or concurrent obstructive lung disease.* A normal range is assumed to be above 80% of predicted. In scoliosis there is a reduction in the TLC > FRC > RV. The RV may be low but within the normal range. In ankylosing spondylitis, the chest wall is relatively fixed at a higher than normal FRC volume. Moving above or below this volume is difficult resulting in a reduced TLC and increased RV. In simple obesity the TLC and RV are typically within the normal range, but the FRC is low normal or reduced. The ERV is the most consistently reduced lung volume. In the obesity hypoventilation syndrome, the TLC is often mildly reduced and the FRC is more severely reduced than in simple obesity. The chest wall behavior is somewhat like scoliosis except that the RV is usually within the normal range. In chronic neuromuscular disorders the TLC is reduced. One might predict a normal FRC but there are chronic changes in the lung that may reduce the FRC. The RV may be normal or increased depending on the pattern of muscle weakness. In cervical spinal cord injury, there is abdominal paralysis resulting in a high RV. Inspiratory muscles are also affected resulting in a reduced TLC. The chest wall can develop rigidity, and this can tend to reduce the TLC. The FRC is variable and depends on the degree of obesity.[58] (Adapted from Bergofsky EH. Respiratory failure in disorders of the thoracic cage. *Am Rev Respir Dis.* 1979;119(4):643-669.)

9. During sleep the $PaCO_2$ rises slightly (alveolar ventilation falls more than the CO_2 production falls) and the PaO_2 falls slightly. Reduction in minute ventilation occurs owing to a reduction in the tidal volume with minimal change in the respiratory rate. The drop in the PaO_2 is associated with only small change in the SaO_2 (1–2 mm Hg) because a normal awake PaO_2 is on the flat portion of the oxygen hemoglobin dissociation curve.

10. The hypercapnic ventilatory response is reduced during normal sleep with the response during REM sleep lower than NREM sleep.

11. The apneic threshold (AT) is the level of $PaCO_2$ below which central apnea occurs during NREM sleep. It is usually near the awake $PaCO_2$ value. Patients with a high hypercapnic respiratory drive have a lower CO_2 reserve (decrease in $PaCO_2$ needed to reach the AT) and are more likely to reach the apneic threshold and have central apnea. An AT does not exist during REM sleep, and patients with central apnea during NREM sleep due to a fall in $PaCO_2$ below the AT usually do not have central apnea during REM sleep.

12. An OVD is characterized by a FEV_1/FVC with normal or increased lung volumes. A decrease in the FVC can occur due to a larger increase in the RV than the TLC. If the VC is reduced, this is secondary to a high RV. The pattern of increased lung volumes in OVD is RV > increase in FRC > increase in TLC. In asthma and chronic bronchitis, the diffusing capacity is normal, whereas a reduced diffusing capacity in a patient with OVD is associated with a significant component of emphysema.

13. A RVD pattern on spirometry is characterized by a normal FEV_1/FVC ratio and a reduced FVC. However, a definitive diagnosis of RVD requires demonstration of a reduced TLC on lung volume testing. An **intrinsic RVD** pattern is characterized by a reduced diffusing capacity and is secondary due to disease of the lung parenchyma (interstitial lung disease), whereas an **extrinsic RVD** pattern is characterized by a normal to decreased diffusing capacity depending on the severity of the reduction in lung volumes and is secondary due to disorders of the thoracic cage (kyphoscoliosis, obesity) or respiratory muscle weakness. In mild to moderate extrinsic RVD the diffusing capacity can be normal or only mildly decreased.

14. The pattern of normal spirometry and a reduced DLco can occur with pulmonary vascular disease, early interstitial lung disease (including drug-associated pneumonitis), emphysema, left-to-right shunt, and anemia (the diffusing capacity should be corrected for alterations in hemoglobin).

15. The most common pulmonary function test abnormality in patients with simple obesity is a reduced ERV (low FRC relative to the RV). Usually the TLC and vital capacity are normal.

Patients with the obesity hypoventilation syndrome usually have a low normal or reduced total lung capacity.

16. Muscle weakness can cause RVD but must be moderate to severe (MIP < 60 cm H_2O). An FVC < 50% or predicted is considered a severe reduction in a patient with neuromuscular disease and an indication for nocturnal noninvasive ventilatory support. However, many clinicians favor using a higher threshold (FVC < 70%).

17. An increased serum CO_2 (HCO_3^-) is a clue that chronic hypoventilation may be present (especially if >27 mEq/L) in the absence of a reason for a metabolic alkalosis. The increased serum CO_2 is secondary to renal compensation.

18. The hydrogen ion concentration (or pH) is determined by the ratio $PaCO_2/HCO_3^-$. *Compensatory mechanisms attempt to normalize the ratio.* A 10 mm Hg increase in the $PaCO_2$ results in an **acute** increase of 1 mEq/L in HCO_3^-, but with chronic compensation the increase in HCO_3^- is 3 to 4 mEq/L.

19. The pre-Bötzinger area is the respiratory pacemaker, and opioid action at mu receptors located in this brain center causes respiratory suppression.

CLINICAL REVIEW QUESTIONS

1. What is the most commonly reduced lung volume in obesity?
   A. ERV (expiratory reserve volume)
   B. FRC (functional residual capacity)
   C. TLC (total lung capacity)
   D. IC (inspiratory capacity)
2. Which of the following changes occur from wake to sleep? (V_T is tidal volume, RR respiratory rate)
   A. Reduced V_T, minimally changed RR
   B. Unchanged V_T, increased RR
   C. Unchanged minute ventilation, increased RR
   D. Unchanged $PaCO_2$, increased RR
3. Assuming an unchanged CO_2 production, which of the following is **always** associated with an increase in $PaCO_2$?
   A. Decreased alveolar ventilation
   B. Increased V_D/V_T ratio
   C. Increased dead space
   D. Decreased tidal volume
4. Which of the following would be most consistent with a stable patient and normal lungs with muscle weakness and hypoventilation?
   A. $PaCO_2 = 55$, $PaO_2 = 50$ mm Hg
   B. $PaCO_2 = 60$, $PaO_2 = 65$ mm Hg
   C. $PaCO_2 = 50$, $PaO_2 = 50$ mm Hg
   D. $PaCO_2 = 50$, $PaO_2 = 55$ mm Hg
5. A patient has significant expiratory muscle weakness but fairly normal inspiratory muscle weakness. Which lung volume would be affected the most?
   A. TLC
   B. FRC
   C. RV
6. A patient has stable hypoventilation with a $PaCO_2$ of 70 mm Hg. What serum HCO_3 would be expected assuming a normal HCO_3^- value is 24 mEq/L?
   A. 26
   B. 28
   C. 34
   D. 40
7. The relative hypercapnic ventilatory response is
   A. Wake > NREM > REM.
   B. Wake > REM > NREM.
   C. Wake > NREM = REM.
8. Chronic metabolic alkalosis is associated with which of the following hypercapnic ventilatory response phenomenon?
   A. Increased baseline $PaCO_2$, no change in slope, shift in hypercapnic ventilatory response line to the right.
   B. Decreased baseline $PaCO_2$, no change in slope, shift in hypercapnic ventilatory response curve to the left.
   C. Increased baseline $PaCO_2$, reduced slope, shift in hypercapnic ventilatory response line to the right.
   D. Decreased baseline $PaCO_2$, increased slope, shift in hypercapnic ventilatory response line to the left.
9. Which of the following would increase periphertal chemoreceptor activity the most?
   A. An SaO_2 of 92%.
   B. A fall in the PaO_2 to below 55 mm Hg.
   C. A decrease in the $PaCO_2$ and increase in the PaO_2.
   D. An increase in the $PaCO_2$ by 4 mm Hg with a PaO_2 of 80 mm Hg.
10. Which of the following is **NOT** true?
    A. The pre-Bötzinger nucleus is the respiratory pacemaker.
    B. The parabrachial complex may be responsible for arousal responses to hypercapnia.
    C. Opioids can suppress respiration by acting at mu receptors in the pre-Bötzinger nucleus.
    D. The pneumotaxic center is in the medulla.
11. The following pulmonary function test results are most consistent with (see below table)
    A. RVD intrinsic.
    B. RVD extrinsic.
    C. OVD-COPD predominant chronic bronchitis.
    D. OVD-COPD with significant emphysema.

	Prebronchodilator	% Predicted	Postbronchodilator	% Change
FEV_1 (L)	1.61	48	1.86	18
FVC (L)	3.32	75	3.93	18
FEV_1/FVC	0.48			
TLC	7.13	111		
FRC	4.71	132		
RV	3.72	188		
DLco	21.85	78		

Assume normal ranges are FEV_1, FVC ≥ 80% of predicted, TLC 80%–120% of predicted, and diffusing capacity ≥ 75% of predicted.

12. The following pulmonary function test was obtained on a patient with hypoventilation of unknown etiology: age 55, male, height 65 inches (165 cm), weight 200 pounds, BMI 32.
Arterial blood gas on room air pH = 7.36, PCO_2 = 52 mm Hg, PO_2 = 74 mm Hg, HCO_3 = 30 mEq/L.
The patient's only medications were vitamins. (see below table)

	Prebronchodilator	% Predicted
FEV_1 (L)	1.72	48
FVC (L)	2.07	52
FEV_1/FVC	0.83	
TLC	3.64	61
FRC	2.401	73
RV	1.66	85
DLco	20.2	76

Assume normal ranges are FEV_1, FVC ≥ 80% of predicted, TLC 80%–120% of predicted, and diffusing capacity ≥ 75% of predicted.

Which of the following is the best description of the patient's condition?
A. COPD with significant emphysema, chronic respiratory acidosis
B. Idiopathic pulmonary fibrosis, chronic respiratory acidosis
C. Neuromuscular disease, chronic hypoventilation
D. Neuromuscular disease, acute hypoventilation

13. A 40-year-old patient was admitted with hypercapnic respiratory failure and treated with BiPAP by mask and supplemental oxygen. He had a history of smoking and a few wheezes were heard on auscultation, but breath sounds were bilaterally diminished. A chest radiograph showed a normal thoracic cage but a possible right lower lobe infiltrate. The patient was treated with antibiotics, inhaled bronchodilators, and corticosteroids for presumed COPD exacerbation with possible pneumonia. He improved dramatically. The patient complained of shortness of breath while recumbent. Before discharge the following arterial blood gas was obtained breathing room air: pH = 7.36, PCO_2 = 52 mm Hg, PO_2 = 74 mm Hg, HCO_3 =30 mEq/L.
Which statement best describes the findings?
A. COPD with an exacerbation worsening hypoventilation
B. Chronic hypoventilation due to muscle weakness
C. Hypoventilation due to pneumonia, now resolving

ANSWERS

1. A. The FRC is below normal in many patients with obesity, but the ERV = FRC − RV is the lung volume most often reduced.
2. A. Some studies have suggested the respiratory rate can be mildly increased.
3. A. Decreased alveolar ventilation. An increased V_D/V_T ratio tends to decrease alveolar ventilation for a given minute ventilation. However, patients with lung disease and an increased V_D/V_T associated with an increased V_D or neuromuscular/chest wall disease with an increased V_D/V_T due to a low V_T may maintain a normal $PaCO_2$ and alveolar ventilation by sufficiently increasing minute ventilation. If the increase in minute ventilation cannot be maintained, hypoventilation occurs. Patients with muscle weakness or a stiff chest wall breathing with a low tidal volume (also increases V_D/V_T) can maintain a normal alveolar ventilation, but this requires a high respiratory rate. [Alveolar ventilation = minute ventilation $(1 - V_D/V_T) = RR \times VT\ (1 - V_D/V_T)$]
4. B. (normal A-a gradient). 150 − 60/0.8 = 75 PAO_2 − PaO_2 = 75 − 60 = 15 mm Hg. The A-a gradient for A is 31.25, C = 37.5, D = 32.5.
5. C. Reaching RV requires expiratory muscle strength.
6. C. The $PaCO_2$ is increased by 30 mm Hg, so the additional HCO_3 would be = 3 × (3 to 4), or an increase in HCO_3 of about 9 to 12 mEq/L. The expected HCO_3 would be around 33 to 36 mEq/L.
7. A.
8. A (see Fig. 13–17).
9. B. The hypoxic ventilatory response depends on the PaO_2, not the SaO_2. In addition, an SaO_2 of 92% would be associated with a PO_2 at or above 60 mm Hg. Therefore a PaO_2 of 55 mm Hg would be associated with the greatest stimulation of the peripheral chemoreceptors.
10. D. The pneumotaxic center is in the pons.
11. C. The pulmonary function test shows an obstructive ventilatory defect with a reduced FEV_1/FVC ratio. There is a large increase in the residual volume (RV) but a normal total lung capacity (TLC). Therefore a restrictive ventilatory defect (RVD) is not present (answers A and B are incorrect). A significant bronchodilator response is noted along with a low normal diffusing capacity. Predominant emphysema would be associated with a reduced diffusing capacity for carbon monoxide. Predominant chronic bronchitis is associated with a normal or near normal diffusing capacity. There may or may not be a significant improvement with inhaled bronchodilator. When there is a significant response, some clinicians use the term *asthmatic bronchitis*.
12. C. Assume a normal HCO_3 is 24 mEq/L. Then a chronic increase in PCO_2 of 12 mm Hg would predict an increase in HCO_3 of 1.2 × 4 = 4.8 mEq/L. Computing the predicted HCO_3: 24 + 4.8 = 28.9 mEq/L, which is close to the actual HCO_3. Or one could simply observe that the pH was only slightly reduced consistent with chronic compensation. Pulmonary function testing shows an extrinsic restrictive defect. A patient with idiopathic pulmonary fibrosis severe enough to cause hypoventilation would be expected to a significantly reduced diffusing capacity. This patient was found to have a neuromuscular disorder with severe respiratory muscle weakness consistent with the findings of an extrinsic RVD. The maximum inspiratory pressure was measured and was −50 cm H_2O (severely reduced).
13. B. The PAO_2 = 150 − (52/0.8) = 85 A-a gradient = 85 − 74 = 11 (normal!). Hypoventilation is not due to lung disease (COPD or pneumonia). Lung disease severe enough to cause hypoventilation would be associated with an increased A-a gradient. The severe orthopnea is likely due to diaphragmatic weakness. The patient was found to have amyotrophic lateral sclerosis with preferential involvement of the diaphragm.

SUGGESTED READING

Dempsey JA. Central sleep apnea: misunderstood and mistreated! *F1000Res.* 2019;8:F1000 Faculty Rev-981.

Dempsey TM, Scanlon PD. Pulmonary function tests for the generalist: a brief review. *Mayo Clin Proc.* 2018;93(6):763-771.

Johnson JD, Theurer WM. A stepwise approach to the interpretation of pulmonary function tests. *Am Fam Physician.* 2014;89(5):359-366.

Lechtzin N, Wiener CM, Shade DM, et al. Spirometry in the supine position improves the detection of diaphragmatic weakness in patients with amyotrophic lateral sclerosis. *Chest.* 2001;121:436-442.

REFERENCES

1. Troester MM, Quan SF, Berry RB, et al; for the American Academy of Sleep Medicine. *The AASM Manual for the Scoring of Sleep and Associated Events: Rules, Terminology and Technical Specifications.* Version 3. American Academy of Sleep Medicine; 2023.
2. Berry RB, Budhiraja R, Gottlieb DJ, et al. Rules for scoring respiratory events in sleep: update of the 2007 AASM Manual for the Scoring of Sleep and Associated Events. Deliberations of the Sleep Apnea Definitions Task Force of the American Academy of Sleep Medicine. *J Clin Sleep Med.* 2012;8(5):597-619.
3. West JB, Wagner P. Ventilation, blood flow, and gas exchange. In: Murray JF, Nadel JA, eds. *Textbook of Respiratory Medicine.* 3rd ed. WB Saunders; 2000:55-89.
4. Sharma S, Hashmi MF, Burns B. Alveolar gas equation. Aug 30, 2021. In: *StatPearls* [Internet]. Treasure Island (FL): StatPearls Publishing; 2022.
5. Harris DE, Massie M. Role of alveolar-arterial gradient in partial pressure of oxygen and PaO2/fraction of inspired oxygen ratio measurements in assessment of pulmonary dysfunction. *AANA J.* 2019;87(3): 214-221.
6. Kanber GJ, King FW, Eshchar YR, Sharp JT. The alveolar-arterial oxygen gradient in young and elderly men during air and oxygen breathing. *Am Rev Respir Dis.* 1968;97(3):376-381.
7. Mellemgaard K. The alveolar-arterial oxygen difference: its size and components in normal man. *Acta Physiol Scand.* 1966;67(1):10-20.
8. Robertson HT. Dead space: the physiology of wasted ventilation. *Eur Respir J.* 2015;45(6):1704-1716. Erratum in: *Eur Respir J.* 2015; 46(4):1226.
9. Miller WF, Scacci R, Gast LR, eds. *Laboratory Evaluation of Pulmonary Function.* JB Lippincott; 1987:468.
10. Hart MC, Orzalesi MM, Cook CD. Relation between anatomic respiratory dead space and body size and lung volume. *J Appl Physiol (1985).* 1963;18(3):519-522.
11. Mohsenin V. Sleep in chronic obstructive pulmonary disease. sleep and respiration. *Semin Respir Crit Care Med.* 2005;26:109-115.
12. Krieger J. Respiratory physiology: breathing in normal subjects. In: Kryger MH, Roth T, Dements WC, eds. *Principles and Practice of Sleep Medicine.* Elsevier; 2005:232-255.
13. Krieger J, Maglasiu N, Sforza E, Kurtz D. Breathing during sleep in normal middle-aged subjects. *Sleep.* 1990;13(2):143-154.
14. Douglas NJ, White DP, Pickett CK, Weil JV, Zwillich CW. Respiration during sleep in normal man. *Thorax.* 1982;37(11):840-844.
15. Gould GA, Gugger M, Molloy J, et al. Breathing pattern and eye movement density during REM sleep in humans. *Am Rev Respir Dis.* 1988; 138:874-877.
16. Wiegand L, Zwillich CW, Wiegand D, White DP. Changes in upper airway muscle activation and ventilation during phasic REM sleep in normal men. *J Appl Physiol (1985).* 1991;71(2):488-497.
17. Hudgel DW, Devadda P. Decrease in functional residual capacity during sleep in normal humans. *J Appl Physiol.* 1984;57:1319-1322.
18. Hudgel DW, Martin RJ, Capehart M, et al. Contribution of hypoventilation to sleep oxygen desaturation in chronic obstructive pulmonary disease. *J Appl Physiol Respir Environ Exerc Physiol.* 1983;55(3):669-677.
19. Dempsey JA, Skatrud JB. A sleep-induced apneic threshold and its consequences. *Am Rev Respir Dis.* 1986;133(6):1163-1170.
20. Dempsey JA. Central sleep apnea: misunderstood and mistreated! *F1000Res.* 2019;8:F1000 Faculty Rev-981.
21. Javaheri S, Dempsey JA. Central sleep apnea. *Compr Physiol.* 2013;3(1): 141-163.
22. Sowho M, Amatoury J, Kirkness JP, Patil SP. Sleep and respiratory physiology in adults. *Clin Chest Med.* 2014;35(3):469-481.
23. Newton K, Malik V, Lee-Chiong T. Sleep and breathing. *Clin Chest Med.* 2014;35(3):451-456.
24. Malik V, Smith D, Lee-Chiong T. Respiratory physiology during sleep. *Sleep Med Clin.* 2012;7:497-505.
25. Kasai T, Motwani SS, Yumino D, et al. Contrasting effects of lower body positive pressure on upper airways resistance and partial pressure of carbon dioxide in men with heart failure and obstructive or central sleep apnea. *J Am Coll Cardiol.* 2013;61(11):1157-1166.
26. Edwards BA, White DP. Control of the pharyngeal musculature during wakefulness and sleep: implications in normal controls and sleep apnea. *Head Neck.* 2011;33(suppl 1):S37-S45.
27. Fenik VB, Penzel T, Malhotra A. Editorial: anatomy of upper airway and neuronal control of pharyngeal muscles in obstructive sleep apnea. *Front Neurol.* 2019;10:733.
28. Grace KP, Hughes SW, Shahabi S, Horner RL. K+ channel modulation causes genioglossus inhibition in REM sleep and is a strategy for reactivation. *Respir Physiol Neurobiol.* 2013;188(3):277-288.
29. Lo YL, Jordan AS, Malhotra A, et al. Influence of wakefulness on pharyngeal airway muscle activity. *Thorax.* 2007;62(9):799-805.
30. Worsnop C, Kay A, Pierce R, Kim Y, Trinder J. Activity of respiratory pump and upper airway muscles during sleep onset. *J Appl Physiol (1985).* 1998;85(3):908-920.
31. Mezzanotte WS, Tangel DJ, White DP. Influence of sleep onset on upper-airway muscle activity in apnea patients versus normal controls. *Am J Respir Crit Care Med.* 1996;153(6 Pt 1):1880-1887.
32. Carberry JC, Jordan AS, White DP, Wellman A, Eckert DJ. Upper airway collapsibility (Pcrit) and pharyngeal dilator muscle activity are sleep stage dependent. *Sleep.* 2016;39(3):511-521.
33. Eckert DJ, Malhotra A, Lo YL, White DP, Jordan AS. The influence of obstructive sleep apnea and gender on genioglossus activity during rapid eye movement sleep. *Chest.* 2009;135(4):957-964.
34. Berry RB, McNellis MI, Kouchi K, Light RW. Upper airway anesthesia reduces phasic genioglossus activity during sleep apnea. *Am J Respir Crit Care Med.* 1997;156(1):127-132.
35. Caruana-Montaldo B, Gleeson K, Zwillich CW. The control of breathing in clinical practice. *Chest.* 2000;117(1):205-225.
36. Montes de Oca M, Celli BR. Mouth occlusion pressure, CO2 response and hypercapnia in severe chronic obstructive pulmonary disease. *Eur Respir J.* 1998;12(3):666-671.
37. Douglas NJ, White DP, Weil JV, Pickett CK, Zwillich CW. Hypercapnic ventilatory response in sleeping adults. *Am Rev Respir Dis.* 1982; 126(5):758-762.
38. Douglas NJ, White DP, Weil JV, et al. Hypoxic ventilatory response decreases during sleep in normal men. *Am Rev Respir Dis.* 1982;125(3):286-289.
39. White DP, Douglas NJ, Pickett CK, Weil JV, Zwillich CW. Hypoxic ventilatory response during sleep in normal premenopausal women. *Am Rev Respir Dis.* 1982;126(3):530-533.
40. Berthon-Jones M, Sullivan CE. Time course of change in ventilatory response to CO2 with long-term CPAP therapy for obstructive sleep apnea. *Am Rev Respir Dis.* 1987;135:144-147.
41. Oren A, Whipp BJ, Wasserman K. Effects of chronic acid-base changes on the rebreathing hypercapnic ventilatory response in man. *Respiration.* 1991;58:181-185.
42. Javaheri S, Shore NS, Burton R, et al. Compensatory hypoventilation in metabolic alkalosis. *Chest.* 1982;81:296-301.
43. Bear RA, Dyck RF. Clinical approach to the diagnosis of acid-base disorders. *Can Med Assoc J.* 1979;120(2):173-182.
44. Haber RJ. A practical approach to acid-base disorders. *West J Med.* 1991;155(2):146-151.
45. Lung function testing: selection of reference values and interpretative strategies. American Thoracic Society. *Am Rev Respir Dis.* 1991;144(5): 1202-1218.
46. Pellegrino R, Viegi G, Brusasco V, Crapo RO, et al. Interpretative strategies for lung function tests. *Eur Respir J.* 2005;26(5):948-968.
47. Dempsey TM, Scanlon PD. Pulmonary function tests for the generalist: a brief review. *Mayo Clin Proc.* 2018;93(6):763-771.
48. Stanojevic S, Kaminsky D, Miller M, et al. ERS/ATS technical standard on interpretive strategies for routine lung function tests. Eur Respir J. 2022;60:21011499. doi:10.1183/ 13993003.01499-2021.
49. Haynes JM, Kaminsky DA, Stanojevic S, Ruppel GL. Pulmonary function reference equations: a brief history to explain all the confusion. *Respir Care.* 2020;65(7):1030-1038.
50. DeCato TW, Hegewald MJ. Breathing red: physiology of an elevated single-breath diffusing capacity of carbon monoxide. *Ann Am Thorac Soc.* 2016;13(11):2087-2092.
51. Sterner JB, Morris MJ, Sill JM, Hayes JA. Inspiratory flow-volume curve evaluation for detecting upper airway disease. *Respir Care.* 2009;54(4): 461-466.

52. Hart N, Cramer D, Ward SP, et al. Effect of pattern and severity of respiratory muscle weakness on carbon monoxide gas transfer and lung volumes. *Eur Respir J*. 2002;20(4):996-1002.
53. Pennock BE, Cottrell JJ, Rogers RM. Pulmonary function testing. What is "normal"? *Arch Intern Med*. 1983;143(11):2123-2127.
54. Rabe KF, Hurd S, Anzueto A, et al; Global Initiative for Chronic Obstructive Lung Disease. Global strategy for the diagnosis, management, and prevention of chronic obstructive pulmonary disease: GOLD executive summary. *Am J Respir Crit Care Med*. 2007;176:532-555.
55. Johnson JD, Theurer WM. A stepwise approach to the interpretation of pulmonary function tests. *Am Fam Physician*. 2014;89(5):359-366.
56. Bergofsky EH. Respiratory failure in disorders of the thoracic cage. *Am Rev Respir Dis*. 1979;119(4):643-669.
57. De Troyer A, Borenstein S, Cordier R. Analysis of lung volume restriction in patients with respiratory muscle weakness. *Thorax*. 1980;35(8):603-610.
58. Stepp EL, Brown R, Tun CG, Gagnon DR, Jain NB, Garshick E. Determinants of lung volumes in chronic spinal cord injury. *Arch Phys Med Rehabil*. 2008;89(8):1499-1506.
59. American Thoracic Society/European Respiratory Society. ATS/ERS statement of respiratory muscle testing. *Am J Respir Crit Care Med*. 2002:166:518-624.
60. American College of Chest Physicians. Clinical indications for noninvasive positive pressure ventilation in chronic respiratory failure due to restrictive lung disease, COPD, and nocturnal hypoventilation. *Chest*. 1999;116:521-534.
61. Lechtzin N, Wiener CM, Shade DM, et al. Spirometry in the supine position improves the detection of diaphragmatic weakness in patients with amyotrophic lateral sclerosis. *Chest*. 2001;121:436-442.
62. Morgan RK, McNally S, Alexander M, et al. Use of sniff nasal-inspiratory force to predict survival in amyotrophic lateral sclerosis. *Am J Respir Crit Care Med*. 2005;171(3):269-274.
63. Renzetti Jr AD, Bleecker ER, Epler GR, Jones RN, Kanner RE, Repsher LH. Evaluation of impairment/disability secondary to respiratory disorders. American Thoracic Society. *Am Rev Respir Dis*. 1986;133(6):1205-1209.

Chapter 14

Cardiac Monitoring During Polysomnography

INTRODUCTION AND ECG NOMENCLATURE

The purpose of this chapter is to discuss the aspects of electrocardiographic (ECG) monitoring relevant to polysomnography. For a detailed discussion of the ECG and related disorders, the reader is referred to comprehensive references.[1,2] The normal ECG recording is composed of several different waveforms. Each waveform represents a different electrical event during the contraction of the heart. The waveforms include the P wave, QRS complex, and T wave (Figure 14–1A). The *P wave* represents atrial depolarization (right atrium followed by left). The *QRS complex* represents ventricular depolarization. Nomenclature of the components of the QRS complex is illustrated in Figure 14–1B. By convention, if the first deflection is negative, the deflection is called a *Q wave.* The first positive deflection is called the *R wave.* The negative deflection after the R wave is called the *S wave.* If a single negative deflection occurs, it is termed the *QS wave.* The second positive deflection after an S wave is called the *R′ wave.* Very small Q, R, and S waves are sometimes labeled q, r, and s, respectively. The entire QRS duration should be **less than** 0.12 second. The *T wave* represents ventricular repolarization. The T wave **direction** is usually concordant with the maximum QRS deflection. The *U wave* is a small wave that follows the T wave. It may be absent or very small and is usually in the same direction as the T wave but approximately 10% of its amplitude. The *PR interval* is the time from the **start** of the P wave to the first part of the QRS complex (see Figure 14–1A). The PR **interval** varies with heart rate (shorter with faster heart rate) but is normally 0.12 to 0.2 second in duration. The PR interval should not be confused with the PR **segment** which extends from the end of the p wave to the start of the QRS complex (Figure 14–1A). The time from the **start** of the QRS until the **end** of the T wave is the *QT interval.* The QT interval is different in different ECG leads and determining the end point of the T waves can be difficult.[3] The QT shortens with increases in heart rate. The *RR interval* is the time between successive QRS complexes. The heart rate in beats per minute (bpm) is 60/RR interval (seconds). The corrected *QT duration (QTc)* is based on heart rate, and there are several QTc formulas. One simple formula is QTc = (QT interval)/RR interval (seconds). Another frequently used QTc formula developed by Bazett replaces the RR interval with the square root of the RR interval.[3] A normal QTc is $<$ 0.44 seconds and a clearly prolonged value exceeds 0.50 seconds (Figure 14–2). A prolonged QT can occur with congenital long QT syndromes and with medications including antibiotics (erythromycin, clarithromycin, levofloxacin); antipsychotics (haloperidol, risperidone); tricyclic antidepressants, trazodone, antiarrhythmic medications (amiodarone, sotalol); and electrolyte abnormalities (hypokalemia, hypomagnesemia). A life-threatening complication of a long QT is the development of polymorphic ventricular tachycardia (torsades de pointes).

The *ST interval* is the time interval from the end of the QRS complex (J point) to the start of the T wave. The ST is usually isoelectric (zero potential as identified by the level at the PQ junction (end of the PR segment) but can change with disease states. The ST may be depressed by ischemia (ST depression) or elevated associated with an acute myocardial infarction or pericarditis. Of note, some references use the T-P line to determine zero potential.

The standard ECG uses 12 leads.[1] In standard ECG recording, electrodes are placed on the right and left arms (RA, LA) and left leg (LL). A ground is placed on the right leg (RL). Leads I, II, and III are then recorded as (I = [(LA+) / (RA–)], II = [(LL+) / (RA–)], III= [(LL+)/LA–)]

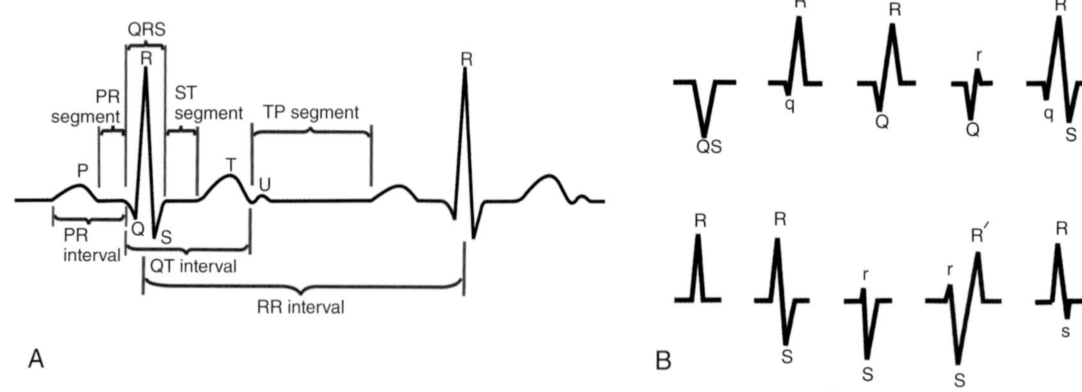

Figure 14–1 (A) Electrocardiographic wave forms and intervals are illustrated. (B) Nomenclature of the components of the QRS complex is illustrated. The Q wave is the initial negative deflection and R-wave the initial positive deflection of the QRS complex. (Adapted from Goldberger AL, Goldberger ZD, Shvilken A. *Goldberger's Clinical Electrocardiography.* 10th ed. Elsevier; 2024:9, 14.)

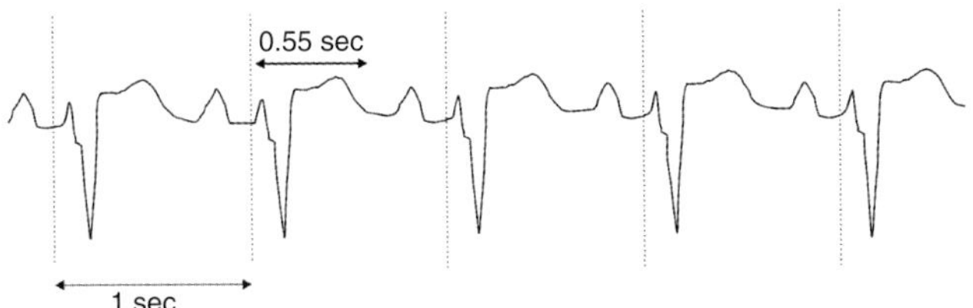

Figure 14–2 Illustration of a tracing with a prolonged QT interval. The RR interval is approximately 1 second so that the QTc is also approximately 550 msec (clearly prolonged). (From Berry RB. *Fundamentals of Sleep Medicine.* 3rd ed. Elsevier; 2012. p 160.)

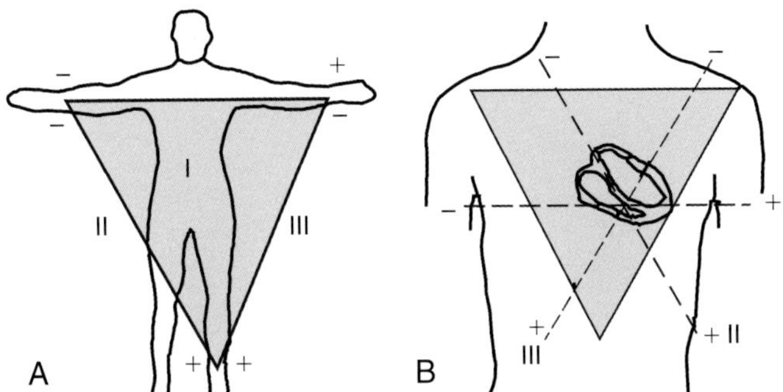

Figure 14–3 (A) Illustration of the ECG leads I, II, and III. (B) The three leads are moved to intersect over the heart. Lead II is in a heart base–to–apex direction. (From Berry RB. *Fundamentals of Sleep Medicine.* 3rd ed. Elsevier; 2012. p 161.)

(Figure 14–3). These are bipolar limb leads. There are also three augmented unipolar leads in which one electrode is referenced against a combination of the other limbs. These additional three frontal plane leads are named aVF, aVR, and aVL (where a is for augmented leads) and are depicted in Figure 14–4. Here each extremity electrode is recorded against the average of the other two extremity electrodes. Remember, RL is ground. Here aVR is right arm, aVL is left arm, and aVF is left leg, where aVR = [(RA+) − ({½(LA + LL)} −)], aVL = [(LA+) − ({½ (RA + LL)} −)], aVF = [(LL+) − ({½ (RA + LA)} −)]. In the standard ECG, transverse plane electrodes are also recorded (precordial leads). The precordial V1 (4th intercostal space to the right of the sternum), V2 (4th intercostal space to the left of the sternum), V3 (midpoint on a straight line between V2 and V4, V4 (5th intercostal space on the midclavicular line), V5 (lateral to V4 and on the anterior axillary line), and V6 (lateral to V5 on the midaxillary line) are depicted in Figure 14–5. Each precordial lead is recorded against linked left arm, left leg, and right arm electrodes, with the right leg as ground. A useful landmark for placement of the precordial electrodes is the angle of Louis which is the junction of the manubrium and sternum and correspond to the second costal cartilage (attached to the second rib) on each side. The second intercostal space is below the second rib.

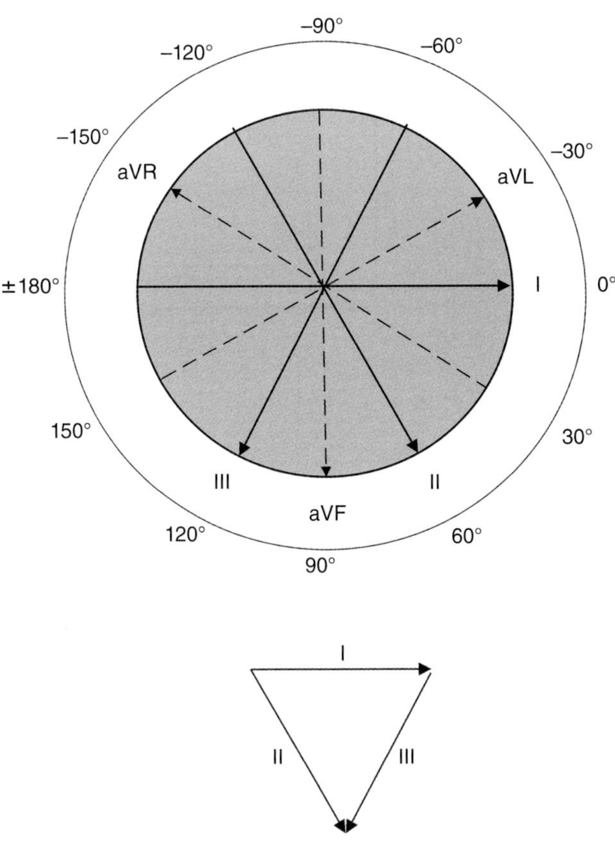

Figure 14–4 Electrographic frontal plane ECG leads. (From Berry RB. *Fundamentals of Sleep Medicine.* 3rd ed. Elsevier; 2012:161.)

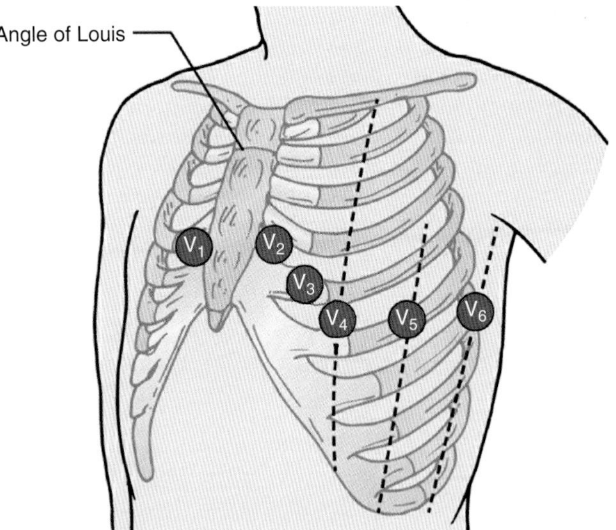

Figure 14–5 Illustration of electrographic precordial lead positions. (Adapted from Goldberger AL, Goldberger ZD, Shvilken A. *Goldberger's Clinical Electrocardiography.* 10th ed. Elsevier; 2024:9, 14.)

ECG RECORDING DURING POLYSOMNOGRAPHY

In most sleep centers, a single ECG lead is recorded during sleep monitoring. Monitoring of a single ECG lead is most useful for determining the cardiac rhythm and the heart rate. Determination of the QRS axis requires multiple frontal plane electrodes. In addition, accurate determination of ST changes requires both frontal and precordial electrodes. The QRS duration in a single lead may not reflect the widest value considering the complete 12-lead ECG. For example, if part of the QRS is isoelectric in a single lead monitoring the ECG, this does not reflect the widest QRS duration. Multiple precordial leads are also needed for differentiation of the causes of wide-complex tachycardia (WCT). Some sleep centers

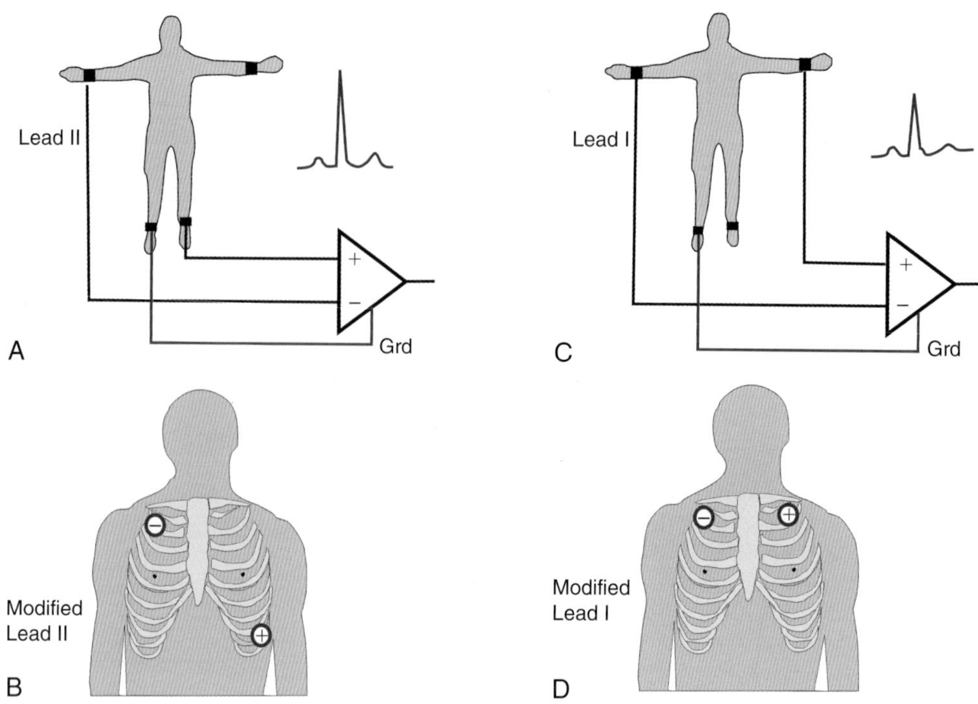

Figure 14–6 (A) The standard ECG lead II. (B) The modified lead II. (C) Standard lead I. (D) Modified lead I.

record three or more cardiac electrodes. Although the standard lead II is derived from electrodes placed on the right arm (−) and left leg (+) with the right leg as ground, the American Academy of Sleep Medicine (AASM) scoring manual[4-6] recommends use of a modified lead II with the negative electrode below the right clavicle at the midclavicular line (ECGneg) and the positive electrode on the left lower chest at the anterior axillary line in the 6th or 7th intercostal space (ECGpos) (Figure 14–6). In ECG monitoring positive is upward, so if negative polarity upward is used as is standard in EEG recording, the correct derivation is (ECGneg − ECG pos). In lead II the p wave, QRS, and T wave are upright (Figure 14–7). Another electrode used in some sleep centers is a modified lead I with the positive electrode below the left clavicle and a negative electrode below the right clavicle with both positioned at the midclavicular line (Figure 14–6). In the days of paper recording with ink writing pens, a paper speed of 30 mm/sec was used for clinical EEG recording (equivalent to a 10-second window) and ECG was recorded at a paper speed of 25 mm/sec. Therefore a 10-second PSG window provides a view similar to a standard ECG and is useful to observe the details of the ECG tracing. Most PSG software also has tools allowing measurement of durations and intervals of interest. The AASM scoring manual recommends that the ECG signal be acquired with a sampling rate of 500/sec (a sampling rate of 200/sec is acceptable). The recommended low- and high-frequency filter settings for display of the signal are 0.3 and 100 Hz, respectively.[6] Previously a high frequency filter setting of 70 Hz was recommended. Using a high-frequency filter setting of 100 Hz may allow better visualization of pacer spikes (Figure 14–8). Note that use of a 60-Hz notch filter also reduces high-frequency components

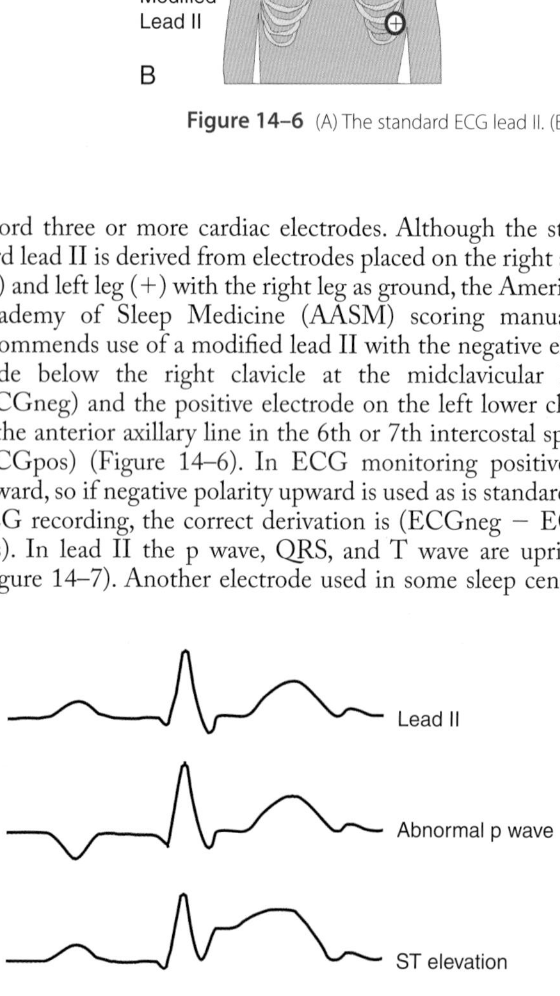

Lead II

Abnormal p wave

ST elevation

Peaked T wave

Figure 14–7 Examples of waveforms. In lead II the p, R, and T waves are upright. An inverted P wave shows that this is not from the sinus node. Examples of ST elevation and a peaked T wave are also noted. (From Berry RB. *Fundamentals of Sleep Medicine.* 3rd ed. Elsevier; 2012:162.)

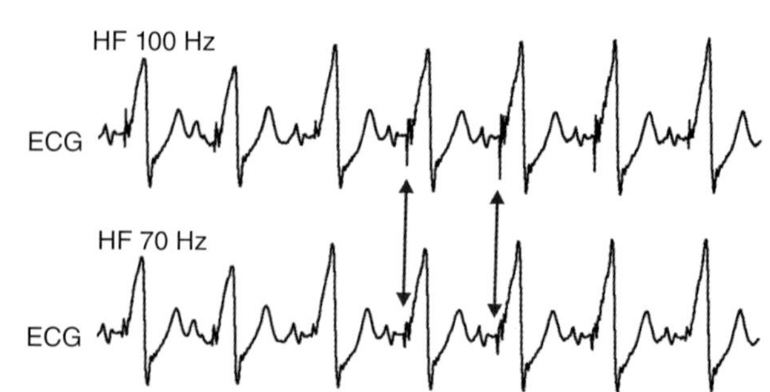

Figure 14–8 Visualization of pacer spikes is improved with use of a 100-Hz high-frequency filter rather than a 70-Hz filter. In both tracings the 60-Hz notch filter is off.

of a signal and should ideally be turned off to visualize pacer spikes. A simple way to estimate heart rate is to count the number of QRS complexes in 10 seconds and then multiply by 6 for bpm. If the rhythm is irregular, a longer interval of 20 to 30 seconds should be used for a more accurate estimate of the average heart rate. Many PSG programs have a channel showing the instantaneous pulse rate based on a moving time average of pulsations in blood flow detected by the oximetry probe. Of note, premature beats (PBs) may fail to produce a sufficient pulsation to be counted, and the "pulse rate" may not equal the ECG heart rate in patients with frequent PBs or atrial fibrillation.

SINUS RHYTHM AND NORMATIVE DATA FOR HEART RATE

As noted above, normal sinus rhythm is associated with an upright P wave, R wave, and T wave in lead II. Each P wave is followed by a QRS complex with a relatively constant PR interval. If there is significant variability in heart rate with respiration, this is often called a sinus arrhythmia (Figure 14–9). In a sinus arrhythmia, the heart rate increases with inspiration and decreases during expiration. Traditionally, sinus bradycardia is defined as a heart rate less than 60 bpm and tachycardia greater than 100 bpm. However, the heart rate normally decreases during sleep. The lowest heart rate in normal adults is usually during non–rapid eye movement (NREM) sleep when there is an increase in parasympathetic tone and a decrease in sympathetic tone. A review of the evidence that formed the basis for the AASM cardiac scoring rules by Caples and coworkers[4] reports unpublished data from the Sleep Heart Health Study cohort of 2067 adult individuals. The individuals in the analysis had an apnea-hypopnea index lower than 5/hr and were not taking cardiac or antihypertensive medications. The 95% confidence interval based on mean ± 2 standard deviations for heart rate during sleep found a minimum normative value of 43 bpm in men and 47.5 bpm in women. The maximum normative values for heart rate were 80.8 bpm for men and 84.7 bpm for women. Based on this information, the AASM cardiac scoring rules define *sinus bradycardia during sleep as a* ***sustained*** *sinus heart rate less than 40 bpm for age 6 through adults*. Here, "sustained" means longer than 30 seconds in duration.[4-6] It should be noted that normal individuals, especially endurance-conditioned athletes, often exhibit heart rates less than 40 bpm during sleep. The AASM cardiac scoring rules also define *sinus tachycardia during sleep in adults as a sustained heart rate greater than 90 bpm*.

Summary for Sinus Tachycardia/Bradycardia During Sleep

- Score *sinus tachycardia during sleep* for a **sustained** (>30 seconds) sinus heart rate > 90 bpm for adults.

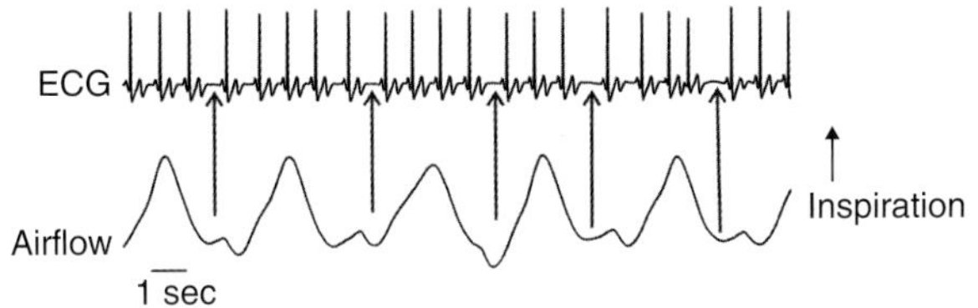

Figure 14–9 An example of sinus arrhythmia. The heart rate speeds up during inspiration and slows during expiration. (From Berry RB, Wagner MH. *Sleep Medicine Pearls*. 3rd ed. Elsevier Saunders; 2015:153.)

- Score *sinus bradycardia during sleep* for a **sustained** (>30 seconds) sinus heart rate < 40 bpm for ages 6 through adult.
- Score *atrial fibrillation* if there is an irregularly irregular ventricular rhythm associated with replacement of consistent P waves by rapid oscillations that vary in size, shape, and timing.
- Score the presence of second- (identify as Mobitz I or Mobitz II) or third-degree atrioventricular (AV) heart block.
- Score the presence of cardiac pacemaker rhythm.

Notes:

1. Sustained sinus bradycardia or tachycardia is defined by >30 seconds of a stable rhythm to distinguish it from transient responses, associated with sleep-disordered breathing events or arousals.
2. Sustained WCT and sustained narrow-complex tachycardia (NCT) are present for >30 seconds.

Defining normal heart rate limits is more complex in children, in whom the heart rate is faster than in adults. The heart rate in normal children during wakefulness undergoes a large decrease with age[7-8] (Figure 14–10, Table 14–1). Scant information is available for normative heart rates in children *during sleep*. As in adults, one would expect a lower heart rate in sleep than during wakefulness. A study analyzed data from the Cleveland Children's Sleep and Health Study and the Tucson Children's Assessment of Sleep Apnea study.[9] The study concluded that sleeping heart rates in children are lower than wake and decrease significantly with age. African American ethnicity, female gender, and obesity were associated with faster heart rates. A later study of the same cohort analyzed an adolescent age group[10] and found a decrease in heart rate during sleep with age. Female individuals had a faster heart rate than males. The AASM scoring manual did not provide rules for scoring the heart rate in children because of the age dependence and more limited normative data. A graphical representation of awake heart rate data[8] and sleep heart rate data[9,10] is shown in Figure 14–11.

CONDUCTION SYSTEM

A brief review of the cardiac conduction system (Figure 14–12) is useful for understanding the terminology of PBs and block. The electrical impulse during normal sinus rhythm starts with an impulse from the sinoatrial (SA) node located high in the right atrium near the entry of the superior vena cava. The SA node is the major cardiac pacemaker because the cells there have the highest intrinsic rate. The impulse is conducted through atrial muscle without special fibers until it reaches the AV node located at the bottom of the right atrium near the interatrial septum. The next part of the specialized conducting system is the bundle of His (common bundle). The bundle splits into a right bundle and a left bundle. The left bundle then splits into left anterior and right posterior fascicles. The Purkinje fibers then transmit the signal to myocardial cells. Purkinje cells have both pacemaking capability and the ability to rapidly conduct electrical impulses. Impulses conducted via the normal pathway produce a narrow QRS complex and coordinated right and left ventricular contraction. Impulses originating in the AV node, or His bundle (together termed the *AV junction*) usually have a rate of 40 bpm and result in a normal QRS duration. Impulses beginning below

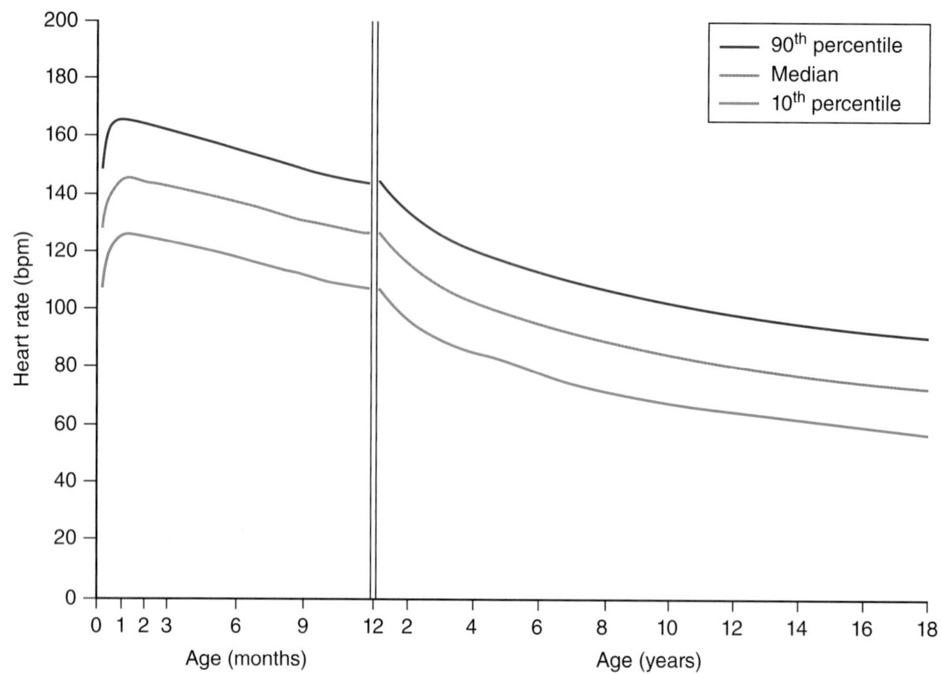

Figure 14–10 The heart rate decreases with age during **wakefulness** in normal children. The median and 10th and 90th percentile values are shown. (From Fleming S, Thompson M, Stevens R, et al. Normal ranges of heart rate and respiratory rate in children from birth to 18 years of age: a systematic review of observational studies. *Lancet.* 2011;377(9770): 1011-1018.)

Table 14–1 Normal Heart Rate During Wakefulness in Children

Age	Minimum	Maximum	Mean	2nd–98th Percentile	No. of Subjects
<1 day	88	168	123	93–154	189
1–2 days	57	170	123	91–159	179
3–6 days	87	166	129	91–166	181
2 wk	96	188	148	107–182	119
1–2 mo	114	204	149	121–179	112
3–5 mo	101	188	141	106–186	109
6–11 mo	100	176	134	109–169	138
1–2 yr	68	165	119	89–151	191
3–4 yr	68	145	108	73–137	210
5–7 yr	60	139	100	65–133	226
8–11 yr	51	145	91	62–130	233
12–15 yr	51	133	85	60–119	247

Adapted from Davignon A, Rautaharju P, Boisselle E. et al. Normal ECG standards for infants and children. *Pediatr Cardiol.* 1980;1:123-131. See also reference[4] (provides data in a table format).

the separation of the common bundle result in wide QRS complexes. Of note, if an impulse reaches the normal AV junction during a relatively refractory period, it may be conducted with a wide QRS (aberrant conduction). If an impulse arrives at the AV junction very early during a refractory period, it may not be conducted at all. This phenomenon does not represent heart block but is simply a reflection that the AV node does have a refractory period that depends on a number of factors including the heart rate. In summary, normally electrical impulses begin in the SA node, traverse the AV node, and are transmitted out to the ventricles by the Purkinje system via the left and right bundles. When the P wave is not present or is not conducted, slower pacemakers in the heart may function to continue regular ventricular rhythm. Rhythms from pacemakers in junctional areas (AV node and His bundle) usually have a narrow QRS complex with a rate of approximately 40 to 60 bpm (junctional or nodal rhythm). If the rhythm originates from a pacemaker in the ventricles, the QRS is wide and the rate is slower, often around 40 bpm (idioventricular rhythm). If the sinus node activity slows sufficiently, one of the other pacemakers may cause ventricular capture (so-called escape rhythms). The junctional and idioventricular rates can increase above the typical values in some circumstances. The terms *accelerated junctional rhythm* and

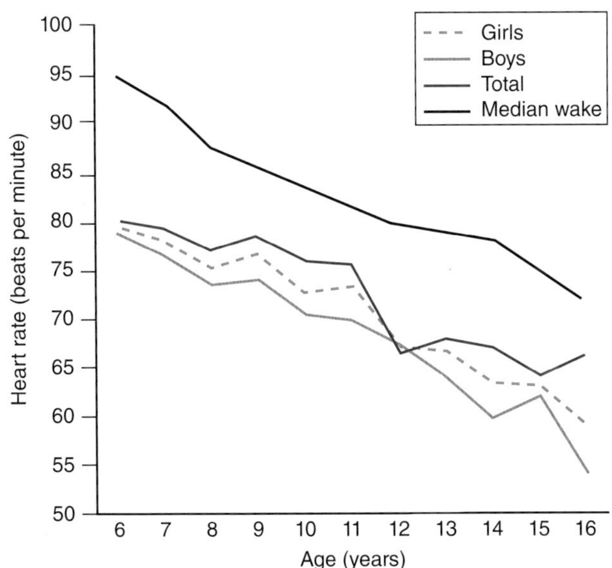

Figure 14–11 Median awake heart rate and mean sleeping heart rate of normal children. The figure is plotted from data in three articles. (median awake heart rate from Fleming S, Thompson M, Stevens R, et al. Normal ranges of heart rate and respiratory rate in children from birth to 18 years of age: a systematic review of observational studies. *Lancet.* 2011;377(9770):1011-1018; mean heart rate data age 6 to 11 years from Archbold KH, Johnson NL, Goodwin JL, et al. Normative heart rate parameters during sleep for children aged 6 to 11 years. *J Clin Sleep Med.* 2010;6:47–50; and mean heart rate data age 12 to 16 years from Hedger-Archbold K, Sorensen ST, Goodwin JL, Quan SF. Average heart rates of Hispanic and Caucasian adolescents during sleep: longitudinal analysis from the TuCASA cohort. *J Clin Sleep Med.* 2014;10(9):991-995.)

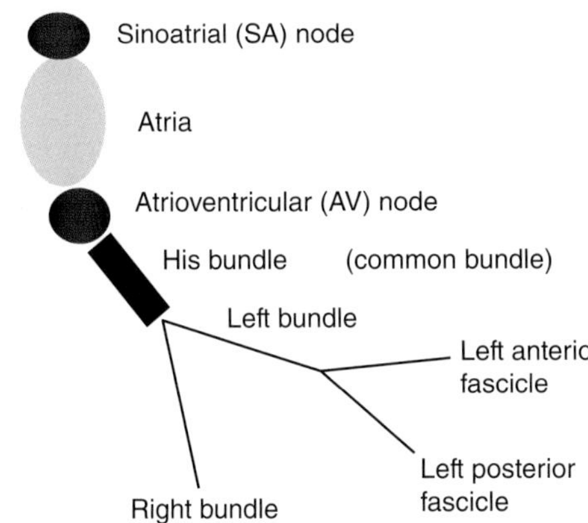

Figure 14–12 Schematic illustration of the cardiac conduction system. (From Berry RB. *Fundamentals of Sleep Medicine.* 3rd ed. Elsevier; 2012:164.)

accelerated idioventricular rhythm are used to describe these rhythms. Bundle branch block (BBB) is due to dysfunction of either the right or the left bundles (RBBB or LBBB) and results in a wide QRS complex. The type of BBB is best identified using a 12-lead ECG. RBBB and LBBB produce characteristic patterns in leads I, V1, and V6. The pattern in lead II is variable. One cannot determine the type of BBB from a modified lead II but can simply report that the QRS is wide (>0.12 second). If one uses a modified lead I (alone or with modified lead II), this allows identification of the type of BBB (Figure 14–13). The morphology in *modified lead I is usually similar to V6 with a wide S wave in RBBB and a wide R wave (often notched or M pattern) in LBBB.* The other common cause

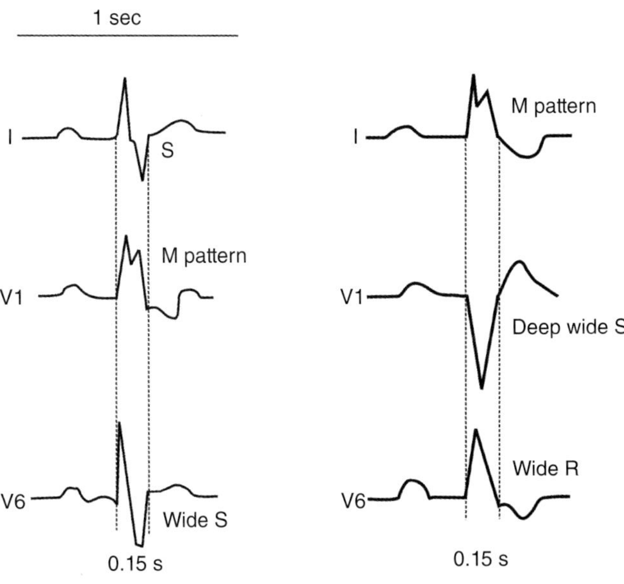

Figure 14–13 Characteristics of right and left bundle branch block (BBB) as seen in leads I, V1, and V2. **The appearance of BBB is variable in lead II.** Using a modified lead I can help identify the likely type of BBB, but definitive diagnosis requires analysis of a 12-lead ECG. Usually, the patient's history will contain useful information about this issue.

of a widened QRS commonly encountered in sleep centers is a ventricular pacemaker with the lead in the right ventricle. This gives a pattern of an LBBB because the right ventricle is depolarized slightly before the left ventricle. In BBB the *T wave usually has the opposite direction from the last part of the QRS* (discordant). In modified lead II the T wave is upright in normal sinus rhythm with a normal QRS duration. BBB is usually associated with an inverted T wave if the terminal part of the wide QRS is upward (Figure 14–13).

BRADYCARDIA AND AV BLOCK DURING SLEEP

Bradycardia During Sleep

The common causes of a slow heart rate during sleep are listed in Table 14–2. A slow heart rate during sleep (sustained heart rate < 40 bpm) can be a normal variant, associated with the effects of medications, due to high parasympathetic tone, or associated with disease of the conduction system (SA node, AV node). If the sinus node fails to trigger a P wave or slows below 40 bpm, escape beats or sustained escape rhythms are usually provided by pacemakers in the nodal area or ventricular areas. Nodal or junctional escape beats/rhythm is characterized

Table 14–2 Causes of a Slow Heart Rate
• Sinus bradycardia
• Sinus pauses (>3 sec)
• Sinus node disorder (sick sinus syndrome)
• AV block
• Medications
• Increased parasympathetic tone

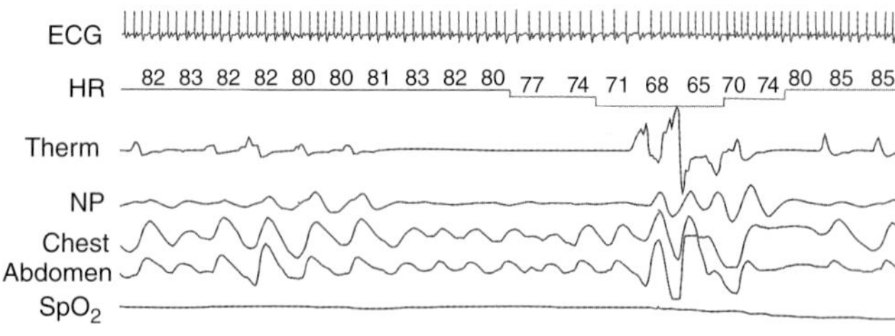

Figure 14–14 The heart rate during an obstructive apnea. The heart rate (HR) signal is the output of the oximeter (a moving time average of the pulse rate) that tends to lag behind the actual change in heart rate. Changes in the heart rate can be noted by changes in the RR interval, which widen at apnea onset and then narrow at apnea termination. *Chest and Abdomen,* Effort belt signals; *ECG,* electrocardiogram; *NP,* nasal pressure; *SpO_2,* pulse oximetry; *Therm,* oronasal thermal airflow. (From Berry RB. Wagner MH. *Sleep Medicine Pearls.* 3rd ed. Elsevier Saunders; 2015:154.)

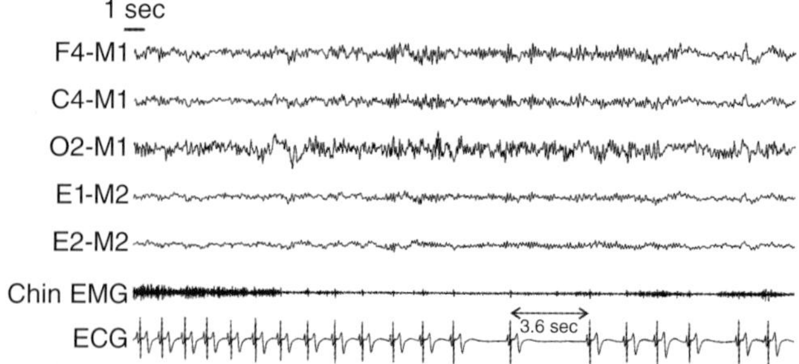

Figure 14–15 A sinus pause of 3.6 seconds is illustrated meeting criteria for asystole. (From Berry RB, Wagner MH. *Sleep Medicine Pearls.* 3rd ed. Elsevier; 2015:154.)

by no p waves, a narrow QRS, regular rhythm, and rate 40–60 bpm). Retrograde p wave (usually negative in leads II, III, aVF) can be noted just before (PR interval usually less than 0.12 sec) or following the QRS. Ventricular escape beats/rhythm is characterized by no p waves, a wide QRS, regular rhythm, and rate 40–50 bpm. The escape ventricular rhythm is sometimes called idioventricular rhythm. Retrograde p waves can also be noted usually inverted compared to sinus p waves and often distortening the last portion of the preceding wide QRS. As previously mentioned, if nodal rhythm is faster (90–100 bpm), this is called accelerated junctional rhythm. Similarly, a ventricular rhythm of 50 to 100 bpm is called an accelerated idioventricular rhythm.

Cyclic increases and decreases in heart rate are commonly associated with untreated obstructive sleep apnea. This phenomenon is often called *tachycardia-bradycardia cycles.* However, in many patients the lower heart rate is typically greater than 40 bpm, and the highest heart rate may not exceed 90 bpm. The heart rate typically accelerates at apnea termination owing to withdrawal of vagal tone (hypoxia-dependent bradycardia overridden by activation of lung stretch receptors with resumption of ventilation) and an increase in sympathetic activity. The slowing of the heart rate at event onset is thought to be due to vagal tone. Typically, the heart rate slows, then speeds up toward the end of the obstructive events with a sudden increase in heart rate at apnea termination (Figure 14–14). However, the change in heart rate during apnea may have other patterns including no change or an increase during apnea in some patients.[11] Some PSG computer programs provide a moving time average heart rate based on the ECG. Others simply record a heart rate output of the oximeter, which is a moving time average of the rate of blood flow pulses reaching the oximetry probe.

Sinus Pause/Asystole

The AASM scoring manual recommends **scoring asystole if a sinus pause is *greater* than 3 seconds in duration for ages 6 years through adult**[4-6] (Figure 14–15). The review paper by the AASM cardiac event scoring task force[4] that provided evidence for the cardiac scoring rules quotes normative data in young healthy subjects that found sinus pauses to be longer in males (range 1.20–2.06 seconds) than in females (1.08–1.92 seconds). In trained athletes, up to 37% had sinus pauses between 2 and 3 seconds. A study of a cohort of 40- to 79-year-old individuals found the longest pause during sleep to be 2 seconds.[12] For this reason, sinus pauses **greater** than 3 seconds are scored as asystole. Of note, a common cause of an unexpected sinus pause (usually much less than 3 seconds) is a nonconducted premature atrial impulse. This is discussed in the section on "Premature Beats." The rapid eye movement (REM)-related bradyarrhythmia syndrome is characterized by absence of structural heart abnormality but periods of asystole or third-degree heart block during REM sleep, often in young asymptomatic patients.[13,14] This is believed to be due to periods of very high vagal tone during REM sleep. This is unusual because REM sleep is associated with high sympathetic tone.

Summary for Asystole:

- Score **asystole** for cardiac pauses during sleep ***greater*** than 3 seconds for ages 6 years through adult.

AV Block

AV block is classified into three types[1,2] based on ECG characteristics that correlate with the location of the abnormality in the conducting system or the influences of changes in autonomic tone.

1. **First-degree AV block** is defined as a prolongation of PR interval longer than 0.20 second (Figure 14–16). The normal PR interval is usually 0.12 to 0.20 second. Studies in normal healthy populations[15] have found a prolonged PR interval in between 0.5% and 1% of individuals. The prolonged PR is more appropriately called prolonged AV conduction rather than "block."
2. **Second-degree AV block** is defined when one or more (but not all) of atrial impulses fail to reach the ventricle because of abnormal conduction.
   a. Mobitz type I (Wenckebach): A pattern of AV block in which there are varying PR intervals. Usually, there is progressive prolongation of the PR interval until a P wave is not conducted (Figure 14–17). This is typical of a block in the AV node, which is capable of variations in conduction time. This type of second-degree AV block is generally thought to be benign.[1]
   b. Mobitz type II: A pattern of AV block in which the PR intervals are nearly constant (Figure 14–18). It is often seen in the setting of BBB.
3. **Third-degree AV block (complete AV block):** None of the atrial impulses are conducted to the ventricles (Figure 14–18). One can often see both P waves and QRS complexes, but they have no fixed relationship (AV dissociation). The term

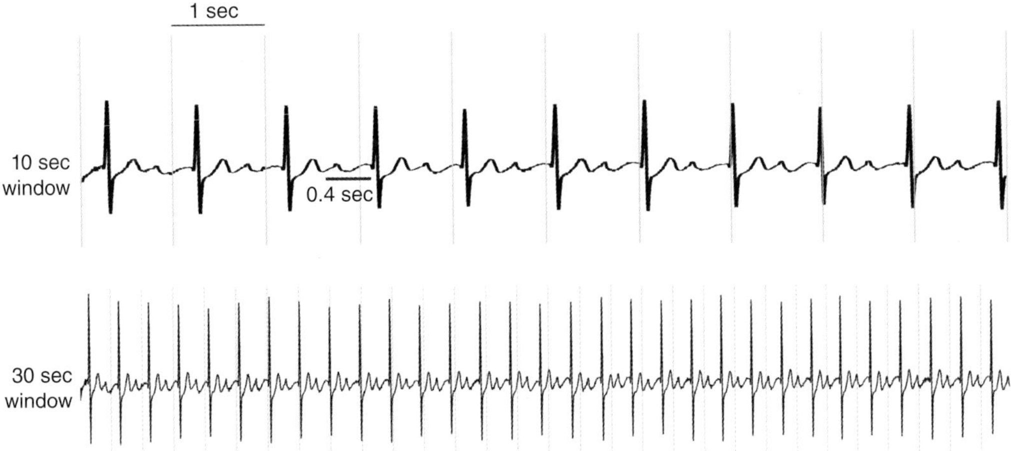

Figure 14–16 An example of first-degree AV block. This may be difficult to recognize in the usual 30-second viewing window. First-degree AV block is defined as a PR interval > 0.2 second.

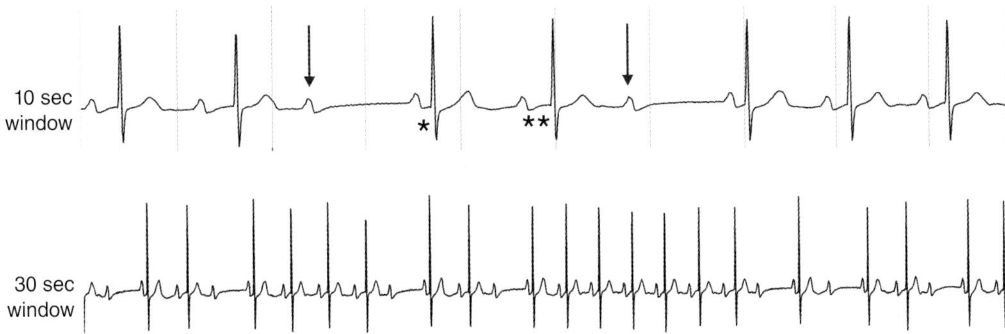

Figure 14–17 An example of second-degree Mobitz type I (Wenckebach) AV block as seen in 10-second and 30-second windows. In a 30-second window this type of block is recognized based on p waves without associated QRS and progressive PR interval progression. A hint is observation of groups of a variable number of QRS complexes preceding the nonconducted p wave. In the 10-second window, * and ** show an increase in the PR interval before the nonconducted p waves *(arrows)*.

AV dissociation means that the atrial and ventricular rhythms have no relationship. This can occur with third-degree block. However, other causes include an intrinsic ventricular rhythm that is faster than the sinus rhythm (RR interval is shorter than PP interval).

Aberrant Conduction

When cardiac tissue responds to a stimulus, the reaction is followed by a refractory period (dormant interval) during which it cannot respond to a similar stimulus. The refractory period of cardiac conducting paths is proportional to the length of the preceding cycle (RR interval). Thus a long preceding cycle in combination with a short immediate cycle predisposes the cardiac conduction system to be in a refractory state. A wide QRS can occur even if the beat originates in a supraventricular location (SA node or AV junction). This occurs for three reasons:[1] (1) a refractory right or left bundle fascicle, (2) an anomalous supraventricular activation, or (3) a paradoxical critical rate.[1] In the first case, the impulse transverses the bundle of His but finds either the right or the left bundle refractory. In the second case, the impulse bypasses the AV node, arises in the AV node in an eccentric location, or is abnormally conducted due to diseased junctional fibers such that the impulse does not reach the left and right fascicles at the same time. In the third case, a critical rate occurs above which part of the ventricular conducting system is refractory. A preceding long RR interval and a short current RR interval increases the chance of aberrant conduction. Figure 14–19 shows a schematic example of a beat with aberrant conduction when the preceding cycle is long and the current cycle is short.

PREMATURE BEATS (PBS)

PBs are QRS complexes not originating in the SA node that occur earlier than the next expected sinus beat. These can occur as a single PB, a pair of PBs (couplet of PBs), or three PBs (by convention, non-sustained tachycardia if the rate is >100 bpm). Narrow and wide complex tachycardia are discussed in the following section. The nomenclature when a PB follows every normal sinus beat is bigeminy, every second sinus beat is trigeminy, or every third sinus beat is quadrigeminy (Table 14–3, Figures 14–20 and 14–21). The characteristics of PBs are listed in Table 14–4. Supraventricular premature beats (SVPBs) are either atrial premature beats (APBs) or junctional premature beats. Although exceptions occur, SVPBs usually have a narrow QRS complex and the QRS morphology

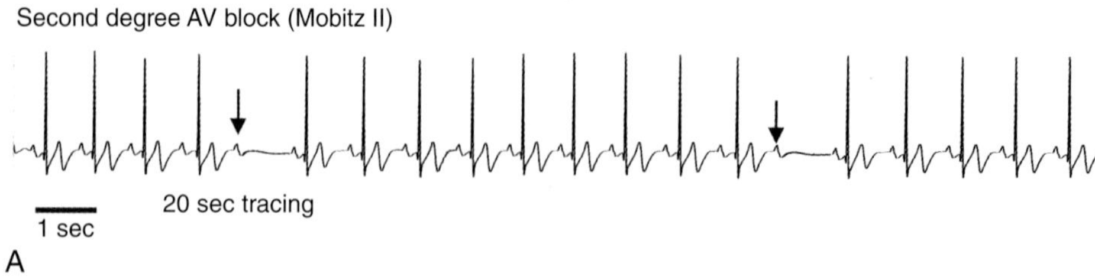

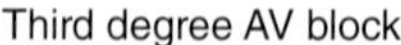

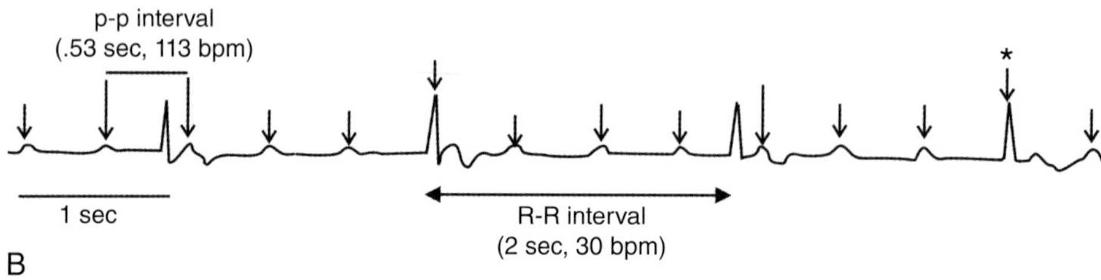

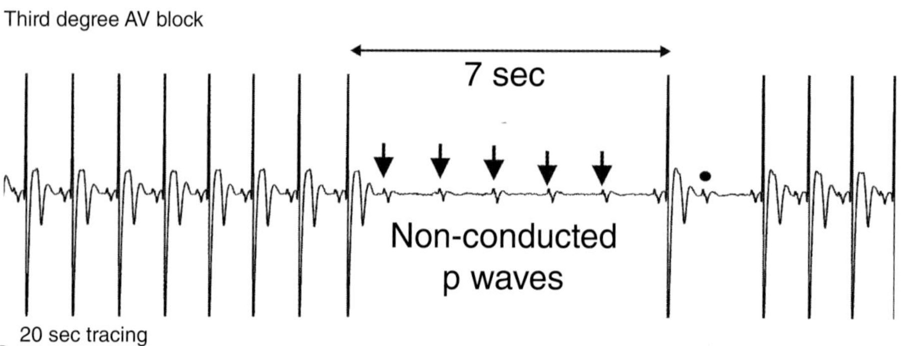

Figure 14–18 Examples of second-degree Mobitz type II block and third-degree AV block. (A) In Mobitz type II there is no increase in PR interval before the nonconducted p wave. (B) In third-degree AV block, p waves are not conducted to the ventricle. Although regular p wave and QRS intervals may be noted, they are not temporally related. The asterisks (*) show the postion of the expected p wave likely obscured by the QRS complex. In (C), there is a long period of asystole due to five nonconducted p waves *(down arrows)*. This patient also exhibited second-degree block *(small black circle)*.

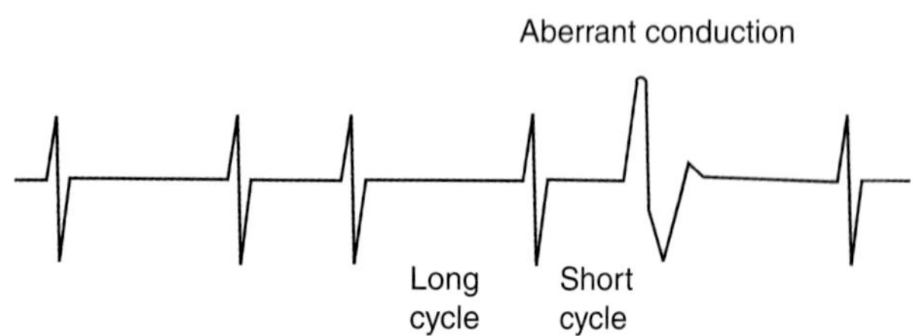

Figure 14–19 A schematic illustrating a patient with atrial fibrillation and aberrant conduction after a short cycle preceded by a long cycle. Aberrant conduction means a supraventricular pulse is not conducted normally and results in a widened QRS complex. (From Berry RB. *Fundamentals of Sleep Medicine*. 3rd ed. Elsevier; 2012:167.)

Table 14–3 Premature Beat (PB) Terminology	
1 beat	A PB
2 beats	A pair or couplet
3 beats	Nonsustained rhythm (non-sustained tachycardia if rate > 100 bpm)
>30 sec	Sustained rhythm
PB follows every normal sinus beat	Bigeminy
PB follows every second sinus beat	Trigeminy
PB follows every third sinus beat	Quadrigeminy

PB, Premature beat.

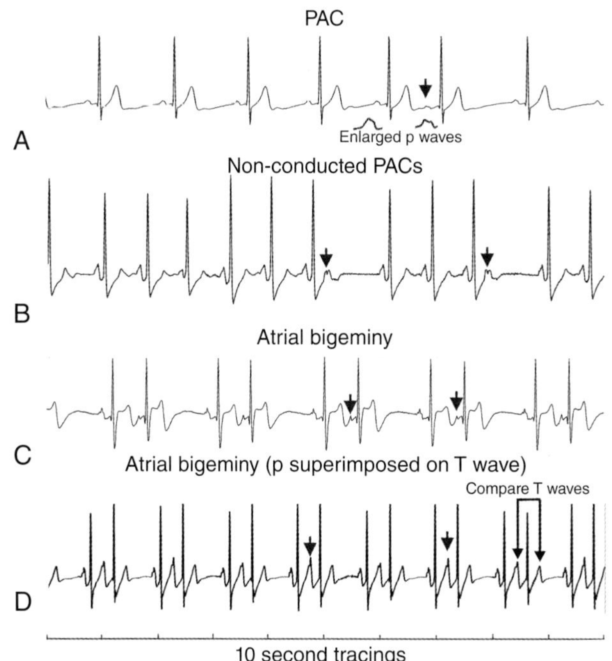

Figure 14–20 Examples of premature atrial contractions/premature atrial beats. The p wave of an atrial premature beat is usually different than the sinus p wave and is earlier than expected based on previous p-to-p intervals. The premature p wave can be hidden in the preceding T wave (or change the shape of the T wave). In tracing A, one can see a premature p wave with slightly different morphology. In tracing B, premature p waves change the T wave shape but are so early that they are not conducted. In tracings C and D, premature atrial beats occur every other beat (atrial bigeminy). In tracing C, the premature p waves are easily recognized *(down arrows)*. In tracing D, the p waves are more difficult to recognize but result in a changed T wave shape *(more peaked, arrows)*.

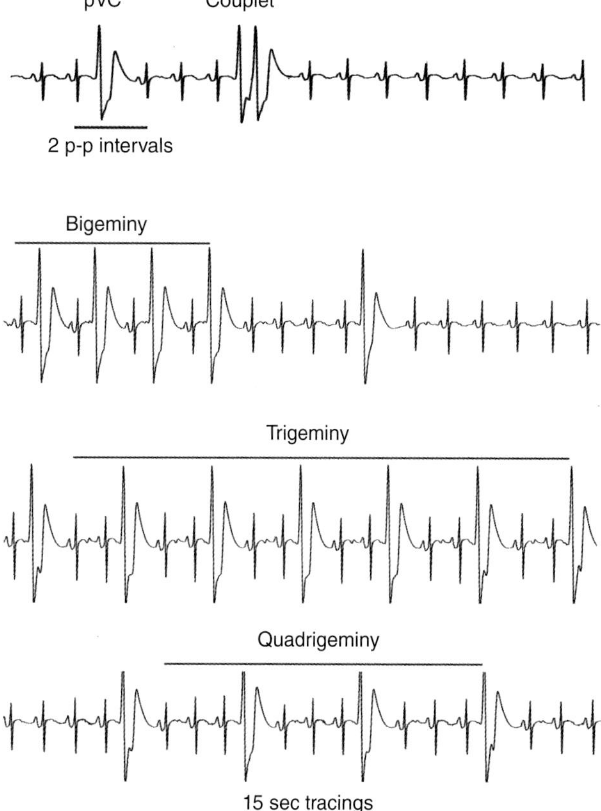

Figure 14–21 Examples of premature ventricular contractions. The QRS is wide and premature (earlier than expected based on the previous p-p interval). This can occur alone, in a couplet, or alternating with one, two, or three sinus beats (bigeminy, trigeminy, or quadrigeminy, respectively).

Table 14–4 Characteristics of Premature Supraventricular and Ventricular Beats

	SVPBs	VPBs (PVCs)
QRS complex	Normal duration (usually), resembles sinus beats Wide QRS can occur (aberrant conduction)	Wide QRS
Source of rhythm	Atria: APB Junctional (AV node + His)	Ventricles
Compensatory pause	No (usually): SA node discharged (reset)	Compensatory pause: sinus node not reset
P wave	Atrial: P wave premature and abnormal Junctional: often none, retrograde p wave can occur	Usually none Retrograde P wave can occur
Exceptions	APB: P wave can be obscured in preceding T wave	May appear <0.12 sec in a given lead if part of wave is isoelectric in that lead

APB, Atrial premature beat; *AV*, atrioventricular; *PVCs*, premature ventricular contractions; *SA*, sinoatrial; *SVPBs*, supraventricular premature beats; *VPBs*, ventricular premature beats.

resembles that of the normal sinus beats. In the case of APBs (also called premature atrial contractions [PACs]), there is usually a visible abnormal P wave (sometimes called *P′*) (Figure 14–20A). The abnormal P wave may be negative in lead II or have a different morphology than the sinus P waves. If premature atrial impulses are very early, they may not be conducted (non conducted PACs) and are a common cause of sinus pauses without an apparent etiology (Figure 14–20B). When PACs occur between normal sinus beats, they produce atrial bigeminy (Figure 14–20C, D). Note that the premature P wave can be hidden in the preceding T wave or distort the T wave shape (Figure 14–20D). Ventricular premature beats (VPBs), also known as premature ventricular contractions (PVCs), invariably are associated with a wide QRS (usually >0.16 second) and are usually not preceded by an abnormal P wave (retrograde p waves can occur) (Figure 14–21). Supraventricular premature beats (SVPBs or PACs) usually reset the SA node and the next sinus beat occurs less than two PP

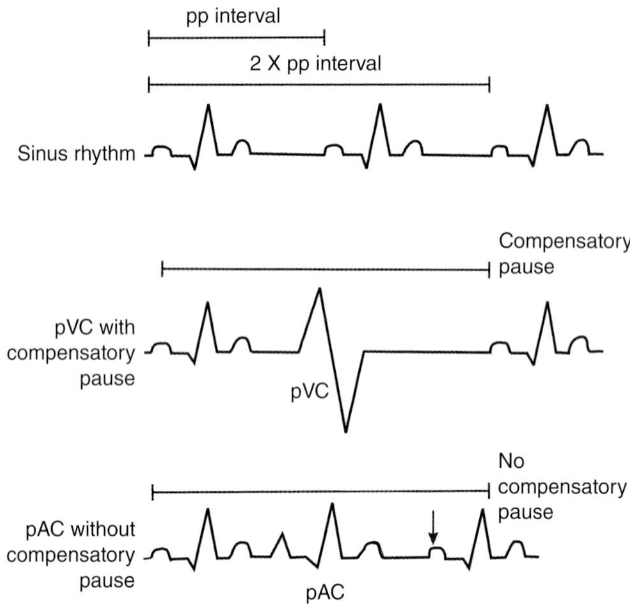

Figure 14–22 A schematic illustrating that the PVCs are usually associated with a compensatory pause; that is, the p-p interval is unchanged as the sinus node is not reset by the PVC. In contrast, a PAC does reset the sinus node, and there is no compensatory pause. This effect could be useful in identifying PACs that are aberrantly conducted (QRS is wider than normal). (From Berry RB. *Fundamentals of Sleep Medicine.* 3rd ed. Elsevier; 2012:169.)

intervals after the last normal P wave (Figure 14–22). If the SVPB is aberrantly conducted, the QRS can be wide. There is usually a **compensatory pause** after the VPB (PVCs) with the next P wave occurring about two PP intervals after the last normal P wave (retrograde p waves can occur) (Figure 14–22). VPBs originate in a ventricular focus and can be conducted retrograde via the AV node to the atria (retrograde p wave). The retrograde P wave can be seen deforming the VPBs or T wave after the beat. When all VPBs have the same morphology, they are said to be unifocal (unimorphic or monomorphic). If VPBs originate from multiple ventricular areas, they are usually of different morphology (polymorphic VPBs).

TACHYCARDIA DURING SLEEP

The scoring criteria for NCT and WCT require that there must be **three or more beats with a rate greater than *100 bpm.*** Note that this differs from sinus tachycardia during sleep, which must have a sustained (>30 second) rate of greater than 90 bpm. **In WCT the QRS duration is > 0.12 second, and in NCT the QRS duration is < 0.12 second.** The common causes of tachycardias seen during sleep studies are shown in Table 14–5. With a single ECG lead, it is not possible to determine whether a WCT originates from a ventricular focus rather than a supraventricular focus with aberrant conduction. Therefore the AASM scoring manual recommends scoring a WCT rather than a ventricular tachycardia (VT). However, most WCTs are VT.

Narrow-Complex Tachycardia

NCT is characterized by a QRS duration **shorter** than 0.12 second, with three or more beats and a heart rate greater than 100 bpm (Figure 14–23). The major types of NCTs are listed in Table 14–5. The term *supraventricular tachycardia (SVT) or paroxysmal SVT (PSVT)* is used to describe a diverse group of rhythms characterized by regular rhythm and narrow QRS, when the morphology does not otherwise allow identification of atrial fibrillation (Afib) or atrial flutter. The etiology of PSVT could be a rapidly firing ectopic focus in the atria or nodal area or via reentrant mechanisms outside the AV nodal area. AV reentrant tachycardia is due to an accessory path outside the AV node (Wolff-Parkinson-White), and AV **nodal**

Table 14–5 Common Tachycardias During Sleep
Sinus Tachycardia During Sleep Rate > 90 sec for ≥30 sec
Narrow-Complex Tachycardias ≥3 consecutive beats, rate > 100 bpm, QRS duration < 0.12 sec

• Supraventricular tachycardia (also called paroxysmal SVT or PSVT): usually regular, rate 120–240 bpm
  • Ectopic atrial tachycardia
  • Ectopic nodal tachycardia
  • AV nodal reentrant tachycardia or AV reentrant tachycardia

• Afib: irregular atrial activity, ventricular activity irregular, rate variable

• Aflutter:
  • Flutter waves 240–330 bpm (usually ~ 300 bpm)
  • Ventricular response is variable
  • (2:1 block ventricular rate ~150 bpm, 4:1 block ventricular rate ~75 bpm)

• MAT: irregular RR intervals, with three or more P wave morphologies (atrial rate 100–250 bpm)
Wide-Complex Tachycardia ≥3 beats, rate > 100 bpm, QRS duration ≥ 0.12 sec
• Ventricular tachycardia: usually regular, can be slightly irregular • SVT with aberrant conduction usually regular • Afib with aberrant conduction: irregular rhythm • Aflutter with aberrant conduction: often irregular, can be regular with fixed block

Afib, Atrial fibrillation; *aflutter* = atrial flutter; *AV,* atrioventricular; *MAT,* multifocal atrial tachycardia; *PSVT,* paroxysmal supraventricular tachycardia.

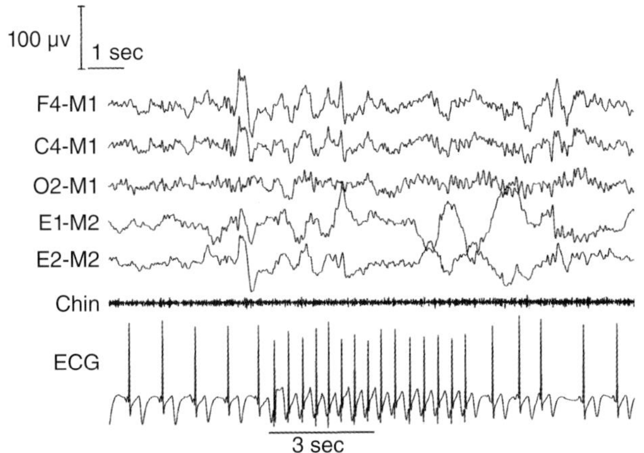

Figure 14–23 An example of narrow-complex tachycardia with a regular R-R interval. The rate is approximately 160 bpm. (From Berry RB, Wagner MH. *Sleep Medicine Pearls.* 3rd ed. Elsevier Saunders; 2015:156.)

reentrant tachycardia is due to a conduction loop through the nodal area. The reader is referred to a comprehensive textbook by Goldberger, Goldberger, and Shvilken[1] for further reading on this topic. PSVT has regular RR intervals, and Afib has irregular RR intervals. Atrial flutter can have regular or irregular RR intervals (variable AV conduction). Both Afib and atrial flutter, which are discussed in the next section, can result in a ventricular rate greater than 100 bpm and narrow QRS complexes. When a burst of NCT is short, it is often not possible to differentiate between PSVT and Afib.

Summary of Narrow- and Wide-Complex Tachycardias

- Score ***NCT*** for a rhythm lasting a minimum of three consecutive beats at a rate >100/min with a QRS duration < 120 msec (0.12 second).
- Score ***WCT*** for a rhythm lasting a minimum of three consecutive beats at a rate >100/min with a QRS duration ≥ 120 msec (0.12 second). (note ≥)

Atrial Fibrillation and Atrial Flutter

Atrial fibrillation (Afib) and atrial flutter can present as either NCT or WCT in the sleep center. However, patients may also exhibit a ventricular rate less than 100 bpm due to the effects of medications on the AV node or intrinsic AV node disease. In the case of Afib with an average ventricular response less than 100 bpm, the rhythm is called *Afib with a controlled ventricular rate.* If the average heart rate exceeds 100 bpm, the rhythm is termed *Afib with a rapid ventricular response (Afib with RVR).* The hallmark of Afib is that it is an irregular rhythm (Figure 14–24). This occurs due to irregular conduction via the AV node. In atrial flutter, the sawtooth-shaped flutter waves (called *F waves*) usually have a frequency of 240 to 330 bpm[1] and are often discernible at slower ventricular rates (Figure 14–25). The ventricular rate can be regular (fixed AV block) or irregular (variable AV conduction). **An NCT of 150 bpm should always trigger the suspicion of atrial flutter with 2:1 block.** In this circumstance, the flutter waves may be hidden by the receding T wave (Figure 14–25A). There may be short periods of increased AV block allowing recognition of the atrial flutter waves (Figure 14–25B). A sinus tachycardia with a heart rate of 150 bpm in the absence of an extreme situation such as hypotension or exercise is unlikely. The

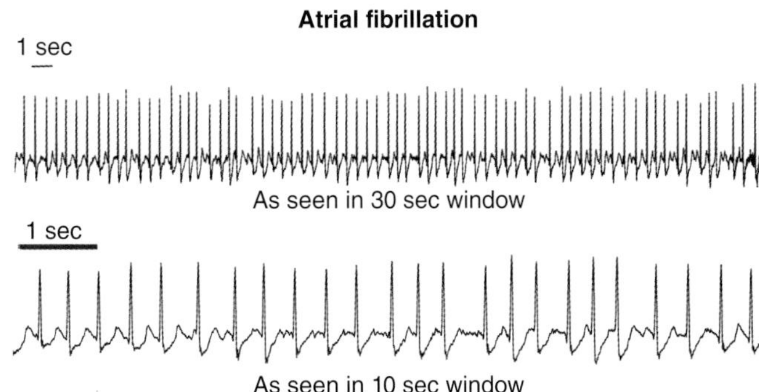

Figure 14–24 An example of atrial fibrillation as seen in 30-second and 10-second windows. An irregular-irregular pattern is seen. (From Berry RB, Wagner MH. *Sleep Medicine Pearls.* 3rd ed. Elsevier Saunders; 2015:157.)

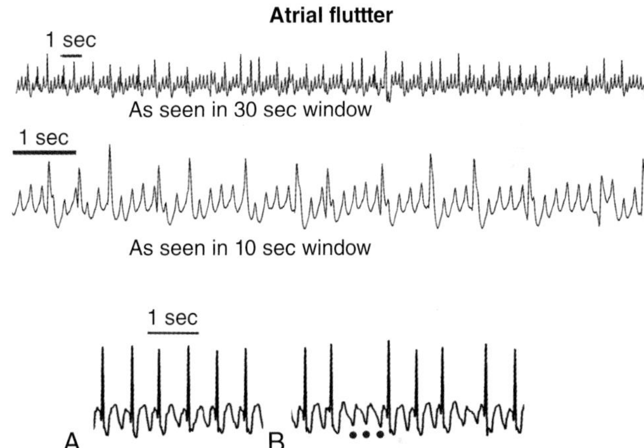

Figure 14–25 Examples of atrial flutter as seen in 30-second and 10-second windows (2 top tracings rows). Distinct flutter waves are seen. In the tracing on the bottom row at A, the flutter waves are hidden at a ventricular rate of 150 bpm (2:1 block), but at B, flutter waves can be seen with a ventricular rate of 75 (4:1 block). Any time the heart rate is approximately 150 bpm, the possibility of atrial flutter should be considered. Sinus rhythm is rarely that fast except during exercise, and certainly not during sleep. (Adapted from Berry RB, Wagner MH. *Sleep Medicine Pearls.* 3rd ed. Elsevier Saunders;

ventricular response of atrial flutter may also be approximately 70-75 bpm (4:1 block). Sometimes, the AV block can be variable resulting in atrial flutter with irregular RR intervals (see Figure 14–25). Although atrial fibrillation and flutter are usually associated with a narrow QRS, the rhythms can occur with a patient with a wide QRS and AV node dysfunction.

Summary of atrial fibrillation and flutter

- Score atrial fibrillation if there are irregularly irregular QRS complexes associated with replacement of consistent p waves by rapid oscillation that vary in size, shape, and timing.
- Atrial flutter is characterized by a rhythm that is associated with atrial flutter waves (240–330 beats perminute) usually with a narrow QRS duration and either a fixed ventricular rate (fixed block usually 2:1, 3:1 or 4:1) or a variable ventricular rate (variable block). Atrial flutter with 2:1 block should always be considered when there is a rhythm characterized by a narrow QRS, regular rhythm, and a rate of approximately 150 beats/min. At rapid rates the flutter waves may be obscured by T waves.

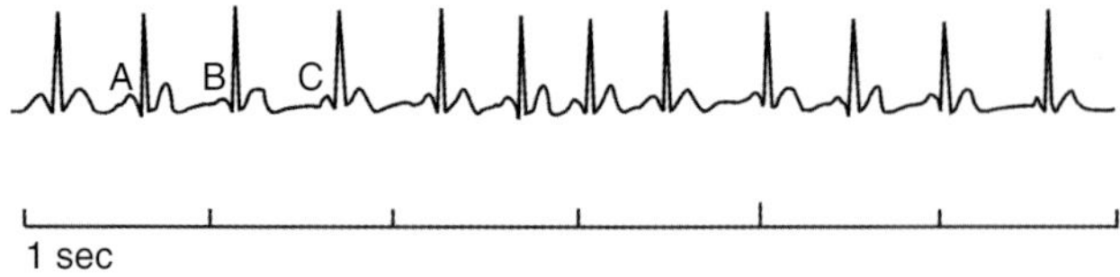

Figure 14–26 A tracing of multiple atrial tachycardia with three or more distinct p waves. A 6 second tracing is shown with a heart rate of 120 bpm.

Multifocal Atrial Tachycardia

Multifocal atrial tachycardia (MAT), also known as *multifocal atrial rhythm if the rate is less than 100 bpm*, is characterized by at least three different P wave morphologies and an irregular PP and RR interval (Figure 14–26). MAT is often seen in association with an exacerbation of chronic obstructive pulmonary disease (therefore it is uncommon in the sleep center). Atrial fibrillation and MAT are the two rhythms characteristically associated with irregular RR intervals.

Wide Complex Tachycardia

WCT is characterized by a QRS of **0.12 second or greater** (Figure 14–27); see also Table 14–5). The two causes of WCT are (1) VT (or Vtach) originating in the ventricles or (2) supraventricular tachycardia with aberrant conduction (SVTAC) originating from the atria or junctional areas. Even with multiple ECG leads, differentiating VT from SVTAC is difficult. The lead V_1 has been used in emergency settings and intensive care units to help distinguish VT from SVTAC. However, discussion of differentiating VT from SVTAC this is beyond the scope of this chapter. *At least three wide complexes are the minimum* to score WCT. **Sustained WCT** is usually defined as longer than 30 seconds and nonsustained WCT as less than 30 seconds. VT accounts for up to 80% of cases of WCT in unselected populations. It accounts for 95% of cases in patients with previous myocardial infarction. **Sustained WCT in the sleep center should be considered VT until proven otherwise.** The sudden appearance of a wide complex rhythm in a patient with a known pacemaker with a rate less than 100 bpm is almost always simply due to ventricular pacing (Figure 14–28). A rhythm cannot be WCT if the "T" (tachycardia) is absent. Pacer spikes may or may not be visible. It is very important for sleep technologists to know if a patient has a pacemaker in place. Fortunately, this is often noted by physical examination during chest monitoring sensor placement.

If **sustained** WCT occurs in the sleep center in an out-of-hospital setting, the emergency medical services (EMS) should be called (911) and emergency equipment including an automated external defibrillator (AED) should be brought to the bedside. If the patient is asleep, they should be gently awakened and assessed for chest pain or shortness of breath. If the sleep center is within the hospital, an emergency code blue is usually called for rapid response. For **nonsustained** ventricular tachycardia (NSVT), the clinical setting and condition of the patient dictate the actions. A symptomatic patient would require EMS activation (outpatient setting) or rapid response team/transfer to the emergency department depending on the severity of the situation. An asymptomatic patient with short and self-limited episodes of sustained ventricular tachycardia would usually require at a minimum notification of the primary physician or physician on call for the sleep center. To be accredited by the AASM, a sleep center must have clearly specified written procedures for handling cardiac emergencies.[16] AEDs should be available close to all monitoring rooms. In some sleep centers, it is a policy to wake the patient up if recurrent NSVT is noted to check for symptoms.[16] Patients with NSVT require a cardiac evaluation if this has not been recently performed. NSVT in patients with structural heart disease has a poor prognosis without intervention. A typical evaluation includes echocardiography

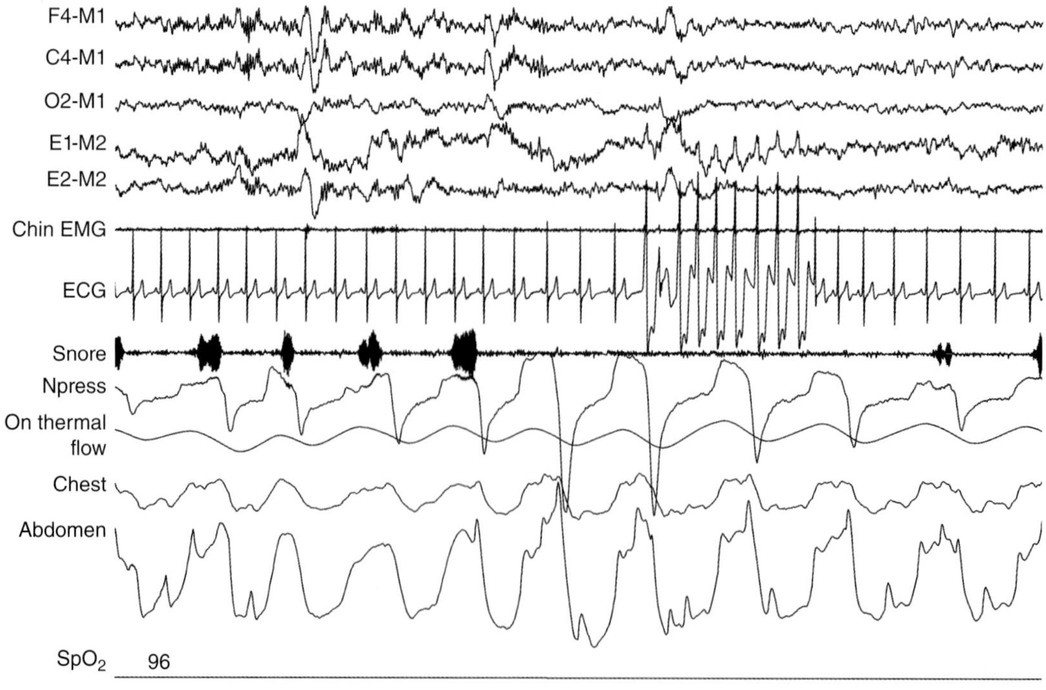

Figure 14–27 A run of wide-complex tachycardia. The patient was asymptomatic.

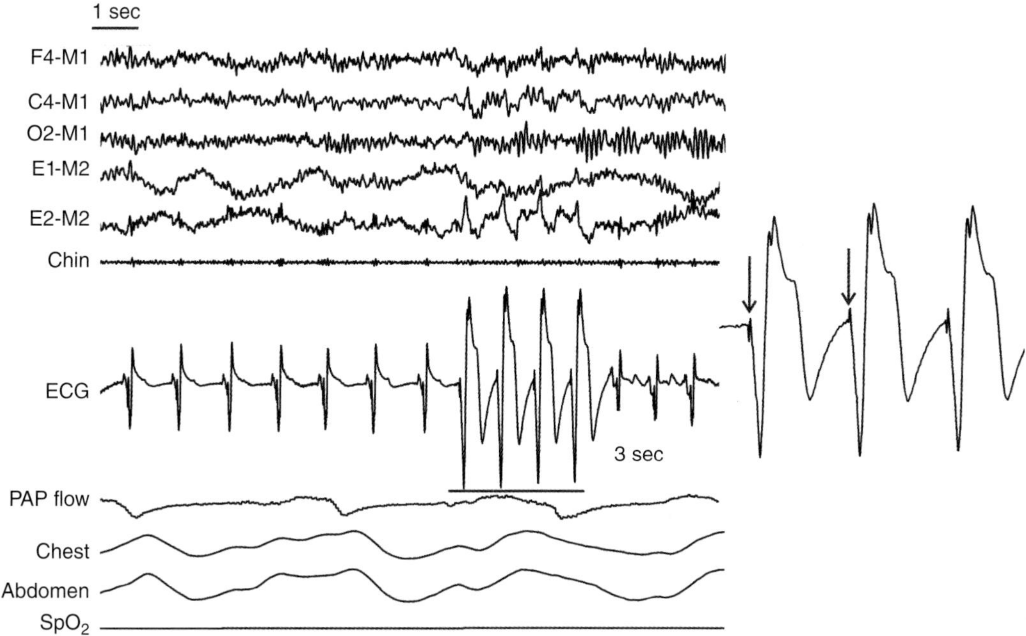

Figure 14–28 The sudden appearance of wide complexes. This is not wide-complex tachycardia as the rate is about 80 bpm. Careful examination (including changing to a 10-second window) shows ventricular pacer spikes (*arrows* in enlargement to the right of the wide complexes). (From Berry RB, Wagner MH. *Sleep Medicine Pearls.* 3rd ed. Elsevier Saunders; 2015:157, 158.)

(evaluation for cardiomyopathy and valvular heart disease), Holter monitoring, cardiac magnetic resonance imaging, and stress testing to rule out coronary artery disease.[16]

ADVERSE EVENTS DURING PSG

An investigation by Mehra and Strohl[17] collected information from 16,084 sleep studies and found that the incidence of serious adverse events during nocturnal PSG was very low at 0.35%, and the incidence of death during or within 2 weeks of an adverse event was 0.006%. There was 1 death due to VT leading to ventricular fibrillation in a patient with coronary artery disease. Excluding this patient there were 56 events. Of the 56 events, 28 events were noted during the study prompting the technologist to ask for immedicate physician evaluation or transfer of the patient to an emergency care facility and another 28 events were noted after the study by the scoring technologist (complex ventricular arrhythmias). In the latter cases, the referring physician was notified of the problem. Of the 28 nonfatal events noted *during the sleep study*, only 1 patient reported chest pain and shortness of breath. In contrast, another review of safety events in the sleep center[18] found them to be uncommon (1/623 studies), and chest pain, falls, and acute neurological changes were more frequent than complex arrhythmias.

WIDE QRS AND PACEMAKERS

Single or dual chamber pacemakers have the ventricular pacing lead in the right ventricle. Ventricular paced beats have the morphology of an LBBB. If all sinus beats have a wide QRS and the patient does not have a pacemaker, the patient likely has a BBB. As mentioned previously, using lead II alone one cannot accurately determine whether a LBBB or RBBB is present. The appearance of BBBs in lead II is variable and changes with the frontal plane QRS axis. If a modified lead I is also recorded, the pattern is usually similar to that in V6 and might allow a tentative identification of a BBB type. In precordial leads, an RBBB (initial activation of the left ventricle) is usually manifested by a QRS with an "M or rSR" pattern (small initial upward deflection, downward deflection, larger upward deflection in V1) as illustrated in Figure 14–13. In leads V6 and I there is a RS pattern with a wide S wave. In LBBB (there is initial activation of the right ventricle) and the pattern in V1 is usually manifested by a "QS or rS" pattern. The "QS" pattern is a single wide downward deflection (see Figure 14–1). The "rS" pattern has a small initial upward deflection followed by a wider downward deflection. In leads V6 and I there is a wide R wave. Accurate diagnosis of a BBB requires a 12-lead ECG. However, one can simply comment in the sleep study report that a wide QRS is present. Often the history included with the sleep study request will include information that the patient has a specific type of BBB.

The sudden appearance of a run of wide complexes on the ECG can cause panic in the sleep center. Sometimes, the fact that the rate is less than 100 (often 60 or 70) is missed in the excitement. However, in the prestudy evaluation, *it is always helpful if the sleep technologist asks the patient whether they have a pacemaker (or notes the presence of a pacemaker while applying ECG electrodes)*. Although a detailed discussion of pacemakers is beyond the scope of this chapter, a few concepts will be discussed. The reader is referred to the discussion by Mond.[19] As mentioned previously, a ventricular pacemaker with the pacing lead in the right ventricle will produce wide-paced beats with an LBBB morphology. Pacer spikes are often difficult to see but using a high-frequency filter of 100 Hz may help in visualizing pacer spikes. Figure 14–28 shows a single chamber ventricular pacemaker in a patient in sinus rhythm and episodes of sinus node dysfunction. When the ventricular rate falls below a cutoff value, the ventricular pacer fires, producing a wide-complex QRS. Dual chamber pacemakers with both atrial and ventricular leads are commonly used today. The common terminology is DDD(R) (Dual chamber, Dual sensing - both leads sensed, Dual pacing - both leads paced, R - adaptive rate control). The top panel in Figure 14–29 shows four possible dual chamber pacemaker patterns. The rhythms that occur in a patient with a DDD pacemaker depend upon the underlying heart rate and AV nodal conduction. A completely normal p and QRS can occur when the p rate is above the atrial pacing threshold (atrial p wave sensed and atrial pacing inhibited) followed by normal AV conduction and a native QRS complex. However, in the second example (p synchronous pacing), there is a native p wave but an intrinsic AV nodal delay that is greater than the AV delay threshold of the pacer, and ventricular pacing occurs at a set AV delay manifested by a ventricular pacer spike and wide QRS. In the third scenario atrial pacing occurs (sinus rate falls below the lower limit set in the pacemaker) followed by a paced p wave and normal AV conduction with a normal QRS complex. In the fourth possibility there is both atrial and ventricular pacing (sinus bradycardia and AV conduction delay). An atrial pacer spike followed by a paced p wave and ventricular pacing (ventricular pacer spike and wide QRS). The bottom panel shows an actual tracing from a patient with a dual chamber pacer. On the left portion of the tracing, only the atrial pacer lead is activated followed by normal AV conduction and a narrow QRS complex (narrow). On the right, both atrial and ventricular leads are pacing. This produces both atrial and ventricular pacing spikes and a wide QRS complex. The paced p wave in this example is not clearly seen. The paced p wave morphology depends on the position of the atrial pacer lead. Modern DDD pacemakers have a number of algorithms to minimize RV pacing and encourage native AV conduction. The algorithms can produce delays that might suggest pacemaker dysfunction. Clearly, the best approach is to send concerning ECG tracings to a cardiologist for review if there is any doubt about pacemaker function.

Patients with significant heart failure often have a biventricular (BiV) pacemaker in place with a RV pacemaker lead and an LV pacemaker wire located in a branch of the coronary sinus vein on the lateral posterior wall of the LV. The

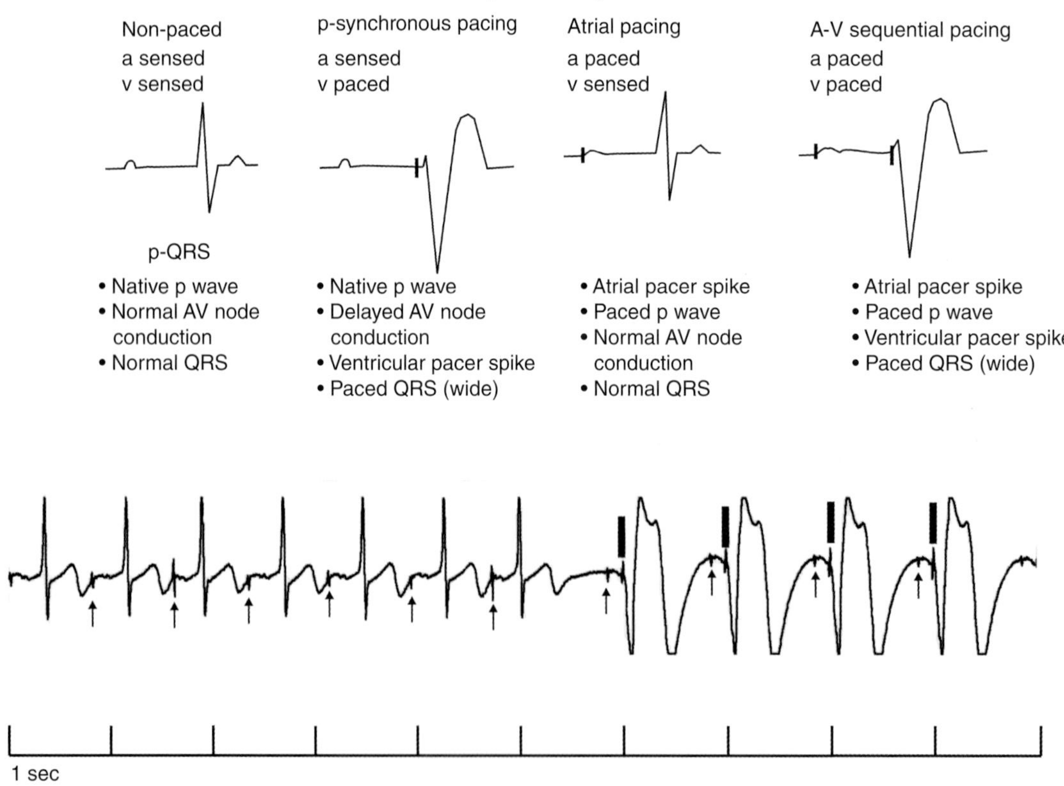

Figure 14–29 *(Top panel)* Some possible patterns in a patient with a dual chamber pacemaker are shown in the upper top panel. In the leftmost pattern the sinus node rate exceeds a minimum rate, and the AV node conducts adequately, resulting in a normal sinus beat. In the second pattern a normal p wave occurs, but AV conduction time exceeds a threshold, resulting in ventricular pacing (wide QRS). In the third pattern the atrial pacer fires followed by a paced p wave but with normal conduction and a normal QRS. In the rightmost pattern there is both atrial and ventricular pacing. Note that if the AV node does not conduct within a minimum time, ventricular pacing occurs with a wide QRS (pacer lead in the right ventricle, so an LBBB pattern). *(Bottom panel)* Timing in seconds is shown below the actual tracing. In the first seven complexes atrial pacer spikes (**up arrows**) are seen with normal conduction and a narrow QRS. In the last four complexes the atrial pacing is not normally conducted, and ventricular pacer spikes (**dark vertical lines**) with a wide QRS occur consistent with ventricular pacing. The p-to-p interval before the last four beats is slightly prolonged, but this is likely due to the pacemaker algorithm encouraging normal atrial activation.

coronary sinus vein drains deoxygenated blood from the heart muscle into the right atrium. The appearance of the QRS depends on the position of the LV pacing wire and the set delay (if any) between RV and LV pacing. When limited to a modified lead II, pacer spikes may or may not be seen and the QRS width is variable (but usually ≥ 0.12 second). In fact, visualized in a 30-second window it may **not** be apparent to the physician reading the study that the patient even has a BiV pacemaker. One should note that these devices automatically check the ability to pace both the RV and LV (usually at 1 or 2 AM) with each individual pacer wire tested.[20] When only the RV or LV is paced, this will cause the appearance of a much wider and different morphology QRS (Figure 14–30). The pattern can be mistaken for WCT (although the rate is usually well below 100 bpm). It is important that sleep technologists know that a BiV pacemaker is present and that changes in the paced QRS can occur during the night associated with pacer function testing.

CARDIAC EVENT REPORTING

The AASM scoring manual recommends reporting the average heart rate during sleep, the lowest and highest heart rates during sleep (and for the recording), the occurrence of bradycardia

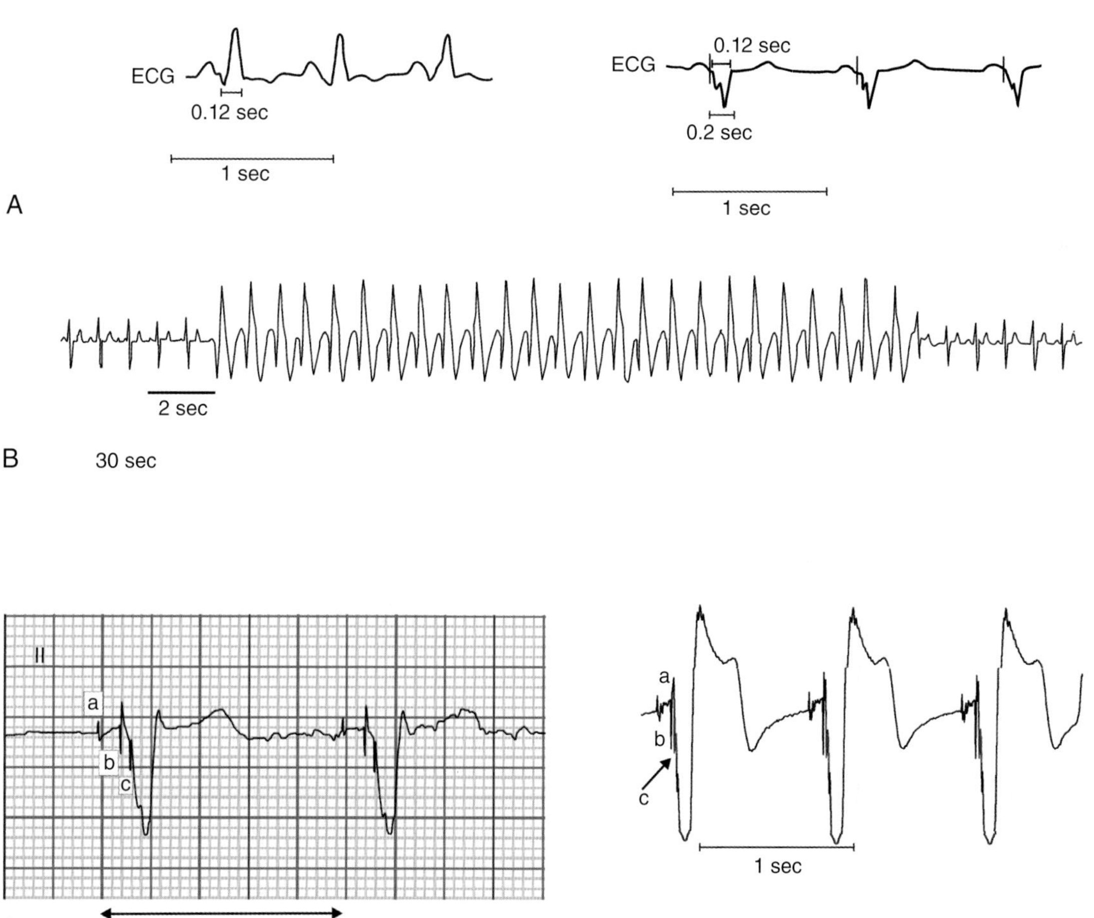

Figure 14–30 (A) Two tracings of the appearance of sinus rhythm with a biventricular (BiV) pacemaker are shown (modified lead II). The wide QRS can be variable from just slightly wider than 0.12 second to an obviously widened QRS complex. The appearance varies based on the position of the pacing leads for right ventricle (RV) and left ventricle (LV) and the timing of pacing of the LV relative to the RV. The QRS duration also depends on order and latency with which each chamber is paced (often called the offset). For example the LV is paced 20 msec before the RV (offset -20 msec). When there is near simultaneous pacing (usually LV first), the QRS can be narrower. Either 1, 2, or no ventricular pacer spikes may be visible in the modified lead II. When viewed in a 30-second or greater time window, the rhythm can appear as normal sinus rhythm. It is important to determine the presence and type of pacemaker from the history. The presence/absence of a pacemaker should be a question in the prestudy patient questionnaire (often omitted from clinic notes). (B) The sudden appearance of a wide complex waveform during a sleep study. This pattern is associated with automatic testing of the LV and RV pacing electrodes normally occurring during the night (autocapture algorithms check one lead at a time). Note that the rate is similar to that of the narrower QRS complexes (in a 30-second window the pre-testing QRS has a normal appearance). This seemingly bizarre pacemaker behavior is frequently observed in the 1 to 2 AM time frame and is one of many automated self-diagnostic or safety assurance algorithms used by implantable cardiac devices. A excellent example of pacemaker electrode testing in a patient during a sleep study has been published[20] (C) An example of a dual chamber BiV pacemaker using traditional ECG timelines is shown on the left. Atrial (a) and two ventricular pacer spikes (b, c) are seen in the ECG (Lead II). When the same patient underwent sleep monitoring the tracing on the right was recorded (3 seconds shown). It is difficult to see the pacer spike c *(red).*

during sleep (if observed, including lowest rate), the occurrence of asystole (if observed, including the longest pause), the occurrence of sinus tachycardia during sleep (if observed and highest heart rate), the occurrence of WCT and NCT (if observed and maximum rates), the occurrence of atrial fibrillation (if observed and associated average heart rate), and any other abnormal rhythms. The occurrence of AV block and the type of block should also be reported. Most physicians would also report paced rhythms. For WCT and NCT the length of episodes (sustained or nonsustained) is also usually reported.

SUMMARY OF KEY POINTS

1. A single modified lead II (negative below the right clavicle in the mid-clavicular line, positive left lower thorax anterior axillary line 6th or 7th intercostal space) is recommended for monitoring ECG rhythm sleep studies with a minimal sampling rate of 200 Hz and low and high filter settings of 0.3 Hz and 100 Hz, respectively. Multiple ECG electrode positions can be recorded referentially. If the right electrode is called EKG1 and the left electrode EKG3 the derivation EKG1-EKG3 will produce an upward p and QRS (G1-G2 produces an upward deflection if G1 is negative with respect to G2, negative polarity up convention). However, the ECG may simply be recorded as a bipolar channel. Recording more ECG electrodes is available on many PSG systems and is useful. For example, both a modified lead I and lead II channels are recorded and displayed.
2. Score sinus tachycardia during sleep for a *sustained* (>30 second) heart rate > 90 bpm for adults.
3. Score sinus bradycardia during sleep for a sustained (>30 second) heart rate < 40 bpm for ages 6 through adult.
4. Score asystole for cardiac pauses >3 seconds for ages 6 through adult.
5. Score WCT for a rhythm lasting a minimum of three consecutive beats at **a rate > 100/min** with a QRS duration ≥ 120 msec (0.12 second).
6. Score NCT for a rhythm lasting a minimum of three consecutive beats at a **rate > 100/min** with a QRS duration < 120 msec (0.12 second).
7. Score Afib if there is an irregularly irregular ventricular rhythm associated with replacement of consistent P waves by rapid oscillations that vary in size, shape, and timing.
8. When the heart rate is ~150 bpm, consider aflutter with 2/1 block. Look for periods of greater block to visualize the flutter waves.
9. Change to 10-second window to better visualize the ECG.
10. Sustained WCT (>30 seconds) should be treated as an emergency, and it is likely VT (especially in patients with known coronary artery disease). Emergency procedures in the sleep center should be activated.
11. In lead II, the P wave should be upright.
12. It is essential that the technologist or ordering physician document the presence of a pacemaker. It is also helpful to know whether the patient has known Afib.
13. A sudden run of wider complex beats < 100 bpm (e.g., 60–70 bpm) is not WCT (by definition >100 bpm) and maybe a pacemaker rhythm.
14. If there is a concern about a run of wide QRS complexes, ask the patient if a pacemaker is in place or consult the medical record. Pacemaker rhythms usually have a rate less than 100 bpm. Pacemaker spikes may be better visualized with a high filter of 100 Hz with the 60-Hz notch filter off.

CLINICAL REVIEW QUESTIONS

1. What cardiac rhythm is shown is Figure 14–31?
2. What cardiac rhythm is shown in Figure 14–32?
3. What cardiac rhythm is shown in Figure 14–33?
4. You notice that the heart rate accelerates to 120 bpm for 10 seconds after an obstructive apnea. Is this sinus tachycardia during sleep?
5. Asystole is defined as:
   A. A 4-second pause in ventricular rhythm
   B. A 4-second pause in atrial rhythm (no p waves)
   C. A 3-second pause in ventricular rhythm
   D. A 3-second pause in atrial rhythm

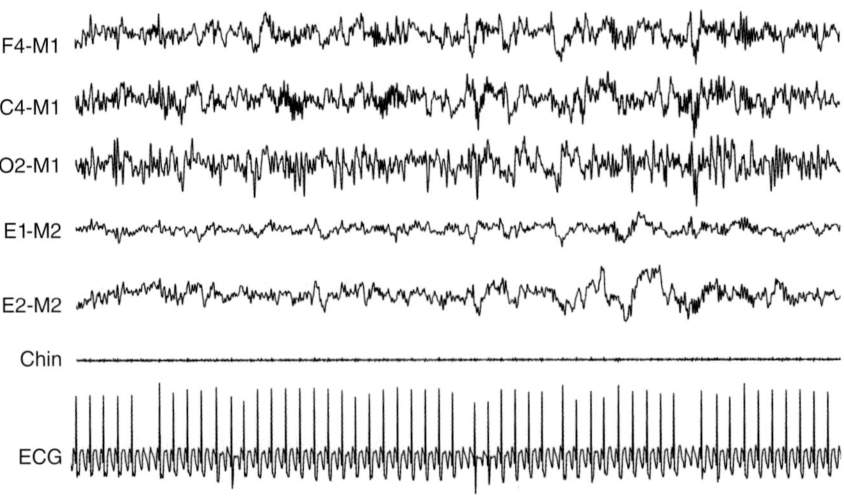

Figure 14–31 A 30-second figure for review question 1.

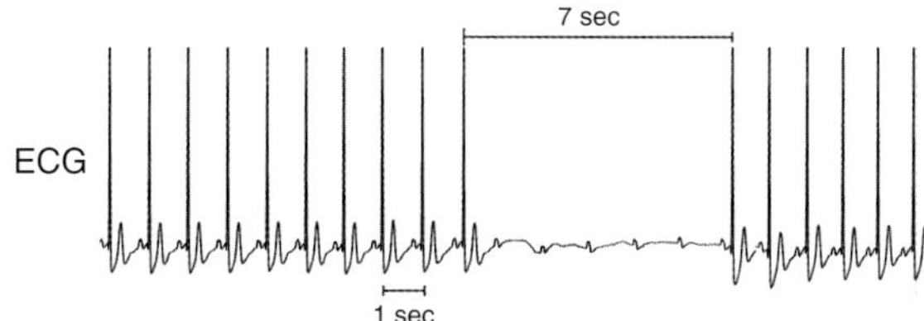

Figure 14–32 A figure for review question 2.

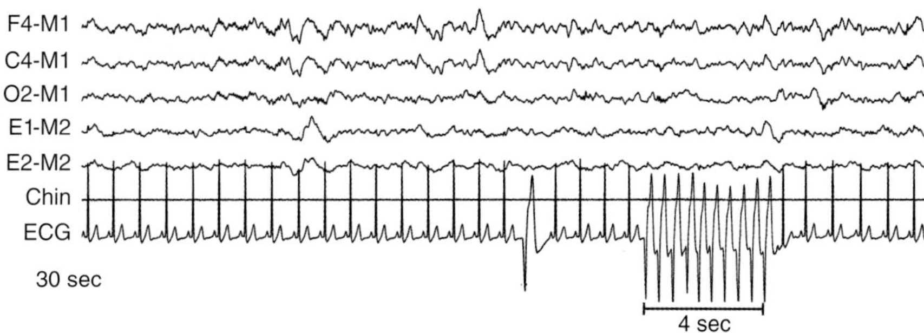

Figure 14–33 Figure for question 3.

6. Wide complex tachycardia requires all of the following properties EXCEPT:
   A. At least three beats
   B. Rate > 90 bpm
   C. QRS width > 0.12 second

ANSWERS

1. Atrial flutter with variable block. On can see flutter waves after the fifth QRS.
2. Third-degree AV block. P waves without an associated QRS complex. This event would also qualify as asystole as there was no ventricular beat for more than 3 seconds.
3. Wide complex tachycardia.
4. No. Sinus tachycardia during sleep requires a sustained increase in heart rate (>30 seconds).
5. C. A systole refers to absence of a ventricular beat for >3 seconds.
6. B. A rate > 100/min is required.

RECOMMENDED READING

Caples SM, Rosen CLK, Shen WK, et al. The scoring of cardiac events during sleep. *J Clin Sleep Med.* 2007;3:147-154.

Goldberger AL, Goldberger ZD, Shvilken A. *Goldberger's Clinical Electrocardiography.* 10th ed. Elsevier; 2024.

Mond HG. Interpreting the normal pacemaker electrocardiograph. *Heart Lung Circ.* 2019;28(2):223-236.

Troester MM, Quan SF, Berry RB, et al; for the American Academy of Sleep Medicine. *The AASM Manual for the Scoring of Sleep and Associated Events: Rules, Terminology and Technical Specifications.* Version 3. American Academy of Sleep Medicine; 2023.

REFERENCES

1. Goldberger AL, Goldberger ZD, Shvilken A. *Goldberger's Clinical Electrocardiography.* 10th ed. Elsevier; 2024.
2. Dubin D. *Rapid Interpretation of EKGs.* 6th ed. Cover Publishing; 2000.
3. Postema PG, Wilde AA. The measurement of the QT interval. *Curr Cardiol Rev.* 2014;10(3):287-294.
4. Caples SM, Rosen CLK, Shen WK, et al. The scoring of cardiac events during sleep. *J Clin Sleep Med.* 2007;3:147-154.
5. Iber C, Israel S, Chesson A, Quan SF; for the American Academy of Sleep Medicine. *The AASM Manual for the Scoring of Sleep and Associated Events: Rules, Terminology and Technical Specification.* American Academy of Sleep Medicine; 2007.
6. Troester MM, Quan SF, Berry RB, et al; for the American Academy of Sleep Medicine. *The AASM Manual for the Scoring of Sleep and Associated Events: Rules, Terminology and Technical Specifications.* Version 3. American Academy of Sleep Medicine; 2023.
7. Davignon A, Rautaharju P, Boisselle E, et al. Normal ECG standards for infants and children. *Pediatr Cardiol.* 1980;1:123-131.
8. Fleming S, Thompson M, Stevens R, et al. Normal ranges of heart rate and respiratory rate in children from birth to 18 years of age: a systematic review of observational studies. *Lancet.* 2011;377(9770):1011-1018.
9. Archbold KH, Johnson NL, Goodwin JL, et al. Normative heart rate parameters during sleep for children aged 6 to 11 years. *J Clin Sleep Med.* 2010;6:47-50.
10. Hedger-Archbold K, Sorensen ST, Goodwin JL, Quan SF. Average heart rates of Hispanic and Caucasian adolescents during sleep: longitudinal analysis from the TuCASA cohort. *J Clin Sleep Med.* 2014;10(9):991-995.
11. Bonsignore MR, Romano S, Marrone O, Chiodi M, Bonsignore G. Different heart rate patterns in obstructive apneas during NREM sleep. *Sleep.* 1997;20(12):1167-1174.
12. Bjerregaard P. Mean 24 hour heart rate and pauses in healthy subjects 40–79 years of age. *Eur Heart J.* 1983;4:44-51.
13. Holty JE, Guilleminault C. REM-related bradyarrhythmia syndrome. *Sleep Med Rev.* 2011;15(3):143-151.
14. Biswas A, Berry RB, Sriram PS, Prasad A. A man with sleep-associated symptomatic bradycardia. *Ann Am Thorac Soc.* 2017;14(4):597-600.
15. Holmqvist F, Daubert JP. First-degree AV block—an entirely benign finding or a potentially curable cause of cardiac disease? *Ann Noninvasive Electrocardiol.* 2013;18(3):215-224.
16. Gamaldo C, Sala RE, Collop NA. Complex arrhythmia during a sleep study—what to do? *J Clin Sleep Med.* 2009;5:171-173.
17. Mehra R, Strohl KP. Incidence of serious adverse events during nocturnal polysomnography. *Sleep.* 2004;27:1379-1383.
18. Kolla BP, Lam E, Olson E, Morgenthaler T. Patient safety incidents during overnight polysomnography: a five-year observational cohort study. *J Clin Sleep Med.* 2013;9(11):1201-1205.
19. Mond HG. Interpreting the normal pacemaker electrocardiograph. *Heart Lung Circ.* 2019;28(2):223-236.
20. Mittal V, Lloyd MS, Collop NA. Polysomnography and implantable cardiac devices: identifying normal and abnormal paced beats. *J Clin Sleep Med.* 2012;8(3):340-342.

Chapter 15

Monitoring of Limb Movements and Other Movements During Sleep

ABBREVIATIONS

PLMSI periodic limb movements in sleep index, PLMSAI periodic limb movements in sleep arousal index

INTRODUCTION

The International Classification of Sleep Disorders, 3rd edition (ICSD-3)-TR[1] lists the sleep-related movement disorders as:

- *Restless legs syndrome*
- *Periodic limb movement disorder*
- *Nocturnal muscle cramps*
- *Sleep-related bruxism*
- *Sleep-related rhythmic movement disorder*
- *Benign sleep myoclonus of infancy*
- *Propriospinal myoclonus at sleep onset*
- *Sleep-related movement disorder due to a medical disorder*
- *Sleep-related movement disorder due to a medication, or substance*

The restless legs syndrome (RLS) and periodic limb movement disorder (PLMD) are discussed in detail in Chapter 31. This chapter discusses monitoring of limb movements (LMs) and the scoring rules for periodic limb movements in sleep (PLMS), bruxism, the sleep-related rhythmic movement disorder (RMD), and scoring REM sleep without atonia. Propriospinal myoclonus at sleep onset and benign infantile spasms will be briefly mentioned. The chapter also covers scoring rules for three LM patterns considered to be benign conditions: alternating leg movement activation (ALMA), hypnagogic foot tremor (HFT), and excessive fragmentary myoclonus (EFM). These three LM patterns are listed in the ICSD-3-TR under "Isolated Symptoms and Normal Variants." The polysomnographic (PSG) finding of PLMS is very common and often not associated with symptoms. However, a majority of patients with the RLS exhibit PLMS during polysomnography (PSG) and PLMS can be associated with disturbed sleep or daytime symptoms in the absence of RLS (the PLMD).

LIMB MONITORING TECHNIQUES

The presence and frequency of limb movements (LMs) during sleep is documented by recording the electromyography (EMG) activity of muscles involved in producing the movement. The EMG activity of the right and left anterior tibialis muscles is routinely monitored. The American Accademy of Sleep Medicine (AASM) Manual for the Scoring of Sleep and Associated Events, Rules, and Technical Specifications hereafter referred to as the AASM scoring manual provides recommendations for monitoring and scoring sleep-related movements.[2] The classic periodic leg movement consists of extension of the big toe, dorsiflexion at the ankle, and sometimes flexion at the knee and hip, similar to the leg movement with the Babinski reflex (see Video 15.1). The PSG finding of increased muscle activity during REM sleep (REM sleep without atonia) is required for the diagnosis of the REM sleep behavior disorder (RBD)[1]. Arm muscle EMG activity is often recorded (Fig. 15–1) if a diagnosis of RBD is being considered. In some patients with RBD, abnormal EMG activity during REM sleep is more prominent in the arms than leg muscles. Some clinicians feel the activity in the arm muscles is more specific for RBD. Monitoring of left and right arm EMG is recommended by the AASM scoring manual[2] for diagnosis of the REM sleep behavior disorder.

Leg EMG activity is recorded using bipolar alternating current (AC) amplifiers with surface electrodes using methods similar to those used to record chin EMG activity. The electrodes should have an impedance less than 10 kΩ, although an impedance $\leq$ 5 kΩ is preferred. The recommended low and high filter display settings are 10 Hz and 100 Hz, respectively.[2,3] Use of a 60-Hz notch filter is not recommended. As discussed later, because voltage amplitude criteria are used to identify candidate LMs, *the relaxed leg EMG activity should be less than* $\pm 5\ \mu V$ (no greater than 10 μV between negative and positive deflections). This requires low electrode impedance. As the high filter setting is 100 Hz, turning off the 60-Hz notch filter will make 60-Hz contamination very prominent unless electrode impedance is low. The leg EMG electrodes are placed longitudinally (along the long axis) and symmetrically in the middle of the anterior tibialis muscle (Fig. 15–1). The AASM scoring manual recommends that the electrodes be placed either 2 to 3 cm apart or one-third the length of the anterior tibialis muscle, whichever is shorter.[2] Both legs should be monitored for the presence of leg movements. Using a separate channel (tracing) for each leg is strongly recommended. The AASM scoring manual[2] states that "combining electrodes from the two legs to give one recorded channel may suffice in some clinical settings, although it should be recognized that this strategy may reduce the number of detected LMs."

The EMG activity of several upper extremity muscles has been recorded in studies evaluating patients for suspected RBD. In one study the highest rates of phasic EMG activity were found in the mentalis muscles, the flexor digitorum superficialis (FDS) muscle (a forearm muscle), and the extensor digitorum brevis (EDB) muscle on upper surface of the foot.[4,5] The location of the FDS is illustrated in Figure 15–1. The EDB is a muscle on the upper surface of the foot that helps extend digits two through four. The extensor digitorum communis is another muscle in the upper extremities showing frequent activity during REM sleep in patients with the REM sleep behavior disorder (RBD). Electrode placement sites for the flexor digitorum

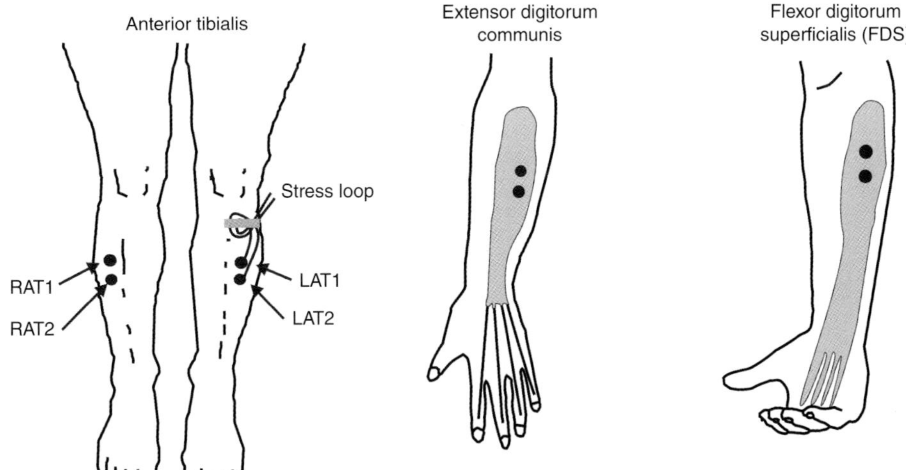

Figure 15–1 Illustration of the electrode positions for monitoring the leg EMG activity of left and right anterior tibialis (*LAT* and *RAT*) muscles and arm EMG activity of the extensor digitorum communis (EDC) and the flexor digitorum superficialis (FDS). Identification of the FDS muscle is improved with muscle activation (flexion at the base of the fingers [metacarpophalangeal joints] while avoiding bending of the fingers). For the EDC extension of the fingers backward without moving the wrist is used for muscle activation. Electrodes are placed parallel to the long axis of the muscles 2 to 3 cm apart. (Adapted from Berry RB, Wagner MH. *Sleep Medicine Pearls.* 3rd ed. Elsevier; 2015:166.)

superficialis (FDS) and the extensor digitorum communis (EDC) are provided in the AASM scoring manual.[2] The same filter settings used for recording the anterior tibialis EMG are also recommended for upper extremity EMG monitoring. Accurate placement of the FDS and EDC electrodes is more precise if the muscle is activated so the muscle can be easily felt. The FDS is located on the medial side of the volar surface of the forearm (Fig. 15–1). For the FDS, flexion at the base of the fingers (MCP joint) (avoiding bending of fingers) will activate the muscle. The EDC is located on the lateral/dorsal aspect of the forearm and is an extensor of the digits (see Fig. 15–1). Placement of the electrodes to monitor the extensor digitorum is along the long axis of the belly of the muscle separated by a few centimeters. Extension of the fingers backward without moving the wrist is used for muscle activation to aid in electrode placement and to verify signal adequacy during biocalibration.

CRITERIA FOR SCORING LEG MOVEMENTS AND PERIODIC LIMB MOVEMENTS

The reader should be aware that the scoring rules for leg movements in the AASM scoring manual differ from those accepted by the World Association of Sleep Medicine (WASM) in collaboration with the International Restless Legs Syndrome Study Group (IRLSSG).[6,7] This alternative set of scoring rules is often used in research publication studying leg movements during sleep. In the following discussion, individual leg (limb) movements are denoted by **LM**, individual periodic leg movements as **PLM,** and the polysomnography finding of periodic limb movements in sleep as **PLMS.** Although leg movements are typically monitored, the term *periodic limb movements* is used to be more inclusive (as periodic arm movements occur in some patients).

Scoring of PLMS

The current criteria for determining a **candidate LM** event[2] (a candidate for inclusion in a PLMS series) includes a duration from **0.5 to 10 seconds** with a **minimum amplitude is an 8 μV increase above the resting leg EMG for at least 0.5 seconds.** The *time of onset* is the time at which the amplitude increased to 8 μV above baseline resting activity, and the *end of the LM (offset)* is defined as the START of a period lasting at least 0.5 second during which the EMG does not exceed 2 μV above resting EMG (Fig. 15–2). A portion of, or the entire, LM event **must occur in an epoch scored as sleep**. As noted earlier, use of voltage criteria based on an absolute increase in microvolts above the resting baseline requires a stable resting EMG for the relaxed anterior tibialis muscle. The AASM scoring manual provides rules for defining a PLMS series, that is, criteria for determining if a candidate LM can be included in a PLMS series. The minimum number of consecutive candidate LMs to define a PLM series is four. The time from onset of one LM to the onset of the next LM is 5 to 90 seconds. LMs on different legs separated by **less than 5 seconds** between LM onsets are counted as a single LM (Fig. 15–3). The period length to the next LM after this group of LMs is measured from the onset of the first LM to the onset of the next leg movement (that is not part of the group). Figure 15–4 presents a 90-second segment of left and right anterior tibial EMG tracings. There are five LMs in this PLMS series. The two LMs at A and C are each considered to be one PLM, but at D there are two LMs as the time from onset to onset is greater than 5 seconds.

Summary for Scoring Leg Movements:

- Candidate leg movement (LM) for inclusion in PLMS series
  - LM duration 0.5 to 10 seconds
  - Minimum amplitude of LM is an increase of 8 μV above resting EMG activity for at least 0.5 seconds
  - Onset: time at which LM amplitude exceeds 8 μV above baseline resting EMG activity
  - Offset: start of a period of at least 0.5 seconds with LM amplitude less than or equal to 2 μV above the resting EMG activity
  - A portion (or entire LM event) occurs in an epoch scored as sleep
- Criteria for candidate leg movement to be included in PLMS series
  - Minimum number of consecutive LMs events is four

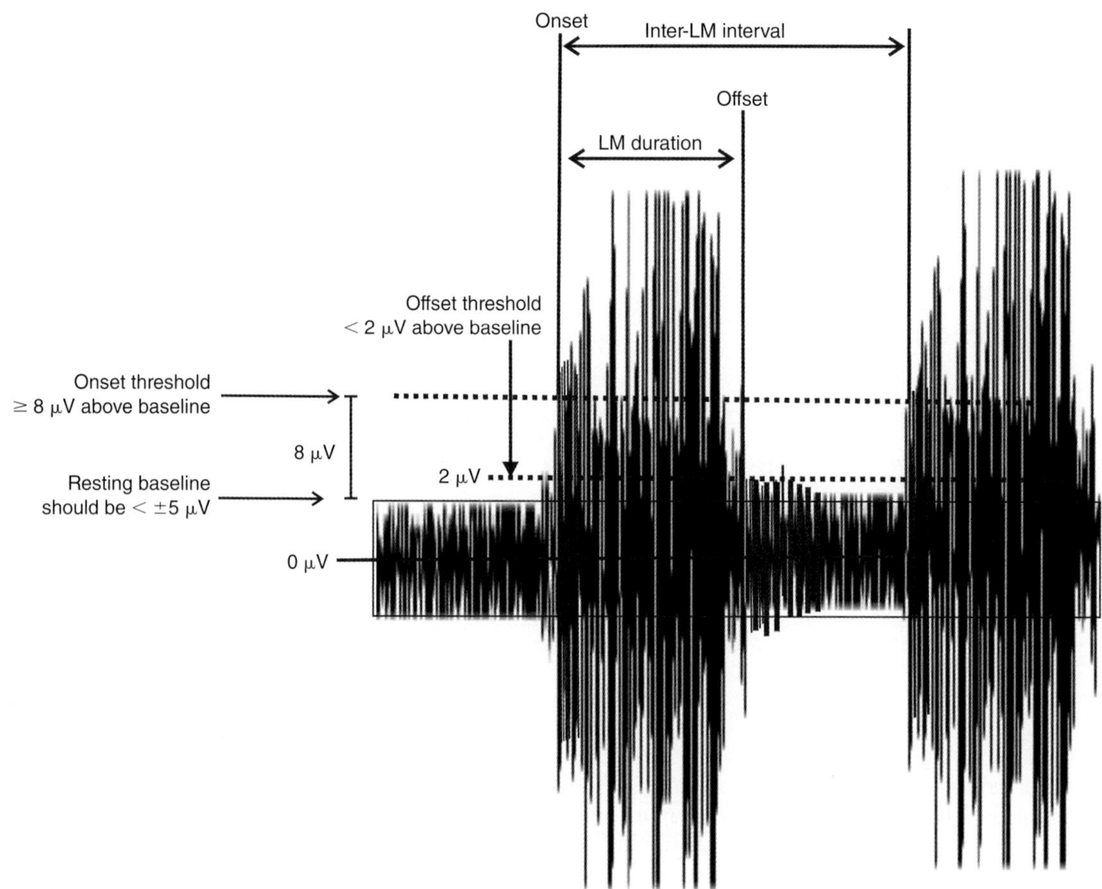

Figure 15–2 Illustration of requirements for identification of a candidate leg movement *(LM)* (a candidate for inclusion in a PLM series). The duration of a candidate LM is 0.5 to 10 seconds with a minimum amplitude of 8 µV above the resting EMG for at least 0.5 seconds. The onset is the point at which its activity is 8 µV above the resting (baseline) and the offset is the START of a period of at least 0.5 seconds when the activity is less than 2 µV above the resting muscle activity.[2]

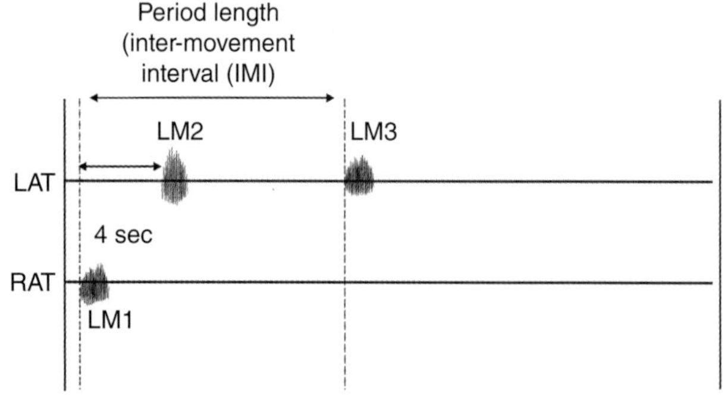

Figure 15–3 Schematic illustration of the combining of leg movements on different legs *(LM1, LM2)* onsets <5 seconds apart as one leg movement. The period length to the next leg movement *(LM3)* is defined based on the start of the first leg movement in the combined group. *LAT,* Left anterior tibialis; *RAT,* right anterior tibialis.

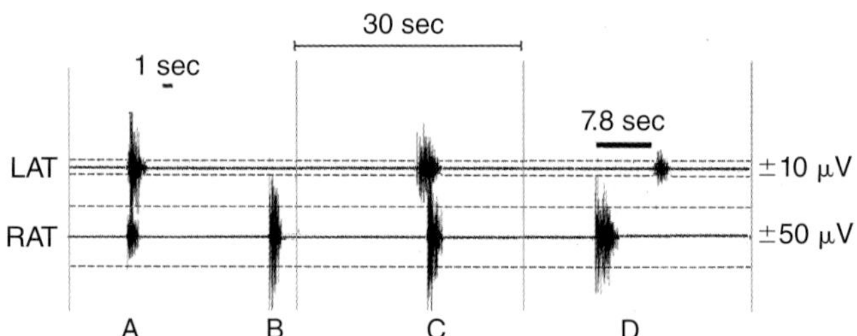

Figure 15–4 Illustration of definition of a periodic limb movements in sleep (PLMS) series. In this 90-second tracing there are five limb movements (LMs) qualifying for a PLMS series. These include one PLM at A (simultaneous LMs), one PLM at B, one PLM at C (combined LMs), and two PLMs at D. The LMs at D have onsets greater than 5 seconds apart and are considered two separate PLMs. The period length of all PLMs is 5 to 90 seconds. (Adapted from Berry RB, Wagner MH. *Sleep Medicine Pearls.* 3rd ed. Elsevier; 2015:168.)

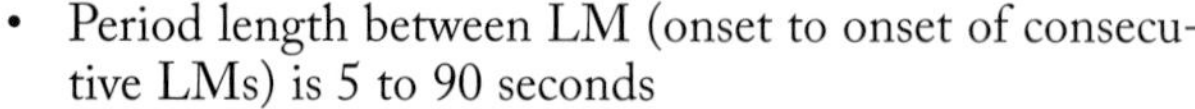

- Period length between LM (onset to onset of consecutive LMs) is 5 to 90 seconds
- Two leg movements on different legs separated by < (not ≤) 5 seconds onset to onset are considered a single LM. The period length to the next LM after this **group of LMs** is measured from the onset of the first LM in the group to the onset of the next candidate LM not part of the group.

The WASM intermovement interval (IMI) criteria for a LM to be a member of a PLMS series is 10 to 90 seconds. The term *IMI* rather than *period length* is used. The reason for this difference compared with AASM criteria is that using a minimum IMI of 10 seconds is more specific for patients with both PLMS and RLS.[8] Analysis of the IMI in controls and patients with RLS shows a bimodal pattern in RLS patients with one IMI group having a peak at 2 to 4 seconds and the

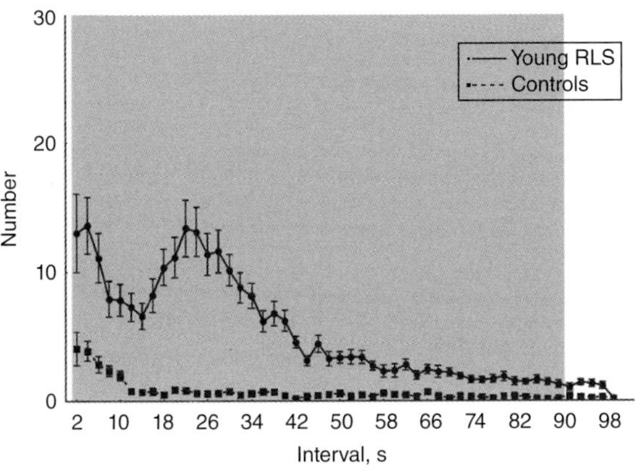

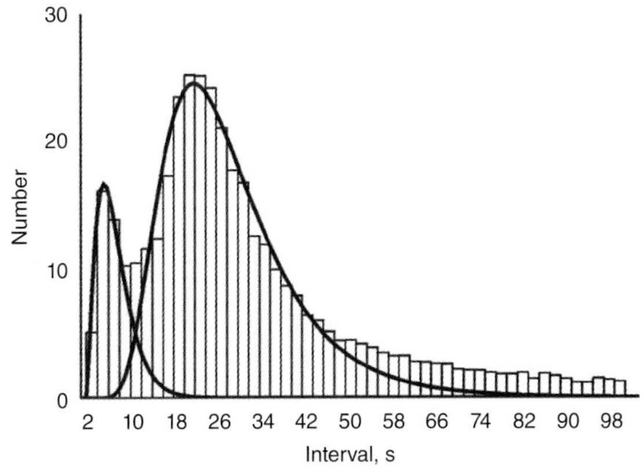

Figure 15–5 *(Left panel)* Inter-movement intervals for leg movements (LMs) for young patients with the restless legs syndrome *(RLS)* and a control group. The normal control group did not have the second peak at 18-26 seconds. *(Right panel)* Bimodal distribution for inter-movement intervals in patients with RLS. An interval of 10 seconds separates the first and second groups of LMs. (From Ferri R, Zucconi M, Manconi M, et al. New approaches to the study of periodic leg movements during sleep in restless legs syndrome. *Sleep.* 2006;29(6):759-769.)

second group with a peak at 18 to 24 seconds (Fig. 15–5). Normal controls do not have the second peak. In addition, leg movements associated with the second peak respond to dopamine agonists, whereas those associated with the first peak do not.[9] A cutoff duration of 10 seconds separates the two groups of leg movements, and therefore a period length (IMI) of 10 seconds to 90 seconds is recommended for inclusion of a LM as part of a PLMS series. However, this changes the criteria for grouping leg movements on different legs that occur close together. The WASM criteria for grouping movements on different legs are more complex than the AASM scoring manual rule. In addition, in the WASM scoring standards there are rules for ending a PLMS series when the next LM has an IMI less than 10 seconds.[7]

Wake and Sleep and PLMS

The "S" of PLMS means that the LMs in the series occur at least partially in an epoch of sleep. Sometimes epochs of wake interrupt a PLMS series. As long as the period length rules are met, LMs before and after the epoch of wake can be included (Fig. 15–6).

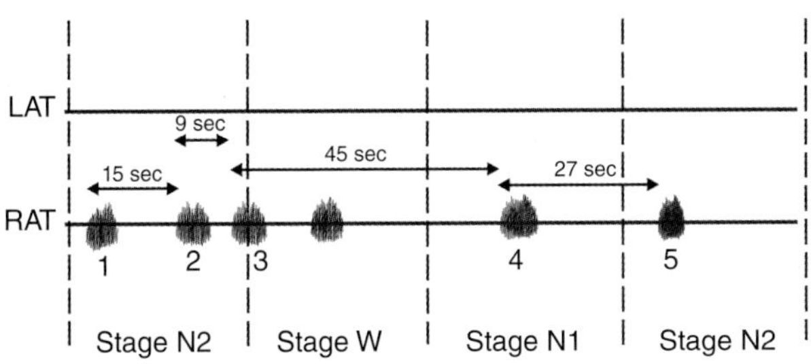

Figure 15–6 This schematic illustrates that inclusion in a PLMS series requires at least a portion of an LM to occur in an epoch scored as sleep, but that one can continue a PLMS series across an epoch of stage W as long as the intermovement intervals meet the 5- to 90-second criterion of an LM to be included in a PLMS series.[2] In this 120-second schematic, five LMs can be included in the PLMS series. Note that LM 3 is partially in an epoch scored as sleep and can be a candidate LM. The next EMG burst is entirely in stage W and is not a candidate LM. Note the LM4 can be included in the PLMS series even if there is an intervening epoch of wakefulness. *LAT,* Left anterior tibialis; *RAT,* right anterior tibialis.

Association of Arousals With an LM in a PLMS Series

According to the AASM scoring manual,[2] an arousal and a LM in PLM series should be considered associated with each other (Fig. 15–7) if they occur simultaneously, overlap, or when there is *less than 0.5 second* between the END of one event and the ONSET of the other event, regardless of which is first. It is important to remember that for EEG activity to be scored as an arousal *it must be preceded by at least 10 seconds of stable sleep.* When periodic limb movements occur with an interval of less than 10 seconds between onsets and each is associated with a ≥3-second change in the EEG/chin EMG meeting criteria for an arousal, only the first EEG/chin EMG change should be scored as an arousal (assuming it is preceded by at least 10 seconds of sleep). Both limb movements may be scored, assuming the onsets are separated by 5 seconds or more, but only one PLM associated with an arousal (and only one arousal) would be scored.[2] This point is illustrated in Figure 15–8.

LMs Associated With Respiratory Events Are Not Scored

An LM should **not** be scored (included in a PLMS series) if it occurs during a **period from 0.5 second before to 0.5 second after an apnea, hypopnea, or respiratory effort-related arousal (RERA).** LMs associated with respiratory events are not scored, that is, included in a PLMS series.[2] It is not uncommon for LMs to be noted at apnea termination even if an associated cortical arousal is not present. In Figure 15–9, the leg EMG bursts associated with respiratory events are not scored as candidate LMs for inclusion in a PLMS series. The reader should know that some experts in the field of sleep-related movements recommend scoring these movements although considering them to be a separate entity. However, there is still controversy about how they should be scored.[10-12]

Summary of Scoring PLMS Associated Arousals and LMs Associated with Respiratory Events:

- An LM that is part of a PLMS series is considered associated with an arousal when they occur simultaneously, overlap, or when there is *less than 0.5 second* between the END of one event and the ONSET of the other event, regardless of which is first.

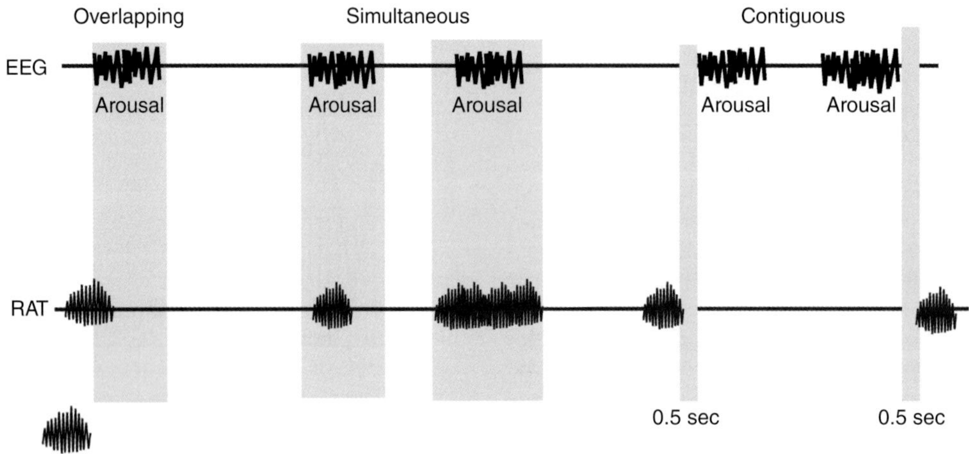

Figure 15–7 This schematic figure illustrates the association of a limb movement (LM) with an arousal. The LM and arousal can be overlapping, simultaneous, or contiguous with offset of the first event to onset of the second less than 0.5 seconds no matter which (LM or arousal) comes first.[2] *EEG,* Electroencephalogram; *PLM,* periodic limb movement; *RAT,* right anterior tibialis.

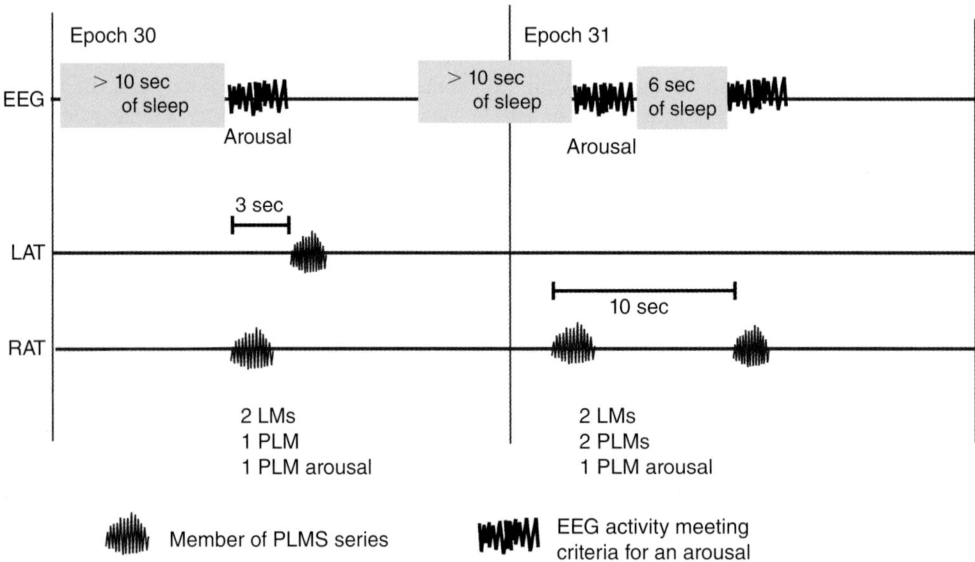

Figure 15–8 Schematic figure illustrating the relationship between limb movements *(LMs)* and arousals. In epoch 30 there are two LMs (one periodic limb movement [PLM] as LM onsets separated by less than 5 seconds) and one PLM arousal. In Epoch 31 there are two EEG changes that could potentially qualify to be scored as an arousal. However, only the first is preceded by ≥10 seconds of sleep and can be scored as an arousal. In summary in Epoch 31 there are two LMs and two PLMs but only one PLM arousal. This figure assumes that the LMs shown are candidate LMs that meet criteria to be included in a PLMS series. *EEG,* Electroencephalogram; *LAT,* left anterior tibialis; *PLM,* periodic limb movement; *RAT,* right anterior tibialis.

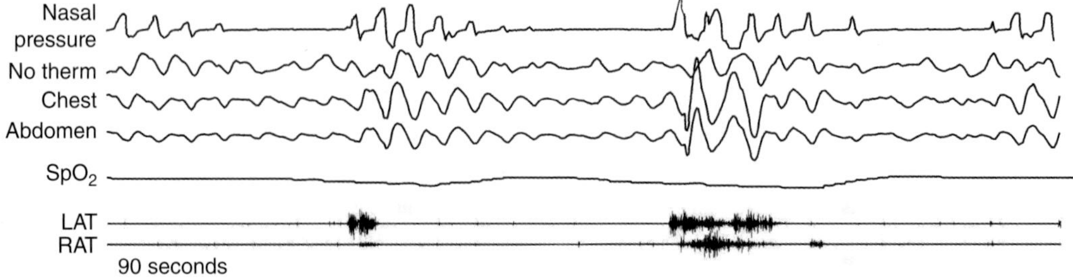

Figure 15–9 This figure shows limb movements that could not be included in a periodic limb movements during sleep series as they occur in the interval from 0.5 seconds before to 0.5 seconds after the duration of the respiratory event. (Adapted from Berry RB, Wagner MH. *Sleep Medicine Pearls.* 3rd ed. Elsevier; 2015:168.)

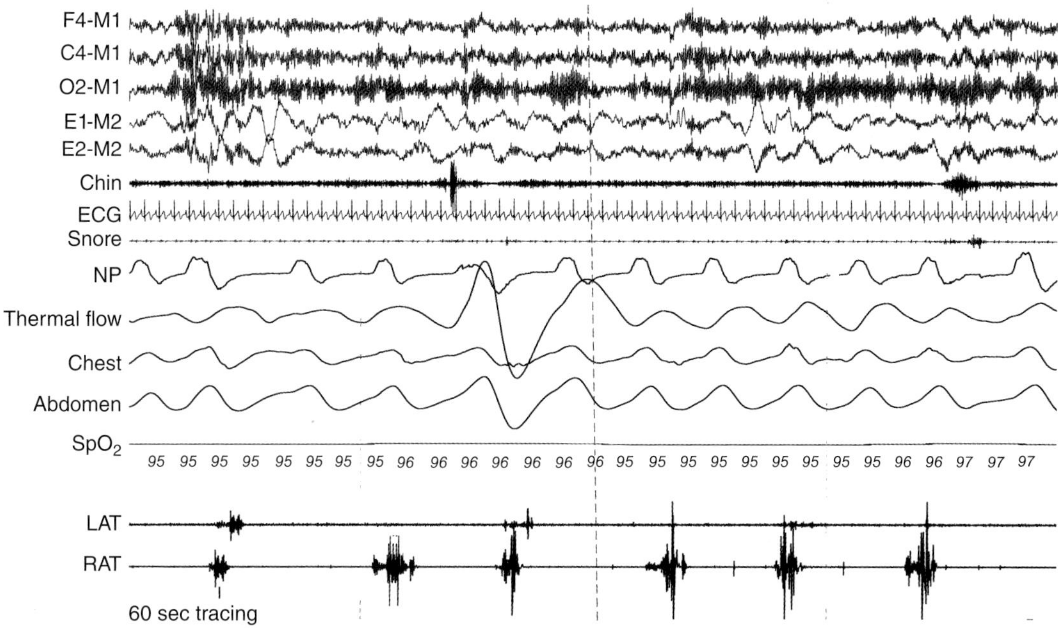

Figure 15–10 An example of limb movements occurring during epochs of wake. There is prominent alpha activity in O2-M1 consistent with stage W. The patient had difficulty falling asleep because of restless legs syndrome symptoms. *LAT and RAT,* Left and right anterior tibial EMG tracings, respectively; *NP,* nasal pressure.

- An LM should not be scored (included in a PLMS series) if it occurs during a period from 0.5 second before to 0.5 second after an apnea, hypopnea, or respiratory effort-related arousal (RERA).

Reporting PLMS

Of note, the term *PLMS* implies that PLMs occur during sleep. The AASM scoring manual[2] recommends reporting the number the periodic limb movement in sleep and the PLMS index (PLMSI) defined as the number of PLMs per hour of sleep. The number of PLMS associated with arousal (PLMSA) and the periodic limb movement in sleep arousal index (PLMSAI) should also be reported. PLMSI = 60 × number of PLMs/TST (min) and the PLMSAI = 60 × number of PLMs with arousal/TST (min).

Periodic Limb Movements in Wake

The AASM scoring manual does not recommend criteria for scoring periodic limb movements during wake (PLMW). The WASM in collaboration with the IRLSSG[6,7] published recommendations for PLMW. The criteria for PLMW events is similar to those for PLMS events except that the patient is awake (Fig. 15–10). The most recent recommendations are that a PLMW series can begin in sleep and continue to wake or vice versa.[8] The *PLMW index* is defined as the number of PLMW events divided by wake time (hr) from lights out to lights on *while the patient is in bed.* That is, the time when the patient is *out of bed or sitting on the side of the bed is not included.* Of note, frequent PLMW events are highly suggestive of the RLS. If PLMW events are noted, the patient history should be reviewed to determine if RLS symptoms are reported.

Suggested Immobilization Test

The Suggested Immobilization Test (SIT) was developed to help make the diagnosis of the RLS.[13] The test detects and counts PLMW. The patient sits with the legs outstretched and attempts to keep the legs still for 30 minutes to an hour. EMG recording of the left and right anterior tibialis muscles is performed. The test is often administered in the evening. The combination of rest and monitoring in the evening worsens RLS. In one study of the SIT, in patients with and without RLS using a PLMW index of 40/hr to diagnose RLS, the sensitivity and specificity were 81% and 81%, respectively (compared with RLS clinical criteria based on history).[13]

Clinical Significance of PLMS

The clinical significance of the polysomnographic finding of PLMS is discussed in more detail in Chapter 31. There are no widely accepted criteria for what constitutes a normal, mildly, moderately, or severely increased PLMSI. The AASM scoring manual does not provide a scheme for grading severity of the PLMS index. The ICSD-3-TR[1] requires a PLM index >15/hr in adults and >5/hr in children as criteria for the diagnosis of the PLMD. A diagnosis of RLS excludes a diagnosis of PLMD. The PLMD requires both PLMS and impairment of sleep and wake (as well as the absence of a clinical diagnosis of RLS). In normal individuals the PLMS index does increase with age.[14] In addition, the PLMS index tends to decrease over the night. Of note, the *finding of PLMS during REM sleep (stage R) is uncommon except in patients with the RBD or narcolepsy.* PLMS during REM sleep should not be confused with transient muscle activity in the leg EMG that can occur during stage R. However, if a patient has both PLMS in REM sleep and transient muscle activity in the leg EMG during stage R, scoring can be challenging.

The percentage of patients with RLS that have PLMS depends on the number of nights monitored and the PLMS index criteria but is over 80%.[15] The percentage of patients with PLMS that have RLS is not well defined but is likely 25% to 30%.

OTHER LMS DURING SLEEP

In the following sections, other identifiable LM patterns are discussed, including alternating leg movement activation (ALMA), hypnagogic foot tremor (HFT), and excessive fragmentary myoclonus (EFM).[16-23] To date, the presence of these patterns does not appear to be associated with a clinically significant disorder. Some have suggested that HFT and ALMA should be grouped into a category known as high-frequency leg movements.[19,20] ALMA and HFT are fairly common and are sometimes confused with PLMs. Of note, the AASM scoring manual states that scoring ALMA, HFT, and EFM is **optional**.

Alternating Leg Muscle Activation

ALMA[2,16-20] is characterized by short EMG bursts that alternate between the legs and are higher in frequency than PLMS (Fig. 15–11). Because there have been no reported clinical consequences of this pattern, it is believed to be a benign finding. ALMA can often occur in association with arousals or at sleep-wake transitions. The usual range of duration of ALMA EMG bursts is 100 to 500 msec. The minimum frequency of ALMAs is 0.5 Hz, meaning that the onsets can be separated by no more than 2 seconds (in contrast, individual PLMs are separated (onset to onset) by a **minimum** of 5 seconds).

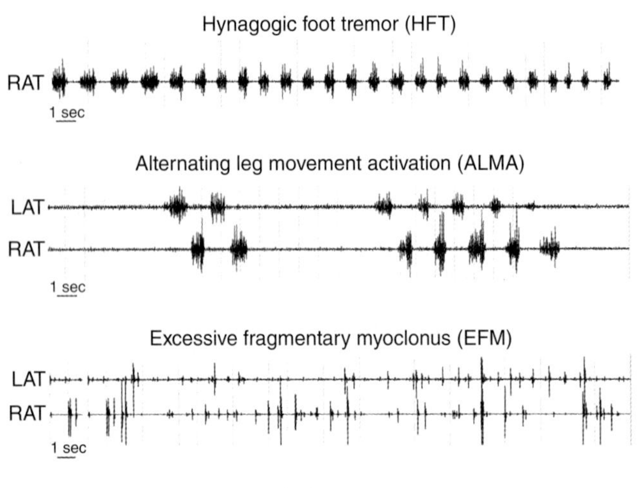

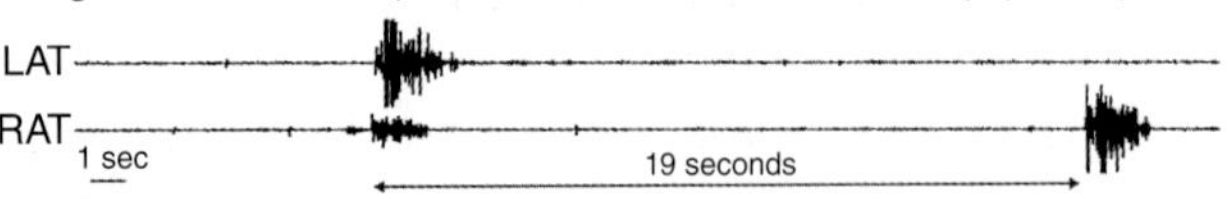

	LM bursts	Sleep required	Burst duration	Frequency (time between bursts)
HFT	Minimum of 4 Not alternating between legs	No	250–1000 msec	0.3 to 4.0 Hz (0.25 to 3.33 sec)
ALMA	Minimum of 4 Alternating between legs	No	100–500 msec	0.5 to 3.0 Hz (0.33 to 2 sec)
PLMS	Minimum of 4 can alternate	Yes	0.5 to 10 sec	(5–90 sec)

Figure 15–11 Thirty-second illustrations of the appearance of hypnogogic foot tremor *(HFT)*, alternating leg movement activation *(ALMA)*, excessive fragmentary myoclonus *(EFM)*, and limb movements *(LMs)* that are part of a periodic limb movements during sleep *(PLMS)* series. The intermovement interval of the HFT and ALMA bursts is much shorter than that of the LMs that are part of a PLMS series (only 2 LMs of the required 4 or more are shown). *LAT and RAT,* Left and right anterior tibial EMG tracings. (Adapted from Berry RB, Wagner MH. *Sleep Medicine Pearls.* 3rd ed. Elsevier; 2015:170.)

Summary of ALMA properties:

- Scoring is optional
- At least four leg EMG bursts and alternating between legs
- Burst duration 100 to 500 msec
- Burst frequency 0.5 to 3 Hz (2 to 0.33 seconds between burst onsets)
- Sequences occur at transitions between wakefulness and sleep or after arousals

Hypnogogic Foot Tremor

Hypnogogic foot tremor (HFT)[2,17,19,20] is a phenomenon characterized by a pattern of leg EMG bursts that is more rapid than those seen with PLMS. The usual range for the duration of HFT bursts is 250 to 1000 msec. The pattern may be seen during wakefulness or associated with arousal from sleep (Fig. 15–11). Unlike ALMA, the *EMG bursts of HFT do not alternate between the legs*. The maximum time period between onset of HFT EMG bursts is 3.3 seconds. Although memorizing the exact frequency criterion may be difficult, the specific patterns of HFT and ALMA on PSG are very characteristic and easy to recognize. HFT is not believed to have any clinical significance. The main issue is not confusing HFT and PLMS.

Summary of HFT:

- Scoring is optional
- Minimum of four bursts **not** alternating between legs
- Burst duration 100 to 500 msec
- Frequency of bursts 0.3 Hz to 4.0 Hz (time between burst onsets is 0.25 to 3.33 seconds)

Excessive Fragmentary Myoclonus

EFM[2,21-23] (Fig. 15–11) is defined by a characteristic EMG pattern in the leg tracings consisting of very brief EMG bursts (<150 msec) that occur at a frequency ≥ 5/min. It is thought to be a benign phenomenon. It most cases, no movements are visible, or if present, they are much like the small twitch-like movements of the fingers and toes seen intermittently during REM sleep in normal individuals. To qualify for EFM, the EMG pattern often seen during REM sleep *must also be seen during non–rapid eye movement (NREM) sleep.* There is overlap between the criteria for transient muscle activity during stage R (0.1 to 5 seconds in duration) and the pattern of EFM (<150 msec). It may be difficult to differentiate EFM during stage R from transient muscle activity. For this reason, the pattern must be present for at least *20 minutes during NREM sleep*. It is not surprising that patients with REM sleep without atonia (RWA) and the REM sleep behavior disorder are believed to have a higher prevalence of EFM than normal control groups.[23]

Summary of EFM Characteristics:

- Scoring is optional
- Maximal burst duration 150 msec
- At least 20 minutes of EFM must be recorded during NREM sleep
- At least 5 EMG bursts/min must be recorded

NOCTURNAL MUSCLE CRAMPS

The ICSD-3-TR[1] changed nomenclature from sleep-related leg cramps to nocturnal muscle cramps (NMC). The change recognizes that the cramps can occur at night during wakefulness and cramps can occur in other areas than the legs. Characteristics of NMC include:

- A painful sensation in a muscle associated with sudden, involuntary muscle hardness or tightness, indicating a strong muscle contraction.
- They occur during time in bed associated with wakefulness or sleep.
- Relief is obtained by stretching the affected muscle.

NMC affecting the legs can be a mimic of RLS as they both occur at rest at night and can improve with activity. However, the improving activity for NMC is usually stretching, and there is a hardness or tightness in the affect leg muscle. A systematic review[24] attempted to identify diagnostic criteria that would help differentiate NMC of the legs and RLS/PLMS. NMC involving the legs is intensely painful, located in calf or foot, not associated with other abnormal sensations or the urge to move (as in RLS) with a duration of seconds to 10 minutes. Pain can persist after the leg cramp resolves.

The best treatment for NMC is not known. Magnesium salts have been recommended as a prophylaxis, but a Cochrane Database review found no firm evidence of efficacy.[25] On the other hand, a recent randomized controlled study[26] did find that magnesium oxide monohydrate was helpful for NMC. The authors emphasized that prolonged treatment (in this study 60 days) is needed to see an effect. Pre-bedtime stretching, avoiding dehydration, vitamins B and E, gabapentin, and calcium channel blockers have been effective in some patients. Quinine appears to be effective but has severe side effects including thrombocytopenia and is generally not recommended except in the most severe cases and then under close medical supervision. The reader is referred to the literature for more in depth discussion.[27]

SLEEP-RELATED BRUXISM

Bruxism is a grinding or clinching of the teeth.[1,2,28] It is associated with characteristic rhythmic muscle artifact in the EEG (rhythmic EMG activity of the scalp muscle underlying the EEG electrodes) and chin EMG activity. During sleep, jaw contractions are either tonic (jaw clinching) or phasic (intermittent bursts of activity) and are termed *rhythmic masticatory muscle activity (RMMA).*

The ICSD-3-TR diagnostic criteria for bruxism include[1]:

- The presence of repetitive jaw-muscle activity characterized by grinding or clinching of the teeth in sleep
- The presence of one or more of the following:
  1. Abnormal tooth wear
  2. Transient morning jaw muscle pain or fatigue or temporal headache

Polysomnography is not required for a diagnosis. Bruxism is prevalent in teenagers (12%), middle-aged adults (8%), and older adults (3%). Bruxism tends to occur in families. Approximately 20% to 50% of patients have at least one family member with a history of bruxism.

Of note, a reliable diagnosis of bruxism on the basis of polysomnography consists of more than detection of RMMA. RMMA refers only to the rhythmic EMG activity observed in the masticatory muscles during sleep, whereas sleep-related bruxism refers to the specific orofacial movements. Rhythmic movements of the mouth or chewing can mimic the EEG pattern associated with bruxism, but no tooth grinding will be heard. Ideally, there must be audible tooth grinding during bruxism episodes. For detecting bruxism, masseter electrodes may be placed (optional in AASM scoring manual). The location of masseter electrodes is shown in Figure 15–12. *Characteristic changes in masseter EMG are often more prominent during bruxism episodes than changes in the chin EMG.* The use of synchronized audio and video may also improve the accuracy of identification of bruxism.

Bruxism can occur in any stage of sleep or at arousal from sleep. It is most common in stages N1 and N2 and least common during REM sleep. As noted above, PSG evidence is NOT required for diagnosis. However, the ICSD-3-TR states that audio-video monitoring and recording of the EMG of at least one masseter muscle during polysomnography increases the reliability of the diagnosis of bruxism.[1]

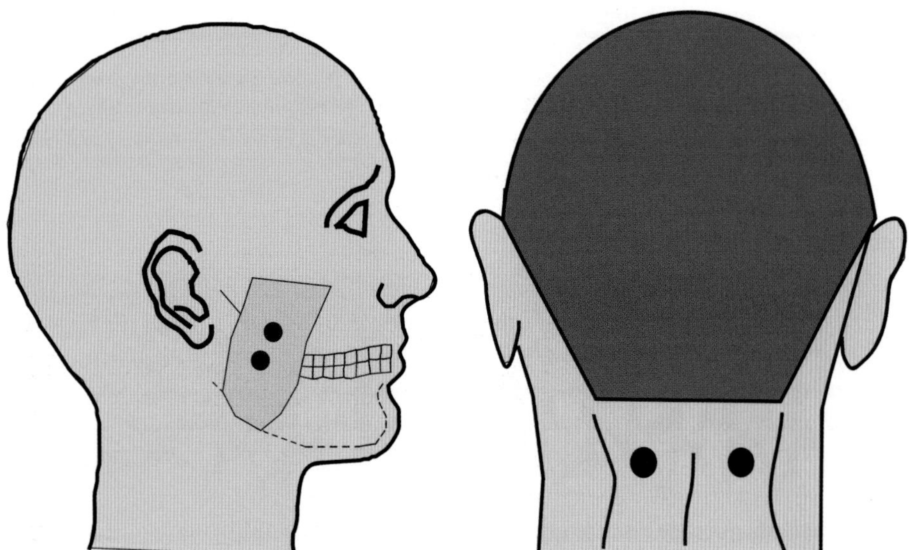

Figure 15–12 *(Left)* Schematic illustration of placement of electrodes to measure masseter EMG activity. One electrode can also be used and if so, is referred to a chin electrode. *(Right)* Placement of electrodes on the paraspinal muscles to assist in detection of rhythmic movements.

The AASM scoring manual[2] provides scoring criteria for bruxism.

- Bruxism may consist of brief (phasic) or sustained (tonic) elevations of chin EMG activity that are at least twice the amplitude of the background chin EMG.
- Brief elevations of chin EMG activity are scored as bruxism if they are 0.25 to 2 seconds in duration and if at least three such elevations occur in a regular sequence.
- Sustained elevations of chin EMG activity are scored as bruxism if the duration is **more than 2 seconds.**
- A period of at least 3 seconds of stable background chin EMG must occur before a new episode of bruxism can be scored.
- Bruxism can be scored reliably by time synchronized video and audio in combination with PSG by *a minimum of two audible tooth grinding episodes per night of polysomnography* (PSG) in the absence of associated epileptic discharges (see Video 15.2).

The scoring rules indicate that the chin EMG activity must be at least twice the amplitude of the background EMG. At least three elevations of EMG activity that are 0.25 to 2 seconds in duration should be present (Fig. 15–13). For **sustained EMG** elevations to be scored as bruxism, the duration must be **more than 2 seconds**. Whereas rhythmic EMG activity in the chin electrodes can often be noted during bruxism episodes, *prominent rhythmic activity may actually be more apparent from muscle artifact in the EEG and electrooculogram (EOG) derivations (overlying scalp muscles) than in the chin EMG.* As previously noted, EMG recording of the masseter muscles is more sensitive for detection of bruxism episodes than the chin EMG. Sleep-related bruxism can be comorbid with several other sleep disorders including obstructive sleep apnea.[29] There are patients who have bruxism episodes associated with obstructive apnea that can potentially improve with treatment of sleep apnea. The literature on bruxism and possible treatments is immense, and discussion of treatment is beyond the scope of this chapter.

RHYTHMIC MOVEMENTS AND THE SLEEP-RELATED RHYTHMIC MOVEMENT DISORDER

Rhythmic movements (RMs) are common in normal infants and children. Without significant evidence of consequences, the movements alone would not be considered a disorder. The term *rhythmic movement* ***disorder*** *(RMD)* implies consequences are present. The ICSD-3-TR terminology is *sleep-related rhythmic movement disorder (SRRMD).*[1,30]

The following is a summary of the ICSD-3-TR diagnostic criteria for the SRRMD:

- Repetitive, stereotyped, and rhythmic motor behaviors involving large muscle groups
- Movements are predominantly sleep related, occur near nap or bedtime, or when the individual appears drowsy or asleep
- **The behaviors result in a significant complaint manifested by at least one of the following:**
  1. Interference with normal sleep
  2. Significant impairment in daytime function
  3. Self-inflicted bodily injury of likelihood of injury if preventive measures are not used
- The rhythmic movements are not better explained by another movement disorder or epilepsy

Associated adverse consequences of the SRRMs is required to make the diagnosis of SRRMD and include interference with normal sleep, daytime sleepiness or sleep disturbance, and bodily injury to the patient (or potential bodily injury if preventive measures were not taken). If clinical consequences of the rhythmic movements are absent, the rhythmic movements are simply noted and the term RMD not used.

Several clinical subtypes of RMD are noted including body rocking type, head banging type, head rolling type, and combined type. An example of body rocking is visible in Video 15.3. As the patient did not report associated dysfunction this is simply sleep related rhythmic movements (no disorder). An example of head rocking is visible in Video 15.4. In this case the patient reported associated insomnia and believed the movements to actually prevent sleep onset. Head banging may occur when the individual is prone and lifts head and forcefully bangs head against pillow or mattress (Video 15.5). Episodes often occur near sleep onset but can occur at any time during the night and even during quiet wakeful activities such as listening to music or traveling in a car. Children are generally amnestic for the activities; adults may be aware and have a volitional component ("it helps me relax"). According to ICSD-3-TR1, at 9 months 59% of all infants have been reported to exhibit one or more of body rocking, head banging, or head rolling. The prevalence decreases to 33% at 18 months and by 5 years to only 5%. *In children there is no gender predominance, but in adults a male predominance has been reported.*[1]

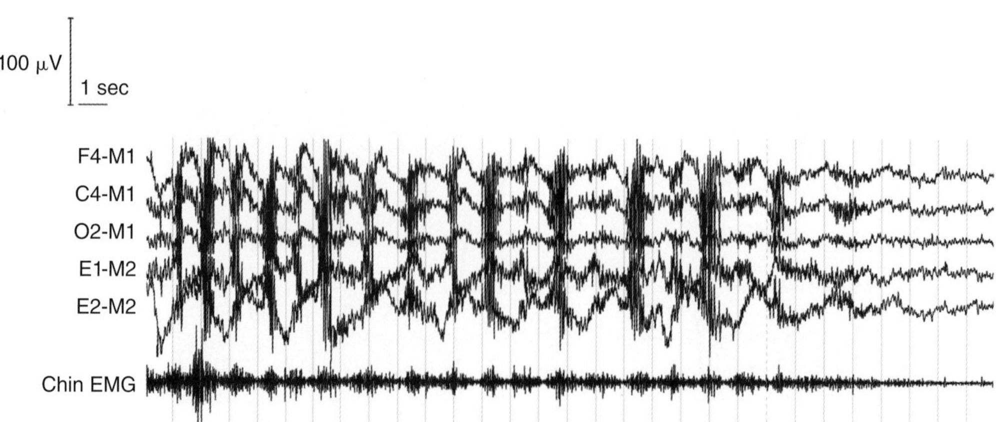

Figure 15–13 A 30-second tracing of an episode of bruxism. Loud tooth griding noise was heard. In this figure EMG artifact is more prominent in the EEG and EOG electrodes than the rhythmic activity (brief elevations) in the Chin EMG. (Adapted from Berry RB, Wagner MH. *Sleep Medicine Pearls.* 3rd ed. Elsevier; 2015:175.)

PSG Findings in RM

Video-PSG studies have shown RM to occur most often in association in stages N1 and N2. However, approximately (46%) occur while falling asleep, 30% during both NREM and REM sleep, and 24% occur only during REM sleep.[1,2,30-33] The literature concerning RM varies with some references stating that RMs occur at sleep-wake transitions, whereas others state that RMs are more common in stage N2. In some patients, RMs occur primarily during sleep-wake transitions. In most patients, the EEG shows normal activity between episodes of rhythmic behavior (although often obscured by movement artifact).

A summary of the AASM scoring manual[2] criteria for scoring RMs includes:

- Frequency of movements is between 0.5 and 2.0 Hz
- At least four movements must be present to define a cluster of RMs
- The minimum amplitude of individual bursts is twice the background EMG activity

An example of sleep-related rhythmic movements is shown in Figure 15–14. The scoring manual recommends that bipolar surface electrodes be placed to record large muscle group involvement (Fig. 15–12). However, time-synchronized video PSG is necessary to make the diagnosis of RMD. For most patients, no treatment for SRRMD is needed. In others with violent movements, bed padding may be necessary. In some studies, an association between RMD and attention deficit hyperactivity disorder has been found in school-age children. The RMD can persist into adulthood[32] and was associated with a group of patients with obstructive sleep apnea in one publication.[33]

PROPRIOSPINAL MYOCLONUS AND HYPNIC JERKS

Propriospinal myoclonus (PSM) consists of sudden jerks mainly of the abdomen, trunk, and neck.[1,34-36] These occur during relaxed wakefulness in the recumbent position during the period before sleep onset. They are inhibited by mental activity and disappear upon the onset of stable sleep. PSM are included in this chapter although the AASM scoring manual does not provide rules for detecting these events.

The ICSD-3-TR1 diagnostic criteria for PSM are as follows:

- The patient complaints of sudden jerks, mainly of the abdomen, trunk, and neck.
- The jerks appear during relaxed wakefulness and drowsiness as the patient attempts to fall asleep.
- The jerks disappear upon mental activity and with onset of stable sleep stage.
- The jerks result in difficulty in initiating sleep.
- The jerks are not better explained by another sleep disorder, medical or neurological disorder, mental disorder, medication use, or substance disorder.

PSM can be associated with sleep onset insomnia. A characteristic pattern is initial central muscle activation with spread rostrally and caudally. Sleep monitoring including the monitoring of the EMG of multiple muscles has demonstrated propagation of muscle activation starting in the abdominal muscles and spreading to upper and lower extremity muscles. The best treatment for PSM is not known but has included clonazepam in some series.

Hypnic jerks (sleep starts) are sudden, brief, simultaneous contractions of the body or one or more body segments

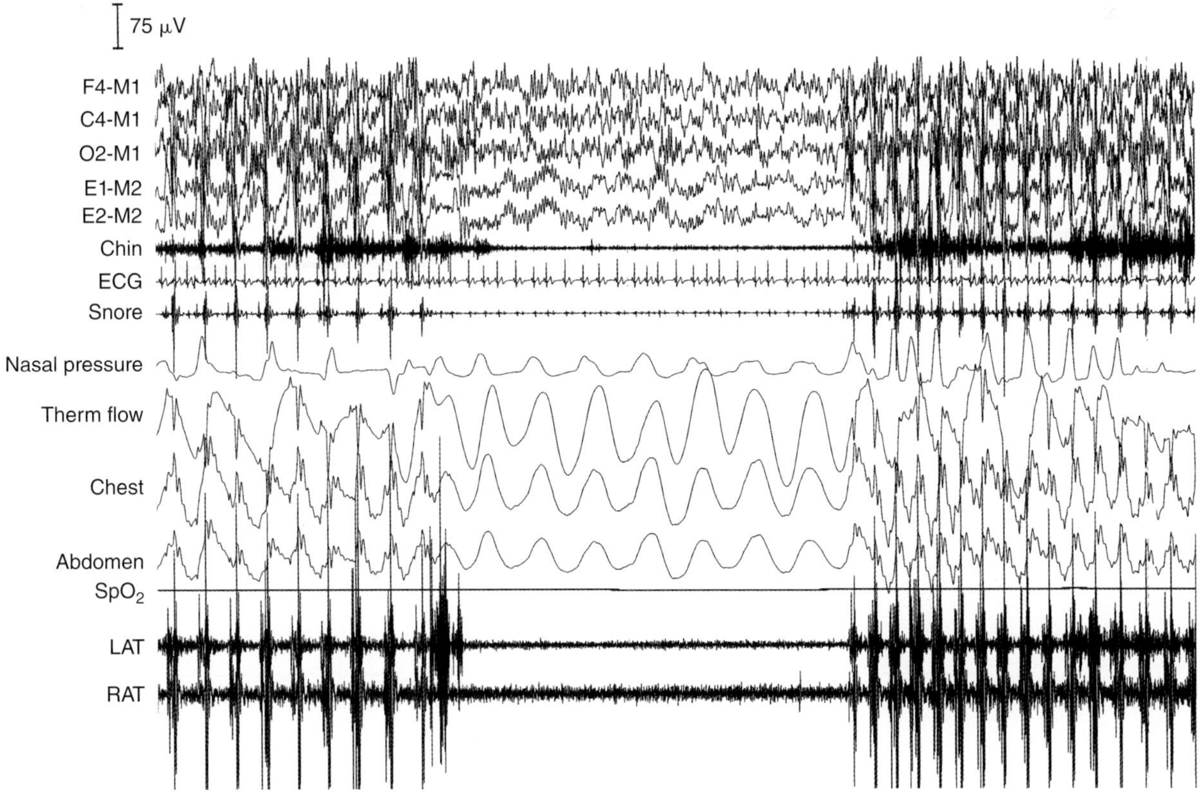

Figure 15–14 A 30-second tracing of a 5-year-old child exhibiting head-banging. This episode appears to occur during sleep. As the child complained of head tenderness in the morning, this was considered to be a manifestation of a sleep-related rhythmic movement disorder. (see Video 15.5).

occurring at sleep onset. The jerk is often associated with a sensation of falling. Hypnic jerks are differentiated from PSM, which *can be prominent while the patient is still awake* and will be abolished by mental activity. Hypnic jerks are very common and rarely cause an issue.

BENIGN SLEEP MYOCLONUS OF INFANCY (BSMI)

BSMI will rarely be encountered in the sleep center unless very young infants are being monitored. The phenomenon consists of jerks involving limbs, trunk, or the entire body that occur *only during sleep*.[1,37] This condition is noted in early infancy, typically from birth to 6 months of age. The movements stop abruptly when the infant is aroused. BSMI is relatively rare and benign but can be confused with epilepsy. Unlike the jerks of myoclonic seizures and myoclonic encephalopathy, *the jerks of BSMI occur only during sleep*. The jerks are typically bilateral and very significant typically involve large muscle groups.

Summary of BSMI characteristics[1]:

- Repetitive myoclonic jerks that involve the limbs, trunk, or whole body
- The movements occur in early infancy, typically from birth to 6 months of age
- *The movements occur only during sleep*
- The movements stop abruptly and consistently when the infant is aroused
- The disorder is not better explained by another sleep disorder, medical or neurological disorder, or medication use

SCORING REM WITHOUT ATONIA(RWA)

A diagnosis of the REM sleep behavior disorder (RBD) requires PSG evidence of RWA and either a video PSG showing dream-enacting behavior or compatible clinical history of episodes of dream-enacting behavior.[1] The REM sleep behavior disorder is discussed in detail in Chapter 36. Several video examples of RBD are included in chapter 36. RWA can occur as an isolated finding without a history of dream enactment, associated with narcolepsy, or associated with certain medications such as selective serotonin reuptake inhibitors or serotonin and norepinephrine reuptake inhibitors.[4,5,38-42] Investigations of the activity of various muscles in patients with the REM sleep behavior disorder have demonstrated the value of monitoring additional muscles aside from the chin and leg EMG.[4,5] Various criteria have been used to identify REM sleep without atonia.[4,5,41,42] The AASM scoring manual has recommended rules for scoring RWA, but scoring RWA is optional.[2] **Excessive sustained muscle activity** (tonic activity) in REM sleep is scored when an epoch of stage R has at least 50% of the epoch with a **chin EMG amplitude** at least two times greater than the stage R atonia level or the lowest amplitude in NREM sleep, if no stage R atonia is present. Multiple chin EMG segments may contribute to the total duration, but each segment must be *greater than 5 seconds*. An example of sustained chin EMG activity during stage R is shown in Figure 15–15. **Excessive transient muscle activity** (phasic activity) is present when at least five 3-second mini-epochs contain bursts of transient muscle **activity in the chin or limb EMG.** That is, a 30-second epoch is divided into 10 sequential mini-epochs each 3 seconds in duration. In RWA, excessive transient muscle activity bursts **are 0.1 to 5 seconds in duration** and at least *two times as high in amplitude* as the stage R atonia level (or lowest amplitude in NREM, if no stage R atonia is present). Although sustained activity tends to have a fairly constant amplitude (sustained) and transient activity has a pattern varying in amplitude ("spiky"), the designation of sustained or transient is based on the *duration of the bursts*. Sometimes it is difficult to determine if the chin EMG increased activity meets criteria for sustained versus phasic activity as determining the duration of an episode of EMG activity is often difficult. Some epochs contain episodes of continuous increased chin activity greater than

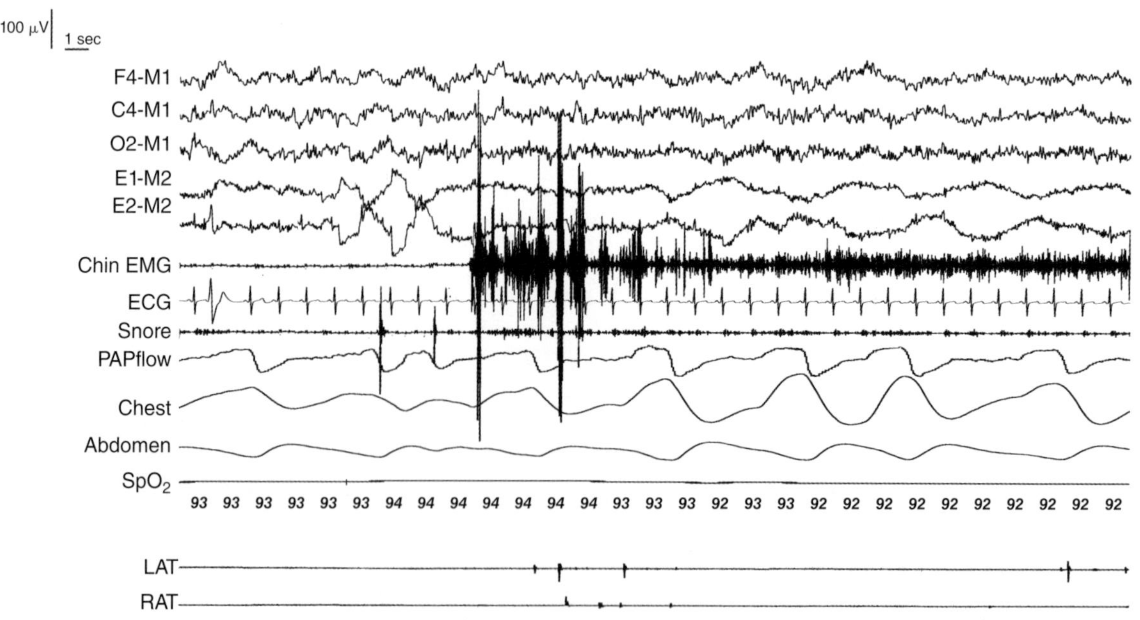

Figure 15–15 A 30-second tracing of an epoch of REM sleep without atonia associated with excessive sustained chin EMG activity for more than 50% of the epoch (requirement is at least 50% of the epoch).

5 seconds (not considered transient muscle activity), but the total duration of the episodes is less than 15 seconds (epoch does not qualify as having excessive sustained activity chin EMG activity). For these reasons a third category has been used. **"Any chin activity"** is defined as chin EMG activity with a minimum amplitude two times greater than the stage R atonia level (or lowest amplitude in NREM sleep if no stage R atonia is present) **without regard to duration of activity** (including bursts from 5 to 15 seconds). Based on these definitions, an *epoch is scored as exhibiting RWA* when one of the following is present:

1. Excessive sustained **chin EMG** activity as defined previously
2. Excessive transient muscle activity in **chin or limb leads** as defined previously
3. At least 50% of the 3-second mini-epochs contain **any chin EMG activity** (minimum amplitude ≥ 2 REM atonia level without regard for duration of activity) or **limb EMG activity** (bursts of 0.1–5 seconds in duration and at least two times as high in amplitude as the stage R atonia level, or the lowest amplitude in NREM if no stage R atonia is present).

The rules for scoring RWA are summarized in Figure 15–16. An example of an epoch with RWA is shown in Figure 15–17. As previously discussed, use of upper extremity EMG monitoring may reveal RWA not present in the chin or leg EMG. Figure 15–18 is an example of an epoch with transient

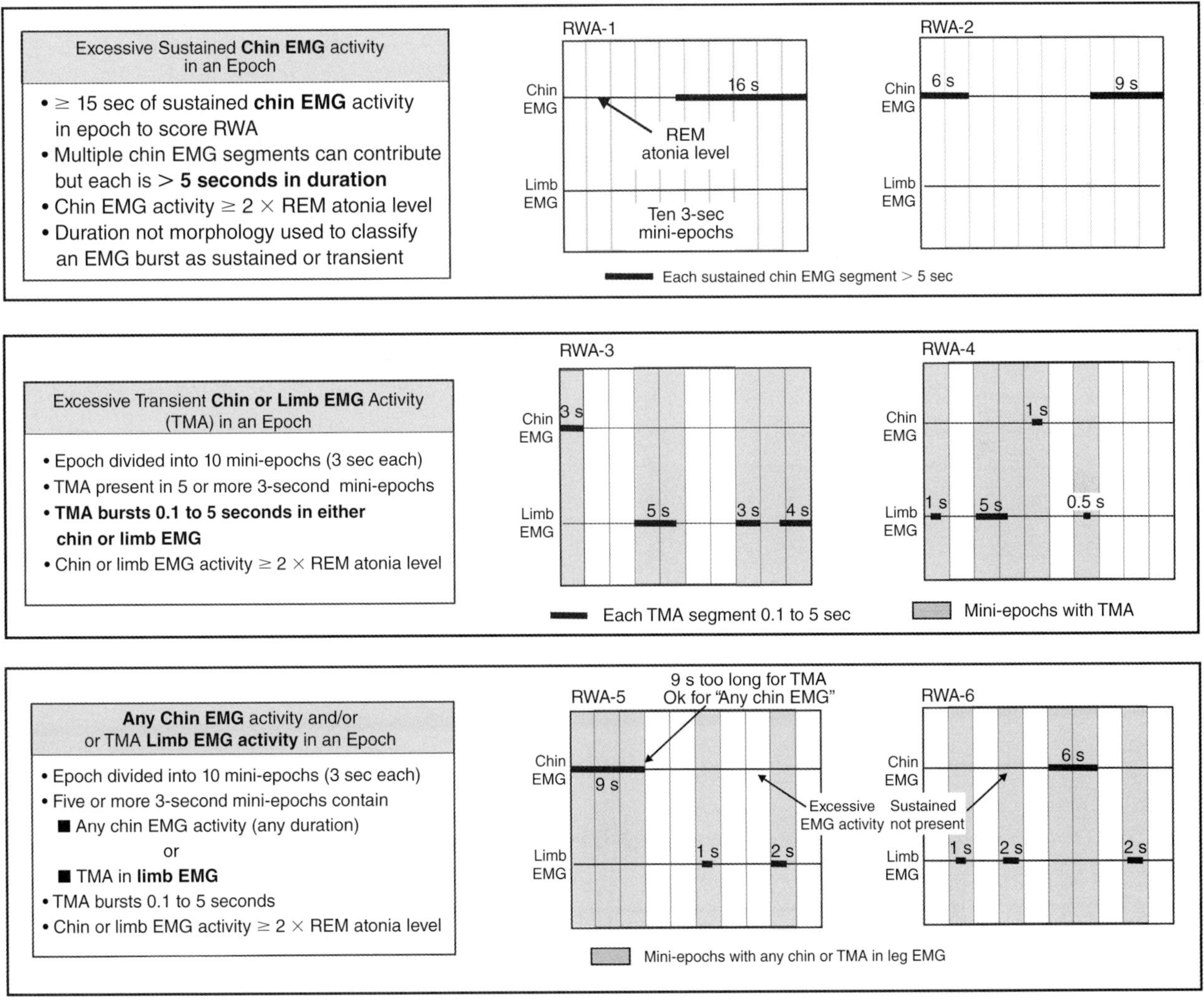

Figure 15–16 A figure summarizing the rules for scoring REM sleep without atonia (RWA). Schematic examples for each of the three categories illustrate the rules. In RWA-1 and RWA-2 excessive sustained chin EMG activity is illustrated. RWA can be scored if 50% or more (≥ 15 seconds) has sustained chin EMG activity during stage R. Each segment must be > 5 seconds in duration. In RWA-3 and RWA-4 excesive transient muscle activity (TMA) in the chin and limb EMG is present. Note that each segment of TMA must be 0.1 to 5 seconds in duration. The 30 second epoch is divided into 10 sequential 3-second mini-epochs. In RWA-3 six 3-sec mini-epochs contain TMA in the chin or leg EMG and in RWA-4 five 3-sec mini-epochs contain TMA in the chin or leg EMG. Therefore both epochs meet criteria for RWA. None of the segments of TMA exceeds 5 seconds in duration. Note that the 4 second segment of TMA in RWA-3 is present in the very last part of the ninth and all of the tenth 3-second mini-epoch. In RWA-5 and RWA-6 scoring RWA based on "any chin EMG activity" and TMA in the limb EMG is illustrated. In RWA-5 the 9 second segment of increased chin EMG activity is too long to qualify as TMA. On the other hand sustained chin EMG is present for only 9 of the 15 seconds needed to score excessive sustained EMG acitivity. However, the 9 seconds qualifies as "any chin EMG activity". There are 5 mini-epochs with either "any chin EMG activity" or TMA in the limb EMG. In RWA-6 the 6 second chin EMG burst is too long for TMA but qualifies and "any chin EMG activity".

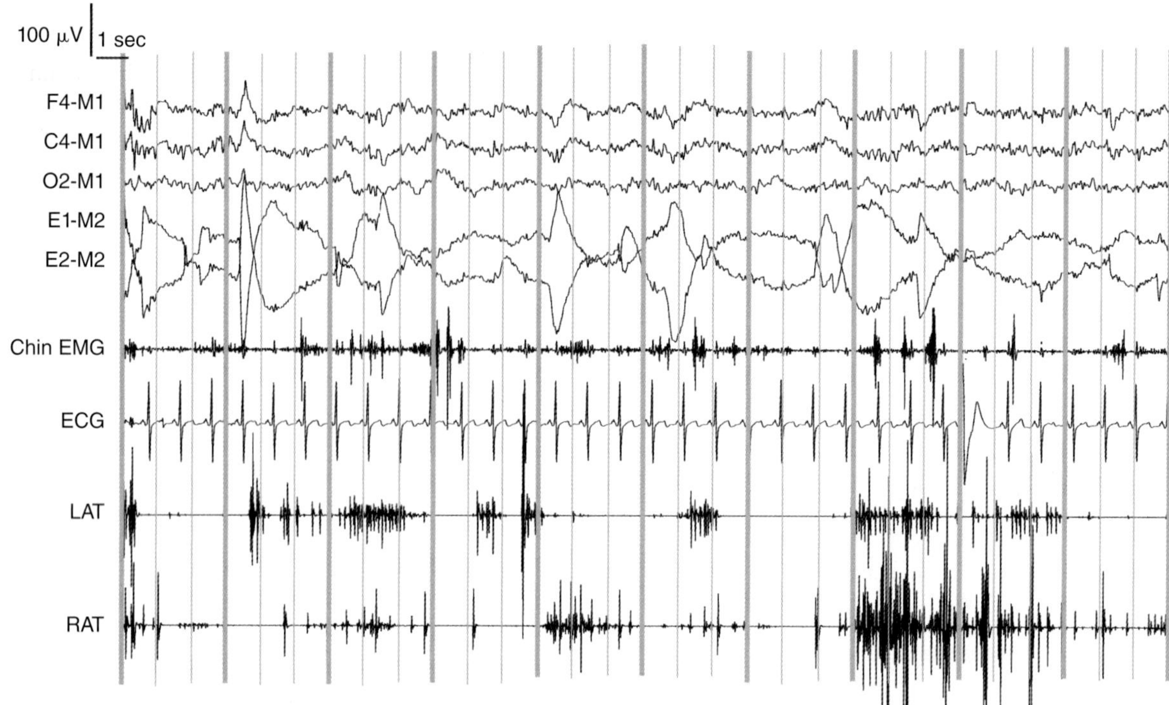

Figure 15–17 A 30-second tracing divided into 10 3-second mini-epochs. Every 3-second mini-epoch contains either "any chin EMG activity" or transient LAT or RAT activity. Therefore, the epoch qualifies as one having REM sleep without atonia. *If reporting REM sleep without atonia it is important to specify which limb muscles were monitored.*

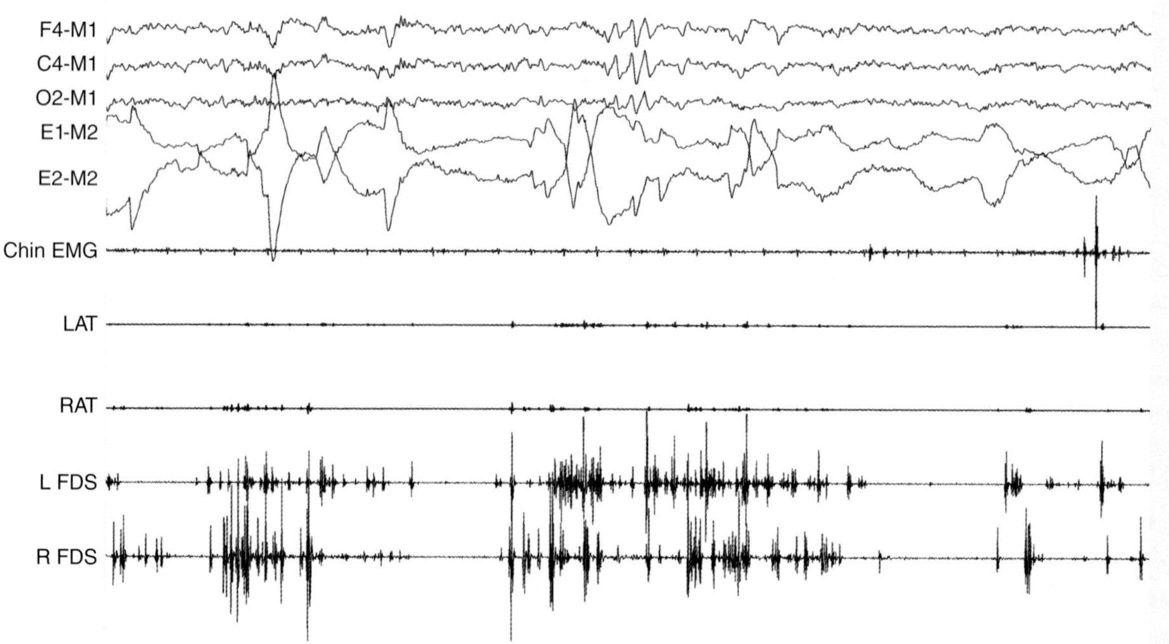

Figure 15–18 A 30-second epoch illustrating minimal activity in the chin and leg EMG channels but significant activity in the left and right flexor digitorum superficialis (FDS) EMGs. When monitoring for possible RBD, including arm EMG monitoring may increase the epochs containing REM sleep without atonia. *If reporting REM sleep without atonia, it is important to specify which limb muscles were monitored.*

muscle activity in the arm EMG (flexor digitorum superficialis) with minimal activity in the chin and legs. It is worth noting that in patients with RBD, epochs can be scored as stage R in the absence of low chin EMG when they otherwise meet criteria for stage R. At times it may be difficult to determine if a patient is awake or asleep in some epochs based on REMs and an elevated chin EMG activity. Looking at the video and observing closed eyelids and the presence of transient muscle activity in the limb EMG is evidence for stage R. When questionable epochs are contiguous with epochs with stage R and typical atonia, this also favors that the questionable epoch is in fact stage R. Finally video evidence of what appears to be dream enactment with the eyes closed is evidence of stage R even if the EMG activity is not low.

The AASM scoring manual provides criteria to determine if a given epoch has sufficient activity in the chin and limb EMGs during REM sleep to be classified as REM sleep without atonia. The REM sleep atonia index (RWAI) is the percentage of stage R epochs that meet criteria for RWA (scoring RWA and reporting a RWAI is optional). However, the RWA index that is considered abnormal (sufficient to support a diagnosis of RBD) is not specified. Studies addressing this issue are discussed in detail in Chapter 36. It is important to note that polysomnographic demonstration of a significant number of epochs with RWA is NOT equivalent to a diagnosis of RBD in the absence of supporting clinical information or video evidence of dream enactment.

SUMMARY OF KEY POINTS

1. The criteria for a candidate leg movement (candidate for inclusion in a PLMS series, that is, a PLM) is a duration of 0.5 to 10 seconds and an amplitude ≥ 8 μV above the baseline EMG for at least 0.5 seconds.
2. The period length from one candidate LM in a PLMS series to the next is 5 to 90 seconds (measured onset to onset). The minimum number of LMs to define a PLMS series is four.
3. Candidate LMs on different legs separated by less than 5 seconds (onset to onset) are considered to be a single LM. The onset of the first, LM in the group is considered to be the onset of the combined LM.
4. LMs from 0.5 seconds before to 0.5 seconds after an apnea, hypopnea, or RERA are not scored (not included in a PLMS series).
5. An arousal and an LM are considered associated if they overlap, are simultaneous, or if the time between the end of one and the beginning of the other is less than 0.5 second irrespective of which comes first.
6. The sleep-related rhythmic movement disorder requires a PSG with synchronized video and audio for a reliable diagnosis. The word "disorder" implies some associated dysfunction.
7. Bruxism can occur in any sleep stage or wakefulness but is most common in stages N1 and N2. Polysomnography is not required for a clinical diagnosis of bruxism but is useful if it includes synchronized video and audio recording.
8. Although the AASM scoring manual provides scoring criteria for bruxism based on the chin EMG activity, the muscle artifact in the EEG and EOG derivations may be more prominent (overlying scalp muscles activated during bruxism episodes). Recording of the masseter EMG is optional but will also show greater activity than the chin EMG during bruxism episodes.
9. The AASM scoring manual states that "bruxism can be scored reliably by time synchronized video and audio in combination with polysomnography by a minimum of two audible tooth grinding episodes per night of polysomnography in the absence of associated epileptic discharges."
10. The nomenclature of sleep-related leg cramps has been changed to nocturnal muscle cramps in the latest edition of the ICSD-3 (ICSD-3-TR).
11. Scoring REM sleep without atonia (RWA) is optional in the AASM scoring manual. However, criteria for scoring an epoch as demonstrating RWA are provided.
12. An *epoch is scored as exhibiting RWA* when one of the following is present:
    a. Excessive sustained **chin** EMG activity (as defined below)
    b. Excessive transient muscle activity in **chin or limb leads (as defined below)**
    c. At least 50% of the 3-second-mini-epochs contain **any chin EMG activity** or **limb EMG activity** (bursts of 0.1 - 5 seconds in duration and at least two times as high in amplitude as the stage R atonia level, or the lowest amplitude in NREM if no stage R atonia is present).
    - **Excessive sustained muscle activity** (tonic activity) in REM sleep is scored when an epoch of stage R has at least 50% of the epoch (≥15 seconds) with a **chin EMG amplitude** at least two times greater than the stage R atonia level or the lowest amplitude in NREM sleep if no stage R atonia is present. *Multiple segments may contribute to the total duration, but each segment must be* ***greater*** *than 5 seconds in duration.*
    - **Excessive transient muscle activity** (phasic activity) is present when at least five 3-second mini-epochs contain bursts of transient muscle **activity in the chin or limb EMG.** That is, a 30-second epoch is divided into 10 sequential mini-epochs each 3 seconds in duration. In RWA, excessive transient muscle activity bursts **are 0.1 to 5 seconds in duration** and at least two times as high in amplitude as the stage R atonia level (or lowest amplitude in NREM, if no stage R atonia is present).
    - **"Any chin activity"** is defined as activity in the chin EMG with a minimum amplitude two times greater than the stage R atonia level (or lowest amplitude in NREM sleep if no stage R atonia is present) without regard to the duration of activity (including bursts from 5 to 15 seconds).

CLINICAL REVIEW QUESTIONS

1. Frequent LMs during wake as documented by the anterior tibial derivations is most suggestive of
   A. PLMD.
   B. PLMS.
   C. RLS.
2. The duration of a candidate LM is
   A. 0.5 to 5 seconds.
   B. 0.5 to 10 seconds.
   C. 1 to 10 seconds.
   D. 0.5 to 15 seconds.
3. According to the AASM scoring manual, the minimum amplitude of a candidate LM is
   A. ≥8 μV above baseline limb EMG activity for at least 0.5 seconds.
   B. ≥8 μV above baseline limb EMG activity of any duration.
   C. ≥10 μV above baseline limb EMG activity of any duration.
   D. ≥10 μV above baseline limb EMG activity for at least 0.5 seconds.
4. LMs on different legs are considered to be a combined LM if the time from onset of the first until the onset of the second is
   A. Equal to or less than 5 seconds.
   B. Less than 5 seconds.
   C. Equal to or less than 10 seconds.
   D. Less than 10 seconds.
5. According to the AASM scoring manual, the time between onsets of consecutive LMs in a PLMS series must be
   A. 10 to 90 seconds.
   B. 5 to 90 seconds.
   C. 5 to 120 seconds.
   D. 10 to 120 seconds.

6. A diagnosis of EFM requires that fragmentary myoclonus be present for at least
   A. 20 minutes of REM sleep.
   B. 10 minutes of NREM sleep.
   C. 20 minutes of NREM sleep.
   D. 10 minutes of REM sleep.
7. A diagnosis of the sleep related rhythmic movement disorder (SRRMD) requires that
   A. Movements must occur during sleep.
   B. Behaviors result in a significant complaint (impaired daytime function, bodily injury, interference with normal sleep).
   C. At least five movements in a cluster must be present.
   D. The minimum frequency of movements is 3 Hz.
8. In which of the following is the use of synchronized video and audio NOT recommended for evaluation?
   A. PLMS
   B. Sleep-related rhythmic disorder
   C. REM sleep behavior disorder
   D. Bruxism
9. What is the minimum number of LMs to define a PLMS series?
   A. Two LMs
   B. Three LMs
   C. Four LMs
   D. Five LMs
10. In Figure 15–19, how many PLMs are noted?
11. In Figure 15–20, what type of leg EMG activity is shown?
12. In Figure 15–21, what type of leg EMG activity is present?
13. Does the epoch in Figure 15–22 meet criteria for REM sleep without atonia?

ANSWERS

1. C
2. B
3. A
4. B

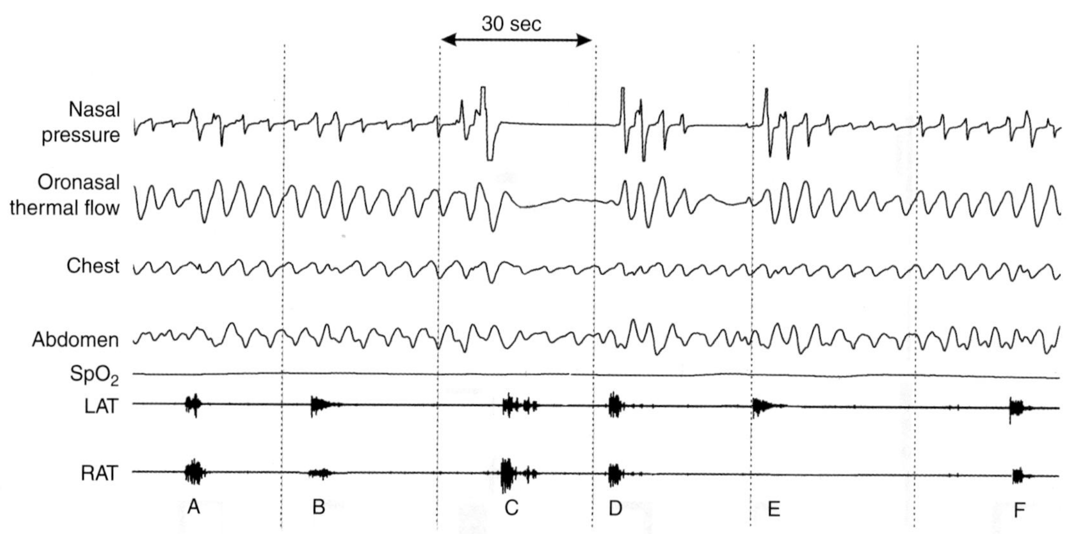

Figure 15–19 This is a 180-second tracing. LAT and RAT are right and left anterior tibial EMG. How many PLMs are shown? (Adapted from Berry RB, Wagner MH. *Sleep Medicine Pearls.* 3rd ed. Elsevier; 2015:174.)

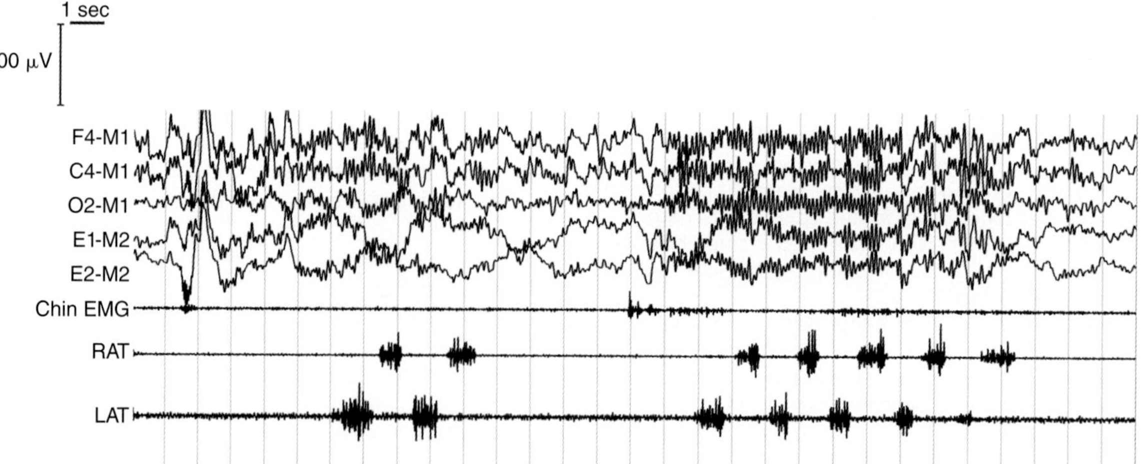

Figure 15–20 This is a 30-second epoch. What leg movement activity is noted. LAT and RAT are the left and right anterior tibial EMG channels. (Adapted from Berry RB, Wagner MH. *Sleep Medicine Pearls.* 3rd ed. Elsevier; 2015:174.)

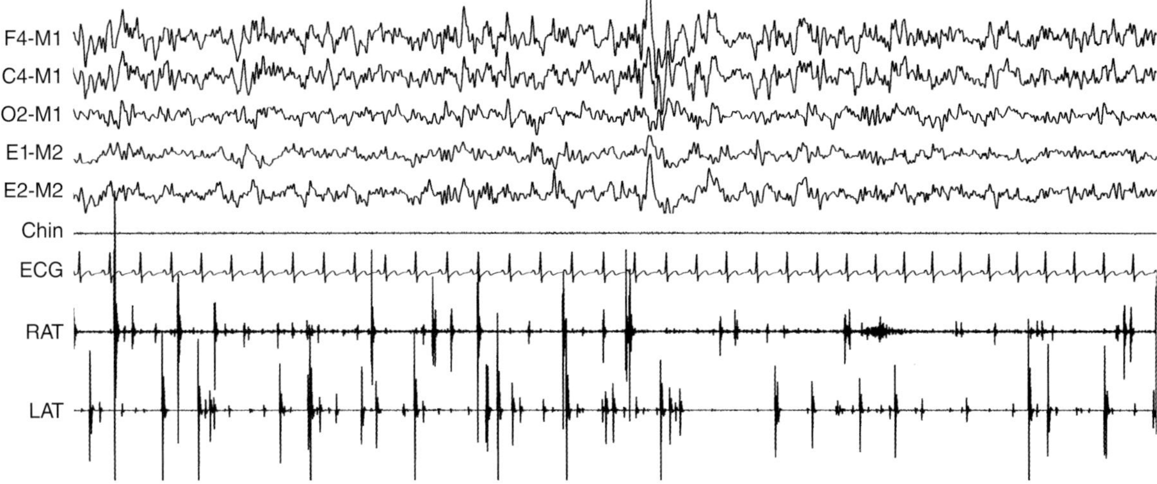

Figure 15–21 A 30-second tracing of NREM sleep. What leg movement activity is shown?

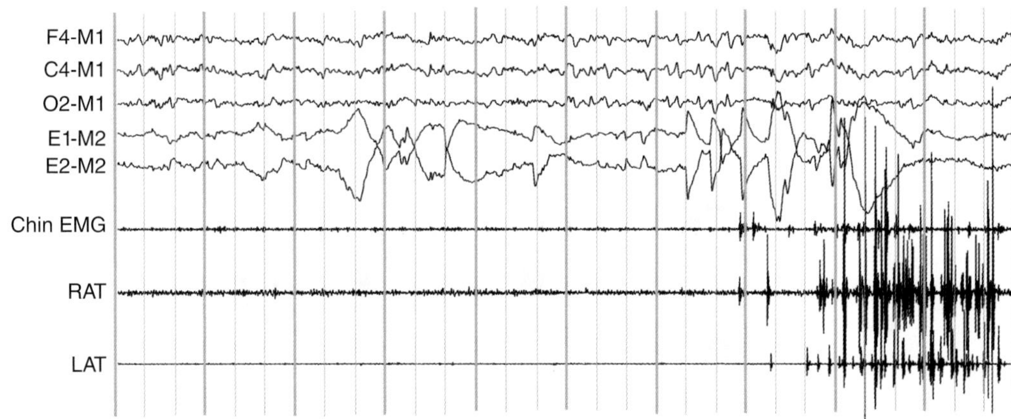

Figure 15–22 Does this 30-second epoch meet criteria for REM sleep without atonia?

5. B
6. C
7. B. A disorder requires a significant complaint including interference of sleep, impairment of daytime function, or self-inflicted injury (or injury if preventive measures are not taken). The minimum number of movements in a cluster is four, and the minimum frequency is 0.5 Hz (movement every 2 seconds).
8. A. Synchronized video/audio is essential for evaluation of bruxism, RBD, and the SRRMD.
9. C. 4 LMs.
10. Three LMs qualify for inclusion in a PLMS series (are PLMs). LMs at C, D, and E are not included in the PLMS series as they occur in the period from 0.5 seconds before an apnea to 0.5 seconds after an apnea. The LMs at A, B, and F are each considered to be one PLM as they occurred simultaneously (therefore three LMs qualify for inclusion in the PLMS series).
11. Alternating Leg Muscle Activation (ALMA). The EMG bursts occur during wakefulness and sleep and the time duration onset to onset is about 1 seconds (frequency about 1 Hz). The duration between LMs that are part of a PLMS series is 5 to 90 seconds.
12. Excessive fragmentary myoclonus
13. Not quite: only four mini-epochs (3 seconds each) contain any chin EMG activity or leg EMG activity twice the REM atonia level.

SUGGESTED READING

American Academy of Sleep Medicine. *International Classification of Sleep Disorders*. 3rd ed. text revision. American Academy of Sleep Medicine; 2023.

Frauscher B, Iranzo A, Gaig C, et al; SINBAR (Sleep Innsbruck Barcelona) Group. Normative EMG values during REM sleep for the diagnosis of REM sleep behavior disorder. *Sleep*. 2012;35(6):835-847.

Troester MM, Quan SF, Berry RB, et al; for the American Academy of Sleep Medicine. *The AASM Manual for the Scoring of Sleep and Associated Events: Rules, Terminology and Technical Specifications*. Version 3. American Academy of Sleep Medicine; 2023.

REFERENCES

1. American Academy of Sleep Medicine. *International Classification of Sleep Disorders*. 3rd ed. text revision. American Academy of Sleep Medicine; 2023.
2. Troester MM, Quan SF, Berry RB, et al; for the American Academy of Sleep Medicine. *The AASM Manual for the Scoring of Sleep and Associated Events: Rules, Terminology and Technical Specifications*. Version 3. American Academy of Sleep Medicine; 2023.
3. Walters AS, Lavigne G, Hening W, et al. The scoring of movements in sleep. *J Clin Sleep Med*. 2007;3:155-167.

4. Frauscher B, Iranzo A, Högl B, et al. Quantification of electromyographic activity during REM sleep in multiple muscles in REM sleep behavior disorder. *Sleep*. 2008;31(5):724-731.
5. Frauscher B, Iranzo A, Gaig C, et al. Normative EMG values during REM sleep for the diagnosis of REM sleep behavior disorder. *Sleep*. 2012;35(6):835-847.
6. Zucconi M, Ferri R, Allen R, et al. International Restless Legs Syndrome Study Group (IRLSSG). The official World Association of Sleep Medicine (WASM) standards for recording and scoring periodic leg movements in sleep (PLMS) and wakefulness (PLMW) developed in collaboration with a task force from the International Restless Legs Syndrome Study Group (IRLSSG). *Sleep Med*. 2006; 7(2):175-183.
7. Ferri R, Fulda S, Allen RP, et al. International and European Restless Legs Syndrome Study Groups (IRLSSG and EURLSSG). World Association of Sleep Medicine (WASM) 2016 standards for recording and scoring leg movements in polysomnograms developed by a joint task force from the International and the European Restless Legs Syndrome Study Groups (IRLSSG and EURLSSG). *Sleep Med*. 2016;26:86-95.
8. Ferri R, Zucconi M, Manconi M. New approaches to the study of periodic leg movements during sleep in restless legs syndrome. *Sleep*. 2006;29(6):759-769.
9. Manconi M, Ferri R, Feroah TR. Defining the boundaries of the response of sleep leg movements to a single dose of dopamine agonist. *Sleep*. 2008;31(9):1229-1237.
10. Manconi M, Zavalko I, Bassetti CL, et al. Respiratory-related leg movements and their relationship with periodic leg movements during sleep. *Sleep*. 2014;37(3):497-504.
11. Manconi M, Zavalko I, Fanfulla F. An evidence-based recommendation for a new definition of respiratory-related leg movements. *Sleep*. 2015;38(2):295-304.
12. Chokroverty S, Bhat S, Gupta D. Respiratory-related leg movements vs periodic limb movements in sleep: a scoring conundrum. an editorial. *Sleep Med*. 2021;81:98-100.
13. Montplaisir J, Boucher S, Nicolas A. Immobilization tests and periodic leg movements in sleep for the diagnosis of restless leg syndrome. *Mov Disord*. 1998;13(2):324-329.
14. Pennestri MH, Whittom S, Adam B. PLMS and PLMW in healthy subjects as a function of age: prevalence and interval distribution. *Sleep*. 2006;29(9):1183-1187.
15. Montplasir J, Boucher S, Poirer G, et al. Clinical, polysomnographic, and genetic characteristics of restless legs syndrome: a study of 133 patients diagnosed with the new standard criteria. *Mov Disord*. 1997;12:61-65.
16. Chervin RD, Consens FB, Kutluay E. Alternating leg muscle activation during sleep and arousals: a new sleep-related motor phenomenon? *Mov Disord*. 2003;18(5):551-559.
17. Berry RB. A woman with rhythmic foot movements. *J Clin Sleep Med*. 2007;3(7):749-751.
18. Cosentino FI, Iero I, Lanuzza B, Tripodi M, Ferri R. The neurophysiology of the alternating leg muscle activation (ALMA) during sleep: study of one patient before and after treatment with pramipexole. *Sleep Med*. 2006;7(1):63-71.
19. Bergmann M, Stefani A, Brandauer E, et al. Hypnagogic foot tremor, alternating leg muscle activation or high frequency leg movements: clinical and phenomenological considerations in two cousins. *Sleep Med*. 2019;54:177-180.
20. Yang C, Winkelman JW. Clinical and polysomnographic characteristics of high frequency leg movements. *J Clin Sleep Med*. 2010;6(5):431-438.
21. Broughton R, Tolentino MA, Krelina M. Excessive fragmentary myoclonus in NREM sleep: a report of 38 cases. *Electroencephalogr Clin Neurophysiol*. 1985;6:123-133.
22. Vetrugno R, Piazzi G, Provini F, et al. Excessive fragmentary hypnic myoclonus: clinical and neurophysiological findings. *Sleep Med*. 2001;3:73-76.
23. Nepozitek J, Dostalova S, Kemlink D, et al. Fragmentary myoclonus in idiopathic rapid eye movement sleep behaviour disorder. *J Sleep Res*. 2019;28(4):e12819.
24. Hallegraeff J, de Greef M, Krijnen W, van der Schans C. Criteria in diagnosing nocturnal leg cramps: a systematic review. *BMC Fam Pract*. 2017;18(1):29.
25. Garrison SR, Korownyk CS, Kolber MR, et al. Magnesium for skeletal muscle cramps. *Cochrane Database Syst Rev*. 2020;9(9):CD009402.
26. Barna O, Lohoida P, Holovchenko Y, et al. A randomized, double-blind, placebo-controlled, multicenter study assessing the efficacy of magnesium oxide monohydrate in the treatment of nocturnal leg cramps. *Nutr J*. 2021;20(1):90.
27. Winkleman JW. *Nocturnal Leg Cramps*. UpToDate. Available at: https://www.uptodate.com/contents/nocturnal-leg-cramps?search=nocturnal%20leg%20cramps§ionRank=1&usage_type=default&anchor=H74260295&source=machineLearning&selectedTitle=1,16&display_rank=1#H74260295. Accessed August 29, 2023.
28. Beddis H, Pemberton M, Davies S. Sleep bruxism: an overview for clinicians. *Br Dent J*. 2018;225(6):497-501.
29. Kuang B, Li D, Lobbezoo F, et al. Associations between sleep bruxism and other sleep-related disorders in adults: a systematic review. *Sleep Med*. 2022;89:31-47.
30. Kohyama J, Matsukura F, Kimura K, Tachibana N. Rhythmic movement disorder: polysomnographic study and summary of reported cases. *Brain Dev*. 2002;24(1):33-38.
31. Mayer G, Wilde-Frenz J, Kurella B. Sleep related rhythmic movement disorder revisited. *J Sleep Res*. 2007;16(1):110-116.
32. Stepanova I, Nevsimalova S, Hanusova J. Rhythmic movement disorder in sleep persisting into childhood and adulthood. *Sleep*. 2005;28(7): 851-857.
33. Chiaro G, Maestri M, Riccardi S, et al. Sleep-related rhythmic movement disorder and obstructive sleep apnea in five adult patients. *J Clin Sleep Med*. 2017;13(10):1213-1217.
34. Baldelli L, Provini F. Fragmentary hypnic myoclonus and other isolated motor phenomena of sleep. *Sleep Med Clin*. 2021;16(2):349-361.
35. Vetrugno R, Montagna P. Sleep-to-wake transition movement disorders. *Sleep Med*. 2011;12(suppl 2):S11-S16.
36. Antelmi E, Provini F. Propriospinal myoclonus: the spectrum of clinical and neurophysiological phenotypes. *Sleep Med Rev*. 2015;22:54-63.
37. Ghossein J, Pohl D. Benign spasms of infancy: a mimicker of infantile epileptic disorders. *Epileptic Disord*. 2019;21(6):585-589.
38. Khalil A, Wright MA, Walker MC, Eriksson SH. Loss of rapid eye movement sleep atonia in patients with REM sleep behavioral disorder, narcolepsy, and isolated loss of REM atonia. *J Clin Sleep Med*. 2013;9(10):1039-1048.
39. Ferri R, Aricò D, Cosentino FII, et al. REM sleep without atonia with REM sleep-related motor events: broadening the spectrum of REM sleep behavior disorder. *Sleep*. 2018;41(12).
40. Lee K, Baron K, Soca R, Attarian H. The prevalence and characteristics of REM sleep without atonia (RSWA) in patients taking antidepressants. *J Clin Sleep Med*. 2016;12(3):351-355.
41. Montplaisir J, Gagnon JF, Fantini ML, et al. Polysomnographic diagnosis of idiopathic REM sleep behavior disorder. *Mov Disord*. 2010;25(13): 2044-2051.
42. McCarter SJ, St Louis EK, Duwell EJ, et al. Diagnostic thresholds for quantitative REM sleep phasic burst duration, phasic and tonic muscle activity, and REM atonia index in REM sleep behavior disorder with and without comorbid obstructive sleep apnea. *Sleep*. 2014;37(10):1649-1662.

Polysomnography, Home Sleep Apnea Testing, and Actigraphy

Chapter 16

POLYSOMNOGRAPHY—PUTTING IT ALL TOGETHER

Previous chapters have discussed monitoring of sleep, respiration, cardiac rate and rhythm, and leg movements. Polysomnography (PSG) is the detailed monitoring of sleep and combines all these elements. Digital PSG systems provide the ability to record many more signals than during the era of paper recording. In Table 16–1 the commonly recorded parameters and purposes are displayed. Digital PSG systems allow one to view all or a portion of the parameters recorded. A channel is a horizontal display of a recorded parameter versus time. The number of channels displayed can be customized. Display time windows of 5, 10, 15, 30, 60, 90, 180, and 240 seconds are typically available. A 10-second window is used for clinical EEG, a 30-second window to stage sleep, and 60 to 300-second windows for viewing and scoring respiratory events or periodic limb movements in sleep (PLMS). Most PSG systems also allow two synchronized windows that can be set at different time windows. For example, channels related to sleep staging in a 30-second window and channels relating to respiration and leg movements in a 90- or 120-second window. The properties of each displayed channel including color, low and high frequency filters, sensitivity, channel

Table 16–1 Polysomnography—Recorded Signals

Parameter	Sensors	Purpose
EEG derivations	F4-M1, C4-M1, O2-M1 (Frontal, central, occipital)	Staging of Sleep
EOG derivations	E1-M2, E2-M2	
Chin EMG	Chin1, Chin2, ChinZ	
ECG	Electrocardiogram	Cardiac rate and rhythm
Airflow (diagnostic study)	Nasal pressure Oronasal thermal flow	Detection of hypopnea Detection of apnea
Airflow (PAP titration)	PAP device flow	Detection of apnea, hypopnea
Snoring	Microphone, piezoelectric sensor	Detection of snoring
Respiratory Effort	Chest and Abdominal RIP bands	Classify apneas as obstructive, mixed, or central
Arterial oxygen saturation (SpO_2)	Pulse Oximetry	Detect arterial oxygen desaturation
Left anterior tibial EMG (LAT)	EMG surface electrodes	Detect Periodic limb movements in sleep
Right anterior tibial EMG (RAT)	EMG surface electrodes	
Heart rate (HR)	Oximeter output	Moving time average estimate of pulse rate
PAP device pressure, leak, tidal volume	Signals from laboratory PAP device (flow and pressure sensors)	Monitor delivered pressure, leak, tidal volume
Optional		
Estimate of tidal volume	RIPsum	Alternate sensor for apnea and hypopnea
Estimate of airflow	RIPflow	Alternate sensor for apnea and hypopnea
Chest wall/diaphragmatic EMG	Right costal EMG electrodes	Detect inspiratory muscle firing (respiratory effort)
End-tidal PCO_2	Diagnostic study (recommended /**not optional in children**)	Detect hypoventilation
Transcutaneous PCO_2	Diagnostic and PAP titration	Detect hypoventilation
Display Window Information:		
Epoch number, Body position, Sleep Stage, CPAP level, oxygen flow rate (if applicable)	Watermark or in Display Window (Body position sensor can be used)	Body position and epoch number

LAT, Left anterior tibial; *PAP,* positive airway pressure; *RAT,* right anterior tibial; *RIP,* respiratory inductance plethysmography.

width, 60-Hz notch filter (on, off) can be changed. In some PSG systems turning on an ECG filter to remove ECG artifact is an option. Default channel properties and the signals to be displayed are saved in montages (sometimes called *workspaces* or *display views*). During review it is also possible to add or remove a signal from the current display view and rearrange the order of the channels. A typical diagnostic montage is shown as seen in a montage editor view in Table 16–2. The settings for each channel can be changed and the display view/montage saved with a specific name for use now and in the future when viewing other studies. As discussed in Chapter 2, a combination of referential, true bipolar, and direct current (DC) recording is used. In most systems the pulse rate is derived from oximetry data. The technology of recording respiratory signals is discussed in chapter 10. Both nasal pressure (without or without a square root transformation) and an oronasal thermal airflow signal are recorded to detect hypopnea and apnea, respectively. Respiratory inductance plethysmography (RIP) chest and abdominal effort belts (calibrated or uncalibrated) are used to detect respiratory effort. The RIPsum (deflections an estimate of tidal volume) is derived from the sum of RIPchest and RIP abdomen signals. The RIPflow (deflections an estimate of airflow) is the time derivative of the RIPsum. The RIPsum and RIPflow as discussed in Chapter 10 are not available on all PSG systems. Some systems use built-in software calibration of the RIPchest and RIPabdomen signal with the result that deflections in the RIPsum and RIPflow are better estimates of the tidal volume and flow. A pulse oximetry signal is used to record the arterial oxygen saturation (SpO_2). Modern PSG systems have an integrated oximeter with automatic calibration and the oximetry probe connects to the head box or bed side PSG amplifier. Low- and high-frequency filters can be applied to DC signals in some PSG systems. The nasal pressure is usually recorded as a DC signal but can be recorded as an AC signal using an appropriate low frequency filter setting (see chapter 10). A typical positive airway pressure (PAP) titration montage is shown in a montage editor view in Table 16–3. DC outputs from the laboratory PAP device including PAP flow (PAP device flow), PAP pressure, and PAP leak are usually recorded. Use of these signals will be discussed in Chapters 23 and 24. In addition to the above recorded parameters, the current epoch number, body position, time of night, the values of PAP and the oxygen flow rate (if applicable) are also displayed either at the bottom of the tracings or a part of a watermark. Some physicians use a montage displaying only the recommended EEG and EOG derivations with each displayed channel having the option to change to an alternative combination of referential electrodes if needed (Diagnostic 1, Table 16–4). Another typical option is to display all the recommended and alternative EEG derivations

Table 16–2 Diagnostic Montage

Channel		G1	G2	Low Filter (Hz)	High Filter (Hz)	Sensitivity* (μV/mm)	Channel Width 100 = default	Notch Filter	Color
1	**R**	F4	M1	0.3	35 Hz	7	100	Off	
2	**R**	C4	M1	0.3	35 Hz	7	100	Off	
3	**R**	O2	M1	0.3	35 Hz	7	100	Off	
4	**R**	F3	M2	0.3	35 Hz	7	100	Off	
3	**R**	C3	M2	0.3	35 Hz	7	100	Off	
5	**R**	O1	M2	0.3	35 Hz	7	100	Off	
6	**R**	E1	M2	0.3	35 Hz	7	100	Off	
7	**R**	E2	M2	0.3	35 Hz	7	100	Off	
8	**R**	Chin1	ChinZ	10	100	7	100	Off	
9	**BP**	ECG		0.3	100	7	100	Off	
10	**DC**	Heart rate (derived)		DC	DC	variable	100	Off	
11	**DC**	Nasal Pressure		None or ≤0.08***	DC or 100 Hz	variable	200	Off	
12	**BP**	Oronasal Thermal Flow		0.1	15	7	200	Off	
13	**BP**	Snoring		10	100	7	100	Off	
14	**BP**	Chest		0.1	15	7	200	Off	
15	**BP**	Abdomen		0.1	15	7	200	Off	
16	**DC**	SpO_2		DC	DC	Automatic cal**	200	Off	
17	**BP**	LAT		10	100	7	100	Off	
18	**BP**	RAT		10	100	7	100	Off	
19	**DC**	Capnogram		DC	DC	DC cal**	100	Off	
20	**DC**	P_{ETCO_2} value		DC	DC	DC cal**	100	Off	

*Sensitivity varies with PSG system, channel width is relative width.
G1, G2 inputs 1 and 2 for referential channels (derivation G1-G2 is displayed); DC calibration: end-tidal PCO_2 (0 to 1 v, 0 to 100 mm Hg).
BP, Bipolar channel; Bipolar channels each have 2 inputs (input-1, input-2); *DC,* direct current channel; *R,* referential channel; ** cal, calibration;*** if recorded as an AC signal; LAT, RAT left and right anterior tibial EMG; P_{ETCO_2} end-tidal PCO_2; Capnogram is exhaled PCO_2 wave form..

Table 16–3 PAP Titration Study Montage

Channel		G1	G2	Low Filter(Hz)	High Filter(Hz)	Sensitivity (μv/mm)	Channel Width	NotchFilter	Color
1	**R**	F4	M1	0.3	35 Hz	7	100	OFF*	
2	**R**	C4	M1	0.3	35 Hz	7	100	OFF	
3	**R**	O2	M1	0.3	35 Hz	7	100	OFF	
4	**R**	F3	M2	0.3	35 Hz	7	100	OFF	
3	**R**	C3	M2	0.3	35 Hz	7	100	OFF	
5	**R**	O1	M2	0.3	35 Hz	7	100	OFF	
6	**R**	E1	M2	0.3	35 Hz	7	100	OFF	
7	**R**	E2	M2	0.3	35 Hz	7	100	OFF	
8	**R**	Chin1	ChinZ	10	100	7	100	OFF	
9	**BP**	ECG		0.3	100	7	100	OFF	
10	**D**	Heart rate (derived)		0.3	DC	DC calibration	100	OFF	
11	**BP**	Snoring		10	100	7	100	OFF	
12	**DC**	PAP Flow		DC	OFF	DC calibration	200	OFF	
13	**BP**	Chest		0.1	15	7	200	OFF	
14	**BP**	Abdomen		0.1	15	7	200	OFF	
15	**DC**	SpO_2		DC	DC	DC calibration	200	OFF	
16	**BP**	Left anterior tibial (input1, input2)		10	100	7	100	OFF*	
17	**BP**	Right anterior tibial		10	100	7	100	OFF	
18	**DC**	PAP pressure		DC	DC	DC calibration	100	OFF	
19	**DC**	PAP leak		DC	DC	DC calibration	100	OFF	
20	**DC**	$PtcPCO_2$		DC	DC	DC calibration	100	OFF	

G1, G2 inputs 1 and 2 for the referential channels (derivation G1-G2 is displayed) ; Typical DC cal: SaO_2 (0 to 1 v, 0 to 100%), PAP flow (–1 to 1 v, -200 to 200 L/min), PAP pressure (0 to 1 v, 0 to 30 cm H_2O), PAPleak (0 to 1 v, 0 to 120 L/min).
DC calibration may vary depending on the manufacturer of the laboratory PAP device. * ON setting is used in review if 60 Hz or ECG artifact is prominent, BP bipolar channels have (input 1, input 2); LAT, RAT left and right right anterior tibial EMG; $PtcCO_2$ Transcutaneous PCO_2.

with the EOG channels at the top of the page (Diagnostic 2, Table 16–4). The Diagnostic 3 montage (Table 16–4) includes the RIPsum and RIPflow signals. The PAP titration montage (Table 16–4) includes typical signals from the laboratory PAP device and a transcutaneous PCO_2 signal.

Of note, although many PSG amplifiers record the ECG signal as true bipolar (two inputs with electrodes positioned as recommended by the American Academy of Sleep Medicine [AASM] scoring manual[1]), it is also possible to record individual ECG electrodes as referential signals. For example, if electrodes ECG1, ECG2, and ECG3 are recorded referentially, this allows visualization of different combinations (e.g., ECG1-ECG3 or ECG1-ECG2). If ECG1 is located below the right clavicle and ECG3 is located on the left lower chest as recommended in the AASM scoring manual, then ECG1-ECG3 is a modified lead II with upward p wave and QRS complex. ECG2 might be placed under the left clavicle or in a precordial location. If ECG2 is placed below the left clavicle, then ECG1-ECG2 is a modified lead[1] (see Chapter 14).

The standard montage is often adjusted to evaluate patients with certain issues. For parasomnias, temporal electrodes (T3 and T4) could be added for improved detection of epileptiform activity (interictal or ictal activity) (see chapter 35). Inspection of the tracings using a 10-second window is often needed to identify epileptiform activity (such as spikes with a duration of 20-70 msec). Turing off the 60 Hz notch filter and using a high filter setting higher than 35 Hz may allow better visualization of spikes. In patients with the suspected REM sleep behavior disorder, arm electromyogram (EMG) electrodes are often added (see Chapter 15). Patients with known or suspected hypoventilation would benefit from transcutaneous PCO_2 or end-tidal PCO_2 monitoring. Of note, monitoring for hypoventilation (typically by end-tidal PCO_2) during diagnostic studies is recommended (required) by the AASM scoring manual[1] for pediatric diagnostic studies but is optional in adults.

All-Night Graphical Trend Summary

A graphical display and summary of parameter values over the night is also available. Body position and PAP values are also displayed. The information (channels) included in the all-night display can be edited by the user. By clicking on a portion of the all-night display, the detailed display view will instantly move to the time of night selected. One can easily move to areas of interest, for example a time when there was supine REM sleep. In Figure 16–1, an example of an all-night

Table 16–4 Sample PSG Display Views (Montages)

Channel	Diagnostic 1	Diagnostic 2	Diagnostic 3	PAP Titration
1	F4-M1	E1-M2	F4-M1	F4-M1
2	C4-M1	E2-M2	C4-M1	C4-M1
3	O2-M1	F4-M1	O2-M1	O2-M1
4	E1-M2	F3-M2	E1-M2	E1-M2
5	E2-M2	C4-M1	E2-M2	E2-M2
6	Chin EMG	C3-M2	Chin EMG	Chin EMG
7	ECG	O2-M1	ECG	ECG
8	Heart rate	O1-M2	Heart rate	Heart rate
9	Snoring	Chin EMG	Snoring	Snoring
10	Nasal pressure	ECG	Nasal pressure	PAP flow
11	Oronasal thermal flow	Heart rate	Oronasal thermal flow	Chest
12	Chest	Snoring	RIPsum	Abdomen
13	Abdomen	Nasal Pressure	RIPflow	SpO_2
14	SpO_2	ON Therm	Chest	LAT
15	LAT	Chest	Abdomen	RAT
16	RAT	Abdomen	SpO_2	PAP leak
17	Exhaled PCO_2 (value)	SpO_2	LAT	PAP pressure
18	End-tidal PCO_2 (waveform)	LAT	RAT	PAP tidal volume
19	Diaphragmatic EMG*	RAT	Diaphragmatic EMG*	$PtcCO_2$

Chest/Abdomen, RIP effort belts; *LAT,* left anterior tibial; *ON Therm,* oronasal thermal airflow; *PAP,* positive airway pressure; *$PtcCO_2$,* transcutaneous PCO_2; *RAT,* right anterior tibial; *RIPsum/RIPflow,* respiratory inductance plethysmography sum and flow. * using surface electrodes.

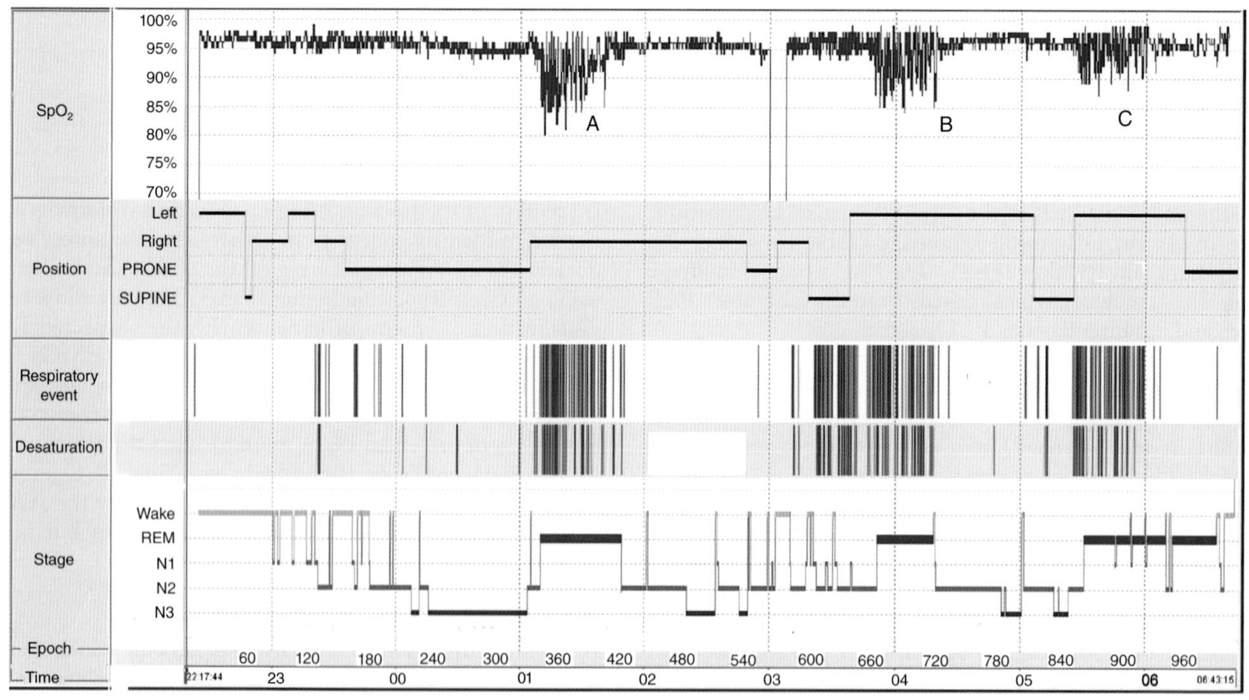

Figure 16–1 An example of an all-night summary (time line) showing key elements of PSG data including sleep stage, SpO_2, body position, respiratory events, and desaturations. This all-night summary clearly shows that respiratory events occur mainly during REM sleep (stage R) at A, B, and C. In addition, one can see that supine REM sleep was not recorded.

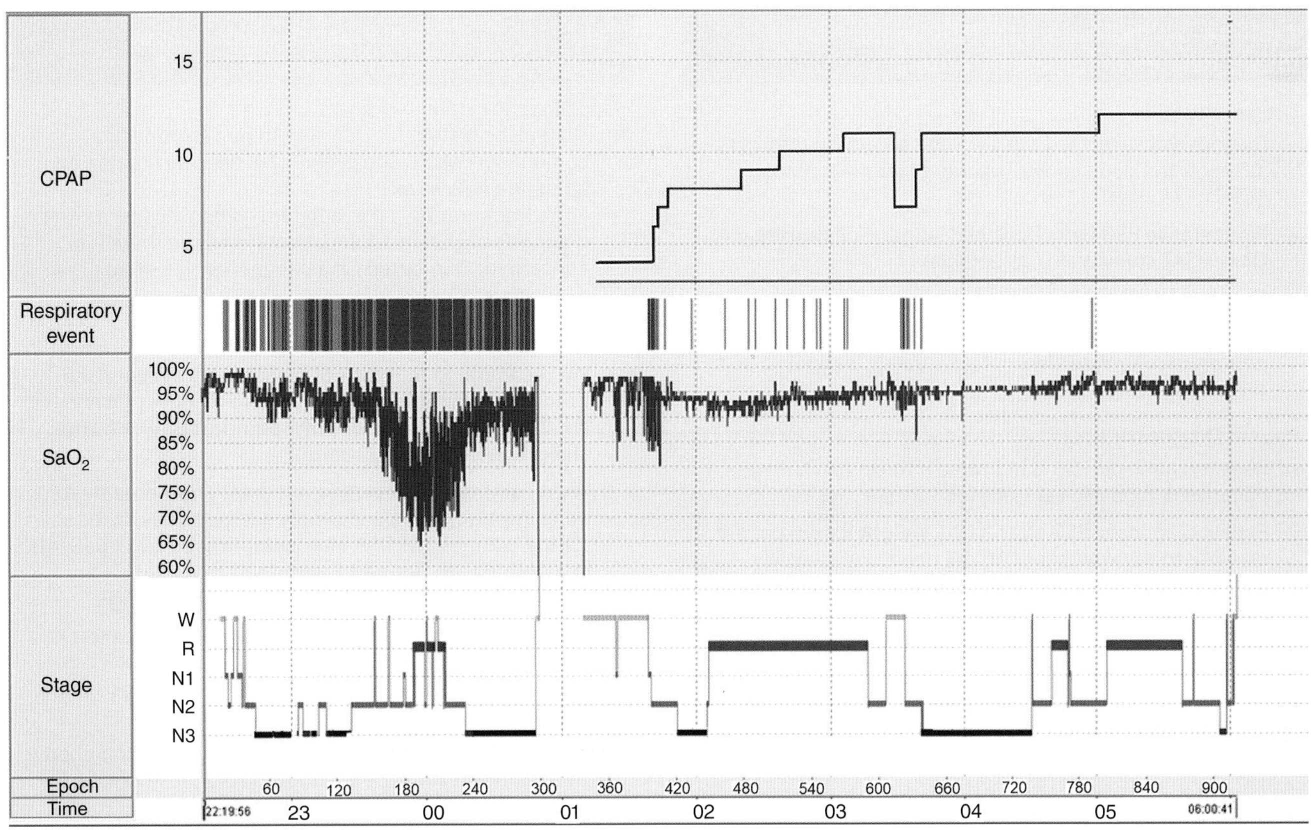

Figure 16–2 An example of an all-night summary from a split sleep study. The first part of the night (diagnostic) shows frequent respiratory events with worse desaturations during REM sleep. The second part of the night (CPAP titration) shows incremental increases in the level of continuous positive airway pressure (CPAP) with resolution of events and long periods of stage N3 and stage R (REM) sleep.

trend display for a diagnostic study is shown. This patient has REM associated sleep apnea. In Figure 16–2 an example of an all-night trend display for a split sleep study is shown (initial portion diagnostic, second portion PAP titration).

Video-Audio PSG

The AASM scoring manual recommends that the digital PSG system being used has the ability to record synchronized simultaneous video and audio signals. This will allow the reviewer to see patient movement corresponding exactly to a given time point in the recorded PSG signals. When the play button is activated, typically a line moves across the tracings to show the time position in the visualized tracings that corresponds to the current video display. For example, one could note facial twitching during a particular EEG pattern. Video PSG is an important development and allows the reviewer to confirm the patient position and document unusual behavior (e.g., parasomnias) during the night. Video-PSG is essential for evaluation of parasomnias or possible nocturnal seizures. Video files are often quite large and are usually compressed (e.g., MPEG4). The size of the file will depend on the quality of the video (10 or 25 frames/sec). Simultaneous audio is also recorded and is very useful for documenting teeth grinding (bruxism), talking during parasomnias, snoring, and other vocal behaviors during the recording. In most sleep centers, PSG/video/audio recording begins when the patient enters the sleep room. This is a quality assurance and safety measure that protects both patient and sleep technologist. Typically, the patient is asked to consent for video recording.

INDICATIONS FOR POLYSOMNOGRAPHY AND HOME SLEEP APNEA TESTING

The AASM practice parameters for PSG,[2] best clinical practice guidelines for Diagnostic Testing for Obstructive Sleep Apnea (OSA),[3] and Use of PSG and HSAT for Longitudinal Management of OSA in adults[4] outline the indications for PSG and home sleep apnea testing (HSAT) in adults. Several other practice parameters and clinical guidelines for the use of PSG in special situations have also been published.[5-18] The AASM has published accreditation standards for PSG and HSAT,[19] and the Centers for Medicare and Medicaid Services (CMS) has also published standards.[20] For Medicare, each Medicare Area Contractor also publishes local area guidance. The recommendations are summarized in Tables 16–5, 16–6, and 16–7. Because the many practice parameters address slightly different issues, all recommendations will be addressed with an attempt to coalesce their information. A detailed discussion of HSAT will follow an initial discussion of PSG. However, some comments concerning the use of HSAT will be made during the discussion of PSG.

Diagnosis and Follow-up

Diagnostic testing for OSA should be performed in conjunction with a comprehensive sleep evaluation and adequate

Table 16–5 Indications for Polysomnography (Sleep-Related Breathing Disorders)

Diagnostic PSG

- Diagnosis of suspected sleep-related breathing disorders (OSA, central sleep apnea, hypoventilation—but not COPD)
- Preoperative PSG before planned surgery for **snoring or OSA** (HSAT study is also acceptable)
- Negative HSAT for diagnosis of OSA
- Evaluation of symptoms of sleep disorders in patients with ***neuromuscular disorders*** not adequately diagnosed with clinical assessment

Repeat Diagnostic PSG

- Repeat diagnostic PSG is indicated if the initial PSG was negative + high clinical suspicion for OSA
- Repeat diagnostic PSG after ≥10% **weight loss** in patient on CPAP to see whether CPAP still needed (if clinically indicated)

Follow-up Diagnostic PSG (Non-PAP Treatment)

- After surgery for OSA—usually 3–6 months after surgery
- After previous surgery for OSA if symptoms return
- After adequate adjustment of an oral appliance (OA) for OSA (all severities*) while wearing the OA
- On OA treatment but symptoms return – while using OA

Diagnostic PSG Not Indicated

- Evaluation of COPD unless OSA suspected

*Mild severity also included in practice parameters for OA[15].

HSAT, Home sleep apnea testing; *OA,* oral appliance; *PAP,* positive airway pressure; *PSG,* polysomnography.

Kushida CA, Littner MR, Morgenthaler T, et al. Practice parameters for the indications for polysomnography and related procedures: an update for 2005. *Sleep.* 2005;28(4):499-521.

follow-up.[3] PSG is the standard diagnostic test for the diagnosis of OSA in adult patients in whom there is a concern for OSA based on a comprehensive evaluation. Clinical tools, questionnaires, and prediction algorithms should not be used **in the absence** of PSG or HSAT. PSG is the standard test for diagnosis of suspected sleep-related breathing disorders (SRBDs), narcolepsy (when combined with a multiple sleep latency test [MSLT]), PAP titration, evaluation of parasomnias (under certain conditions), determining the efficacy of prior surgical treatment for OSA, determining the efficacy of oral appliance (OA) treatment for OSA (PSG while wearing the OA),[2-4] and can allow an opportunity to adjust the voltage range for hypoglossal nerve stimulation[21] (Tables 16–5 and 16–6).

Whereas PSG is the recommended test for diagnosis of OSA,[3-5] HSAT is indicated for diagnosis of OSA in certain circumstances[3,4,16] (see Table 16–6 recommendation 4) and will be discussed in a later section. All PSG and HSAT studies should be preceded by a comprehensive physician evaluation documenting the medical indication for the study. The CMS and private insurance providers require documentation of symptoms (including the Epworth sleepiness scale), as well as elements of the physical examination including the body mass index (BMI), neck circumference, and a focused upper airway

Table 16–6 Clinical Practice Guideline for Diagnostic Testing for Adult OSA

Good Practice Statements:

- Diagnostic testing for OSA should be performed in conjunction with a comprehensive sleep evaluation and adequate follow-up.
- Polysomnography is the standard diagnostic test for the diagnosis of OSA in adult patients in whom there is a concern for OSA based on a comprehensive sleep evaluation.

Recommendations:

1. We recommend that clinical tools, questionnaires, and prediction algorithms not be used to diagnose OSA in adults, in **the absence of polysomnography or home sleep apnea testing**. (Strong)
2. We recommend that polysomnography, or home sleep apnea testing with a technically adequate device, be used for the diagnosis of OSA in **uncomplicated** adult patients presenting with signs and symptoms that indicate an increased risk of moderate to severe OSA. (Strong)
3. We recommend that if a single home sleep apnea test is negative, inconclusive, or technically inadequate, **polysomnography** be performed for the diagnosis of OSA. (Strong)
4. We recommend that polysomnography, rather than home sleep apnea testing, be used for the diagnosis of OSA in patients (Strong) with:
   (1) significant cardiorespiratory disease
   (2) potential respiratory muscle weakness due to neuromuscular condition
   (3) awake hypoventilation or suspicion of sleep related hypoventilation
   (4) chronic opioid medication use
   (5) history of stroke
   (6) severe insomnia
5. We suggest that, if clinically appropriate, a split-night diagnostic protocol, rather than a full-night diagnostic protocol for polysomnography be used for the diagnosis of OSA. (Weak) When these criteria are met:
   (1) A moderate to severe degree of OSA is observed during a minimum of 2 hours of **recording** time on the diagnostic PSG—AND
   (2) At least 3 hours are available to complete CPAP titration.
6. We suggest that when the initial polysomnogram is negative and clinical suspicion for OSA remains, a second polysomnogram be considered for the diagnosis of OSA. (Weak)

Other Recommendations:

Perform **PSG** or **HSAT** by an accredited sleep center under the supervision of a board-certified sleep physician

Adequate HSAT device: HSAT devices that incorporate a minimum of the following sensors: [nasal pressure, chest and abdominal respiratory inductance plethysmography (RIP) and oximetry] or [peripheral arterial tonometry (PAT) with oximetry and actigraphy].

Adequate HSAT study: A technically adequate HSAT includes a minimum of 4 hours of technically adequate oximetry and flow data, obtained during a recording attempt that encompasses the habitual sleep period.

Kapur VK, Auckley DH, Chowdhuri S, et al. Clinical practice guideline for diagnostic testing for adult obstructive sleep apnea: an American Academy of Sleep Medicine clinical practice guideline. *J Clin Sleep Med.* 2017;13(3):479-504.

exam (Mallampati score, see Chapter 18). The AASM sleep center accreditation standards[19] require that the sleep center medical director review all sleep study requests that are submitted by physicians not on staff at the sleep center to ensure the study is indicated and that the proper study is ordered.

PSG is the standard initial diagnostic study for evaluation of suspected obstructive or central sleep apnea.[2-5] A diagnostic study may be repeated if the initial study is negative for sleep apnea and there is a clinical suspicion for this disorder (Table 16–5). If the initial diagnostic evaluation using a single HSAT is negative, inconclusive, or of poor technical quality, a PSG should be performed.[4,5,16] That is, rather than repeat the HSAT, a PSG is recommended. A PSG should be performed preoperatively for planned surgery to treat snoring or suspected OSA.[2,3,13] Even if the surgery is planned for treatment of snoring alone, screening questions or physical examination are not sufficient to eliminate the possibility of OSA. If OSA is present, this may change treatment. A PSG is indicated after surgery for OSA (after surgical healing) to document effectiveness.[2,3,13] The 2005 practice parameters[2] specify "in moderate to severe OSA," although 2010 practice parameters for surgical treatment of OSA[13] recommended postsurgical objective determination of efficacy without specifying the severity of OSA. HSAT can also be used to document the efficacy of surgery.[4,5] Most clinicians would perform a PSG or HSAT after surgical healing *for all severities of OSA.* A PSG is indicated after adjustment of an OA for OSA (not for primary snoring) to document efficacy. The 2005 practice parameters for PSG recommended a sleep study *with the patient using an OA* (after adjustment) for treatment of moderate to severe OSA to document efficacy.[2,14] In a subsequent practice parameter on OA treatment of OSA, a PSG to document efficacy was recommended for OSA of all severities.[15] However an HSAT is another option to document efficacy of an OA (while patient is wearing the OA).[4] In 2021 guidelines for the use of PSG and HSAT for the longitudinal management of adult patient with OSA were published. Although similar to previous recommendations for the use of PSG and HSAT, the guidelines address new situations including a change in cardiovascular disease or concerning findings on a PAP device data download.

Guidelines for the **longitudinal management** of adult OSA using follow-up PSG or HSAT state the following:[4]

Follow-up PSG or HSAT recommendations

- Not recommended for asymptomatic OSA patients on PAP
- Can be used to reassess patients with *recurrent or persistent symptoms,* despite good PAP adherence
- Recommended to assess response to treatment with non-PAP interventions
- May be used if clinically significant *weight gain or loss* has occurred since diagnosis of OSA or treatment initiation
- May be used if treated OSA patients *develop or have a change in cardiovascular disease*

Follow-up PSG only recommendations:

- Follow-up PSG may be used for reassessment of sleep-related hypoxemia and/or hypoventilation after initiation of treatment for OSA
- Follow-up PSG may be used in patients with unexplained PAP device-generated data

PSG or HSAT is recommended to assess response to treatment with non-PAP interventions.[4] These would include surgery, an OA, a positioning device, or newer treatments such as neuromuscular stimulation. For patients with prior effective surgical treatment (documented by PSG or HSAT), the *PSG or HSAT may be repeated* at a later time *if symptoms of sleep apnea return.* For a patient using an OA as treatment for OSA, the PSG may also be repeated *while the patient wears the device if symptoms return.* An HSAT is another option in this situation. A ***diagnostic*** PSG is sometimes performed in a patient currently using continuous positive airway pressure (CPAP) after weight loss (typically by more than 10%) to determine if continued CPAP treatment is needed. If the study does NOT confirm the continued presence of significant OSA, withdrawal of CPAP could be considered. However, if symptoms return, usually this may require a return to CPAP or another treatment. As noted above, recent guidance states that a follow-up PSG may be used for reassessment of sleep-related hypoxemia and/or sleep-related hypoventilation after initiation of treatment.[4] If hypoventilation is suspected, monitoring of CO_2 (end-tidal or transcutaneous) should be performed (if available). In considering diagnosis and treatment of patients with known or suspected hypoventilation from neuromuscular disorders, a knowledge of the requirements for securing a bilevel PAP device with a backup rate is essential (see Chapter 24). There are situations where a diagnostic PSG may not be needed (neuromuscular disease) to qualify a patient for a bilevel PAP device with a backup rate and a PAP titration study might be a better choice than a diagnostic study.[22] A repeat PSG or HSAT may be used in patients being treated for OSA who develop or have a change in cardiovascular disease.[4] For example, a patient developing atrial fibrillation can have an increased apnea-hypopnea index (AHI) due to central sleep apnea. For a patient using PAP treatment a device download might show increased periodic breathing or an abrupt increase in the device-determined AHI. If the patient is on PAP, then a PAP PSG is the indicated test if nocturnal symptoms have worsened. *Recent guidance also recommends a follow-up PSG (titration) for patients with unexplained PAP device-generated data*[4] (e.g., an increase in the device determined AHI after development of heart failure or a high number of apneas classified as central). *One should be aware that the device-determined increase in AHI is not always accurate.* If the amount of leak is very high, the first intervention would be to reduce the leak. The device determined AHI may not accurate when there is high leak. High leak can also reduce PAP effectiveness. A PSG or HSAT may be used after clinically significant weight gain or loss. A patient with mild OSA not currently on PAP treatment could have worsening of disease after substantial weight gain, informing decision making about future appropriate treatment. This is especially true if there has been an increase in symptoms possibly due to worsening sleep apnea.

Split Sleep Studies and Positive Airway Pressure PSG Titration

The indications for use of PSG for PAP titration are shown in Table 16–7. A PSG is the standard method for PAP titration[2,10,11] and is useful for determining optimal noninvasive PAP treatment in patients with hypoventilation.[12] In patients undergoing a planned split PSG (diagnostic portion followed by PAP titration), the 2005 AASM practice parameters specify

Table 16–7 Indications for Polysomnography (PAP Titration and Treatment)

PAP Titration

- After a diagnostic study with results: AHI ≥15/hr with or without symptoms, AHI ≥5/hr with symptoms
  A. Full night of PSG titration
  B. Split study (2005 guidelines)*
    (1) AHI ≥ 40/hr during minimum of 2 hours of monitoring in the initial diagnostic portion
    (2) AHI 20–40/hr in special clinical circumstances (long apnea/severe desaturation)
    (3) 3 hours remain for PAP titration
    (4) Repeat PSG for PAP titration if inadequate PAP titration portion of study
  C. Split study (2017 guidelines)**: we suggest if clinically appropriate, a split-night diagnostic protocol, rather than a full-night diagnostic protocol for polysomnography, be used for the diagnosis of OSA. When these criteria are met:
    (1) A moderate to severe degree of OSA is observed during a minimum of 2 hours of **recording** time on the diagnostic PSG—AND
    (2) At least 3 hours are available to complete CPAP titration.

Repeat PSG PAP Titration—Patient on CPAP

- After ≥10% weight loss to determine if previously titrated CPAP is needed (a lower pressure may suffice)
- After ≥10% weight gain of an adherent patient on CPAP who is again *symptomatic*—to determine if CPAP adjustment is needed (higher pressure).
- Clinical symptoms return in patient on CPAP (consider PSG + MSLT if narcolepsy suspected). Optimize mask fit, adherence before ordering PSG
- See also Guidelines for the Longitudinal Management of patients with OSA using follow-up PSG or HSAT presented in the text in the section on Diagnosis and Follow-up

Repeat PSG on CPAP NOT Indicated

- Routine follow-up of a patient doing well on PAP treatment.

*Adapted from Kushida CA, Littner MR, Morgenthaler T, et al. Practice parameters for the indications for polysomnography and related procedures: an update for 2005. *Sleep.* 2005;28(4):499-521.
**Adapted from Kapur VK, Auckley DH, Chowdhuri S, et al. Clinical practice guideline for diagnostic testing for adult obstructive sleep apnea: an American Academy of Sleep Medicine clinical practice guideline. *J Clin Sleep Med.* 2017;13(3):479-504.
PAP, positive airway pressure; *PSG,* polysomnography.

criteria for proceeding with the titration portion based on the diagnostic portion.[2] The diagnostic AHI should be ≥40/hr or 20 to 40/hr for special circumstances such as severe desaturation.[2,10] A least 3 hours should remain for the PAP titration. The more recent recommendations for diagnostic testing for OSA in adults recommend a split sleep study over a diagnostic sleep study when the following criteria are met: (1) moderate to severe OSA on at least 2 hours of recording (not 2 hours of sleep); and (2) at least 3 hours remained for the PAP titration.[3] Thus, patients with an AHI of ≥15/hr could qualify for a split sleep study. The newer recommendation is more in line with actual practice. In some settings a split sleep study must be performed because of financial or patient-related issues. Requiring two studies (diagnostic followed by a PSG PAP titration) will delay treatment. It is also important to note that reimbursement for PAP treatment generally requires either 2 hours of sleep on the diagnostic study or the number of events associated with a given AHI that would be expected from 2 hours of sleep. For example, to meet a ≥5/hr AHI target, at least 10 events should be recorded. *If a PAP titration during a split night study is not considered adequate, a subsequent PSG PAP titration is indicated.* Treatment with auto-adjusting PAP (APAP) rather than a PAP titration is an alternative to a PAP titration sleep study in uncomplicated patients.[23] APAP devices can be used in auto-titrating PAP mode to perform an unattended PAP titration at home to select an effective level of CPAP for chronic treatment rather than a PSG PAP titration. The devices can also be used as auto-adjusting PAP for chronic treatment without the need for a PSG titration or when a PSG titration is not adequate and a repeat PSG PAP titration is not acceptable to the patient or would cause a concerning delay in treatment. Use of APAP is discussed in chapter 23.

*A routine follow-up PSG (using CPAP) is **NOT** recommended in patients on CPAP treatment who are doing well.*[2-4] If the patient is being treated on CPAP and is NOT doing well (recurrence of persistent symptoms) *despite good PAP adherence,* a repeat PSG study on CPAP is indicated.[4,11] However, before this expensive procedure, it is essential to *document adequate objective adherence and to optimize treatment and the mask interface (intervention for increased leak).* If a patient on CPAP loses more than 10% of body weight, a PSG titration study is indicated to determine if the previously titrated pressure is still needed (lower pressure may suffice). Most clinicians would reserve this intervention for patients who might benefit from a lower pressure (mask leak, bloating, or pressure intolerance issues). Today most patients are treated with APAP devices that should adapt to modest weight gain or loss but might require changing the upper and lower pressure limits. A PSG titration study is also indicated if a patient on CPAP gains more than 10% of body weight and is ***symptomatic*** to determine if the pressure is adequate (a higher pressure could be needed). Current PAP devices provide an estimate of AHI, and the clinician may choose not to perform a PSG if the AHI is at goal and the patient is doing well clinically even with recent weight gain (or perhaps empirically slightly increase the pressure). A repeat PSG on PAP followed by an MSLT[2,6,7] (on PAP) can be performed for persistent sleepiness when narcolepsy is suspected in an OSA patient using PAP treatment. However, adequate adherence and optimization of PAP treatment should occur before these procedures.

As mentioned above a repeat PAP PSG may be used in patients with sleep-related hypoxemia or hypercapnia after initiation on PAP treatment; for example, a patient with borderline oxygenation on the highest pressure used during a previous titration or a patient with worsening daytime hypercapnia despite good PAP adherence. A PAP titration study is also needed to qualify a patient for the addition of supplemental oxygen to PAP. Persistent hypoxemia on an effective level of PAP must be demonstrated (see chapter 23). Although noninvasive positive pressure ventilation (NPPV) treatment of patients with stable chronic hypoventilation can be started on an outpatient basis without a preceding PAP titration study, best clinical practice guidelines have been published.[12] A PSG NPPV titration has many advantages including the ability to try several different mask interfaces under pressure, selecting a level of expiratory positive airway pressure (EPAP) to address upper airway obstruction, and the ability to adjust treatment based on monitoring of transcutaneous PCO_2 (if available). See chapter 24 for more information on starting NPPV (also known as noninvasive ventilation or NIV).

Patients at High Risk for OSA

The 2005 practice parameters for PSG also mentioned circumstances in which SRBDs are very common.[2] However, PSG is NOT routinely indicated in those circumstances unless a clinical evaluation reveals a **reasonable suspicion** for SRBD. It should be noted that a significant number of individuals with these disorders have OSA and are asymptomatic. Thus, a high clinical index of suspicion is needed. The disorders identified in the practice parameters as high risk conditions include patients with systolic or diastolic heart failure, coronary artery disease, recent or past stroke or transient ischemic attack, and tachyarrhythmias or bradyarrhythmias. Most clinicians would also place resistant hypertension or pulmonary hypertension of unknown etiology in this category as well. The practice parameters also list neuromuscular diseases as a group of disorders in which PSG is indicated for *evaluation of sleep-related symptoms*. Routine evaluation of chronic lung disease is not an indication for PSG unless coexistent OSA is suspected. Nocturnal oximetry is a useful tool for determining whether nocturnal oxygen desaturation is occurring in a patient with chronic obstructive pulmonary disease. A sawtooth pattern is suggestive of sleep apnea and should prompt a PSG if clinically indicated.

Nonrespiratory Disorders Including Parasomnias

PSG is indicated for evaluation narcolepsy (combined with MSLT)[2,6,7] and other nonrespiratory disorders under certain conditions (Tables 16–8, 16–9). In general, a PSG is not indicated for routine evaluation of patients with nonrespiratory disorders (with the exception of narcolepsy) unless comorbid sleep apnea is suspected.

A PSG is **not** needed for evaluation of uncomplicated parasomnia presenting to sleep clinic. NREM parasomnias including sleep walking or night terrors are common in children and young adults. A PSG is indicated if sleep apnea is suspected or the parasomnia is complicated.[2] A parasomnia would be considered complicated if (1) the nocturnal behavior is possibly due to seizures; (2) atypical parasomnia behavior is present (frequent episodes each night, stereotypic behavior, or

Table 16–8 Indications for Diagnostic Polysomnography (Nonrespiratory Sleep Disorders Part I)

Narcolepsy:

PSG Indicated:
- Before MSLT for diagnosis of suspected narcolepsy

Parasomnias or Seizure Disorder

PSG Indicated:
- Nocturnal seizure is suspected (undiagnosed).
- Presumed parasomnia/nocturnal seizure disorder does not respond to conventional treatment.
- Presumed parasomnia is injurious to the patient or others (or is potentially injurious) or follows trauma or with forensic (legal) implications.
- Presumed parasomnia has atypical features (stereotypic behavior, frequent events in the same night, atypical age of onset).

PSG Not Indicated:
- Typical parasomnia, noninjurious behavior for which clinical evaluation is sufficient.
- Known seizure disorder patient without nocturnal complaints.

Sleep-Related Movement Disorder:

PSG Indicated
- For suspected periodic limb movement disorder.

PSG Not Indicated
- Evaluation and treatment of RLS.

MSLT, Multiple sleep latency test; *RLS,* restless legs syndrome.

Table 16–9 Indications for Diagnostic Polysomnography (Nonrespiratory Sleep Disorders Part II)

Insomnia

PSG Not Indicated
- Routine evaluation of transient insomnia, chronic insomnia, or insomnia associated with psychiatric disorders

PSG Indicated
- Sleep-related breathing disorder is suspected.
- Periodic limb movement disorder is suspected.
- Initial diagnosis is uncertain.
- Treatment of insomnia fails.
- Precipitous arousals occur with violent or dangerous behavior.

Depression

PSG Not indicated
- Diagnosis of depression (unless sleep apnea is suspected)

Circadian Rhythm Sleep-Wake Disorders

PSG Not indicated
- Diagnosis of circadian rhythm sleep-wake disorders

Table adapted from: Kushida CA, Littner MR, Morgenthaler T, et al. Practice parameters for the indications for polysomnography and related procedures: an update for 2005. *Sleep.* 2005;28(4):499-521.
Standards of Practice Committee of the American Academy of Sleep Medicine. Practice parameters for using polysomnography to evaluate insomnia: an update for 2002. *Sleep.* 2003;26(6):754-760.

Table 16–10 Summary of Circumstances in Which Polysomnography Is NOT Indicated

- Routine evaluation of a patient doing well on CPAP treatment
- Evaluation of asthma or chronic lung disease (unless OSA is suspected)
- Routine evaluation of insomnia
- Evaluation and treatment of RLS (unless the periodic limb movement disorder is suspected)
- Evaluation of depression
- Evaluation of uncomplicated parasomnias for which a clinical diagnosis is sufficient
- Evaluation of a circadian rhythm sleep-wake disorder

CPAP, Continuous positive airway pressure; *OSA,* obstructive sleep apnea; *RLS,* restless legs syndrome.
Kushida CA, Littner MR, Morgenthaler T, et al. Practice parameters for the indications for polysomnography and related procedures: an update for 2005. *Sleep.* 2005;28(4):499-521.

behavior unusual for age); (3) nocturnal behavior/parasomnia has resulted in injury to the patient or others (or has the potential to do so); (4) presumed parasomnia or nocturnal seizure disorder does not respond to conventional treatment; or (5) legal/forensic implications of nocturnal behavior. Of note, PSG for patients with a known seizure disorder is not indicated unless there are nocturnal complaints or behavior that require further evaluation.

A summary of circumstances where PSG is NOT indicated is shown in Table 16–10. As noted above, PSG is not indicated for follow-up of patients doing well on CPAP. A PSG is not indicated for diagnosis of restless legs syndrome (RLS) (a clinical diagnosis) but would be indicated for if the periodic limb movement disorder (PLMD) is suspected. According to the practice parameter for use of PSG for evaluation of insomnia,[8] PSG is not indicated for the routine evaluation of transient insomnia, chronic insomnia, or insomnia associated with psychiatric disorders. PSG is indicated in patients with a complaint of insomnia[8] when *"a sleep-related breathing disorder or periodic limb movement disorder is suspected, initial diagnosis is uncertain, treatment fails, or precipitous arousals occur with violent or injurious behavior."* Of note, insomnia is often a symptom of untreated OSA in women. PSG is also not indicated for evaluation of asthma or chronic lung disease (unless OSA is suspected) and not indicated for evaluation of circadian rhythm sleep-wake disorders.

POLYSOMNOGRAPHY REPORT AND INTERPRETATION

The AASM scoring manual[1] specifies the parameters that should be reported in the PSG report (Tables 16–11 and 16–12). These parameters frequently change with updated versions of the AASM scoring manual and the reader should examine the newest version. The exact format of sleep data reporting varies between sleep centers and depends on the type of sleep study (diagnostic, PAP titration, split study) and the software. Usually, the physician interpretation is much shorter than the total data generated by the software. The interpretation may consist entirely of prose containing the values of each entity discussed or a combination of tabular data and prose commenting on the significance of the tabular data.

Table 16–11 Parameters to Appear in PSG Report

Parameter	Explanation, Definition
Sleep Scoring Data (Recommended)	
Lights out (hrs:min)	Recording (analysis) starts*
Lights on (hrs:min)	Recording (analysis) ends
Total Sleep Time (TST)	Minutes of N1 + N2 + N3 + R
Total Recording Time (TRT)	Time for lights out to lights on, in min
Sleep Efficiency (%)	TST × 100/TRT (%)
Sleep Latency (min) (SL)	Time lights out to first epoch of sleep
REM Latency (min) (RL)	Time from sleep onset to first stage R
WASO (min)	Stage W from sleep onset to lights on**
Stages N1, N2, N3, R	Each stage in **minutes and %TST**
Arousal number (Ar #)	Number of arousals
Arousal index (ArI)	Ar I = Ar # X 60/TST in min
Respiratory Events (Recommended)	
# OA, #CA, #MA (Apn = apnea)	Obstruct., mixed, central Apn
# of Apneas (# Apn)	#OA + #MA + #CA
Apnea index (AI) (#/hr)	(# of apneas) X 60/TST in min
# of Hypopneas (#Hyp)	Specify hypopnea definition
Hypopnea index (HI) (#/hr)	(# hypopneas) X 60/TST min
A + H (#)	# of Apneas+ Hypopneas
Apnea hypopnea index (AHI)	(# Ap + # Hyp) X 60/TST in min
Mean SaO_2 during sleep	SaO_2 oxygen saturation
Minimum SaO_2 during sleep	
Time $SaO_2 \leq$ threshold, min	Threshold often 88% or 90%
Occurrence of hypoventilation	Diagnostic study children
Occurrence of CSB	Adults
Occurrence of Periodic breathing	Children

#number, WASO wake after sleep onset, Obstr. Obstructive; CSB Cheyne-Stokes Breathing
*recording starts when patient- technologist interaction begins in many sleep centers, but analysis starts at Lights out and ends at lights on
**TRT=TST+SL+WASO

The diagnostic impression and recommendations are especially important, as this is what non–sleep MDs tend to read. If a finding is important, it should be always mentioned in the impression and the significance explained. Recommendations for treatment are important, but to be useful to the referring physician they should be specific to the patient rather than providing a long list of generic recommendations.

Sleep Study Parameters

Sleep reports begin with the date of the study, patient demographics, the names of the recording and scoring technologists (and their credentials). Next there is a section describing

Table 16–12 Parameters to Appear in PSG Report (Continued from Table 16–11)

Parameter	Explanation, Definition
Respiratory Events (Optional)	
# Obstructive Hypopneas	No. Obstr. Hypopneas
# Central Hypopneas	# Central Hypn
Obstructive AHI	(#OA + #MA + #Hypn) × 60/ TST (min)
Central AI	(# Apn) X 60/TST (min)
Central AHI	(# CA + # Central Hypn) × 60/ TST min
#Respiratory Related Arousals	# RERAs
RERA index	#RERAs X 60/ TST (min)
RDI	AHI + RERA index
Occurrence of hypoventilation	Adults (diagnostic, PAP PSG)
Occurrence of hypoventilation	Children (PAP PSG)
Duration of CSB	(absolute time or % TST), # CSB events
# O_2 Desaturations	(≥ 3% or ≥ 4% or both), specify
O_2 Desaturation index (ODI)	(#Oxy Desats) X 60/TST(min)
Cardiac Events (Recommended)	
Average Heart Rate during Sleep	Report #
Bradycardia during sleep (if noted)	Report lowest heart rate
Asystole (if noted)	Report longest value
Sinus tachycardia during sleep*	Report highest HR
Narrow Complex Tachycardia*	Report highest HR
Wide Complex Tachycardia*	Report highest HR
Atrial fibrillation*	Report average HR
Other arrhythmias	List type
Cardiac Events (Optional)	
Highest and lowest HR	During sleep and during Recording
Movement Events (Recommended)	
Number of PLMS	# PLMS
PLMS index	# PLMS × X 60/TST (min)
Number of PLMS arousals	# PLMS Ar
PLMS arousal index	(PLMS Arl) = (# PLMS Ar) X 60/ TST (min)
Movement Events (Optional)	
REM sleep without atonia	If observed, # of epochs
RWSA Index (RWSAI)	# RWSA epochs x 100/Epochs of stage R

CSB, Cheyne-Stokes Breathing; # number; RWSA REM sleep without atonia, O_2 oxygen, * if noted; PSG polysomnography

what parameters were recorded, and scoring criteria. For example "sleep was manually scored in 30 second epochs" and "all scoring followed the guidelines of the AASM scoring manual including hypopneas scored with an associated ≥3% oxygen desaturation or arousal."

Standard *sleep architecture parameters* that should be included in every report are listed in Table 16–11. These were discussed in the chapter on sleep architecture (chapter 6) but will be defined briefly here for convenience. With the publication of the new AASM scoring manual,[1] reporting of hypopneas scored on the basis of an associated ≥3% desaturation or arousal and an AHI based on this hypopnea definition is recommended (must be reported). Reporting of hypopneas based on ≥4% oxygen desaturation and the associated AHI is an option. Most sleep centers will report both, and an example of such a report is in Table 16–13. One can see the difference the two hypopnea definitions make with respect to the AHI and number of desaturations. An example of a **diagnostic PSG tabular report** is shown in Table 16–13

A **PSG PAP titration tabular report** would be similar to the diagnostic PSG report (same sleep architecture information) with the addition of information about the CPAP treatment results usually displayed in a treatment table (Table 16–14). A **split sleep study report** is shown in Tables 16–15 and 16–16. For simplicity a single hypopnea definition is shown. Lights-out and lights-on are the actual clock time **analysis** of the recording started and ended. In many sleep centers, recording is also performed during hookup (software/human scoring only analyzes data between lights-out and lights-on). It is important *to notice if the period of recording is atypical or does not match the patient's reported sleep period.* A long sleep latency might simply be due to a lights-out time several hours before the typical bedtime for the patient. An early lights-on time (study termination) can occur at the patient's request (to report to their job on time) or because they feel they can no longer sleep. The total recording time (TRT) is the time in minutes from lights-out to lights-on (period of time analyzed). The total sleep time (TST) is minutes of stages N1, N2, N3, and R. The sleep efficiency (%) is TST × 100/TRT (min). Sleep latency is the time (minutes) from lights-out to the first epoch of sleep. Sleep onset is defined as the first epoch of sleep. The REM latency (stage R latency) is the time from the first epoch of sleep until the first epoch of stage R. A sleep latency greater than 30 minutes is typical of patients with sleep onset insomnia. A short REM latency can be seen with narcolepsy, depression, OSA, prior sleep restriction, and withdrawal of REM-suppressing medications. A long REM latency is often seen due to difficulty adapting to the monitoring environment or medications suppressing REM sleep (many antidepressants). Wake after sleep onset (WASO) is the total minutes of stage W after the first epoch of sleep until lights-on including the time out of bed (disconnected). Of note, TRT = sleep latency +WASO + TST.

The duration of each sleep stage is typically presented in minutes and as a percentage of TST. The number of arousals and arousal index is typically reported with other sleep parameters. Arousals can be separated into those associated with respiratory events, periodic limb movements, snoring/respiratory effort–related arousals, and spontaneous arousals. However, the AASM scoring manual specifies that the only *specific* type of arousal that must be reported is the PLMS

Table 16–13 Diagnostic Sleep Report (Tabular)

Patient	John Doe	DOB: 5/18/1969	Medical Record #	xxxx
Date of Study	1/3/2023	Age: 58 Gender: Male	BMI	40
Tech: Tech 1 RPSGT	Scorer: Tech 2 RPSGT	Referring MD: Dr. X	Neck size	15 in
Monitoring: Frontal, Central, Occipital EEG, EOG, chin EMG, ECG, Airflow (nasal pressure + nasal-oral thermal sensor, Respiratory effort (RIP), SpO_2, R/L leg EMG. Sleep scored in 30 second epochs. Hypopneas scored by both associated (≥3% desat or arousal) and ≥4%				
Lights out:	9:58 PM	Lights on:	6:50 AM	
Sleep Architecture				Normal Range
Total Recording Time	(min)	531		(420–514)
Total Sleep Time	(min)	474		(396–460)
Sleep Efficiency	(%)	89%		(80–90)
Sleep Latency	(min)	5		(7–17)
REM Latency	(min)	75		(65–100)
Sleep Stages				
Wake After Sleep Onset	(min)	51		(10–55)
			(%TST)	
Stage N1	(min)	38.5	8.1	(5–10)
Stage N2	(min)	219.5	46.3	(50–65)
Stage N3	(min)	114.0	24.0	(5–17)
Stage REM	(min)	102.0	21.5	(19–24)
Arousal index (ArI) Summary (#/hr)				
Total ArI	Apn + Hyp ArI	Snore ArI	PLM ArI	Spontaneous ArI
11.1	3.5	0.0	0.0	7.6
Respiratory Events (hypopneas scored with ≥3% Desat or arousal			**AHI = Apnea + Hypopnea Index**	
AHI (#/hr)	13.9	Obstructive Apneas (#)	52	
AI (#/hr)	6.8	Mixed Apneas (#)	0	
HI (#/hr)	7.1	Central Apneas (#)	2	
AHI NREM (#/hr)	10.0	Hypopneas (#)	56	
AHI REM (#/hr)	28.2	Apneas + Hypopneas (#)	110	
AHI Supine (#/hr)	24.2	% TST on Back (/hr)	52.6	
AHI Nonsupine (#/hr)	2.4			
Respiratory Events (hypopneas scored with ≥4% Desat				
AHI (/hr)	11.1	Obstructive Apneas (#)	52	
HI (#/hr)	4.3	Mixed Apneas (#)	0	
AHI NREM (#/hr)	7.7	Central Apneas (#)	2	
AHI REM (#/hr)	23.5	Hypopneas (#)	34	
AHI Supine (#/hr)	20.2	Apneas + Hypopneas (#)	88	
AHI Nonsupine (#/hr)	1.1	% TST on Back (/hr)	52.6	
Oximetry during Sleep (SaO_2 = arterial oxygen saturation)				
Min SaO_2 NREM (%)	79.0	Avg SaO_2 at ≥3% Desat (%)	93.0	
Min SaO_2 REM (%)	88.0	Avg SaO_2 at ≥4% Desat (%)	92.0	
≥3% Desaturations (#)	92	NREM SaO_2 ≤ 88% (min)	1.1	
≥4% Desaturations (#)	66	REM SaO_2 ≤ 88% (min)	0.3	
Average SaO_2 (%)	94			

Table 16–13 Diagnostic Sleep Report (Tabular)—cont'd

Patient	John Doe	DOB: 5/18/1969	Medical Record #	xxxx
Periodic Limb Movements in Sleep (PLMS)				
PLMS (#)	20	PLMS Index (/hr)	2.5	
PLMS Arousals (#)	3	PLMS AI (/hr)	0.4	
Heart Rate (HR) Analysis		Wake	NREM	REM
Avg HR (BPM)		76	66	69
Min HR (BPM)		57	55	58
Max HR (BPM)		94	92	79

Table 16–14 CPAP/BPAP Treatment Table

PAP Level	TST	REM	TST sup	AHI	AHI-REM	OA	MA	CA	HYP	AvgSpO$_2$
(cm H$_2$0)	(min)	(min)	(min)	(#/hr)	(#/hr)	(#)	(#)	(#)	(#)	(%)
4	12.6	0	12.6	76.3	0	2	0	0	14	92
6	25.6	0	25.6	25.7	0	0	0	0	11	93
7	21.1	3.9	21.1	19.9	91.9	0	0	0	7	94
8	14.6	14.6	14.6	16.4	16.4	0	0	0	4	96
9	22.2	22.2	22.2	8.1	8.1	0	0	0	3	96
10	156.7	42.3	0	1.5	5.7	0	0	4	0	96
11	150.5	65.5	0	0	0	0	0	0	0	96

This table illustrates that no supine sleep was recorded on pressures 10 and 11 cm H_2O.; *PAP*, positive airway pressure in cm H_2O; *TSTsup*, total sleep time in the supine position; *OA*, obstructive apnea; *MA*, mixed apnea; *CA*, central apnea; *HYP*, hypopnea; *AvgSpO$_2$*, average saturation on this pressure. For simplicity only one hypopnea definition is shown..

arousal number and the PLMS arousal index (number of PLMS arousals × 60/ TST(min).

Although not included in the AASM scoring manual, it is important to report the *% of TST in the supine position.* OSA is typically more severe during REM sleep and in the supine position. There is an interaction between these two factors, and the circumstance with the *highest AHI is typically supine REM sleep*. Some software reports provide much more detailed information including the number of respiratory events of each type in NREM sleep, REM sleep, in each body position, as well as the mean duration of each type of event. A common approach is to report the total number of each respiratory event type, as well as the AHI during NREM and REM sleep and in the supine and nonsupine positions (and the percentage of sleep in the supine position). From these data one can determine the effects of NREM versus REM sleep and the supine versus nonsupine position of the AHI. An example of a tabular display of respiratory data from a diagnostic study is shown in Table 16–17. This table shows the AHIsupine and the AHInonsupine, as well as the % of TST in the supine position. In the table one can see that the AHI is much higher during REM sleep compared with NREM sleep. If central apneas are present, it is important to comment if they meet criteria for Cheyne-Stokes breathing (CSB).[1] Either the duration of CSB (absolute value in minutes or %TST) or the number of CSB events can be reported (optional in the AASM scoring manual). It is useful clinically to report the average (or typical) total cycle time as a longer cycle time is associated with worse cardiac function.

The AASM scoring manual recommends reporting the average arterial oxygen saturation, the minimum oxygen saturation and the time below an oxygen saturation threshold (often ≤ 88%). Reporting the number of oxygen desaturation (≥ 3%, ≥ 4%, or both) and the oxygen desaturation index (ODI, # of desaturations per hour of sleep) are optional but are included in most sleep study reports. Limb (leg movement) events to be reported include the number of PLMS, the PLMS index, the number of PLMS arousals, and the PLMS arousal index.[1]

The results of the PAP titration are included in the data reported in PAP titration sleep studies and split sleep studies.[1,12] The titration results are often presented in tabular format (Table 16–14, Table 16–16) or in prose. If using prose, the optimal pressure, whether or not supine REM sleep was recorded on the optimal pressure, the residual AHI on the final pressure and some index of oxygenation on the optimal/final pressure should be reported. It is ideal if the mask type used is also included somewhere in the report (technologist notes). Many sleep centers use a PAP treatment table showing each level of pressure used and the amount of sleep, REM sleep, supine sleep, residual AHI, number of events (number of obstructive apneas, mixed apneas, central

Table 16–15 Split Sleep Study Tabular Format

Lights Out:	09:34 PM	Lights On:	06:26 AM		
Sleep Architecture:		**Total Night**	**Range**	**Range**	
Total Recording Time	(min)	531.6	(414–455)	(414–455)	
Total Sleep Time	(min)	504.0	(400–443)	(400–443)	
Sleep Efficiency	(%)	94.8	(95–99)	(95–99)	
Sleep Latency	(min)	1.5	(2–10)	(2–10)	
REM Latency	(min)	138.5	(70–100)	(70–100)	
Sleep Stages					
Awake (WASO):	(min)	26.1		(0–13)	
			%TST		
Stage N1:	(min)	31.5	6.3	(2–9) (%)	
Stage N2:	(min)	204.5	40.6	(50–64) (%)	
Stage N3:	(min)	95.0	18.8	(7–18) (%)	
Stage R:	(min)	173.0	34.3	(20–27) (%)	
Arousals					
Arousal Index (#/hr)	Total:	Apnea + Hyp:	Snore:	PLM:	
Diagnostic	99.8	99.8	0.0	0.0	
Treatment	5.4	3.8	0.0	0.0	
Respiratory Events	**Diagnostic**	**Treatment**		**Diagnostic**	**Treatment**
Monitoring Time (min)	171.4	360.2	Obstr. Apnea (#):	194	14
TST (min)	160	344	Mixed Apnea (#):	40	0
REM (min)	10.5	162.5	Central Apnea (#)	0	4
AHI = Apnea + Hypopnea Index			Hypopneas (#):	42	57
AHI (#/hr)	102.8	12.9	Hyp ≥3% desat or arousal		
AHI NREM (#/hr)	105.3	15.0			
AHI REM (#/hr)	82.3	10.4			
AHI supine (#/hr):	102.8	12.9			
AHI nonsupine (#/hr):	0	0			
% TST on Back:	100.0	100.0			
Oxygen Saturation (SaO_2)	**Diagnostic**	**Treatment**	**Time ≤88% (min)**	**NREM**	**REM**
Low SaO_2 (%) NREM	58	80	(Total Night)	25	35
Low SaO_2 (%) REM	57	95			
Desaturations (≥3%) (no.)	276	77			
Avg SaO_2 at Desat (%)	69.2	87.8			
Time SaO_2 ≤ 88% (min)	40	20			
PLMS Summary	**Diagnostic**	**Treatment**	**Total Night**		
PLMS Number	0	0	0		
PLM Index (#/hr)	0	0	0		
PLMS Arousal Number:	0	0	0		
PLMS Arousal Index (#/hr):	0.0	0.0	0.0		
Heart Rate	**Wake**	**NREM**	**REM**		
Average Heart Rate (BPM)	85	82	80		
Minimum Heart Rate (BPM)	64	59	59		
Maximum Heart Rate (BPM)	107	107	100		
CPAP Titration Table: see Table 16–16					

For simplicity what paramer were recorded is omitted from the report and only hypopnea using the recommended definition is reported

Table 16–16 CPAP/Bilevel Positive Airway Pressure Treatment

Technologist note summary: An XXX full face mask size small and heated humidity were used during the titration study. High leak was a problem and the mask had to be adjusted during the study.

PAP	TST	REM	TST sup	AHI	AHI-REM	OA	MA	CA	HYP
(cm H_2O)	(min)	(min)	(min)	(#/hr)	(#/hr)	(#)	(#)	(#)	(#)
6	11.5	0	11.5	93.9	0	6	0	1	11
8	15.5	0	15.5	27.1	0	0	0	0	7
9	19.5	3	19.5	12.3	40	1	0	0	3
10	74.5	73	74.5	17.7	18.1	0	0	3	19
11	81.5	38	81.5	2.2	4.7	0	0	0	3
12	**56.5**	**48.5**	**56.5.5**	**3.2**	1.1	0	0	0	3

PAP is pressure in cm H_2O. *Sup*, supine; *OA*, obstructive apnea; *MA*, mixed apnea; *CA*, central apnea; *HYP*, hypopnea. For simplicity data using only one hypopnea defintion is displayed.

Table 16–17 Respiratory Event Table

Respiratory Events			Number	Index
AHI(/hr)	38.9	Obstructive Apneas	59	8.4
AHI NREM	28.1	Mixed Apneas	0	0
AHI REM	**77.4**	Central Apneas	0	0
AHI supine (/hr)	38.9	Apneas	59	8.4
AHI nonsupine (/hr)	0.0	Hypopneas	212	30.4
% TST on Back	100%	Apneas+ Hypopneas	271	38.9

apneas, and hypopneas) along with an average and/or minimum or oxygen saturation for each level of PAP (Tables 16–14 and 16–16). Note that in Table 16–14 that on CPAP of 10 cm H_2O REM sleep but no supine sleep was recorded. In Table 16–16 CPAP of 12 cm H_2O is seen to be effective during supine REM sleep. Of note if supplemental oxygen was added to PAP treatment, this can also appear in the treatment table. If the technologist notes are extensive, the interpreting physician can summarize the most important information in a section labeled technologist notes. This might include the mask inferface(s) used (type, brand, and size) and whether or not humidity was used during the titration.

Sleep reports should also include basic cardiac data which typically includes the average heart rate, the minimum heart rate, and the maximum heart rate. The AASM scoring manual recommends reporting the average heart rate during sleep. Reporting the highest and lowest heart rate during sleep, and the highest and lowest heart rate during recording is optional.[1] The cardiac rhythm and the presence of any abnormality should also be reported (see Chapter 14). Abnormal video/audio findings should also be reported, as well as excessive sustained or transient muscle activity during stage R. Reporting the number of stage R epochs meeting criteria for REM sleep without atonia (RWA) and an RWA index (the % of the total REM epochs with RWA) is optional.[1] As discussed in chapter 15, the type of EMG recording used to determine RWA should be reported (for example the right and left anterior tibial EMG, chin EMG, right and left flexor digitorum superficialis EMG).

In the split sleep study report (Table 16–15) one can see the overall sleep architecture and the TST and amount of REM sleep in both the diagnostic and treatment portions. A PAP treatment table would also be included in the split study report.

Approach to Reading the PSG

Using Clinical History, Technologist Comments, All-Night Trend Summary, and Biocalibrations

Before and during reading of a PSG there are important historical elements to review (Table 16–18). A review of the clinical history with special attention to symptoms of sleep apnea, narcolepsy, RLS, and medications taken by the patient is very useful. The amount of chronic alcohol or use of a potent opioid use and the medications taken before the sleep study should be noted (and reported). The presence of underlying lung disease may help explain a low awake arterial oxygen saturation by oximetry (SpO_2) or low baseline sleeping SpO_2. A clinical history of pacemaker insertion or known atrial fibrillation is also very helpful in providing a useful interpretation of ECG findings. If a PAP titration is planned for a patient *currently using CPAP*, the current treatment pressure level and mask interface type should be noted (if the information is available). Review of technologist notes and comments are very valuable and often provide information otherwise unavailable to the reading physician.

Technologist comments often report abnormal EEG, ECG patterns and the epoch when the abnormality occurred. Mention of abnormal body movements is also important to

Table 16–18 Historical Elements to Review Based on Polysomnography Findings

Finding	Historical Elements to Consult
EEG/EOG/Chin EMG	
• Long sleep latency	• History of sleep onset insomnia? • Delayed habitual bedtime compared with lights-out time?
• Short REM latency	• History or symptoms of narcolepsy, cataplexy, or depression?
• Alpha sleep (prominent alpha in NREM)	• Chronic pain syndrome or psychiatric disorder?
• Persistent eye movements during stage N2	• SSRI medication?
• Increased sleep spindle activity	• BZ/BZ receptor agonists?
• Increased sustained/transient chin EMG activity during stage R	• SSRI treatment, history of dream enactment?
• Arousal from stage N3 with confusion or screaming	• History of NREM parasomnia?
• Body movement and speech during REM sleep	• History suggestive of dream enactment/RBD?
Respiration	
• Low awake SpO_2 • Low sleeping baseline SaO_2	• Presence of lung disease? • Previous ABG showing hypoventilation?
• Cheyne-Stokes breathing	• History of congestive heart failure?
• Ataxic breathing, low respiratory rate, central apnea	• History of using potent opiates?
• Delay in SpO_2 nadir after respiratory events	• Decreased cardiac output, CHF?
Limb Monitoring	
• Frequent LMs during wake	• Symptoms of RLS?
• High PLMS index—can occur with OSA, PAP titration, RLS	• Symptoms of RLS?
• Increased transient muscle activity during REM sleep	• ? SSRI medications, history of dream enactment?
ECG Findings	
• Tachycardia in sleep (>90 bpm)	• Anxiety, stimulants, obesity?
• Bradycardia in sleep (<40 bpm)	• Beta blocker, AV block, cardiac disorder?
• Wide complex QRS with normal rate (e.g., 60–80)	• Pacemaker?
• Atrial fibrillation	• Previously documented?

BZ, Benzodiazepine; *ECG,* electrocardiogram; *EEG,* electroencephalogram; *EMG,* electromyogram; *EOG,* electrooculogram; *LMs,* limb movements; *NREM,* non–rapid eye movement; *PAP,* positive airway pressure; *PLM,* periodic limb movement; *RBD,* rapid eye movement sleep behavior disorder; *REM,* rapid eye movement; *RLS,* restless legs syndrome; *SpO_2,* arterial oxygen saturation by oximetry; *SSRI,* selective serotonin reuptake inhibitor.

note. Special attention to portions of the tracings or video with reported abnormalities is indicated. In PAP titrations, the masks used, use of chin straps, use of humidity, and rationale for changes of PAP pressure are important. For example, on might wonder why 14 cm H_2O did not work previously but later seemed to be effective. One explanation might be a change of mask interface and/or lower mask leak. *It is also important to review which medications the patient took immediately before the sleep study*. These should be documented in the technologist notes and relevant portions included in the sleep report either as technologist notes or as part of the physician report.

Review of the *overnight summary/trend* can be very helpful. For example, it may be obvious that respiratory events were much more prevalent in the supine position or during stage R. A long sleep latency or long periods of wake during the night may be recognized when viewing the overnight summary. The *biocalibration procedure* (see chapter 2) is often helpful in noting the appearance of eyes-open wake in each patient and if the patient produced a posterior dominant (alpha) rhythm in the occipital EEG derivations with eye closure. This information can be useful in differentiating eyes-open wake from REM sleep (the chin EMG activity is usually higher during wakefulness). The biocalibration procedure is discussed in detail in Chapter 2. During the reading of the PSG, a return to the clinical history may be helpful, as PSG findings might prompt a review of specific details in the history (Table 16–18). For example, review of the presence or absence of RLS symptoms in a patient with an elevated PLMS index. An orderly approach to reviewing the raw data is useful to avoid missing an important finding.

Diagnostic Sleep Study Interpretation

Some of the important elements to include in a diagnostic PSG interpretation are shown in Table 16–19. The interpretation usually includes sections on history and indication for the sleep study and comments about the sleep architecture including arousals, respiration, oxygenation, cardiac findings (including the basic rhythm and mention of abnormalities if present), leg movement activity, abnormal video findings, impression, and recommendations. If the patient took medications before the study, this should be reported. The use of an oral appliance (OA) during the study or use of supplemental oxygen (and what liter flow rate) should also be mentioned in the report. In some centers the interpretation simply provides the data in Table 16–14 in prose. In others the data is displayed in tables and then the report discusses each section in prose. Abnormalities in sleep architecture are emphasized, and if the *technical quality of the tracings or artifact is prominent*, that should also be mentioned. The presence of abnormal EEG activity or REM sleep without atonia should also be reported, and unusual video or audio findings such as parasomnia should be discussed. The severity of the AHI and information on the type of central apneas if present (CSB) should be detailed. A much higher AHI during REM sleep or in the supine position should be mentioned. If minimal supine sleep or REM sleep were recorded, this should be mentioned as this could result in a study that underestimates the severity of sleep apnea. Some reports list event durations, but if this is not presented the report should mention the duration of particularly long apneas and hypopneas. *There is an occasional patient with a relatively low AHI but a significant time*

Table 16–19 Important Elements of the Diagnostic PSG Physician Interpretation

Indication for sleep study and important historical elements (e.g., pacemaker)
What was monitored (if not included elsewhere):
Frontal, central, occipital EEG, EOG, chin EMG, chin EMG, ECG, snore sensor, nasal pressure, oronasal thermal flow, chest and abdominal RIP effort belts, SpO_2, left and right anterior tibial EMG + additional (end tidal PCO_2)
Medications taken before the study, special circumstances
Sleep, respiration, oximetry, cardiac, limb movement data if not in tabular form (Table 16–12)

Sleep architecture comments:
- Significant abnormalities (increased sleep latency, decreased total sleep time)
- Absence or reduced amounts of stage R or supine sleep
- EEG abnormalities
- Sleep fragmentation
- Increased sustained or transient chin EMG activity during stage R

Respiration comments:
- Severity of AHI
- Effect of stage R and supine sleep on AHI
- If increased central apneas, type of central apneas
- Duration of long apneas or hypopneas
- Severity of desaturation (awake $\mathbf{SaO_2}$, number of desaturations, minimum SpO_2 and time below SaO_2 threshold)

Cardiac comments:
- Presence of sinus tachycardia or bradycardia during sleep, high average HR
- Abnormalities in rate or rhythm (premature beats, AV block, NCT, WCT, atrial fibrillation)

Leg movement analysis comments:
- Assessment of PLMS (± history of RLS if increased PLMS index)
- Excessive transient Leg EMG activity during stage R

Video/audio
- Abnormal body movements, sounds

Impression
Recommendations

with the SpO_2 ≤88%. Of course, an inaccurate SpO_2 signal is one explanation. However, the presence of lung disease or long periods of severe airflow limitation (very flattened nasal pressure signal and snoring) could be present. Therefore, it is important to note BOTH the minimum SpO_2 and the time with the SpO_2 ≤88% (or 90% in some sleep centers). If the nadir in the SpO_2 signal after respiratory events is delayed, this suggests a long circulation time (and should be mentioned). The significance of the PLMS index and PLMS arousal index should be addressed. If elevated (PLMS index ≥15/hr in adults and ≥5/hour), the presence or absence of RLS complaints in the history should be mentioned. If there is no information on RLS in the history, a recommendation to question the patient about leg symptoms is important. Of note, most sleep centers have patients complete a prestudy focused sleep history questionnaire. This is especially important if the sleep study was ordered by a physician not associated with the sleep center. Most sleep centers also have the patient complete a poststudy questionnaire about their experience in the sleep center, how the sleep compared with that at home, and if PAP was tried how that was tolerated and a question about their willingness to use PAP for treatment. If relevant, patient comments should be mentioned in the sleep study interpretation.

Positive Pressure Titration Interpretation

The PAP titration interpretation includes the information provided in the diagnostic study interpretation, as well as information specific to the titration. Some of the important information to include is summarized in Table 16–20. The PAP titration report typically shows the overall sleep architecture and respiratory events summary as noted in diagnostic PSG reports. Relevant to the sleep architecture, if there is a large increase in stage R or stage N3 (evidence of rebound in stage R stage N3) on PAP, this should be mentioned and usually implies a good treatment effect. On the other hand a reduction in stage R or TST may be due to poor tolerance of PAP or an inadequate titration. The major difference between a diagnostic sleep study and PAP titration interpretation is a discussion of the results of the titration. As noted previously the PSG titration report usually includes a *PAP treatment table* showing various pressures used and the amount of sleep (total, REM, supine) and the AHI on each pressure. Although the titration table(s) provide a useful summary, the physician interpretation can provide very useful additional information. For example, the table may provide the AHI during REM sleep and supine sleep but not display if **supine REM sleep** was recorded. A comment of the efficacy of PAP during supine REM sleep for on the final pressures used can be useful. If large leak is present, this should be mentioned. The reason for changes in interface is important to note; for example, change from a nasal to an oronasal mask because of nasal congestion or mouth leak. If the patient was changed from CPAP to bilevel pressure (BPAP) or if oxygen was added, this should also be addressed. *It is important to describe the most effective (optimal) pressure and the AHI and oxygenation on that pressure.* If efficacy was (was not) documented in supine REM sleep (usually the highest pressure required), this should also be mentioned. If no supine or REM sleep were recorded, it is important to address this issue as pressure higher than used during the titration could be needed for treatment at home. If the residual AHI was above goal (usually ≥10/hr) or the SaO_2 on the final pressure was lower than desired, this fact should also be addressed. Classification of the PAP titration as optimal, adequate, or inadequate is discussed in Chapter 23. *Finally, the treatment recommended based on the study should be specified, including the pressure, mode, interface type, humidity, and comfort measures (expiratory pressure relief). The interpreting physician may not agree with the need for pressure increases during the study.* If the final pressure was CPAP of 16 cm H_2O, the physician may recommend **a lower pressure if this was effective.** It is not enough to look at the treatment table; one must look at the tracings to select a treatment pressure for recommendation. If the titration was not successful, a repeat titration should be recommended and possible causes of the inadequate titration be addressed, including inadequate pressure or excessive mask leak. Recommending the approach on a repeat titration is very useful to avoid a new technologist not learning from a prior titration. For example, if the patient clearly needs pressure higher than 12 cm H_2O, starting the titration at 4 cm H_2O wastes valuable time. When the recommendation involves a PAP device with a backup rate based on

Table 16–20 Elements in the PAP Titration Interpretation

Quality of sleep on CPAP:

- Decreased TST or amount of stage R may represent a poor response to PAP
- Large increase in stage N3 or stage R, may represent a good treatment response
- Mask interface(s) used (technologist notes or physician report)
- If CPAP changed to BPAP why?, Was expiratory pressure relief used?
- Use of humidity
- Was supplementay oxygen used, if so why?, what flow rate?
- AHI and SpO_2 at optimal pressure
- Significant amount and nature of central apneas (?Cheyne-Stokes)
- Interface and leak issues
- Issues with patient PAP tolerance (pressure?, mask?)
- Optimal PAP pressure (was an effective pressure for supine REM sleep documented?)
- If flexible pressure was used, document the type and level (for example, for Res Med devices expiratory Pressure relief (EPR) 1,2, or 3).

Recommendations:

- Recommended PAP pressure, interface options, humidity options
- Should a repeat titration be performed? (If so, should a different mode of PAP be used? Should a higher starting pressure be used?)
- Need for nocturnal oximetry at home on PAP to rule out persistent desaturation

a diagnosis of complex sleep apnea, it is important to summarize the data qualifying the patient under respiratory assist device (RAD) criteria[22] (see Chapters 24 and 30). For example, to qualify for bilevel positive airway pressure (BPAP) with a backup rate on the basis of a complex sleep apnea pattern, either in tabular format or prose, it must be demonstrated that after obstructive events are controlled with CPAP or BPAP without a backup rate (obstructive AHI < 5/hr) and that central events persist or emerged (central AHI ≥ 5/hr with $\geq 50\%$ of residual events being central in nature).[22]

Split Sleep Study Interpretation

Split sleep study reports and interpretations generally use two general formats. In one format the diagnostic portion is completely described using information provided in a diagnostic sleep study report and interpretation followed by a separate PAP titration report providing information about this portion of the study. That is, the split study report is a diagnostic study report followed by a PAP titration report. At the end of the reports the overall physician interpretation and recommendations based on the two portions of the study are presented. The other format is to provide information about both study portions in a table with text interpretation of the significance of findings. In Table 16–15 one can see that very little REM sleep was recorded in the **diagnostic** portion (10.5 minutes). *Minimal or no REM sleep in the diagnostic portion of a split sleep study can result in an underestimation of the severity of sleep apnea.* The AHI and desaturations are much more severe during REM sleep in most patients. However, as the largest amount of REM sleep occurs in the second half of the night, often minimal REM sleep is recorded in the diagnostic portion. For example, the sleep report may give the impression of a moderately increased AHI and mild arterial oxygen desaturation based on the diagnostic portion of the split study when minimal REM sleep was recorded. Physicians reading the sleep report may not be aware that his *may underestimate the true severity of sleep apnea unless this possibility is discussed.* A large amount of wake during the titration portion may occur with poor tolerance of PAP. A large amount of stage R in the titration portion may represent REM rebound and suggest a good treatment effect with PAP. In Table 16–15 there is evidence of REM rebound with a large amount of REM during the titration (162.5 min). A summary of respiratory events in each portion of the study is presented either in prose or tabular format. The overall AHI on PAP may not reflect the efficacy of optimal pressure but may still provide important information about the overall PAP titration. In some patients many central apneas may be present on the titration but not during the diagnostic portion. The type of central apnea should be reported. The criteria for diagnosis of treatment emergent central apnea are discussed in Chapter 30. Some reports list event durations but if this is not presented the report should mention particularly long apneas and hypopneas. Leg movement number and indices are usually provided for each portion of the study. Some individuals may exhibit few events in the diagnostic portion but frequent leg movements during the titration. The opposite pattern also occurs. As mentioned previously if the impression mentions an elevated limb movement index, then the presence or absence of a history of RLS should be addressed. An elevated PLMS index is a PSG finding and not a diagnosis of a disorder. A discussion of the results of the PAP titration should cover the elements mentioned in the section on PAP titration studies.

POLYSOMNOGRAPHY IN CHILDREN

PSG in children differs from adults in many respects. Split *sleep studies are not recommended, and use of exhaled PCO2 monitoring is recommended (required) for diagnostic studies. PSG in children is challenging as often sensors are removed or displaced during the study.* Depending on the age of the child, the parent and child may sleep in the same bed. For very young children, nursing or bottle feeding during the night is routine and the child may sleep in a crib. As nostrils are smaller, a single catheter to monitor nasal pressure and exhaled PCO_2 is frequently used.

Indications for Polysomnography in Children (Nonrespiratory Disorders)

The indications for PSG for nonrespiratory PSG in children[17] are listed in Table 16–21. A PSG is indicated for evaluation of suspected PLMD and for suspected RLS when supportive data is needed (demonstration of PLMS). PSG with MSLT is indicated for suspected narcolepsy or for evaluation of hypersomnia (and to differentiate from narcolepsy). PSG is also indicated in children with atypical or potentially injurious parasomnias to differentiate from sleep-related epilepsy (extended EEG monitoring recommended). If OSA is suspected in children with frequent parasomnias, epilepsy, or *nocturnal enuresis* PSG is indicated as sleep apnea can complicate these

Table 16–21 Nonrespiratory Indications for PSG and MSLT in Children

Recommendations FOR Use of PSG in Children

- Suspected periodic limb movement disorder (PLMD) for diagnosing PLMD. (Standard)
- Preceding the MSLT as part of the evaluation for suspected narcolepsy. (Standard)
- For suspected OSA or PLMD in children with frequent NREM parasomnias, epilepsy, or nocturnal enuresis. (Guideline)
- Preceding the MSLT in children suspected of having hypersomnia from causes other than narcolepsy to assess excessive sleepiness and to aid in differentiation from narcolepsy. (Option)
- PSG using an expanded EEG montage is indicated in children to confirm the diagnosis of an atypical or potentially injurious parasomnia or differentiate a parasomnia from sleep-related epilepsy. (Option)
- PSG is indicated in children suspected of having RLS who require supportive data for diagnosing RLS. (Option)

Recommendations AGAINST Use of PSG in Children

- Polysomnography is not routinely indicated for evaluation of children with sleep-related bruxism. (Standard)

From Aurora RN, Lamm CI, Zak RS, et al. Practice parameters for the non-respiratory indications for polysomnography and multiple sleep latency testing for children. *Sleep.* 2012;35(11):1467-1473.

disorders increasing the frequency or impairing response to treatment. PSG is not routinely indicated for evaluation of children with sleep-related bruxism (unless OSA suspected).

Indications for Polysomnography in Children (Respiratory Disorders)

The indications for PSG in children with respiratory disorders[18] are listed in Table 16–22. In children neither the use of split sleep studies nor or HSAT is currently recommended. PSG is the study to make a diagnosis of OSA. PSG is indicated for evaluation of children being considered for adenotonsillectomy (AT). The requirement for a PSG before AT surgery varies with the otolaryngologist (ENT surgeon), the patient, and the community. This issue will be discussed in chapter 27 on pediatric OSA. A PSG after AT is indicated in patients with mild OSA pre-surgery *if residual symptoms are present* and is indicated *in all patients with moderate to severe OSA presurgery* and for patients at risk for significant residual OSA (see Table 16–22). PSG is indicated for assessment of residual disease after rapid maxillary expansion and for PAP titration. Follow-up PAP PSG is indicated to determine if pressure requirements have changed as a result of growth and development, with recurrent symptoms on PAP, or after additional or alternative treatment has been started. PSG is also indicated with children wearing their OA if being treated with this device to document efficacy. PSG is indicated for noninvasive positive pressure ventilation (NIPPV) titration in children with other sleep related breathing disorders (SRBDs). Children treated with mechanical ventilation may benefit from periodic evaluation to adjust ventilator settings. PSG is also indicated for suspected congenital central alveolar hypoventilation syndrome or suspected hypoventilation due to neuromuscular disorders or chest wall deformities, as well as selected case of primary sleep apnea of infancy. Monitoring of PCO_2 would definitely be needed. Children treated with tracheostomy for SRBDs benefit from PSG as part of the evaluation before decannulation. These children should be followed clinically after decannulation to assess for recurrence of symptoms of SRBDs. PSG is indicated in the following disorders only if there is a clinical suspicion for an accompanying SRBD: chronic asthma, cystic fibrosis, pulmonary hypertension, bronchopulmonary dysplasia, or chest wall abnormality such as kyphoscoliosis.

HOME SLEEP APNEA TESTING (HSAT)

Several names have been used for home sleep apnea test (HSAT) studies including portable monitoring (PM), a home sleep test (HST), a limited channel sleep test (LCST), and an out of center test (OCST).[1,4,5,16,20,24-31] HSAT studies are usually performed unattended in the home but can be performed as attended or unattended studies in the hospital or sleep center. In general, an HSAT is acceptable for diagnosis of OSA in patients with high pretest probability of moderate to severe OSA in the absence of certain comorbidities and for determining the adequacy of prior surgery for OSA or effectiveness of current OA treatment for OSA.[3,4,16] HSAT devices usually do not record EEG, EOG, or EMG derivations and therefore cannot determine the amount of sleep recorded.

Classification of Sleep Testing/Testing and Devices

There is a wide spectrum of HSAT devices. The commonly used general classification of sleep apnea testing was proposed by Ferber et al.[24] in a 1994 American Sleep Disorders Association review (Table 16–23). This classification used the terminology Levels I, II, III, and IV. This terminology was later modified to Types 1, 2, 3 and 4 (or Types I, II, III, and IV).[25,26] In 2008 the CMS issued a decision to allow HSAT to qualify an adult patient for CPAP.[27-29] The national carrier determination (NCD) for coverage of CPAP is 240.4. The designation for a HSAT study used by CMS is a home sleep test (HST) and the types of sleep diagnostic testing are defined slightly differently (Table 16–24) than that of Ferber et al.[24] The major difference is that CMS type IV test must include a minimum of three channels. One of the three channels must airflow as specified in some CMS publications[30] (including the current local carrier determination (LCD) for polysomnography and sleep testing).[20] CMS also created G-codes (G0398, G0399, and G0400) to describe HST services (Table 16–24).[29,31,32] The G-codes are found in the Healthcare Common Procedure Coding System Level II codebook and are maintained and valued by CMS. G-codes are procedure codes developed by CMS to identify products, supplies, and services that do not have an assigned Current Procedural Terminology (CPT) code for which there is a programmatic operating need to separately identify them on a national level. Reimbursement for the HST G codes is determined regionally by the specific local coverage determination (LCD). Later HSAT studies were assigned CPT codes 95800, 95801, and 95806 (Table 16–25). CPT codes are copyrighted and maintained by the American Medical Association. Although CPT codes now exist for HSAT studies, many insurance providers still require use of G-codes for billing. The AASM scoring manual uses the HSAT CPT codes in their recommended standards for home sleep apnea testing.[1,32] Note that the CPT classification of HSAT studies differs somewhat from the G-code classification. However, the G code (G0399) or

Table 16–22 Respiratory Indications for Polysomnography in Children

Recommendations FOR Use of Polysomnography

- Interpret PSG in accordance with the recommendations of the *AASM Manual for the Scoring of Sleep and Associated Events.* (Standard)
- Diagnosis of obstructive sleep apnea syndrome (OSAS) in children. (Standard)
- Children with mild OSAS preoperatively should have clinical evaluation after adenotonsillectomy to assess for residual symptoms. If there are residual symptoms of OSAS, polysomnography should be performed. (Standard)
- After adenotonsillectomy to assess for residual OSAS in children with **preoperative evidence for moderate to severe OSAS, obesity, craniofacial anomalies that obstruct the upper airway, and neurologic disorders (e.g., Down syndrome, Prader-Willi syndrome, and myelomeningocele).** (Standard)
- Positive airway pressure (PAP) titration in children with obstructive sleep apnea syndrome. (Standard)
- When clinical assessment suggests the diagnosis of congenital central alveolar hypoventilation syndrome or sleep related hypoventilation due to neuromuscular disorders or chest wall deformities. It is indicated in selected cases of primary sleep apnea of infancy. (Guideline)
- When there is clinical evidence of a sleep-related breathing disorder (SRBD) in infants who have experienced an apparent life-threatening event (ALTE). (Guideline)
- Polysomnography is indicated in children being considered for adenotonsillectomy to treat OSAS. (Guideline)
- Follow-up PSG in children on chronic PAP support is indicated to determine whether pressure requirements have changed as a result of the child's growth and development, if symptoms recur while on PAP, or if additional or alternate treatment is instituted. (Guideline)
- PSG indicated after treatment of children for OSAS with rapid maxillary expansion to assess for the level of residual disease and to determine whether additional treatment is necessary. (Option)
- Children with OSAS treated with an oral appliance should have clinical follow-up and polysomnography to assess response to treatment. (Option)
- PSG indicated for noninvasive positive pressure ventilation (NIPPV) titration in children with other SRBDs. (Option)
- Children treated with mechanical ventilation may benefit from periodic evaluation with polysomnography to adjust ventilator settings. (Option)
- Children treated with tracheostomy for SRBDs benefit from polysomnography as part of the evaluation before decannulation. These children should be followed clinically after decannulation to assess for recurrence of symptoms of SRBDs. (Option)
- PSG in the following respiratory disorders only if there is a clinical suspicion for an accompanying SRBD: chronic asthma, cystic fibrosis, pulmonary hypertension, bronchopulmonary dysplasia, or chest wall abnormality such as kyphoscoliosis. (Option)

Recommendation AGAINST Use of Polysomnography

- Nap (abbreviated) polysomnography is not recommended for the evaluation of obstructive sleep apnea syndrome in children. (Option)
- Children considered for treatment with supplemental oxygen do not routinely require polysomnography for management of oxygen therapy. (Option)

Level of recommendation: Standard > Guideline > Option. *OSAS*, Obstructive sleep apnea syndrome.
From Aurora RN, Zak RS, Karippot A, et al. Practice parameters for the respiratory indications for polysomnography in children. *Sleep.* 2011;34(3):379-388.

Table 16–23 Classification of Sleep Testing

	Level I (Type 1 or I)	Level II (Type 2 or II)	Level III (Type 3 or III)	Level IV (Type 4 or IV)
	Attended PSG	**Unattended** PSG	Cardiorespiratory monitoring	Continuous single or dual bioparameter recording
Measures (channels)	Minimum of 7 channels including EEG, EOG, chin EMG, **ECG**, airflow, respiratory effort, oxygen saturation	Minimum of 7 channels including EEG, EOG, chin ***EMG, ECG or heart rate***, airflow, respiratory effort, oxygen saturation	Minimum of 4, including ventilation (at least 2 channels of respiratory movement or respiratory movement and airflow), **heart rate or ECG**, and oxygen saturation	Minimum of 1 oxygen saturation, flow, or chest movement
Body position	Documented or objectively measured	Optional (may be objectively measured)	Optional (may be objectively measured)	Not measured
Leg Movement	EMG or motion sensor desirable but optional	EMG or motion sensor desirable but optional	Optional (may be recorded)	Not recorded
Personnel	In constant attendance	Not in attendance	Not in attendance	Not in attendance
Interventions	Possible	No	No	No

The original terminology of Level I–IV was used but recent terminology is Type I–IV or Type 1–4.
Based on Ferber et al Reference 24

Table 16–24 CMS Classification of Sleep Testing and G-Codes

Code	Type	Setting	Monitoring
N/A	I	In facility attended	See Table 16-23
G0398	II	Unattended in or out of a sleep lab facility or attended in a sleep lab facility	Minimum of **seven** channels including EEG, EOG, EMG, **ECG or/Heart rate**, airflow, breathing/respiratory effort, oxygen saturation
G0399	III	Unattended in or out of a sleep lab facility or attended in a sleep lab facility	Minimum of **four channels** and must record ventilation, oximetry, and ECG or heart rate
G0400	IV	Unattended in or out of a sleep lab facility or attended in a sleep lab facility	Minimum of **three channels***
No code**		Unattended in or out of a sleep lab facility or attended in a sleep lab facility	Minimum of three channels including peripheral arterial tonometry, actigraphy, and oximetry

*The current LCD for Polysomnography and Sleep Testing (L33405)[20] specifies that one of the Type IV channels be airflow. However, this is not required in the corresponding G code G0400[29,32]).
**Can use G0400 if CPT codes not allowed.
G codes are Healthcare Common Procedure Coding System (HCPCS) codes that are used to identify temporary procedures and professional services. The codes are still used for HSAT in some locales.
CMS, Center for Medicare and Medicaid Services.[29,31]

Table 16–25 Current Procedural Terminology (CPT) Codes for PSG and HSAT

Code	Description
95782	Polysomnography; younger than 6 years, sleep staging with 4 or more additional parameters of sleep, attended by a technologist
95783	Polysomnography: younger than 6 years, sleep staging with 4 or more additional parameters of sleep, with initiation of continuous positive airway pressure therapy or bilevel ventilation, attended by a technologist
95810	Polysomnography: age 6 years or older, sleep staging with 4 or more additional parameters of sleep, attended by a technologist
95811	Polysomnography: age 6 years or older, sleep staging with 4 or more additional parameters of sleep, with initiation of continuous positive airway pressure therapy or bilevel ventilation, attended by a technologist
95800	Sleep study, **unattended,** simultaneous recording; heart rate, oxygen saturation, respiratory analysis (e.g., by airflow or peripheral arterial tone) **and sleep time**
95801	Sleep study, **unattended,** simultaneous recording; minimum of heart rate, oxygen saturation and respiratory analysis (e.g., by airflow or peripheral arterial tone)
95806	Sleep study, **unattended,** simultaneous recording of heart rate, oxygen saturation, respiratory airflow and respiratory effort (e.g., thoracoabdominal movement).

Note: Use the Technical Component (TC) modifier when only the technical component is billed and the 26 (professional component) modifier when only the professional component is billed.

CPT code 95806 describes most Type 3 (III) devices (measuring airflow, effort, oximetry, and a derived pulse rate). Sleep testing using peripheral arterial tonometry (PAT), actigraphy, and oximetry was also approved for HST by CMS, but a G-code was not specifically assigned to this type of testing.[29-31] Studies with these devices are usually coded with CPT code 95800 or 95801. If CPT codes are not accepted, G4000 can be used. In CPT code 95800 the method of determining sleep time is not specified. Presumably, a HSAT device with EEG/EOG monitoring or estimates of sleep using a PAT device (see below) would qualify. Another classification of HSAT devices termed SCOPER (Sleep, Cardiovascular, Oximetry, Position, Effort, and Respiratory) was used in a review of device technology and was published in an attempt to improve the classification of the wide variety of devices.[25]

The result of HSAT testing is often called the AHI, although the denominator of the metric is monitoring time rather than TST. The AASM scoring manual[1] uses the designation *respiratory event index* (REI) for the number of apneas and hypopneas divided by monitoring time, and CMS uses the term respiratory disturbance index (RDI). In contrast, the AASM scoring manual defines the RDI as the AHI + RERA index where RERAs are respiratory effort related arousals. Since publication of the 2008 revision of the **national coverage determination (NCD** 240.4) on CPAP treatment,[27-29] CMS and private insurers now allow patients to qualify for PAP treatment based on a HSAT study (as noted above the CMS term is HST) provided certain guidelines are followed. Subsequent to the revision of NCD 240.4 by CMS a number of local carrier determinations (LCDs) by regional Durable Medical Equipment Medicare Administrative Contractors (DME-MAC, or DMACs) or private insurance providers were published further defining requirements for the performance of HST (HSAT) (Table 16–26). Medicare and most private insurance providers also now pay for HSAT,[20,30-32] and many private insurance plans require HSAT for initial diagnostic testing of OSA unless certain comorbidities are present. In some locales HSAT is required by certain private insurance plans as initial testing for nearly all patients. The specific rules vary according to LCDs.

The AASM published the *Clinical Guidelines for the Use of Unattended Portable Monitors in the Diagnosis of OSA in Adults (CGPM)*[16] and more recently clinical practice guidelines for diagnostic testing of adult sleep apnea.[3] The AASM scoring manual also provides guidance on the components

Table 16–26 Typical Requirements for Reimbursement for Home Sleep Apnea Testing

- Treating physician who orders the study must perform a face-to-face evaluation. Evaluation must include the following:
  1. Sleep history and symptoms including, but not limited to, snoring, daytime sleepiness, observed apneas, choking or gasping during sleep, and morning headaches
  2. Epworth Sleepiness Scale
  3. Physical examination documents body mass index, neck circumference, and a focused cardiopulmonary and upper airway evaluation (Mallampati scale)
- Sleep center performing home sleep apnea testing study must be accredited by the AASM or JC or ACHC
- Sleep technicians or technologists attending PSG or sleep studies affiliated with HSAT (HST) must have appropriate personnel certification. Examples of certification in PSG and sleep technology for technologists are
  - Registered Polysomnography Technologist (RPSGT)
  - Registered Electroencephalographic technologist (R. EEG T.) – Polysomnography
  - Certified Respiratory Therapist Sleep Disorders Specialist (CRT-SDS)
  - Registered Respiratory Therapist Sleep Disorders Specialist (RRT-SDS)
  - American Board of Sleep Medicine Registered Sleep Technologist (RST)*

The raw data from all sleep tests must be reviewed and the tests must be interpreted by either:
1. A diplomate of the ABSM OR
2. A physician board certified in sleep medicine by a member board of the ABMS OR
3. An osteopathic physician board certified in sleep medicine by a member board of the AOA OR
4. An active physician staff member of an AASM-accredited sleep center or sleep laboratory OR
5. An active physician staff member of a JC-accredited sleep laboratory OR
6. An active physician staff member of an ACHC-accredited sleep laboratory OR
7. A diplomate of the ABFM with CAQ in sleep medicine

Adapted from CMS requirements: local coverage determination L33405.
AASM, American Academy of Sleep Medicine; *ABFM*, American Board of Family Medicine; *ABMS*, American Board of Medical Specialties; *ABSM*, American Board of Sleep Medicine; *AOA*, American Osteopathic Association; *CAQ*, Certificate of Added Qualifications; *JC*, The Joint Commission; *ACHC*, Accreditation Commission for Health Care.
*ABSM-RT examination is no longer offered, Recertification exams will be offered through 2032.

of the HSAT report.[1] In addition, the AASM accreditation standards provide HSAT study guidance[19] to assure the studies are performed and scored according to high standards. The accreditation standards change frequently, and the reader should review the most current version. The indication and conditions for use of unattended HSAT are summarized in Table 16–27.

HSAT Equipment Standards

The AASM scoring manual[1], AASM sleep center accreditation standards,[19] and AASM guidelines for diagnostic testing for sleep apnea[3] specify standards for HSAT devices and studies. The major recommendations are listed here. The reader should consult the above documents for complete information and the latest revisions for updates and changes.

For monitoring using airflow (or tidal volume) HSAT devices must be cleared or approved by the U.S. Food and Drug Administration (FDA) with a unique identifier for each unit and meet CPT criteria for 95800, 95801, or 95806. The devices must monitor at least three parameters (airflow, effort, oximetry or [peripheral arterial tonometry/actigraphy/oximetry]). The HSAT unit must have the ability to record oximetry and a measure of heart rate (usually pulse rate from oximeter) and the ability to determine an average heart rate (recommended), and minimum and maximum heart rate (optional). HSAT computer software must have the ability to display raw data for review, allow manual scoring and/or editing of automated scoring. The devices and software must have the ability to calculate an REI as a surrogate for the AHI determined by PSG. Here the REI is the number of respiratory events per hour of monitoring time. The AASM scoring manual defines monitoring time as the recording time minus time with artifact or time the patient is awake based on actigraphy, body position, respiratory pattern, or patient diary *The AASM scoring manual defines*. For devices recording EEG, an AHI based on TST is reported. For devices monitoring airflow, apneas and hypopneas are scored. Ideally, apneas can be classified as obstructive, central, or mixed (optional). Hypopneas must be scored and reported using an associated ≥3% desaturation although there is an option to **ALSO** determine hypopneas with a ≥4% oxygen desaturation (in this case hypopneas meeting the two defintions are both reported). The criteria used for scoring hypopneas should be specified.

If airflow is used to determine respiratory events and an REI, at least one of the following should be used to detect airflow: nasal pressure, oronasal thermal airflow sensor, or an alternative sensor. Alternative sensors include respiratory inductance plethysmography (RIP)sum or RIPflow (recommended) or polyvinylidene (PVDF) sum (acceptable). For detection of respiratory effort, dual RIP effort belts are recommended, and acceptable methods include a single RIP belt, single or dual PVDF effort belt(s), single or dual piezoelectric effort belt(s), and a single pneumatic belt. Oximetry and a measure of heart rate are also required. Although not required, *HSAT devices ideally should be able to detect body position* (REI supine and nonsupine can be determined), and most provide a snore signal (measure or derived). Of note, the *AASM clinical practice guideline for diagnostic testing of adult OSA published in 2017 recommended dual effort belts*,[3] and dual belts are required for reimbursement in some locales.

Standards for HSAT Devices NOT Monitoring Airflow and Effort

At the time of writing, there has been an explosion of devices FDA cleared for the diagnosis of OSA using novel measurements. In this chapter only the most commonly used device

Table 16–27 Summary of Indications and Conditions for HSAT (AASM)

Indications:

- Home sleep apnea testing with a technically adequate device, can be used for the diagnosis of OSA in ***uncomplicated*** adult patients presenting with signs and symptoms that indicate **an increased risk of moderate to severe OSA**
- Diagnosis of OSA in patients in whom laboratory PSG is not possible by virtue of immobility, safety, or critical illness
- To document the efficacy of non-PAP treatments for OSA (oral appliances, upper airway surgery, weight loss)

Conditions:

- HSAT must be performed in conjunction with a **comprehensive sleep evaluation** supervised by a BC/BE sleep physician
- **No comorbid medical conditions** that may degrade HSAT accuracy are present
  - Severe pulmonary disease
  - Neuromuscular disease (potential respiratory muscle weakness)
  - Congestive heart failure
  - Chronic opioid medication use
  - Awake or suspected sleep-related hypoventilation (obesity hypoventilation syndrome)
  - History of CVA
  - Severe insomnia
- **No clinical suspicion of other sleep disorders**
  - Central sleep apnea
  - Narcolepsy
  - PLMD
  - Parasomnias
  - Circadian rhythm sleep disorders
- Not for screening asymptomatic populations

Methods:

- **Use of an acceptable device:**
  a Minimum of airflow, effort, oximetry[16]
  b Minimum of airflow, dual thoraco-abdominal effort belts, oximetry[3]
  c Meets definitions for CPT codes 95800, 95801, 95806 (see Table 16–25)[1]
- Methodology conforms to AASM Scoring Manual[1] and Accreditation Standards[19]
- Study read by BC/BE sleep physician with review of raw data
- If HSAT negative or technically inadequate, a PSG should be ordered

CVA, cerebrovascular accident; *HSAT*, home sleep apnea test; *OSA*, obstructive sleep apnea; *PAP*, positive airway pressure; *PSG*, polysomnography; *AASM*, American Academy of Sleep Medicine.
Troester MM, Quan SF, Berry RB, et al; for the American Academy of Sleep Medicine. The AASM Manual for the Scoring of Sleep and Associated Events: Rules, Terminology and Technical Specifications. Version 3.Darien, IL: American Academy of Sleep Medicine; 2023.

employing peripheral arterial tonometry will be discussed (WatchPAT – Zoll). The AASM scoring manual provides guidance for use of the PAT device.[1] As with traditional HSAT devices the type of device, serial number, and signals used (PAT, actigraphy, oximetry) should be reported, as well as the fact that the device provides sleep/wake and REM estimates, and a measure of heart rate. In addition, if body position and snoring are recorded that should be reported.

Recording data to be reported include recording start and stop time, duration of recording, estimated sleep time, and estimated % REM sleep. Heart rate [average (recommended) and, highest and lowesst heart rate (optional)] should be reported. The pAHI, which is the surrogate of the AHI used in PAT devices, should be reported based on apnea-hypopnea events associated with a ≥3% desaturation. There is an option to ALSO report a pAHI based on *≥4% desaturation as well. There is an option to report the oxygen desaturation index (ODI) and whether the ODI this is based on ≥3% or ≥4% desaturation should be specified (should be the same as used for determining the pAHI).*

HSAT Reports

The AASM scoring manual recommends information to be reported from HSAT.[1] A sample report for a device monitoring flow is shown in Table 16–28. Both recording time and monitoring time should be reported and the method used to determine monitoring time specified; for example, the time from lights-out to lights-on from a patient diary. As noted above, the AASM scoring manual defines *monitoring time as the recording time minus time with artifact or time the patient is awake based on actigraphy, body position, respiratory pattern, or patient diary*. If actigraphy is used to identify periods of wake (and eliminate them from the monitoring time), that should be specified. Some devices have a *chain of custody option* so that the intended patient is actually monitored (preventing fraudulent recording of an individual other than the one intended). The REI should be reported, and reporting a central apnea index and or snoring quality is optional. At least one of the following measures of the SpO_2 must be reported, including mean value, maximum value, and minimum value, the time below a SpO_2 threshold, or ODI based either on ≥3% or

Table 16–28 Sample HSAT Report (Device Measuring Airflow)

Home Sleep Apnea Test		Best Sleep Center	101 Highway X, City, State XXXX	Telephone #: XXX	Fax: XXX
Name	John Doe	DOB	1/1/1970	Age	50
Study date	1/3/2023	Medical Record #	XXXX	Gender	Male
Referring MD	Dr. Good	Device used	XXXX	Height	69 in
Tech	Tech 1 RPSGT	Serial #	XXX	Weight (pounds	280
Scorer	Tech 1 RPSGT			BMI (kg/m2)	41
				Neck Size/ESS	17/12
Equipment: Type 3: monitoring airflow by nasal pressure, effort by respiratory inductance plethysmography belts, oxygen saturation and pulse by oximetry, body position. **Procedure**: The patient was educated on sensor application by a RPSGT who downloaded study, manually scored study or edited study and ran report. Hypopneas scored with both ≥3% and 4% desaturation. Monitoring time based on patient diary.					
Recording start		Lights out	1/23/2023 10:00 PM	Recording Time	780 min
Recording stop		Lights on	1/24/2023 6:30 AM	Monitoring Time	480
≥3% Desaturation Respiratory Events		REI respiratory event index = REI events/monitoring time (hr)			
Apneas	40	REI (AHI) (#/hr)	30	Awake SpO_2 (%)	94
OA (#)	20	REI (AHI) (#/hr) supine	50	Lowest SpO_2 (%)	86
MA (#)	1	REI (AHI) (#/hr) nonsupine	20.6	≥3% desaturations (#)	240
CA (#)	19	% supine	32	ODI (#/hr)	30
Hypopneas (#)	200			Time (min) with $SaO_2 \leq 88\%$	4.7
≥4% Desaturation Respiratory Events		REI Respiratory Event Index = REI Events/Monitoring Time (hr)			
Apneas	40	REI (AHI) (#/hr)	20	Awake SpO_2 (%)	94
OA (#)	20	REI (AHI) (#/hr) supine	50	Lowest SpO_2 (%)	86
MA (#)	1	REI (AHI) (#/hr) nonsupine	5.9	≥3% desaturations (#)	160
CA (#)	19	% supine	32	ODI (#/hr)	20
Hypopneas (#)	120			Time (min) with $SaO_2 \leq 88\%$	4.7
Heart rate (pulse rate)					
Mean rate (bpm)	77	Maximum rate (bpm)	105	Minimum rate (bpm)	63
Indication for study: snoring, witnessed apnea, mild daytime sleepiness. Medical problems: hypertension. Medications: losartan. **Physician statement:** I reviewed the raw tracings in detail and the summary report. The technical quality was adequate. **Impression:** 1. Obstructive sleep apnea (G47.33) **severe** in frequency by REI (AHI) (based on hypopneas scored with ≥3% desaturations) with mild desaturation **Recommendations:** A CPAP titration is recommended for this patient. Weight loss may also be helpful. The patient should avoid driving if sleepy.					
Interpretation Date. XXXX	Signature: Dr john Doe Diplomate ABIM sleep Medicine				

≥4%—the one used to determine hypopneas. In practice, most sleep centers will report the number of hypopneas based on both ≥3% and ≥4% desaturations, as well as the ODI3% and ODI4% (as they will likely report an REI based on both ≥3% and ≥4% desaturations). Most sleep centers will report time the minimum SpO_2 and the time at or below a SpO_2 threshold (commonly 88%) If available REI values in the supine and nonsupine positions and during NREM and REM sleep (if available) should be reported (optional).

Physician Interpretation

The physician reading the HSAT should *state that they have reviewed the raw data*, comment on the technical adequacy of the data (or if not adequate, document why), provide a diagnosis of OSA (or not), the severity of OSA, and recommendations based on AASM treatment guidelines.

The physician reading the study should also review the raw data to document that the scoring is accurate. The reading physician should inform the physician who ordered the study that HSAT tends to underestimate the severity of sleep apnea. HSAT recommendations should include a statement (if indicated) that home sleep apnea tests that are negative or technically inadequate should be followed by PSG. Quite often insurance providers are willing to pay for a PSG if the initial HSAT is negative. Of note, a PSG rather than a repeat HSAT is recommended.

Reimbursement of HSAT: Indications, Reading Physician

The CGPM recommended that HSAT be performed in conjunction with a comprehensive sleep evaluation supervised by a board-certified/board-eligible (BC/BE) sleep physician. However, CMS and private insurers allow any treating physician to order HSAT as long as they document certain items including symptoms, an Epworth sleepiness scale score, and an upper airway examination (Mallampati score and neck circumference) (Table 16–26). The CGPM and the AASM guidelines for diagnosis of OSA recommend HSAT for patients at increased risk of **moderate to severe OSA.**[3,16] However, private insurance providers and CMS do not limit testing based on suspected severity. The AASM guidelines also lists comorbid conditions (Tables 16–6 and 16–27) that should exclude an HSAT in favor of a PSG. However, some private insurers require HSAT as the first study in virtually all patients. The AASM Scoring Manual,[1] CGPM,[16] and AASM accreditation standards[19] suggest who should perform HSAT, who should interpret HSAT studies, and quality assurance measures. The required proper training certification for sleep technologists attaching HSAT sensors, instructing the patient, or scoring of the study is also specified (e.g., a registered PSG technologist). CMS and private insurance providers do require that an HSAT is read by a *BC/BE sleep physician or a staff member of an accredited sleep* center (AASM, The Joint Commission, or Accreditation Commission for Health Care). Some LCDs have other specific requirements. The AASM website provides guidance on both sleep medicine codes and billing for sleep studies.[32]

Potential Advantages and Limitations of Home Sleep Apnea Testing

HSAT has some advantages compared with PSG (Table 16–29).[33] The patient can sleep in their normal environment with fewer attached sensors (and thus may sleep better). For patients with immobility, claustrophobia, or those who have obligations requiring them to stay at home at night, HSAT may be more convenient. The availability of HSAT is not limited by the number of monitoring rooms in the sleep center (shorter wait time). The devices are less expensive and require less expertise in applying them to patients and less time and expertise for scoring studies.

HSAT also has *disadvantages* compared with PSG. Less information is obtained, and the REI may underestimate the

Table 16–29 Potential Advantages and Disadvantages for HSAT Compared With PSG

Advantages

- Sleep in normal home environment (patients may sleep better)
- Some patients may find HSAT more comfortable than PSG (fewer monitoring leads)
- Good for patients who are immobile or who might find PSG challenging (claustrophobia)
- Flexible setting: home, hospital room, hotel
- HSAT monitoring less technically complex than PSG
- Each device less costly than PSG equipment
- Less expertise needed to setup HSAT device and sensors
- Less expertise needed to score and interpret HSAT studies than PSG
- Virtual sleep center—number of patients who can be studied is not limited by the size of a sleep center
- In some locales HSAT may decrease wait time for diagnosis and treatment (depends on availability of PSG)
- Multiple night testing can be performed (only one night is reimbursed)
- Mulitple night testing capability available on many HSAT devices

Disadvantages

- Some patients very anxious about becoming disconnected without someone available for reconnection
- Unattended—so potential for monitoring leads becoming unhooked or technically inadequate study
- 10%–15% technically inadequate studies (up to 30% in some studies if patient places the sensors)
- TST and amounts of different sleep stages are not documented by most devices (was TST and amount of REM sleep adequate?)
- AHI underestimated because of division by monitoring time that is greater than TST
- May not determine amount of supine monitoring time (some HSAT devices)
- HSAT device loss or damage can be a significant problem
- Good-quality HSAT studies require trained personnel and have substantial costs (education, setup, download, cleaning units, analysis, report generation)
- Less cost to perform HSAT but much less reimbursement
- Need to perform PSG for negative studies in most patients
- If diagnosis of significant obstructive sleep apnea is made—still need to perform PSG CPAP titration in most patients unless alternate approach used (APAP titration, APAP treatment, empiric CPAP level)
- Cannot detect arrhythmias if pulse rate by oximetry rather than electrocardiogram recorded

AHI, Apnea-hypopnea index; *CPAP,* continuous positive airway pressure; *HSAT,* home sleep apnea test; *PSG,* polysomnography; *REM,* rapid eye movement; *TST,* total sleep time.

severity of sleep apnea. Technical failure can occur if monitoring sensors are disconnected. The devices are less costly, but the reimbursement is much less. If HSAT is negative, most patients will require a subsequent PSG unless the clinical suspicion for OSA is very low. The AASM recommends a PSG following a negative HSAT for all patients. Device loss can occur, and the devices need cleaning. Some HSAT devices cannot determine body position, and most cannot determine the amount of sleep (or REM sleep) that occurred during the recording time. In patients with insomnia, if minimal sleep or REM sleep occurred during testing, this will not be apparent from results, and the REI will very likely underestimate the true severity of OSA. The heart rate is based on oximetry, and no ECG is available to detect arrhythmias. A diagnosis of OSA often results in a PSG PAP titration; the many moderate to severe patients would save money with a single split sleep study (versus HSAT followed by a PSG PAP titration study).

HSAT Protocols

There are a number of methods to perform HSAT and deliver HSAT devices.[33] One procedure is to have patients come to the sleep center to receive the device and for education on use of the device. In some centers the device is placed on the patient and all or most of the sensors applied. This method can reduce the number of technically inadequate studies. Many devices have an automatic start time to eliminate the need for the patient to activate the device at bedtime. HSAT devices can be returned in person or by mail. Another approach is to mail the HSAT device directly to the patient who applies the device (typically instructions with illustrations or video instructions are available) with return of the device by mail. When devices are returned to the sleep center, the recorded information is extracted and the device cleaned, batteries recharged or replaced, and the device initialized for recording the next patient. Most devices have the option of disposable effort belts and oximetry probes. Recently use of disposable HSAT devices has gained popularity with the recorded information sent to central cloud-based platforms using smartphones or internet devices. This eliminates the need for return of the device and cleaning before the next patient uses the device.

Types of HSAT Devices

There are numerous devices available for HSAT monitoring (Figure 16–3). Devices having more sensors provide more information (including backup sensors if one fails) but are more difficult for patients to apply. It is always a trade-off between the amount of information versus the complexity of sensor application. Some sleep centers using the more complex devices have a technologist attach the sensors in the sleep center on the day of the study. In contrast, the patient often attaches the sensors on simpler HSAT devices. The simpler devices are often mailed to the patient with detailed instruction including instructional videos. Most HSAT devices monitor airflow using a nasal cannula for monitoring nasal pressure (with or without a square root transformation). A snore signal is usually derived from nasal pressure, or a separate snore sensor may be used. Some HSAT devices can simultaneously record oral/nasal thermal flow along with nasal pressure. Respiratory effort is typically detected with one or more piezoelectric, PVDF, or RIP effort belts. Some HSAT devices use reusable effort belts, whereas others have the option of disposable effort belts. Cleaning of devices between patient use is an important consideration, as well as the cost of expendables. Arterial oxygen saturation and pulse rate are typically determined by pulse oximetry. Several oximetry probe options are available, including clip or adhesive wrap probes (either reusable or disposable). The reusable wrap approach is cheaper but more difficult for the patient to apply. As noted above, many HSAT devices also have the capability of recording body position and movement (actigraphy). Actigraphy is used by some devices to exclude portions of the tracing from analysis when there is considerable patient movement (assumes the patient is awake).

Examples of HSAT Devices

A few typical HSAT devices will be discussed. This does not represent an endorsement. The Philips Respironics (Murrysville, PA) Alice NightOne and ResMed (Poway, CA) ApneaLink Plus (or recently ApneaLink Air) are examples of relatively simple devices that the patient can attach at home (Figure 16–3). They both would qualify as a Type 3 device (or 95806/G39809). These monitors use nasal pressure to detect airflow and snoring, a single effort belt, and oximetry (SaO_2 and pulse rate). The Alice NightOne uses a single thoracic respiratory inductance belt that also holds the monitor in place, and the ResMed device uses a pneumatic effort belt. The NightOne also has a body position sensor and could record data via a Bluetooth connection from older versions of Philips Respironics PAP device (flow, pressure, leak) instead of nasal pressure. A tracing from the Alice NightOne device is shown in Figure 16–4.

The Nox T3 (Nox Medical) is an example of a more complex HSAT device. Nasal pressure is used to detect airflow and respiratory effort is detected by dual RIP thoracoabdominal belts. There is a microphone to record snoring, a body position sensor, and actigraphy. The oximetry uses a probe

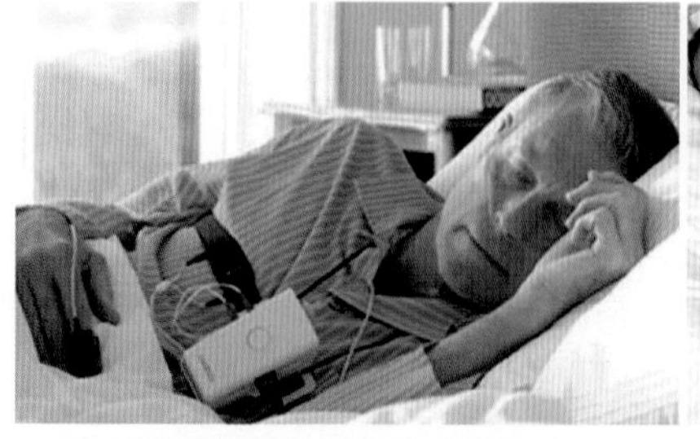
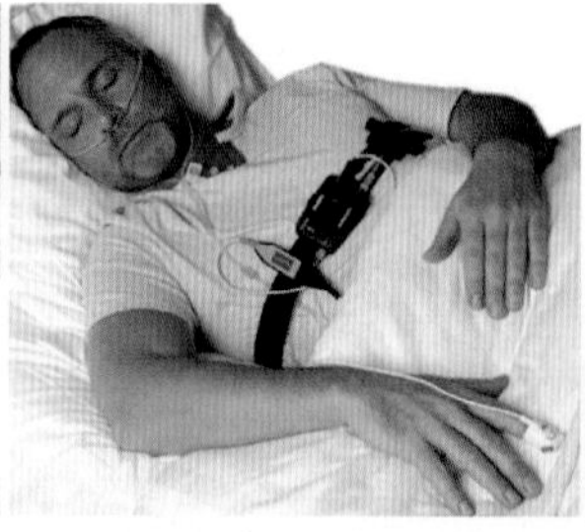
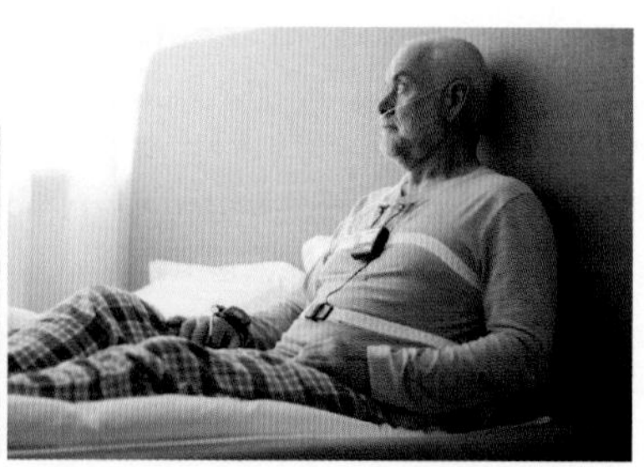

Figure 16–3 Three home sleep apnea testing devices. The left panel shows the Alice NightOne device (Philips Respironics), the middle panel the ApneaLink Air (ResMed), and the right panel the Nox T3 (Nox Medical).

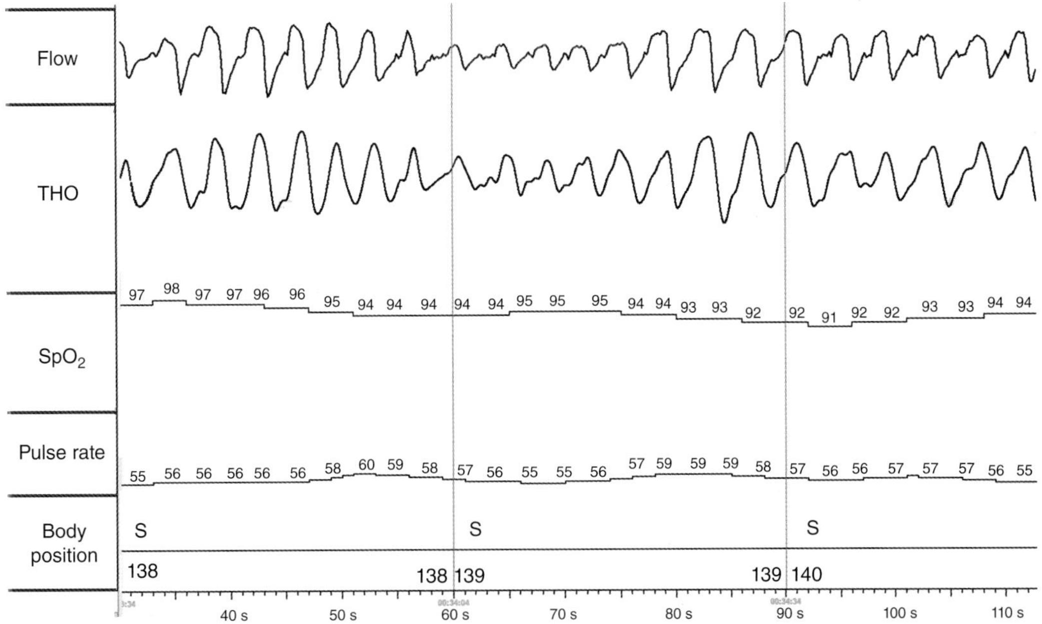

Figure 16–4 A 90-second tracing from the Alice NightOne device (Philips Respironics) showing a hypopnea with a ≥4% arterial oxygen desaturation. Channels include nasal pressure (Flow), thoracic effort using a respiratory inductance plethysmography belt (THO), SpO_2, and pulse rate, as well as body position (S = supine).

attached to a watch-like oximetry monitor that communicates with the main unit recording data via Bluetooth. This avoids the long cable connecting the main monitoring unit to the oximetry probe. Both RIP sum (estimate of tidal volume) and RIP flow (estimate of flow) are calculated and provide a backup signal to detect apnea or hypopnea (Figure 16–5) should the nasal pressure signal not be adequate in quality. Use of RIPflow avoids the need for an oronasal thermal sensor. In the case of mouth breathing the nasal pressure signal could be flat but the RIPsum or RIPflow signals would continue to display deflections. A sample HSAT report using a Type 3 device (nasal pressure, oronasal thermal sensor, chest and abdominal RIP effort belts, oximetry, body position sensor) is shown in Table 16–28.

The WatchPAT (Itamar Medical, Caesarea, Israel) is a unique device based on peripheral arterial tonometry (PAT) that

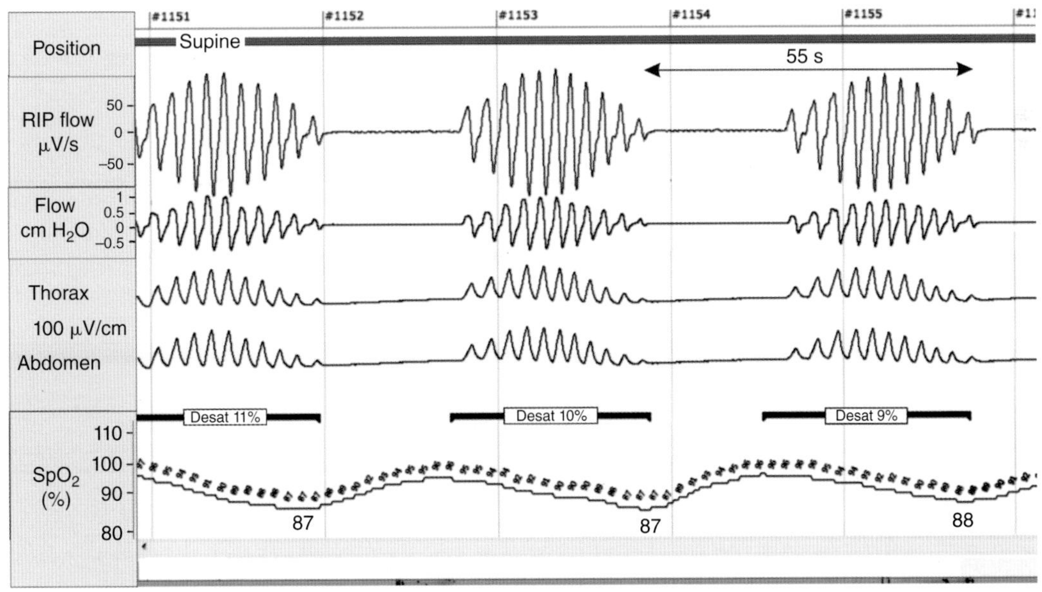

Figure 16–5 A 150-second tracing from the Nox T3 home sleep apnea testing device (Nox Medical). Channels include the RIPflow (estimate of flow), flow derived from nasal pressure, thoracic and abdominal respiratory inductance plethysmography (RIP) effort belt signals, and the pulse oximetry SpO_2 tracing. The tracings shows central apneas with Cheyne-Stokes breathing (CSB). The RIPflow is the time derivative of the RIPsum (estimate of tidal volume) derived from the sum of the thoracic and abdominal RIP belt signals. A tracing of pulse rate is also vailable (not shown). The cycle length of CSB is 55 seconds in this patient and the nadir in the SpO_2 is delayed following the central apneas (long circulation time).

detects respiratory events by recording changes in sympathetic tone (rather than airflow).[34-45] The device using this technology is worn on the wrist (Figure 16–6). The current WatchPAT device (WatchPAT 300) has a single PAT/oximetry probe and an optional sensor placed on the chest below the sternal notch. This optional sensor records snoring and is used to determine body position. The snoring/body position sensor also senses chest movement, and the WatchPAT now offers a central option[41] that can classify respiratory events as obstructive (Figure 16–7) and central (Figure 16–8) based on movement of the chest sensor, variation in the upstroke of the PAT signal associated with intrathoracic pressure changes, and snoring. The PAT signal is a measure of the blood volume in the digit. When sympathetic tone increases, stimulation of alpha receptors causes vasoconstriction of the blood vessels in the digit, which decreases the fingertip volume and the PAT signal. As surges in sympathetic tone follows respiratory event termination, the combination of a decrease in PAT signal, a fall in SpO_2 followed by an increase, and an increase in heart rate allow determination of respiratory events (Figure 16–7). These events are termed apnea/hypopnea (A/H) events as no airflow is measured and differentiation between apneas and hypopneas is not possible. Nonrespiratory arousals could reduce the PAT signal but would not reduce the SpO_2. The device results include an estimate of the AHI and REI (the pAHI) based on estimated TST. One can specify if the pAHI is to be based on apnea/hypopnea events requiring a ≥3% or ≥4% desaturation. The device also specifies a pRDI that includes events not meeting criteria for an A/H event but associated with changes in the PAT signal, heart rate, and changes in the SpO_2 less than required for an A/H event.

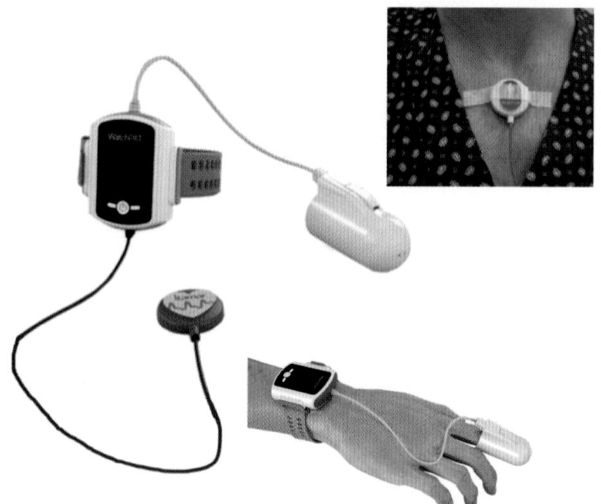

Figure 16–6 The WatchPAT 300 (Itamar Medical). The device is worn on the wrist and has a single combined PAT and oximetry probe. An attached sensor placed below the suprasternal notch records snoring intensity, body position, and detects chest movement (used to classify events as obstructive or central). PAT, peripheral arterial tonometry.

As noted above the atchPAT device can now provide a central AHI estimate (pAHIc) and detect CSB using the motion of the chest sensor.[41] If the snore/body position/respiratory movement sensor positioned below the sternal notch is not

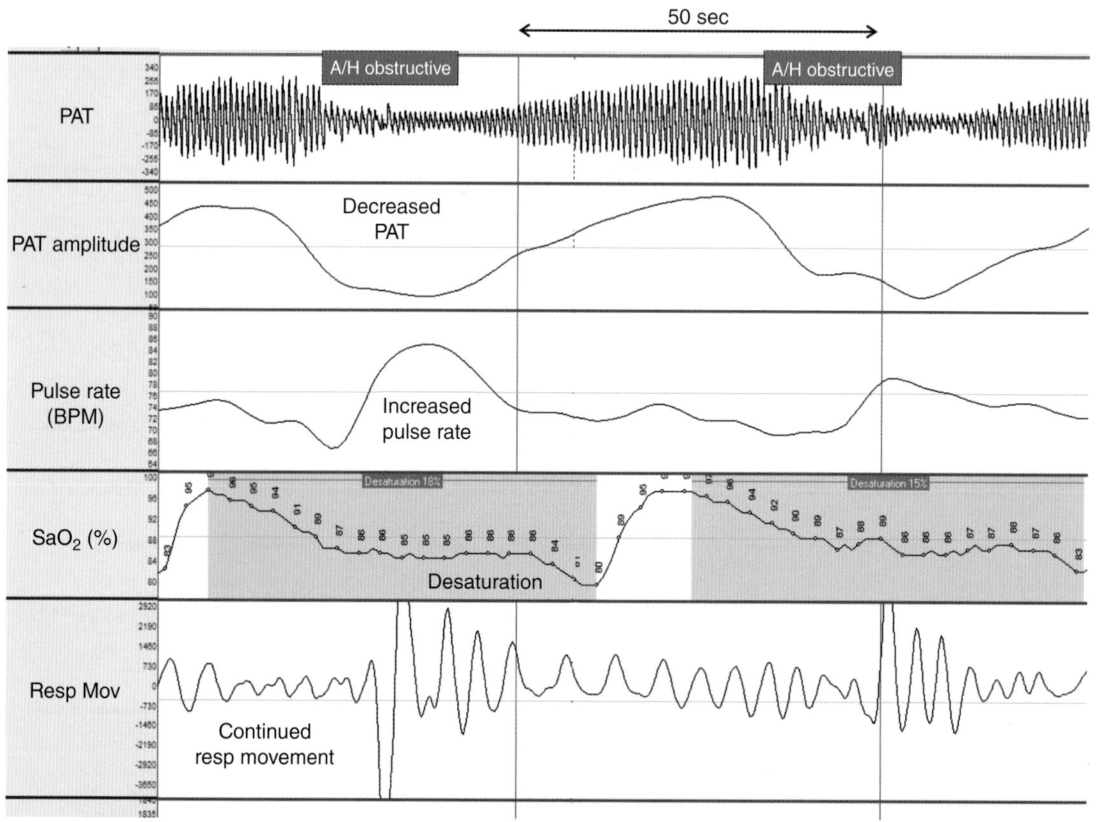

Figure 16–7 Two obstructive apnea/hypopnea (A/H) events using the WatchPAT device. The A/H event is based on a decrease in the peripheral arterial tonometry (PAT) amplitude (increased sympathetic tone), desaturation, and increased then decreased pulse rate. The obstructive nature is based on continued respiratory movement (effort). Remember that the changes in the PAT signal follow the respiratory event. Resp Mov is respiratory movement.

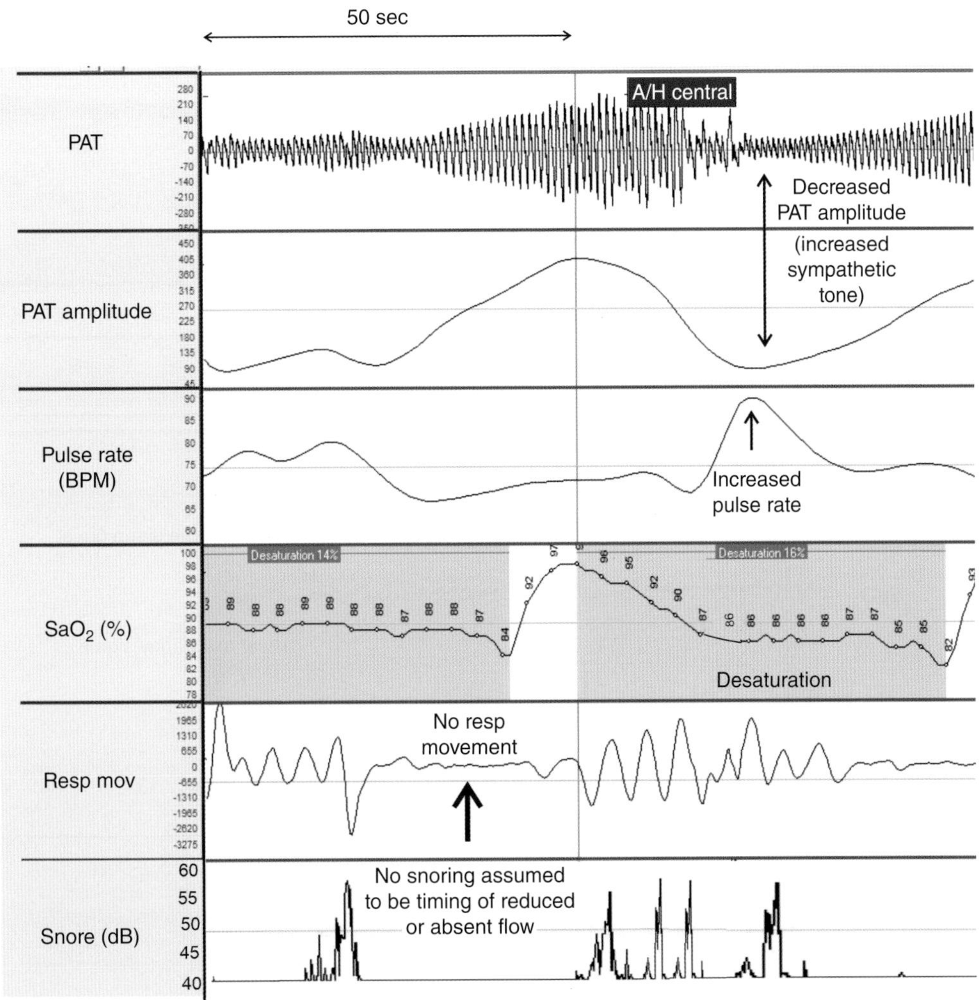

Figure 16–8 A central A/H event using the WatchPAT device. This has a similar pattern as an obstructive event, but no respiratory movement was noted. Note that the nadir in the PAT signal follows the actual change in flow, but because a flow signal is not recorded, the relationship in time between the apnea/hypopnea and the PAT signal is hard to visualize. However, looking at the snoring channel one can see snoring at the beginning and end of the event, which allows one to estimate the position of the apnea/hypopnea. Here one can see absent respiratory movement during the period of absent snoring.

recording body movements accurately the detection of A/H as "central" is often not accurate. However, the reviewing physician can convert all central events to "an obstructive event" with a single command and the pAHIc will be 0/hr. An ODI, which is the number of desaturations per hour based on the number of ≥4% desaturations is also provided. New versions of software now allow an ODI based on a ≥3% desaturation. The PAT device has built in actigraphy and novel algorithms designed for patients with sleep apnea to help with estimation of sleep.[37-40] The combination of actigraphy and the PAT signal has been used to determine estimates of wakefulness, light NREM, deep NREM, and REM sleep as the sympathetic tone characteristics of these sleep stages differ[37-40] (Figure 16–9). In the study by Hedner and coworkers,[40] the agreement with PSG was around 85% for detection of wake versus sleep and 88% for detection of NREM versus REM sleep. However, the kappa values were in the moderate range. The PAT device provides at total pAHI as well as pAHI values during estimated NREM and REM sleep. Using the optional combined body position, snore, and motion sensor, the device provides pAHI values for supine and nonsupine positions. Thus, the effect of body position can be determined. When the central option is not used, all events are assumed to be obstructive. A plot of PAT events, arterial oxygen saturation, snoring, and estimated sleep stages is shown in Figure 16–10. One can see that this patient has severe REM associated sleep apnea as severe desaturation occurs when the device detects REM sleep. In Figure 16–11(A) a portion of a report is displayed showing the pAHI, which is a surrogate for the AHI. Values for the pAHI during NREM and NREM sleep are also shown along with the effect of body position. In this study the pAHI was determined based on a ≥4% desaturation. The pAHIc is an estimate of a central event index. In Figure 16–11B a new format showing the pAHI and ODI determined using both ≥3% and ≥4% oxygen desaturations is shown. The software has options to change the report appearance.

The PAT devices have been well validated by studies comparing the results with PSG. A metaanalysis showed a high correlation between the PSG AHI and the WatchPAT pAHI.[36] However, in individual patients the difference between the PSG AHI and WatchPAT pAHI values can be over 10/hr. Another study comparing WatchPAT with PSG found

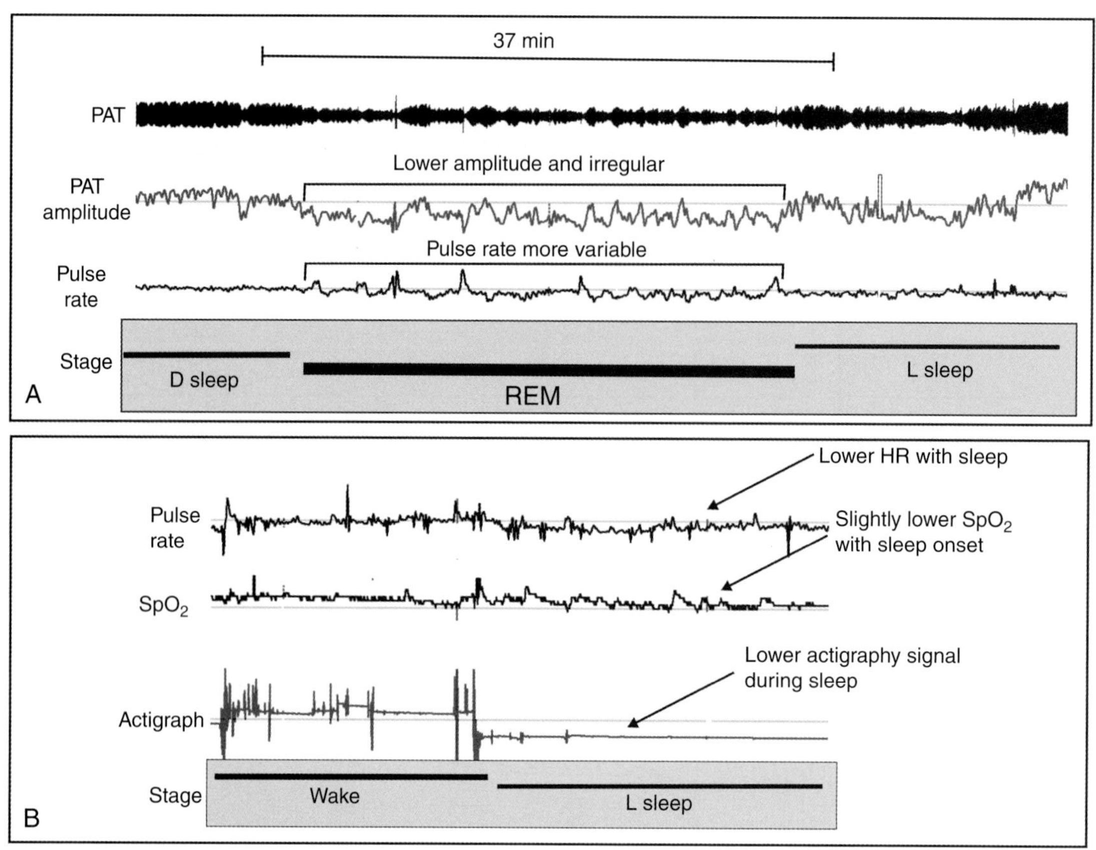

Figure 16–9 Sleep staging with the WatchPAT device provides estimates of Wake, light sleep (L Sleep), deep sleep (D Sleep), and stage R (REM) based on actigraphy, the PAT morphology, pulse rate variability and the SpO_2. In (A) a period of REM sleep is illustrated with a low amplitude and variable PAT signal. Deep sleep is associated with a steady amplitude of the PAT signal. Light sleep is associated with a variable PAT amplitude that is not substantially reduced. In (B) the transition from wake to light sleep is illustrated. During light sleep, actigraphy shows little movement and the oxygen saturation (SpO_2) is slightly lower than during wake.

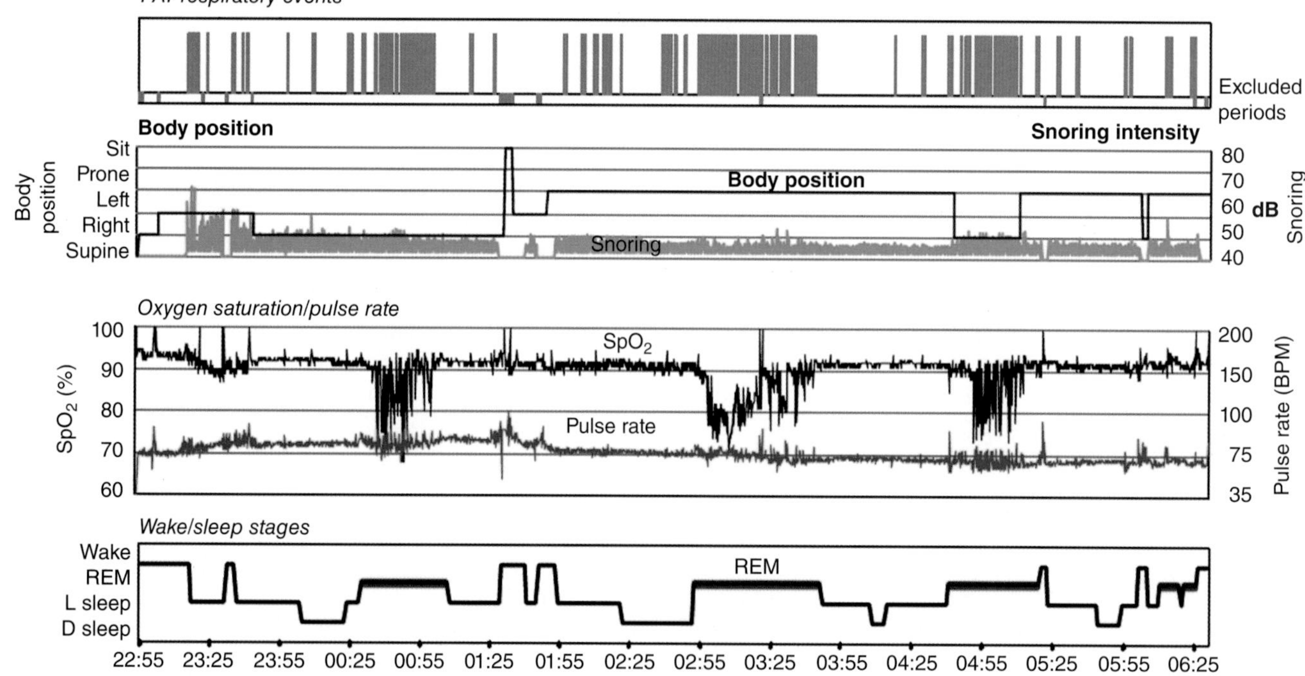

Figure 16–10 An all-night summary of WatchPAT findings show PAT respiratory events, the oxygen saturation, pulse rate, and estimated sleep stage. The snoring amplitude and body position are also displayed. Note that the periods of REM sleep detected by the WatchPAT corresponds closely to the periods of significant desaturation in this patient with sleep apnea associated with REM sleep.

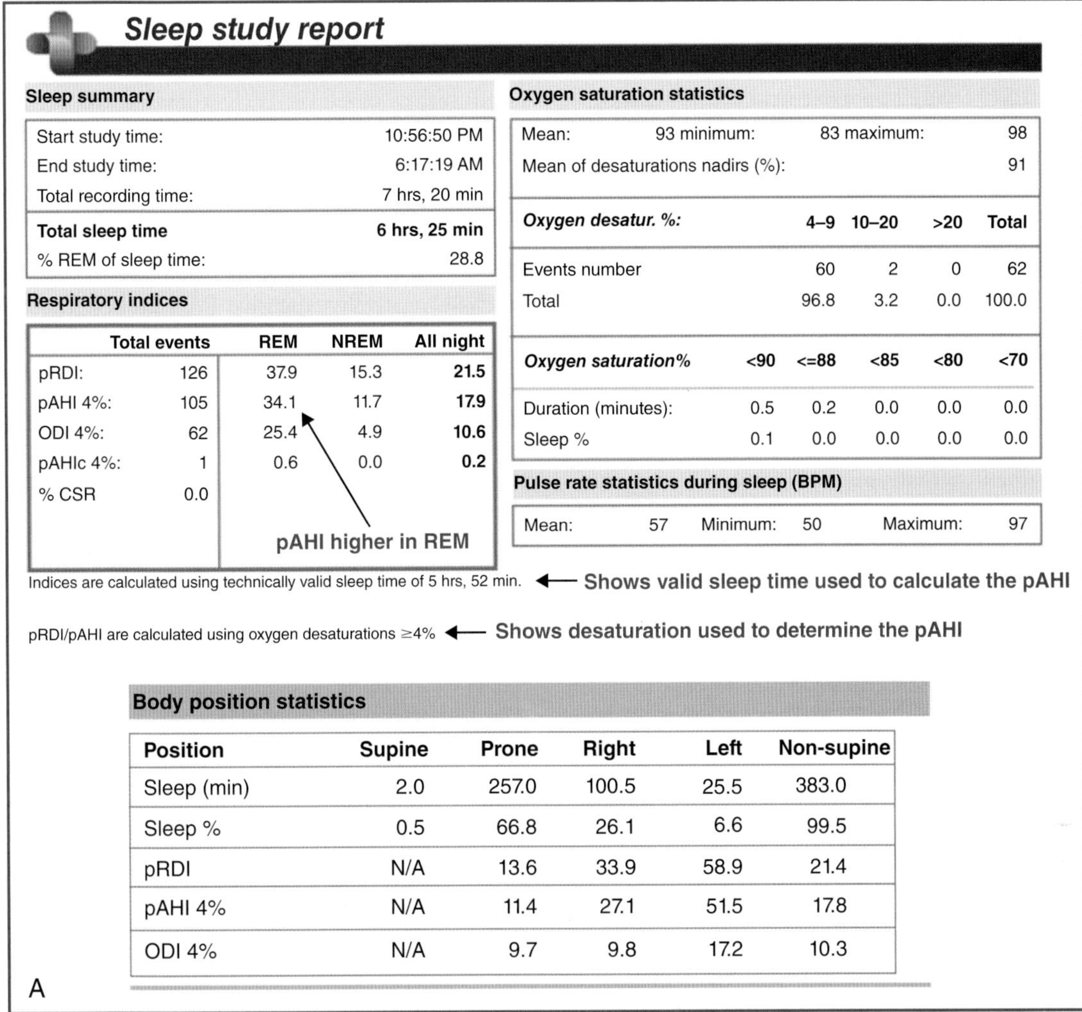

Sleep study report

Sleep summary

Start study time:	10:56:50 PM
End study time:	6:17:19 AM
Total recording time:	7 hrs, 20 min
Total sleep time	**6 hrs, 25 min**
% REM of sleep time:	28.8

Respiratory indices

	Total events	REM	NREM	All night
pRDI:	126	37.9	15.3	**21.5**
pAHI 4%:	105	34.1	11.7	**17.9**
ODI 4%:	62	25.4	4.9	**10.6**
pAHIc 4%:	1	0.6	0.0	**0.2**
% CSR	0.0			

pAHI higher in REM

Oxygen saturation statistics

Mean:	93 minimum:	83 maximum:			98
Mean of desaturations nadirs (%):					91

Oxygen desatur. %:	4–9	10–20	>20	Total
Events number	60	2	0	62
Total	96.8	3.2	0.0	100.0

Oxygen saturation%	<90	<=88	<85	<80	<70
Duration (minutes):	0.5	0.2	0.0	0.0	0.0
Sleep %	0.1	0.0	0.0	0.0	0.0

Pulse rate statistics during sleep (BPM)

Mean:	57	Minimum:	50	Maximum:	97

Indices are calculated using technically valid sleep time of 5 hrs, 52 min. ← Shows valid sleep time used to calculate the pAHI

pRDI/pAHI are calculated using oxygen desaturations ≥4% ← Shows desaturation used to determine the pAHI

Body position statistics

Position	Supine	Prone	Right	Left	Non-supine
Sleep (min)	2.0	257.0	100.5	25.5	383.0
Sleep %	0.5	66.8	26.1	6.6	99.5
pRDI	N/A	13.6	33.9	58.9	21.4
pAHI 4%	N/A	11.4	27.1	51.5	17.8
ODI 4%	N/A	9.7	9.8	17.2	10.3

A

Another patient with format showing pAHI and ODI based on ≥3% or ≥ 4% desaturations

	Total events	REM	NREM	All night
pRDI:	41	15.2	5.7	**8.7**
pAHI 3%:	25	10.6	2.8	**5.3**
ODI 3%:	27	11.2	3.1	**5.7**
pAHIc 3%:	0	0.0	0.0	**0.0**
% CSR:	0.0			
pAHI 4%:	4			**0.9**
ODI 4%:	5			**1.1**

B

Figure 16–11 (A) A sample report from the WatchPAT device showing the overall pAHI and the NREM and REM pAHI. At the bottom of the report the effect of body position is shown. The oxygen desaturation index (≥4%) is shown and information on the individual desaturations. This device has central A/H capability and a central pAHI (pAHIc 4%) is shown (0.2/hr). It is possible to have the device score respiratory events based on a ≥4% or ≥3% arterial oxygen desaturation. In the past the oxygen desaturation index (ODI) was based on 4% desaturations but in the latest software and ODI 3% or ODI 4% can be determined. The N/A values in the supine position occur as there was less than 15 minutes in the supine position. (B) One can also show the pAHI based on both ≥3% and ≥4% desaturations). It is possible to review the raw tracings, and one can delete events or change A/H events from central to obstructive events. When limited supine or REM sleep is detected N/A is provided by the program. Note the estimated total sleep time and estimate REM sleep % are provided as well as the "valid" total sleep time used to compute the pAHI.

misclassification in a significant proportion of the patients.[42] In this study there were false-positive and false-negative WatchPAT studies. A recent meta-analysis of studies comparing the WatchPAT with PSG focused on agreement rather than correlation and found significant differences between the AHI using the WatchPAT and PSG.[43] Of note, the pAHI often exceeds the ODI, which means the scoring algorithm can score pAHI events without associated desaturation if other factors are present (proprietary algorithm). Even when scoring events by airflow the AHI and ODI can differ as scoring apneas does not require a desaturation. For example, a patient has many short obstructive apneas each with minimal drops in the SpO_2. In any case the physician reviewing the study *should compare the pAHI and ODI*. A large divergence between the pAHI and ODI would cast doubt on the accuracy of the pAHI. A patient with frequent periodic leg movements associated with increased in sympathetic activity might result in an abnormal pAHI with minimal desaturation. There always should be a concern about a false positive study if the ODI is not ≥5/hr. The raw data is available for viewing and editing. The software automatically excludes portions of the data felt to contain artifact. Additional portions can be manually marked as artifact. As noted above it is possible for the reviewing technologist or physician to review the raw data and edit the automatic scoring of the WatchPAT. Algorithms have been proposed to improve the accuracy of the device (better agreement with PSG).[44] At a minimum, physicians reviewing WatchPAT studies should review the raw data to determine if it is technically adequate. Ideally, they should learn how to edit the autoscoring and run a new report. As noted above it is important to compare the pAHI and ODI. The WatchPAT device is one of the easier HSAT devices for patients to apply. With proper education there are relatively few technical failures. The device cannot be used in patients on alpha-blockers (e.g., Terazosin) but beta-blockers are permitted. In the past the device was not recommended for patients in atrial fibrillation but can function in these patients unless they have a predominantly paced rhythm.[45] The main downside to using the device is that the PAT probes are relatively expensive. The WatchPAT device is acceptable to CMS and the recent AASM clinical guidelines listed devices based on PAT, oximetry, and actigraphy as acceptable for diagnosis of OSA.[3] There is now a disposable version of the WatchPAT (WatchPAT One). A new HSAT device based on changes in the oximetry photoplethysmography that reflect changes in sympathetic tone (NightOwl)[46] has been developed using the same general approach as the WatchPAT. Although less well validated, it avoids the need to purchase relatively expensive PAT probes. The utility of this and similar devices remains to be determined.

Multiple Night Testing

There is known night-to-night variability in testing results in patients with mild to moderate OSA whether using HSAT or PSG.[47,48] Multiple night testing with PSG is too costly for widespread application, but multiple night testing is possible with several HSAT devices. Some studies suggest using an average of the multiple night values may improve the diagnostic utility of testing of HSAT. However, there is no firm consensus of what result to use. Should one use the average, the lowest, or the highest AHI? This night-to-night variability is more of a problem for milder OSA. In such patients the amount or supine and REM sleep can determine if the AHI is above or below 5/hr.

What to Do After HSAT

Many of the insurance providers that mandate an HSAT rather than PSG on the majority of patients may also decline a PSG titration in favor of treatment with APAP. Whereas this approach may work for uncomplicated patients, those with comorbidities such as a substantial amount of central apnea, congestive heart failure, treatment with potent opioids, and suspicion for hypoventilation are not good candidates for APAP treatment.[23] The use of APAP will be discussed in chapter 23, but clinical pathways for diagnosis and treatment are presented in Figure 16–12.

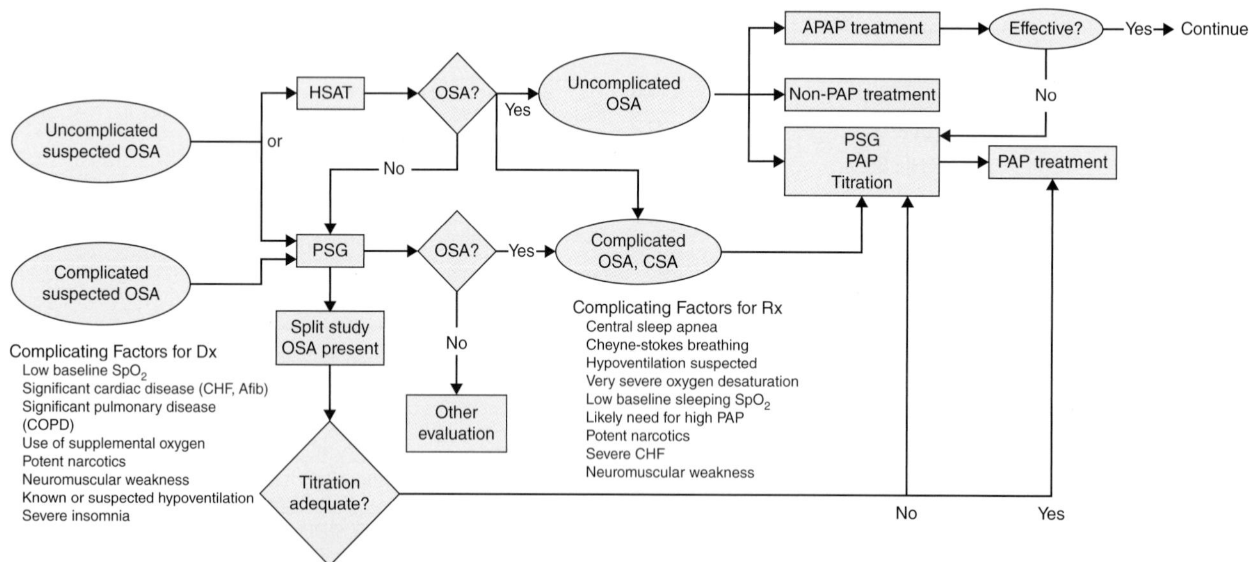

Figure 16–12 Algorithm for integration of HSAT and PSG into overall treatment pathways. Uncomplicated patients may be handled with HSAT followed by treatment with APAP (auto-adjusting positive airway pressure device). However, those with complex problems identified by history (before a diagnostic study) or identified based on the HSAT (or a diagnostic PSG) should undergo a polysomnography PAP titration.

ACTIGRAPHY

Actigraphy uses a portable device (the actigraph) usually worn on the wrist that records movement over an extended period (Figure 16–13). Sleep-wake patterns are estimated from the pattern of movement. Algorithms (software) estimates the TST, sleep latency, and wake time for each day from the data. The estimates of TST and wake time (WASO) are more accurate in normal individuals than in patients with sleep disorders. However, information from actigraphy is extremely valuable in documenting patterns of sleep and wake. This information is useful for evaluation of patients with insomnia and circadian rhythm sleep-wake disorders. *Of note, actigraphy is not recommended for the "routine" evaluation of insomnia.* However, when patients either do not reliably complete sleep logs or the information is not plausible, actigraphy can be helpful. In 2008 actigraphy transitioned from a CPT category III (emerging technology) to a category I (95893), which is a stand-alone code. Actigraphy should be performed for a minimum of 72 hours to a maximum of 14 days consecutive days to be billed. Currently the procedure is not reimbursed by most private insurance payors or Medicare. A suitable diagnosis must be submitted when billing 95893, such the delayed sleep phase disorder. In fact, for clinical accuracy actigraphy should be performed for a minimum of 7 days, ideally 14 days, for evaluation of most patients with insomnia and especially circadian rhythm disorders. A sleep log (diary) is also completed noting time in bed, time trying to sleep, estimates of periods of sleep and wake during the night, final wake time, and final out of bed time. Time with the device off can also be noted. More information on actigraphy for evaluation of insomnia and circadian sleep-wake rhythm disorders is available in Chapters 33 and 34.

The AASM practice parameters for the use of actigraphy were published in 2005 and 2007.[49,50] In 2018, a clinical practice guideline for use of actigraphy for the evaluation of sleep

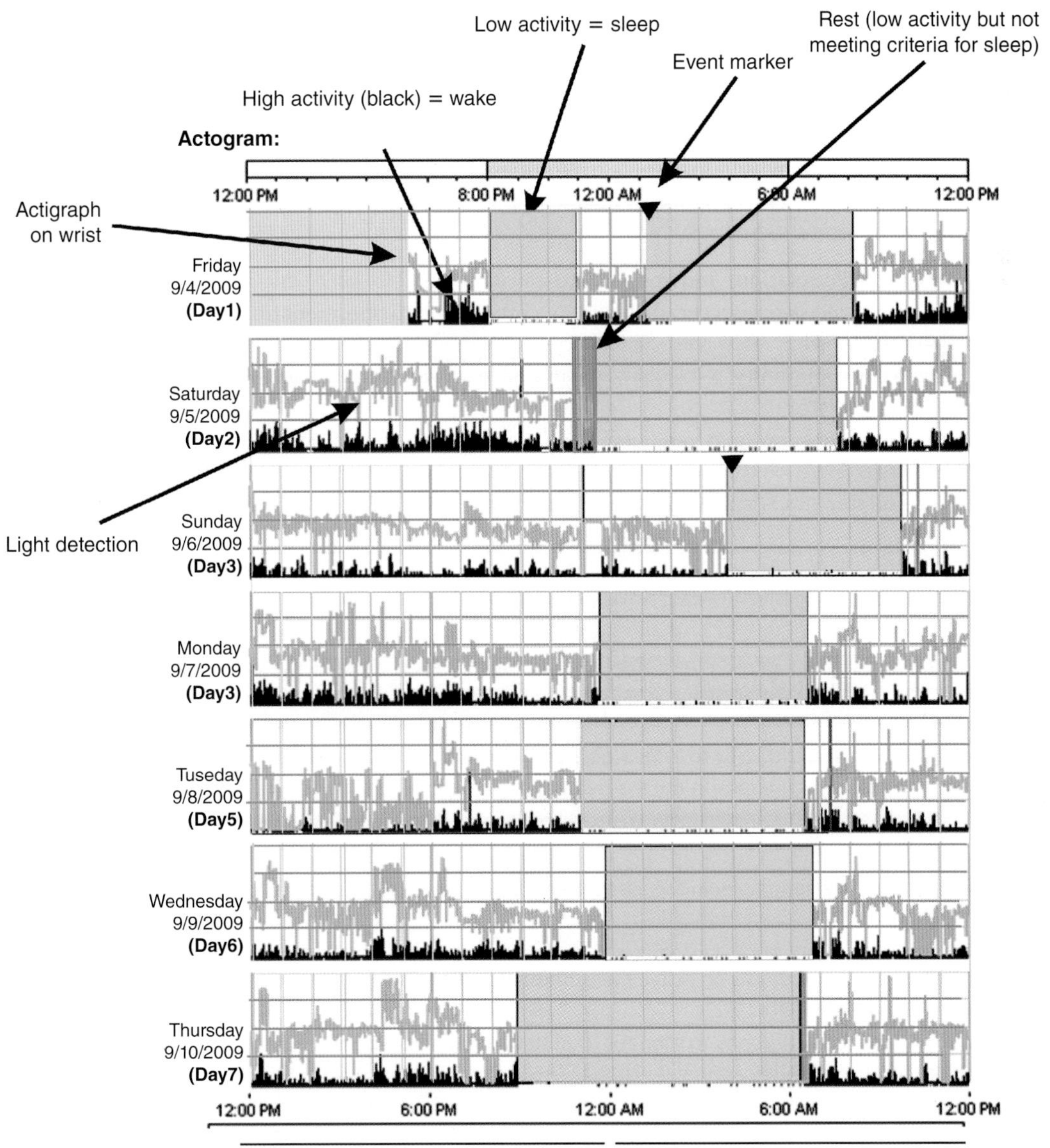

Figure 16–13 Actigraphy over 1 week in a patient with insomnia complaints. Variable sleep onset and duration are noted. The dark activity is wake and pale blue is sleep. The green box is rest (not meeting criteria for sleep). The light gray tracing is detected light (a light-detecting sensor is built into this actigraph). Midnight is the center of the graphs.

disorders and circadian rhythm sleep-wake disorders in adult and pediatric patients was published along with a review of the evidence (meta-analysis).[51,52]

A summary of the 2007 recommendations is presented in Table 16–30 along with the level of recommendation. Actigraphy was recommended to assess sleep-wake patterns in normal populations and patients with circadian rhythm sleep-wake disorders (including response to treatment), patients with insomnia, and patients complaining of hypersomnia (to rule out insufficient sleep). A standard recommendation was given to use of actigraphy in OSA to improve accuracy of HSAT. Note the recommendation is to assess the sleep-wake pattern and not TST, sleep latency and other measures of sleep duration. The recommendations from the 2018 clinical guideline for the use of actigraphy for evaluation of sleep disorders and circadian rhythm sleep-wake disorders are

Table 16–30 Summary of 2007 Practice Parameters for Use of Actigraphy

Use of Actigraphy in Evaluation of Sleep Disorders

- Determining sleep patterns in normal, healthy adult populations (Standard), and in certain suspected sleep disorders (Option-Guideline-Standard depending on disorder).
- Evaluation of suspected of advanced sleep-wake phase disorder (ASWPD), delayed sleep-wake phase disorder (DSWPD), shift work sleep disorder (Guideline), jet lag and non–24-hour sleep-wake rhythm disorder [including that associated with blindness]. (Option)
- When PSG is not available, actigraphy is indicated to estimate total sleep time in patients with obstructive sleep apnea syndrome. Combined with a validated way of monitoring respiratory events, use of actigraphy may improve accuracy in assessing the severity of obstructive sleep apnea compared with using time in bed. (Standard)
- Characterize circadian rhythm patterns or sleep disturbances in individuals with insomnia, including insomnia associated with depression. (Option)
- Determine circadian pattern and estimate average daily sleep time in individuals complaining of hypersomnia. (Option)

Use of Actigraphy in Assessing the Response to Therapy of Sleep Disorders

- Actigraphy is useful as an outcome measure in evaluating the response to treatment for circadian rhythm sleep-wake disorders. (Guideline)
- Actigraphy is useful for evaluating the response to treatment for patients with insomnia, including insomnia associated with depressive sleep-wake disorders. (Guideline)

Use of Actigraphy in Special Populations and Special Situations

- Characterizing and monitoring sleep and circadian rhythm patterns and to document treatment outcome (in terms of sleep patterns and circadian rhythms).
- **Older adults living in the community**, particularly when used in conjunction with other measures such as sleep diaries and/or caregiver observations. (Guideline)
- **Older nursing home residents** (in whom traditional sleep monitoring by polysomnography can be difficult to perform and/or interpret). (Guideline)
- **Normal infants and children** (traditional PSG can be difficult to perform and/or interpret), and in special pediatric populations. (Guideline)

Adapted from references 45 and 46 level of recommendation.
From References 49, 50. Level of Recommendation Standard > Guideline > Option , Circadian disorder terminology updated.

Table 16–31 Summary of 2018 AASM Clinical Practice Guideline for the Use of Actigraphy for the Evaluation of Sleep Disorders and Circadian Rhythm Sleep-Wake Disorders

1. We suggest that clinicians use actigraphy to *estimate sleep parameters* in adult patients with insomnia disorder. (Conditional)
2. We suggest that clinicians use actigraphy in the assessment of pediatric patients with insomnia disorder. (Conditional)
3. We suggest that clinicians use actigraphy in the assessment of adult patients with circadian rhythm sleep-wake disorders. (Conditional)
4. We suggest that clinicians use actigraphy in the assessment of pediatric patients with circadian rhythm sleep-wake disorders. (Conditional)
5. We suggest that clinicians use actigraphy integrated with home sleep apnea test devices to estimate total sleep time during recording (in the absence of alternative objective measurements of total sleep time) in adult patients suspected of sleep-disordered breathing. (Conditional)
6. We suggest that clinicians use actigraphy to monitor total sleep time before testing with the multiple sleep latency test in adult and pediatric patients with suspected central disorders of hypersomnolence. (Conditional)
7. We suggest that clinicians use actigraphy to estimate total sleep time in adult patients with suspected insufficient sleep syndrome. (Conditional)
8. We recommend that clinicians NOT use actigraphy in place of electromyography for the diagnosis of periodic limb movement disorder in adult and pediatric patients. (Strong)

Adapted from reference 52

shown in Table 16–31. The level of recommendation in the clinical guidelines was "conditional" for all the positive recommendations. It was suggested that clinicians use actigraphy for evaluation of adult and pediatric patients with insomnia disorder and circadian rhythm sleep-wake disorders. It was also suggested that clinicians could use information from actigraphy when integrated in a home-sleep monitoring device to provide an estimate of TST and hopefully improve the accuracy of the derived AHI (dividing by estimated TST rather than monitoring time or recording time). Use of actigraphy to estimate sleep duration and timing of the habitual sleep period in the weeks before a planned PSG to be followed by an MSLT is suggested in adult and pediatric patients. Bradshaw and coworkers[53] compared patient-reported estimated sleep duration, sleep duration obtained from sleep logs, and sleep duration based on actigraphy. Both estimated sleep duration and sleep log–determined sleep duration significantly exceeded the sleep duration by actigraphy. Only the actigraphy sleep duration correlated with the mean sleep latency on the MSLT. Finally, use of actigraphy was suggested to estimate TST in patients believed to have insufficient sleep. The evidence was "strong" for the recommendation to NOT use actigraphy for the diagnosis of the PLMD (adult and pediatric patients). The use of actigraphy to complement a sleep log in the period before testing with PSG followed by MSLT is a relatively new recommendation but is consistent with recommendations for testing in the ICSD-3-TR for the diagnosis of narcolepsy.[54]

The best use of actigraphy in patients with insomnia and circadian rhythm sleep-wake disorders is to document the pattern of wake and sleep periods. Some actigraphy devices have a built-in light sensor that can detect exposure to light. As noted above in the 2008 practice parameters, actigraphy was recommended for determining the response to therapy in patients with circadian rhythm disorders. Although not precisely recommended in the 2018 practice guideline recommendations, in the text of the article there was a statement that meta-analysis results "show that actigraphy is useful in the assessment of sleep onset and offset times and in the evaluation of treatment outcomes in some patients with circadian rhythm sleep-wake disorders (CRSWD)."

The accompanying evidence review for the actigraphy guidelines published in 2018 as a companion article included a meta-analysis of studies performed in adult and pediatric

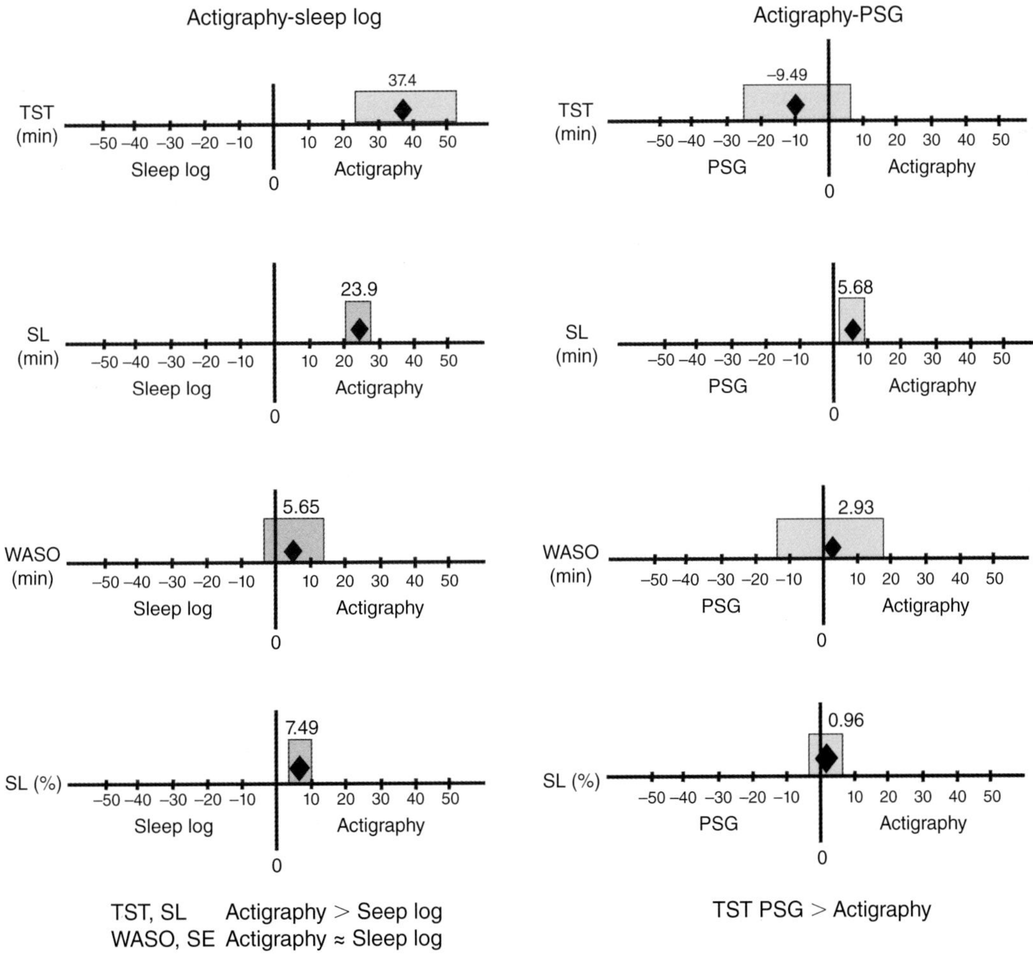

Figure 16–14 Plots of the results of a meta-analysis comparing actigraphy, PSG, and sleep logs. These plots are from patients with known or suspected insomnia in adult populations. For actigraphy versus sleep logs, actigraphy found higher total sleep time (TST) and longer sleep latency (SL) but similar wake after sleep onset (WASO) and sleep efficiency (SE). Compared with PSG, actigraphy found slightly less total sleep time, but similar sleep latency, wake after sleep onset, and sleep efficiency. Grey Boxes are 95% confidence intervals. (Plotted using data from Smith MT, McCrae CS, Cheung J, et al. Use of actigraphy for the evaluation of sleep disorders and circadian rhythm sleep-wake disorders: an American Academy of Sleep Medicine systematic review, meta-analysis, and GRADE assessment. J Clin Sleep Med. 2018;14[7]:1209–1230. [Supplementary figures S1a,S1b, S2a, S2b,S3a, S3b, S4a, S4b.])

patients with **known or suspected insomnia** comparing sleep logs versus actigraphy or actigraphy versus PSG.[51] The parameters TST, sleep latency (SL), WASO, and sleep efficiency (SE) were analyzed. Actigraphy overestimated TST and sleep latency compared with sleep logs by an average of 37.4 and 23.9 minutes, respectively (Figure 16–14). The conclusion was that actigraphy provides information that is often "unique" from patient-reported sleep logs. In summary, the information from actigraphy and sleep logs is complementary. As noted previously, it is standard practice to have patients fill out a sleep log while wearing the actigraph device. The differences comparing PSG and actigraphy were relatively small. Actigraphy underestimated total sleep time compared to PSG by about 9.5 minutes. Actigraphy overestimated the sleep latency compared to PSG by about 5.7 minutes.

A detailed discussion of reading actograms is beyond the scope of this chapter.[55-56] However, Figure 16–13 illustrates some essential elements actogram. This is an example of the 24-hour format with noon in the center of the plot. The jagged black areas represents activity level. The software first determines periods of "rest" and then the periods of rest that meet criteria for sleep. Event markers can be used by the patient to signal trying to sleep. Many actigraphy devices can detect light. Thus, one can determine "lights-out" from this information. The actogram in Figure 16–14 is an example of an individual with highly variable sleep onset times and wake times. A middle of the sleep period awakening was noted on day 1 for over 2 hours, and one can see that the patient turned the lights on during this awakening. A confusing issue for those new to actigraphy is use of the double plot (Figure 16–15). Each line consists of two 24-hour periods with the center of each line being midnight separating the two 24-hour periods. The last 24 hours of one line is repeated on the first part of the next line. This type of plot allows visualization of many nights on a single page thus showing visualization of trends over a longer time duration. In the actogram in Figure 16–16, there is a progressive delay in the onset of sleep. This is characteristic of a patient with non-24-hour circadian rhythm sleep-wake disorder. More detailed discussion is provided in the chapter on circadian rhythm sleep-wake disorders (Chapter 34).

There has been an explosion in wearable, bedside, bed pad, and video technology providing estimates of TST and sleep quality. Some devices even report that amount and pattern of light, deep, and stage R sleep.[57] To date accuracy at estimating sleep time is better than determining sleep stages. The AASM published a useful position statement that provides advice for the clinician when discussing the results of wearable technology estimates of sleep.[58] This is an important issue as patients voice anxious concern that "I am not getting enough REM sleep" when the technology being used is unlikely to accurately define the amount of REM sleep.

SUMMARY OF KEY POINTS

1. PSG is indicated for the diagnosis of OSA, PAP titration, documenting efficacy of non-PAP treatments (after weight loss, after surgery, or while wearing an OA), preceding MSLT, and for evaluation of complicated parasomnias. PSG is indicated before any surgical procedure (even for snoring).
2. Repeat PSG is indicated if a previous false-negative study is suspected or if the prior study was technically inadequate. Repeat PAP titration is not routinely indicated for patients doing well on treatment but is indicated if symptoms return or are not well controlled, or if PAP device download

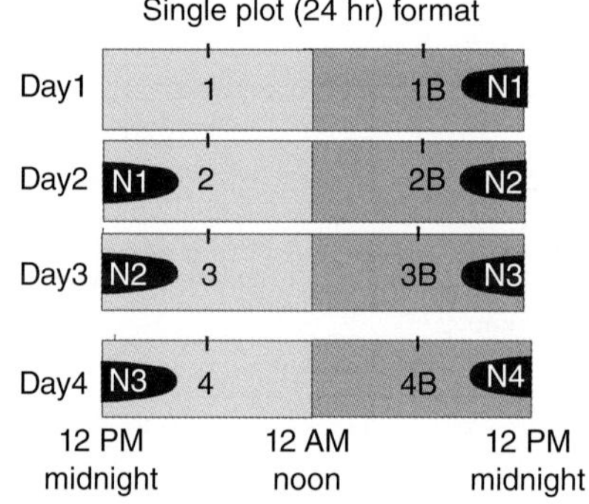

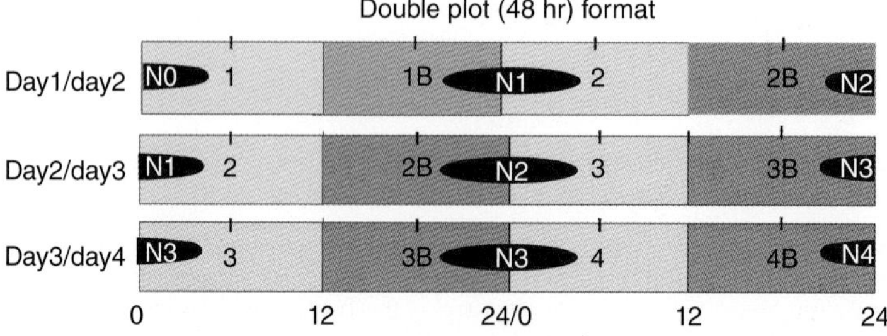

Figure 16–15 A schematic of single and double plot formats. In the single plot each line is 24 hours starting at midnight. Noon is at the middle of the plot. At the bottom a double plot is shown. Each line is 48 hours. Midnight is at the center of the plot. The second 24 hours on one line is repeated as the first 24 hours on the next line. This allows entire nights to be compared at the center of the plot. In addition, more nights can be covered with fewer lines.

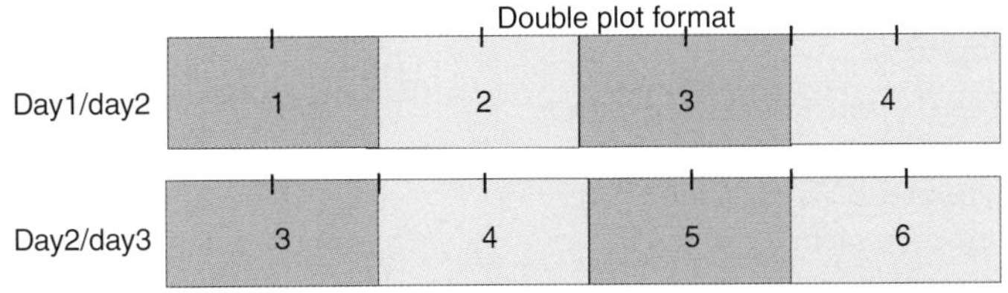

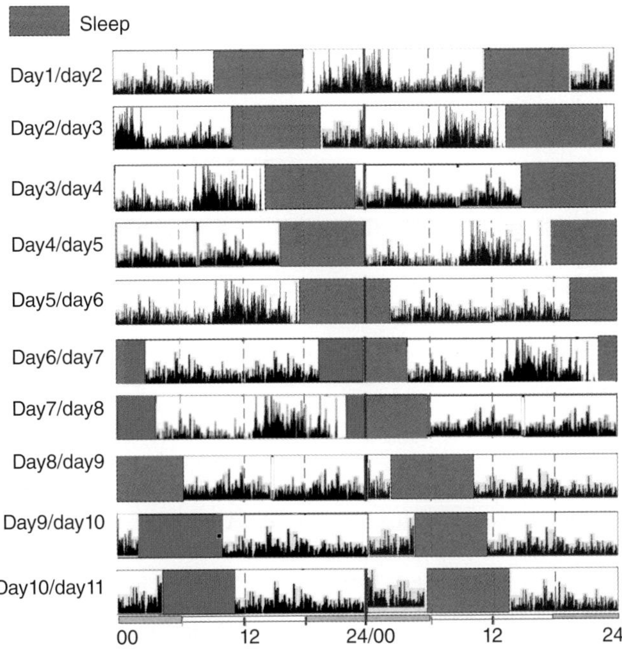

Figure 16–16 An idealized double plot of a patient with non–24-hour circadian rhythm sleep-wake disorder (previously called free running). The sleep onset time and wake time are progressively delayed.

information suggests treatment is not effective. Repeat PSG is indicated in patients with prior surgery or weight loss if symptoms return and is indicated while wearing an OA if symptoms return on OA treatment.

3. PSG is not indicated for patients doing well on CPAP or for evaluation of insomnia or uncomplicated parasomnias, in patients with a known seizure disorder, for depression, and in patients with RLS unless a diagnosis of OSA is suspected. PSG is indicated to assist in making a diagnosis of PLMD (recall a diagnosis of RLS excludes a diagnosis of PLMD).
4. HSAT is indicated in patients with a high probability of having moderate to severe obstructive sleep apnea in the absence of comorbidities mandating the use of PSG, including known or suspected hypoventilation, use of supplemental oxygen, evaluation for a parasomnia, significant chronic lung disease, or congestive heart failure. HSAT can be used to assess the effectiveness of non-PAP treatments (after surgery, using an OA). If a single HSAT is technically inadequate or negative, a PSG should be ordered.
5. HSAT devices measuring airflow (but not EEG for sleep staging) provide a respiratory event index (REI) as a surrogate of the AHI. The REI = (number of apneas and hypopneas) × 60 / monitoring time in minutes. The monitoring time may equal the recording time, but in most sleep centers the monitoring time is based on lights-on and lights-off time using a patient diary. The monitoring time equals the recording time minus time with artifact or time awake based on actigraphy, body position, or patient diary.
6. Interpretation of HSAT requires review of the raw data to verify adequate technical quality of a study and to determine whether the respiratory events were properly scored. An HSAT device must have at a minimum recording of airflow, respiratory effort, and oxygen saturation or PAT/oximetry and actigraphy. For HSAT devices measuring flow or tidal volume, ideally respiratory effort should be monitored by dual RIP thoracoabdominal belts. Qualified providers should either place the HSAT sensors or instruct the patients to avoid a high proportion of technically inadequate studies (or provide video instructions).
7. Selection of the HSAT device should consider the setting in which it will be used and whether the patient will place the sensors without assistance at home. More complex devices have backup sensors, whereas simple devices are easier to place.
8. Multiple night testing is ideal as there is considerable night-to-night variability in the AHI (REI)—especially in patients with milder OSA.
9. Actigraphy is useful for establishing the sleep-wake pattern of patients with insomnia and circadian rhythm sleep-wake disorders. Whereas it is not routinely indicated for evaluation of patients with insomnia, it can be very useful in individuals unable to keep an accurate sleep log. It is helpful in documenting insufficient sleep and potentially very helpful in the weeks before MSLT to document the amount and pattern of sleep. A sleep log is always collected with actigraphy. The sleep log and actigraphy data are complementary.

CLINICAL REVIEW QUESTIONS

1. A 45-year-old man is referred to the sleep laboratory with a long history of snoring, witnessed apnea, and daytime sleepiness. The physical examination shows a BMI of 31 kg/m^2, very crowded upper airway, and neck circumference of 17 inches. An unattended PM (type 3) sleep study found an AHI of 3.5 events/hr with the lowest SaO_2 being 89%. The patient reports he did not sleep that well (worried about pulling out wires from PM device). Which of the following would you do next?
   A. Repeat HSAT
   B. PSG
   C. Tell the patient that he doesn't have OSA
   D. Refer him for an OA or upper airway surgery to treat primary snoring
2. A 40-year-old man was referred to the sleep center with a long history of loud snoring, witnessed apnea, and daytime sleepiness. The physical examination shows a BMI of 31 kg/m^2 and a very long, swollen uvula. His neck is 18 inches in circumference. The patient is otherwise healthy. Which of the following would you do next?
   A. HSAT (type 3 with monitoring airflow, effort, SaO_2)
   B. Attended PSG
   C. Nocturnal oximetry
   D. Treatment with APAP
   E. Refer him for an OA or surgery to treat primary snoring
3. A 40-year-old man was referred to the sleep center with a history of loud snoring that bothers his wife. The patient denies daytime sleepiness. His wife has never noted breathing pauses. The patient has been evaluated by an ear-nose-throat (ENT) physician who recommends upper airway surgery for snoring. On examination, he has a long uvula but a minimally crowded upper airway. His neck circumference is 15 inches and his BMI is 22 kg/m^2. Which of the following do you recommend?
   A. Proceed to have the upper airway surgery for snoring
   B. Schedule for a PSG
   C. Schedule for oximetry
   D. Schedule HSAT with type 3 device
4. You are asked to follow a 50-year-old woman who was diagnosed with OSA about 2 years ago at another sleep and has been using CPAP regularly. Her body weight is stable and her husband reports that she does not snore when using CPAP. A download of the device shows excellent adherence and a device estimated AHI is 2/hr. The patient denies daytime sleepiness and is happy with her sleep quality. What do you suggest?
   A. CPAP titration to check the adequacy of current treatment
   B. Ongoing follow-up to document adherence and a good symptomatic response
   C. A diagnostic PSG to determine if CPAP treatment is still needed
   D. No follow-up needed
5. A 35-year-old man with OSA had palatal surgery performed 3 months ago for OSA (preoperative AHI was 25/hr). He reports that his snoring is much improved and that his daytime sleepiness is better as well. Physical examination shows a well-healed palatal scar. Which of the following do you recommend?
   A. PSG or HSAT
   B. As his symptoms have improved, clinical follow-up only
   C. PSG if symptoms return
   D. Oximetry
6. A 55-year-old man with known diastolic heart failure (normal ejection fraction) has been using CPAP regularly for years. Recently a return of atrial fibrillation has been noted after a previous ablation procedure. He is undecided if he should have another cardioversion and attempt at ablation. A download of his CPAP shows an AHI of 20/hr (previously 5/hr), and some of the events were classified as clear airway apneas. Periodic breathing was present in 20% of the night. Which of the following do you recommend?
   A. Empiric increase in CPAP
   B. PAP titration study
   C. No changes until his cardiac status improves
   D. Nocturnal oximetry
7. A 75-year-old man recently had a left-sided cerebrovascular accident (CVA) and now has mild right hemiparesis. Per his spouse, there is no snoring or witnessed apnea. He complains of insomnia and frequent nocturnal arousals. Physical examination is notable for the hemiparesis and moderate obesity. Which of the following do you recommend?
   A. Screening oximetry
   B. PSG
   C. HSAT
   D. Cognitive behavior therapy for insomnia
   E. Empirical trial of a hypnotic
8. A 16-year-old boy with Duchenne muscular dystrophy complains of frequent episodes of nocturnal dyspnea and frequent awakenings. He is wheelchair bound. Physical examination shows diffuse muscle atrophy and weakness, obesity. An awake SaO_2 is 94% breathing room air. Which of the following do you recommend?
   A. Oximetry, and nocturnal supplemental oxygen if indicated
   B. HSAT
   C. PSG with end-tidal PCO_2 monitoring
   D. Hypnotic
9. A 45-year-old woman has complaints of poor sleep with frequent nocturnal arousals and daytime sleepiness. Her husband says that she kicks her legs at night. Only mild snoring and no witnessed apneas are reported. The patient DENIES symptoms of the RLS. Which of the following is recommended?
   A. PSG
   B. HSAT
   C. Sleep diary for 2 weeks
   D. Empirical treatment with a hypnotic
   E. Actigraphy
10. A 60-year-old woman is complaining of severe difficulty initiating and maintaining sleep. This has not improved with several hypnotics and cognitive behavioral therapy for insomnia. Her husband reports mild snoring and no breathing pauses. She has coronary artery disease and has recently undergone an angioplasty with two stents. The patient also has a long history of hypertension and diabetes mellitus. Her medications include clopidogrel and aspirin. Physical examination shows moderate obesity and a slightly crowded oropharynx. Which of the following do you recommend?
    A. Actigraphy
    B. PSG
    C. HSAT
    D. Trazodone

11. A HSAT test is performed for insomnia and the results are listed here. The HSAT device signals included nasal pressure, RIPflow, chest and abdominal RIP effort belt signals and oximetry. The patient reports loud snoring but no daytime sleepiness. What do you recommend?
Monitoring time: 7 hours
AHI (based on monitoring time) = 3/hr
Events: 13 obstructive apneas, 8 hypopneas
Desaturations: 70, with ODI of 15/hr, lowest SpO_2 = 83%
A. PSG.
B. Evaluate raw tracings.
C. Treatment for snoring.
D. Inform the patient that OSA is not present.

ANSWERS

1. B. A negative HSAT should be followed by a PSG, especially when there is a significant clinical suspicion of OSA. Technically inadequate study (<4 good hours of data) is another indication for PSG. Ideally HSAT is indicated when there is a high risk of moderate to severe OSA. This patient has a high risk of having OSA based on snoring, witnessed apnea, and an upper airway exam. In this case a PSG is needed to rule out a false-negative HSAT.
2. A or B. This patient has a high risk of moderate OSA without any conditions precluding HSAT. However, a PSG is still the test of choice. Empiric treatment without a diagnosis is not recommended. Patients with planned upper airway surgery (even for "snoring") should always have either PSG or HSAT.
3. B. Testing should always be performed even if surgery is planned only to treat snoring. In this case the patient has a normal BMI, no witnessed apnea, and no symptoms other than snoring. A PSG is ideal as there is not a high risk of moderate to severe OSA. However, an HSAT may be required by insurance plans as the patient has no comorbidity making HSAT contraindicated.
4. B. A diagnostic PSG would not be indicated unless the patient wanted to stop treatment or after a 10% or greater weight loss. A CPAP titration is not indicated in a patient doing well on treatment. Ongoing follow-up is needed to ensure adequate adherence, a low device AHI estimate, and continued symptomatic response.
5. A. After upper airway surgery for OSA, a PSG or HSAT is indicated routinely to assess treatment results (after surgical healing). Improvement in symptoms is not a reliable indicator of an adequate response to treatment. An acceptable HSAT device rather than oximetry should be used.
6. B. The recent guidelines for longitudinal follow-up of patients with OSA state that testing is indicated based on concerning data from the PAP device or if there is a change in the cardiac status of a patient. There is a reasonable chance that central apnea is now present. Although it is true that restoration of sinus rhythm may be the best treatment, it is not known when this will occur. In addition, PSG findings may provide some guidance on the need for optimization of the patient's cardiac status.
7. B. A patient with a recent CVA is in a high-risk group for OSA, and given the frequent arousals, evaluation is indicated. He has a comorbidity that makes PSG the best choice.
8. C. HSAT is not indicated in patients with neuromuscular weakness or suspected hypoventilation. Although oximetry might provide useful information, a PSG is the definitive study to detect OSA and evidence of nocturnal hypoxemia and hypoventilation. One could argue that because the patient has a neuromuscular disorder, documentation of significant desaturation would qualify him for a RAD with a backup rate, and that the best sleep study would be a PAP titration. However, nocturnal supplemental oxygen would not be the treatment if there is a finding of nocturnal desaturation. See Chapter 24 for more discussion of qualification for RADs.
9. A. This patient has a lower risk for moderate to severe OSA and the etiology of the kicking is of interest. OSA may present as insomnia in women. Most patients with isolated insomnia do not complain of daytime sleepiness. The is also a concern that the PLMD might be present.
10. B. A PSG is not indicated for most cases of insomnia. However, this patient has failed several attempts at insomnia treatment and has coronary artery disease. HSAT would not be the most appropriate study in a patient with significant insomnia. However, some insurance plans might mandate an HSAT. If the HSAT is negative, there is a reasonable chance that a PSG will be reimbursed.
11. B. The ODI and AHI are not consistent. Either the airflow signal or the oximetry signal might not be reliable. In this case review of the tracings showed a poor nasal pressure signal that was used by autoscoring to detect apneas or hypopneas. Unfortunately, the study was not properly edited. If manual scoring of the study using an alternate flow signal (RIPflow) is not technically possible or the results not reliable, a PSG should be ordered.

SELECTED REFERENCES

Caples SM, Anderson WM, Calero K, Howell M, Hashmi SD. Use of polysomnography and home sleep apnea tests for the longitudinal management of obstructive sleep apnea in adults: an American Academy of Sleep Medicine clinical guidance statement. J Clin Sleep Med. 2021;17(6):1287-1293.

Kapur VK, Auckley DH, Chowdhuri S, et al. Clinical practice guideline for diagnostic testing for adult obstructive sleep apnea: an American Academy of Sleep Medicine clinical practice guideline. *J Clin Sleep Med.* 2017;13(3):479-504.

Purdy S, Berry R. Home sleep apnea testing. In: Mattice C, Brooks R, Lee-Chiong T, eds. *Fundamentals of Sleep Technology*. 3rd ed. Wolters Kluwer Health; 2020.

Smith MT, McCrae CS, Cheung J, et al. Use of actigraphy for the evaluation of sleep disorders and circadian rhythm sleep-wake disorders: an American Academy of Sleep Medicine clinical practice guideline. *J Clin Sleep Med.* 2018;14(7):1231-1237.

REFERENCES

1. Troester MM, Quan SF, Berry RB, et al; for the American Academy of Sleep Medicine. *The AASM Manual for the Scoring of Sleep and Associated Events: Rules, Terminology and Technical Specifications*. Version 3. American Academy of Sleep Medicine; 2023.
2. Kushida CA, Littner MR, Morgenthaler T, Alessi CA. Practice parameters for the indications for polysomnography and related procedures: an update for 2005. *Sleep*. 2005;28:499-521.
3. Kapur VK, Auckley DH, Chowdhuri S, et al. Clinical Practice Guideline for diagnostic testing for adult obstructive sleep apnea: an American Academy of Sleep Medicine clinical practice guideline. *J Clin Sleep Med.* 2017;13(3):479-504.

4. Caples SM, Anderson WM, Calero K, et al. Use of polysomnography and home sleep apnea tests for the longitudinal management of obstructive sleep apnea in adults: an American Academy of Sleep Medicine clinical guidance statement. *J Clin Sleep Med.* 2021;17(6):1287-1293.
5. Epstein LJ, Kristo D, Strollo Jr PJ, et al. Adult Obstructive Sleep Apnea Task Force of the American Academy of Sleep Medicine. Clinical guideline for the evaluation, management and long-term care of obstructive sleep apnea in adults. *J Clin Sleep Med.* 2009;5(3):263-276.
6. Littner MR, Kushida C, Wise M, et al. Practice parameters for clinical use of the multiple sleep latency test and the maintenance of wakefulness test. *Sleep.* 2005;28:113-121.
7. Krahn LE, Arand DL, Avidan AY, et al. Recommended protocols for the Multiple Sleep Latency Test and Maintenance of Wakefulness Test in adults: guidance from the American Academy of Sleep Medicine. *J Clin Sleep Med.* 2021;17(12):2489-2498.
8. Littner M, Kramer M, Kapen S, et al. Practice parameters for using polysomnography to evaluate insomnia: an update. *Sleep.* 2003;26:754-760.
9. Morgenthaler TI, Lee-Chiong T, Alessi C, et al. Practice parameters for the clinical evaluation and treatment of circadian rhythm sleep disorders. *Sleep.* 2007;30:1445-1459.
10. Kushida CA. Littner MR, Hirshkowitz M, et al. Practice parameters for the use of continuous and bilevel positive airway pressure devices to treat adult patients with sleep-related breathing disorders. *Sleep.* 2006;29: 375-380.
11. Kushida CA, Chediak A, Berry RB, et al; Positive Airway Pressure Titration Task Force; American Academy of Sleep Medicine. Clinical guidelines for the manual titration of positive airway pressure in patients with obstructive sleep apnea. *J Clin Sleep Med.* 2008;4(2):157-171.
12. Berry RB, Chediak A, Brown LK, et al; NPPV Titration Task Force of the American Academy of Sleep Medicine. Best clinical practices for the sleep center adjustment of noninvasive positive pressure ventilation (NPPV) in stable chronic alveolar hypoventilation syndromes. *J Clin Sleep Med.* 2010;6(5):491-509.
13. Aurora RN, Casey KR, Kristo D, et al; American Academy of Sleep Medicine. Practice parameters for the surgical modifications of the upper airway for obstructive sleep apnea in adults. *Sleep.* 2010;33(10):1408-1413.
14. Kushida CA, Morgenthaler T, Littner MR, et al. Practice parameters for the treatment of snoring and obstructive sleep apnea with oral appliances: an update for 2005. *Sleep.* 2006;29:240-243.
15. Ramar K, Dort LC, Katz SG, et al. Clinical practice guideline for the treatment of obstructive sleep apnea and snoring with oral appliance therapy: an update for 2015. *J Clin Sleep Med.* 2015;11(7):773-827.
16. Collop NA, Anderson, WM, Boehlecke B, et al. Clinical guidelines for the use of unattended portable monitors in the diagnosis of obstructive sleep apnea in adult patients. Portable Monitoring Task Force of the American Academy of Sleep Medicine. *J Clin Sleep Med.* 2007;3:737-747.
17. Aurora RN, Lamm CI, Zak RS, et al. Practice parameters for the nonrespiratory indications for polysomnography and multiple sleep latency testing for children. *Sleep.* 2012;35(11):1467-1473.
18. Aurora RN, Zak RS, Karippot A, et al; American Academy of Sleep Medicine. Practice parameters for the respiratory indications for polysomnography in children. *Sleep.* 2011;34(3):379-388.
19. AASM-Facility-Standards-for-Accreditation-8.2020.pdf (netdna-ssl.com). https://aasm.org/wp-content/uploads/2022/07/AASM-facility-standards-accreditation.pdf. Accessed July 25, 2021.
20. Department of Health and Human Services Centers for Medicare and Medicaid Services. *Polysomnography and Sleep Testing.* LCD L33405. Available at: https://www.cms.gov/medicare-coverage-database/view/lcd.aspx?LCDId=33405&ver=25&Date=&DocID=L33405&bc=iAAAABAAgAAA&. Accessed August 29, 2023.
21. Soose RJ, Faber K, Greenberg H, et al. Post-implant care pathway: lessons learned and recommendations after 5 years of clinical implementation of hypoglossal nerve stimulation therapy. *Sleep.* 2021;44(suppl 1): S4-S10.
22. Department of Health and Human Services Centers for Medicare and Medicaid Services. *Respiratory Assist Devices.* L33800. Available at: https://www.cms.gov/medicare-coverage-database/view/lcd.aspx?LCDId=33800. Accessed August 29, 2023.
23. Patil SP, Ayappa IA, Caples SM, et al. Treatment of adult obstructive sleep apnea with positive airway pressure: an American Academy of Sleep Medicine clinical practice guideline. *J Clin Sleep Med.* 2019;15(2): 335-343.
24. Ferber R, Millman R, Coppola M, et al. ASDA standards of practice: portable recording in the assessment of obstructive sleep apnea. *Sleep.* 1994;17:378-392.
25. Collop NA, Tracy SL, Kapur V, et al. Obstructive sleep apnea devices for out-of-center (OOC) testing: technology evaluation. *J Clin Sleep Med.* 2011;7(5):531-548.
26. Flemons WW, Littner MR, Rowley JA, et al. Home diagnosis of sleep apnea: a systematic review of the literature: an evidence review cosponsored by the American Academy of Sleep Medicine, the American College of Chest Physicians, and the American Thoracic Society. *Chest.* 2003;124:1543-1579.
27. Department of Health and Human Services Centers for Medicare and Medicaid Services. *National Coverage Determination (NCD) for Continuous Positive Airway Pressure (CPAP) Therapy for Obstructive Sleep Apnea (OSA)* 240.4. 2008. Available at: https://www.cms.gov/medicare-coverage-database/details/ncd-details.aspx?NCDId=226&ncdver=3&NCAId=204&keyword=cpap&keywordType=starts&areaId=all&docType=NCA%2cCAL%2cNCD%2cMEDCAC%2cTA%2cMCD%2c6%2c3%2c5%2c1%2cF%2cP&contractOption=all&sortBy=relevance&KeyWordLookUp=Doc&KeyWordSearchType=Exact&bc=AAAAAAQACAAA&. Accessed August 29, 2023.
28. Department of Health and Human Services Centers for Medicare and Medicaid Services. *CMS Decision Memo for Continuous Positive Airway Pressure (CPAP) Therapy for Obstructive Sleep Apnea (OSA).* CAG-0093R2. March 2008. Available at: https://www.cms.gov/medicare-coverage-database/details/nca-decision-memo.aspx?NCAId=204&NCDId=226&ncdver=3&keyword=cpap&keywordType=starts&areaId=all&docType=NCA%2cCAL%2cNCD%2cMEDCAC%2cTA%2cMCD%2c6%2c3%2c5%2c1%2cF%2cP&contractOption=all&sortBy=relevance&KeyWordLookUp=Doc&KeyWordSearchType=Exact&bc=AAAAAAQACAAA&. Accessed August 29, 2023.
29. Department of Health and Human Services Centers for Medicare and Medicaid Services. *Continuous Positive Airway Pressure (CPAP) Therapy for Obstructive Sleep Apnea.* Communication R86NCD. July 3, 2008. Available at: www.cms.gov/regulations-and-guidance/guidance/transmittals/downloads/r86ncd.pdf. Assessed December 24, 2023.
30. Department of Health and Human Services Centers for Medicare and Medicaid Services. *CMS Decision Memo for Sleep Testing for Obstructive Sleep Apnea (OSA).* CAG-00405N. March 2009. Availale at: https://www.cms.gov/medicare-coverage-database/details/nca-decision-memo.aspx?NCAId=227&keyword=sleep+testing&keywordType=starts&areaId=all&docType=NCA%2cCAL%2cNCD%2cMEDCAC%2cTA%2cMCD%2c6%2c3%2c5%2c1%2cF%2cP&contractOption=all&sortBy=relevance&KeyWordLookUp=Doc&KeyWordSearchType=Exact&bc=AAAAAAQACAAA&. Accessed August 29, 2023.
31. Department of Health and Human Services Centers for Medicare and Medicaid Services. *Billing and Coding: Polysomnography.* A56995. Available at: https://www.cms.gov/medicare-coverage-database/view/article.aspx?articleid=56995. Accessed August 29, 2023.
32. American Academy of Sleep Medicine. *Sleep Medicine Codes.* Available at: https://aasm.org/clinical-resources/coding-reimbursement/sleep-medicine-codes/. Accessed August 29, 2023.
33. Purdy S, Berry R. Home sleep apnea testing. In: Mattice C, Brooks R, Lee-Chiong T, eds. *Fundamentals of Sleep Technology.* 3rd ed. Wolters Kluwer Health; 2020.
34. Bar A, Pillar G, Dvir I, et al. Evaluation of a portable device based on peripheral arterial tone for unattended home sleep studies. *Chest.* 2003;123:695-703.
35. Ayas NT, Pittman S, MacDonald M, White DP. Assessment of a wrist-worn device in the detection of obstructive sleep apnea. *Sleep Med.* 2003;4:435-442.
36. Yalamanchali S, Farajian V, Hamilton C, et al. Diagnosis of obstructive sleep apnea by peripheral arterial tonometry: meta-analysis. *JAMA Otolaryngol Head Neck Surg.* 2013;139(12):1343-1350.
37. Hedner J, Pillar G, Pittman SD, et al. A novel adaptive wrist actigraphy algorithm for sleep-wake assessment in sleep apnea patients. *Sleep.* 2004; 27:1560-1566.
38. Herscovici S, Pe'er A, Papyan S, Lavie P. Detecting REM sleep from the finger: an automatic REM sleep algorithm based on peripheral arterial tone (PAT) and actigraphy. *Physiol Meas.* 2007;28(2):129-140.
39. Bresler M, Sheffy K, Pillar G, Preiszler M, Herscovici S. Differentiating between light and deep sleep stages using an ambulatory device based on peripheral arterial tonometry. *Physiol Meas.* 2008;29(5):571-584.
40. Hedner J, White DP, Malhotra A, et al. Sleep staging based on autonomic signals: a multi-center validation study. *J Clin Sleep Med.* 2011;7(3):301-306.
41. Pillar G, Berall M, Berry R, et al. Detecting central sleep apnea in adult patients using WatchPAT—a multicenter validation study. *Sleep Breath.* 2020;24(1):387-398.

42. Ioachimescu OC, Allam JS, Samarghandi A, et al. Performance of peripheral arterial tonometry-based testing for the diagnosis of obstructive sleep apnea in a large sleep clinic cohort. *J Clin Sleep Med.* 2020;16(10): 1663-1674.
43. Iftikhar IH, Finch CE, Shah AS, et al. A meta-analysis of diagnostic test performance of peripheral arterial tonometry studies. *J Clin Sleep Med.* 2022;18(4):1093-1102.
44. Zhang Z, Sowho M, Otvos T, et al. A comparison of automated and manual sleep staging and respiratory event recognition in a portable sleep diagnostic device with in-lab sleep study. *J Clin Sleep Med.* 2020;16(4): 563-573.
45. Tauman R, Berall M, Berry R, et al. Watch-PAT is useful in the diagnosis of sleep apnea in patients with atrial fibrillation. *Nat Sci Sleep.* 2020;12:1115-1121.
46. Massie F, Mendes de Almeida D, Dreesen P, et al. An evaluation of the NightOwl home sleep apnea testing system. *J Clin Sleep Med.* 2018; 14(10):1791-1796.
47. Tschopp S, Wimmer W, Caversaccio M, et al. Night-to-night variability in obstructive sleep apnea using peripheral arterial tonometry: a case for multiple night testing. *J Clin Sleep Med.* 2021;17(9):1751-1758.
48. Punjabi NM, Patil S, Crainiceanu C, Aurora RN. Variability and misclassification of sleep apnea severity based on multi-night testing. *Chest.* 2020;158(1):365-373.
49. Littner MR, Kushida DA, Anderson WM, et al. Standards of Practice Committee of the American Academy of Sleep Medicine: practice parameters for the role of actigraphy in the study of sleep and circadian rhythms: an update for 2002. *Sleep.* 2003;26:337-341.
50. Morgenthaler T, Alessi C, Friedman L, et al. Practice parameters for the use of actigraphy in the assessment of sleep and sleep disorders: an update for 2007. *Sleep.* 2007;30:519-529.
51. Smith MT, McCrae CS, Cheung J, et al. Use of actigraphy for the evaluation of sleep disorders and circadian rhythm sleep-wake disorders: an American Academy of Sleep Medicine systematic review, meta-analysis, and GRADE assessment. *J Clin Sleep Med.* 2018;14(7):1209-1230.
52. Smith MT, McCrae CS, Cheung J, et al. Use of actigraphy for the evaluation of sleep disorders and circadian rhythm sleep-wake disorders: an American Academy of Sleep Medicine clinical practice guideline. *J Clin Sleep Med.* 2018;14(7):1231-1237.
53. Bradshaw DA, Yanagi MA, Pak ES, et al. Nightly sleep duration in the 2-week period preceding multiple sleep latency testing. *J Clin Sleep Med.* 2007;3(6):613-619.
54. American Academy of Sleep Medicine. *International Classification of Sleep Disorders.* 3rd ed, text revison. Darien, IL: Amererican Academcy of Sleep Medicine; 2023.
55. Ancoli-Israel S, Martin JL, Blackwell T, et al. The SBSM Guide to Actigraphy Monitoring: clinical and research applications. *Behav Sleep Med.* 2015;13(suppl 1):S4-S38.
56. Martin JL, Hakim AD. Wrist actigraphy. *Chest.* 2011;139(6):1514-1527.
57. Baron KG, Duffecy J, Berendsen MA, et al. Feeling validated yet? A scoping review of the use of consumer-targeted wearable and mobile technology to measure and improve sleep. *Sleep Med Rev.* 2018;40:151-159.
58. Khosla S, Deak MC, Gault D, et al. Consumer sleep technology: an American Academy of Sleep Medicine position statement. *J Clin Sleep Med.* 2018;14(5):877-880.

Chapter 17

Subjective and Objective Measures of Sleepiness

EXCESSIVE DAYTIME SLEEPINESS

Excessive daytime sleepiness (EDS) is defined as sleepiness that occurs in a situation when an individual would usually be expected to be awake and alert. EDS is a common symptom in the general population. The prevalence ranges from 5% to 30% in several epidemiological studies[1] and varies considerably depending on the EDS definition (severity, duration, frequency/days per week, and impact on daily living). Given the epidemic of reduction in sleep time,[2] it is estimated that up to 33% of the U.S. population experiences some degree of daytime sleepiness.[3] Habitual EDS with impairment of daytime function is said to affect at least 5% of the general population with about 2% due to disorders of hypersomnolence and the other 3% due to insufficient sleep or medications. Causes of EDS include sleep deprivation/inadequate sleep, a number of sleep disorders (obstructive sleep apnea [OSA], narcolepsy, idiopathic hypersomnia, periodic limb movement disorder), sleep disturbance from medical conditions, medication side effects, and depression (usually complaints of insomnia > hypersomnia). A consensus panel made a recommendation[4] for 7 or more hours of sleep for adults for optimal health. Surveys suggest that 35% to 40% of the adult U.S. population report sleeping less than 7 hours on weekday nights, whereas about 15% report to sleep less than 6 hours.[5] Thus, behaviorally induced inadequate sleep is likely the most common cause of daytime sleepiness in the general population. The degree of sleepiness can be assessed by subjective and objective measures of sleepiness. Subjective measures include the Stanford Sleepiness Scale,[6,7] the Epworth Sleepiness Scale (ESS),[8-11] and the Karolinska Sleepiness Scale.[12,13] The Multiple Sleep Latency Test (MSLT)[14-18] and Maintenance of Wakefulness Test (MWT)[16-18] are objective measures of sleepiness and the ability to stay awake (alertness), respectively. New guidance recommending protocols for performance of the MSLT and MWT was published in 2021.[18]

SUBJECTIVE MEASURES

Questionnaires such as the Stanford Sleepiness Scale,[6,7] the ESS,[8-12] and the Karolinska Sleepiness Scale[12,13] are measures of self-rated symptoms of sleepiness. The Stanford Sleepiness Scale[6,7] (Table 17–1) measures subjective feelings of sleepiness ("fogginess, beginning to lose interest in staying awake"). A score greater than 3 is considered sleepy. In contrast, the ESS measures self-rated average sleep propensity (chance of dozing) over eight common situations that almost everyone encounters. The propensity to fall asleep is rated as 0, 1, 2, or 3, where 0 corresponds to never and 3 to a high chance of dozing (Table 17–2). The maximum score is 24, and normal is assumed to be 10 or less. ESS scores of 16 or greater are associated with severe sleepiness. It is common for patients with narcolepsy to report ESS scores of 20 or greater.

The correlation between the ESS and objective measures of sleepiness is low. The MSLT,[14-18] an objective measure of sleepiness, determines a **mean sleep latency (MSL)** during four or five naps spread across the daytime hours (short latency = greater sleepiness). A higher ESS is correlated with a lower MSL in some[8] but not all studies.[19,20] The ESS correlates roughly with the severity of OSA[8,21] and improves (lower score) after continuous positive airway pressure (CPAP) treatment.[22] The minimal clinically important improvement in the ESS with treatment is thought to be a change of −2 to −3.[23,24] In one study[8] the mean ESS values in mild, moderate, and severe OSA were 9.5, 11.5, and 16.0, respectively. However, the range of values was wide and included the normal range in all severities of sleep apnea. While not a perfect metric, the ESS is easy to administer, a standard part of the evaluation of patients in sleep clinic, and is repeated at each clinic visit for patients on positive airway pressure (PAP) treatment.

The Karolinska Sleepiness Scale (Table 17–3) is a 9-point (or 10 in some versions) scale in which the level of sleepiness in the last 5 to 10 minutes is reported. The scale is a sensitive indicator of insufficient sleep and impaired waking function.[12,13] Of note, the group of disorders with central causes of

Table 17–1 Stanford Sleepiness Scale

Degree of Sleepiness	Scale Rating
Feeling active, vital, alert, or wide awake	1
Functioning at high levels, but not at peak; able to concentrate	2
Awake, but relaxed; responsive but not fully alert	3
Somewhat foggy, let down	4
Foggy; losing interest in remaining awake; slowed down	5
Sleepy, woozy, fighting sleep; prefer to lie down	6
No longer fighting sleep, sleep onset soon; having dreamlike thoughts	7
Asleep	X

Table 17–2 Epworth Sleepiness Scale

Situation: "Usual Way of Life in Recent Times"	Chance of Dozing Score 0, 1, 2, 3*
Sitting and reading	0–3
Watching TV	0–3
Sitting, inactive in a public place (e.g., a theater or a meeting)	0–3
As a passenger in a car for an hour without a break	0–3
Lying down to rest in the afternoon when circumstances permit	0–3
Sitting talking to someone	0–3
Sitting quietly after a lunch without alcohol	0–3
In a car, while stopped for a few minutes in traffic	0–3
Total	0–24 (0 - 10 normal)
*0 = would ***NEVER*** doze 1 = ***SLIGHT*** chance of dozing 2 = ***MODERATE*** chance of dozing 3 = ***HIGH*** chance of dozing	

Johns MW. A new method for measuring daytime sleepiness: the Epworth Sleepiness Scale. *Sleep.* 1991;14:540-545.

Table 17–3 Karolinska Sleepiness Scale

Choose the appropriate level of sleepiness in the last 5 to 10 minutes

1. Extremely alert
2. Very alert
3. Alert
4. Rather alert
5. Neither alert nor sleepy
6. Some signs of sleepiness
7. Sleepy, but no effort to keep awake
8. Sleepy, but some effort to keep awake
9. Very sleepy, great effort to keep awake, fighting sleep

Some versions contain #10

10. Extremely sleepy, can't keep awake

From Akerstedt T, Gillberg M. Subjective and objective sleepiness in the active individual. *Int J Neurosci.* 1990;52(1-2):29-37.

daytime sleepiness is classified as disorders of central hypersomnolence versus hypersomnia. Technically speaking, hypersomnia means "a lot of sleep or the need for a lot of sleep." Hypersomnolence is the sensation of feeling sleepy. However, both terms are often used to mean excessive sleepiness.

OBJECTIVE MEASURES OF SLEEPINESS OR THE ABILITY TO STAY AWAKE

Multiple Sleep Latency Test

The MSLT (Box 17–1) is an objective measure of daytime sleepiness and is used to support a diagnosis of narcolepsy.[14-18]

Box 17–1 ESSENTIAL MSLT FACTS

- Follows nocturnal PSG by 1.5 to 3 hours
- Four or five naps starting every 2 hours
- Sleep latency is the time from lights out to the first epoch of sleep
- If no sleep occurs in 20 minutes, the nap is terminated (sleep latency = 20 minutes)
- Monitoring continues for 15 minutes of **clock time** after the first epoch of sleep to detect sleep onset REM sleep (a sleep onset REM period, SOREMP)
- Major findings include
  - MSL an objective measure of sleepiness (lower value = sleepier)
  - Number of sleep onset REM periods (REM latency ≤ 15 minutes)

- **PSG /MSLT criteria for narcolepsy with cataplexy (NT1)[28]**
  - PSG SOREMP

  OR
  - MSLT MSL ≤ 8 minutes and MSLT showing two or more SOREMPs
- **PSG/MSLT criteria for narcolepsy without cataplexy (NT2)[28]**
  - MSLT MSL ≤ 8 minutes and MSLT showing two or more SOREMPs. A PSG SOREMP can replace one of the required MSLT SOREMPs.

MSL, Mean sleep latency; *MSLT,* Multiple Sleep Latency Test; *PSG,* polysomnography; *REM,* rapid eye movement; *SOREMP,* sleep onset rapid eye movement period. From Krahn LE, Arand DL, Avidan AY, et al. Recommended protocols for the Multiple Sleep Latency Test and Maintenance of Wakefulness Test in adults: guidance from the American Academy of Sleep Medicine. *J Clin Sleep Med.* 2021;17(12):2489–2498.

The two main MSLT findings are the MSL and the number of sleep onset rapid eye movement (REM) periods (SOREMPs). The sleep latency is the time from lights out to the beginning of the first epoch of any stage of sleep. This is an objective measure of daytime sleepiness, and the shorter the sleep latency, the sleepier the individual. SOREMPs on the MSLT are defined as REM sleep within 15 minutes of clock time after sleep onset. Normal individuals are expected to have zero or one SOREMP. The MSLT must be preceded by polysomnography (PSG) during the patient's normal sleep period to document an adequate amount of nocturnal sleep (minimum total sleep time [TST] = 360 minutes) and the absence of another sleep disorder that may explain daytime sleepiness and abnormal MSLT findings.[14-18] Many factors can alter the findings of the MSLT, and considerable clinical judgment is needed to avoid an error in interpretation (false-positive or false-negative results).

Mean Sleep Latency Findings From the MSLT

In the original guidelines for performance of the MSLT, an MSL < 5 minutes was said to represent pathological daytime sleepiness.[14] A later MSLT guideline specified MSL severity ranges as MSL (minutes): <5 severe, 5 to 10 moderate, and 10 to 15 mild sleepiness with a normal range of 10 to 20 minutes.[15,25] An MSL < 5 minutes was a diagnostic criterion for narcolepsy in the first edition of the *International Classification of Sleep Disorders* (ICSD).[25] However, in the second and third editions (ICSD-2, ICSD-3, ICSD-TR)[26-28] an MSL ≤ 8 minutes is one of the MSLT diagnostic criteria for narcolepsy. The higher MSL cutoff was felt to increase the sensitivity of the test.[29] However, as seen in Table 17–4, up to

Table 17–4 MSLT Mean Sleep Latency Findings

	MSL (min) (mean ± SD)
Normal	10.4 ± 4.3 (four naps) 11.6 ± 5.2 (five naps) **16% MSL < 5 min**
Narcolepsy	3.1 ± 2.9 (diagnostic criteria ≤ 8 min) **16% MSL > 5 min**
Idiopathic hypersomnia	6.2 ± 3.0 (diagnostic criteria ≤ 8 min)
Sleep apnea	7.2 ± 6.0
Traditional MSL ranges	<5 min: severe sleepiness 5 – 10 min: moderate sleepiness >10 to 15 min: mild (borderline) sleepiness

MSL, Mean sleep latency; *MSLT*, Multiple Sleep Latency Test.
As the MSL increases with age, the normal value depends on the age composition sampled.
From Arand D, Bonnet M, Hurwitz T, et al. A review by the MSLT and MWT Task Force of the Standards of Practice Committee of the AASM. The clinical use of the MSLT and MWT. *Sleep.* 2005;28:123-144; and Standards of Practice Committee of the American Academy of Sleep Medicine. Practice parameters for clinical use of the Multiple Sleep Latency Test and the Maintenance of Wakefulness Test. *Sleep.* 2005;28(1):113-121; and Littner MR, Kushida C, Wise M, et al. Standards of Practice Committee of the American Academy of Sleep Medicine. Practice parameters for clinical use of the multiple sleep latency test and the maintenance of wakefulness test. Sleep. 2005;28:113-121.

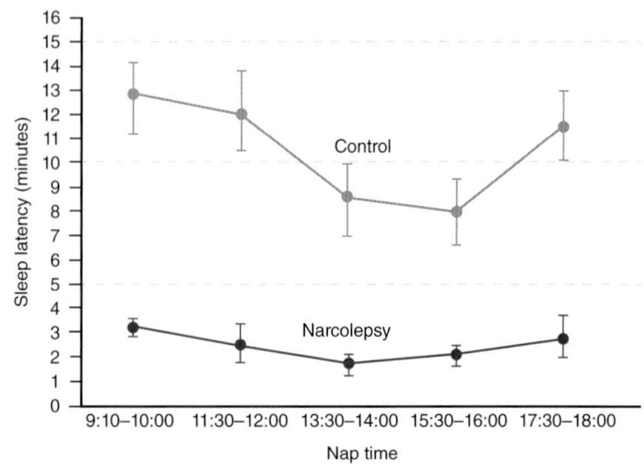

Figure 17–1 Variation of the sleep latency over the five naps in the Multiple Sleep Latency Test in normal individuals and patients with narcolepsy. In this study the shortest sleep latency was noted on naps 3 and 4. There was less variability from nap to nap in the patients with narcolepsy. (From Richardson GS, Carskadon MA, Flagg W, Van den Hoed J, Dement WC, Mitler MM. Excessive daytime sleepiness in man: multiple sleep latency measurement in narcoleptic and control subjects. *Electroencephalogr Clin Neurophysiol.* 1978; 45[5]:621-627.)

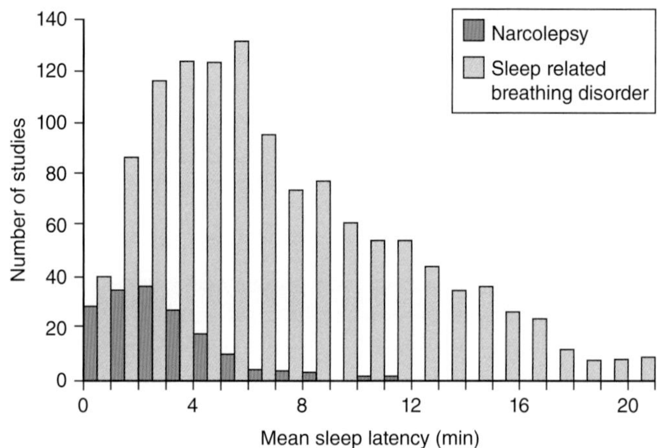

Figure 17–2 The mean sleep latency in patients with narcolepsy is very low, although there is some overlap with results from patients with sleep related breathing disorders. (From Aldrich MS, Chervin RD, Malow BA. Value of the Multiple Sleep Latency Test [MSLT] for the diagnosis of narcolepsy. *Sleep.* 1997;20:620-629.)

16% of normal individuals have an MSL < 5 minutes.[17] The distribution of MSL values in normal populations approximates a normal distribution and using a mean of 11.6 minutes and a standard deviation of 5.2 min (normal value for 5 nap MSLT) about 24% of normal individuals would have a MSL ≤ 8 minutes. Patients with *narcolepsy* often have a very short MSL (on average around 3 minutes), but up to 16% have an MSL > 5 minutes. Patients with idiopathic hypersomnia and OSA have moderate sleepiness on the average, but there is a wide range of MSL values in these groups.

Factors influencing the MSL on the MSLT are presented in Box 17–2. Prior sleep deprivation can affect the MSLT (reduce the MSL) for days.[30] *The MSL increases with age.* Stimulant medications increase the MSL, and sedatives decrease the MSL. Of note, the shortest sleep latency tends to occur during naps 3 or 4 on the MSLT[31,32] (Figure 17–1). The mean MSL on five-nap MSLT studies is slightly longer (less sleepiness) than on four-nap studies. It should be appreciated that the MSL in most patients with narcolepsy is very low compared with other disorders such as OSA (Figure 17–2).

Box 17–2 FACTORS INFLUENCING THE MEAN SLEEP LATENCY

- Age (MSL longer in older individuals)
- Shortest sleep latency on naps 3 or 4 in the MSLT
- MSL on five nap MSLT is longer compared with a four nap MSLT
- Prior sleep restriction or sleep deprivation (decrease the MSL)
- Circadian factors: (can decrease the MSL)
  1. Shift work
  2. Chronically delayed sleep period
  3. Delayed Sleep Wake Phase Disorder
- Medications:
  - Stimulants – increase MSL
  - Sedatives – decrease MSL

MSL, Mean sleep latency; *MSLT*, Multiple Sleep Latency Test.

Sleep Onset REM Periods

As previously noted, a SOREMP is defined as REM sleep within 15 minutes (clocktime) of sleep onset. Early studies found zero or one SOREMP during the MSLT in normal individuals.[31] However, two population-based studies have found the prevalence of two or more SOREMPs was present in 13.1% males and 5.6% of females in the first study[33] and 3.9% with male predominance in the second study.[34] In a third population-based study Goldbart and coworkers[35] found two or more SOREMPs in 7% of the population, an MSL ≤ 8 minutes in 22%, and a "positive MSLT" (MSL ≤ 8 minutes and two or more SOREMPs) in 3.4%. Correlates for a positive MSLT were *short sleep time and shift work.* The propensity

Box 17–3 CAUSES OF SLEEP ONSET REM PERIOD (MSLT NAP)

- Narcolepsy
- Untreated obstructive sleep apnea
- Depression
- Prior sleep and REM sleep reduction/fragmentation
- Withdrawal of REM-suppressing medications (SSRIs, lithium, SNRI, TCAs)
- Delayed circadian phase
    - shift work
    - chronically delayed sleep period
    - Delayed Sleep-Wake Phase Disorder

MSLT, Multiple Sleep Latency Test; *REM,* Rapid eye movement; *SNRI,* serotonin-norepinephrine reuptake inhibitor; *SSRI,* selective serotonin reuptake inhibitor; *TCA,* tricyclic antidepressant.

for REM sleep is strongly related to the circadian clock. The MSLT is not an appropriate tool for evaluation of narcolepsy in shift workers.[28] About 5% of patients evaluated for OSA (untreated) have *two or more SOREMPs* if an MSLT is performed.[29,36] The common causes of SOREMPs are listed in Box 17–3. In general, *the number of SOREMPs increases as the MSL decreases*. The presence of two or more SOREMPs is more specific for the diagnosis of narcolepsy than a short sleep latency.[17] A nocturnal SOREMP on the PSG preceding the MSLT occurs in only about 30% to 50% of patients with narcolepsy but when present has a high positive predictive value.[29,37,38] A **PSG** SOREMP in untreated OSA is very rare (1% or less).[29] Given these findings, the ICSD-3 specified that a **PSG** SOREMP could be used as one of the two or more SOREMPs required for the diagnosis of narcolepsy.[27] However, in the ICSD-3-TR[28] the finding of a PSG SOREMP alone supports a diagnosis of narcolepsy with cataplexy (NT1), and in the absence of a PSG SOREMP, two or more SOREMPs on the MSLT are required to support a diagnosis of narcolepsy with cataplexy. The MSLT criteria for diagnosis of NT2 are the same in the ICSD-3 and ICSD-3-TR (Box 17-1).

Patients with narcolpesy with cataplexy tend to have a higher number of SOREMPs on the MSLT than patients with narcolepsy without cataplexy.[38] The sleep stage sequence preceding sleep onset REM appears to provide additional information. In a study by Drakatos et al[39] patients with hypocretin deficient narcolepsy (narcolepsy with cataplexy) tend to enter the first period of stage R (FREMP) on the **nocturnal PSG** from wake or stage N1.[39] This was true even if the FREMP was not a SOREMP. A smaller percentage of individuals with narcolepsy without cataplexy show this pattern. Patients with idiopathic hypersomnia or insufficient sleep usually do not exhibit a SOREMP on the nocturnal PSG. Another study found that if a SOREMP occurs on the MSLT in patients with narcolepsy with cataplexy entry into stage R is usually via stage N1. In contrast in patients with insufficient sleep or idiopathic hypersomnia, entry into stage R is usually from stage N2 sleep.[40] In this study in patients with narcolepsy with cataplexy, 75% of MSLT SOREMPs arose from stage N1 (21% stage N2). In narcolepsy without cataplexy the the percentage of SOREMPs arising from stage N1 52%.[40] Dietmann and coworkers found that three or more SOREMPs during the MSLT had a very high positive predictive value for narcolepsy.[38] In general, narcolepsy patients with cataplexy (type 1) have more frequent MSLT SOREMPs and a shorter sleep

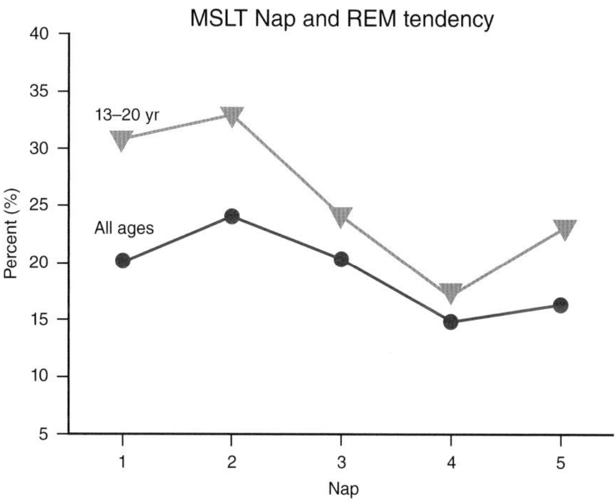

Figure 17–3 The tendency for a sleep onset rapid eye movement (REM) period (SOREMP) was highest in nap 2 and lowest in nap 4. The tendency of SOREMPs in adolescents is highest in the first two naps. Of note, the SOREMPs analyzed were not confined to patients with MSLT findings consistent with a diagnosis of narcolepsy (16.3% of studies consistent with narcolepsy). In the 13-20 year old age group the finding of greater SOREMPs in the first two naps illustrates the difficulty of differentiating patients with narcolepsy from individuals without narcolepsy who have SOREMPs due to a delay in the chronic sleep period. *MSLT,* Multiple Sleep Latency Test. (Adapted from Cairns A, Trotti LM, Bogan R. Demographic and nap-related variance of the MSLT: results from 2,498 suspected hypersomnia patients: clinical MSLT variance. *Sleep Med.* 2019;55:115-123.)

latency than patients with narcolepsy without cataplexy (type 2). There is variation in the probability of a SOREMP over the five naps. Studies vary but all have found a *lower likelihood* of a SOREMP on nap 4.[41-43] Younger patients tend to have a higher tendency for SOREMPs in the first two naps (Figure 17–3). In a study by Cairns et al[42] in the 13-20 year old age group 27% had "ambiguous" MSLT results (either ≥ 2 SOREMPs or 1 SOREMP both combined with a MSL > 8 minutes).

MSLT Protocol

New American Academy of Sleep Medicine (AASM) guidelines for performance of the MSLT[18] were published in 2021. The preceding guidelines were published in 2005.[16] The protocol and standards for MSLT reporting are now included in the AASM scoring manual.[44] MSLT clinical guidance for *patient preparation for testing* includes the following:

- Adequate sleep should be documented by sleep diary and, when available, actigraphy for 2 weeks before testing.
- Treatments for existing sleep disorders are well established and effective. For PAP treatment of OSA, review of downloaded data (documenting adequate adherence) or self-report for non-PAP treatments. The patient should use PAP and/or non-PAP therapy during the PSG on the night before the MSLT. The same treatment ins used during the MSLT.
- In general, medications with alerting, sedating, and/or REM sleep-modulating properties should be stopped at least 2 weeks before the MSLT. Clinical judgment should be used regarding changes to medications that could impair patient safety. A plan for handling over-the-counter agents, herbal remedies, and other substances should be in place.
- Acceptable caffeine consumption before testing to avoid confounding the MSLT results is recommended while avoiding caffeine withdrawal symptoms on the day of the test. The goal should be abstinence, and when necessary, withdrawal should be preceded by a taper.

It is important that the patient obtain an adequate amount of sleep with regular timing before testing. Sleep deprivation can result in false-positive results. Adequate sleep should be documented by sleep diary or, if available, actigraphy for 2 weeks before testing. The new MSLT guidelines mandate a sleep diary or actigraphy, whereas the previous guidelines stated that such information "may" be obtained. Sleep diary documentation ideally should include two weekends and at least 7 days before testing. Bradshaw and coworkers[45] found sleep duration by actigraphy to correlate with the MSL on the MSLT, whereas the sleep diary information or patient estimates did not correlate with the sleep latency. The mean actigraphy sleep duration in the 2 weeks before the MSLT was less than the sleep diary sleep duration. If a patient has OSA and suspected narcolepsy, adequate treatment and adherence with either PAP or non-PAP treatment should be documented. The patient should be clinically stable and the effectiveness of treatment for OSA clearly established. For PAP treatment this includes objective adherence monitoring. Of note, although adherence to PAP is often defined based on ≥70% of nights ≥4 hours, actually at least 6 hours is needed for maximum benefit.[46] *The patient should use PAP and/or non-PAP therapy during PSG on the night before the MSLT. The same treatment should be used during the MSLT.* This recommendation is an important clarification that was missing in the previous guidelines. Of note, an MSLT after a split sleep study or a PAP titration is NOT allowed.

In general, medications with alerting, sedating, and/or REM sleep-modulating properties should be stopped at least 2 weeks before the MSLT. Clinical judgment should be used regarding changes to medications that could impair patient safety. An acceptable level of caffeine consumption before testing should be established. In particular, caffeine withdrawal symptoms should be avoided (pre-study weaning of caffeine). The new MSLT protocol guidelines provide a table listing typical medications of interest with respect to the MSLT.[18] *Gradual withdrawal rather than abrupt cessation* is recommended for many medications and, for patients with depression, checking with the patient's psychiatric provider is essential. Some medications such as fluoxetine have a very long half-life, and the usual recommendation is to stop medications for at least the duration of five times a medication's half-life (for fluoxetine, 6 weeks). A study by Kolla and coworkers[47] found that advance taper of antidepressants before the MSLT increased the number of SOREMPs and reduced the MSL. This approach should make the test more sensitive for the diagnosis of narcolepsy but *may not be possible in all patients.* Many stimulants have a relative short half-life, and patients may have great difficulty withdrawing these medications for 2 weeks. The new AASM MSLT guidelines state that "in the case of medications with very short half-lives, consideration could be given to a washout of <2 weeks, particularly in patients in whom a longer time off medication would negatively impact patient safety." This is especially relevant for stimulant medications. An abrupt withdrawal of a REM sleep-suppressing medication close to the MSLT date can increase the likelihood of SOREMPs and should be avoided. Medical and recreational marijuana use is increasing. Both acute and chronic tetrahydrocannabinol (THC) use have been reported to induce sleep. *Recent discontinuation of THC can result in REM sleep rebound.*[48] Thus, similar to other medications that can affect sleep-wake and MSLT results,

MSLT Protocol Part 1

1. The MSLT should be performed after an attended PSG
   - Minimum 7 hours time in bed with a least 6 hours of sleep
   - Timing that corresponds with patient's major sleep period
   - Should NOT follow a PAP titration or split night study

2. The patient's clothing should be comfortable, appropriate to the environment, and not interfere with testing
   - No requirement to change clothes between PSG and MSLT

3. Abstain from alcohol, caffeine, marijuana, and other sedating or alerting medications
   - Nicotine discouraged, but if necessary stop 30 min before each nap trial

4. Patients on PAP or non-PAP treatment for OSA should use the treatment during the PSG and MSLT
   - PAP settings/mask should match those used at home

5. The recording montage for the MSLT should at a minimum include 3 EEG recording leads with 1 each for frontal (F3-M2 or F4-M1), central (C3-M2 or C4-M1), and occipital (O1- M2 or O2-M1) derivations, left and right eye EOG derivations, chin EMG, and EKG.
   - Other sensors used for the PSG are unnecessary and should be removed for patient comfort.

6. Audiovisual recordings must be made during the nap trials and be accessible to interpreting clinicians. The patient must be audiovisually monitored throughout the day, but retention of recordings made between nap trials is discretionary.

7. The MSLT should consist of 5 nap trials.
   - The initial trial should begin 1.5–3 hours after termination of the nocturnal recording.
   - Each subsequent trial should begin 2 hours after the start of the prior trial.

Only when the results are clearly diagnostic of narcolepsy after 4 naps with mean latency ≤ 8 minutes and 2 or more SOREMPs have occurred (either because of 2 or more SOREMPs during the nap trials or 1 in the nap trials and 1 during the PSG) should a shorter 4-nap trial test be performed.

Figure 17–4 Multiple Sleep Latency Test Protocol (Part 1). (Data from Krahn LE, Arand DL, Avidan AY, Davila DG, et al. Recommended protocols for the Multiple Sleep Latency Test and Maintenance of Wakefulness Test in adults: guidance from the American Academy of Sleep Medicine. *J Clin Sleep Med.* 2021;17[12]:2489-2498.)

THC substances should either be withdrawn 2 weeks before the MSLT or, if used, continued at a stable dose to avoid withdrawal effects.

MSLT protocol recommendations for testing, data acquisition, and reporting are listed in Figures 17–4 and 17–5. *The MSLT should be performed after an attended PSG, which allows a minimum 7 hours of time in bed with at least 6 hours of sleep*, with timing that corresponds with the patient's major sleep period. The ICSD-3-TR[28] states that the MSLT should not be used in shift workers. The MSLT should NOT be performed during the night, as no data are available to guide the interpretation. The best approach for patients with an "unusual" chronic sleep period is to ask the patient to follow a "normal schedule" during the 2 weeks before testing. This can sometimes be done during vacation time but is not always possible. Ideally actigraphy would be needed to document adequate sleep duration and timing. However, in the absence

MSLT Protocol Part 2

8. Before each nap trial, the patient should be offered the use of the restroom and queried regarding other requirements for comfort.

9. Sleep rooms should be dark, quiet, and at a comfortable temperature during testing.

10. The patient should be lying in bed for all nap trials.

11. Patient bio-calibrations should be conducted before starting each nap trial.
    Standard instructions include:
    (1) "lie quietly with your eyes open for 30 seconds";
    (2) "close both eyes for 30 seconds";
    (3) "without moving your head, look to the right, then left, then right, then left, right and then left";
    (4) "blink eyes slowly for 5 times"; and
    (5) "clench or grit your teeth tightly together."

12. At the start of each nap trial, the patient should be instructed as follows:
    "Please lie quietly, assume a comfortable position, keep your eyes closed, and allow yourself to fall asleep."
    - Testing starts immediately after instructions are given, and bedroom lights are turned off.

13. Each nap trial is ended if the patient does not fall asleep in 20 minutes.
    - If sleep onset occurs, the trial is continued for an additional 15 minutes, regardless of the amount of intervening sleep or wake.
    - Sleep onset is defined as the start of the first epoch scored as any stage of sleep.

14. Stimulating activities such as the use of electronic devices and the use of cell phones should end at least 30 minutes before each nap trial. Vigorous physical activity and prolonged exposure to sunlight/bright artificial light should be avoided all day.

15. Between nap trials, the patient should be out of bed and not permitted to sleep.

16. A light breakfast at least 1 hour before the first trial and a light lunch immediately after **ther termination of the second nap trial are recommended.**

17. Urine drug screening should be employed when indicated to ensure that the MSLT results are not confounded by inadvertent, **intentional, or illicit medication or substance use.**

Figure 17–5 Multiple Sleep Latency Test Protocol (Part 2). (Data from Krahn LE, Arand DL, Avidan AY, Davila DG, et al. Recommended protocols for the Multiple Sleep Latency Test and Maintenance of Wakefulness Test in adults: guidance from the American Academy of Sleep Medicine. *J Clin Sleep Med.* 2021;17[12]:2489-2498.)

of typical cataplexy or a low CSF hypocretin-1 level a positive MSLT result would still be problematic in shift workers as a diagnosis of NT2 requires exclusion of other causes of excessive sleepiness.[28] As noted above, an MSLT should not follow a split night or PAP titration PSG.

Although not addressed in the 2005 MSLT standard of practice guideline, prior guidelines specified that the patient change to daytime attire after awakening from the PSG. *Current guidelines do NOT require a change of clothes* between the PSG and the MSLT and stipulate only that clothing should be comfortable and appropriate to the environment. The patient should abstain from alcohol, caffeine, marijuana, and other sedating or alerting agents on the day of the test. Nicotine use is discouraged but if unavoidable should be terminated at least 30 minutes before a nap trial. Stimulating activities such as the use of electronic devices and the use of cell phones should end at *least 30 minutes before each nap trial.* Vigorous physical activity and prolonged exposure to sunlight/bright artificial light should be avoided all day. Bonnet and Arand found that walking or watching television affected MSLT results.[49] Monitoring rooms should be quiet, dark, and comfortable. The patient is offered a bathroom break before each nap and testing is performed with patients lying in bed. *However, patients should be out of bed between naps and not allowed to sleep.*

The MSLT consists of five naps started every 2 hours (after the start of the previous nap) with the first nap started about 1.5 to 3 hours after the end of the nocturnal PSG (Figures 17–4 and 17–5).[18] Ideally, the nocturnal sleep period should end with a spontaneous awakening. A forced awakening at a time based on the sleep center schedule (e.g., 6 a.m.) may result in sleep deprivation in some individuals. The new MSLT guidelines mandate use of a recording montage consistent with that recommended in the AASM scoring manual (see Chapters 1 and 3), including the standard frontal, central, occipital, electrooculography, chin electromyography monitoring (as well as an electrocardiography channel). The use of additional monitoring leads is not recommended, as this may reduce patient comfort. *Biocalibration before each nap is recommended. A light breakfast is recommended at least 1 hour before the first nap and a light lunch after the second nap.* At the start of the MSLT the standard instruction is *"Please lie quietly, assume a comfortable position, keep your eyes closed, and try to fall asleep."* Each MSLT nap is terminated if no sleep occurs within 20 minutes following lights out (sleep latency is 20 minutes). If sleep occurs, the MSLT continues for another 15 minutes of clock time *after* the first epoch of sleep. If REM sleep occurs within this time period, a SOREMP is said to have occurred. Therefore, the total MSLT duration is between 20 and 35 minutes. Figure 17–6 displays a schematic illustration of sleep staging during an MSLT nap. Figure 17–7 shows the very unusual circumstance that the first epoch of stage R was in the last 30 seconds of the 15-minute monitoring time to detect REM sleep. As noted above, between naps the individual stays out of bed and is prevented from sleeping. New in the current guidelines is the recommendation that *audiovisual recordings be made during the nap trials and accessible to interpreting physicians. Continuous audiovisual monitoring* is needed during the entire day, but retention of recordings between naps is optional. The 2021 guidelines state, "Urine drug screening should be employed when indicated to ensure that the MSLT results are not confounded by inadvertent, intentional, or illicit medication or substance use." If a urine drug screen is performed, the type of test and the results should appear in the MSLT report. Of note, some urine drug screens detect amphetamines but not methylphenidate. A study by Anniss and coworkers[50] found a high percentage of drug screen tests to reveal an unexpected substance. Of 69 studies (43 MSLT and 26 MWT), 16% of patients had positive urinary drug screening (7 MSLT and 4 MWT). Drugs detected included amphetamines, cannabinoids, opiates, and benzodiazepines. No patient self-reported use of these medications before testing.

Recommendations for MSLT reporting are listed in Figure 17–8. MSLT reports should include a summary of the history (daytime sleepiness, presence/absence of cataplexy), medications (including ones stopped and when), summary of

LO at end of epoch 30				Nap 1					
Epoch	30	31	32	33	34	35	36	37	38	39
Stage	LO	W	W	W	N1	N1	N1	N2	N2	N2
Epoch	40	41	42	43	44	45	46	47	48	49
Stage	N1	N2	N2	R	R	R	R	R	R	W
Epoch	50	51	52	53	54	55	56	57	58	59
Stage	W	W	N1	N1	N2	N2	N2	R	R	R
Epoch	60	61	62	63	64	65	66	67	68	69
Stage	R	R	R	R	R					

Figure 17–6 Schematic illustration of sleep stage scoring during a nap in a Multiple Sleep Latency Test. The sleep latency is the time from lights out (LO) to the start of the first epoch of any stage of sleep. Lights out (LO) was at the *end of epoch 30*. In this example, the sleep latency is three epochs (1.5 minutes). The three stage W epochs are labeled with *light gray boxes*. The REM latency is the time from the start of the first epoch of sleep (any stage) to the start of the first epoch of stage R, labeled with *dark gray boxes*. In this case the REM latency is nine epochs (4.5 minutes). *After* the first epoch of sleep, monitoring is continued for another 15 minutes of clock time (30 epochs, *dark horizontal line*). Monitoring during the 15 minutes of clock time does NOT stop even if stage R (REM sleep) is noted.

LO at end of epoch 30				Nap					
Epoch	30	31	32	33	34	35	36	37	38	39
Stage	LO	W	W	W	N1	N2	N2	N2	N2	N2
Epoch	40	41	42	43	44	45	46	47	48	49
Stage	N2	N2	N2	N2	N2	N2	N2	N2	N2	N2
Epoch	50	51	52	53	54	55	56	57	58	59
Stage	W	W	N1	N1	N2	N2	N2	N2	N2	N2
Epoch	60	61	62	63	64	65	66	67	68	69
Stage	W	N1	N2	N2	R					

Figure 17–7 An example of the occurrence of stage R in the last epoch of the 30 epochs (15 minutes) after the first epoch of sleep. Note that although the 15-minute monitoring period *(dark bar)* follows the end of the first epoch of sleep, the REM latency is 15 minutes *(darker gray boxes)*, the time from start of epoch 34 to start of epoch 64. *LO*, Lights out is at the end of epoch 30.

MSLT Report

1. Patient demographics (name, DOB, test date, BMI, medical record number).

2. Names of referring clinician, sleep specialist, and sleep technologist.

3. Documentation of medications used within 24 hours of and during the MSLT and changes to medications within last 2 weeks. If performed, the type of drug screening (and results) should be documented

4. Documentation of available pre-study data including *sleep diary, actigraphy, and PAP download.*

5. Recording parameters of each trial including
   - Start time
   - End time
   - Total sleep time
   - Sleep latency
   - REM sleep latency of each trial.

6. Mean sleep latency, number of SOREMPs during naps, and *whether SOREMP occurred on the PSG.* If no sleep occurs on a trial, 20 minutes is used for the sleep latency value and in the calculation of the mean sleep latency.

7. Deviations from ideal testing times and conditions (e.g., caffeine, nicotine, napping, cell phone, fire alarms, or other stimulating activities) should be documented by the sleep technologist.

8. Interpretation of study findings with signature of board-certified sleep medicine specialist.

Figure 17–8 Recommended components of the Multiple Sleep Latency Test Report. (Data from Krahn LE, Arand DL, Avidan AY, Davila DG, et al. Recommended protocols for the Multiple Sleep Latency Test and Maintenance of Wakefulness Test in adults: guidance from the American Academy of Sleep Medicine. *J Clin Sleep Med.* 2021;17[12]:2489-2498.)

the sleep diary (and actigraphy if performed) information, urine drug screen results, and relevant PSG findings. Information about each nap should include start time, end time, TST, sleep latency, and REM latency. The MSLT report should also include a summary of the overall MSLT findings (MSL and number of SOREMPs—including if one was noted on the nocturnal PSG), adiagnostic impression, and recommendations. If a patient on CPAP is being studied, recent adherence data should also be included in the report.

Indications for the MSLT

The indications for an MSLT[16] are listed in Table 17–5. The MSLT is used to support a diagnosis of narcolepsy in a patient with complaints of daytime sleepiness. The test is not indicated to determine the degree of sleepiness in patients with sleep apnea (treated or untreated), neurological diseases (other than narcolepsy), or insomnia. A repeat MSLT is indicated if an initial study was negative and there is a high clinical suspicion for narcolepsy, if appropriate study conditions were not present (unusual extraneous conditions), or if ambiguous or uninterpretable results are present. A small study confirmed benefits of repeating a nondiagnostic MSLT when the initial results are negative.[51] However, MSLT findings tend to be repeatable for narcolepsy type 1 (with cataplexy) but not with narcolepsy type 2 (no cataplexy).[52,53] The MSLT protocol recommends either four or five naps. Often, the need for the fifth nap is questioned. Goddard and coworkers[43] examined this issue and recommended a fifth nap if the cumulative MSL is 5 to 10 minutes after four naps or if only two SOREMPs (including the PSG) have been detected after four naps. The rationale is that with an MSL in this range, the MSL on the fifth nap might determine if the overall average MSL was ≤ 8 minutes. The recommendation for patients with two SOREMPs after four naps was based on the idea that there might be disagreement over the scoring of one SOREMP between technologist and physician reading the study. They found that most patients with a SOREMP on the fifth nap had two or more SOREMPs after four naps. One might wonder why not recommend the fifth nap if only one SOREMP was found after four naps (including the PSG)? However, in their study a SOREMP was noted in only 7% of fifth naps, and most occurrences were for patients who had already satisfied or in some cases exceeded the criteria for narcolepsy after four naps. Overall, with respect to SOREMPs, adding the fifth nap changed results in only 2 of 122 patients. However, given the cost of the entire enterprise, one could make a case for five naps in patients with a high clinical suspicion for narcolepsy or those with more challenging circumstances (withdrawal of antidepressants before the study) unless unequivocal results are present after four naps.

Table 17–5 When Is the MSLT Indicated?

MSLT Indicated
- Confirmation of suspected narcolepsy (Standard)
- Suspected idiopathic hypersomnia (Option)—to help differentiate idiopathic hypersomnia from narcolepsy

MSLT Not indicated
- Routine evaluation of patients with OSA
- Change in sleepiness in OSA after CPAP treatment
- Evaluation of sleepiness in medical or neurologic conditions (other than narcolepsy)
- Evaluation of sleepiness in insomnia

Repeat MSLT Indicated (Standard)
- Initial MSLT affected by extraneous/unusual conditions
- Appropriate study conditions were not present during initial testing
- Ambiguous or uninterpretable findings
- Clinical suspicion of narcolepsy not confirmed by an earlier MSLT

MSLT, Multiple Sleep Latency Test.
From Littner MR, Kushida C, Wise M, et al. Practice parameters for clinical use of the Multiple Sleep Latency Test and the Maintenance of Wakefulness Test. *Sleep.* 2005;28:113-121.

Diagnosis of Narcolepsy With the MSLT

The MSLT criteria to support a diagnosis of narcolepsy[27] have included an MSL ≤ 8 minutes and two or more SOREMPs on the MSLT. In the ICSD-3[27] published in 2014, a SOREMP on the nocturnal PSG could be used as one of the two required SOREMPs. One should note that studies published before 2014 typically required two SOREMPs on the MSLT without regard for the presence or absence of a PSG SOREMP. The ICSD-3-TR specifies that a nocturnal SOREMP **alone** can be used to support a diagnosis of narcolepsy **with cataplexy (type 1).**[28] The 2014 diagnostic criteria for narcolepsy without cataplexy (type 2) have not changed (Box 17–1). Although a PSG SOREMP would be suggestive of either type of narcolepsy, the best evidence was for patients with narcolepsy and cataplexy. In the discussion to follow, narcolepsy type 1 (cataplexy present, hypocretin deficiency) is abbreviated NT1, and narcolepsy type 2 (cataplexy absent) is abbreviated as NT2. Pediatric considerations for use of the MSLT are discussed in a later section.

Interpretation of MSLT. The requirement of two or more SOREMPs is much more *specific for narcolepsy* than a short MSL (about 20%–30% of normal individuals have an MSL ≤ 8 minutes). Causes of a "false-positive MSLT" include untreated/inadequately treated sleep apnea (see Table 17–6), a habitually delayed sleep period, shift work, prior sleep deprivation or restriction, and recent withdrawal of a REM-suppressing medication. A retrospective study of patients evaluated for OSA undergoing an MSLT found two SOREMPs to be present in only about 5% of patients.[36] However, untreated sleep apnea could also shorten the MSL, and daytime sleepiness often resolves with adequate treatment of sleep apnea (MSLT not needed unless narcolepsy suspected). The standard of practice is to treat significant OSA before proceeding with an evaluation for narcolepsy with an MSLT. *A SOREMP on the PSG is very uncommon in patients with OSA without comorbid narcolepsy*. The finding of a nocturnal SOREMP or a history of cataplexy would raise the clinical suspicion that both OSA and narcolepsy could be present. A minimum of 360 minutes of sleep should be recorded on the nocturnal PSG for the MSLT results to be considered reliable. Ideally, patients should have a spontaneous awakening in the morning rather than a forced awakening at 6 a.m. An inadequate duration of sleep during the weeks preceding an MSLT can cause a false positive study.[30] A very high sleep efficiency, long total sleep time, or increased amount of REM sleep on the PSG preceding the MSLT would raise a concern for insufficient sleep. A chronically delayed sleep period may also result in a short sleep latency and SOREMPs in the early MSLT naps. If only the first two naps have SOREMPs, one should always consider the possibility that these are due to a normally delayed awakening time (typical in adolescents). As previoulsy noted, the *ICSD-3-TR states that the MSLT should not be used in patients with shift work to support a diagnosis of narcolepsy*. In addition, a sleep diary for at least 1 week (2 weeks optimum) or actigraphy if possible is recommended.[28] Kizawa and coworkers[54] selected 12 hypersomnolent patients to undergo a second MSLT *after supervised extended sleep in the hospital for three nights*. The individuals studied had a high sleep efficiency on the PSG before the first MSLT, had a sleep duration on the sleep log pre-MSLT less than 6 hours, or had a sleep duration on the PSG before first MSLT that exceeded 7.5 hours. Repeat testing showed a normal sleep latency in 5 of the 12 individuals studied. Although hospitalization is not practical in nonresearch settings, the study illustrates the *important of adequate sleep pre-MSLT*.

False-negative MSLTs can occur with the concurrent use of a REM-suppressant medication or for no obvious reason in a patient with a high clinical suspicion for the diagnosis of narcolepsy (Table 17–6). Note that in the absence of a documented low cerebrospinal fluid (CSF) hypocretin level, the ICSD-3-TR diagnosis of NT1 requires **both** the presence of cataplexy and a PSG/MSLT meeting diagnostic criteria (PSG SOREMP or [MSL ≤ 8 minutes + two or more SOREMPs on the MSLT]).[28] Therefore, a negative PSG/MSLT in a patient with a history of cataplexy would require a repeat PSG/MSLT to confirm the diagnosis. In the setting of a history of cataplexy but a negative PSG/MSLT, a **negative** HLA-DQB1*06:02 antigen test would imply that true cataplexy was not present (essentially all NT1 patients are positive for this antigen). Similarly obtaining a CSF hypocretin-1 level would not be useful (unlikely to be positive if the HLA-DQB1*06:02 antigen test is negative). As noted above, a small retrospective study[51] found that a repeat MSLT confirmed the diagnosis of narcolepsy in 20% of patients undergoing repeat testing for a nonconfirmatory first MSLT. This study provides support for a repeat MSLT in cases where clinical suspicion for narcolepsy is high despite a negative first test. However, as previously noted, two retrospective studies found that the results of an MSLT were repeatable in NT1 but not NT2 patients.[52,53] Thus, in patients without cataplexy, a positive repeat MSLT result should be viewed with some caution. For NT2 the ICSD-3-TR[28] specifies that a positive PSG/MSLT alone is not sufficient for a diagnosis. *Insufficient sleep should be ruled out, as well as other medical or psychiatric disorders or the use of drugs or medications that could explain the MSLT findings.*

The sensitivity and specificity of the MSLT to diagnose narcolepsy have varied between studies and depend on the study population and the criteria used for the gold standard. In a study by Aldrich and coworkers[29] published in 1997 combining patients with NT1 and NT2, the sensitivity was 0.78 and specificity of 95% (MSL < 8 minutes and two or more MSLT SOREMPs). In that study a diagnosis of NT1 was based on a clinical history of sleepiness and cataplexy. A false-negative MSLT for NT2 implies that there was a repeat MSLT meeting diagnostic criteria. In a large meta-analysis published in 2005 by Arand and coworkers on the ability of the MSLT to diagnose narcolepsy, *two more MSLT SOREMPs* (not including MSL criteria) had a sensitivity of 0.78 and specificity of 0.93 for the diagnosis of narcolepsy.[16,17] In general, the MSLT sensitivity is higher for NT1 patients. Andlauer and coworkers[37] analyzed a sample of 254 successive patients with hypersomnia referred to the sleep clinic for daytime sleepiness not due to sleep apnea and having undergone a nocturnal PSG and MSLT. The gold standard diagnosis of NT1 was based on a low CSF hypocretin-1 level or with typical cataplexy and HLA-DQB1*06:02 positivity (making false-positive cataplexy less likely). The MSLT sensitivity and specificity for diagnosis of NT1 were 92% and 71%. However, the population analyzed may not reflect one typically seen in

Table 17–6 False-Positive and False-Negative MSLTs

False-Positive MSLT
- Circadian factors (chronically delayed sleep period)
- Prior sleep restriction/deprivation
- Untreated/poorly treated OSA
- Recent withdrawal of a REM-suppressing medication
- Short/inadequate sleep on the preceding PSG

False-Negative MSLT
- Medications that suppress REM sleep
- Stimulants
- Anxiety
- Noise during recording

MSLT, Multiple Sleep Latency Test; *OSA*, obstructive sleep apnea; *PSG*, polysomnography; *REM*, rapid eye movement.

most community sleep centers. The low specificity is possibly due to false-positive patients having NT2 (NT1 was the target for diagnosis). The ICSD-3-TR[28] specifies the characteristics of "typical" cataplexy including precipitation by positive emotion, bilateral involvement (although not necessarily symmetric), and brief duration (less than 2–3 minutes).

In summary, both false-positive and false-negative MSLT results are not rare. Proper interpretation of the MSLT requires careful attention to causes of false-positive and false-negative results. The difficulty in making a diagnosis of NT2 narcolepsy using the MSLT was discussed by Baumann and coworkers[55] who emphasized the improtance of excluding sleep deprivation, shift work, or circadian disorders with actigraphy or sleep logs. A trial of sleep extension is warranted if there is a suspicion of insufficient sleep. The authors also discussed the utility of obtaining a CSF hypocretin-1 level (as long as the patient is HLA-DQB1*06:02 positive) as 10 to 30% of patients with narcolepsy without cataplexy have low to intermediate levels. Murer et al[56] determined characteristics of the MSLT assisting with a diagnosis of narcolepsy. One goal was to avoid false positive SOREMPs. However, the study did not use conventional MSLT definitions or methods. Naps were terminated 20 minutes after light out (without respect to recorded sleep) and a SOREMP was defined as the occurrence of stage R during the 20 minute nap. Nearly all REM periods did meet the standard SOREMP definition. When analyzing all naps containing REM sleep, the **combination** of a stage R latency ≤ 5 minutes on the MSLT (measured from lights out to the first epoch of stage R, not the standard definition) and ≥50% of of the 20 minute in stage R sleep was highly specific but not sensitive for narcolepsy (sensitivity 50%, specificity 99%).[56] Patients with narcolepsy entered stage R earlier and stayed in stage R for a greater percentage of time. Patients with narcolepsy also achieved REM sleep before stage N2.

The presence of a SOREMP on the preceding PSG is present about 30% to 50% of the time in patients with confirmed narcolepsy. While this finding can occur with disorders other than narcolepsy, it is very rare. In the study of Aldrich and coworkers[29] a nocturnal SOREMP was present 33% of the time in NT1 and 24% of the time in NT2 but only 1% of the time in patients with sleep-related breathing disorders (Table 17–7). A review of PSG data of 79,651 patients having PSG without MSLT[57] found a nocturnal SOREMP to be present in less than 1%. Evaluating a group of patients with PSG followed by MSLT, the presence of a nocturnal SOREMP was highly specific but not sensitive for narcolepsy. It should be noted that this study did not count a nocturnal SOREMP as one of the two required SOREMPs on the MSLT. In the study of Andlauer and coworkers[37] the finding of a *nocturnal SOREMP had a high positive predictive value for NT1* but was present only about 50% of the time.

As previously mentioned, NT1 patients usually have SOREMPs arising from stage N1.[40] Drakatos and coworkers found that SOREMPs in patients with idiopathic hypersomnia or insufficient sleep arose out of stage N2. In contrast 75% of SOREMPs arose out of stage N1 in NT1 and 52% in in NT2 patients.[40] Pizza and coworkers[58] compared the traditional sleep latency and a sustained sleep latency (time to three epochs of stage N1 or one epoch of another sleep stage) in a group of patients with NT1, NT2, and idopathic hypersomnia. The study found a smaller difference between the traditional sleep latency and the sustained sleep latency was associated with narcolepsy (usually <1 epoch). Patients with idiopathic hypersomnia oscillated between wake and sleep for a longer period of time before achieving sustained sleep.

Diagnosis of Narcolepsy in a Patient With OSA. The approach to patients with OSA and persistent sleepiness on what appears to be adequate CPAP (or other treatment) is challenging.[59] The use of the MSLT in a patient with sleep apnea has been discussed. However, when to proceed with MSLT evaluation is a challenging question. Residual daytime sleepiness can occur in OSA patients with adequate CPAP treatment (hypersomnia due to medical disorder)[28,59] in the absence of another sleep disorder. Alerting agents are approved by the U.S. Food and Drug Administration (FDA) for treatment of excessive sleepiness in this situation. Some patients will also respond to off-label use of a stimulant. A caveat is that the first approach should always be ensuring adequate nightly use of CPAP (6 hours may not be long enough) using objective adherence monitoring. A trial of sleep extension on CPAP is an initial reasonable approach, as well as identification of other conditions impairing sleep or alertness. One could argue that pursuing a diagnosis of narcolepsy would be most useful if it would change treatment. A lifelong history of severe sleepiness (before onset of sleep apnea), the symptom of cataplexy, a SOREMP on PSG, and failure to improve on alerting agents FDA approved for residual sleepiness in OSA patients (or stimulants) are reasons to rule out narcolepsy comorbid

Table 17–7 MSLT Findings in Patients Evaluated for Daytime Sleepiness

Criteria	Narcolepsy With Cataplexy*	Narcolepsy Without Cataplexy**	Sleep-Related Breathing Disorder
≥2 SOREMP + MSL < 5 min	67%	75%	4%
≥2 SOREMP + MSL < 8 min	71%	91%	6%
≥ 2 SOREMPs on MSLT	74%	91%	7%
2 SOREMPs on MSLT	24%	45%	5%
SOREMP on **PSG**	33%	24%	1%

*Narcolepsy diagnosed on basis of cataplexy even if MSLT did not meet criteria.
**Diagnosed by repeat MSLT if necessary.
Data from Aldrich MS, Chervin RD, Malow BA. Value of the Multiple Sleep Latency Test (MSLT) for the diagnosis of narcolepsy. *Sleep.* 1997;20:620-629.
MSL, Mean sleep latency; *MSLT,* Multiple Sleep Latency Test; *SOREMP,* sleep onset rapid eye movement period; *PSG,* polysomnography.

with OSA. A PSG on CPAP (or other treatment) followed by an MSLT on CPAP (or using other treatment) is the correct approach. As noted earlier, a reasonable period of PAP treatment (6 weeks to 2 months) and objective measures of good adherence should precede the MSLT. It is recommended that the *MSLT* ***report*** *contain documentation of the objective PAP adherence.*

Clinical Examples of Use of the MSLT. Case 1: A 25-year-old woman was referred for a second opinion about her diagnosis of narcolepsy with cataplexy. The patient was convinced that she did not have narcolepsy. About 2 years prior, the patient had a syncopal episode. No cardiovascular abnormality was documented and after referral to a neurologist, sleep testing was performed, as the patient reported daytime sleepiness and there was concern that the syncopal episode was cataplexy. A PSG and MSLT were performed, and the results are displayed in Table 17–8. The patient was taking no medications at the time of testing. The PSG showed a normal REM latency and no evidence of sleep apnea. Of interest, the high sleep efficiency and high % REM sleep both suggest prior sleep restriction. The MSLT met criteria for narcolepsy. The ESS was 6 at the current clinic visit. The patient denied current daytime sleepiness or cataplexy and was sleeping 7 hours per night. Physical examination was unremarkable. The circumstances associated with prior testing were discussed. At the time of testing, the patient was the sole caregiver for an 8-month-old infant, as her husband had been deployed overseas as part of his military duties. Her mother provided childcare during her testing. Although the patient could not remember exact details of her typical sleep during that time period, she recalled rarely getting more than 6 hours of sleep each night (and sometimes less). Given the history of inadequate sleep before testing and absence of current daytime sleepiness, the assessment was that narcolepsy was NOT present and that the prior test results were due to inadequate sleep.

Table 17–8 Clinical Example 1

PSG Summary:		
Total sleep time	440 min	
Sleep efficiency	98%	
REM % TST	28%	
Sleep latency	1 min	
REM latency	80 min	
AHI	0/hour	
MSLT Summary:		
	Sleep Latency	SOREMP
Nap 1	5	0
Nap 2	5	Yes
Nap 3	5	Yes
Nap 4	6	0
Nap 5	8	0
Mean SL	5.8	2/5

AHI, Apnea-hypopnea index; *MSLT*, Multiple Sleep Latency Test; *PSG*, polysomnography; *REM*, rapid eye movement; *SL*, sleep latency; *SOREMP*, sleep onset rapid eye movement period; *TST*, total sleep time.

Case 2: A 30-year-old male with a prior sleep study showing moderate sleep apnea was evaluated for difficulty using CPAP and severe daytime sleepiness. On the prior diagnostic test, the REM latency was 5 minutes (a PSG SOREMP), and the apnea-hypopnea index (AHI) was 20/hour. The patient denied cataplexy and admitted to poor CPAP use, as this did not improve his severe sleepiness. His treating physician refused to add an alerting medication, given his poor CPAP use. The current ESS was 20. Physical examination was unremarkable except for a Mallampati 4 upper airway examination. After discussion the patient agreed to nightly use of CPAP for at least 7 hours followed by testing for narcolepsy. Prior to testing, a CPAP download revealed 60/60 days' use with average daily use of 6 hours and 45 minutes and a residual AHI estimate of 2/hour. A PSG using CPAP was followed by an MSLT on CPAP. The PSG showed adequate sleep, a normal REM latency, no evidence of REM sleep rebound, and an AHI of 1/hour. The MSLT (while using CPAP) documented three SOREMPs and an MSL of 2.5 minutes. A diagnosis of narcolepsy without cataplexy was made (in addition to OSA). The patient was treated with modafinil (an alerting medication) and continued CPAP (objectively confirmed adherence) with resolution of his daytime sleepiness.

Maintenance of Wakefulness Test

The MWT was designed to test the patient's ability to stay awake.[16,17,18,60-63] The test differs from the MSLT in a number of ways (Table 17–9). Although the MWT has been used in both the 20-minute and the 40-minute versions,[60-67] the 40-minute test is recommended by the 2005 and 2021 AASM guidelines.[16,18] Treatment of patients with excessive daytime sleepiness may result in improvement in the sleep latency on MWT but not the MSL on MSLT testing.[60-63] The MWT has often been used to assess the effects of medication treatment on the ability of patients with sleep disorders to stay awake as reflected by the MSL (longer MSL = better ability to stay awake).[16,18,61,62]

Specific Indications for the Use of the MWT

The AASM practice parameters for the use of the MWT list specific indications.[16]

1. The MWT 40-minute protocol may be used to assess an individual's ability to remain awake when their ability to remain awake constitutes a public or personal safety issue. (Option)
2. The MWT may be indicated in patients with excessive sleepiness to assess response to treatment. (Guideline)

MWT Protocol

The recommended 40-minute MWT protocol is outlined by the 2021 AASM guidelines.[18] In preparation for the MWT the clinician and patient should define goals for adequate sleep (duration and timing). Adequate sleep should be documented by a sleep diary and whenever possible, actigraphy for 2 weeks before testing. The MWT should be performed during a period of medical stability and when treatments for known sleep disorders are established and effective. For patients with OSA a PAP download showing adequate adherence and efficacy is essential. For non-PAP treatment of OSA self report of adequate adherence is also needed. Patients should use PAP or non-PAP treatments for OSA on the night before the MWT. If a PSG on PAP precedes the

Table 17–9 Comparison of MSLT and MWT

	MSLT	MWT
Preceding PSG	Required	Optional
Naps/trials	4 or 5	4
Timing	• 1–3 hours after PSG ends • Naps every 2 hours	To 3 hours after wakeup time Wake trials every 2 hours
Posture	Lying in bed Dark room	Sitting in bed or in recliner Dim light to side of patient
Biocalibration	• Yes	• Yes
Recommended montage	• Yes	• Yes
Instruction	• Please lie quietly, assume a comfortable position, keep your eyes closed, and allow yourself to fall asleep.	• Please sit still and remain awake for as long as possible. Look directly ahead of you, and do not look directly at the light.
Nap termination	• 20 min if no sleep • 15 min of **clock time** after first epoch of sleep	• 40 min in no sleep • After three consecutive epochs of stage N1 or an epoch of any other stage of sleep (N2, N3, R)
Sleep latency	Time from lights out to first epoch of sleep	Same
REM latency	Time from start of first epoch of sleep until start of first epoch of stage R	n/a
Results	Mean sleep latency, number of SOREMPs	Mean sleep latency
Sleep logs, actigraphy	For 2 weeks preceding testing	same
Audio-visual recorded	Recommended	Same
Prenap activity	Stop stimulating activity 30 min before nap	Stop stimulating activity 30 min before wake trial
Urine drug screen	If indicated	If indicated

MSLT, Multiple Sleep Latency Test; *MWT*, Maintenance of Wakefulness Test; *PSG*, polysomnography; *REM*, rapid eye movement; *SOREMP*, sleep onset rapid eye movement period.

MWT, the mask and pressure should match those used at home. However, in contrast to the MSLT, patients *do not use the treatment for OSA during the MWT*. For both OSA and other disorders of hypersomnolence, the current daytime medications used to maintain alertness can be used during the MWT to document the efficacy of treatment.

As shown in Figures 17–9 and 17–10, using a four-nap protocol is standard. Relevant clinical data such as preceding sleep schedules, adherence to PAP or other treatments, and medications should be available for the interpreting physician. The performance of a *PSG on the night before the MWT is optional* (left up to the clinician). The MWT should be performed after the patient's habitual major sleep period. Note that the sleep latency is defined as the time from lights out to the start of any epoch of sleep. If a PSG is performed before the MWT, a change in clothing between in the PSG and MWT is not required. The patient should abstain from alcohol, marijuana, and other sedating substances on the day of testing. The recording montage for the MWT is similar to that of the MSLT. Audiovisual recording must be made during wake trials and be accessible to the interpreting physician. The patient must be audiovisually monitored throughout the day, but retention of recordings made between trials is discretionary. Stimulating activities such as consuming nicotine and the use of electronic devices and cell phones should end at least 30 minutes before each wake trial. Vigorous physical activity and prolonged exposures to sunlight/bright artificial light should be avoided all day. As previously noted, in contrast to the MSLT, individuals with a known hypersomnia undergoing a MWT often take the alerting medication they are using for outpatient treatment. That is, the ability of current treatment to maintain alertness is being tested. The dose and timing of the alerting medication should be documented.

The MWT consists of four 40-minute wake trials. The initial trial should begin 1.5 to 3 hours after termination of the preceding night's sleep at home (or the preceding PSG), and subsequent trials should begin 2 hours after the start of the prior trial. Use of the bathroom should be offered to the patient before each wake trial. In contrast to the MSLT, *the patient should be seated in a bed or reclining chair with the back and head comfortably supported.* The option for use of a recliner is new in the 2021 guidelines. Sleep rooms should be dimly lit, quiet, and at a comfortable temperature during testing. The light source should deliver an illuminance of 0.1 to 0.13 lux at the corneal level (such as a 7.5-watt nightlight) placed 12 inches off the floor and 3 feet lateral to the patient's head. Biocalibrations similar to that for the MSLT are performed before each wake trial. At the start of each wake trial, the patient should be instructed as follows: "*Please sit still and remain awake for as long as possible.* Look directly ahead of you, and do not look directly at the light." Testing starts immediately after instructions are given, and bedroom lights are turned off.

Each MWT nap lasts a maximum of 40 minutes after lights out. Each wake trial is ended once the patient has three consecutive epochs of stage N1 sleep or one epoch of any other sleep stage or after 40 minutes. Of note, it is essential

MWT Protocol (part 1)

1. Relevant clinical data such as preceding sleep schedules, PAP adherence, or other therapies should be available to the interpreting clinician. The MWT should be performed after the patient's major sleep period. Performance of a PSG before the MWT is at the discretion of the sleep clinician.

2. The patient's clothing should be comfortable, be appropriate to the environment, and not interfere with the performance of tests. If a PSG is performed, then a change in clothing is **not** required between the PSG and the MWT.

3. The patient should abstain from alcohol, marijuana, and other sedating substances on the day of the test.

4. Patients on PAP/non-PAP therapies for sleep-disordered breathing should use them the night before **(but not during)** the MWT. If a PSG is performed, then the PAP settings and mask interface should match those used at home.

5. The recording montage for the MWT should, at a minimum, include 3 EEG recording leads with 1 each for frontal (F3-M2 or F4-M1), central (C3-M2 or C4-M1), and occipital (O1-M2 or O2-M1) derivations, left and right eye EOG derivtions, mental/submental EMG, and EKG.

6. Audiovisual recordings must be made during the wake trials and be accessible to interpreting sleep specialists. The patient must be audiovisually monitored throughout the day, but retention of recordings made between trials is discretionary.

7. The MWT should consist of four **40-minute wake trials.** The initial trial should begin **1.5–3 hours after termination of the preceding night's sleep at home,** and a subsequent trial should begin **2 hours after the start of the prior trial.**

8. Before each wake trial, the patient should be offered the use of the restroom and queried regarding other requirements for comfort.

9. Sleep rooms should be dimly lit, quiet, and at a comfortable temperature during testing. The light source should deliver an illuminance of 0.1–0.13 lux at the corneal level (such as a 7.5-watt nightlight) placed 12 inches off the floor and 3 feet lateral to the patient's head. The patient should be given sufficient time to acclimate to the recording room before the start of the first trial.

10. The patient should be seated in a bed or reclining chair with the back and head comfortably supported. This should be the same for all wake trials.

Figure 17–9 Recommended Maintenance of Wakefulness Test Protocol (part 1). (Data from Krahn LE, Arand DL, Avidan AY, Davila DG, et al. Recommended protocols for the Multiple Sleep Latency Test and Maintenance of Wakefulness Test in adults: guidance from the American Academy of Sleep Medicine. *J Clin Sleep Med.* 2021;17[12]:2489-2498.)

MWT Protocol (part 2)

11. Patient biocalibrations should be conducted before starting each wake trial.
    Standard instructions include:
    (1) "sit quietly with your eyes open for 30 seconds";
    (2) "close both eyes for 30 seconds"
    (3) "without moving your head, look to the right, then left, then right, then left, right and then left"
    (4) "blink eyes slowly for 5 times"; and
    (5) "clench or grit your teeth tightly together."
    Before the trials, patients should be instructed to refrain from activities and vocalizations that promote wakefulness such as fidgeting or singing.

12. At the start of each wake trial, the patient should be instructed as follows: "Please sit still and remain awake for as long as possible. Look directly ahead of you, and do not look directly at the light." Testing starts immediately after instructions are given, and bedroom lights are turned off.

13. Each wake trial is ended once the patient has **3 consecutive epochs of stage N1 sleep or 1 epoch of any other sleep stage or after 40 minutes.**

14. Stimulating activities such as consuming nicotine and the use of electronic devices and cell phones should end at least 30 minutes before each wake trial. Vigorous physical activity and prolonged exposures to sunlight/bright artificial light should be avoided all day.

15. Between wake trials, the patient should be out of bed and not permitted to sleep.

16. A light breakfast at least 1 hour before the first wake trial and a light lunch immediately after the termination of the second wake trial are recommended.

17. Urine drug screening should be employed when indicated to ensure that the MWT results are not confounded by inadvertent, intentional, or illicit medication or substance use.

Figure 17–10 Recommended Maintenance of Wakefulness Test Protocol (part 2). (Data from Krahn LE, Arand DL, Avidan AY, Davila DG, et al. Recommended protocols for the Multiple Sleep Latency Test and Maintenance of Wakefulness Test in adults: guidance from the American Academy of Sleep Medicine. *J Clin Sleep Med.* 2021;17(12):2489-2498.)

that during testing visual observation is continuous, as the individual being tested is not allowed to use extreme measures (hitting, moving in bed) to maintain alertness. Between wake trials, the patient should be out of bed and not permitted to sleep. A light breakfast at least 1 hour before the first wake trial and a light lunch immediately after the termination of the second wake trial are recommended. Stimulating activities such as consuming nicotine and the use of electronic devices and cell phones should end at least 30 minutes before each wake trial. Vigorous physical activity and prolonged exposures to sunlight/bright artificial light should be avoided all day. Urine drug screening should be employed when indicated to ensure that the MWT results are not confounded by inadvertent, intentional, or illicit medication or substance use. When patients are taking their usual stimulant medication, a positive drug screen might be expected if the type of medication being taken is detected by the type of drug screen being used.

Elements to be contained in the MWT report are listed in Figure 17–11. The history and reason for testing should be documented. Any information on preceding sleep (sleep diaries) should be discussed, as well as PSG findings (if PSG is performed). *Documentation of medications used within 24 hours of and during the MWT and any changes to medications within the last 2 weeks should be reported.* If performed, the type of drug screening (and results) should be documented. Recording parameters that should be reported include the start time, end time, TST, and sleep latency of each wake trial. **Sleep latency** is defined as the time from lights out until the start of the first epoch of any stage of sleep (an epoch of N1, N2, N3, or R). *Note that this differs from the criteria to end a nap trial.* An MSL averaged over the four wake trials is determined. If no sleep occurs on a trial, then 40 minutes is used as the sleep latency and in the calculation of the MSL. An interpretation

MWT Reporting

1. Patient demographics (name, DOB, test date, BMI, medical record number).

2. Names of referring clinician, sleep specialist, and sleep technologist.

3. Documentation of medications used within 24 hours of and during the MWT and any changes to medications within last 2 weeks.
   - If performed, the type of drug screening should be documented.

4. Documentation of available pre-study data including sleep diary, actigraphy, and PAP download.

5. Recording parameters for each wake trial including
   - Start time
   - End time
   - Total sleep time
   - Sleep latency of each wake trial

   Sleep latency is defined as the time from lights out until the start of the first epoch of any stage of sleep (an epoch of N1, N2, N3, or R).

6. Mean sleep latency averaged over the 4 wake trials.
   - If no sleep occurs on a trial, then 40 minutes is used as the sleep latency and in the calculation of the mean sleep latency.

7. Deviations from ideal testing times and conditions (e.g., nicotine, caffeine, napping, cell phone, fire alarms, or other stimulating activities) should be documented by the sleep technologist.

8. Interpretation of study findings with signature of board-certified sleep medicine physician.

Figure 17–11 Recommended information to include in a Maintenance of Wakefulness Test Report. (Data from Krahn LE, Arand DL, Avidan AY, Davila DG, et al. Recommended protocols for the Multiple Sleep Latency Test and Maintenance of Wakefulness Test in adults: guidance from the American Academy of Sleep Medicine. *J Clin Sleep Med.* 2021;17[12]:2489-2498.)

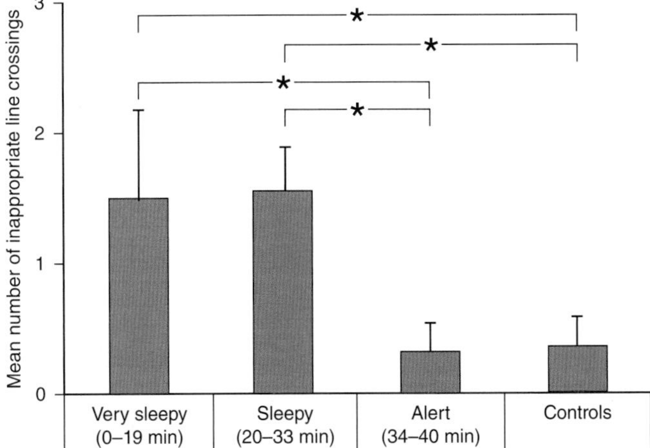

Figure 17–12 A Maintenance of Wakefulness Test mean sleep latency over 33 minutes was associated with a normal incidence of inappropriate lane crossings during actual driving. (From Philip P, Sagaspe P, Taillard J, et al. Maintenance of Wakefulness Test, obstructive sleep apnea syndrome and driving risk. *Ann Neurol.* 2008;64:410-416.)

of the findings is made along with recommendations. Most physicians include a disclaimer that the MWT findings do not guarantee alertness or fitness of duty, as these depend on the recent amount of sleep and adherence to treatment (CPAP and medications).

MWT Normative Data

Normative data for the MWT from a systematic review of MWT studies[17] are displayed in Table 17–10. Using the 40-minute MWT, 59% of patients were able to stay awake for 40 minutes on each nap. The lower 95% confidence limit was 8 minutes (97.5% had MSL > 8 minutes). Another study by Banks and coworkers[65] evaluated normal subjects and found an MSL to the first epoch of unequivocal sleep during the 40-minute trial MWT was 36.9 ± 5.4 minutes. The lower normal limit, defined as 2 standard deviations (SDs) below the mean, was therefore 26.1 minutes. In this study the SD was much lower than in the systematic review. While of interest, these data do little to set a standard for individuals in whom alertness is essential for personal and public safety. Certainly, staying awake for all trials is an appropriate expectation for individuals requiring the highest level of safety. Therefore, whereas an MSL less than 8 minutes is abnormal, an MSL of 8 to 40 minutes is of uncertain significance. A "normal" MWT finding is no guarantee of what will happen in the work environment. The ability to maintain alertness (different than the ability to maintain wakefulness) may depend on adherence to treatment, prior TST, medication side effects, and circadian factors. A study of patients with OSA during actual 90-minute driving sessions on the road with a driving instructor intervening, if necessary, determined inappropriate line crossing[66] (determined by video recording). Two groups "very sleepy" with an MWT MSL less than 19 minutes and "sleepy" with an MSL of 20 to 33 minutes had significantly higher line crossings than controls and patients with mild sleepiness (MWT MSL of 34–40 minutes) (Figure 17–12). This study suggests that an MSL ≤ 33 minutes is consistent with impaired alertness to perform a task such as driving. Of note, the sleep latency on the MWT increases with age similar to the sleep latency on the MSLT.[17] Another study of MWT and self-reported driving history[67] found patients with MWT latency between 19 and 33 minutes had a 3.2-fold increase in risk of reporting a near-miss accident compared with patients with a MWT latency greater than 33 minutes. Patients with a MWT latency less than 19 minutes had an approximately fivefold increased risk.

Table 17–10 Normative Data for the MWT

MSL (mean ± SD)	30.4 ± 11.2 min
MSL upper limit (95% CI)	40 min
MSL lower limit	8 min
MSL > 8 min	97.5% of normal individuals
MSL = 40 min (stay awake in all naps)	59% of normal individuals

CI, confidence interval; *MSL*, mean sleep latency; *SD*, standard deviation. Adapted from Arand D, Bonnet M, Hurwitz T, et al. A review by the MSLT and MWT Task Force of the Standards of Practice Committee of the AASM. The clinical use of the MSLT and MWT. *Sleep.* 2005;28:123-144.

Relationship Between the MSLT and the MWT

The MWT tests different characteristics than the MSLT. For example, some patients with a short MSLT sleep latency may

Table 17–11 Comparison of MSLT and MWT in Sleep Apnea Patients (N= 170)*

Sleep Apnea	(MWT MSL) Low	(MWT MSL) High
(MSLT MSL) **High**	15%	34%
(MSLT MSL) **Low**	36%	**15%**

*Cutoff low and high MSLT and MWT based on median values for the studies (7.5-min MSL on the MSLT and 30-min MSL on the MWT).

Note: 15% of patients were in the sleepiest group by MSLT (MSLT MSL Low) but by MWT were in the group better at maintaining wake (MWT MSL high). *MSL,* Mean sleep latency; *MSLT,* Multiple Sleep Latency Test; *MWT,* Maintenance of Wakefulness Test.

From Sangal RB, Thomas L, Mitler MM. Maintenance of Wakefulness Test and Multiple Sleep Latency Test: measurements of different abilities in patients with sleep disorders. *Chest.* 1992;101:898-902.

have a high MWT sleep latency. When Sangal and associates[62] administered both the MSLT and the MWT to a group of patients with excessive daytime sleepiness, the correlation between the MSL on the two tests was significant but low (r = 0.41, P < .001). Several individuals did not fall asleep during the MWT but had some degree of daytime sleepiness as assessed by the MSLT. Table 17–11 illustrates classifications of the group of OSA patients by MSL (low or high) on a four-nap MSLT and MWT. The study found that 15% of the patients were sleepy (MSLT low) but able to stay awake (MWT high). In research studies the MWT is commonly used to demonstrate alerting medication efficacy, as the test measures the ability to stay awake.

EVALUATING SLEEPINESS IN CHILDREN

Studies of sleep duration in normal children before the age of widespread use of personal electronics by children found the normal 50 percentile sleep duration for children aged 5, 10, and 15 years to be approximately 11, 10, and 8.5 hours (see Chapter 7).[68] If school wake-up time is at 6 a.m., a 10-year-old child should go to bed at 8 to 9 p.m. An AASM consensus statement[69] on recommended sleep duration in infants and children was published and the recommendations are listed in Table 17–12. The consensus statement stated that the benefits of an adequate sleep duration include "improved attention, behavior, learning, memory, emotional regulation, quality of life, and mental and physical health. Regularly sleeping fewer than the number of recommended hours is associated with attention, behavior, and learning problems. Insufficient sleep also increases the risk of accidents, injuries, hypertension, obesity, diabetes, and depression. Insufficient sleep in teenagers is associated with increased risk of self-harm, suicidal thoughts, and suicide attempts." Another very important consideration is that although the normal sleep needs of children are greater than in adults, *this fact may not be comprehended by a majority of parents.*[70] Survey results suggest that many parents' knowledge about the sleep needs of their children is limited. In one survey study, 23% of children did not have a consistent bedtime, 25% had a bedtime later than 9 p.m., 23% had at least one electronic device in the bedroom, and 56% frequently fell asleep with an adult present. Both positive and negative sleep habits tended to cluster together. Children who had irregular and late bedtimes were more than twice as likely to obtain insufficient sleep that those with regular and early bedtimes. While 25% of children were getting less than the recommended sleep amount for age, just 13% of parents believed that their child was getting insufficient sleep.[70]

Table 17–12 Recommended Sleep Duration in Infants and Children

Age	Recommended Sleep Duration
Infants 4 months to 12 months	12 to 16 hours per 24 hours (including naps)
Children 1 to 2 years	11 to 14 hours per 24 hours (including naps)
Children 3 to 5 years	10 to 13 hours per 24 hours (including naps)
Children 6 to 12 years	9 to 12 hours per 24 hours
Adolescents 13 to 18 years	8 to 10 hours per 24 hours

Adapted from Paruthi S, Brooks LJ, D'Ambrosio C, Hall WA, et al. Consensus statement of the American Academy of Sleep Medicine on the recommended amount of sleep for healthy children: methodology and discussion. *J Clin Sleep Med.* 2016;12(11):1549-1561.

Prepubertal pediatric patients are less likely to complain of symptoms of sleepiness compared with adults with sleep disorders or sleep restriction. In disorders such as childhood OSA, daytime sleepiness is rarely the most prominent complaint unless sleep apnea is accompanied by sleep restriction. The manifestations of sleepiness may *include inattention, learning difficulty, and behavioral problems.* In young children a daytime nap provides a portion of the recommended sleep duration. Nap duration (or number) starts to decrease about 3 years of age, is uncommon after 5 years of age, and is rare at 7 years.[68,71] A return to napping in a child who was previously nap free could be a manifestation of excessive sleepiness.

Screening Tools and Subjective Sleepiness

The "BEARS" screening tool has been used as a guide for primary physicians but is also useful for the sleep physician[72] (BEARS is an acronym representing B = bedtime issues, E = excessive daytime sleepiness, A = awakenings, R= regularity and duration of sleep, and S = Snoring).

For older children and adolescents, a modified ESS has been developed (ESS-CHAD for children and adolescents).[72] The chance of dozing or falling asleep in the following 8 situations is assesed (new modfied situations in italics, wording varies slightly in some versions): 1. sitting and reading, 2. watching TV or a video, 3. *sitting in a classroom at school during the morning*, 4. sitting as a passenger in a car or bus for about half an hour, 5. lying down to rest in the afternoon, 6. sitting and talking to someone, 7. *sitting quietly by yourself after lunch*, 8. *sitting and eating a meal.* As in adults each situation receives a score of 0,1,2,or 3 (see Table 17-1) with the total scoring ranging from 0 to 24. A total a score of 10 or less is usually considered normal. A four-item Pediatric Sleep Questionnaire has also been used[73] (Table 17–13). The parent answers but is encouraged to ask the child for help. In one study, the test distinguished children with sleep-disordered breathing from controls.

Objective Sleepiness: The MSLT in Children

The AASM practice parameters for the nonrespiratory indications for PSG and multiple sleep latency testing for children[74]

Table 17–13 Pediatric Sleep Questionnaire (PSQ-SS)

1. Does your child wake up feeling unrefreshed in the morning?
2. Does your child have a problem with sleepiness during the day?
3. Does your child appear sleepy during the day according to comments of a teacher or other supervisor?
4. Is your child hard to wake up in the morning?

Responses are *Yes*, *No*, or *Don't Know*. If at least two of the four are positive, the child is classified as subjectively sleepy.

From Chervin RD, Hedger KM, Dillon JE, Pituch KJ. Pediatric Sleep Questionnaire (PSQ): validity and reliability of scales for sleep-disordered breathing, snoring, sleepiness, and behavioral problems. *Sleep Med.* 2000;1:21-32.

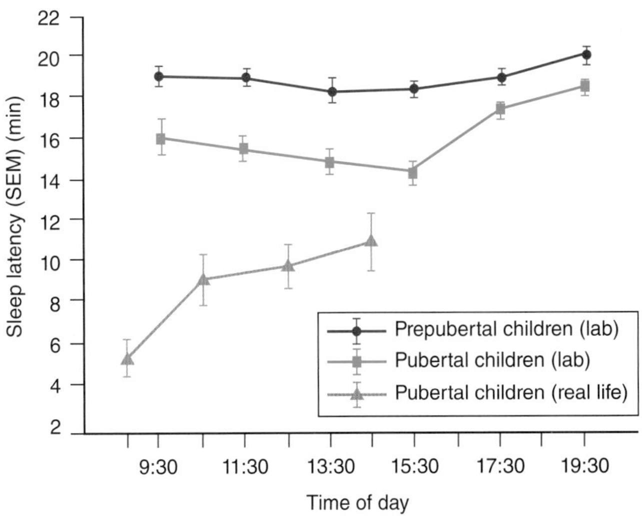

Figure 17–13 Mean sleep latency of groups of children over the day on the Maintenance of Wakefulness Test. Prepubertal children had a mean sleep latency 18 to 20 minutes. The sleep latency of pubertal children when studied in the lab with regular bedtimes and adequate sleep was shorter than the prepubertal group. In real life, because of sleep restriction the mean sleep latency in pubertal individuals was much shorter. (From Jenni OG and Carskadon MA. Sleep behavior and sleep regulation from infancy through adolescence: normative aspects. *Sleep Med Clin.* 2007;2(3):321-329.)

state that "the collective evidence demonstrated that the MSLT is technically feasible and can provide meaningful results in developmentally normal children aged 5 years and older." The practice parameters give the following recommendations concerning the MSLT. No recommendations were made for the MWT.

1. The MSLT, preceded by nocturnal PSG, is indicated in children as part of the evaluation for suspected narcolepsy. (Standard)
2. The MSLT, preceded by nocturnal PSG, is indicated in children suspected of having hypersomnia from causes other than narcolepsy to assess excessive sleepiness and to aid in differentiation from narcolepsy. (Option)

The MSLT studies in children (Table 17–14, Figure 17–13) have shown long sleep latencies in prepubertal children (18 to 20 minutes, or no sleep on any nap).[75,76] In *pubertal children* (9th and 10th grades) the MSL was lower (16 minutes) even when adequate sleep time was enforced (bedtime 11 p.m., wake time 8 a.m. in the lab).[77,78] Dim light melatonin onset, a circadian marker, was later in the 10th grade compared with the 9th grade (delay in circadian rhythm). A part of the study that evaluated real-world conditions using home actigraphy[77] documented that an earlier wake time (school) was not associated with an earlier bedtime with the result that TST was decreased, and the sleep latency was much shorter. In addition, a *significant percentage of pubertal children had SOREMPs.* One SOREMP was noted in 48% and two sleep onset periods in 16%. *Thus, the clinician should exercise caution in interpreting SOREMPs on the MSLT in adolescents.* This is especially true if the only SOREMPs are in the first two naps.

Given the high MSL in prepubertal children, use of an MSL ≤ 8 minutes for the diagnosis of narcolepsy could potentially be problematic. Some investigators have suggested that an MSL ≤ 12 minutes be considered as abnormal.[79] However, studies of children with narcolepsy have in fact found very low MSL values well below 8 minutes. In a study by Aran and coworkers,[80] the MSL in pediatric patients with narcolepsy was 2.5 minutes.

In general, the MSLT and MWT protocols for children and adolescents are similar to adults. One exception is that for younger children parental involvement is often necessary and sleep technologists with experience studying children are preferred. For adolescent patients the urine drug screen is very important. In a retrospective study[81] of urine drug screening performed the morning before MSLT in 383 patients less than 21 years old referred for excessive daytime sleepiness, the urine drug screen was positive in 10%, and 43% of patients that had positive urine drug screens for THC met MSLT criteria for narcolepsy versus 24% with negative drug screens meeting criteria for narcolepsy. No drug screen was positive in patients aged less than 13 years. *The authors concluded that drug screening is important in interpreting MSLT findings for children 13 years or older.*

As in adults, the use of REM-suppressing antidepressants in children and inadequate sleep are important factors to consider in interpreting the MSLT. A retrospective study of MSLT testing in children and adolescents[82] found that patients taking REM-suppressing antidepressants at initial evaluation had fewer SOREMPs but not different sleep latencies on a subsequent MSLT. About half (8/17) on antidepressants were able to discontinue the medications before testing. This group had more SOREMPs, but the difference was not statistically significant (likely because of small numbers).

Table 17–14 Multiple Sleep Latency Findings in Children and Adolescents

Stage of Development	Mean Sleep Latency (min)	Standard Deviation (min)
Tanner stage 1	19.0	1.8
Tanner stage 2	18.5	2.1
Tanner stage 3	16.5	2.8
Tanner stage 4	15.5	3.3
Tanner stage 5	16.1	1.5
Older adolescents	15.7	3.5

From Carskadon M. The second decade. In Gulleminault C, ed. *Sleeping and Waking Disorders—Indications and Techniques.* Butterworths; 1982:99-125.

Table 17–15 Summary of Clinical Case 3

PSG1				PSG2			
Lights out	21:41			Lights out	21:07		
Lights on	**04:17**			Lights on	06:25		
Total sleep time (min)	375			Total sleep time (min)	522		
REM latency (min)	84.5			REM latency (min)	80.0		
AHI (no/hour)	2.6			AHI (no/hour)	3.5		
MSLT	Start of Nap	Sleep Latency (min)	SOREMP	MSLT	Start of Nap	Sleep Latency (min)	SOREMP
Nap 1	06:13 AM	8.5	Yes	Nap 1	8:10 AM<	8	No
Nap 2	07:33 AM	7.0	No	Nap 2	10:10 AM	11	No
Nap 3	09:02 AM	4.5	Yes	Nap 3	12:10 PM	10	No
Nap 4	10:19 AM	5.0	No	Nap 4	2:10 PM	10	No
Nap 5	–	–	–	Nap 5	4:10 PM	15	No
	Mean	6	2/4		Mean	10.7	0/5

AHI, Apnea-hypopnea index; *MSLT,* Multiple Sleep Latency Test; *PSG,* polysomnography; *REM,* rapid eye movement; *SOREMP,* sleep onset rapid eye movement period.
(Adapted From Reference[85])

Longer time in bed by actigraphy but not a longer self-reported sleep duration was associated with a greater MSL. Time in bed on actigraphy was a better predictor than TST. As in adults, children taking REM-suppressing medications are problematic with respect to detecting SOREMPs, and actigraphy is useful to detect inadequate sleep in the weeks before testing.

Altered Sleep in Children With Narcolepsy

As in adults, studies have evaluated various sleep parameters to improve detection of narcolepsy in children. Nocturnal (PSG) SOREMPs in children were found to be highly suggestive of narcolepsy with cataplexy.[83] The specificity was 97% but the sensitivity was only 54.8%. Maski and coworkers developed an index of disrupted nighttime sleep. The wake/N1 index was the number of transitions from any sleep stage to awake or N1 (normalized by TST) was found to be associated with objective daytime sleepiness, daytime SOREMPs, self-reported disturbed sleep, and low CSF hypocretin levels.[84]

Clinical MSLT Example 3

An 11-year-old child was sent for a second opinion concerning a diagnosis of narcolepsy made at a community sleep center. A modified ESS was 13, and there was no history of cataplexy, hypnogogic hallucinations, or sleep paralysis. Loud snoring but no witnessed apnea were reported by the parents. The normal sleep period for the child was 11 p.m. to 7 a.m. The physical examination was normal except for enlarged tonsils. Salient features of the PSG and MSLT data are shown (PSG1) in Table 17–15. The most concerning feature of the prior evaluation was the *early termination of the PSG* at 4:17 a.m. and the short TST. The timing of the MSLT was very early at a time when the patient likely was experiencing REM sleep at home. The PSG and MSLT were repeated, and the results are shown as PSG2 in Table 17–15. An AHI of 3.5/hour on the PSG was noted (clinically significant for age 11). On the MSLT, the MSL was 10.7 minutes and no SOREMPs were noted. The daytime sleepiness was thought to be due to untreated OSA. The patient underwent tonsillectomy and adenoidectomy with resolution of sleepiness.

SUMMARY OF KEY POINTS

1. The Epworth sleepiness scale (ESS) measures self-rated average sleep propensity (chance of dozing) over eight common situations. The scale ranges from 0 to 24 with 10 or less being considered normal.
2. The Multiple Sleep Latency Test (MSLT) determines the mean sleep latency (an objective measure of daytime sleepiness, tendency to fall asleep) and the presence of sleep onset REM periods (SOREMPs).
3. The MSLT consists of four or five naps spaced every 2 hours beginning about 1.5 to 3 hours after the wake-up time after a preceding polysomnography (PSG). The time of onset of each subsequent nap is 2 hours after the start of the preceding nap. For example if nap 1 starts at 7:45AM, nap 2 would start at 9:45AM.
4. A short MSL on the MSLT provides evidence of excessive sleepiness but there is considerable overlap between normal populations and patients with sleep disorders.
5. An MSLT nap is terminated after 20 minutes if no sleep is recorded (sleep latency = 20 minutes). The nap continues for 15 minutes of clock time *after* the first epoch of sleep. The nap duration varies from 20 to 35 minutes. The mean sleep latency for the naps and the number of SOREMPs is determined.
6. The MSLT should be preceded by a PSG to detect causes of sleepiness such as sleep apnea and to verify adequate sleep before the MSLT. MSLT findings are **not** considered reliable if less than 360 minutes of sleep are recorded.
7. Audiovisual monitoring is recommended during and between naps.

8. Medications that can affect sleepiness or REM sleep should be withdrawn 2 weeks before MSLT date (or at least five times the drug half-life).
9. Stimulant withdrawal, ideally for 2 weeks, may be shortened if necessary based on the potential impact on patient safety and societal requirements.
10. MSLT diagnostic criteria for narcolepsy were formerly an MSL $\leq$ 8 minutes and two or more SOREMPs. A SOREMP on the nocturnal PSG could be used as one of the qualifying SOREMPs. In the recent of ICSD-3-TR diagnostic criteria for NT1 are a *either* a SOREMP on the PSG *or* a MSL $\leq$ 8 minutes and two or more SOREMPs on the MSLT. For NT2 the criteria are an MSL $\leq$ 8 min combined with two or more SOREMPs during the MSLT. A SOREMP on the PSG can be counted as one of the two MSLT SOREMPs (see Chapter 32).
11. A sleep diary 2 weeks before testing (or actigraphy if possible) should be performed to help document sufficient duration and pattern of sleep.
12. A urine drug screen is optional, but most clinicians feel this is essential given the high number of unexpected positive results.
13. MSLT testing in a patient with obstructive sleep apnea (narcolepsy in addition to sleep apnea is suspected) requires adequate OSA treatment (including documented adherence) before testing. The PSG is performed using the usual treatment, and the MSLT is also performed using the usual treatment. For example, the PSG is on CPAP and the MSLT is performed on CPAP.
14. The Maintenance of Wakefulness Test (MWT) objectively quantifies a patient's ability to remain awake in a situation predisposing to sleep (dimly lighted room, sitting on a bed or in recliner). The use of four naps of up to 40 minutes in duration is recommended. The MWT assesses the ability to stay awake. However, a definite sleep latency defining normal alertness has not been defined. *Some studies of driving suggest a value greater than 33 minutes could be considered normal alertness.*
15. A PSG preceding the MWT is optional. However, adequate sleep is essential.
16. The MWT consists of four wake trials separated by 2 hours and starting 1.5 to 3 hours after awakening from sleep.
17. Each MWT nap is terminated after 40 minutes of no sleep (sleep latency = 40 minutes) or three consecutive epochs of stage N1 or a single epoch of any other stage of sleep. The sleep latency is the time from lights out to the start of an epoch of any stage of sleep (including one epoch of stage N1).
18. During the MWT the patient sits upright in bed or in a recliner with the head comfortably supported in a dark room. The light source should deliver an illuminance of 0.1–0.13 lux at the corneal level (such as a 7.5-watt nightlight placed 12 inches off the floor and 3 feet lateral to the patient's head).
19. The MSLT and MWT measure different things. It is possible to have short MSL by MSLT but a long MSL by MWT. That is, a patient can be sleepy but be able to maintain alertness.
20. Sleepiness in children may manifest itself by inattentive, impulsive, and aggressive behavior.
21. Normal prepubertal children have very long sleep latencies and may not fall asleep on any MSLT nap. The MSL during an MSLT for prepubertal children is 18 to 20 minutes. However, the mean sleep latency of children with narcolepsy is usually less than 5 minutes.
22. Adolescents have a shorter sleep latency than prepubertal children, a delayed sleep phase, and a tendency for SOREMPs on early MSLT naps. A delayed sleep period can cause a false positive MSLT. Caution is advised if the only SOREMPs are on the first two MSLT naps.
23. Taking naps usually ceases by age 5 to 7 years. A return to napping is an indication of daytime sleepiness in children.
24. Children 6 to 12 years of age need 9 to 12 hours of sleep. If wake-up time is 6 a.m. during school days, bedtime should be 8 to 9 p.m to obtain 9 hours of sleep or bedtime should be 7 to 8 PM to obtain 10 hours of sleep.

CLINICAL REVIEW QUESTIONS

1. Which of the following are the MSLT diagnostic criteria for **narcolepsy with cataplexy**? (MSL = mean sleep latency, PSG = polysomnography performed before the MSLT)
   A. MSL < 8 minutes and two or more SOREMPs during the MSLT. A PSG SOREMP can count as one of the SOREMPs during the MSLT.
   B. MSL $\leq$ 8 minutes and two or more SOREMPs during the MSLT. A PSG SOREMP can count as one of the SOREMPs during the MSLT.
   C. A PSG SOREMP OR (MSL < 8 minutes and two or more SOREMPs on the MSLT).
   D. A PSG SOREMP OR (MSL $\leq$ 8 minutes and two or more SOREMPs on the MSLT).
2. After the first epoch of sleep occurs, how many minutes are recorded before the MSLT is terminated?
   A. 15 minutes of clock time
   B. 15 minutes of sleep
   C. Until the first epoch of unequivocal REM sleep
   D. 20 minutes of clock time
3. After lights out, an MSLT nap is terminated if no sleep occurs in how many minutes (maximum possible sleep latency)?
   A. 15 minutes
   B. 20 minutes
   C. 10 minutes
   D. 35 minutes
4. Which of the following is true concerning the MWT?
   A. Naps are terminated after the first epoch of any sleep stage.
   B. A PSG must precede testing.
   C. A 40-minute test is recommended.
   D. The patient is supine during testing.
5. Which of the following is **NOT** true about the recommended MSLT protocol?
   A. PSG the night before the MSLT (required)
   B. Patient out of bed between naps and observed to prevent sleep
   C. Sleep diary for 2 weeks before MSLT
   D. Use of CPAP during the PSG but **not** the MSLT (for patients with OSA on CPAP treatment)
6. About what percentage of **normal individuals** will have an MSL < 5 minutes?
   A. 10%
   B. 16%
   C. 30%
   D. 40%
7. An 18-year-old male is evaluated for daytime sleepiness. He falls asleep in morning classes routinely but denies cataplexy

(emotionally induced muscle weakness). The patient's normal sleep period is from midnight to 1 a.m. (or later on weekends) until approximately 7 a.m. (weekdays) and 10 to 11 a.m. on weekends. The preceding PSG with lights out at 10 p.m. and lights on at 6:00 a.m. showed a nocturnal sleep latency of 40 minutes, and 400 minutes of sleep was recorded. The REM latency on the PSG was normal. An MSLT is performed with naps at 8 a.m., 10 a.m., 12 noon, 2 p.m., and 4 p.m. The results include an MSL of 8 minutes and two SOREMPs (8 a.m. and 10 a.m. naps). The patient was off from school for 1 week before the sleep study and was asked to get at least 7 hours of sleep. What is the most likely diagnosis?
A. Narcolepsy without cataplexy
B. Idiopathic hypersomnia
C. Insufficient sleep syndrome
D. Insufficient sleep syndrome and delayed sleep phase

8. A nap (wake trial) of a MWT is shown in Figure 17–14. What is the sleep latency? Why was the nap terminated at epoch 58? In this patient the average sleep latency on four naps was 15 minutes. Should the patient be driving?
9. A 7-year-old undergoes an MSLT for suspected narcolepsy. No SOREMPs were noted, and the sleep latency was 9 minutes. Is there objective evidence of daytime sleepiness? Parents report bedtime at 10:30 p.m. and wake time at 6 a.m. during school days. Is this sufficient sleep?
10. A 8-year-old child stopped napping about age 5 but recently has been taking naps when not at school. Is this normal?
11. What is considered the minimum acceptable time in bed (TIB or total recording time) and total sleep time (TST) on the PSG preceding the MSLT?
    A. TIB 8 hours, TST 7 hours
    B. TIB 7 hours, TST 6 hours
    C. TIB 7 hours, TST 5 hours
12. What is NOT true concerning REM-suppressing medications and performance of the MSLT?
    A. Should be weaned and stopped 2 weeks before testing or five times the half-life
    B. Must always be stopped
    C. Abrupt withdrawal is contraindicated near the MSLT date
    D. Consultation with the physician prescribing the REM-suppressing medication is essential for patient safety and continuity of care
13. What is the sleep latency and REM latency based on the tracings from the MSLT nap in Figure 17–15?

ANSWERS

1. D. The diagnostic criteria for narcolepsy with cataplexy in the ICSD-3-TR state that either a PSG SOREMP OR (MSL ≤ 8 minutes and two or more SOREMPs on the MSLT) support a diagnosis of narcolepsy with cataplexy. For narcolepsy without cataplexy, answer B would be correct. That is, the MSLT diagnostic criteria have only changed for narcolepsy with cataplexy (NT1) but not for NT2.
2. A. 15 minutes of clock time.
3. B. 20 minutes.
4. C. Naps are terminated after three consecutive epochs of stage N1 or a single epoch of any other sleep stage (N2, N3, R). The tested individual sits up in bed or in a recliner.
5. D. If the patient has been using CPAP treatment for OSA, the device is used at the same pressure and mask as used at home during *both* the PSG and the MSLT.
6. B. About 16% of normal individuals will have an MSL < 5 minutes, and 16% of narcolepsy patients have an MSL > 5 minutes.
7. D. The fact that only the morning naps show SOREMPs and the history of a delayed sleep phase suggest that

LO at end of epoch 30					Nap 1					
Epoch	30	31	32	33	34	35	36	37	38	39
Stage	LO	W	W	W	W	W	W	W	W	W
Epoch	40	41	42	43	44	45	46	47	48	49
Stage	W	W	W	W	W	W	W	W	W	W
Epoch	50	51	52	53	54	55	56	57	58	59
Stage	W	W	W	W	N1	N1	W	N1	N2	

Figure 17–14 Question 8: Nap 1 (Wake trial 1) of a Maintenance of Wakefulness Test in a patient with narcolepsy taking modafinil. What is the sleep latency? Why was the nap terminated at epoch 58? *LO*, Lights out at the end of epoch 30.

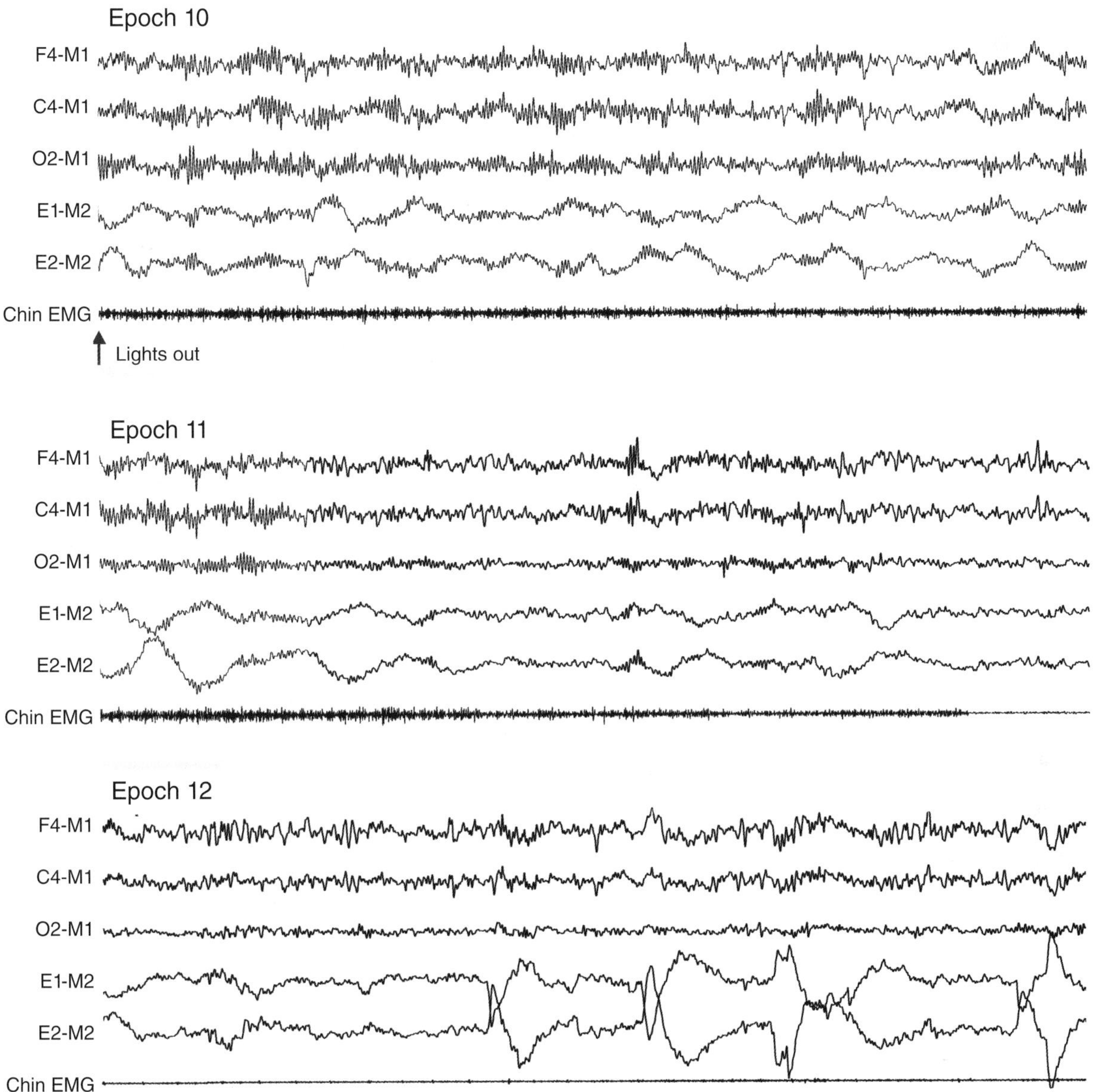

Figure 17–15 Question 13: What is the sleep latency and rapid eye movement latency in this patient?

the SOREMPs are due to a circadian phase delay. The patient likely was sleeping for 6 hours or less on weeknights at home. The MSL of 8 minutes was longer than expected, as the patient likely obtained more sleep when not waking up early to attend school.

8. 23 epochs or 11.5 minutes. The nap was terminated at epoch 58 because this meets the criteria of three consecutive epochs of stage N1 or any single epoch of another sleep stage. While the three consecutive epochs of stage N1 or a single epoch of any other sleep stage is needed to terminate an MWT nap, the *sleep latency is defined as the time from lights out to the start of the first epoch* of any sleep stage (including stage N1). Three consecutive epochs of N1 are not required in determining the sleep latency. The sleep latency criteria for adequate alertness on the MWT have not been defined. However, based on published studies showing adequate alertness in during driving longer than 33 minutes, this study would **not** be considered evidence to support sufficient alertness for driving.

9. Yes, there is evidence of excessive sleepiness. The sleep latency of prepubertal children is usually above 15 minutes, with many children failing to fall asleep on any nap. A 7-year-old child should be getting 9 to 12 hours of sleep. An earlier bedtime is needed. Of note, when children have narcolepsy, the average sleep latency is less than 5 minutes.

10. No. Napping is uncommon after 5 years, and a return to napping is suggestive of daytime sleepiness.

11. B. However, even 6 hours of sleep may not be sufficient in some patients.

12. B. In some patients REM-suppressing medications cannot be stopped because of the potential for significant adverse consequences. Ideally, REM-suppressing medications should be weaned and stopped 2 weeks before the MSLT *if this is safe and with the approval of the physician prescribing the medication*. For medications with a long half-life, a longer period of withdrawal (five times the half-life) is optimal (fluoxetine, 6 weeks).

13. Epoch 10 is stage W (Wakefulness), epoch 11 is stage N1, and epoch 12 stage R. Epoch 11 is not stage R as there are slow eye movements after sleep onset and the chin EMG is higher for most of the epoch than epoch 12 (see Chapter 3). The sleep latency is 0.5 minutes and the REM latency is 0.5 minutes.

SELECTED REFERENCES

Arand D, Bonnet M, Hurwitz T, et al. A review by the MSLT and MWT Task Force of the Standards of Practice Committee of the AASM. The clinical use of the MSLT and MWT. *Sleep*. 2005;28:123-144.

Johns MW. A new method for measuring daytime sleepiness: the Epworth Sleepiness Scale. *Sleep*. 1991;14:540-545.

Krahn LE, Arand DL, Avidan AY, et al. Recommended protocols for the Multiple Sleep Latency Test and Maintenance of Wakefulness Test in adults: guidance from the American Academy of Sleep Medicine. *J Clin Sleep Med*. 2021;17(12):2489-2498.

Littner MR, Kushida C, Wise M, et al. Practice parameters for clinical use of the Multiple Sleep Latency Test and the Maintenance of Wakefulness Test. *Sleep*. 2005;28:113-121.

REFERENCES

1. Ohayon MM, Dauvilliers Y, Reynolds CF III. Operational definitions and algorithms for excessive sleepiness in the general population: implications for DSM-5 nosology. *Arch Gen Psychiatry*. 2012;69(1):71-79.
2. Ford ES, Cunningham TJ, Croft JB. Trends in self-reported sleep duration among US adults from 1985 to 2012. *Sleep*. 2015;38:829-832.
3. Kolla BP, He J-P, Mansukhani MP, Frye MA, Merikangas K. Excessive sleepiness and associated symptoms in the US adult population: prevalence, correlates, and comorbidity. *Sleep Health*. 2020;6(1):79-87.
4. Watson NF, Badr MS, Belenky G, et al. Recommended amount of sleep for a healthy adult: a joint consensus statement of the American Academy of Sleep Medicine and Sleep Research Society. *Sleep*. 2015;38(6):843-844.
5. Centers for Disease Control and Prevention. Effect of short sleep duration on daily activities—United States, 2005–2008. *MMWR Morb Mortal Wkly Rep*. 2011;60(8):239-242.
6. Hoddes E, Zarcone V, Smythe H, Philips R, Dement WC. Quantification of sleepiness: a new approach. *Psychophysiol*. 1973;10:431-436.
7. Dement W, Zarcone V. The development and use of the Stanford Sleepiness Scale (SSS). *Psychophysiol*. 1972;9:150.
8. Johns MW. A new method for measuring daytime sleepiness: the Epworth Sleepiness Scale. *Sleep*. 1991;14:540-545.
9. Johns MW. Reliability and factor analysis of the Epworth Sleepiness Scale. *Sleep*. 1992;15(4):376-381.
10. Johns MW. Daytime sleepiness, snoring, and obstructive sleep apnea. The Epworth Sleepiness Scale. *Chest*. 1993;103(1):30-36.
11. Lok R, Zeitzer JM. Physiological correlates of the Epworth Sleepiness Scale reveal different dimensions of daytime sleepiness. *Sleep Adv*. 2021;2(1):zpab008.
12. Akerstedt T, Gillberg M. Subjective and objective sleepiness in the active individual. *Int J Neurosci*. 1990;52(1-2):29-37.
13. Akerstedt T, Anund A, Axelsson J, Kecklund G. Subjective sleepiness is a sensitive indicator of insufficient sleep and impaired waking function. *J Sleep Res*. 2014;23(3):240-252.
14. Carskadon MA. Guidelines for the Multiple Sleep Latency Test. *Sleep*. 1986;9:519-524.
15. Thorpy MJ. The clinical use of the Multiple Sleep Latency Test. The Standards of Practice Committee of the American Sleep Disorders Association. *Sleep*. 1992;15:268-276.
16. Littner MR, Kushida C, Wise M, et al. Practice parameters for clinical use of the Multiple Sleep Latency Test and the Maintenance of Wakefulness Test. *Sleep*. 2005;28:113-121.
17. Arand D, Bonnet M, Hurwitz T, et al. A review by the MSLT and MWT Task Force of the Standards of Practice Committee of the AASM. The clinical use of the MSLT and MWT. *Sleep*. 2005;28:123-144.
18. Krahn LE, Arand DL, Avidan AY, et al. Recommended protocols for the Multiple Sleep Latency Test and Maintenance of Wakefulness Test in adults: guidance from the American Academy of Sleep Medicine. *J Clin Sleep Med*. 2021;17(12):2489-2498.
19. Kendzerska TB, Smith PM, Brignardello-Petersen R, et al. Evaluation of the measurement properties of the Epworth Sleepiness Scale: a systematic review. *Sleep Med Rev*. 2014;18(4):321-331.
20. Benbadis SR, Mascha E, Perry MC, et al. Association between the Epworth Sleepiness Scale and the Multiple Sleep Latency Test in a clinical population. *Ann Intern Med*. 1999;130:289-292.
21. Gottlieb DJ, Whitney CW, Bonekat WH, et al. Relation of sleepiness to respiratory disturbance index. *Am J Respir Crit Care Med*. 1999;159:502-507.
22. Patel SR, White DP, Malhotra A, et al. Continuous positive airway pressure therapy in a diverse population with obstructive sleep apnea. *Arch Intern Med*. 2003;163:565-571.
23. Crook S, Sievi NA, Bloch KE, et al. Minimum important difference of the Epworth Sleepiness Scale in obstructive sleep apnoea: estimation from three randomised controlled trials. *Thorax*. 2019;74(4):390-396.
24. Patel S, Kon SSC, Nolan CM, et al. The Epworth Sleepiness Scale: minimum clinically important difference in obstructive sleep apnea. *Am J Respir Crit Care Med*. 2018;197(7):961-963.
25. ICSD-Diagnostic Classification Committee, Thorpy MJ, Chairman. *International Classification of Sleep Disorders: Diagnostic and Coding Manual*. American Sleep Disorders Association; 1990.
26. American Academy of Sleep Medicine. *International Classification of Sleep Disorders: Diagnostic and Coding Manual*. 2nd ed. American Academy of Sleep Medicine; 2005.
27. American Academy of Sleep Medicine. *International Classification of Sleep Disorders*. 3rd ed. American Academy of Sleep Medicine; 2014.
28. American Academy of Sleep Medicine. *International Classification of Sleep Disorders*. 3rd ed. text revision. American Academy of Sleep Medicine; 2023.
29. Aldrich MS, Chervin RD, Malow BA. Value of the Multiple Sleep Latency Test (MSLT) for the diagnosis of narcolepsy. *Sleep*. 1997;20:620-629.
30. Janjua T, Samp T, Cramer-Bornemann M, Hannon H, Mahowald MW. Clinical caveat: prior sleep deprivation can affect the MSLT for days. *Sleep Med*. 2003;4(1):69-72.
31. Richardson GS, Carskadon MA, Flagg W, Van den Hoed J, Dement WC, Mitler MM. Excessive daytime sleepiness in man: multiple sleep latency measurement in narcoleptic and control subjects. *Electroencephalogr Clin Neurophysiol*. 1978;45(5):621-627.
32. Clodoré M, Benoit O, Foret J, Bouard G. The Multiple Sleep Latency Test: individual variability and time of day effect in normal young adults. *Sleep*. 1990;13(5):385-394.
33. Mignot E, Lin L, Finn L, et al. Correlates of sleep-onset REM periods during the Multiple Sleep Latency Test in community adults. *Brain*. 2006;129:1609-1623.
34. Singh M, Drake CL, Roth T. The prevalence of multiple sleep-onset REM periods in a population-based sample. *Sleep*. 2006;29(7):890-895.
35. Goldbart A, Peppard P, Finn L, et al. Narcolepsy and predictors of positive MSLTs in the Wisconsin Sleep Cohort. *Sleep*. 2014;37(6):1043-1051.
36. Chervin RD, Aldrich MS. Sleep onset REM periods during Multiple Sleep Latency Tests in patients evaluated for sleep apnea. *Am J Respir Crit Care Med*. 2000;161:426-431.
37. Andlauer O, Moore H, Jouhier L, et al. Nocturnal rapid eye movement sleep latency for identifying patients with narcolepsy/hypocretin deficiency. *JAMA Neurol*. 2013;70(7):891-902. Published correction appears in *JAMA Neurol*. 2013;70(10):1332.
38. Dietmann A, Gallino C, Wenz E, Mathis J, Bassetti CLA. Multiple sleep latency test and polysomnography in patients with central disorders of hypersomnolence. *Sleep Med*. 2021;79:6-10.
39. Drakatos P, Kosky CA, Higgins SE, et al. First rapid eye movement sleep periods and sleep-onset rapid eye movement periods in sleep-stage sequencing of hypersomnias. *Sleep Med*. 2013;14(9):897-901.
40. Drakatos P, Suri A, Higgins SE, et al. Sleep stage sequence analysis of sleep onset REM periods in the hypersomnias. *J Neurol Neurosurg Psychiatry*. 2013;84(2):223-227.
41. Sansa G, Falup-Pecurariu C, Salamero M, Iranzo A, Santamaria J. Non-random temporal distribution of sleep onset REM periods in the MSLT in narcolepsy. *J Neurol Sci*. 2014;341(1-2):136-138.
42. Cairns A, Trotti LM, Bogan R. Demographic and nap-related variance of the MSLT: results from 2,498 suspected hypersomnia patients: clinical MSLT variance. *Sleep Med*. 2019;55:115-123.
43. Goddard J, Tay G, Fry J, Davis M, Curtin D, Szollosi I. Multiple Sleep Latency Test: when are 4 naps enough? *J Clin Sleep Med*. 2021;17(3):491-497.
44. Troester MM, Quan SF, Berry RB, et al. For the American Academy of Sleep Medicine. *The AASM Manual for the Scoring of Sleep and Associated Events: Rules, Terminology and Technical Specifications. Version 3*. American Academy of Sleep Medicine; 2023.
45. Bradshaw DA, Yanagi MA, Pak ES, Peery TS, Ruff GA. Nightly sleep duration in the 2-week period preceding multiple sleep latency testing. *J Clin Sleep Med*. 2007;3(6):613-619.

46. Budhiraja R, Kushida CA, Nichols DA, et al. Predictors of sleepiness in obstructive sleep apnoea at baseline and after 6 months of continuous positive airway pressure therapy. *Eur Respir J.* 2017;50(5):1700348.
47. Kolla BP, Jahani Kondori M, Silber MH, et al. Advance taper of antidepressants prior to multiple sleep latency testing increases the number of sleep-onset rapid eye movement periods and reduces mean sleep latency. *J Clin Sleep Med.* 2020;16(11):1921-1927.
48. Schierenbeck T, Riemann D, Berger M, Hornyak M. Effect of illicit recreational drugs upon sleep: cocaine, ecstasy and marijuana. *Sleep Med Rev.* 2008;12(5):381-389.
49. Bonnet MH, Arand DL. Sleepiness as measured by modified multiple sleep latency testing varies as a function of preceding activity. *Sleep.* 1998;21(5):477-483.
50. Anniss AM, Young A, O'Driscoll DM. Importance of urinary drug screening in the Multiple Sleep Latency Test and Maintenance of Wakefulness Test. *J Clin Sleep Med.* 2016;12(12):1633-1640.
51. Coelho FM, Georgsson H, Murray BJ. Benefit of repeat multiple sleep latency testing in confirming a possible narcolepsy diagnosis. *J Clin Neurophysiol.* 2011;28(4):412-414.
52. Ruoff C, Pizza F, Trotti LM, et al. The MSLT is repeatable in narcolepsy type 1 but not narcolepsy type 2: a retrospective patient study. *J Clin Sleep Med.* 2018;14(1):65-74.
53. Lopez R, Doukkali A, Barateau L, et al. Test-retest reliability of the Multiple Sleep Latency Test in central disorders of hypersomnolence. *Sleep.* 2017;40(12).
54. Kizawa T, Hosokawa K, Nishijima T, et al. False-positive cases in Multiple Sleep Latency Test by accumulated sleep debt. *Neuropsychopharmacol Rep.* 2021;41(2):192-198.
55. Baumann CR, Mignot E, Lammers GJ, et al. Challenges in diagnosing narcolepsy without cataplexy: a consensus statement. *Sleep.* 2014; 37(6):1035-1042.
56. Murer T, Imbach LL, Hackius M, et al. Optimizing MSLT specificity in narcolepsy with cataplexy. *Sleep.* 2017;40(12).
57. Cairns A, Bogan R. Prevalence and clinical correlates of a short onset REM period (SOREMP) during routine PSG. *Sleep.* 2015;38(10): 1575-1581.
58. Pizza F, Vandi S, Detto S, et al. Different sleep onset criteria at the Multiple Sleep Latency Test (MSLT): an additional marker to differentiate central nervous system (CNS) hypersomnias. *J Sleep Res.* 2011;20(1 Pt 2):250-256.
59. Javaheri S, Javaheri S. Update on persistent excessive daytime sleepiness in OSA. *Chest.* 2020;158(2):776-786.
60. Mitler MM, Gujavarty KS, Browman CP. Maintenance of Wakefulness Test: a polysomnographic technique for evaluation treatment efficacy in patients with excessive somnolence. *Electroencephalogr Clin Neurophysiol.* 1982;53(6):658-661.
61. Sangal RB, Thomas L, Mitler M. Disorders of excessive sleepiness: treatment improves the ability to stay awake but does not reduce sleepiness. *Chest.* 1992;102:699-703.
62. Sangal RB, Thomas L, Mitler MM. Maintenance of Wakefulness Test and Multiple Sleep Latency Test. Measurement of different abilities in patients with sleep disorders. *Chest.* 1992;101(4):898-902.
63. Sangal RB, Mitler MM, Sangal JM. Subjective sleepiness ratings (Epworth Sleepiness Scale) do not reflect the same parameter of sleepiness as objective sleepiness (Maintenance of Wakefulness Test) in patients with narcolepsy. *Clin Neurophysiol.* 1999;110(12):2131-2135.
64. Doghramji K, Mitler MM, Sangal RB, et al. A normative study of the Maintenance of Wakefulness Test (MWT). *Electroencephalogr Clin Neurophysiol.* 1997;103:554-562.
65. Banks S, Barnes M, Tarquinio N, et al. The Maintenance of Wakefulness Test in normal healthy subjects. *Sleep.* 2004;27(4):799-802.
66. Philip P, Sagaspe P, Taillard J, et al. Maintenance of Wakefulness Test, obstructive sleep apnea syndrome and driving risk. *Ann Neurol.* 2008;64(4):410-416.
67. Philip P, Guichard K, Strauss M, et al. Maintenance of wakefulness test: how does it predict accident risk in patients with sleep disorders? *Sleep Med.* 2021;77:249-255.
68. Iglowstein I, Jenni OG, Molinari L, Largo RH. Sleep duration from infancy to adolescence: reference values and generational trends. *Pediatrics.* 2003;111:302-307.
69. Paruthi S, Brooks LJ, D'Ambrosio C, et al. Consensus statement of the American Academy of Sleep Medicine on the recommended amount of sleep for healthy children: methodology and discussion. *J Clin Sleep Med.* 2016;12(11):1549-1561.
70. Owens JA, Jones C, Nash R. Caregivers' knowledge, behavior, and attitudes regarding healthy sleep in young children. *J Clin Sleep Med.* 2011;7(4):345-350.
71. Owens JA, Dalzell V. Use of the "BEARS" sleep screening tool in a pediatric residents' continuity clinic: a pilot study. *Sleep Med.* 2005; 6(1):63-69.
72. Wang YG, Benmedjahed K, Lambert J, Evans CJ, Hwang S, Black J, Johns MW. Assessing narcolepsy with cataplexy in children and adolescents: development of a cataplexy diary and the ESS-CHAD. *Nat Sci Sleep.* 2017 Aug 14;9:201-211.
73. Chervin RD, Hedger KM, Dillon JE, Pituch KJ. Pediatric Sleep Questionnaire (PSQ): validity and reliability of scales for sleep-disordered breathing, snoring, sleepiness, and behavioral problems. *Sleep Med.* 2000;1:21-32.
74. Aurora RN, Lamm CI, Zak RS, et al. Practice parameters for the non-respiratory indications for polysomnography and multiple sleep latency testing for children. *Sleep.* 2012;35(11):1467-1473.
75. Carskadon MA, Harvey K, Duke P, et al. Pubertal changes in daytime sleepiness. *Sleep.* 1980;2:453-460.
76. Carskadon M. The second decade. In: Gulleminault C, ed. *Sleeping and Waking Disorders—Indications and Techniques.* Butterworths; 1982:99-125.
77. Carskadon MA, Wolfson AR, Acebo C, Tzischinsky O, Seifer R. Adolescent sleep patterns, circadian timing, and sleepiness at a transition to early school days. *Sleep.* 1998;21(8):871-881.
78. Jenni OG, Carskadon MA. Sleep behavior and sleep regulation from infancy through adolescence: normative aspects. *Sleep Med Clin.* 2007;2(3):321-329.
79. Gozal D, Kheirandish-Gozal L. Obesity and excessive daytime sleepiness in prepubertal children with obstructive sleep apnea. *Pediatrics.* 2009;123(1):13-18.
80. Aran A, Einen M, Lin L, et al. Clinical and therapeutic aspects of childhood narcolepsy-cataplexy: a retrospective study of 51 children. *Sleep.* 2010;33(11):1457-1464.
81. Dzodzomenyo S, Stolfi A, Splaingard D, et al. Urine toxicology screen in Multiple Sleep Latency Test: the correlation of positive tetrahydrocannabinol, drug negative patients, and narcolepsy. *J Clin Sleep Med.* 2015;11(2):93-99.
82. Mansukhani MP, Dhankikar S, Kotagal S, Kolla BP. The influence of antidepressants and actigraphy-derived sleep characteristics on pediatric multiple sleep latency testing. *J Clin Sleep Med.* 2021;17(11):2179-2185.
83. Reiter J, Katz E, Scammell TE, Maski K. Usefulness of a nocturnal SOREMP for diagnosing narcolepsy with cataplexy in a pediatric population. *Sleep.* 2015;38(6):859-865.
84. Maski K, Pizza F, Liu S, et al. Defining disrupted nighttime sleep and assessing its diagnostic utility for pediatric narcolepsy type 1. *Sleep.* 2020;43(10):zsaa066.
85. Ryals S, Berry RB, Girdhar A, Wagner M. Second opinion: does this patient really have narcolepsy? *J Clin Sleep Med.* 2015;11(7):831-833.

Chapter 18

Obstructive Sleep Apnea Syndrome in Adults—Diagnosis, Epidemiology, Variants

HISTORY AND DEFINITIONS

The obstructive sleep apnea (OSA) syndrome was first recognized as a significant health problem over the last half of the 20th century. In 1956, Burwell and coworkers[1] used the term *pickwickian syndrome* to describe individuals with obesity, hypersomnolence, hypercapnia, cor pulmonale, and erythrocytosis. The term *pickwickian* was based on the character Fat Boy Joe from Charles Dickens' *The Posthumous Papers of the Pickwick Club* (1837), who was markedly obese and tended to fall asleep uncontrollably during the day. The current terminology describing such individuals is the *obesity hypoventilation syndrome (OHS).* We now know that such patients represent only 10% to 15% of the total number of patients with OSA. Guilleminault and colleagues[2] described the OSA syndrome in patients with daytime sleepiness and obstructive apneas on polysomnography (PSG). An apnea index of 5/hour or greater was considered abnormal.[3] An *apnea* was defined as absent airflow at the nose and mouth for 10 seconds or more. Obstructive apneas are secondary to airway closure at a supraglottic location that reverses at apnea termination often associated with a brief awakening (arousal).[4] Obstructive apneas are followed by a fall in arterial oxygen saturation (SaO_2) of varying severity. Hypopnea were first described by Block and coworkers to characterize events associated with a reduction in airflow and associated arterial oxygen desaturation.[5] It was soon realized the episodes of reduced airflow and tidal volume (hypopneas) that are the result of upper airway narrowing are also clinically significant.[5,6] Patients with primarily hypopneas had the same symptoms, arousals, and arterial oxygen desaturation as patients with obstructive apneas. The term *obstructive sleep apnea hypopnea syndrome (OSAHS)* has been used to be more inclusive. However, many clinicians still use the term *OSA* to refer to the syndrome, and it is used in this chapter with the understanding that patients may have variable amounts of apneas and hypopneas. As discussed in Chapter 11, the definition of hypopnea has varied considerably.[7-10] The American Academy of Sleep Medicine (AASM) scoring manual[11-14] recommends scoring apnea using an oronasal thermal sensor and hypopnea using nasal pressure monitoring (diagnostic study) or positive airway pressure (PAP) device flow for both apnea and hypopnea (PAP titration studies). An apnea is scored when there is a ≥90% drop in the oronasal thermal sensor signal from baseline for ≥10 seconds. The current recommended hypopnea definition (diagnostic study) requires a ≥30% or greater reduction in the nasal pressure signal from baseline for ≥10 seconds associated with either an arousal or a ≥3% arterial oxygen desaturation[14]. In former versions of the AASM scoring manual[13] the **acceptable** hypopnea definition required a ≥30% reduction in nasal pressure signal for ≥10 seconds in association with a ≥4% arterial oxygen desaturation. However, in the newest version of the scoring manual there is only one hypopnea definition (the recommended one) that must be used and reported. There is an option to also report hypopneas using what was formerly called the acceptable definition.[14] For more details on scoring respiratory events in adults, see Chapter 11. Patients with OSA have predominantly obstructive apneas but often have some mixed and central apneas as well as hypopneas. However, the majority of respiratory events are obstructive apneas or hypopnea.

ADULT OSA—DIAGNOSTIC CRITERIA

The apnea-hypopnea index (AHI), defined as the number of apneas and hypopneas per hour of sleep, is the main metric used for the diagnosis of OSA and for assessment of severity.[14,15] The metric is useful but has limitations.[15] Sometimes the respiratory disturbance index (RDI) is also used as a synonym for the AHI, but the meaning of this metric has varied between sleep centers. The AASM scoring manual[13,14] defines the RDI as the number of apneas, hypopneas, and respiratory effort-related arousals (RERAs) per hour of sleep (RDI = AHI + RERA index).

The *International Classification of Sleep Disorders,* 3rd edition text revision (ICSD-3-TR) criteria for a diagnosis of the OSA syndrome in adults[16] based on PSG or home sleep apnea testing (HSAT) include the following (A+B or C) and D:

A. Five or more predominately obstructive respiratory events (obstructive and mixed apneas, hypopneas, or RERAs) per hour of sleep during a PSG or monitoring time on a HSAT.

B. The presence of one or more of the following:
   1. The patient complains of sleepiness, insomnia, fatigue, or other symptoms leading to impaired sleep-related quality of life.
   2. The patient wakes with breath-holding, gasping, or choking
   3. The bed partner (or other observer) reports habitual snoring or breathing interruptions during the patient's sleep

C. Fifteen or more predominantly obstructive respiratory events (obstructive and mixed apneas, hypopneas, or RERAs) per hour of sleep during a PSG or monitoring time on a HSAT

D. The symptoms are not better explained by another current sleep disorder, medical disorder, medication, or substance use.

As electroencephalography (EEG) is not recorded by most HSAT devices, determining total sleep time and scoring arousals and RERAs is not possible. For HSAT devices the terminology for the AHI is the respiratory event index (REI) which is equal to the number of apneas and hypopneas per hour of monitoring time (see chapter 16)[1]. The ICSD-3-TR criteria allow a diagnosis of OSA even without symptoms or manifestation if moderate to severe OSA is present (AHI≥ 15/hour). The ICSD-3[17] diagnostic criteria for mild OSA required the presence of **either** symptoms or comorbidities (hypertension, a mood disorder, cognitive dysfunction, coronary heart disease, stroke, congestive heart failure, atrial fibrillation, or type 2 diabetes mellitus). The rationale for inclusion of co-morbidities in the diagnostic criteria was that asymptomatic patients with mild OSA and comorbidities might benefit from treatment. The new ICSD-3-TR eliminates comorbidities in the diagnostic criteria with the thought that using comorbidities without symptoms would result in the diagnosis of an excessive proportion of individuals. Many clinicians do not agree with this decision, and unless the insurance providers change their requirements for PAP reimbursement, certain comorbidities may still be used to justify a diagnosis and treatment for patients with an AHI or REI in the mild range. The continued inclusion of bed partner observation of habitual snoring or breathing interruptions in the ICSD-3-TR criteria also allows most patients with an AHI in the mild range to meet diagnostic criteria even if they do not report symptoms. The word "predominately" is used because patients may have some central apneas or central hypopneas, but obstructive events predominate. The Centers for Medicare and Medicaid Services (CMS)[18] uses slightly different criteria for an OSA diagnosis qualifying patients for coverage of continuous positive airway pressure (CPAP) and other treatments (Box 18–1). The AHI is defined as the number of apneas and hypopneas **per hour of sleep** using a hypopnea definition based on a ≥4% desaturation. The term RDI is defined as the number of apnea and hypopneas **per hour of recording** and is used for HSAT. Home sleep testing (HST) is the CMS nomenclature for HSAT. The hypopnea definition is a reduction in airflow associated with ≥4% desaturation. As noted above the AASM nomenclature for the AHI determined by HSAT is the respiratory event index (REI), which is the number of events per hour of monitoring time. The AASM recommended hypopnea definition is a decrease in airflow and ≥3% desaturation or an arouasl. CMS requires the AHI (RDI) to be ≥15/hour (minimum of 30 events). If the AHI (RDI) is 5 to ≤14/hour, CMS requires the documentation of the presence of symptoms of excessive daytime sleepiness, impaired cognition, mood disorders or insomnia, or certain comorbidities (hypertension, ischemic heart disease, or history of stroke) to make the diagnosis of OSA and qualify a patient for CPAP treatment. This list of qualifying conditions in mild OSA is less inclusive than used in the ICSD-3 (which also included atrial fibrillation, congestive heart failure [CHF], and diabetes mellitus). However, as noted above, the ICSD-3-TR no longer includes comorbidity in the diagnostic criteria for OSA.

EVALUATION OF PATIENTS

The AASM has published clinical guidelines for the diagnostic evaluation of OSA,[19,20] as well as evaluation, management, and long-term care of OSA in adults.[21] Table 18–1 summarizes diagnostic consideration in a patient suspected of having OSA.

Box 18–1 CMS* DIAGNOSTIC CRITERIA FOR OSA AND QUALIFICATION FOR PAP TREATMENT

Definitions

Apnea cessation of airflow for ≥10 seconds.

Hypopnea is defined as an abnormal respiratory event lasting ≥10 seconds associated with ≥30% reduction in thoracoabdominal movement or airflow as compared with baseline, and with ≥4% decrease in oxygen saturation.

AHI is defined as the average number of episodes of apnea and hypopnea **per hour of sleep** without the use of a positive airway pressure device. For purposes of this policy, **RERAs are not included** in the calculation of the AHI. Sleep time can only be measured in a Type I (facility-based PSG) or Type II sleep study.

The **RDI** is defined as the average number of apneas plus hypopneas **per hour of recording** without the use of a positive airway pressure device. For purposes of this policy, RERAs are not included in the calculation of the RDI. The RDI is reported in Type III, Type IV, and other home sleep studies.

An E0601 device is covered for the treatment of OSA if criteria A–C are met:

A. The beneficiary has an in-person clinical evaluation by the treating practitioner prior to the sleep test to assess the beneficiary for obstructive sleep apnea.
B. The beneficiary has a sleep test (as defined below) that meets either of the following criteria (1 or 2):
   1. The AHI or RDI is ≥15 events per hour with ≥30 events; or,
   2. The AHI or RDI is ≥ 5 and ≤ 14 events per hour with ≥10 events and documentation of:
      a. Excessive daytime sleepiness, impaired cognition, mood disorders, or insomnia; or,
      b. Hypertension, ischemic heart disease, or history of stroke.
C. The beneficiary and/or their caregiver has received instruction from the supplier of the device in the proper use and care of the equipment.

An E0470 device (BPAP **without** a backup rate) is covered for those beneficiaries with OSA who meet criteria A–C above, in addition to criterion D:

D. An E0601 has been tried and proven ineffective based on a therapeutic trial conducted in either a facility or in a home setting.

Ineffective is defined as documented failure to meet therapeutic goals using an E0601 during the titration portion of a facility-based study or during home use despite optimal therapy (i.e., proper mask selection and fitting and appropriate pressure settings)

If an E0601 device is tried and found ineffective during the initial facility-based titration or home trial, substitution of an E0470 does not require a new initial in-person clinical evaluation or a new sleep test.

If an E0601 device has been used for more than 3 months and the beneficiary is switched to an E0470, a new initial in-person clinical evaluation is required, but a new sleep test is not required. A new 3 month trial would begin for use of the E0470.

*Centers for Medicare and Medicaid Services. PAP Devices for treatment of OSA. Excerpt from L33718. https://www.cms.gov/medicare-coverage-database/view/lcd.aspx?lcdid=33718&ver=48&= assessed 12/10/2023

AHI, Apnea-hypopnea index; *BPAP*, bilevel positive airway pressure; *CMS*, Centers for Medicare and Medicaid Services; *OSA*, obstructive sleep apnea; *PSG*, polysomnography; *RDI*, respiratory disturbance index; *RERA*, respiratory effort-related arousal.

E0601 CPAP, E0470 Bilevel PAP without a backup rate.

Table 18–1 Diagnostic Considerations in Patient Suspected of Having OSA

Important Historical Information

- Snoring?
- Witnessed apneas/ breathing pauses?
- Gasping/choking at night?
- Nonrefreshing sleep?
- Total sleep duration
- Sleepiness? (ESS)
- Nocturia?
- Morning headaches?
- Morning dry mouth?
- Decreased concentration?
- Memory loss?
- Decreased libido/erectile dysfunction?
- Irritability?
- Hypertension?

Physical Examination

- Increased neck circumference (>17 inches in men, >16 inches in women)?
- Increased BMI?
- Retrognathia?
- Nasal obstruction?
- Narrow oropharynx?
- High Mallampati/Friedman Score?*
- High arched palate?
- Evidence of cor pulmonale?

At High-Risk for OSA

- Obesity (BMI > 35)
- Congestive heart failure
- Atrial fibrillation
- Refractory hypertension
- Nocturnal arrhythmia
- CVA
- Pulmonary hypertension
- High risk driving populations
- Pre-operative for bariatric surgery
- Type 2 diabetes

BMI, (kg/m²) body mass index; *CVA,* cerebrovascular accident; *ESS,* Epworth sleepiness scale; *OSA,* obstructive sleep apnea.

*Mallampati or Friedman score on upper airway examination is discussed below.

Modified from Epstein LJ, Kristo D, Strollo PJ, et al. Clinical guideline for the evaluation, management, and long-term care of obstructive sleep apnea in adults. *J Clin Sleep Med.* 2009;5:263-276.

An in-person evaluation is needed before ordering a sleep study. The CMS criteria for testing include "the beneficiary has an in-person clinical evaluation by the treating practitioner prior to the sleep test to assess the beneficiary for obstructive sleep apnea." A review by Gottlieb and Punjabi provides a concise overview of the methods and challenges of making a diagnosis of sleep apnea.[22]

OSA Symptoms and Key Historical Points

Key historical information and physical examination findings in the evaluation of a patient with suspected OSA are listed in Table 18–1. The patient or bed partner frequently reports excessive daytime sleepiness, loud habitual snoring, gasping/choking or witnessed apnea, personality change, morning headache, nocturia, or nonrestorative sleep. A typical patient with severe OSA is shown Video 18-1. The Epworth Sleepiness Scale[23] (ESS), a subjective estimate of the propensity to doze off in eight situations, is often (but not invariably) increased. The range of the scale is 0 to 24 with greater than 10 indicating excessive daytime sleepiness (see Chapter 17). There is only a weak correlation between the AHI and either subjective or objective sleepiness. A substantial percentage (40%–60%) of patients with OSA do not report daytime sleepiness, and the absence of sleepiness should not discourage further evaluation. However, patients with more severe OSA do have, on average, greater daytime sleepiness (Figure 18–1).[24,25] Other symptoms such as frequent awakenings or nonrestorative sleep may be more prominent than daytime sleepiness in some patients. In a study by Gottlieb and coworkers[24] of community dwelling adults in the Sleep Heart Health Study, the mean ESS for the categories of normal, mild, moderate, and severe AHI were 7.2, 7.8, 8.3, and 9.3, respectively. Sleep clinic populations are likely to be more sleepy as symptoms usually are the reason for referral. Although men and women with OSA generally report the same symptoms, women may report *more insomnia and less witnessed apnea*. Women with OSA are more likely to complain of depression, insomnia, morning headache, awakenings, and fatigue (Box 18–2).[26-28] They tend to have hypopneas rather than apneas and often have obstructive events predominantly during rapid eye movement sleep. One study suggested women are more likely **NOT** to be eligible for CPAP treatment (not diagnosed with OSA) using a hypopnea definition based on ≥4% desaturation compared with one based on ≥3% desaturation or an associated arousal.[29]

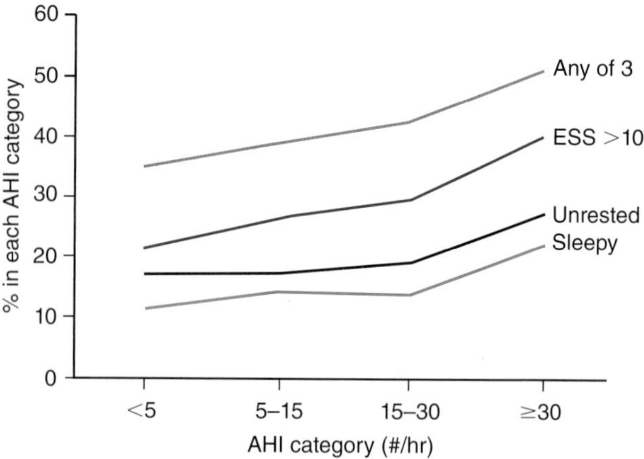

Figure 18–1 The percentage of individuals with an Epworth Sleepiness Scale (ESS) > 10, reports of feeling sleepy, unrested, or any of the three increases with worsening obstructive sleep apnea (OSA) severity as measured by the apnea-hypopnea index (AHI). Note the relatively low percentage of symptoms of sleepiness or poor sleep even with severe OSA. These results are from a population-based study. Sleep clinic populations may manifest greater sleepiness. (Figure plotted from data from Kapur VK, Baldwin CM, Resnick HE, et al. Sleepiness in patients with moderate to severe sleep-disordered breathing. *Sleep.* 2005;28(4):472-477.)

Box 18–2 CHARACTERISTICS OF OSA IN WOMEN

- More prominent symptoms of insomnia, impaired mood, daytime fatigue/lack of energy, morning headache, nightmares
- Less prominent symptoms of snoring and apnea
- Lower AHI for the same BMI (compared with men)
- Prevalence of OSA doubles after menopause
- Prevalence peaks at a greater age compared with men
- More likely to have REM-associated OSA
- Tend to have shorter apneas, more likely to have hypopneas, long periods of partial airway obstruction
- Greater symptoms than men for a given AHI
- Diagnosed at later age and greater BMI

AHI, Apnea-hypopnea index; *BMI,* body mass index; *OSA,* obstructive sleep apnea; *REM,* rapid eye movement.

At-Risk Populations

It is recommended that patients in high-risk populations for the presence of OSA be questioned in detail concerning symptoms of OSA. A number of populations with a high prevalence of OSA have been identified, including patients with refractory hypertension, CHF, and recent or past cerebrovascular accident or transient ischemic attack (Table 18–1). However, automatic testing of these high-risk patients is not recommended without a clinical evaluation documenting the need for testing. However, the clinician should be aware that a high proportion of patients with OSA and these disorders are asymptomatic.

Physical Examination

The physical examination of patients with suspected OSA should include measurement of the body mass index (BMI) and systemic blood pressure, as well as careful examination of the nose, ears, and oropharynx. Observation of the oropharynx usually reveals a crowded upper airway, and *examination of the patient's face in profile may reveal retrognathia.* The Mallampati (MP) score of the upper airway was developed to predict the risk of difficult endotracheal intubation (Figure 18–2).[30] The patient's oropharynx is examined with tongue protruded. The modified Mallampati score (MMP), also called the Friedman score,[31] is performed *without the tongue protruded.* A high MP or MMP score (3 or 4) is associated with a greater risk of having OSA, as well as OSA of greater severity (Figure 18–2). Scalloping of the tongue implies a relatively large tongue for a given mandibular size. The nose should also be examined for evidence of narrowing due to septal deviation or turbinate hypertrophy. Treatment of nasal obstruction may be essential for good CPAP adherence. Measurement of neck circumference and

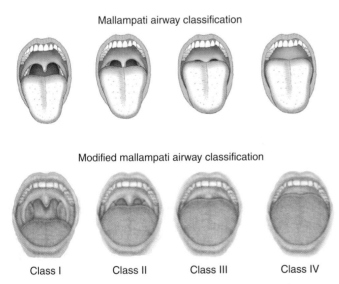

Figure 18–2 Mallampati and Modified Mallampati Airway Classification. In the Mallampati maneuver, patients are instructed not to emit sounds but to open the mouth as wide as possible and protrude the tongue as far as possible. In the modified Mallampati, the patient is instructed to open the mouth as wide as possible without emitting sounds and **without** tongue protrusion. (Mallampati figure reproduced with permission from Friedman M, Tanyeri H, La Rosa M, et al. Clinical predictors of obstructive sleep apnea. *Laryngoscope.* 1999;109:1901-1907; Modified Mallampati reproduced with permission from Nuckton TJ, Glidden DV, Browner WS, Claman DM. Physical examination: Mallampati score as an independent predictor of obstructive sleep apnea. *Sleep.* 2006;29:903-908.)

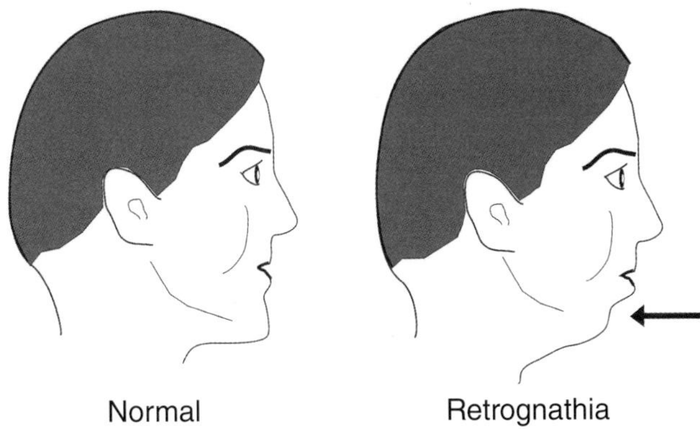

Figure 18–3 This drawing illustrates the appearance of a patient with significant retrognathia *(arrow).* The mandible is small and displaced posteriorly and is associated with a narrow upper airway and increased propensity for sleep apnea.

observation of signs of right heart failure may also be revealing. A greater neck circumference increases the risk of having OSA. A neck size greater than 17 inches (43 cm) in men and 16 inches in women suggests the possibility of OSA.[32,33] However, a normal MP/MMP score and/or thin neck does not rule out OSA. It is important to note that retrognathia (Figure 18–3) or a high arched palate (lateral narrowing) can also predispose a patient to OSA.

Laboratory Testing in OSA

Laboratory testing in patients with OSA is usually not indicated apart from routine health maintenance unless a particular problem such as hypothyroidism is suspected. In patients with severe nocturnal hypoxemia, polycythemia (increased hematocrit) may be present. An unexplained elevation in the serum CO_2 (composed primarily of HCO_3^-) on electrolyte testing is suggestive of chronic compensation for hypercapnia (in the absence of evidence for causes of metabolic alkalosis). A value $\geq$27 mmol/L should alert the clinician to the possibility of the presence of the OHS (daytime hypercapnia, obesity, and usually severe OSA). This screening tool is sensitive but not specific.[34] Therefore, determination of the arterial PCO_2 ($PaCO_2$) during wakefulness is needed to document daytime hypoventilation. Use of the serum CO_2 for detection of the OHS is discussed in more detail in the section on the OHS. If the index of suspicion for OHS is high based on severe obesity or a high AHI, arterial blood gas testing is recommended irrespective of the value of HCO_3^- or CO_2. Pulmonary function testing, chest radiography, and arterial blood gas testing are indicated in patients with a low awake SaO_2 or suspected hypoventilation to determine the role of lung disease as a cause of impaired gas exchange and to document daytime hypoventilation.

Prediction of the Presence of OSA

Several clinical indices and questionnaires have been developed to predict the presence of OSA based on symptoms, signs, and measurements. Although they have some success, they are neither satisfactorily sensitive nor specific enough to be a substitute for objective documentation of the presence of OSA by a sleep study. An adaptation of a prediction rule developed by Flemons and coworkers uses an adjusted neck circumference[32,33] to classify patients as low, moderate, or high probability (Table 18–2). Netzer and colleagues[35] studied the

Table 18–2 Prediction of OSA Using Adjusted Neck Circumference

Measured Neck Circufmerence = MNC (cm)	Adjustment of MNC
A. If hypertension present	+4
B. If habitual snoring present	+3
C. If gasping or choking present	+3
Adjusted MNC = MNC + A + B+ C	
<43 cm (17 inches) = low probability of OSA	
43–48 cm (17–19 inches) = moderate probability of OSA	
>48 cm (19 inches) = high probability of OSA	

MNC, Measured neck circumference; *NC*, neck circumference; *OSA*, obstructive sleep apnea.
Adapted from Flemons WW. Obstructive sleep apnea. *N Engl J Med.* 2002; 347:498-504.

utility of the Berlin Questionnaire to predict whether patients were high or low risk for having OSA. The questionnaire consists of three categories: category 1 concerns snoring and witnessed apnea, category 2 concerns being sleepy/tired/fatigued more than three or four times a week or nodding off while driving a vehicle, and category 3 concerns the presence of hypertension or a BMI greater than 30. After questionnaire completion, patients were studied by HSAT. The Berlin Questionnaire identified patients with an AHI > 5/hour (based on assignment to the high-risk group) with a sensitivity of 0.86 and a specificity of 0.77.

The STOP-BANG (**S**noring, **T**ired, **O**bserved apnea, elevated blood **P**ressure, increased **B**ody mass index, older **A**ge, larger **N**eck circumference, and the male **G**ender) Questionnaire is a screening tool that has been used for preoperative evaluation to detect sleep apnea (Table 18–3).

Table 18–3 STOP-BANG Scoring Model

1. **S**noring	Do you snore loudly (louder than talking or loud enough to be heard through closed doors)?	Yes / No
2. **T**ired	Do you often feel tired, fatigued, or sleepy during daytime?	Yes / No
3. **O**bserved Apnea	Has anyone observed you stop breathing during your sleep?	Yes / No
4. Blood **P**ressure	Have you have been or are you being treated for high blood pressure?	Yes / No
5. **B**MI	BMI > 35 kg/m²?	Yes / No
6. **A**ge	Age older than 50 years?	Yes / No
7. **N**eck circumference	Neck circumference > 40 cm?	Yes / No
8. **G**ender	Male?	Yes / No

High risk of OSA: answering yes to three or more items.
Low risk of OSA: answering yes to less than three items.
BMI, Body mass index.
Chung F, Abdullah HR, Liao P. STOP-Bang Questionnaire: A Practical Approach to Screen for Obstructive Sleep Apnea. *Chest.* 2016;149(3):631-638.

A study of 2467 patients found sensitivities of 84%, 92%, and 100% for AHI cutoffs of greater than 5/hour, 15/hour, and 30/hour, respectively.[36] In populations characterized by older obese males, a STOP-BANG cut-off score higher than 3 is needed for improved specificity. However, screening tools are of limited clinical utility in high-risk populations.

Diagnostic Testing for Suspected Sleep Apnea

PSG and HSAT are discussed in Chapter 16. However, some important concepts will be repeated here. Attended PSG is the gold standard to determine whether OSA is present and to classify the severity.[19,20,37] An entire night of diagnostic monitoring or the initial diagnostic portion of a split (partial night) study can be used. The second part of a split study is used as a PAP titration. The CMS formerly required a minimum of 2 hours of sleep during the diagnostic portion to qualify a patient for reimbursement of CPAP treatment.[18] Currently, if less than 2 hours of monitoring is performed, the number of events to qualify the patient should be the same as if 2 hours of sleep had been recorded. The minimum number of respiratory events is 10 (equivalent to an AHI of 5/hour with 2 hours of monitoring). If an AHI of 15/hour qualifies a patient for CPAP (symptoms not required), the total number of apneas and hypopneas must equal 30 or more. The second part of the night typically has a greater proportion of REM sleep (stage R). Obstructive apneas and hypopneas are more frequent and arterial oxygen desaturation more severe during stage R.[38] An entire night of diagnosis is usually needed for patients with milder OSA, who frequently have OSA primarily during REM sleep. However, even in more severe patients, *the diagnostic portion of a split study can underestimate the severity by AHI* and the degree of arterial oxygen desaturation because relatively little REM sleep is recorded in the first part of the night. The 2005 recommended criteria for performing a split study are (1) AHI ≥ 40/hour or AHI ≥ 20/hour with severe desaturation, (2) at least 3 hours remaining for a PAP titration.[19]

Updated recommendations for diagnostic testing for suspected OSA published in 2017 recommended use of a split night protocol rather than a full night diagnostic study if clinically appropriate. A split night study is recommended if (1) moderate to severe OSA is observed during a minimum of 2 hours of recording time on the diagnostic PSG portion AND (2) at least 3 hours are available for the CPAP titration.[20] The patient's insurance may mandate that a split study be ordered.

The classic PSG findings in patients with OSA are listed in Box 18–3. A typical obstructive apnea is shown in Figure 18–4. The degree of abnormality in the sleep architecture varies with severity. Patients with severe OSA usually have a high arousal index, increased wake after sleep onset (WASO), increased stage N1 sleep, and decreased stage N3 or stage R sleep. A typical classification of OSA severity based on the AHI (or RDI in some sleep centers) is 5 to <15/hour = mild, 15 to 30 = moderate, and >30 = severe OSA.[8] Whereas the AHI (RDI) is the most widely used index for classification of severity, it is also important to characterize the severity of arterial oxygen desaturation. The most severe drops in the SaO_2 and longest respiratory events usually occur during REM sleep.[38]

Factors important for determining the severity of desaturation are listed in Box 18–4. Obesity and lung disease play an important role in the severity of desaturation. A widely

Box 18–3 PSG FINDINGS IN ADULT OSA

Sleep Architecture Findings

- Increased WASO and stage N1
- Reduced stage N3
- Reduced stage R (REM sleep)
- Increased respiratory arousals

Respiratory Findings

- Snoring
- Obstructive, mixed, and central apneas
- Obstructive hypopneas
- AHI: mild 5 to <15/hour, moderate 15–30/hour, severe >30/hour
- Postural OSA = AHI supine > 2 × AHI nonsupine
- AHI REM > AHI NREM (common finding)
- AHI-supine-REM > AHI-supine-NREM >AHI-non-supine-REM > AHI-non-supine-NREM
- Apnea duration REM > NREM
- Arterial oxygen desaturation
    - Lowest SaO_2 during REM sleep
    - Longest REM periods in the early morning hours typically associates with the lowest SaO_2

Cardiac Findings

- Cyclic variation in heart rate

AHI, Apnea-hypopnea index; *EEG*, electroencephalogram; *NREM*, non-rapid eye movement; *OSA*, obstructive sleep apnea; *REM*, rapid eye movement; *SaO_2*, arterial oxygen saturation; *WASO*, wake after sleep onset.

Box 18–4 SEVERITY OF ASSOCIATED ARTERIAL OXYGEN DESATURATION

Factors Associated With Severe Desaturation

Low awake SaO_2
Long apnea/hypopnea time/Short ventilatory phase between events
Decreased ERV (FRC-RV)

- Low FRC (obesity)
- High RV (obstructive lung disease)

Groups With Severe Desaturation

Severe obesity
Obesity hypoventilation syndrome (daytime hypercapnia)
OSA + COPD (overlap syndrome, can have daytime hypercapnia)

COPD, Chronic obstructive pulmonary disease; *ERV*, expiratory reserve volume; *FRC*, functional residual capacity; *OSA*, obstructive sleep apnea; *RV*, residual volume; *SaO2*, arterial oxygen desaturation.

accepted standard for the characterization of the severity of desaturation does not exist. It is common to present the number of desaturations (usually defined as a drop in the SaO_2 $\geq$ 3% or 4% from pre-event baseline), the lowest SaO_2, the average SaO_2 at desaturation, and the time below various saturations. For example, a commonly used metric is the time at or below an SaO_2 of 88%. The recommended and optional oxygenation parameters to appear in a sleep study report are discussed in chapter 16. Recently, use of the hypoxic burden

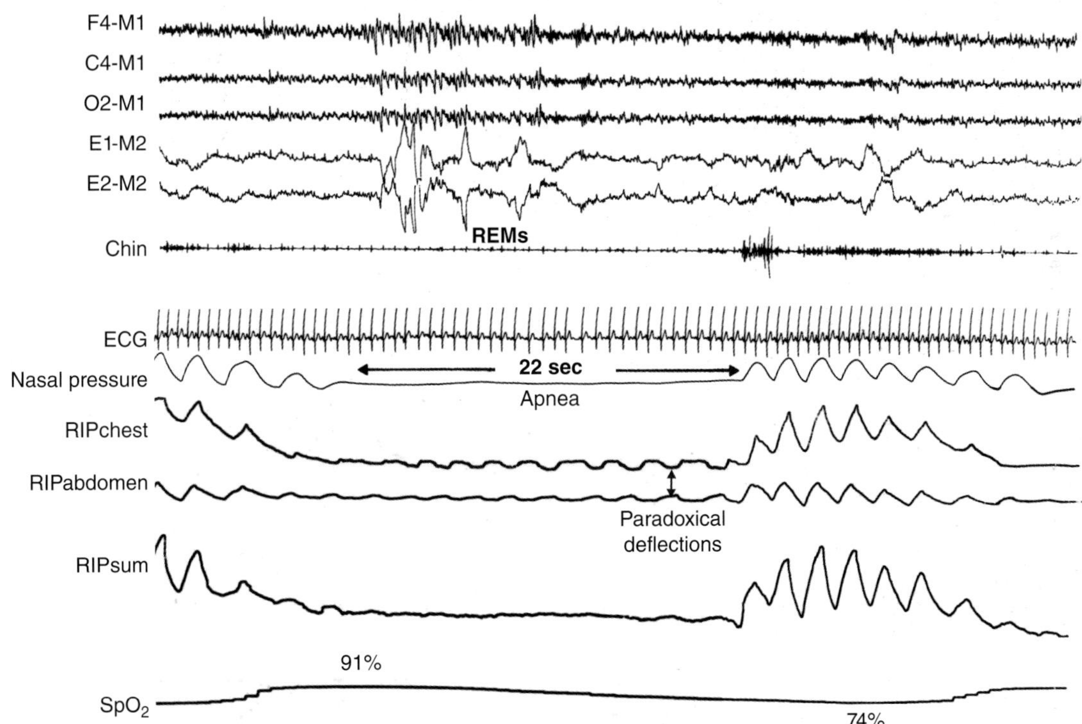

Figure 18–4 An obstructive apnea during REM sleep is illustrated. Note the paradoxical RIPchest and RIPabdomen tracings during the apnea. Looking at the R to R interval in the ECG, one can see a slowing during initial portion of the apnea followed by an increase in heart rate (shorter RR interval) slightly before and after apnea termination. Here, the RIPsum is substituted for the usual oronasal thermal flow sensor. The RIPsum is the sum of the RIPchest and RIPabdomen signals, and deflections are estimates of tidal volume. The signal will detect changes in tidal volume with either nasal or oral breathing. *RIP*, respiratory inductance plethysmography.

appears to improve prediction of the risk of cardiovascular morbidity and mortality.[39,40] The sleep apnea-specific hypoxic burden is the area under the SaO_2 curve compared with baseline pre-event desaturation (see chapter 19 for more information on determination of the hypoxic burden).

Because the AHI is often higher in the supine position[41,42] and during REM sleep,[43,44] presentation of the AHI for those conditions in the sleep study report may be useful (Table 18–4). The overall AHI can be mild even if severely increased in the supine position and during REM sleep. The diagnosis of positional OSA (POSA) is usually made when the AHI supine is greater than twice the AHI nonsupine (some clinicians also require the AHI nonsupine to be normal (or less than 10/hour)—a condition termed *exclusive POSA*). Rapid eye movement (REM)-associated OSA can be defined as a normal AHI during non-REM (NREM) sleep associated with an elevated AHI during REM sleep. However, clinicians also use the term to denote patients with a relatively mild AHI in NREM but moderate to severe elevation in AHI during REM sleep. REM-associated OSA is discussed as a variant of OSA in a subsequent section. There is also an interaction between body position and sleep stage. *The AHI tends to be higher during supine REM than nonsupine REM sleep.*[44] The *longest respiratory events and most severe desaturation are usually present during supine REM sleep.*[38,44] An all-night summary graphic for a patient with REM-associated OSA is shown in Figure 18–5. One can see from the graphic that respiratory events and desaturations are mostly confined to REM sleep. As mentioned earlier, there is an interaction between REM sleep and body position. The most severe desaturations occur during supine REM sleep, as shown in Figure 18–6.

It is important to note that in milder OSA patients the total night AHI can vary depending on the amounts of supine or REM sleep recorded. Because REM sleep usually composes 20% or less of the total sleep time, large changes in the REM AHI result in relatively small changes in the entire night AHI. For a patient with milder OSA, this may change an AHI from "normal" (e.g., 4/hour) to mild OSA (7–8/hour). The amount of supine sleep can have a larger impact on the entire night AHI. For the patient whose data is listed in Table 18–4, the AHI would be much higher if more supine sleep was recorded. Note that although the AHI was high in REM sleep, this had only a smaller effect on the total AHI, as

Table 18–4 Typical PSG Report Presentation of Respiratory Events

	Total	Supine	Nonsupine	NREM	REM
TST (min)	360	60	300	290	70
OA	19	15	4	4	15
MA	0	0	0	0	0
CA	1	1	0	1	0
Hypopnea	40	25	15	20	20
Total events	60	41	19	25	35
AHI	10.0	41.0	3.8	5.2	30.0
% TST supine	16%				

AHI, Apnea-hypopnea index; *CA*, central apnea; *MA*, mixed apnea; *NREM*, nonrapid eye movement sleep; *OA*, obstructive apnea; *REM*, rapid eye movement sleep; *TST*, total sleep time.

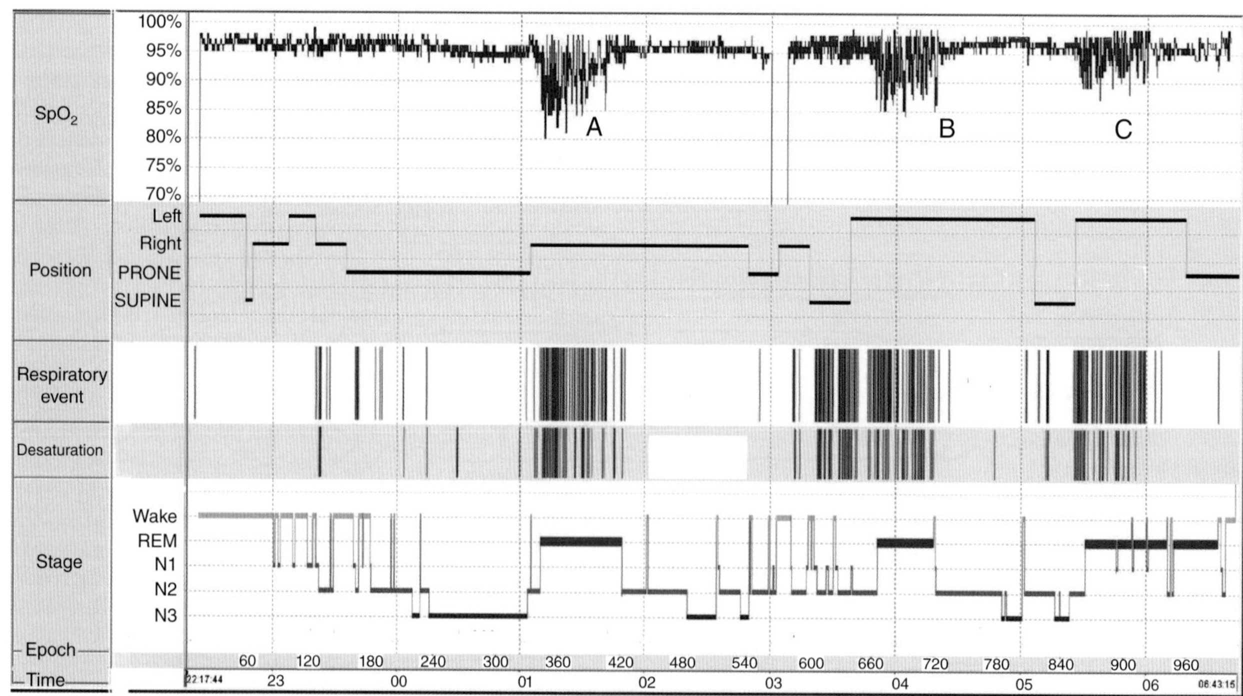

Figure 18–5 An all-night display illustrating REM-associated sleep apnea (A, B, C). The patient had limited supine sleep, but some respiratory events were noted in the supine position during NREM sleep. The periods of REM sleep were all in the lateral positions. Just before REM period B the patient was supine and had frequent respiratory events during NREM sleep but during the subsequent REM sleep in the left position (B) the arterial oxygen desaturation was more severe. (From Berry RB. *Fundamentals of Sleep Medicine*, first edition, Elsevier, Philadelphia 2013; pg 245.)

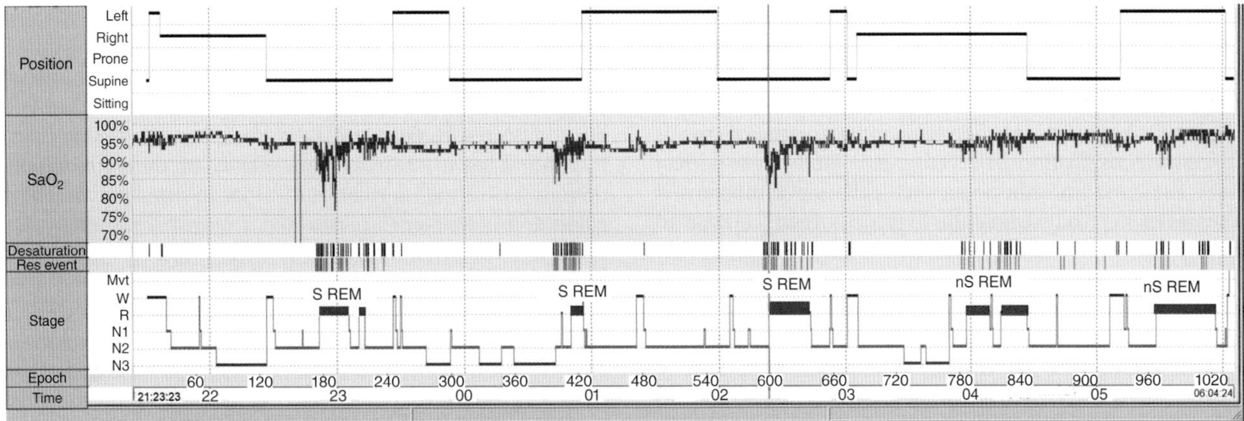

Figure 18–6 An all-night display of selected respiratory events. The tracings show the interaction between REM sleep and body position. The three supine REM episodes (S REM) were associated with more severe arterial oxygen desaturation than the final two REM periods in the lateral position (nS REM).

REM sleep made up only about 19% of the total sleep time. There is night-to-night variability in the AHI, especially in milder patients. Use of multiple nights of testing may give a better estimate of the true severity of sleep apnea.[45,46,47] One issue to resolve is whether one should use the median, average, or maximum AHI value from the multiple nights of testing.

Cyclic variation in heart rate is typically noted during the repeated episodes of obstructive events.[48] The heart rate slows at the start of apnea, may remain decreased or begin to increase during the final portions of apnea, and significantly increases in rate following event termination. Often, the heart rate remains between 60 and 100 bpm. A standard part of most PSG reports is to present the maximum, minimum, and average heart rate along with notations of abnormalities (premature ventricular contractions, atrial fibrillation, sinus pauses). The AASM recommended and optional heart rate parameters to be included in the sleep report[1] are discussed in chapter 16. There is increasing interest in looking at the postapnea response in heart rate and blood pressure to assess the impact of OSA on the cardiovascular system.[49]

Table 18–5 Use of HSAT Versus PSG

HSAT Acceptable	PSG Needed

• Immobility or safety issues
• Delay in obtaining PSG
• Moderate to high probability of OSA
• Absent comorbidities
• Absent indication for PSG (parasomnia)
	• Low probability of OSA
	• Comorbidities present
	  • Central sleep apnea suspected
	  • CHF
	  • Hypoventilation
	  • Neuromuscular weakness
	  • Supplemental oxygen
	  • Potent narcotics
	• Parasomnia suspected
	• Previous negative HSAT

CHF, Congestive heart failure; *HSAT*, home sleep apnea testing; *OSA*, obstructive sleep apnea; *PSG*, polysomnography.

Adapted from Kapur VK, Auckley DH, Chowdhuri S, et al. Clinical practice guideline for diagnostic testing for adult obstructive sleep apnea: an American Academy of Sleep Medicine clinical practice guideline. *J Clin Sleep Med.* 2017;13(3):479-504; and Collop NA, Anderson WM, Boehlecke B, et al. Portable Monitoring Task Force of the American Academy of Sleep Medicine. Clinical guidelines for the use of unattended portable monitors in the diagnosis of obstructive sleep apnea in adult patients. Portable Monitoring Task Force of the American Academy of Sleep Medicine. *J Clin Sleep Med.* 2007;3(7):737-747.

Home Sleep Apnea Testing

The use of HSAT—also known as out of center sleep testing (OCST), portable monitoring (PM), home sleep testing (HST), or limited-channel sleep testing (LCST)—is discussed in detail in Chapter 16. Use of HSAT for the diagnosis of OSA is most appropriate when PSG is difficult because of immobility or safety issues, when there is a delay in obtaining a PSG owing to access or availability and the clinical situation is urgent, when there is a high probability of OSA, when complicated comorbidities are not present, and when coexisting sleep disorders that may benefit from PSG are **NOT** present (Table 18–5).[20,37] Of note, the AHI derived from testing without EEG provides the number of events per hour of monitoring time, not total sleep time. Some sleep centers report both a recording time (device acquiring data) and a monitoring time (based on estimated lights out/lights on). The AASM scoring manual defines the REI as the number or apneas and hypopneas per hour of monitoring time.[13,14] As noted earlier, CMS uses the nomenclature RDI for the AHI determined by HSAT (the CMS term is HST). The use of monitoring time (or recording time) versus total sleep time reduces the AHI. For example, if PSG and HSAT both identify 100 events, the total sleep time is 6 hours, and the monitoring time is 7 hours, then the AHI PSG = 100/6 and the REI HSAT = 100/7. Therefore, the REI (AHI) by HSAT will be less than by PSG even if similar numbers of respiratory events are detected. The possibility of a false-negative HSAT should always be considered. This could occur if the patient does not sleep well during the HSAT, with the result that monitoring time greatly exceeds total sleep time or if minimal REM sleep occurred The AASM clinical practice guidelines for diagnostic testing for OSA recommend that if a HSAT is negative, inconclusive, or technically inadequate, a PSG should be performed for the diagnosis of OSA.[20,37] In patients with mild to moderate sleep apnea, one night of HSAT can lead to misclassification of disease severity, given the substantial night-to-night variability in the AHI.[45,46,47] Many HSAT devices now have the ability to monitor multiple nights.

Limitations of the AHI

Although the AHI remains the major index for the diagnosis of OSA and classification of severity, it is far from a perfect metric.[15] The correlation between the AHI and symptoms is low. Indices of hypoxia such as the hypoxic burden[40] appear to be better predictors of cardiovascular mortality. This and other indices that capture not only the frequency but the depth and duration of sleep-related drop in oxygen saturation are important disease characterizing features. Efforts to use the PSG for more than determining an AHI are attempting to determine endotypes (physiology) and phenotypes (clinic presentation) such as patients with a low arousal threshold and ventilatory control instability (high loop gain).[50] There is also work attempting to define phenotypes that are based on symptoms, such as clusters of patients with excessive sleepiness or complaints of fragmented sleep[51] Another issues with the AHI is defining what is normal. Depending on the definition of hypopnea, there can be a large difference in the percentage of normal populations with an AHI ≥ 5/hour.[9,52,53]

EPIDEMIOLOGY OF ADULT OSA

Prevalence and Progression

The epidemiology of OSA is an ever-changing topic given the epidemic of obesity and the aging population.[22,54-59] Prevalence is defined as the proportion of a population with a condition. The prevalence of OSA depends on the defining RDI or AHI criteria, the definition of hypopnea (as noted above), the method used to detect airflow, and the presence or absence of a requirement that symptoms or comorbidity be present.[17,52,53,54] The landmark Wisconsin-based cohort study of state employees younger than 65 years of age found a prevalence of sleep-disordered breathing (SDB) defined as an AHI ≥ 5/hour (with hypopneas based on a definition of discernible change in airflow and ≥4% desaturation) to be 9% in women and 24% in men.[54] The OSA *syndrome*, defined as the presence of both an increased AHI and self-reported sleepiness, was present in 2% of women and 4% of men. The prevalence of OSA syndrome is likely to be higher in clinic populations.

There is evidence that a large fraction of patients with OSA remain undiagnosed. In 1997 it was estimated that in Western countries up to 5% of the population have an undiagnosed OSA syndrome (elevated AHI and symptoms).[56] However, given the worldwide high prevalence of OSA in countries with limited health resources, it is likely that the majority of patients with OSA world wide remain undiagnosed.[58]

OSA severity can progress with time. Analysis of 8-year follow-up in 282 participants in the Wisconsin cohort study showed a mean increase in the AHI from 2.6/hour to 5.1/hour.[55] However, not all studies have shown clear-cut progression, and progressive weight gain with age may be a confounding variable. Peppard and coworkers[59] developed a model based on longitudinal study of the Wisconsin population-based cohort based on age, sex, and BMI. Extrapolating to the current prevalence of obesity, *the model predicted prevalence estimates for an AHI ≥ 15/hour (moderate to severe sleep apnea) in 50- to 70 year-old individuals to be 17% in men and 9% in women.* A recent assessment of the global burden of sleep apnea estimated worldwide prevalence of sleep apnea[58] using AHI threshold values of ≥5/hour and ≥15/hour, estimated that 936 million adults aged 30 to 69 years (men and women) have mild to severe OSA, and 425 million adults aged 30 to 69 years have moderate to severe OSA globally. The number of affected individuals was highest in China, followed by the United States, Brazil, and India.[58]

Studies have evaluated the effects of different hypopnea definitions on the prevalence of OSA in *clinic populations.* Rueland and coworkers[60] performed a retrospective analysis of a clinical population studied in two sleep centers using a AHIRec—based on a hypopnea definition requiring a ≥4% desaturation and an AHIalt based on a hypopnea definition requiring a *50% drop in airflow* and ≥3% desaturation or arousal. The percentage of the patients classified as having an AHI ≥ 5/hour using AHIRec was 59% and using the alternative 76%. Note that in the 2007 version of the AASM scoring manual[11] the alternative hypopnea definition required a 50% drop in airflow associated with a ≥3% desaturation or arousal, whereas the current AASM recommended hypopnea definition requires a >= 30% drop in airflow. Analysis of a population-based cohort (HypnoLaus) aged 35 to 75 years recruited from a random sample of age-eligible adults living in Lausanne, Switzerland, was performed by Hirotsu and coworkers[51] using different hypopnea definitions (Figure 18–7). Individuals were studied with home PSG with a standard EEG and electrooculogram montage. Airflow was monitored with nasal pressure. Using the more stringent hypopnea definition of a ≥ 30% drop in airflow associated with a ≥ 4% desaturaion or arousal (CMS, current AASM optional definition), 46.9% of the population had an AHI ≥ 5/hour. Using the less stringent hypopnea definition based on a ≥30% drop in airflow associated with a ≥3% desaturation or arousal, 72% of the population had an AHI ≥ 5/hour. These findings suggest using a higher AHI threshold for the diagnosis of OSA might be indicated. Using either hypopnea definition the prevalence of OSA is very high. It is also important to note that for a milder AHI, the ICSD-3-TR (and CMS)[17,18] require that symptoms (ICSD-3-TR and CMS) and/or comorbidity (CMS) be present for a diagnosis of OSA. In an early evaluation of the HypnoLaus cohort,[53] about 40% of men had an AHI in the mild range using the hypopnea definition based on ≥4% desaturation, but only about 6% also had an ESS score > 10. *Thus, requiring associated symptoms reduces the percentage diagnosed with the OSA syndrome.*

Risk Factors for OSA

Several population-based studies have documented risk factors for the presence of OSA (Table 18–6).[54-57] Of these, the most consistent findings have been the presence of obesity and the male gender.

Obesity

An association between AHI and obesity has been documented in many studies. *About 60% of patients with OSA are obese.* Peppard and coworkers[61] found that a 10% increase in weight was associated with a sixfold increase in the risk of developing moderate to severe OSA. Other studies have documented a decrease in the AHI with weight loss.[62] Whether the type of obesity or areas of excess fat (neck vs. abdomen) are important is currently under investigation. Prediction models for OSA have used neck circumference as a predictor.[33] However, one study found neck circumference to correlate best with AHI in women, whereas abdominal obesity (girth) correlated better with the AHI in men.[63]

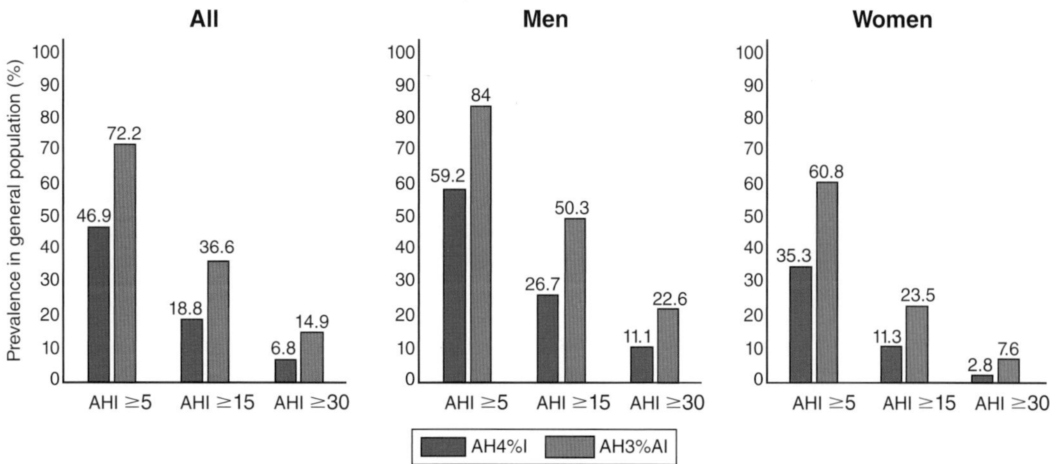

Figure 18–7 The figure illustrates the apnea-hypopnea index (AHI) values for a large population study using two hypopnea definitions. The AH4%I requires hypopneas be associated wth a ≥4% desaturation in addition to a drop in airflow. The AH3%AI uses a hypopnea definition that requires a drop in airflow with either a ≥3% desaturation or an arousal. Even with the more stringent hypopnea definition a very large proportion of individuals have an AHI ≥ 5/hour. It should be noted that not all the individuals with mild obstructive sleep apnea reported symptoms or necessarily needed treatment. (Adapted from Hirotsu C, Haba-Rubio J, Andries D, Tobback N, et al. Effect of three hypopnea scoring criteria on OSA prevalence and associated comorbidities in the general population. *J Clin Sleep Med.* 2019;15[2]:183-194.)

Table 18–6 Risk Factors for OSA

Risk Factor	Evidence
Obesity—present in roughly 60%–70% of OSA	+++
Male sex	+++
Aging	++
Postmenopausal state	++
Black race	+ (some studies)
Alcohol, smoking, hypothyroidism, acromegaly	±

OSA, Obstructive sleep apnea.

Adapted from Malhotra A, White DP. Obstructive sleep apnea. *Lancet.* 2002;360:237-245.

Gender

The Wisconsin cohort study by Young and coworkers[54] found men to have twice the incidence of the OSA **syndrome** (AHI ≥ 5/hour and symptoms) compared with women (4% vs. 2%). Analysis of the Sleep Heart Health data also showed the risk of OSA in men was greater (odds ratio 1.5).[64] Several other studies have evaluated the impact of gender.[65-69] Of interest, a study by Tishler and coworkers[66] suggests that after age 50 the risk of OSA for men and women is similar. As previously noted, there are a number of differences in the presentation of OSA in women compared with men[26,27] and PSG findings[68] (see Box 18–2).

Age

The prevalence of OSA appears to be higher in the elderly than in middle-aged populations. There is evidence from the Sleep Heart Health Study that the SDB prevalence increases from age 40 to around 60 years.[55] After that, the prevalence appears to plateau. Huang and coworkers[69] also found evidence of a plateau in the prevalence of OSA at the 60- to 70-year range. However, in men, Bixler and coworkers[70] found that based on the AHI *alone* that prevalence increased monotonically with age. However, using the criteria of AHI > 10/hour and daytime symptoms, the prevalence of the OSA syndrome peaked in middle age. In addition, the clinical significance (severity) of apnea decreases with age. In older adults, the AHI may be less correlated with excessive sleepiness and increased cardiovascular risk. Fietze and coworkers[71] found that the AHI continued to increase with age without evidence of a plateau. In a study of an urban population, Tishler and coworkers found that increasing age affects both the male predominance in OSA, as well as the effect of obesity.[66] By age 50 the prevalence of OSA in men and women was similar, and after age 60 an increased BMI (obesity) was negligible as a risk factor for OSA. Some have suggested that OSA in the elderly is a different disease. Enright and coworkers studied reported snoring and found it to be less common after age 70 and not associated with cardiovascular disease.[72] Endeshaw[73] found that *nocturia was a common complaint in the elderly with OSA.*

Postmenopausal Status

Although the factors of age and higher BMI complicate the analysis of the effect of postmenopausal status on the risk for OSA, it appears that postmenopausal women are at increased risk of developing OSA if they are not on hormone replacement treatment (HRT).[74,75] Young and coworkers analyzed[74] the Wisconsin Sleep Cohort and found that compared with premenopausal women, *post-menopausal women were 2.6 times more likely to have SDB defined as AHI ≥ 5/hour and 3.5 times more likely using an AHI ≥ 15/hour.* There was a slight protective effect with the use of HRT, but this did not reach statistical significance. Shahar and coworkers[75] analyzed the Sleep Heart Health cohort and found that in postmenopausal women on HRT, the prevalence of moderate to severe OSA (AHI ≥ 15/hour) was about half that of those not on HRT even when adjusting for confounding factors. Bixler and coworkers[76] also found a higher prevalence of OSA in postmenopausal women not on HRT compared with those on HRT. The study concluded that menopause is a significant risk factor for sleep apnea and that hormone replacement was associated with a reduced risk. *Does treatment with HRT in postmenopausal women not currently on HRT reduce the severity of sleep apnea?* Manber studied the effects of estrogen replacement and estrogen + progesterone replacement on sleep apnea in postmenopausal women with a small pilot study. Estrogen but not estrogen-progesterone was beneficial.[77] In contrast, in a prospective short-term placebo-controlled study of medroxyprogesterone, there was no benefit.[78] In summary, postmenopausal women (especially if not on HRT) have an increased risk of having OSA compared to premenopausal women. However, the benefits of adding HRT to postmenopausal women for improvement in sleep apnea are not well documented and likely depend on the type of hormonal replacement, the timing, and possibly the duration of treatment. At this time the addition of HRT solely for reduction of OSA risk cannot be recommended.

Race

There has been conflicting evidence concerning the possibility that OSA is more common in African American than White populations. An investigation by Redline and associates[79] found an increase in the risk of having OSA to be greater in African Americans than in Whites only for those younger than age 25 years. Ip and coworkers[80] found a similar prevalence of OSA in a Chinese population as in Whites. The fact that OSA is common in Asian areas where obesity is much less common than in the United States has led to the hypothesis that craniofacial characteristics of the Asian population might predispose this group to OSA.[81]

Smoking and Alcohol

The evidence for an association between smoking and OSA is conflicting.[82-84] Wetter and coworkers[82] found a dose relationship between smoking and the severity of sleep apnea. Current smokers had greater odds of having moderate or severe OSA compared with nonsmokers. In contrast, analysis of data from the Sleep Heart Health study found a greater percentage of nonsmokers at each level of AHI compared with current smokers.[83] The possible mechanisms by which smoking could increase the likelihood of OSA are reviewed in detail by Krishnan and coworkers.[84] Chronic alcohol consumption has been found to be associated with OSA in some studies.[85] Some but not all studies have found an association between acromegaly[86,87] or hypothyroidism[88] and OSA. If a patient with OSA is found to have hypothyroidism, they should be treated, as restoration of normal thyroid levels does not ensure resolution of OSA. Similarly if a patient with acromegaly has OSA, OSA treatment is indicated even if treatment for acromegaly is underway. In summary, a few studies have suggested that smoking and alcohol consumption are associated with an increased risk of OSA, but the evidence is not considered to be strong, as no large convincing studies are available. Hypothroidism and acromegaly may increase the risk of OSA but effective treatment of OSA is indicated unless resolution of OSA is proven after effective treatment of these endocrine disorders.

VARIANTS OF OSA

Some of the common variants of snoring and OSA are listed in Table 18–7. Some patients may fit into more than one category. The importance of primary snoring continues to be

Table 18–7 Snoring and OSA Variants

Primary snoring	• AHI < 5/hour, no daytime sleepiness
UARS	• RERAs with few desaturations, in ICSD-3 a subtype of OSA • AHI < 5/hour when hypopnea definition requires ≥4% desaturation, but RDI ≥ 5/hour • AHI ≥ 5/hour using recommended hypopnea definition but <5/hour using a hypopnea definition requiring a ≥4% desaturation
POSA	• AHIsupine > 2 × AHInonsupine • If AHInonsupine < 5–10/hour = "exclusive POSA"
REM-associated OSA	• AHI-REM > 2 × AHI-NREM, additional criteria are **normal NREM AHI**, or NREM-AHI ≤ 15/hour. • Depending on definition about 25%–30% of patients being studied for OSA. • More common in milder OSA, and women • AHI-REM associated with risk of hypertension and non-dipping nocturnal blood pressure • Even if the total AHI is mild, these patients may benefit from treatment
OHS	• Obesity • Daytime PCO_2 > 45 mm Hg (≥ 45 mmHg in many references)[16] • Hypoventilation not explained by lower airway or parenchymal lung disease, a thoracic cage disorder (other than obesity), or a neuromuscular disorder • 80%–90% have OSA, others daytime hypercapnia worsened during sleep • High morbidity and mortality if not treated • CO_2 (HCO_3^-) > 27 mEq/L in an obese patient with OSA = a clue to evaluate with an ABG; if high suspicion, order ABG, even if HCO_3^- < 27 mEq/L • If severe obesity and AHI, obtaining an ABG (or surrogate) is recommended to evaluate daytime $PaCO_2$
OLS	• OSA + chronic obstructive pulmonary disease • More severe nocturnal desaturation (especially if low awake SaO_2) • Daytime hypercapnia can be present with only mild reductions in the FEV_1

ABG, Arterial blood gas; *AHI,* apnea-hypopnea index; *FEV_1,* forced expiratory volume in 1 second; *ICSD-3, International Classification of Sleep Disorders,* version 3; *OHS,* obesity hypoventilation syndrome; *OLS,* overlap syndrome; *OSA,* obstructive sleep apnea; *POSA,* positional obstructive sleep apnea; *RDI,* respiratory disturbance index (AHI + RERA index); *REM,* rapid eye movement; *RERA,* respiratory effort-related arousal; *UARS,* upper airway resistance syndrome.

controversial.[89] The upper airway resistance syndrome (UARS) is listed as a subtype of OSA in the ICSD-3-TR. The OHS and overlap syndrome (OLS) are important clinically. The OHS is characterized by daytime hypoventilation and may not be recognized until a patient is hospitalized for hypercapnic respiratory failure. Optimal treatment of the OLS requires effective treatment of both chronic obstructive pulmonary disease (COPD) and OSA. Observational studies suggest a decreased survival in patients with the OLS not treated with CPAP compared with those who receive this treatment. Treatment with nocturnal supplemental oxygen alone is not the treatment of choice.

Primary Snoring and Long Periods of Airflow Limitation

Snoring may be defined as a vibratory, sonorous noise made during inspiration and, less commonly, expiration. Factors believed to worsen snoring include nasal congestion, the supine posture, and ethanol. Risk factors for snoring include gender (men > women) and increasing age. Some studies have suggested that up to 60% of men and 40% of women older than age 40 years have some snoring.[89] Whereas snoring is a cardinal symptom of OSA, not all snorers have OSA. Simple or primary snoring is defined as the presence of snoring without associated symptoms of insomnia, daytime sleepiness, or sleep disruption. Although a PSG is not necessary unless OSA is suspected, the PSG characteristics of simple snoring would include evidence of snoring on the PSG as detected by audio recording, a snore sensor, or vibration in the nasal pressure signal (or technologist report of snoring) AND the absence of a significant AHI. A study by Lee and associates[90] found that heavy snoring (defined as the presence of snoring for >50% of the nights) was associated with increased carotid atherosclerosis independent of other risk factors such as nocturnal hypoxemia and OSA severity. However, other studies to date have not confirmed the finding. In addition, patients with heavy snoring are at risk for developing OSA as they age or if significant weight gain occurs. Although not every snorer needs a sleep study, evaluation is recommended if the patient has a moderate to high likelihood of having OSA, is symptomatic, or if a surgical intervention for snoring is being considered. A PSG is also needed before an oral appliance is made for snoring to rule out significant OSA. If significant sleep apnea is present, this may change the treatment approach. The treatments for snoring are similar to those for mild OSA (oral appliance, positional treatment, and some types of palatal surgery (Pillar procedure). However, the costs of these treatments are not usually covered by insurance.

An entity in which patients have long periods of snoring and airflow limitation, sometimes without sufficient events to qualify for a diagnosis of OSA, is occasionally seen.[91] A similar presentation occurs when the AHI meets criteria for a diagnosis of very mild OSA, but the patient has a low baseline sleeping SaO_2 during the airflow limitation, such as an AHI of 6/hour but 30 to 60 minutes with a $SaO_2 \leq 88\%$. Most of these patients will have improved oxygenation on CPAP. The importance of recognizing the pattern of long severe airflow limitation is that the AHI may underestimate the impact of sleep apnea, and patients may have symptoms more severe than would be expected on the basis of a very low AHI. The situation is similar to that in children with OSA who have periods of obstructive hypoventilation and increased end-tidal PCO_2 but low AHI values. Monitoring of end-tidal PCO_2 is recommended for pediatric diagnostic studies but is uncommonly performed in adult diagnostic PSG. It is possible that end-tidal PCO_2 monitoring would be helpful in adults with long periods of upper airway narrowing with few discrete apneas or hypopneas.

Upper Airway Resistance Syndrome

Guilleminault and coworkers[92] identified a group of patients who complained of sleepiness or fatigue but did not have an AHI ≥ 5/hour (thermal devices measured airflow, hypopneas required a desaturation). The group was defined by having a *respiratory arousal index* greater than 10/hour using esophageal pressure monitoring. The symptoms responded to CPAP or other treatments. The mean arousal index of the group was 33/hour (range 16–52), and the mean maximally negative esophageal pressure nadir was −37 cm H_2O. The patients were said to have the upper airway resistance syndrome (UARS). There has been controversy as to whether the UARS is a distinct entity or simply a milder form of OSA. The UARS is considered a subtype of OSA in the ICSD-3 and ICSD-3-TR. Use of nasal pressure to detect more subtle decreases in airflow as well as airflow limitation (flattening of the inspiratory NP waveform) has increased the ability to diagnose patients with milder OSA. If a hypopnea definition requiring a drop in airflow + ≥4% desaturation is used, most UARS patients with an AHI < 5/hour will have an RDI = AHI + RERA index ≥ 5/hour. Furthermore, if hypopneas are scored based on the recommended hypopnea definition requiring either an associated ≥3% desaturation OR an arousal, most events previously scored as RERAs (based on ≥4% desaturations) will now be classified as hypopneas.[93,94]

REM-Associated OSA (REM-OSA)

Some patients have episodes of OSA primarily during REM sleep.[95-102] These patients may report symptoms typical of OSA, although the overall AHI is only mildly increased. The worsening of OSA during REM can be manifested in a number of ways, including more frequent events, events of longer duration, and greater oxygen desaturation associated with events. A typical finding is that the overall AHI may be low with a low or normal AHI during NREM sleep but a moderately to severely increased AHI during REM sleep. Other OSA patients will have an elevated AHI during both NREM and REM sleep with a much higher AHI and more severe desaturation during REM sleep. Definitions vary but one can define REM predominant OSA based on an AHI-REM/AHI-NREM ≥ 2 but an AHI-NREM > 15/hour. That is, the AHI is much high during REM sleep but also significant during NREM sleep. The overall AHI is moderate to severe in frequency. REM-associated/related OSA can be defined as REM-AHI/NREM-AHI ≥ 2 and a NREM-AHI < 15/hour. In this case the overall AHI is usually less than 15/hour while the AHI-REM is in the moderate to severe range. A retrospective review by Conwell and coworkers[96] used the following definitions. Definition #1) required an overall AHI ≥ 5/hr and AHI-REM/AHI-NREM ≥ 2. Definition #2) was defined as an overall AHI ≥ 5/hr, AHI-REM/AHI-NREM ≥ 2, and AHI-NREM < 15/hr. Definition-3) was defined as an overall AHI ≥ 5/hr, AHI-REM/AHI-NREM ≥ 2, and an AHI-NREM < 8/hr and at least 10.5 min of REM sleep duration. The study found that about 37% of patients met Definition#1 and 24% met Definition#2 (that is REM-associated OSA). Therefore, depending on the exact definition and population studied, REM-associated OSA accounts for about 25% of the patients evaluated in sleep centers for suspected OSA. Patients with REM-associated OSA tend to be women and have similar symptoms of daytime sleepiness as patients with non-sleep stage-specific OSA. In *population* studies the degree of sleepiness correlates with the NREM-AHI but not the REM-AHI.[99-101] In a *clinic-based study* of patients with excessive daytime sleepiness and an overall AHI < 10, Kass and coworkers[97] found that the REM-AHI correlated with daytime sleepiness, explaining 35% of the variance in sleep latency ($P < .001$) on the multiple sleep latency test (MSLT). A REM-AHI greater than 15/hour was predictive of reduced sleep latency on MSLT. This finding suggests, that an elevated AHI during REM sleep alone may justify treatment if the patient is symptomatic even if the overall AHI is barely increased. Chervin and coworkers analyzed a clinic group of patients with OSA undergoing the MSLT.[98] In linear regression models, the AHI explained 11.0% of the variance in MSLT results, the AHI in NREM sleep explained 10.8%, and the AHI in REM sleep explained only 6.0% ($P \leq .0001$ for each).

Thus, even using the entire-night AHI, the correlation between the AHI and subjective or objective measures of sleepiness is low. Su and coworkers[102] studied the outcome of PAP treatment in groups with and without REM-associated OSA. REM-associated OSA was defined as AHI-REM/AHI-NREM > 2 and NREM-AHI < 15/hour. All functional outcomes improved significantly after PAP therapy in both groups. The groups did not differ in the improvement in outcomes after PAP treatment. The authors concluded that improvement in functional outcomes in patients with REM-associated OSA after treatment with PAP therapy was comparable to that observed in patients with OSA without REM-associated OSA. REM-associated OSA patients appear to have similar symptoms, equal CPAP adherence, and benefit from CPAP treatment as those with NREM on non-sleep stage-specific OSA.[102] Thus, the etiology of symptoms in patients with a low or normal AHI during NREM sleep but an increased REM-AHI remains unknown. Findings in *population cohort studies* with many normal individuals may not correlate with findings in clinic populations. In addition symptoms of non-restorative sleep or daytime fatigue may be prominent even if a patient denies daytime sleepiness.

There is evidence that an elevated-REM-AHI has important cardiovascular manifestations. An extended follow-up of the Wisconsin sleep cohort found that REM-associated OSA (REM-AHI > 15/hour and NREM-AHI < 5/hour) was independently associated with an increase in prevalent and incident hypertension,[103,104] as well as with nondipping of the nocturnal blood pressure.[104] In these studies, there was *no association between hypertension and the NREM-AHI.* Appleton and coworkers also found that hypertension was associated with undiagnosed OSA during REM sleep.[105] Aurora and coworkers studied a subgroup of patients (Sleep Heart Health cohort) with a NREM AHI < 5/hour. Using those patients with a **REM-AHI** < 5/hour, as the reference group, patients with a **REM-AHI** > 30/hour had an increased risk (compared to the reference group) of having a composite cardiovascular endpoint (defined as the occurrence of nonfatal or fatal events, including myocardial infarction, coronary artery revascularization, CHF, and stroke).[106] There is also evidence that REM-OSA is associated with neurocognitive dysfunction and may present with insomnia and nightmares and could affect cognitive function and mood.[107] These studies suggest untreated REM-associated OSA may have important consequences.

The etiology of the worsening of OSA during REM sleep remains controversial. Traditional thinking explains worsening OSA during REM sleep as due to upper airway muscle hypotonia. During bursts of eye movements there is decreased phasic activity in the upper airway muscles and the diaphragm.[108] In addition to the general loss of upper airway muscle tone during sleep, there is also cholinergic inhibition of hypoglossal motor neuron activity.[109] At least during phasic REM sleep (REM sleep with the presence of REMs), one could expect a more collapsible upper airway that does not respond to increases in upper airway pressure. However, two studies of the upper airway found similar collapsibility during NREM and REM sleep (passive P_{CRIT}, critical pressure).[110,111] However, using a large group of participants and measurement of "active P_{CRIT}," Carberry and coworkers demonstrated increased collapsibility during REM sleep.[112] Critical closing pressure (P_{CRIT}) is discussed in more detail in Chapter 19. REM sleep is not homogeneous, and upper airway muscle tone is often lowest during bursts of phasic eye movements.[108] The frequency of eye movements increases in the later REM periods of the night. Periods of decreased ventilation are also more common and longer during REM sleep in the later part of the night. As in normal individuals, the periods of stage R are longer in the last part of the night. Thus, it is not surprising that the most severe desaturation often occurs during the last REM periods of the night. Hypercapnic and hypoxic ventilatory drives are lower in REM than NREM sleep.[113] This might be of benefit in patients with instability of ventilatory control (high loop gain). Joosten and coworkers[114] found patients with REM-associated OSA tend to have increased upper airway collapsibility, and those with NREM-OSA are more likely to have ventilatory control instability (increased loop gain). A study by Messineo et al found evidence that withdrawal of ventilatory drive to BOTH the upper airway and pump muscles results in respiratory events during REM sleep without a preferential decrease in genioglossus activity or compensation.[115] There also was no evidence of increased upper airway collapsibility during REM sleep which is not consistent with the findings of Carberry et al[112] who assessed collapsibility by measuring P_{CRIT}. The methods of assessing collapsibility in these studies were quite different. Of interest, in the study by Messineo et al there was evidence of a lower arousal threshold during REM sleep. However, this finding is not consistent with the common finding of longer respiratory events and more severe arterial oxygen desaturations during REM sleep. In contrast, experimental mask occlusion in normal individuals has found that subjects arouse more quickly during REM than NREM sleep. Thus, reason for the longer events during REM sleep in OSA patients is unknown. There is also an interaction between REM sleep and posture. The AHI is usually higher during supine than lateral REM sleep. Oksenberg and coworkers[44] found that the order of AHI severity was

AHI-REM supine > AHI-NREM supine > AHI-REM lateral > AHI-NREM lateral

For the REM-related and non-REM-related OSA patients, the interaction between supine posture and REM sleep led to the highest AHI during supine REM sleep.

However, the average length of apnea and hypopneas during REM sleep was similar in the supine and lateral postures.[42]

In summary, the importance of treatment of REM-associated OSA remains controversial, but in a symptomatic patient without other causes of daytime sleepiness, most clinicians would proceed with a trial of CPAP or other treatment. Symptomatic patients with REM-OSA are as likely to benefit from treatment as other patients with symptomatic patients with milder OSA. The mechanisms causing a higher AHI during REM sleep with longer events are still under investigation. However, any discussion of mechanisms should acknowledge the interaction between the supine position and REM sleep.

Obesity Hypoventilation Syndrome

The majority of patients with OSA do not have daytime hypoventilation. Two groups of OSA patients who do present with daytime hypoventilation include those with OHS and the overlap syndrome (OLS, a combination of OSA and COPD). Some important points concerning the OHS are listed in Box 18–5.

Diagnostic criteria for OHS include:[16]

- Presence of hypoventilation during wakefulness ($PaCO_2 \geq 45$ mm Hg) as measured by arterial PCO_2, end-tidal PCO_2, or transcutaneous PCO_2
- Presence of obesity (BMI $\geq 30 kg/m^2$, $\geq$ 95 percentile for age and sex for children
- Hypoventilation is not primarily due to lung parenchymal or airway disease, chest wall disorder (other than mass loading from obesity), medication use, neurologic disorder, muscle weakness, or a known congenital or idiopathic central alveolar hypoventilation syndrome.

Patients with OHS were previously referred to as "pickwickian." Today, use of this term is discouraged. Note that previously, the ICSD-3[17] used a daytime $PaCO_2$ >45 mm Hg but the ICSD3-TR uses $PaCO_2 \geq 45$ mm Hg, as do many references (a review of OHS by Masa and coworkers used $PaCO_2 \geq 45$ mm Hg).[117] New in the text revision of the ICSD-3 (ICSD-3-TR) is that documentation of hypoventilation is allowed by end-tidal PCO_2 and transcutaneous PCO_2. Randerath and coworkers[118] proposed a staging system for patients with obesity and hypercapnia, with stage 0 being no hypercapnia; stage 1 being intermittent nocturnal hypercapnia ($PaCO_2$ greater in morning compared with evening, HCO_3^- < 27 mmol/L); stage 2 being sustained nocturnal hypercapnia and HCO_3^- > 27 mmol/L; stage 3 being daytime hypercapnia but no cardiometabolic comorbidity; and stage 4 being daytime hypercapnia and cardiometabolic comorbidity. Patients with isolated nocturnal hypoventilation likely retain HCO_3^- during sleep and on awakening reduce the $PaCO_2$ to normal levels, resulting in an increased base excess.

Box 18–5 OBESITY HYPOVENTILATION SYNDROME (OHS) KEY POINTS

- Obesity (BMI > 30 kg/m^2, or >95th percentile for age and sex in children)
- Daytime hypoventilation
- Lung airway/parenchymal disease, thoracic cage abnormalities (other than obesity), neuromuscular weakness are **excluded as major cause of hypoventilation**
- Male = female prevalence
- 90% have OSA, others daytime hypercapnia that worsens at night
- 70%–80% have severe OSA
- High mortality if not treated, especially after hospitalization for respiratory failure
- Episodes of respiratory failure often mistaken for a COPD exacerbation
- NIV needed for hospitalization with respiratory failure
- Stable outpatient OHS with severe OSA responds to CPAP/BPAP without a backup rate if good adherence
- Stable outpatient OHS **without** severe OSA will often need NIV for improvement in hypoventilation

BPAP, Bilevel positive airway pressure; *COPD,* chronic obstructive pulmonary disease; *CPAP,* continuous positive airway pressure; *NIV,* noninvasive ventilation; *OSA,* obstructive sleep apnea.

The incidence of OHS in populations evaluated for sleep apnea varies from about 8% to 20%.[117] Unlike OSA, there is **NO gender predominance** for patients with OHS (prevalence in men ≈ women). Usually, OHS patients with hypercapnia are more obese than OSA patients without hypercapnia. The severity of OSA and the impairment of respiratory system mechanics are closely associated with the degree of obesity. Specifically, lower forced expiratory volume in 1 second (FEV_1), lower vital capacity (VC), lower total lung capacity, lower minimum overnight SpO_2, and higher AHI and BMI are associated with hypercapnia.[119] Approximately 90% of patients with the OHS have OSA (AHI ≥ 5/hour), and about 70% have severe OSA. Those OHS patients without OSA simply have daytime hypercapnia and worsening hypoventilation during sleep without many discrete apneas or hypopneas. Daytime hypercapnia worsens during sleep in all OHS patients (with or without OSA) and is often associated with severe arterial oxygen desaturation. Hypoventilation is usually worse during REM compared with NREM sleep. Those OHS patients without significant OSA exhibit sustained or episodic periods of shallow breathing during sleep associated with worsening hypoventilation and hypoxemia.

Berger and coworkers[120] described a spectrum of patients with OHS. As discussed by Masa and coworkers,[117] two phenotypes have been identified: OHS with severe OSA and OHS with milder OSA and predominant hypoventilation. A tracing of a patient with an AHI of 10/hour and predominantly long periods of hypoventilation is shown in Figure 18–8. Those patients with coexistent severe OSA tend to be younger, predominantly male, more obese and have more significant daytime sleepiness, worse gas exchange, and a lower prevalence of cardiovascular comorbidity. This group also tends to be hospitalized less (fewer days) compared with OHS *without* severe OSA. Both groups can present with acute respiratory failure (acute superimposed on chronic) be identified during evaluation for suspected OSA.[121]

Diagnosis and treating patients with OHS is very important. Patients with untreated OHS are at increased risk for cardiovascular and respiratory morbidity, mortality, and health care usage compared with patients with eucapnic OSA or eucapnic obesity, as discussed later.

Clinical Presentation of OHS

Patients with OHS may present with a hospitalization for acute superimposed on chronic respiratory failure[121-123] or present to sleep clinic for evaluation of OSA with stable chronic hypercapnia (which is often unrecognized). They may

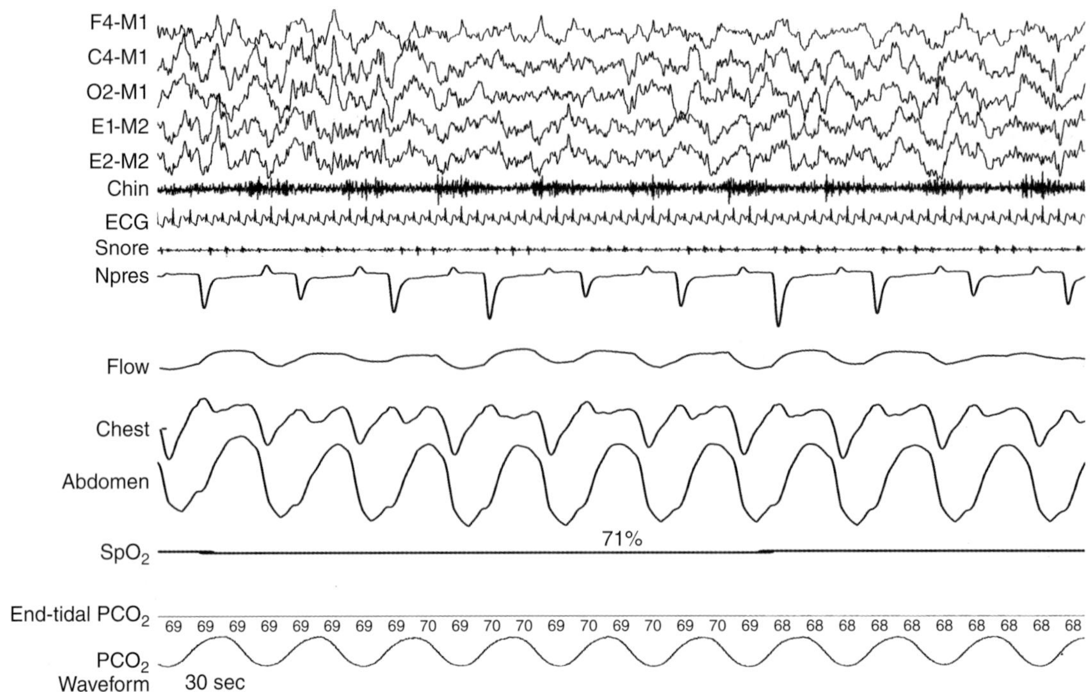

Figure 18–8 A 30-second tracing of a patient with obesity hypoventilation syndrome and severe hypoventilation and oxygen desaturation during sleep, but relatively few discrete respiratory events. This type of patient will need noninvasive positive airway pressure ventilation to both maintain an open airway and reduce the severe nocturnal hypercapnia. The addition of supplemental oxygen could be needed. In fact, the patient was titrated with high levels of bilevel positive airway pressure and supplemental oxygen was used. An end-tidal PCO_2 is shown in this tracing during the diagnostic portion of the study, but during the titration transcutaneous PCO_2 monitoring was performed. If the patient does not improve, BPAP with a back-up rate may be needed. If the PCO_2 improves with chronic treatment, supplemental oxygen may no longer be needed.

have few, if any, sleep complaints, or may present with considerable sleep disturbance including reduced sleep efficiency and frequent awakenings. Hypercapnia and hypoxemia may remain unnoticed for quite some time until sudden deterioration with cardiopulmonary arrest or severe decompensation (acute or chronic hypercapnic respiratory failure) develops. Patients with OHS may develop evidence of cor pulmonale and right ventricular hypertrophy. As will be discussed in detail later, they have a high mortality if not identified and treated.

Marik and Desai[122] evaluated patients admitted to the intensive care unit with "malignant OHS" and excluded patients with neuromuscular disorders or known CHF. This patient group had frequent admissions to the hospital, and *up to 75% were misdiagnosed as having a COPD exacerbation and/or treated for presumed CHF.* Indeed, patients with severe OHS may have right heart failure and volume overload. Patients are sometimes discharged on supplemental oxygen alone (not with PAP), and this can worsen hypercapnia.[123] Nowbar and coworkers[124] evaluated 4,332 consecutive patients admitted to the hospital, 277 of whom were severely obese. Of these, 150 met inclusion criteria and agreed to participate. Of the 150 obese participants, 45 (31%) were hypercapnic. Therapy for hypoventilation at discharge was initiated in only 6 (13%) of the patients with obesity-associated hypoventilation. At 18 months after hospital discharge, the mortality was 23% in the group with obesity associated with hypoventilation as compared with 9% in the group with simple obesity. Thus, hospitalized obese patients with hypercapnia have a poor prognosis and are usually discharged without treatment. As previously noted, such patients are often diagnosed as having a COPD exacerbation but never have a confirmation of this disorder by spirometry when stable. In contrast to the poor prognosis of untreated OHS, a study of the long-term effectiveness of noninvasive ventilation (NIV) started acutely or in chronic stable patients by Priou and coworkers[125] showed 1-, 2-, 3-, and 5-year survival rates of 97.5%, 93%, 88.3%, and 77.3%, respectively. The patients started on NIV on an acute or chronic basis did not differ in outcomes. Of interest is the fact that those patients treated with *supplemental oxygen as well as NPPV had a worse prognosis.*[125] This could simply identify them as having a component of lung disease or having more severe OHS. Another interpretation might be that the NIV was not sufficiently titrated such that supplemental oxygen was needed. Budweiser and coworkers[126] performed a retrospective analysis of patients started on NIV for OHS and found improved rates of survival. Gas exchange improved and hypoxemia was associated with a worse prognosis. *The average inspiratory (IPAP) and expiratory positive airway pressure (EPAP) used were approximately 26 cm H_2O and 6 cm H_2O, respectively.* The average backup rate was 19 bpm. Optimal NIV in OHS patients requires high IPAP and ideally a backup rate. When titrating such patients for **treatment of OSA**, higher EPAP is usually used. However, lowering the EPAP when large pressure support is used evidently maintains an open airway. Very severe patients may require temporary endotracheal intubation and mechanical ventilation.[121]

Tracheostomy can be lifesaving in patients noncompliant with PAP treatment who have repeated bouts of severe hypercapnic respiratory failure.

When stable patients with OHS are evaluated for OSA, it is not unusual for the presence of daytime hypercapnia to go unrecognized with patients simply characterized as having severe OSA. An arterial blood gas (ABG) test is the definitive test to demonstrate an obese patient has daytime hypoventilation and OHS. Pulmonary function testing can rule out a significant component of lung disease. Patients with OHS often have near normal spirometry but can have a reduced VC and total lung capacity (restrictive ventilatory defect). In a study to characterize predictors of OHS, Mokhlesi and associates[34] found that 20% of 410 patients referred to a sleep center to rule out OSA had OHS. In this study, only 3% of OHS patients had a HCO_3^- < 27 mEq/L. However, only 50% of patients with a HCO_3^- of ≥ 27 mEq/L had OHS. That is, the HCO_3^- cutoff (or electrolyte CO_2) of 27 mEq/L is sensitive but not specific for identifying OHS.[34] The authors concluded that patients with both OSA and a HCO_3^- ≥ 27 mEq/L should undergo arterial blood gas testing. Other clues that OHS may be present include a borderline awake SaO_2 (90%–92%) or evidence of significant cor pulmonale. Recent American Thoracic Society (ATS) guidelines for evaluation and treatment of OHS suggest an ABG if there is a high suspicion of OHS *irrespective of the level of* HCO_3^-.[127] If there is a lower suspicion for OHS, the serum HCO_3^- should be assessed. If CO_2 is less than 27 mEq/L, OHS is unlikely, but if the HCO_3^- is ≥ 27 mEq/L, an ABG should be performed (Figure 18–9). A low awake SpO_2 might be another clue suggesting that the OHS is present. Measuring oximetry in the supine position could conceivably be more sensitive. Chung and coworkers[128] studied the utility of the awake supine SpO_2 to detect OHS in a group of morbidly obese individuals. An SpO_2 < 91% was very specific for detection of OHS but not very sensitive. Another approach would be to measure end-tidal PCO_2 in clinic. As noted above it is important to recognize whether or not a patient has OHS in addition to OSA, because this group has a high incidence of complications and increased mortality if not properly treated.

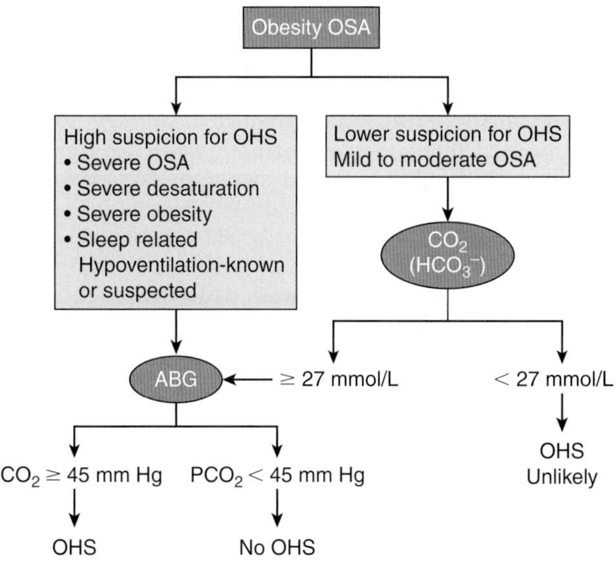

Figure 18–9 Algorithm for screening obese patients with obstructive sleep apnea (OSA) for the presence of obesity hypoventilation syndrome (OHS). If the suspicion for OHS is high, an **awake** arterial blood gas (ABG) is indicated. If the suspicion is lower, screening with the HCO_3^- (CO_2 on routine electrolytes) is recommended. However, if the CO_2 or HCO_3^- is ≥ 27 mmol/ L, an ABG is indicated for confirmation. Of note for CO_2 1 mmol/L = 1 meq/L)

Pathogenesis of OHS

The pathophysiology of OHS is related to three mechanisms: (1) obesity-related change in the respiratory system, (2) alterations in respiratory drive, and (3) breathing abnormalities during sleep (reduced ventilatory drive and apneas and hypopneas).[129] A comparison between eucapnic obese and OHS patients is listed in Table 18–8. Kaw and coworkers[119] performed a meta-analysis of cohort studies of obese patients to determine predictors of hypercapnia. They found daytime hypercapnia was associated with severe OSA, greater obesity (BMI), and greater chest wall restriction (lower FVC and total lung capacity). The eucapnic obese tended to have low normal total lung capacity. Overnight oximetry showed worse hypoxemia in the hypercapnic group. Obesity results in mass loading of the abdomen and chest wall resulting in a reduction in the expiratory reserve volume (ERV) and functional residual capacity (FRC) and reduced respiratory system compliance. Breathing at low lung volumes increases ventilation perfusion mismatch. OHS patients exhibit a greater impairment in respiratory mechanics than the morbidly obese without OHS, often associated with weakness of the respiratory muscles.[129] Overall, there is an increase in the work required for breathing that needs to be compensated by elevated drive from the respiratory centers to the respiratory muscles. Obesity also increases CO_2 production, requiring

Table 18–8 Comparison of Normocapnic Obesity and the OHS

	Normocapnic Obesity	OHS
Lung volumes		
FRC	↓	↓
ERV	↓	↓↓
TLC	Normal	Normal to ↓
$PaCO_2$ awake	Normal	↑ or ↑↑
Respiratory compliance	↓	↓↓
Respiratory drive	↑↑	Normal
Hypercapnic ventilatory response	Normal to ↑	↓↓
P0.1 hypercapnic ventilatory drive*	↑	↓↓
Hypoxic ventilatory response	Normal to ↑	↓↓
Respiratory muscle strength (PImax)	Normal to ↓	↓↓

ERV, Expiratory reserve volume; *FRC,* functional reserve capacity; *OHS,* obesity hypoventilation syndrome; *TLC,* total lung capacity.
*P0.1 is the pressure 0.1 seconds after airway occlusion. A measure of ventilatory drive not affected by decreased chest wall compliance
Verbraecken J, McNicholas WT. Respiratory mechanics and ventilatory control in overlap syndrome and obesity hypoventilation. *Respir Res.* 2013;14(1):132.

higher alveolar ventilation for the same $PaCO_2$. *Lack of increased compensatory drive is one explanation for CO_2 retention.* Leptin is a ventilatory stimulant (and appetite suppressant), and leptin levels are increased in obesity.[130] Obese patients are thought to have leptin resistance. High leptin levels might increase ventilatory drive to compensate for obesity. However, obese patients with hypercapnia have higher leptin than obese individuals without hypercapnia.[131] This suggests resistance to the effects of leptin. Another study found that leptin levels were lower in OHS patients without OSA than a group of eucapnic obese individuals but increased after effective NIV treatment with an associated increase in ventilatory drive (change in the occlusion pressure [P0.1] versus PCO_2).[132] P0.1 is the pressure generated in the first 100 msec after airway occlusion and is not affected by increased resistance (no flow with occlusion) or decreased compliance due to impaired chest wall mechanics. Of note, in both obese groups leptin levels were higher than normal controls. In contrast, another study found treatment of OHS reduced leptin levels.[133] However, this patient group contained patients with OSA (some were treated with CPAP). The role of leptin in the control of ventilation in OHS patients is complex and may vary between patients. Leptin resistance further complicates the picture.

Although it is known that OSA is worse during REM sleep, this sleep stage also worsens hypoventilation. REM sleep hypoventilation is severe in patients with OHS without severe OSA, as ventilation depends on the diaphragm because of REM-associated muscle hypotonia. Ventilatory drive is reduced during REM sleep even in normal individuals. A reduced leptin effect (low levels or leptin resistance) is thought to exacerbate this situation.

The OHS group with severe OSA develops nocturnal hypercapnia due to inability to excrete CO_2 due to repetitive apneas with limited ventilation between events. High upper airway resistance may also reduce the ability to maintain an adequate level of ventilation.[134,135] With nightly nocturnal hypoventilation there is a retention in HCO_3^- and likely a rightward shift in the ventilatory response to hypercapnia with a higher set point for PCO_2.[133,134] CPAP treatment shifted the response to the left without changing the slope in one study,[136] and in the other both the set point and slope of the P0.1 versus PCO_2 response improved, and daytime $PaCO_2$ normalized in some individuals.[137] The P0.1 is a better measure of ventilatory drive in patients with high upper or lower airway resistance or decreased respiratory system compliance. Chronic hypoxemia at night may also impair ventilatory drive. In some patients with OHS, effective treatment will normalize the daytime $PaCO_2$. If a patient with OHS has resolution of daytime hypoventilation—do they still have the OHS? One approach would be to consider them as having OHS in remission due to treatment, as daytime hypercapnia could return if PAP treatment was stopped or other exacerbating factors became an issue. In summary, the effects of obesity on the respiratory system are more severe in OHS patients than the eucapnic obese. OHS patients with OSA have impaired ability to maintain CO_2 homeostasis due to repetitive apneas and hypopneas. With time, isolated nocturnal hypoventilation extends to the daytime. The group of OHS patients that manifests hypoventilation without significant OSA is likely to have abnormal ventilatory control or very decreased respiratory system compliance (and increased work of breathing) because of massive obesity. Alterations in the ability of leptin to enhance ventilatory drive may also play a role in hypoventilation. This could occur due to reduced leptin levels or a reduced ventilatory response to leptin. The relative importance of OSA, abnormal ventilatory control, and decreased respiratory system compliance (mass loading from obesity) likely varies between individuals with OHS. One might assume that if untreated severe OSA is present, then treatment to open the upper airway during sleep might have a significant effect on nighttime and daytime hypercapnia. On the other hand, if OSA were milder, factors other than OSA might be more important and overall the hypercapnia might be less likely to respond to simply maintaining an open airway during sleep. Treatments aimed at augmenting nocturnal ventilation (normalizing) might have a greater benefit than simply treating the OSA. In fact, this thinking about the relative importance of the presence or absence of significant OSA in a given patient has implications for treatment.

Treatment of OHS

Treatment of OHS is discussed in detail in Chapters 21 and 24. The approach depends on the presence or absence of severe OSA and the severity of the current condition (stable outpatient vs. hospitalized patients with hypercapnic respiratory failure).[127] A brief summary of the current recommended approach is presented. In stable patients with severe OSA, treatment with CPAP is as effective as bilevel positive airway pressure (BPAP) or NIV for improving long-term outcomes (resolution or improvement in hypercapnia). In these patients, maintaining an open airway during sleep improves daytime and sleep-related hypoventilation. Elimination of hypoxia at night and improvement in volume status with diuresis results in a normalization of the daytime $PaCO_2$ (or at least an improvement) if they are adherent to PAP treatment. Good PAP adherence is essential for improvement in daytime $PaCO_2$. The ATS has published recommendations for the diagnosis and treatment of OHS.

A brief summary of the ATS recommendations[127] is as follows:

- Clinicians should use a serum bicarbonate level < 27 mmol/L to exclude the diagnosis of OHS in OSA patients when the suspicion for OHS is not very high ($<20\%$) but should measure arterial blood gases in patients strongly suspected of having OHS.
- Clinicians should not use the awake SpO_2 to decide if the $PaCO_2$ should be measured.
- Stable ambulatory patients with OHS should receive PAP.
- CPAP rather than NIV should be offered as the first-line treatment to stable ambulatory patients with OHS and concomitant severe OSA (AHI $\geq$ 30/hour).
- Patients hospitalized with respiratory failure and suspected of having OHS should be discharged with NIV until they undergo outpatient diagnostic procedures and PAP titration in the sleep laboratory (ideally within the first 2–3 months after discharge).
- Patients with OHS should use weight-loss interventions that produce sustained weight loss of 25% to 30% of body weight. This level of weight loss is likely required to achieve resolution of OHS.

The outpatient diagnostic procedures would include a diagnostic PSG if indicated (presence and severity of OSA) and pulmonary function testing if needed to rule out lung disease as a cause of hypoventilation). The guidelines, though very useful, do not address several issues. The first is that CPAP is touted over bilevel positive airway pressure (BPAP) in stable OHS patients with severe OSA. Indeed, BPAP is not more effective at opening the upper airway than CPAP in most patients. However, the maximum pressure of CPAP devices is 20 cm H_2O while the maximum pressure of BPAP devices without a backup rate is 25 cm H_2O. If a patient needs higher pressure than 20 cm H_2O, BPAP can be useful. Resolution of hypercapnia on PAP depends on good adherence. If a patient has pressure intolerance to high levels of CPAP, bloating, or mouth or mask leak, they might do better on BPAP than CPAP. Some patients with OHS have residual hypoxemia on CPAP that may respond to BPAP. This is a better option than adding supplemental oxygen.[123,125] In addition, there are patients with very severe hypoventilation (or severe oxygen desaturation) confined to REM sleep, and they may be better treated with BPAP. Some of the studies comparing CPAP with BPAP excluded patients with very severe hypoventilation or severe REM hypoventilation and hypoxemia.[116]

OHS patients hospitalized with acute respiratory failure (often acute superimposed on chronic) usually need NIV regardless of the presence or absence of severe OSA (often not known). NIV is best provided with some form of BPAP (usually with capacity to deliver IPAP up to 30 cm H_2O) and a backup rate. A backup rate is useful as acute reductions in severe hypercapnia can trigger central apneas in some patients, and other patients may not trigger the device during REM sleep. Some patients require a backup rate to deliver adequate ventilation when a device rate higher than the native respiratory rate is needed. Using NIV in the hospital is not an issue. *On the other hand, supplying an effective device at discharge is a major issue.*[138] Unfortunately, obtaining a BPAP with a backup rate (a respiratory assist device [RAD] with a backup rate) for an OHS patient is not always possible.[139] As discussed in Chapter 24, qualifying a patient for BPAP with a backup rate for initial treatment of hypoventilation is often difficult because of RAD criteria, which mandate an initial trial of BPAP without a backup rate (see Table 18–9).[139] Therefore, in some patients, NIV as an outpatient means BPAP *without a backup rate* for initial treatment (see chapter 24 for additional discussion of RAD critiera). After significant clinical improvement on NIV in the hospital, BPAP without a backup rate (but set to augment ventilation with optimal pressure support) may be adequate. If a patient is discharged on BPAP without a backup rate but this is proven inadequate on an outpatient titration, this might qualify them for a BPAP device with a backup rate. However, the titration should try to meet the qualifications for a backup rate. Evidence supporting a need for BPAP with a backup rate is as follows: "A **facility-based PSG or HST demonstrates oxygen saturation** ≤ 88% for ≥5 minutes of nocturnal recording time (minimum recording time of 2 hours) that is not caused by obstructive upper airway events (i.e., AHI < 5/hour while using BPAP without a backup rate)" (Table 18-9). If an OHS patient discharged on NIV has severe OSA, they can often be transitioned to BPAP without a backup rate (or CPAP) after clinical improvement. Ideally, this would occur after a PSG titration confirms the effectiveness of non-NIV PAP.

The reader should consult the references[127,138] for published recommended algorithms. A similar but slightly different approach is shown in Figure 18–10. There is a separation

Table 18–9 Respiratory Assist Devices

Hypoventilation Syndrome

E0470 is covered if:

- An initial arterial blood gas $PaCO_2$, done while awake, and breathing the beneficiary's prescribed FIO_2 is ≥45 mm Hg; and
- Spirometry shows an FEV1/FVC ≥ 70% and an FEV1 ≥ 50% of predicted (refer to RAD criteria for severe COPD[139] for information about device coverage for beneficiaries with FEV1/FVC ≤ 70% or FEV1 ≤ 50% of predicted); and

Beneficiary's condition also meets one of the following:

- An ABG $PaCO_2$, done during sleep or immediately upon awakening, and breathing the beneficiary's prescribed FIO_2, shows the beneficiary's $PaCO_2$ worsened ≥ 7 mm Hg compared with the original result in criterion 1 (above); or
- A **facility-based PSG or HST demonstrates oxygen saturation** ≤ 88% for ≥5 minutes of nocturnal recording time (minimum recording time of 2 hours) that is not caused by obstructive upper airway events (i.e., AHI < 5/hour).

E0471 is covered if:

- A covered E0470 is being used; **and**
- Spirometry shows an FEV1/FVC ≥ 70% and an FEV1 ≥ 50% of predicted (otherwise refer to COPD coverage); **and**

One of the following criteria are being met:

- An ABG $PaCO_2$, done while awake, and breathing the beneficiary's prescribed FIO_2, shows that the beneficiary's $PaCO_2$ worsens ≥7 mm HG compared with the ABG result performed to qualify the beneficiary for the E0470 device; or
- A facility-based PSG or HST demonstrates oxygen saturation ≤ 88% for ≥ 5 minutes of nocturnal recording time (minimum recording time of 2 hours) that is not caused by obstructive upper airway events (i.e., AHI ≤ 5 while using an E0470 device).

Continued Coverage (Beyond the First Three Months of Therapy):

The medical record contains a reevaluation **on or after the 61st day of therapy.** The reevaluation records the progress of relevant symptoms, and

- The reevaluation documents beneficiary usage of the device up to that time.
- The supplier's file includes a signed and dated statement completed by the treating physician no sooner than 61 days after initiating use of the device.
  - The statement declares that the beneficiary compliantly uses the device (an average of 4 hours per 24-hour period); and
  - The statement confirms that the beneficiary is benefiting from its use.

ABG, Arterial blood gas; *AHI*, apnea-hypopnea index; *COPD*, chronic obstructive pulmonary disease; *FEV1*, forced expiratory volume in 1 second; *FVC*, forced vital capacity; *HST*, home sleep testing; *PSG*, polysomnography. E0470 BPAP without backup rate, E0471 BPAP with backup rate
Adapted from: LCD:L33800 Respiratory Assist Devices (RADs) https://www.cms.gov/medicare-coverage-database/view/lcd.aspx?lcdid=33800&ver=26&KeyWord=respiratory+assis&KeyWordLookUp=Title&KeyWordSearchType=Exact&bc=CAAAAAAAAAAA. Assessed 12/10/2023.

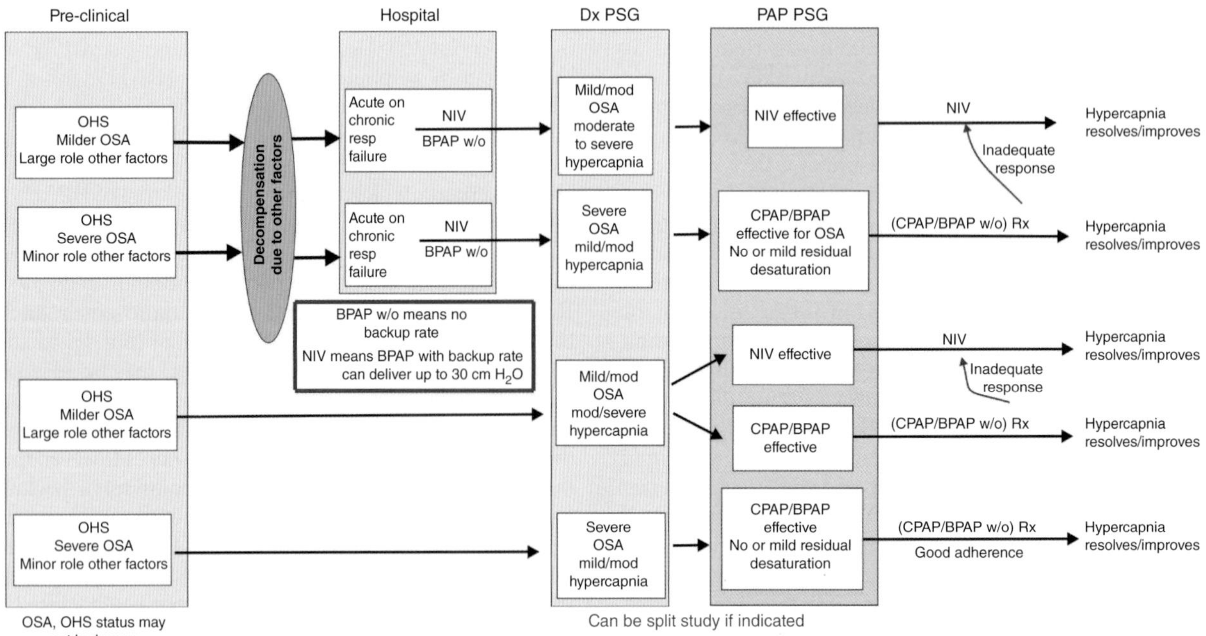

Figure 18–10 An algorithm of the approach to treatment of the obesity hypoventilation syndrome (OHS) in hospitalized patients and stable outpatients. Treatment type depends on the presence or absence of severe obstructive sleep apnea (OSA). Hospitalized OHS patients will likely need noninvasive ventilation (NIV) but might be discharged on NIV or bilevel positive airway pressure (BPAP) without a backup rate with high pressure support. Those with severe OSA may be transitioned to continuous positive airway pressure (CPAP)/BPAP at the time of an outpatient titration if they are clinically improved. Those without severe OSA may need long-term NIV. Stable patients with OHS and severe OSA can be treated with CPAP or BPAP without a backup rate. Treatment of OSA usually results in clinical improvement if PAP adherence is adequate. Stable OHS patients **without** severe OSA may need long-term NIV, but some may be transitioned to BPAP without a backup rate set to augment ventilation (high-pressure support).

between stable OHS patients and those hospitalized with respiratory failure. The general concept is that similar to the ATS guidelines, treating severe OSA is likely to be effective in OHS patients unless NIV is needed initially (as in decompensated hypercapnic respiratory failure). As discussed above, NIV (BPAP with a backup rate) is generally needed for all OHS patients hospitalized with severe hypercapnia. After clinical improvement some patients can be discharged on BPAP without a backup rate, whereas others will need NIV at home. If a hospitalized patient does have severe OSA and is discharged on NIV, they can often be transitioned to BPAP without a backup rate or CPAP as an outpatient after a PSG titration. Hospitalized OHS patients **without** severe OSA often need continued NIV as a long-term treatment for resolution of hypercapnia although some may be treated with BPAP without a backup rate. It should be appreciated that BPAP of 16/12 cm H_2O might be effective for treating OSA, but use of higher-pressure support would be needed if the goal is treatment of nocturnal hypoventilation. For example use of inspiratory positive airway pressure (IPAP) of 20 to 24 cm H_2O with expiratory positive airway pressure (EPAP) of 10 to 12 cm H_2O. In studies using a very high IPAP (eg 22-24 cm H_2O) lower EPAP was effective. NIV treatment of hypoventilation will be discussed in Chapter 24. **Stable OHS patients** with severe OSA (about 70% to 80%) can be treated with a device targeting the OSA usually without the need to provide high-pressure support. The optimal treatment should be determined during the PSG PAP titration.

Overlap Syndrome

Patients with the combination of OSA and COPD (the OLS) may have severe nocturnal oxygen desaturation and/or awake hypoventilation.[140-143] This topic is discussed in more detail in chapter 29. An overlap between OSA and asthma has also been described. An epidemiologic study found that patients with mild COPD have NO higher incidence of OSA than the general population.[143] However, because both COPD and OSA are common, the combination is common even if by chance. Of interest, those patients with both airway obstruction and sleep apnea in this study had more severe arterial oxygen desaturation. Patients with COPD alone rarely retain CO_2 until the FEV1 is below 1.0 L or 40% of predicted. However, patients with the OSA and mild to moderate COPD may retain CO_2.[144] Patients with the OLS tend to have particularly severe arterial oxygen desaturation at night. They are often assumed to simply have COPD and are treated with nocturnal oxygen alone. This may incompletely reverse the nocturnal hypoxemia and worsen the CO_2 retention during sleep.[145,146] The long-term outcome of patients with the OLS may worsen if upper airway obstruction is not addressed.[147-149] As nocturnal oximetry is always needed to document nocturnal desaturation and qualify COPD patients for nocturnal oxygen, the OLS should be suspected when there is a sawtooth pattern in the oximetry tracings, which is the result of individual apneas and hypopneas.[145] Proper treatment of patients with the OLS usually requires adequate treatment of both the COPD (smoking cessation and bronchodilators) and OSA (CPAP or BPAP and supplemental oxygen if needed).[150] The daytime PCO_2 may improve in some patients with adequate treatment of upper airway obstruction during sleep. Aggressive treatment of the component of COPD with bronchodilators and smoking cessation may also be helpful in improving gas exchange both during the day and at night. Observational studies have found worse survival in OLS patients not treated for OSA.[147-149] Adequate CPAP adherence is needed to receive benefit from treatment. Use of oxygen alone can worsen hypoventilation and is not sufficient treatment.

SUMMARY OF KEY POINTS

1. A significant proportion of patients diagnosed with OSA do not complain of daytime sleepiness. Although the majority of patients are obese, lack of obesity should not discourage evaluation for OSA.
2. Women with OSA may have more prominent symptoms of insomnia and fatigue compared with men. They are likely to have REM-associated OSA (often associated with a mild overall AHI).
3. A high Mallampati (or modified Mallampati) score for the upper airway is a predictor of the presence of OSA.
4. Patients with habitual snoring, witnessed apnea or gasping, hypertension, and a large neck circumference are at increased risk for having obstructive sleep apnea.
5. Questionnaires are not sufficiently sensitive or specific to obviate the need for objective testing to determine the presence or absence of OSA. However, they may be useful in alerting providers that evaluation for OSA is needed.
6. In patients with milder OSA the amount of supine and REM sleep may determine if the overall AHI is in the normal range or elevated (AHI $\geq$ 5/hour). For patients with moderate to severe OSA, lack of a supine and/or a normal amount of REM sleep may result in an AHI that underestimates the true severity of the disorder.
7. The severity of OSA may be underestimated by the AHI and lowest SaO_2 values obtained during the **diagnostic portion of a split sleep study.** The majority of REM sleep occurs in the second part of the night.
8. The correlation between the AHI and symptoms is low. In determining the need for treatment of the patients OSA, consideration of symptoms and comorbid conditions rather than the AHI alone is suggested. Consideration of the degree of oxygen desaturation is also important. Indices of the time with the $SpO_2 \leq$ 88% or 90% or newer indices such as the **hypoxic burden** may be more predictive of cardiovascular risk associated with untreated OSA.
9. If home sleep apnea testing (HSAT) is negative in a patient with a suspicion of OSA, a PSG is needed to rule out a false-negative result. HSAT results also underestimate the severity of OSA.
10. There is high night-to-night variability in the AHI of patients with mild to moderate OSA. Multiple nights of monitoring may prevent incorrect classification of patients.
11. Risk factors for the presence of obstructive sleep apnea include obesity, male sex, older age, and postmenopausal status (not on hormonal replacement therapy). Hypothyroidism, acromegaly, cigarette smoking, and chronic alcohol usage are also considered possible risk factors, but the evidence is much less compelling.
12. The two groups of patients with OSA that have daytime hypercapnia are those with the OHS and the overlap syndrome (OLS) defined as a combination of obstructive airways disease (COPD) and OSA.
13. The obesity hypoventilation syndrome (OHS) requires 1. obesity (BMI >30 kg/m^2), 2. daytime hypoventilation ($PaCO^2 \geq$ 45 mm Hg, 3. 3. the hypoventilation cannot be explained by lung disease, chest wall disease (other than obesity), or a neuromuscular disorder.
14. About 10% to 20% of patients presenting to sleep clinic for evaluation of OSA have the OHS (a commonly missed diagnosis). The possibility that the OHS syndrome is present should always be considered in patients with obesity and severe OSA. Findings of a low normal or decreased daytime SaO_2 or an elevated HCO_3^- (CO_2) > 27 mmol/L on electrolyte testing (reflecting compensation for hypercapnia) is suggestive of OHS. The use of the HCO_3^- (CO_2) $\geq$ 27 mmol/L was sensitive but not specific in screening for OHS. The definitive test is an ABG documenting an awake $PaCO_2$ $\geq$ 45 mm Hg, and this test (or an acceptable surrogate) should be performed in all patients with a high suspicion of OHS *irrespective of the level of the* HCO_3^-.
15. Approximately 80% to 90% of patients with the OHS have obstructive sleep apnea. The other 10% to 20% have daytime hypercapnia and sleep-related worsening of daytime hypercapnia and hypoxemia with relatively few discrete apneas or hypopneas. Approximately 70% of OHS patients have severe OSA. In these patients, adequate treatment of OSA (CPAP or BPAP without a backup rate) usually normalizes or improves the daytime $PaCO_2$. Those without severe OSA may need NIV to improve the daytime PCO_2.
16. Untreated OHS patients have a poor prognosis, especially if requiring hospitalization for acute superimposed on chronic hypercapnic respiratory failure. Obese patients admitted with hypercapnic respiratory failure are frequently misdiagnosed as having a COPD or CHF exacerbation. A definitive diagnosis of COPD requires spirometry. One approach is to discharge patients with residual hypercapnia/hypoxia after stabilization on empiric NIV (with oxygen if needed) with a plan for polysomnography (diagnostic PSG if needed and PAP titration PSG) when they are stable. Treatment with supplemental oxygen alone is not adequate treatment and could potentially worsen hypoventilation if timely PAP treatment is not started as an outpatient. Based on the polysomnography as an outpatient, patients may be transitioned to CPAP or BPAP without a backup rate and supplemental oxygen (if being used) may no longer be needed.
17. For **stable** OHS patients with severe OSA, the recommended treatment is CPAP (or BPAP without a backup rate if pressure intolerance is present or high pressures are needed to treat OSA). In these patients, adequate treatment of OSA improves daytime and nocturnal $PaCO_2$ and oxygenation. For OHS patients with acute respiratory failure/severe hypercapnia or those **without** severe OSA, treatment with NIV is recommended. BPAP devices with a backup rate are ideal for delivering NIV, and high levels of pressure support are needed for optimal normalization of nocturnal and daytime $PaCO_2$.
18. Patients with OSA and obstructive airway disease (COPD) may have severe arterial oxygen desaturation during sleep and daytime hypercapnia. There may be a milder reduction in the forced expiratory volume in 1 second (FEV_1) than typically seen in COPD patients with daytime hypercapnia that do not have comorbid OSA. *A hint that OSA in addition to COPD is present is when nocturnal oximetry exhibits a saw-tooth pattern associated with discrete respiratory events.*
19. Optimal treatment of overlap syndrome consists of both treatment of COPD and OSA. Nocturnal oxygen without PAP is not adequate treatment. Use of CPAP (or BPAP) and nocturnal oxygen if needed is the treatment of choice. In observational studies adequate treatment of OSA with PAP (with oxygen if needed) was associated with improved survival compared with patients not treated with PAP.

CLINICAL REVIEW QUESTIONS

1. Of the following, what is the best documented risk factor for OSA?
A. Cigarette smoking
B. Alcohol consumption
C. Postmenopausal status
D. Obesity

2. Which of the following is NOT always true about patients with the OHS?
A. Daytime $PCO_2 >$ (or $\geq$) 45 mm Hg
B. BMI > 30 kg/m^2
C. Worsening PCO_2 and PO_2 with sleep
D. AHI $\geq$ 5/hour

3. Which of the following is the best description of the ICSD-3-TR criterion for diagnosis of OSA in adults?
A. (Obstructive and mixed apneas + hypopneas + RERAs)/hour $\geq$ 5/hour
B. (Obstructive and mixed apneas + hypopneas + RERAs)/hour $\geq$ 15/hour
C. (Obstructive and mixed apneas + hypopneas + RERAs)/hour = $\geq$ 5/hour + symptoms + associated comorbidity*
D. (Obstructive and mixed apneas + hypopneas + RERAs)/hour = 5/hour + symptoms
OR (obstructive and mixed apneas + hypopneas + RERAs)/hour $\geq$ 15/hour

4. Which of the following group of symptoms in a patient would indicate a good candidate for home sleep apnea testing?
A. Snoring, witnessed apnea, daytime sleepiness, hypertension
B. Snoring, witnessed apnea, congestive heart failure, daytime sleepiness
C. Snoring, no witnessed apnea, nonrestorative sleep, no daytime sleepiness
D. Snoring, daytime sleepiness, neuromuscular disorder

5. Which of the following is **NOT** true about the prevalence of OSA in a given population?
A. Depends on hypopnea definition and presence of a requirement for associated symptoms
B. A majority of worldwide patients with OSA are undiagnosed
C. Prevalence is lower in Asian countries with a thinner population than in the United States
D. Postmenopausal status not on hormone replacement therapy increases the risk of having OSA

6. Which of the following statements concerning OSA in women is true?
A. They have more apneas than hypopneas.
B. REM-associated OSA is uncommon.
C. Insomnia or non-restorative sleep can be a presenting symptom.
D. For a given BMI they have a higher AHI compared with men.
E. They have a lower prevalence of the OHS.

7. An oximetry performed on a patient with mild to moderate COPD shows 3 hours of a $SaO_2 \leq 88\%$ and a sawtooth pattern in the tracings for the majority of the night. Which of the following is **NOT** true?
A. A PSG should be ordered.
B. Daytime hypercapnia could be present.
C. The addition of nocturnal oxygen is the best treatment for the hypoxemia.
D. Optimized treatment of COPD is indicated.

8. An obese female patient is admitted with hypercapnic respiratory failure with a diagnosis of a COPD exacerbation. The patient smokes but has not had pulmonary function testing. Which of the following is **NOT** true?
A. If OHS is not recognized and treated, the long-term risk of mortality is high.
B. A diagnosis of COPD should be confirmed by pulmonary function testing.
C. The female gender is associated with lower risk of OHS.
D. If severe OSA is present, effective long-term PAP treatment can result in resolution or improvement of daytime hypercapnia.

ANSWERS

1. D. Obesity is the best documented risk factor of those listed.

2. D. Approximately 10% to 20% of OHS patients do not have OSA but simply have daytime hypoventilation that worsens during sleep.

3. D. This option completely describes the criteria for adult OSA.

4. A. This describes a patient with a high probability of moderate to severe OSA who does not have a comorbid medical disorder such as CHF or a neuromuscular disorder. The patient in C may well have sleep apnea but is not considered to have a high probability of having OSA based on lack of witnessed apnea. PSG rather than HSAT is the best diagnostic option.

5. C. The prevalence of OSA in Japan and the United States is similar. Obesity is not the only risk factor for OSA. A normal BMI does not rule out the presence of OSA.

6. C. Insomnia or nonrestorative sleep is more often a presenting complaint in women with OSA compared with men. Women tend to have more hypopneas than apneas, REM-associated OSA is common, and women have a lower AHI for a given BMI compared with men. In addition, in the OHS there is no male predominance.

7. C. This patient almost certainly has the OLS. A sawtooth pattern means discrete events are present, and sleep apnea is almost certainly present. Most oximetry reports also provide an oxygen desaturation index, which is a rough estimate of the expected AHI. Daytime hypercapnia can occur with only mild to moderate COPD in patients with the OLS. Supplemental oxygen alone can worsen nighttime hypercapnia, and the long-term prognosis is unfavorable if the patient is not treated with both positive airway pressure and supplemental oxygen (if needed).

8. C. There is no gender predominance in the OHS. Studies have shown that a large percentage of obese patients admitted with hypercapnic respiratory failure are incorrectly diagnosed as having a COPD exacerbation. That is , later pulmonary function testing testing did not confirm a diagnosis of COPD. A diagnosis of COPD should be confirmed by pulmonary function testing if not previously performed. If OHS is not recognized as the cause of hypercapnic respriatory failure and treated appropriately, there is a high mortality risk.

SUGGESTED READING

American Academy of Sleep Medicine. *International Classification of Sleep Disorders*. 3rd ed. text revision. American Academy of Sleep Medicine; 2023.

Kapur VK, Auckley DH, Chowdhuri S, et al. Clinical practice guideline for diagnostic testing for adult obstructive sleep apnea: an American Academy of Sleep Medicine clinical practice guideline. *J Clin Sleep Med*. 2017;13(3):479-504.

Malhotra A, Ayappa I, Ayas N, et al. Metrics of sleep apnea severity: beyond the apnea-hypopnea index. *Sleep*. 2021;44(7):zsab030.

Mokhlesi B, Masa JF, Brozek JL, et al. Evaluation and management of obesity hypoventilation syndrome. An Official American Thoracic Society Clinical

Practice Guideline. *Am J Respir Crit Care Med.* 2019;200(3):e6-e24. Erratum in: *Am J Respir Crit Care Med.* 2019;200(10):1326.

Owens RL, Macrea MM, Teodorescu M. The overlaps of asthma or COPD with OSA: a focused review. *Respirology.* 2017;22(6):1073-1083.

Troester MM, Quan SF, Berry RB, et al.; for the American Academy of Sleep Medicine. *The AASM Manual for the Scoring of Sleep and Associated Events: Rules, Terminology and Technical Specifications.* Version 3. American Academy of Sleep Medicine; 2023.

REFERENCES

1. Burwell C, Robin E, Whaley R, Bickelman A. Extreme obesity associated with alveolar hypoventilation- a pickwickian syndrome. *Am J Med.* 1956;21:811-818.
2. Guilleminault C, Tilkian A, Dement WC. The sleep apnea syndromes. *Annu Rev Med.* 1976;27:465-484.
3. Guilleminault C. Obstructive sleep apnea: the clinical syndrome and historical perspective. *Med Clin North Am.* 1985;69:1187-1203.
4. Remmers JE, Degroot WJ, Sauerland EK, et al. Pathogenesis of upper airway occlusion during sleep. *J Appl Physiol.* 1978;44:931-938.
5. Block AJ, Boysen PG, Wynne JW, Hunt LA. Sleep apnea, hypopnea, and oxygen desaturation in normal subjects. *N Engl J Med.* 1979;300:513-517.
6. Gould GA, Whyte KF, Rhind GB, et al. The sleep hypopnea syndrome. *Am Rev Respir Dis.* 1988;137:895-888.
7. Redline S, Sanders M. Hypopnea, a floating metric: implications for prevalence, morbidity estimates, and case finding. *Sleep.* 1997;20:1209-1217.
8. Sleep-related breathing disorders in adults: recommendations for syndrome definition and measurement techniques in clinical research. The Report of an American Academy of Sleep Medicine Task Force. *Sleep.* 1999;22(5):667-689.
9. Redline S, Kapur VK, Sanders MH, et al. Effects of varying approaches for identifying respiratory disturbances on sleep apnea assessment. *Am J Respir Crit Care Med.* 2000;161:369-374.
10. Berry RB, Abreu AR, Krishnan V, Quan SF, Strollo PJ, Malhotra RK. A transition to the American Academy of Sleep Medicine-recommended hypopnea definition in adults: initiatives of the Hypopnea Scoring Rule Task Force. *J Clin Sleep Med.* 2022;18(5):1419-1425.
11. Iber C, Ancoli-Israel S, Chesson A, Quan SF; for the American Academy of Sleep Medicine: *The AASM Manual for Scoring of Sleep and Associated Events: Rules, Terminology and Technical Specifications.* American Academy of Sleep Medicine; 2007.
12. Berry RB, Budhiraja R, Gottlieb DJ, et al. American Academy of Sleep Medicine. Rules for scoring respiratory events in sleep: update of the 2007 *AASM Manual for the Scoring of Sleep and Associated Events.* Deliberations of the Sleep Apnea Definitions Task Force of the American Academy of Sleep Medicine. *J Clin Sleep Med.* 2012;8(5):597-619.
13. Berry RB, Quan SF, Abreu AR, et al.; for the American Academy of Sleep Medicine. *The AASM Manual for the Scoring of Sleep and Associated Events: Rules, Terminology and Technical Specifications.* Version 2.6. American Academy of Sleep Medicine; 2020.
14. Troester MM, Quan SF, Berry RB, et al.; for the American Academy of Sleep Medicine. *The AASM Manual for the Scoring of Sleep and Associated Events: Rules, Terminology and Technical Specifications.* Version 3. American Academy of Sleep Medicine; 2023.
15. Malhotra A, Ayappa I, Ayas N, et al. Metrics of sleep apnea severity: beyond the apnea-hypopnea index. *Sleep.* 2021;44(7):zsab030.
16. American Academy of Sleep Medicine. *International Classification of Sleep Disorders.* 3rd ed. text revision. American Academy of Sleep Medicine; 2023.
17. American Academy of Sleep Medicine. *International Classification of Sleep Disorders.* 3rd ed. American Academy of Sleep Medicine; 2014.
18. Centers for Medicare and Medicaid Services. *PAP Devices for treatment of OSA. Excerpt from L33718.* Available at: https://www.cms.gov/medicare-coverage-database/view/lcd.aspx?lcdid=33718&ver=48&=. Accessed December 10, 2023.
19. Kushida CA, Littner MR, Morgenthaler T, et al. Practice parameters for the indications for polysomnography and related procedures. An update for 2005. *Sleep.* 2005;28:499-521.
20. Kapur VK, Auckley DH, Chowdhuri S, et al. Clinical practice guideline for diagnostic testing for adult obstructive sleep apnea: an American Academy of Sleep Medicine clinical practice guideline. *J Clin Sleep Med.* 2017;13(3):479-504.
21. Epstein LJ, Kristo D, Strollo PJ, et al. Clinical guideline for the evaluation, management, and long-term care of obstructive sleep apnea in adults. *J Clin Sleep Med.* 2009;5:263-276.
22. Gottlieb DJ, Punjabi NM. Diagnosis and management of obstructive sleep apnea: a review. *JAMA.* 2020;323(14):1389-1400.
23. Johns MW. Daytime sleepiness, snoring, and obstructive sleep apnea. The Epworth Sleepiness Scale. *Chest.* 1993;103:30-36.
24. Gottlieb DJ, Whitney CW, Bonekat WH, et al. Relation of sleepiness to respiratory disturbance index. *Am J Respir Crit Care Med.* 1999;159:502-507.
25. Kapur VK, Baldwin CM, Resnick HE, et al. Sleepiness in patients with moderate to severe sleep-disordered breathing. *Sleep.* 2005;28(4):472-477.
26. Shepertycky MR, Bano K, Kryger MH. Differences between men and women in the clinical presentation of patients diagnosed with obstructive sleep apnea syndrome. *Sleep.* 2005;28:309-314.
27. Wimms A, Woehrle H, Ketheeswaran S, Ramanan D, Armitstead J. Obstructive sleep apnea in women: specific issues and interventions. *Biomed Res Int.* 2016;2016:1764837.
28. Kapsimalis F, Kryger MH. Gender and obstructive sleep apnea syndrome, part 1: clinical features. *Sleep.* 2002;25(4):412-419.
29. Khalid F, Ayache M, Auckley D. The differential impact of respiratory event scoring criteria on CPAP eligibility in women and men. *J Clin Sleep Med.* 2021;17(12):2409-2414.
30. Nuckton TJ, Glidden DV, Browner WS, Claman DM. Physical examination: Mallampati score as an independent predictor of obstructive sleep apnea. *Sleep.* 2006;29:903-908.
31. Friedman M, Tanyeri H, La Rosa M, et al. Clinical predictors of obstructive sleep apnea. *Laryngoscope.* 1999;109(12):1901-1907.
32. Flemons WW. Clinical practice. Obstructive sleep apnea. *N Engl J Med.* 2002;347(7):498-504.
33. Flemons W, Whitelaw WA, Bryant R, Remmers JE. Likelihood ratios for a sleep apnea clinical prediction rule. *Am J Respir Care Med.* 1994;150:1279-1285.
34. Mokhlesi B, Tulaimat A, Faibussowitsch I, Wang Y, Evans AT. Obesity hypoventilation syndrome: prevalence and predictors in patients with obstructive sleep apnea. *Sleep Breath.* 2007;11(2):117-124.
35. Netzer NC, Stoohs RA, Netzer CM, et al. Using the Berlin questionnaire to identify patients at risk for the sleep apnea syndrome. *Ann Intern Med.* 1999;131:485-491.
36. Chung F, Abdullah HR, Liao P. STOP-Bang Questionnaire: a practical approach to screen for obstructive sleep apnea. *Chest.* 2016;149(3):631-638.
37. Collop NA, Anderson WM, Boehlecke B, et al.; Portable Monitoring Task Force of the American Academy of Sleep Medicine. Clinical guidelines for the use of unattended portable monitors in the diagnosis of obstructive sleep apnea in adult patients. Portable Monitoring Task Force of the American Academy of Sleep Medicine. *J Clin Sleep Med.* 2007; 3(7):737-747.
38. Findley LJ, Wilhoit SC, Suratt PM. Apnea duration and hypoxemia during REM sleep in patients with obstructive sleep apnea. *Chest.* 1985; 87(4):432-436.
39. Azarbarzin A, Sands SA, Stone KL, et al. The hypoxic burden of sleep apnoea predicts cardiovascular disease-related mortality: the Osteoporotic Fractures in Men Study and the Sleep Heart Health Study. *Eur Heart J.* 2019;40(14):1149-1157. Erratum in: *Eur Heart J.* 2019; 40(14):1157.
40. Azarbarzin A, Sands SA, Taranto-Montemurro L, et al. The sleep apnea-specific hypoxic burden predicts incident heart failure. *Chest.* 2020;158(2): 739-750.
41. Oksenberg A, Khamaysi I, Silverberg DS, Tarasiuk A. Association of body position with severity of apneic events in patients with severe nonpositional obstructive sleep apnea. *Chest.* 2000;118(4):1018-1024.
42. Oksenberg A, Silverberg DS, Arons E, Radwan H. Positional vs. nonpositional obstructive sleep apnea patients: anthropomorphic, nocturnal polysomnographic, and multiple sleep latency test data. *Chest.* 1997;112(3):629-639.
43. Haba-Rubio J, Janssens JP, Rochat T, Sforza E. Rapid eye movement-related disordered breathing: clinical and polysomnographic features. *Chest.* 2005;128(5):3350-3357.
44. Oksenberg A, Arons E, Nasser K, Vander T, Radwan H. REM-related obstructive sleep apnea: the effect of body position. *J Clin Sleep Med.* 2010;6(4):343-348.
45. Punjabi NM, Patil S, Crainiceanu C, Aurora RN. Variability and misclassification of sleep apnea severity based on multi-night testing. *Chest.* 2020;158(1):365-373.
46. Dzierzewski JM, Dautovich ND, Rybarczyk B, Taylor SA. Night-to-night fluctuations in sleep apnea severity: diagnostic and treatment implications. *J Clin Sleep Med.* 2020;16(4):539-544.
47. Tschopp S, Wimmer W, Caversaccio M, Borner U, Tschopp K. Night-to-night variability in obstructive sleep apnea using peripheral arterial tonometry: a case for multiple night testing. *J Clin Sleep Med.* 2021; 17(9):1751-1758.
48. Bonsignore MR, Romano S, Marrone O, Chiodi M, Bonsignore G. Different heart rate patterns in obstructive apneas during NREM sleep. *Sleep.* 1997;20(12):1167-1174.
49. Azarbarzin A, Sands SA, Younes M, et al. The sleep apnea-specific pulse-rate response predicts cardiovascular morbidity and mortality. *Am J Respir Crit Care Med.* 2021;203(12):1546-1555.

50. Eckert D, White D, Jordan A, et al. Defining phenotypic causes of obstructive sleep apnea. Am J Respir Crit Care Med. 2013;188(8): 996–1004.
51. Zinchuk A, Yaggi HK. Phenotypic subtypes of OSA: a challenge and opportunity for precision medicine. *Chest*. 2020;157(2):403-420.
52. Hirotsu C, Haba-Rubio J, Andries D, et al. Effect of three hypopnea scoring criteria on OSA prevalence and associated comorbidities in the general population. *J Clin Sleep Med*. 2019;15(2):183-194.
53. Heinzer R, Vat S, Marques-Vidal P, et al. Prevalence of sleep-disordered breathing in the general population: the HypnoLaus study. *Lancet Respir Med*. 2015;3(4):310-318.
54. Young T, Palta M, Dempsey J, Skatrud J, Weber S, Badr S. The occurrence of sleep-disordered breathing among middle-aged adults. *N Engl J Med*. 1993;328(17):1230-1235.
55. Young T, Peppard PE, Gottlieb DJ. Epidemiology of obstructive sleep apnea: a population health perspective. *Am J Respir Crit Care Med*. 2002;165(9):1217-1239.
56. Young T, Evans L, Finn L, Palta M. Estimation of the clinically diagnosed proportion of sleep apnea syndrome in middle-aged men and women. *Sleep*. 1997;20(9):705-706.
57. Punjabi NM. The epidemiology of adult obstructive sleep apnea. *Proc Am Thorac Soc*. 2008;5(2):136-143.
58. Benjafield AV, Ayas NT, Eastwood PR, et al. Estimation of the global prevalence and burden of obstructive sleep apnoea: a literature-based analysis. *Lancet Respir Med*. 2019;7(8):687-698.
59. Peppard PE, Young T, Barnet JH, Palta M, Hagen EW, Hla KM. Increased prevalence of sleep-disordered breathing in adults. *Am J Epidemiol*. 2013;177(9):1006-1014.
60. Ruehland WR, Rochford PD, O'Donoghue FJ, Pierce RJ, Singh P, Thornton AT. The new AASM criteria for scoring hypopneas: impact on the apnea hypopnea index. *Sleep*. 2009;32(2):150-157.
61. Peppard PE, Young T, Palta M, Dempsey J, Skatrud J. Longitudinal study of moderate weight change and sleep-disordered breathing. *JAMA*. 2000;284(23):3015-3021.
62. Smith PL, Gold AR, Meyers DA, Haponik EF, Bleecker ER. Weight loss in mildly to moderately obese patients with obstructive sleep apnea. *Ann Intern Med*. 1985;103(6 Pt 1):850-855.
63. Simpson L, Mukherjee S, Cooper MN, et al. Sex differences in the association of regional fat distribution with the severity of obstructive sleep apnea. *Sleep*. 2010;33(4):467-474. Erratum in: *Sleep*. 2010;33(8).
64. Young T, Shahar E, Nieto FJ, et al.; Sleep Heart Health Study Research Group. Predictors of sleep-disordered breathing in community-dwelling adults: the Sleep Heart Health Study. *Arch Intern Med*. 2002;162(8):893-900.
65. Bixler EO, Vgontzas AN, Lin HM, et al. Prevalence of sleep-disordered breathing in women: effects of gender. *Am J Respir Crit Care Med*. 2001; 163(3 Pt 1):608-613.
66. Tishler PV, Larkin EK, Schluchter MD, Redline S. Incidence of sleep-disordered breathing in an urban adult population: the relative importance of risk factors in the development of sleep-disordered breathing. *JAMA*. 2003;289(17):2230-2237.
67. Bonsignore MR, Saaresranta T, Riha RL. Sex differences in obstructive sleep apnoea. *Eur Respir Rev*. 2019;28(154):190030.
68. O'Connor C, Thornley KS, Hanly PJ. Gender differences in the polysomnographic features of obstructive sleep apnea. *Am J Respir Crit Care Med*. 2000;161(5):1465-1472.
69. Huang T, Lin BM, Markt SC, et al. Sex differences in the associations of obstructive sleep apnoea with epidemiological factors. *Eur Respir J*. 2018; 51(3):1702421.
70. Bixler EO, Vgontzas AN, Ten Have T, Tyson K, Kales A. Effects of age on sleep apnea in men: I. Prevalence and severity. *Am J Respir Crit Care Med*. 1998;157(1):144-148.
71. Fietze I, Laharnar N, Obst A, et al. Prevalence and association analysis of obstructive sleep apnea with gender and age differences—results of SHIP-Trend. *J Sleep Res*. 2019;28(5):e12770.
72. Enright PL, Newman AB, Wahl PW, Manolio TA, Haponik EF, Boyle PJ. Prevalence and correlates of snoring and observed apneas in 5,201 older adults. *Sleep*. 1996;19(7):531-538.
73. Endeshaw Y. Clinical characteristics of obstructive sleep apnea in community-dwelling older adults. *J Am Geriatr Soc*. 2006;54(11):1740-1744.
74. Young T, Finn L, Austin D, Peterson A. Menopausal status and sleep-disordered breathing in the Wisconsin Sleep Cohort Study. *Am J Respir Crit Care Med*. 2003;167(9):1181-1185.
75. Shahar E, Redline S, Young T, et al. Hormone replacement therapy and sleep-disordered breathing. *Am J Respir Crit Care Med*. 2003;167(9):1186-1192.
76. Bixler EO, Vgontzas AN, Lin HM, et al. Prevalence of sleep-disordered breathing in women: effects of gender. *Am J Respir Crit Care Med*. 2001;163(3 Pt 1):608-613.
77. Manber R, Kuo TF, Cataldo N, Colrain IM. The effects of hormone replacement therapy on sleep-disordered breathing in postmenopausal women: a pilot study. *Sleep*. 2003;26(2):163-168.
78. Anttalainen U, Saaresranta T, Vahlberg T, Polo O. Short-term medroxyprogesterone acetate in postmenopausal women with sleep-disordered breathing: a placebo-controlled, randomized, double-blind, parallel-group study. *Menopause*. 2014;21(4):361-368.
79. Redline S, Tishler PV, Hans MG, et al. Racial differences in sleep-disordered breathing in African-Americans and Caucasians. *Am J Respir Crit Care Med*. 1997;155(1):186-192. Erratum in: *Am J Respir Crit Care Med*. 1997;155(5):1820.
80. Ip MS, Lam B, Lauder IJ, et al. A community study of sleep-disordered breathing in middle-aged Chinese men in Hong Kong. *Chest*. 2001; 119(1):62-96.
81. Li KK, Kushida C, Powell NB, Riley RW, Guilleminault C. Obstructive sleep apnea syndrome: a comparison between Far-East Asian and white men. *Laryngoscope*. 2000;110(10 Pt 1):1689-1693.
82. Wetter DW, Young TB, Bidwell TR, Badr MS, Palta M. Smoking as a risk factor for sleep-disordered breathing. *Arch Intern Med*. 1994; 154(19):2219-2224.
83. Nieto FJ, Young TB, Lind BK, et al. Association of sleep-disordered breathing, sleep apnea, and hypertension in a large community based study. Sleep Heart Health Study. *JAMA*. 2000;283(1):1829-1836.
84. Krishnan V, Dixon-Williams S, Thornton JD. Where there is smoke ... there is sleep apnea: exploring the relationship between smoking and sleep apnea. *Chest*. 2014;146(6):1673-1680.
85. Burgos-Sanchez C, Jones NN, Avillion M, et al. Impact of alcohol consumption on snoring and sleep apnea: a systematic review and meta-analysis. *Otolaryngol Head Neck Surg*. 2020;163(6):1078-1086.
86. Giustina A, Barkan A, Beckers A, et al. A consensus on the diagnosis and treatment of acromegaly comorbidities: an update. *J Clin Endocrinol Metab*. 2020;105(4):dgz096.
87. Parolin M, Dassie F, Alessio L, et al. Obstructive sleep apnea in acromegaly and the effect of treatment: a systematic review and meta-analysis. *J Clin Endocrinol Metab*. 2020;105(3):dgz116.
88. Thavaraputta S, Dennis JA, Laoveeravat P, Nugent K, Rivas AM. Hypothyroidism and its association with sleep apnea among adults in the United States: NHANES 2007–2008. *J Clin Endocrinol Metab*. 2019;104(11):4990-4997.
89. De Meyer MMD, Jacquet W, Vanderveken OM, Marks LAM. Systematic review of the different aspects of primary snoring. *Sleep Med Rev*. 2019;45:88-94.
90. Lee SA, Amis TC, Byth K, et al. Heavy snoring as a cause of carotid artery atherosclerosis. *Sleep*. 2008;31(9):1207-1213.
91. Anttalainen U, Tenhunen M, Rimpilä V, et al. Prolonged partial upper airway obstruction during sleep an underdiagnosed phenotype of sleep-disordered breathing. *Eur Clin Respir J*. 2016;3:31806.
92. Guilleminault C, Stoohs R, Clerk A, Cetel M, Maistros P. A cause of excessive daytime sleepiness. The upper airway resistance syndrome. *Chest*. 1993;104(3):781-787.
93. Masa JF, Corral J, Teran J, et al. Apnoeic and obstructive nonapnoeic sleep respiratory events. *Eur Respir J*. 2009;34(1):156-161.
94. Cracowski C, Pépin JL, Wuyam B, Lévy P. Characterization of obstructive nonapneic respiratory events in moderate sleep apnea syndrome. *Am J Respir Crit Care Med*. 2001;164(6):944-948.
95. Varga AW, Mokhlesi B. REM obstructive sleep apnea: risk for adverse health outcomes and novel treatments. *Sleep Breath*. 2019;23(2): 413-423.
96. Conwell W, Patel B, Doeing D, et al. Prevalence, clinical features, and CPAP adherence in REM-related sleep-disordered breathing: a cross-sectional analysis of a large clinical population. *Sleep Breath*. 2012;16(2):519-526.
97. Kass JE, Akers SM, Bartter TC, et al. REM-specific sleep-disordered breathing: a possible cause of excessive daytime sleepiness. *Am J Respir Crit Care Med*. 1996;154:167-169.
98. Chervin RD, Aldrich MS. The relation between multiple sleep latency test findings and the frequency of apneic events in REM and non-REM sleep. *Chest*. 1998;113(4):980-984.
99. Khan A, Harrison SL, Kezirian EJ, et al.; Osteoporotic Fractures in Men (MrOS) Study Research Group. Obstructive sleep apnea during rapid eye movement sleep, daytime sleepiness, and quality of life in older men in Osteoporotic Fractures in Men (MrOS) Sleep Study. *J Clin Sleep Med*. 2013;9(3):191-198.
100. Blackwell T, Yaffe K, Ancoli-Israel S, et al.; Osteoporotic Fractures in Men Study Group. Associations between sleep architecture and sleep-disordered breathing and cognition in older community-dwelling men: the Osteoporotic Fractures in Men Sleep Study. *J Am Geriatr Soc*. 2011;59(12):2217-2225.

101. Chami HA, Baldwin CM, Silverman A, et al. Sleepiness, quality of life, and sleep maintenance in REM versus non-REM sleep-disordered breathing. *Am J Respir Crit Care Med*. 2010;181(9):997-1002.
102. Su CS, Liu KT, Panjapornpon K, Andrews N, Foldvary-Schaefer N. Functional outcomes in patients with REM-related obstructive sleep apnea treated with positive airway pressure therapy. *J Clin Sleep Med*. 2012;8(3):243-247.
103. Mokhlesi B, Finn LA, Hagen EW, et al. Obstructive sleep apnea during REM sleep and hypertension. Results of the Wisconsin Sleep Cohort. *Am J Respir Crit Care Med*. 2014;190(10):1158-1167.
104. Mokhlesi B, Hagen EW, Finn LA, et al. Obstructive sleep apnoea during REM sleep and incident non-dipping of nocturnal blood pressure: a longitudinal analysis of the Wisconsin Sleep Cohort. *Thorax*. 2015;70:1062-1069.
105. Appleton SL, Vakulin A, Martin SA, et al. Hypertension is associated with undiagnosed OSA during rapid eye movement sleep. *Chest*. 2016;150:495-505.
106. Aurora RN, Crainiceanu C, Gottlieb DJ, et al. Obstructive sleep apnea during REM sleep and cardiovascular disease. *Am J Respir Crit Care Med*. 2018;197(5):653-660.
107. BaHammam AS, Pirzada AR, Pandi-Perumal SR. Neurocognitive, mood changes, and sleepiness in patients with REM-predominant obstructive sleep apnea. *Sleep Breath*. 2023;27(1):57-66.
108. Wiegand L, Zwillich CW, Wiegand D, White DP. Changes in upper airway muscle activation and ventilation during phasic REM sleep in normal men. *J Appl Physiol (1985)*. 1991;71(2):488-497.
109. Grace KP, Hughes SW, Horner RL. Identification of the mechanism mediating genioglossus muscle suppression in REM sleep. *Am J Respir Crit Care Med*. 2013;187(3):311-319.
110. Penzel T, Moeller M, Becker HF. Effects of sleep position and sleep stage on collapsibility of the upper airways in sleep apnea. *Sleep*. 2001;24:90-95.
111. Boudewyns A, Punjabi N, Van de Heyning PH, et al. Abbreviated method for assessing upper airway function in obstructive sleep apnea. *Chest*. 2000;118:1031-1041.
112. Carberry JC, Jordan AS, White DP, et al. Upper airway collapsibility (PCRIT) and pharyngeal dilator muscle activity are sleep stage dependent. *Sleep*. 2016;39(3):511-521.
113. Douglas NJ, White DP, Weil JV, et al. Hypercapnic ventilatory response in sleeping adults. *Am Rev Respir Dis*. 1982;126(5):758-762.
114. Joosten SA, Landry SA, Wong A-M, et al. Assessing the physiologic endotypes responsible for REM- and NREM-based OSA. *Chest*. 2021;159(5):1998-2007.
115. Messineo L, Eckert DJ, Taranto-Montemurro L, et al. Ventilatory drive withdrawal rather than reduced genioglossus compensation as a mechanism of obstructive sleep apnea in REM sleep. *Am J Respir Crit Care Med*. 2022;205(2):219-232.
116. Piper AJ, Grunstein RR. Obesity hypoventilation syndrome: mechanisms and management. *Am J Respir Crit Care Med*. 2011;183(3):292-298.
117. Masa JF, Pépin JL, Borel JC, et al. Obesity hypoventilation syndrome. *Eur Respir Rev*. 2019;28(151):180097.
118. Randerath W, Verbraecken J, Andreas S, et al. Definition, discrimination, diagnosis and treatment of central breathing disturbances during sleep. *Eur Respir J*. 2017;49(1):1600959.
119. Kaw R, Hernandez AV, Walker E, et al. Determinants of hypercapnia in obese patients with obstructive sleep apnea: a systematic review and meta analysis of cohort studies. *Chest*. 2009;136(3):787-796.
120. Berger KI, Ayappa I, Chatr-Amontri B, et al. Obesity hypoventilation syndrome as a spectrum of respiratory disturbances during sleep. *Chest*. 2001;120(4):1231-1238.
121. Shivaram U, Cash ME, Beal A. Nasal continuous positive airway pressure in decompensated hypercapnic respiratory failure as a complication of sleep apnea. *Chest*. 1993;104(3):770-774.
122. Marik PE, Desai H. Characteristics of patients with the "malignant obesity hypoventilation syndrome" admitted to an ICU. *J Intensive Care Med*. 2013;28(2):124-130.
123. Hollier CA, Harmer AR, Maxwell LJ, et al. Moderate concentrations of supplemental oxygen worsen hypercapnia in obesity hypoventilation syndrome: a randomised crossover study. *Thorax*. 2014;69(4):346-353.
124. Nowbar S, Burkart KM, Gonzales R, et al. Obesity-associated hypoventilation in hospitalized patients: prevalence, effects, and outcome. *Am J Med*. 2004;116(1):1-7.
125. Priou P, Hamel JF, Person C, et al. Long-term outcome of noninvasive positive pressure ventilation for obesity hypoventilation syndrome. *Chest*. 2010;138(1):84-90.
126. Budweiser S, Riedl SG, Jörres RA, Heinemann F, Pfeifer M. Mortality and prognostic factors in patients with obesity-hypoventilation syndrome undergoing noninvasive ventilation. *J Intern Med*. 2007;261(4):375-383.
127. Mokhlesi B, Masa JF, Brozek JL, et al. Evaluation and management of obesity hypoventilation syndrome. An official American Thoracic Society clinical practice guideline. *Am J Respir Crit Care Med*. 2019;200(3):e6-e24. Erratum in: *Am J Respir Crit Care Med*. 2019;200(10):1326.
128. Chung Y, Garden FL, Jee AS, et al. Supine awake oximetry as a screening tool for daytime hypercapnia in super-obese patients. *Intern Med J*. 2017;47(10):1136-1141.
129. Verbraecken J, McNicholas WT. Respiratory mechanics and ventilatory control in overlap syndrome and obesity hypoventilation. *Respir Res*. 2013;14(1):132.
130. Phipps PR, Starritt E, Caterson I, Grunstein RR. Association of serum leptin with hypoventilation in human obesity. *Thorax*. 2002;57(1):75-76.
131. Fitzpatrick M. Leptin and the obesity hypoventilation syndrome: a leap of faith? *Thorax*. 2002;57(1):1-2.
132. Redolfi S, Corda L, La Piana G, Spandrio S, Prometti P, Tantucci C. Long-term non-invasive ventilation increases chemosensitivity and leptin in obesity-hypoventilation syndrome. *Respir Med*. 2007;101(6):1191-1195.
133. Yee BJ, Cheung J, Phipps P, et al. Treatment of obesity hypoventilation syndrome and serum leptin. *Respiration*. 2006;73(2):209-212.
134. Berger KI, Ayappa I, Sorkin IB, et al. CO(2) homeostasis during periodic breathing in obstructive sleep apnea. *J Appl Physiol (1985)*. 2000;88(1):257-264.
135. Berger KI, Ayappa I, Sorkin IB, et al. Postevent ventilation as a function of CO2 load during respiratory events in obstructive sleep apnea. *J Appl Physiol (1985)*. 2002;93(3):917-924.
136. Berthon-Jones M, Sullivan CE. Time course of change in ventilatory response to CO2 with long-term CPAP therapy for obstructive sleep apnea. *Am Rev Respir Dis*. 1987;135(1):144-147.
137. Lin CC. Effect of nasal CPAP on ventilatory drive in normocapnic and hypercapnic patients with obstructive sleep apnoea syndrome. *Eur Respir J*. 1994;7(11):2005-2010.
138. Mokhlesi B, Won CH, Make BJ, et al.; ONMAP Technical Expert Panel. Optimal NIV Medicare access promotion: patients with hypoventilation syndromes: a technical expert panel report from the American College of Chest Physicians, the American Association for Respiratory Care, the American Academy of Sleep Medicine, and the American Thoracic Society. *Chest*. 2021;160(5):e377-e387.
139. Centers for Medicare and Medicaid Services. Respiratory Assist Devices. https://www.cms.gov/medicare-coverage-database/view/lcd.aspx?lcdid=33800&ver=26&KeyWord=respiratory+assis&KeyWordLookUp=Title&KeyWordSearchType=Exact&bc=CAAAAAAAAAAA. [Accessed 10 December 2023].
140. Weitzenblum E, Chaouat A, Kessler R, Canuet M. Overlap syndrome. Obstructive sleep apnea syndrome in patients with chronic obstructive pulmonary disease. *Proc Thorac Soc*. 2008;5:237-241.
141. McNicholas WT. COPD-OSA overlap syndrome: evolving evidence regarding epidemiology, clinical consequences, and management. *Chest*. 2017;152(6):1318-1326.
142. Owens RL, Macrea MM, Teodorescu M. The overlaps of asthma or COPD with OSA: a focused review. *Respirology*. 2017;22(6):1073-1083.
143. Sanders MH, Newman AB, Haggerty CL, et al. Sleep and sleep disordered breathing in adults with predominantly mild obstructive airway disease. *Am J Respir Crit Care Med*. 2003;167:7-14.
144. Resta O, Foschino Barbaro MP, Brindicci C, et al. Hypercapnia in overlap syndrome: possible determinant factors. *Sleep Breath*. 2002;6(1):11-18.
145. Goldstein RS, Ramcharan V, Bowes G, et al. Effect of supplemental nocturnal oxygen on gas exchange in patients with severe obstructive lung disease. *N Engl J Med*. 1984;310:425-429.
146. Fletcher EC, Schaaf JW, Miller J, Fletcher JG. Long-term cardiopulmonary sequelae in patients with sleep apnea and chronic lung disease. *Am Rev Respir Dis*. 1987;135:525-533.
147. Machado MCL, Vollmer WM, Togeiro SM, et al. CPAP and survival in moderate to severe obstructive sleep apnea syndrome and hypoxemic COPD. *Eur Respir J*. 2010;35:132-137.
148. Marin JM, Soriano JB, Carrizo SJ, et al. Outcomes in patients with chronic obstructive pulmonary disease and obstructive sleep apnea. *Am J Respir Crit Care Med*. 2010;182:325-331.
149. Stanchina ML, Welicky LM, Donat W, et al. Impact of CPAP use and age on mortality in patients with combined COPD and obstructive sleep apnea: the overlap syndrome. *J Clin Sleep Med*. 2013;9(8):767-772.
150. Sampol G, Sagalés MT, Roca A, de la Calzada MD, Bofill JM, Morell F. Nasal continuous positive airway pressure with supplemental oxygen in coexistent sleep apnoea-hypopnoea syndrome and severe chronic obstructive pulmonary disease. *Eur Respir J*. 1996;9(1):111-116.

Chapter 19

Pathophysiology of Obstructive Sleep Apnea

PATHOGENESIS OF UPPER AIRWAY OBSTRUCTION

Obstructive sleep apnea (OSA) is a heterogeneous disease,[1-9] both from the standpoint of underlying mechanisms (endotypes)[2,4,7,8] and clinical expression (phenotypes). However, many clinicians use the term *phenotype* for both mechanisms and clinical expression. This chapter will consider underlying mechanisms. Since a landmark study by Remmers and colleagues[10] published in 1978, a tremendous number of studies have sought to understand the pathogenesis of upper airway narrowing or occlusion in patients with OSA. Multiple factors determine upper airway patency during sleep (Table 19–1). Different factors may be more or less important in each individual. The major factors include unfavorable upper airway anatomy (small or collapsible), ineffective upper airway muscle responsiveness (to chemical and negative pressure stimuli), instability of ventilatory control (high loop gain), and a low arousal threshold.[1-9] A low arousal threshold may prevent long respiratory events, but it fragments sleep and does not allow sufficient time for upper airway muscle augmentation to stabilize the airway. The arousals may also contribute to the ventilatory control instability. Although obesity is a major risk factor for OSA, only about 50% of OSA patients are obese, and not all obese individuals have sleep apnea. A study to determine the frequency of endotypes in OSA[4] found that 36% of OSA patients had reduced upper airway muscle responsiveness, 37% had a low arousal threshold, and 36% had a high loop gain. Further, 28% had multiple nonanatomical features. Of interest, 19% had a noncollapsible upper airway similar to individuals without OSA. Nonanatomical features were thought to play a significant role in 56% of patients with OSA. It should also be recognized that the endotype factors do not act independently, and *targeting only one factor may not result in clinical improvement*.

Upper Airway Size and Collapsibility

Most patients with OSA have small and collapsible upper airways. However, in some patients nonanatomical factors are the main cause of sleep apnea. In the following sections characteristics of the upper airway predisposing patients for the development of sleep apnea, including size and collapsibility, will be discussed. In most studies of upper airway characteristics there is an *overlap between OSA patients and normal individuals*. It is not unusual for a patient to have some degree of both anatomical and nonanatomical factors.

Anatomical Factors

About 50% of patients with OSA are obese, and obesity can narrow the upper airway. However, nonobese patients can still have an anatomically narrow upper airway. The anatomy of the upper airway of patients with OSA has been studied using cephalometric measurement (traditional radiology),[11,12] computed tomography (CT) scans,[13,14] static and dynamic magnetic resonance imaging (MRI),[15,16] optical coherence tonometry,[17] video endoscopy (and determination of cross-sectional area),[18] and recently, three-dimensional photography (scanning).[19] An important limitation of most of these studies is that the patients were awake, and sleep could change the findings. The upper airway shape as well as the size may be important.[20] Leiter hypothesized that an airway with the long axis horizontally would benefit the most from an increase in the anterior-posterior dimension.[20] However, different levels of the upper airway may have different shapes and findings may apply to one level of the upper airway but not another

Table 19–1 Factors Determining Upper Airway Patency

Open Upper Airway	Closed Upper Airway
Passive Factors	
• Larger, stiffer upper airway (zero or negative P_{CRIT}) • Large bony enclosure • Less soft tissue (including fat) surrounding the upper airway. Thinner lateral pharyngeal walls, smaller tongue) • Higher lung volume • Lateral decubitus posture • Less negative intraluminal pressure	• Smaller, more compliant upper airway (positive P_{CRIT}) • Small bony enclosure • More soft tissue (including fat) surrounding the upper airway. Thicker lateral pharyngeal wall, larger tongue • Lower lung volume • Supine posture • More negative intraluminal pressure • Longer upper airway
Upper Airway Muscle Factors	
• High upper airway muscle activity • Large upper airway muscle response to negative pressure	• Low upper airway muscle activity • Low upper airway muscle response to negative upper airway pressure
Ventilatory Control Stability	
• Stable ventilatory drive • Low loop gain (low controller gain, low plant gain)	• Fluctuating ventilatory drive • High loop gain (high controller gain, high plant gain)
Arousal Threshold	
• High arousal threshold	• Low arousal threshold

P_{CRIT}, Pharyngeal closing pressure of the upper airway.

(velopharyngeal versus hypopharyngeal). The results of the studies are not consistent with respect to upper airway size or shape, likely because of variability in the OSA patients studied and the techniques. In addition, as noted previously, nearly all studies were performed while subjects were awake, and the size or shape of the upper airway may be different during sleep. Some studies also determined changes in airway size in the supine versus lateral positions.[13,14] Findings could differ in patients with or without positional sleep apnea (AHI-supine > 2 × AHI-non-supine). Patients with OSA generally tend to have small upper airways compared with weight-matched normal subjects either secondary to a small bony enclosure[11] or because of increased soft tissue (including fat) surrounding the airway.[15,16] In general, a short and posteriorly placed mandible, a narrow maxilla or a laterally narrow palatal bone structure, a long dependent palate, a large tongue (scalloped or increased tongue fat), a long distance from the hyoid bone to the mandibular plane, nasal obstruction, and thick lateral pharyngeal walls/pharyngeal fat all predispose to upper airway narrowing and collapse during sleep. Whereas some studies found the shape of the upper airways of OSA patients to differ from that of normal individuals (narrower in the lateral dimension),[15,16] others found upper airway shapes narrower in the anterior-posterior dimension.[13,17] A study comparing the passive properties of the upper airway during general anesthesia in normal individuals with those of OSA patients found that the upper airways of OSA patients are narrower and more collapsible.[18] Although some patients have a large parapharyngeal fat pad, tongue fat is also important. Wang and coworkers found that improvement in the apnea-hypopnea index (AHI) after weight loss was associated with *loss of tongue fat*.[21]

Airflow Limitation

Airflow through the pharynx shows various degrees of airflow limitation during sleep. Inspiratory flow limitation is defined by an increase in the pressure drop across the upper airway (more negative supraglottic and intrathoracic pressure) without a corresponding increase in flow rate (Fig. 19–1). This pressure-flow relationship during inspiration is commonly caused by narrowing of a hypotonic upper airway in response to the loss of upper airway muscle tone and increasingly negative intraluminal pressure developed during inspiration.[22,23] However, at sleep onset intraluminal pressure may not be more negative and airway narrowing can be primarily passive, simply due to a reduction in upper muscle activity. A transition from wake to sleep is shown in Figure 19–2A. The first two breaths do *not* show airflow limitation, and inspiratory airflow has a round shape. The third breath, which occurs after sleep onset, demonstrates airflow limitation with a constant flow during the time when the inspiratory pressure (supraglottic pressure) is becoming more negative (increased pressure difference across the upper airway). Note the fall in inspiratory effort at sleep onset (a smaller supraglottic pressure deflection) and a fall in genioglossus (GG) activity (tongue protrusion). Later breaths might reveal increased effort as the respiratory system responds to increases in the arterial partial pressure of carbon dioxide ($PaCO_2$) resulting from a reduction in ventilation (tidal volume [V_T]). In other patients, airflow limitation occurs at sleep onset without a fall

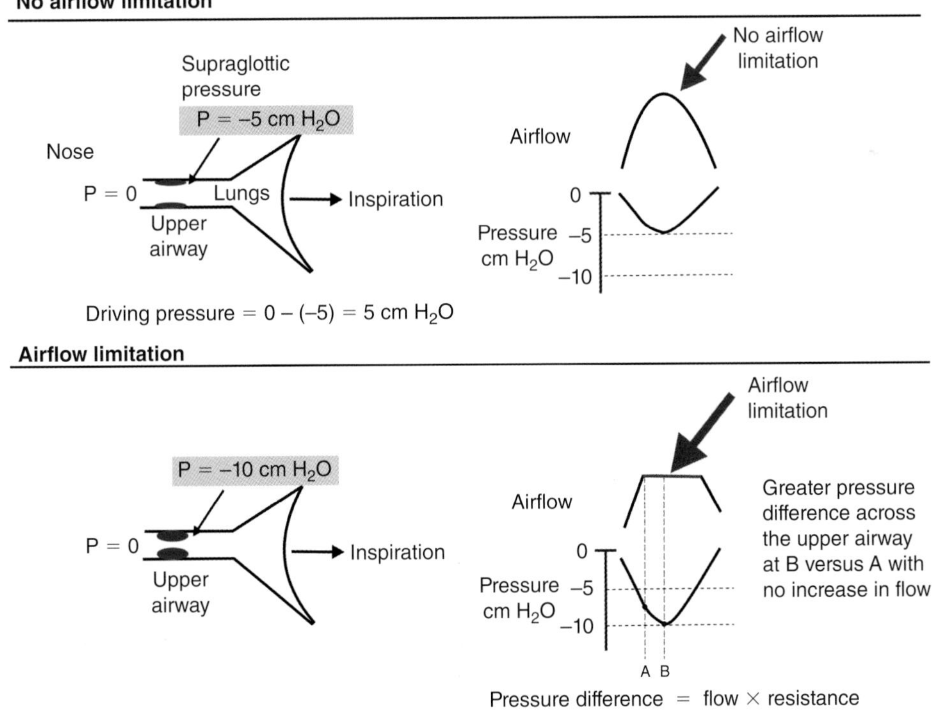

Figure 19–1 *(Top panel)* Normal airflow without flow limitation. The inspiratory waveform is round. *(Bottom panel)* An example of airflow limitation. There is a plateau (constant flow) while the driving pressure across the airway increases. The pressure difference across the upper airway increases from A to B (supraglottic pressure more negative), but flow does not increase. The effective resistance (pressure difference/flow) has increased based on constant airflow associated with more negative supraglottic pressure (higher driving pressure).

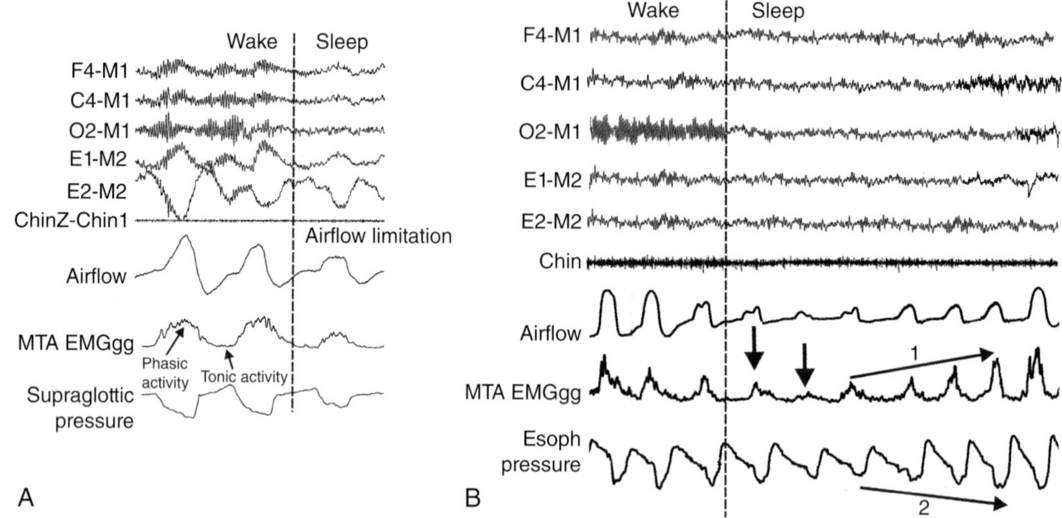

Figure 19–2 **(A)** A transition from wake to sleep with loss of the wakefulness stimulus and decreased genioglossus (GG) EMG activity associated with airflow limitation is shown. In this case the supraglottic pressure deflection also decreased at sleep onset. MTA EMGgg is the moving time average of GG EMG; airflow is measured by a pneumotachograph in a mask over the nose and mouth. **(B)** Transition from wake to sleep with a decrease in the GG activity initially (down arrows) accompanied by airflow limitation. However, over time the GG activity increases stimulated by increasing ventilatory drive, as manifested by increasing esophageal pressure deflections (downsloping arrow at 2). Increasingly negative upper airway pressure also helps increase GG activity. There was improvement in airflow and GG activity *(upsloping arrow at 1)*. Airflow is measured by a pneumotachograph in a mask over the nose and mouth.

or increase in inspiratory effort. In this figure MTA EMGgg is the moving time average of the GG electromyogram (EMG), and airflow is measured using a pneumotachograph in a mask covering the nose and mouth. Figure 19–2B is another example of changes in airflow, GG activity, and esophageal pressure at sleep onset (posterior dominant rhythm/alpha activity in O2-M1 ceases). The first several breaths show airflow limitation, but there is an augmentation in respiratory effort (esophageal pressure deflections) and an increase in GG activity with recovery of airflow.

Upper Airway Collapsibility

The pharynx is not rigid and pharyngeal resistance is not constant. The nonrigid portions of the pharynx tend to become increasingly narrow with more negative inspiratory pressure (Fig. 19–1). In portion of the upper airway with OSA there can be multiple sites of upper airway narrowing (retropalatal, retroglossal, and diffusely with inward collapse of the lateral pharyngeal walls). The portion of the upper airway with the smallest cross-sectional area may change during the inspiration. The collapsibility of the upper airway and tendency for closure can be defined by the pharyngeal critical closing pressure (P_{CRIT}).[23-30]

The P_{CRIT} is determined by applying various positive or negative mask pressures and determining the inspiratory flow rate (Fig. 19–3A).[23-30] This process begins with stable breathing using a level of positive airway pressure (holding pressure) associated with normal flow and minimal upper airway muscle activity and proceeds with a sudden pressure dial down

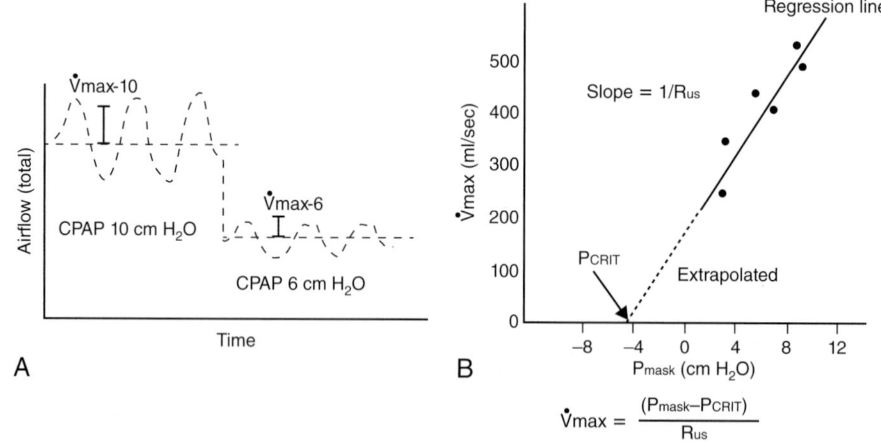

Figure 19–3 **(A)** Schematic of determination of P_{CRIT} by determining changes in airflow associated with a CPAP dial down of pressure (here 10 to 6 cm H_2O). **(B)** Individual airflow measurements at each mask pressure are plotted, and a regression line is extrapolated to a flow of zero. The intercept with the *x*-axis is the P_{CRIT}. The slope of the regression line is (1/Rus).

from stable sleep at the holding pressure with measurement of flow at each dial-down pressure (progressively lower pressure). The inspiratory flow decreases as mask pressure decreases from a more positive pressure (Fig. 19–3B). After each measurement, the level of continuous positive airway pressure (CPAP) is returned to the holding pressure, and after stable sleep occurs there is another abrupt dial down to a different CPAP level. Measurements are made of airflow at different levels of CPAP below the holding pressure. Values of mask pressure and flow are plotted. The mask pressure at which flow is zero is P_{CRIT} (determined by extrapolation of a regression line to zero flow). The relationship between flow and mask pressure is given by Equation 19-1.

$$\dot{V}max = (Pmask - P_{CRIT})/Rus \qquad \text{Equation 19–1}$$

Here, Rus is upstream resistance, and Pmask is the mask pressure. The inverse of the slope of the regression line (1/Rus) is the effective resistance (Δ pressure/Δ flow) and is called the *upstream resistance (Rus)*. The P_{CRIT} values for normal individuals, snorers, obstructive hypopnea (mild to moderate sleep apnea), and obstructive apnea (moderate to severe apnea) are plotted in Figure 19–4.[23,24] During sleep, a positive pressure is needed to keep the airway open ($P_{CRIT} > 0$) in patients with sleep apnea. P_{CRIT} values differ between studies, but a $P_{CRIT} \geq 5$ cm H_2O indicates a highly collapsible upper airway. In normal individuals, the airway does not collapse unless a negative mask pressure is applied (-5 to -8 cm H_2O or more negative) with a gray zone of approximately 0 to -5 cm H_2O (0 to -8 cm H_2O in some studies, Fig. 19–4). In the range 0 to -5 cm H_2O there is overlap between patients with snoring only and patients with OSA. Up to 20% of OSA patients have a similar P_{CRIT} as those individuals without OSA.[4]

The relationship between flow and mask pressure can be modeled using a Starling resistor (Fig. 19–5). This consists of a collapsible segment between rigid tubes.[23] As long as the intraluminal pressure within any point of the collapsible segment is less than P_{CRIT}, the relationship in Figure 19–5C will hold. Creating more negative pressure downstream from the collapsible segment will not increase flow. When the intraluminal pressure along the entire collapsible segment is less than the P_{CRIT}, no flow occurs. The actual breaths after the CPAP dial down used for computation of P_{CRIT} (measurement of inspiratory flow) vary between studies. When P_{CRIT} is determined using the first few breaths (breaths 1 to 3), it is termed "passive P_{CRIT}," and after several breaths and the upper airway muscles have a chance to respond (measuring breaths 3 to 5), the value is considered "active" P_{CRIT}.[30] Whereas different methods have been used to define an active P_{CRIT},[27] a truly passive P_{CRIT} can be determined with anesthesia during drug-induced sleep endoscopy, but this procedure is reserved for research studies or patients in whom upper airway surgery is planned. There is a correlation between P_{CRIT} and the effective CPAP pressure (higher P_{CRIT} associated with higher CPAP), but there is considerable variability (range of effective CPAP pressure for a given P_{CRIT}).[31] The collapsibility of the upper airway can be estimated by procedures during wakefulness, and this is a topic of ongoing research.[32-35] Note that the collapsibility of the upper airway is reduced by breathing at higher lung volumes or sleep in the lateral position, as will be discussed below. Several studies did not show a sleep stage dependence for P_{CRIT} (P_{CRIT} not higher in rapid eye movement [REM] sleep compared with non-rapid eye movement [NREM] sleep).[26,28,29] However, Carberry and coworkers[30] found the upper airway to be more collapsible during REM sleep (higher "active" P_{CRIT}). The authors believe this result depended on studying a larger group of individuals but also may have been due to measurement of airflow several breaths after the CPAP dial down.

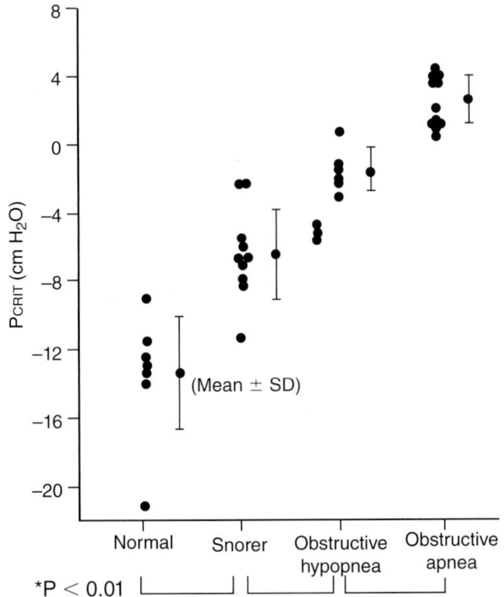

Figure 19–4 Values of P_{CRIT} in normal individuals, snorers, patients with predominantly obstructive hypopnea, and patients with predominantly obstructive apnea (severe). In severe OSA a positive pressure must be present in the upper airway to prevent collapse. Values differ between publications but in general, a value >5 cm H_2O is associated with severe OSA, and 0 to -5 cm H_2O is an overlap region between snorers and milder OSA. A P_{CRIT} < -8 cm H_2O is noted in normal individuals in this study. (Reprinted with permission from Schwartz AR, Smith PL, Kashima HK, et al. Respiratory function of the upper airways. In: Murray JF, Nadel JA, eds. Textbook of respiratory medicine. 2nd ed. Philadelphia: WB Saunders, 1994; 1451-1470.)

Lung Volume, Sleeping Position, and Rostral Fluid Shifts

Upper airway size also has a dependence on lung volume with decreasing airway size as lung volume decreases.[36,37] The upper airways of patients with OSA may have greater lung volume dependence than normal individuals. The lung volume dependence of the upper airway may be mediated via passive distending forces due to a downward tension on upper airway structures during inspiration ("tracheal tug").[38,39] Another way of thinking of the tracheal tug is a decrease in extramural pressure surrounding the airway. Using dynamic MRI, Tong and colleagues[39] found that tracheal displacement during quiet breathing was larger in individuals with more severe sleep apnea. The explanation might be more displaceable upper airway structures or more negative intrathoracic pressure change during tidal breathing. Any fall in end-expiratory volume (functional residual capacity [FRC]) would then reduce upper airway size during tidal breathing during sleep. FRC is known to decrease during sleep,[40] and this would tend to predispose to airway closure. Avraam and colleagues documented a greater decrease in FRC in *overweight* compared with normal weight individuals in the supine position during NREM sleep.[41] No further worsening during REM sleep or differences between men and women was detected. Jordan and colleagues[42] did not

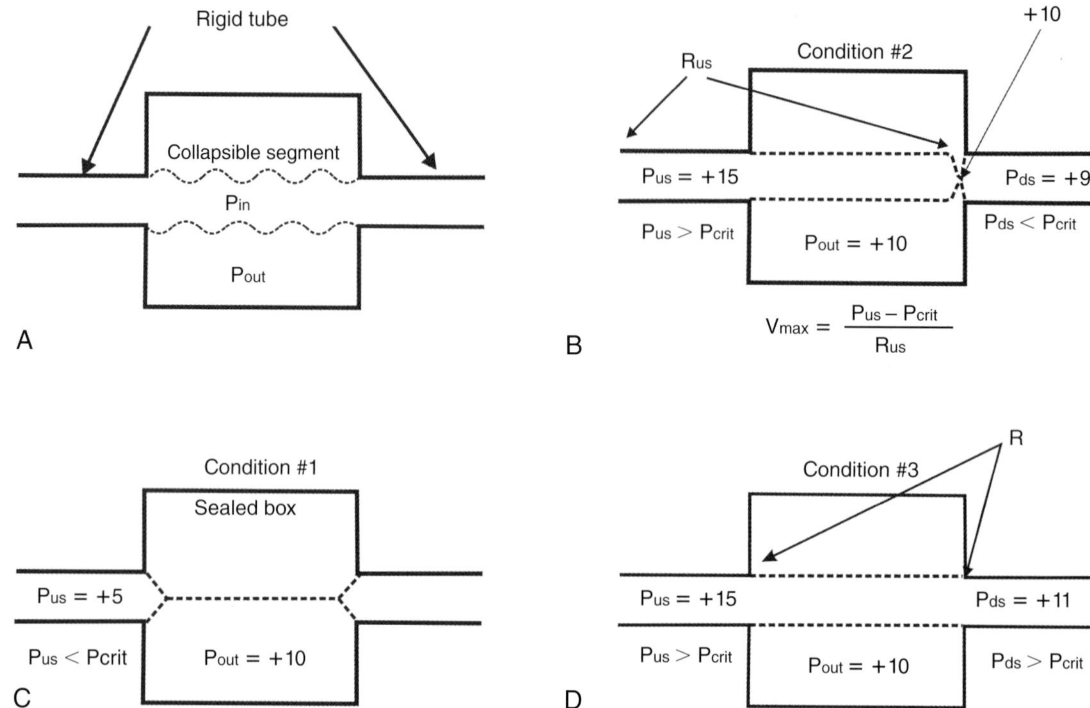

Figure 19–5 (A) Starling resistor model with pharynx assumed to be a collapsible segment with rigid tubes on the upstream and downstream sides. Vmax is the maximum flow. The intraluminal pressure (P_{in}) and extraluminal pressure (P_{out}) are shown. (B) The upstream pressure Pus = 5 cm H_2O and (P_{us}) < P_{out}; as Pin < P_{out} the collapsible segment remains collapsed and occluded. No airflow occurs. Here the pharyngeal critical pressure (P_{crit}) = P_{out}. (C) The mask pressure is 15 cm H_2O. P_{us} > P_{crit}, and airflow depends on the resistance of the upstream resistance (R_{us}). The pressure downstream (P_{ds}) from the collapsible segment is less than P_{crit}. The collapsible segment collapses or flutters to maintain the intraluminal pressure at its downstream end at 10 cm H_2O. If flow increases slightly above Vmax, the pressure at the end of the collapsible segment is slightly less than 10 cm H_2O and the segment collapses. However, if flow stops, the pressure along the entire collapsible segment becomes 15 cm H_2O and flow temporarily resumes. (D) The R_{us} is lower, such that the pressure drop across the collapsible segment is less than P_{crit} (P_{ds} > P_{crit}), and flow is not limited by the collapsible segment but depends on the resistance of the entire tube (R). (Adapted from Gold AR, Schwartz AR. The pharyngeal critical pressure. *Chest.* 1996;100:1077-1088.)

find a difference in end-expiratory lung volume between stable stage N2 sleep and REM sleep using magnetometers in a group of OSA patients. However, other studies suggest that lung volume may fall during hypopneic breathing episodes associated with phasic REM sleep.[43] Squier and colleagues[44] documented a more favorable P_{CRIT} (more negative) as end-expiratory lung volume increased in sleeping normal individuals. Morrell and coworkers[45] demonstrated a progressive fall in end-expiratory retropalatal cross-sectional area, as well as end-expiratory lung volume in the breaths leading up to obstructive apnea. Heinzer and colleagues[46] found that an increase in lung volume (induced by extrathoracic pressure) resulted in a lower level of CPAP required to prevent airflow limitation. In summary, a decrease in FRC occurs on transition from wake to sleep and might be expected to be greater with obesity. Falls in end-expiratory lung volume may contribute to upper airway narrowing in OSA patients. Higher end-expiratory lung volume is associated with a more stable upper airway, but the relative importance (compared to other factors) of a lower FRC during sleep in obese OSA patients causing upper airway narrowing remains to be determined.

Sleeping position also has important effects on airway patency, and some patients with OSA have apnea or hypopnea only in the supine position. Studies have found that 30% to 60% of OSA patients have position-dependent sleep apnea (AHI supine > 2 × AHI non-supine).[47] The literature attempting to document changes in upper airway size or shape in the lateral versus supine position is difficult to read given the variability in the study techniques, patient groups being studied, and the method of comparison (controls versus OSA, nonpositional OSA versus positional OSA). Walsh and colleagues[17] found no difference in cross-sectional area between the supine and lateral positions (using optical coherence tonometry) in awake age, and body mass index (BMI) matched normal and OSA groups and found no difference in cross-sectional area with body position in either group. However, they found airway shape to change from elliptical with a narrower anterior posterior dimension and longer lateral dimension in the supine position to a rounder shape in the lateral position. Kim and coworkers[14] using CT found that moving from the supine to lateral position increased airway size only in the retroglossal but not retropalatal space. However, the subjects were awake in these studies. One study of patients with OSA using video endoscopy[48] found that the effect of body position on upper airway patency was determined by the site of obstruction. The greatest increase in upper airway patency with lateral sleep was in patients with epiglottic collapse, a modest improvement in patients with nontongue obstruction (palatal or lateral wall collapse) and no effect on those with tongue obstruction. In the lateral position the tongue remained posteriorly located, although it did move laterally. The study findings refute the notion that the tongue falls back when supine because of gravitational effects, but additional studies are needed for confirmation. An advantage of this study was that it was performed during "natural sleep." Joosten and coworkers[49] studied 20 patients with OSA using CPAP dial downs and found for the entire group that *lateral positioning significantly improved the critical closing pressure* (lower critical closing pressure), the ability of the airway to stiffen and dilate, and increased the awake FRC without changing loop gain or the arousal threshold. The subgroup with position-dependent OSA (higher supine AHI compared to lateral AHI) had a lower critical pressure (less collapsible airway) in the lateral position (supine position 3 cm H_2O, lateral -4.63 cm H_2O). Penzel[29] also found a significant improvement in P_{CRIT} in the lateral compared with the supine position but did not find an effect of sleep stage. However, the number of subjects with sleep in all of the four combinations of NREM versus REM and supine versus non-supine was small. Another study[50] using multi-dimensional CT scanning of control, positional (supine) OSA, and REM-related OSA patients found that the supine OSA group demonstrated a significant decrease in FRC of 340 mL when moving from the lateral to supine position, which was significantly greater than the much smaller change in the controls. Interestingly, no differences between groups in upper airway size and shape were found. However, all groups showed a significant change in airway shape in the supine position with the velopharyngeal airway adopting a more ellipsoid shape (with the long axis laterally oriented), with reduced anteroposterior diameter (similar to the study by Walsh and colleagues[17]). The relevance of some of the above studies is limited by the fact that the participants were awake, and all studies had relatively few participants in the groups being compared. In summary, the effect of transitioning from the supine to lateral position may not change the upper airway size but may change the shape. There may be a greater decrease in the FRC moving from lateral to supine position in position-dependent OSA patients compared with normal individuals. *The most consistent finding is that the upper airway is less likely to collapse in the lateral position.* Changes in the upper airway with a move from supine to the lateral position may also depend on the site of obstruction. Ultimately, it is not the *change in the airway* moving from the supine to the lateral position but rather the *state of the upper airway in the lateral position* that will determine if the AHI is much lower in that posture.

There is an important interaction between the effects of the supine sleeping position and REM sleep. Oksenberg and coworkers[51] documented an interaction between the position and sleep stage factors. The following order was noted: AHI-REM/supine > AHI-NREM/supine > AHI-REM/nonsupine > AHI-NREM/nonsupine. The average length of apneas and hypopneas during REM sleep was similar in the supine and nonsupine positions. Clinicians often carefully consider if sufficient REM sleep was recorded, but this study suggests that *the amount of REM sleep in the supine position is also important.*

On transition from the upright awake to the recumbent sleeping posture, there is a potential for fluid shifts, especially in individuals with leg edema to the neck and upper airway. The redistribution could be more prominent toward the end of the night. This process can increase neck size and contribute to upper airway narrowing and worsening OSA.[52,53] The importance of these fluid shifts on OSA remains to be documented but could be significant in edematous patients. Careful attention to volume status or use of compression stockings in some individuals could minimize the effect.

Upper Airway Muscle Activity

The major upper airway muscles relevant to sleep include the GG, which protrudes the tongue, the tensor palatini that tenses the palate, the levator palatini that elevates the palate and pulls in backward, and the palatoglossus (PG) that elevates the posterior tongue and brings the soft palate inferiorly narrowing the diameter of the oropharyngeal isthmus. The GG, LP, and PG all have increased activity during inspiration (phasic activity; see Fig. 19–2 for the GG), but the TP has tonic (constant) activity (Fig. 19–6).[52-58] Activation of phasic

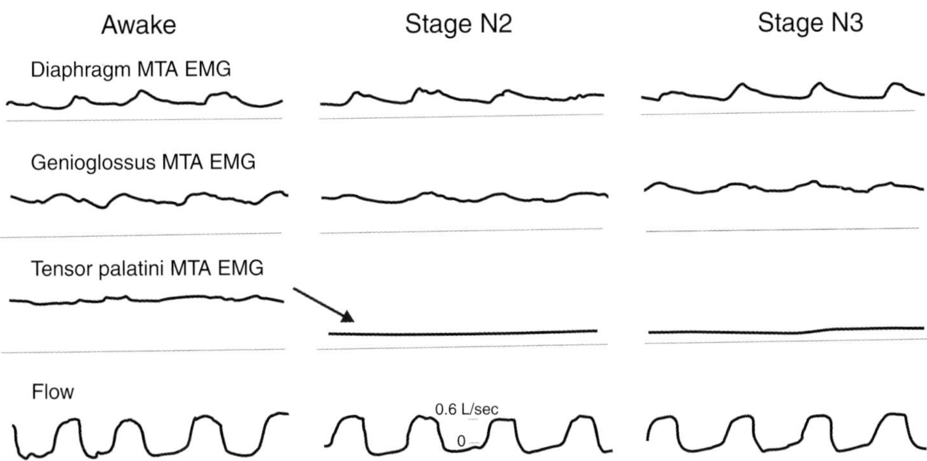

Figure 19–6 Moving time average (MTA) of the EMG of the diaphragm, genioglossus, and tensor palatini during wake, stage N2, and stage N3 sleep. The genioglossus and diaphragm show inspiratory activity (phasic) that is maintained during NREM sleep. The tensor palatini shows only tonic activity, which decreased significantly from wake to sleep. (From Tangel DJ, Mezzanotte WS, Sandberg EJ, White DP. Influences of NREM sleep on the activity of tonic vs. inspiratory phasic muscles in normal men. *J Appl Physiol (1985).* 1992;73[3]:1058-1066.)

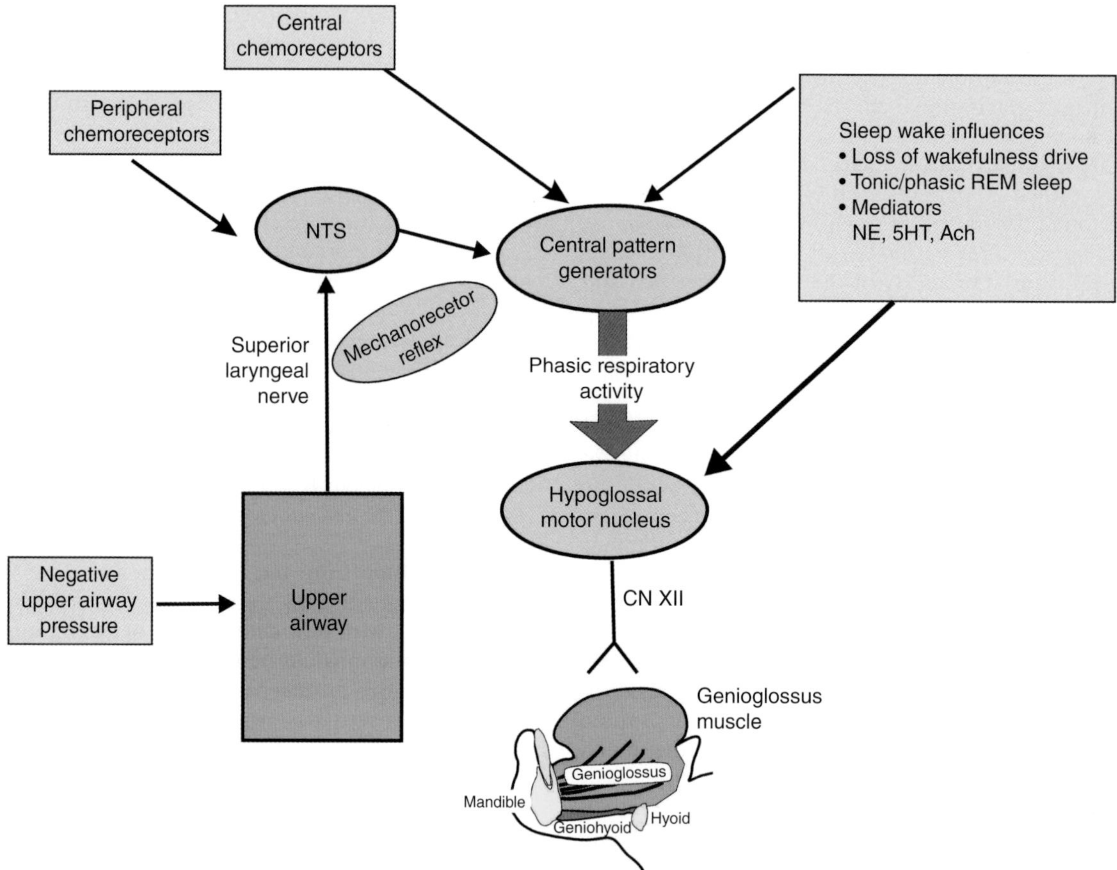

Figure 19–7 Simplified schematic illustrating the major sources of input to the genioglossus (GG) muscle across wake-sleep states. These include mechanoreceptor reflexes (negative pressure), phasic respiratory inputs from central pattern generator neurons (under the influence of chemoreceptor input), and wake sleep-sensitive neural systems. *NTS*, nucleus of the solitary tract.

upper airway muscles is triggered slightly before the muscles of the respiratory pump. This allows for a stable upper airway during inspiratory flow.

The GG is the most frequently studied upper airway muscle and is innervated by the hypoglossal nerve (cranial nerve 12). The inspiratory activity of the GG muscle is affected by (1) negative intraluminal pressure via effects on upper airway mechanoreceptors mainly in the laryngeal area, (2) central pattern generators in the brainstem (responding to PCO_2 and PO_2), and (3) influences of sleep state (wakefulness stimulus, REM sleep) (Fig. 19–7).[1,6,54] The activity of the phasic upper airway muscles (GG) but not the tonic palatal muscles (tensor palatini [TP]) is closely related to pharyngeal pressure.[55] As the intraluminal pressure becomes more negative, there is greater phasic activity. The activity of tonic upper airway muscles such as the TP appears to be more sleep state dependent (decreasing on transition from wake to NREM sleep[30,57,58] with studies showing no further decrease from NREM to REM sleep).[30,54]

Wake to Sleep Transition, NREM and REM Influences

The loss of the "wakefulness stimulus," a term describing the excitatory influence of wakefulness on respiratory function, has important influences on upper airway muscle activity, but the mechanisms are still under intensive study. It is important to remember that upper airway muscles have functions in addition to respiration, and modulation by non-respiratory neurons is important for the overall upper airway motor neuron activity.[59] Withdrawal of noradrenergic > serotonergic excitation of the hypoglossal motor neurons reduces GG activity during NREM sleep.[59-61] During REM sleep a decrease in GG tonic activity occurs with additional episodic decreases in phasic (inspiratory) activity occurring associated with the influences of non-respiratory inputs to the hypoglossal motor nucleus associated with REM sleep phasic activity (usually during bursts of REMs).[59,62] That is, the hypoglossal motor neurons receive additional modulation associated with the phasic phenomenon of REM sleep independent of chemical drive. The reduction in hypoglossal activity during REM sleep is likely due to monoaminergic dysfacilitation (less norepinephrine) and muscarinic inhibition mediated through specific potassium channels (G-protein-coupled inwardly rectifying potassium channels [GIRK channels]) resulting in membrane hyperpolarization and reduced neuronal excitability.[63,64] In support of the importance of loss of noradrenergic facilitation and cholinergic inhibition of hypoglossal nerve activity, a study found that the combination of atomoxetine (increased norepinephrine) and oxybutynin (anticholinergic) was effective in reducing the AHI in OSA.[65]

GG tonic activity decreases on entry into REM sleep (Fig. 19–8), and periods of increased and decreased GG phasic activity are also noted during periods of phasic REM sleep

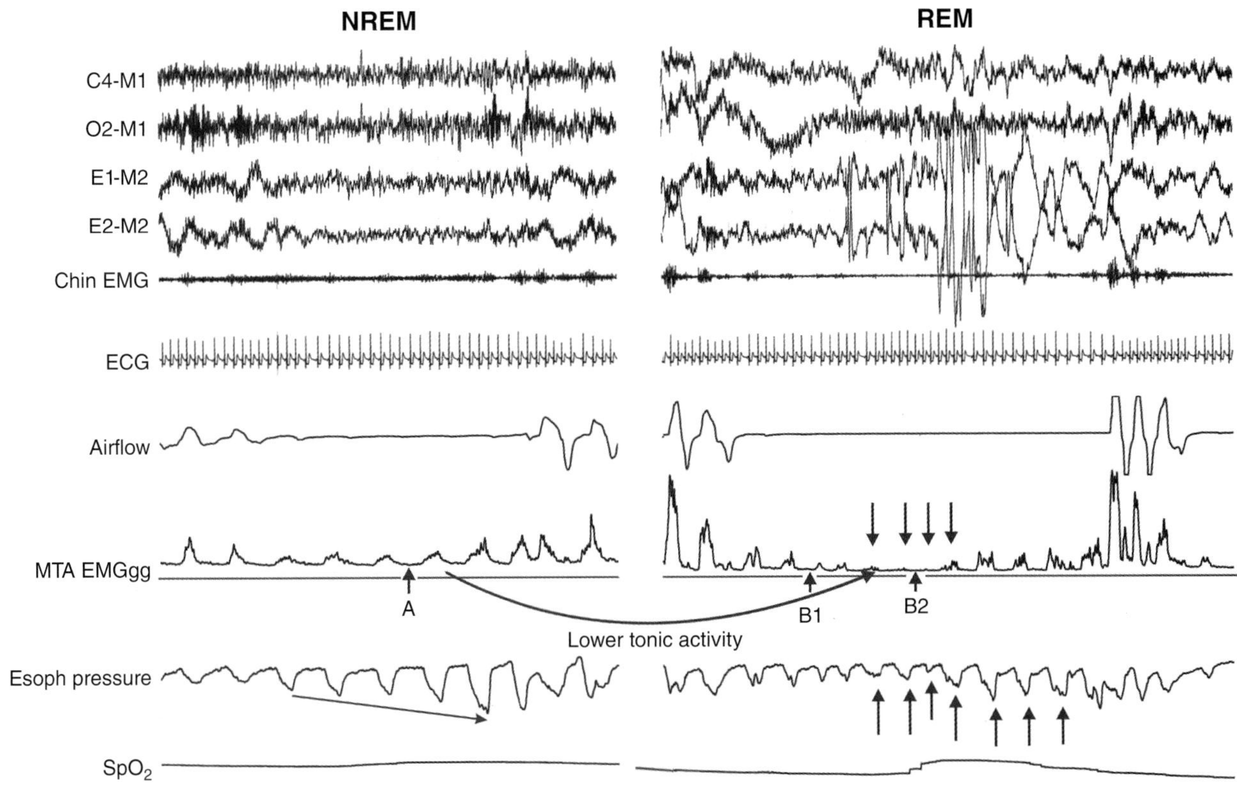

Figure 19–8 Tracings from contiguous periods of NREM and phasic REM sleep with the patient in the same body position. Two obstructive apneas are illustrated. There is a decrease in tonic GG EMG activity on transition to REM sleep (A to B1), as well as a decrease in phasic activity (down arrows) and further decrease in tonic acitivty (A to B2) during bursts of REMs. Note that the pattern of esophageal pressure deflections during apnea is quite different between NREM and REM sleep. In NREM sleep there is a steady increase in esophageal pressure deflections *(down sloping arrow)*, whereas in REM sleep the activity is more chaotic without a clear-cut progressive increase in esophageal pressure deflections. Esophageal deflections reflecting phrenic nerve activity are often decreased or irregular (up arrows) associated with the phasic activity of REM sleep (associated with REMs).

(REMs present). Neuromodulation of hypoglossal motor neuron activity by medullary non-respiratory REM phasic neurons changes the effects of stimulation from respiratory pattern generators with respect to both tonic and phasic activity (Fig. 19–9).[66,67] REM phasic non-respiratory neurons also may act on the premotor respiratory neurons causing periods of excitation or inhibition *independent of chemical drive* (Figure 19–10). While baseline phrenic nerve tonic activity is not significantly affected by REM sleep (tonic REM sleep), phasic REM sleep is associated with irregular inspiratory phrenic motor neuron activity (increased and decreased diaphragmatic EMG acitivity and esophageal pressure deflections) associated with rapid eye movements (REMs). Non-respiratory brainstem neuron activity during REM sleep results in presynaptic neuromodulation of respiratory motor neuron activity via changes in the motor neuron membrane properties and neuronal excitability (Figure 19–9). An extreme case would be an apparent central apnea during REM sleep due to a reduction in the phrenic motor neuron excitability due to the influences of non-respiratory motor neurons. Although the $PaCO_2$ may not be reduced and inspiratory respiratory input is still present there is absent phrenic motor neuron inspiratory activity due to very decreased motor neuronal excitability mediated by REM sleep phenomenon[67]. In contrast to phrenic motor neurons the tonic activity of hypoglossal motor neurons is reduced during tonic REM sleep. Further reductions in tonic and phasic genioglossus EMG activity can occur associated with bursts of REMs (Figure 19–8).

As noted above, non-respiratory neurons active during phasic REM sleep can also influence the diaphragm activity and the pattern of ventilation. Their activity during REM sleep can also modulate the output of medullary premotor neurons supplying rhythmic excitatory respiratory drive to the phrenic motor neurons, as well as direct influences on the phrenic motor neurons. A model of competing excitatory (facilitation) and inhibitory (dysfacilitation) modulation is shown in Figure 19–10.[66,67] These non-respiratory influences "compete" for control of respiration with information from chemoreceptors and other afferent input to the ventilatory control centers. The result is *periods of irregular ventilation during phasic REM sleep* (increased and decreased ventilation). That is, ventilation is not completely controlled by chemical stimulation (hypercapnia and hypoxia). The periods of decrements in ventilatory drive to the diaphragm decrease upper airway negative pressure (-10 instead of -20 cm H_2O), thus indirectly decreasing upper airway muscle activity. Of note, as perviously mentioned, *the tonic activity of the diaphragm is not significantly reduced during REM sleep (in the absence of phasic REM changes), whereas the tonic activity of upper airway muscles, intercostal muscles, and accessory muscles of respiration is decreased. During REM sleep there is an increased dependence on the diaphragm for maintenance of ventilation.*

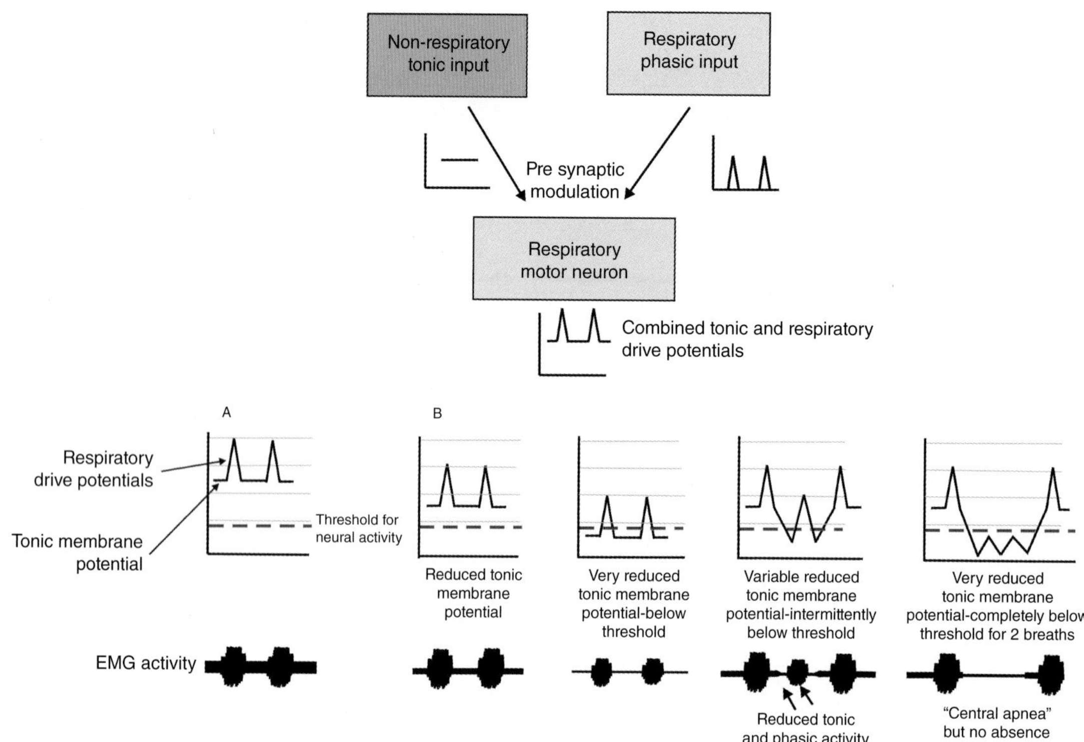

Figure 19–9 Schematic illustrating that both tonic non-respiratory neuron input and phasic respiratory input (under chemoreceptor influence) combine to determine the output of respiratory motor neurons including upper airway neurons. The activity of phasic REM non-respiratory neurons can affect *both the tonic and phasic activity* of upper airway motor neurons such as the genioglossus. Periods of excitation or inhibition usually occur associated with bursts of REMs and in parallel with changes in diaphragmatic activity or esophageal pressure deflections (see Figure 19–13). A decrease in tonic input such as at the wake to sleep transition can reduce EMG tonic activity. If the non-respiratory neuron mediated reduction in the tonic respiratory motor neuron membrane voltage is sufficiently large, the tonic and phasic activity of the respiratory motor neuron can be reduced. (Based on Horner RL. Central neural control of respiratory neurons and motoneurons during sleep. In: Kryger MH, Goldstein C, Roth T, eds. *Principles and Practice of Sleep Medicine.* Elsevier; 2021:238.)

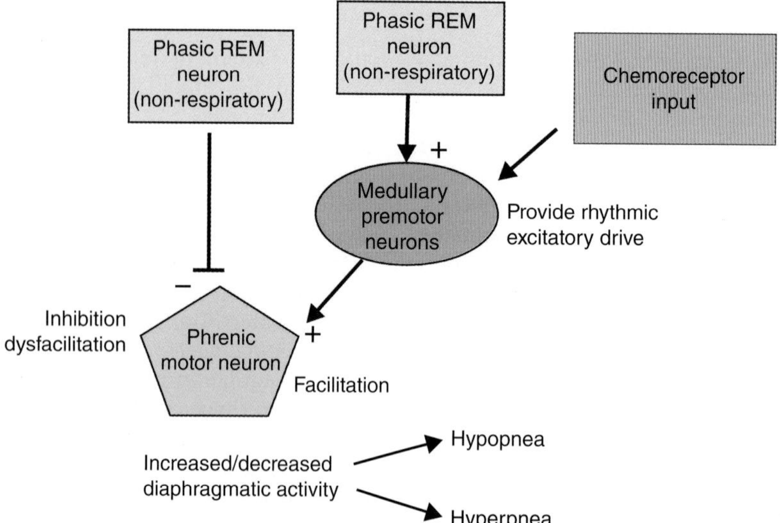

Figure 19–10 Schematic of a model illustrating possible modulating effects of non-respiratory phasic REM neurons on premotor respiratory neurons and phrenic motor neurons. There is both facilitation and inhibition of phrenic motor neuron activity independent from the influence of chemoreceptor input. The result are periods of decreased and increased ventilation not totally under control of information from chemoreceptors. Thus, there can be periods of decreased diaphragmatic activity during REM sleep *despite continuing and often increased input from premotor respiratory neurons driven by hypoxia or hypercapnia.* (Adapted from Orem J. Neuronal mechanisms of respiration in REM sleep. *Sleep.* 1980;3[3/4]:251-267.)

Upper Airway Muscle Activity During Wake and at the Sleep Transition

During wakefulness, upper airway muscle activity maintains an open upper airway even if the airway is anatomically narrow. In fact, patients with OSA tend to have higher upper airway activity than normal controls during wake as compensation.[42,68,69] Despite evidence for higher basal upper airway muscle activity during wakefulness, the upper airways of OSA patients are still more collapsible during wake than those of normal persons.[33] Obese individuals without obstructive sleep also have enhanced upper airway activity.[70] A study by Fogel and colleagues found that the higher GG activity during wake in OSA patients compared with normal controls appears to be due to increased tonic activation and the response to higher negative pressure.[69] Patients with apnea generated a more negative epiglottic pressure (P_{epi}) on a breath-by-breath basis reflecting a higher upper airway resistance. In this study, the slope of the GG versus negative pressure did not differ between normal controls and patients with OSA. However, during sleep, some OSA patients have impaired augmentation of upper airway muscles as a response to upper airway narrowing. During wake the GG muscle in OSA patients has normal (or increased) strength but decreased endurance.[71] For this reason, neurostimulation during wakefulness to increase endurance fibers in the GG is being used to treat snoring and mild OSA.[72] In both OSA and normal individuals, upper airway muscle activity falls at sleep onset because of withdrawal of the wakefulness stimulus. On transition to sleep GG activity falls (Fig. 19–2), and the change may be greater in OSA than normal individuals, given the higher compensatory activity during wake in OSA.[73,74] There may be an associated reduction in airflow and tidal volume (V_T). However, after the initial fall at sleep onset, GG activity increases to normal or higher levels to maintain an open airway in normal individuals[73] (Figs. 19–2B and 19–11). The recovery of upper airway muscle activity is in response to negative upper airway pressure and increased stimulation from chemoreceptors (increased PCO_2, decreased PO_2). In patients with OSA, apnea or hypopnea may occur because of unfavorable upper airway anatomy *before increased upper airway muscle activity can compensate.* During the event the GG activity increases and at apnea termination (with or without arousal) the increased ventilation results in a fall in ventilatory drive and the return to sleep reduces upper airway muscle activity. The result is continued cycles of decreased (during the the initial portion of the obstructive event) and increased (before and following the event termination) GG activity. However, many patients with OSA have some periods of stable breathing that occurs with augmentation of the GG.[42] This requires an effective GG response to chemical stimuli and negative airway pressure and a sufficiently high arousal threshold time to allow time for augmentation to occur.[1,4,7,42]

Changes in Upper Airway and Ventilation During REM Sleep

As noted previously, REM sleep is not homogenous and often divided into periods with bursts of REMs (phasic REM sleep) or periods without REMs (tonic REM sleep). During phasic REM sleep, ventilation is irregular even in normal persons and there are periods with reduced airflow, tidal volume (V_T), and respiratory effort associated with a reduction in diaphragmatic and GG activity.[62,75–77] The REM bursts are markers of brainstem phasic REM activity that affects respiration.[66,67,75] Because periods of REM sleep are longest and the REM density (number of eye movements per time) highest during the early morning hours, it is not surprising that this is the time of the greatest changes in ventilation during sleep in patients with lung disease and OSA. A study in normal individuals did not find a significant change in ventilation between early and late

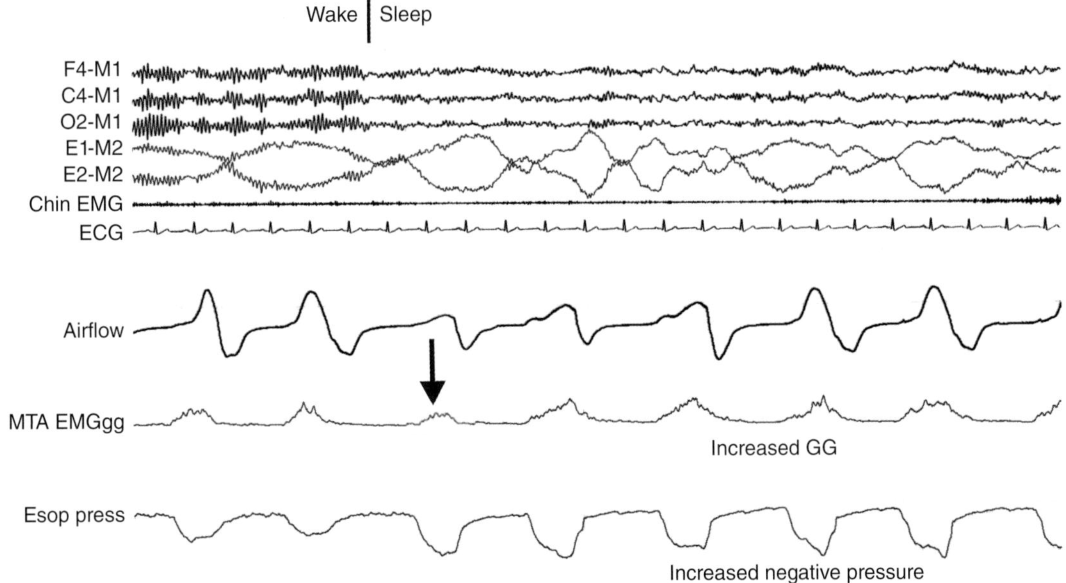

Figure 19–11 A transition from wake to sleep. With loss of alpha activity (onset of stage N1 sleep) there is a decrease in genioglossus (GG) activity *(arrow)* and airflow. As respiratory effort increases (higher esophageal pressure deflections reflecting increased ventilatory drive), the GG activity increases to above the level in wake as compensation to maintain an open upper airway with airflow. In this case the inspiratory shape of the airflow becomes round, typical of unobstructed breathing. In other patients there is persistent airflow limitation. MTA EMGgg is the moving time average of the GG EMG. Esoph Press is esophageal pressure. Airflow is the signal from a pneumotachograph inserted in the opening of a mask covering the nose and mouth. Inspiration is upward.

REM sleep periods because an increase in respiratory rate compensated for fall in V_T.[76] However, patients with OSA or lung disease are more susceptible to the phasic changes of REM sleep and V_T falls with either no change in respiratory rate or an increase insufficient to maintain ventilation.[78] During REM sleep, there is generalized muscle hypotonia and the muscles of respiration other than the diaphragm are less active. Although the diaphragm is not affected by the generalized tonic muscle hypotonia of REM sleep, as noted previously, periodic decrements in diaphragmatic activity (inspiratory effort) do occur during phasic REM sleep and are associated with reduced airflow (V_T) (Fig. 19–12).[66,75,77] There can also be periods of increased diaphragmatic activity during REM sleep (even in the absence of arousal). These changes in diaphragmatic EMG activity are due to modulation of both the tonic and respiratory related inputs to respiratory motor neurons by non-respiratory neuron activity associated with the phasic REM sleep. As noted above, upper airway muscles are also affected during REM sleep. In normal persons tonic GG activity is reduced on transition from NREM to REM sleep. In addition, GG phasic activity is variable showing periods of decrement in parallel to decreases in diaphragmatic activity (esophageal pressure deflections) associated with bursts of REMs (Fig. 19–13).[62] Note that at the end of the tracings in Figure 19–12 both esophageal pressure and GG activity are increased. This is illustrates that REM sleep is associated with both increase and decreases in diaphragmatic and genioglossus activity (irregular ventilation during REM sleep).

In many patients with OSA the AHI is much higher during REM sleep, and in some OSA patients apnea and hypopnea are confined primarily to REM sleep (REM-related OSA). As previously mentioned, several studies found no greater collapsibility (P_{CRIT}) of the upper airway during REM than NREM sleep.[26,28,29] On the other hand a study of a larger number of subjects did find a higher P_{CRIT} (more collapsible airway) during REM sleep.[30] McSharry and colleagues[79] measured single motor unit EMG of the GG and found reductions from NREM to REM with especially low activity during phasic REM sleep. Eckert and colleagues[80] found that when the upper airway was stabilized with CPAP, peak GG EMG activity dropped from NREM to tonic REM to phasic REM, but there was no difference between OSA patients and controls of either gender. Jordan and coworkers[42] studied OSA patients who could maintain upper airway patency during some periods of NREM sleep. Stable breathing during stage N2 was compared with cyclic REM sleep (with apneas). The end-expiratory lung volume and peak GG EMG did not differ between stage N2 and stage R. During REM sleep, the relationship between the negative epiglottic pressure (P_{epi}) and the phasic GG activity also did not differ from stage N2 sleep. However, P_{epi} was much less negative, and the tonic GG activity was lower during REM sleep. The simultaneous fall in drive to both the GG and the diaphragm would result in less negative upper airway pressure (indirectly decreasing GG activity). During these periods of reduced upper airway and diaphragm activity,

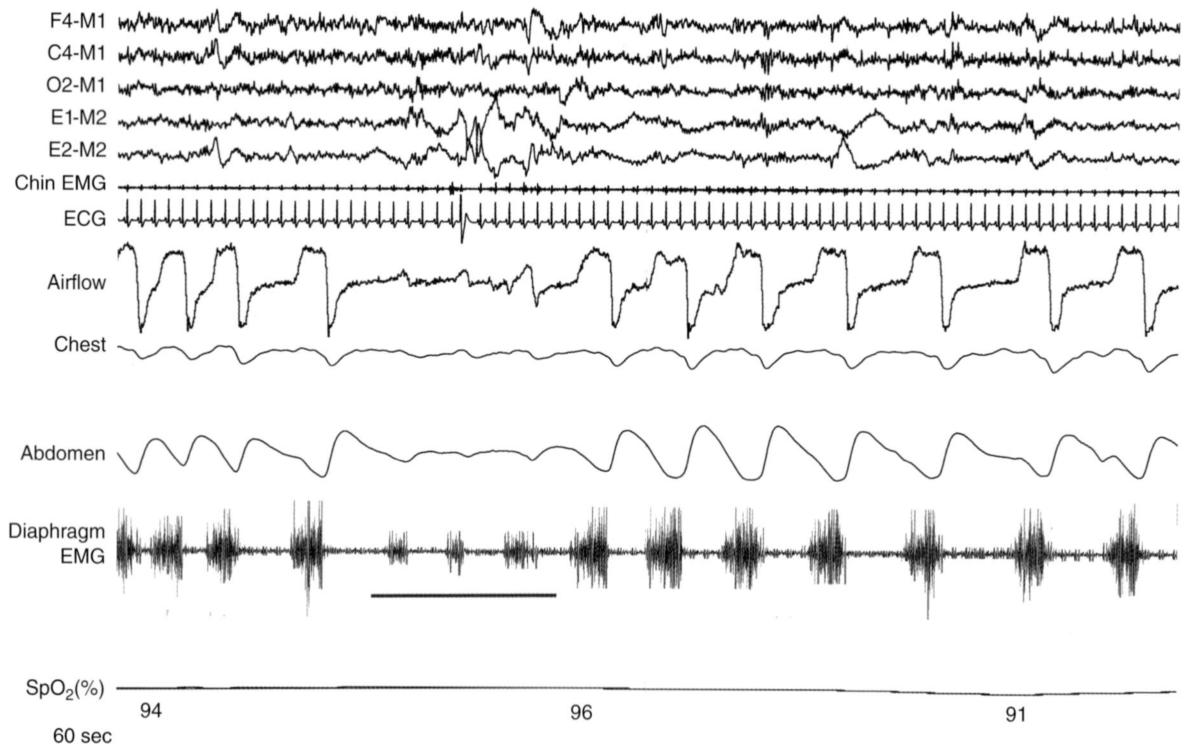

Figure 19–12 A 60-second tracing of a period of inhibition of the diaphragm (reduced diaphragmatic EMG, *dark horizontal line*) during phasic REM sleep associated with a burst of REMs. During this period there is a decrease in chest and abdominal movements and a dramatic decrease in airflow. Note that the respiratory rate is somewhat irregular, which is typical of REM sleep. Here, airflow was measured using a pneumotachograph inserted in the opening of a mask over the nose and mouth. Inspiration is upward. The diaphragm EMG was recorded using surface electrodes with removal of ECG artifact. Note compared with the baseline diaphragmatic EMG bursts (in the first two bursts) there are also periods of increased activity (breaths to right of the horizontal line).

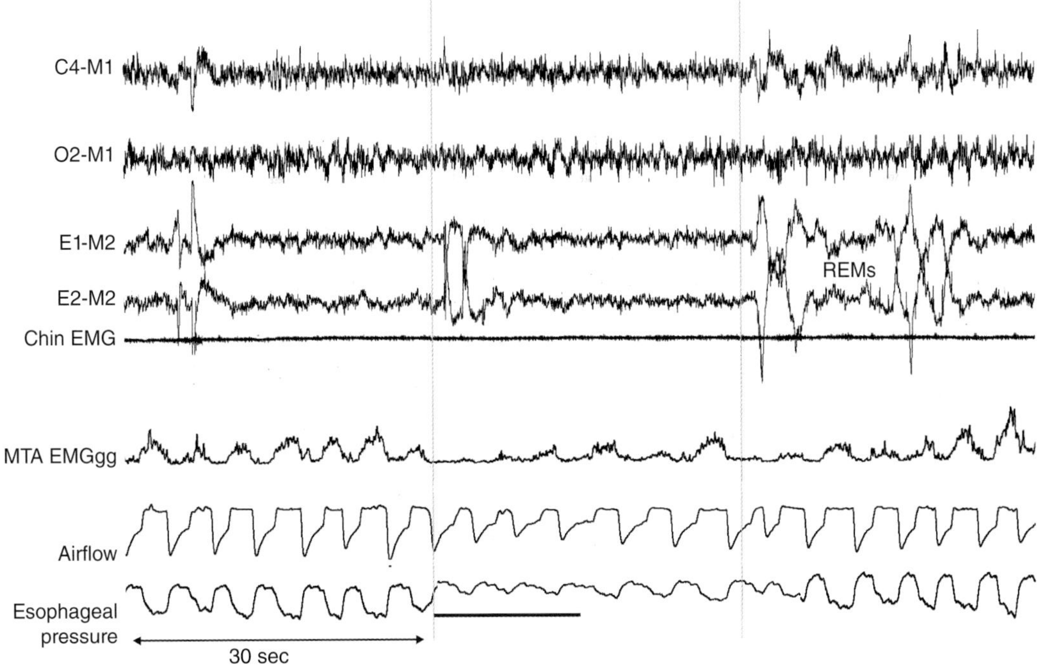

Figure 19–13 A 90-second tracing of irregular breathing during phasic REM sleep. Note the period of inhibition of drive (reduced esophageal pressure deflections, *dark horizontal line*) associated with decreased airflow and reduced moving time average genioglossus EMG activity (MTA EMGgg). The GG EMG activity is not uniformly decreased in this patient *with periods of increased and intermediate amplitude activity*. Here, airflow was measured using a pneumotachograph in a mask over the nose and mouth. Inspiration is upward.

end-expiratory lung volume could fall;[40] this, coupled with the decrease in tonic activity, would make the upper airway more collapsible. Jordan and colleagues[42] did not find a decrease in end-expiratory volume or peak GG activity in REM sleep versus stage N2, but this finding likely relates to REM sleep as a whole rather than periods of hypopneic breathing. As noted above, one study did document a higher P_{CRIT} during REM sleep.[30] Of interest, a recent study found evidence that worsening of apnea during REM sleep is due to a withdrawal of ventilatory drive rather than reduced GG compensation.[81] This is consistent with the finding of Jordan and colleagues that the relationship of GG activity to upper airway negative pressure was similar in stage N2 and stage R. It appears that OSA patients have changes in upper airway and diaphragmatic activity during phasic REM that are similar to normal individuals, but the underlying upper airway abnormality results in apnea and hypopnea. In addition, there is no evidence of a preferential impairment of the GG to respond to negative pressure during REM sleep. OSA patients depend on higher GG activity (and other upper airway muscle activity) to maintain patency of an unfavorable upper airway and that the typical REM-associated reduction in airway muscle activity has greater impact in OSA. A decreased drive (or effective drive from neuromodulation from phasic REM neurons) to both the diaphragm and the GG muscle during phasic REM sleep without a preferential GG dysfunction is likely the etiology of increased apnea and hypopnea during REM sleep. Relevant to the OSA endotypes a study found that individuals with REM predominant OSA have a more collapsible upper airway during REM compared to NREM sleep while those with NREM predominant OSA had higher loop gain during NREM than REM sleep.[9] In addition to a higher AHI, respiratory events are longer and desaturation more severe during REM sleep.[82] The mechanisms of arousal will be discussed later, but the reason respiratory events are longer during REM sleep is not known.

REM Sleep and Hypocapnic Central Sleep Apnea

Patients with hypocapnic central sleep apnea (primary sleep apnea, central sleep apnea with Cheyne-Stokes breathing, and treatment-emergent central sleep apnea) that occurs because the $PaCO_2$ falls below an *apneic threshold* often exhibit a resolution of central apnea during REM sleep. Often, the AHI in NREM sleep is much greater than in REM sleep in these patients with hypocapnic central sleep apnea. There are two likely explanations of this phenomenon. First, ventilatory responses to increased PCO_2 and decreased PO_2 are lower in REM than NREM sleep, minimizing the tendency to reduce the $PaCO_2$ below the apneic threshold. Second, as discussed above, phrenic motor neuron activity is driven by both chemostimulation and presynaptic modulation of phrenic and respiratory premotor neurons by phasic REM-related activity of nonrespiratory neurons (Fig. 19–10). The result are periods of inhibition and excitation of diaphragmatic activity *independent of input from chemoreceptors*. Thus breathing (often rapid and irregular) can occur even when the PCO_2 is low (at a level that would trigger a central apnea in NREM sleep). For these reasons, central apnea due to hypocapnia does not occur during REM sleep.

Awake Tests of Genioglossus Function

A negative pressure reflex of the GG can be assessed by application of a sudden negative pressure pulse with determination

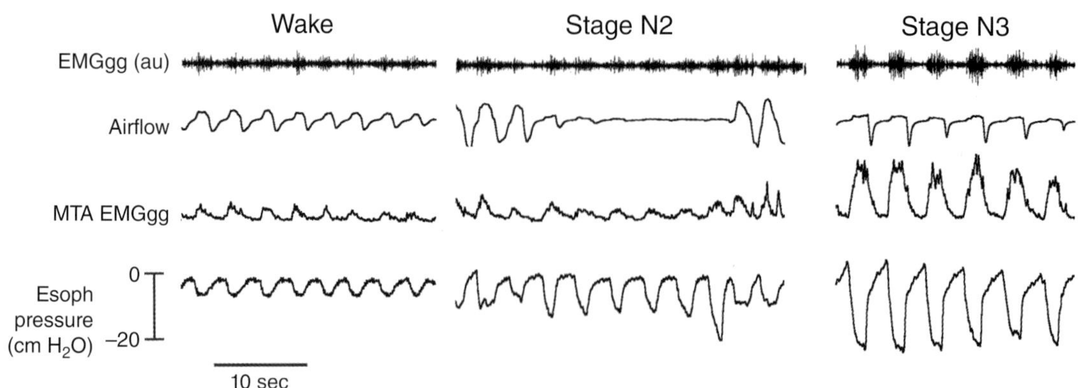

Figure 19–14 Selected segments for airflow, esophageal pressure, and GG activity during wake, stage N2, and stage N3 sleep. This patient had obstructive apnea during stage N2 but when reaching stage N3 had long periods of stable breathing with airflow limitation and very increased GG EMG activity (much higher than the wakefulness level) to maintain an open airway (although narrowed). The esophageal pressure deflections were very increased during stage N3 consistent with a high upper airway resistance. Most patients with OSA have some periods of stable breathing often during stage N3 sleep or in the lateral position. After arousal from N3 sleep, this patient again had back-to-back apneas in stage N1 and N2 sleep. EMGgg is the raw genioglossus EMG signal, and MTA EMGgg is the moving time average of the genioglossus EMG signal. Airflow was measured using a pneumotachograph in a mask over the nose and mouth. Inspiration is upward. au, arbitrary units.

of the GG response before cortical influences.[83,84] During wakefulness the GG response to negative pressure is greater in OSA patients than normal individuals,[84] likely as compensation for a narrow upper airway. A reflex activation can also be demonstrated with the levator palatini (LP) and palatoglossus (PG) which are palatal muscles with inspiratory activity[85] and the tensor palatini a muscle with tonic activity[88] during wakefulness. In contrast to the GG, the awake response of the LP and PG to negative pressure was impaired in the OSA patients compared to normal individuals[85]. Sleep reduces the effect of negative pressure on both the GG and palatal muscles.[86-88] During NREM sleep the response of the GG to the negative pressure associated with airway narrowing in OSA patients varies considerably between individuals with the disorder. As previously discussed, those patients with a robust GG response to negative pressure and increased chemical drive often have periods of the night with regular breathing, often with high negative upper airway pressure (−30 cm H_2O versus −15 cm H_2O) and augmented GG activity[42] (Fig. 19–14).

Negative Pharyngeal Pressure and Mechanoreceptors

The effects of negative upper airway pressure on the GG are mediated through a reflex neural pathway. The pathway starts with upper airway mechanoreceptors (both supraglottic and subglottic) and travels through the trigeminal, superior laryngeal, and glossopharyngeal nerves to sensory brainstem nuclei (nucleus of the solitary tract [NTS]). Neurons in the NTS then stimulate hypoglossal motor neurons in the brainstem that innervate the GG via the hypoglossal nerve.[89] During periods of increasingly negative upper airway pressure, GG inspiratory activity is increased. The importance of upper airway mechanoreceptor mediation of the effect of negative upper airway pressure on GG activity has been studied by applying topical upper airway anesthesia to supraglottic and subglottic areas, which reduced the GG response to a negative pressure pulse in awake normal individuals[89] and the response to negative supraglottic pressure during obstructive apnea in OSA patients.[90] The reduction in GG activity is thought secondary to lidocaine impairment of upper airway mechanoreceptor function with a decreased mechnoreceptor response to negative upper airway pressure. Of note, even during obstructive apnea, there is still mechanoreceptor stimulation from increasingly negative pressure below the site of obstruction. In Figure 19–15, the top panel (prelidocaine) show a progressive increase in GG activity during apnea. After topical lidocaine anesthesia of the upper airway, the GG activity is markedly diminished (middle panel). With time the effects of anesthesia were no longer present with restoration of GG activity (bottom panel). The findings imply that mechanoreceptor stimulation from increasingly negative pressure below the site of obstruction results in significant augmentation of GG activity and that lidocaine impairs the response. As noted previously, during sleep the GG but not tonic palatal muscles relate closely to negative pressure. The TP (tonic) palatal muscle activity is primarily state dependent, falling on the transition from wakefulness to sleep.

Hypoxia and hypercapnia can also increase upper airway muscle activity directly via effects on the central pattern generators (Figure 19–7) or indirectly by augmenting ventilatory drive/inspiratory effort generating more negative upper airway pressure (higher suction pressure). There appears to be an interaction between the effects of chemostimulation and negative pressure, but both can increase upper airway muscle activity alone. Pillar and colleagues[91] administered exogeneous CO_2 to normal individuals during NREM sleep and found no significant augmentation of GG activity. The epiglottic negative pressure was not significantly different between baseline and CO_2 inhalation. This study was performed with subjects in the lateral sleep position. In contrast, during monitoring in the supine position, Lo and co-workers[92] did find that exogenous CO_2 administration augmented GG activity. The response of the GG to CO_2 was affected by the amount of negative pressure (greater in the supine position).

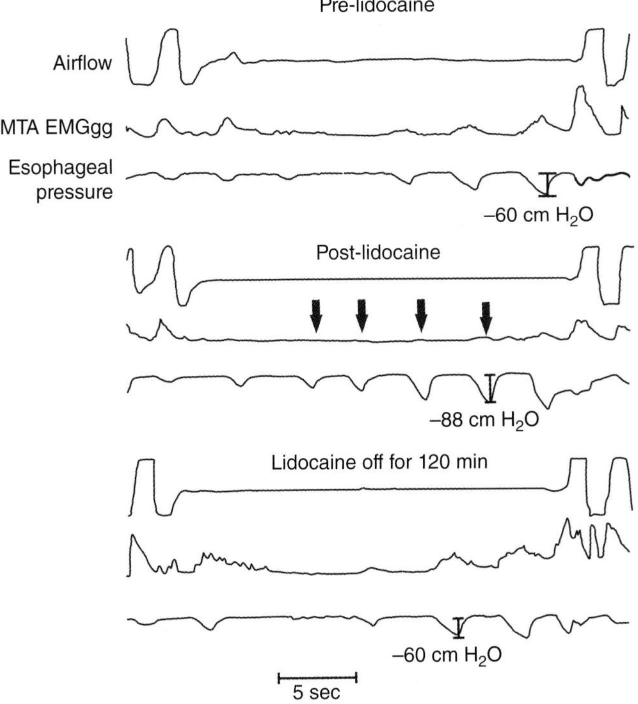

Figure 19–15 This figure shows genioglossus (GG) activity during obstructive apnea prelidocaine (topical) in the throat and upper airway, postlidocaine, and 120 minutes after lidocaine administration. The GG activity is reduced by lidocaine *(downward arrows)*, presumably due to reduced mechanoreceptor function, suggesting that the negative pressure reflex plays an important role in determining GG activity, at least during obstructive apnea. Note the very negative esophageal pressure deflections in a patient with severe obstructive sleep apnea. MTA EMGgg is the moving time average of the genioglossus EMG. Airflow was measured using a pneumotachograph in a mask over the nose and mouth. Inspiration is upward. (Reprinted with permission of the American Thoracic Society. Copyright © 2023 American Thoracic Society. All rights reserved. From Berry RB, McNellis M, Kouchi K, Light RW: Upper airway anesthesia reduces genioglossus activity during sleep apnea. Am J Respir Crit Care Med 1997;156:127–132. The American Journal of Respiratory and Critical Care Medicine is an official journal of the American Thoracic Society.)

UPPER AIRWAY ACTIVITY DURING APNEA AND HYPOPNEA

Augmentation of the GG during upper airway narrowing occurs due to increasing negative upper airway pressure and chemical stimulation. If increased activity has compensatory effectiveness, stable ventilation can occur. During stable stage N3 sleep, the GG activity can be much higher than during wakefulness (Fig. 19–14). In patients with OSA owing to unfavorable anatomy, the upper airway activity is not sufficient to maintain an open upper airway in OSA patients, and the result is apnea or hypopnea. In Figures 19–16 and 19–17, a fall in GG activity as the patient returns to sleep is associated with an obstructive apnea. Compensatory effectiveness requires a sufficient increase in upper airway muscle activity (stimulated by hypercapnia and negative upper airway pressure) and that the associated increase in muscle activity is effective in maintaining (or restoring) upper airway patency. This process depends on the maintenance of stable sleep to allow time for adequate recruitment of upper airway muscle activity. In individuals who arouse quickly due to stimuli associated with high respiratory effort, adequate time for upper airway muscle recruitment does not occur. In those OSA patients who exhibit some periods of regular breathing, recruitment of upper airway muscle enables maintaining an open airway (although often with snoring). This is most likely to occur in lateral NREM sleep and in patients who have a high threshold for arousal (maintain sleep even during high ventilatory drive).

During upper airway obstruction, phasic GG activity increases proportionately to esophageal pressure deflections (reflecting increased respiratory drive) (see Figs. 19–16 and 19–17). Stimulation of chemoreceptors by hypoxia and hypercapnia increase inspiratory drive, and esophageal pressure deflections increase. If an arousal occurs, both GG and palatal muscles are augmented, and the upper airway opens.[7,10] However, as discussed later, the termination of a substantial

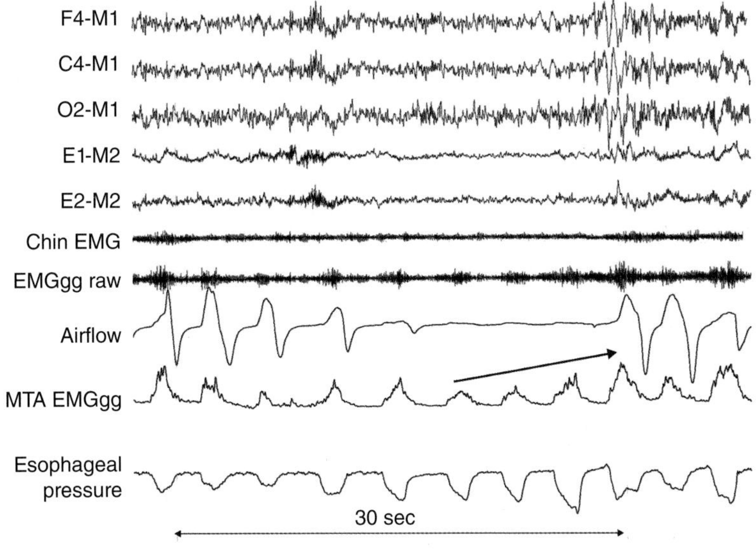

Figure 19–16 A 30-second tracing showing resolution of obstructive apnea by augmentation of upper airway activity (here, the genioglossus [GG]) without the need for arousal. MTA EMGgg is the moving time average of the GG EMG. Airflow is from a pneumotachograph inserted into the front opening of a mask covering the nose and mouth.

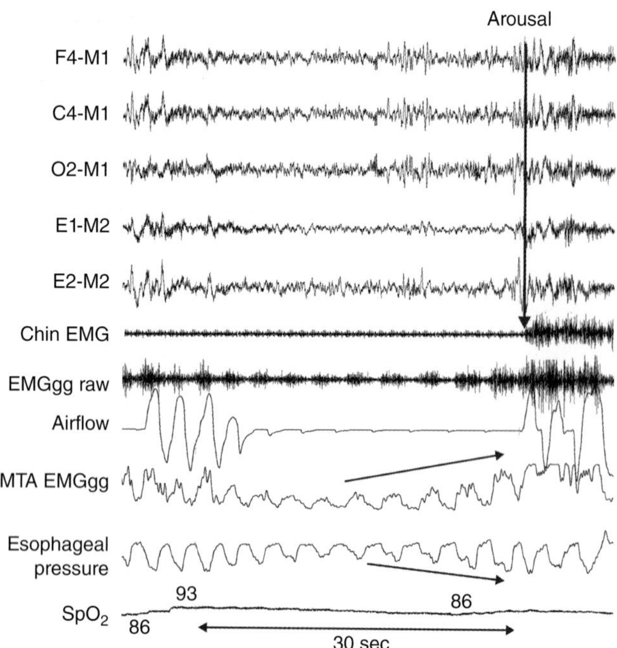

Figure 19–17 A 30-second tracing showing resolution of the obstructive apnea that required arousal for event termination even though there was brisk recruitment of the genioglossus EMG activity. MTA EMGgg is the moving time average of the genioglossus EMG. Airflow was measured using a pneumotachograph in a mask over the nose and mouth. Inspiration is upward.

fraction of obstructive apneas and hypopneas is not associated with cortical arousal. In this case once upper airway muscle activity reaches a threshold for airway opening (airway opening threshold [AOT]), this terminates the apnea or hypopnea (Fig. 19–16).[7,93] On the other hand, some events are terminated only after cortical arousal occurs (Fig. 19–17). It is important to remember that the GG is just one of many muscles maintaining an open airway. Tonic upper airway muscles are state dependent and may increase activity only after arousal. Activation of upper airway muscles other than the genioglossus during apnea and hypopnea is likely very important for upper airway opening.[7,94]

Traditionally, the concept of a balance between negative inspiratory pressure tending to collapse the airway and upper airway muscle dilating forces was assumed to determine the state of the airway.[10] However, more recently, the concept of passive collapse at sleep onset has gained favor. In fact, at sleep onset, the ventilatory drive decreases and supraglottic pressure may initially decrease (less negative) in some patients (although resistance increases). Upper airway closure has also been documented during central apnea in which there is no inspiratory effort or negative pressure collapsing forces.[95] Therefore, suction pressure during obstruction may help keep the airway closed but is not necessary for the onset of airway occlusion. Cyclic variations in ventilatory drive can induce obstructive or central apneas at the nadir in drive.[96] Thus, when ventilatory drive to the respiratory pump muscles decreases, the simultaneous reduction of neural drive to the upper airway muscles in patients with unfavorable upper airway anatomy results in airway narrowing or collapse. As discussed later, ventilatory instability results in continuing cycles of reduced breathing (apnea, hypopnea) and postevent hyperventilation.

Ventilatory Control and Loop Gain

Ventilatory instability tends to occur when there is high ventilatory drive. Hypoxia and hypercapnia from apnea coupled with arousal at apnea termination result in ventilation greater than needed for eucapnia (hyperventilation). This reduces the $PaCO_2$, and this coupled with a return to sleep reduces ventilatory drive. The cycles of increased and decreased ventilatory drive predispose to subsequent upper airway closure and help perpetuate repetitive cycles of increased respiration followed by apnea.[96-100] As ventilatory drive fluctuates, both upper airway muscle and diaphragmatic activity may fluctuate, with apnea or hypopnea tending to occur at the nadir of ventilatory drive. If the patient falls asleep rapidly after arousal, the $PaCO_2$ may be near or below the apneic threshold, the level of $PaCO_2$ below which ventilation is no longer triggered during sleep, and central apnea will occur.[101] There can be upper airway closure during central apnea.[95] If the upper airway is closed at the time of resumption of inspiratory effort, an obstructive apnea will occur. This is the etiology of mixed apnea (initial central portion, terminal obstructive portion).[102] Alternatively, an obstructive hypopnea or obstructive apnea may occur as ventilatory drive and upper airway muscle activity fall, but the $PaCO_2$ remains above the apneic threshold.[103] Patients with a small difference between the sleeping $PaCO_2$ and the apneic threshold would be more likely to have a central apnea on return to sleep.[98,99,101,104] However, the tendency for an overshoot in ventilation is also important and will be discussed below. The other factor is the time it takes for the effects of changes in ventilation to reach ventilatory control centers. If the circulation time is long, blood reaching the chemoreceptors may provide delayed information pre-disposing to ventilation that is not appropriate for the current $PaCO_2$ and PaO_2.

The concept of loop gain has been applied to explain ventilatory instability. Loop gain is also discussed in Chapter 30. Loop gain characterizes the response to a perturbation (Fig. 19–18).[2,97-99] The loop gain is equal to the controller gain × plant gain (Equation 19-2, Fig. 19–19). The controller gain is the change in ventilation divided by the change in the $PaCO_2$ reaching the chemoreceptors. The plant gain is the change in $PaCO_2$ divided by the change in ventilation. Examples of the effects of changes in controller gain and plant gain are illustrated in chapters 13 and 30. Sometimes a mixing factor is added to the loop gain equation to account for the time delay of the change in the $PaCO_2$ to reach the chemoreceptors. Patients with high loop gain are predisposed to ventilatory instability. For example, a patient with a high loop gain may respond to a mild elevation in $PaCO_2$ with inappropriately increased ventilation resulting in hypocapnia rather than simply bringing the system back to the original state (eucapnia). High loop gain may be due to high controller gain (high hypercapnic ventilatory response) or high plant gain (large decrease in $PaCO_2$ for a given increase in ventilation). Plant gain is increased when there is hypercapnia, a low dead space, and a low FRC.[2,97-99] At low lung volumes the lung stores of PCO_2 are smaller and an increase in ventilation causes a greater drop in the $PaCO_2$. A lower dead space also increases alveolar ventilation for a given amount of minute ventilation and increases plant gain. Conversely, hypocapnia reduces loop gain because of the hyperbolic relationship between ventilation and PCO_2. The position of a low baseline sleeping $PaCO_2$ is on the steep portion of the isometabolic hyperbola

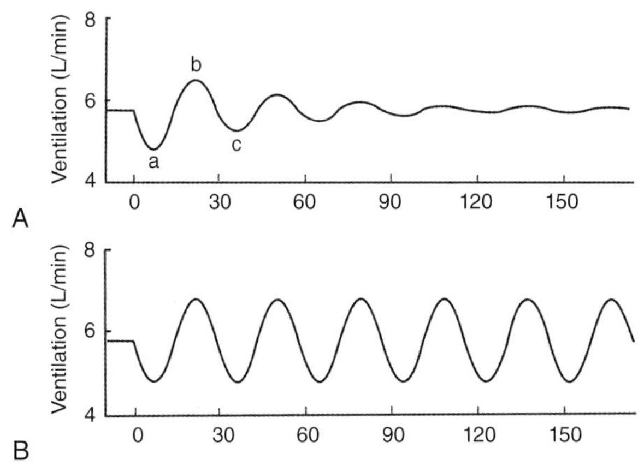

Figure 19–18 Loop gain (LG) is the ventilatory response to the ventilatory disturbance ratio. (A) Example of an LG of 0.72. The ventilatory control system is disturbed with a transient reduction in ventilation (a). This produces a response (b) in the opposite direction that is 72% as large as the disturbance. The next response (c) will also be 72% as large as (b), and so on. Thus, an LG of 0.72 produces transient fluctuations in ventilation, but ventilation eventually returns to baseline. (B) A LG of 1 will produce a response that is equal in magnitude to the disturbance. Therefore, ventilation oscillates without returning to baseline. The system in B is highly unstable. The closer LG is to zero, the smaller the fluctuations in ventilation, and thus the more stable the system. Note that the graph is *magnitude of ventilation (increasing and decreasing) and NOT an airflow tracing. The short, straight line at the beginning of each ventilation graph is the stable ventilation that is disturbed by a reduction in ventilation (at a, e.g., a hypopnea).* (From Wellman A, Malhotra A, Jordan AS, Stevenson KE, Gautam S, White DP. Effect of oxygen in obstructive sleep apnea: role of loop gain. *Respir Physiol Neurobiol.* 2008;162[2]:144-151.)

(alveolar ventilation versus $PaCO_2$ relationship) results in a given increase in ventilation being associated with a smaller drop in the $PaCO_2$.

Loop gain = response to disturbance/the disturbance   Equation 19–2

Loop gain = controller gain (chemosensitivity) × plant gain

Controller gain = change in ventilation per change in $PaCO_2$ (reaching chemoreceptors)

Plant gain = change in $PaCO_2$ per change in ventilation

Arousal after upper airway events has the potential to increase ventilatory overshoot by augmentation of ventilation. Although arousal may be needed for termination of some respiratory events, it destabilizes breathing control.[7,93,104] A low arousal threshold could result in shorter respiratory events with less severe arterial oxygen desaturation. On the other hand, a low arousal threshold can result in sleep fragmentation, destabilize breathing control, and not provide time for upper airway muscle recruitment.

Younes and associates[100] found that chemical control is more unstable in patients with severe OSA than those with milder OSA. Wellman and colleagues[97] subsequently reported that loop gain measured during NREM sleep was an important predictor of apnea severity (respiratory disturbance index), but only in patients with intermediate collapsibility of the pharyngeal airway. Individuals with extreme airway collapsibility will have obstructive events regardless of loop gain. It is unclear if the ventilatory instability in OSA patients is inherent or acquired.[2] It should also be noted that increased upper airway resistance can reduce effective controller gain by reducing the change in ventilation for a given change in $PaCO_2$. That is, the actual increase in ventilation for a given increase in neural drive is reduced by an increase in resistance. Normalization of upper airway narrowing can increase the effective controller gain and unmask underlying ventilatory instability. Treatment with CPAP or upper airway surgery may allow manifestation of the underlying ventilatory control instability and result in treatment emergent central apnea. Both treatments have been associated with treatment emergent central sleep apnea.[98,99] Thus, it would appear that ventilatory control instability may play an important role in the pathophysiology of airway obstruction in some patients with OSA either before or after treatment.[97-99] As discussed later, interventions can target the issue of high loop gain.

Arousal Threshold and Apnea/Hypopnea Termination

Obstructive apnea or hypopnea termination is often associated with cortical arousals. The relationship between these two phenomena (event termination and arousal) is still the subject of investigation.[7,93,105-108] During obstructive apnea or hypopnea during NREM sleep, upper airway muscle activity increases proportional to inspiratory effort. Studies by Remmers and coworkers[10] suggested that airway opening does not occur until there is a preferential increase in upper airway muscle activity (compared with the diaphragm). The preferential increase in upper airway muscle activity was believed to be due to associated arousal. One problem with this concept is that not all event terminations are associated with cortical arousal (e.g., 60%–80% of event terminations are associated with arousal). Sometimes obstructive event termination is associated with signs of cortical activation that may not meet the electroencephalogram (EEG) change criteria to score an arousal as defined by the American Academy of Sleep Medicine Scoring Manual criteria.[109] For example, a delta burst may be seen at apnea termination. Even when cortical arousal cannot be detected, some have hypothesized a state change occurs at the level of the brainstem. These "brainstem arousals" are sometimes referred to as subcortical or autonomic arousals because changes in sympathetic tone, heart rate, or blood pressure can be detected in the absence of cortical changes meeting criteria for arousal. Younes[93] challenged the concept that arousal is an essential component of upper airway opening. His work found that arousal may precede, coincide with, follow, or not occur with upper airway opening. Thus, in this view, arousal may be associated with event termination, but what opens the airway is a sufficient augmentation of upper airway muscle activity by chemical and mechanical stimuli. Thus, Younes hypothesized that airway opening and arousal are two separate independent phenomena that occur in parallel with similar time courses during obstructive respiratory events. Upper airway muscle activity is progressively augmented until an upper airway opening threshold (AOT) is reached and the airway opens. Likewise, during obstructive events, the arousal stimulus (proportional to the level of inspiratory effort[105-107]) increases until the arousal threshold is reached and arousal occurs. If augmentation of upper airway muscle activity is brisk, the required degree of muscle augmentation is not excessive, and the arousal threshold is high, the airway can reopen without arousal (the patient remains asleep) (Fig. 19–16). Evidence for this concept is that most patients with OSA have some periods of the night without events and, thus, are able to maintain upper airway patency without

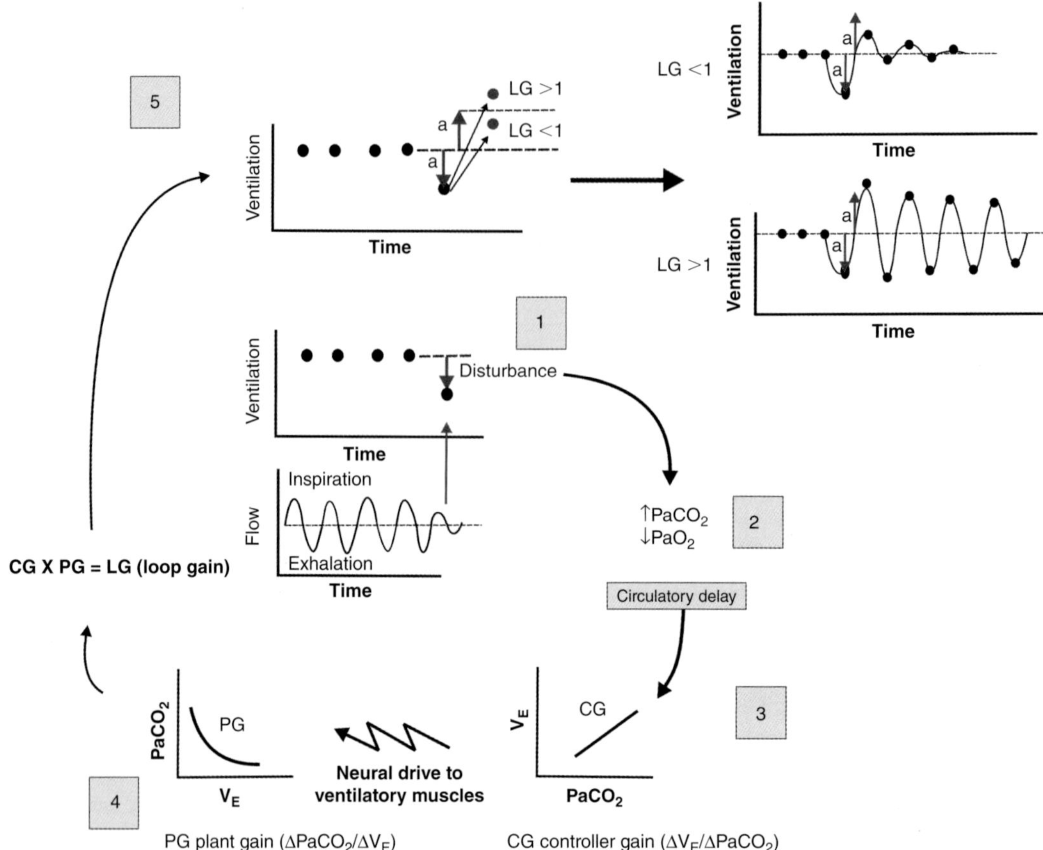

Figure 19–19 Schematic of ventilatory loop gain (LG). (1) A disturbance to breathing causes a reduction in ventilation below eupnea (down red arrow at 1). (2) Reduced ventilation increases the arterial CO_2 ($PaCO_2$) and reduces arterial O_2 (PaO_2). (3) Controller gain (CG) reflects the sensitivity of the peripheral and central chemoreceptors to blood gases and dictates the magnitude of the increase in neural drive to ventilatory muscles ($\Delta VE/\Delta PaCO_2$). (4) Plant gain (PG) represents the effectiveness of the lungs to change blood gases ($\Delta PaCO_2/\Delta VE$). (5) The product of CG and PG determines overall LG. If LG $<$ 1, the fluctuations in ventilation will dampen out and breathing will stabilize. If LG $>$ 1, the fluctuations in ventilation will increase in amplitude and instability will be self-perpetuating. For simplicity, the effect of delay of the information concerning changes in the PCO_2 and PO_2 from reaching the chemoreceptors (also called mixing gain) is not included in the calculation of the loop gain. (Adapted from Deacon-Diaz N, Malhotra A. Inherent vs. induced loop gain abnormalities in obstructive sleep apnea. *Front Neurol.* 2018;9:896.)

arousal. However, this concept does not explain event termination during REM sleep when upper airway muscles do not necessarily augment during the event (Fig. 19–8) or in patients with poor augmentation of upper airway activity. In addition, whereas phasic upper airway muscles augment with increasing inspiratory drive (and more negative upper airway pressure), tonic upper airway muscles usually do not. Tonic muscles increase their activity with a state change (arousal). Thus, arousal may play a role in termination of some obstructive events. Amatoury and colleagues[94] induced arousal by CPAP dial down in OSA patients and found that about 65% of arousals associated with respiratory events occur during inspiration and about 35% during expiration. Expiratory arousals occurred predominantly in early expiration and followed resumption of airflow. Peak TP EMG was higher in prearousal breaths preceding expiratory arousals, whereas GG and tonic TP activities were similar in inspiratory and expiratory arousals. Although the TP is generally thought to have mainly tonic activity, it can display phasic activity when stimulated with high negative pressure. The authors hypothesized that non-pressure threshold mechanisms may enhance TP neuromuscular compensation, for example, a state change in the medulla before evidence of a cortical arousal. In any case, the relationship of respiratory event termination and arousal is the subject of ongoing investigation.

Even if arousal is not essential to upper airway opening, repeated arousals are thought to contribute to daytime sleepiness (along with the associated hypoxemia).[110] In addition, arousals might destabilize breathing tending to perpetuate respiratory events. Jordan and colleagues[111] studied apneas and hypopneas terminated with and without cortical arousals. Respiratory events that were terminated with arousal were more severely flow-limited, had enhanced hyperventilation after event termination, *and were more often followed by secondary events than those not terminated with arousal.* However, secondary events were not associated with low dilator muscle activity, and airflow was improved after both types of apnea termination. There seems little doubt that respiratory events with a termination associated with arousals have enhanced hyperventilation after event termination, as well as an increased chance of secondary events, but this may **not** be due to reduced upper airway muscle activity postarousal. Cori and coworkers[112] performed an analysis of the effects arousals associated with event termination with measurement of end-tidal PCO_2. Arousal-induced hypocapnia did not result in reduced dilator muscle activity after return to sleep, and the authors concluded that hypocapnia may not contribute to further obstructions via this mechanism. They hypothesized that elevated dilator muscle activity postarousal is likely driven by non-CO_2-related stimuli. In a subsequent study,[113] arousal from acoustic stimuli was induced in normal subjects while breathing on bilevel positive airway pressure. Prearousal end-tidal PCO_2 was manipulated by changes in pressure support and addition of CO_2. After-discharge, defined as an increase in GG activity above prearousal levels, occurred after the return to sleep following an induced arousal. This phenomenon was minimally affected by the prearousal PCO_2. The results suggest that after-discharge is the mechanism preventing a drop in GG activity after arousal even if hypocapnia is present. In any case, preservation of upper airway muscle activity (at least the GG) does not prevent secondary events. Therefore, the cause of the secondary events is still not well understood.

The mechanisms that contribute to respiratory arousal are also of interest. Whereas hypercapnia and hypoxia drive the increase in respiratory effort, the level of effort rather than individual values of hypoxia or hypercapnia seems to trigger arousal.[105-108] Thus, the level of effort is an index of the combined arousal stimulus. Studies have suggested that information from upper airway mechanoreceptors may contribute to the arousal stimulus.[114,115] In NREM sleep, arousal appears to occur when inspiratory effort reaches an "arousal threshold." Normal subjects tend to arouse during mask occlusion when suction pressure reaches −20 to −40 cm H_2O.[116] In contrast, patients with severe OSA and long respiratory events arouse only after the nadir in esophageal pressure deflections reache −60 to −80 cm H_2O.[117] The increased arousal threshold in some OSA patients is probably due in part to chronic sleep deprivation or the long-term effects of hypoxemia (intermittent hypoxemia) on areas of the brain important for the arousal response. Withdrawal of CPAP for even 3 nights has been shown to increase the arousal threshold in OSA.[117] Haba-Rubio and colleagues found that CPAP treatment reduced the arousal threshold without a change in event duration due to a decrease in the ramp of respiratory effort during apnea.[118] However, chronic CPAP treatment does not restore the arousal threshold to normal in many OSA patients. Patients with OSA could have an intrinsically increased respiratory arousal threshold. As studies have suggested that information from upper airway mechanoreceptors may contribute to the arousal stimulus, damage to mechanoreceptors from years of snoring or to chemoreceptors from repetitive nightly stimulation could contribute to development of a higher arousal threshold.[107] A study of respiratory-related evoked potentials (RREPs) in patients with mild OSA suggested that there is a sleep-specific blunted cortical response to inspiratory occlusion.[119] At least in these milder patients, there was no evidence of impaired mechanoreceptor function because the RREP was normal during wakefulness.[119] Kimoff and colleagues[120] found two-point and vibratory sensory detection to be impaired in untreated but not CPAP-treated OSA patients and hypothesized that untreated patients have impairment of detection of mechanical stimuli.

A study by Charbonneau and coworkers found that apnea duration lengthened over the night.[121] A follow-up study found that the prolongation in event duration that occurs overnight in patients with OSA is secondary to a blunting of the cortical response as the level of inspiratory effort at apnea termination increased during the night.[122] However, another study found that the within-night variation in the arousal threshold followed the cycles of NREM sleep[123] with a higher arousal threshold associated with higher EEG delta power (deeper sleep). Sforza and colleagues[124] studied the within-night changes in the arousal threshold associated with respiratory events and found that the arousal threshold tended to peak during the first 3 hours of sleep, plateau, and then decrease slightly in the last hour of sleep. They did find a mild increase in apnea duration over the night. The authors concluded that their findings showed the arousal threshold was **not** dependent on sleep fragmentation (which should have continued to worsen). When looking at changes in arousal over the entire night, it is important to note that arousal mechanisms during REM sleep may be different from NREM.[125] It is also worth noting that the apnea duration (time to arousal) depends on both the arousal threshold and the rate of increase in inspiratory effort over the event (respiratory response to airway occlusion).[107] Hence, Haba-Rubio found that CPAP decreased the arousal threshold, but apnea event duration was unchanged because of a decrease in the ramp of respiratory effort during respiratory events.[118] For example, the acute addition of supplemental oxygen results in longer apneas (reduction in rate of augmentation in inspiratory effort), but event termination occurs at similar levels of esophageal pressure (similar arousal threshold).[106,107] In summary, studies have found different patterns of changes in the arousal threshold over the night, and more investigations are needed. The causes of overnight changes in the arousal threshold are also unknown. If airway opening is independent of arousal, a similar scheme can still be invoked with the determinants of event duration being the rate of upper airway muscle augmentation and the airway opening threshold (AOT).

Defining the arousal threshold based on esophageal pressure deflections limits the ability to assess this clinically, although one could assume that longer events means an increased threshold. Edwards and colleagues[126] developed clinical predictors of a low arousal threshold based on standard polysomnography (PSG) parameters. The score included the addition of 1 for every criteria met: AHI $<$ 30 events/hour, nadir oxygen saturation as measured by pulse oximetry $>$ 82.5%, and fraction of hypopneas $>$ 58.3%. A score of 2 or 3 correctly predicted a low arousal threshold in 84.1% of participants with a sensitivity of 80.4% and a specificity of 88.0%. Sands and colleagues[127] developed a sophisticated approach using computer modeling of regular PSG data, but this approach is not widely available. An arousal threshold can also be determined as a ventilation (reflecting an amount of ventilatory drive). For example, baseline ventilation is 6 L/min but falls to 2 L/min with hypopnea; an arousal might require (be associated with) a higher than normal ventilation of 8 L/min. The brain centers involved in arousal from apnea and hypopnea are not known. There is evidence that arousal from hypercapnia is mediated by neurons in the parabrachial nucleus, which has projections to higher brain centers.[128]

In REM sleep, the arousal mechanisms are even less well understood than during NREM sleep. Esophageal pressure deflections do not always show a steady increase during apnea in REM sleep (see Fig. 19–8).[125] In addition, normal subjects arouse more quickly from mask occlusion during REM sleep than during NREM sleep.[116] In one study using ventilation to define the arousal threshold, the arousal threshold was actually lower in REM than in NREM sleep[81]. In contrast, patients with OSA have the longest apneas and most severe desaturation during REM sleep.[82] The reasons for the delayed arousal during REM sleep in OSA patients are not known.

GENDER AND OSA

A number of investigations have sought to determine the pathophysiology of the higher incidence of OSA in men than in women. *Men have a longer upper airway, and this is believed to predispose them to pharyngeal collapse.*[129] Of note, postmenopausal women have longer upper airways than premenopausal women.[130] Many studies have demonstrated no clear gender differences in loop gain, upper airway collapsibility (P_{CRIT}), or pharyngeal muscle activation.[131,132] Pillar and associates[133] found that men developed more hypopnea due to resistive loading. Because no difference in upper airway muscle activation was noted, the increased tendency for male upper airway narrowing was believed to be due to anatomic factors. One issue with the previous studies of gender is that the number of subjects may be underpowered to find a difference. In a study of 2057 subjects, moderate to severe OSA was found in 41% of men and 21% women.[134] Using advanced computerized analysis of routine polysomnographic data endotyping was performed. Women *demonstrated lower loop gain, less airway collapsibility, and lower arousal threshold* during NREM sleep than men ($P < .0005$). Endotypes based on airway collapsibility, loop gain, and arousal threshold explained 30% of the relative sex differences in NREM using hypopnea scored on the basis of a ≥4% desaturation. Thus, more studies in large data sets may help explain the lower incidence of OSA in women. Loop gain is not the only possible difference in ventilatory control between genders. There has been evidence of a difference in susceptibility to hypocapnia. As noted previously, the apneic threshold is the sleeping PCO_2 at which ventilation is no longer triggered. A study found that men and postmenopausal women had a *smaller difference* between their sleeping $PaCO_2$ and the apneic threshold compared with premenopausal women, predisposing the former groups to central apnea or hypopnea after periods of hyperventilation.[104] In another study premenopausal women were less susceptible to hypocapnic central apnea during NREM sleep than men.[135] This effect was not explained by progesterone. Preservation of ventilatory motor output during hypocapnia may explain the gender difference in sleep apnea. In summary, study of the reasons for gender differences in the prevalence of sleep apnea is ongoing. Anatomic differences (shorter upper airway length), lower loop gain, a less collapsible upper airway, and reduced susceptibility to falling ventilatory drive in women may explain the reduced risk of OSA in women, especially premenopausal women. In contrast a lower arousal threshdold in women would predispose them to developing OSA.

ARTERIAL OXYGEN DESATURATION IN OSA

Patients with a similar AHI may have vastly different degrees of arterial oxygen desaturation. Box 19–1 lists factors determining the severity of arterial oxygen desaturation. Studies of breath-holding in normal subjects suggest that the rate of fall in the SaO_2 is inversely proportional to the baseline SaO_2 and to the lung volume (oxygen stores) at the start of breath-hold.[136] The rate of fall is disproportionately higher at low lung volumes secondary to increases in ventilation/perfusion mismatch. A study of OSA patients by Bradley and associates[137] found that the severity of nocturnal arterial oxygen desaturation was related to several factors, including the awake supine arterial partial pressure of oxygen (PaO_2), the percentage of sleep time spent in apnea, and the expiratory reserve volume (ERV = FRC − RV). Patients with a baseline PaO_2 of 55 to 60 mm Hg are on the steep part of the oxyhemoglobin saturation curve. A small fall in PaO_2 results in significant desaturation. Although apnea duration is an obvious factor in the severity of desaturation, the length of the ventilatory period between events also is important. Some patients do not completely resaturate between events as they quickly return to sleep, and the airway closes again. Long event duration and short periods between apneas result in a high percentage of total sleep time spent in apnea. A small ERV is associated with more severe arterial oxygen desaturation during respiratory events. The ERV is the difference between the FRC (end-expiratory volume) and the residual volume (RV). A small ERV is usually due to a low FRC, a high RV, or both. In obesity the ERV is reduced mainly owing to a reduction in the FRC. A lower FRC is associated with lower oxygen stores pre-respiratory event. Tidal breathing at low lung volumes results in substantial small airway closure (below the closing volume). This increases the amount of ventilation perfusion mismatch (no ventilation reaches some alveoli). A high RV is usually due to air-trapping associated with obstructive airway disease. The presence of obstructive airway disease is also associated with more ventilation perfusion mismatch. Low oxygen stores at the start of apnea and ventilation perfusion mismatch both contribute to a more rapid and more severe drop in the arterial oxygen saturation during apnea or reduced ventilation (hypopnea) when the ERV is low.

Clinically, the groups of OSA patients with severe desaturation include patients with a awake low PaO_2 for any reason (severe obesity, daytime hypoventilation, and chronic obstructive pulmonary disease [COPD]). In fact, some patients can

Box 19–1 FACTORS ASSOCIATED WITH MORE SEVERE ARTERIAL OXYGEN DESATURATION

- Higher BMI—more effect during REM than NREM sleep
- Lower baseline awake supine PaO_2 or SaO_2
  - Lower ERV (FRC − RV)
  - Low FRC—obesity
  - High RV—obstructive airway disease (COPD)
- Longer event duration/shorter ventilation period between events
- Greater change in V_T (hypopnea)
- REM sleep vs. NREM sleep (REM events are also longer)
- Higher BMI, especially during REM sleep
- Supine vs. lateral position
- Men vs. women

BMI, Body mass index; *COPD,* chronic obstructive pulmonary disease; *ERV,* expiratory reserve volume; *FRC,* functional residual capacity; *NREM,* non-rapid eye movement; *PaO_2,* arterial partial pressure of oxygen; *REM,* rapid eye movement; *RV,* residual volume; *SaO2,* arterial oxygen saturation; *VT,* tidal volume.

have significant desaturation after events as short as 10 to 15 seconds. The severity of desaturation also depends on sleep stage. As noted previously, in most OSA patients, the longest apneas and most severe desaturations occur in REM sleep.[82] Some studies also have suggested that at equivalent apnea length, the severity of desaturation is worsened in obstructive compared with central apnea.[138] A large study of the Wisconsin cohort found that a higher BMI was associated with more severe arterial oxygen desaturation independent of age, gender, sleeping position, baseline SaO_2, and event duration.[139] A higher BMI had a *greater effect on desaturation in REM than in NREM sleep*. In addition, a fall in V_T had a greater effect on arterial oxygen desaturation when the BMI was higher. The predicted fall in the SaO_2 with apnea or hypopnea was also higher in the supine position than in the lateral position, in men compared than in women, and in smokers than in nonsmokers. Another study found that obstructive events in the supine position tended to be longer, were associated with more severe desaturation, and were more likely to be associated with an arousal at event termination.[140]

The number of arterial oxygen desaturations and the low SaO_2 are standard parameters in most sleep reports. The time with an SaO_2 below a threshold (<90% or ≤88%) is also commonly reported. The hypoxic burden (also known as the sleep apnea-specific hypoxic burden [SASHB]) determines the area between a threshold and the SaO_2 curve (Fig. 19–20) and therefore accounts for both the time and severity of desaturation (units are % hours).[141] In one study the hypoxic burden due to sleep apnea predicted cardiovascular disease mortality in two cohorts of patients (while the AHI was not predictive).[141] In another study the hypoxic burden was associated with incident heart failure.[142] A different group defined a desaturation severity index slightly differently but found this desaturation index reflected daytime sleepiness better than the AHI.[143]

ENDOTYPES OF OBSTRUCTIVE SLEEP APNEA

As discussed at the start of the chapter, certain endotypes define risk factors for developing OSA (Table 19–2). These include (1) a compromised upper airway anatomy, (2) decreased upper airway muscle responsiveness, (3) instability in ventilatory control (high loop gain), and (4) a low arousal threshold (easily aroused from sleep).[7,8] For example, factors contributing to OSA vary between a very obese male with a very narrow and collapsible upper airway and a thin woman with a relatively normal upper airway anatomically. A mixture of the risk factors is also possible, but there may be a predominant one. However, auxiliary factors can be very important if a treatment reduces one factor. For example, if CPAP normalizes anatomic factors uncovering a high loop gain resulting in treatment emergent central apneas. There has been great interest in defining endotypes of OSA with the thought that various endotypes might respond to different treatment modalities. That is, different treatment options might be beneficial for specific endotypes.[144-146] A patient with a narrow upper airway might benefit from weight loss, treatment with CPAP, upper airway surgery, or an oral appliance. Patients with volume overload and significant nocturnal redistribution of fluid to the upper airway might benefit from diuresis.[52] A patient with a high loop gain might benefit from acetazolamide[147,148] or oxygen[149,150] (both lower loop gain). Supplemental oxygen decreases controller gain,[149,150] and acetazolamide decreases plant gain.[147,148] A low arousal index might be treated with a hypnotic,[150-152] although different hypnotics might have different effects. Knowing the patient has a high

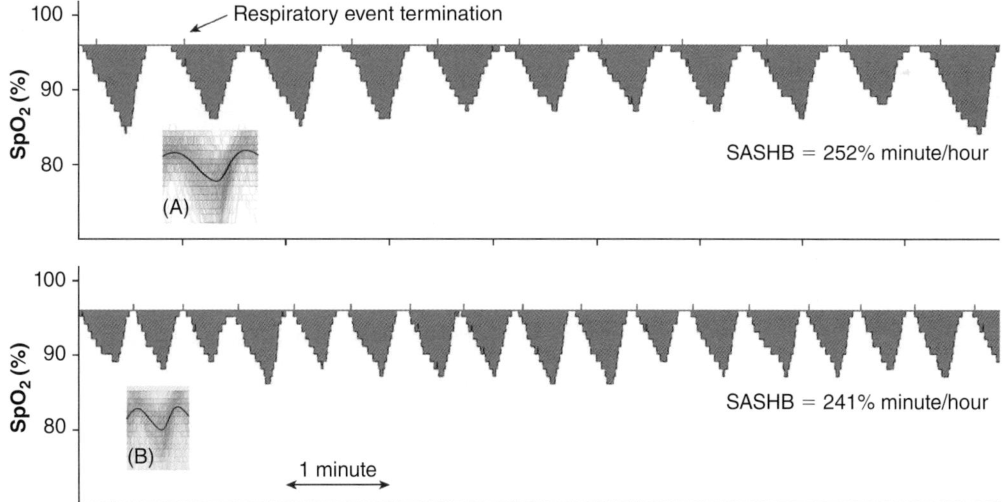

Figure 19–20 Examples of sleep apnea-specific hypoxic burden (SASHB) for two individuals with different desaturation patterns and similar SASHBs. A and B show the overlaid oxygen saturation signals (SpO_2) associated with all respiratory events for these two individuals. These signals were ensemble averaged to obtain subject-specific search window to calculate the individual areas under desaturation curves. SASHB was the sum of individual areas divided by total sleep time. As shown, different patterns of desaturation (e.g., longer, deeper, and less frequent desaturations) (*top tracings* and A) versus shorter, milder, and more frequent desaturations (*bottom tracings* and B) could result in similar SASHBs. SASHB was defined as the area under the desaturation curve (below the preevent SpO_2 baseline) associated with respiratory events. Units of SASHB are % min/hour (a SASHB of 50% min/h corresponds to a 5% reduction in SpO_2 below baseline for 10 minutes for every hour of sleep). (From Azarbarzin A, Sands SA, Taranto-Montemurro L, et al. The sleep apnea-specific hypoxic burden predicts incident heart failure. *Chest.* 2020;158[2]:739-750.)

Table 19–2 Endotypes, Factors, Evaluations, and Potential Interventions

Endotypes	Factors	Evaluations	Potential Interventions

Unfavorable upper airway anatomy (small/narrow upper airway)
Increased upper airway collapsibility
	• Skeletal
	  • High arched bony palate
	  • Small, posteriorly placed mandible
	  • Short chin-to-hyoid distance
	  • Narrow nasal passages
	• Tissue
	  • Long, dependent palate
	  • Increased upper airway fat (tongue or lateral walls)
	  • Large tongue
	• Other
	  • Low lung volume
	  • Supine posture
	  • Rostral fluid redistribution
		• Upper airway imaging
		• Drug-induced sleep endoscopy
		• P_{CRIT} (passive)
			• Weight loss (dietary, surgery, medications)
			• Avoid supine position
			• Oral appliances
			• CPAP
			• Upper airway surgery
			• Diuretics if volume overload[52,53]

Impaired pharyngeal dilator muscle activity Poor upper airway muscle response	• Neuromuscular disorders • Reduced genioglossus endurance[71]	• Absent periods of stable ventilation • High percentage of apneas	• Noradrenergic/antimuscarinic medications[64,65] (atomoxetine/oxybutynin) • Muscle training[72] • Hypoglossal nerve stimulation
Ventilatory control stability	• High loop gain	• Tendency for NREM AHI > REM AHI[9] • Treatment emergent central apnea • Reduced central apnea in nonsupine positions[153]	• Acetazolamide[147,148] • Oxygen[149,150,149]
Arousal threshold	Low arousal threshold—early awakening with respiratory disturbance	• Shorter respiratory events • Prediction equations[126]	Hypnotics[150,151]

AHI, Apnea-*hypopnea* index; *CPAP*, continuous positive airway pressure; *NREM*, non-rapid eye movement; P_{CRIT}, pharyngeal closing pressure of the upper airway; *REM*, rapid eye movement.

Adapted from Eckert DJ. Phenotypic approaches to obstructive sleep apnoea—new pathways for targeted therapy. *Sleep Med Rev.* 2018;37:45-59; Eckert DJ, White DP, Jordan AS, Malhotra A, Wellman A. Defining phenotypic causes of obstructive sleep apnea. Identification of novel therapeutic targets. *Am J Respir Crit Care Med.* 2013;188(8):996-1004; and Osman AM, Carter SG, Carberry JC, Eckert DJ. Obstructive sleep apnea: current perspectives. *Nat Sci Sleep.* 2018;10:21-34.

loop gain might predict a tendency to develop central apneas on CPAP treatment, after upper airway surgery, or with an oral appliance.[144] Sleeping in the lateral position results in lower dynamic loop gain than sleep in the supine position, and this might explain the reduction in central apnea with supine position avoidance.[153] For patients with inadequate upper airway muscle response, a noradrenergic/antimuscarinic medication such as the combination of atomoxetine and oxybutynin might help.[65] Training upper airway muscles[72] or hypoglossal nerve stimulation might be other approaches. A detailed discussion of the many studies addressing treatment of specific components of OSA endotypes is beyond the scope of this chapter. The reader is referred to the listed references. Currently, many of the proposed interventions would be considered investigational. However, treatment options for OSA based on endotype will likely expand in the future and allow personalized and precision treatment of OSA.

Table 19–3 Traits Contributing to Obstructive Sleep Apnea

Anatomic/Physiologic Trait	Apnea Predisposition
Upper airway anatomy	Small or collapsible upper airway
Upper airway motor control	Poor upper airway muscle response during sleep
Ventilatory control stability	High loop gain
Arousal threshold	Low arousal threshold

SUMMARY OF KEY POINTS

1. Patients with OSA have obstructive apnea and hypopnea during sleep because of a variable combination of unfavorable upper airway anatomy, inadequate upper airway muscle compensation, instability in ventilatory control (high loop gain), and a low arousal threshold (Table 19–3). Whereas a high arousal threshold may prolong respiratory events, a low arousal threshold fragments sleep, results in insufficient time for augmentation of upper airway muscle activity to increase sufficiently to stabilize the upper airway, and predisposes to instability in ventilatory control.
2. The upper airway of patients with OSA is smaller than in normal individuals due to a small bony enclosure or increased soft tissue (including fat) surrounding the airway. A short and posteriorly placed mandible, a long dependent palate, a large tongue, nasal obstruction, and thick lateral

pharyngeal walls and/or tongue and pharyngeal fat all predispose to upper airway collapse during sleep.

3. The upper airway of patients with OSA is more collapsible (higher P_{CRIT}) than in normal subjects. However, about 20% of OSA patients have a P_{CRIT} in the gray zone overlapping with normal individuals.

4. The reasons for the greater prevalence of OSA in men than women are incompletely understood. Men have a longer upper airway, and this may predispose to upper airway collapse. They also may be more susceptible to airway closure during hypocapnia or falling ventilatory drive. Women have shorter upper airways then men which would make the airway less collapsible. No clear difference in P_{CRIT} or upper airway muscle activation between men and women has been demonstrated. Using endotyping techniques women appear to have less collapsible upper airways and lower loop gain than men consistent with a lower risk of OSA. On the other hand they have a lower arousal thresold during NREM sleep. This would predispose them to have OSA. One study found that endotyping explained only 30% of the sex difference in the AHI during NREM sleep. Therefore, our current understanding of gender differences the prevalence of OSA is incomplete.

5. The activity of phasic upper airway muscles (e.g., GG [tongue protruder]) increases with each inspiration. At sleep onset with loss of the wakefulness stimulus, there is decrease in tonic and phasic GG activity but phasic activity recovers with the development of more negative upper airway pressure and increased chemical drive. The activity of tonic upper airway muscles is constant (does not vary with respiration) but does vary with sleep state (wake > NREM ? > REM). For example, the activity of the tensor palatini (a palatal muscle with tonic activity) decreases from wakefulness to NREM sleep but a further decrease from NREM to REM sleep has not been demonstrated by several studies.

6. The GG (tongue protrusion) has both inspiratory (phasic) activity and tonic activity. The GG activity is controlled by central pattern generators, chemostimulation (hypercapnia, hypoxia) via effect on central pattern generators, sleep state (loss of the wakefulness stimuli and the effects of REM sleep), and negative pressure stimulation of upper airway mechanoreceptors. More negative upper airway pressure is associated with increased GG inspiratory activity.

7. The GG (and other upper airway muscles) activity falls with sleep onset (loss of the wakefulness stimulus), and the decrease is greater in patients with OSA compared with normal individuals. During wake, increased upper airway muscle activity in patients with OSA compensates for unfavorable anatomy.

8. In most studies, obstructive apnea/hypopnea termination is associated with arousal in 60% to 80% of the events. Termination of apnea and hypopnea can occur with augmentation of respiratory muscle activity without an arousal. However, some patients lack effective upper airway muscle compensation.

9. Loss of the wakefulness stimulus may be explained at least in part by loss of noradrenergic facilitation of hypoglossal motor neurons during NREM sleep and loss of noradrenergic facilitation and muscarinic (cholinergic) inhibition during REM sleep.

10. During phasic REM sleep, the activity of non-respiratory phasic neurons modulates the activity of respiratory motor neurons (including upper airway motor neurons). This results in periods of inhibition of phasic diaphragmatic activity and tonic and phasic upper airway muscle activity (depending on the muscle) independent of the current chemical drive. That is, EMG activity may fall, although chemical drive is increasing.

11. At sleep onset, loss of the wakefulness stimuli results in a fall in GG muscle activity and ventilatory drive. Upper airway resistance increases, and there is an initial fall in airflow. Increased negative upper airway pressure and chemostimulation increase upper airway muscle activity, and there may be recovery of airflow and ventilation (although lower than during wake). In patients with unfavorable anatomy or inadequate (decreased) upper airway muscle compensation, apnea or hypopnea may occur before stabilization can occur.

12. During REM sleep, GG activity is controlled by input from both respiratory premotor neurons (inspiratory activity) and non-respiratory phasic REM sleep neurons, which can reduce the tonic and phasic (inspiratory activity) of the GG. During REM sleep, with bursts of REMs there are periods of decreased GG and diaphragmatic activity even in normal individuals. In patients with OSA and unfavorable anatomy, obstructive apnea and hypopnea can occur.

13. In the past, airway opening (event termination) was thought to depend on arousal from sleep and an associated large preferential increase in upper airway muscle activity. However, recent evidence suggests arousal and airway opening may be two independent phenomena with similar time courses. Arousal may not occur, or it may precede or follow airway opening. In this view, increasing chemostimulation (hypoxemia and hypercapnia) and mechanoreceptor simulation (negative upper airway pressure) progressively augment upper airway muscle activity until "an airway opening threshold (AOT)" is reached and the airway opens (independent of arousal). However, in some situations restoration of upper airway patency does depend on arousal.

14. The arousal stimulus during obstructive apnea and hypopnea in NREM sleep appears to be proportional to the magnitude of inspiratory effort (esophageal pressure excursions). Hypercapnia and hypoxemia may cause increasing respiratory effort, but arousal occurs when the level of effort reaches an arousal threshold. Input from chemoreceptors, mechanoreceptors, and sleep state may influence the arousal threshold.

15. The arousal threshold to respiratory stimuli during NREM sleep is increased in patients with OSA compared with normal individuals (higher inspiratory effort is needed to trigger arousal). CPAP treatment may lower (improve) the arousal threshold but does not restore the threshold to normal levels in most OSA patients.

16. Obstructive apneas and hypopneas are longer during REM than NREM sleep. In contrast, normal individuals arouse from experimental mask occlusion more rapidly in REM than NREM sleep. The pathophysiology of the longer obstructive apneas in REM sleep is not understood. During REM sleep there is often a slow or no clear-cut progressive increase in respiratory effort during airway occlusion.

17. Factors associated with more severe arterial oxygen desaturation include a higher BMI, low awake SaO_2 or PaO_2, longer respiratory events/shorter period of ventilation between events, and a smaller ERV. A small ERV is due to a low FRC and/or a high RV. A low FRC is associated with lower oxygen stores and more ventilation-perfusion mismatch. A high RV is usually due to air-trapping from obstructive airway disease, which is also associated with more ventilation-perfusion mismatch.

18. New indices of hypoxemia such as the sleep apnea specific hypoxic burden (SASHB) may predict daytime sleepiness or cardiovascular morbidity in OSA patient better than the AHI.

CLINICAL REVIEW QUESTIONS

1. Which of the following factors may help explain the greater prevalence of OSA in men than women?
   A. Longer upper airway length in men
   B. Lower P_{CRIT} (more negative) in men
   C. Less pharyngeal muscle activation
   D. Lower loop gain in men than women
2. Breathing through the nose rather than the mouth causes more negative supraglottic airway pressure during inspiration (e.g., −6 cm H_2O with nasal breathing, −2 cm H_2O with oral breathing). Which route of breathing is associated with greater phasic activity of the GG muscle?
   A. Oral breathing route
   B. Nasal breathing route
3. Which of the following would predispose to upper airway narrowing or closure?
   A. NREM > REM
   B. Higher FRC
   C. More negative upper airway pressure (−10 vs. −6 cm H_2O)
   D. Higher P_{CRIT}
4. Which of the following is **NOT** associated with worse arterial oxygen desaturation during sleep in OSA patients?
   A. REM > NREM
   B. Lower ERV
   C. Low baseline SpO_2
   D. Longer respiratory events
   E. Lateral position > supine
   F. Higher BMI
5. Which of the following statements about arousal and respiratory event termination is **NOT** true?
   A. Lower arousal threshold is associated with a shorter duration respiratory event but may cause instability in ventilatory control.
   B. Arousal is necessary for respiratory event termination.
   C. The arousal threshold is higher than normal in many patients with OSA.
   D. A higher arousal threshold may prolong respiratory events but can allow respiratory muscle time to stabilize the upper airway.

ANSWERS

1. A. Longer upper airway length in men. Studies have also found a smaller difference between the sleeping PCO_2 and the apneic threshold in men. A higher (more postive) P_{CRIT} in men would be associated with a more collaspible upper airway, However, no clear differences between men and women in the P_{CRIT} or upper airway muscle activation have been demonstrated. A study of a large group of patients using advanced computer endotyping analysis of routine polysomnography did suggest that the upper airway of women is less collapsible than men and women. Women tend to have lower (not higher) loopgain than men. However, women have a lower arousal threshold.
2. B. Nasal. Negative upper airway pressure augments phasic upper airway muscle activity.
3. D. A higher P_{CRIT} is associated with a more collapsible upper airway. Upper airway volume decreases with lower lung volume. A higher FRC would not predispose to airway closure or narrowing. More negative upper airway pressure increases upper airway muscle activity. The AHI is higher during REM sleep in many patients, and some have OSA only during REM sleep.
4. E. Supine body position is associated with worse desaturation. REM > NREM, men > women, higher BMI, lower ERV, and low baseline SaO_2 increase the severity of desaturation. Of note, the greatest effect of a high BMI on worsening oxygen desaturation is during REM sleep.
5. B. Depending on the patient, respiratory event terminations are associated with arousal in only about 60% to 80% of events. Arousal may occur before, simultaneous with, or after apnea/hypopnea termination.

REFERENCES

1. Eckert DJ, Malhotra A. Pathophysiology of adult obstructive sleep apnea. *Proc Am Thorac Soc.* 2008;5:144-153.
2. Deacon-Diaz N, Malhotra A. Inherent vs. induced loop gain abnormalities in obstructive sleep apnea. *Front Neurol.* 2018;9:896.
3. Eckert DJ. Phenotypic approaches to obstructive sleep apnoea—new pathways for targeted therapy. *Sleep Med Rev.* 2018;37:45-59.
4. Eckert DJ, White DP, Jordan AS, Malhotra A, Wellman A. Defining phenotypic causes of obstructive sleep apnea. Identification of novel therapeutic targets. *Am J Respir Crit Care Med.* 2013;188(8):996-1004.
5. Carberry JC, Amatoury J, Eckert DJ. Personalized management approach for OSA. *Chest.* 2018;153(3):744-755.
6. Jordan AS, White DP. Pharyngeal motor control and pathogenesis of obstructive sleep apnea. *Respir Physiol Neurobiol.* 2008;160:1-7.
7. Osman AM, Carter SG, Carberry JC, Eckert DJ. Obstructive sleep apnea: current perspectives. *Nat Sci Sleep.* 2018;10:21-34.
8. Malhotra A, Mesarwi O, Pepin JL, Owens RL. Endotypes and phenotypes in obstructive sleep apnea. *Curr Opin Pulm Med.* 2020;26(6):609-614.
9. Joosten SA, Landry SA, Wong AM, et al. Assessing the physiologic endotypes responsible for REM and NREM-based OSA. *Chest.* 2021;159(5):1998-2007.
10. Remmers JE, Degroot WJ, Sauerland EK, and colleagues. Pathogenesis of upper airway occlusion during sleep. *J Appl Physiol.* 1978;44:931-938.
11. Neelapu BC, Kharbanda OP, Sardana HK, et al. Craniofacial and upper airway morphology in adult obstructive sleep apnea patients: a systematic review and meta-analysis of cephalometric studies. *Sleep Med Rev.* 2017;31:79-90.
12. Sforza E, Bacon W, Weiss T, Thibault A, Petiau C, Krieger J. Upper airway collapsibility and cephalometric variables in patients with obstructive sleep apnea. *Am J Respir Crit Care Med.* 2000;161(2 Pt 1):347-352.
13. Joosten SA, Sands SA, Edwards BA, et al. Evaluation of the role of lung volume and airway size and shape in supine-predominant obstructive sleep apnoea patients. *Respirology.* 2015;20(5):819-827.
14. Kim WY, Hong SN, Yang SK, et al. The effect of body position on airway patency in obstructive sleep apnea: CT imaging analysis. *Sleep Breath.* 2019;23(3):911-916.
15. Schwab RJ, Gefter WB, Hoffman EA, et al. Dynamic upper airway imaging during wake respiration in normal subjects and patients with sleep disordered breathing. *Am Rev Respir Dis.* 1993;148:1385-1400.
16. Schwab RJ, Pasirstein M, Pierson R, et al. Identification of upper airway anatomic risk factors for obstructive sleep apnea with volumetric magnetic resonance imaging. *Am J Respir Crit Care Med.* 2003;168:522-530.
17. Walsh JH, Leigh MS, Paduch A, et al. Effect of body posture on pharyngeal shape and size in adults with and without obstructive sleep apnea. *Sleep.* 2008;31:1543-1549.
18. Isono S, Remmers JE, Tanaka A, et al. Anatomy of pharynx in patients with obstructive sleep apnea and normal subjects. *J Appl Physiol.* 1997;82:1319-1326.
19. Eastwood P, Gilani SZ, McArdle N, et al. Predicting sleep apnea from three-dimensional face photography. *J Clin Sleep Med.* 2020;16(4):493-502.
20. Leiter JC. Upper airway shape: is it important in the pathogenesis of obstructive sleep apnea? *Am J Respir Crit Care Med.* 1996;153:894-898.

21. Wang SH, Keenan BT, Wiemken A, et al. Effect of weight loss on upper airway anatomy and the apnea-hypopnea index. The importance of tongue fat. *Am J Respir Crit Care Med*. 2020;201:718-727.
22. Clark SA, Wilson CR, Satoh M, et al. Assessment of inspiratory flow limitation invasively and noninvasively during sleep. *Am Respir Crit Care Med.* 1998;158:713-722.
23. Gold AR, Schwartz AR. The pharyngeal critical pressure. *Chest*. 1996;100:1077-1088.
24. Gleadhill IC, Schwartz AR, Schubert N, et al. Upper airway collapsibility in snorers and in patients with obstructive hypopnea and apnea. *Am Rev Respir Dis*. 1991;143:1300-1303.
25. Smith PL, Wise RA, Gold AR, Schwartz AR, Permutt S. Upper airway pressure-flow relationships in obstructive sleep apnea. *J Appl Physiol (1985)*. 1988;64(2):789-795.
26. Schwartz AR, O'Donnell CP, Baron J, et al. The hypotonic upper airway in obstructive sleep apnea: role of structures and neuromuscular activity. *Am J Respir Crit Care Med*. 1998;157(4 Pt 1):1051-1057.
27. Patil SP, Schneider H, Marx JJ, Gladmon E, Schwartz AR, Smith PL. Neuromechanical control of upper airway patency during sleep. *J Appl Physiol (1985)*. 2007;102(2):547-556.
28. Boudewyns A, Punjabi N, Van de Heyning PH, et al. Abbreviated method for assessing upper airway function in obstructive sleep apnea. *Chest*. 2000;118(4):1031-1041.
29. Penzel T, Moller M, Becker HF, et al. Effect of sleep position and sleep stage on the collapsibility of the upper airways in patients with sleep apnea. *Sleep*. 2001;24:90-95.
30. Carberry JC, Jordan AS, White DP, Wellman A, Eckert DJ. Upper airway collapsibility (Pcrit) and pharyngeal dilator muscle activity are sleep stage dependent. *Sleep*. 2016;39(3):511-521.
31. Landry SA, Joosten SA, Eckert DJ, et al. Therapeutic CPAP level predicts upper airway collapsibility in patients with obstructive sleep apnea. *Sleep*. 2017;40(6):zsx056.
32. Osman AM, Tong BK, Landry SA, et al. An assessment of a simple clinical technique to estimate pharyngeal collapsibility in people with obstructive sleep apnea. *Sleep*. 2020;43(10):zsaa067.
33. Malhotra A, Pillar G, Edwards J, et al. Upper airway collapsibility: measurement and sleep effects. *Chest*. 2001;120:156-161.
34. Azarbarzin A, Sands SA, Taranto-Montemurro L, et al. Estimation of pharyngeal collapsibility during sleep by peak inspiratory airflow. *Sleep*. 2017;40(1):zsw005.
35. Osman AM, Carberry JC, Burke PGR, et al. Upper airway collapsibility measured using a simple wakefulness test closely relates to the pharyngeal critical closing pressure during sleep in obstructive sleep apnea. *Sleep*. 2019;42(7):zsz080.
36. Hoffstein V, Zamel N, Phillipson EA. Lung volume dependence of cross-sectional area in patients with obstructive sleep apnea. *Am Rev Respir Dis*. 1984;130:175-178.
37. Stanchina ML, Malhotra A, Fogel RB, et al. The influence of lung volume on pharyngeal mechanics, collapsibility, and genioglossus muscle activation during sleep. *Sleep*. 2003;26:851-856.
38. Van de Graaff WB. Thoracic influences on upper airway patency. *J Appl Physiol*. 1988;65:2124-2131.
39. Tong J, Jugé L, Burke PG, et al. Respiratory-related displacement of the trachea in obstructive sleep apnea. *J Appl Physiol (1985)*. 2019;127(5): 1307-1316.
40. Hudgel DW, Devadatta P. Decrease in functional residual capacity during sleep in normal humans. *J Appl Physiol*. 1984;57:1319-1322.
41. Avraam J, Dawson A, Rochford PD, et al. The effect of sex and body weight on lung volumes during sleep. *Sleep*. 2019;42(10):zsz141.
42. Jordan AS, White DP, Lo YL, et al. Airway dilator muscle activity and lung volume during stable breathing in obstructive sleep apnea. *Sleep*. 2009;32:361-368.
43. Hudgel DW, Martin RJ, Capehart M, Johnson B, Hill P. Contribution of hypoventilation to sleep oxygen desaturation in chronic obstructive pulmonary disease. *J Appl Physiol Respir Environ Exerc Physiol*. 1983;55(3): 669-677.
44. Squier SB, Patil SP, Schneider H, et al. Effect of end-expiratory lung volume on upper airway collapsibility in sleeping men and women. *J Appl Physiol (1985)*. 2010;109(4):977-985.
45. Morrell MJ, Arabi Y, Zahn B, Badr MS. Progressive retropalatal narrowing preceding obstructive apnea. *Am J Respir Crit Care Med*. 1998; 158:1974-1981.
46. Heinzer RC, Stanchina ML, Malhotra A, et al. Lung volume and continuous positive airway pressure requirement in obstructive sleep apnea. *Am J Respir Crit Care Med*. 2005;172:114-117.
47. Mador MJ, Kufel TJ, Magalang UJ, Rajesh SK, Watwe V, Grant BJ. Prevalence of positional sleep apnea in patients undergoing polysomnography. *Chest*. 2005;128(4):2130-2137.
48. Marques M, Genta PR, Sands SA, et al. Effect of sleeping position on upper airway patency in obstructive sleep apnea is determined by the pharyngeal structure causing collapse. *Sleep*. 2017;40(3):zsx005.
49. Joosten SA, Edwards BA, Wellman A, et al. The effect of body position on physiological factors that contribute to obstructive sleep apnea. *Sleep*. 2015;38(9):1469-1478.
50. Joosten SA, Sands SA, Edwards BA, et al. Evaluation of the role of lung volume and airway size and shape in supine-predominant obstructive sleep apnoea patients. *Respirology*. 2015;20(5):819-827.
51. Oksenberg A, Arons E, Nasser K, et al. REM-related obstructive sleep apnea: the effect of body position. *J Clin Sleep Med*. 2010;6:343-348.
52. White LH, Bradley TD. Role of nocturnal rostral fluid shift in the pathogenesis of obstructive and central sleep apnoea. *J Physiol*. 2013;591(5):1179-1193.
53. Perger E, Jutant EM, Redolfi S. Targeting volume overload and overnight rostral fluid shift: a new perspective to treat sleep apnea. *Sleep Med Rev*. 2018;42:160-170.
54. Lo YL, Jordan AS, Malhotra A, et al. Influence of wakefulness on pharyngeal airway muscle activity. *Thorax*. 2007;62(9):799-805.
55. Malhotra A, Pillar G, Fogel RB, et al. Genioglossal but not palatal muscle activity relates closely to pharyngeal pressure. *Am J Respir Crit Care Med*. 2000;162:1058-1062.
56. Tangel DJ, Mezzanotte WS, White DP. Influences of NREM sleep on activity of palatoglossus and levator palatini muscles in normal men. *J Appl Physiol*. 1995;78:689-695.
57. Tangel DJ, Mezzanotte WS, Sandberg EJ, White DP. Influences of NREM sleep on activity of tonic vs. inspiratory phasic muscles in normal men. *J Appl Physiol*. 1992;73:1058-1066.
58. Tangel DJ, Mezzanotte WS, White DP. Influence of sleep on tensor palatini EMG and upper airway resistance in normal men. *J Appl Physiol (1985)*. 1991;70(6):2574-2581.
59. Horner RL, Hughes SW, Malhotra A. State-dependent and reflex drives to the upper airway: basic physiology with clinical implications. *J Appl Physiol (1985)*. 2014;116(3):325-336.
60. Fenik VB, Penzel T, Malhotra A. Editorial: anatomy of upper airway and neuronal control of pharyngeal muscles in obstructive sleep apnea. *Front Neurol*. 2019;10:733.
61. Fenik VB. Contribution of neurochemical inputs to the decrease of motoneuron excitability during non-REM and REM sleep: a systematic review. *Front Neurol*. 2018;9:629.
62. Wiegand L, Zwillich CW, Wiegand D, White DP. Changes in upper airway muscle activation and ventilation during phasic REM sleep in normal men. *J Appl Physiol*. 1991;71:488-497.
63. Grace KP, Hughes SW, Horner RL. Identification of the mechanism mediating genioglossus muscle suppression in REM sleep. *Am J Respir Crit Care Med*. 2013;187(3):311-319.
64. Grace KP, Hughes SW, Shahabi S, Horner RL. K+ channel modulation causes genioglossus inhibition in REM sleep and is a strategy for reactivation. *Respir Physiol Neurobiol*. 2013;188(3):277-288.
65. Taranto-Montemurro L, Messineo L, Sands SA, et al. The combination of atomoxetine and oxybutynin greatly reduces obstructive sleep apnea severity. A randomized, placebo-controlled, double-blind crossover trial. *Am J Respir Crit Care Med*. 2019;199(10):1267-1276.
66. Orem J. Neuronal mechanisms of respiration in REM sleep. *Sleep*. 1980; 3(3-4):251-267.
67. Horner RL. Central neural control of respiratory neurons and motoneurons during sleep. In: Kryger MH, Goldstein CA, Roth T, eds. *Principles and Practice of Sleep Medicine*. 7th ed. Elsevier; 2022.
68. Mezzanotte WS, Tangel DJ, White DP. Waking genioglossal electromyogram in sleep apnea patients versus normal controls (a neuromuscular compensatory mechanism). *J Clin Invest*. 1992;89:1571-1579.
69. Fogel RB, Malhotra A, Pillar G, et al. Genioglossal activation in patients with obstructive sleep apnea versus control subjects. *Am J Respir Crit Care Med*. 2001;164:2025-2030.
70. Sands SA, Eckert DJ, Jordan AS, et al. Enhanced upper-airway muscle responsiveness is a distinct feature of overweight/obese individuals without sleep apnea. *Am J Respir Crit Care Med*. 2014;190:930-937.
71. Eckert DJ, Lo YL, Saboisky JP, Jordan AS, White DP, Malhotra A. Sensorimotor function of the upper-airway muscles and respiratory sensory processing in untreated obstructive sleep apnea. *J Appl Physiol (1985)*. 2011;111(6):1644-1653.
72. Baptista PM, Martínez Ruiz de Apodaca P, Carrasco M, et al. Daytime neuromuscular electrical therapy of tongue muscles in improving snoring

in individuals with primary snoring and mild obstructive sleep apnea. *J Clin Med.* 2021;10(9):1883.
73. Worsnop C, Kay C, Pierce R, et al. Activity of respiratory pump and upper airway muscles during sleep onset. *J Appl Physiol.* 1998;85:908-920.
74. Mezzanotte WS, Tangel DJ, White DP. Influence of sleep onset on upper-airway muscle activity in apnea patients versus normal controls. *Am J Respir Crit Care Med.* 1996;153:1880-1887.
75. Gould GA, Gugger M, Molloy J, et al. Breathing pattern and eye movement density during REM sleep in humans. *Am Rev Respir Dis.* 1988;138:874-877.
76. Neilly JB, Gaipa EA, Maislin G, Pack A. Ventilation during early and later rapid-eye-movement sleep. *J Appl Physiol.* 1991;71:1201-1215.
77. Kline LR, Hendricks JC, Davies RO, Pack AI. Control of activity of the diaphragm in rapid-eye-movement sleep. *J Appl Physiol (1985).* 1986;61(4):1293-1300.
78. Becker HF, Piper AJ, Flynn WE, et al. Breathing during sleep in patients with nocturnal desaturation. *Am J Respir Crit Care Med.* 1999;159(1):112-118.
79. McSharry DG, Saboisky JP, Deyoung P, et al. Physiological mechanisms of upper airway hypotonia during REM sleep. *Sleep.* 2014;37(3):561-569.
80. Eckert DJ, Malhotra A, Lo YL, White DP, Jordan AS. The influence of obstructive sleep apnea and gender on genioglossus activity during rapid eye movement sleep. *Chest.* 2009;135(4):957-964.
81. Messineo L, Eckert DJ, Taranto-Montemurro L, et al. Ventilatory drive withdrawal rather than reduced genioglossus compensation as a mechanism of obstructive sleep apnea in REM sleep. *Am J Respir Crit Care Med.* 2022;205(2):219-232.
82. Findley LJ, Wilhoit SC, Suratt PM. Apnea duration and hypoxemia during REM sleep in patients with obstructive sleep apnea. *Chest.* 1985;87(4):432-436.
83. Horner RL, Innes JA, Murphy K, Guz A. Evidence for reflex upper airway dilator muscle activation by sudden negative airway pressure in man. *J Physiol.* 1991;436:15-29.
84. Berry RB, White DP, Roper J, et al. Awake negative pressure reflex response of the genioglossus in OSA patients and normal subjects. *J Appl Physiol.* 2003;94:1875-1882.
85. Mortimore IL, Douglas NJ. Palatal muscle EMG response to negative pressure in awake sleep apneic and control subjects. *Am J Respir Crit Care Med.* 1997;156:867-873.
86. Wheatley JR, Tangel DJ, Mezzanotte WS, White DP. Influence of sleep on response to negative airway pressure of tensor palatini muscle and retropalatal airway. *J Appl Physiol.* 1993;75:2117-2124.
87. Horner RL, Innes JA, Morrell MJ, et al. The effect of sleep on reflex genioglossus muscle activation by stimuli of negative airway pressure in humans. *J Physiol (Lond).* 1994;476:141-151.
88. Wheatley JR, Mezzanotte WS, Tangel DJ, White DP. The influence of sleep on genioglossal muscle activation by negative pressure in normal men. *Am Rev Respir Dis.* 1993;148:597-605.
89. Horner RL, Innes JA, Holden HB, Guz A. Afferent pathway(s) for pharyngeal dilator reflex to negative pressure in man: a study using upper airway anesthesia. *J Physiol.* 1991;436:31-44.
90. Berry RB, McNellis M, Kouchi K, Light RW. Upper airway anesthesia reduces genioglossus activity during sleep apnea. *Am J Respir Crit Care Med.* 1997;156:127-132.
91. Pillar G, Malhotra A, Fogel RB, et al. Upper airway muscle responsiveness to rising PCO_2 during NREM sleep. *J Appl Physiol.* 2000;89:1275-1282.
92. Lo YL, Jordan AS, Malhotra A, et al. Genioglossal muscle response to CO_2 stimulation during NREM sleep. *Sleep.* 2006;29(4):470-477.
93. Younes M. Role of arousals in the pathogenesis of obstructive sleep apnea. *Am J Respir Crit Care Med.* 2004;169(5):623-633.
94. Amatoury J, Jordan AS, Toson B, Nguyen C, Wellman A, Eckert DJ. New insights into the timing and potential mechanisms of respiratory-induced cortical arousals in obstructive sleep apnea. *Sleep.* 2018;41(11):zsy160.
95. Badr MS, Toiber F, Skatrud JB, Dempsey J. Pharyngeal narrowing/occlusion during central sleep apnea. *J Appl Physiol (1985).* 1995;78(5):1806-1815.
96. Onal E, Lopata M. Periodic breathing and the pathogenesis of occlusive sleep apneas. *Am Rev Respir Dis.* 1982;126(4):676-680.
97. Wellman A, Jordan AS, Malhotra A, et al. Ventilatory control and airway anatomy in obstructive sleep apnea. *Am J Respir Crit Care Med.* 2004;170:1225-1232.
98. Orr JE, Malhotra A, Sands SA. Pathogenesis of central and complex sleep apnoea. *Respirology.* 2017;22(1):43-52.
99. Roberts EG, Raphelson JR, Orr JE, LaBuzetta JN, Malhotra A. The pathogenesis of central and complex sleep apnea. *Curr Neurol Neurosci Rep.* 2022;22(7):405-412.
100. Younes M, Ostrowski M, Thompson W, et al. Chemical control stability in patients with obstructive sleep apnea. *Am J Respir Crit Care Med.* 2001;163:1181-1190.
101. Dempsey J. Crossing the apneic threshold. Causes and consequences. *Exp Physiol.* 2004;90:13-24.
102. Iber C, Davies SF, Chapman RC, Mahowald MM. A possible mechanism for mixed apnea in obstructive sleep apnea. *Chest.* 1986;89:800-805.
103. Badr MS, Kawak A. Post-hyperventilation hypopnea in humans during NREM sleep. *Respir Physiol.* 1996;103:137-145.
104. Rowley JA, Zhou XS, Diamond MP, Badr MS. The determinants of the apnea threshold during NREM sleep in normal subjects. *Sleep.* 2006;29:95-103.
105. Eckert DJ, Younes MK. Arousal from sleep: implications for obstructive sleep apnea pathogenesis and treatment. *J Appl Physiol (1985).* 2014;116(3):302-313.
106. Gleeson K, Zwillich CW, White DP. The influence of increasing ventilatory effort on arousal from sleep. *Am Rev Respir Dis.* 1990;142:295-300.
107. Berry RB, Gleeson K. Respiratory arousal from sleep. Mechanisms and significance. *Sleep.* 1997;20:654-675.
108. Kimoff RJ, Cheong TH, Olha AE, et al. Mechanisms of apnea termination in obstructive sleep apnea. Role of chemoreceptor and mechanoreceptor stimuli. *Am J Respir Crit Care Med.* 1994;149:707-714.
109. Berry RB, Quan SF, Abreu AR, et al. *The AASM Manual for the Scoring of Sleep and Associated Events: Rules, Terminology and Technical Specifications.* Version 2.6. American Academy of Sleep Medicine; 2020.
110. Roehrs T, Zorick F, Wittig R, Conway W, Roth T. Predictors of objective level of daytime sleepiness in patients with sleep-related breathing disorders. *Chest.* 1989;95:1202-1206.
111. Jordan AS, Eckert DJ, Wellman A, et al. Termination of respiratory events with and without cortical arousal in obstructive sleep apnea. *Am J Respir Crit Care Med.* 2011;184(10):1183-1191.
112. Cori JM, Thornton T, O'Donoghue FJ, et al. Arousal-induced hypocapnia does not reduce genioglossus activity in obstructive sleep apnea. *Sleep.* 2017;40(6):zsx057.
113. Cori JM, Rochford PD, O'Donoghue FJ, Trinder J, Jordan AS. The influence of CO2 on genioglossus muscle after-discharge following arousal from sleep. *Sleep.* 2017;40(11). doi:10.1093/sleep/zsx160.
114. Berry RB, Kouchi KG, Bower JL, Light RW. Effect of upper airway anesthesia on obstructive sleep apnea. *Am J Respir Crit Care Med.* 1995;151:1857-1861.
115. Cala SJ, Sliwinski P, Cosio MG, Kimoff RJ. Effect of topical upper airway anesthesia on apnea duration through the night in obstructive sleep apnea. *J Appl Physiol.* 1996;81:2618-2626.
116. Issa FG, Sullivan CE. Arousal and breathing responses to airway occlusion in healthy sleeping adults. *J Appl Physiol.* 1983;55:1113-1119.
117. Berry RB, Kouchi KG, Der DE, Dickel MJ, Light RW. Sleep apnea impairs the arousal response to airway occlusion. *Chest.* 1996;109(6):1490-1496.
118. Haba-Rubio J, Sforza E, Weiss T, Schröder C, Krieger J. Effect of CPAP treatment on inspiratory arousal threshold during NREM sleep in OSAS. *Sleep Breath.* 2005;9(1):12-19.
119. Gora J, Trinder J, Pierce R, Colrain IM. Evidence of a sleep specific blunted cortical response to inspiratory occlusions in mild obstructive sleep apnea syndrome. *Am J Respir Crit Care Med.* 2002;166:1225-1234.
120. Kimoff RJ, Sforza E, Champagne V, et al. Upper airway sensation in snoring and obstructive sleep apnea. *Am J Respir Crit Care Med.* 2001;164:250-255.
121. Charbonneau M, Marin JM, Olha A, Kimoff RJ, Levy RD, Cosio MG. Changes in obstructive sleep apnea characteristics through the night. *Chest.* 1994;106(6):1695-1701.
122. Montserrat JM, Kosmas EN, Cosio MG, Kimoff RJ. Mechanism of apnea lengthening across the night in obstructive sleep apnea. *Am J Respir Crit Care Med.* 1996;154:988-993.
123. Berry RB, Asyali MA, McNellis MI, Khoo MC. Within-night variation in respiratory effort preceding apnea termination and EEG delta power in sleep apnea. *J Appl Physiol.* 1998;85:1434-1441.
124. Sforza E, Krieger J, Petiau C. Arousal threshold to respiratory stimuli in OSA patients: evidence for a sleep-dependent temporal rhythm. *Sleep.* 1999;22(1):69-75.
125. Berry RB. Dreaming about an open upper airway. *Sleep.* 2006;29(4):429-431.

126. Edwards BA, Eckert DJ, McSharry DG, et al. Clinical predictors of the respiratory arousal threshold in patients with obstructive sleep apnea. *Am J Respir Crit Care Med.* 2014;190(11):1293-1300.
127. Sands SA, Terrill PI, Edwards BA, et al. Quantifying the arousal threshold using polysomnography in obstructive sleep apnea. *Sleep.* 2018;41(1):zsx183.
128. Chamberlin NL. Brain circuitry mediating arousal from obstructive sleep apnea. *Curr Opin Neurobiol.* 2013;23(5):774-779.
129. Malhotra A, Huang Y, Fogel RB, et al. The male predisposition to pharyngeal collapse: importance of airway length. *Am J Respir Crit Care Med.* 2002;166:1388-1395.
130. Malhotra A, Huang Y, Fogel R, et al. Aging influences on pharyngeal anatomy and physiology: the predisposition to pharyngeal collapse. *Am J Med.* 2006;119:72.e9-72.e14.
131. Jordan AS, Wellman A, Edwards JK, et al. Respiratory control stability and upper airway collapsibility in men and women with obstructive sleep apnea. *J Appl Physiol.* 2005;99:2020-2027.
132. Rowley JA, Zhou X, Vergine I, et al. Influence of gender on upper airway mechanics: upper airway resistance and Pcrit. *J Appl Physiol.* 2001;91:2248-2254.
133. Pillar G, Malhotra A, Fogel R, et al. Airway mechanics and ventilation in response to resistive loading during sleep: influence of gender. *Am J Respir Crit Care Med.* 2000;162:1627-1632.
134. Won CHJ, Reid M, Sofer T, et al. Sex differences in obstructive sleep apnea phenotypes, the multi-ethnic study of atherosclerosis. *Sleep.* 2020; 43(5):zsz274.
135. Zhou XS, Shahabuddin S, Zahn BR, et al. Effect of gender on the development of hypocapnic apnea/hypopnea during NREM sleep. *J Appl Physiol.* 2000;89:192-199.
136. Findley LJ, Ries AL, Tisi GM, Wagner PD. Hypoxemia during apnea in normal subjects: mechanisms and impact of lung volume. *J Appl Physiol.* 1983;55:1777-1783.
137. Bradley TD, Martinez D, Rutherford R, et al. Physiological determinants of nocturnal arterial oxygenation in patients with obstructive sleep apnea. *J Appl Physiol.* 1985;59:1364-1368.
138. Sériès F, Cormier Y, La Forge J. Influence of apnea type and sleep stage on nocturnal postapneic desaturation. *Am Rev Respir Dis.* 1990;141:1522-1526.
139. Peppard PE, Ward NR, Morrell MJ. The impact of obesity on oxygen desaturation during sleep disordered breathing. *Am J Respir Crit Care Med.* 2009;180:788-793.
140. Oksenberg A, Khamaysi I, Silverberg DS, Tarasiuk A. Association of body position with severity of apneic events in patients with severe nonpositional obstructive sleep apnea. *Chest.* 2000;118:1018-1024.
141. Azarbarzin A, Sands SA, Stone KL, et al. The hypoxic burden of sleep apnoea predicts cardiovascular disease-related mortality: the Osteoporotic Fractures in Men Study and the Sleep Heart Health Study. *Eur Heart J.* 2019;40(14):1149-1157.
142. Azarbarzin A, Sands SA, Taranto-Montemurro L, et al. The sleep apnea-specific hypoxic burden predicts incident heart failure. *Chest.* 2020; 158(2):739-750.
143. Kainulainen S, Töyräs J, Oksenberg A, et al. Severity of desaturations reflects OSA-related daytime sleepiness better than AHI. *J Clin Sleep Med.* 2019;15(8):1135-1142.
144. Owens RL, Edwards BA, Eckert DJ, et al. An integrative model of physiological traits can be used to predict obstructive sleep apnea and response to non-positive airway pressure therapy. *Sleep.* 2015;38(6):961-970.
145. Taranto-Montemurro L, Messineo L, Wellman A. Targeting endotypic traits with medications for the pharmacological treatment of obstructive sleep apnea. A review of the current literature. *J Clin Med.* 2019;8(11):1846.
146. Dutta R, Delaney G, Toson B, et al. A novel model to estimate key obstructive sleep apnea endotypes from standard polysomnography and clinical data and their contribution to obstructive sleep apnea severity. *Ann Am Thorac Soc.* 2021;18(4):656-667.
147. Edwards BA, Sands SA, Eckert DJ, et al. Acetazolamide improves loop gain but not the other physiological traits causing obstructive sleep apnoea. *J Physiol.* 2012;590(5):1199-1211.
148. Schmickl CN, Landry S, Orr JE, et al. Effects of acetazolamide on control of breathing in sleep apnea patients: mechanistic insights using meta-analyses and physiological model simulations. *Physiol Rep.* 2021; 9(20):e15071.
149. Wellman A, Malhotra A, Jordan AS, Stevenson KE, Gautam S, White DP. Effect of oxygen in obstructive sleep apnea: role of loop gain. *Respir Physiol Neurobiol.* 2008;162(2):144-151.
150. Edwards BA, Sands SA, Owens RL, et al. The combination of supplemental oxygen and a hypnotic markedly improves obstructive sleep apnea in patients with a mild to moderate upper airway collapsibility. *Sleep.* 2016;39(11):1973-1983.
151. Carter SG, Eckert DJ. Effects of hypnotics on obstructive sleep apnea endotypes and severity: novel insights into pathophysiology and treatment. *Sleep Med Rev.* 2021;58:101492.
152. Messineo L, Eckert DJ, Lim R, et al. Zolpidem increases sleep efficiency and the respiratory arousal threshold without changing sleep apnoea severity and pharyngeal muscle activity. *J Physiol.* 2020;598(20):4681-4692.
153. Joosten SA, Landry SA, Sands SA, et al. Dynamic loop gain increases upon adopting the supine body position during sleep in patients with obstructive sleep apnoea. *Respirology.* 2017;22(8):1662-1669.

Chapter 20

Clinical Consequences of Obstructive Sleep Apnea and Benefits of Treatment

INTRODUCTION

This chapter reviews the consequences of untreated adult obstructive sleep apnea (OSA) and the benefits of treatment. Prominent consequences of OSA are listed in Table 20–1.[1-5] Many of the studies discussed in this chapter are cross-sectional population-based investigations looking for associations between the *prevalence* of disorders (amount of disease in a population) at a given time with the severity/presence of OSA (various levels of apnea-hypopnea index [AHI]). Others follow a population over a period of time and determine the number of new cases (*incidence* of a given disease). These studies determine the risk of developing consequences at various levels of the AHI. The results of population-based studies may vary depending on the group being evaluated (age, proportions of men and women). It is also worth noting that investigations of *clinic-based* versus *population-based* studies could find different associations or benefits from treatment.[6] From another perspective, one might ask how often do patients with a given **cardiovascular (CV)** disorder have OSA? The result will depend on the AHI used to define the presence of OSA3. However, Figure 20–1 shows estimates for common CV disorders.

Considering the effects of continuous positive airway pressure (CPAP) treatment on consequences of untreated OSA, it is important to understand that observational studies are less convincing than randomized controlled trials (RCTs). There is always the concern that patients who adhered to CPAP treatment are somehow more compliant with other medical therapy as well; therefore, they are more likely to have better outcomes. A study by Platt and colleagues[7] found CPAP users were more adherent in taking lipid-lowering medications. However, another study by Villar and coworkers[8] found that participants adherent or nonadherent to CPAP did not differ in their adherence to medication. Both studies relied on prescriptions filled or patient report, so actual medication use could differ. There are several ethical and experimental considerations that make designing a study to prove a benefit of CPAP treatment on CV outcomes very difficult. With the widespread knowledge of CPAP, it is difficult to design a study with effective blinding and a satisfactory control treatment (e.g., sub-therapeutic CPAP).[9] Two other important issues to consider when evaluating the results of RCTs of CPAP treatment are (1) many RCTs **excluded** the sleepiest OSA patients, and some studies suggest that this group may have a higher risk for CV disorders and the most potential benefit from CPAP, and (2) CPAP adherence was low (3–4 hours per night).[10,11] Some of the RCTs recruited patients who did not present to sleep clinics with symptoms and may not represent populations seen in sleep clinics.[6] Longitudinal analysis in a community-based cohort (Wisconsin Sleep Cohort) revealed a significant association between rapid eye movement (REM) AHI categories and the development of hypertension (HTN), whereas the non-rapid eye movement (NREM) AHI was not a significant predictor of the development of HTN.[12] Analysis of the Sleep Heart Health Study (SHHS) cohort revealed that severe OSA that occurs primarily during REM sleep was associated with a higher incidence of a composite CV endpoint, but only in those with prevalent cardiovascular disease (CVD).[13] Therefore, not using positive airway pressure (PAP) the entire night will not treat OSA during REM sleep, as the majority of this sleep stage occurs in the last half of the night. Thus, an average use of CPAP of 3 to 4 hours may not be enough for CV benefit.

PATHOPHYSIOLOGY OF THE ADVERSE EFFECTS OF OSA

During normal NREM sleep, there is a decrease in metabolic rate, sympathetic nerve activity, blood pressure (BP), and heart rate, whereas vagal tone increases during NREM sleep compared with wakefulness. OSA changes this normal pattern considerably[3,14-16] (Fig. 20–2). Cycles of hypoxia and CO_2

Table 20–1 Consequences of Obstructive Sleep Apnea

Cardiovascular
• Mortality
• Hypertension (especially resistant) (P, I)
• Congestive heart failure (P, I men)
• Coronary artery disease (P, I men <70 years)
• Pulmonary hypertension (P)
• Atrial fibrillation (P, I*)
• Stroke (P, I)
Metabolic/Endocrine
• Independent risk factor for development of diabetes type 2
• Risk factor for fatty liver
Neurological
• Excessive daytime sleepiness
• Increased risk of motor vehicle accidents
Urological
• Nocturia
• Erectile dysfunction
Gastrointestinal
• Gastroesophageal reflux

P Prevalence; *I* incidence.
*Atrial fibrillation (AF) has a higher prevalence and incidence in OSA than normal poulations but OSA is not an independent risk factor for AF. Increasing agė, obesity, nocturnal oxygen desaturation, and central sleep apnea are indepent risk factors in some studies.

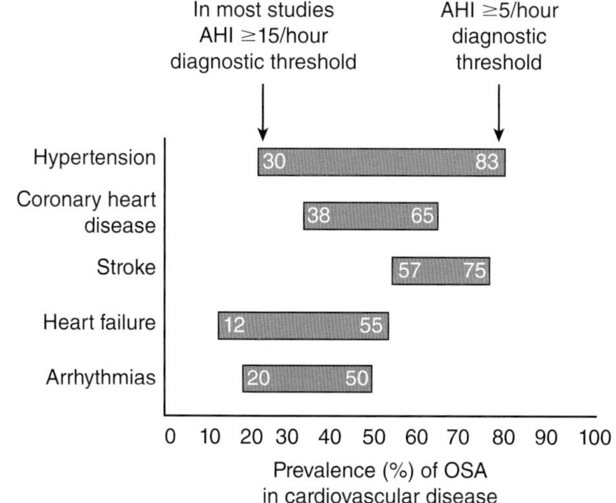

Figure 20–1 Estimates of the prevalence of OSA in major cardiovascular disorders. The lower ranges are invariably using a diagnostic threshold for OSA of AHI ≥ 15/hour and the upper ranges are using a diagnostic threshold of AHI ≥ 5/hour. (From Javaheri S, Barbe F, Campos-Rodriguez F, et al. Sleep apnea: types, mechanisms, and clinical cardiovascular consequences. *J Am Coll Cardiol.* 2017;69[7]:841-858.)

retention elicit changes in sympathetic and parasympathetic activity. Hypoxia and hypercapnia increase ventilatory drive and obstructed inspiratory efforts create negative intrathoracic pressure (sometimes reaching −80 cm H_2O). The negative pressure increases venous return to the right side of the heart (increased right ventricular [RV] preload), and the hypoxia causes pulmonary vasoconstriction (increased RV afterload). The right ventricle may dilate and the septum bulge into the left ventricle, impairing left ventricular (LV) filling and decreasing stroke volume. Negative intrathoracic pressure increases the transmural pressure across the left ventricle walls and increases the effective left ventricular afterload. The cycles of increased sympathetic tone[15] (Fig. 20–3) increase systemic vascular resistance which also increases left ventricular afterload. Arousal at apnea termination is associated with a large increase in sympathetic tone and decreased vagal tone (with resumption of airflow), with the result that BP and heart rate increase following apnea termination. In patients with OSA, high sympathetic tone is still present during wakefulness (see Fig. 20–3) and is associated with impaired vagally mediated heart rate variability (sympathetic rather than parasympathetic influence). Intermittent hypoxia causes oxygen free radical production and activates inflammatory pathways that can predispose to atherosclerosis

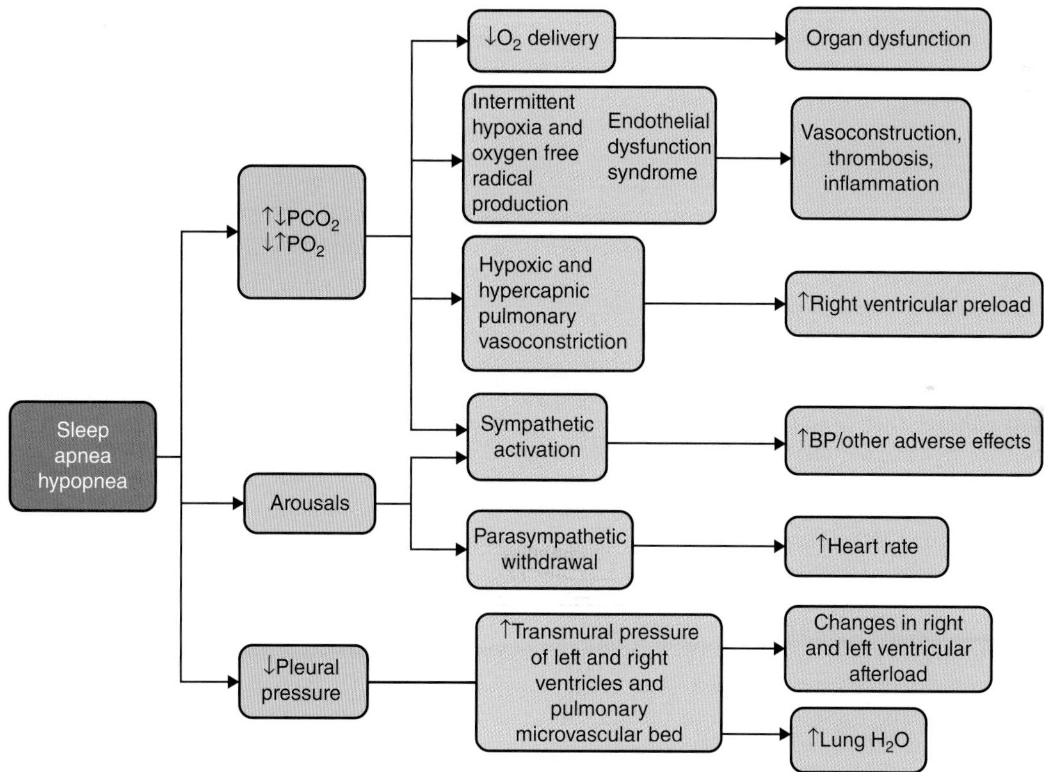

Figure 20–2 Pathophysiologic consequences of sleep apnea and hypopnea mediating adverse cardiovascular consequences. Acutely, OSA is associated with a number of adverse consequences including alterations in PO_2 and PCO_2 resulting in intermittent hypoxia, large negative swings in intrathoracic pressure and arousals, collectively imposing hemodynamic consequences, neurohormonal activation, oxidative stress, biochemical and cellular abnormalities, release of inflammatory mediators such as cytokines, and increased expression of adhesion molecules (resulting in attachment of white blood cells to endothelial cells and their transmigration). These reactions underlie the pathologic processes involved in endothelial dysfunction syndrome and are the underlying pathophysiologic mechanisms for atherosclerosis, hypertension, stroke, HF, and coronary artery disease. Pleural pressure is a surrogate of the pressure surrounding the heart and other vascular structures. ↑, Increased; ↓, decreased; BP, blood pressure; O_2, oxygen; PCO_2, partial pressure of carbon dioxide in the blood; PO2, partial pressure of oxygen in the blood. (With permission from Javaheri S. Cardiovascular diseases. In: Kryger MH, Avidan AY, Berry RB, eds. *Atlas of Clinical Sleep Medicine.* 2nd ed. Saunders; 2014:316-328.)

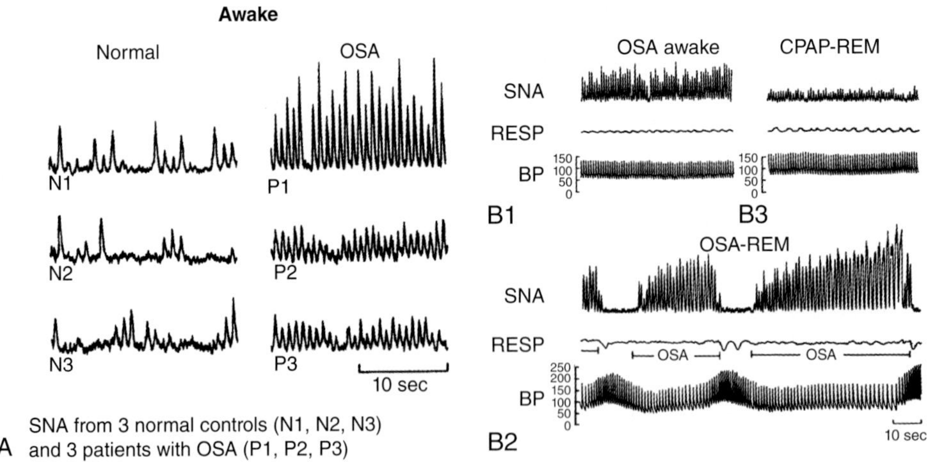

Figure 20–3 A. Recordings of sympathetic nerve activity (SNA) during wakefulness in patients with obstructive sleep apnea (OSA) (P1, P2, P3) and matched controls (N1, N2, N3) The tracings show high levels of SNA in **awake** patients with sleep apnea. Tracings **B1, B2, and B3 show** recordings of sympathetic nerve activity (SNA), respiration (RESP), and arterial blood pressure (BP) in a patient with OSA. At **B1** a tracing while the patient is awake shows high SNA. At **B2** a tracing during REM sleep shows two apneas with very high SNA. At **B3** a tracing shows the same patient during REM sleep while wearing continuous positive airway pressure (CPAP) with resolution of apneas and reduced SNA. (From Somers VK, Dyken ME, Clary MP, Abboud FM. Sympathetic neural mechanisms in obstructive sleep apnea. *J Clin Invest.* 1995;96:1897-1904.)

and thrombosis.[17-19] Decreased oxygen delivery can cause organ dysfunction. Sleep fragmentation, hypoxia, and long-term changes in brain centers responsible for maintaining wake and alertness are believed to result in daytime sleepiness.

MORTALITY

In patients with OSA, frequent coexisting conditions such as HTN and obesity make analysis of the impact of OSA on survival difficult. It is unlikely that a randomized long-term trial of treatment of OSA versus observation is possible now for ethical reasons. Most of the information we have about mortality and OSA is from retrospective studies or prospective observational studies (Table 20–2). Some of the studies are from **clinical cohorts** that would be expected to have a higher prevalence of disease, but such studies are subject to referral bias. Other studies are from large population-based cohorts are free of referral bias but have a relatively low number of patients with severe OSA. Some studies have analyzed all-cause mortality and others looked at CV mortality.

An early retrospective study by He and associates[20] showed a decreased survival in untreated patients with an apnea index (AI) greater than 20/hour. Patients with an AI greater than 20/hour who were treated with tracheostomy or CPAP did not have a decreased survival. The causes of death in the patients were not documented. Lavie and coworkers[21] reviewed the results on 1620 patients diagnosed with OSA between 1976 and 1988. Fifty-seven patients had died by 1990 with 53% of the deaths due to respiratory and CV causes. Excess mortality was noted in *men* of *30 to 50 years of age* with OSA but not in patients older than 70 years of age. Lavie and colleagues[22] later published results of a sleep clinic cohort (1991–2000) consisting of 14,589 patients and found that the hazard of mortality was higher in patients with *moderate and severe OSA* compared with the general population. *The results were significant for patients younger than 50 years of age.* Another analysis of the cohort sought to determine the factors associated with mortality in OSA patients. The study found that the risk of mortality in patients with OSA was increased by the presence of comorbidities. For patients younger than 62 years, increased mortality was associated with the presence of heart failure or diabetes mellitus (DM). For OSA patients older than 62 years, predicators of increased mortality included chronic obstructive pulmonary disease (COPD), congestive heart failure (CHF), and DM.[23] Older patients with OSA appear to be resistant to the adverse effects of OSA on mortality.[24] This effect could be due to "survivor" bias. Marshall and associates[25] found an increase in *all-cause mortality* associated with *moderate to severe OSA* in a population-based study. Marin and coworkers[26] studied a *clinic population of* ***men*** and found an increase of fatal and nonfatal CV events for severe untreated OSA patients compared with healthy individuals, snorers, patients with mild to moderate OSA, and patients with OSA on CPAP treatment (Fig. 20–4). The AHI of the group on CPAP did not differ from the AHI of the severe untreated OSA group. Yaggi and colleagues[27] published data on another cohort referred to a sleep clinic and found an increased mortality in severe OSA patients. Young and associates[28] published results from the Wisconsin Sleep Cohort and found that severe OSA patients had an increased risk of all-cause mortality. The results of this study were adjusted for gender. Punjabi and coworkers[29] published results on a large population cohort from the SHHS. There was an increase in mortality for the severe OSA patients who were *male and aged 40 to 70 years*. In this study, statistical corrections for the effects of age, body mass index (BMI), and gender (when appropriate) were performed. Using a prospective observational cohort study design, Campos-Rodriguez and coworkers[30] found *severe OSA* to be associated with *CV death in women*. Gami and colleagues[31] studied 10,701 consecutive adults undergoing their first diagnostic polysomnogram with a follow-up duration as long as 15 years. The incidence of resuscitated or fatal sudden cardiac death (SCD) was determined in relation to the presence of OSA and physiological data including the AHI, nocturnal oxygen saturation, and relevant comorbidities.

Table 20–2 Increased Mortality and Obstructive Sleep Apnea

Author	Selection	Participants	Findings
Punjabi, 2009[29] Population-based	Sleep Heart Health Cohort	6441 patients Average f/u 8.2 yr Severe OSA $N = 341$	Severe OSA AHI ≥ 30/hour associated with increased mortality only in men 40–70 yr. Measures of sleep-related hypoxemia but not sleep fragmentation were associated with increased mortality.
Marin, 2005[26] Clinical cohort—sleep clinic recruited	Snorers, OSA, and a healthy group (BMI matched to untreated severe OSA)	Men only Groups (G) G1: 264 healthy men G2: 337 simple snorers G3: 403 untreated mild to moderate OSA G4: 235 severe OSA untreated G5: 372 OSA treated with CPAP	Men with severe OSA AHI > 30/hour untreated (G4) had increased incidence of fatal (MI, CVA) and nonfatal adverse cardiovascular events (MI, CVA, CABPG, coronary angiography) compared with groups G1, G2, G3, G5. OSA patient group treated with CPAP (G5) did not have increased risk compared with G1 and G2. Odds ratio fatal CVE 2.87. Odds ratio nonfatal CVE 3.17.
Yaggi, 2005[27] Clinical cohort	1. Patients referred to sleep clinic 2. PSG 3. Adjustments for age, sex, race, smoking status, BMI, DM, AF, HTN	1022 patients (77% male) 697 had OSA	OSA (AHI ≥ 5/hour) was associated with increased risk of death from any cause.
Lavie, 2005[22] Clinical cohort	Patients referred to sleep clinic	$N = 14{,}589$ 372 deaths after median f/u of 4.6 yr	RDI > 30/hour males had higher mortality but only in males < 50 yr.
Young, 2008[28] Population-based	1. 18 year mortality f/u 2. PSG at baseline 3. Adjustments for age, gender, BMI, DM, cholesterol, mean BP	$N = 1522$ Severe OSA $N = 63$	All-cause mortality higher in severe OSA (AHI ≥ 30/hour) vs. no OSA even when CPAP-treated patients eliminated. The results were not changed based on the presence or absence of sleepiness.
Marshall, 2008[25] (Busselton Health Study) Population-based	1. Prospective observational 2. Home sleep testing 3. 14-yr f/u 4. Adjustments for age, gender, BMI, DM, cholesterol, mean BP	397 participants moderate to severe OSA $N = 18$ 380 free from MI and CVA at baseline 18 AHI > 15/hour 77 AHI 5 to <15/hour 285 no OSA	Moderate to severe OSA (AHI ≥ 15/hour) had greater risk of all-cause mortality compared with no OSA. Mild OSA had no increased risk.

AF, Atrial fibrillation; *AHI,* apnea-hypopnea index; *BMI,* body mass index; *BP,* blood pressure; *CABPG,* coronary artery bypass grafting; *CPAP,* continuous positive airway pressure; *CVA,* cerebrovascular accident; *CVE,* complex ventricular event; *DM,* diabetes mellitus; *f/u,* follow-up; *HTN,* hypertension; *MI,* myocardial infarction; *OSA,* obstructive sleep apnea; *PSG,* polysomnography; *RDI,* respiratory distress index.

During an average follow-up of 5.3 years, 142 patients were resuscitated or had fatal SCD (annual rate 0.27%). In multivariate analysis, independent risk factors for SCD were age, HTN, coronary artery disease (CAD), cardiomyopathy or heart failure, ventricular ectopy or nonsustained ventricular tachycardia (VT), and the lowest nocturnal oxygen saturation. SCD was best predicted (hazard ratio [HR], all $P < .0001$) by age > 60 years (HR: 5.53), AHI > 20 (HR: 1.60), mean nocturnal oxygen saturation < 93% (HR: 2.93), and lowest nocturnal arterial oxygen saturation (SaO_2) < 78% (HR: 2.60). *Nocturnal hypoxemia strongly predicted SCD independently of well-established risk factors.* Of note, 68% of those studied were male, but gender was not an independent predictor of SCD.

In summary, analysis of mortality in community and clinic populations provides strong evidence for an increase in mortality in untreated *middle-aged male patients with severe OSA* (Table 20–2). Indeed, two clinic-based population studies included only or predominantly men. Conversely, the Wisconsin Cohort data **did not** show a sex difference in the increased mortality associated with severe OSA. However, relatively few patients had severe OSA in this study. The observational study of Campos and coworkers[30] found an increased CV mortality in women with untreated severe OSA. Thus, untreated severe OSA in women is likely also associated with increased CV risk but less well documented than in men.

The time of sudden death appears to be different for patients with OSA. Gami and colleagues[32] found that for patients with OSA, the relative risk of sudden death from cardiac causes from *midnight to 6 a.m.* was 2.57 (95% confidence interval (CI) 1.87–3.52) compared with other times during the day. People with OSA have a peak in sudden death from cardiac causes during the sleeping hours, which contrasts strikingly with the nadir of sudden death from cardiac causes during this period in people without OSA and in the general population. In patients ***without*** *sleep apnea*, the risk of sudden death was greatest in the morning hours **after awakening** (Fig. 20–5).[32]

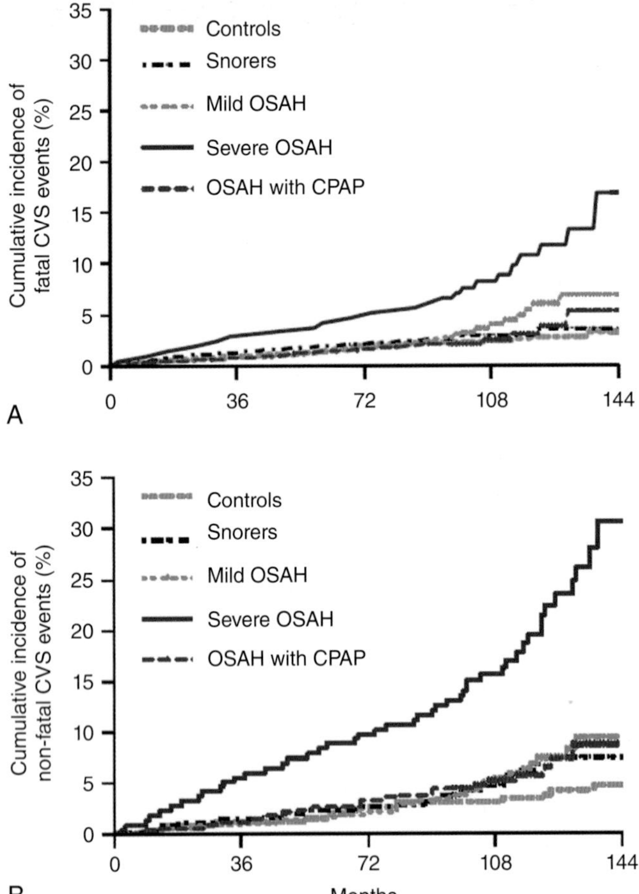

Figure 20–4 Cumulative incidence of fatal **(A)** and nonfatal **(B)** cardiovascular events (CVS) in controls, snorers, patients with untreated mild to moderate obstructive sleep apnea (OSA), patients with untreated severe OSA, and OSA patients on CPAP treatment. Patients with severe OSA had increased cumulative adverse events compared to the other groups. If OSA was treated with CPAP outcomes were similar to snoring patients and the control group. OSAH = obstructive sleep apnea-hypopnea. (From Marin JM, Carrizo S, Vicente E, Agusti AGN. Long term cardiovascular outcomes in men with obstructive sleep apnea-hypopnea with or without treatment with continuous positive airway pressure: an observational study. *Lancet.* 2005;365:1046-1053.)

OSA AND RELATED CARDIOVASCULAR DISEASE/ EFFECT OF CPAP

OSA is strongly associated with an increased prevalence of CVDs including HTN (especially resistant HTN), pulmonary hypertension (PH), heart failure, stroke, atrial fibrillation (AF), and CAD (Table 20–3). The presence of OSA is also associated with the risk of **incident** CVD (Table 20–4). In most studies statistical significance was present when comparing the ***most severe** OSA group to a no OSA or mild OSA group*. When severe, OSA is associated with all-cause and CV mortality (best evidence for middle-aged men). As noted previously, the mechanisms by which untreated OSA worsening CVD include increased *sympathetic nerve activity, oxidative stress, vascular endothelial dysfunction, intermittent hypoxia, and metabolic dysregulation*. These factors have interactions; for example, intermittent hypoxia and reoxygenation result in oxidative stress. The large negative swings in intrathoracic pressure increase LV afterload, increase oxygen consumption, and decrease stroke volume. Stretching of the left atrial walls may facilitate development of atrial arrhythmias and is associated with secretion of atrial natriuretic peptide (ANP), which is one cause of nocturia. CPAP treatment of OSA can reduce sympathetic overactivity (and secretion of norepinephrine).[33]

Observational studies have demonstrated a benefit from CPAP treatment. A study by Marin and colleagues[26] found severe OSA in men (compared with healthy controls, snorers, and mild to moderate OSA) to be associated with an increased risk of fatal and nonfatal CV events, and CPAP treatment reduced the risk (Fig. 20–4). Wu and colleagues[34] found that patients with untreated moderate to severe OSA who had undergone percutaneous coronary intervention had an increased risk of the need for revascularization compared with a CPAP-treated, moderate to severe OSA group, but there was no difference in mortality. Another study compared mortality with and without CPAP and found that CPAP reduced mortality but only in certain age groups and only in men.[35] Using a prospective observational cohort study design, Campos-Rodriguez and coworkers[30] found that CPAP reduced the risk of CV death in women.

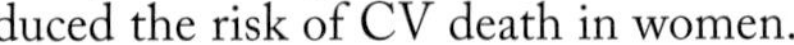

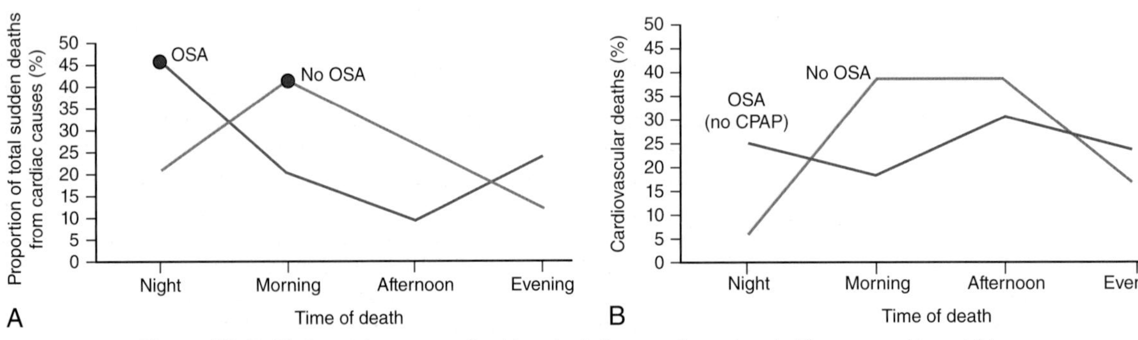

Figure 20–5 **(A)** Day-night pattern of sudden death from cardiac causes in 78 persons with and 34 persons without obstructive sleep apnea (OSA). For OSA patients the most common time of sudden death is during the sleep period. In normal individuals the most common time of sudden death is in the morning. **(B)** Another study of the day-night pattern of cardiovascular death in non-OSA patients and OSA patients not using CPAP. The study found disrupted day-night pattern of cardiovascular death in obstructive apnea. However, analysis of data found that there was not a clear cut increase in nocturnal deaths, but the patients failed to have the normal pattern of increased death in the morning hours. (A, Plotted from data from Gami AS, Howard DE, Olson EJ, Somers VK. Day-night pattern of sudden death in obstructive sleep apnea. *N Engl J Med.* 2005;352:1206-1214. B, Plotted from data from Martins EF, Martinez D, Sabino da Silva FAB, et al. Disrupted day-night pattern of cardiovascular death in obstructive sleep apnea. *Sleep Med.* 2017;38:144-150.)

Table 20–3 Cardiovascular Disease and Obstructive Sleep Apnea

Sleep Heart Health Study*—Risk of Self-Reported CVD (Prevalence)						
Quartile	I	II	III	IV		*P*
AHI (/hour)	0–1.3	1.4–4.4	4.5–11.0	>11.0		
CAD*	1.0	0.92 (0.71–1.20)	1.20 (0.93–1.54)	1.27 (0.99–1.62)		.004
CHF*	1.0	1.13 (0.54–2.39)	1.95 (0.99–3.83)	2.38 (1.22–4.62)		.002
Stroke*	1.0	1.15 (0.72–1.83)	1.42 (0.91–2.21)	1.58 (1.02–2.46)		.03
Sleep Heart Health Study†—Prevalence of Hypertension‡						
AHI category	1	2	3	4	5	
AHI	<1.5	1.5–4.9	5–14.9	15–29.9	≥30	
HTN risk (OR)	1.0	1.07 (0.91–1.26)	1.20 (1.01–1.42)	1.25 (1.0–1.56)	1.37 (1.03–1.83)	.005

*Shahar E, Whitney CW, Redline S, et al. Sleep-disordered breathing and cardiovascular disease. *Am J Respir Crit Care Med.* 2001;163:19-25.
†Nieto FJ, Young TB, Lind BK, et al. Association of sleep disordered breathing, sleep apnea, and hypertension in a large community-based study. *JAMA.* 2000;283:1829-1836.
‡Blood pressure ≥ 140/90 mm Hg or current antihypertensive treatment.
Values are risk (95% confidence interval) relative to quartile I.
AHI, Apnea-hypopnea index; *CAD,* coronary artery disease; *CHF,* congestive heart failure; *HTN,* hypertension; *OR,* odds ratio.

Table 20–4 Studies Showing an Increased Risk of *Incident* Cardiovascular Disease in OSA

Stroke	Yaggi et al.,[27] Redline et al.[235]
Hypertension	Peppard et al.,[97] Marin et al.[98]
Coronary artery disease	Gottlieb et al.[190] (men <70 years)
Congestive heart failure	Gottlieb et al.[190] (men)

RCTs have yet to demonstrate that CPAP treatment of OSA patients (Table 20–5) is associated with decreased CV mortality or reduced incidence of major adverse cardiovascular events (MACEs). The Continuous Positive Airway Pressure Treatment of Obstructive Sleep Apnea to Prevent Cardiovascular Disease study[36] enrolled 2717 nonsleepy or mildly sleepy (Epworth Sleepiness Scale [ESS] < 15) patients aged 45 to 75 years, with a **prior** history of coronary or cerebrovascular disease and OSA, defined by an *oxygen desaturation index ≥ 12/hour, diagnosed by means of a two-channel screening device*. Patients were allocated to CPAP or usual-care treatment for a mean of 3.7 years. The primary composite end point was death from CV causes, myocardial infarction (MI), stroke, or hospitalization for unstable angina, heart failure, or transient ischemic attack (TIA). The incidence of a composite CV outcome was similar in the CPAP and control groups. In the CPAP group, the mean duration of adherence to CPAP therapy was 3.3 hours per night, and the mean AHI (the number of apnea or hypopnea events per hour of recording) decreased from 29.0 events per hour at baseline to 3.7 events per hour during follow-up. The authors concluded that therapy with CPAP plus usual care, as compared with usual care alone, did not prevent CV events in patients with moderate to severe OSA and established CVD. The study has a number of limitations including use of a two-channel recorder for diagnosis, inclusion of recruited patients rather than clinic patients, exclusion of sleepy patients (ESS > 15), and poor CPAP adherence. One-to-one propensity-score matching was performed to compare 561 patients who were adherent to CPAP therapy with 561 patients in the usual-care group. In this sensitivity analysis, a lower risk of a composite end point *of **cerebral*** events was found in the group of patients who used CPAP for at least 4 hours per day. Barbé and coworkers[37] performed an RCT to determine *the effect of CPAP on the incidence of HTN* in *nonsleepy* OSA patients. In patients with OSA ***without*** *daytime sleepiness*, the prescription of CPAP compared with usual care did not result in a statistically significant reduction in the incidence of HTN or CV events. However, the study may have had limited power to detect a significant difference. Peker and colleagues[38] randomized nonsleepy (ESS < 10) patients with newly *revascularized CAD and moderate to severe OSA (AHI ≥ 15/hour)* to autotitrating PAP or no PAP for a median of 57 months (the Randomized Intervention with Continuous Positive Airway Pressure in CAD and OSA [RICCADSA] trial). The incidence of the primary composite CV endpoint did not differ between the two groups. However, adjusted on treatment analysis showed a significant CV risk reduction in those who used CPAP for >4 hours, compared with those who used the device <4 hours per night or did not receive treatment. There was a significant reduction in risk after adjustment for baseline comorbidities and compliance with treatment. The Impact of Sleep Apnea syndrome in the evolution of Acute Coronary syndrome and Effect of intervention with CPAP (ISAACC) study was a randomized controlled trial determining the effect of OSA and CPAP treatment on the prevalence of cardiovascular events in *nonsleepy patients with an acute coronary syndrome* (ACS) found that the presence of OSA was not associated with an increased prevalence of CV events in patients with OSA compared with ACS patients without OSA. Treatment of OSA with CPAP did not significantly reduce this prevalence.[39] Yu and coworkers performed a meta-analysis of the RCTs of CPAP and CV outcomes.[40] They found that the use of PAP,

Table 20–5 Studies of the Effects of Continuous Positive Airway Pressure on Cardiovascular Outcomes

Study	Subjects/Interventions	Primary Outcomes	Main Findings
CPAP for prevention of cardiovascular events in obsructive sleep apnea (the SAVE study)[36]	2717 nonsleepy or mildly sleepy (ESS $<$ 15) patients aged 45–75 years, prior history of coronary or cerebrovascular disease OSA, defined by an oxygen desaturation index $\geq$ 12/hour, diagnosed by means of a two-channel screening device Intervention: CPAP plus usual care (CPAP group) or usual care alone	Primary composite end point was death from CV causes, MI, stroke, or hospitalization for unstable angina, heart failure, or TIA. Mean CPAP adherence 3.3 hours.	No significant effect on any individual or other composite CV endpoint was observed. CPAP significantly reduced snoring and daytime sleepiness and improved health-related quality of life and mood. The propensity score-matched analysis patients adherent to CPAP therapy had a lower risk of stroke than those in the usual-care group and lower risk of the non-prespecified composite end point of cerebral events; results were not adjusted for multiple testing.
Effect of OSA and CPAP Treatment on Cardiovascular Outcomes in Acute Coronary Syndrome in the RICCADSA Trial[38]	Nonsleepy (ESS $<$ 10) patients with newly revascularized coronary artery disease and moderate to severe OSA (AHI $\geq$ 15/hour) Intervention: APAP (n = 86) or no PAP (n = 85) for a median of 57 months	MACCE in patients with ACS.	No difference autotitrating PAP vs. standard care. Adjusted on treatment analysis showed a significant CV risk reduction in those who used CPAP for $>$4 hours. OSA is an independent risk factor for adverse CV outcomes in patients with ACS. CPAP treatment may reduce this risk if the device is used at least 4 hours/day.
Effect of OSA and its treatment with CPAP on the **prevalence** of CV events in patients with ACS (ISAACC study)[39]	Nonsleepy patients with an ACS and the presence of OSA (AHI $\geq$ 15/hr) RCT CPAP vs. no CPAP Group without OSA was control group	The primary endpoint was the prevalence of a composite of CV events (CV death or nonfatal events [acute MI, nonfatal stroke, hospital admission for heart failure, and new hospitalizations for unstable angina or TIA]) in patients followed up for a minimum of 1 year.	Among nonsleepy patients with ACS, the presence of OSA was not associated with an increased prevalence of CV events, and treatment with CPAP did not significantly reduce this prevalence.
Effect of CPAP on Blood Pressure in Patients with OSA and Resistant Hypertension (HIPARCO study)[43]	194 patients with resistance HTN and AHI $\geq$ 15/hour Intervention: CPAP or no CPAP while maintaining usual BP control	The primary endpoint as the change in 24-hour mean BP after 12 weeks. Secondary end points included changes in other BP values and changes in nocturnal BP. Both ITT and per-protocol analyses were performed. CPAP group had greater decrease in 24-hour mean BP and diastolic BP with greater decrease in dipper pattern on CPAP. 72% $\geq$ 4 hours of nightly CPAP use.	CPAP reduced 24-hour mean and diastolic BP and increased the dipping pattern.
Effect of CPAP on the Incidence of HTN and Cardiovascular Events in Nonsleepy Patients with OSA[37]	Parallel group AHI $\geq$ 20/hour and ESS $\leq$ 10 N = 357 CPAP, N = 366 control group analyzed CPAP vs. no CPAP	Incidence of HTN defined as taking BP medications, $>$ BP / 140/90, or CV events.	The prescription of CPAP compared with usual care did not result in a statistically significant reduction in the incidence of HTN or CV events. However, the study may have had limited power to detect a significant difference.

ACS, Acute coronary syndrome; *AHI*, apnea-hypopnea index; *APAP*, automatic (auto-adjusting) positive airway pressure; *BP*, blood pressure; *CPAP*, continuous positive airway pressure; *CV*, cardiovascular; *ESS*, Epworth Sleepiness Scale; *HTN*, hypertension; *ITT*, intention to treat; *MACCE*, major adverse cardiovascular and cerebrovascular event; *MI*, myocardial infarction; *OSA*, obstructive sleep apnea; *PAP*, positive airway pressure; *RCT*, randomized controlled trial; *TIA*, transient ischemic attack; *RICCADSA*, Randomized Intervention with Continuous Positive Airway Pressure in CAD and OSA; *ISAACC*, Impact of Sleep Apnea syndrome in the evolution of Acute Coronary syndrome.

compared with no treatment or sham, was did **NOT** find reduced risks of CV outcomes or death for patients with sleep apnea. Although there are other benefits of treatment with PAP for sleep apnea, these findings do not support treatment with PAP with a goal of prevention of these outcomes. There were similar findings in another 2020 meta-analysis.[41] More recently, Javaheri and colleagues[42] performed a meta-analysis of data from five RCTs of CPAP and CV outcomes looking at the individuals with *greater than 4 hours of CPAP use nightly*. The primary outcome was a composite of stroke, cerebrovascular or cardiac death, and acute MI. Secondary outcomes were a cerebrovascular composite outcome (TIA, stroke, and cerebrovascular death) and a cardiac composite outcome (revascularization, angina, acute MI, and cardiac death). The overall composite score showed a significant lowering of risk with CPAP. However, the most interesting findings were the secondary outcomes. CPAP treatment significantly lowered the risk for cerebrovascular events but not cardiac outcomes. Thus, it is likely that improvement in the overall composite score depended on improvement in cerebrovascular disease. The authors felt that a RCT evaluating the effect of PAP treatment (with good PAP adherence) on cerebrovascular outcomes was indicated.

In contrast to the non-significant results of the above RCTs, an RCT of CPAP treatment in resistant HTN showed improvement with CPAP.[43] This is an important finding as *more than 70% of patients with resistant HTN have OSA*.

In summary, although observational studies suggest that CPAP treatment can improve CV outcomes in patients with moderate to severe OSA, most RCTs have failed to document a beneficial effect of CPAP on outcomes. Subgroup analysis of CPAP adherent patients in some of the studies demonstrated a benefit for **cerebrovascular** outcomes, but this analysis is not solid evidence of a CPAP benefit. As noted earlier, the RCT studies all had significant limitations.[3,10,44] As previously noted, an analysis by Reynor and colleagues[6] showed that the populations studied in most randomized trials (often nonsleepy) were very different from the typical sleep clinic population. Therefore, the results of the negative RCTs may not generalize to typical sleep clinic populations.

SYMPTOM AND POLYSOMNOGRAPHY SUBTYPES AND CARDIOVASCULAR RISK

Mazzotti and coworkers[11] analyzed a cohort of OSA patients and defined four symptom subtypes: *disturbed sleep, minimally symptomatic, excessively sleepy, and moderately sleepy*. When compared with individuals without sleep apnea, increased risk for prevalent and incident CV events was observed mostly in the *excessively sleepy* subtype. On the other hand, a previous study of the Wisconsin Sleep Cohort found OSA to be associated with increased mortality in 40- to 70-year old men without regard for the presence or absence of excessive sleepiness.[28] Analysis of event duration in the SHHS cohort[45] found that a shorter duration was associated with greater mortality in men and women after adjustment for demographic factors, smoking, prevalent CVD, and AHI. Of interest, a higher AHI (alone) was associated with greater mortality in men but not women. The authors hypothesized a shorter duration was associated with a lower arousal threshold or augmented autonomic nervous system responses to OSA. However, it should be emphasized that the quartile with the longest event duration was associated with the highest mortality before adjustment for AHI and other factors. Shorter event duration usually is associated with milder arterial oxygen desaturation and more severe sleep fragmentation. However, a previous analysis of SHHS cohort[29] data found an association between the total sleep time in which the oxygen saturation was ≤90% and mortality in men with OSA younger than 70 years. No association between mortality risk and the arousal index was found. Analysis of two large cohorts of patients (Outcomes of Sleep Disorders in Older Men [MrOS] and SHHS) found that *unlike the AHI*, the hypoxic burden predicted CV mortality and all-cause mortality (MrOS only).[46] The hypoxic burden was determined by measuring the respiratory event-associated area under the desaturation curve from preevent baseline. In another study, the change in heart rate with respiratory events (ΔHR) was also found to be predictive of CV morbidity and mortality.[47] Of interest, Trzepizur and coworkers found that hypoxic burden and not symptom subtypes was associated with increased CV risk.[48] However, the group analyzed was somewhat different than those undergoing the previous cluster analysis, suggesting a relationship between daytime sleepiness and CV risk.[49]

The three factors (daytime sleepiness, event duration, and severity of desaturation) are not independent of each other. For example, a study found daytime sleepiness to have a greater association with the severity of desaturation than the AHI.[50] In summary, it seems likely that daytime sleepiness, a short event duration, or severe oxygen desaturation due to OSA all are markers of increased risk of CV morbidity and all-cause mortality depending on the population being studied. A short event duration and greater hypoxic burden appear to be better predictors of mortality than the AHI.

EXCESSIVE DAYTIME SLEEPINESS AND NEUROCOGNITIVE DYSFUNCTION

Excessive daytime sleepiness (EDS) is a cardinal manifestation of OSA. However, the severity of this symptom is extremely variable, and the correlation with the AHI is very low. In fact, 30% to 50% of patients with OSA do not report significant daytime sleepiness. The study by Mazzotti and colleagues[11] that categorized patients with OSA by prominent symptom found that about *55% of the patients were characterized as having moderate to excessive sleepiness*. Chronic sleep deprivation and/or fragmentation from respiratory events is believed to be the major cause of sleepiness, although hypoxemia may also play a role. Normal individuals subjected to experimental sleep fragmentation without hypoxemia develop subjective and objective daytime sleepiness.[51,52] Attempts at finding abnormalities demonstrated on polysomnography (PSG) that correlate highly with subjective or objective sleepiness have not been very successful. Johns[53] found the ESS (subjective sleepiness) to correlate with the respiratory disturbance index (RDI) in a group of 165 patients with OSA ($r = 0.439$) and slightly less with the minimum SaO_2 ($r = -0.404$). Guilleminault and associates[54] found no polysomnographic variable to be significantly correlated with sleepiness as assessed by the Multiple Sleep Latency Test (MSLT). Roehrs and coworkers[52] analyzed data from 466 patients using multiple regression analysis and found daytime sleepiness as assessed by the MSLT had a slightly higher correlation with the respiratory arousal index ($r = -0.36$) than indices of hypoxemia ($r = -0.34$). Cheshire and colleagues found the arousal index to correlate with impaired cognitive function testing but not objective daytime sleepiness.[55] Bennett and associates[56] found that the AHI, cortical arousal index (central and frontal electroencephalogram [EEG]), sleep disturbance based on a neural network model, and a body movement index correlated with objective daytime sleepiness. The correlation between excessive sleepiness and the *indices of sleep disturbance* was only slightly higher than the correlation between sleepiness and the AHI.

Routine EEG analysis based on sleep staging or EEG arousals may not be sensitive enough to detect all the adverse effects of respiratory disturbance. For example, noncortical arousals from respiratory events or other causes may result in daytime sleepiness.[57] New indices of sleep depth have been developed, such as the Odds Ratio Product.[58] Using this index of sleep depth, a study found that individuals who return to deeper sleep quickly after arousals tend to have a greater average depth of NREM sleep.[59] Therefore, the impact of a given arousal index could be very different in individuals who return to sleep quickly compared with those with a slow return to sleep. It may also be possible that long periods of airflow limitation with high respiratory effort without discrete arousal could be associated with symptoms. This pattern commonly occurs in children with OSA[60,61] who develop behavioral changes and impaired school performance without frequent discrete arousals. Findings from the SHHS show an increase in sleepiness with higher AHI, but the relationship is weak.[62] There is also evidence from several studies that hypoxemia may be a factor associated with impaired cognition in patients with OSA.[63] As noted earlier,[50] one study found a greater association between OSA-induced oxygen desaturation and daytime sleepiness than the AHI. For many patients, a number of factors other than OSA also contribute to daytime sleepiness, including insufficient sleep and medication side effects. There is also considerable individual variability in the ability to tolerate sleep fragmentation. Therefore, it should not be surprising that there is only a modest correlation between the AHI and subjective or objective measures of daytime sleepiness. Of note, studies of heart failure patients with OSA often show that a large proportion do not complain of daytime sleepiness.[64] CPAP is very effective at reducing daytime sleepiness if patients are adherent. Some patients need nightly use up to 7 hours for maximum benefit. Typically, the ESS improves by 4 or more points,[65] and this can occur in patients with mild OSA.[66]

It should also be noted that effective treatment of sleepy OSA patients (e.g., CPAP) does not always abolish daytime sleepiness in 20% or more of treated patients. Javaheri and Javaheri hypothesized[67] that when all known causes of EDS are excluded in adequately treated subjects, the mechanisms that could explain residual sleepiness relate to long-term exposure to the OSA-related sleep fragmentation, sleep deprivation, and hypoxic injury to the arousal system, as well as shifts in melatonin secretion or altered microbiome. For example, Zhu and colleagues[68] showed irreversible injury in wake-promoting dopaminergic neurons in the ventral periaqueductal gray area and noradrenergic neurons in the locus coeruleus 6 months after recovery from an 8-week exposure to hypoxia/reoxygenation in an animal model of OSA. Other studies have shown white matter changes in OSA patients, and the degree of changes correlated with disease severity.[69] Some studies have shown abnormal pattern secretion of melatonin across 24 hours in OSA patients. For example, studies found serum melatonin levels remain flat into morning[70] and elevated in the afternoon hours[71] in some patients with OSA, which could cause daytime sleepiness.

Can OSA impair neurocognitive function in addition to causing daytime sleepiness, and if so, can CPAP treatment improve functioning? This question was addressed by the Apnea Positive Pressure Long-term Efficacy Study.[72] The group studied was about 50 years of age and recruited from sleep clinics. The AHI was ≥10/hour (average AHI about 40/hour). Prior treatment of OSA was an exclusion. Subjects were randomized to CPAP or sham CPAP. At baseline weak correlations were found for both the AHI and several indices of oxygen desaturation and neurocognitive performance in unadjusted analyses. After adjustment for level of education, ethnicity, and gender, there was no association between the AHI and neurocognitive performance. However, severity of oxygen desaturation was weakly associated with worse neurocognitive performance on some measures of intelligence, attention, and processing speed. The authors concluded that the impact of OSA on neurocognitive performance is small for many individuals with this condition and is most related to the severity of hypoxemia. On CPAP treatment daytime sleepiness improved both subjectively and objectively measured sleepiness, especially in individuals with severe OSA (AHI > 30). CPAP use resulted in mild, transient improvement in the most sensitive measures of executive and frontal-lobe function for those with severe disease, which suggests the existence of a complex OSA-neurocognitive relationship.[73]

Can CPAP treatment slow the deterioration in cognitive abilities in elderly patients with mild cognitive impairment and OSA? A detailed discussion is beyond the scope of this chapter, and the reader is referred to the review by Mullins and colleagues[74] There is evidence that CPAP treatment may slow cognitive decline in older adults with OSA and cognitive impairment.[75] Further studies are needed.

AUTOMOBILE ACCIDENTS AND SLEEP APNEA

Does untreated sleep apnea increase the risk of a motor vehicle accident (MVA)? The answer is yes, but the degree of increased risk is not known and certainly varies between patients. Published studies have found a two to three times greater risk of an MVA in untreated patients with OSA.[76-78] Clearly, not all patients with sleep apnea are at high risk of having an MVA. It appears that the presence of sleep apnea plus a history of a previous accident (or a history of frequently falling asleep at the wheel) identifies a group of patients with especially high risk. The decision of whether to report a patient with OSA to a motor vehicle licensing agency is a difficult one. In some states patients with an episode of loss of awareness are supposed to **self report** (although the physician should educate the patient about this situation and document the conversation in the medical record. A balance between patient confidentiality and protection of the public is required. A committee of the American Thoracic Society issued the following recommendations in 1994:[79]

> *In those jurisdictions in which conditions such as EDS caused by sleep apnea may be construed as reportable events, we recommend reporting to licensing bureaus if: (a) the patient has EDS, sleep apnea, and a history of a MVA or equivalent level of clinical concern; and (b) one of the following circumstances exists: (i) the patient's condition is untreatable or is not amenable to expeditious treatment (within 2 months of diagnosis); or (ii) the patient is not*

willing to accept treatment or is unwilling to restrict driving until effective treatment has been instituted.

The committee also noted that it is the physician's responsibility to notify every patient with sleep apnea that driving when sleepy is unsafe. Some form of written documentation that the patient understands this warning is prudent. Commercial motor vehicle (CMV) drivers are a high concern considering that accidents involving large vehicles often involve multiple fatalities. No regulatory mandate exists in the United States for comprehensive OSA risk assessment and stratification for CMV drivers. Current Federal Motor Carrier Safety Administration (FMCSA) requirements still do not reflect advice from several groups convened to assess the issue. The recommendations of several groups were reviewed by Colvin and Collop,[80] who outlined the historical facts concerning those recommendations. A statement concerning sleep apnea and CMV operators by a joint task force of the American College of Chest Physicians, the American College of Occupational and Environmental Medicine, and the National Sleep Foundation[81] provided guidance concerning the evaluation, treatment, and return to work of drivers with suspected or known OSA. A medical expert panel convened to advise the FMCSA made recommendations in 2008 with a subsequent revision in 2011. Finally in 2012 recommendations were made to the FMCSA jointly by the Medical Review Board and the Motor Carrier Safety Advisory Committee[80]. Proposed revised regulations by the FMCSA were published in 2012 for public comment, but were later withdrawn. Congress passed laws in 2013 requiring the secretary of transportation to only implement or enforce a requirement pertaining to OSA pursuant to formal rulemaking procedures. This effectively stopped progress on the initiative. In 2017 a recommendation concerning management of OSA in CVM operators was published by the American Academy of Sleep Medicine Sleep and Transportation Safety Awareness Task Force.[82] Major conclusions include:

(1) moderate-to-severe OSA is common among commercial motor vehicle operators (CMVOs) and contributes to an increased risk of crashes; (2) objective screening methods are available and preferred for identifying at-risk drivers, with the most commonly used indicator being body mass index; (3) treatment in the form of continuous positive airway pressure (CPAP) is effective and reduces crashes; (4) CPAP is economically viable; (5) guidelines are available to assist medical examiners in determining whether CMVOs with moderate-to-severe OSA should continue to work without restrictions, with conditional certification, or be disqualified from operating commercial motor vehicles.

The most current recommendations[82] advise treatment before certification for driving if the AHI > 20/hour, and drivers may be certified with AHI ≤ 20/hour if there is no EDS. A history of sleepiness at the wheel or history of an MVA associated with sleepiness usually mandates evaluation and treatment before certification. CMV certification requires evaluation by medical examiners meeting specified standards who often refer patients with suspected sleep apnea to sleep specialists for evaluation. In addition, patients with known OSA on CPAP treatment are often referred for yearly evaluation and verification of adequate PAP adherence. The process of certification and a registry of certified U.S. Department of Transportation examiners is available on the FMCSA website.[83] The process for identification of OSA in drivers depends entirely on the *diligence of the occupational medical examiners in screening for sleep apnea.* CMV operators rarely volunteer that they are sleepy or have symptoms of sleep apnea.

It is concerning that large financial tort settlements have been brought successfully against some physicians for failure to report a person with a medical condition who was subsequently involved in a serious traffic accident. Each state has its own laws, and local medical societies have guidelines. As noted above, in some states the patient is required to self report. However, in the end, the decision rests with the judgment of the treating physician. In some states, reporting is done to a health agency rather than directly to the motor vehicle licensing agency. Note that reporting does not always result in the loss of the patient's license.

To date, there is no objective test that can quantify a patient's degree of driving impairment. The maintenance of wakefulness test (MWT) is the appropriate test to assess the ability to stay awake. However, MWT results may not generalize to the real world in which sleep deprivation and other factors are operative. There have been promising attempts at developing protocols using driving simulators,[84] but results in a simulator may not correlate with driving performance on the road. A study of untreated OSA patients[84] found a MWT mean sleep latency (MSL) < 19 minutes was associated with impairment on a driving simulator. The same group extended this work by testing patients with OSA during actual 90-minute driving sessions on the road with a driving instructor intervening if necessary (the test car had two steering wheels).[85] Inappropriate line crossing was determined by video recording. Two groups "very sleepy" with a MWT MSL < 19 minutes and "sleepy" with a MSL 20 to 33 minutes had significantly more line crossings than controls and patients with mild sleepiness (MWT MSL 34–40 minutes). In the future, more complex measures of the awake EEG may inform the degree of alertness. For example, an investigation found that sleep depth coherence between the hemispheres predicts driving safety in sleep apnea.[86] Sleep deprivation causes decreased coherence.

Studies have shown improved performance on driver simulators after CPAP treatment of OSA.[87] The risk of traffic accidents does appear to be reduced with nasal CPAP therapy (if patients are compliant).[88-91] Data from the first large-scale, employer-mandated program to screen, diagnose, and monitor OSA treatment adherence in the U.S. trucking industry[92] found non-treatment-adherent OSA-positive drivers had a fivefold greater risk of serious preventable crashes. Non-treatment adherent drivers were discharged or quit rapidly, being retained only one-third as long as other drivers. Thus, the mandated program removed risky non-treatment-adherent drivers and retained adherent drivers. Unfortunately, due to privacy concerns there was no mechanism in place to prevent the non-adherent drivers from being hired by other trucking companies. Despite this limitation, it seems likely that *employer-mandated programs* are the best hope for improving safety in commercial drivers given the political pressure on Congress not to follow the advice of multiple expert panels.

ARTERIAL HYPERTENSION

Normal persons and many patients with HTN but without sleep apnea have a nocturnal fall in blood pressure (BP). However, 20%

to 40% of patients with OSA fail to have the normal nocturnal fall in systemic blood pressure (SBP) ("nondippers").[93] There are also patients with higher nocturnal than daytime HTN ("risers"). During obstructive apnea, BP tends to rise slightly and then to rise abruptly at apnea termination (Fig. 20–6) secondary to arousal from sleep and restoration of breathing associated with sympathetic activation and parasympathetic withdrawal. Key points about HTN and OSA are listed in Box 20–1.

Untreated OSA can definitely cause **nocturnal** HTN and nondipping. Can untreated OSA cause or contribute to daytime HTN? Animal models of simulated OSA suggest untreated sleep apnea can cause daytime HTN.[94] Several studies have found that OSA is very common in adult populations with HTN (>30%–40%).[2,3] This association does not prove causality because patients with HTN and OSA share common, potentially causative, factors such as obesity. Carlson and coworkers[95] found that age, obesity, and sleep apnea were independent and additive risk factors for the presence of HTN. That is, there was a high prevalence of HTN in OSA patients independent of obesity. The SHHS, a large population-based investigation, found an increased risk of having **prevalent** HTN when OSA was present (Table 20–3).[96] A prospective study of the Wisconsin cohort found an increase in AHI predicted the *development of HTN* in the following 4 years (*increased incidence*) after adjusting for confounding factors such as obesity, age, and smoking (Table 20–4).[97] Marin and coworkers[98] also documented that untreated OSA was associated with an increased risk of incident HTN. In contrast to these findings, an analysis of the SHHS data found that there was no relationship between the AHI and the risk of **incident** HTN (risk of developing HTN in the next 5 years) when the risk was adjusted for obesity.[99] There was a trend for a relationship when the AHI was greater than 30/hour. One problem with the SHHS is that the population *contained relatively few patients with severe OSA*. The current consensus is that *severe OSA* is associated with an increased risk of prevalent and incident HTN.

The importance of the REM AHI for the association of OSA with HTN has been noted. Appleton and colleagues[100] found that in men not considered to have OSA (AHI < 10), HTN was associated with OSA during REM sleep (REM AHI > 20/hour). In a study of the Wisconsin sleep cohort,[12] **prevalent and incident** HTN was associated with the REM AHI *and not the NREM AHI*. In individuals with NREM AHI ≤ 5, a twofold increase in REM AHI was associated with 24% higher odds of HTN (odds ratio [OR] 1.24). Another study found the REM AHI was associated with development of a nondipping pattern.[101] In summary, patients with OSA are at risk of developing HTN. The risk is most significant with severe OSA, and the risk is confounded by the presence of obesity. Recent data suggests that an increased risk for prevalent and incident HTN is associated with the REM AHI but not the NREM AHI. This fact is very pertinent for CPAP treatment, as most REM sleep occurs in the second part of the night, so CPAP adherence of 4 hours likely leaves OSA in REM sleep largely untreated. This suggests that one would expect CPAP to improve BP if used for 6 or more hours per night. The issues with measurement of BP during sleep are discussed later. On the other hand, heart rate is easily assessed. Studies on nondipping *heart rate*[102] suggest that this finding may have similar prognostic importance as nondipping BP.

The presence of sleep apnea may worsen the impact of HTN or impair treatment efficacy. For example, Verdecchia and coworkers[103] found that hypertensive patients who failed

Box 20–1 KEY POINTS ABOUT OBSTRUCTIVE SLEEP APNEA AND HYPERTENSION

- OSA is an independent risk factor for prevalent and incident hypertension.
- Hypertension is very prevalent in OSA (30%–40% or higher).
- Randomized controlled trials have documented about a 2 mmHg decrease in 24 hour systolic and diastolic blood pressure and a greater decrease in blood pressure resistant hypertension.
- A 2 mm Hg decrease in blood pressure has been associated with a 10% drop in the risk of mortality from stroke and a 7% drop in mortality from ischemic heart disease.[114]
- Nondipping blood pressure is associated with increased mortality.
- REM AHI but not NREM AHI is associated with prevalent and incident hypertension and non-dipping.
- A very high percentage of patients with resistant hypertension have OSA (50%–70%) treatment of OSA may improve blood pressure control.

AHI, Apnea-hypopnea index; *NREM,* non-rapid eye movement; *OSA,* obstructive sleep apnea; *REM,* rapid eye movement.

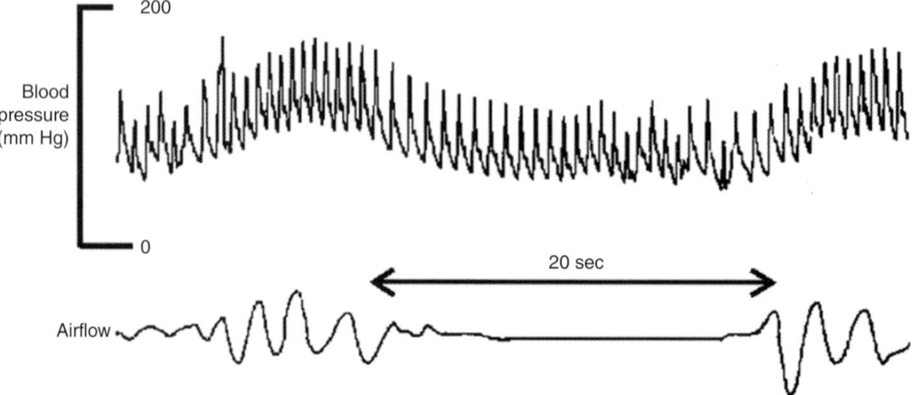

Figure 20–6 This tracing shows the swings in arterial blood pressure associated with obstructive sleep apnea (respiratory effort tracing not shown). At apnea termination, there is a steep increase in blood pressure that coincides with increased sympathetic activity. (From Berry RB. *Sleep Medicine Pearls.* 2nd ed. Hanley & Belfus; 2003:191.)

to have a 10% nocturnal fall in BP had greater LV hypertrophy. Studies have also documented an increase in all cause mortality among nondippers.[104] Studies of populations with resistant HTN have found a high prevalence of OSA.[105] Therefore, the possibility of the presence of OSA should be considered in all patients with resistant HTN. Several studies have confirmed that CPAP treatment is helpful in patients with resistant HTN who have OSA.[43,106,107]

Studies have documented that treatment of OSA with CPAP improves daytime or 24-hour BP. Becker and colleagues[108] found that effective treatment of sleep apnea with nasal CPAP for 9 weeks or more lowered both *nocturnal and daytime* BP by approximately 10 mm Hg using a placebo-controlled (sham CPAP) study design (Fig. 20–7). Other investigations have shown smaller[109,110] or no effects on daytime BP.[111,112] These conflicting results may reflect inadequate CPAP treatment (poor adherence), too short a treatment interval, or less severe sleep apnea populations. Several meta-analysis have confirmed a benefit. For example, one meta-analysis of 12 randomized trials of the effect of CPAP on BP found that CPAP did significantly reduce 24-hour BP by about 2 mm Hg. Results were largest in patients with more severe OSA and better use of CPAP.[113] Although a 2–mm Hg change may not seem very impressive, this has been associated with a 10% drop in the risk of mortality from stroke and a 7% drop in mortality from ischemic heart disease.[114] Of note, ambulatory BP monitoring (intermittent cuff inflation) can cause awakenings and can change what it is trying to measure.[115] The study of Becker and colleagues[108] used beat-to-beat BP with a finger probe rather than a periodically inflating a cuff (often causing arousal). Continuous measurements of BP using pulse transit time have also been studied and have shown periods of extreme BP elevations during periods of severe desaturations in patients with OSA.[116] However, the accuracy of the measurements using this method is still debated. Javaheri and colleagues[3] reviewed data before 2017[113,117-122] and found that CPAP treatment resulted

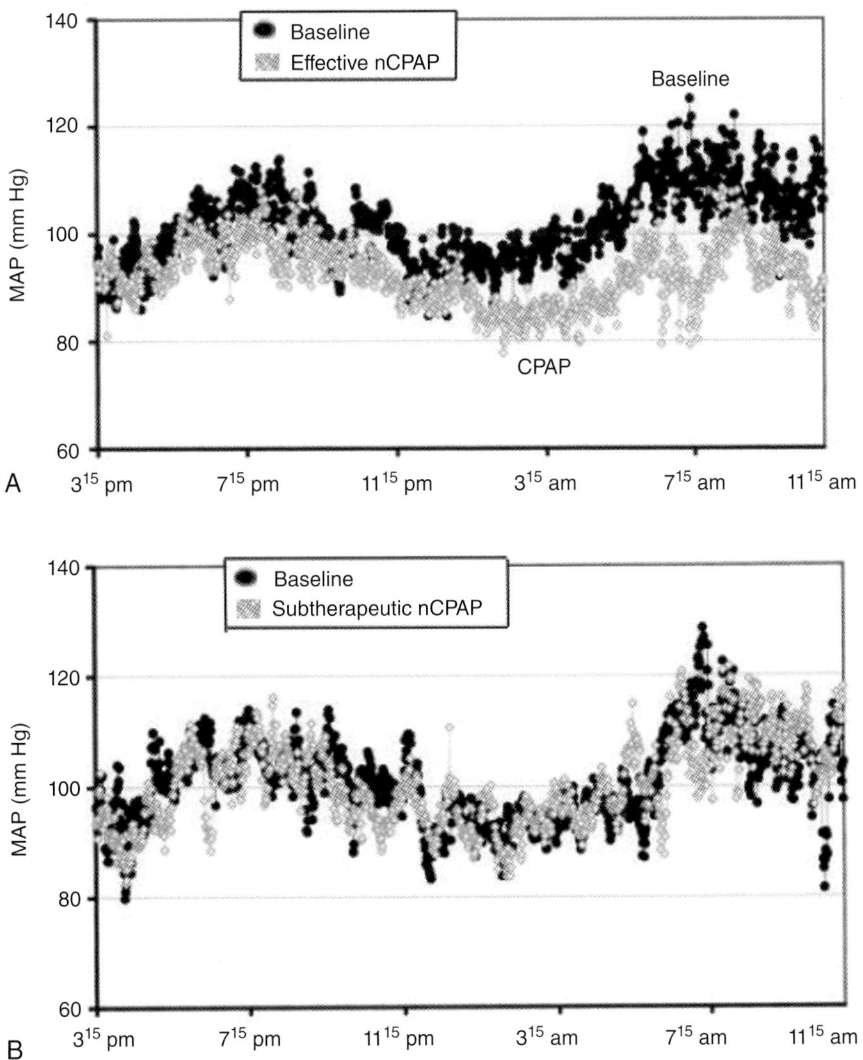

Figure 20–7 A. Time course of mean arterial blood pressure (MAP) before *(closed circles)* and on treatment *(open circles)* with therapeutic nasal continuous positive airway pressure (nCPAP). On average, 7.2 hours were recorded during the night. **B.** Time course of MAP before *(closed circles)* and on treatment *(open circles)* with subtherapeutic nasal CPAP. Note the decreased blood pressure on effective CPAP (A) but not on sub-therapeutic CPAP (B). (From Becker HF, Jerrentrup A, Ploch T, et al. Effect of nasal continuous positive airway pressure treatment on blood pressure in patients with obstructive sleep apnea. *Circulation.* 2003;107:68-73.)

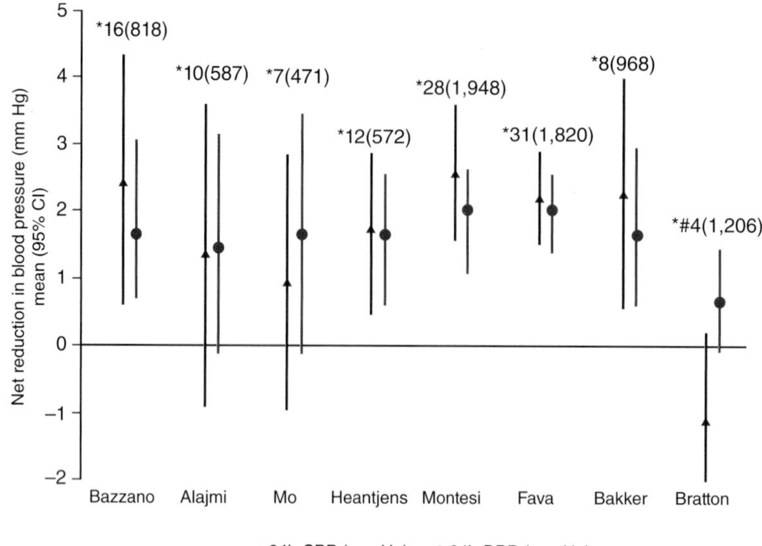

Figure 20–8 Summary of different meta-analysis on the effect of CPAP on 24 hour blood pressure in OSA patients. The mean reduction in 24 hour systolic and diastolic blood pressure on CPAP compared with controls in eight meta-analysis publications is shown. Overall, there was about a 2-mm Hg decrease. * number of studies, (number of patients studied), # patients without daytime sleepiness (all individuals in the study by Bratton et al were minimally symptomatic). (From Javaheri S, Barbe F, Campos-Rodriguez F, et al. Sleep apnea: types, mechanisms, and clinical cardiovascular consequences. *J Am Coll Cardiol.* 2017;69[7]:841-858.)

in a 2– to 2.5–mm Hg decrease in SBP and a 1.5– to 2–mm Hg decrease in diastolic blood pressure (DBP) (Fig. 20–8). For patients with resistant HTN, SBP fell by 4.7 to 7.2 mm Hg, and DBP fell by 2.0 to 4.9 mm Hg.[43,107,123-127] CPAP treatment can also reverse the nondipper pattern. CPAP adherence is an important confounder in CPAP treatment studies. Kohler and colleagues[128] used a CPAP withdrawal design (all patients adherent on CPAP and then randomized to therapeutic or subtherapeutic CPAP for 2 weeks). Compared with continuing CPAP, 2 weeks of CPAP withdrawal was associated with a significant increase in morning SBP (mean difference in change, +8.5 mm Hg) and morning DBP (mean difference in change, +6.9 mm Hg). The CPAP withdrawal design was therefore associated with a more robust effect of CPAP on BP. In general, most hypertensive patients with sleep apnea will still continue to require antihypertensive medications when treated with CPAP. However, 24-hour control of BP may improve on CPAP treatment. In one study, losartan with the addition of CPAP in patients with OSA did significantly reduce 24-hour BP but only in those using CPAP longer than 4 hours.[129] Investigators have sought characteristics that would predict a good response to CPAP in patients with resistant HTN. Of interest, a study found a singular pre-CPAP treatment cluster of three plasma microribonucleic acid profiles to predict a BP response to CPAP treatment in patients with RH and OSA.[130] The significance of this interesting finding remains to be determined, but more research to identify characteristics of patients with a BP response to CPAP is needed.

PULMONARY HYPERTENSION (PH)

PH is currently defined as a **mean** pulmonary arterial pressure > 20 mm Hg (previous criterion of ≥25 mm Hg). It is important to recognize PH, as this can result in RV failure over time. A recent classification of PH organized patients into five groups[131] (Table 20–6). The group associated with OSA is group 3 (mechanism is hypoxia). The term pulmonary **arterial** hypertension (PAH) is reserved for disorders of the *pulmonary arteries* that result in PH. PAH is associated with an increase in the pulmonary vascular resistance (PVR). Of note, diastolic dysfunction (high pulmonary venous pressures and LV end diastolic pressure) also results in increased pulmonary arterial pressure, and diastolic dysfunction (stiff left ventricle) is common in OSA patients. The pulmonary artery wedge pressure is increased but the pulmonary resistance is normal if PH is due to left ventrriuclar dsyfunction. However, mixed patterns can occur in OSA patients (increased PVR and increased wedge pressure). Left atrial enlargement is a clue that diastolic dysfunction may be present. Both hypoxemia and acidosis cause constriction of the pulmonary arteries. Hence, *it* is not surprising that episodes of nocturnal PH occur during obstructive apnea and hypopneas in patients with OSA (Fig. 20–9). For OSA patients with a normal daytime arterial partial pressure of oxygen (PaO_2), the pulmonary pressures usually return to normal in most patients. *However, daytime hypoxemia is not necessary for daytime pulmonary artery hypertension in OSA.*[132] Long-term vascular remodeling may result in daytime PH in the absence of daytime hypoxemia. Some key points concerning PH and OSA are listed in Box 20–2. Initial evaluations of pulmonary pressure in patients with OSA found PH mainly in those with coexistent lung disease or severe obesity with daytime hypoxemia[133] (likely obesity hypoventilation syndrome [OHS] resulting in daytime hypoxemia or hypercapnia). Sajkov and coworkers[134] evaluated a group of OSA patients *without lung or primary cardiac disease* and found mild PH (defined as a mean pulmonary artery pressure ≤ 26 mm Hg) in 41%. The groups with and without PH did not differ in BMI or AHI, but the PH group had lower (albeit normal) daytime PaO_2. The authors hypothesized that some patients had a more significant response to episodic nocturnal

Table 20–6 New Classification of Pulmonary Hypertension

Groups	Subgroups (Selected Disorders)
1. Pulmonary arterial HTN (PAH)	Idiopathic; heritable; drug toxin induced; associated with connective tissue diseases, HIV infection, portal HTN, congenital heart disease, and schistosomiasis
2. PH due to left heart disease	Pulmonary venous HTN, **increased PCWP**, diastolic dysfunction
3. PH secondary to lung disease and/or hypoxia	Obstructive lung disease, restrictive lung disease, lung disease with mixed obstructive/restrictive pattern
4. PH due to pulmonary artery obstruction	Chronic thromboembolic PH
5. PH due to unclear or multifactorial mechanisms	Hematology disorders, complex congenital heart disease
Hemodynamic Definitions	
Precapillary PH	mPAP > 20 mm Hg PAWP ≤ 15 mm Hg PVR ≥ 3 WU Groups 1, 3, 4, and 5
Isolated postcapillary PH (IpcPH)	mPAP > 20 mm Hg PAWP > 15 mm Hg PVR < 3 WU Groups 2 and 5
Combined pre- and postcapillary PH (CpcPH)	mPAP > 20 mm Hg PAWP > 15 mm Hg PVR ≥ 3 WU Groups 2 and 5

Some define PH as a mPAP ≥ 20 mm Hg (rather than >20 mm Hg).

HTN, Hypertension; *mPAP*, mean pulmonary arterial pressure; *PAWP*, pulmonary arterial wedge pressure; *PCWP*, pulmonary capillary wedge pressure; *PH*, pulmonary hypertension; *PVR*, pulmonary venous resistance; *WU*, Woods units.

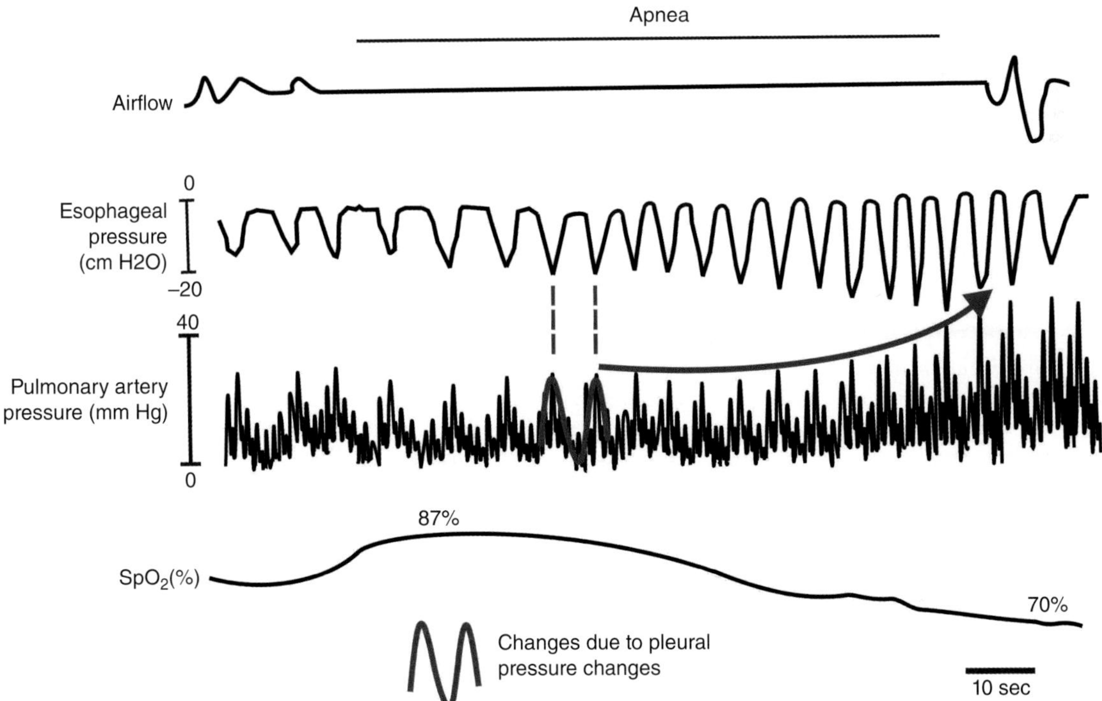

Figure 20–9 A schematic illustrating changes in pulmonary artery pressure during obstructive apnea. Note the progressively negative esophageal pressure. There is cyclic variation in the pulmonary artery pressure (red) due to cycles of negative pressure in the chest, but the overall trend is upward *(red arrow) due to pulmonary artery vasoconstriction.* Hypoxemia and acidosis (hypercapnia) cause pulmonary arterial vasoconstriction. SpO_2 = arterial oxygen saturation.

Box 20–2 KEY POINTS PULMONARY HYPERTENSION

- Mild PH can occur in OSA in the absence of lung disease or hypoventilation (about 30% of OSA patients have PH).
- Moderate to severe PH in OSA can occur with comorbid lung disease, heart disease (diastolic dysfunction), and OHS.
- A sleep study to rule out OSA is recommended in patients with PH.
- If OSA is present but PH is moderate to severe, evaluation of complicating factors is indicated (if not obvious). Determining if PAH is present (elevated PVR) and the severity maybe indicated.
- Treatment of OSA usually improves PH.

OHS, Obesity hypoventilation syndrome; *OSA*, obstructive sleep apnea; *PAH*, pulmonary arterial hypertension; *PH*, pulmonary hypertension; *PVR*, pulmonary vascular resistance.

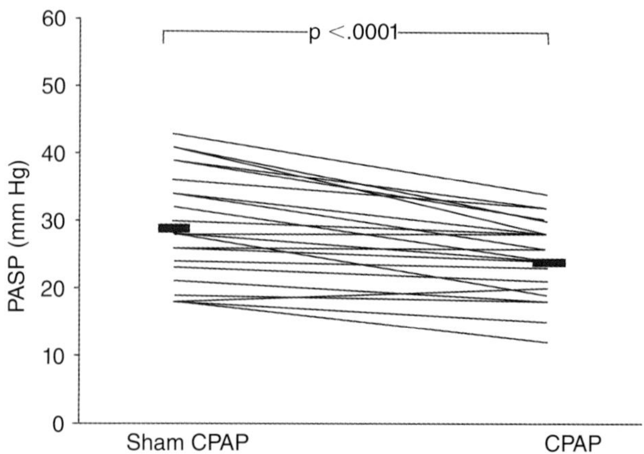

Figure 20–10 A reduction in pulmonary arterial systolic pressure (PASP) (Doppler Echo) after 3 months of continuous positive airway pressure (CPAP) treatment in CPAP versus sham CPAP. This was a randomized crossover trial. (From Arias MA, García-Río F, Alonso-Fernández A, et al. Pulmonary hypertension in obstructive sleep apnoea: effects of continuous positive airway pressure: a randomized, controlled cross-over study. *Eur Heart J.* 2006;27:1106-1113.)

hypoxemia and respiratory acidosis with subsequent pulmonary vascular remodeling. Most studies have found that OSA patients with normal daytime blood gases usually have normal or only *mildly increased daytime pulmonary artery pressures.*[134-141] The presence of coexistent COPD or LV diastolic dysfunction does appear to *increase the prevalence* and severity of daytime PH. However, the *presence of COPD is not obligatory* for mild daytime PH.[134-136] Patients with OSA without lung disease or daytime hypoxemia may develop PH because of an increased vascular response to nocturnal episode acidosis and hypoxemia. In the absence of lung disease or elevated LV end-diastolic pressure, Sajkov and McEvoy estimated the incidence of PH in OSA patients to be 20% to 40%.[136] In a study to explore characteristics of OSA patients with PH,[135] a study group with OSA and normal lung function were divided into a PH subgroup with mean pulmonary artery (PA) pressure ≥ 20 mm Hg and a subgroup without PH. The participants received dobutamine to increase cardiac output and also were challenged with isocapnic hypoxia. The PH group had a larger increase in PA pressure to both challenges. The authors felt these findings supported the idea that patients with OSA and PH had a greater response to hypoxemia and probably remodeling of the pulmonary vascular bed. Of note, tracings of pulmonary pressure in patients with OSA during apnea show faster changes associated with changes in intrathoracic pressure and slower changes over the course of the apnea due to hypoxia (and/or hypercapnia) (Fig. 20–9).[137] Combining the results of previous studies and excluding patients with significant lung or heart disease, a recent review estimated that the incidence of precapillary PH in OSA (normal wedge pressure) is 28%.[142]

Several studies have determined the response of OSA patients with PH to CPAP treatment.[143-146] One long-term case series study by Chaouat and colleagues showed that patients with OSA and PH had stable pulmonary pressures over 5 years when treated with CPAP.[143] Another study found that CPAP improved pulmonary arterial pressure and vascular reactivity in OSA.[144] Alchanatis and colleagues[145] found mild daytime PH in a group of OSA patients without lung disease that reversed after 6 months of CPAP. Arias and coworkers[146] performed a randomized crossover trial (sham or effective CPAP) for 12 weeks. CPAP resulted in lower pulmonary arterial SBP compared with sham (Fig. 20–10).

Patients found to have an increased PA pressure on echocardiography are often referred to the sleep clinic to rule out OSA as the cause. An American College of Cardiology Foundation Task Force recommended evaluation of OSA in all patients with PH.[147] The evaluation for OSA is reasonable, and OSA treatment may help PH even if other causes of PH are present. However, as stated in the consensus recommendations:[147] "Generally, the magnitude of the pressure elevation is modest even in severe cases of sleep apnea. Accordingly, if a patient with sleep disordere breathing is found to have severe PH, a complete diagnostic evaluation should be undertaken to assess for other possible etiologies of the PH". One would not feel comfortable explaining moderate to severe PH by the presence of OSA *alone* in the absence of daytime hypoxemia or comorbid lung disease. Other etiologies of PH should be explored. Some degree of diastolic dysfunction is often present in patients with PH and OSA and may improve with treatment of OSA. Treatment of systemic HTN or diastolic dsyfunction may also improve PH. In contrast, to the usual mild PH in OSA, patients with the moderate to severe OHS with daytime hypoxemia and hypercarbia can have significant PH and right heart failure. *It should also be noted that echocardiogram-Doppler estimates of PA pressure can be very inaccurate.* The gold standard is right heart catheterization, and this procedure can confirm PH is present, assess the severity, and determine if the issue is PAH or PH due to pulmonary venous HTN. However, this invasive procedure is reserved for moderate to severe PH cases when it is likely to affect therapy (vasodilator testing).

In summary, SDB, especially when accompanied by frequent and severe hypoxemia, can produce PH without comorbid conditions. Generally, the magnitude of the pressure elevation is mild even in severe cases of sleep apnea. Accordingly, if a patient with OSA is found to have severe PH, a complete diagnostic evaluation should be undertaken to assess for other possible etiologies of the PH. At the same time, all patients with PH should be evaluated and treated (if indicated) for OSA to limit the adverse pulmonary vascular effects of the of untreated OSA.

Sleep Disorders in Patients With PH

How frequently do patients with known PH have OSA or other sleep-related breathing disorders? The exact frequency varies widely depending on the definition of OSA (8%–89%).[142,148-150]

OSA is also prevalent in patients with precapillary PHs, such as in idiopathic PAH and chronic thromboembolic PH, which may be part of pathophysiologic processes through perturbations of gas exchange, hemodynamics, and metabolic pathways. One study found that unexpected nocturnal desaturation was common in patients with precapillary PH.[150] As noted earlier, guidelines recommend evaluation for OSA in all patients with PH.[147]

ARRHYTHMIAS

In normal individuals, the heart rate is lower during NREM sleep than during wakefulness. This is thought to be due to parasympathetic predominance during sleep (especially NREM sleep).[3,14] During REM sleep there are sympathetic surges and variability in heart rate. In patients with OSA, the heart rate varies in cycles: slowing with apnea onset, increasing slightly, staying the same, or decreasing during apnea, and increasing in the postapneic period[151-153] (Fig. 20–11). Early studies attributed the slowing of heart rate during apnea to increased vagal tone and hypoxia.[151] The slowing was diminished by atropine and supplemental oxygen. Later studies[152-154] have not consistently found a reduction in heart rate in the last part of apnea. The increased vagal tone during apnea is the result of hypoxic stimulation of the carotid body **during absent ventilation.**[155] Hypoxia by increasing sympathetic tone can cause tachycardia. However, in the absence of breathing, hypoxia is associated with bradycardia. With resumption of respiration, inflation of the lungs decreases vagal tone, and the hypoxic influences on sympathetic tone are unmasked (tachycardia).[155] Bonsignore and coworkers[152] found that the heart rate during apnea could increase, stay the same, or decrease depending on relative amounts of parasympathetic and sympathetic tone. One investigation suggested that the individual differences in the effect of apnea on heart rate may be secondary to differences in the response of the carotid body to hypoxia.[155] Although the cyclic changes in heart rate are sometimes referred to as *brady-tachycardia,* the heart rate often remains between 60 and 90 bpm in most patients. In a study of patients with OSA taking beta-blockers, cyclic changes in heart rate were still present, but the mean R–R interval change was reduced.[156] In this study no severe bradycardia or heart block was noted.

Patients with untreated OSA have increased sympathetic activity both day and night.[15] Heart rate variability has been used as a tool to study the balance of parasympathetic and sympathetic tone in patients with OSA. During wakefulness, OSA patients show less heart rate variability than normal individuals. This is thought to be secondary to the increase in sympathetic tone that is still present during the day. After successful treatment with CPAP, the heart rate variability may increase, suggesting a drop in sympathetic activity. Khoo and coworkers[157] found that CPAP treatment of OSA improved vagal heart rate control and that the degree of improvement varied directly with the amount of adherence to CPAP treatment.

Arrhythmia Prevalence in OSA

A wide spectrum of arrythmias and conduction disturbances have been found in OSA patients.[158-172] Guilleminault and colleagues[162] reported on 400 patients with sleep apnea. These patients had severe OSA with a mean AHI of 42.8/hour. Forty-eight percent had some type of arrhythmia. Twenty percent had more than two premature ventricular contractions (PVCs)/min during sleep, 7% had severe bradycardia to <30 bpm, 3% had nonsustained VT, and 5% and 3% had Mobitz type I and type II second-degree HB, respectively. Sinus arrest from 2.5 to 13 seconds was noted in 11%. A previous investigation reported on similar arrythmias during sleep in OSA and their resolution with tracheostomy.[163] A prospective study of 45 recently diagnosed OSA patients used Holter monitoring for 18 hours after diagnosis and again after 2 to 3 days of CPAP.[164] Only 8 of the 45 had significant rhythm disturbances including VT, AF, supraventricular tachycardia, and second- or third-degree heart block (HB). In 7 of these 8 patients, CPAP resulted in the abolition of rhythm disturbances. A major limitation of this study is the small number of OSA patients studied.

Mehra and coworkers[165] evaluated a cohort of older men and found that sleep-disordered breathing (SDB) was associated with atrial fibrillation (AF) and complex ventricular events (CVEs). The prevalence of CVE was associated with OSA and

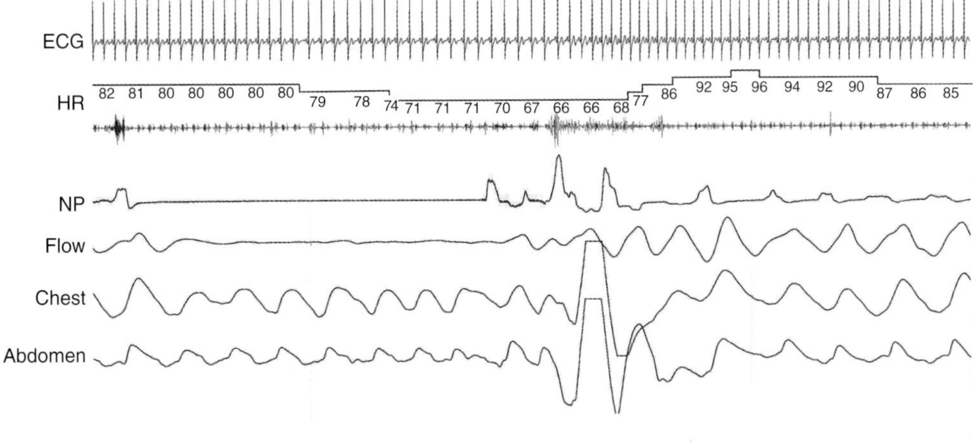

Figure 20–11 Changes in heart rate during an obstructive apnea. HR is the moving time average of the pulse rate from oximetry, which lags the changes in the ECG rate. Note that during the apnea, the R-R interval increased (slower heart rate) but then increases after event termination. With consecutive apneas, a cyclic pattern of varying heart rate occurs. NP nasal pressure, Flow is oronasal thermal sensor flow. HR for heart rate is really pulse rate derived from oximetry.

hypoxemia, whereas AF was associated with central sleep apnea (CSA). Another analysis[166] found that the odds of an arrhythmia after a respiratory disturbance were nearly 18 times the odds of an arrhythmia occurring after normal breathing.

Bradycardia and Heart Block

Atrioventricular (AV) conduction can worsen during obstructive apnea, and severe bradycardia or asystole can occur. The parasympathetic predominance during apnea may have little significance in most OSA patients, but in a few individuals this can cause or worsen significant bradycardia or HB. As noted earlier, a study of 400 patients with OSA[162] found Mobitz type I (5%) and type II second-degree HB (3%), respectively, and sinus arrest from 2.5 to 13 seconds was noted in 11%. A study by Becker and coworkers documented a reversal of AV conduction block on CPAP treatment.[167] Koehler and coworkers evaluated patients with HB during sleep in whom previous electrophysiological tests of the sinus and AV nodes were normal.[168] The majority of the HB episodes occurred during REM sleep (88% REM, 12% in NREM) and were associated with a ≥4% desaturation. This is surprising given the parasympathetic predominance during NREM sleep with REM sleep associated with sympathetic predominance. However, *surges in vagal tone* can also occur during REM sleep.[169,170] With nasal CPAP/nasal BiPAP therapy, the AHI decreased from 75.5 to 3.0/hour and the number of arrhythmias from 651 to 72 ($P < .01$). Grimm and colleagues[171] studied patients with OSA and HB with testing of sinus and AV node function and found that they had either normal or only slightly impaired function, implying OSA rather than intrinsic heart problems was the cause of the HB. An example of third-degree HB (followed by second-degree HB) during an obstructive apnea during REM sleep is shown in Figure 20–12.

Ventricular Arrhythmias

PVCs are not uncommon in patients with OSA patients. In the study of 400 OSA patients[162], 20% had ≥2 PVCs per hour. However, in some patients, the PVC frequency is actually lower during sleep. Shepard and associates[172] found no correlation between the SaO_2 at desaturation and PVC frequency during sleep unless the SaO_2 was less than 60%. Ryan and coworkers[173] performed a small (18 patients) RCT of CPAP treatment in patients with OSA and *heart failure* with >10 PVCs per hour to determine whether PVCs (also known as ventricular premature beats, VPBs) would decrease. The study found that CPAP did reduce VPB frequency (58% reduction) during sleep. The urinary norepinephrine concentration also decreased. No changes were noted in the control group. In contrast, Craig and coworkers found that CPAP reduced the heart rate in OSA patients but did not affect dysrhythmias.[174] The effect of CPAP probably depends on the population studied and the incidence of arrhythmias in the population. Gerçek and coworkers performed a retrospective study that analyzed VT burden, the rate of antitachycardia pacing, and the number of shocks delivered in patients with heart failure and an implantable cardioverter-defibrillator (ICD), as well as moderate

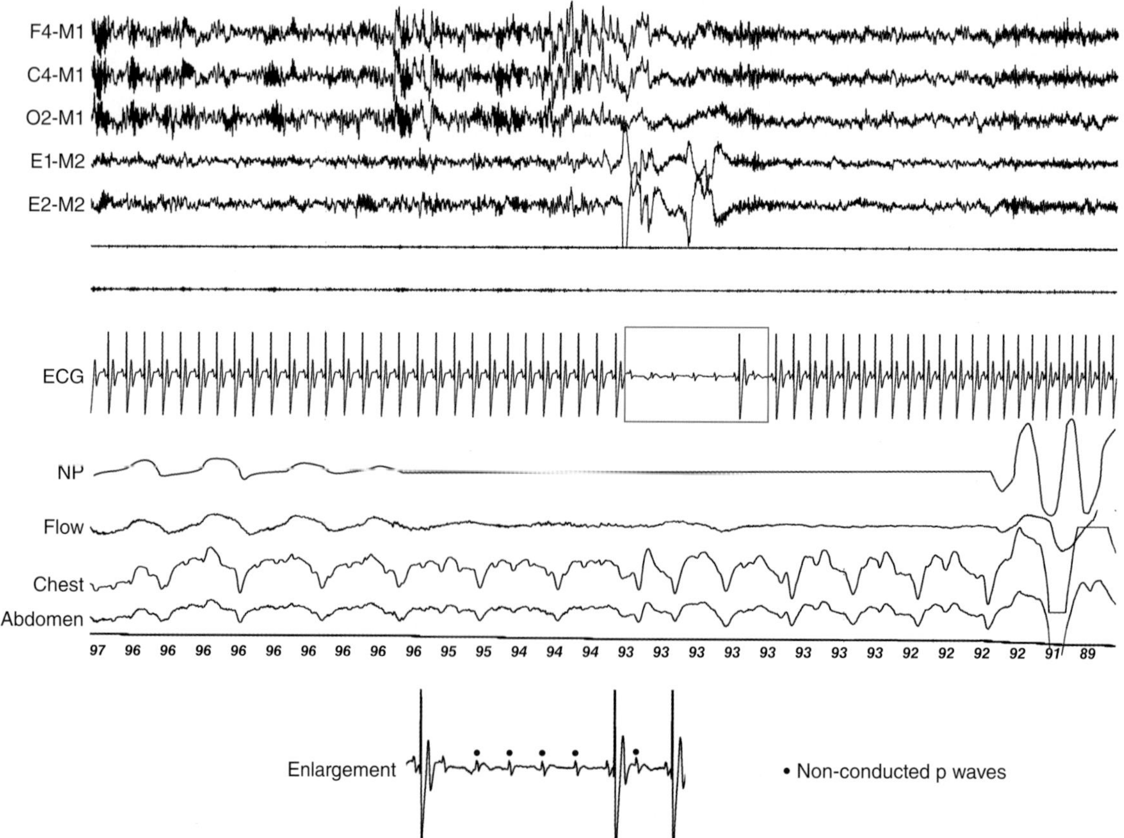

Figure 20–12 An example of third degree heart block during and obstructive apnea during REM sleep. In the red rectangle nonconducted p waves (dark circles) are followed by one conducted beat followed by a nonconducted p wave (second-degree block).

sleep apnea.[175] The study compared propensity score-matched cohort of patients with and without CPAP. The results showed that CPAP treatment in heart failure patients with an ICD in place was associated with significant improvement in VT burden, atrial tachycardia pacing, and shock therapy. In most studies ventricular arrhythmias in patients with OSA occur mainly associated with respiratory events.[176] Ryan and colleagues[177] found that in patients with heart failure, nocturnal ventricular ectopy oscillates in time with oscillations in ventilation, with VPBs occurring predominantly during apneas in patients with OSA but during hyperpnea in patients with CSA. Do patients with ventricular arrhythmias have an increased prevalence of sleep apnea? An evaluation of patients with ventricular arrhythmias and a normal ejection fraction found a high prevalence of OSA, and 60% of patients had at least mild OSA and 35% moderate to severe OSA.[178]

Atrial Fibrillation (AF)

AF is the most common sustained arrhythmia in adults. Key points about AF and OSA are listed in Box 20–3. Additional information about AF and sleep is presented in Chapter 28. The prevalence of AF in OSA patients is estimated to be about 4.8% compared to 0.9% in the general population. On the other hand the prevalence of OSA in AF patients is estimated to be 21% to 74%.[160] Gami and colleagues[179] found that the presence of OSA was predictive of *incident AF* in individuals < 65 years of age. However using a multivariant analysis the independent factors associated with incident AF in individuals with an age < 65 years were increased age, higher BMI, the male gender, coronary artery disease, and the severity of nocturnal desaturation (but not an AHI ≥ 5/hour). For individuals over 65 years of age only congestive heart failure was assosicate with incident AF. In a analysis of individuals in the Sleep Heart Health Study, Mehra et al found sleep disordered breathing to be associated with an increase risk of AF (OSA versus central sleep apnea was not specified).[180] Another analsysis by Tung and coworkers[181] of same population found central sleep apnea rather than OSA to be associated with an increased risk of incident AF[181]. In summary while an increased prevalence and incidence of AF is associated with OSA, the presence of OSA does not appear to be an independent predictor of AF. In some studies central sleep apnea but not OSA was associated with incident AF.

Untreated OSA is common in patients with AF and appears to worsen arrhythmia control. As previously noted, an

Box 20–3 KEY POINTS ABOUT ATRIAL FIBRILLATION AND OBSTRUCTIVE SLEEP APNEA

- OSA prevalence in patients with AF is 21%–74%[160].
- Atrial fibrillation prevalence:
  - General population: 0.9%
  - OSA patients 4.8%
- OSA associated with increased prevalence and incidence of AF. However, OSA is not an independent risk factor. Other factors associated with OSA such as increased age, high BMI, male gender, and nocturnal desaturation are independent risk factors.
- AF recurrence after cardioversion
  - AF: 53%
  - AF+OSA: 82%
- AF recurrence after PVI
  - AF: 23–27%
  - AF+OSA: 31–35%
- Observational studies show CPAP treatment of OSA decreases AF recurrence after cardioversion or PVI.
- To date, randomized controlled trials have not shown a benefit of CPAP treatment on AF recurrence after cardioversion or PVI.

AF, Atrial fibrillation; *PVI*, pulmonary vein isolation.

Data from Linz D, McEvoy RD, Cowie MR, et al. Associations of obstructive sleep apnea with atrial fibrillation and continuous positive airway pressure treatment: a review. *JAMA Cardiol.* 2018;3(6):532-540.

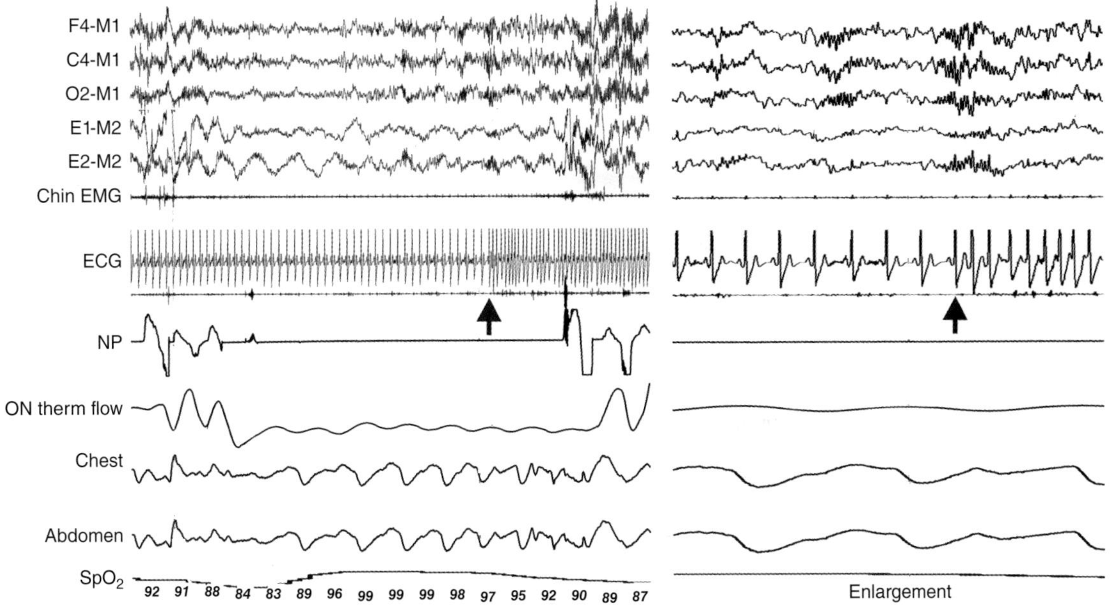

Figure 20–13 Transition from sinus rhythm to atrial fibrillation during an obstructive apnea (arrow). On the right an enlargement is shown. ON Therm flow is the oral-nasal thermal flow sensor signal. NP nasal pressure. Inspiration is upward.

evaluation of the SHHS cohort found that, although the rate of arrhythmias was low, the relative risk of AF or nonsustained VT was much higher after respiratory events.[165] In Figure 20–13, a patient with OSA changes from sinus rhythm to AF during an apnea. *Observational studies* have shown that CPAP reduced the risk of recurrence of AF after cardioversion or ablative treatments. Kanagala and associates[182] found that patients with untreated OSA had a higher recurrence of AF after cardioversion than patients without a polysomnographic diagnosis of sleep apnea. Appropriate treatment with CPAP in OSA was associated with a lower recurrence of AF. After this study, several other studies have documented an increased risk of recurrence of AF after cardioversion or ablation if untreated OSA is present and an improvement in restoration of sinus rhythm if OSA is treated with CPAP.[183-184] A consensus document on treatment of AF stated that OSA was a risk factor for AF recurrence and recommended evaluation if OSA was suspected and treatment of confirmed OSA.[185] As many of these patients with OSA and AF have relatively few symptoms associated with sleep apnea, a high clinical index of suspicion is necessary to avoid missing unsuspected OSA. However, although observational studies found a reduced risk with CPAP treatment of recurrence of AF after cardioversion or ablation procedures, a recent RCT was unable to show a benefit.[186] The study has been criticized for its low power and low incidence of recurrence in the entire study.

CORONARY ARTERY DISEASE

The periods of tachycardia and elevated BP postapnea increase myocardial oxygen demand at the same time that hypoxemia exists, predisposing to ischemia and possibly tachyarrhythmias. In normal individuals, sleep usually is a time of reduced tachyarrhythmias and ischemia. Patients with OSA may not enjoy the same protection. Sleep apneic events induce a state of increased cardiac oxygen demand, which occurs together with a reduction in oxygen supply because of a lack of ventilation, which may trigger nocturnal angina in patients with CAD. The risk of experiencing angina pectoris or an acute coronary syndrome (ACS), such as unstable angina or acute MI increases during the late hours of sleep or in the early morning hours soon after awakening.[187] Key points concerning CAD and OSA are shown in Box 20–4.

Box 20–4 KEY POINTS CORONARY ARTERY DISEASE AND OBSTRUCTIVE SLEEP APNEA

- The presence of OSA is a risk factor for prevalent and incident (men < 70 years) CAD.
- CAD patients with OSA have increased risk for MACCEs compared with CAD patients without OSA.
- **Observational studies** have shown that CPAP treatment of OSA in patients with CAD lowers need for revascularization or MACEs (including recurrent MI).
- In patients admitted with STEMI or who have bypass surgery, the presence of OSA is associated with a worse prognosis.
- RCTs have not demonstrated a benefit in CV outcomes with CPAP treatment of patients with CAD and OSA, but CPAP adherence was low.

CAD, Coronary artery disease; *CPAP,* continuous positive airway pressure; *MACCEs,* major adverse cardiovascular and cerebrovascular events; *MACEs,* major adverse cardiovascular events; *OSA,* obstructive sleep apnea; *RCT,* randomized controlled trial; *STEMI,* ST-elevation myocardial infarction.

Analysis of a large prospective cohort of patients (the SHHS cohort) found evidence of a slight increase in risk of having self-reported CAD at even low levels of sleep apnea (prevalence).[188] Peker and colleagues[189] found an increase in mortality in patients with CAD who had untreated OSA. Gottlieb and associates evaluated the SHHS cohort data and found an increased risk of **incident** CAD was associated with the presence of OSA in *men younger than 70 years of age*.[190] The association was strongest for severe OSA. The ongoing multicentric European Sleep Apnea Cohort, which prospectively recruits adults with a new diagnosis of OSA, reported a CAD prevalence of 8.7% among 6616 patients. There was a dose-response relationship between AHI (no OSA [AHI < 5 events/hour], mild [AHI 5–15 events/hour], moderate [AHI 15–30 events/hour], severe OSA [AHI ≥ 30 events/hour]), and the occurrence of CAD (5%, 8%, 11%, and 12%, respectively; $P < .001$).[191]

The presence of OSA in patients with CAD also worsens the prognosis. A study of patients with CAD and OSA found an increased risk of coronary events or CV death even when with adjustment for BMI and HTN.[192] Koo and colleagues found that the presence of OSA in patients undergoing nonemergent coronary artery bypass grafting (CABG) inferred an increased risk of major adverse cardiac and cerebrovascular events (*MACCEs*).[193] A prospective study[194] found that 42% of the patients admitted with ST-elevation myocardial infarction have undiagnosed severe OSA. The investigators also found that the presence of severe OSA carries a negative prognostic impact for this group of patients. It was associated with a lower event-free survival rate at 18-month follow-up. Xie and coworkers found that nocturnal hypoxemia in OSA is an important predictor of poor prognosis for patients after MI. They concluded that their findings suggest that routine use of low-cost nocturnal oximetry may be an economical and practical approach to stratify risk in post-MI patients.[195]

Does CPAP treatment of OSA reduce the risk of poor outcomes in CAD patients? Milleron and coworkers[196] found CPAP treatment of patients with OSA and CAD improved event-free survival (Fig. 20–14). The endpoint was a composite of CV death, ACS, hospitalization for CHF, or need for coronary revascularization. The control group comprised patients

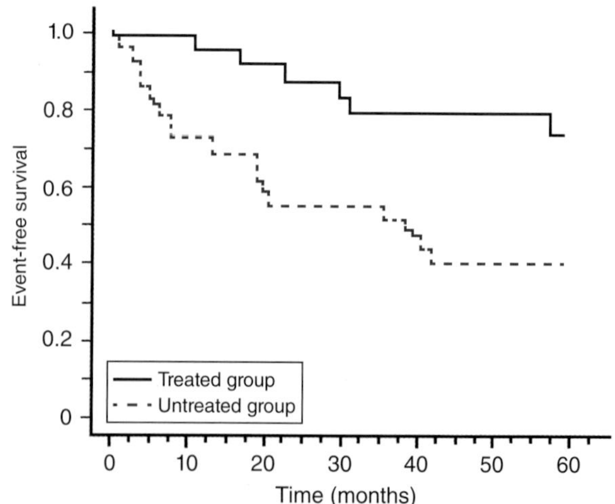

Figure 20–14 Patients with coronary artery disease (CAD) and OSA. Those treated with CPAP had improved survival compared with untreated patients. (From Milleron O, Pillière R, Foucher A, et al. Benefits of obstructive sleep apnoea treatment in coronary artery disease: a long-term follow-up study. *Eur Heart J*. 2004;25:728-734.)

who declined CPAP (not a randomized trial). The mean follow-up was 86 months. The primary endpoint was the first event of repeat revascularization, MI, stroke, or CV mortality. Cassar and coworkers[197] analyzed a *retrospective cohort of patients* with OSA diagnosed with PSG between 1992 and 2004 (AHI ≥ 15) who subsequently underwent a percutaneous coronary intervention (PCI). Patients (n = 371) were stratified according to whether they were treated for OSA (n = 175) or not (n = 196). The main outcome measures were cardiac death, general mortality, MACE (severe angina, MI, PCI, CABG, or death), and a MACCE. Treatment of OSA was associated with a reduction in the number of cardiac deaths, but not in MACE or MACCE, after PCI. The authors concluded that screening for and treating OSA in patients with CAD who may undergo PCI may result in decreased cardiac death. Chen and coworkers[198] performed a meta-analysis to assess the benefit of CPAP in patients with CAD. They concluded that compared with usual care, CPAP was associated with reduced risk of adverse CV outcomes or death in patients with OSA and CAD, particularly in the subgroup with AHI *less* than 30 events/hour. The reason benefits could be greater in patients with less severe sleep apnea is unclear. A prospective observational study followed 196 CAD patients after acute MI for 6 years[199]. The CAD patients had sleep studies and were offered CPAP. They were allowed to keep CPAP only if adherent. Thus, three groups (no OSA, OSA-no CPAP, OSA-CPAP) were followed with the end point being recurrent MI or need of revascularization. After adjustment for confounding factors, treated OSA patients had a lower risk of recurrent MI and revascularization than untreated OSA patients, and similar to non-OSA patients (Fig. 20–15).

The most rigorous studies of CPAP in OSA patients with CAD are the RICCADSA and the ISAACA studies. Neither study found a benefit from CPAP in the intention to treat cohorts. The RICCADSA study[38] was a single-center, prospective, randomized, controlled, open-label, blinded evaluation trial in consecutive patients with newly revascularized CAD and OSA (AHI ≥ 15/hour) without daytime sleepiness (ESS < 10). This study was discussed previously, but a few details will be repeated. Patients were randomized to autotitrating CPAP (n = 122) or no PAP (n = 122). Routine prescription of CPAP to patients with CAD with nonsleepy OSA did not significantly reduce long-term adverse CV outcomes in the intention-to-treat population. There was a significant reduction after adjustment for baseline comorbidities and compliance with the treatment. At 3 months the average CPAP use was 5.1/hour, but PAP was only used 73% of nights. Many patients with CAD and OSA are not sleepy, and in the RICCADSA study 44% of the patients initially evaluated for inclusion in the study were not sleepy. The sleepy patients were not included in the study but were offered CPAP. At 12 months, 63% of nonsleepy patients and 78% of the sleepy patients were still on CPAP. A *parallel observational arm* of the RICCADSA RCT[200] offered CPAP to revascularized CAD patients with moderate to severe OSA and daytime sleepiness (ESS ≥ 10). Those without OSA served as controls. The incidence of MACCEs was 23.2% in OSA patients on CPAP versus 16.1% in those with no OSA[200]. This finding is consistent with equal risk (adjusted HR 0.96, 95% CI 0.40–2.31; P = .923). Therefore, CPAP treatment eliminated the additional risk of having OSA.

Patients with moderate to severe OSA and CAD and adequate CPAP adherence might benefit from CPAP, but PAP adherence is an issue, especially in nonsleepy patients. The ISAACC study of nonsleepy patients with an ACS did NOT find an increased prevalence of CV events in patients without OSA compared with CPAP did not significantly reduce this prevalence.[39]

If CPAP does not improve the prognosis of patients with OSA and CAD, would treatment provide symptomatic benefit by reducing nocturnal angina? A related question is the

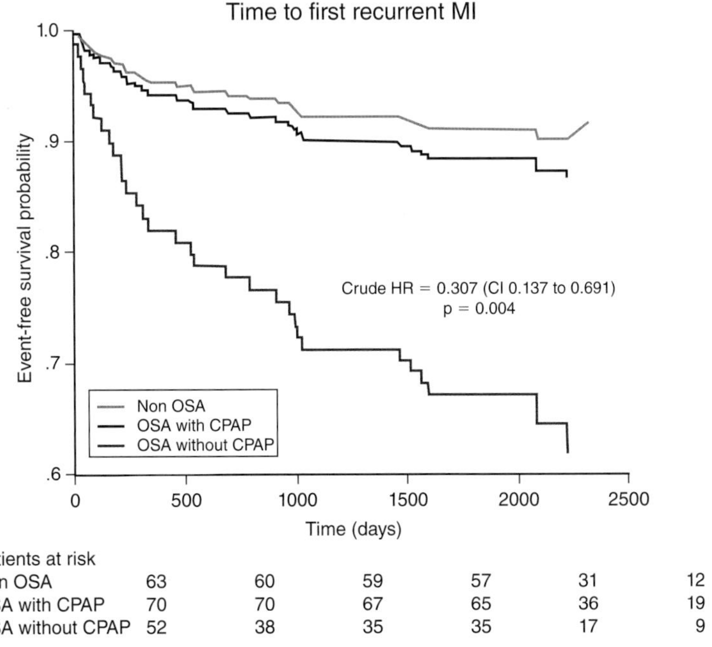

Patients at risk						
Non OSA	63	60	59	57	31	12
OSA with CPAP	70	70	67	65	36	19
OSA without CPAP	52	38	35	35	17	9

Figure 20–15 Patients with myocardial infarction underwent a sleep study and those with sleep apnea were offered treatment with CPAP. Three groups were followed for 6 years: no OSA, OSA no CPAP, OSA CPAP. The risk of current MI in those using CPAP was much less than OSA with no CPAP and similar to those with no OSA. (From Garcia-Rio F, Alonso-Fernandez A, Armada E, et al. CPAP effect on recurrent episodes in patients with sleep apnea and myocardial infarction. *Int J Cardiol.* 2013;168:1328-1335.)

frequency of an association between ischemia and obstructive apneas and hypopneas. A study monitoring the electrocardiogram (ECG) for ST-segment depression in a group of patients with OSA and nocturnal angina found depressions occurred in 59%. ST depressions were noted within 2 minutes of a respiratory event in 12% of events but was more tightly associated with more severe desaturations.[201] The authors concluded that episodes of nocturnal myocardial ischemia are common in patients with angina pectoris. However, a temporal relationship between sleep-disordered breathing and myocardial ischemia is present only in a minority of the patients, but it occurs more frequently in men and in more severely disordered breathing.

A study with a small number of participants with nocturnal angina and sleep apnea was found in 9 of 10 patients, nocturnal angina diminished during treatment of sleep apnea by CPAP, and the number of nocturnal myocardial ischemic events measured by computerized vector-cardiography was reduced.[202] Similar evaluations in a larger group of patients are needed. Why is CPAP not more effective in improving CAD outcomes (at least in randomized trials)? One explanation is that OSA-related hypoxemia could favor the development of coronary collaterals, thereby exerting a protective effect.[203] Another possibility is that hypoxic preconditioning may improve coronary artery disease outcomes, and while on CPAP this preconditioning is not present.[19,204]

INFLAMMATION, ATHEROSCLEROSIS, THROMBOSIS, AND ENDOTHELIAL DYSFUNCTION

There has also been a growing number of studies showing changes in blood components or indicators of inflammation in OSA that may be associated with an increased risk of atherosclerosis or thrombosis. However, obesity also causes changes in inflammatory markers, and the studies have usually been in a small number of selected patients and often with conflicting results. In OSA, there is an increase in the early-morning hematocrit[205] and fibrinogen levels[206] in untreated OSA that decrease after CPAP treatment.[207] A retrospective cohort study by H*ong and colleagues*[208] *found that* patients with moderate to severe OSA had elevated blood coagulability markers compared with healthy individuals, which may contribute to the occurrence of cardiovascular complications. OSA patients *had a lower prothrombin time (PT)* and a lower international normalized ratio *(INR)*. Vascular endothelial growth factor (VEGF), a potent angiogenic cytokine regulated by hypoxia-inducible factor, is thought to stimulate the progression of CVD. Some (but not all studies) have found an increase in the levels of VEGF in OSA.[209] A meta-analysis found that VEGF is decreased after CPAP treatment.[210] There is also evidence of platelet activation in OSA patients due to intermittent hypoxia.[211] A small preliminary study found that CPAP reduced this activation.[212] The white blood cells of OSA patients are believed to be activated and release reactive oxygen species.[213] Inflammation is now believed to play a role in atherosclerosis or plaque rupture. Nadeem and coworkers[214] performed a meta-analysis and found that levels of C-reactive protein (CRP, a marker of inflammation), tumor necrosis factor alpha (TNF-α), interleukin (IL)-6, IL-8, intercellular adhesion molecule, vascular cell adhesion molecule, and selectins were all increased in OSA patients compared with controls. Some studies have demonstrated a reduction in CRP with CPAP treatment. For example, Ishida and colleagues found decreases in CRP after CPAP treatment but only in those patients with good CPAP compliance and with elevated CRP levels at baseline.[215] Therefore, results may vary depending on the characteristics of the patients at baseline and the compliance with CPAP treatment. Note that not all studies have found an elevated CRP in OSA and in some the CRP elevations were thought to be due to obesity and not OSA. Fei and colleagues[216] defined OSA phenotypes and compared inflammatory markers in OSA patients with and without the phenotype of obesity. The phenotypes of obesity, HTN, heart disease, and metabolic syndrome were defined. For each phenotype, OSA patients were compared. CRP was increased in all phenotypes, whereas TNF-α was increased only in the obese and HTN phenotypes. This study illustrates that the degree of increase in inflammatory markers likely varies considerably between OSA patients based on the presence or absence of other factors such as obesity, and this likely explains the different findings in studies. Intermittent hypoxia (hypoxia-reoxygenation) is believed to selectively activate several inflammatory pathways.[217] For example, TNF-α and IL-8 are elevated in untreated OSA but decrease with CPAP treatment.[218] TNF-α can also cause daytime sleepiness. In the study by Bayram and colleagues higher TNF-α levels were associated with higher ESS scores and worsened arterial oxygen desaturation. Endothelial function is impaired in many OSA patient (specifically nitric oxide-dependent flow-mediated dilatation), and studies suggest improvement after CPAP.[219] In studies comparing inflammatory markers in OSA patients with normal subjects, using an appropriate control group is essential. For example, it is often difficult to match groups for obesity. Trials of the effects of CPAP do not require a *normal* control group. However, many of the previously discussed studies of effects of CPAP on inflammatory changes in OSA patients were not RCTs. Therefore, the results need to be confirmed by controlled trials. For example, a recent RCT of CPAP found no change in several inflammatory mediators after 4 weeks of CPAP.[220] In summary, the role of inflammation and endothelial dysfunction likely varies between OSA patients and likely depends on associated obesity or the severity of intermittent hypoxia. The effects of CPAP depend both on CPAP adherence and baseline characteristics of the patient.

CONGESTIVE HEART FAILURE (CHF)

In-depth discussion of CHF can be found in Chapter 28 as both OSA and CSA are associated with CHF. Often patients have variable amounts of OSA and CSA on any one night. In this chapter **OSA** and CHF will be discussed. Shahar and colleagues analyzed the SHHS cohort[188] and found that the presence of OSA *increases the risk* of having CHF (Table 20–3). On the other hand, studies have suggested that sleep-disordered breathing is common in patients with CHF.[221,222] Oldenburg and coworkers[221] evaluated 700 patients with symptomatic heart failure and found sleep apnea in 76% (40% Central sleep apnea [CSA], 36% OSA). CSA patients were more symptomatic and had a lower LV ejection fraction. One should not assume that complaints of disturbed nocturnal sleep are simply secondary to heart failure. Sin and colleagues[223] retrospectively evaluated a group of patients with significant LV failure referred to the sleep laboratory and found that risk factors for CSA were male gender, AF, age > 60 years, and hypocapnia. The risk factors for **OSA** differed by gender and were an increased BMI for men and increased age for women. In patients with CHF and OSA, negative intrathoracic pressure, hypoxemia, and increased sympathetic tone associated with the apneas are believed to negatively affect ventricular function.[224] Nocturnal hypoxemia is associated with increased mortality in stable heart failure patients and is a better predictor of mortality than the AHI.[225] Heart failure is often divided into (1) a group with a normal ejection fraction (>50%) but diastolic dysfunction due to stiff left ventricle also known as HFpEF (heart failure with preserved ejection fraction), and (2) another group with reduced ejection fraction (EF < 40%, HFrEF), that is both systolic and diastolic heart failure. HFpEF is the more common type of heart failure in elderly patients. *The prevalence of moderate to severe OSA is similar in both types of heart failure (about 20% HFrEF and 23% HFpEF)*[3]. Treatment of OSA with nasal CPAP in patients with CHF and predominant OSA has been found to improve the ejection fraction and symptoms in a number of studies.[226-227] This appears to occur because of *a reduction in sympathetic tone and a decrease in ventricular afterload*.[222] A multicenter randomized trial of CPAP versus sham CPAP in a mixed group of CHF patients[228] (some with OSA, some with Cheyne-Stokes breathing [CSB]) found an improvement in the ejection fraction only in patients with a baseline LV ejection fraction > 37. Those with OSA only did have an improvement as well. *However, the improvements were very modest*. To date, no RCT has confirmed a reduction in mortality in CHF patients using PAP treatment. Randomized trials treatment of CHF with CPAP[229] and adaptive servoventilation[230] have targeted mainly patients with predominant central apnea and are discussed in Chapter 28. Adaptive servoventilation (ASV) is effective in HFpEF[231] and is effective for both central and obstructive events (see Chapter 24). ASV also effectively reduces the AHI in HFrEF. However, this type of treatment is currently felt to be contraindicated in CHF patients with a low ejection fraction.[230] New preliminary findings concerning this issue are discussed in Chapter 28.

STROKE AND OSA

A number of studies have shown a high prevalence of sleep-disordered breathing in patients soon after a cerebrovascular accident (CVA).[232,233] Some key points concerning stroke and OSA are listed in Box 20–5. Although the predominant form of sleep-disordered breathing after stroke is OSA, CSA with CSB can also occur.[232-234] The CSA-CSB is believed to occur early in the post-CVA period and then usually resolves. In contrast, OSA seems to persist after a CVA. However, the temporal relationship between OSA and stroke is not well defined. It is not known whether brain damage from a CVA causes sleep apnea or if sleep apnea preceded the stroke. If sleep apnea precedes the stroke, is the presence of sleep apnea an independent risk factor for the development of a CVA? The SHHS showed an increased risk of having a self-reported CVA (prevalence) if OSA is present (Table 20–2).[188] In another study, Redline and associates[235] evaluated the SHHS data and found an increased risk for *incident* ischemic stroke in men with mild to moderate OSA (Table 20–4). In this study, data were adjusted for a number of confounders that complicated the analysis including obesity. If there is a causal role for OSA in stroke, what are the mechanisms? OSA may predispose to atherosclerosis, HTN, and early-morning hemoconcentration. These factors increase the risk of stroke. During sleep apnea, there are increases in intracranial pressure (ICP)[236] and decreases in cerebral blood

Box 20–5 KEY POINTS ABOUT STROKE AND OBSTRUCTIVE SLEEP APNEA

- OSA is an independent risk factor for incident stroke (about twofold increased risk).
- Sleep apnea is present in a high percentage of patients after stroke (up to 70% in some studies).
- OSA is the most common form of sleep apnea, but CSA can occur (including Cheyne-Stokes breathing).
- The presence of OSA after a CVA is associated with a worse prognosis.
- The presence of OSA after stroke is a risk factor for **recurrent** stroke.
- Commonly used screening tools for OSA are not effective in poststroke patients.
- PSG is the gold standard study, but HSAT can be considered.
- Attempts at PAP treatment in poststroke patients show low adherence.
- **Observational studies** show PAP treatment may improve stroke outcomes. However, to date an intention to treat analysis of RCTs of CPAP treatment of patients with moderate to severe OSA and cerebrovascular diease has not documented improved outcomes. However, secondary analysis of RCTs of CPAP treatment considering only CPAP adherent patients has found evidence of cerebrovascular outome benefit.

CSA, Central sleep apnea; *CVA*, cerebrovascular accident; *HSAT*, home sleep apnea testing; *OSA*, obstructive sleep apnea; *PAP*, positive airway pressure; *PSG*, polysomnography.

flow.[237] There is an increase in ICP with each apneic event, and the rise tends to be correlated with the length of apnea. The increase in ICP is thought to be secondary to increases in central venous pressure, systemic pressure, and cerebral vasodilatation from increases in $PaCO_2$ during respiratory events. Because cerebral perfusion is proportional to the mean arterial pressure (MAP) minus ICP, increases in ICP may reduce perfusion pressure even if MAP also rises. Studies of cerebral blood flow velocity using Doppler monitoring have shown that flow velocity increases in early apnea and then has approximately a 25% fall below baseline at end apnea.[237]

There is evidence that the presence of OSA in patients who have suffered a CVA is a bad prognostic sign regardless of whether OSA precedes or follows the CVA. Good and coworkers[238] found that the Barthel Index (a multifaceted scale measuring mobility and activities of daily living that is used to assess patients after stroke) was significantly lower (more impaired) in patients with OSA and CVA compared with those with no evidence of OSA after CVA. The presence of OSA was determined at discharge, and the Barthel Index was lower at 3 and 12 months in the OSA-CVA group.

A 2014 meta-analysis investigated the effect of OSA on incident ischemic and "hemorrhagic stroke" across 10 prospective community-based, population-based, or clinic-based studies, including patients with and without a history of prior stroke.[239] Across all 10 studies, *OSA was associated with a twofold increased risk of incident stroke* (relative risk 2.10; 95% CI 1.50–2.93). *Thus, sleep apnea is best described as a well-established independent risk factor for stroke that confers an approximately twofold increased risk.*

Can treatment with OSA reduce the risk of CVA or improve outcomes in patients with OSA and known cerebrovascular disease?

A prospsective observational study by Martinez-Garcia and colleagues[240] found that CPAP treatment reduced the mortality after ischemic stroke in patients with concomitant OSA. However adherence to CPAP in patients started on CPAP following a recent CVA tends to be low.

The 2016 Sleep Apnea Cardiovascular Endpoints RCT (SAVE study)[36] investigated stroke incidence (as a secondary end point and a component of the primary endpoint) in 2717 participants aged 45 to 75 years who had CAD or cerebrovascular disease and moderate to severe sleep apnea. Half of the participants were assigned to receive CPAP plus usual care, and half of the participants were assigned to usual care alone. After a mean follow-up of 3.7 years, no difference was observed in stroke incidence between the CPAP group and the usual care group. However, interpretation of the study's results is complicated by an Asian predominant study population, as well as by the exclusion of patients with severe daytime sleepiness or recent stroke, factors that limit the generalizability of the results. Others have noted that only 42% of the CPAP group had good adherence to treatment (≥4 hours of CPAP use per night) during follow-up, with an overall mean of 3.3 hours of nightly use in the intervention. Therefore, because of the limitations of this study, the generalizability of the findings is questionable. A secondary propensity score-matched analysis of the study's data showed that the patients who were adherent to CPAP therapy did have a lower risk of stroke than those in the usual-care group (HR, 0.56; 95% CI 0.32 to 1.00; $P = .05$), but these results were not adjusted statistically for multiple comparisons. The meta-analysis by Javaheri and colleagues[42] of RCTs determining if CPAP can reduce MACEs considering only patients with good adherence did find a benefit in cerebrovascular disease (but not cardiac disease). Therefore, there is reason to believe that CPAP treatment could reduce cerebrovascular events. Thus, with good PAP adherence, there may be a benefit in OSA patients with respect to the risk of cerebrovascular events.

Catalan-Serra and colleagues studied the role of CPAP on incident stroke risk[241] in a population of participants age > 65 years using a post hoc analysis of a *prospective observational study*. Four groups were analyzed. These included a reference group (AHI < 15), untreated mild to moderate OSA, untreated severe OSA, and a CPAP-treated group with moderate to severe OSA and good CPAP adherence. An association between i*ncident stroke and untreated severe OSA* (but not for untreated mild to moderate OSA) was found. No association between the CPAP-treated group and incident stroke was found. The findings suggest a role for CPAP in severe OSA in older patients for prevention of stroke but the observational and post hoc nature of the study limits the conclusions. How often is OSA found after stroke or TIA? This question was addressed by Seiler and coworkers[242] who performed a meta-analysis of 89 studies including 7096 patients and found that the prevalence of sleep apnea (AHI > 5/hour) after stroke or TIA was 71%. Lisabeth and colleagues[243] performed a population-based study of 995 ischemic stroke patients; the presence of sleep apnea was determined by a limited channel device soon after stroke, and outcomes were evaluated at 90 days. The presence of sleep apnea was associated with worse functional and cognitive outcomes at 90 days poststroke. In summary, sleep apnea is a well-established independent risk factor for stroke that confers an approximately twofold increased risk of incident stroke. Sleep apnea is highly prevalent poststroke and is associated with worse outcomes after stroke. Sleep apnea is an attractive target for research addressing secondary stroke prevention and recovery.[244]

Can CPAP treatment after stroke reduce the recurrence rate or improve outcomes? This question was addressed by Brill and coworkers[245] who performed a meta-analysis of randomized trials. Ten trials with 564 participants were included in the analysis. Two studies compared CPAP with sham CPAP; eight compared CPAP with usual care. Mean CPAP use across the trials was 4.53 hours per night. Two trials of early CPAP use found no differences between the CPAP and non-CPAP groups in recurrent TIA, stroke, MI, hospitalization for CHF, and death, but the trials were of short duration and underpowered. The combined analysis of two neurofunctional scales (National Institutes of Health Stroke Scale and Canadian Neurological Scale) showed an overall neurofunctional improvement with CPAP, but the heterogeneity in study results limited the confidence in the findings. Bravata and coworkers[246] reported results of an RCT of OSA with CPAP in *acute ischemic stroke and TIA*. Groups included control group, standard CPAP intervention, and *enhanced intervention to improve PAP adherence*. No differences in CPAP use and no differences in outcomes were found. However, CPAP was only used on 50% of the nights. This result is disappointing but shows the difficulty of using CPAP to improve stroke outcomes.

Wake-up Stroke and Sleep Apnea

Wake-up strokes are those whose symptoms begin during sleep, and therefore they have an uncertain time of onset. Historically, patients with wake-up stroke have been excluded from acute stroke therapies because of an unclear last known normal time, despite some evidence that stroke is more common in the morning hours shortly before awakening. Several small studies have explored the relationship between sleep apnea and wake-up strokes, and the results have generally suggested a higher prevalence or severity of sleep apnea in patients with wake-up stroke than in patients with non-wake-up stroke. A study by Koo and colleagues of 164 participants observed a relationship between sleep apnea and wake-up stroke in men but not women.[247]

A larger study in 466 **women**[248] who presented with wake-up stroke determined the presence or absence of OSA by home sleep apnea testing. When the prevalence was adjusted for age and HTN and other confounders, there was no association with OSA. The findings are consistent with the aforementioned small study that observed a relationship between sleep apnea and wake-up stroke in men but not in women and raise the possibility of an interesting sex-specific relationship between sleep apnea and wake-up stroke.

Given the importance of OSA in stroke, it is concerning that stroke patients are rarely screened for OSA. In one study of 981 patients at 90 days poststroke, only 55 (6%) recalled being offered PSG.[249] Questionnaires for identifying sleep apnea in acute and subacute stroke patients tend to be sensitive but not specific and are of limited utility in the poststroke population.[250] The American Heart Association/American Stroke Association guideline[251] states: "A sleep study might be considered for patients with an ischemic stroke or TIA on the basis of the very high prevalence of sleep apnea in this population and the strength of the evidence that the treatment of sleep apnea improves outcomes in the general population."

DIABETES AND OSA

Obesity is a major confounding factor in the analysis of the interactions between diabetes mellitus (DM) and OSA because both are worsened with obesity. Studies suggest that more than half of patients with diabetes also have OSA and, conversely, diabetes is present in 15% to 30% of patients with OSA.[252] Their coexistence may be strongly related to the presence of obesity, a key risk factor for both conditions.

However, there is evidence that the presence of sleep apnea increases the risk of developing diabetes, independent of other risk factors.[253–255] Among patients with more severe sleep apnea, regular PAP use may attenuate this risk.[253] A study by Appleton and coworkers[254] concluded that severe undiagnosed OSA and nocturnal intermittent hypoxemia were independently associated with the recent development of diabetes in a community sample of middle-aged and older men. Weight loss can produce clinically relevant improvements in OSA among obese patients with diabetes, improvements that are sustained at 4 years. A reduction in the burden of undiagnosed OSA and undiagnosed diabetes is likely to occur if patients presenting with one disorder are assessed for the other. In a retrospective analysis from a clinical cohort, severe OSA (AHI ≥ 30/hour) and oxygen saturation less than 90% for > 6.4 minutes were independently associated with the development of diabetes.[255] Another study, compared with patients with and without sleep apnea found that moderate to severe OSA was significantly associated with abnormal fasting glucose in African Americans (OR 2.14; 95% CI 1.12–4.08) and White participants (OR 2.85; 95% CI 1.20–6.75), but not among Chinese or Hispanic subjects, after adjusting for site, age, sex, waist circumference, and sleep duration ($P = .06$ for ethnicity-by-OSA severity interaction).[256] In contrast, sleep duration was not significantly associated with abnormal fasting glucose after considering the influence of OSA.

Punjabi and Beamer[257] found that independent of adiposity, sleep-disordered breathing was associated with impairment of insulin sensitivity, glucose effectiveness, and pancreatic beta cell function. Harsch and associates[258] found the CPAP rapidly improved insulin sensitivity, although the greatest results were in nonobese patients. Babu and coworkers[259] found that in diabetic OSA patients with a hemoglobin A1C greater than 7%, CPAP treatment reduced the A1C. Lam and colleagues[260] compared sham CPAP and effective CPAP in patients with OSA and found that 1 week of CPAP improved insulin sensitivity in nondiabetic males, and the improvement was maintained for 12 weeks of treatment in those with moderate obesity. Conversely, West and associates[261] were not able to show an improvement insulin resistance with CPAP treatment. Although these studies do suggest that OSA independent of obesity impairs glucose metabolism, the effect may be more pronounced in nonobese patients. The impact of treatment of OSA on long-term diabetes and the diabetic complications remains to be determined.

Can CPAP treatment in a patient with OSA and prediabetes improve glucose control? Three RCTs[262-264] have demonstrated that treatment of OSA with CPAP improves insulin sensitivity. In one RCT by Pamidi and coworkers,[262] supervised CPAP treatment for 8 hours over 2 weeks nightly significantly improved insulin sensitivity and glucose response in intravenous and oral glucose tolerance tests in a group of patients with *prediabetes and OSA*. In another RCT of prediabetic patients with moderate to severe OSA, the insulin sensitivity index improved significantly in those with severe OSA treated with CPAP,[263] and there was a significant correlation between hours of CPAP use and improvement in insulin sensitivity, emphasizing the critical importance of adherence. Salford and colleagues evaluated CPAP versus control in patients with morbid obesity and severe OSA and found that CPAP improved insulin resistance.[264] Thus, current evidence suggests that OSA is associated with insulin resistance, and CPAP treatment may improve insulin sensitivity in prediabetic patients. The effects of CPAP therapy of OSA on full-blown diabetes remain to be elucidated.[265]

NONALCOHOLIC LIVER DISEASE

Nonalcoholic fatty liver disease (NAFLD) is one of the most common liver disorders and consists of a spectrum of disease including (1) hepatic steatosis and (2) nonalcoholic steatohepatitis (NASH).[266,267] In hepatic steatosis, also known as nonalcoholic fatty liver (NAFL), there is macrovascular accumulation of triglyceride in hepatocytes that develops in the absence of secondary causes (e.g., medications, excessive alcohol consumption, or certain heritable conditions). NASH is the inflammatory subtype of NAFLD consisting of both steatosis and evidence of hepatocyte injury (ballooning) and inflammation, with or without fibrosis. Although often clinically silent, with time NASH can progress to cirrhosis, end-stage liver disease, or the need for a liver transplant. Steatosis has a much lower rate of progression to cirrhosis (≈4%). Patients with NASH are often asymptomatic or complain of bloating. Evaluation for elevated aminotransferases with a hepatic ultrasound showing steatosis is often the way the disorder is discovered. However, not all individuals with NAFL have elevated aminotransferases. Race is an important factor in the development of NASH with higher risk in Hispanics, intermediate risk in Whites, and the lowest risk in Blacks in several studies. *Studies have documented that severe OSA is associated with the development and evolution of NAFL independent of obesity or other shared risk factors.*[267] *Some studies have found an association with the AHI and others the hypoxic burden.* A study of patients undergoing liver biopsy for bariatric surgery found an association between OSA and elevated aminotransferases, the presence of NASH, steatosis grade, and the fibrosis scale.[268] An association does not imply causality. Studies have found conflicting results concerning the benefit of CPAP treatment of OSA with respect to NASH.[269,270] For example, a retrospective analysis found a benefit from CPAP treatment[269], whereas an RCT[270] failed to document a benefit. Issues with comparing CPAP trials include different pathological and clinical definitions, the need for a liver biopsy, racial confounders, and the fact that weight loss alone is often beneficial.

ERECTILE DYSFUNCTION

An association between erectile dysfunction (ED) and sleep disorders appears to exist in survey studies relying on self-report and in small case series.[271,272] Hormonal, neural, and endothelial mechanisms have been implicated in linking sleep disorders with ED. OSA, insomnia, shift work disorder, and restless legs syndrome are all common sleep disorders and are associated with ED and/or other urological disorders. Therefore, careful attention should be paid to the diagnosis and treatment of concomitant sleep disorders in patients with sexual dysfunction. Observational studies suggest that treatment of sleep disorders, specifically sleep apnea with CPAP, has been shown to improve patient erectile function.[273-275]

NOCTURIA

It has been a common clinical observation that many patients with OSA who start CPAP treatment report fewer awakenings to urinate. Hajduk and coworkers[276] found a high incidence of pathologic nocturia (PN) (defined as ≥2 urination events per night) in OSA patients. The percentage of PN was 47.8% in a cohort of OSA patients; age, arousal index, AHI, and measures of oxygenation were predictors of the presence of PN. Some of the reported effects of CPAP treatment could be due to better sleep. However, studies have shown a reduced sodium excretion in OSA patients treated with CPAP. Krieger and colleagues[277] found that OSA patients had greater urinary flows and greater urinary sodium excretion compared with controls. Nasal CPAP resulted in a reduction in urinary flow and sodium and chloride excretion. A second study by the same group found evidence of increased guanosine 3′5′-cyclic monophosphate excretion in untreated OSA patients, which reflects ANP release. The authors hypothesized that atrial stretch during sleep apnea induced release of ANP, which caused increased sodium excretion.[278] Umlauf and associates[279] also found increased nocturia and elevated urinary ANP when the AHI was ≥15/hour. Fitzgerald and coworkers[280] did a retrospective review of sleep studies and found the fraction of patients with nocturia to be similar in patients with and without OSA. However, in those with nocturia, the *frequency of nocturia episodes* was related to age, diabetes, and the severity of OSA. Patients with OSA and nocturia who were treated with CPAP demonstrated a significant decrease in nocturic frequency ($P < .001$). Parthasarathy and colleagues performed a retrospective analysis of the SHHS cohort and found nocturia to be independently associated with sleep-disordered breathing.[281] After adjusting for SDB, there was association between nocturia and CV morbidity. A meta-analysis of studies assessing the frequency of nocturia found that the presence of OSA increased the risk of nocturia in men but not women.[282] Miyauchi and coworkers found that CPAP decreased episodes of nocturia, nocturnal urinary frequency, and sodium excretion.[283] There is evidence that nocturia is a core symptom of sleep apnea in the elderly.[284] In summary, nocturia is a manifestation of untreated OSA, can be a common complaint of elderly patients with OSA, and can improve with CPAP treatment.

SUMMARY OF KEY POINTS

1. The nocturnal physiological consequences of OSA vary with the frequency of the events and severity of desaturations. Possible changes include episodic hypercapnia, hypoxia, negative intrathoracic pressure, increases in pulmonary and systemic pressure, cyclic slowing then speeding of heart rate, and surges of sympathetic tone at event termination. Most studies show that the cardiovascular (CV) consequences are most closely related to the severity of hypoxemia. The hypoxic burden is a better predictor of morbidity than the AHI.
2. Patients with daytime sleepiness, short duration events, or increased hypoxic burden have the greatest risk of mortality and morbidity.
3. Patients with untreated OSA have elevated sympathetic tone during day and night, as well as decreased heart rate variability.
4. Populations studies have documented an increase in prevalence of CAD, CHF, Stroke, and HTN in patients with **severe OSA** compared to patients with no or mild OSA. Studies have also found an increased incidence of stroke, HTN, CAD (men < 70 years), and CHF (men) in severe OSA.
5. There is an increased prevalence of OSA in populations with stroke, HTN, CAD, CHF, and arrhythmias.
6. Patients with untreated OSA often have nondipping nocturnal BP, elevated morning BP, high daytime sympathetic tone, and decreased heart rate variability.
7. The best evidence of increased mortality in untreated OSA is for men with severe OSA, with an approximate age range of 30 to 50 years (40–70 in some studies). The time of sudden death is **midnight to 6 a.m.** in contrast to normal populations with a peak risk in the morning after awakening.
8. Observational studies suggest that OSA patients treated with CPAP have normal survival, all other factors being equal. No RCT of CPAP treatment of OSA has documented improvement in CV or cerebrovascular outcomes. The studies targeted nonsleepy patients who differed from the typical sleep clinic patient and whose CPAP adherence was very poor.
9. The severity of daytime sleepiness increases with higher AHI, but there is substantial variability. Other polysomnographic indices such as the arousal index do not have significantly higher correlations with subjective or objective sleepiness than the AHI. Daytime sleepiness is believed to be due to both sleep fragmentation and hypoxia. New metrics of sleep depth may provide better assessment of sleep quality.
10. OSA patients are at increased risk for MVAs (especially if there is a history of sleepiness at the wheel or a near miss/accident associated with sleepiness). Effective CPAP treatment can reduce the risk of MVAs.
11. Patients with OSA may fail to have a fall in BP with sleep (nondippers). Clinical cohorts with HTN or resistant HTN have a high prevalence of OSA. Effective treatment with CPAP is associated with small decreases in the 24-hour SBP and DBP. However, even small decreases reduce the risk of CV morbidity and mortality. CPAP results in a larger decrease in BP in patients with resistant HTN.
12. OSA in the *absence of lung disease or diastolic dysfunction* is associated with **daytime** PH in 20% to 40% of patients. The PH is usually of a mild nature (unless other factors are present). If moderate to severe PH is present, OSA should be treated, but other causes of PH should be explored.
13. Untreated OSA is associated with nocturnal arrhythmias, although the incidence is low. In some cases, effective treatment will improve arrhythmias.
14. Untreated OSA is associated with an increased incidence of recurrence of AF after cardioversion or catheter ablation. Several observational studies have found that CPAP treatment lowers the risk of recurrence of AF after cardioversion or ablation. However, this benefit has not been confirmed by a randomized controlled trial (RCT).
15. Observational studies suggest that untreated OSA is associated with a higher risk of adverse outcomes in patients with CAD. Some observational studies suggest a benefit from CPAP treatment, but to date no RCT has shown benefit.
16. A high percentage of patients after a stroke have some type of sleep apnea (up to 70%). The great majority of sleep apnea is obstructive, but in the early poststroke period central apneas can occur. The presence of OSA after stroke is a risk factor for recurrent stroke.
17. Untreated OSA is associated with a higher incidence of stroke. In stroke patients, observational studies suggest CPAP treatment of OSA can reduce mortality and improve outcomes (including reduced recurrence of stroke). A meta-analysis of RCTs of OSA patients using CPAP >4 hours a night found improved cerebrovascular outcomes. Confirmation is needed by a RCT with intention to treat analysis showing improved cerebrovascular outcomes in patients with patients with OSA.
18. Untreated OSA can worsen nocturia, and CPAP treatment can improve this manifestation.

CLINICAL REVIEW QUESTIONS

1. OSA is associated with all of the following EXCEPT
   A. Increased **daytime** sympathetic tone.
   B. Increased heart rate variability.
   C. Endothelial dysfunction.
   D. Increased nocturnal sodium excretion.
2. During sleep patients with OSA experience
   A. Decreased venous return.
   B. More negative intrathoracic pressure (-15 cm H_2O versus -10 cm H_2O).
   C. Decreased systemic afterload.
   D. Higher than normal parasympathetic tone.
3. All of the following are associated **with increased mortality in OSA** EXCEPT
   A. Severe arterial oxygen desaturation.
   B. Age > 60 years.
   C. Severe versus mild OSA.
   D. Comorbid conditions (diabetes, CHF, COPD).
4. All of the following are true concerning patients with a recent stroke **who have sleep apnea** EXCEPT
   A. CSA more common than OSA.
   B. A worse prognosis than patients without sleep apnea.
   C. Improved prognosis with CPAP treatment.
   D. Low adherence to CPAP treatment.
5. Untreated OSA is associated with all of the following EXCEPT
   A. Increased risk of thrombosis.
   B. Decreased CRP.
   C. Increased morning hematocrit.
   D. Increased VEGF.
6. Which of the following is the best predictor of atrial fibrillation?
   A. A high AHI
   B. Severe arterial oxygen desaturation at night
   C. Male gender
7. In OSA the most common time of death is
   A. Noon to 6 p.m.
   B. 6 p.m. to midnight.
   C. Midnight to 6 a.m.
   D. 6 a.m. to noon.

ANSWERS

1. B. Untreated OSA is associated with *decreased* heart rate variability. This is thought to be due to higher sympathetic compared with parasympathetic tone.
2. B. Obstructive apneas are associated with more negative intrathoracic pressure. Answer C is not correct, as afterload is **increased** because of negative intrathoracic pressure associated with an obstructive apnea and hypopnea as well as increased systemic vascular resistance because of high sympathetic tone. Answer D is not correct, as OSA patients have increased sympathetic tone rather than parasympathetic tone.
3. B. Most of the available evidence suggests an increased mortality risk with **severe OSA** for middle-aged as compared with older patients.
4. A. Although both obstructive and central apnea can occur after stroke, obstructive sleep apnea is much more common. Observational studies suggest that the presence of sleep apnea is associated with a worse prognosis and that CPAP treatment improves outcome. However, adherence with CPAP treatment is problematic.
5. B. Most studies have found an increase in CRP in OSA, although in some studies the level correlated better with the degree of obesity than the AHI.
6. B. The best predictor of incident atrial fibrillation is nocturnal oxygen desaturation.
7. C. The time of highest risk of sudden death in OSA is during the night. In the general population it is after awakening in the early morning.

SUGGESTED READING

Javaheri S, Barbe F, Campos-Rodriguez F, et al. Sleep apnea: types, mechanisms, and clinical cardiovascular consequences. *J Am Coll Cardiol.* 2017;69(7):841-858.

Javaheri S, Martinez-Garcia MA, Campos-Rodriguez F, Muriel A, Peker Y. Continuous positive airway pressure adherence for prevention of major adverse cerebrovascular and cardiovascular events in obstructive sleep apnea. *Am J Respir Crit Care Med.* 2020;201(5):607-610.

Linz D, McEvoy RD, Cowie MR, et al. Associations of obstructive sleep apnea with atrial fibrillation and continuous positive airway pressure treatment: a review. *JAMA Cardiol.* 2018;3(6):532-540.

McDermott M, Brown DL. Sleep apnea and stroke. *Curr Opin Neurol.* 2020;33(1):4-9.

McEvoy RD, Antic NA, Heeley E, et al. CPAP for prevention of cardiovascular events in obstructive sleep apnea. *N Engl J Med.* 2016;375(10): 919-931.

Reutrakul S, Mokhlesi B. Obstructive sleep apnea and diabetes: a state of the art review. *Chest.* 2017;152(5):1070-1086.

Simonneau G, Montani D, Celermajer DS, et al. Haemodynamic definitions and updated clinical classification of pulmonary hypertension. *Eur Respir J.* 2019;53(1):1801913.

REFERENCES

1. Gottlieb DJ, Punjabi NM. Diagnosis and management of obstructive sleep apnea: a review. *JAMA.* 2020;323(14):1389-1400.
2. Yeghiazarians Y, Jneid H, Tietjens JR, et al. Obstructive sleep apnea and cardiovascular disease: a scientific statement from the American Heart Association. *Circulation.* 2021;144(3):e56-e67.
3. Javaheri S, Barbe F, Campos-Rodriguez F, et al. Sleep apnea: types, mechanisms, and clinical cardiovascular consequences. *J Am Coll Cardiol.* 2017;69(7):841-858.
4. Cowie MR, Linz D, Redline S, Somers VK, Simonds AK. Sleep disordered breathing and cardiovascular disease: JACC state-of-the-art review. *J Am Coll Cardiol.* 2021;78(6):608-624.
5. Reutrakul S, Mokhlesi B. Obstructive sleep apnea and diabetes: a state of the art review. *Chest.* 2017;152(5):1070-1086.
6. Reynor A, McArdle N, Shenoy B, et al. Continuous positive airway pressure and adverse cardiovascular events in obstructive sleep apnea: are participants of randomized trials representative of sleep clinic patients? *Sleep.* 2022;45(4):zsab264.
7. Platt AB, Kuna ST, Field SH, et al. Adherence to sleep apnea therapy and use of lipid-lowering drugs: a study of the healthy-user effect. *Chest.* 2010;137:102-108.
8. Villar I, Izuel M, Carrizo S, et al. Medication adherence and persistence in severe obstructive sleep apnea. *Sleep.* 2009;32:623-628.
9. Brown DL, Anderson CS, Chervin RD, et al. Ethical issues in the conduct of clinical trials in obstructive sleep apnea. *J Clin Sleep Med.* 2011; 7:103-108.
10. Pack AI, Magalang UJ, Singh B, Kuna ST, Keenan BT, Maislin G. Randomized clinical trials of cardiovascular disease in obstructive sleep apnea: understanding and overcoming bias. *Sleep.* 2021;44(2):zsaa229.
11. Mazzotti DR, Keenan BT, Lim DC, Gottlieb DJ, Kim J, Pack AI. Symptom subtypes of obstructive sleep apnea predict incidence of cardiovascular outcomes. *Am J Respir Crit Care Med.* 2019;200(4):493-506.
12. Mokhlesi B, Finn LA, Hagen EW, et al. Obstructive sleep apnea during REM sleep and hypertension. Results of the Wisconsin Sleep Cohort. *Am J Respir Crit Care Med.* 2014;190(10):1158-1167.
13. Aurora RN, Crainiceanu C, Gottlieb DJ, et al. Obstructive sleep apnea during REM sleep and cardiovascular disease. *Am J Respir Crit Care Med.* 2018;197(5):653-660.

14. Mehra R. Sleep apnea and the heart. *Cleve Clin J Med.* 2019;86(9 Suppl 1):10-18.
15. Somers VK, Dyken ME, Clary MP, Abboud FM. Sympathetic neural mechanisms in obstructive sleep apnea. *J Clin Invest.* 1995;96:1897-1904.
16. Bradley TD, Floras JS. Obstructive sleep apnea and its cardiovascular consequences. *Lancet.* 2009;373;82-93.
17. Maniaci A, Iannella G, Cocuzza S, et al. Oxidative stress and inflammation biomarker expression in obstructive sleep apnea patients. *J Clin Med.* 2021;10(2):277.
18. Bikov A, Meszaros M, Schwarz EI. Coagulation and fibrinolysis in obstructive sleep apnoea. *Int J Mol Sci.* 2021;22(6):2834.
19. Labarca G, Gower J, Lamperti L, Dreyse J, Jorquera J. Chronic intermittent hypoxia in obstructive sleep apnea: a narrative review from pathophysiological pathways to a precision clinical approach. *Sleep Breath.* 2020;24(2):751-760.
20. He J, Kryger MH, Zorick FJ, et al. Mortality and apnea index in obstructive sleep apnea. *Chest.* 1988;94:9-14.
21. Lavie P, Herer P, Peled R, et al. Mortality in sleep apnea patients: a multivariate analysis of risk factors. *Sleep.* 1995;18:149-157.
22. Lavie P, Lavie L, Herer P. All-cause mortality in males with sleep apnea syndrome: declining mortality rates with age. *Eur Respir J.* 2005;25:514-520.
23. Lavie P, Herer P, Lavie L. Mortality risk factors in sleep apnoea: a matched case-control study. *J Sleep Res.* 2007;16:128-134.
24. Lavie P, Lavie L. Unexpected survival advantage in elderly people with moderate sleep apnoea. *J Sleep Res.* 2009;18:397-403.
25. Marshall NS, Wong KK, Liu PY, et al. Sleep apnea as an independent risk factor for all-cause mortality: the Busselton Health Study. *Sleep.* 2008;31:1079-1085.
26. Marin JM, Carrizo S, Vicente E, Agusti AGN. Long-term cardiovascular outcomes in men with obstructive sleep apnoea-hypopnoea with or without treatment with continuous positive airway pressure: an observational study. *Lancet.* 2005;365:1046-1053.
27. Yaggi HK, Concato J, Kernan WN, et al. Obstructive sleep apnea as a risk factor for stroke and death. *N Engl J Med.* 2005;353:2034-2041.
28. Young T, Finn L, Peppard PE, et al. Sleep disordered breathing and mortality: eighteen-year follow-up of the Wisconsin Sleep Cohort. *Sleep.* 2008;31:1071-1078.
29. Punjabi N, Caffo BS, Goodwin JL, et al. Sleep-disordered breathing and mortality: a prospective cohort study. *PLoS Med.* 2009;6:e1000132.
30. Campos-Rodriguez F, Martinez-Garcia MA, de la Cruz-Moron I, et al. Cardiovascular mortality in women with obstructive sleep apnea with or without continuous positive airway pressure treatment: a cohort study. *Ann Intern Med.* 2012;156:115-122.
31. Gami AS, Olson EJ, Shen WK, et al. Obstructive sleep apnea and the risk of sudden cardiac death: a longitudinal study of 10,701 adults. *J Am Coll Cardiol.* 2013;62:610-616.
32. Gami AS, Howard DE, Olson EJ, Somers VK. Day-night pattern of sudden death in obstructive sleep apnea. *N Engl J Med.* 2005;352:1206-1214.
33. Imadojemu VA, Mawji Z, Kunselman A, et al. Sympathetic chemoreflex responses in obstructive sleep apnea and effects of continuous positive airway pressure therapy. *Chest.* 2007;131(5):1406-1413.
34. Wu X, Lv S, Yu X, et al. Treatment of OSA reduces the risk of repeat revascularization after percutaneous coronary intervention. *Chest.* 2015; 147:708-718.
35. Jennum P, Tønnesen P, Ibsen R, Kjellberg J. All-cause mortality from obstructive sleep apnea in male and female patients with and without continuous positive airway pressure treatment: a registry study with 10 years of follow-up. *Nat Sci Sleep.* 2015;7:43-50.
36. McEvoy RD, Antic NA, Heeley E, et al. CPAP for prevention of cardiovascular events in obstructive sleep apnea. *N Engl J Med.* 2016; 375(10):919-931.
37. Barbé F, Durán-Cantolla J, Sánchez-de-la-Torre M, et al. Effect of continuous positive airway pressure on the incidence of hypertension and cardiovascular events in nonsleepy patients with obstructive sleep apnea: a randomized controlled trial. *JAMA.* 2012;307(20):2161-2168.
38. Peker Y, Thunström E, Glantz H, Eulenburg C, Wegscheider K, Herliz J. Effect of positive airway pressure on cardiovascular outcomes in coronary artery disease patients with nonsleepy obstructive sleep apnea: the RICCADSA randomized controlled trial. *Am J Respir Crit Care Med.* 2016;194:613-620.
39. Sánchez-de-la-Torre M, Sánchez-de-la-Torre A, Bertran S, et al. Effect of obstructive sleep apnoea and its treatment with continuous positive airway pressure on the prevalence of cardiovascular events in patients with acute coronary syndrome (ISAACC study): a randomised controlled trial. *Lancet Respir Med.* 2020;8(4):359-367.
40. Yu J, Zhou Z, McEvoy RD, et al. Association of positive airway pressure with cardiovascular events and death in adults with sleep apnea: a systematic review and meta-analysis. *JAMA.* 2017;318(2):156-166.
41. Labarca G, Dreyse J, Drake L, Jorquera J, Barbe F. Efficacy of continuous positive airway pressure (CPAP) in the prevention of cardiovascular events in patients with obstructive sleep apnea: systematic review and meta-analysis. *Sleep Med Rev.* 2020;52:101312.
42. Javaheri S, Martinez-Garcia MA, Campos-Rodriguez F, et al. Continuous positive airway pressure adherence for prevention of major adverse cerebrovascular and cardiovascular events in obstructive sleep apnea. *Am J Respir Crit Care Med.* 2020;201(5):607-610.
43. Martínez-García MA, Capote F, Campos-Rodríguez F, et al. Effect of CPAP on blood pressure in patients with obstructive sleep apnea and resistant hypertension: the HIPARCO randomized clinical trial. *JAMA.* 2013;310(22):2407-2415.
44. Drager LF, McEvoy RD, Barbe F, Lorenzi-Filho G, Redline S. Sleep apnea and cardiovascular disease: lessons from recent trials and need for team science. *Circulation.* 2017;136(19):1840-1850.
45. Butler MP, Emch JT, Rueschman M, et al. Apnea-hypopnea event duration predicts mortality in men and women in the sleep heart health study. *Am J Respir Crit Care Med.* 2019;199(7):903-912.
46. Azarbarzin A, Sands SA, Stone KL, et al. The hypoxic burden of sleep apnoea predicts cardiovascular disease-related mortality: the Osteoporotic Fractures in Men Study and the Sleep Heart Health Study. *Eur Heart J.* 2019;40(14):1149-1157.
47. Azarbarzin A, Sands SA, Younes M, et al. The sleep apnea-specific pulse-rate response predicts cardiovascular morbidity and mortality. *Am J Respir Crit Care Med.* 2021;203(12):1546-1555.
48. Trzepizur W, Blanchard M, Ganem T, et al. Sleep apnea-specific hypoxic burden, symptom subtypes, and risk of cardiovascular events and all-cause mortality. *Am J Respir Crit Care Med.* 2022;205(1):108-117.
49. Keenan BT, Magalang UJ, Mazzotti DR, et al. Obstructive sleep apnea symptom subtypes and cardiovascular risk: conflicting evidence to an important question. *Am J Respir Crit Care Med.* 2022;205(6):729-730.
50. Kainulainen S, Töyräs J, Oksenberg A, et al. Severity of desaturations reflects OSA-related daytime sleepiness better than AHI. *J Clin Sleep Med.* 2019;15(8):1135-1142.
51. Bonnet MH. Performance and sleepiness as a function of frequency and placement of sleep disruption. *Psychophysiology.* 1986;3:263-271.
52. Roehrs T, Merlotti L, Petrucelli N, et al. Experimental sleep fragmentation. *Sleep.* 1994;17:438-443.
53. Johns MW. Daytime sleepiness, snoring, and obstructive sleep apnea. The Epworth Sleepiness Scale. *Chest.* 1993;103:30-36.
54. Christian G, Markka P, Quera-Salva MA, et al. Determinants of daytime sleepiness in obstructive sleep apnea. *Chest.* 1988;94:32-37.
55. Cheshire K, Engleman H, Deary I, et al. Factors impairing daytime performance in patients with sleep apnea/hypopnea syndrome. *Arch Intern Med.* 1992;152:538-541.
56. Bennett LS, Langford BA, Stradling JR. Sleep fragmentation indices as predictors of daytime sleepiness and nCPAP response in obstructive sleep apnea. *Am J Respir Crit Care Med.* 1998;158:778-786.
57. Martin SE, Wraith PK, Deary IJ, Douglas NJ. The effect of nonvisible sleep fragmentation on daytime function. *Am J Respir Crit Care Med.* 1997;155:1596-1601.
58. Younes M, Ostrowski M, Soiferman M, et al. Odds ratio product of sleep EEG as a continuous measure of sleep state. *Sleep.* 2015;38(4):641-654.
59. Younes M, Hanly PJ. Immediate postarousal sleep dynamics: an important determinant of sleep stability in obstructive sleep apnea. *J Appl Physiol (1985).* 2016;120(7):801-808.
60. Marcus CL. Sleep-disordered breathing in children. *Am J Respir Crit Care Med.* 2001;164:16-30.
61. Capdevila OS, Kheirandish-Gozal L, Dayyat E, Gozal D. Pediatric obstructive sleep apnea: complications, management, and long-term outcomes. *Proc Am Thorac Soc.* 2008;5:274-282.
62. Gottlieb DJ, Whitney CW, Bonekat WH, et al. Relation of sleepiness to respiratory disturbance index: the Sleep Heart Health Study. *Am J Respir Crit Care Med.* 1999;159:502-507.
63. Findley LJ, Barth JT, Powers DC, et al. Cognitive impairment in patients with obstructive sleep apnea and associated hypoxemia. *Chest.* 1986;90:686-690.
64. Arzt M, Young T, Finn L, et al. Sleepiness and sleep in patients with both systolic heart failure and obstructive sleep apnea. *Arch Intern Med.* 2006;166:1716-1722.
65. Berry RB, Sriram P. Auto-adjusting positive airway pressure treatment for sleep apnea diagnosed by home sleep testing. *J Clin Sleep Med.* 2014;10(12):1269-1275.

66. Wimms AJ, Kelly JL, Turnbull CD, et al. Continuous positive airway pressure versus standard care for the treatment of people with mild obstructive sleep apnoea (MERGE): a multicentre, randomised controlled trial. *Lancet Respir Med.* 2020;8(4):349-358.
67. Javaheri S, Javaheri S. Update on persistent excessive daytime sleepiness in OSA. *Chest.* 2020;158(2):776-786.
68. Zhu Y, Fenik P, Zhan G, et al. Selective loss of catecholaminergic wake active neurons in a murine sleep apnea model. *J Neurosci.* 2007; 27(37):10060-10071.
69. Chen HL, Lu CH, Lin HC, et al. White matter damage and systemic inflammation in obstructive sleep apnea. *Sleep.* 2015;38(3):361-370.
70. Hernández C, Abreu J, Abreu P, Castro A, Jiménez A. Nocturnal melatonin plasma levels in patients with OSAS: the effect of CPAP. *Eur Respir J.* 2007;30(3):496-500.
71. Ulfberg J, Micic S, Strøm J. Afternoon serum-melatonin in sleep disordered breathing. *J Intern Med.* 1998;244(2):163-168.
72. Quan SF, Chan CS, Dement WC, et al. The association between obstructive sleep apnea and neurocognitive performance—the Apnea Positive Pressure Long-term Efficacy Study (APPLES). *Sleep.* 2011;34(3): 303-314B.
73. Kushida CA, Nichols DA, Holmes TH, et al. Effects of continuous positive airway pressure on neurocognitive function in obstructive sleep apnea patients: the Apnea Positive Pressure Long-term Efficacy Study (APPLES). *Sleep.* 2012;35(12):1593-1602. [Erratum in: *Sleep.* 2016; 39(7):1483].
74. Mullins AE, Kam K, Parekh A, et al. Obstructive sleep apnea and its treatment in aging: effects on Alzheimer's disease biomarkers, cognition, brain structure and neurophysiology. *Neurobiol Dis.* 2020;145:105054.
75. Richards KC, Gooneratne N, Dicicco B, et al. CPAP adherence may slow 1-year cognitive decline in older adults with mild cognitive impairment and apnea. *J Am Geriatr Soc.* 2019;67(3):558-564.
76. Findley LJ, Unverzagt ME, Suratt PM. Automobile accidents involving patients with obstructive sleep apnea. *Am Rev Respir Dis.* 1988;138:337-340.
77. Cassel W, Ploch C, Becker D, et al. Risk of traffic accidents in patients with sleep disordered breathing: reduction with nasal CPAP. *Eur Respir J.* 1996;9:2602-2611.
78. Tregear S, Reston J, Schoelles K, Phillips B. Obstructive sleep apnea and risk of motor vehicle crash: systematic review and meta-analysis. *J Clin Sleep Med.* 2009;5:573-581.
79. Sleep apnea, sleepiness, and driving risk. American Thoracic Society. *Am J Respir Crit Care Med.* 1994;150:1463-1473.
80. Colvin LJ, Collop NA. Commercial motor vehicle driver obstructive sleep apnea screening and treatment in the United States: an update and recommendation overview. *J Clin Sleep Med.* 2016;12(1):113-125.
81. Hartenbaum N, Collop N, Rosen IM, et al. Sleep apnea and commercial motor vehicle operators: statement from the joint task force of the American College of Chest Physicians, the American College of Occupational and Environmental Medicine, and the National Sleep Foundation. *Chest.* 2006;130:902-905.
82. Gurubhagavatula I, Sullivan S, Meoli A, et al. Management of obstructive sleep apnea in commercial motor vehicle operators: recommendations of the AASM Sleep and Transportation Safety Awareness Task Force. *J Clin Sleep Med.* 2017;13(5):745-758.
83. Federal Motor Carrier Safety Administration. *Driver Physical Qualification.* Updated February 23, 2023. Accessed September 4, 2023. Available at: https://www.fmcsa.dot.gov/medical/driver-medical-requirements/driver-medical-fitness-duty.
84. Sagaspe P, Taillard J, Chaumet G, et al. Maintenance of wakefulness test as a predictor of driving performance in patients with untreated obstructive sleep apnea. *Sleep.* 2007;30:327-330.
85. Philip P, Sagaspe P, Taillard J, et al. Maintenance of wakefulness test, obstructive sleep apnea syndrome and driving risk. *Ann Neurol.* 2008; 64:410-416.
86. Azarbarzin A, Younes M, Sands SA, et al. Interhemispheric sleep depth coherence predicts driving safety in sleep apnea. *J Sleep Res.* 2021;30:e13092.
87. Hack M, Davies RJ, Mullins R, et al. Randomised prospective parallel trial of therapeutic versus subtherapeutic nasal continuous positive airway pressure on simulated steering performance in patients with obstructive sleep apnoea. *Thorax.* 2000;55:224-231.
88. George CF. Reduction in motor-vehicle collisions following treatment of sleep apnea with nasal CPAP. *Thorax.* 2001;56:508-512.
89. Tregear S, Reston J, Schoelles K, Phillips B. Continuous positive airway pressure reduces risk of motor vehicle crash among drivers with obstructive sleep apnea: systematic review and meta-analysis. *Sleep.* 2010; 33(10):1373-1380.
90. Karimi M, Hedner J, Häbel H, Nerman O, Grote L. Sleep apnea-related risk of motor vehicle accidents is reduced by continuous positive airway pressure: Swedish Traffic Accident Registry data. *Sleep.* 2015;38(3): 341-349.
91. Myllylä M, Anttalainen U, Saaresranta T, Laitinen T. Motor vehicle accidents in CPAP-compliant obstructive sleep apnea patients—a long-term observational study. *Sleep Breath.* 2020;24(3):1089-1095.
92. Burks SV, Anderson JE, Bombyk M, et al. Nonadherence with employer-mandated sleep apnea treatment and increased risk of serious truck crashes. *Sleep.* 2016;39(5):967-975.
93. Suzuki M, Guilleminault G, Otsuka K, Shimomi T. Blood pressure "dipping" and "non-dipping" in obstructive sleep apnea syndrome patients. *Sleep.* 1996;19:382-387.
94. Brooks D, Horner RL, Kozar LF, et al. Obstructive sleep apnea as a cause of systemic hypertension. Evidence from a canine model. *J Clin Invest.* 1997;99:106-109.
95. Carlson JT, Hedner JA, Ejnell H, Peterson LE. High prevalence of hypertension in sleep apnea patients independent of obesity. *Am J Respir Crit Care Med.* 1994;150:72-77.
96. Nieto FJ, Young TB, Lind BK, et al. Association of sleep-disordered breathing, sleep apnea, and hypertension in a large community-based study. Sleep Heart Health Study. *JAMA.* 2000;283:1829-1836.
97. Peppard PE, Young T, Palta M, Skatrud J. Prospective study of the association between sleep-disordered breathing and hypertension. *N Engl J Med.* 2000;342:1378-1384.
98. Marin JM, Agusti A, Villar I, et al. Association between treated and untreated obstructive sleep apnea and risk of hypertension. *JAMA.* 2012;307(20):2169-2176.
99. O'Connor GT, Caffo B, Newman AB, et al. Prospective study of sleep disordered breathing and hypertension. *Am J Respir Crit Care Med.* 2009;179:1159-1164.
100. Appleton SL, Vakulin A, Martin SA, et al. Hypertension is associated with undiagnosed OSA during rapid eye movement sleep. *Chest.* 2016;150(3):495-505.
101. Mokhlesi B, Hagen EW, Finn LA, et al. Obstructive sleep apnoea during REM sleep and incident non-dipping of nocturnal blood pressure: a longitudinal analysis of the Wisconsin Sleep Cohort. *Thorax.* 2015;70:1062-1069.
102. Nakagawa N, Sato N. Potential impact of non-dipping pulse rate pattern and nocturnal high pulse rate variability on target organ damage in patients with cardiovascular risk. *Hypertens Res.* 2023;46(4):1054-1055.
103. Verdecchia P, Schillaci G, Guerrieri M, et al. Circadian blood pressure changes and left ventricular hypertrophy in essential hypertension. *Circulation.* 1990;81:528-536.
104. Brotman DJ, Davidson MB, Boumitri M, Vidt DG. Impaired diurnal blood pressure variation and all-cause mortality. *Am J Hypertens.* 2008;21:92-97.
105. Gonzaga CC, Gaddam KK, Ahmed MI, et al. Severity of obstructive sleep apnea is related to aldosterone status in subjects with resistant hypertension. *J Clin Sleep Med.* 2010;6:363-368.
106. Labarca G, Schmidt A, Dreyse J, et al. Efficacy of continuous positive airway pressure (CPAP) in patients with obstructive sleep apnea (OSA) and resistant hypertension (RH): systematic review and meta-analysis. *Sleep Med Rev.* 2021;58:101446.
107. Lozano L, Tovar JL, Sampol G, et al. Continuous positive airway pressure treatment in sleep apnea patients with resistant hypertension: a randomized, controlled trial. *J Hypertens.* 2010;28:2161-2168.
108. Becker HF, Jerrentrup A, Ploch T, et al. Effect of nasal continuous positive airway pressure treatment on blood pressure in patients with obstructive sleep apnea. *Circulation.* 2003;107:68-73.
109. Pepperell JCT, Ramdassingh-Dow S, Crosthwaite N, et al. Ambulatory blood pressure after therapeutic and subtherapeutic nasal continuous positive airway pressure for obstructive sleep apnea: a randomised parallel trial. *Lancet.* 2002;359:204-210.
110. Faccendia J, Mackay TW, Bood NA, Douglas NJ. Randomized placebo-controlled trial of continuous positive airway pressure on blood pressure in the sleep apnea-hypopnea syndrome. *Am J Respir Crit Care Med.* 2001;163:344-348.
111. Engleman HM, Gough K, Martin SE, et al. Ambulatory blood pressure on and off continuous positive airway pressure therapy for the sleep apnea/hypopnea syndrome: effects in "non-dippers." *Sleep.* 1996;19:378-381.
112. Dimsdale JE, Loredo JS, Profant J. Effect of continuous positive pressure on blood pressure placebo trial. *Hypertension.* 2000;35:144-147.
113. Haentjens P, Van Meerhaeghe A, Moscariello A, et al. The impact of continuous positive airway pressure on blood pressure in patients with obstructive sleep apnea syndrome: evidence from a meta-analysis of placebo-controlled randomized trials. *Arch Intern Med.* 2007;167(8):757-764.

114. Lewington S, Clarke R, Qizilbash N, Peto R, Collins R. Age-specific relevance of usual blood pressure to vascular mortality: a meta-analysis of individual data for one million adults in 61 prospective studies. *Lancet*. 2002;360(9349):1903-1913.
115. Heude E, Bourgin P, Feigel P, et al. Ambulatory monitoring of blood pressure disturbs sleep and raises systolic pressure at night in patients suspected of suffering from sleep-disordered breathing. *Clin Sci (Colch)*. 1996;91:45-50.
116. Gehring J, Gesche H, Drewniok G, Küchler G, Patzak A. Nocturnal blood pressure fluctuations measured by using pulse transit time in patients with severe obstructive sleep apnea syndrome. *Sleep Breath*. 2018;22(2):337-343.
117. Bakker JP, Edwards BA, Gautam SP, et al. Blood pressure improvement with continuous positive airway pressure is independent of obstructive sleep apnea severity. *J Clin Sleep Med*. 2014;10(4):365-369. [Erratum in: *J Clin Sleep Med*. 2014;10(6):711].
118. Alajmi M, Mulgrew AT, Fox J, et al. Impact of continuous positive airway pressure therapy on blood pressure in patients with obstructive sleep apnea hypopnea: a meta-analysis of randomized controlled trials. *Lung*. 2007;185(2):67-72.
119. Fava C, Dorigoni S, Dalle Vedove F, et al. Effect of CPAP on blood pressure in patients with OSA/hypopnea: a systematic review and meta-analysis. *Chest*. 2014;145(4):762-771.
120. Montesi SB, Edwards BA, Malhotra A, Bakker JP. The effect of continuous positive airway pressure treatment on blood pressure: a systematic review and meta-analysis of randomized controlled trials. *J Clin Sleep Med*. 2012;8(5):587-596.
121. Bazzano LA, Khan Z, Reynolds K, He J. Effect of nocturnal nasal continuous positive airway pressure on blood pressure in obstructive sleep apnea. *Hypertension*. 2007;50(2):417-423.
122. Bratton DJ, Stradling JR, Barbé F, Kohler M. Effect of CPAP on blood pressure in patients with minimally symptomatic obstructive sleep apnoea: a meta-analysis using individual patient data from four randomised controlled trials. *Thorax*. 2014;69(12):1128-1135.
123. Liu L, Cao Q, Guo Z, Dai Q. Continuous positive airway pressure in patients with obstructive sleep apnea and resistant hypertension: a meta-analysis of randomized controlled trials. *J Clin Hypertens (Greenwich)*. 2016;18(2):153-158.
124. de Oliveira AC, Martinez D, Massierer D, et al. The antihypertensive effect of positive airway pressure on resistant hypertension of patients with obstructive sleep apnea: a randomized, double-blind, clinical trial. *Am J Respir Crit Care Med*. 2014;190(3):345-347.
125. Muxfeldt ES, Margallo V, Costa LM, et al. Effects of continuous positive airway pressure treatment on clinic and ambulatory blood pressures in patients with obstructive sleep apnea and resistant hypertension: a randomized controlled trial. *Hypertension*. 2015;65(4):736-742.
126. Pedrosa RP, Drager LF, de Paula LKG, et al. Effects of OSA treatment on BP in patients with resistant hypertension: a randomized trial. *Chest*. 2013;144(5):1487-1494.
127. Iftikhar IH, Valentine CW, Bittencourt LR, et al. Effects of continuous positive airway pressure on blood pressure in patients with resistant hypertension and obstructive sleep apnea: a meta-analysis. *J Hypertens*. 2014;32(12):2341-2350.
128. Kohler M, Stoewhas A-C, Ayers L, et al. Effects of continuous positive airway pressure therapy withdrawal in patients with obstructive sleep apnea: a randomized controlled trial. *Am J Respir Crit Care Med*. 2011; 184(10):1192-1199.
129. Thunström E, Manhem K, Rosengren A, Peker Y. Blood pressure response to losartan and continuous positive airway pressure in hypertension and obstructive sleep apnea. *Am J Respir Crit Care Med*. 2016;193(3):310-320.
130. Sánchez-de-la-Torre M, Khalyfa A, Sánchez-de-la-Torre A, et al. Precision medicine in patients with resistant hypertension and obstructive sleep apnea: blood pressure response to continuous positive airway pressure treatment. *J Am Coll Cardiol*. 2015;66:1023-1032.
131. Simonneau G, Montani D, Celermajer DS, et al. Haemodynamic definitions and updated clinical classification of pulmonary hypertension. *Eur Respir J*. 2019;53(1):1801913.
132. Laks L, Lehrhaft B, Grunstein RR, Sullivan CE. Pulmonary hypertension in obstructive sleep apnoea. *Eur Respir J*. 1995;8(4):537-541.
133. Weitzenblum E, Krieger J, Apprill M, et al. Daytime pulmonary hypertension in patients with obstructive sleep apnea syndrome. *Am Rev Respir Dis*. 1988;138(2):345-349.
134. Sajkov D, Cowie RJ, Thornton AT, Espinoza HA, McEvoy RD. Pulmonary hypertension and hypoxemia in obstructive sleep apnea syndrome. *Am J Respir Crit Care Med*. 1994;149(2 Pt 1):416-422.
135. Sajkov D, Wang T, Saunders NA, et al. Daytime pulmonary hemodynamics in patients with obstructive sleep apnea without lung disease. *Am J Respir Crit Care Med*. 1999;159:1518-1526.
136. Sajkov D, McEvoy RD. Obstructive sleep apnea and pulmonary hypertension. *Prog Cardiovasc Dis*. 2009;51(5):363-370.
137. Marrone O, Bonsignore MR, Romano S, Bonsignore G. Slow and fast changes in transmural pulmonary artery pressure in obstructive sleep apnoea. *Eur Respir J*. 1994;7(12):2192-2198.
138. Chaouat A, Weitzenblum E, Krieger J, Oswald M, Kessler R. Pulmonary hemodynamics in the obstructive sleep apnea syndrome. Results in 220 consecutive patients. *Chest*. 1996;109(2):380-386.
139. Bady E, Achkar A, Pascal S, Orvoen-Frija E, Laaban JP. Pulmonary arterial hypertension in patients with sleep apnoea syndrome. *Thorax*. 2000;55(11):934-939.
140. Sanner BM, Doberauer C, Konermann M, Sturm A, Zidek W. Pulmonary hypertension in patients with obstructive sleep apnea syndrome. *Arch Intern Med*. 1997;157(21):2483-2487.
141. Minai OA, Ricaurte B, Kaw R, et al. Frequency and impact of pulmonary hypertension in patients with obstructive sleep apnea syndrome. *Am J Cardiol*. 2009;104(9):1300-1306.
142. Rodriguez F, Martínez-García MA, Mohsenin V, Javaheri S. Systemic and pulmonary hypertension in OSA. In: Kryger MH, Goldstein C, Roth T, eds. *Principles and Practice of Sleep Medicine*. 7th ed. Elsevier; 2022;1440-1452.
143. Chaouat A, Weitzenblum E, Kessler R, et al. Five-year effects of nasal continuous positive airway pressure in obstructive sleep apnoea syndrome. *Eur Respir J*. 1997;10:2578-2582.
144. Sajkov D, Wang T, Saunders NA, et al. Continuous positive airway pressure treatment improves pulmonary hemodynamics in patients with obstructive sleep apnea. *Am J Respir Crit Care Med*. 2002;165:152-158.
145. Alchanatis M, Tourkohoriti G, Kakouros S, et al. Daytime pulmonary hypertension in patients with obstructive sleep apnea: the effect of continuous positive airway pressure on pulmonary hemodynamics. *Respiration*. 2001;68(6):566-572.
146. Arias MA, García-Río F, Alonso-Fernández A, et al. Pulmonary hypertension in obstructive sleep apnoea: effects of continuous positive airway pressure: a randomized, controlled cross-over study. *Eur Heart J*. 2006;27:1106-1113.
147. McLaughlin VV, Archer SL, Badesch DB, et al. ACCF/AHA 2009 expert consensus document on pulmonary hypertension—a report of the American College of Cardiology Foundation Task Force on Expert Consensus Documents and the American Heart Association developed in collaboration with the American College of Chest Physicians; American Thoracic Society, Inc.; and the Pulmonary Hypertension Association. *J Am Coll Cardiol*. 2009;53(17):1573-1619.
148. Dumitrascu R, Tiede H, Eckermann J, et al. Sleep apnea in precapillary pulmonary hypertension. *Sleep Med*. 2013;14(3):247-251.
149. Jilwan FN, Escourrou P, Garcia G, et al. High occurrence of hypoxemic sleep respiratory disorders in precapillary pulmonary hypertension and mechanisms. *Chest*. 2013;143(1):47-55.
150. Rafanan AL, Golish JA, Dinner DS, Hague LK, Arroliga AC. Nocturnal hypoxemia is common in primary pulmonary hypertension. *Chest*. 2001;120(3):894-899.
151. Zwillich C, Devlin T, White D, et al. Bradycardia during sleep apnea. Characteristics and mechanisms. *J Clin Invest*. 1982;69:1286-1292.
152. Bonsignore MR, Romano S, Marrone O, et al. Different heart rate patterns in obstructive sleep apnea during NREM sleep. *Sleep*. 1997;20:1167-1174.
153. Weiss JW, Remsburg S, Garpestad E, et al. Hemodynamic consequences of obstructive sleep apnea. *Sleep*. 1996;19:388-397.
154. Sato F, Nishimura M, Sinano H, et al. Heart rate during obstructive sleep apnea depends on individual hypoxic chemosensitivity of the carotid body. *Circulation*. 1997;96:274-281.
155. Leung RS. Sleep-disordered breathing: autonomic mechanisms and arrhythmias. *Prog Cardiovasc Dis*. 2009;51(4):324-338.
156. Lombardi C, Faini A, Mariani D, et al. Nocturnal arrhythmias and heart-rate swings in patients with obstructive sleep apnea syndrome treated with beta blockers. *J Am Heart Assoc*. 2020;9(21):e015926.
157. Khoo MC, Belozeroff V, Berry RB, Sassoon CSH. Cardiac autonomic control in obstructive sleep apnea: effects of long-term CPAP therapy. *Am J Respir Crit Care Med*. 2001;164:807-812.
158. Geovanini GR, Lorenzi-Filho G. Cardiac rhythm disorders in obstructive sleep apnea. *J Thorac Dis*. 2018;10(suppl 34):S4221-S4230.
159. Laczay B, Faulx MD. Obstructive sleep apnea and cardiac arrhythmias: a contemporary review. *J Clin Med*. 2021;10(17):3785.
160. Linz D, McEvoy RD, Cowie MR, et al. Associations of obstructive sleep apnea with atrial fibrillation and continuous positive airway pressure treatment: a review. *JAMA Cardiol*. 2018;3(6):532-540.

161. Riaz S, Bhatti H, Sampat PJ, Dhamoon A. The converging pathologies of obstructive sleep apnea and atrial arrhythmias. *Cureus*. 2020;12(7):e9388.
162. Guilleminault C, Connolly SJ, Winkle RA. Cardiac arrhythmia and conduction disturbances during sleep in 400 patients with sleep apnea syndrome. *Am J Cardiol*. 1983;52:490-494.
163. Tilkian AG, Guilleminault C, Schroeder JS, Lehrman KL, Simmons FB, Dement WC. Sleep-induced apnea syndrome. Prevalence of cardiac arrhythmias and their reversal after tracheostomy. *Am J Med*. 1977;63(3):348-358.
164. Harbison J, O'Reilly P, McNicholas WT. Cardiac rhythm disturbances in obstructive sleep apnea syndrome: effects of nasal continuous positive airway pressure therapy. *Chest*. 2000;118:591-595.
165. Mehra R, Stone KL, Varosy PD, et al. Nocturnal arrhythmias across a spectrum of obstructive and central sleep-disordered breathing in older men: outcomes of sleep disorders in older men (MrOS sleep) study. *Arch Intern Med*. 2009;169:1147-1155.
166. Monahan K, Storfer-Isser A, Mehra R, et al. Triggering of nocturnal arrhythmias by sleep-disordered breathing events. *J Am Coll Cardiol*. 2009;54:1797-1804.
167. Becker H, Brandenburg U, Peter JH, et al. Reversal of sinus arrest and atrioventricular conduction block in sleep apnea during nasal continuous positive airway pressure. *Am J Respir Crit Care Med*. 1995;151:215-218.
168. Koehler U, Fus E, Grimm W, et al. Heart block in patients with obstructive sleep apnoea: pathogenetic factors and effects of treatment. *Eur Respir J*. 1998;11(2):434-439.
169. Janssens W, Willems R, Pevernagie D, Buyse B. REM sleep-related brady-arrhythmia syndrome. *Sleep Breath*. 2007;11(3):195-199.
170. Biswas A, Berry RB, Sriram PS, Prasad A. A man with sleep-associated symptomatic bradycardia. *Ann Am Thorac Soc*. 2017;14(4):597-600.
171. Grimm W, Hoffmann J, Menz V, et al. Electrophysiologic evaluation of sinus node function and atrioventricular conduction in patients with prolonged ventricular asystole during obstructive sleep apnea. *Am J Cardiol*. 1996;77(15):1310-1314.
172. Shepard JW Jr, Garrison MW, Grither DA, et al. Relationship of ventricular ectopy to oxyhemoglobin desaturation in patients with obstructive sleep apnea. *Chest*. 1985;88:335-340.
173. Ryan CM, Usui K, Floras JS, Bradley TD. Effect of continuous positive airway pressure on ventricular ectopy in heart failure patients with obstructive sleep apnea. *Thorax*. 2005;60:781-785.
174. Craig S, Pepperell JC, Kohler M, Crosthwaite N, Davies RJ, Stradling JR. Continuous positive airway pressure treatment for obstructive sleep apnoea reduces resting heart rate but does not affect dysrhythmias: a randomised controlled trial. *J Sleep Res*. 2009;18(3):329-336.
175. Gerçek M, Gerçek M, Alzein K, et al. Impact of sleep-disordered breathing treatment on ventricular tachycardia in patients with heart failure. *J Clin Med*. 2022;11(15):4567.
176. Marinheiro R, Parreira L, Amador P, et al. Ventricular arrhythmias in patients with obstructive sleep apnea. *Curr Cardiol Rev*. 2019;15(1):64-74.
177. Ryan CM, Juvet S, Leung R, Bradley TD. Timing of nocturnal ventricular ectopy in heart failure patients with sleep apnea. *Chest*. 2008;133(4):934-940.
178. Koshino Y, Satoh M, Katayose Y, et al. Association of sleep-disordered breathing and ventricular arrhythmias in patients without heart failure. *Am J Cardiol*. 2008;101(6):882-886.
179. Gami AS, Hodge DO, Herges RM, et al. Obstructive sleep apnea, obesity, and the risk of incident atrial fibrillation. *J Am Coll Cardiol*. 2007;49:565-571.
180. Mehra R, Benjamin E, Shahar E, et al. Association of nocturnal arrhythmias with sleep-disordered breathing: The Sleep Heart Health Study. *Am J Crit Care Med*. 2006;173(8):910–916.
181. Tung P, Levitzky Y, Wang R, et al. Obstructive and Central Sleep Apnea and the Risk of Incident Atrial Fibrillation in a Community Cohort of Men and Women. *J Am Heart Assoc*. 2017;6(7):e004500.
182. Kanagala R, Murali NS, Friedman PA, et al. Obstructive sleep apnea and the recurrence of atrial fibrillation. *Circulation*. 2003;107:2589-2594.
183. Qureshi WT, Nasir UB, Alqalyoobi S, et al. Meta-analysis of continuous positive airway pressure as a therapy of atrial fibrillation in obstructive sleep apnea. *Am J Cardiol*. 2015;116(11):1767-1773.
184. Li L, Wang ZW, Li J, et al. Efficacy of catheter ablation of atrial fibrillation in patients with obstructive sleep apnoea with and without continuous positive airway pressure treatment: a meta-analysis of observational studies. *Europace*. 2014;16(9):1309-1314.
185. Calkins H, Kuck KH, Cappato R, et al. 2012 HRS/EHRA/ECAS expert consensus statement on catheter and surgical ablation of atrial fibrillation: recommendations for patient selection, procedural techniques, patient management and follow-up, definitions, endpoints, and research trial design: a report of the Heart Rhythm Society (HRS) Task Force on Catheter and Surgical Ablation of Atrial Fibrillation. *Heart Rhythm*. 2012;9:632-696.e21.
186. Hunt T-E, Traaen GM, Aakerøy L, et al. Effect of continuous positive airway pressure therapy on recurrence of atrial fibrillation after pulmonary vein isolation in patients with obstructive sleep apnea: a randomized controlled trial. *Heart Rhythm*. 2022;19(9):1433-1441.
187. Muller JE, Tofler GH, Stone PH. Circadian variation and triggers of onset of acute cardiovascular disease. *Circulation*. 1989;79(4):733-743.
188. Shahar E, Whitney CW, Redline S, et al. Sleep-disordered breathing and cardiovascular disease: cross-sectional results of the Sleep Heart Health Study. *Am J Respir Crit Care Med*. 2001;163:19-25.
189. Peker Y, Hender J, Kraiczi H, Loth S. Respiratory disturbance index: an independent predictor of mortality in coronary artery disease. *Am J Respir Crit Care Med*. 2000;162:81-86.
190. Gottlieb DJ, Yenokyan G, Newman AB, et al. Prospective study of obstructive sleep apnea and incident coronary heart disease and heart failure: the Sleep Heart Health Study. *Circulation*. 2010;122:352-360.
191. Kent BD, Grote L, Ryan S, et al. Diabetes mellitus prevalence and control in sleep-disordered breathing: the European Sleep Apnea Cohort (ESADA) study. *Chest*. 2014;146(4):982-990.
192. Shah NA, Yaggi HK, Concato J, Mohsenin V. Obstructive sleep apnea as a risk factor for coronary events or cardiovascular death. *Sleep Breath*. 2010;14:131-136.
193. Koo CY, Aung AT, Chen Z, et al. Sleep apnoea and cardiovascular outcomes after coronary artery bypass grafting. *Heart*. 2020;106(19):1495-1502.
194. Lee CH, Khoo SM, Chan MY, et al. Severe obstructive sleep apnea and outcomes following myocardial infarction. *J Clin Sleep Med*. 2011;7:616-621.
195. Xie J, Sert Kuniyoshi FH, Covassin N, et al. Nocturnal hypoxemia due to obstructive sleep apnea is an independent predictor of poor prognosis after myocardial infarction. *J Am Heart Assoc*. 2016;5(8):e003162.
196. Milleron O, Pillière R, Foucher A, et al. Benefits of obstructive sleep apnoea treatment in coronary artery disease: a long-term follow-up study. *Eur Heart J*. 2004;25:728-734.
197. Cassar A, Morgenthaler TI, Lennon RJ, et al. Treatment of obstructive sleep apnea is associated with decreased cardiac death after percutaneous coronary intervention. *J Am Coll Cardiol*. 2007;50:1310-1314.
198. Chen Y, Chen Y, Wen F, et al. Does continuous positive airway pressure therapy benefit patients with coronary artery disease and obstructive sleep apnea? A systematic review and meta-analysis. *Clin Cardiol*. 2021;44(8):1041-1049.
199. Peker Y, Thunström E, Glantz H, et al. Outcomes in coronary artery disease patients with sleepy obstructive sleep apnoea on CPAP. *Eur Respir J*. 2017;50(6):1700749.
200. Garcia-Rio F, Alonso-Fernandez A, Armada E, et al. CPAP effect on recurrent episodes in patients with sleep apnea and myocardial infarction. *Int J Cardiol*. 2013;168:1328-1335.
201. Mooe T, Franklin KA, Wiklund U, et al. Sleep-disordered breathing and myocardial ischemia in patients with coronary artery disease. *Chest*. 2000;117:1597-1602.
202. Franklin KA, Nilsson JB, Sahlin C, Naslund U. Sleep apnoea and nocturnal angina. *Lancet*. 1995;345(8957):1085-1087.
203. Randerath W, Bonsignore MR, Herkenrath S. Obstructive sleep apnoea in acute coronary syndrome. *Eur Respir Rev*. 2019;28(153):180114.
204. Mallet RT, Manukhina EB, Ruelas SS, et al. Cardioprotection by intermittent hypoxia conditioning: evidence, mechanisms, and therapeutic potential. *Am J Physiol Heart Circ. Physiol*. 2018;315(2):H216-H232.
205. Kreiger J, Sforza E, Barthelmebs M, et al. Overnight decrease in hematocrit after nasal CPAP in patients with OSA. *Chest*. 1990;97:729-730.
206. Lu F, Jiang T, Wang W, Hu S, Shi Y, Lin Y. Circulating fibrinogen levels are elevated in patients with obstructive sleep apnea: a systemic review and meta-analysis. *Sleep Med*. 2020;68:115-123.
207. Lin J, Hu S, Shi Y, Lu F, Luo W, Lin Y. Effects of continuous positive airway pressure on plasma fibrinogen levels in obstructive sleep apnea patients: a systemic review and meta-analysis. *Biosci Rep*. 2021;41(1):BSR20203856.
208. Hong SN, Yun HC, Yoo JH, Lee SH. Association between hypercoagulability and severe obstructive sleep apnea. *JAMA Otolaryngol Head Neck Surg*. 2017;143(10):996-1002.
209. Lavie L, Kraiczi H, Hefetz A, et al. Plasma vascular endothelial growth factor in sleep apnea syndrome: effects of nasal continuous positive air pressure treatment. *Am J Respir Crit Care Med*. 2002;165(12):1624-1628.

210. Qi JC, Zhang L, Li H, et al. Impact of continuous positive airway pressure on vascular endothelial growth factor in patients with obstructive sleep apnea: a meta-analysis. *Sleep Breath.* 2019;23(1):5-12.
211. Krieger AC, Anand R, Hernandez-Rosa E, et al. Increased platelet activation in sleep apnea subjects with intermittent hypoxemia. *Sleep Breath.* 2020;24(4):1537-1547.
212. Bokinsky G, Miller M, Ault K, Husband P, Mitchell J. Spontaneous platelet activation and aggregation during obstructive sleep apnea and its response to therapy with nasal continuous positive airway pressure. A preliminary investigation. *Chest.* 1995;108(3):625-630.
213. Dyugovskaya L, Lavie P, Lavie L. Increased adhesion molecules expression and production of reactive oxygen species in leukocytes of sleep apnea patients. *Am J Respir Crit Care Med.* 2002;165(7):934-939.
214. Nadeem R, Molnar J, Madbouly EM, et al. Serum inflammatory markers in obstructive sleep apnea: a meta-analysis. *J Clin Sleep Med.* 2013;9(10):1003-1012.
215. Ishida K, Kato M, Kato Y, et al. Appropriate use of nasal continuous positive airway pressure decreases elevated C reactive protein in patients with obstructive sleep apnea. *Chest.* 2009;136:125-129.
216. Fei Q, Tan Y, Yi M, Zhao W, Zhang Y. Associations between cardiometabolic phenotypes and levels of TNF-α, CRP, and interleukins in obstructive sleep apnea. *Sleep Breath.* 2023;27(3):1033-1042.
217. Ryan S, Taylor CT, McNicholas WT. Selective activation of inflammatory pathways by intermittent hypoxia in obstructive sleep apnea syndrome. *Circulation.* 2005;112:2660-2667.
218. Ryan S, Taylor CT, McNicholas WT. Predictors of elevated nuclear factor-κB-dependent genes in obstructive sleep apnea syndrome. *Am J Respir Crit Care Med.* 2006;174:824-830.
219. Bayram NA, Ciftci B, Keles T, et al. Endothelial function in normotensive men with obstructive sleep apnea before and 6 months after CPAP treatment. *Sleep.* 2009;32:1257-1263.
220. Kohler M, Ayers L, Pepperell JC, et al. Effects of continuous positive airway pressure on systemic inflammation in patients with moderate to severe obstructive sleep apnoea: a randomised controlled trial. *Thorax.* 2009;64:67-73.
221. Oldenburg O, Lamp B, Faber L, et al. Sleep-disordered breathing in patients with symptomatic heart failure: a contemporary study of prevalence in and characteristics of 700 patients. *Eur J Heart Fail.* 2007;9(3):251-257.
222. Leung RST, Bradley TD. Sleep apnea and cardiovascular disease. *Am J Respir Crit Care Med.* 2001;164:2147-2165.
223. Sin D, Fitzgerald F, Parker J. Risk factors for central and obstructive sleep apnea in 450 men and women with congestive heart failure. *Am J Respir Crit Care Med.* 1999;160:1101-1106.
224. Khattak HK, Hayat F, Pamboukian SV, et al. Obstructive sleep apnea in heart failure: review of prevalence, treatment with continuous positive airway pressure, and prognosis. *Tex Heart Inst J.* 2018;45(3):151-161.
225. Oldenburg O, Wellmann B, Buchholz A, et al. Nocturnal hypoxaemia is associated with increased mortality in stable heart failure patients. *Eur Heart J.* 2016;37(21):1695-1703.
226. Kaneko Y, Floras JS, Usui K, et al. Cardiovascular effects of continuous positive airway pressure in patients with heart failure and obstructive sleep apnea. *N Engl J Med.* 2003;348:1233-1241.
227. Mansfield DR, Gollogly NC, Kaye DM, et al. Controlled trial of continuous positive airway pressure in obstructive sleep apnea and heart failure. *Am J Respir Crit Care Med.* 2004;169(3):361-366.
228. Egea CJ, Aizpuru F, Pinto JA, et al. Cardiac function after CPAP therapy in patients with chronic heart failure and sleep apnea: a multicenter study. *Sleep Med.* 2008;9(6):660-666.
229. Bradley TD, Logan AG, Kimoff RJ, et al. Continuous positive airway pressure for central sleep apnea and heart failure. *N Engl J Med.* 2005;353(19):2025-2033.
230. Cowie MR, Woehrle H, Wegscheider K, et al. Adaptive servo-ventilation for central sleep apnea in systolic heart failure. *N Engl J Med.* 2015;373(12):1095-1105.
231. Bitter T, Westerheide N, Faber L, et al. Adaptive servoventilation in diastolic heart failure and Cheyne-Stokes respiration. *Eur Respir J.* 2010;36(2):385-392.
232. Turkington P, Bamfor J, Wanklyn P, et al. Prevalence and predictors of upper airway obstruction in the first 24 hours after acute stroke. *Stroke.* 2002;33:2037-2041.
233. Para O, Arboix A, Bechichi S, et al. Time course of sleep-related breathing disorders in first-ever stroke or transient ischemic attack. *Am J Respir Crit Care Med.* 2000;161:375-380.
234. Siccoli MM, Valko PO, Hermann DM, Bassetti CL. Central periodic breathing during sleep in 7 patients with acute ischemic stroke—neurogenic and cardiogenic factors. *J Neurol.* 2008;255:1687-1692.
235. Redline S, Yenokyan G, Gottlieb DJ, et al. Obstructive sleep apnea-hypopnea and incident stroke: the Sleep Heart Health study. *Am J Respir Crit Care Med.* 2010;182:269-277.
236. Sugita Y, Susami I, Yoshio T, et al. Marked episodic elevation of cerebral spinal fluid pressure during nocturnal sleep in patients with sleep apnea hypersomnia syndrome. *Electroencephalgr Clin Neurophysiol.* 1985;60:214-219.
237. Balfors EM. Impairment of cerebral perfusion during obstructive sleep apneas. *Am J Respir Crit Care Med.* 1994;150:1587-1591.
238. Good DC, Henkle JQ, Gelber D, et al. Sleep disordered breathing and poor functional outcome after stroke. *Stroke.* 1996;27:252-259.
239. Li M, Hou WS, Zhang XW, Tang ZY. Obstructive sleep apnea and risk of stroke: a meta-analysis of prospective studies. *Int J Cardiol.* 2014;172(2):466-469.
240. Martinez-Garcia MA, Soler-Cataluna JJ, Ejarque-Martinez L, et al. Continuous positive airway pressure treatment reduces mortality in patients with ischemic stroke and obstructive sleep apnea: a five-year follow-up. *Am J Respir Crit Care Med.* 2008;180:36-41.
241. Catalan-Serra P, Campos-Rodriguez F, Reyes-Nunez N, et al. Increased incidence of stroke, but not coronary heart disease in elderly patients with sleep apnea. *Stroke.* 2019;50:491-494.
242. Seiler A, Camilo M, Korostovtseva L, et al. Prevalence of sleep-disordered breathing after stroke and TIA: a meta-analysis. *Neurology.* 2019;92:e648-e654.
243. Lisabeth LD, Sanchez BN, Lim D, et al. Sleep-disordered breathing and poststroke outcomes. *Ann Neurol.* 2019;86:241-250.
244. McDermott M, Brown DL. Sleep apnea and stroke. *Curr Opin Neurol.* 2020;33(1):4-9.
245. Brill AK, Horvath T, Seiler A, et al. CPAP as treatment of sleep apnea after stroke: a meta-analysis of randomized trials. *Neurology.* 2018;90:e1222-e1230.
246. Bravata DM, Sico J, Vaz Fragoso CA, et al. Diagnosing and treating sleep apnea in patients with acute cerebrovascular disease. *J Am Heart Assoc.* 2018;7:e008841.
247. Koo BB, Bravata DM, Tobias LA, et al. Observational study of obstructive sleep apnea in wake-up stroke: the SLEEP TIGHT study. *Cerebrovasc Dis.* 2016;41(5-6):233-241.
248. Brown DL, Li C, Chervin RD, Case E, et al. Wake-up stroke is not associated with sleep-disordered breathing in women. *Neurol Clin Pract.* 2018;8:8-14.
249. Brown DL, Jiang X, Li C, et al. Sleep apnea screening is uncommon after stroke. *Sleep Med.* 2019;59:90-93.
250. Takala M, Puustinen J, Rauhala E, Holm A. Prescreening of sleep-disordered breathing after stroke: a systematic review. *Brain Behav.* 2018;8:e01146.
251. Kernan WN, Ovbiagele B, Black HR, et al. Guidelines for the prevention of stroke in patients with stroke and transient ischemic attack: a guideline for healthcare professionals from the American Heart Association/American Stroke Association. *Stroke.* 2014;45:2160-2236.
252. Pamidi S, Tasali E. Obstructive sleep apnea and type 2 diabetes: is there a link? *Front Neurol.* 2012;3:126.
253. Botros N, Concato J, Mohsenin V, et al. Obstructive sleep apnea as a risk factor for type 2 diabetes. *Am J Med.* 2009;122(12):1122-1127.
254. Appleton SL, Vakulin A, McEvoy RD, et al. Nocturnal hypoxemia and severe obstructive sleep apnea are associated with incident type 2 diabetes in a population cohort of men. *J Clin Sleep Med.* 2015;11(6):609-614.
255. Kendzerska T, Gershon AS, Hawker G, et al. Obstructive sleep apnea and incident diabetes. A historical cohort study. *Am J Respir Crit Care Med.* 2014;190:218-225.
256. Bakker JP, Weng J, Wang R, Redline S, Punjabi NM, Patel SR. Associations between obstructive sleep apnea, sleep duration, and abnormal fasting glucose. The multi-ethnic study of atherosclerosis. *Am J Respir Crit Care Med.* 2015;192(6):745-753.
257. Punjabi N, Beamer BA. Alterations in glucose disposal in sleep-disordered breathing. *Am J Respir Crit Care Med.* 2009;179:235-240.
258. Harsch IA, Schahin SP, Radespiel-Tröger M, et al. Continuous positive airway pressure treatment rapidly improves insulin sensitivity in patients with obstructive sleep apnea syndrome. *Am J Respir Crit Care Med.* 2004;169:156-162.
259. Babu AR, Herdegen J, Fogelfeld L, et al. Type 2 diabetes, glycemic control, and continuous positive airway pressure in obstructive sleep apnea. *Arch Intern Med.* 2005;165:447-452.

260. Lam JC, Lam B, Yao TJ, et al. A randomized controlled trial of nasal positive airway pressure on insulin sensitivity in obstructive sleep apnea. *Eur Respir J*. 2010;35:138-145.
261. West SD, Nicoll DJ, Wallace DM, et al. Effect of CPAP on insulin resistance and HbA1c in men with obstructive sleep apnea and type 2 diabetes. *Thorax*. 2007;62:969-974.
262. Pamidi S, Wroblewski K, Stepien M, et al. Eight hours of nightly continuous positive airway pressure treatment of obstructive sleep apnea improves glucose metabolism in patients with prediabetes. A randomized controlled trial. *Am J Respir Crit Care Med*. 2015;192:96-105.
263. Weinstock TG, Wang X, Rueschman M, et al. A controlled trial of CPAP therapy on metabolic control in individuals with impaired glucose tolerance and sleep apnea. *Sleep*. 2012;35:617-625B.
264. Salord N, Fortuna AM, Monasterio C, et al. A randomized controlled trial of continuous positive airway pressure on glucose tolerance in obese patients with obstructive sleep apnea. *Sleep*. 2016;39:35-41.
265. Pamidi S, Tasali E. Continuous positive airway pressure for improving glycemic control in type 2 diabetes: where do we stand? *Am J Respir Crit Care Med*. 2016;194:397-399.
266. Sheka AC, Adeyi O, Thompson J, et al. Nonalcoholic steatohepatitis: a review. *JAMA*. 2020;323(12):1175-1183. [Erratum in: *JAMA*. 2020;323(16):1619].
267. Mesarwi OA, Loomba R, Malhotra A. Obstructive sleep apnea, hypoxia, and nonalcoholic fatty liver disease. *Am J Respir Crit Care Med*. 2019;199(7):830-841.
268. Corey KE, Misdraji J, Gelrud L, et al. Obstructive sleep apnea is associated with nonalcoholic steatohepatitis and advanced liver histology. *Dig Dis Sci*. 2015;60(8):2523-2528.
269. Kim D, Ahmed A, Kushida C. Continuous positive airway pressure therapy on nonalcoholic fatty liver disease in patients with obstructive sleep apnea. *J Clin Sleep Med*. 2018;14(8):1315-1322.
270. Ng SSS, Wong VWS, Wong GLH, et al. Continuous positive airway pressure does not improve nonalcoholic fatty liver disease in patients with obstructive sleep apnea. A randomized clinical trial. *Am J Respir Crit Care Med*. 2021;203(4):493-501.
271. Cho JW, Duffy JF. Sleep, sleep disorders, and sexual dysfunction. *World J Mens Health*. 2019;37(3):261-275.
272. Jankowski JT, Seftel AD, Strohl KP. Erectile dysfunction and sleep related disorders. *J Urol*. 2008;179:837-841.
273. Gonçalves MA, Guilleminault C, Ramos E, et al. Erectile dysfunction, obstructive sleep apnea syndrome and nasal CPAP treatment. *Sleep Med*. 2005;6:333-339.
274. Schulz R, Bischof F, Galetke W, et al. CPAP therapy improves erectile function in patients with severe obstructive sleep apnea. *Sleep Med*. 2019;53:189-194.
275. Budweiser S, Luigart R, Jörres RA, et al. Long-term changes of sexual function in men with obstructive sleep apnea after initiation of continuous positive airway pressure. *J Sex Med*. 2013;10(2):524-531.
276. Hajduk IA, Strollo PJ, Jasani RR, et al. Prevalence and predictors of nocturia in obstructive sleep apnea hypopnea syndrome—a retrospective study. *Sleep*. 2003;26:61-64.
277. Krieger J, Imbs JL, Schmidt M, Kurtz D. Renal function in patients with obstructive sleep apnea. Effects of nasal continuous positive airway pressure. *Arch Intern Med*. 1988;148:1337-1340.
278. Krieger J, Schmidt M, Sforza E, et al. Urinary excretion of guanosine 3′:5′-cyclic monophosphate during sleep in obstructive sleep apnea patients with and without nasal continuous positive airway pressure. *Clin Sci (Lond)*. 1989;76:31-37.
279. Umlauf MG, Chasens ER, Greevy RA, et al. Obstructive sleep apnea, nocturia and polyuria in older adults. *Sleep*. 2004;27:139-144.
280. Fitzgerald MP, Mulligan M, Parthasarathy S. Nocturic frequency is related to severity of obstructive sleep apnea, improves with continuous positive airways treatment. *Am J Obstet Gynecol*. 2006;194: 1399-1403.
281. Parthasarathy S, Fitzgerald M, Goodwin JL, Unruh M, Guerra S, Quan SF. Nocturia, sleep-disordered breathing, and cardiovascular morbidity in a community-based cohort. *PloS One*. 2012;7(2):e30969.
282. Zhou J, Xia S, Li T, Liu R. Association between obstructive sleep apnea syndrome and nocturia: a meta-analysis. *Sleep Breath*. 2020; 24(4):1293-1298.
283. Miyauchi Y, Okazoe H, Okujyo M, et al. Effect of the continuous positive airway pressure on the nocturnal urine volume or night-time frequency in patients with obstructive sleep apnea syndrome. *Urology*. 2015;85(2):333-336.
284. Endeshaw YW, Johnson TM, Kutner MH, et al. Sleep-disordered breathing and nocturia in older adults. *J Am Geriatr Soc*. 2004;52(6): 957-960.

Chapter 21

Obstructive Sleep Apnea and Obesity Hypoventilation Syndrome Treatment Overview

INTRODUCTION

This chapter will present an overview of treatment options for obstructive sleep apnea (OSA) and the obesity hypoventilation syndrome (OHS) in adults. Treatment of OSA in children is discussed in Chapter 27. Various treatments are discussed in more detail in other chapters, and only a general overview will be presented here.

TREATMENT OF OBSTRUCTIVE SLEEP APNEA

Decision to Treat Obstructive Sleep Apnea

There are several considerations affecting the decision to treat a patient with OSA as well as the selection of the type of treatment (Figure 21–1). The first to be considered includes the severity of OSA as based on the apnea-hypopnea index (AHI), the severity of arterial oxygen desaturation, and the association of significant arrhythmias with obstructive events.[1,2] The AHI is an imperfect metric and may not capture the effect of sleep apnea in many cases.[3-5] The diagnostic AHI may not reflect typical AHI severity due to poor sleep or decreased supine or rapid eye movement (REM) sleep during the diagnostic study. The diagnostic AHI and degree of oxygen desaturation from the diagnostic portion of a split sleep study are often based on a limited amount of supine or REM sleep. Due to night-to-night variability, the severity on one night may not represent the typical findings.[6,7] Home sleep apnea testing (HSAT) may underestimate the AHI if the actual total sleep time is much less than the monitoring time. These factors should be considered before classifying a patient with a 20-inch neck as having "mild" OSA. In the past, there has been no standardized method to assess the severity of arterial oxygen desaturation. Azarbarzin et al found that the "hypoxic burden," determined by measuring the area between the pre-event baseline and the saturation curve associated with respiratory events,[8] was predictive of mortality related to cardiovascular disease, while the AHI was not predictive. There is also evidence that the REM AHI may have a better association with cardiovascular disorders than the non-REM (NREM) AHI.[9,10]

The second consideration is the presence or absence of symptoms. In fact, the presence of symptoms *believed to be due to untreated sleep apnea* may be the most convincing reason to treat patients until future randomized controlled trials (RCTs) document the benefit of treatment of OSA on cardiovascular morbidity and mortality.[11,12] Excessive daytime sleepiness, non-restorative sleep, nocturia, morning headache, and impaired quality of life (vitality) often improve with adequate treatment, even in patients with mild OSA.[13] Symptomatic OSA should usually be treated, but the choice of treatment may vary. Symptoms often do not correlate with the AHI, and the dictum "treat the patient, not the AHI" should be considered. In some patients with comorbid depression or insomnia,[14] it may be difficult to determine the degree to which untreated OSA is responsible for the patient's symptoms. Symptoms may not improve until both the comorbid conditions and OSA are addressed.[14] Cognitive behavioral treatment of insomnia before CPAP treatment may improve CPAP adherence.[15] This issue is discussed in more detail in a separate section of this chapter.

The third consideration is the effect of OSA on the sleep of the patient's bed partner and marital satisfaction. Loud snoring and apnea may cause marital discord and impair the sleep of the patient's bed partner.[16] Significant others may leave the bedroom to ensure restorative sleep. A caveat is that

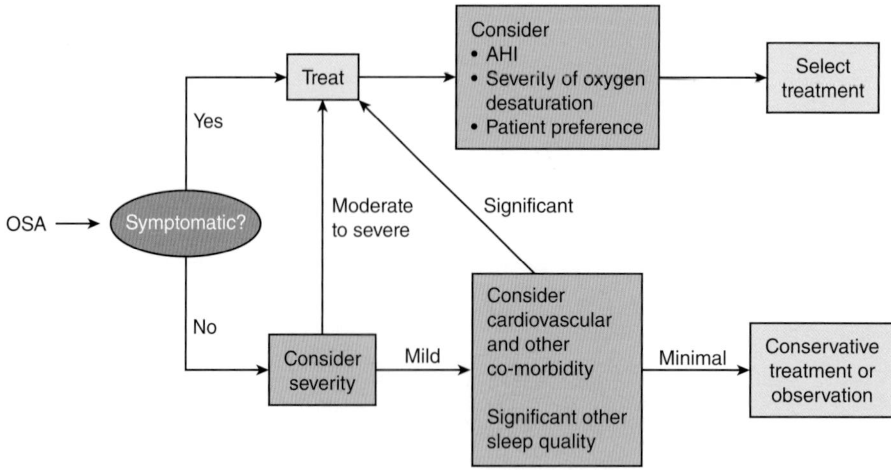

Figure 21–1 Schematic Approach for Decision to Treat or Not Treat Obstructive Sleep Apnea. *AHI,* apnea-hypopnea index.

some bed partners may not like CPAP or other treatments. The fourth consideration is the potential increased risk of death or adverse cardiovascular morbidity from untreated OSA. The evidence for increased risk is *strongest for severe OSA* (AHI >30 events/hour) and in men who are 40 to 70 years of age.[17,18] The evidence is less clear for mild-to-moderate OSA and for women. However, the presence of certain comorbid conditions such as coronary artery disease, cerebrovascular disease, arrhythmias, or congestive heart failure may increase the mortality risk, even from untreated milder degrees of sleep apnea. Given that positive airway pressure (PAP) treatment is a safe and noninvasive treatment, many clinicians feel that even asymptomatic patients with moderate-to-severe OSA and comorbid cardiovascular issues should be treated, with the goal of improving cardiovascular outcomes (morbidity and mortality). Observational studies have documented improvements in mortality and composite cardiovascular outcomes (major adverse cardiovascular or cerebrovascular events, MACCEs) with CPAP treatment.[19,20] However, RCTs have not documented that PAP treatment improves cardiovascular outcomes except in patients with resistant hypertension.[11,12] While the negative RCT results could be due to exclusion of sleepy patients and poor PAP adherence, many clinicians now question if it is good medical practice to convince asymptomatic patients to undergo treatment solely for the unproven potential benefit with respect to cardiovascular mortality and morbidity.[11] Proponents of PAP treatment contend that 4 hours of PAP use a night, which is typical adherence in most of the RCTs, is insufficient for cardiovascular benefit. There is evidence that the REM AHI may be more predictive of the effect of OSA on disorders such as hypertension.[10] If PAP is not used during the final hours of the night when the majority of REM sleep occurs, this may reduce the effect of treatment. Some studies suggest that sleepy patients receive the most cardiovascular benefit from PAP treatment, but they were excluded from the RCTs for safety considerations.[12] However, at least in treatment-adherent patients, there is evidence from secondary analysis of RCTs that a benefit from CPAP may be present (especially for cerebrovascular events)[20] (see Chapter 20). In any case, many physicians still offer treatment to patients with moderate-to-severe OSA in the absence of symptoms, especially if significant comorbid cardiovascular disease is present.[19,20] In summary, the most convincing evidence for OSA treatment involves improvement in symptoms, including measures of daytime sleepiness and quality of life. Patient motivation is an important determinant of the success of any treatment. Patient education about the potential benefits of treatment is essential. It is also important for the patient to have realistic expectations. CPAP treatment might be expected to have a more dramatic and rapid benefit when symptoms and the AHI are severe. However, it can take time for adaptation to CPAP and finding the optimal mask and treatment pressure.

When reviewing the evidence of the utility of various treatments, the concepts of efficacy and effectiveness should be considered. *Efficacy* is defined as the ability of treatment to reduce the AHI or improve oxygenation. *Effectiveness* considers the impact of a given treatment on the actual nightly AHI and oxygenation. If CPAP reduces the AHI from 40 to 4 events/hour but CPAP is used on average for only 50% of the night, the average AHI is 22 events/hour. This is equivalent to the effect of an oral appliance (OA) that reduces the AHI from 40 to 20 events/hour but is used for 90% of the night ($20 \times 0.9 + 40 \times 0.1$). Some have recommended use of the *mean disease alleviation*[21] metric, [(% reduction in baseline AHI on treatment) × (% of night treatment used)] to compare treatment effectiveness (Figure 21–2). The % reduction in the baseline AHI on treatment = {[(baseline AHI − treatment AHI) × 100] / baseline AHI}. For example, crossover studies comparing CPAP and an OA have shown similar improvement in daytime sleepiness and quality of life measures, although CPAP was more effective at reducing the AHI.[22] This finding may be explained by greater adherence with the OA (by patient report). New technology may allow objective adherence monitoring during OA treatment.[21] Of note, use of the mean disease alleviation metric assumes that use of CPAP for 4 hours has no effect on OSA during the second part of the night. This assumption may not be correct, as some patients may experience a "carryover effect." In addition, there is evidence that many patients do benefit from even 4 hours of use. More investigations are needed concerning this topic. Adherence is not an issue for surgical treatment of sleep apnea. A meta-analysis of surgery for OSA found evidence of improved outcomes such as daytime sleepiness, although the AHI was often not reduced to <10 events/hour.[23]

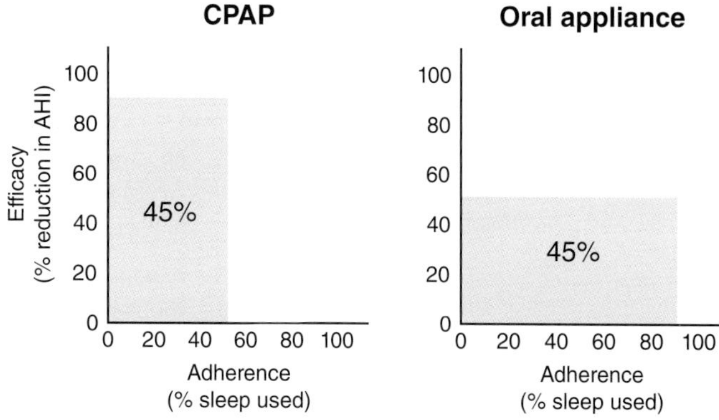

Figure 21–2 Examples of Mean Disease Alleviation Plots. The y axis shows efficacy (% reduction in apnea-hypopnea index [AHI]); the x axis shows adherence (% of sleep treatment is used). On left is an example of good continuous positive airway pressure (CPAP) efficacy but poor adherence. On the right is an oral appliance with fair efficacy but excellent adherence. Here, the areas (mean disease alleviation scores) are the same. Both efficacy and adherence determine the effectiveness of a treatment.

Choosing Treatment

The choice of treatment is based on the severity of OSA and patient characteristics and preferences (Table 21–1). Correction of insufficient sleep is an important intervention for all severities of OSA. For most levels of OSA severity, noninvasive treatments are given priority, although individual patients may prefer surgical options. Separate chapters address medical therapy (weight loss, positional treatment, upper-airway muscle training, and alerting agents for residual sleepiness) (Chapter 22), PAP treatment (Chapter 23 & Chapter 24), surgical treatment including hypoglossal nerve stimulation (Chapter 26), and OA treatment (Chapter 25). Practice parameters or clinical practice guidelines have been published on the use of medical therapy,[24] PAP,[25,26] OAs,[27,28] and upper-airway surgery.[29,30] Guidelines for the use of polysomnography (PSG) and HSAT to monitoring treatment efficacy have also been published.[31] A summary of the

Table 21–1 Treatment of Obstructive Sleep Apnea by Severity

	Snoring	Mild OSA	Moderate OSA	Severe OSA
AHI	AHI <5 events/hr	5 to <15 events/hr	15 to 30 events/hr	>30 events/hr
Primary	• Observation • Treat nasal congestion • Avoid supine sleep	• Observation (if asymptomatic) • Avoid supine sleep position* • Oral appliance or • PAP (if symptomatic and motivated)	• PAP	• PAP
Secondary	• Oral appliance or • Upper airway surgery[(A)] • Upper airway muscle training***	• Upper airway surgery[(B)] • Upper airway muscle training***	• Oral appliance or • Upper airway surgery[(B)] or • Avoid supine sleep position*	• Upper airway surgery[(C)] or • Oral appliance
Adjunctive	• Weight loss	• Weight loss	• Weight loss • Avoid supine sleep position*	• Weight loss • Avoid supine sleep position*

*Positional OSA present. *FDA*, Federal Drug Administration.
[(A)]Upper airway surgery: Palatal implants, Uvulopalatopharyngoplasty (UPPP), laser assisted uvuloplasty. However, insurance usually does not pay for surgery for snoring.
[(B)]Upper airway surgery: Modified UPPP ± GAHM, modified UPPP + tongue base procedure, or hypoglossal nerve stimulation (surgical implantation and stimulation).
[(C)]Upper airway surgery: Maxillomandibular advancement (MMA), hypoglossal nerve stimulation.
***Daytime neurostimulation device (ExciteOSA) is FDA cleared for snoring and mild OSA, but limited data are available.
AHI, apnea-hypopnea index; *OSA*, obstructive sleep apnea; *PAP*, positive airway pressure; *GAHM*, genioglossus advancement and hyoid myotomy.

recommendations for use of PSG and HSAT to follow or reassess patients on treatment include:

- PSG or HSAT **is NOT recommended** for routine reassessment of asymptomatic patients with OSA on PAP therapy.
- PSG or HSAT can be used to reassess patients with recurrent or persistent symptoms despite good PAP adherence. For patients on CPAP, the PSG is on CPAP treatment (with adjustment of the level of CPAP if indicated). HSAT is rarely used in this setting as this would require an adaptation to monitor airflow on CPAP.
- PSG or HSAT **may be used** if clinically significant weight gain/loss has occurred since diagnosis of OSA or the start of treatment.
- PSG or HSAT may be used in patients being treated for OSA who develop or have a change in cardiovascular disease.
- PSG or HSAT is **recommended** to assess response to treatment with non-PAP interventions. This recommendation includes studies at treatment initiation to document efficacy or while a patient is on chronic treatment if symptoms return.

Overview of Major Treatment Options

Weight Loss. Even loss of 10% to 15% of body weight can improve the AHI. Weight loss is included as an adjunctive treatment in every OSA severity category in Table 21–1; as weight loss requires time, the benefit varies among individuals, and weight-loss maintenance is an issue. Both a structured diet with heathy lifestyle interventions and bariatric surgery can result in significant weight loss, although surgery is associated with a greater change in weight. More effective medication treatments for weight loss are now available but weight gain usually occurs when medications are stopped. In patients with severe obesity, bariatric surgery is effective for weight loss and usually improves the AHI considerably.[32,33] However, residual sleep apnea is present in the majority of patients after weight loss. In one prospective study, the prevalence of OSA decreased from 71% at baseline to 44% at 12 months after surgery. OSA was cured in 45% and cured or improved in 78% of the patients, but moderate or severe OSA persisted in 20% of the patients after the operation.[34] Of note, the baseline AHI was 29.8 events/hour in this study. Other studies have found lower cure rates. For example, a study of very severe OSA (51 events/hour) found only 4% of patients were cured. However, the required CPAP was reduced after weight loss. The best predictor of the posttreatment AHI was the pretreatment AHI.[35] Patient reports of improvement in symptoms ("I don't need CPAP anymore") are often not consistent with objective findings. PSG or HSAT is needed after weight stabilizes to determine if treatment beyond weight loss is needed.[31]

Positive Airway Pressure. CPAP and the variations autoCPAP and bilevel PAP (BPAP) are the treatments of choice for moderate-to-severe OSA, as they are safe and reliably reduce the AHI, typically to 5 events or less/hour.[26] The American Academy of Sleep Medicine (AASM) clinical guidelines for PAP treatment[26] recommend use of PAP to treat adults with excessive sleepiness (strong), impaired quality of life (conditional), and comorbid hypertension (conditional). Note that no recommendation was given concerning treatment of adults with cardiovascular comorbidity. While the short-term adherence to CPAP among patients in one big data study[36] was 75%, long-term adherence is around 50% in many studies. Pretreatment daytime sleepiness and improvement of sleepiness with PAP treatment are predictors of good adherence, but the type of PAP device or pressure level does not affect adherence.[37] Some studies suggest that adherence can be improved with objective adherence monitoring via telemonitoring/telemedicine,[38] rapid interventions, and improved patient engagement using smartphone applications.[39]

Emerging Airway Pressure Treatments. There are a number of new positive or negative airway pressure treatments available as an alternative to CPAP (Figure 21–3). Nasal expiratory PAP has been used to treat sleep apnea. The original device (Provent) was a single-use, disposable item held in place in the nostrils by adhesive that is no longer manufactured.[40] Two newer devices are being sold. The Bongo (AirAvant)[41,42] is a treatment cleared by the U.S. Food and Drug Administration (FDA) for mild-to-moderate OSA consisting of reusable valves that fit in the nostrils. The valves for the two nostrils are attached by a soft connection, and the part inserted into the nostrils expands, holding the device in place. Inhalation is not obstructed, but exhalation through the valves provides back pressure. The ULTepap (BRxYGGS Medical)[42] is another FDA-cleared device for treatment of mild-to-moderate OSA consisting of two nasal pillow-like structures held in place by a head strap. The device is reusable, and exhalation induces back pressure caused by narrowing of the passage by a flexible, thin-walled shell that extends into the air passage (Rashidi-Sleeper valve) during exhalation. An oral negative pressure device, the iNAP (Somnics),[43] is cleared by the FDA for treatment of all severities of OSA. The device consists of a soft oral interface fitting over the tongue and a suction device with a saliva trap. The induced negative pressure sucks the palate and tongue forward (Figure 21–3C), permitting unobstructed nasal breathing. All of these devices require a physician's prescription but are not currently reimbursed by most insurance plans.

Positional Treatment. Patients with exclusive positional OSA (ePOSA), defined as an AHI supine greater than two times the AHI non-supine **and** an AHI non-supine less than 5 to 10 events/hour, may potentially be treated by avoidance of the supine position.[44] Traditional positioning devices prevent sleep in the supine position by using cushions or a "tennis ball" in a pocket on the back of a shirt. These devices can be effective but are uncomfortable, and adherence is low. New smaller smart devices that monitor patient position and vibrate until the patient moves from the supine position are now available. The devices also track adherence and efficacy at preventing supine sleep, and this data is available to both the patient and physician. Two smart devices (NightBalance [NB],[45] NightShift[46]) and one cushion device (Zzoma)[47] are approved by the FDA for treatment of sleep apnea and require a physician's prescription (Chapter 22). Recently the Centers for Medicare and Medicaid Services (CMS) announced that electronic positioning devices for treatment of sleep apnea will be covered. The total reimbursement over 13 months is about $334 (this could change over time). The Healthcare Common Procedure Coding System (HCPCS) code is 0530 (Electronic positional obstructive sleep apnea treatment). Unfortunately Philips Respironics will no longer sell the NB device. However, the NB will be discussed here and in Chapter 22 as it is a model for future devices. The NightShift - LE device by Advanced Brain Monitoring is still available for about $500 at the time of writing and has

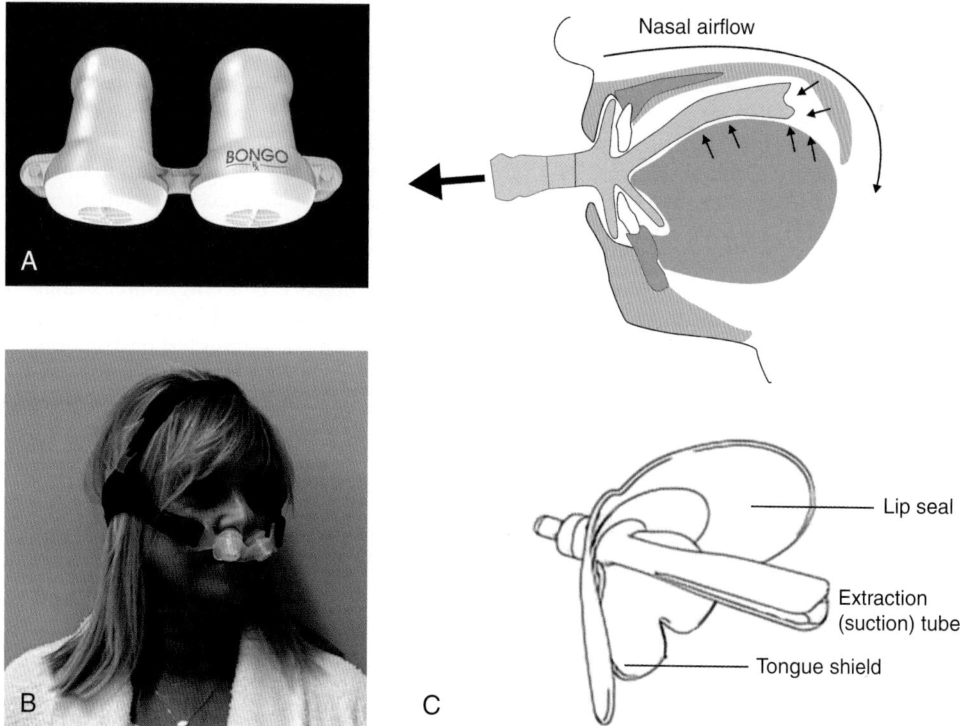

Figure 21–3 **Three Emerging Treatment Options for Obstructive Sleep Apnea.** **(A)** The Bongo (AirAvant) is a reusable nasal pillows device with valves providing expiratory positive airway pressure (EPAP). The pillows expand when placed in the nostrils stabilizing the device (an optional head strap is available). **(B)** The ULTepap is a reusable nasal pillows device providing EPAP and held in place by head straps. **(C)** The iNAP (Somnics) provides suction pressure to the palate and tongue, allowing unobstructed nasal breathing. ([A] From AirAvant.com [B] BRYGGS Medical, Avon, Ohio. [C] From https://www.inapsleep.online/user-guide/.)

many of the same features as the NB. A randomized crossover trial of the NB (vibrates in the supine position) versus autoCPAP in treatment-naïve patients with ePOSA found a higher AHI with the NB than with autoCPAP (7.3 events/hour vs. 3.7 events/hour), but also higher nightly adherence with NB (345 minutes vs. 287 minutes).[45] At the end of the study, about 50% preferred positional treatment. One study of position-device adherence at 1 year after starting treatment found 9 of 58 patients had stopped using the device.[48] More studies of the long-term adherence and efficacy of positioning devices are needed. Use of a positioning device that is capable of objective use monitoring is needed to ensure long-term adherence. Given the CMS decision to cover electronic positioning devices for treatment of OSA, hopefully this will stimulate the development of more electronic positioning devices.

Oral Appliances. Treatment with OA devices is recommended for mild-to-moderate OSA and can work in patients with severe OSA.[27,28,49] The 2015 AASM clinical guidelines[28] state, "We recommend that sleep physicians consider prescription of OAs, rather than no treatment, for adult patients with obstructive sleep apnea who are intolerant of CPAP therapy or prefer alternate therapy (Standard)." The 2006 AASM practice parameters for use of OAs for treatment of adult OSA state, "Although not as efficacious as CPAP, OAs are indicated for use in patients with mild to moderate OSA who prefer OAs to CPAP, or who do not respond to CPAP, are not appropriate candidates for CPAP, or who fail treatment attempts with CPAP or treatment with behavioral measures such as weight loss or sleep position change (Guideline)." The 2006 publication and the 2015 updated guidelines for OA treatment of OSA[28] recommended follow-up sleep testing while patients wear the OA (after final adjustment). This recommendation to document efficacy applies to patients with OSA of all severities. The 2019 AASM practice parameters for surgical treatment of OSA state, "Those with moderate OSA should initially be offered either PAP therapy or OAs rather than surgery." The OA devices can lower the AHI by 50% to less than 10 events/hour in about 50% of patients (Table 21–2).[49] However, a higher proportion have improvement in symptoms. The patient must have adequate dentition for a mandibular advancing device (eight teeth per dental arch), but more teeth are optimal for good retention. As of now, it is not possible to predict who will respond, but patients with all severities of OSA can see a significant improvement. Additional description of patient characteristics associated with a good response to OA treatment is included in the section on clusters, endotypes, and phenotypes as the end of this chapter and in chapter 25. One issue is that the custom devices (impressions of the upper and lower arches are obtained), while more comfortable and effective, can be expensive, with variable insurance coverage. However, lower-priced "semi-custom" devices with adjustable protrusion are now available. In the past, adjustment (the amount of protrusion) relied on patient report (improved snoring); the use of monitoring at home has increasingly been used for OA adjustment. Another option would be an OA titration PSG, which is possible with some devices. PSG or HSAT after optimal OA adjustment should document efficacy. As previously noted, some studies comparing CPAP treatment to OA treatment found that OAs reduced the AHI less reliably, but they often reported adherence was better than with CPAP. In addition, improvements in daytime sleepiness or quality of life did not differ from those of individuals receiving CPAP treatment.[22] New methods for monitoring objective adherence during OA treatment using heat sensors are available.[21] In the future, objective adherence monitoring may be more widely available. As with CPAP, long-term OA adherence tends to decrease with time. OA treatment can move teeth, but sometimes occlusion is improved. Long-term follow-up with both a sleep physician to ensure OSA is adequately treated (treatment efficacy and adherence) and the dentist who constructed the device is indicated. Dental follow-up is needed to ensure the OA is in good repair and to monitor for dental side effects.[27,28] More information about OA treatment is provided in Chapter 25.

Surgery. A wide variety of surgical techniques are available, including newer non-ablative palate procedures, genioglossus advancement with or without hypoid suspension, tongue-base procedures, and maxillomandibular advancement (MMA). Chapter 26 describes patient selection for the different procedures. Depending on the definition of success, around 50% of patients with palate procedures, a higher percentage with multilevel procedures, and 80%–90% with MMA are effectively treated. While the AHI is not as effectively reduced as with CPAP, adherence is a non-issue. A meta-analysis by Kent et al.[23] demonstrated that surgery, as an initial treatment for adults with major anatomical obstruction, results in a clinically significant reduction in the AHI/respiratory disturbance index (RDI), sleepiness, snoring, blood pressure, and oxygen desaturation index; and an increase in the lowest arterial oxygen

Table 21–2 Example of the Efficacy of an Oral Appliance

Outcome	Criteria	All OSA	Mild	Moderate	Severe
Complete response	AHI <5 events/hr	36.5%	52.2%	38.3%	23.6%
Near complete response	AHI <10 events/hr and ≥50% reduction in AHI	52.2%	52.2%	59.6%	42.1%
Partial response	≥50% reduction in AHI	63.8%	52.2%	64.8%	70%

These data show OA efficacy variation with regard to a sample of 425 patients with OSA treated with a two-piece customized device set to the maximum comfortable protrusive limit. These data represent an individual-level analysis of research participants in studies from a single research center. No upper limits for AHI or body mass index (BMI) were set as entry criteria for the studies. Proportions of responders are shown for three commonly used definitions based on changes in AHI.
AHI, apnoea-hypopnea index; *OA*; oral appliances; *OSA*, obstructive sleep apnoea.
Data from Sutherland K, Takaya H, Qian J, Petocz P, Ng AT, Cistulli PA. Oral Appliance Treatment Response and Polysomnographic Phenotypes of Obstructive Sleep Apnea. *J Clin Sleep Med.* 2015;11(8):861-868.

saturation. Upper airway surgery can be effective in mild OSA, but proper patient selection is essential. In one study of uvulopalatopharyngoplasty (UPPP) in unselected patients with mild OSA, only 40% saw a reduction in AHI by 50% or more.[50] Hypoglossal nerve stimulation (HNS) is an option for patients with moderate-to-severe OSA (AHI of 15 to 100 events/hour, FDA indication) who do not tolerate or accept PAP treatment.[51] Some insurance providers use an upper AHI limit of ≤ 65 events/hour. In the past, a weight limit (body mass index [BMI] ≤32 kg/m^2) was required; currently, some insurance providers use a BMI limit of ≤40 kg/m^2. The qualifications for HNS often change, the most current guidelines should be reviewed. Drug-induced sleep endoscopy (DISE) is performed presurgery, and the pattern of circumferential collapse is considered a contraindication to the procedure. While patient adherence and satisfaction are good, up to a third of patients experience some residual OSA.[51,52] In the ADHERE study, at post-titration (after stimulation voltage optimization), an AHI of ≤5 events/hour, ≤10 events/hour, or ≤15 events/hour was achieved in 53%, 79%, and 94% of patients, respectively.[52] A study of endotypes found a high arousal threshold was associated with a better response.[53] In some cases, an adequate result can be obtained with avoidance of the supine position (combination treatment). If the AHI response is not adequate or the required voltage is not comfortable, using a different electrode configuration or adjusting the stimulation characteristics may improve efficacy and tolerance.[54]

Muscle Training. Muscle training alternatives include inspiratory muscle training (IMT), orofacial myofunctional therapy (OMT), and daytime neurostimulation. IMT using 75% of maximal inspiratory pressure effectively reduced the AHI in one study.[55] OMT is a treatment consisting of isotonic and isometric exercises that target oral (lip, tongue) and oropharyngeal (soft palate, lateral pharyngeal wall) structures. An RTC assigned patients to 3 months of daily (30 minutes) sham therapy or oropharyngeal exercises for the tongue, soft palate, and lateral pharyngeal wall.[56] A reduction in the AHI was noted. However, another study of a customized tongue-training device was unable to show a benefit.[57] A neurostimulation device (ExciteOSA, Signifier Medical)[58] for training the tongue to improve endurance is cleared by the FDA for the treatment of snoring and mild OSA. Training is performed daily for 20 minutes and consists of electrical stimulation of varying frequencies and voltage amplitudes to improve genioglossus muscle endurance. A smartphone application follows adherence and allows the patient to adjust voltage levels with the goal of progressive increases. While promising, more studies are needed to determine long-term effectiveness. The device is not usually covered by insurance and is relatively expensive (approximately $1700 USD at the time of writing). In summary, muscle training may prove effective for snoring and mild OSA in some patients. This type of treatment requires motivation and long-term commitment to continue exercises. A smartphone application to monitor adherence and provide feedback is ideal and likely essential for success.

Oxygen. Currently, insurance providers do not provide coverage (reimbursement) for oxygen as a treatment for OSA. The only exception is when a titration demonstrates persistent desaturation when the AHI has been normalized. Use of oxygen in OSA treatment is discussed in Chapter 22. The combination of supplemental oxygen and CPAP is often needed in patients with OSA and significant lung disease.

Choosing Treatment Based on Severity

For mild asymptomatic OSA extension of sleep duration (in mild OSA sleepy patients tend to have a shorter nightly sleep duration than non-sleepy patients), an OA, positional therapy (if positional OSA is present), or upper-airway surgery can be effective. An OA is preferred over surgery, as it avoids an invasive procedure. Non-ablative palatal surgery (modified UPPP and others) results in less morbidity than traditional UPPP and would be effective in patients with obstruction mainly at the palatal areas. PAP can also be effective if acceptable to the patient with mild OSA[13]. Many patients with mild OSA will decline surgery, and the lack of reimbursement for the cost of OAs by insurance providers or poor dentition may render this option unacceptable for many patients (although more lower cost adjustable OA devices are now available). Therefore, CPAP is ultimately tried for treatment of mild OSA and can be quite effective in symptomatic, motivated patients.[13]

For moderate OSA, PAP is the treatment of choice; OAs and upper airway surgery are secondary treatments. Both can be effective in selected patients, although success is less reliable than with PAP. However, successful PAP treatment requires adherence. The 2010 practice parameters for surgical treatment of OSA recommended PAP or an OA be offered before surgery.[29] For unselected patients, 50% or less will have an acceptable result with palate surgery. Many patients with moderate OSA will require multilevel surgery for the best result. As noted, nonablative palatal procedures are associated with fewer side effects than traditional UPPP and can be combined with procedures that address retroglossal obstruction. Further discussion of surgical options is provided in Chapter 26. Hypoglossal nerve stimulation with a surgically implanted stimulator and stimulation lead position around the hypoglossal nerve is another option for patients with moderate-to-severe OSA (if they meet selection criteria) who are unable to accept or tolerate PAP treatment. Although, as mentioned previously, even with careful selection, up to 20% to 30% of these patients hypoglossal nerve stimulation have residual sleep apnea.[52,53]

For severe OSA, PAP is the treatment of choice. Although effective, long-term adherence is approximately 50%; this percentage can be higher with good support.[37] Tracheostomy reliably bypasses upper airway obstruction but is not acceptable to most patients. This procedure is reserved for patients with very severe OSA who will not adhere to PAP when effective treatment is urgently needed (e.g., recurrent hypercapnic respiratory failure) and the patient is not a candidate for maxillary mandibular advancement. Complex upper airway surgery such as maxillary mandibular advancement can be effective in 80% to 90% of patients. Hypoglossal nerve stimulation can be effective in patients with severe OSA, although the AHI may remain over 10 events/hour. It is indicated in patients who do not accept or tolerate PAP treatments. An OA can be effective in severe OSA but rarely reduces the AHI to less than 10 events/hour. However, OA treatment can have benefits on blood pressure, daytime sleepiness, and quality of life, and it can certainly be better than no treatment at all.[28] As noted previously, when comparing treatment effectiveness, one must consider both efficacy and adherence.

Comorbid Insomnia and Depression

Comorbid insomnia and depression are often present along with variable severities of OSA.[14,15] In fact, complaints of fatigue, nonrestorative sleep, and difficulty initiating and maintaining sleep are often the reasons for referral to a sleep center. In general, patients with these complaints tend to have milder AHI values, and it is often difficult to determine if OSA is really the cause of the symptoms. Cognitive behavioral treatment of insomnia is the treatment of choice in this situation and can improve CPAP adherence.[15] Adequate treatment of depression is essential, and use of a low-dose sedating antidepressant along with an effective antidepressant may be helpful in some patients with depression and insomnia. Cognitive behavioral treatment of insomnia (CBTI) is the treatment of choice for insomnia, including insomnia comorbid with OSA with or without anxiety and depression. A recent study showed CBTI is effective even if anxiety or depression are present and may improve CPAP adherence.[59] Ultimately, successful treatment of comorbid insomnia and sleep apnea (COMISA) requires adequate treatment of both insomnia and OSA.

Patient Education Before Treatment

After PSG or HSAT, the physician ordering the study should discuss the findings and the consequences of untreated sleep apnea with the patient.[1] The factors that can exacerbate OSA, including weight gain, insufficient sleep, medications, and alcohol consumption, should also be addressed. The available treatment options and the pros and cons of each should be discussed. Whereas most patients look to the physician for ultimate recommendations, involving the patient and spouse in decision making is essential to improve treatment outcomes. Drowsy-driving counseling should be performed and documented. Many patients have comorbid conditions such as depression, insomnia, restless legs syndrome (RLS), or chronic pain that will make compliance with PAP or other treatments more difficult. These conditions should be evaluated and treated.

Follow-up and Outcomes Assessment

After treatment initiation, careful follow-up is essential, because OSA is a chronic disease.[1,31] A titration PSG is not recommended for patients doing well on PAP treatment but can be considered if symptoms worsen or if the device-supplied AHI estimate or leak estimates are concerning. HSAT or PSG is recommended with all non-PAP treatments to document efficacy. Testing after surgical healing is recommended for all severities of OSA. PSG or HSAT is recommended after final adjustment of an OA used as treatment for all severities of OSA.[1,31] Testing of patients after surgery or while wearing an OA is indicated if symptoms return. It is important that patients understand that, if one treatment does not work, there are other options that are much better than no treatment at all. It is not uncommon for patients who dislike CPAP to both stop treatment and *cancel follow-up sleep-clinic appointments*. Patient education about alternative OSA treatments even if PAP is selected as the initial treatment is essential to prevent "drop outs" from sleep clinic. For PAP treatment, objective adherence should be assessed at every clinic visit; usually, patients complete an Epworth Sleepiness Scale and answer questions about sleep habits and issues with PAP.

Clusters, Endotypes, and Phenotypes

Precision medicine requires choosing the treatment most suitable for a given patient. OSA is a heterogeneous syndrome with varied predisposing factors, pathophysiological mechanisms, clinical presentations, and consequences of respiratory events. Of note, the efficacy of OSA treatment and its effect on outcomes may also vary depending on these characteristics. Finding clusters of patients with common characteristics is one approach to avoiding a "one size fits all" treatment approach. Often, the term *phenotype* is used for a particular cluster of patients with common symptoms or manifestations.

A review by Taranto-Montemurro et al.[60] details the many studies that have assessed treatment of one of the four primary targets: unfavorable (small) upper airway size and increased collapsibility, impaired upper airway muscle compensation, high loop gain, and low arousal threshold (see Chapter 19 for a discussion of the pathophysiology of OSA). For example, interventions for small upper airway size and increased collapsibility might include weight loss, diuresis, CPAP, avoidance of the supine position, upper airway surgery, and an OA. For high loop gain, interventions might include oxygen or acetazolamide. For impaired muscle responsiveness, they may include atomoxetine and oxybutynin[60] (although presently still experimental). Finally, a number of sedatives and hypnotics have been tried to increase the arousal threshold. However, endotype determination is still not widely available and treatment with acetazolamide and oxygen to reduce loop gain and hypnotics to reduce the arousal threshold have not reached the mainstream of clinical practice. Obtaining reimbursement for oxygen in the private sector to treat obstructive sleep apnea is also difficult and usually requires demonstration of residual hypoxemia after normalization of the AHI by PAP-treatment. However, more treatment options will be available in the future, and the concept of precision treatment of OSA is an important innovation.

A review of studies of cluster analysis in sleep apnea by Zinchuk and Yaggi[61] provides an informative discussion of the studies on clusters of patients with OSA based on symptoms and pathophysiology. As discussed in their review, an example of a phenotype would be patients with OSA with a lack of concentric upper airway collapse during drug-induced sleep endoscopy; this helps identify responders to hypoglossal nerve stimulation. Phenotyping strategies can be grouped into two analytic approaches: hypothesis-driven (or supervised) and hypothesis-generating (or unsupervised) learning methods. Mathematic tools can be used to identify clusters of similar characteristics using methods such as hierarchical, K means, or latent class analysis.[61]

The term *endotype* has been used to describe groups with different pathophysiology (high loop gain, low arousal threshold), and phenotype has been used to describe symptom clusters. However, in the literature, the term phenotype has been used for both pathophysiological characteristics and symptoms. Possible phenotype categories are listed in Table 21–3. Different studies have identified different clusters or phenotypes based on prominent symptoms, PSG characteristics, and cardiovascular risk. In Table 21–4, clusters from two of the initial cluster analysis studies are shown.[62,63] For example, Ye et al.[62] analyzed an Icelandic cohort and found three clusters (disturbed sleep, minimally symptomatic, and excessively sleepy) commonly seen in sleep clinic populations. In contrast to other studies, the excessively sleepy group had a

Table 21–3 Phenotype Categories

Symptom
- Sleepy
- Non-sleepy, disturbed sleep
- Insomnia

Demographics
- Age
- Gender

Polysomnography Phenotypes
- Short respiratory event duration, low hypoxic burden
- High AHI, long events, high hypoxic burden
- Positional OSA
- REM-predominant OSA

CVD Risk
- High prevalence
- Low prevalence
- High incident
- Low Incident

Comorbidities
- Few
- Many

CPAP Adherence
- Good, high benefit
- Low, low benefit

Pathophysiological Subtypes (Endotypes)
- Small collapsible upper airway
- Inadequate upper airway muscle compensation
- High loop gain (unstable ventilatory control)
- Low arousal threshold

AHI, apnea-hypopnea index; *CPAP*, continuous positive airway pressure; *CVD*, cardiovascular disease; *OSA*, obstructive sleep apnea; *REM*, rapid eye movement.

Table 21–4 Examples of Clusters (Phenotypes) from Two Studies

Study	Clusters	Comments
Ye et al.	1. Disturbed sleep (33%)	• Insomnia symptoms • Frequent awakenings • Non-restorative sleep
	2. Minimally symptomatic (25%)	• Higher risk of comorbidity (hypertension, cardiovascular disease)
	3. Excessively sleepy (42%)	• Higher ESS score • Drowsy driving, younger • Lower risk of cardiovascular morbidity
Comments: Icelandic cohort, clusters did not differ in AHI, BMI, gender		
Mazzotti et al.	1. Disturbed sleep (12%)	• ESS = 7.0 • Predominant insomnia symptoms
	2. Minimally symptomatic (33%)	• ESS = 4.5 • Lowest symptom burden of all clusters • Less likely to respond to CPAP (not addressed in the study)
	3. Excessively sleepy (17%)	• ESS = 13 • Predominant sleepy, involuntary sleep, drowsy driving • Threefold increased risk of prevalent heart failure compared to other subtypes • Increased risk of prevalent and incident CVD or cardiovascular death vs. patients with no OSA
	4. Moderately sleepy (39%)	• ESS = 10.6 • Snoring, napping
Comments: All patients had AHI ≥ 15 events/hr		

CPAP, continuous positive airway pressure; *CVD*, cardiovascular disease; *ESS*, Epworth Sleepiness Scale.
Ye L, Pien GW, Ratcliffe SJ, et al. The different clinical faces of obstructive sleep apnoea: a cluster analysis. *Eur Respir J*. 2014;44(6):1600-1607.
Mazzotti DR, Keenan BT, Lim DC, Gottlieb DJ, Kim J, Pack AI. Symptom subtypes of obstructive sleep apnea predict incidence of cardiovascular outcomes. *Am J Respir Crit Care Med*. 2019;200(4):493-506.

lower risk of cardiovascular comorbidity. Mazzotti and coworkers[63] found the excessively sleepy cluster to have an increased risk of prevalent heart failure compared to the other three groups (disturbed sleep, minimally symptomatic, and moderately sleepy). The excessively sleepy group was the only group with an increased risk of prevalent and incident cardiovascular disease when compared to a group without OSA. In Table 21–5, clusters proposed by Zinchuk and Yaggi are displayed, along with comments regarding risks and possible treatments. As an example of phenotyping efforts, there have been quite a few studies trying to predict which patients will respond to an OA.[49] Multiple methods, including drug-induced sleep endoscopy, upper-airway imaging, and prediction equations based on AHI, BMI, and the presence or absence of positional OSA, have not proven to reliably predict the response to OAs. In a study of 93 participants, Bamagoos and coworkers[64] found that greater OA efficacy was associated with favorable nonpharyngeal traits (lower loop gain, higher arousal threshold, and lower response to arousal), moderate (non-mild, non-severe) pharyngeal collapsibility, and weaker muscle compensation. Predicted responders (n = 54), when compared with predicted non-responders (n = 39), exhibited a greater reduction in AHI from baseline (73% vs. 51%) and a lower treatment AHI. However, the prediction equation still explained a relatively low amount of variability in response to OA treatment. Edwards et al.[65] studied 14 patients and concluded that OA therapy improved upper-airway collapsibility under passive and active conditions. A greater response to therapy occurred in those with a mild anatomic compromise and a lower loop gain.[65] Marques and coworkers[66] used a combination of upper-airway endoscopy during natural sleep and endotyping using PSG. Patients with posteriorly located tongues (vallecula not visible or vocal cords not visible when viewed from below the palate) exhibited greater improvement in pharyngeal collapsibility with OA therapy. Patients with the combination of a posteriorly located tongue and less-severe collapsibility experienced greater OA efficacy. While these studies are of interest, they used techniques not widely available to most clinicians. In the future, there will likely be

Table 21–5 OSA Subtypes

Subtype	PSG	Symptoms	Risks	Treatment
A. Classic (younger age, male, low comorbidity)	• AHI high • T90 medium	• Excessive sleepiness • Involuntary sleep	• Drowsy driving • Incident CVD	• CPAP • Highest CPAP benefit
B. Oldest, comorbid (oldest, male, highest comorbidity)	• AHI medium • T90 high	• Naps, snoring disturbs partner	• Low CPAP adherence • High prevalent CVD • Low incident CVD	• Lowest CPAP benefit • Optimal treatment includes manage-ment (treatment) of comorbidity?
C. Female, insomnia (middle age, female, medium comorbidity)	• AHI medium • T90 medium	• Insomnia symptoms	• Low CPAP adherence • Possible CVD risk	• Medium CPAP benefit • CPAP +possibly CBTI
D. Youngest, upper airway symptoms (Youngest, male)	• AHI high • T90 low	• Snoring • Sudden awakening • ESS low • ± Insomnia	• Low CPAP adherence • Unknown CVD risk	• Medium CPAP benefit (QOL) • Oral appliances • Possible benefit (hypnotics/CBTI) if insomnia
E. Severe, hypoxemic (younger, male)	• AHI high, T90 high	• Sleepy, severely obese	• Incident CVD	• CPAP
F. Severe, non-hypoxemic (older, male, lowest comorbidity)	• AHI high, short events, T90 low, min SaO_2 high	• Less sleepy, obese	• Low CPAP adherence • Possible neurocogni-tive dysfunction	• CPAP or OA, plus hypnotics/CBTI • (if high loop gain, consider acetazol-amide or oxygen)

AHI, apnea-hypopnea index; *CBTI*, cognitive behavioral treatment of insomnia; *CPAP*, continuous positive airway pressure; *CVD*, cardiovascular disease; *OA*, oral appliance; *OSA*, obstructive sleep apnea; *PSG*, polysomnography; *QOL*, quality of life; *T90*, time below SaO_2 of 90%; *ESS*, Epworth Sleepiness Scale.
Data from Zinchuk A, Yaggi HK. Phenotypic subtypes of OSA: A challenge and opportunity for precision medicine. *Chest.* 2020;157(2):403-420. PMID: 31539538.

greater availability of endotyping software. In a study by Landry et al.,[67] a therapeutic CPAP level ≤8.0 cm H_2O was sensitive (89%) and specific (84%) for detecting a mildly collapsible upper airway. This suggests that, given two patients with similar AHI values, the one with a lower optimal CPAP would be more likely to respond to OA treatment.

TREATMENT OF THE OBESITY HYPOVENTILATION SYNDROME

Diagnosis of OHS is discussed in Chapter 18 and requires demonstration of daytime hypoventilation (partial pressure of carbon dioxide [$PaCO_2$] >45 mm Hg or $PaCO_2$ ≥45 mm Hg in many definitions) in an obese patient (BMI ≥30 kg/m^2) with an absence of other conditions believed to cause hypoventilation (chronic obstructive pulmonary disease [COPD], neuromuscular weakness, respiratory depressant medication, chest wall disease other than obesity). The possibility of OHS should be considered in every obese individual referred for suspected OSA. Patients with OHS are at high risk of morbidity and mortality if not appropriately treated. Approximately 90% of patients with OHS have OSA, defined by an AHI of ≥ 5 events/hour. Nearly 70% of patients with OHS have concomitant severe OSA (AHI >30 events/hour).[68,69] The American Thoracic Society (ATS) has published recommendations for the diagnosis and treatment of OHS.[68,69] The first recommendation concerns the method to identify OHS. A serum bicarbonate level (CO_2 on routine electrolytes, which consist mainly of bicarbonate and a small amount of dissolved CO_2) <27 mmol/L can be used to exclude the diagnosis of OHS in obese patients with OSA *when the suspicion of OHS is low*. A CO_2 value ≥27 mmol/L would trigger ordering an arterial blood gas (ABG) test, as an elevation of CO_2 at or above the 27 mmolEq/L cutoff is not specific for OHS. However, if there is a moderate-to-high suspicion of OHS (severe obesity, mild daytime hypoxemia [SaO_2 91%–93%], very severe OSA, severe nocturnal desaturation, nocturnal hypoventilation), obtaining an ABG test is recommended irrespective of the HCO^-_3/CO_2 level.

The recommended approach to OHS treatment depends on the presence or absence of severe OSA and the severity of the current condition (stable outpatient vs. hospitalized patient with acute or chronic hypercapnic respiratory failure).[68,69]

In the following discussion BPAP-S refers to a, bilevel PAP (BPAP) device without a backup rate and a maximum pressure of 25 cm H2O. The S in BPAP-S refers to the spontaneous or S mode in which the patient spontaneously triggers all breaths.) BPAP-ST devices (ST for spontaneous timed) have a backup rate and a maximum pressure of 30 cm H_2O. Breaths can be triggered by the patient (spontaneous) or by the device (timed, based on the backup rate). The term non-invasive ventilation (NIV) for outpatients generally means BPAP-ST delivered via a mask interface, although home ventilators can provide additional options, including volume ventilation via mask or tracheostomy (see Chapter 24).

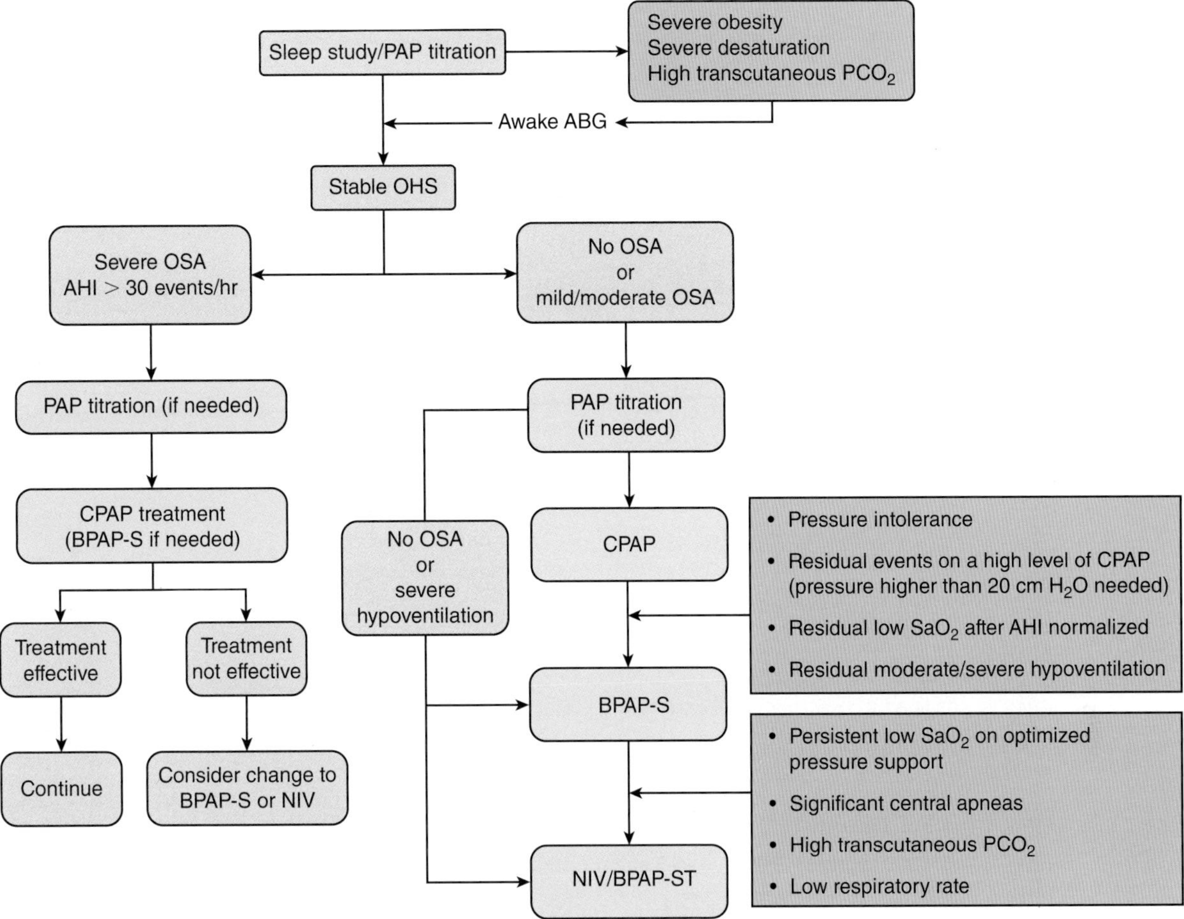

Figure 21–4 An Algorithm for Treatment of Stable Patients with the Obesity Hypoventilation Syndrome (OHS). This assumes *a diagnostic sleep study has been performed to document the presence of obstructive sleep apnea (OSA)* and its severity. Some individuals may have been evaluated with a split sleep study (diagnostic/titration) rather than a diagnostic study. An awake ABG confirms the suspicion of OHS and no other cause of hypoventilation is identified. Patients with severe OSA can usually be treated effectively with continuous positive airway pressure (CPAP) (or BPAP-S bilevel PAP without backup rate, if needed). If hypercapnia does not resolve or improve with adequate treatment (assuming adequate adherence), a change from CPAP to BPAP-S or noninvasive ventilation (NIV) is indicated. In those patients with no OSA or mild-to-moderate OSA, a different approach is usually needed. A PAP titration will establish the effective mode of treatment. Often, BPAP-S or NIV is needed for optimal treatment. The titration should still start with CPAP (unless no OSA is present) and then change to BPAP-S and finally BPAP with a backup rate as needed based on the response of the patient to the different forms of treatment. Supplemental oxygen can be added if necessary, but ideally, hypoventilation should be adequately addressed before supplemental oxygen is added. Use of transcutaneous PCO_2 may aid in optimizing ventilation if this is available. In all cases, weight loss is indicated, and bariatric surgery should be considered. *AHI*, apnea-hypopnea index.

The ATS guidelines for treatment of OHS include a treatment algorithm for stable OHS patients based on the presence or absence of severe OSA. CPAP is recommended if severe OSA is present and NIV if severe OSA is not present. A slightly different algorithm for the treatment of stable OHS is displayed in Figure 21–4. This algorithm assumes that most stable obese patients are not diagnosed with OHS until after an initial sleep study usually showing severe OSA and/or severe desaturation. Treatment with CPAP (or BPAP-S if needed) will normalize or improve daytime hypoventilation in most patients with severe OSA if they are adherent to treatment. The algorithm differs from the ATS algorithm that recommends NIV for OHS patients without severe OSA. The treatment pathways in Figure 21–4 recognizes that the best treatment for OHS patients with no OSA or mild to moderate OSA varies and is best determined by a PAP titration. Not all of these patients require NIV. Treatment of stable OHS patients without OSA is discussed below.

The ATS guidelines for OHS treatment of stable patients are based on data from multiple studies,[70-73] and summaries are available in two meta-analyses.[74,75]

In Table 21–6, results from four RCTs of CPAP versus NIV[70-73] in stable patients with OHS and severe OSA are shown with baseline BMI, $PaCO_2$, and AHI, as well as the treatment settings (CPAP or NIV). Piper et al.[70] used BPAP-S rather than BPAP with a backup rate. The first three studies were short-term, and at 2 to 3 months, groups treated with CPAP and NIV (or BPAP-S) had similar outcomes with respect to improvement in daytime $PaCO_2$. No difference in average adherence rates was also noted between

Table 21–6 Randomized Controlled Trials of BPAP or NIV versus CPAP in OHS

Study	(1) Piper et al.[70] 2008*		(2) Masa et al.[72] 2015 (short-term)		(3) Howard et al.[71] 2017		(4) Masa et al.[73] 2019 (long-term)	
Treatment Modes	CPAP versus BPAP-S		CPAP versus NIV, VAPS (volume target with BUR)		CPAP versus NIV, BPAP-ST		CPAP versus NIV, VAPS (volume target with BUR)	
Treatment pressures								
CPAP (mean, cm H_2O)	14		11		15. 2		10.7	
BPAP-S or NIV	IPAP 16 cm H_2O EPAP 10 cm H_2O		Target volume: 5–6 ml/kg actual body weight IPAP 20 cm H_2O EPAP 7.8 cm H_2O Rate 14 breaths/minute		IPAP 19.3 cm H_2O EPAP 11.9 cm H_2O Rate 15 breaths/minute		Target tidal volume: 5–6 ml/kg actual body weight IPAP 19.7 cm H_2O EPAP 8.2 cm H_2O Rate 14 breaths/minute	
Subject characteristics								
BMI (kg/m²)	CPAP	52	CPAP	45	CPAP	54.5	CPAP	42.7
	BPAP-S	54	NIV	43	NIV	55.5	NIV	42.9
PCO_2 baseline (cm H_2O)	CPAP	52	CPAP	50	CPAP	59.1	CPAP	49
	BPAP-S	49	NIV	51	NIV	60.1	NIV	51
AHI	CPAP	93 N/61 R	CPAP	71	CPAP+ NIV	80	CPAP	68.2
	BPAP-S	70 N/48 R	NIV	68	No difference between groups		NIV	68.7
Results								
Change in PCO_2 (mmHg)	CPAP	-5.8 at 3 months	CPAP	-3.7 at 2 months	CPAP	-6.7 at 3 months	CPAP	-6.4 at 5.4 years
	BPAP-S	-6.9 at 3 months	NIV	-5.5 at 2 months	NIV	-5.9 at 3 months	NIV	-7.5 at 5.6 years
Adherence (hours)	CPAP	5.8	CPAP	5.3	CPAP	5.0	CPAP	6.0 median
	BPAP-S	6.1	NIV	5.3	NIV	5.3	NIV	6.0 median
Hospitalizations (days/year)							CPAP	1.63
							NIV	1.44

*After exclusion of patients with persisting severe nocturnal hypoxemia ($SpO_2 < 80\%$ for >10 min) or acute rise carbon dioxide retention (>10 mm Hg) during REM sleep despite optimal CPAP.

Average values are displayed. *AHI*, apnea-hypopnea index; *BMI*, body mass index; *BPAP*, bilevel positive airway pressure; *BUR*, backup rate; *CPAP*, continuous positive airway pressure; *EPAP*, expiratory positive airway pressure; *IPAP*, inspiratory positive airway pressure; *NIV*, noninvasive ventilation; *OHS*, obesity hypoventilation syndrome; *REM*, rapid eye movement; *R*, REM sleep; *N*, NREM; *S*, spontaneous; *ST*, spontaneous timed; *VAPS*, volume assured pressure support.

CPAP and NIV. A long-term study also demonstrated similar outcomes, including no difference in the number of days hospitalized.[73] Results of the study by Howard et al.[72] are shown in Figure 21–5. For the stable severe OSA group treated with CPAP, average values over the four studies ranged from 11 to 15 cm H_2O. However, with severe obesity, up to 20 cm H_2O was needed. When BPAP without a backup rate was used, the average pressure was 16/10 cm H_2O.[70] This setting provides only 6 cm H_2O of pressure support. While pressure support of 4 to 6 cm H_2O is commonly used to treat OSA, higher levels are typically needed to augment ventilation. Higher levels of expiratory PAP (EPAP) (8 to 12 cm H_2O) are often needed for very obese individuals. Volume-assured pressure support (a form of BPAP in which pressure support varies to attain a target tidal volume) was used in two studies.[72,73] The target tidal volume was 5 to 6 ml/kg of **actual body weight,** and average inspiratory PAP (IPAP) and EPAP values were approximately 20 and 8 cm H_2O, respectively. When a backup rate was used (in three of the four studies), the average rate was either 14 or 15 breaths per minute. At times, the addition of supplemental oxygen was needed. These study results suggest that, for stable outpatients with the OHS, CPAP is as effective as NIV for improvement in hypoventilation when results were assessed after short term treatment (2-3 months). The finding of equivalent adherence is important. Other studies have documented the importance of good adherence for improvement or resolution of daytime hypercapnia (Figure 21–6).[76,77]

Patients With Stable OHS and Severe OSA

Based on the available data, the ATS OHS treatment guidelines[68] recommend CPAP rather than NIV should be the first treatment in ambulatory patients with stable OHS and severe OSA. The response to CPAP means reversal of OSA alone is effective for improvement in hypoventilation, although resolution usually occurs over several months. While the guideline for use of CPAP over NIV in patients with stable OHS and

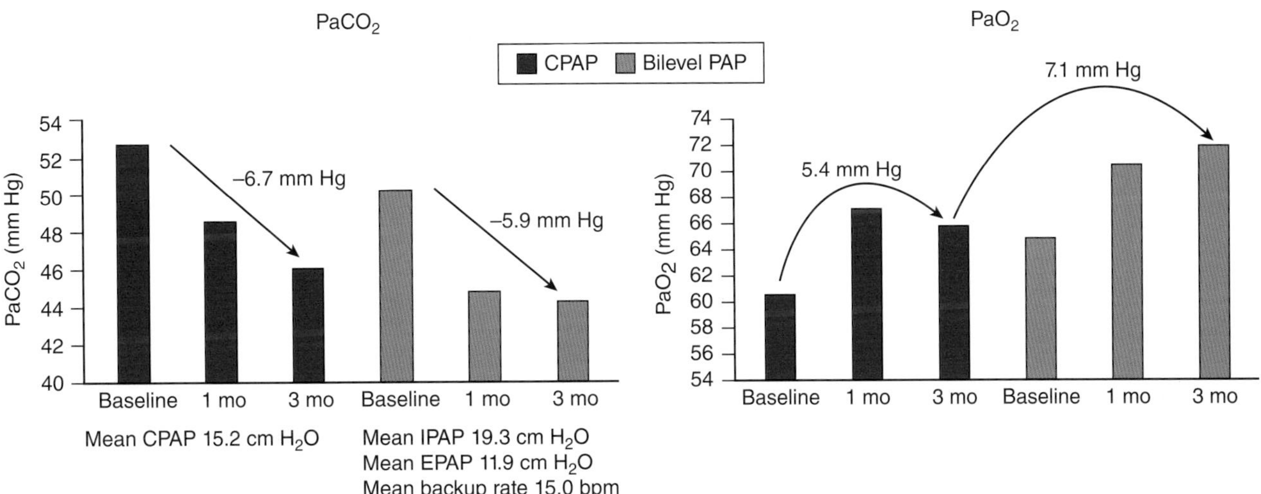

Figure 21–5 **Results of a Study Comparing Continuous Positive Airway Pressure (CPAP) and Bilevel PAP (BPAP with a backup rate) for Patients With Obesity Hypoventilation Syndrome.** This was a randomized controlled study of stable patients with obesity hypoventilation syndrome (OHS). A diagnostic sleep study was not required for entry into the study, but the apnea-hypopnea index (AHI) was 46.15 events/hour for the entire group (reported only in supplementary material). The body mass index (BMI) in the CPAP group was 54.5 kg/m^2 and 55.3 kg/m^2 in the BPAP group. At 3 months, the reduction in daytime $PaCO_2$ or improvement in PaO_2 did not differ between the treatment groups. At 1 month, there was a trend for a lower awake $PaCO_2$ with BPAP treatment. The awake PaO_2 also improved in both groups. BPAP with a backup rate was used in this study. *CPAP*, continuous positive airway pressure; *BPAP*, bilevel positive airway presure; *IPAP*, inspiratory positive airway pressure; *EPAP*, expiratory positive airway pressure; *bpm*, breaths per minute. (Figure drawn using data from Howard ME, Piper AJ, Stevens B, et al. A randomised controlled trial of CPAP versus non-invasive ventilation for initial treatment of obesity hypoventilation syndrome. *Thorax.* 2017;72[5]:437-444.)

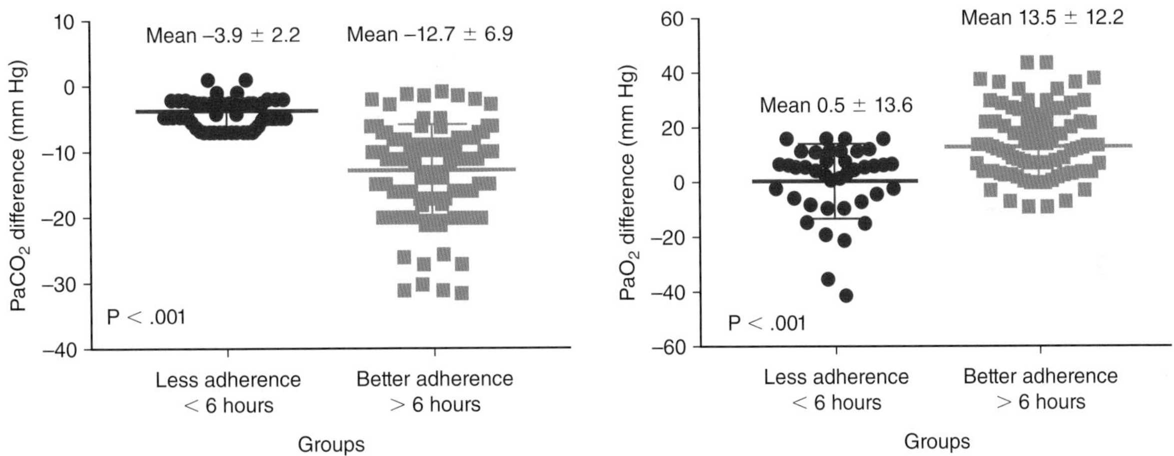

Figure 21–6 **The Importance of Good Adherence for Improvement in the $PaCO_2$ and PaO_2 in Patients Receiving Treatment for Obesity Hypoventilation Syndrome.** Use for longer than 6 hours was associated with much better improvement in gas exchange (greater decrease in $PaCO_2$ and increase in PaO_2). (From Bouloukaki I, Mermigkis C, Michelakis S, et al. The association between adherence to positive airway pressure therapy and long-term outcomes in patients with obesity hypoventilation syndrome: a prospective observational study. *J Clin Sleep Med.* 2018;14[9]:1539-1550.)

severe OSA is supported by research findings, there are situations in which using BPAP **without** a backup rate (BPAP-S) rather than CPAP is useful. BPAP is not more effective than CPAP at opening the upper airway in most patients. However, the maximum pressure of CPAP devices is 20 cm H_2O; that of routine BPAP-S devices is 25 cm H_2O. If a patient requires pressure higher than 20 cm H_2O, BPAP can be useful. As mentioned, resolution of hypercapnia on PAP depends on good adherence.[76,77] If a patient has pressure intolerance to high levels of CPAP, bloating, or mouth or mask leak, they might do better on BPAP-S than on CPAP. Some patients with OHS have residual hypoxemia on CPAP that may respond to BPAP-S. In Figure 21–7, mild hypoxemia was present on CPAP 19 cm H_2O but resolved on BPAP 22/14 cm H_2O. With the goal of improving hypoventilation, BPAP (rather than CPAP) is a better option than adding supplemental oxygen.[78] In addition, there are patients with OHS with both severe OSA and very severe hypoventilation confined to REM sleep that may be better treated with BPAP than CPAP.[70]

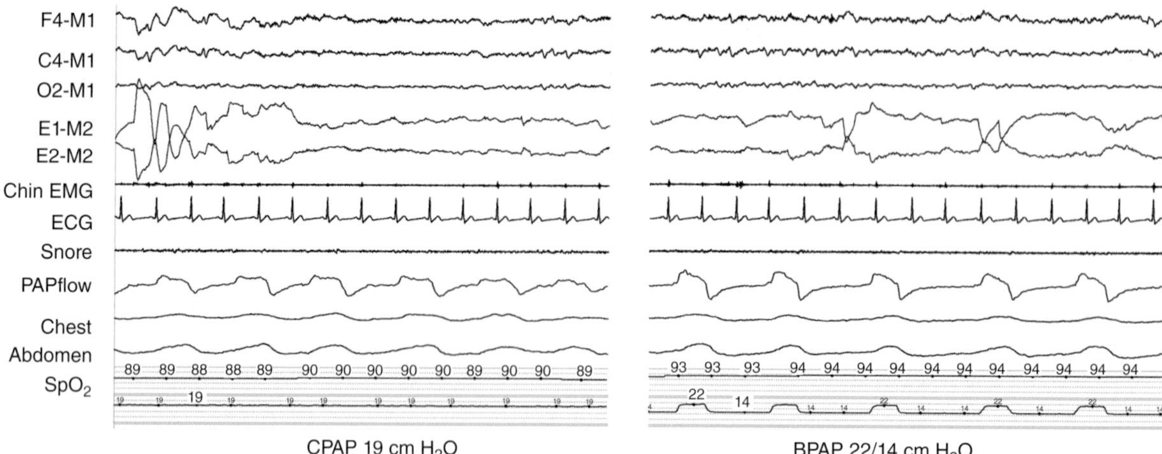

Figure 21–7 This patient with obesity hypoventilation syndrome (OHS) underwent a positive airway pressure (PAP) titration, but on continuous PAP (CPAP) of 19 cm H_2O, there was persistent mild desaturation. The patient was changed to bilevel PAP (BPAP) 22/14 cm H_2O, and the oxygen saturation improved. SpO_2 arterial oxygen saturation was measured by pulse oximetry. BPAP 22/14 is inspiratory pressure (IPAP) = 22 and expiratory positive airway pressure (EPAP) = 14.

Obese Patients (Presumed OHS) Hospitalized for Respiratory Failure

In this group, NIV is needed for initial treatment, irrespective of the presence or absence of severe OSA (often not known). A backup rate is essential to address central apneas that may occur with the treatment-induced reduction in $PaCO_2$, for patients not triggering breaths during REM sleep, or in those better treated with a respiratory rate higher than their native respiratory rate. The utility of a backup rate for hypoventilation treatment is discussed in Chapter 24. The ATS recommendations state that obese patients hospitalized for respiratory failure (presumed OHS) should be discharged on NIV using appropriate settings (some patients may require the addition of supplemental oxygen) until they undergo an outpatient evaluation for hypoventilation (including a diagnostic sleep study if needed) and PAP titration in the sleep laboratory (after stabilization, but ideally within 2 to 3 months). The diagnostic study can determine whether OSA is present and its severity. The PAP titration can document the type of treatment needed for ongoing therapy. Many patients discharged on NIV are found to have severe OSA on diagnostic testing 2 to 3 months after discharge from the hospital and can be treated with CPAP or BPAP without a backup rate. Other patients (severe OSA usually not present) will require long-term NIV. In those **without** severe OSA on the diagnostic study, the NIV settings and supplemental oxygen can be fine-tuned by the PSG PAP titration. Often, supplemental oxygen will no longer be needed. Some patients **without** severe OSA can be adequately treated with a BPAP device without a backup rate. An algorithm for treatment of obese patients hospitalized for hypercapnic respiratory failure (adapted from ATS guideline for treatment of the OHS) is shown in Figure 21–8.

Unfortunately, obtaining a BPAP device with a backup rate at hospital discharge for the indication of hypoventilation is often difficult.[79,80] BPAP devices with and without a backup rate, when used for hypoventilation, are considered respiratory assist devices (RADs). Medicare and other insurance providers initially require use of BPAP without a backup rate (E0470) with later qualification for a BPAP with a backup rate (E0471) dependent on demonstration of failure of improvements with the E0470[79] (Table 21–7). Fortunately, many patients at the time of discharge have improved enough that a BPAP device without a backup rate (set using hospital settings) is sufficient. In patients with severe hypoventilation still present at the time of discharge, treatment with a home ventilator (has a backup rate) under the diagnosis of respiratory failure is an option if they qualify (see discussion in the RAD criteria section to follow). Another option is an expedited PAP titration study as an outpatient documenting the failure of BPAP without a backup rate. For example, showing persistent desaturation on BPAP-S once the AHI is normalized (Table 21–7).

Patients With Stable OHS Without Severe OSA

As discussed, hospitalized patients with unstable OHS and hypercapnic respiratory failure (with or without severe OSA) require NIV, at least initially. What about patients with stable OHS without severe OSA? A long-term study of NIV treatment in patients with stable OHS without severe sleep apnea was stopped due to low enrollment (the majority of patients with OHS have severe OSA).[81] Analysis of the data revealed the NIV treatment did not lower long-term hospital days per year compared to lifestyle modification. The NIV group had a mean nightly adherence of only 3.7 hours. The low adherence might explain the findings and also illustrates that NIV treatment requires intensive follow-up to ensure adequate adherence. In any case, firm evidence supporting the best treatment for stable OHS without severe OSA does not exist. However, the ATS guidelines recommend NIV treatment for OHS without severe sleep apnea with the caveat that treatment should be individualized. Do patients with stable OHS but without severe OSA really need NIV treatment? BaHammam and coworkers[82] studied patients with stable OHS but without severe OSA. There was an initial CPAP titration, and if the SaO_2 was ≤90% for 20% or more of the night, the patient underwent a second titration with BPAP. The results of the first titration showed that seventy percent of the patients could be treated with CPAP alone, and the adherence was acceptable (and no different than in the BPAP

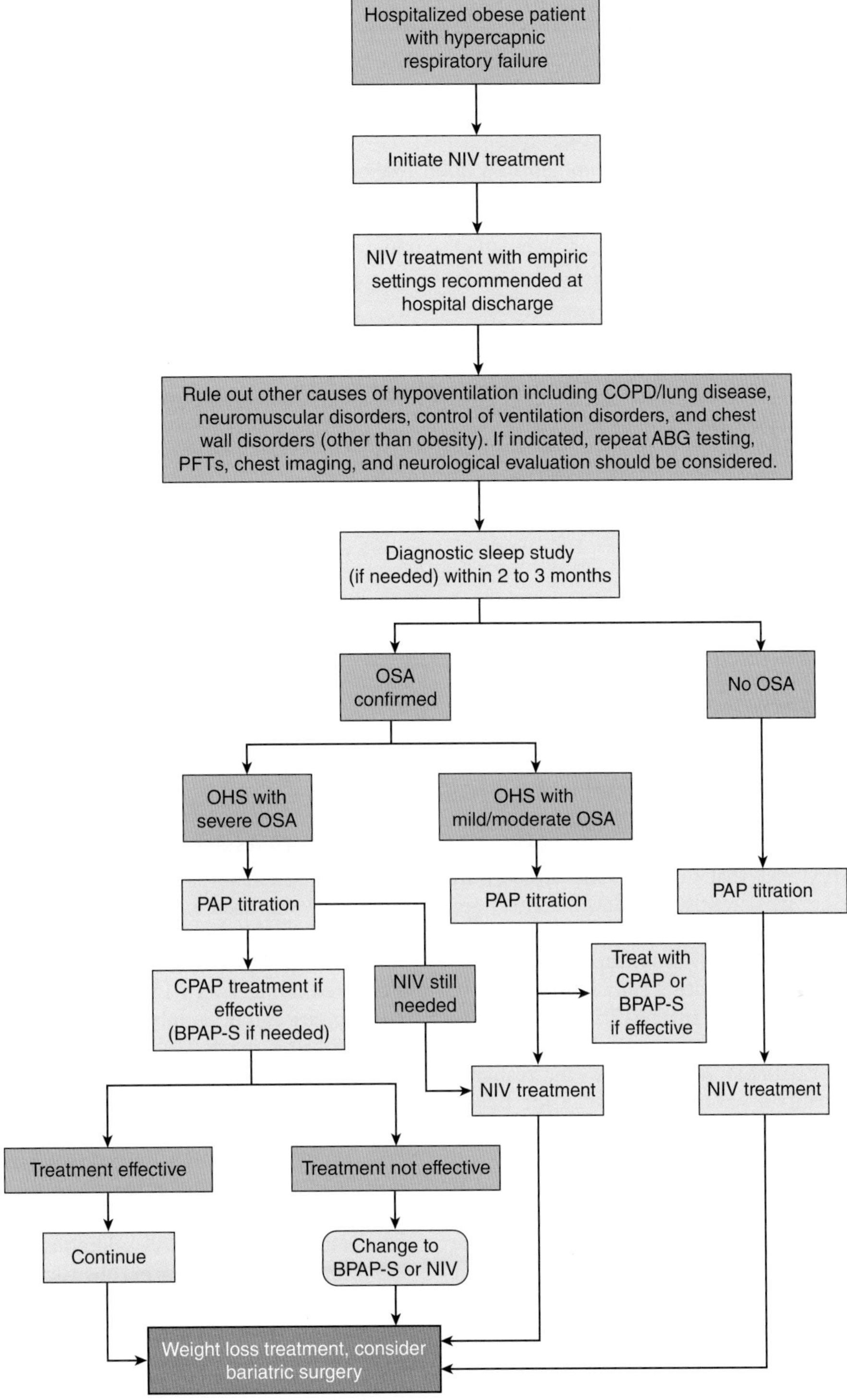

Figure 21–8 Algorithm for Evaluation and Treatment of Obese Patients Hospitalized for Hypercapnic Respiratory Failure (adapted from ATS guidelines[68]). Some form of noninvasive ventilation is typically used in the hospital. The American Thoracic Society (ATS) guidelines recommend that, after stabilization, that patients be discharged on noninvasive ventilation (NIV) using empiric settings similar to those used in the hospital. Other evaluation as an outpatient is often indicated to clarify the etiology of the hypoventilation (for example pulmonary function testing). A diagnostic sleep study is performed 2 to 3 months later to establish the presence of obstructive sleep apnea (OSA) and its severity. This assumes the OSA status is not already known from previous testing. Then, a positive airway pressure (PAP) titration is performed. Patients with severe OSA may be adequately treated with continuous PAP (CPAP) or bilevel PAP (BPAP) without a backup rate (BPAP-S), and this treatment rather than NIV can be used for ongoing treatment. In others (especially if severe hypercapnia/hypoxemia is still present), continued NIV treatment is needed. Patients with no OSA (rare finding) or mild-to-moderate OSA will often require ongoing NIV treatment, but some patients in this category can also be effectively treated with CPAP or BPAP-S. When NIV is needed in patients with obesity hypoventilation syndrome (OHS), the PAP titration can be useful in optimizing settings. Use of transcutaneous PCO_2 monitoring can be helpful, if available. In all cases, weight loss is indicated, and bariatric surgery should be considered. *PFT*, pulmonary function testing; *BPAP-S*, BPAP without a backup rate.

Table 21–7 Respiratory Assistance Device Reimbursement (Hypoventilation Syndrome): *Excerpt from LCD L33800**

E0470* is covered if:**

A. An initial ABG test $PaCO_2$, done while awake and breathing the beneficiary's prescribed FIO_2, is ≥45 mm Hg; **and**
B. Spirometry shows an FEV_1/FVC ≥70% and an FEV_1 ≥50% of predicted** **and**

The beneficiary's condition also meets one of the following:

C. An ABG test $PaCO_2$, done during sleep or immediately upon awakening and while breathing the beneficiary's prescribed FIO_2, shows the beneficiary's $PaCO_2$ worsened ≥7 mm Hg compared to the original result in criterion A (above); **or**
D. A facility-based PSG or HST demonstrates oxygen saturation ≤88% or ≥5 minutes of nocturnal recording time (minimum recording time of 2 hours) that is not caused by obstructive upper airway events—i.e., AHI <5 events/hour.

E0471 is covered if:

A. A covered E0470 is being used; and
B. Spirometry shows an FEV1/FVC ≥70% and an FEV1 ≥50% of predicted (otherwise, refer to Severe COPD coverage); **and**

One of the following criteria are being met:

C. An ABG test $PaCO_2$, done while awake and breathing the beneficiary's prescribed FIO_2, shows that the beneficiary's $PaCO_2$ **worsened ≥7 mm Hg** compared to the ABG result performed to qualify the beneficiary for the E0470 device; **or**
D. A facility-based PSG or HST demonstrates oxygen saturation ≤88% for ≥5 minutes of nocturnal recording time (minimum recording time of 2 hours) that is not caused by obstructive upper-airway events—i.e., AHI <5 events/hour while using an E0470 device.

E0601 CPAP, E0470 BPAP without a backup rate, E0471 BPAP with a backup rate.
*LCD L33800 Respiratory Assist Devices. (cms.gov) https://www.cms.gov/medicare-coverage-database/view/lcd.aspx?lcdid=33800&ver=26&bc=CAAAAAAAAAAA Accessed 12/23/2021.
**Refer to RAD criteria for severe COPD in L33800 if FEV1/FVC< 70% of predicted.
***Refer to criteria for qualification of patients with OSA to receive BPAP (L33718).
LCD - Positive Airway Pressure (PAP) Devices for the Treatment of Obstructive Sleep Apnea (L33718) (cms.gov) https://www.cms.gov/medicare-coverage-database/view/lcd.aspx?LCDId=33718. Accessed 9/11/2021.
ABG, arterial blood gas; *AHI*, apnoea-hypopnea index; *COPD*, chronic obstructive pulmonary disease; *FEV1*, forced expiratory volume in the first sec; *FIO_2*, fraction of inspired oxygen; *FEV1*, forced expiratory volume in one second; *FVC*, forced vital capacity; *HST*, home sleep apnea testing; *OSA*, obstructive sleep apnea; *$PaCO_2$*, partial pressure of carbon dioxide; *PSG*, polysomnography; *mm Hg*, millimeters of mercury.

group). The second titration with BPAP started in the spontaneous mode, and BPAP-ST (backup rate) was added only for ineffective triggering, persistently low SaO_2, central apneas, or low respiratory rate. Supplemental oxygen was added only if BPAP alone (including with a backup rate) was not successful. A treatment algorithm with a similar approach for stable patients with OHS without severe OSA is shown in Figure 21–4. This prevents the need for more expensive NIV in a substantial group of patients. As discussed, the reality is that it is difficult to qualify a patient with OHS for BPAP with a backup rate with hypoventilation as an indication. In patients with OHS but without severe OSA, many will have severe OSA during REM sleep with severe hypoxia. Some of these patients will require BPAP-S, at minimum, and may need NIV. It is worth noting that some of the "CPAP failures" in the study by BaHammam et al.[82] may not have required BPAP. That is, chronic treatment with CPAP may result in improvement in gas exchange to the point that BPAP or supplemental oxygen is no longer needed.[83] *Acute CPAP failure is not equivalent to long-term CPAP failure.* Patients with modest residual hypoxemia on CPAP can often be treated with CPAP alone and close follow-up of oxygenation. A PAP titration of a patient with OHS and some degree of OSA can qualify them for the addition of supplemental oxygen if residual hypoxemia persists despite an adequate reduction of the AHI with CPAP (or BPAP).[84] For these patients, there is an option to use CPAP or BPAP with oxygen, if indicated (especially if use of BPAP-ST is not an option). However, the use of supplemental oxygen was associated with a worse prognosis in one study.[78] Optimizing the nocturnal PCO_2 with NIV (or BPAP without a backup rate, if necessary) rather than adding supplemental oxygen is preferred, if possible.

Respiratory Assistance Device (RAD) Criteria

In most RCTs comparing CPAP with NIV (Table 21–6), the term NIV was used to mean BPAP with a backup rate. BPAP without a backup rate (E0470, BPAP-S) can be reimbursed under the diagnosis of OSA if CPAP has been tried but demonstrated ineffective.[84] In the United States, BPAP *without* a backup rate can be reimbursed for the indication of hypoventilation using the RAD criteria (Table 21–7).[79] If an awake ABG test documents hypoventilation ($PaCO_2$ ≥45 mmHg) and spirometry does not show evidence of severe COPD, then a E0470 device is covered if one of the following is present: (a) an ABG test during sleep or soon after awakening shows a $PaCO_2$ ≥7 mm Hg higher than the awake PCO_2 OR, (b) a facility-based PSG or HST (Centers of Medicare and Medicaid term for HSAT) demonstrates a SaO_2 ≤88% for ≥5 minutes not caused by obstructive upper-airway events (AHI <5 events/hour). BPAP with a backup rate (E0471) can only be obtained if, *after using an E0470 device*, a daytime ABG test documents worsening of the $PaCO_2$ (≥7 mm Hg) compared to the value qualifying the patient for an E0470 OR a facility-based PSG or HST demonstrates oxygen saturation ≤88% for ≥5 minutes of nocturnal recording time (minimum recording time of 2 hours) that is not caused by obstructive upper-airway events—i.e., AHI less than 5 events/hour *while using an E0470 device*. The difficulty of obtaining a BPAP with a backup rate upon discharge from the hospital is obvious. For patients with a neuromuscular disorder, thoracic cage disorder, or COPD, a home ventilator with a backup rate can often be obtained using a diagnosis of acute or chronic respiratory failure (see Chapter 24). However, OHS is not a qualifying diagnosis. Of course, the etiology of hypoventilation is often not known for hospitalized patients (no prior

PFTs), so a diagnosis of respiratory failure associated with lung disease is not unreasonable. This difficulty of providing optimal treatment for OHS patients was addressed in a recent publication suggesting changes in Medicare RAD requirements to improve patient care.[80] If a patient was discharged on BPAP without a backup rate, titration after stabilization might be an opportunity to document the need for a backup rate.

Weight Loss and OHS

The ATS guidelines made a conditional (i.e., weak) recommendation suggesting weight-loss intervention for patients with OHS, targeting a sustained weight loss of 25% to 30% of actual body weight (including consideration of bariatric surgery).[68,85] This recommendation was based on very low-quality evidence. However, many super-obese patients with OHS would benefit greatly from bariatric surgery, which may improve diabetes and other associated medical problems as well.

NIV/BPAP Settings

If BPAP without a backup rate is to be used to augment ventilation, what values are typically used in patients with OHS? As is discussed in Chapter 24, volume target goals are typically 8 cc/kg ideal body weight or 6 cc/kg initially to allow for adaptation. In studies 2 and 4 in Table 21–6, a target tidal volume of 5 to 6 ml/kg **actual body weight** was used with an average backup rate of 14 breaths per minute. Average IPAP and EPAP values were in the ranges of 20 and 8 cm H_2O, respectively. EPAP is used to treat or prevent obstructive apnea, and the required EPAP can vary from 8 to 14 cm H_2O, depending on the patient. The lowest EPAP that will work should be used to allow provision of adequate pressure support without excessive IPAP. When converting from CPAP to BPAP, one should not use EPAP = CPAP. That is, CPAP of 16 might be converted to 20/12 (4 up and 4 down from 16) but not 24/16 unless the high EPAP is really needed. Of note, Murphy and coworkers[86] found that use of a *tidal volume of 10 ml/kg ideal body weight* produced better improvement in daytime $PaCO_2$ with chronic NIV treatment of patients with OHS. However, one must also keep in mind that adherence is probably just as important as a higher tidal volume. Starting with a lower tidal volume goal and increasing as tolerated to 10 ml/kg ideal body weight is one approach.

There is often uncertainty about which NIV settings an obese hypercapnic patient (presumed OHS) should use at home after discharge. In this setting, volume-assured pressure support (VAPS) might provide an advantage. That is, one can avoid the need to use empirically fixed IPAP and EPAP settings. Studies have compared VAPS and BPAP-ST in patients with OHS.[86-88] If the BPAP settings are chosen based on good titrations in patients with stable OHS, there is usually no advantage to VAPS over BPAP-ST. The real benefit of VAPS is to provide adequate NIV until a dedicated titration can be performed. VAPS is discussed in detail in Chapter 24. Of note, in the United States, the available VAPS devices (except for home ventilators) do not have the ability to automatically determine an optimum EPAP. Therefore, an empirically selected EPAP is required until a titration can be performed.

Close follow-up of patients with OHS started on NIV is essential to document good adherence and intervene for mask or pressure issues. In one study of patients undergoing an NIV titration in the hospital,[89] 54% of nonadherent and 20.7% of adherent patients were readmitted within 90 days. If a patient with OHS is discharged on NIV, it is imperative that they be followed closely over the first 1 to 3 months after discharge to ensure that adherence to treatment is adequate.

SUMMARY OF KEY POINTS

1. Once a diagnosis of OSA is made, two questions must be answered:
   1. Should the patient be offered treatment?
   2. What treatment is appropriate?
2. Based on the current state of evidence, the most convincing reason to treat a patient with OSA is the presence of symptoms that can be improved with treatment. These include daytime sleepiness, nonrestorative sleep, nocturia, morning headache, impaired quality of life (vitality), and bed-partner sleep and concern. The effectiveness of a given treatment depends on both efficacy (ability to lower the AHI) and adherence.
3. For mild OSA treatments include observation (if the patients is asymptomatic), positional treatment if positional OSA is present, an oral appliance or upper airway surgery. PAP can also be effective if appropriate. Weight loss is considered an adjunctive therapy if obesity is present.
4. For moderate OSA, PAP is the treatment choice but an oral appliance or surgery (including hypoglossal nerve stimulation) should be offered to the patient if PAP is not acceptable or tolerated.
5. For severe OSA PAP is the treatment of choice, but surgery is an option if PAP is not acceptable or not tolerated. Surgical options appropriate for the severity of OSA should offered. OA treatment is effective in about 25% of patients and is better than no treatment at all.
6. Observational studies and secondary analysis of RCTs (when only CPAP-adherent patients were included) examining the effect of CPAP treatment on major adverse cardiovascular and cerebrovascular events (MACCEs) have shown benefit from CPAP. RCTs with an intention to treat analysis have not documented a benefit from CPAP on MACCEs, but sleepy patients were excluded, and CPAP adherence was inadequate. A trial of patients with resistant hypertension did show a benefit, and a large meta-analysis showed a benefit from CPAP on hypertension (although the amount of reduction in blood pressure was small). Chapter 20 discusses the evidence for benefit of CPAP treatment in OSA with respect to cardiovascular and cerebrovascular outcomes.
7. Previous recommendations to treat all patients with moderate-to-severe OSA, even if asymptomatic (with a goal of reducing MACCEs), have been called into question. Many physicians still offer treatment to these patients, but they should be informed of the current state of the evidence.
8. In choosing treatment, the following should be considered: the AHI, type of study (HSAT or diagnostic portion of a split study), severity of desaturation, patient symptoms and complaints, patient preference, motivation, and financial burden. Most physicians would also consider comorbid cardiovascular conditions an indication for CPAP treatment, even if RCT evidence has not shown benefit from this therapy.
9. The effectiveness of treatment depends on both the efficacy (reduction in AHI) and the adherence. OA treatment has been shown to be as equally effective as CPAP with respect to symptomatic endpoints in mild to moderate OSA, likely due to better adherence, even though the reduction in AHI was not as reliable as that with CPAP.

10. A high index of suspicion for a possible diagnosis of OHS is indicated in all obese patients with severe OSA or severe nocturnal desaturation. A daytime ABG test is recommended ($PaCO_2$) if there is high clinical suspicion. If there is lower suspicion, a diagnosis of OHS can be ruled out by a HCO^-_3 (CO_2 on electrolytes) <27 mEq/L (or mmol/L). If the value is ≥27 mEq/L, an ABG test is recommended as this metric is sensitive but not specific for a diagnosis of OHS.

11. If a patient with **stable** OHS has severe OSA, treatment with CPAP is as effective as NIV for long-term improvement in daytime and nocturnal hypoventilation (assumes adequate adherence). Some patients may benefit from BPAP-S (no backup rate) if they have pressure intolerance or require a higher level of pressure than can be supplied by a CPAP device.

12. In unstable obese patients admitted with hypercapnic respiratory failure, NIV (BPAP-ST) during hospitalization and at discharge is recommended. After 2 to 3 months and stabilization, a diagnostic sleep study (if not previously performed) can determine whether OSA is present (and if so, the severity). The severity of hypoventilation during wakefulness and sleep can also be documented. A positive airway pressure titration should document an effective treatment for ongoing therapy. Some patients with severe OSA can be changed to treatment with CPAP or BPAP without a backup rate. Others will require continued NIV. Of patients with stable OHS and mild-to-moderate OSA, NIV treatment is recommended in the ATS guidelines. However, many of these patients will respond to CPAP or BPAP without a backup rate. In all patients with OHS, qualifying them for BPAP with a backup rate is difficult under hypoventilation RAD criteria.

13. RCTs of NIV versus CPAP in patients with OHS used target tidal volumes *of 5 to 6 ml/**actual** body weight*. Another approach would be 8 to 10 ml/kg ideal body weight (based on height). A backup rate of 14 to 15 breaths per minute was used in the RCTs.

14. CPAP "failures" of OHS treatment have been characterized as persistent hypoxemia when respiratory events have been eliminated. While many physicians treat with CPAP and supplemental oxygen, patients should be assessed after effective treatment for several months, as many will no longer require supplemental oxygen. Another approach would be to try BPAP rather than CPAP, during PAP titraton with the goal of avoiding the need for supplemental oxygen. This is especially true if significant hypoventilation is present on CPAP.

15. Adequate adherence to PAP (or NIV) treatment in patients with OHS is essential for normalization or improvement in daytime (as well as nocturnal) hypoventilation.

CLINICAL REVIEW QUESTIONS

1. A diagnostic sleep study shows an AHI of 40 events/hour and severe desaturation in a patient with a BMI of 50 kg/m^2 and an awake ABG test shows a $PaCO_2$ of 55 mm Hg and a PaO_2 of 65 mm Hg. A PAP titration shows adequate treatment at CPAP 18 cm H_2O. On this pressure, the average oxygen saturation by pulse oximetry on the final pressure was 92%. Which of the following statements is true?
   A. NIV should be used.
   B. CPAP (BPAP-ST) should be effective if adherence is adequate.
   C. If NIV is used, VAPS with a backup rate will be more effective than BPAP-ST.
   D. The addition of supplemental oxygen to PAP will likely be needed.
2. An obese male patient was hospitalized with hypercapnic respiratory failure, which was considered to be caused by OHS. He was treated with NIV with normalization of the pH, but his PCO_2 remained elevated (60 mm Hg), and he was discharged on NIV with the setting used in the hospital (BPAP 18/10 cm H_2O with a backup rate). At 3 months, he underwent a split sleep study. The patient had been adherent, and his weight had decreased by 20 pounds, with improvement of daytime $PaCO_2$ to 50 mm Hg. During the diagnostic portion, the AHI was 40 events/hour with severe desaturation. What do you recommend for the titration?
   A. Start CPAP of 10 to 12 cm H_2O with upward titration as needed.
   B. Start BPAP (IPAP/EPAP) of 12/8 cm H_2O with upward titration as needed.
   C. Start with the settings and backup rate used for outpatient treatment.
3. Which of the following statements about COMISA is **incorrect**?
   A. CBTI may improve CPAP adherence.
   B. CBTI will not be effective if depression and anxiety are present.
   C. CPAP alone is unlikely to completely address insomnia.
   D. Untreated insomnia may prevent CPAP from improving sleep quality.
4. A patient with OSA and a BMI of 33 kg/m^2 had a PSG showing an overall AHI of 20 events/hour. The AHI supine was 30 events/hour, and the AHI non-supine was 15 events/hour. He has not tolerated CPAP ("I hate CPAP."), and he declines surgical consultation. What do you recommend?
   A. A positioning device
   B. An OA, if dentition is appropriate
   C. Another trial of PAP with BPAP
   D. Weight loss
5. An obese 30-year-old salesman had an AHI of 20 events/hour on a recent PSG and has severe daytime sleepiness and hypertension. Nocturia is also an issue. He asks why you recommend CPAP treatment. The best answer is which of the following?
   A. CPAP will help you live longer.
   B. CPAP will improve your daytime sleepiness.
   C. CPAP will reduce your risk of a major adverse cardiovascular event.
   D. If you lose weight, you will not need any treatment at all.
6. A sleep study (PSG or HSAT) is indicated for all of the following **except**:
   A. After a UPPP for moderate sleep apnea.
   B. After adjustment of an OA for mild sleep apnea.
   C. After bariatric surgery, though the patient reports that he no longer snores or has breathing interruptions during sleep.
   D. In a patient doing well on CPAP treatment who has not gained weight but has not had a sleep study for 5 years.

ANSWERS

1. B. The patient has severe OSA and did well on CPAP. While the SaO_2 is lower than ideal, it will likely improve with good adherence. One could perform oximetry on CPAP at home if there is a concern that significant residual

desaturation is present on home treatment. VAPS is not more effective than BPAP-ST when a PAP titration has determined optimal settings. VAPS can be useful if the appropriate pressure settings are not known. Use of BPAP without a backup rate would be an option during the titration to improve the baseline sleeping oxygen saturation. Treatment of residual hypoventilation (trranscutaneous PCO_2) rather than addition of supplemental oxygen is preferred.

2. A. The goal of the titration is to determine whether NIV is still needed and, if so, to select an effective treatment. There are patients who may be treated effectively with CPAP if severe OSA is present. Therefore, starting with CPAP would be appropriate. If increases in CPAP (if needed) are not effective or tolerated, a change to BPAP or BPAP-ST would be appropriate. One could argue that the patient is doing well on NIV and that an NIV titration is appropriate. In reality, the device used for ongoing treatment may depend on PAP device reimbursement. If the current PAP device has already been paid for by insurance, ongoing treatment with that device (possibly at altered settings) would be the best available choice. However, the intent of the ATS guidelines would be a change to CPAP if this is adequate treatment.

3. B. A study by Sweetman et al.[59] found that CBTI in COMISA was still effective if anxiety and depression were present.

4. B. An oral appliance. The non-supine AHI is higher than acceptable for position treatment as the primary intervention. Another try of PAP treatment with BPAP would not be unreasonable, but the patient dislikes PAP. Weight loss is also reasonable but takes time and would not be a good primary treatment. Hypoglossal nerve stimulation may also be a reasonable treatment option.

5. B. Improvement in symptoms is the best documented benefit to CPAP treatment. Mortality risk due to untreated OSA is greatest in middle-aged men with severe OSA (this patient's is moderate). While weight loss would be helpful, one cannot predict how much this will improve his sleep apnea. The current scientific evidence (although flawed) has not documented that CPAP reduces the risk of a major adverse cardiovascular event.

6. D. PSG and HSAT are indicated on OA treatment (after adjustment) for all severities of sleep apnea. A patient doing well on CPAP does not need a study unless there is a clinical indication, such as worsening symptoms, snoring on CPAP, or a high residual AHI on download (machine estimate). Significant OSA is present in many patients after bariatric surgery, and PSG or HSAT is indicated.

SUGGESTED READING

1. Zinchuk A, Yaggi HK. Phenotypic subtypes of OSA: a challenge and opportunity for precision medicine. *Chest*. 2020;157(2):403-420.
2. Mokhlesi B, Masa JF, Brozek JL, et al. Evaluation and management of obesity hypoventilation syndrome. An official American Thoracic Society clinical practice guideline. *Am J Respir Crit Care Med*. 2019;200(3): e6-e24. Erratum in: *Am J Respir Crit Care Med*. 2019;200(10):1326.
3. Caples SM, Anderson WM, Calero K, Howell M, Hashmi SD. Use of polysomnography and home sleep apnea tests for the longitudinal management of obstructive sleep apnea in adults: an American Academy of Sleep Medicine clinical guidance statement. *J Clin Sleep Med*. 2021;17(6): 1287-1293.
4. Sweetman A, Lack L, Catcheside PG, et al. Cognitive and behavioral therapy for insomnia increases the use of continuous positive airway pressure therapy in obstructive sleep apnea participants with comorbid insomnia: a randomized clinical trial. *Sleep*. 2019;42(12):zsz178.
5. Sutherland K, Cistulli PA. Oral appliance therapy for obstructive sleep apnoea: state of the art. *J Clin Med*. 2019;8(12):2121.
6. Javaheri S, Martinez-Garcia MA, Campos-Rodriguez F, Muriel A, Peker Y. Continuous positive airway pressure adherence for prevention of major adverse cerebrovascular and cardiovascular events in obstructive sleep apnea. *Am J Respir Crit Care Med*. 2020;201(5):607-610.

REFERENCES

1. Epstein LJ, Kristo D, Strollo PJ Jr, et al. Adult Obstructive Sleep Apnea Task Force of the American Academy of Sleep Medicine: clinical guideline for the evaluation, management, and long-term care of obstructive sleep apnea in adults. *J Clin Sleep Med*. 2009;5:263-276.
2. Gottlieb DJ, Punjabi NM. Diagnosis and management of obstructive sleep apnea: a review. *JAMA*. 2020;323(14):1389-1400.
3. Malhotra A, Ayappa I, Ayas N, et al. Metrics of sleep apnea severity: beyond the apnea-hypopnea index. *Sleep*. 2021;44(7):zsab030.
4. Edwards BA, Redline S, Sands SA, Owens RL. More than the sum of the respiratory events: personalized medicine approaches for obstructive sleep apnea. *Am J Respir Crit Care Med*. 2019;200(6):691-703.
5. Bianchi MT, Alameddine Y, Mojica J. Apnea burden: efficacy versus effectiveness in patients using positive airway pressure. *Sleep Med*. 2014; 15(12):1579-1581.
6. Dzierzewski JM, Dautovich ND, Rybarczyk B, Taylor SA. Night-to-night fluctuations in sleep apnea severity: diagnostic and treatment implications. *J Clin Sleep Med*. 2020;16(4):539-544.
7. Punjabi NM, Patil S, Crainiceanu C, Aurora RN. Variability and misclassification of sleep apnea severity based on multi-night testing. *Chest*. 2020;158(1):365-373.
8. Azarbarzin A, Sands SA, Taranto-Montemurro L, et al. The sleep apnea-specific hypoxic burden predicts incident heart failure. *Chest*. 2020;158(2): 739-750.
9. Varga AW, Mokhlesi B. REM obstructive sleep apnea: risk for adverse health outcomes and novel treatments. *Sleep Breath*. 2019;23(2): 413-423.
10. Mokhlesi B, Finn LA, Hagen EW, et al. Obstructive sleep apnea during REM sleep and hypertension. Results of the Wisconsin Sleep Cohort. *Am J Respir Crit Care Med*. 2014;190(10):1158-1167.
11. Yu J, Zhou Z, McEvoy RD, et al. Association of positive airway pressure with cardiovascular events and death in adults with sleep apnea: a systematic review and meta-analysis. *JAMA*. 2017;318(2):156-166.
12. Pack AI, Magalang UJ, Singh B, Kuna ST, Keenan BT, Maislin G. Randomized clinical trials of cardiovascular disease in obstructive sleep apnea: understanding and overcoming bias. *Sleep*. 2021;44(2):zsaa229.
13. Wimms AJ, Kelly JL, Turnbull CD, MERGE trial investigators, et al. Continuous positive airway pressure versus standard care for the treatment of people with mild obstructive sleep apnoea (MERGE): a multicentre, randomised controlled trial. *Lancet Respir Med*. 2020;8(4):349-358.
14. Ong JC, Crawford MR, Wallace DM. Sleep apnea and insomnia: emerging evidence for effective clinical management. *Chest*. 2021;159(5): 2020-2028.
15. Sweetman A, Lack L, Catcheside PG, et al. Cognitive and behavioral therapy for insomnia increases the use of continuous positive airway pressure therapy in obstructive sleep apnea participants with comorbid insomnia: a randomized clinical trial. *Sleep*. 2019;42(12):zsz178.
16. Beninati W, Harris CD, Herold DL, Shepard JW Jr. The effect of snoring and obstructive sleep apnea on the sleep quality of bed partners. *Mayo Clin Proc*. 1999;74:955-958.
17. Punjabi NM, Caffo BS, Goodwin JL, et al. Sleep-disordered breathing and mortality: a prospective cohort study. *PloS Med*. 2009;6:e1000132.
18. Marin JM, Carrizo S, Vicente E, Agusti AGN. Long-term cardiovascular outcomes in men with obstructive sleep apnea-hypopnea with or without treatment with continuous positive airway pressure: an observational study. *Lancet*. 2005;365:1046-1053.
19. Javaheri S, Barbe F, Campos-Rodriguez F, et al. Sleep apnea: types, mechanisms, and clinical cardiovascular consequences. *J Am Coll Cardiol*. 2017;69(7):841-858.
20. Javaheri S, Martinez-Garcia MA, Campos-Rodriguez F, Muriel A, Peker Y. Continuous positive airway pressure adherence for prevention of major adverse cerebrovascular and cardiovascular events in obstructive sleep apnea. *Am J Respir Crit Care Med*. 2020;201(5):607-610.

21. Vanderveken OM, Dieltjens M, Wouters K, et al. Objective measurement of compliance during oral appliance therapy for sleep-disordered breathing. *Thorax*. 2013;68(1):91-96.
22. Phillips CL, Grunstein RR, Darendeliler MA, et al. Health outcomes of continuous positive airway pressure versus oral appliance treatment for obstructive sleep apnea: a randomized controlled trial. *Am J Respir Crit Care Med*. 2013;187(8):879-887.
23. Kent D, Stanley J, Aurora RN, et al. Referral of adults with obstructive sleep apnea for surgical consultation: an American Academy of Sleep Medicine systematic review, meta-analysis, and GRADE assessment. *J Clin Sleep Med*. 2021;17(12):2507-2531.
24. Morgenthaler TI, Kapen S, Lee-Chiong T, et al. Practice parameters for the medical therapy of obstructive sleep apnea. *Sleep*. 2006;29:1031-1035.
25. Kushida CA, Littner MR, Hirshkowitz M, et al. American Academy of Sleep Medicine Practice parameters for the use of continuous and bilevel positive airway pressure devices to treat adult patients with sleep-related breathing disorders. *Sleep*. 2006;29:375-380.
26. Patil SP, Ayappa IA, Caples SM, Kimoff RJ, Patel SR, Harrod CG. Treatment of adult obstructive sleep apnea with positive airway pressure: an American Academy of Sleep Medicine clinical practice guideline. *J Clin Sleep Med*. 2019;15(2):335-343.
27. Kushida CA, Morgenthaler TI, Littner MR, et al. American Academy of Sleep Medicine practice parameters for the treatment of snoring and obstructive sleep apnea with oral appliances: an update for 2005. *Sleep*. 2006;29:240-243.
28. Ramar K, Dort LC, Katz SG, et al. Clinical practice guideline for the treatment of obstructive sleep apnea and snoring with oral appliance therapy: an update for 2015. *J Clin Sleep Med*. 2015;11(7):773-827.
29. Aurora RN, Casey KR, Kristo D, et al. Practice parameters for the surgical modifications of the upper airway for obstructive sleep apnea in adults. *Sleep*. 2010;33:1408-1413.
30. Kent D, Stanley J, Aurora RN, et al. Referral of adults with obstructive sleep apnea for surgical consultation: an American Academy of Sleep Medicine clinical practice guideline. *J Clin Sleep Med*. 2021;17(12):2499-2505.
31. Caples SM, Anderson WM, Calero K, Howell M, Hashmi SD. Use of polysomnography and home sleep apnea tests for the longitudinal management of obstructive sleep apnea in adults: an American Academy of Sleep Medicine clinical guidance statement. *J Clin Sleep Med*. 2021;17(6):1287-1293.
32. Arterburn DE, Telem DA, Kushner RF, Courcoulas AP. Benefits and risks of bariatric surgery in adults: a review. *JAMA*. 2020;324(9):879-887.
33. Ashrafian H, Toma T, Rowland SP, et al. Bariatric surgery or non-surgical weight loss for obstructive sleep apnoea? A systematic review and comparison of meta-analyses. *Obes Surg*. 2015;25(7):1239-1250.
34. Peromaa-Haavisto P, Tuomilehto H, Kössi J, et al. Obstructive sleep apnea: the effect of bariatric surgery after 12 months. A prospective multicenter trial. *Sleep Med*. 2017;35:85-90.
35. Lettieri CJ, Eliasson AH, Greenburg DL. Persistence of obstructive sleep apnea after surgical weight loss. *J Clin Sleep Med*. 2008;4(4):333-338.
36. Cistulli PA, Armitstead J, Pepin J-L, et al. Short-term CPAP adherence in obstructive sleep apnea: a big data analysis using real world data. *Sleep Med*. 2019;59:114-116.
37. Sunwoo BY, Light M, Malhotra A. Strategies to augment adherence in the management of sleep-disordered breathing. *Respirology*. 2020;25(4):363-371.
38. Hwang D, Chang JW, Benjafield AV, et al. Effect of telemedicine education and telemonitoring on continuous positive airway pressure adherence. The Tele-OSA randomized trial. *Am J Respir Crit Care Med*. 2018;197(1):117-126.
39. Malhotra A, Crocker ME, Willes L, et al. Patient engagement using new technology to improve adherence to positive airway pressure therapy: a retrospective analysis. *Chest*. 2018;153(4):843-850.
40. Berry RB, Kryger MH, Massie CA. A novel nasal expiratory positive airway pressure (EPAP) device for the treatment of obstructive sleep apnea: a randomized controlled trial. *Sleep*. 2011;34(4):479-485.
41. Gay P, Lankford A, Diesem R, Richard R. A comparison of two nasal expiratory PAP devices for the treatment of OSA. *Chest*. 2019;156(4):A1063-A1064.
42. Sleeper G, Rashidi M, Strohl KP, et al. Comparison of expiratory pressures generated by four different EPAP devices in a laboratory bench setting. *Sleep Med*. 2022;96:87-92.
43. Hung TC, Liu TJ, Hsieh WY, et al. A novel intermittent negative air pressure device ameliorates obstructive sleep apnea syndrome in adults. *Sleep Breath*. 2019;23:849-856.
44. Omobomi O, Quan SF. Positional therapy in the management of positional obstructive sleep apnea—a review of the current literature. *Sleep Breath*. 2018;22(2):297-304.
45. Berry RB, Uhles ML, Abaluck BK, et al. NightBalance sleep position treatment device versus auto-adjusting positive airway pressure for treatment of positional obstructive sleep apnea. *J Clin Sleep Med*. 2019;15(7):947-956.
46. Levendowski DJ, Seagraves S, Popovic D, Westbrook PR. Assessment of a neck-based treatment and monitoring device for positional obstructive sleep apnea. *J Clin Sleep Med*. 2014;10(8):863-871.
47. Permut I, Diaz-Abad M, Eissam C, et al. Comparison of positional therapy to CPAP in patients with positional obstructive sleep apnea. *J Clin Sleep Med*. 2010;6:238-243.
48. Beyers J, Vanderveken OM, Kastoer C, et al. Treatment of sleep-disordered breathing with positional therapy: long-term results. *Sleep Breath*. 2019;23(4):1141-1149.
49. Sutherland K, Cistulli PA. Oral appliance therapy for obstructive sleep apnoea: state of the art. *J Clin Med*. 2019;8(12):2121.
50. Senior BA, Rosenthal L, Lumley A, Gerhardstein R, Day R. Efficacy of uvulopalatopharyngoplasty in unselected patients with mild obstructive sleep apnea. *Otolaryngol Head Neck Surg*. 2000;123(3):179-182.
51. Olson MD, Junna MR. Hypoglossal nerve stimulation therapy for the treatment of obstructive sleep apnea. *Neurotherapeutics*. 2021;18(1):91-99.
52. Heiser C, Steffen A, Boon M, et al. ADHERE registry investigators. Post-approval upper airway stimulation predictors of treatment effectiveness in the ADHERE registry. *Eur Respir J*. 2019;53(1):1801405.
53. Op de Beeck S, Wellman A, Dieltjens M, STAR Trial Investigators, et al. Endotypic mechanisms of successful hypoglossal nerve stimulation for obstructive sleep apnea. *Am J Respir Crit Care Med*. 2021;203(6):746-755.
54. Heiser C, Thaler E, Soose RJ, Woodson BT, Boon M. Technical tips during implantation of selective upper airway stimulation. *Laryngoscope*. 2018;128(3):756-762.
55. Nóbrega-Júnior JCN, de Andrade AD, de Andrade EAM, et al. Inspiratory muscle training in the severity of obstructive sleep apnea, sleep quality and excessive daytime sleepiness: a placebo-controlled, randomized trial. *Nat Sci Sleep*. 2020;12:1105-1113.
56. Guimarães KC, Drager LF, Genta PR, Marcondes BF, Lorenzi-Filho G. Effects of oropharyngeal exercises on patients with moderate obstructive sleep apnea syndrome. *Am J Respir Crit Care Med*. 2009;179(10):962-966.
57. Maghsoudipour M, Nokes B, Bosompra N-O, et al. A pilot randomized controlled trial of effect of genioglossus muscle strengthening on obstructive sleep apnea outcomes. *J Clin Med*. 2021;10(19):4554.
58. Baptista PM, de Apodaca PMR, Carrasco M, et al. Daytime neuromuscular electrical therapy of tongue muscles in improving snoring in individuals with primary snoring and mild obstructive sleep apnea. *J Clin Med*. 2021;10(9):1883.
59. Sweetman A, Lack L, McEvoy RD, et al. Effect of depression, anxiety, and stress symptoms on response to cognitive behavioral therapy for insomnia in patients with comorbid insomnia and sleep apnea: a randomized controlled trial. *J Clin Sleep Med*. 2021;17(3):545-554.
60. Taranto-Montemurro L, Messineo L, Wellman A. Targeting endotypic traits with medications for the pharmacological treatment of obstructive sleep apnea. A review of the current literature. *J Clin Med*. 2019;8(11):1846.
61. Zinchuk A, Yaggi HK. Phenotypic subtypes of OSA: a challenge and opportunity for precision medicine. *Chest*. 2020;157(2):403-420.
62. Ye L, Pien GW, Ratcliffe SJ, et al. The different clinical faces of obstructive sleep apnoea: a cluster analysis. *Eur Respir J*. 2014;44(6):1600-1607.
63. Mazzotti DR, Keenan BT, Lim DC, Gottlieb DJ, Kim J, Pack AI. Symptom subtypes of obstructive sleep apnea predict incidence of cardiovascular outcomes. *Am J Respir Crit Care Med*. 2019;200(4):493-506.
64. Bamagoos AA, Cistulli PA, Sutherland K, et al. Polysomnographic endotyping to select patients with obstructive sleep apnea for oral appliances. *Ann Am Thorac Soc*. 2019;16(11):1422-1431.
65. Edwards BA, Andara C, Landry S, et al. Upper-airway collapsibility and loop gain predict the response to oral appliance therapy in patients with obstructive sleep apnea. *Am J Respir Crit Care Med*. 2016;194(11):1413-1422.
66. Marques M, Genta PR, Azarbarzin A, et al. Structure and severity of pharyngeal obstruction determine oral appliance efficacy in sleep apnoea. *J Physiol*. 2019;597(22):5399-5410.
67. Landry SA, Joosten SA, Eckert DJ, et al. Therapeutic CPAP level predicts upper airway collapsibility in patients with obstructive sleep apnea. *Sleep*. 2017;40(6):zsx056.
68. Mokhlesi B, Masa JF, Brozek JL, et al. Evaluation and management of obesity hypoventilation syndrome. An official American Thoracic Society clinical practice guideline. *Am J Respir Crit Care Med*. 2019;200(3):e6-e24. Erratum in: *Am J Respir Crit Care Med*. 2019;200(10):1326.
69. Gómez de Terreros FJ, Cooksey JA, Sunwoo BY, et al. Clinical practice guideline summary for clinicians: evaluation and management of obesity hypoventilation syndrome. *Ann Am Thorac Soc*. 2020;17(1):11-15.

70. Piper AJ, Wang D, Yee BJ, Barnes DJ, Grunstein RR. Randomised trial of CPAP vs bilevel support in the treatment of obesity hypoventilation syndrome without severe nocturnal desaturation. *Thorax*. 2008;63(5):395-401.
71. Howard ME, Piper AJ, Stevens B, et al. A randomized controlled trial of CPAP versus non-invasive ventilation for initial treatment of obesity hypoventilation syndrome. *Thorax*. 2017;72(5):437-444.
72. Masa JF, Corral J, Alonso ML, et al.; Spanish Sleep Network. Efficacy of different treatment alternatives for obesity hypoventilation syndrome. Pickwick study. *Am J Respir Crit Care Med*. 2015;192(1):86-95.
73. Masa JF, Mokhlesi B, Benítez I, et al.; Spanish Sleep Network. Long-term clinical effectiveness of continuous positive airway pressure therapy versus non-invasive ventilation therapy in patients with obesity hypoventilation syndrome: a multicentre, open-label, randomized controlled trial. *Lancet*. 2019;393(10182):1721-1732.
74. Soghier I, Brożek JL, Afshar M, et al. Noninvasive ventilation versus CPAP as initial treatment of obesity hypoventilation syndrome. *Ann Am Thorac Soc*. 2019;16(10):1295-1303.
75. Afshar M, Brozek JL, Soghier I, et al. The role of positive airway pressure therapy in adults with obesity hypoventilation syndrome. A systematic review and meta-analysis. *Ann Am Thorac Soc*. 2020;17(3):344-360.
76. Bouloukaki I, Mermigkis C, Michelakis S, et al. The association between adherence to positive airway pressure therapy and long-term outcomes in patients with obesity hypoventilation syndrome: a prospective observational study. *J Clin Sleep Med*. 2018;14(9):1539-1550.
77. Mokhlesi B, Tulaimat A, Evans AT, et al. Impact of adherence with positive airway pressure therapy on hypercapnia in obstructive sleep apnea. *J Clin Sleep Med*. 2006;2(1):57-62.
78. Priou P, Hamel JF, Person C, et al. Long-term outcome of noninvasive positive pressure ventilation for obesity hypoventilation syndrome. *Chest*. 2010 Jul;138(1):84-90.
79. *LCD L33800 Respiratory Assist Devices*. cms.gov. Available at: https://www.cms.gov/medicare-coverage-database/view/lcd.aspx? lcdid=33800&ver=26&bc=CAAAAAAAAAAA. Accessed December 23, 2021.
80. Mokhlesi B, Won CH, Make BJ, Selim BJ, Sunwoo BY; ONMAP Technical Expert Panel. Optimal NIV Medicare access promotion: patients with hypoventilation syndromes: a technical expert panel report from the American College of Chest Physicians, the American Association for Respiratory Care, the American Academy of Sleep Medicine, and the American Thoracic Society. *Chest*. 2021;160(5):e377-e387.
81. Masa JF, Benítez I, Sánchez-Quiroga MÁ, et al.; Spanish Sleep Network. Long-term noninvasive ventilation in obesity hypoventilation syndrome without severe OSA: the Pickwick randomized controlled trial. *Chest*. 2020;158(3):1176-1186.
82. BaHammam AS, Aleissi SA, Nashwan SZ, Olaish AH, Almeneessier AS. Results of CPAP titration and short-term adherence rates in patients with obesity hypoventilation syndrome and mild/moderate obstructive sleep apnea. *Nat Sci Sleep*. 2022;14:1137-1148.
83. Lastra AC, Masa JF, Mokhlesi B. CPAP titration failure is not equivalent to long-term CPAP treatment failure in patients with obesity hypoventilation syndrome: a case series. *J Clin Sleep Med*. 2020;16(11):1975-1981.
84. LCD – Positive Airway Pressure (PAP) Devices for the Treatment of Obstructive Sleep Apnea (L33718). Available at: https://www.cms.gov/medicare-coverage-database/view/lcd.aspx?LCDId=33718. Accessed September 11, 2021.
85. Kakazu MT, Soghier I, Afshar M, et al. Weight loss interventions as treatment of obesity hypoventilation syndrome. A systematic review. *Ann Am Thorac Soc*. 2020;17(4):492-502.
86. Murphy PB, Davidson C, Hind MD, et al. Volume targeted versus pressure support non-invasive ventilation in patients with super obesity and chronic respiratory failure: a randomised controlled trial. *Thorax*. 2012;67(8):727-734.
87. Storre JH, Seuthe B, Fiechter R, et al. Average volume-assured pressure support in obesity hypoventilation: a randomized crossover trial. *Chest*. 2006;130(3):815-821.
88. Patout M, Gagnadoux F, Rabec C, et al. AVAPS-AE versus ST mode: a randomized controlled trial in patients with obesity hypoventilation syndrome. *Respirology*. 2020;25(10):1073-1081.
89. Johnson KG, Rastegar V, Scuderi N, Johnson DC, Visintainer P. PAP therapy and readmission rates after in-hospital laboratory titration polysomnography in patients with hypoventilation. *J Clin Sleep Med*. 2022;18(7):1739-1748.

Chapter 22

Medical Treatment of Obstructive Sleep Apnea Including Treatment of Residual Sleepiness With Medications

INTRODUCTION

In this chapter, we will discuss medical, positional, and upper airway muscle training treatment of obstructive sleep apnea (OSA). The use of medications to treat residual daytime sleepiness in OSA patients being treated with CPAP will also be discussed. Bariatric surgery is also included in this chapter. The American Academy of Sleep Medicine (AASM) published practice parameters for the medical treatment of OSA in 2006[1] (Table 22–1) and a clinical guideline for the evaluation, management, and long-term care of OSA in adults in 2007.[2] The treatments discussed include weight loss, oxygen, treatments for nasal patency, postural (positional) treatment, and medications for persistent sleepiness on continuous positive airway pressure (CPAP). Since these practice parameters were published, new devices and medications have become available.

WEIGHT LOSS

Obesity is a major risk factor for the development of OSA. A body mass index (BMI) of 25.0 to 29.9 kg/m^2 is considered overweight, greater than 30 is considered obesity, and greater than 40 is considered severe obesity. In some studies, approximately 70% of patients with OSA were obese (body weight > 120% of predicted). Peppard and colleagues[3] followed the effects of weight change on the apnea-hypopnea index (AHI). A 10% weight gain predicted an approximate 32% increase in the AHI. A 10% weight loss predicted a 26% reduction in the AHI. A 10% increase in weight was associated with a sixfold increase in the risk of developing moderate to severe OSA. Many studies have documented that weight loss of even modest proportions (5%–10%) can produce significant improvement in sleep apnea[4-11] and decrease upper airway collapsibility.[12] Although some patients with even mild obesity (110%–115% of ideal body weight) can benefit from weight reduction, the effectiveness of weight loss in reducing the AHI varies considerably among patients. This may be because a given amount of weight loss may have more of an effect on upper body obesity or upper airway anatomy in one individual than in another. Weight loss may also be less effective in reducing the AHI if skeletal abnormalities play a more prominent role in the pathogenesis of OSA in a given patient. An investigation by Wang and coworkers found the *loss of fat in the tongue* during weight reduction played an important role in the benefits of weight loss on the upper airway.[13]

Behavioral, surgical, and pharmacologic approaches to weight loss have all been successful in selected groups of patients. The reader is referred to the article by Saunders et al.[14] that provides a concise discussion of medications and surgical procedures used for weight loss. A major problem for behavioral, medication, and surgical weight loss has been *maintenance of weight loss*. Behavioral techniques have included low-calorie diets[5,6] and life-style intervention (healthy diet and exercise).[7-11]

Table 22–1 American Academy of Sleep Medicine Practice Parameter Recommendations for Medical Treatment of Obstructive Sleep Apnea[1]

Weight Reduction
• Successful dietary weight loss may improve the AHI in obese patients with OSA. (Guideline)
• Dietary weight loss should be combined with primary treatment of OSA. (Option)
• Bariatric surgery may be adjunctive in treatment of OSA in obese patients. (Option)
Positional Therapies
• Positional therapy, a method that keeps the patient in a nonsupine position, is an effective secondary therapy or can be a supplement to primary therapies for OSA in patients who have a low AHI in the nonsupine vs. the supine position. (Guideline)
Oxygen Supplementation
• Oxygen supplementation is not recommended as a primary treatment for OSA. (Option)
Nasal Corticosteroids
• Topical nasal corticosteroids may improve the AHI in patients with OSA and concurrent rhinitis and thus may be a useful adjunct to primary therapies for OSA. (Guideline)
Modafinil, Armodafinil
• Modafinil and Armodafinil* are recommended for treatment of residual excessive sleepiness in patients with OSA who have sleepiness despite effective PAP treatment and are lacking any other identifiable cause for their sleepiness. (Standard)
Other Treatments—Not Recommended
• Protriptyline, SSRIs, aminophylline, estrogen preparations with or without progesterone, and short-acting decongestants.

AHI, Apnea-hypopnea index; *OSA,* obstructive sleep apnea; *PAP,* positive airway pressure; *SSRIs,* selective serotonin reuptake inhibitors; *armodafinil not available until after publication of practice parameters.

A randomized controlled study of a very low-energy diet for 9 weeks in a group of patients with moderate to severe OSA and moderate obesity[5] found a decrease in body weight of 18.7 kg in the intervention group and an increase of 1.1 kg in the control group (normal diet), with corresponding decreases in the AHI of 25/hour and 2/hour (Table 22–2). The individual values for each patient are shown in Figure 22–1. In the intervention group, the percentage of body fat decreased by about 8%, and the neck circumference decreased by about 4 cm. Bariatric surgery has been proven to reliably induce weight loss, but many patients have a significant amount of residual sleep apnea.[14-18] A meta-analysis by Greenburg et al.[15] found that bariatric surgery decreased the BMI from 55.3 to 37.7 kg/m^2 and the AHI from 54.7/hour to 15.8/hour. However, 62% had a residual AHI ≥ 5/hour. The results from five studies in which individual patient data were available are shown in Table 22–3. In this group of studies, 25% of individuals treated with weight loss had normalization of the AHI. The required level of CPAP fell from 14.8 to 9.2 cm H_2O. *Of note, OSA may return even if patients maintain their body weight.*[19] The AASM practice parameters for use of medical treatments for OSA recommend that weight loss be combined with a primary treatment for OSA[1] (see Table 22–1). This recommendation is based on several facts: weight loss takes time, results vary among patients, and OSA can recur even if initially improved by weight loss. It was stated that bariatric surgery "may" be adjunctive in treatment of OSA in obese patients. Given the variable improvement in the AHI, this statement falls short of recommending bariatric surgery as a primary treatment for OSA. The American Thoracic Society also published a clinical guideline regarding the role of weight reduction in the treatment of adult OSA.[20] The panel strongly recommended that patients with OSA who are overweight or obese be treated with comprehensive lifestyle intervention consisting of (1) a reduced-calorie diet, (2) exercise or increased physical activity, and (3) behavioral guidance. Conditional recommendations were made regarding a reduced-calorie diet and exercise/increased physical activity as separate management tools. The guideline states that pharmacological therapy and bariatric surgery are appropriate for selected patients who require further assistance with weight loss. New medications to assist with weight reduction have been studied in OSA. Winslow et al.[21] evaluated the combination of phentermine 15 mg and extended release topiramate 92 mg versus placebo for 28 weeks. The treatment group had a decrease in AHI of 31.5/hour, whereas this value for the placebo group was 16.6/hour. New glucagon-like peptide-1 agonists are an effective adjunctive measure for weight loss and treatment of type 2 diabetes. The major mechanism of action is decreased appetite and energy intake. Blackman et al.[22] compared liraglutide 3.0 mg weekly versus placebo as adjunct to dietary weight loss and increased physical activity (both groups were treated with diet

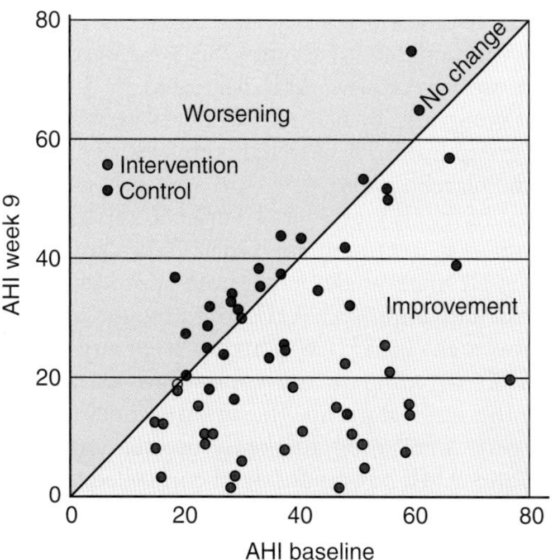

Figure 22–1 The change in the apnea-hypopnea index (AHI) after 9 weeks of control versus very-low-energy (calorie) diet. Each circle is one individual. The intervention group showed a large improvement. However, some in the control group also had some improvement. The control group saw a mean decrease in the AHI of 2/hour with small average weight gain of 1.1 kg. The intervention group had a decrease in the average AHI of 25/hour with an average weight loss of 18.7 kg. In this study, patients were randomized to a very low calorie diet or their usual diet. The order from left to right of individual patients is by increasing prestudy AHI. (Figure plotted using data from Johansson K, Neovius M, Lagerros YT, et al. Effect of a very low-energy diet on moderate and severe obstructive sleep apnoea in obese men: a randomised controlled trial. *BMJ.* 2009;339:b4609.)

Table 22–2 Very-Low-Energy Diet for 9 Weeks in Moderate to Severe OSA

	Intervention	Control
	N = 30	*N* = 33
Age (years)		
BMI (baseline) (Kg/m^2)	34.4 (2.9)	34.8 (2.9)
Change in BMI (Kg/m^2)	−5.7 (1.1)	+0.3 (0.6)*
Body weight (baseline) (Kg)	113.4 (14.8)	111.7 (13.7)
Change in body weight from baseline (kg)	−18.7 (4.1)	+1.1 (1.9)*
AHI (baseline) (events/hr)	37 (17)	37 (14)
AHI 9 weeks (events/hr)	12 (7)	35 (14)*
Change in AHI from baseline (events/hr)	−25 (17)	−2 (11)*

2.3 MJ liquid diet = about 550 kcal (or 550 dietary calories).
Results mean (standard deviation), *$P < 0.001$ intervention vs. controls.
AHI, Apnea-hypopnea index; *BMI,* body mass index.
Data from Johansson K, Neovius M, Lagerros YT, et al. Effect of a very low energy diet on moderate and severe sleep apnea in obese men: a randomised controlled trial. *BMJ.* 2009;339:b4609.

Table 22–3 Meta-analysis of Bariatric Surgery: *Data From Five Studies With Individual Data Available*

	Baseline		Follow-up	
	N	Value	*N*	Value
Weight (kg)	54	227	54	147
BMI (kg/m^2)	47	49.7	47	32.8
AHI (#/hr)	80	67.8	80	18.4
CPAP (cm H_2O)	32	14.8 (4.5)	28	9.2 (5.0)
AHI < 5 events/hr*	80			25%
AHI < 10 events/hr*	80			44%

AHI, Apnea-hypopnea index; *BMI,* body mass index; *CPAP,* continuous positive airway pressure; *following weight loss.
From Greenburg DL, Lettieri CJ, Eliasson AH. Effects of surgical weight loss on measures of obstructive sleep apnea: a meta-analysis. *Am J Med.* 2009; 122:535-542.

and increased physical activity) for 32 weeks in nondiabetic patients with moderate to severe OSA who were unwilling or unable to use CPAP. The AHI decreased by 12/hour in the treatment group and by 6.1/hour in the placebo group. The liraglutide group lost 5.7% of initial body weight compared with 4.2% in the placebo group.

Studies have also evaluated surgical versus nonsurgical weight loss as a treatment for OSA. Ashrafian et al.[23] concluded in their meta-analysis that both approaches resulted in weight loss and improved AHI. The amount of weight loss and improvement in AHI was higher after surgery. However, it is difficult to compare the approaches, as the BMI was higher in the surgical group. The authors concluded that bariatric surgery "may" offer markedly greater improvement in the BMI and AHI, but randomized controlled and comparative trials are needed. Dixon and coworkers[24] randomized patients with OSA to medical weight loss and surgery groups. The surgical group lost more weight and had a greater fall in AHI. However, the decrease in AHI was not statistically significant between the medical and surgical weight loss groups.

In the months after bariatric surgery, studies suggest CPAP adherence in patients treated with CPAP preoperatively is poor, and poor adherence to CPAP is associated with weight gain.[25] Therefore, close follow-up by the sleep physician is needed. If a sleep study after significant weight loss documents a "cure," stopping primary treatment could be considered. If significant OSA is still present, a lower level of CPAP may be effective. A PSG or HSAT is recommended after stabilization of weight loss rather than reliance on patient report of improved symptoms. Consistent with the analysis of Greenburg et al.,[15] Lettieri and associates[16] reported a reduction in required CPAP from 11.5 to 8.4 cm H_2O after weight loss (BMI dropped from 51 to 32 kg/m^2) in a group of patients undergoing bariatric surgery. However, the magnitude of this effect can vary significantly among patients. If CPAP or other treatment for OSA is stopped, patients should be followed closely for signs and symptoms of recurrence. As mentioned, OSA can return in the absence of weight gain. Of note, *weight loss may convert a patient from nonpositional OSA to positional OSA* (see discussion of positional treatment of OSA below) making positional treatment an option.[26] In one study following weight loss, a significant proportion (22%) of patients with obesity showed normalization of the nonsupine AHI. For these patients, avoidance of supine sleep may cure their OSA.

BARIATRIC SURGERY INDICATIONS AND PRECAUTIONS

As sleep physicians are often involved in the care of patients being evaluated for bariatric surgery, some familiarity with the indications and types of procedures is important. The reader is referred to the review of benefits and risks of bariatric surgery by Arterburn et al.[27] The 1991 National Institutes of Health guidelines recommend consideration of bariatric surgery in patients with a BMI of 40 kg/m^2 or higher or 35 kg/m^2 or higher with serious obesity-related comorbidities. Type 2 diabetes that has not responded to medical therapy often responds to bariatric surgery. There is increasing evidence for surgery in patients with a BMI 30 to 35 kg/m^2 if hyperglycemia cannot be controlled by medical therapy. Substantial evidence indicates that surgery results in greater improvements in weight loss and type 2 diabetes outcomes when compared with nonsurgical interventions, regardless of the type of procedures used. The two most common procedures used at the time of this writing, the sleeve gastrectomy and gastric bypass, have similar 5-year effects on weight loss, diabetes outcomes, and safety. Perioperative mortality rates range from 0.03% to 0.2%. Consensus anesthesia guidelines for patients with OSA undergoing bariatric surgery have been published.[28] "It is recommended that all bariatric patients should be screened for OSA and obesity hypoventilation syndrome (OHS) to reduce the risk of perioperative complications." Intraoperative precautions include preoxygenation, induction and intubation in ramped position, CPAP and positive end-expiratory pressure during induction, maintenance of low tidal volumes during surgery, multimodal anesthesia and analgesia with avoidance of opioids, and extubation when patients are free of neuromuscular blockage (and fully awake). CPAP therapy and continuous monitoring with a minimum of pulse oximetry is recommended in the early postoperative period. In most bariatric surgery programs, because of the high probability of the presence of OSA in obese patients, a sleep study is routinely obtained in patients being evaluated for bariatric surgery to assess the presence and severity of sleep apnea. If significant sleep apnea is present, the patient is started on PAP treatment; if this is successful and the patient is adherent, they are usually cleared for surgery with the proviso of postoperative use of PAP as soon as practical (typically with the patient's CPAP and mask), monitoring of oxygen saturation, and minimizing opioids or sedatives.[28] Patients who are CPAP naïve often do not tolerate the imposition of postoperative CPAP when apnea or desaturation are observed in the postoperative period. For this reason, identifying OSA and starting CPAP before surgery is essential. *There is evidence that CPAP mitigates opioid worsening of OSA early after bariatric surgery.*[29] Although supplemental oxygen can be used postoperatively for episodic desaturations due to OSA, this may *mask detection of the development of hypoventilation* by oximetry (depends on detection of desaturation accompanying hypoventilation). Elevation of the head of the bed may assist in maintaining an open airway. Patients with known OSA undergoing bariatric surgery should be given an effective treatment (usually CPAP) in the postoperative period and during weight loss. Patients with untreated (or unrecognized) OSA undergoing surgery could be given postoperative CPAP but may not tolerate this intervention. However, with proper monitoring, head elevation, and the minimization of sedatives, poor outcomes are rare, even in patients with untreated OSA. Some patients may require transfer to a higher level of care after periods of apnea or hypoxemia are observed. Patients with OHS are at much higher risk and often need noninvasive ventilation postoperatively and a high level of postoperative monitoring.

POSTURE AND POSITIONAL TREATMENT

The importance of sleeping position as a major factor determining the severity of OSA has been recognized for more than 25 years.[30] Positional OSA (POSA) is usually defined as a supine apnea-hypopnea index (sAHI) at least two times the nonsupine AHI (nsAHI) (Box 22–1). In studies of large groups of patients with sleep apnea about 50% had POSA,[30-32] including some with severe sleep apnea.[31] An entire night summary of a patient with positional sleep apnea is shown in Figure 22–2. In this patient, relatively few events were noted in nonsupine positions, whereas very frequent events were noted in the supine position. Note that in this patient, body position (rather than non-REM [NREM] vs. REM sleep) was

Box 22–1 POSITIONAL TREATMENT FOR SLEEP APNEA

Positional OSA defined by AHI-sup > 2 × AHI-ns
- 50%–60% of patients with OSA in some studies

- **Exclusive POSA** defined by AHI-sup > 2 × AHI ns *and* AHI-ns < 5 or 10 events/hour
  - 25%–30% of patients with OSA in some studies
- **Lateral position or elevation of the head of bed** can lower required CPAP: 3–5 cm H_2O
- **Positional Treatment** Devices
  - Bumper belt (foam or inflatable cushions), tennis ball or foam cylinder in backpack to make supine sleep uncomfortable
  - Smart devices: vibration until the patient moves from supine position, ability to track effectiveness and adherence, portal for physicians, smartphone applications for patients
  - Elevation of head of bed (can lower required CPAP level)
- **POSA device studies**
  - Devices effective in POSA (but not as effective as CPAP)
  - Better adherence than PAP in some studies
  - Long-term adherence unknown
- **Potential for combined treatment** with oral appliances, CPAP, hypoglossal nerve stimulation

AHI-sup, AHI-ns are AHI supine and nonsupine

the most important factor. A subgroup of patients with POSA have an nsAHI less than 5 or 10 events/hour (definitions vary) and are classified as having exclusive POSA (ePOSA). The prevalence of ePOSA has been estimated to be 25% to 30% and decreases with greater OSA severity and BMI. Mador and coworkers[32] found ePOSA (nsAHI < 5/hour) to be present in 49.5% of patients with mild OSA, 19.4% with moderate OSA, and 6.5% with severe OSA. A population-based study revealed that ePOSA, defined as an nsAHI < 5 events/hour, was present in 36% of individuals with OSA.[33] Positional therapy is potentially a very effective treatment for ePOSA and would benefit a substantial portion of patients with OSA.

The lateral or sitting sleeping positions have been found to reduce the AHI as well as the required effective level of CPAP.[34,35] Oksenberg et al. found the difference in optimal CPAP between the supine and lateral body postures ranged from 2.30 to 2.66 cm H_2O.[34] Neill and associates[35] found that elevation of the head by 30 degrees improved airway stability (compared with the supine position) in patients with OSA as measured by airway occlusion during sleep. In this study, the lateral sleep positioning had less of a stabilizing effect than elevation of the head. This suggests that sleeping with the head elevated may reduce the AHI more in some patients than sleeping in the lateral position.[40] In the same study, CPAP was also progressively elevated until apneas and hypopneas were abolished. The mean effective pressure was 10.4 cm H_2O in the supine position, 5.3 cm H_2O with the head elevated, and 5.5 cm H_2O in the lateral position. McEvoy and associates[36] also found a lower AHI, better oxygen saturation, and better sleep quality in the seated sleeping posture (60 degrees) compared with the supine position, and the AHI was even normalized in a significant number of patients. However, a recent randomized trial in postoperative patients did not find that the semiupright posture reduced the AHI. However, the apnea index was reduced.[37] It is important to note that there is an interaction between body position and the effect of NREM versus REM sleep on the severity of sleep apnea.[38] The highest level of CPAP is needed in the REM-supine condition. In

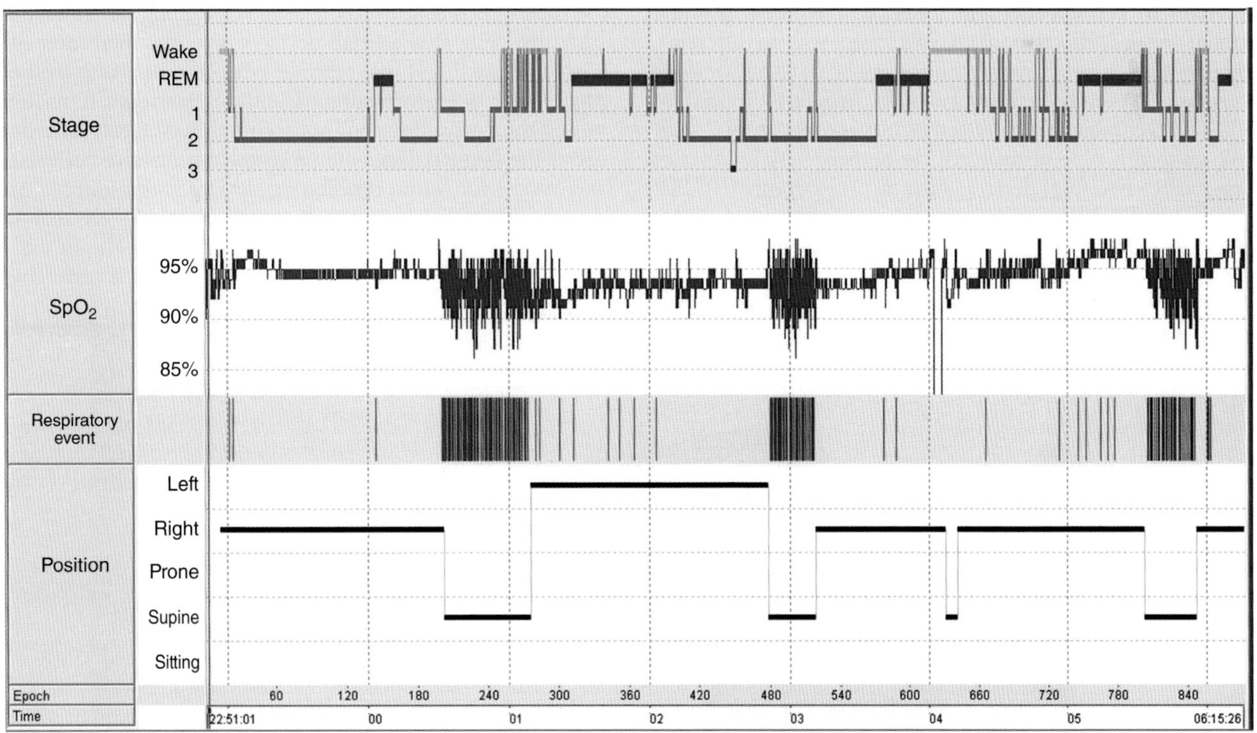

Figure 22–2 An entire night summary of a patient with exclusive positional obstructive sleep apnea. Respiratory events were much more frequent during three periods of supine sleep in which the apnea-hypopnea index (AHI) was quite increased. A few events were noted in the nonsupine positions (especially during REM sleep). Note that the supine position had a much larger influence on the arterial oxygen desaturation than periods of REM sleep.

general, the AHI is higher as follows: REM-supine > NREM-supine > REM nonsupine > > NREM-nonsupine. The physiological reason for improvement in lateral sleep in some patients is still unclear, and studies have found conflicting results, likely because of the methods used and the patient groups studied. The effect of the lateral versus supine position on upper airway size and function are discussed in chapter 19. Some, but not all, studies have found differences in upper airway size (smaller) or shape in the supine sleeping position when compared with the lateral sleeping position in patients with OSA or supine-predominant OSA. Possible worsening in upper airway patency could be due to the effect of gravity on the tissue surrounding the upper airway or to posterior movement of the tongue in the supine position. However, another study found no evidence for a movement in the tongue position to a more anterior location in the lateral versus supine position, but the upper airway was less collapsible in the lateral position.[39] Reductions in lung volume (functional residual capacity) in the supine position may also reduce upper airway size in patients with supine-predominant sleep apnea.[40]

Treatment of POSA and Positioning Devices

A growing body of literature has documented the effectiveness of positional therapy in patients with POSA.[41,42] However, *long-term* studies documenting adherence and effectiveness are needed. Very simple positioning devices can be constructed by patients from backpacks containing foam balls or cylinders. A growing number of commercial positioning devices are available for purchase (to date, none have been paid for by health insurance). The more complex devices require a physician prescription and are more expensive. A number of simple devices are available without prescription, including night shirts or straps with foam balls or cushions that prevent comfortable supine sleep.[43-45] A crossover study compared CPAP and postural treatment (foam balls in a backpack) and found that whereas postural treatment was less effective than CPAP, there was no difference in improvement in the Epworth Sleepiness Scale (ESS) or sleep architecture.[43] A study by Eijsvogel and coworkers[44] found the "tennis ball technique" to be effective, but another study found adherence to this type of treatment to be poor.[45] A number of commercially available devices such as the slumberBUMP (info@slumberBUMP.com, approximately $80) and Rematee (sold by Sleep Solutions for approximately $130 using inflatable cushions) are sold as antisnoring devices; they are probably more comfortable than the tennis ball technique but are still somewhat bulky. The best-studied positional bumper belt device making supine sleep uncomfortable is the Zzoma (Figure 22-3), manufactured by 2Z Medical (Sleep Specialists LLC), is cleared by the U.S. Food and Drug Administration (FDA) for treatment of mild to moderate sleep apnea and is available by prescription only for approximately $200. The device is a large foam block covered with a washable outer fabric that is placed on the body with a Velcro strap. Its outer surface is uneven with a large prominence that, when centered over the back, makes it uncomfortable to stay in that position. The device is assigned a Healthcare Common Procedure Coding System (HCPCS) code of E0190 (Positioning cushion/pillow/wedge, any shape or size, includes all components and accessories), but is not paid for by health insurance. However, it is a relatively inexpensive device that has been demonstrated to be effective in a randomized trial. Permut and colleagues[46] found positional treatment (Zzoma cushion device) to be as effective as CPAP as assessed by one night of polysomnography (PSG) in a group of patients with mild OSA and POSA. In this group, the overall baseline AHI was 13/hour, supine AHI was 31/hour, and nonsupine AHI was 2/hour. The proportion of patients that was able to normalize their AHI to fewer than 5 events/hour was equivalent with the positioning device (92%) and CPAP therapy (97%), Discomfort and lack of the ability to provide the clinician with information about adherence and the efficacy of the device in maintaining nonsupine sleep are two problems limiting the use of mechanical positioning devices. A new generation of devices for positional treatment is designed to address these limitations.[42,47-51] Positioning devices have been developed with the ability to buzz or vibrate when the patient assumes the supine position. The buzzing/vibration prompts the patient to change to the lateral posture. These devices can also measure adherence, and some also measure snoring intensity.[47-50]

The NightBalance (NB, a sleep positioning device manufactured by Philips) is a small device worn over the center of the chest (Figure 22-4) that vibrates when the wearer is in the supine position. Unfortunately Philips Respironics is no longer selling the device in its current form. However, extensive details about the NightBalance are presented here as the device serves as a model for future positioning devices and a number of the devices are currently in use by patients. It is likely that some version of the device will likely be available in the future. The device sold for $450 to $900 depending on the source. The de-

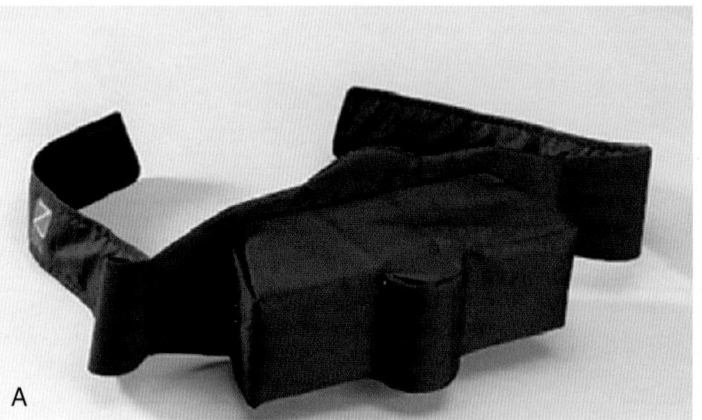

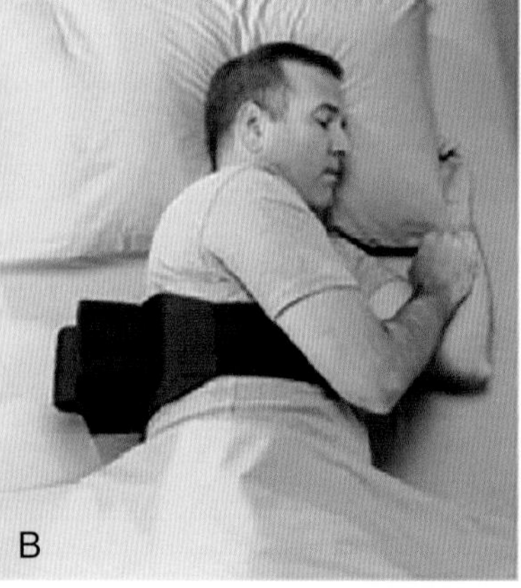

Figure 22–3 The Zzoma (Sleep Specialists, LLC, Abington, PA) is a positional treatment device consisting of a large cushion held in place by a belt. (Used with the permission of © Zzoma.)

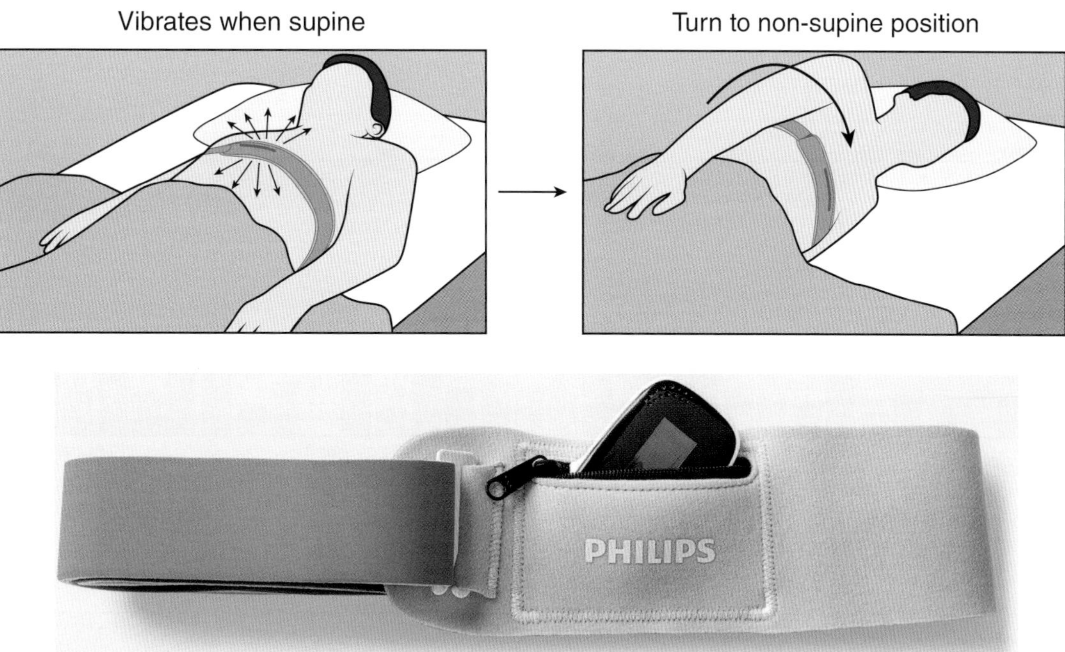

Figure 22–4 The NightBalance (Philips Respironics, Murrysville PA) device consists of a small unit held in a pocket on a belt. When the patient is in the supine position, the device vibrates until the patient moves to a non-supine position. ("Courtesy of Philips RS North America LLC." All rights reserved).

vice is placed in a pocket in a soft belt and has advanced capabilities including 2 nights of body position monitoring without vibration followed by 5 nights of a slow increase in vibration intensity (adaptation period). During the treatment period, the device delivers escalating stimulation if the supine position is maintained. The adherence time and the residual amount of time in the supine position is stored, and information is sent to a cloud portal the clinician can access (Figure 22-5). There is also a smartphone application allowing patients to follow their adherence. The cloud-based portal allows the treating physician to assess the nightly adherence (a thermal sensor in the device allows documentation of actual use versus simply turning the device on) as well as the amount of residual supine sleep (see Figure 22-5). The effectiveness of the NB has been documented in several clinical trials.[44,50,51] A randomized crossover study in patients with exclusive POSA comparing auto CPAP (APAP) and the NB (6 weeks of treatment with each device) found better adherence (345 min vs. 287 min) and noninferior efficacy (defined as an AHI noninferiority margin of 5/hour) with NB, although APAP was more effective at lowering the AHI (NB 7.3/hour vs. APAP 3.7/hour).[50] At the end of the study, about 53% of patients reported a preference for the NB. Long-term (12-month) adherence of NB treatment has been studied, and the NB adherence decreased at 12 months[51,52] but was similar to an oral appliance in one study.[51] Another study found that objective use of more than 4 hours over 6 months was 64% but a significant number of participants were lost to follow-up.[53]

The NightShift Sleep positioner (Figure 22-6) is a device manufactured by Advanced Brain Monitoring[48,49] worn around the neck or chest that vibrates when the wearer is in the supine position. The device is a "smart device" and can track adherence. The device also records snoring intensity and estimates sleep based on movement. The device information can be visualized via a smart telephone application or via a web based portal. The effectiveness of the device has been documented by clinical trials.[48,49] The Night Shift LE costs approximately $400 and requires a physician prescription. The option to wear it around the neck is because of the observation that head orientation (straight ahead vs. turned laterally) is as important as body position in some patients. The Centers for Medicare and Medicaid Services CMS has announced that it will provide reimbursement for electronic positioning devices for the treatment of sleep apnea. The HCPCS code for "Electronic Positional Obstructive Sleep Apnea Treatment" is E0530 and the total reimbursement is approximately $334 over a 13 month period. This decision will certainly stimulate the development of additional positioning treatment options in the future.

The combination of positional treatment and other treatments for OSA is a promising approach for patients with residual events after primary treatment (PAP, surgery, or an oral appliance). The approach would be especially important in those exhibiting POSA during/after the primary treatment.[54,55] As previously noted, weight loss can convert a patient from nonpositional to positional OSA. Postural interventions can be used to improve CPAP treatment. An increase in the required CPAP pressure to maintain upper airway patency is commonly required in the supine position when compared with the lateral body position. As previously noted, Oksenberg and colleagues[33] documented about a 3-cm H_2O difference in the required CPAP between supine and nonsupine postures, and Neill and associates[34] noted that significantly lower PAP was needed in the lateral position or with the head elevated. In pressure-intolerant patients undergoing CPAP treatment, one approach might be to lower the pressure to one effective in the lateral position and encourage patients to sleep in that position (or use a device to discourage supine sleep), at least during the PAP-treatment adaptation period.[55] The use of positional change is also an option during PAP titrations when

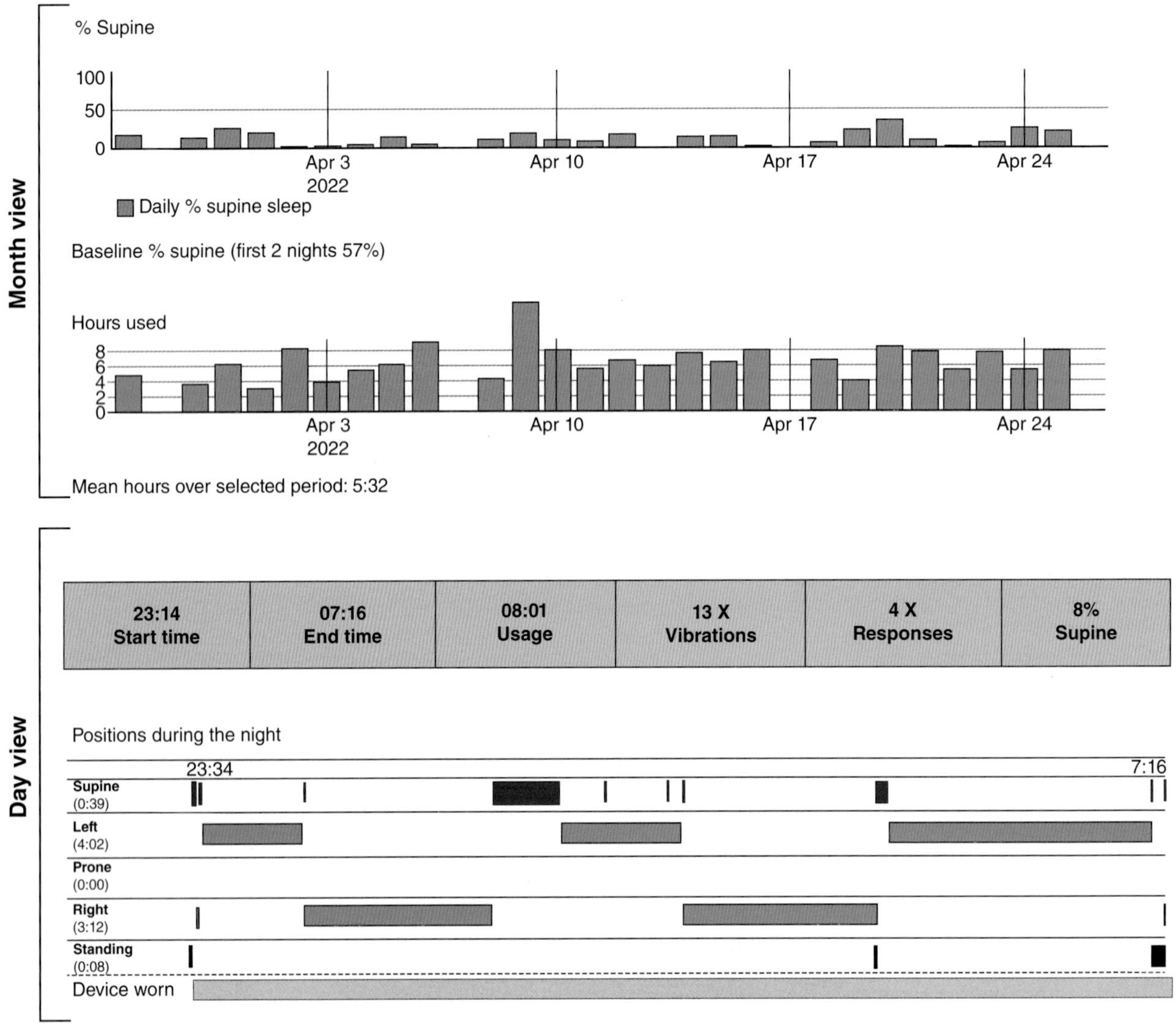

Month view

% Supine

100
50
0
Apr 3 2022
Apr 10
Apr 17
Apr 24

Daily % supine sleep

Baseline % supine (first 2 nights 57%)

Hours used

8
6
4
2
0
Apr 3 2022
Apr 10
Apr 17
Apr 24

Mean hours over selected period: 5:32

Day view

23:14 Start time	07:16 End time	08:01 Usage	13 X Vibrations	4 X Responses	8% Supine

Positions during the night

23:34
7:16
Supine (0:39)
Left (4:02)
Prone (0:00)
Right (3:12)
Standing (0:08)
Device worn

Figure 22–5 Sample information downloaded from the NightBalance portal showing tracking of adherence with both a month view and a single night detail of the body positions and the number of times the device vibrated. In this patient, adherence was good, and the amount of supine sleep was low (on the night in question, 8% of the monitoring time).

patients fail PAP titration in the supine position or do not tolerate the required pressure.[56]

To date, the addition of positional treatment to other therapy for central sleep apnea has not been evaluated by controlled studies. However, studies have noted that both primary central sleep apnea and central sleep apnea with Cheyne-Stokes respiration are worse in the supine position.[57-60] Therefore, the effect is not entirely due to alterations in patients with heart failure. The supine position appears to worsen hypoxemia after apnea,[61] which can increase ventilatory drive. Plant gain also increases in the supine position. Both of these conditions result in increased loop gain, predisposing the individual to an overshoot of ventilation and central apnea on return to sleep when the PCO_2 falls below the apneic threshold (see Chapter 30).

Medical Therapies to Improve Nasal Patency

The AASM practice parameters for medical treatments[1] of OSA do not recommend use of short-acting nasal decongestants (see Table 22–1). The major consideration is the development of rhinitis medicamentosa.[62] A study by Kiely and associates,[63] using a placebo-controlled, randomized, crossover

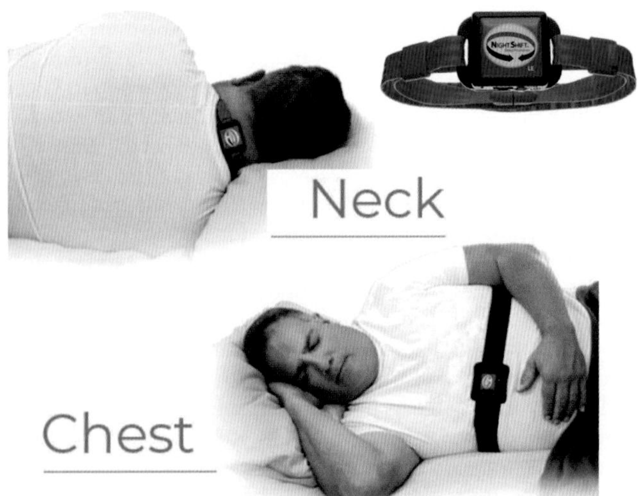

Figure 22–6 The Night Shift Sleep Positioner (Advanced Brain Monitoring, Inc). This device vibrates if the patient is in the supine position. It may be worn around the neck or attached to a belt around the chest.

design, found a modest reduction in AHI in a group of apneic snorers with intranasal fluticasone but no reduction in snoring noise in nonapneic snorers. There was no improvement in objective sleep quality. Of interest, the improvement in AHI was correlated with a reduction in nasal resistance. A treatment effect is likely only if intranasal steroids improve nasal resistance, and this change may not occur in all patients. A meta-analysis of the effect of nasal surgery on CPAP treatment found evidence of a lower required therapeutic pressure and at least short-term improvement in CPAP adherence in some patients.[64] In the absence of significant daytime symptoms due to nasal obstruction, nasal surgery is usually undertaken only in those who have failed aggressive medical treatment and in whom nasal obstruction is a cause of significant difficulty using CPAP. There may be a lower threshold for less complex procedures, such as turbinate reduction. When medical treatment of nasal obstruction is not successful, referral for otolaryngology evaluation is a reasonable option, especially if there are significant daytime symptoms due to nasal congestion.

MUSCLE TRAINING BY EXERCISE OR STIMULATION

Training the upper airway muscles to improve strength or endurance has the potential to treat OSA in patients with snoring and sleep apnea on the milder spectrum. A study by Eckert et al. of patients with untreated OSA found that **genioglossus strength was actually increased** compared with controls, but there was early fatigue, suggesting issues with endurance.[65] It should be appreciated that most forms of training target a diffuse group of upper airway muscles. Small studies have suggested that playing a wind instrument or singing may have a beneficial effect on sleep apnea. The didgeridoo is a wind instrument developed by aboriginal peoples of northern Australia that is played by continuously vibrating the lips to produce a continuous drone while using a special breathing technique called circular breathing. One controlled study found a reduction in sleep apnea and daytime sleepiness in patients playing the digeridoo.[66] Studies have evaluated the effects of inspiratory muscle training (IMT) or targeted oropharyngeal training on snoring and sleep apnea. A controlled trial of IMT for 8 weeks using 75% inspiratory maximal pressure found a small but significant reduction in the AHI.[67]

Orofacial Myofunctional Therapy

Orofacial myofunctional therapy (OMT) consists of isotonic and isometric exercises that target oral (lip, tongue) and oropharyngeal structures (soft palate, lateral pharyngeal wall).[68] A randomized controlled trial assigned patients to 3 months of daily (30-min) sham therapy or oropharyngeal exercises involving the tongue, soft palate, and lateral pharyngeal wall.[69] There was a reduction in the AHI (22.4 events/hour vs. 13.7 events/hour) and improvement in daytime sleepiness. It is likely that ongoing exercise (perhaps with reduced frequency) would be needed to maintain results. However, another study comparing IMT and OMT found that neither reduced the AHI.[70] Careful patient selection (snoring and milder OSA) and *patient motivation* are essential. Documentation/monitoring of treatment adherence (for example, using a smartphone application) is important for the success of either IMT or OMT and serves as both a reminder and motivational tool. A smartphone application has been developed for OMT.[71]

Neuromuscular Electrical Stimulation

Daytime neuromuscular electrical stimulation (NMES) of the tongue to target improvement in genioglossus endurance has also been developed, and a device has been cleared by the FDA for treatment of snoring and mild sleep apnea (ExciteOSA). The patient use a smartphone application to control stimulation for 20 minutes a day, with progressive increases over weeks in the stimulation intensity. The stimulation device fits under the tongue (Figure 22-7). A prospective cohort study[72] found that 6 weeks of training (20 min/day) reduced snoring intensity, and in a subgroup of patients with mild OSA, it reduced the AHI from 9.8 events/hour to 4.7 events/hour and the ESS from 9.1 to 5.1. Another study of NMES[73] found a reduction in snoring in

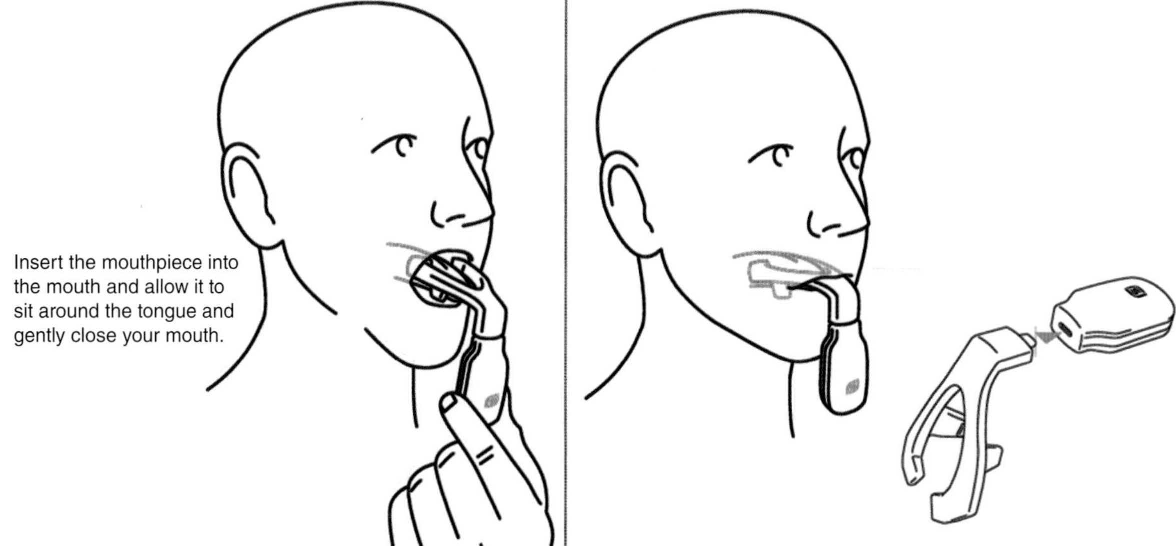

Insert the mouthpiece into
the mouth and allow it to
sit around the tongue and
gently close your mouth.

Figure 22–7 A schematic illustrating tongue training by the ExciteOSA neurostimulation device that is used 20 minutes a day to improve tongue muscle endurance. The stimulator is controlled by an application on a smartphone. The smartphone application can track adherence.

a group with snoring and mild OSA. Further clinical trials are expected in the future. The device is not currently covered by insurance plans and costs about $1700. A prescription from a physician is required. At one time dental metal bridges were a contraindication to NMES but this limitation has been removed.

In summary, muscle training of the upper airway muscles either through exercise or stimulation is promising but will likely be most beneficial for highly compliant and motivated patients with snoring and mild OSA.

SUPPLEMENTAL OXYGEN

Supplemental oxygen can improve nocturnal oxygenation in patients with OSA but has not been shown to improve daytime sleepiness or blood pressure (BP). In a study by Smith and coworkers,[74] nocturnal supplemental oxygen did not improve objective daytime sleepiness but did improve nocturnal oxygenation in a group of patients with OSA. Caution is advised in patients with hypercapnic OSA, because some may develop worsening hypercapnia, especially on high flow rates of oxygen.[75,76] In some studies, acute administration of oxygen caused prolongation of apneas.[75,77,78] In addition, supplemental oxygen, even at fairly high flow rates, may not completely prevent nocturnal desaturation (Figure 22-8). Supplemental oxygen tends to convert central and mixed apneas to obstructive apneas.[79] Loredo and colleagues[80] compared oxygen with CPAP treatment in OSA. CPAP improved sleep quality, but supplemental oxygen improved only nocturnal oxygenation. In a study by Gottlieb et al.[81] of patients with cardiovascular disease or multiple cardiovascular risk factors, the treatment of OSA with CPAP, but not with nocturnal supplemental oxygen, resulted in a significant reduction in BP. As mentioned above, supplemental oxygen often improves but does not normalize nocturnal oxygen saturation in patients with severe drops in arterial oxygen saturation.[75] In contrast to the above findings with lower flow rates of oxygen, a randomized controlled trial of high-flow supplemental oxygen (5 lpm) for 2 weeks in patients withdrawn from CPAP treatment found that oxygen abolished the early-morning rise in BP compared with sham oxygen.[82] A high flow of oxygen was chosen because other studies demonstrated an incomplete reduction in hypoxemia with a flow rate of 3 lpm. The difference in findings between this study and previous studies of oxygen in OSA could be due to the high flow rate of oxygen or the difference in the study population (patients with brief discontinuation of CPAP vs. patients with untreated OSA). The morning rise in BP in patients with well-treated OSA could be different from those with chronic untreated sleep apnea. The latter might have long-term changes in baroreceptors or other chronic changes. In addition, the study only evaluated early-morning and late-morning BP. The effect of nocturnal oxygen on 24-hour BP is unknown. As oxygen had no effect on the AHI or arousal index when not using CPAP, the authors concluded that intermittent hypoxia rather than arousals caused the morning rise in BP. The HEARTBEAT study[83] showed that CPAP had a greater improvement on most quality-of-life measures compared with nocturnal oxygen in a group of patients with known cardiovascular disease or cardiac risk factors. Some aspects of physical function improved more on oxygen, but the clinical significance is unknown. A meta-analysis of studies of the effect of oxygen in patients with OSA revealed improvement in nocturnal oxygen and a very slight improvement in AHI with a prolongation of respiratory events.[84] Supplemental oxygen can reduce the increase in ventilatory drive that occurs secondary to hypoxia from respiratory events. Supplemental oxygen has been shown to reduce loop gain and the AHI in patients with high loop gain and mild upper airway collapsibility.[85] However, although interesting, the place of oxygen in the treatment of patients with increased loop gain in routine clinical practice remains uncertain.

In summary, supplemental nocturnal oxygen is not routinely indicated for the treatment of OSA. It is possible that individual

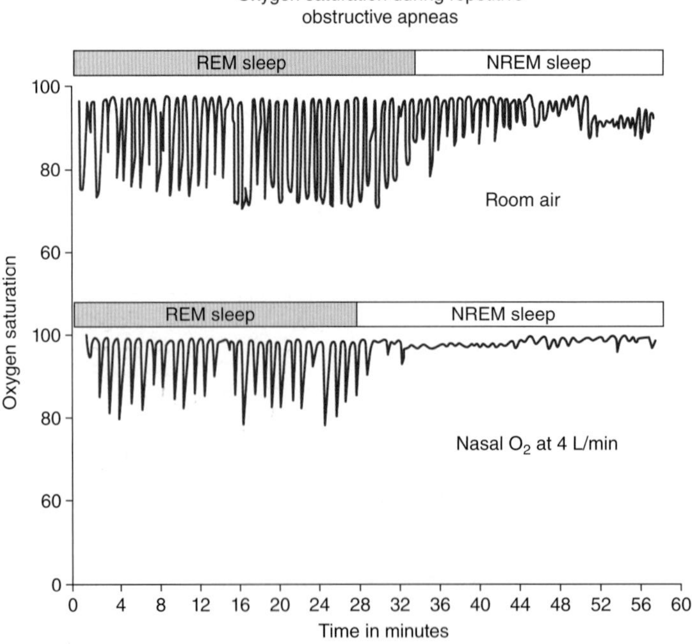

Figure 22–8 This figure illustrates the effect of high-flow supplemental oxygen in a patient with sleep apnea and chronic obstructive pulmonary disease. Even at high flow rates, significant oxygen desaturation was still present during REM sleep. The events were longer (wider individual desaturations) on supplemental oxygen during REM sleep. (From Alford NJ, Fletcher EC, Nickeson D. Acute oxygen in patients with sleep apnea and COPD. *Chest.* 1986;89[1]:30-38.)

patients might be of benefit if all other treatment options fail. The AASM practice parameters for medical treatment of OSA state that supplemental oxygen is not indicated for treatment of OSA.[1] In addition, Medicare and most insurance plans will not cover oxygen as a stand-alone treatment for sleep apnea. Even in patients on CPAP, oxygen is not covered unless a PAP titration shows that oxygen desaturation persists after reduction in the AHI to less than 5/hour by optimal PAP treatment. Requirements for coverage of the addition of supplemental oxygen to the PAP treatment of OSA is discussed in chapter 23.

PERSISTENT DAYTIME SLEEPINESS ON CPAP

A substantial number of patients with OSA continue to have residual excessive daytime sleepiness (rEDS) despite adequate PAP treatment.[86-92] In population studies, rEDS is reported in 6 % to 22% of CPAP-treated patients.[86-92] A large 6-month randomized controlled trial reported 22% of patients (overall) had rEDS after 6 months of CPAP treatment; the rate was higher among patients with CPAP use $<$ 4 hours/night (31%) compared with those with CPAP use $\geq$ 4 hours/night (18%; $P = 0.003$).[91] In those with good CPAP adherence and rEDS, only greater pretreatment subjective (higher ESS) or objective sleepiness (shorter mean sleep latency on the maintenance of wakefulness test) were predictive of rEDS. In patients with residual sleepiness, the first steps are to document adequate objective PAP adherence, document effective treatment, and to try sleep extension, if indicated.[90-93] The ICSD-3-TR[92] defines residual sleepiness in patients with adequately treated OSA as a subtype of hypersomnia due to a medical disorder.

The diagnostic criteria for Hypersomnia Due to a Medical Disorder (1 to 3 must be met) include: (1) daily periods of irrepressible need to sleep or daytime lapses in drowsiness or sleep occur for at least 3 months, (2) the daytime sleepiness occurs as a consequence of a significant underlying medical or neurological condition, and (3) symptoms and signs are not better explained by chronic insufficient sleep, a circadian rhythm sleep-wake disorder, or other current sleep disorder, mental disorder, or medication/substance use or withdrawal.

It is important to consider other causes of persistent daytime sleepiness despite adequate PAP treatment. These include inadequate sleep duration, sedating medications, depression, and other sleep disorders (narcolepsy, periodic limb movement disorder, idiopathic hypersomnia) (Box 22–2). Other sleep disorders should be ruled out if clinically indicated. Patients should be questioned about cataplexy. A long history of daytime sleepiness that began long before snoring and apnea were noted would suggest that another hypersomnia disorder is present in addition to OSA. A diagnosis of narcolepsy as well as OSA can be made by a PSG on CPAP documenting good treatment and a multiple sleep latency test (MSLT) on CPAP the following day. Objective documentation of adequate CPAP adherence before testing is essential. This approach is discussed in Chapters 17 and 32. Comorbid insomnia is an important cause of inadequate sleep duration in some patients with OSA. Referral for cognitive behavioral treatment of insomnia or pharmacological treatment is indicated (see Chapter 33). In addition, some antidepressants may cause sleep disturbance. Questions about mood and coordinating care with a patient's psychiatrist can be helpful. Effective CPAP treatment can improve mood.

Of note, although some might assume 6 hours of nightly CPAP adherence to be "good adherence," in patients with continued daytime sleepiness, the first step would be an attempt at

Box 22–2 CAUSES OF PERSISTENT EXCESSIVE DAYTIME SLEEPINESS IN TREATED OSA (HYPERSOMNIA DUE TO MEDICAL DISORDER)

- Continuous positive airway pressure (CPAP) issues: inadequate adherence, mask leak, suboptimal pressure, treatment emergent central sleep apnea
- Behaviorally insufficient sleep
- Insomnia
- Restless legs syndrome
- Narcolepsy or idiopathic hypersomnia
- Obesity
- Sedating medications
- Circadian rhythm disorders (shift work)
- Depression and anxiety

Adapted from reference by Javaheri S., Javaheri S. Update on persistent excessive sleepiness in OSA. *Chest.* 2020;158(2):776-786.

sleep extension to 7 hours.[90-93] The ESS continues to improve with increased CPAP use duration from 6 to 7 hours (Figure 22-9).[94] *The need for daytime naps should raise suspicion of inadequate sleep at night.* The burden of sleep apnea may increase as the night progresses, particularly in patients with REM-predominant OSA. One study found that, despite having two times lower overall AHI, patients with REM-predominant OSA present with similar daytime sleepiness as those with REM-independent OSA[95]. Daily sleepiness may be more strongly associated with apneas/hypopneas occurring in REM sleep than those occurring in NREM sleep. The length of apneas or hypoxic burden may increase during REM sleep.[96] Some patients, therefore, may have undertreated REM-predominant OSA if they remove their CPAP partway through the night and are untreated in the final portion of the night when REM sleep predominates. They may be achieving adequate PAP use to satisfy insurance adherence criteria, yet undertreated REM-predominant OSA could contribute to EDS. Adequacy of pressure should also be documented, because a surprisingly high percentage of patients remain inadequately treated.[97] Many PAP devices give an estimate of the residual AHI. However, the estimated AHI is not always accurate. An empirical increase in pressure or a repeat PAP titration is indicated if

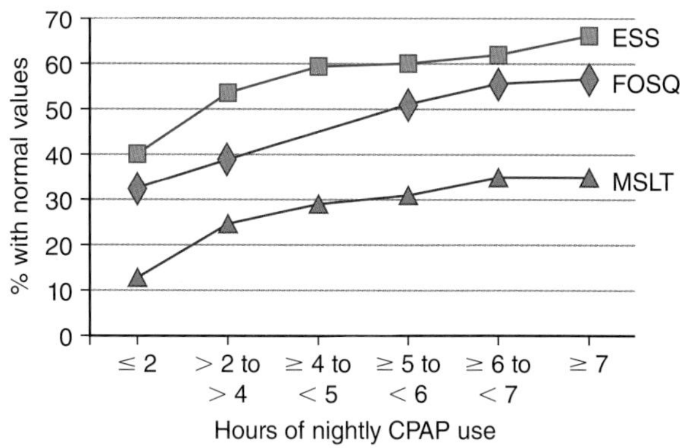

Figure 22–9 Improvements in the Epworth Sleepiness Scale (ESS), the multiple sleep latency test (MSLT; longer latency better), and functional outcomes of sleep questionnaire (FOSQ) showing continued improvement over the range of average nightly CPAP use. While significant improvement occurred with 4 hours of use, maximal benefit required 6 to 7 hours of adherence. (From Weaver TE, Maislin G, Dinges DF, et al. Relationship between hours of CPAP use and achieving normal levels of sleepiness and daily functioning. *Sleep.* 2007;30[6]:711-719.)

there is any suspicion that the current level of CPAP is not effective. A PAP titration may also be useful for identifying other factors, such as mouth leak or mask leak, that reduce the restorative nature of sleep by causing repeated arousals.

The cause of the residual sleepiness in CPAP-treated patients without another explanation for the sleepiness is unknown. One study found that obesity alone without sleep apnea can cause daytime sleepiness.[98] Possible causes include damage to wake/alerting brain areas by long-term intermittent hypoxia, leading to activation of the inflammatory cascade, oxidative stress, and sleep fragmentation; this results in apoptosis/gliosis in the neurons of the arousal system.[87,99] Shifts in melatonin secretion and alteration in the microbiome are also hypothesized to be causes of persistent sleepiness in CPAP-treated patients with OSA.[86] One study found changes in the brain white matter in patients with rEDS.[99]

Koutsourelakis et al.[100] found predictors of residual sleepiness after adequate CPAP treatment to include higher pretreatment EDS, diabetes, heart disease, and a lower AHI at baseline. The finding that a lower AHI was associated with rEDS may seem counterintuitive, but this may simply mean that the daytime sleepiness is not due entirely to OSA and therefore may not respond to CPAP. Many patients with narcolepsy and idiopathic hypersomnia have very mild OSA, which is often an incidental finding. A study by Vernet et al.[101] compared patients on CPAP with and without rEDS. The patients with rEDS had more fatigue, lower stage N3 percentages, more periodic leg movements (without arousals), lower mean sleep latencies, and longer daytime sleep periods.

TREATMENT OF RESIDUAL SLEEPINESS IN OSA PATIENTS ON CPAP

Modafinil, Armodafinil, Solriamfetol, and Stimulants

If daytime sleepiness persists on optimized OSA treatment (usually CPAP) and there is no identifiable additional sleep disorder/cause of sleepiness, treatment with an alerting agent is indicated. There are now three FDA-approved medications for this indication (these are also approved for treatment of sleepiness due to narcolepsy): modafinil, armodafinil, and solriamfetol (Table 22–4). These medications are Schedule IV controlled substances (refills are allowed). Additional discussion of these

Table 22–4 Alerting Medications

Drug	Tmax	Half-life	Metabolism	Elimination/ Excretion	Mechanism of Action	Drug Interactions	Side Effects
Modafinil (Schedule IV)	2–4 hrs	15 hrs*	Hepatic amide hydrolysis and CYP P450 enzymes Reduce dose in hepatic impairment	Elimination mainly by hepatic metabolism Renal (only 10% of parent drug and about 80% of metabolites are excreted in the urine	Dopamine reuptake inhibitor	Hormonal contraceptive and other medications metabolized by CYP3A4†	Headache, nausea, diarrhea, dizziness, anxiety, serious drug rash (Stevens-Johnson)
Armodafinil (Schedule IV)	Same	15 hrs	Same	Same	Same	Same	Same as modafinil and insomnia
Solriamfetol (Schedule IV)	2 hrs fasted 3 hrs high-fat meal	7.1 hrs	Primarily excreted unchanged	Renal Reduce dose with renal insufficiency Do not use in end-stage renal disease	Dopamine and norepinephrine reuptake inhibitor	Contraindicated with MAOIs No other significant interactions	Increased HR and BP, headache, nausea, decreased appetite, anxiety, diarrhea, dry mouth
Pitolisant‡ (no schedule)	3 hrs	10–12 hrs	CYP P450 enzymes CYP3A4, CYP2D6	Extensive hepatic metabolism, renal excretion of inactive metabolite, reduce dose with hepatic impairment	Antagonist/ inverse agonist at presynaptic H3 autoreceptors	Hormonal contraceptive and other medications metabolized by CYP3A4	Increased QT interval insomnia, anxiety, nausea

*L-Modafinil half-life 3–4 hrs; R-modafinil 10–14 hrs.

†The clearance of drugs that are substrates for CYP3A4/5 (e.g., steroidal contraceptives, cyclosporine, midazolam, and triazolam) may be increased by modafinil (or armodafinil) via induction of metabolic enzymes, which results in lower systemic exposure. The effectiveness of steroidal contraceptives may be reduced when used with modafinil and for 1 month after discontinuation of therapy. Alternative or concomitant methods of contraception are recommended for patients taking steroidal contraceptives (e.g., ethinyl estradiol) when treated concomitantly with modafinil and for 1 month after discontinuation of armodafinil treatment. Elimination of drugs that are substrates for CYP2C19 (e.g., phenytoin, diazepam, propranolol, omeprazole, and clomipramine) may be prolonged by armodafinil via inhibition of metabolic enzymes, with resultant higher systemic exposure.

‡Not currently approved for residual sleepiness in OSA.

BP, Blood pressure; *HR,* heart rate; *MAOIs,* monoamine oxidase inhibitors.

Adapted from Javaheri S, Javaheri S. Update on persistent excessive sleepiness in OSA. *Chest.* 2020;158(2):776-786.

medications is available in Chapter 32. The brand names are Provigil for modafinil, Nuvigil for armodafinil and Sunosi for solriamfetol. Generic versions of modafinil and armodafinil are available. Solriamfetol is only available in the brand name formulation (Sunosi). If a patient does not respond to one medication, another in this group should be tried. If patients do not respond to these medications, traditional stimulants can be used off-label. Pitolisant (Wakix) is another nonstimulant medication potentially useful for persistent sleepiness in OSA. The medication is approved by the FDA for sleepiness and cataplexy in narcolepsy, but at the time of writing it is not currently approved for residual sleepiness in adequately treated OSA patients in the United States. Pitolisant is not available in a generic form.

Modafinil (racemic contains L and R enantiomers) and armodafinil (R enantiomer) are dopamine reuptake inhibitors, and solriamfetol is both a dopamine and norepinephrine reuptake inhibitor. Modafinil and armodafinil are approved by the FDA for narcolepsy, residual sleepiness in OSA, and sleepiness in shift-work disorder. Modafinil can be dosed once daily, but many patients do better with a split dose (morning and early afternoon). The L enantiomer is rapidly metabolized, whereas the R enantiomer has a long duration of action and a three-times greater affinity for the dopamine transporter than the L enantiomer.[102] Armodafinil is the longer-acting R enantiomer of modafinil and is dosed once daily. There are patients who respond to armodafinil after treatment failure with modafinil. Generic formulations of armodafinil are now available in the US.

Randomized controlled trials have demonstrated that both modafinil and armodafinil improve subjective alertness (lower ESS) or objective sleepiness (longer sleep latency on the maintenance of wakefulness test [MWT] or the MSLT) in patients with OSA still sleepy on CPAP.[103-116] While treating patients with OSA using modafinil or armodafinil, it is essential to document continued adequate adherence to PAP treatment. In a randomized study comparing modafinil and placebo in patients using CPAP, Kingshott et al. found a small decrease in CPAP adherence (12 min) among patients randomized to modafinil.[109] Patients with OSA who are adherent to PAP treatment will sometimes not be able to use CPAP for various reasons. A study by Williams and coworkers[114] documented that use of modafinil did help patients to function in that circumstance. Unfortunately, the addition of modafinil has minimal or modest benefits in a significant number of patients with OSA who are still sleepy on PAP treatment. Kingshott and colleagues[109] found no improvement in ESS or MSLT with modafinil but did find an improvement in MWT sleep latency. The European Medicines Agency has restricted the use of modafinil to treatment of narcolepsy—not for persistent sleepiness in OSA.[103] The decision was made based on the risk-benefit ratio after review of a limited number of studies.[104-106] The most common side effects from modafinil include headache, nausea, dizziness, anxiety, indigestion, or nasal symptoms. Stevens-Johnson syndrome, a potentially life-threatening skin and mucosal condition, rarely can occur with modafinil use. Patients should stop the medication at the first sign of a rash. The medication alters the function of certain hepatic enzymes and can change the metabolism of components of oral contraceptives. Patients taking modafinil or armodafinil should not rely on oral contraceptives alone for birth control (for up to 1 month after stopping modafinil or armodafinil). Modafinil is available in 100 mg and 200 mg tablets. *The FDA recommended dose for modafinil is 200 mg in the morning.* The FDA prescribing information states, "Doses up to 400 mg/day, given as a single dose, have been well tolerated, but there is no consistent evidence that this dose confers additional benefit beyond that of the 200 mg dose." However, some patients benefit from the higher dose. Figure 22–10 shows the effects of 200 mg and 400 mg doses of modafinil on the ESS (subjective sleepiness) and sleep latency on the MWT (objective sleepiness) in a group of patients with OSA and residual sleepiness on CPAP.[104] Both doses improved subjective and objective sleepiness compared with placebo, but there was no difference between the two doses. Some insurance providers will only pay for 200 mg daily. However, as noted above, some patients will respond better to 400 mg daily. Splitting the dose may work better in some patients. This is likely due to rapid metabolism of the R enantiomer in some patients. Therefore, 100 mg two times daily or 200 mg two times daily, with the second dose given in the early afternoon, may be more effective in some patients.[117] Now that generic armodafinil is available, use of this medication rather than a split does of modafinil may be a better option. Modafinil can increase the levels of citalopram or escitalopram, but as escitalopram is used at a lower dose, this is less of an issue. High levels of citalopram can increase the QT interval. Armodafinil comes in 50 mg, 150 mg, 200 mg, and 250 mg tablets, and the usual dose is 150 to 250 mg daily.[111-113] In a meta-analysis of studies of modafinil and armodafinil, Kuan and

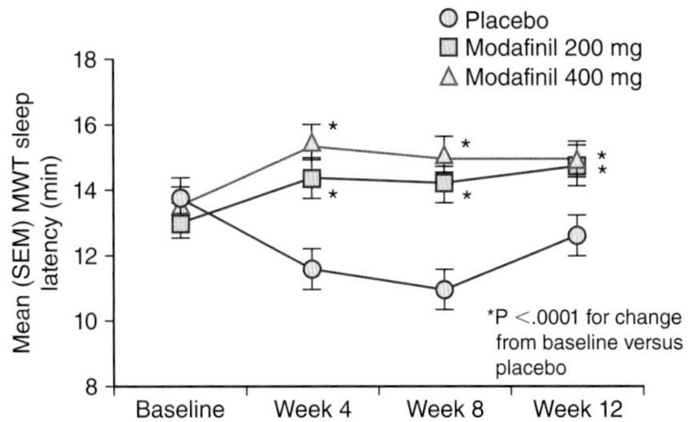

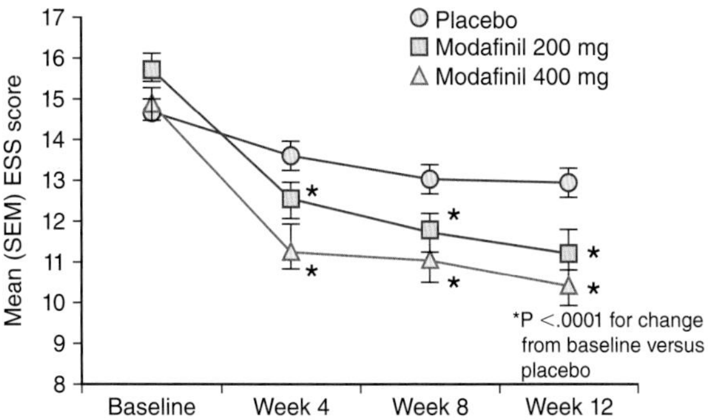

Figure 22–10 The effects of two doses of modafinil on subjective sleepiness (Epworth Sleepiness Score [ESS], lower value better) and objective sleepiness (sleep latency on the maintenance of wakefulness test [MWT], higher value better) in a group of patients with obstructive sleep apnea and residual sleepiness on CPAP. Both doses improved subjective and objective sleepiness compared to placebo, but there was no significant difference between doses. *SEM*, standard error of the mean. (From Black JE, Hirshkowitz M. Modafinil for treatment of residual excessive sleepiness in nasal continuous positive airway pressure-treated obstructive sleep apnea/hypopnea syndrome. *Sleep.* 2005;28[4]:464-471.)

coworkers[115] found that the medications reduced the ESS when compared with placebo by about 3 points (Figure 22-11) and increased sleep latency on the MWT when compared with placebo by about 2.5 minutes (Figure 22-12). The effects of 200 mg and 400 mg of modafinil were similar. Other meta-analyses of the effects of armodafinil and modafinil have found similar results.[103,116]

Solriamfetol

Solriamfetol (Sunosi) is a dopamine/norepinephrine reuptake inhibitor approved by the FDA for treatment of sleepiness in narcolepsy and OSA with residual sleepiness. It has been demonstrated to effectively improve subjective (ESS) and objective sleepiness (MWT latency) and quality-of-life measures in both short-term and long-term studies.[118,119] The medication is available in 75 mg scored tablets and 150 mg tablets. For sleep apnea, the starting dose for OSA is 37.5 mg (75 mg in narcolepsy), and the dose can be increased in ≥3-day intervals to 150 mg. Meta-analysis of the effects of solriamfetol have shown a 4- to 5-point improvement in the ESS (compared with placebo) (see Figure 22-11) and about a 10-minute increase in sleep latency on the MWT (see Figure 22-12). Meta-analyses of modafinil, armodafinil, and solriamfetol studies (indirect comparison) have documented a greater decrease in the ESS and greater increase in MWT sleep latency with solriamfetol than with modafinil or armodafinil.[120] A retrospective analysis of clinical trials[121] showed that about 71% of patients with OSA taking the 150 mg dose of solriamfetol achieved a normal ESS (≤10) compared with 38% taking placebo (baseline ESS about 16). In a study of modafinil 200 mg, Black et al.[105] found that 38% of patients with OSA achieved an ESS < 10 (compared with 17% taking placebo, baseline ESS about 16). *No studies have directly compared the two medications.* Studies have not shown a reduction in PAP use to be associated with use of solriamfetol. However, the previous finding of a lower PAP compliance with modafinil was small and not clinically significant. The most common side effects of solriamfetol include headache, nausea, decreased appetite, anxiety, diarrhea, and dry mouth. **Use of the medication is contraindicated in patients on a monoamine oxidase inhibitor (MAOI) or within 14 days of discontinuing the MAOI medication.** The medication is primarily excreted renally. No dosage adjustment is recommended in patients with mild renal disease but is needed for moderate impairment. *Use of solriamfetol is not recommend in end-stage renal disease.* An average of 21% of solriamfetol is removed by hemodialysis. Caution is indicated in patients with mental disorders. Solriamfetol can increase BP and heart rate, and the effects of the medication should be monitored. *The renal excretion is an advantage over modafinil, armodafinil, and pitolisant, which have a number of potential drug interactions due to P450 hepatic enzyme alterations* (e.g., oral contraceptives). Solriamfetol does not affect the metabolism of oral contraceptives. If a patient does not respond to modafinil or armodafinil, then a trial of solriamfetol is indicated. The major downside of solriamfetol use is the greater cost (no generic formulation available).

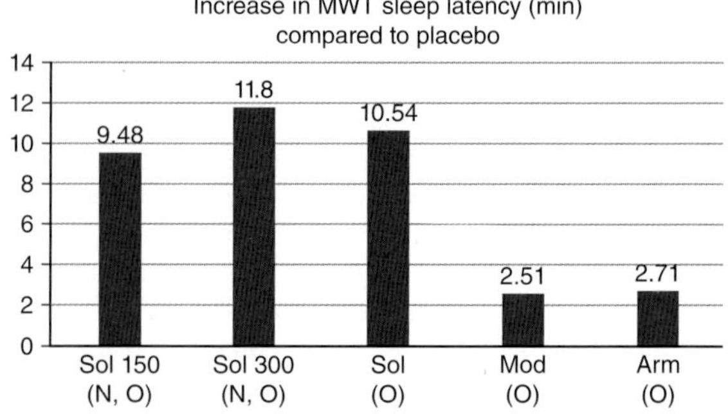

Figure 22–12 Increases in the sleep latency on maintenance of wakefulness testing (MWT) compared to placebo on solriamfetol (Sol), modafinil (Mod) and armodafinil (Arm) for patients with sleep apnea and residual sleepiness on CPAP (O) and narcolepsy (N). [Sol 150 (N,O)] is the result for 150 mg of solriamfetol from a meta-analysis of studies of (O) and (N) patients. [Sol 300 (N,O)] is the result for 300 mg of solriamfetol from meta-analysis of studies of (O) and (N) patients. [Sol (O)] is the result of a meta-analysis of studies of (O) patients on multiple doses of solriamfetol (37.5, 75, 150, and 300 mg). [Mod (O)] is from a meta-analysis of studies of (O) patients using 200 mg or 400 mg of modafinil or both. [Arm (O)] is from a meta-analysis of studies of (O) patients using multiple doses (150, 200, and 250 mg) of armodafinil. Note that the maximum FDA-approved dose for solriamfetol is 150 mg. (Modafinil and armodafinil data from Kuan YC, Wu D, Huang KW, et al. Effects of modafinil and armodafinil in patients with obstructive sleep apnea: a meta-analysis of randomized controlled trials. *Clin Ther.* 2016;38[4]:874-888; solriamfetol data from Subedi R, Singh R, Thakur RK, K C B, Jha D, Ray BK. Efficacy and safety of solriamfetol for excessive daytime sleepiness in narcolepsy and obstructive sleep apnea: a systematic review and meta-analysis of clinical trials. *Sleep Med.* 2020;75:510-521.)

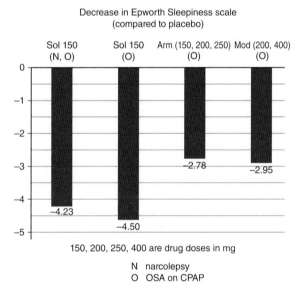

Figure 22–11 Decrease in Epworth Sleepiness Scale (ESS) compared to placebo with solriamfetol (Sol), armodafinil (Arm), and modafinil (Mod) in patients with residual sleepiness on CPAP (O) and narcolepsy (N). The [Sol 150 (N,O)] result is from a meta-analysis of studies using 150 mg of solriamfetol in (N) and (O) patients. The [Sol 150 (O)] result is from a study using 150 mg of solriamfetol in a group of (O) patients. The [Arm 150,200 250 (O)] and [Mod 200,400 (O)] results are from a meta-analysis of the effects of armodafinil and modafinil in (O) patients at the doses shown. The meta-analysis of armodafinil and modafinil combined studies with multiple doses. Most studies have shown minimal difference in the effect on the ESS between 200 mg and 400 mg modafinil doses. (Modafinil and Armodafinil data from Kuan YC, Wu D, Huang KW, et al. Effects of modafinil and armodafinil in patients with obstructive sleep apnea: a meta-analysis of randomized controlled trials. *Clin Ther.* 2016;38(4):874-888; Sol 150 mg (N, O) data for patients with narcolepsy and OSA from Subedi R, Singh R, Thakur RK, K C B, Jha D, Ray BK. Efficacy and safety of solriamfetol for excessive daytime sleepiness in narcolepsy and obstructive sleep apnea: a systematic review and meta-analysis of clinical trials. *Sleep Med.* 2020;75:510-521; Sol 150 mg (O) data for patients with OSA from Schweitzer PK, Rosenberg R, Zammit GK, et al. Solriamfetol for excessive sleepiness in obstructive sleep apnea (TONES 3). A randomized controlled trial. *Am J Respir Crit Care Med.* 2019;199[11]:1421-1431.)

Pitolisant

As noted above, pitolisant (Wakix) is a medication approved by the FDA for treatment of sleepiness and cataplexy in narcolepsy. Some studies suggest the medication may improve sleepiness in OSA as an adjunct to CPAP,[122-125] but the medication is NOT approved by the FDA for that indication. It is approved by European Medicine Agency for treatment of sleepiness in OSA in Europe. The medication is supplied in 4.45 mg and 17.8 mg tablets. Recommended dosing in narcolepsy is as follows: week 1 (8.9 mg daily), week 2 (increase to 17.8 mg daily), week 3 (may increase to maximum recommended dose of 35.6 mg daily). Pitolisant is a selective H3-receptor antagonist/inverse agonist that binds with the H3 receptor, an inhibitory autoreceptor on the presynaptic neurons of the tuberomammillary nuclei, increasing histamine synthesis and release. The medication also binds heteroreceptors (autoreceptors on other monoamine neurons). It may also result in an increase in other excitatory neurotransmitters. It differs from the other medications mentioned in that *it has low abuse potential and is not a controlled substance.* The medication could potentially be used in a patient with OSA and a history of drug abuse. The medication is hepatically metabolized and has potential drug interactions with medications undergoing hepatic metabolism (including oral contraceptives). Side effects include mild headache (16%), insomnia (8%), anxiety (4%), depression (2%), hallucinations (2%), and vertigo (1%). *Pitolisant may reduce the efficacy of hormonal contraception, including up to 21 days after its discontinuation.* In addition, pitolisant can increase the QT interval and it should not be recommended in patients with a long QT interval; it should be used with caution in patients already taking medications that can increase the QT interval. It may be prudent to check the QT interval in patients using the medication. Pitolisant should not be used in individuals with severe hepatic impairment. In patients with moderate hepatic impairment use 8.9 mg of pitolisant for the initial dose with titration to maximum of 17.8 mg after 14 days. In patients with moderate to severe renal impairment start at 8.9 mg to maximum of 17.8 mg after 7 days. Pitolisant is not recommended for patients with end-stage renal disease.

Armodafinil, modafinil, solriamfetol, and pitolisant are not recommended for use during pregnancy. Although stimulants (methylphenidate, dextroamphetamine) are not approved by the FDA nor recommended in the AASM practice parameters for treatment of persistent sleepiness in OSA, there are individual patients with persistent daytime sleepiness despite adequate PAP treatment who will respond better to stimulants than to modafinil or armodafinil. In this situation, either solriamfetol or traditional stimulants ("off-label") could be tried. If clinically indicated, the possibility of coexistent narcolepsy should be ruled out. Stimulants have a higher risk of abuse (Schedule II medications), and refills are not allowed. Patients should be educated about the side effects and risks involved with these medications. Further discussion of methylphenidate and amphetamines is provided in Chapter 32.

FUTURE MEDICAL INTERVENTIONS FOR SLEEP APNEA

Research studies have explored the use of interventions to target some of the endotypes of OSA.[126-133] In general, a narrow and collapsible upper airway, high loop gain, a low arousal threshold, and poor upper airway muscle responsiveness to negative upper airway pressure and/or a large decrease in genioglossus and other upper airway muscle activity on transition from wakefulness to sleep are major factors in the pathogenesis of sleep apnea. For example, acetazolamide and oxygen have been used to lower loop gain.[127,128] For a decreased arousal threshold, trazodone and benzodiazepines have been explored.[128,129] For decreased upper airway muscle responses, combinations of medications increasing norepinephrine signaling and decreasing cholinergic inhibition during REM sleep (atomoxetine combined with oxybutynin or aroxybutnin) have been tried.[130-132] A narrow and collapsible upper airway could be targeted by weight loss, avoidance of the supine position (positional therapy), and minimizing rostral fluid shift in the recumbent position. Studies suggest that there is a rostral fluid shift (from the extremities to the neck) in the recumbent position that could cause edema in the area around the upper airway, which could produce narrowing.[133] Use of diuretics or other methods to reduce the rostral fluid shift from the lower extremities (compression stockings worn during the day) might improve sleep apnea in selected patients. Combination treatment such as use of positional treatment with an oral appliance is another potential approach to therapy for OSA. A detailed discussion of the new investigational treatments for sleep apnea is beyond the scope of this chapter, but the reader should be aware of the ongoing research on medications and other interventions to target specific causes of sleep apnea that may be more prominent in a given individual (precision medicine).

SUMMARY OF KEY POINTS

1. Mild to moderate weight loss can reduce the AHI, but weight loss takes time and has variable effects on different patients. Weight loss is considered adjunctive therapy for OSA. Maintenance of weight loss is an important issue.
2. Bariatric surgery results in significant weight loss that can significantly reduce the AHI. However, the majority of patients with presurgery OSA continue to require treatment after weight loss stabilizes. Normalization of the AHI must be objectively proven (sleep study) before treatment is discontinued. If OSA persists, the required level of CPAP is often lower. OSA can return, even in the absence of weight gain.
3. Positional therapy can be effective in patients with POSA, and new devices are more comfortable and can track adherence. However, long-term studies of adherence and effectiveness are lacking. Sleep in the lateral position or with the head elevated can reduce the level of CPAP required to keep the airway open. There is some evidence that avoiding the supine position may be helpful in central sleep apnea.
4. Oxygen is not recommended as a stand-alone treatment for OSA. Some patients may need the addition of oxygen to PAP, but this should be documented by a PAP titration showing persistent hypoxia after PAP is optimized. In severe OSA, administration of oxygen alone may not eliminate desaturation and may lengthen respiratory events or worsen hypoventilation.
5. Modafinil, armodafinil, and solriamfetol are FDA approved for treatment of rEDS in patients with OSA on effective CPAP treatment (good adherence and residual AHI at goal). Some OSA patients require 7 hours of nightly use of CPAP for maximal benefit. Other sleep disorders, including insufficient sleep, must be ruled out. Stimulants can be effective but are off-label for treatment of residual sleepiness in OSA patients on CPAP.
6. Seven hours of nightly CPAP use may be needed for maximal improvement in daytime sleepiness. Continued adherence to CPAP should be documented after starting an alerting agent.

7. If narcolepsy is suspected after effective treatment of OSA is documented, a PSG on effective CPAP followed by an MSLT on CPAP can be used to document the presence of narcolepsy in addition to OSA.
8. Treatment with solriamfetol, a dual dopamine and norepinephrine reuptake inhibitor, results in significant improvement in subjective and objective daytime sleepiness. The medication is mainly excreted renally and avoids the drug interactions (effect on hepatic enzymes) noted with modafinil and armodafinil. Solriamfetol, unlike modafinil, armodafinil, or pitolisant, has no interactions with oral contraceptives. Current or recent use of an MAOI with solriamfetol is contraindicated.
9. Modafinil (racemic R, L enantiomers) and armodafinil (R enantiomer) can improve residual daytime sleepiness in patients on effective PAP treatment. Although studies have not shown a benefit of 400 mg of modafinil daily over 200 mg, some patients will benefit from the higher dose or from a split dose (in the morning and in the early afternoon). Armodafinil results in effective levels of medication over a much longer period of time, and once a day dosing is effective. Both medications can reduce the effectiveness of oral contraceptives up to 1 month after the medications have been stopped. An alternative method of contraception should be used (or used in addition to an oral contraceptive). Stevens-Johnson syndrome is a very rare but potentially fatal side effect of modafinil and armodafinil. Patients developing a rash should stop the medication and notify their physician.
10. Pitolisant is approved by the FDA for treatment of daytime sleepiness and cataplexy in narcolepsy. Studies have documented effectiveness for residual daytime sleepiness in OSA, but the medication is **not** currently approved by the FDA for that indication. The medication is not scheduled (low abuse potential) and is potentially useful in patients with a history of substance abuse or dependence. It can also reduce the effectiveness of oral contraceptives and can increase the QT interval. Pitolisant acts on H3 presynaptic inhibitory autoreceptors as an antagonist and inverse agonist. Binding results in increased histamine release, and actions on heteroreceptors on other neurons may increase levels of serotonin and norepinephrine.

CLINICAL REVIEW QUESTIONS

1. Which of the following medications does not alter the hepatic metabolism of other medications (including oral contraceptives)?
A. Modafinil
B. Armodafinil
C. Solriamfetol
D. Pitolisant

2. A patient with OSA is adherent to CPAP treatment but has persistent daytime sleepiness. A download of his CPAP data reveals an estimated AHI of 1 event/hour, no large leak, 100% of days with >4 hours of use, and an average nightly use of 6 hours. Which of the following is most appropriate?
A. Addition of modafinil
B. Addition of solriamfetol
C. A PAP titration
D. Increase PAP use to >7 hours nightly

3. A patient with moderate OSA on CPAP treatment has a decrease in BMI from 40 kg/m^2 to 30 kg/m^2 after bariatric surgery. He returns to the clinic and says he has stopped using CPAP. He reports sleeping well without snoring while not using CPAP. The patient requests termination of PAP treatment. Which of the following is **incorrect**?
A. PSG or home sleep apnea testing (HSAT) should document the resolution of OSA before stopping treatment.
B. The majority of patients with OSA are "cured" (AHI < 5 events/hour) after significant weight loss from bariatric surgery.
C. The required level of CPAP may be lower after bariatric surgery.
D. Patients with OSA cured by bariatric surgery can experience a return of OSA in the absence of weight gain.

4. A 40-year-old man recently started on CPAP reports persistent severe daytime sleepiness (ESS 15/24) despite good adherence to CPAP of 10 cm H_2O (average nightly use of 6 hrs). A sleep study 1 year ago showed an AHI of 2 events/hour on CPAP of 10 cm H_2O during supine REM sleep. The patient's wife reports no snoring or apnea on treatment. He is taking fluoxetine 20 mg for depression and denies symptoms of cataplexy. Symptoms of depression improved when he was started on fluoxetine about 12 months ago. What do you recommend?
A. CPAP titration
B. PSG on CPAP followed by MSLT on CPAP
C. Sleep extension followed by modafinil, if needed
D. Change fluoxetine to bupropion

5. A patient with a BMI of 32 kg/m^2 was intolerant of CPAP and stopped using this treatment. He was effectively treated with upper airway surgery when his BMI was 29 kg/m^2. His symptoms have returned, and his HSAT results are listed in the table below.

Home Sleep Apnea Test Results			
Monitoring Time	6 hrs 30 min		
AHI	19	Obstructive apnea	10
AHI supine	30	Central apnea	0
AHI nonsupine	3	Mixed apnea	0
% Supine monitoring time	60%	Hypopneas	115
Desaturations	90	Low SaO_2	80%

What do you recommend?
A. AutoCPAP
B. Weight loss with structured program
C. Evaluation for further upper airway surgery
D. Positional treatment

6. Which of the following medications is not scheduled (no abuse potential) but can increase the QT interval?
A. Solriamfetol
B. Modafinil
C. Pitolisant
D. Dextroamphetamine

ANSWERS

1. C. Solriamfetol is mainly renally excreted and does not alter hepatic enzymes.

2. D. Increase nightly CPAP use to >7 hours. If this is not possible, the other options could be considered. In one study of patients with mild OSA, sleepy patients compared to non-sleepy patients tended to report less nightly sleep on weekdays and longer sleep or naps on the weekends. On PSG they had a longer sleep duration. Oksenberg A, Goizman V, Eitan E, et al. How do sleepy patients differ from non-sleepy patients in mild obstructive sleep apnea? J Sleep Res. 2022 Feb;31(1):e13431.

3. B. The majority of patients with OSA are not cured after bariatric surgery; although the AHI is usually decreased, the reduction is not to less than 5 events/hour in the majority of patients.
4. C. Although a case can be made for all the options, C is probably the best answer. A recent CPAP titration showed the current pressure level was effective, a repeat titration is unlikely to be useful. There is no history of cataplexy; fluoxetine would need to be withdrawn (if possible) to avoid a false negative MSLT (fluoxetine suppresses REM sleep), and mood had responded to fluoxetine. Fluoxetine can cause sleepiness and bupropion is activating, but the patient responded to fluoxetine.
5. D. Positional treatment. The patient has exclusive positional sleep apnea (ePOSA). Ideally, a device that monitors adherence should be used. Of note, it is important for the amount of nonsupine sleep to be long enough to accurately reflect the AHI in that position. That is, nonsupine sleep should ideally contain both NREM and REM sleep. From an HSAT, sleep and sleep staging are not available, but in this patient, about 40% of the monitoring time was in nonsupine positions. Weight loss should be recommended but is considered adjunctive treatment. If the patient does start position treatment, a repeat home sleep apnea test while the patient is wearing the position device would be indicated to document efficacy. The patient did not tolerate CPAP previously, but if positional treatment is not successful, another trial of CPAP is an option.
6. C. Pitolisant is not scheduled (not a controlled substance) and can increase the QT interval. Modafinil can decrease metabolism (by hepatic enzymes) of some medications that can increase the QT interval (citalopram). Therefore indirectly modafinil can affect the QT interval.

SUGGESTED READING

Morgenthaler TI, Kapen S, Lee-Chiong T, et al. Practice parameters for the medical therapy of obstructive sleep apnea. *Sleep*. 2006;29:1031-1035.

Epstein LJ, Kristo D, Strollo Jr PJ, et al. Adult Obstructive Sleep Apnea Task Force of the American Academy of Sleep Medicine. Clinical guideline for the evaluation, management, and long-term care of obstructive sleep apnea in adults. *J Clin Sleep Med*. 2009;5(3):263-276.

Saunders KH, Igel LI, Tchang BG. Surgical and nonsurgical weight loss for patients with obstructive sleep apnea. *Otolaryngol Clin North Am*. 2020;53(3):409-420.

Greenburg DL, Lettieri CJ, Eliasson AH. Effects of surgical weight loss on measures of obstructive sleep apnea: a meta-analysis. *Am J Med*. 2009; 122:535-542.

Oksenberg A, Gadoth N, Töyräs J, Leppänen T. Prevalence and characteristics of positional obstructive sleep apnea (POSA) in patients with severe OSA. *Sleep Breath*. 2020;24(2):551-559.

Mador MJ, Kufel TJ, Magalang UJ, et al. Prevalence of positional sleep apnea in patients undergoing polysomnography. *Chest*. 2005;128(4):2130-2137.

Berry RB, Uhles ML, Abaluck BK, et al. NightBalance sleep position treatment device versus auto-adjusting positive airway pressure for treatment of positional obstructive sleep apnea. *J Clin Sleep Med*. 2019;15(7):947-956.

Javaheri S, Javaheri S. Update on persistent excessive daytime sleepiness in OSA. *Chest*. 2020;158(2):776-786.

Guimarães KC, Drager LF, Genta PR, Marcondes BF, Lorenzi-Filho G. Effects of oropharyngeal exercises on patients with moderate obstructive sleep apnea syndrome. *Am J Respir Crit Care Med*. 2009;179(10):962-966.

REFERENCES

1. Morgenthaler TI, Kapen S, Lee-Chiong T, et al. Practice parameters for the medical therapy of obstructive sleep apnea. *Sleep*. 2006;29:1031-1035.
2. Epstein LJ, Kristo D, Strollo Jr PJ, et al. Adult Obstructive Sleep Apnea Task Force of the American Academy of Sleep Medicine. Clinical guideline for the evaluation, management, and long-term care of obstructive sleep apnea in adults. *J Clin Sleep Med*. 2009;5(3):263-276.
3. Peppard PE, Young T, Palta M, et al. Longitudinal study of moderate weight change and sleep disordered breathing. *JAMA*. 2000;284: 3015-3021.
4. Smith PL, Gold AR, Meyers DA, et al. Weight loss in mildly to moderately obese patients with obstructive sleep apnea. *Ann Intern Med*. 1985;103:850-855.
5. Johansson K, Neovius M, Lagerros YT, et al. Effect of a very low energy diet on moderate and severe sleep apnea in obese men: a randomised controlled trial. *BMJ*. 2009;339:b4609.
6. Tuomilehto HPI, Seppa JM, Partine MM, et al. Lifestyle intervention with weight reduction first-line treatment in mild obstructive sleep apnea. *Am J Respir Crit Care Med*. 2009;179:320-327.
7. Spörndly-Nees S, Åsenlöf P, Lindberg E, Emtner M, Igelström H. Effects on obstructive sleep apnea severity following a tailored behavioral sleep medicine intervention aimed at increased physical activity and sound eating: an 18-month follow-up of a randomized controlled trial. *J Clin Sleep Med*. 2020;16(5):705-713.
8. Kuna ST, Reboussin DM, Strotmeyer ES, et al. Sleep AHEAD Research Subgroup of the Look AHEAD Research Group. Effects of weight loss on obstructive sleep apnea severity. Ten-year results of the Sleep AHEAD Study. *Am J Respir Crit Care Med*. 2021;203(2):221-229.
9. Carneiro-Barrera A, Díaz-Román A, Guillén-Riquelme A, Buela-Casal G. Weight loss and lifestyle interventions for obstructive sleep apnoea in adults: systematic review and meta-analysis. *Obes Rev*. 2019;20(5):750-762.
10. Araghi MH, Chen YF, Jagielski A, et al. Effectiveness of lifestyle interventions on obstructive sleep apnea (OSA): systematic review and meta-analysis. *Sleep*. 2013;36(10):1553-1562, 1562A-1562E.
11. Edwards BA, Bristow C, O'Driscoll DM, et al. Assessing the impact of diet, exercise and the combination of the two as a treatment for OSA: a systematic review and meta-analysis. *Respirology*. 2019;24(8):740-751.
12. Schwartz AR, Gold AR, Schubert N, et al. Effect of weight loss on upper airway collapsibility in obstructive sleep apnea. *Am Rev Respir Dis*. 1991; 144(3 Pt 1):494-498.
13. Wang SH, Keenan BT, Wiemken A, et al. Effect of weight loss on upper airway anatomy and the apnea-hypopnea index. The importance of tongue fat. *Am J Respir Crit Care Med*. 2020;201(6):718-727.
14. Saunders KH, Igel LI, Tchang BG. Surgical and nonsurgical weight loss for patients with obstructive sleep apnea. *Otolaryngol Clin North Am*. 2020;53(3):409-420.
15. Greenburg DL, Lettieri CJ, Eliasson AH. Effects of surgical weight loss on measures of obstructive sleep apnea: a meta-analysis. *Am J Med*. 2009;122:535-542.
16. Lettieri CJ, Eliasson AH, Greenburg DL. Persistence of obstructive sleep apnea after surgical weight loss. *J Clin Sleep Med*. 2008;4:333-338.
17. Dong Z, Hong BY, Yu AM, Cathey J, Shariful Islam SM, Wang C. Weight loss surgery for obstructive sleep apnoea with obesity in adults: a systematic review and meta-analysis protocol. *BMJ Open*. 2018;8(8):e020876.
18. Peromaa-Haavisto P, Tuomilehto H, Kössi J, et al. Obstructive sleep apnea: the effect of bariatric surgery after 12 months. A prospective multicenter trial. *Sleep Med*. 2017;35:85-90.
19. Pillar G, Peled R, Lavie P. Recurrence of sleep apnea without concomitant weight increase 7.5 years after weight reduction surgery. *Chest*. 1994;106:1702-1704.
20. Hudgel DW, Patel SR, Ahasic AM, et al. American Thoracic Society Assembly on Sleep and Respiratory Neurobiology. The role of weight management in the treatment of adult obstructive sleep apnea. An official American Thoracic Society clinical practice guideline. *Am J Respir Crit Care Med*. 2018;198(6):e70-e87.
21. Winslow DH, Bowden CH, DiDonato KP, McCullough PA. A randomized, double-blind, placebo-controlled study of an oral, extended-release formulation of phentermine/topiramate for the treatment of obstructive sleep apnea in obese adults. *Sleep*. 2012;35(11):1529-1539.

22. Blackman A, Foster GD, Zammit G, et al. Effect of liraglutide 3.0 mg in individuals with obesity and moderate or severe obstructive sleep apnea: the SCALE Sleep Apnea randomized clinical trial. *Int J Obes (Lond)*. 2016;40(8):1310-1319.
23. Ashrafian H, Toma T, Rowland SP, et al. Bariatric surgery or non-surgical weight loss for obstructive sleep apnoea? A systematic review and comparison of meta-analyses. *Obes Surg*. 2015;25(7):1239-1250.
24. Dixon JB, Schachter LM, O'Brien PE, et al. Surgical vs. conventional therapy for weight loss treatment of obstructive sleep apnea: a randomized controlled trial. *JAMA*. 2012;308(11):1142-1149.
25. Collen J, Lettieri CJ, Eliasson A. Postoperative CPAP use impacts long-term weight loss following bariatric surgery. *J Clin Sleep Med*. 2015;11(3):213-217.
26. Joosten SA, Khoo JK, Edwards BA, et al. Improvement in obstructive sleep apnea with weight loss is dependent on body position during sleep. *Sleep*. 2017;40(5).
27. Arterburn DE, Telem DA, Kushner RF, Courcoulas AP. Benefits and risks of bariatric surgery in adults: a review. *JAMA*. 2020;324(9):879-887.
28. de Raaff CAL, de Vries N, van Wagensveld BA. Obstructive sleep apnea and bariatric surgical guidelines: summary and update. *Curr Opin Anaesthesiol*. 2018;31(1):104-109.
29. Zaremba S, Shin CH, Hutter MM, et al. Continuous positive airway pressure mitigates opioid-induced worsening of sleep-disordered breathing early after bariatric surgery. *Anesthesiology*. 2016;125:92-104.
30. Oksenberg A, Silverberg DS, Arons E, Radwan H. Positional vs nonpositional obstructive sleep apnea patients: anthropomorphic, nocturnal polysomnographic, and multiple sleep latency test data. *Chest*. 1997;112(3):629-639.
31. Oksenberg A, Gadoth N, Töyräs J, Leppänen T. Prevalence and characteristics of positional obstructive sleep apnea (POSA) in patients with severe OSA. *Sleep Breath*. 2020;24(2):551-559.
32. Mador MJ, Kufel TJ, Magalang UJ, et al. Prevalence of positional sleep apnea in patients undergoing polysomnography. *Chest*. 2005; 128(4):2130-2137.
33. Heinzer R, Petitpierre NJ, Marti-Soler H, Haba-Rubio J. Prevalence and characteristics of positional sleep apnea in the HypnoLaus population-based cohort. *Sleep Med*. 2018;48:157-162.
34. Oksenberg A, Silverberg DS, Arons E, et al. The sleep supine position has a major effect on optimal nasal CPAP. *Chest*. 1999;116:1000-1006.
35. Neill AM, Angus SM, Sajkov D, McEvoy RD. Effects of sleep posture on upper airway stability in patients with obstructive sleep apnea. *Am J Respir Crit Care Med*. 1997;155:199-204.
36. McEvoy RD, Sharp DJ, Thornton AT. The effects of posture on obstructive sleep apnea. *Am Rev Respir Dis*. 1986;133(4):662-666.
37. Lukachan GA, Yadollahi A, Auckley D, et al. The impact of semi-upright position on severity of sleep disordered breathing in patients with obstructive sleep apnea: a two-arm, prospective, randomized controlled trial. *BMC Anesthesiol*. 2023;23(1):236.
38. Oksenberg A, Arons E, Nasser K, Vander T, Radwan H. REM-related obstructive sleep apnea: the effect of body position. *J Clin Sleep Med*. 2010;6(4):343-348.
39. Marques M, Genta PR, Sands SA, et al. Effect of Sleeping Position on Upper Airway Patency in Obstructive Sleep Apnea Is Determined by the Pharyngeal Structure Causing Collapse. *Sleep*. 2017;40(3). doi:10.1093/sleep/zsx005.
40. Joosten SA, Sands SA, Edwards BA, et al. Evaluation of the role of lung volume and airway size and shape in supine-predominant obstructive sleep apnoea patients. *Respirology*. 2015;20(5):819-827.
41. Omobomi O, Quan SF. Positional therapy in the management of positional obstructive sleep apnea a review of the current literature. *Sleep Breath*. 2018;22(2):297-304.
42. Ravesloot MJL, White D, Heinzer R, Oksenberg A, Pépin JL. Efficacy of the new generation of devices for positional therapy for patients with positional obstructive sleep apnea: a systematic review of the literature and meta-analysis. *J Clin Sleep Med*. 2017;13(6):813-824.
43. Jokic R, Klimaszewski A, Crossley M, et al. Positional treatment vs. continuous positive airway pressure in patients with positional obstructive sleep apnea syndrome. *Chest*. 1999;115:771-781.
44. Eijsvogel MM, Ubbink R, Dekker J, et al. Sleep position trainer versus tennis ball technique in positional obstructive sleep apnea syndrome. *J Clin Sleep Med*. 2015;11(2):139-147.
45. Bignold JJ, Deans-Costi G, Goldsworthy MR, et al. Poor long-term patient compliance with the tennis ball technique for treating positional obstructive sleep apnea. *J Clin Sleep Med*. 2009;5:428-430.
46. Permut I, Diaz-Abad M, Eissam C, et al. Comparison of positional therapy to CPAP in patients with positional obstructive sleep apnea. *J Clin Sleep Med*. 2010;6:238-243.
47. Bignold JJ, Mercer JD, Antic NA, McEvoy RD, Catcheside PG. Accurate position monitoring and improved supine-dependent obstructive sleep apnea with a new position recording and supine avoidance device. *J Clin Sleep Med*. 2011;7(4):376-383.
48. Levendowski DJ, Seagraves S, Popovic D, Westbrook PR. Assessment of a neck-based treatment and monitoring device for positional obstructive sleep apnea. *J Clin Sleep Med*. 2014;10(8):863-871.
49. Levendowski D, Cunnington D, Swieca J, Westbrook P. User compliance and behavioral adaptation associated with supine avoidance therapy. *Behav Sleep Med*. 2018;16(1):27-37.
50. Berry RB, Uhles ML, Abaluck BK, et al. NightBalance sleep position treatment device versus auto-adjusting positive airway pressure for treatment of positional obstructive sleep apnea. *J Clin Sleep Med*. 2019;15(7):947-956.
51. de Ruiter MHT, Benoist LBL, de Vries N, de Lange J. Durability of treatment effects of the Sleep Position Trainer versus oral appliance therapy in positional OSA: 12-month follow-up of a randomized controlled trial. *Sleep Breath*. 2018;22(2):441-450.
52. Beyers J, Vanderveken OM, Kastoer C, et al. Treatment of sleep-disordered breathing with positional therapy: long-term results. *Sleep Breath*. 2019;23(4):1141-1149.
53. van Maanen JP, de Vries N. Long-term effectiveness and compliance of positional therapy with the Sleep Position Trainer in the treatment of positional obstructive sleep apnea syndrome. *Sleep*. 2014;37(7):1209-1215.
54. Benoist LBL, Verhagen M, Torensma B, van Maanen JP, de Vries N. Positional therapy in patients with residual positional obstructive sleep apnea after upper airway surgery. *Sleep Breath*. 2017;21(2):279-288.
55. Dieltjens M, Vroegop AV, Verbruggen AE, et al. A promising concept of combination therapy for positional obstructive sleep apnea. *Sleep Breath*. 2015;19(2):637-644.
56. Goyal A, Pakhare A, Subhedar R, Khurana A, Chaudhary P. Combination of positional therapy with positive airway pressure for titration in patients with difficult to treat obstructive sleep apnea. *Sleep Breath*. 2021;25(4):1867-1873.
57. Joho S, Oda Y, Hirai T, Inoue H. Impact of sleeping position on central sleep apnea/Cheyne-Stokes respiration in patients with heart failure. *Sleep Med*. 2010;11(2):143-148.
58. Oktay Arslan B, Ucar Hosgor ZZ, Ekinci S, Cetinkol I. Evaluation of the impact of body position on primary central sleep apnea syndrome. *Arch Bronconeumol*. 2021;57(6):393-398.
59. Szollosi I, Roebuck T, Thompson B, Naughton MT. Lateral sleeping position reduces severity of central sleep apnea/Cheyne-Stokes respiration. *Sleep*. 2006;29(8):1045-1051.
60. Sahlin C, Svanborg E, Stenlund H, Franklin KA. Cheyne-Stokes respiration and supine dependency. *Eur Respir J*. 2005;25(5):829-833.
61. Sériès F, Cormier Y, La Forge J. Influence of apnea type and sleep stage on nocturnal postapneic desaturation. *Am Rev Respir Dis*. 1990; 141(6):1522-1526.
62. Doshi J. *Rhinitis medicamentosa*: what an otolaryngologist needs to know. *Eur Arch Otolaryngol*. 2009;266:623-625.
63. Kiely JL, Nolan P, McNicholas WT. Intranasal corticosteroid therapy for obstructive sleep apnea in patients with co-existing rhinitis. *Thorax*. 2004;59:35-55.
64. Camacho M, Riaz M, Capasso R, et al. The effect of nasal surgery on continuous positive airway pressure device use and therapeutic treatment pressures: a systematic review and meta-analysis. *Sleep*. 2015;38(2): 279-286.
65. Eckert DJ, Lo YL, Saboisky JP, Jordan AS, White DP, Malhotra A. Sensorimotor function of the upper-airway muscles and respiratory sensory processing in untreated obstructive sleep apnea. *J Appl Physiol (1985)*. 2011;111(6):1644-1653.
66. Puhan MA, Suarez A, Lo Cascio C, Zahn A, Heitz M, Braendli O. Didgeridoo playing as alternative treatment for obstructive sleep apnoea syndrome: randomised controlled trial. *BMJ*. 2006;332(7536):266-270.
67. Nóbrega-Júnior JCN, Dornelas de Andrade A, de Andrade EAM, et al. Inspiratory muscle training in the severity of obstructive sleep apnea, sleep quality and excessive daytime sleepiness: a placebo-controlled, randomized trial. *Nat Sci Sleep*. 2020;12:1105-1113.
68. Camacho M, Certal V, Abdullatif J, et al. Myofunctional therapy to treat obstructive sleep apnea: a systematic review and meta-analysis. *Sleep*. 2015;38(5):669-675.
69. Guimarães KC, Drager LF, Genta PR, Marcondes BF, Lorenzi-Filho G. Effects of oropharyngeal exercises on patients with moderate obstructive sleep apnea syndrome. *Am J Respir Crit Care Med*. 2009;179(10): 962-966.
70. Erturk N, Calik-Kutukcu E, Arikan H, et al. The effectiveness of oropharyngeal exercises compared to inspiratory muscle training in obstructive

sleep apnea: a randomized controlled trial. *Heart Lung*. 2020;49(6): 940-948.
71. O'Connor-Reina C, Ignacio Garcia JM, Rodriguez Ruiz E, et al. Myofunctional therapy app for severe apnea-hypopnea sleep obstructive syndrome: pilot randomized controlled trial. *JMIR Mhealth Uhealth*. 2020;8(11):e23123.
72. Kotecha B, Wong PY, Zhang H, Hassaan A. A novel intraoral neuromuscular stimulation device for treating sleep-disordered breathing. *Sleep Breath*. 2021;25(4):2083-2090.
73. Baptista PM, Martínez Ruiz de Apodaca P, Carrasco M, et al. Daytime neuromuscular electrical therapy of tongue muscles in improving snoring in individuals with primary snoring and mild obstructive sleep apnea. *J Clin Med*. 2021;10(9):1883.
74. Smith PL, Haponik EF, Bleecker ER. The effects of oxygen in patients with sleep apnea. *Am Rev Respir Dis*. 1984;130:958-963.
75. Alford NJ, Fletcher EC, Nickeson D. Acute oxygen in patients with sleep apnea and COPD. *Chest*. 1986;89:30-38.
76. Fletcher E, Munafo DA. Role of nocturnal oxygen therapy in obstructive sleep apnea. Should it be used? *Chest*. 1990;98:1497-1504.
77. Martin RJ, Sander MH, Gray BA, Pennock BE. Acute and long-term ventilatory effects in adult sleep apnea. *Am Rev Respir Dis*. 1982;125:175-180.
78. Gold AR, Schwartz AR Bleecker ER, Smith PL. The effect of chronic nocturnal oxygen administration upon sleep apnea. *Am Rev Respir Dis*. 1986;134:925-929.
79. Gold AR, Bleecker ER, Smith PL. A shift from central and mixed sleep apnea to obstructive sleep apnea resulting from low flow oxygen. *Am Rev Respir Dis*. 1985;132:220-223.
80. Loredo JS, Ancoli-Israel S, Kim E, et al. Effect of continuous positive airway pressure versus supplemental oxygen on sleep quality in obstructive sleep apnea: a placebo-CPAP-controlled study. *Sleep*. 2006;29:564-571.
81. Gottlieb DJ, Punjabi NM, Mehra R, et al. CPAP versus oxygen in obstructive sleep apnea. *N Engl J Med*. 2014;370:2276-2285.
82. Turnbull CD, Sen D, Kohler M, Petousi N, Stradling JR. Effect of supplemental oxygen on blood pressure in obstructive sleep apnea (SOX). A randomized continuous positive airway pressure withdrawal trial. *Am J Respir Crit Care Med*. 2019;199(2):211-219.
83. Lewis EF, Wang R, Punjabi N, et al. Impact of continuous positive airway pressure and oxygen on health status in patients with coronary heart disease, cardiovascular risk factors, and obstructive sleep apnea: a Heart Biomarker Evaluation in Apnea Treatment (HEARTBEAT) analysis. *Am Heart J*. 2017;189:59-67.
84. Mehta V, Vasu TS, Phillips B, Chung F. Obstructive sleep apnea and oxygen therapy: a systematic review of the literature and meta-analysis. *J Clin Sleep Med*. 2013;9(3):271-279.
85. Wellman A, Malhotra A, Jordan AS, Stevenson KE, Gautam S, White DP. Effect of oxygen in obstructive sleep apnea: role of loop gain. *Respir Physiol Neurobiol*. 2008;162:144-151.
86. Javaheri S, Javaheri S. Update on persistent excessive daytime sleepiness in OSA. *Chest*. 2020;158(2):776-786.
87. Lal C, Weaver TE, Bae CJ, Strohl KP. Excessive daytime sleepiness in obstructive sleep apnea. Mechanisms and clinical management. *Ann Am Thorac Soc*. 2021;18(5):757-768.
88. Gasa M, Tamisier R, Launois SH, et al. Scientific Council of the Sleep Registry of the French Federation of Pneumology–FFP. Residual sleepiness in sleep apnea patients treated by continuous positive airway pressure. *J Sleep Res*. 2013;22:389-397.
89. Pépin JL, Viot-Blanc V, Escourrou P, et al. Prevalence of residual excessive sleepiness in CPAP-treated sleep apnoea patients: the French multicentre study. *Eur Respir J*. 2009;33(5):1062-1067.
90. Craig S, Pépin JL, Randerath W, et al. Investigation and management of residual sleepiness in CPAP-treated patients with obstructive sleep apnoea: the European view. *Eur Respir Rev*. 2022;31(164):210230.
91. Budhiraja R, Kushida CA, Nichols DA, et al. Predictors of sleepiness in obstructive sleep apnoea at baseline and after 6 months of continuous positive airway pressure therapy. *Eur Respir J*. 2017;50(5):1700348.
92. American Academy of Sleep Medicine. *International Classification of Sleep Disorders*. 3rd ed., text revision. American Academy of Sleep Medicine; 2023.
93. Kapur VK, Donovan LM. Taking care of persistent sleepiness in patients with sleep apnea. *Am J Respir Crit Care Med*. 2019;199(11):1310-1311.
94. Weaver TE, Maislin G, Dinges DF, et al. Relationship between hours of CPAP use and achieving normal levels of sleepiness and daily functioning. *Sleep*. 2007;30(6):711-719.
95. Gabryelska A, Białasiewicz P. Association between excessive daytime sleepiness, REM phenotype and severity of obstructive sleep apnea. *Sci Rep*. 2020;10(1):34.
96. Findley LJ, Wilhoit SC, Suratt PM. Apnea duration and hypoxemia during REM sleep in patients with obstructive sleep apnea. *Chest*. 1985;87(4):432-436.
97. Pittman SD, Pillar G, Berry RB, Malhotra A, MacDonald MM, White DP. Follow-up assessment of CPAP efficacy in patients with obstructive sleep apnea using an ambulatory device based on peripheral arterial tonometry. *Sleep Breath*. 2006;10(3):123-131.
98. Vgontzas AN, Bixler EO, Tan TL, Kantner D, Martin LF, Kales A. Obesity without sleep apnea is associated with daytime sleepiness. *Arch Intern Med*. 1998;158(12):1333-1337.
99. Zhang J, Weaver TE, Zhong Z, et al. White matter structural differences in OSA patients experiencing residual daytime sleepiness with high CPAP use: a non-Gaussian diffusion MRI study. *Sleep Med*. 2019;53:51-59.
100. Koutsourelakis I, Perraki E, Economou NT, et al. Predictors of residual sleepiness in adequately treated obstructive sleep apnoea patients. *Eur Respir J*. 2009;34(3):687-693.
101. Vernet C, Redolfi S, Attali V, et al. Residual sleepiness in obstructive sleep apnoea: phenotype and related symptoms. *Eur Respir J*. 2011;38(1):98-105.
102. Loland CJ, Mereu M, Okunola OM, et al. R-modafinil (armodafinil): a unique dopamine uptake inhibitor and potential medication for psychostimulant abuse. *Biol Psychiatry*. 2012;72(5):405-413.
103. Chapman JL, Vakulin A, Hedner J, Yee BJ, Marshall NS. Modafinil/armodafinil in obstructive sleep apnoea: a systematic review and meta-analysis. *Eur Respir J*. 2016;47(5):1420-1428.
104. Pack AI, Black JE, Schwartz JR, Matheson JK. Modafinil as adjunct therapy for daytime sleepiness in obstructive sleep apnea. *Am J Respir Crit Care Med*. 2001;164:1675-1681.
105. Black JE, Hirshkowitz M. Modafinil for treatment of residual excessive sleepiness in nasal continuous positive airway pressure-treated obstructive sleep apnea/hypopnea syndrome. *Sleep*. 2005;28(4):464-471.
106. Dinges DF, Weaver TE. Effects of modafinil on sustained attention performance and quality of life in OSA patients with residual sleepiness while being treated with nCPAP. *Sleep Med*. 2003;4(5):393-402.
107. Schwartz JR, Hirshkowitz M, Erman MK, Schmidt-Nowara W. Modafinil as adjunct therapy for daytime sleepiness in obstructive sleep apnea: a 12-week, open-label study. *Chest*. 2003;124(6):2192-2199.
108. Inoue Y, Takasaki Y, Yamashiro Y. Efficacy and safety of adjunctive modafinil treatment on residual excessive daytime sleepiness among nasal continuous positive airway pressure-treated Japanese patients with obstructive sleep apnea syndrome: a double-blind placebo-controlled study. *J Clin Sleep Med*. 2013;9(8):751-757.
109. Kingshott RN, Vennelle M, Coleman EL, Engleman HM, Mackay TW, Douglas NJ. Randomized, double-blind, placebo-controlled crossover trial of modafinil in the treatment of residual excessive daytime sleepiness in the sleep apnea/hypopnea syndrome. *Am J Respir Crit Care Med*. 2001;163(4):918-923.
110. Bittencourt LR, Lucchesi LM, Rueda AD, et al. Placebo and modafinil effect on sleepiness in obstructive sleep apnea. *Prog Neuropsychopharmacol Biol Psychiatry*. 2008;32(2):552-559.
111. Krystal AD, Harsh JR, Yang R, Rippon GA, Lankford DA. A double-blind, placebo-controlled study of armodafinil for excessive sleepiness in patients with treated obstructive sleep apnea and comorbid depression. *J Clin Psychiatry*. 2010;71(1):32-40. Erratum in *J Clin Psychiatry*. 2011;72(8):1157.
112. Greve DN, Duntley SP, Larson-Prior L, et al. Effect of armodafinil on cortical activity and working memory in patients with residual excessive sleepiness associated with CPAP-treated OSA: a multicenter fMRI study. *J Clin Sleep Med*. 2014;10(2):143-153.
113. Roth T, White D, Schmidt-Nowara W, et al. Effects of armodafinil in the treatment of residual excessive sleepiness associated with obstructive sleep apnea/hypopnea syndrome: a 12-week, multicenter, double-blind, randomized, placebo-controlled study in nCPAP-adherent adults. *Clin Ther*. 2006;28(5):689-706.
114. Williams SC, Marshall NS, Kennerson M, et al. Modafinil effects during acute continuous positive airway pressure withdrawal: a randomized crossover double-blind placebo-controlled trial. *Am J Respir Crit Care Med*. 2010;181:825-831.
115. Kuan YC, Wu D, Huang KW, et al. Effects of modafinil and armodafinil in patients with obstructive sleep apnea: a meta-analysis of randomized controlled trials. *Clin Ther*. 2016;38(4):874-888.
116. Sukhal S, Khalid M, Tulaimat A. Effect of wakefulness-promoting agents on sleepiness in patients with sleep apnea treated with CPAP: a meta-analysis. *J Clin Sleep Med*. 2015;11(10):1179-1186.
117. Schwartz JR, Feldman NT, Bogan RK, Nelson MT, Hughes RJ. Dosing regimen effects of modafinil for improving daytime wakefulness in patients with narcolepsy. *Clin Neuropharmacol*. 2003;26(5):252-257.

118. Schweitzer PK, Rosenberg R, Zammit GK, et al; TONES 3 Study Investigators. Solriamfetol for excessive sleepiness in obstructive sleep apnea (TONES 3). A randomized controlled trial. *Am J Respir Crit Care Med.* 2019;199(11):1421-1431.
119. Malhotra A, Shapiro C, Pepin JL, et al. Long-term study of the safety and maintenance of efficacy of solriamfetol (JZP-110) in the treatment of excessive sleepiness in participants with narcolepsy or obstructive sleep apnea. *Sleep.* 2020;43(2):zsz220.
120. Ronnebaum S, Bron M, Patel D, et al. Indirect treatment comparison of solriamfetol, modafinil, and armodafinil for excessive daytime sleepiness in obstructive sleep apnea. *J Clin Sleep Med.* 2021;17(12):2543-2555.
121. Rosenberg R, Baladi M, Bron M. Clinically relevant effects of solriamfetol on excessive daytime sleepiness: a posthoc analysis of the magnitude of change in clinical trials in adults with narcolepsy or obstructive sleep apnea. *J Clin Sleep Med.* 2021;17(4):711-717. Erratum in *J Clin Sleep Med.* 2021;17(11):2343.
122. Herring WJ, Liu K, Hutzelmann J, et al. Alertness and psychomotor performance effects of the histamine-3 inverse agonist MK-0249 in obstructive sleep apnea patients on continuous positive airway pressure therapy with excessive daytime sleepiness: a randomized adaptive crossover study. *Sleep Med.* 2013;14(10):955-963.
123. Pépin JL, Georgiev O, Tiholov R, et al. HAROSA I Study Group. Pitolisant for residual excessive daytime sleepiness in OSA patients adhering to CPAP: a randomized trial. *Chest.* 2021;159(4):1598-1609.
124. Dauvilliers Y, Verbraecken J, Partinen M, et al; HAROSA II Study Group Collaborators. Pitolisant for daytime sleepiness in patients with obstructive sleep apnea who refuse continuous positive airway pressure treatment. A randomized trial. *Am J Respir Crit Care Med.* 2020; 201(9):1135-1145.
125. Wang J, Li X, Yang S, et al. Pitolisant versus placebo for excessive daytime sleepiness in narcolepsy and obstructive sleep apnea: a meta-analysis from randomized controlled trials. *Pharmacol Res.* 2021;167:105522.
126. Taranto-Montemurro L, Messineo L, Wellman A. Targeting endotypic traits with medications for the pharmacological treatment of obstructive sleep apnea. A review of the current literature. *J Clin Med.* 2019;8(11):1846.
127. Ni YN, Yang H, Thomas RJ. The role of acetazolamide in sleep apnea at sea level: a systematic review and meta-analysis. *J Clin Sleep Med.* 2021;17(6):1295-1304.
128. Edwards BA, Sands SA, Owens RL, et al. The combination of supplemental oxygen and a hypnotic markedly improves obstructive sleep apnea in patients with a mild to moderate upper airway collapsibility. *Sleep.* 2016;39(11):1973-1983.
129. Carter SG, Eckert DJ. Effects of hypnotics on obstructive sleep apnea endotypes and severity: novel insights into pathophysiology and treatment. *Sleep Med Rev.* 2021;58:101492.
130. Taranto-Montemurro L, Messineo L, Sands SA, et al. The combination of atomoxetine and oxybutynin greatly reduces obstructive sleep apnea severity. A randomized, placebo-controlled, double-blind crossover trial. *Am J Respir Crit Care Med.* 2019;199(10):1267-1276.
131. Schweitzer PK, Taranto-Montemurro L, Ojile JM, et al. The combination of aroxybutynin and atomoxetine in the treatment of obstructive sleep apnea (MARIPOSA): a randomized controlled trial. *Am J Respir Crit Care Med.* 2023. doi:10.1164/rccm.202306-1036OC.
132. Aishah A, Lim R, Sands SA, et al. Different antimuscarinics when combined with atomoxetine have differential effects on obstructive sleep apnea severity. *J Appl Physiol (1985).* 2021;130(5):1373-1382. Erratum in *J Appl Physiol (1985).* 2023;134(1):84.
133. Redolfi S, Yumino D, Ruttanaumpawan P, et al. Relationship between overnight rostral fluid shift and obstructive sleep apnea in nonobese men. *Am J Respir Crit Care Med.* 2009;179(3):241-246.

Chapter 23

Positive Airway Pressure Treatment

INTRODUCTION

Since the original description of continuous positive airway pressure (CPAP) treatment for obstructive sleep apnea (OSA) by Sullivan, Issa, and Berthon-Jones in 1981,[1] positive airway pressure (PAP) remains the mainstay of treatment for moderate to severe OSA in adults.[2-6] It is also an effective treatment for mild OSA if patients are symptomatic and motivated.[7] Whereas CPAP maintains a single positive pressure during inspiration and expiration (Figure 23–1), a device with separately adjustable inspiratory PAP (IPAP) and expiratory PAP (EPAP) was subsequently developed (bilevel PAP or BPAP).[8] Both CPAP and BPAP devices have traditionally required a polysomnography (PSG) titration study to determine the optimal treatment pressure(s). The American Academy of Sleep Medicine (AASM) has published clinical practice guidelines for PSG titration.[9] Subsequently, automatically adjusting/titrating CPAP (APAP) devices and BPAP devices (auto BPAP) were developed.[5,10] These automatic devices can be used unattended at home to select effective CPAP and BPAP settings (autotitration) without the need for PSG titration in uncomplicated patients. The automatic devices can also be used for chronic treatment (without a prior titration study). In today's pandemic world, chronic treatment with an APAP or autoBPAP is the norm rather than autotitration with a titration device used by multiple patients. However, an APAP or autoBPAP device can be used in an individual patient in the APAP or autoBPAP mode to select a level(s) of CPAP or BPAP for that patient. That is, an APAP/autoBPAP device can be used in the fixed CPAP or BPAP mode based after one or more weeks of autotitration with the device to determine effective pressures. The 90th (Philips Respironics, PR) or 95th (ResMed) percentile pressure can be used as the level of CPAP. BPAP devices with a backup rate (spontaneous timed mode, adaptive servoventilation, and volume-assured pressure support [PS]) can also be used to treat central sleep apnea and hypoventilation syndromes.[11] The use of these advanced devices is discussed in Chapter 24. Despite advances in the technology of PAP devices, the major challenge facing clinicians is improving adherence to PAP treatment.[5,12,13] That is, PAP is efficacious (reduces the apnea-hypopnea index [AHI] when used), but is effective only if patient use is adequate. For example, if CPAP reduces the AHI from 30 to 5/hour but is only used for 50% of the night, the average AHI for the entire night is 17.5/hour ($0.5 \times 30 + 0.5 \times 5$). In the following discussion, references to features on representative devices are made. However, options change among device versions, and the physician should consult the most recent device clinical manual for the latest options and recommended settings. It should be noted that at the time of writing PR has decided not to sell CPAP or BPAP units in the US after the recall on their devices is completed. Refurbished Dreamstation 1 devices and new Dreamstation 2 devices will continue to be provided as part of the recall process until the recall is completed. Many patients in the US will continue to use PR devices for several years until their insurance plans will pay for a new non-Philips PAP device. However refurbished devices (Dreamstation 1) or devices not under recall (Dreamstation 2) have been supplied as replacement devices and are currently in use by many patients. CPAP and APAP devices from other manufacturers than PR and ResMed are available and the reader should consult the clinical device manuals for details of their operation.

MECHANISM OF ACTION

PAP works by splinting the upper airway open during sleep.[14,15] Studies have shown CPAP to increase upper airway size, especially in the lateral dimension (Figure 23–2). Positive intraluminal pressure expands the upper airway (pneumatic splint). This is a passive process, as upper airway muscle activity is reduced by CPAP.[16] Although the pneumatic splint is the main mechanism of action, an increase in lung volume due to CPAP may also increase upper airway size and/or stiffen the upper airway walls, making them less collapsible. In general, upper airway size increases with lung volume.[17] This is thought to be due to a downward pull on upper airway structures during lung expansion ("tracheal tug").[18]

EFFICACY OF PAP

Numerous studies have shown that PAP can bring the AHI down to below 5 to 10 events/hour in the majority of patients.[2-5] The virtual elimination of apnea and hypopnea improves arterial oxygen saturation and decreases respiratory arousals. In some patients, PAP treatment can also increase the amount of stage N3 and stage R (REM) sleep during the PAP portion of a split sleep study or during a separate titration study.[19,20] An occasional patient with severe apnea will have a very large increase in the amount of stage N3 or REM sleep (stage N3 or R rebound). As discussed here, the *effectiveness* of PAP depends on adherence as well as efficacy.

INDICATIONS FOR PAP TREATMENT

An AASM clinical practice guideline for PAP treatment of adult patients (PAP-CPG) (Table 23–1) was published in 2019 along with an accompanying systemic review of the published evidence.[4,5] The guideline recommends PAP treatment be based on diagnostic testing: that is, a diagnosis of OSA based on objective testing should precede treatment. If empiric treatment based on clinical suspicion is started in the hospital in emergent situations, a diagnostic test and a PAP titration (if indicated) should be performed as an outpatient. The guideline states that "adequate follow-up, including

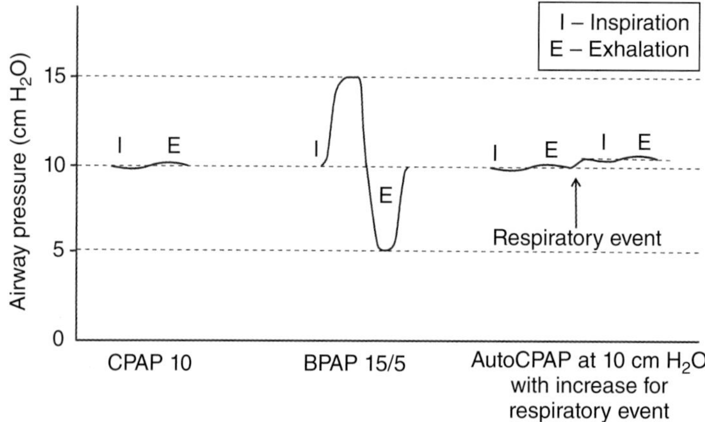

Figure 23–1 Schematic illustrating three modes of positive airway pressure: continuous positive airway pressure (CPAP), bilevel PAP (BPAP), and autoPAP (APAP). I is the inspiratory phase and E the expiratory phase. In AutoCPAP, a pressure increase in response to a respiratory event is noted (up arrow).

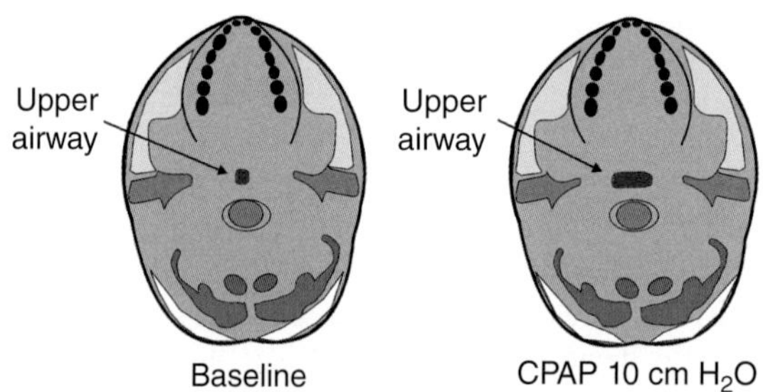

Figure 23–2 A schematic of an axial slice of an MRI of the head showing changes in upper airway shape with application of continuous positive airway pressure (CPAP). There is an increase in the lateral dimensions of the upper airway when comparing baseline (no CPAP) with CPAP of 10 cm H_2O. The change could vary among individuals depending on their upper airway structure.

troubleshooting and monitoring of objective efficacy and usage data to ensure adequate treatment and adherence, should occur following PAP therapy initiation and during treatment of OSA."[5] OSA is a chronic disease and requires significant physician involvement, especially at treatment initiation.[12,13] Chronic follow-up is important to reinforce ongoing adherence and provide interventions for mask and equipment issues. The importance of regular change of filters and mask cushions can also be emphasized. The PAP-CPG recommends PAP treatment for daytime sleepiness (standard), sleep-related quality-of-life issues (conditional), and comorbid hypertension (conditional). There was insufficient evidence to recommend treatment to reduce overall mortality or improve comorbid medical and neurological comorbidities (no recommendation).[5] The quality-of-life conditions include snoring, sleep-related choking, insomnia, disruption of bedpartner's sleep, morning headaches, nocturia, impairments in productivity or social functioning, and daytime fatigue.

PAP is considered the treatment of choice for moderate to severe OSA and may also be effective for mild OSA in motivated and symptomatic patients. In making treatment decisions in milder OSA, one must "treat the patient, not the AHI." The diagnostic AHI may not represent the typical severity of OSA at home. Studies have shown significant night-to-night variability in testing.[21] The same AHI can have a very different clinical impact on different patients. The International Classification of Sleep Disorders, 3rd Edition, Text Revision (ICSD-3-TR) criteria for the diagnosis of adult OSA[22] are listed below. For mildly increased AHI values, symptoms or manifestations are required. The diagnostic criteria (A+B+D) or (C+D) are required.

A. The presence of one or more of the following:
   1. The patient complains of sleepiness, nonrestorative sleep, fatigue, or insomnia symptoms
   2. The patient wakes with breath holding, gasping, or choking
   3. The bedpartner or other observer reports habitual snoring, breathing interruptions, or both during the patient's sleep
B. **Polysomnography** (PSG) or **home sleep apnea testing** (HSAT) demonstrates:
   - Five or more predominantly obstructive respiratory events (obstructive and mixed apneas, hypopneas, or respiratory effort related arousals [RERAs]) per hour of sleep during a PSG or per hour of monitoring (HSAT)
C. PSG or HSAT demonstrates:
   - Fifteen or more predominantly obstructive respiratory events (apneas, hypopneas, or RERAs) per hour of sleep during a PSG or per hour of monitoring (HSAT)
D. Symptoms are not better explained by another current sleep disorder, medical disorder, medication or substance use

Table 23–1 AASM Task Force Clinical Practice Guideline for PAP Treatment of Adults With OSA

Good Practice

- PAP treatment should be based on objective diagnostic testing
- Adequate follow-up, including troubleshooting and monitoring of objective efficacy and usage data to ensure adequate treatment and adherence, should occur after PAP therapy initiation and during treatment of OSA

Indications

Use PAP (compared with no treatment) for OSA patients with:

- Excessive sleepiness (Strong)
- Impaired sleep related quality of life* (Conditional)
- Comorbid hypertension (Conditional)
- Cardiovascular morbidity (no recommendation)

Treatment Initiation

- Provide education interventions before PAP initiation (Strong)
- Initiation using APAP in the home in patients with no comorbidities** or after a laboratory PSG PAP titration in all patients is recommended (Strong)

Treatment Mode

- Use APAP or CPAP for ongoing treatment of OSA (Strong)
- APAP or CPAP rather than BPAP for routine treatment (Conditional)
- Nasal or intranasal masks over oronasal masksfor routine OSA treatment (no level of recommendation specified)

Adherence Interventions

- Education interventions with initiation of PAP treatment (Strong)
- Use behavioral and/or troubleshooting interventions during initial period of PAP treatment (Conditional)
- Use telemonitoring-guided interventions during initial period of PAP treatment (Conditional)

Additional Meta-analysis Findings

- Modified pressure profile PAP (expiratory pressure reflief): No evidence for increased adherence
- Mask interface: Higher adherence rates with nasal versus oronasal masks (no difference in daytime sleepiness).
- Humidified PAP: significant reduction in side effects (dry mouth, nasal discharge, nasal congestion, dry nose, bleeding nose, sinus pain or headache, sore throat, hoarse voice, and reduced smell). No difference in adherence, sleepiness, or quality of life

*Snoring, sleep-related choking, insomnia, disruption of bedpartner's sleep, morning headaches, nocturia, impairments in productivity or social functioning, and daytime fatigue.

**Patients with congestive heart failure, chronic opiate use, significant lung disease (such as chronic obstructive pulmonary disease), neuromuscular disease, history of uvulopalatopharyngoplasty, sleep-related oxygen requirements, or expectation for nocturnal arterial oxyhemoglobin desaturation resulting from conditions other than OSA, including hypoventilation syndromes and central sleep apnea syndromes should have PSG titration polysomnography.

APAP, Automatically adjusting *PAP; BPAP,* bilevel PAP; *CPAP,* continuous PAP; *OSA,* obstructive sleep apnea; *PAP,* positive airway pressure; *PSG,* polysomnography.

Adapted from Patil SP, Ayappa IA, Caples SM, Kimoff RJ, Patel SR, Harrod CG. Treatment of adult obstructive sleep apnea with positive airway pressure: an American Academy of Sleep Medicine clinical practice guideline. *J Clin Sleep Med.* 2019;15(2):335-343.

During HSAT a respiratory event index (REI) based on monitoring time is used rather than an AHI, as EEG is not usually recorded (total sleep time not determined). In addition, one cannot score cortical arousals or RERAs. HSAT tends to underestimate the severity of sleep apnea.

The Centers for Medicare and Medicaid Services (CMS) criteria for reimbursement for CPAP (Table 23–2) include either an AHI ≥ 15 events/hour (moderate to severe OSA) OR an AHI 5 to ≤14 events/hour (mild, ≤ 14 rather than < 15 events per hour is the actual wording), accompanied by one or more of the following symptoms/comorbid conditions: excessive daytime sleepiness, impaired cognition, mood disorders, insomnia, hypertension, ischemic heart disease, or history of stroke.[23] However, other symptoms and comorbid conditions may also improve with PAP treatment.[24] The respiratory disturbance index (RDI) is the nomenclature used by CMS (REI by the AASM) for the AHI determined with home sleep apnea testing (when total sleep time is not determined). The previous version of the ICSD-3[25] added congestive heart failure, atrial fibrillation, or type 2 diabetes mellitus to the comorbid conditions listed by CMS to qualify a patient with mild OSA for CPAP treatment. However, the ICSD-3-TR does not include comorbid conditions in the diagnostic criteria.[22] It is useful to characterize PAP indications into three categories: daytime sleepiness, sleep-related quality-of-life issues, and cardiovascular or other medical comorbidities. Sleep-related quality-of-life issues include, but are not limited to, snoring, nocturnal choking, insomnia, disruption of the partner's sleep, morning headaches, nocturia, impairments in productivity or social functioning, and daytime fatigue.[5] Before addressing sleepiness and sleep-related quality-of-life issues with PAP treatment, the clinician should assess whether untreated OSA is the major (or a significant) contributor. This is especially true if the AHI is mildly increased. For example, treatment of depression or *extension of total sleep time* could have more benefit than CPAP treatment of mild OSA. Studies have found that in patients with mild OSA, sleepy patients report less nightly sleep duration than non-sleepy patients and often take naps on the weekend. As PAP is safe and there is limited harm to an unsuccessful trial of PAP therapy, treatment is often tried even if there is uncertainty concerning the role of untreated OSA in causing symptoms (if the patient is motivated). The famous

Table 23–2 Excerpt From L33718: Positive Airway Pressure Treatment of Obstructive Sleep Apnea

Definitions

- **Apnea** is cessation of airflow for at least 10 seconds.
- **Hypopnea** is an abnormal respiratory event lasting at least 10 seconds associated with at least a 30% reduction in thoracoabdominal movement or airflow as compared with baseline and with at least a 4% decrease in oxygen saturation.
- **Apnea-hypopnea index (AHI)** is the average number of episodes of apnea and hypopnea **per hour of sleep** without the use of a positive airway pressure device. For purposes of this policy, **respiratory effort related arousals (RERAs) are not included** in the calculation of the AHI. Sleep time can only be measured in a Type I (facility-based polysomnography [PSG]) or Type II sleep study (attended or unattended measuring a minimum of 7 channels (EEG, EOG, EMG, ECG-heart rate, airflow, breathing/respiratory effort, SaO_2).
- The **respiratory disturbance index (RDI)** is the average number of apneas plus hypopneas **per hour of recording** without the use of a positive airway pressure device. For purposes of this policy, RERAs are not included in the calculation of the RDI. The RDI is reported in Type III, Type IV, and other home sleep studies.

An E0601 device is covered for the treatment of obstructive sleep apnea (OSA) if criteria A through C are met:

A. The beneficiary has an in-person clinical evaluation by the treating practitioner prior to the sleep test to assess the beneficiary for obstructive sleep apnea.

B. The beneficiary has a sleep test that meets either of the following criteria (1 or 2):

1. The AHI or RDI is ≥15 events/hour with a minimum of 30 events; or,
2. The AHI or RDI is ≥5 and ≤14 events/hour* with a minimum of 10 events and documentation of:
   a. Excessive daytime sleepiness, impaired cognition, mood disorders, or insomnia; or,
   b. Hypertension, ischemic heart disease, or history of stroke.

C. The beneficiary and/or the caregiver has received instruction from the supplier of the device in the proper use and care of the equipment.

Coverage beyond the initial three months of therapy requires an in-person clinical re-evaluation by the treating practitioner no sooner than the 31st day or later than the 91s day after initiation of therapy documenting benefit (symptoms of sleep apnea have improved) and objective adherence (30 consecutive day period with use ≥ 4hrs on ≥ 70% of nights).

An E0470 device (BPAP without a backup rate) is covered for those beneficiaries with OSA who meet criteria A–C above, in addition to criterion D:

D. An E0601 has been tried and proven ineffective based on a therapeutic trial conducted in either a facility or in a home setting.

Ineffective is defined as documented failure to meet therapeutic goals using an E0601 during the titration portion of a facility-based study or during home use, despite optimal therapy (i.e., proper mask selection and fitting and appropriate pressure settings).

If an E0601 device is tried and found ineffective during the initial facility-based titration or home trial, substitution of an E0470 does not require a new initial in-person clinical evaluation or a new sleep test. If more than 30 days are left in the initial 90 day trial period a clinical re-evaluation visit should occur on day 31 to 91 days since starting the E0601 and objective adherence must be documented prior to the 91st day follow initiation of the E0601. If less than 30 days remain in the initial trial period the re-evaluation and objective documentation of adherence must occur before the 120th day following initiation of the E0601.

If an E0601 device has been used for more than 3 months and the beneficiary is switched to an E0470, a new initial in-person clinical evaluation is required, but a new sleep test is not. A new 3-month trial would begin for use of the E0470.

*≤ 14 is the actual wording, although < 15 would be more appropriate.
For more details, including definitions of sleep tests (see chapter 16): CMS Centers for Medicare and Medicaid Services. LCD—Positive airway pressure (PAP) devices for the treatment of obstructive sleep apnea (L33718). Accessed November 1, 2023. https://www.cms.gov/medicare-coverage-database/view/lcd.aspx?LCDId=33718

quote credited to Dr. Philip Westbrook—"when in doubt, pressurize the snout"—often influences clinician decisions. However, it is imperative to also address non-OSA conditions contributing to the patient's complaints, including insomnia and the restless legs syndrome. If these are not addressed, sleep may not improve, and patients may discontinue PAP treatment due to a lack of perceived benefit.

In most categories of cardiovascular and cerebrovascular disorders, *observational studies* have shown benefit from PAP treatment.[26] However, large, randomized trials have failed to show consistent benefit for cardiovascular outcomes, likely due in part to the exclusion of sleepy patients and poor PAP adherence.[27,28] Subanalysis of PAP-adherent patients often showed benefit, but post hoc analysis is not definitive proof of treatment benefit. A randomized controlled trial of CPAP for resistant hypertension did document a benefit.[29] A discussion of the evidence supporting a benefit of PAP in cardiovascular, cerebrovascular, and metabolic disorders and the difficulties in performing randomized controlled trials of CPAP is included in Chapter 20. The PAP-CPG makes no recommendation concerning cardiovascular disease as an indication for PAP treatment.[5]

PAP TECHNOLOGY AND DEVICE FLOW AND LEAK

PAP devices have evolved from a single flow-rate blower and external spring-adjusted pressure threshold values to sophisticated devices with variable flow rates and sophisticated algorithms that use information from accurate internal flow and pressure sensors to adjust flow and maintain the desired airway pressure profile despite variable leaks (Figure 23–3). Most current devices control pressure entirely by variations in flow and do not use an internal pressure valve. The PAP circuit uses a single hose and masks with nonrebreathing orifices that wash

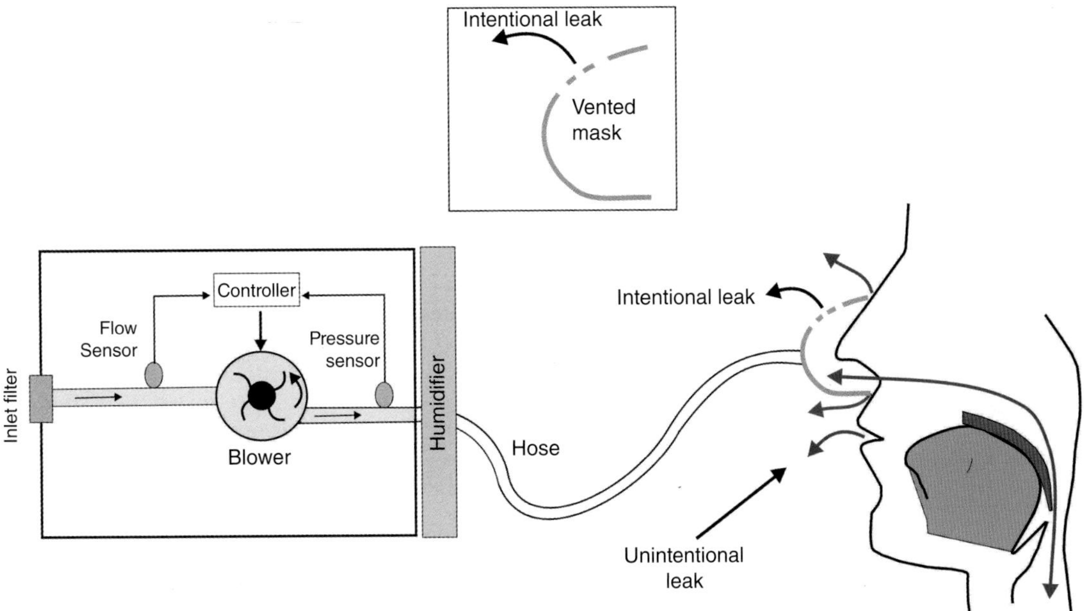

Figure 23–3 Schematic of a positive airway pressure (PAP) device and circuit illustrating intentional and unintentional leak. Most modern PAP devices control pressure with changes in flow (blower speed).

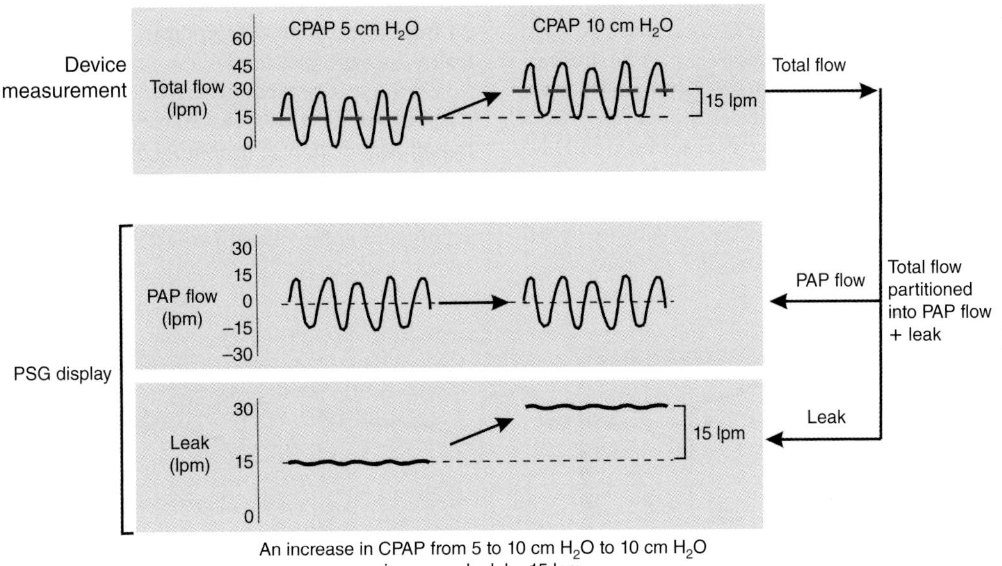

Figure 23–4 Schematic illustrating the partitioning of total flow into positive airway pressure (PAP) device flow and bias flow (leak). Here leak it the total leak and includes intentional and unintentional leak). In this example, when continuous positive airway pressure (CPAP) increases from 5 cm H_2O to 10 cm H_2O, total flow increases due to increased leak (intentional and unintentional). PAP flow (variation in patient flow with respiration) is similar, but leak has increased. *PSG*, polysomnography.

out the exhaled CO_2 (the intentional leak). The total leak is the intentional leak and unintentional leak (mouth and/or mask). The devices are leak tolerant and vary the flow rate to maintain the desired pressure to compensate for variable leaks. Complex algorithms provide specified pressure profiles, including BPAP and drops in pressure with exhalation (flexible PAP). The devices use the internal flow sensor to determine the appropriate timing of changes in pressure (e.g., transitions between IPAP and EPAP). As total flow varies with pressure and leak, total flow is partitioned into PAP flow due to patient respiration and leak (bias flow) (Figure 23–4). The intentional leak can be estimated based on pressure and mask type (Figure 23–5); the unintentional leak can be computed as the difference between total leak and expected (intentional) leak. As will be discussed in later sections, *laboratory PAP devices* can output device PAP flow, leak, and PAP device pressure signals that can be recorded during PSG titration studies[11] (Figure 23–6). As pressure increases, the leak increases, because the intentional mask leak (and total flow) increases as higher pressure results in greater flow through the mask non rebreathing orifices.

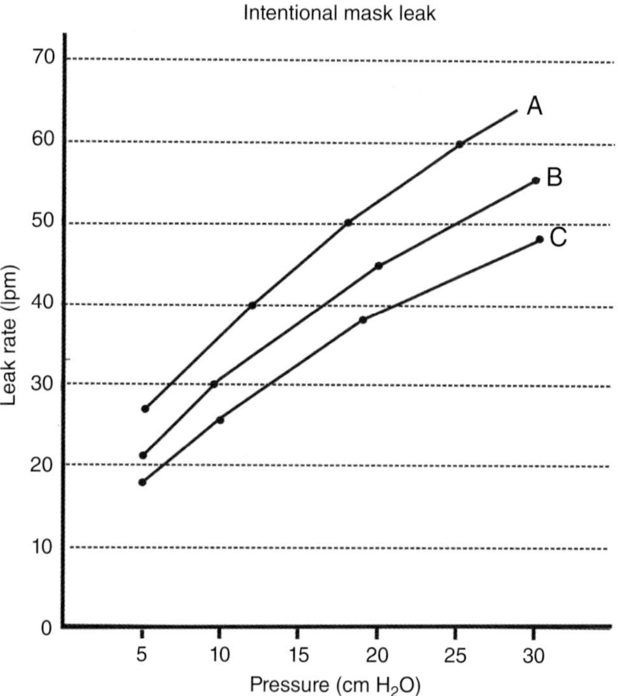

Figure 23–5 Intentional mask leak. Examples of typical mask leak (intentional) from mask exhalation ports (nonrebreathing orifices) for different mask types (A–C) at different pressures. The exact leak depends on the manufacturer and mask type as well as the current treatment pressure. The nonrebreathing mask vents must be large enough to produce a sufficient leak at low pressure to wash out the exhaled CO_2.

PAP devices used by patients for chronic treatment use the PAP flow (measured by the internal flow sensor) to determine an estimate of residual events (based on flow amplitude, flow shape [flattening/airflow limitation], and vibration [snoring]). This information, along with information about pressure, leak, and usage is stored in the device (see Figure 23–7) and is available via download (data card) or sent by modem to cloud-based data storage. The information can then be assessed by physicians and other health care providers. Philips Respironics (PR) PAP devices usually provide total leak information (time in large leak or % of time in large leak). A large leak is one that is at least twice the expected leak for a given pressure and mask. Some newer PR PAP devices provide information on unintentional leak. Note that blower time not associated with pressure changes is not considered use time and is NOT included in the calculation of large leak time. If mask leak is very high, mask pressure changes are minimal (even if the patient is actually using the device) and the time during very high leak is not considered use time. For example, a blower time of 8 hours and a use time of 1 hour means the device was on for 7 hours during which time it did not detect pressure changes. The leak value determined by ResMed PAP devices represents only the unintentional leak. These devices compute an estimated intentional leak from the pressure and mask type (specified in the clinical menu) and then subtract this from the total leak. Usually, an unintentional leak of less than 24 lpm is considered acceptable, and median, mean, and 95% leak values are provided.

During active treatment APAP and autoBPAP devices use the device-identified respiratory event information (apnea, hypopnea, airflow limitation, airflow vibration/snoring) to make decisions regarding changes in pressure using proprietary algorithms. Premium CPAP devices also detect residual events and store this information. However, the information

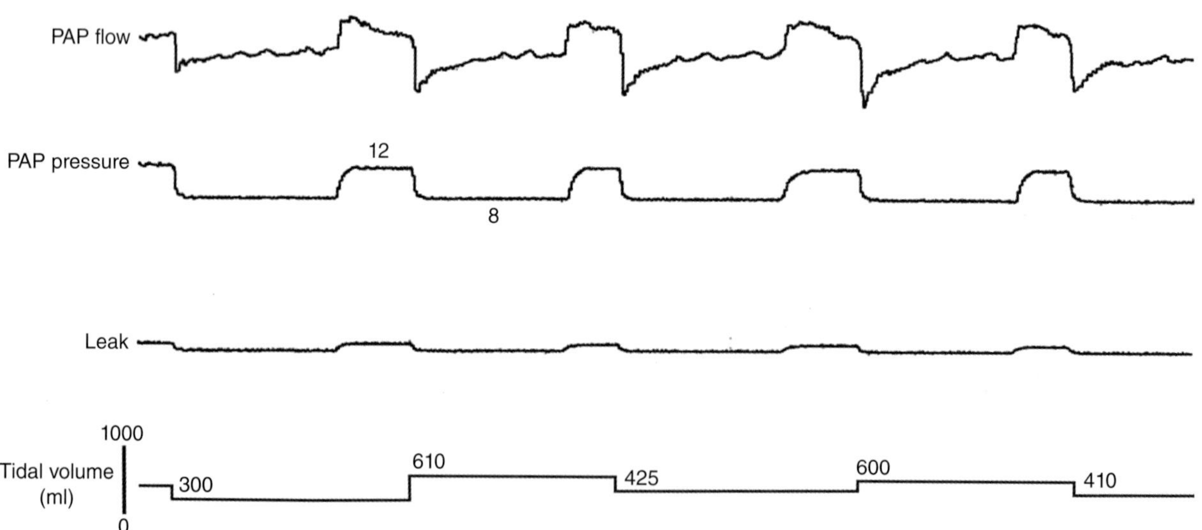

Figure 23–6 Tracings of typical signals from a positive airway pressure (PAP) device that can be recorded during polysomnography. The PAP flow signal is used to score respiratory events. The PAP pressure signal (cm H_2O) shows the current treatment pressure. Here the patient is on bilevel PAP (IPAP/EPAP) of 12/8 cm H_2O. The leak signal in lpm shows the current estimated leak (in this case total leak). The tidal volume signal is useful for determining an optimal treatment in patients with hypoventilation (*tidal volume depends on both peak flow and inspiratory time*). The tidal volume is calculated by integration of the flow signal during inspiration.

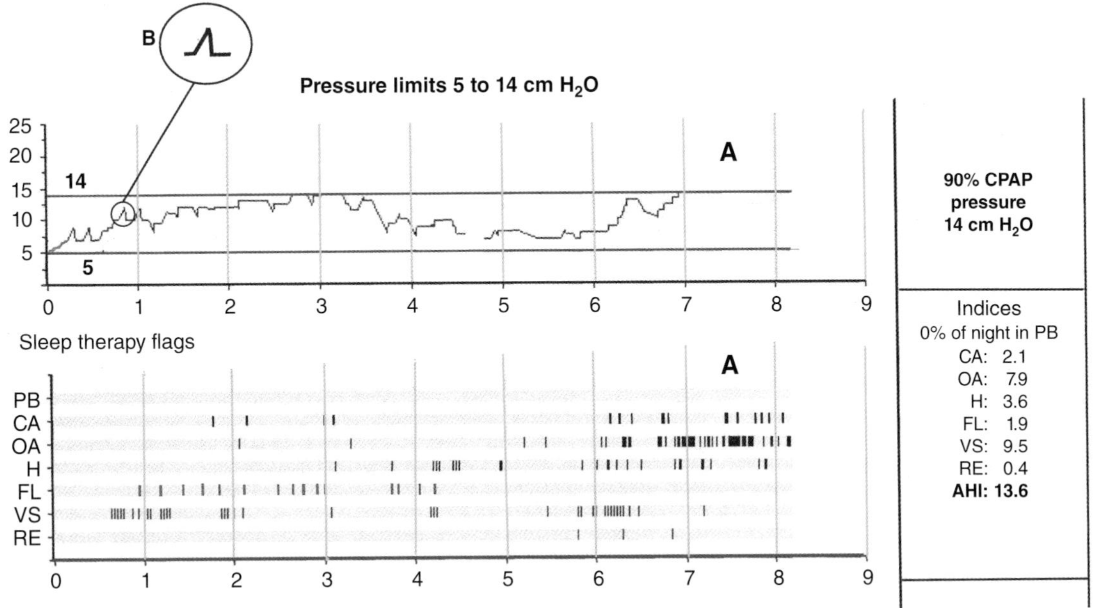

Figure 23–7 Single-night detail showing changes in the delivered positive airway pressure (PAP) between limits of 5 and 14 cm H_2O by the automatic positive airway pressure (APAP) device. The bottom panel shows sleep therapy flags, which are the respiratory events identified by the device. At A, the pressure increases in response to airway events but is *constrained by the upper pressure limit.* The overall AHI is increased. This patient would benefit from an increase in the upper pressure limit. Here the 90% pressure is equal to the upper pressure limit. An example of the APAP algorithm is shown at B, with a temporary increase in pressure to determine if the airway status would benefit from higher pressure. Note that summary information on adherence and delivered pressure, leak, and residual AHI as well as single-night detailed information is stored in the device memory of PAP units used for treatment and transferred by modem to data storage in the cloud. The information can also be accessed via data-card transfer to a computer program, or assessing the data stored in the cloud by a web-based computer program specific to different brands of devices. *AHI,* Apnea-hypopnea index; *CA,* clear airway apnea; *CPAP,* continuous positive airway pressure; *FL,* flow limitation; *H,* hypopnea; *OA,* obstructed airway apnea; *PB,* periodic breathing; *RERA,* respiratory effort related arousal; *RE,* RERA event; *VS,* vibratory snoring.

is not used to change the delivered pressure. Pressure and flow information is used for delivery of drops in pressure during early exhalation (flexible CPAP or expiratory pressure relief). Modified pressure profile PAP (flexible PAP) is discussed in a later section.

BASIC PAP MODES

As previously noted, several basic modes of delivering PAP exist (Table 23–3). CPAP delivers a predetermined constant pressure during both inspiration and exhalation (Figure 23–1). APAP devices deliver an effective level of CPAP in response to respiratory events. APAP devices may also be used for unattended titration (autotitration) to determine an effective level of CPAP. As noted above, the 90% pressure (PR) or 95% pressure (ResMed) from several nights of APAP treatment is chosen for CPAP treatment. A 90% pressure would indicate the pressure exceeded only 10% of the time. The PAP-CPG recommends APAP or CPAP for ongoing treatment of OSA (strong level of recommendation).[5]

BPAP

BPAP delivers separately adjustable higher IPAP and lower EPAP.[8] In the spontaneous (S) mode, the patient determines the respiratory rate (triggering the EPAP to IPAP transition), and the device cycles from IPAP to EPAP based on proprietary algorithms detecting reduced flow. The BPAP mode in PR BPAP devices is called BiPAP, and in ResMed BPAP devices VPAP. As will be discussed in chapter 24, the trigger and cycle sensitivity of ResMed BPAP devices can be adjusted. In unselected patients, BPAP treatment does not result in rates of adherence higher than those of CPAP.[5,30,31] A Cochrane database analysis of six studies and 285 participants found no significant difference in usage with BPAP compared with CPAP.[31] It should be noted that patients were adherent in most comparison studies, and studies *of nonadherent* patients may provide different results. The 2019 evidence-based review of published information did not find evidence that BPAP increased adherence when compared with CPAP or APAP.[4] The PAP-CPG recommends CPAP or APAP rather than BPAP for *routine* treatment.[5] However, some patients failing CPAP due to ineffectiveness of CPAP (high residual AHI or desaturation) or issues related to pressure (pressure intolerance, difficulty exhaling, bloating, mouth leak) can be effectively treated with BPAP.[32-34] Some patients with chronic obstructive pulmonary disease (COPD) may also tolerate BPAP better than CPAP. It is worth noting that routine BPAP devices have a maximum pressure of 25 cm H_2O, whereas CPAP devices have a maximum pressure of 20 cm H_2O. During a PAP PSG titration, a patient may be changed from CPAP to BPAP for pressure intolerance or ineffectiveness of the maximal level of CPAP (or the maximum CPAP tolerated).[32] For example, patients might be treated successfully with BPAP 25/21 cm H_2O when they have significant residual events or arterial oxygen desaturation on CPAP of 20 cm H_2O. A retrospective analysis found that patients

Table 23–3 Basic Modes of Positive Airway Pressure Devices

PAP Mode	Method	Uses
CPAP	• Continuous pressure during inhalation and exhalation	• OSA • Some patients with central apnea
APAP (autotitrating, autoadjusting PAP)	• Titrates between maximum and minimum pressure limits to prevent apnea, hypopnea, airway vibration, and airflow limitation**	• PAP treatment without titration PSG • Autotitration (determine optimal CPAP treatment pressure) • Pressure intolerance
BPAP S (spontaneous mode—no backup rate)	• IPAP (inspiratory PAP) • EPAP (expiratory PAP) • PS (pressure support) = IPAP − EPAP	• Maximum pressure 25 cm H_2O vs. 20 cm H_2O CPAP devices—may be useful in patients requiring very high pressure • Pressure intolerance • OHS, combined OSA + COPD • Bloating, mouth leak
Flexible PAP*	• Pressure falls in early exhalation • Returns to set pressure at end-exhalation	• Pressure intolerance • Mouth leak
AutoBPAP	• Titrates IPAP and EPAP between EPAPmin and IPAPmax (using either PS [Res Med] or PSmin to PSmax [PR] algorithms vary	• BPAP treatment without titration PSG • Pressure intolerance • Nonadherent patients

*Flexible PAP includes expiratory pressure relief (EPR, ResMed) and Cflex, Cflex+, Aflex, or Flex (PR devices).
**ResMed APAP devices respond to apnea, airflow limitation, and snoring.
APAP, Autoadjusting (autotitrating) positive airway pressure; *BPAP,* bilevel positive airway pressure; *COPD,* chronic obstructive pulmonary disease; *CPAP,* continuous positive airway pressure; *EPAP,* expiratory positive airway pressure; *EPR,* expiratory pressure relief; *IPAP,* inspiratory positive airway pressure; *OHS,* obesity hypoventilation syndrome; *PAP,* positive airway pressure; *PR,* Philips Respironics; *PSG,* Polysomnogram; *PS,* pressure support; *S mode,* spontaneous mode.

started on BPAP or changed to from CPAP to BPAP tended to have higher AHI, body mass index (BMI), and partial pressure of carbon dioxide (PCO_2) values and lower SaO_2 values.[33]

Of note, the Centers for Medicare and Medicaid Services (CMS) and most insurance providers will not continue to pay for CPAP/APAP beyond 90 days unless use is ≥4 hours for ≥70% for 1 month in the first 90 days.[23] Patients who fail the trial period are termed "non-adherent" and usually require another study (diagnostic, titration or split study) to qualify for another 90-day trial period.[23] The study is usually a titration study. Most insurance providers, including CMS, will not pay for BPAP unless CPAP is tried first and found to be ineffective. This can happen during a PAP titration (intolerance or ineffectiveness must be documented) or in the first 90 days of CPAP treatment (with documentation in the medical record). Once switched to BPAP, patients are required to meet adherence criteria within the initial 90 days after CPAP initiation (unless fewer than 30 days remain, then adherence must be met within 120 days from the start CPAP treatment).[23] The rules for CPAP reimbursement are constantly changing and may vary with locale. The reader should review the most current information applicable to their location and the patient's insurance coverage. CMS refers to CPAP and BPAP devices without a backup rate using the Healthcare Common Procedure Coding System codes E0601 (CPAP) and E0470 (BPAP without backup rate), respectively.

There is evidence that BPAP can be used to "rescue" nonadherent patients. Ballard et al.[34] studied a group of patients still nonadherent after aggressive interventions who underwent PSG titration to identify effective levels of CPAP and flexible BPAP (BPAP with Biflex, see Figure 23–8). In flexible BPAP, after transition from IPAP to the start of EPAP, there is an additional fall in pressure during exhalation, returning to the EPAP level at the end of exhalation.[34,35] Flexible PAP will be discussed in more detail in a later section. Patients were then randomized to 90 days of treatment with CPAP or flexible BPAP at the pressure demonstrated to be effective during the titration. Of the 53 patients randomized to CPAP, adherence criteria were met in 28%. Of the 51 patients randomized to flexible BPAP, adherence criteria were met in 49% (CPAP vs. flexible BPAP, $P = 0.03$). As flexible pressure has not been demonstrated to improve adherence,[4,35] the improvement in adherence was likely due to the change to BPAP and not the addition of flexible pressure. Benjafield et al.[36] analyzed a large telemonitoring database of studies on individuals changed from CPAP/APAP to BPAP (or autoBPAP). The improvement in average adherence was about 1 hour, and 56.8% met adherence criteria after the change to BPAP. However, it should be noted that many patients tolerate high levels of CPAP quite well, and BPAP is no more effective at maintaining an open airway than properly adjusted CPAP.

BPAP delivers pressure support (PS = IPAP − EPAP) that is useful for augmenting ventilation in patients with OSA and concomitant hypoventilation. When the goal is augmentation of ventilation, the IPAP − EPAP difference needs to be greater than the typical value of 4 cm H_2O used to maintain upper airway patency (e.g., 8–10 cm H_2O or higher).[11] Patients with OSA and daytime hypoventilation include those with obesity hypoventilation syndrome (OHS) and the "overlap syndrome" (OSA + COPD). The PAP treatment of OHS patients is discussed in Chapters 18 and, 21. In brief, **stable** patients with OHS and severe OSA can be effectively treated with CPAP.[37-39] Effective treatment of severe OSA with CPAP improves hypoventilation in most patients if they are adherent to treatment. BPAP in the S mode (no backup rate) can be used in this situation if there is pressure intolerance or the need for pressures higher than 20 cm H_2O. For patients admitted with acute worsening of chronic hypoventilation or stable OHS patients **without** severe OSA, treatment with noninvasive ventilation (BPAP with a backup rate) is recommended.[38,40] However,

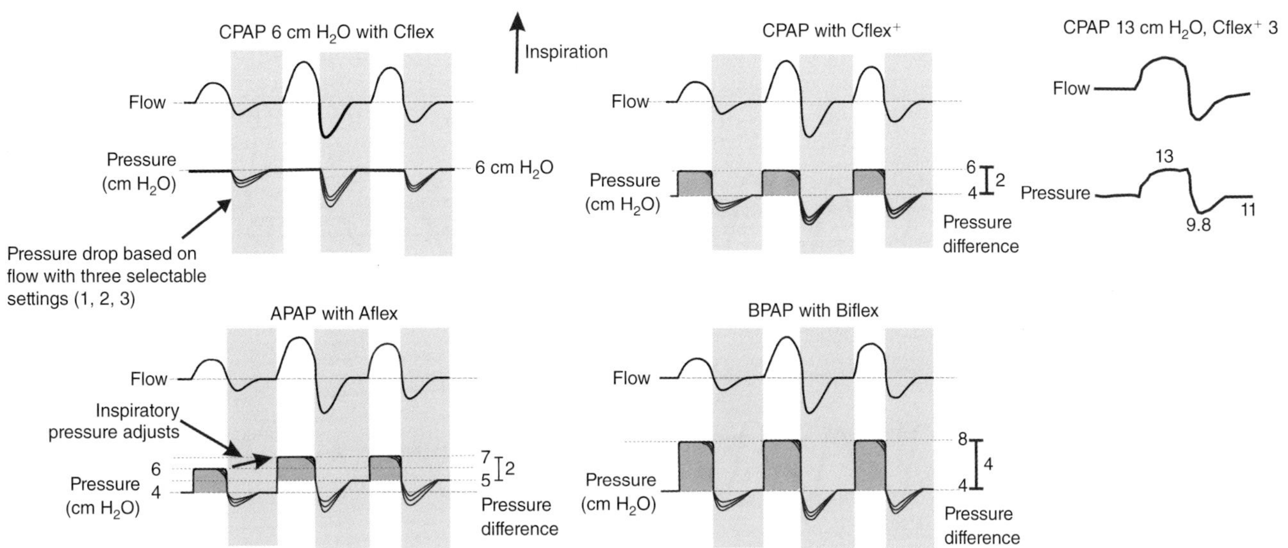

Figure 23–8 Schematic of the types of flexible positive airway pressure in Philips Respironics devices. The top left panel shows continuous positive airway pressure (CPAP) with Cflex. There is a pressure drop based on expiratory flow with three selectable levels. The pressure returns to the CPAP level at the end of exhalation. In the top right panel, Cflex+ is illustrated. There is a 2 cm H_2O difference between inspiratory and expiratory pressure, with further drop, as in Cflex, during exhalation. In the bottom left panel, Aflex is illustrated. This is similar to Cflex+, except the the inspiratory pressure changes in response to respiratory events. In the bottom right panel, bilevel pressure with Biflex is illustrated. There is a set difference between inspiratory positive airway pressure (IPAP) and expiratory positive airway pressure (EPAP), with a futher drop during exhalation, as in Cflex. Note that in Cflex+, Aflex, and Biflex, there is a smoothing of the transition from inspiration to expiration, with the magnitude depending on the flex setting. Cflex, Cflex+, Aflex, and Biflex are trademarks of Philips Respironics. *In the most recent iteration of the PR devices, the term Flex refers to Cflex+ in the CPAP mode and Aflex in the automatic positive airway pressure (APAP) mode.*

some stable OHS patients without severe OSA can be effectively treated with CPAP or BPAP-S if hypoventilation is not severe. In patients with hypoventilation in the overlap group (OSA and COPD), effective treatment of the OSA with CPAP often improves the hypoventilation. BPAP may be better tolerated by some patients and may be more effective if hypoventilation is significant. Trials compared CPAP and BPAP in this group have not been performed. Treatment of the overlap group is discussed in Chapters 18 and 29.

APAP

APAP devices vary the delivered pressure between upper and lower pressure limits to eliminate apnea, hypopnea (some devices), snoring, and airflow limitation (Figure 23–7).[10,41,42] If no events are noted, the autoadjusting devices lower pressure gradually until events reoccur, at which time the pressure again increases. These devices constantly search for the lowest effective pressure in any circumstance. The exact algorithms are proprietary. In APAP devices from PR, changes in pressure are periodically performed to see if there is improvement in flow or other parameters. That is, the algorithm is preemptive, trying to make pressure changes before events occur. As noted previously, APAP devices can be used for autotitration to define an effective level of CPAP or for chronic treatment (titration sleep study not required).[10,41,42] The **average** pressure using an APAP device is typically only 2 to 3 cm H_2O lower than the fixed pressure that would be effective during the entire night, but the average pressure can be up to 6 cm H_2O lower than the 90% or 95% pressure.[43] This is likely due to variable effects of REM sleep and the supine position on the pressure required to keep the upper airway patent. APAP device algorithms differ among manufacturers and the algorithms can change over time.[44] For example, ResMed devices respond to apnea, airflow limitation (flattening of the inspiratory flow profile), and airway vibration, but not to hypopnea. A different algorithm for women has been designed to address the large amount of airflow limitation and REM-associated sleep apnea.[45] As previously noted, in some APAP algorithms, pressure is increased slightly every few minutes to determine if this improves upper airway function and thus proactively attempts to prevent future airway obstruction. If the monitored parameters do not improve, pressure is lowered to the original pressure (Figure 23–7 at B). Ideally, pressure should not be increased for central apnea. However, detecting central apnea without a measure of patient respiratory effort has been a challenge for APAP algorithms. Currently, APAP devices attempt to classify apneas as clear-airway (open-airway) or obstructive-airway apneas, and treatment algorithms do not increase pressure if the airway is open. The PAP devices monitor pressure and flow, but not respiratory effort, and have no method of determining whether inspiratory effort is present during an apnea. Hence terms have been developed such as obstructive airway apnea (OAA) and clear airway apnea (CAA) to describe these events versus obstructive and central apneas (inspiratory effort measured). Here the abbreviations OAA and CAA are used to refer to the state of the airway versus the presence or absence of inspiratory effort. However, the abbreviations actually used in device reports are OA and CA. It is important to note that a closed airway can occur with some central apneas.[46] Thus, an apnea classified as obstructive (OAA) might actually be a closed airway central apnea. Technology used by PR attempts to differentiate CAA apneas from OAA apneas by delivering a small pressure pulse (1 to 2 cm H_2O) after approximately 4 seconds of a >80% reduction in airflow (Figure 23–9A). If the pressure pulse does produce an increase in flow, this is compatible with a

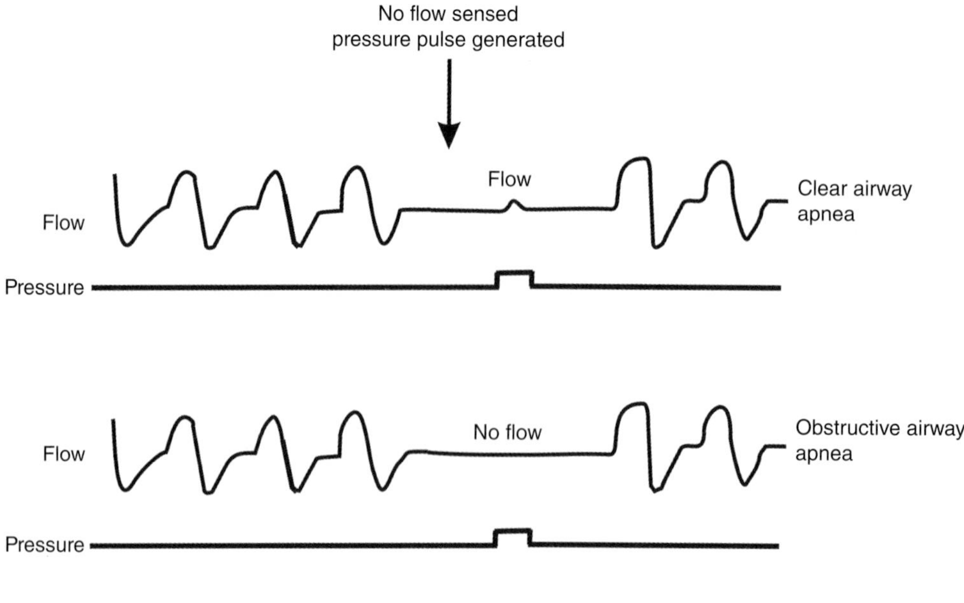

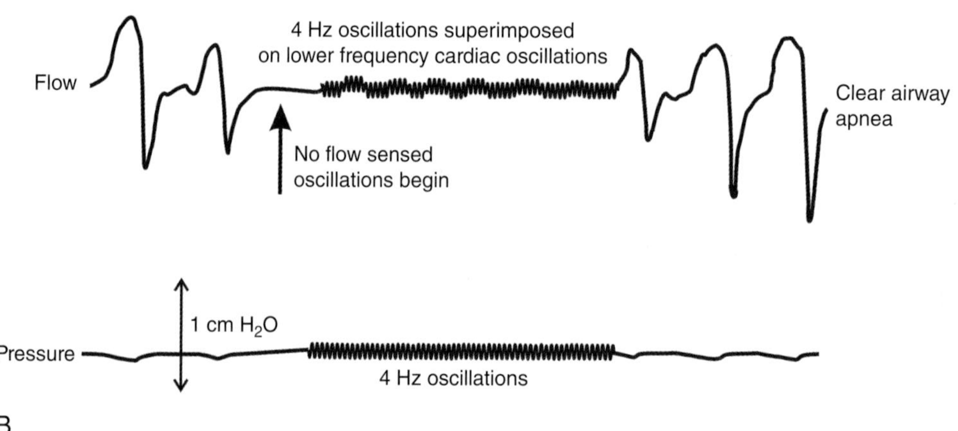

Figure 23–9 Schematic showing detection of clear or obstructive airway apneas using two different technologies. At the top (A), a small pressure pulse is delivered when no airflow is sensed. If a change in flow is noted, this is consistent with a clear airway apnea. If there is no change in flow, the event is classified as an obstructive airway apnea. This method is used by Philips Respironics devices. In the bottom tracings (B), a forced oscillation technique is used to document a clear airway apnea. This method is used by ResMed devices.

clear airway apnea (CAA or open airway). If the pressure pulse does not increase flow, the airway is assumed to be closed (obstructed airway apnea). The APAP device does not increase pressure for CAA events. ResMed PAP devices use a forced oscillation technique (1 cm H_2O at 4 Hz) that begins about 4 seconds after the detection of an absence of airflow to determine whether the upper airway is open or closed (Figure 23–9B).

Although airway property technology is helpful for adjustment of pressure, the results are not always correct. In a study by Li et al.,[47] only 62% of events device-scored as clear airway apneas (CAA) were scored as central apneas by PSG. Some of the CAA events were scored as RERAs, hypopneas, or even obstructive apneas (16%) using PSG tracings. Of note the detected events are stored in memory to provide information to the clinician. It should be noted that events are detected *based only on flow* (amplitude, flow contour/airflow limitation, and flow vibration/snoring). PSG events are scored on the basis of flow, respiratory effort, and oximetry. It is not surprising that the device AHI and PSG AHI may not agree.

As noted previously, APAP devices may be used for chronic treatment without the need for PSG titration with the advantage of delivering the lowest effective pressure in any circumstance.[5,10] The price point of APAP devices is near that of CPAP devices, and chronic APAP treatment, rather than APAP titration followed by CPAP treatment, is a common practice and is effective in carefully selected patients.[5,48] Autotitration studies unattended at home are not reimbursed, and cleaning APAP units between patients being titrated is also problematic. A clinical pathway of diagnosis by a home study and APAP treatment versus diagnosis by PSG and a PSG PAP titration followed by CPAP treatment found similar adherence and effectiveness in both approaches.[48] One study found that APAP treatment was less effective with lower adherence in the presence of excessive leak.[49] This is not surprising, as the APAP algorithms depend on accurate flow measurement and identification of events. High and variable leak may reduce the efficacy of the algorithms. The PAP-CPG recommends treatment initiation at home with APAP without a titration in patients with **uncomplicated OSA** or after a PSG PAP titration in all patients (Table 23–1). Complicated patients may require advanced PAP modes or the addition of supplemental oxygen. These interventions are possible during an attended PSG PAP titration sleep study. Of note, some uncomplicated patients may also benefit from an attended titration, and this is still the standard in some locales. When APAP is used for chronic treatment without a preceding titration, lower and upper pressure limits can be set as 4 to 20 cm H_2O, respectively, then adjusted by monitoring the 90th and 95th percentile pressures after use of the device over days to weeks. Larger patients are often more comfortable on a lower pressure limit of 6 to 8 cm H_2O. Some APAP units have an option that automatically adjusts the lower pressure limit based on initial results. There are patients in whom CPAP is more effective than APAP, especially those with persistent large or intermittent leak. APAP units do not always appropriately titrate, and maintaining a constant treatment pressure is beneficial in some patients.

When APAP was developed, it was hypothesized that it might improve adherence to PAP. For unselected patients, studies have **NOT** documented a clinically significant improvement in usage when compared with that of CPAP.[4,31,50,51] A large meta-analysis of 30 studies and 1136 participants by Smith and Lasserson found a statistically significant difference in machine usage of 0.21 hours (12 min) only in studies with a crossover design.[31] This is not a clinically significant difference. A more recent analysis[51] found similar results, including an insignificant difference between CPAP and APAP for reducing the AHI (very slightly lower AHI with CPAP) and slightly improved diastolic blood pressure with CPAP compared with that with APAP. However, individual patients may tolerate APAP better than CPAP. Hukins et al.[52] found greater adherence with APAP than with CPAP *in patients reporting side effects*, and leak was lower. In contrast, another study found no difference in leak between APAP and CPAP.[53] Shirlaw and coworkers studied patients complaining of aerophagia and found APAP improved symptoms without affecting adherence.[54] In summary, APAP may be more comfortable than CPAP for many patients, but it may not improve adherence. APAP could be tried for pressure intolerance, bloating, or leak, including mask or mouth leak. As previously noted, CPAP could be more effective than APAP at reducing the AHI in some individuals. For example, a sudden transition from NREM to REM sleep might require a significant increase in pressure, but APAP devices ramp up pressure slowly. In this case, using a pressure effective during REM sleep for the entire night (CPAP) would eliminate this issue.

AUTOBPAP

AutoBPAP devices adjust the delivered IPAP and EPAP to maintain an open airway[34] (Figure 23–10). The devices manufactured by PR (DreamStation auto BiPAP) vary both IPAP and EPAP between pressure limits (EPAPmin, IPAPmax). The minimum and maximum PS can be set (PSmin and PSmax). Older versions of PR BPAP devices did not have the option of setting the PSmin. Typical initial settings include an IPAPmax of 25 cm H_2O and an EPAPmin set based on the previous CPAP treatment and/or BMI and neck circumference. For example, 4 cm H_2O in a smaller, pressure-intolerant individual or 6 to 8 cm H_2O if previous CPAP was >10 cm H_2O or in patients with significant obesity or a large neck circumference (≥17 in.). Typical values for PSmin and PSmax are 4 and 8 cm H_2O, respectively (maximum available value is 8 cm H_2O). The autoBPAP device from ResMed (Aircurve 10 Vauto) varies the EPAP using a single fixed PS that is set by the clinician (typically 4 to 6 cm H_2O; maximum PS value is 10 cm H_2O).

AutoBPAP is useful for delivery of BPAP treatment without the need for a titration or for chronic treatment in very pressure-intolerant patients. For example, a patient who requires relatively high pressure but is pressure intolerant could benefit from autoBPAP treatment.[34,55,56] Gentina et al.[55]

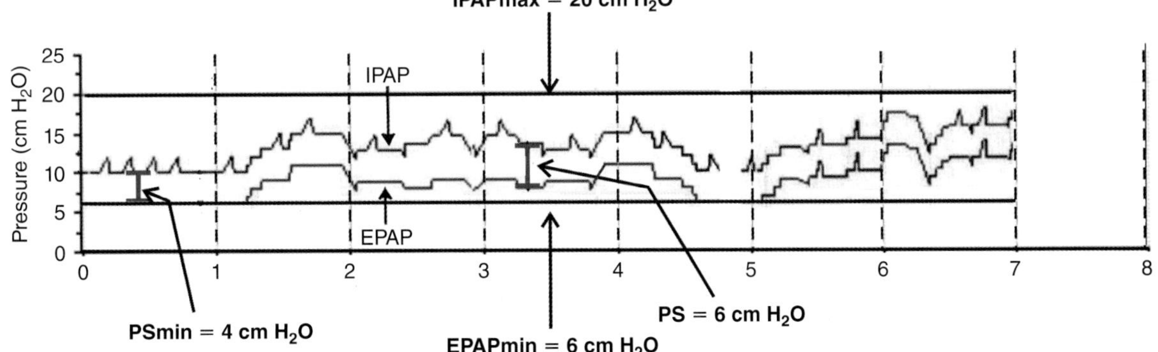

Figure 23–10 An example of a single-night titration with autoBPAP using a Philips Respironics device. Both the EPAP and IPAP vary between minimum EPAP (EPAPmin, here 6 cm H_2O) and maximum IPAP (IPAPmax, here 20 cm H_2O) with pressure support (PS = IPAP − EPAP) that can vary between minimum PS (PSmin) and maximum PS (PSmax). Here, PSmin is 4 cm H_2O and PSmax 8 cm H_2O. Between hours 3 and 4, the device delivered EPAP and IPAP with a PS of 6 cm H_2O. Note that, at the start of the night, EPAP was 6 cm H_2O and IPAP was 10 cm H_2O (PSmin + EPAPmin). Note that for ResMed autoBPAP devices there is a single specified pressure support and only the delivered EPAP varies to address respiratory events. *BPAP,* Bilevel positive airway pressure; *EPAP,* expiratory positive airway pressure; *IPAP,* inspiratory positive airway pressure; *PS,* pressure support.

changed a group of patients with poor CPAP adherence to flexible autoBPAP and noted an improvement in adherence and excessive sleepiness. Those with CPAP > 10 cm H_2O benefited the most. However, a randomized controlled pilot study[56] of patients with a poor initial CPAP experience found no advantage to autoBPAP compared with CPAP. In this study, after a pressure titration, patients were randomized to CPAP or flexible autoBPAP. The adherence in both groups was similar, with the CMS adherence standard met by 62% in the autoBPAP group and by 54% in the CPAP group. The study may have been under powered to detect a difference in adherence, but even if statistically significant, this difference in adherence would be of marginal clinical significance. *Both groups likely benefited from the good clinical care that was part of the protocol and from a repeat titration sleep study.* Carlucci and coworkers[57] found autoBPAP useful *during a PAP titration* in those not responding to or tolerating CPAP. However, most sleep centers would use a conventional BPAP titration and not autoBPAP in this circumstance. Of note, if using autoBPAP for titration to select fixed BPAP pressure, one could use the 90% IPAP and 90% EPAP levels in PR devices or, in ResMed devices, the 95th percentile EPAP and an IPAP equal to 95% EPAP + the PS used during the titration with autoBPAP. For example, after a period of treatment with PS of 4 cm H_2O and an EPAP at the 95th percentile of 10 cm H_2O, one could use a fixed BPAP of 14/10 cm H_2O. However, chronic treatment with autoBPAP, rather than fixed BPAP, is an attractive option if covered by insurance. As with APAP and CPAP, BPAP-S (no backup rate) and autoBPAP-S devices often have similar price points.

COMFORT MEASURES

Modified Pressure Profile PAP

Several manufactures of PAP devices have developed modified pressure profile PAP (flexible PAP) with the goal of improving patient comfort and adherence. These algorithms drop expiratory pressure but return to the inspiratory pressure at end exhalation. For simplicity, only pressure modifications for PR and ResMed devices will be discussed here. In the past, PR devices provided the comfort options Cflex and Cflex+ (for CPAP devices) and Aflex (for APAP devices) (Figure 23–8).[35,57,58] In these modes, pressure drops in early exhalation and returns to the inspiratory baseline at end exhalation. The amount of pressure drop using Cflex depends on expiratory flow (greater flow associated with a greater pressure drop using a proprietary algorithm) and on the setting (1, 2, or 3). Of greater clinical significance in the Cflex+ or Aflex modes, the expiratory pressure drops 2 cm H_2O below that of current inspiration, with further drops as in Cflex. That is, the difference between Aflex and Cflex+ is that the former is used with the APAP mode and the latter with CPAP. With Aflex using the APAP mode, the inspiratory pressure varies according to the APAP algorithm, but in exhalation, there is a 2 cm H_2O pressure drop combined with further drops due to the flex setting during exhalation. Of note, with Cflex+ and Aflex, the expiratory pressure cannot drop below 4 cm H_2O, which is the lowest pressure the devices can deliver. In both Cflex+ and Aflex, there is also a smoothing of the transition from inhalation to exhalation, and the degree of smoothing depends on the flex setting. *However, in the latest models of PR APAP and CPAP DreamStation 2 devices, only the "flex" option (0, 1, 2, 3) is provided.* In the CPAP mode, flex is equivalent to Cflex+; in APAP mode, it is equivalent to Aflex. This change reflects the fact that the 2 cm H_2O drop in pressure during exhalation is much more apparent to users and clinically significant than the additional drops with the flex portion (1, 2, 3). Flexible drops in expiratory pressure (Biflex) are available on the PR BPAP devices (BiPAP). ResMed CPAP and APAP devices offer expiratory pressure relief (EPR). In this mode, an EPR setting of 1, 2, or 3 results in a drop in expiratory pressure of 1, 2 or 3 cm H_2O, respectively. EPR can be turned off, used only during the ramp period or used full-time. The ramp option is discussed below, and is a time period when the device increases from a ramp start pressure to either the set level of CPAP or the lower pressure limit of APAP.

An initial study found that flexible PAP improved adherence by about half an hour using a cross-over design.[58] Several subsequent studies of patients on CPAP[51,59-63] or APAP[64] did not find an increase in adherence with flexible PAP. A meta-analysis[51] and review of the literature by an AASM PAP-treatment task force[4,5] also found no evidence for improvement in adherence with pressure profile modifications.

In summary, although the idea of flexible PAP (pressure profile modifications) is appealing, there are no convincing data indicating flexible PAP options improve adherence in unselected patients. However, dropping the exhalation pressure 2 cm H_2O or more in PR devices or 1, 2, or 3 cm H_2O in ResMed devices during exhalation could be considered "mini BPAP," and flexible PAP is potentially useful in some patients with *pressure intolerance, bloating, or expiratory mouth leak* (if using a nasal interface).

Ramp

Most PAP devices allow the patient the ability of using a ramp option at the start of treatment. The ramp option allows a slow increase in pressure at the start of treatment from a lower initial pressure than used for treatment. In some devices, there is a separate ramp button (to initiate a ramp period). In others, the ramp can be turned on/off and the ramp time set (15, 30, or 45 min) using a device menu. The starting ramp pressure can be set by the clinician or the patient, depending on the device and the options allowed for patient modification. For CPAP devices, this means the pressure falls to the set ramp pressure, then slowly increases to the set CPAP level over the ramp time. For APAP devices, the pressure increases from the starting ramp pressure to the minimum pressure setting, then pressure is adjusted per the APAP algorithm. On newer PR PAP devices, the "ramp plus" option allows the user to set both the ramp time (15, 30, or 45 min) and the starting ramp pressure (4 to 10 cm H_2O, or off). The ramp can be activated by tapping an icon on the touchscreen, and the pressure can be changed during use up or down by hitting + or −. Once set, the ramp plus will automatically be activated at the start of future treatment settings using the latest pressure and ramp-time settings. For ResMed CPAP and APAP devices, ramp time can be set to off, 5 to 45 minutes, or auto. In the auto ramp option, the pressure starts at the ramp pressure (can be set) with a default ramp time of 30 minutes. If the device "detects sleep" during the 30-minute period, the pressure increases by 1 cm H_2O per minute to the minimum pressure setting. However, if sleep onset is not detected the device will reach the target pressure within 30 minutes. The ramp option is appealing and can be used during middle-of-the night awakenings to help the individual return to sleep. However, no study has shown that the ramp option increases adherence. The advanced PAP options are changed periodically and the reader is referred to the latest device manual.

Humidification

Complaints of nasal congestion and nasal or oral dryness are common in PAP users.[65] Most PAP devices have an integrated heated humidification system (although the patient can choose not to use humidity). The devices can be used in cool humidity mode, if desired. Heated humidity (HH, warm air) can deliver a greater level of moisture than cool humidity and may be especially useful in patients with mouth leak or nasal congestion. Some important facts concerning PAP and heated humidification are listed in Box 23–1. PAP humidifiers consist of a water chamber sitting on a heating element ("hot plate"). The temperature of the heating element and air in the humidifier chamber are increased so that the air can hold more moisture (higher setting, higher heat, warmer air). Absolute humidity is the amount of water vapor in the air regardless of the temperature. Absolute humidity (g/m^3) increases at higher humidifier settings. Relative humidity is the absolute humidity as a percentage of maximum water vapor the air can hold at a given temperature. The temperature at which a given absolute humidity is 100% of the capacity of air to hold water vapor, relative humidity= 100%) of the relative humidity is called the dew point, the point at which water can condense. As the temperature in the patient's bedroom is lower than the temperature of the air in the humidifier, there is a potential for condensation in the tube and mask ("rain out").

It is important to realize the connection between mask or mouth leak and complaints of dryness. The increased airflow needed to maintain pressure to compensate for increased leak removes moisture (humidity) from the mask/tube system, lowers humidity at the mask, and causes dryness. Increased airflow also evaporates more water, reducing the level of water left in the humidifier chamber. Mouth leak can cause a dramatic fall in relative humidity[65] and a loss of humidity from the upper airway/CPAP system, thus drying the nasal or oral mucosa. In Figurere 23–11, the reduction in humidity during mouth leak is minimized by the use of humidity. Drying of the nasal mucosa increases nasal resistance,[66,67] and this is minimized by use of HH (Figure 23–12).[67] Interventions for complaints of dryness *should always include addressing mask or mouth leak* as well as adjustment of humidification. An oronasal (full face) mask can reduce the loss of humidity associated with mouth leak. However, getting a good mask seal is more difficult and loss of humidity can actually be greater with the use of a oronasal mask due to high mask leak (compared to a nasal mask) in some patients.

Box 23–1 PAP HUMIDIFICATION FACTS

- Heated humidity (HH) provides an increased amount of moisture (warmer than room air) compared with cool (pass-over) humidification.
- HH improves symptoms of dryness and nasal congestion in many patients.*
- No increase in adherence with HH in unselected patients.*
- May improve adherence in selected patients with nasal or dryness symptoms.
- Water condensation in the hose (can produce thumping sound) or mask is common if higher levels of humidity are provided (especially with low room temperature).
- Interventions for water condensation include lowering the humidity setting, change to adaptive humidification, hose insulation, avoiding a very cool room temperature, lowering the PAP device to a level below bed, and use of a heated hose.
- Adaptive humidification modes reduce "rain out" when compared with nonadaptive modes by monitoring the room temperature to determine the relative humidity at the mask and avoid delivery of levels of moisture which would result in condensation. The adaptive modes deliver lower levels of moisture compared to a fixed mode (*unless a heated tube is used*).
- Heated tubes are the most effective method for preventing water condensation in the tube and mask ("rain out") and allow the delivery of higher levels of moisture. When heated tubes are attached one can adjust the both the humidity level and tube temperature.
- The current PR Dreamstation 2 CPAP/APAP devices features only adaptive humidification but can supply more moisture when used with a heated tube. When a heated tube is attached one can select both a humidity setting and a tube temperature setting. When a heated tube is attached to ResMed devices one can select manual or auto. With the manual option the level of humidity and tube termpature can be set. Using the auto option the tube temperature can be set to auto or a tube temperature can be specified. The humidity setting is automatically controlled based on the tube temperature.**
- If humidification results in variable abmount of water being used this suggests a variable amount of leak (assuming humiidty settings are not changed). Reducing leak may improve symptoms of dryness without changing same level of humidity. Interventions for a complaint of dryness should include both addressing high leak and changing the humidification (if needed).

*AASM PAP clinical guidelines[5] recommend use of HH to improve symptoms, but AASM did not find evidence that HH improved PAP adherence.
** If "rain out" occurs with a heated tube either reduce the humidity setting or increase the tube temperature.
AASM, American Academy of Sleep Medicine; *HH,* heated humidity; *PAP,* positive airway pressure.

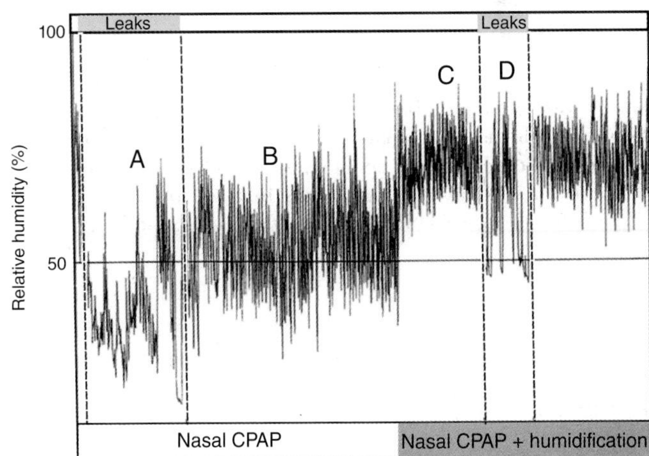

Figure 23–11 Change in relative humidity during treatment with nasal continuous positive airway pressure (CPAP). On the left, nasal CPAP alone; on the right, nasal CPAP with humidification. A fall in humidity with airleak is shown at the left (A), with return to baseline after the leak is resolved (B). With humidification, the relative humidity increases, even with baseline breathing on nasal CPAP (C). With humidification the mask relative humidity is maintained above 50% even with a fall in relative humidity during a period of leak (D). (From Martins de Araujo MT, Vieira SB, Vasquez EC, Fleury B. Heated humidification or face mask to prevent upper airway dryness during continuous positive airway pressure therapy. *Chest.* 2000;117:142-147.)

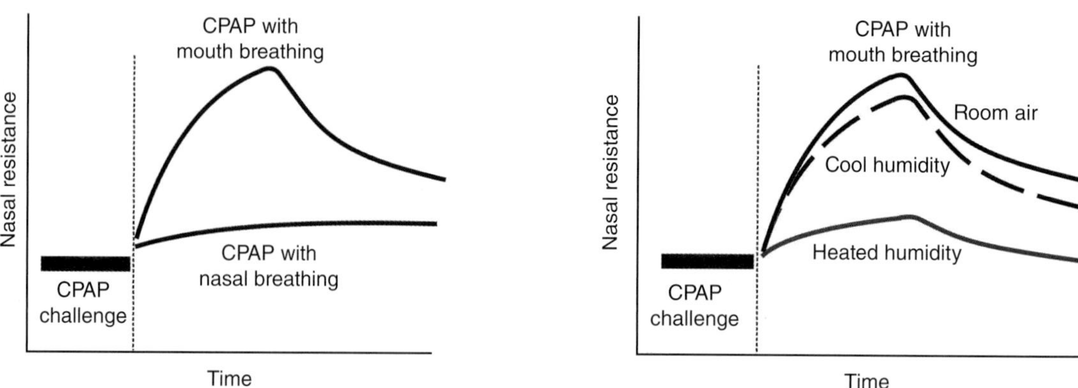

Figure 23–12 Schematic showing effects of (left) changes in nasal resistance after a 10-minute challenge with CPAP with nasal breathing or with mouth breathing (simulating mouth leak). Loss of humidity through the mouth causes mucosal drying and an increase in nasal resistance. (Right) Use of heated humidification during a 10-minute CPAP challenge with mouth breathing delivers sufficient humidification to minimize the increase in nasal resistance by preventing drying of the nasal mucosa even with loss of humidity via the mouth. The amount of humidity delivered by cool humidity was not sufficient to prevent a large increase in nasal resistance. (Schematic based on data from Richards GN, Cistulli PA, Ungar RG, et al. Mouth leak with nasal continuous positive airway pressure increases nasal airway resistance. *Am J Respir Crit Care Med.* 1996;154:182-186.)

Rain out (water condensation in mask and tubing) is a major issue with the use of HH. There is always a balance between controlling symptoms of dryness and avoiding excessive condensation ("my CPAP spit water at me"). As with modes of pressure, there has been an increase in the complexity of humidity settings. PAP devices may offer both fixed and adaptive humidity modes. In the fixed mode a given amount of absolute humidity (moisture) is delivered (based on the humidity setting/temperature of the air in the humidifier chamber). Adaptive humidity modes monitor room temperature and adjust the absolute humidity output so that the relative humidity at the mask and distal tubing (mask temperature is approximately room temperature) is less than 100% (usually around 80–85%, to prevent rain out). The Philips Dreamstation 1 PAP devices in the fixed (classic) mode delivers high humidity but often this is often associated with "rain out" at the higher settings. The settings are 0 and 1 to 5 with a higher setting associated with more humidity. The adaptive humidity mode prevents water condensation but may deliver an inadequate amount of moisture. The solution is using the heated tube mode that can deliver higher humidity without rain out (temperature higher than room temperature). The Philips Dreamstation 2 PAP devices have only an adaptive humidity mode and a heated tube is the best option if a higher amount of moisture is needed. A number of interventions for rain out, such as increasing bedroom temperature, use of a cloth tube insulator, and lowering the PAP unit below bed level (tube water runs back into humidifier chamber due to gravity), were recommended but often with inadequate control of condensation. Today, heated tubes are the best option if high humidity is needed. In ResMed devices without a heated tube, the humidity can be set to Off or levels 1 to 8 using a menu. The humidifier works in a fixed mode (a given setting associated with a given absolute humidity). If a heated tube is attached the climate control options are available (manual or auto). In the manual mode the level of humidity and tube temperature may be set. The tube temperature range is 60 to 86°F; default setting is 81°F. The humidity setting (1-8) is can be specified. In the auto mode the tube temperature may be set to auto or the tube temperature specified as in the manual mode. In the auto mode the humidity adjusts automatically based on the tube temperature. The goal is a relative humidity of about 85%. The heated tube has a temperature sensor near the connection of the tube to the mask. In the manual mode if rain out occurs with a humidity setting of 6 and a heated tube setting of 72 degrees Fahrenheit, the heated tube temperature should be increased or the humidity setting decreased. In both PR and ResMed devices *heated tube options do not appear in the menu unless the heated tube is attached.* It is also important to note that substantial water in the tube can result in disturbing noises, including gurgling, percolating, or thumping sounds. Adequate cleaning of the humidifier chamber and hoses (usually with non-antibacterial soap and water) does require extra patient effort.

The two factors that determine the amount of water removed from the humidifier chamber are the humidity setting and the flow across the water (evaporation). PAP devices are leak tolerant and maintain pressure in the face of higher leak by simply increasing flow. *Note that, when a patient reports a variable amount of water use* without *changing the humidity settings, this means the flow across the water was different (higher flow with higher leak and more water used). If no pressure settings were changed, this means higher unintentional leak.* In circumstances with high humidity settings and high leak, it is possible to completely use all the water in the chamber during one night.

An initial study found that use of HH, when compared with use of cool humidity and no humidity, improved CPAP adherence.[68] Subsequent studies did not find improvements in either acceptance of CPAP (after titration) or long-term adherence to CPAP treatment.[4,69,70] Another investigation could not document a benefit from the "prophylactic" use of HH for titration.[71] However, if dryness causes severe nasal congestion, this may increase the chance of titration failure or cause a full face mask to be used. In the 2003 AASM practice parameters for PAP treatment, use of HH was recommended to improve CPAP usage (not necessarily routine use).[3] An AASM systematic review by Patil et al. concluded there was no evidence that HH improved PAP adherence.[4] *There was evidence that HH improved symptoms such as dryness and nasal congestion.* A criticism of many humidity-adherence studies is that patients with baseline nasal congestion or dryness were not targeted. It seems reasonable to use humidity in patients with complaints of nasal congestion or mouth breathing at baseline. Certainly, in some patients, use of HH is crucial; in others, it may improve satisfaction or not be needed at all. It is common practice to order a PAP device with a humidifier (many devices have a mandatory humidifier chamber integrated into the design), providing the HH option if needed. Some patients only use HH during winter months when household air is dry. As noted, reduction in mouth or mask leak along with adjustment of humidification is important to improve symptoms of dryness or nasal congestion. *Nasal congestion that worsens overnight with PAP use is suggestive of nasal drying (inadequate humidity or excessive leak).*

MASK INTERFACES

When CPAP devices became available commercially, the first interfaces were nasal masks. Today, a large and ever-increasing variety of interfaces is available (Box 23–2). Nasal masks (including masks with cradle cushions), nasal pillow (prongs) masks, oronasal (full face) triangular masks, and full face masks consisting of cushions that cover the mouth but with a nasal cradles or nasal pillows at the top of the cushion are available (Figures 23–13 and 23–14).[72] However, it is still difficult to obtain a good mask fit in many patients.[72-75] *Repeated mask leaks can cause nonrestorative sleep as well as residual events.*[76] An American Thoracic Society (ATS) workshop report by Genta et al. provided a comprehensive review of published evidence concerning mask selection.[74] Mask selection was also evaluated in an AASM systematic review by Patil et al.[4] New technology using facial scanning with more mask size options or customized masks will allow more personalization of mask fitting.[77,78] Rather than three sizes of masks, there may be five or more to allow a personalized mask with improved fit. It is common for a small size to be too small and a medium size to be too large. PR and ResMed have developed facial scanning and mask selector programs, but as might be expected, they recommend one of their own masks. Other facial scanning software is available, and some smartphone applications allow patient-centered involvement in mask selection (https://www.maskfitar.com and others). Some applications are also available online for use in telemedicine visits. There are several *nasal mask* options including triangular masks over the nose (Figure 23–13A, D), nasal pillow masks (Figure 23–13B), and masks with an under-the-nose opening/cradle (Figure 23–13 C, E). Nasal pillow masks are often better tolerated than traditional nasal masks by patients with claustrophobia, nasal bridge abrasion/difficulty sealing in the nasal bridge area, a mustache, and absent upper teeth (no support for the upper lip).[72] Nasal pillow masks obviate the need for a seal on the nasal bridge and may be helpful if patients complain of air leaking into the eyes. It is essential to use a pillow size large enough to provide a good seal. Although it is said that nasal pillow masks are not suitable for high pressures, this is not always the case. Zhu et al. found pillows to work as well as other masks at pressures >12 cm H_2O.[79] There is a significant pressure drop across the nasal inlet during inspiration. Flexible nasal pillows under pressure dilate the nasal inlet and reduce the pressure drop in some patients. This can result in a sensation of higher pressure using nasal pillows, and in fact, a lower level of CPAP might be more comfortable and as effective as the existing pressure level with a traditional nasal mask.

A popular version of several masks allows the tubing to come off the top of the head. Other patients may prefer a quick release option at the front of the mask (nocturnal bathroom trips). Some masks utilize magnetic clips which are very convenient Figure 23–13 A, D. However, at the time of writing these masks are under recall. There is a concern that the magnetic fields can change the function of certain medical devices (e.g. pacemakers) or adversely affect patients with metallic implants. One can expect non-magnetic clip versions to be available in the future. The reader should check the Philips Respironics and ResMed websites for that latest information. At the time of writing PR and ResMed masks with magnetic clips may be used if the contraindications and concerns are addressed. In general masks with magnetic clips are not recommended for use in patients with pacemakers or other devices in whom a magnetic field can impair function.

For patients who have severe nasal congestion or open their mouths during PAP treatment, oronasal masks[80-82] and oral interfaces[83] are available. Oral interfaces are rarely used because of the need for very aggressive humidification. Mouth leak can be addressed by adding a chin strap[84] (variably effective and not always well accepted by patients) to a nasal interface or by using an oronasal mask. Other mouthpiece options have been developed to reduce mouth leak.[85] Various types of mouth tapes or soft shields between the teeth and lips are available.

Box 23–2 KEY POINTS ABOUT PAP INTERFACES

Nasal Interfaces

- Triangular cushions, nasal pillow cushions (prongs), under the nose cradles with various opening configurations
- Options for masks with hose attachment to the front of the mask or on top of the head
- Recommended initial interface
- Chin strap may be needed for mouth leak
- Difficulty breathing through the nose suggests an oronasal mask may be needed, at least initially
- Aggressive treatment with humidity, nasal steroids, or nasal surgery may reduce mouth leak or allow a switch from full face (oronasal) to a nasal interface

Oronasal (Full Face) Masks

- Only option for some patients with nasal congestion or mouth leak
- Treatment of nasal congestion or addition of a chin strap can allow some patients to convert to a nasal interface
- Oronasal masks are associated with increased leak, lower adherence, and a higher pressure requirement compared with nasal masks

Mask Fitting

- Careful fitting and education on adjustment are helpful (videos)
- Cushion should be cleaned daily and replaced monthly
- 3D-scanning applications becoming available with increased cushion sizes to personalize mask fit
- Trial of multiple masks is often needed
- Patient preference should be considered

2019 AASM PAP Clinical Guidelines and Evidence[5]

- Nasal interface recommended for treatment initiation
- PAP adherence greater with nasal than with oronasal interfaces

PAP, Positive airway pressure.

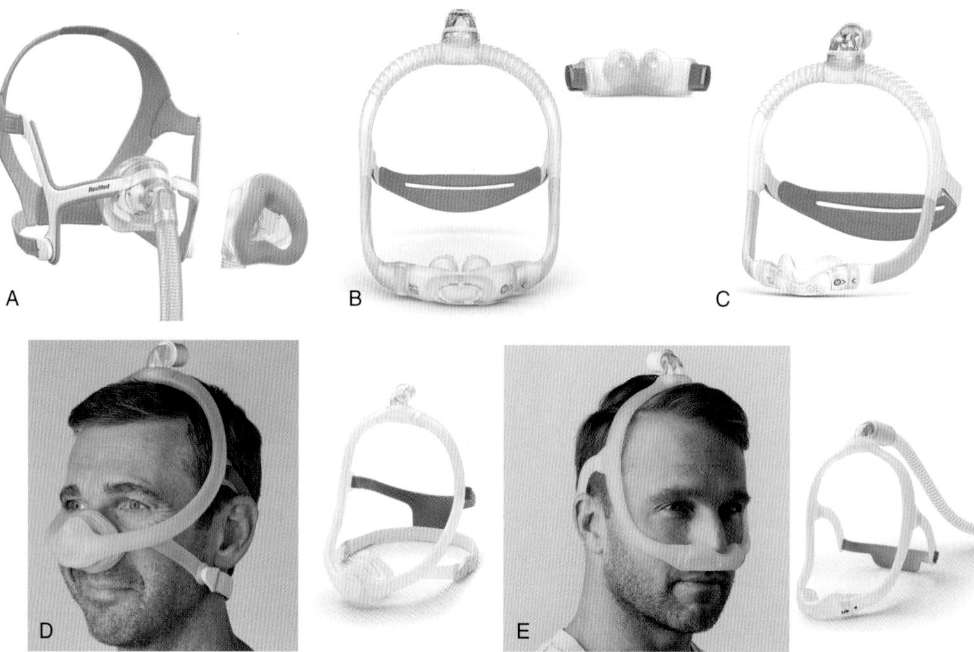

Figure 23–13 Examples of currently available nasal interface options. (A) AirTouch N20 (nasal mask with memory foam cushion) (© ResMed. All rights reserved.); (B) P30i (nasal pillows with hose attached to the top of the head) (© ResMed. All rights reserved.); (C) N30i nasal cradle mask (© ResMed. All rights reserved.); (D) DreamWisp nasal mask ("Courtesy of Philips RS North America LLC." All rights reserved.); (E) Dreamwear nasal cradle mask ("Courtesy of Philips RS North America LLC." All rights reserved.) Whereas most CPAP mask cushions are made of silicone, AirTouch cushions are made from UltraSoft memory foam material. Of note all masks with magnetic clips (A and D) are under "recall" at the time of writing. There is a concern that the magnetic fields can change the function of certain medical devices or adversely affect patients with metallic implants. Non-magnetic clip versions will likely be available in the future. At the time of writing Philips Respironics mask should not be used in patients with pacemakers or other metallic devices listed in the mask packaging. ResMed masks may be used if the proper patient warning is inserted in the packaging and contraindications (should not be used in patients with pacemakers or metallic implants) and cautions are observed. If magnetic clips are more than 6 inches away from medical devices the masks are felt to be safe. The reader should consult the latest information on Philips Respironics and ResMed websites as the recommendations often change.

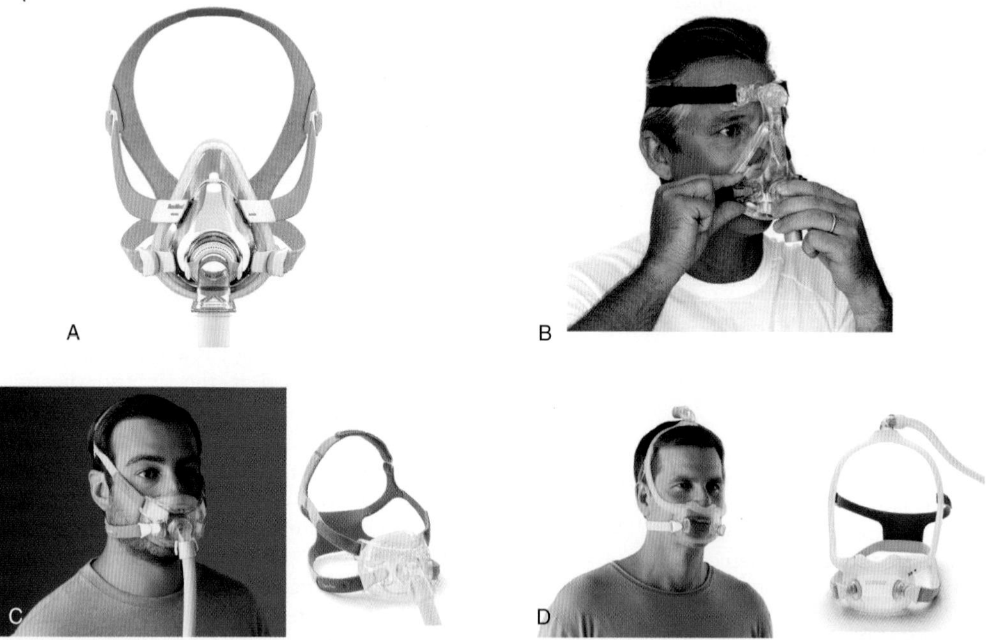

Figure 23–14 Examples of oronasal full face masks. (A) AirTouch F20 (© ResMed. All rights reserved.); (B) Mirage Quattro (© ResMed. All rights reserved.); (C) Amara View ("Courtesy of Philips RS North America LLC." All rights reserved.); (D) DreamWear Full ("Courtesy of Philips RS North America LLC." All rights reserved.). Of note all masks with magnetic clips (A, C, and D) are under "recall" at the time of writing. See the legend in Figure 23-13 for additional information. The reader should consult the Philips Respironics and ResMed websites for the latest information.

Oronasal masks (Figure 23–14) must seal over a large area, and this makes finding a good fit very difficult in some patients. In edentulous patients, oronasal masks may also compress the soft tissues or actually move the mandible, posteriorly narrowing the airway. In fact, one study found the oronasal mask caused posterior displacement of the mandible, and use of a mandibular advancement device improved this issue.[86] A case report found that events with an oronasal mask were noted **only in the supine position**, even with high pressure (CPAP of 16 cm H_2O), suggesting *body position may affect the efficacy of oronasal masks.* Subsequent titration with a nasal mask found resolution of events in all body positions at a much lower pressure (7 cm H_2O).[87] Several studies have found that oronasal masks (when compared with nasal interfaces) resulted in lower adherence, higher leak, and higher required treatment pressures.[4,74,88-93] The results of numerous studies were concisely reviewed by Genta et al.[74] Therefore, treatment initiation with a nasal interface is recommended unless not tolerated by the patient. The 2019 AASM evidenced-based review concluded that PAP adherence was higher with nasal interfaces when compared with oronasal (full face) interfaces.[4] *The 2019 PAP-CPG recommends routine use of nasal or intranasal interfaces as the first treatment option.*[5] As obtaining a good seal at the nasal bridge is difficult, as mentioned previously, several nasal masks use nasal pillows (prongs) or feature a cradle-shaped cushion with openings "under the nose," with the cushion covering only the lower part of the nose. Some oronasal masks cover the nose and mouth (Figure 23–14 A, B). However, under-the-nose options also exist (Figure 23–14 C, D). Of note, under-the-nose oronasal masks may be better tolerated by patients with claustrophobia.[94,95] Patients having difficulty obtaining a good seal with an oronasal mask may benefit from a change to a nasal mask (without or without a chin strap), and often, a slightly lower treatment pressure is effective[74] and improves mask seal or oral venting. It is possible that pressure modifications allowing a drop in pressure during exhalation (BPAP, EPR, Flex) can reduce expiratory oral venting. *The fact that an oronasal mask was used in the PSG titration should not prevent consideration for use of a nasal interface for chronic treatment.* If nasal congestion was the issue, medical treatment of nasal symptoms may allow use of a nasal interface. If the required PAP seems high given a relatively small neck circumference or BMI in a patient using an oronasal mask, then a change to a nasal interface should be considered.

THE IMPORTANCE OF LEAK

Leak (mouth and/or mask) is an important issue for both PAP titration studies and chronic treatment. High leak can prevent PAP from being effective. Although the devices are leak tolerant, adequate pressure at the mask may not be maintained with high leak. Leak removes humidity from the system and cause dryness, even with the use of HH. Intermittent leak into the eyes or intermittent mouth leak can cause repeated arousals. Recording of the leak signal is useful for the physician reviewing a PAP titration. Lebret et al.[96,97] performed a systematic review of the literature for determinants of leak and identified nasal obstruction (likely increasing mouth opening), the male sex, older age, high BMI and central fat distribution (likely requiring higher pressure or higher work of breathing), and oronasal masks as associated with higher unintentional leak. No PAP modality was associated with higher leak. Increased risk of high leak with older age may be associated with loss of teeth (less mask support), changes in skin elasticity, and a decrease in subcutaneous fat (wrinkles). If an edentulous patient sleeps without dentures in place, this can also increase leak (less mask support). Body positions other than the supine position (i.e., lateral position) and REM sleep (vs. non-REM [NREM] sleep) can increase leak. Transition from the supine to the lateral position may require a readjustment of straps and pillows can press on the mask/tubing causing displacement. Oronasal masks tended to reduce the risk of unintentional leak during mouth opening and REM sleep. However, for PAP treatment in general, nasal masks are associated with lower unintentional leak than oronasal masks. There is limited data on the efficacy of chin straps for reducing unintentional leak,[84] though individual patients may benefit. If a chin strap or oronasal mask is not successful at addressing mouth leak, a nasal interface with lower pressure or PAP modes that lower pressure in exhalation can be tried. *It is important to remember that PAP titrations often overestimate the required pressure*[98] *and that nasal masks may be effective at lower pressure.* There is also an option to use positional treatment as an adjunctive therapy, as many patients require much lower pressure in the lateral sleeping position.

INTERVENTIONS FOR PAP SIDE EFFECTS

It is essential for the patient to quickly communicate difficulties when starting PAP or during PAP treatment. Establishing a good patient-provider relationship and enthusiastically addressing concerns is important. Realistic expectations should also be set. Patients may expect an instant "miracle," so informing them that the need for multiple mask changes and pressure and humidity adjustments is common avoids discouragement. Numerous side effects of PAP treatment have been described (Table 23–4), including mask discomfort, mask leaks, air leak into the eyes, dryness, nasal congestion, claustrophobia, disturbance of sleep, excessive pressure, aerophagia/bloating, and difficulty exhaling. Some patients remove the mask for a bathroom visit but do not restart treatment. Although for unselected patients the number of side effects does not correlate with adherence, individual patients may have a large improvement in adherence with an aggressive approach to handling problems.[34] The 2019 AASM PAP-CPG recommends troubleshooting interventions during PAP initiation.[5] The accompanying evidence review found that education combined with troubleshooting can improve adherence. Finding a comfortable and well-fitting mask interface is one of the biggest challenges in PAP treatment.[4] Interventions for mask side effects, including dry eye, discomfort, mask leaks, and skin breakdown are commonly needed. Proper sizing and mask strap adjustment are essential; they should be checked at every visit to the physician or respiratory therapist providing PAP support. Interventions for mask issues will be discussed in more detail later in this chapter. For bloating or pressure intolerance, a reduction in pressure (or upper pressure limit when using APAP), use of flexible PAP options, education on the ramp option, and a change to BPAP are options. Often, a reduction in pressure by a few centimeters of water is very helpful and often does not impair treatment efficacy. Accepting a mild increase in the AHI is better than the patient abandoning treatment. Patients with claustrophobia may benefit from a nasal pillow mask, an under-the-nose mask, or referral to psychology for behavioral therapy (mask

Table 23–4 Common PAP Treatment Side Effects and Interventions

Positive Pressure Side Effects	Interventions
Mask Side Effects (See Also Table 23-5)	
• Mask discomfort • Skin breakdown (especially on nasal bridge)	• Avoid overtightening—intervene for mask leaks • Alternate between different mask types • Nasal prongs/pillows—eliminate trauma to nasal bridge • Tape barrier for skin protection

• Air leaks
  • Conjunctivitis
  • Discomfort
  • Noise
	• Proper mask fitting
	• Proper mask application (education)
	• Different brand/type of mask
	• Monthly change of mask cushion

• Mouth leak • Mouth dryness	• Treat nasal congestion if present (see below) • Chin strap • Heated humidity • Full face (oronasal) mask • Consider BPAP, flexible PAP, lower pressure, APAP
• Mask claustrophobia	• Nasal pillows/prongs interface • Desensitization
• Unintentional mask removal	• Address mask and pressure issues • Consider increase or decrease in pressure
Nasal Symptoms	
• Congestion/obstruction	• Nasal steroid inhaler • Antihistamines (if allergic component) • Nasal saline • Humidification (heated) • Full face (oronasal) mask—eliminating mouth leak may reduce dryness • ENT referral for possible surgical intervention to improve PAP treatment
• Epistaxis	• Nasal saline • Humidification (heated) • Reduce nasal steroid dose • ENT referral if intractable
• Nostril pain with nasal pillows	• Saline gel just inside nostril entry • Change nasal pillows size
• Rhinitis/rhinorrhea	• Nasal ipratropium bromide
Other Problems	
• Water in the mask and/or hose	• Reduce humidity setting, use adaptive mode • Tube insulator • Order a heated tube
• Pressure intolerance	• Ramp • Flexible PAP • BPAP • APAP • Lower prescription pressure (lower pressure than used in titration may be effective) • Lower pressure + adjunctive measures (elevated head of bed, side sleeping position, weight loss)
• Aerophagia/bloating	• BPAP, flexible PAP (Flex PR, EPR ResMed), reduce pressure
• Bedpartner dissatisfaction	• Education on importance of treatment • Intervention for noisy leaks or other concerns

AHI, Apnea-hypopnea index; *APAP*, autoadjusting positive airway pressure; *BPAP*, bilevel positive airway pressure; *ENT*, ear, nose, and throat; *EPR*, expiratory pressure relief; *PAP*, positive airway pressure; *RAMP*, period of lower pressure before treatment with prescription pressure; *ENT*, otolaryngologist.

desensitization).[94,95] Unintentional mask removal can occur as a result of nasal congestion, mask discomfort, or leaks but can also occur because of inadequate pressure. For example, APAP devices may not increase pressure rapidly enough at the transition from NREM to REM sleep, with resulting respiratory events, choking, arousal, and mask removal. Nasal congestion can be a significant issue that may be addressed with nasal steroids, antihistamines (oral or topical), increased humidity, or reduced mask leak (tends to remove humidity from the system). As noted, studies have demonstrated that *loss of humidity via a leak can dramatically increase nasal resistance* (Figure 23–12).[67] Increased nasal resistance increases oral breathing, which can increase mouth leaks in a patient using a nasal mask or result in a patient stopping treatment. A patient report of nasal congestion worsening as the night progresses suggests leak or inadequate humidification. Epistaxis often responds to increased humidity, nasal saline, or reduction in nasal steroids. If nasal bleeding continues, a referral to otolaryngology is needed. Sometimes mucosal vasculature needs to be cauterized. Excessive rhinorrhea in the morning may be a cholinergic-mediated reflex and responds to nasal ipratropium bromide. If nasal symptoms are intractable, referral to otolaryngology is recommended. PAP treatment/satisfaction in some patients may improve with inferior turbinate reduction or repair of septal deviation. A retrospective analysis of nonadherent PAP patients with ear, nose, and throat (ENT) issues found that otolaryngology intervention can improve CPAP adherence in select patients.[99] If mouth leak is occurring, a chin strap or oronasal mask can be used, but these options are not always acceptable to the patient. Some patients can tolerate leak if the amount of humidification is increased.

Bloating may respond to lowering of pressure or a switch to APAP or BPAP.[54] For pressure intolerance, use of a lower pressure, the addition of flexible CPAP, a change to APAP or BPAP, and education regarding using the ramp setting are all options. It is also worth emphasizing that, if all else fails, using a lower treatment pressure with a mild elevation in the residual AHI is preferred compared with no PAP treatment ("a lower pressure vs. no pressure at all"). As noted, titration studies overestimate CPAP requirements.[98] Weight loss, nonsupine sleep, and elevation of the head of the bed may also lower pressure requirements.

The attitude of the bedpartner is important for treatment success. Including the significant other in clinic visits and education on the importance of treatment are helpful. Bedpartners may report snoring or mouth or mask leak, which can help identify problems the patient does not report. Bedpartner complaints of noisy treatment usually mean there are mask or equipment issues.

Interventions for Mask and Leak Issues

Interventions for common mask issues are summarized in Tables 23–4 and 23–5. A trial of several masks is often needed to find one that a patient can use comfortably. This is one situation in which trying several different types of masks in the sleep center before and during the PSG titration can be useful. When trying a new mask, it is best to try the mask on with some level of PAP (if feasible) to determine whether the seal is adequate. When troubleshooting, have the patient apply the mask with education on proper strap adjustment if needed. Patients tend to overtighten masks, and this can cause damage to the nasal bridge or impair the mask's ability to seal. Modern mask designs have flexible cushions that balloon out against the face for a better seal, and overtightening prevents this process. The mask size should be checked. Patients with long faces may be better treated using masks with a more elongated cushion. Gel pads for the nasal bridge are available but are not a good long-term solution. If there is nasal abrasion or difficulty obtaining a seal at the nasal bridge, a change to a nasal pillow mask or under-the-nose cradle mask may solve the issue. Patients with intractable leaks using oronasal masks can be switched to a nasal interface after addressing nasal congestion or addition of a chin strap. In some patients, lower pressure using a nasal interface may be effective. Contact with the mask cushion can cause dermatitis.[100] Several brands of cloth mask liners are available. A change to another brand or type of mask (different cushion material) may resolve issues. Patients should avoid mask-cleaning wipes with allergenic chemicals. For nasal congestion, increased humidification, medical treatment of rhinitis, and addressing mask or mouth leak are options.

Table 23–5 Interventions for Mask Issues

Issue	Interventions
• Leak into eyes • Nasal bridge abrasion	• Nasal pillow mask better nasal mask fit • Nasal cradle or pillows mask • Minimask not touching nasal bridge
• Skin irritation	• Change mask type (different cushion material) • Cloth mask liner • Use nonallergenic mask cleaner
• Severe nasal congestion	• Aggressive medical treatment • Humidification • Oronasal mask • Consider ENT referral
• Mouth leak	• Chin strap • Humidification • Treat nasal congestion • Reduced pressure in exhalation (BPAP, Flex) • Reduced pressure • Oronasal (full face) mask
• Mask movement causing leaks	• Proper mask headgear size and adjustment • Use mask with a more stable headgear (or hose connection on the top of the head) • CPAP hose caddy (swivel arm holds hose above bed)
• Moisture in mask	• Reduce humidity setting or change to adaptive mode • Heated tube • Hose insulator, avoid very cool room temperature, level of PAP device below bed level
• Mask leaks in lateral position	• Pillow with lateral indentations so mask not displaced by pillow, different mask • Patient education
• Intractable mask leak	• Monthly cushion replacement • Adjust headgear, assure proper cushion size • Change mask type • Change from oronasal mask to nasal interface • Use 3D scanner to recommend mask • Try slightly lower treatment pressure

CPAP, Continuous positive airway pressure; *ENT,* ears, nose and throat (otolaryngology); *PAP,* positive airway pressure.

Adequate care and timely replacement of masks (and mask cushions) are also essential to maximize their ability to seal. Removing facial oils from the mask cushion (with a wet towel or nonantibacterial soap) daily will extend the life of the cushion. Most insurance plans allow monthly replacement of mask cushions. One study found patients who changed their masks/equipment frequently had better adherence.[101] If a patient gets up to use the bathroom during the night, we encourage disconnection of the hose from the mask rather than taking off the mask. Many masks have a quick release option where the hose attaches to the mask. Masks that are removed in the middle of the night often are not replaced (or replaced incorrectly). Of note, for unselected patients, the **type of nasal interface** does not seem to affect adherence. However, as noted, oronasal masks were associated with lower adherence than nasal interfaces but are sometime the only option acceptable to patients. To avoid patient discouragement, it is worth informing them that it is normal for patients to try many masks before finding a suitable interface. Some patients report difficulty keeping a good mask seal when in the lateral sleeping position. Often, pulling the mask away from the face and repositioning the mask will work better than tightening the straps. There are commercially available special "CPAP pillows" with an indentation on each side so the pillow does not push up on the mask. As a last resort, one could try a slightly lower treatment pressure, as some masks will seal much better after a reduction of only 1 or 2 cm H_2O. As noted, patients can often be treated effectively at pressures below the final pressure used in titration studies.[98] The upper airway displays a type of hysteresis, and a lower pressure than one used to open the airway can maintain an open airway. Some titration protocols lower the pressure once the airway is stabilized to see if a lower pressure will work. Changing from CPAP to APAP may lower the average treatment pressure in some patients.

If the tubing pulling on the mask is a source of difficulty, CPAP hose caddy devices are available that position the hose above the mask, with the hose attached to an arm that swivels with movement from the supine to lateral position to avoid the hose pulling on the mask. *Masks with a tube connection/swivel on the top of the head* might also reduce difficulty with the hose pulling on the mask.

Less Common Complications of PAP Treatment

Some uncommon complications of PAP treatment are worth noting. Patients can develop periorbital swelling (either bilateral or unilateral)[102,103] and air leak up the nasal lacrimal duct (carries tears from the lacrimal sac of the eye into the nasal cavity).[104-106] In one case report,[103] switching to a nasal pillow interface that did not compress the area over the zygomatic arch resolved the issues (hypothesized interference with venous or lymphatic drainage). In another case, a fracture of the orbital bone was found.[102] Leak up the lacrimal duct can be associated with unexplained dry eyes unresponsive to mask changes.[104,105] Leak can be documented by the "bubbling test," with a few drops of saline applied at the medial eye. CPAP is then initiated; one eye is tested at a time. Bubbling through the saline from the lower lacrimal punctum is diagnostic for CPAP-associated retrograde air escape via the nasolacrimal system.[106] A discussion of possible treatments can be found in the article by Ryals et al.[105] A change to non-CPAP treatment (if an option) is associated with resolution of the problem. Alternobaric vertigo is a sensation that can occur with aviation or diving; it can sometimes occur with CPAP use in association with decreased hearing.[107] The etiology is expansion of trapped air within the middle ear space due to the inability of the eustachian tubes to equalize the middle-ear pressure with ambient pressure. The positive middle-ear pressure results in the sudden movement of the stapes at the oval window, causing excess vestibular stimulation. When the pressures in both ears reach ambient levels, symptoms resolve. Precipitant factors for alternobaric vertigo include allergic rhinitis or recent upper airway infection, both of which can affect the patency of the eustachian tube. This condition has been described with CPAP use. Lowering of the level of CPAP used for treatment or improvement with withdrawal of treatment with rechallenge using gradual pressure increments has also been reported.[107] Tympanic membrane perforation associated with CPAP treatment or air leak out of an existing perforation can also occur during CPAP treatment via air passage up the eustachian tube.[108] There was a report of a patient with masseter muscle pain due to repeated attempts during sleep to prevent mouth leak while using a nasal mask.[109] As mentioned, contact dermatitis can occur from facial skin contact with mask cushion material.[100] A change in type of cushion (different mask manufacture or type) or use of a cloth mask liner may resolve this issue. Treatment with low potency topical steroids or topical calcineurin inhibitors such as pimecrolimus or tacrolimus, which decrease the immune response at the site of the dermatitis, has also been described.

Sanner et al. retrospectively reviewed CPAP-treated patients for infectious complications and found an increase in infectious complications with CPAP, especially in those using heated humidification who inadequately cleaned the devices.[110] Ortolano and coworkers recovered bacteria from CPAP hoses when the same bacteria were introduced into heated humidifier water and found no contamination when bacterial filters were fitted between the hose and humidifier.[111] However, another study found no significant difference in the prevalence of rhinosinusitis, lower respiratory tract infections, and hospital admissions for pneumonia between CPAP and non-CPAP treated patients. The presence of a humidifier did not influence the prevalence of infections. Nasal swab cultures from both groups found similar bacterial isolates. The authors concluded that use of humidifiers have no significant effect on infections or microorganisms residing in the nose.[112] However, adequate cleaning of humidifiers and other CPAP equipment is recommended and may be *important in patients susceptible to recurrent sinus infections*. This concern has resulted in a number of CPAP cleaning devices. However, those using ozone can damage CPAP equipment. Deterioration of sound abatement foam from ozone exposure has been reported. The U.S. Food and Drug Administration has not cleared devices producing ozone or ultraviolet light for cleaning CPAP equipment.[113] We have seen a few patients with recurrent sinus infection on PAP improve with *complete cessation of humidity* and have observed a preference for some residual dryness rather than repeated infections. The mechanism is unknown, but some patients using humidity with CPAP complain of a sensation of wetness in the nose and sinuses.

ADHERENCE—DEFINITIONS AND MEASUREMENT

The major challenge of PAP treatment is to ensure that a patient's adherence to treatment is adequate.[12,114-119] Despite the excellent efficacy of PAP devices for reducing the AHI, as previously noted, the actual effectiveness can be much lower. Some important facts about PAP adherence are summarized in Box 23–3. The pattern of PAP use is established early,[119] and objective adherence (not a patient's report) is essential to guide treatment.[12,114-119] Patient reports are not reliable and consistently overestimate actual use (in one study by 69 minutes).[117] PAP devices can record both blower hours and time at pressure (actual use). Detailed daily information can show important patterns (e.g., consistent mask removal at 5 a.m.). As most REM sleep occurs in the last hours of the night (when OSA is usually the most severe), wearing the CPAP

Box 23–3 PAP ADHERENCE FACTS

- Thresholds of adherence (nightly use) for benefit
  - Decreased subjective daytime sleepiness (ESS) ≈ 4 hrs or longer
  - Decreased Objective sleepiness (MSLT) ≈ 6 hrs
  - Improved quality of life ≈ 7-7.5 hrs
- Even suboptimal adherence may bring benefits.
- Some patients need longer than 3 months to meet adherence standards.
- CMS standard (≥4 hours for ≥70% of nights over 30 days in the first 90 days after treatment initiation). However, 4 hours use is too low for maximal PAP benefit.
- Objective adherence monitoring is essential. Patient report overestimates use.
- Early adherence predicts long-term adherence.

CMS, Centers for Medicare and Medicaid Services; *ESS*, Epworth Sleepiness Scale; *MSLT*, multiple sleep latency test; *PAP*, positive airway pressure.

device the entire night is important for maximal benefit. The data obtained from PAP devices often also includes useful information on leak and an estimate of the residual AHI. Today, PAP machines have both internal memory and removable memory (smart cards, SD cards, flash drives). The removable media can store extensive information on adherence and patterns of use. The recorded device information can be assessed by direct machine interrogation (internal memory) or by transferring the information to a computer. Modern PAP devices contain wireless modems that send information to a central location (cloud based). The physician or durable medical equipment (DME) company can assess the information from the central server. Information about patient adherence is provided during the critical first weeks of use without requiring the patient to come into the clinic or a DME company office (telemonitoring). Modern devices usually include a Bluetooth option that can communicate with smartphone patient applications and provide the patient with direct daily feedback on use, mask fit, and efficacy.[120] Most PAP devices provide information on use and the quality of mask fit on the PAP device screen (smiling face indicates good mask fit).

Adherence rates are defined in many ways. Most devices compute the percentage of days used, the average use all days (averaging in zeros for days not used), average nightly use (days used), and the percentage of nights used for more than 4 hours. An early paper reporting measurement of objective adherence by Kribbs and coworkers[117] defined regular users as those who used CPAP at least 4 hours/day on at least 70% of nights. In their study, only 46% of patients met these criteria. CMS and most private insurers have accepted this adherence standard. For Medicare, the patient must have 30 consecutive days over the first 3 months with ≥4 hours of use on ≥70% of nights.[23] Some private insurers use CMS guidelines, whereas others use a portion of the initial 90-day window to address adherence. An adherence visit is required 31 to 91 days after starting PAP for the physician to document benefit and adherence. Payment for PAP will end after 3 months if adherence criteria are not met. If the patient is evaluated by the provider and has another sleep study (usually a titration study), this qualifies the patient for another 3-month trial. The requirements for another sleep study are excessive (and costly). A face-to-face interaction with the physician to address the adherence issue (often with mask fitting or adjustment of pressure) is more effective and less costly.[24] In the future, insurers will likely move away from the strict requirements for another sleep study. Naik et al.[121] analyzed APAP use in a Veterans Health Administration (VA) setting over 9 months after treatment initiation using telemonitoring data and found that, of the adherent patients over the first 3 months, 31% became nonadherent in the following 9 months; of the nonadherent patients at 1 month, 30% became adherent. That is, **early nonadherence does not rule outet long-term adherence** in almost a third of the nonadherent patients. Therefore, restricting the trial of CPAP to 3 months eliminates potential benefit in a significant fraction of patients. Another investigation of a group of nonadherent patients (average use 3–4 hrs) randomized patients to continued CPAP or sham CPAP groups. The sham CPAP group had an increase in Epworth Sleepiness Scale (ESS) score and worsening of quality of life as measured by the Functional Outcomes of Sleep Questionnaire (FOSQ) compared with the group continuing CPAP.[122] *Thus, even suboptimal use of PAP is associated with patient benefit.* A recent technical advisory panel published recommendations for changing the current CMS guidelines for PAP reimbursement. Some patients receive benefit even from suboptimal adherence, some will meet adherence if given longer than 90 days, and a repeat sleep/titration study is expensive and rarely beneficial. Evidence of physician assessment of PAP issues with interventions (with or without a clinic visit) is more cost-effective.[24]

RATES OF ADHERENCE AND FACTORS INFLUENCING ADHERENCE

There has been tremendous variability in the reported rates of PAP adherence.[123-128] This is a result of several factors, including different populations (moderate to severe OSA vs. all patients), different definitions of adherence, different length of follow-up, and different algorithms for initiating PAP treatment and following patients. CPAP nonadherence rates from 29% to 83% have been reported.[4,114] One of the largest studies of long-term adherence with nasal CPAP by McArdle and coworkers reported 68% of patients were still using CPAP at 5 years.[124] Pepin et al. found 79% of patients using CPAP for >4 hours on 70% of nights at 3 months.[125] Sin and coworkers followed patients with an AHI of >20 events/hour and found >85% were using the device > 3.5 hours/night at 6 months.[126] Kohler et al. found that 81% of patients were using CPAP at 5 years.[127] A study using big data from cloud-based storage found average **short-term** PAP adherence (use ≥ 4 hours on ≥70% of nights) to be 75%.[128] A study using new technology to enhance patient engagement found up to 87% adherence.[120] Most (but not all) long-term studies report a significant decrement in adherence with time.

Factors Influencing Adherence and Importance of Early Adherence

Adherence studies vary widely in the factors associated with improved or decreased adherence to PAP as well as those not affecting adherence.[114,118-130] The most frequently documented factors are shown in Table 23–6. Age, gender, and marital status do not consistently affect adherence, although one study found older age to be associated with better adherence and a decreased importance of adverse effects of CPAP use on sexual intimacy to impair adherence.[119] Some studies have found the African American race to be associated with lower

Table 23–6 Factors Associated With Good or Poor Adherence

Good Adherence	Poor Adherence	No Effect
• Pretreatment daytime sleepiness • Subjective benefit • High AHI (some studies) • High oxygen desaturation index • Good early adherence	• Spouse referral • Anatomical factors (high nasal resistance*, epiglottic collapse) • High mask leak • Poor early adherence • Adverse effect on sexual intimacy • ±Race (Black) • Lower socioeconomic group • Distressed personality type • Claustrophobia • Use of oronasal mask	• Age, gender (most studies) • Level of pressure • Type of nasal mask • Mode of pressure • Heated humidification • Modified pressure profile (Flex, EPR)

*Sugiura T, Noda A, Nakata S, et al. Influence of nasal resistance on initial acceptance of continuous positive airway pressure in treatment for obstructive sleep apnea syndrome. *Respiration.* 2007;74(1):56–60.
AHI, Apnea-hypopnea index; *EPR,* expiratory pressure relief.

adherence, but this may be better explained by lower socioeconomic status. A retrospective study of PAP adherence in a VA population found better adherence in patients living in a high socioeconomic neighborhood.[129] Several factors do not seem to affect adherence. The technology used to diagnose and treat OSA, such as the PAP device, HH, and mask interface, does not seem to affect adherence (except for lower adherence with oronasal masks). Psychological factors, including personality type and the presence of claustrophobia, affect adherence, but the presence of depression does not. A type D (distressed) personality (negative affect, social inhibition, increased perceived side effects) and low self-efficacy are associated with worse adherence.[130] *The AHI was a significant factor (higher AHI associated with better adherence) in only a few studies.*[124] However, the amount of pretreatment sleepiness and the amount of improvement after treatment have significant effects on adherence. McArdle et al.[124] found an ESS score of >10 to be associated with better adherence, whereas Sin and coworkers [126] found an improvement in sleepiness to be associated with better long-term adherence.

Factors not affecting PAP adherence are listed in Table 23–6. As noted, the level of pressure, use of flexible PAP (pressure profile modification), and pressure mode of treatment (CPAP, APAP, BPAP) do not seem to be important determinants of adherence [4,114] in unselected patients. Individual patients, including those *not meeting adherence requirements*, may benefit from a change in treatment mode. Whether patients had a split-night sleep study or a separate diagnostic and PAP titration PSG did not seem to be a determinant of adherence. In uncomplicated patients, an HSAT and autotitration before CPAP treatment did not affect adherence; in one study, a clinical pathway using HSAT had higher adherence compared with traditional treatment initiation with PSG.[131] Similarly, HSAT followed by APAP treatment had similar adherence to treatment initiation compared with a PSG for diagnosis and PAP titration.[48] Although about two-thirds of PAP users report side effects, there is no evidence that the number of side effects predicts PAP use.[12] HH is effective for reducing nasal symptoms and dryness but does not increase adherence.[4] Finding an appropriate mask interface is one of the most challenging parts of providing PAP treatment. However, there is no evidence for the superiority of any type of **nasal** interface.[4] As noted, oronasal masks had lower adherence rates than nasal interfaces in several studies.[4,74]

Factors associated with poor adherence are listed in Table 23–6. These include poor early adherence,[115,119] a high amount of mask leak,[132] anatomical factors such as a high nasal resistance[114] or epiglottic collapse,[133] impaired sexual intimacy,[134] high residual AHI,[134] use of oronasal masks (compared with nasal interfaces),[4,74] claustrophobia,[93,94] the African American race,[119,134] lower socioeconomic group,[117] and spouse referral.[135]

A major motivation for seeking treatment may be spouse complaints about snoring or apnea. However, the patient must be convinced CPAP treatment is needed for their health in addition to calming the concerns of their bedmate. Involving the spouse or significant other in the treatment process has been a part of many PAP programs. If the spouse understands the health risks of untreated sleep apnea, they may encourage better CPAP use. However, the underlying relationship dynamics often determine the benefit or decrement of spousal involvement in determining CPAP adherence. Gentina et al.[136] found that marital quality was a significant moderator of these interactions, meaning a spouse's/partner's engagement improved adherence only when the quality of marriage was high. Noisy leaks that disturb the sleep of the bed partner can reduce satisfaction with treatment.[124,126]

How Much Adherence Is Enough?

Weaver and associates[137] studied patients before and after 3 months of therapy and correlated objective adherence with improvement in functioning. Duration thresholds of nightly PAP use above which significant improvement was noted for the following outcomes, include ≈4 hrs for the ESS, ≈6 hrs for improvement in the multiple sleep latency test (MSLT), and ≈7.5 hrs for optimal improvement in the Functional Outcomes of Sleep Questionnaire (FOSQ) results (Figure 23–15). Thus, as average nightly usage increased, subjective sleepiness, objective sleepiness, and then quality-of-life measures improved. The necessary amount of PAP usage depends on which outcome is being evaluated. In reading published adherence study results it is helpful to know what improvement is clinically significant (not just statistically significant). The minimum clinically significant reduction in ESS score is considered to be a decrease by 2.[138]

The current CMS guidelines state that devices will be reimbursed after 12 weeks only if objective adherence for a period of at least 1 month in the first 3 months shows ≥4 hours use per night for 70% or more of nights and the treating physician

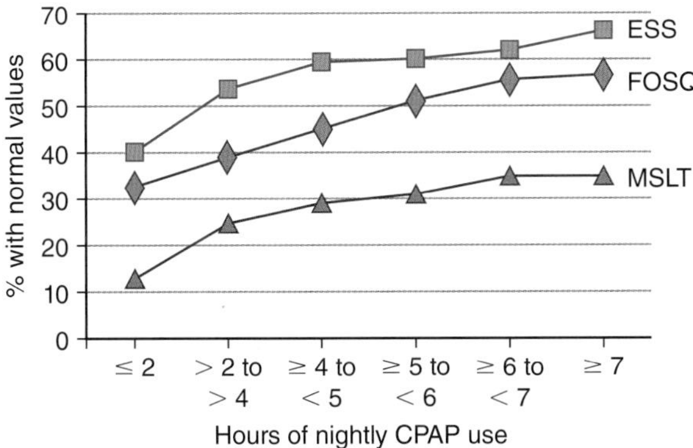

Figure 23–15 Measurements of the Epworth Sleepiness Scale (ESS, measure of subjective sleepiness), Function Outcomes of Sleep Questionnaire (FOSQ, quality of life), and sleep latency on the multiple sleep latency test (MSLT, objective sleepiness) at various hours of nightly continuous positive airway pressure (CPAP) use. Note the values are percentages of normal values rather than raw values. The ESS rises to a higher percentage of normal (less sleepy) as the amount of CPAP increases. The FOSQ (higher score, better quality of life) increases with nightly use. The sleep latency (lower score is better) improves with longer nightly use of CPAP. Note that, although significant benefit occurs with nightly use of 4 hours, the improvement in all parameters continues to increase (especially the FOSQ) as sleep duration on CPAP increases above 4 hours/night. (From Weaver TE, Maislin G, Dinges DF, et al. Relationship between hours of CPAP use and achieving normal levels of sleepiness and daily functioning. *Sleep.* 2007;30:711-719.)

documents in a face-to-face meeting that the patient is benefiting from PAP treatment.[23] For most patients, an average of 4 hours use is not enough PAP use for optimal benefit. Campos-Rodriguez and coworkers[139] followed a historical cohort of 871 patients with OSA for a mean of 48 months. The 5-year cumulative survival was highest in the group of patients who used PAP therapy >6 hours/night on average (96.4% survival), compared with patients who used PAP from 1 to 6 hours/night (91.3% survival) and patients who used PAP <1 hour/night (85.5%). The same group conducted a prospective cohort study of 55 patients with hypertension.[140] Patients with average use >5.3 hours/day and hypertension at entry to the study had a drop in mean arterial blood pressure of about 4 mm Hg. Numerous other studies of the effect of CPAP on cardiovascular disorders found better adherence was associated with better outcomes. However, as noted, suboptimal adherence to PAP treatment may still be of benefit to patients.[122]

Interventions to Improve Adherence

Given the importance of PAP adherence, there have been a large number of studies using different interventions or combinations of interventions with comparison to standard care. Recommended interventions are listed in Box 23–4. The AASM systematic review and meta-analysis[4] showed that evidence existed for pretreatment education (either alone or with troubleshooting), troubleshooting, and telemonitoring at treatment initiation to enhance adherence. There was no evidence for adherence enhancement with any mode of PAP treatment or HH. A Cochrane meta-analysis suggests that education-only interventions have a small effect on adherence, supportive interventions are associated with a mild improvement in PAP use, and behavioral interventions result in the largest improvement in adherence.[141] Hwang et al.[142] compared adherence outcomes between usual care, web-based OSA education (Tel-Ed added), CPAP telemonitoring with automated feedback

Box 23–4 INTERVENTIONS TO IMPROVE ADHERENCE

- OSA and PAP education pretreatment
- Mask fitting and mask education, humidity education (if humidity is to be used), interventions for nasal congestion
- Behavioral interventions to enhance treatment
- Attention to early adherence
- Monitoring objective adherence and treatment efficacy (residual AHI, leak)
- Telemonitoring (especially at PAP initiation to assess adherence and efficacy)
- CPAP help line, secure messaging for patient complaints
- Troubleshooting with interventions
- Patient smartphone applications (patient facing, daily patient feedback)
- Telemedicine—especially for patients with transportation issues

AHI, Apnea-hypopnea index; *CPAP,* continuous positive airway pressure; *OSA,* obstructive sleep apnea; *PAP,* positive airway pressure.

(Tel-TM), and both (Tel-both = Tel-Ed and Tel-TM). The CMS adherence rates for 90 days were as follows: usual care (53.5%), Tel-Ed (61.0%), Tel-TM (65.6%), and Tel-both (73.2%). Both Tel-TM and Tel-both were significantly higher than usual care, but Tel-Ed was not. This study demonstrates that education alone is the least effective intervention but can have an additive benefit to other interventions.

Hoy et al. used an intensive program with several interventions to improve adherence.[135] A study by Ballard et al.[34] showed that an aggressive approach salvaged a significant proportion of patients who initially had poor adherence. It is difficult to determine which interventions are the most useful in promoting adherence, as many interventional studies had several components.[12,114,135] Comprehensive programs of education (patient and bed partner), early contact with interventions,[135] a simple CPAP help line, or group education have improved adherence in some studies. As the PAP adherence pattern is determined early, intensive monitoring and interventions are important in the weeks after treatment initiation. A study at a VA medical center[143] found that cloud-based sleep coaches improved early adherence when compared with usual care employing motivational techniques and early interventions for problems. Cognitive behavioral therapy (CBT) interventions have shown promise.[144,145] Richards et al. used a CBT program including 2-hour sessions with patient and partner that provided education promoting the benefits of PAP ("sleep safely using CPAP") and videos of real-life CPAP users (role models) discussing their personal experiences dealing with CPAP issues and how CPAP use was an important benefit. CBT interventions are especially pertinent to patients with comorbid insomnia or claustrophobia.[94,95] The use of telemonitoring (use of cloud based storage of adherence data) has been beneficial[116,119,143,146] and is recommended in the AASM PAP-CPG.[4,5] The use of wireless modems allows the provider to view daily adherence, leak, and residual AHI and to change pressure settings. The AASM PAP task force recommended the use of telemonitoring during PAP initiation. Telemonitoring was an important component of a VA study of enhanced early interventions (use of sleep coaches) in improving early adherence.[143] However, having adherence information alone cannot improve adherence unless combined with a structured approach for patient interaction (reinforcing benefits of CPAP use) and early intervention.[116,119,143] A PAP hotline and quick access/walk-in clinics for PAP problems can be helpful. Although telemonitoring can provide information on the residual AHI on treatment as well as adherence and leak information, an ATS statement on the use of telemonitoring emphasized the limitations on the accuracy of the device determined AHI.[146] The statement suggests that the device determine AHI be labeled as the AHIflow, as it is based mainly on device flow.

The ability of patients to easily communicate PAP problems to providers is essential. The increasing use of secure messaging in the electronic medical record prevents long waits on hold or telephone tag. Smartphone applications and computer programs supplied by PAP manufacturers allow patients to view their adherence and detect problems with mask fit.[120] Patient engagement with smart phone applications has been shown to increased adherence.[120] In general, increased patient engagement with treatment is beneficial. Some PAP devices remind patients to change the filter and/or mask after a certain period of use.

Telemedicine is increasingly used in sleep medicine and is convenient for patients and providers.[147,148] Detailed PAP information is available from cloud-based sources, and barriers to adherence can be discussed with the patient. The only downside is that mask fitting really requires the presence of the patient, but this can be arranged by the local DME provider that started the patient on PAP. Use of smartphone facial-scanning applications may help address the issue of mask fitting interventions via telemedicine.

COMORBID INSOMNIA, HYPNOTICS

Patients with both insomnia and OSA pose a difficult problem. In addition, some patients who normally have no problems with insomnia will have problems falling asleep or staying asleep on CPAP. The importance of comorbid insomnia in patients with OSA (COMISA) has been increasingly recognized.[149] Unless insomnia is addressed, there is a high likelihood of PAP treatment failure. Some clinicians have been hesitant to prescribe hypnotics, believing it may reduce the effectiveness of CPAP. One study found that zolpidem, a commonly used hypnotic, did not impair efficacy of a given level of CPAP.[150] On the other hand, it has been hypothesized that using a hypnotic might improve adherence to PAP in some patients. A study by Bradshaw and colleagues[151] using zolpidem did not find an improvement. In contrast, Lettieri and associates[152,153] found improvement during CPAP titration (sleep quality) and long-term adherence with eszopiclone (a hypnotic with a longer duration of action than zolpidem). It is possible that a longer-acting medication is needed to improve CPAP adherence. A meta-analysis of studies of the use of nonbenzodiazepine hypnotics and CPAP adherence concluded the best evidence of improvement in adherence was with eszopiclone.[154] Note that these studies did not specifically target patients with comorbid insomnia. Although the routine use of a hypnotic to aid in CPAP treatment cannot currently be recommended, temporary use of a hypnotic should be considered if insomnia is a major obstacle to CPAP use. A better option is referral for CBT treatment of insomnia (CBTI). A study by Sweetman et al.[155] found that CBTI improved PAP adherence in patients with both insomnia and OSA. In a VA population, CBTI with a PAP adherence program provided by a "sleep coach" (with behavioral sleep medicine supervision) improved adherence compared with a sleep education control intervention.[156] CBTI can also work in individuals with insomnia and severe OSA.[157] However, Ong and coworkers[158] found that whereas CBTI and PAP improved insomnia complaints more than PAP alone, there was no improvement in CPAP adherence. In summary, the addition of hypnotics has not consistently improved adherence, though the "Z" drugs appear safe to use if the patient is using PAP. This assumes the patient does not have risk factors potentially impairing breathing during sleep, such as severe lung disease or current opioid or alcohol use. CBTI alone or when combined with a behavioral PAP adherence program appears to improve CPAP adherence in some patients with OSA and insomnia. However, more confirmation of a benefit on PAP adherence is needed. Clearly, *PAP alone is unlikely to improve insomnia complaints unless combined with treatment specific for insomnia.*

PAP Adherence in Pediatric Patients

Special interventions are needed to improve acceptance of PAP treatment and adherence in pediatric patients.[159-161] Behavioral techniques such as desensitization (allowing children to play with masks before a sleep study), a system of rewards for good adherence, and a team approach using social workers and psychologists are helpful. Educating parents on the importance of treatment and providing them techniques for encouraging adherence are essential. The use of a DME company with experience dealing with children is also important. More discussion of PAP treatment of pediatric patients can be found in Chapter 27. There has been some interest in the use of APAP in children with OSA. Certainly, starting PAP without a titration in uncomplicated cases or in patients in whom a sleep study might be difficult due to caregiver issues could be useful. Khaytin and coworkers[162] reviewed their experience with APAP in children. They found that APAP-derived optimal CPAP pressure correlated well with optimal CPAP levels determined by PSG (although there were substantial differences in some children). At least for older children, APAP treatment might be an option, but more data is needed.

PAP TITRATION AND AUTOTITRATION

PSG is the standard method for PAP titration (to determine optimal pressure) and is usually accomplished either as the second part of a split-night study or during an entire night after a previous diagnostic PSG study (or diagnostic HSAT). The practice parameters provide guidance regarding when a split study is acceptable.[3] A split study was recommended only if the AHI was greater than 40 events/hour (or 20 events/hour with severe desaturation or arrhythmia) and 2 hours of monitoring had occurred. At least an additional 3 hours of monitoring time must be available for the PAP titration. If an adequate titration is not obtained, a repeat PSG titration is indicated. Of note, these recommendations for a split study are based on limited data. A more recent clinical practice guideline for diagnostic testing of OSA[163] stated, "We suggest that, if clinically appropriate, a split-night diagnostic protocol, rather than a full-night diagnostic protocol for PSG, be used for the diagnosis of OSA." The guideline assumes a split-night protocol that initiates CPAP titration only when the following criteria are met: (1) moderate to severe OSA is observed with a minimum of 2 hours of recording time on the diagnostic PSG, and (2) at least 3 hours are available for CPAP titration. Sometimes, use of a split study is required for reimbursement. The CMS guidelines[23] for qualifying a patient for PAP have been revised to state that if less than 2 hours of sleep are recorded, the minimum number of apneas and hypopneas must equal the number that would have been required if 2 hours of sleep had been recorded. For example, to meet a cutoff AHI of 15 events/hour, a total of 30 apneas and/or hypopneas must be recorded in the diagnostic portion of a study.

General Titration Considerations

Before a PAP titration, the patient should be educated about OSA, PAP treatment, and the PAP titration process.[9] They should be given mask interface options, and they should try on one or more interfaces while breathing on low pressure (CPAP practice) before the study begins. If a split study has been ordered, these events should take place *before any diagnostic monitoring begins*. Several interfaces should be available (nasal, oronasal, oral, pillows). HH should be available as well as a source of supplemental oxygen.

Pediatric PAP Titration Considerations

PAP titrations in children require some extra considerations. Children are often given a mask to play with and try on during the day for at least a week before scheduled study. The child should be desensitized to the mask during the day by wearing it for increasing periods while engaging in a fun activity (e.g., watching a favorite video). Split-night studies are not recommended for children. If a child without previous mask desensitization undergoes a split-night study, this may frighten the child and make subsequent CPAP use unlikely. Pediatric-sized masks should be available. DME providers and sleep technologists skilled and willing to provide care for pediatric patients should be used. Studies have shown that structured behavioral interventions that help with compliance include graduated exposure, positive reinforcement, dealing with escape and avoidance behavior, and praising distracting activities that allow the child to wear a mask successfully.

Monitoring During Positive-Pressure Titration

As previously noted, PAP devices used in a sleep disorder center can provide several analog or digital outputs that can be recorded, including the PAP flow, leak, pressure, and tidal volume (Table 23–7 and Figure 23–6). The total flow delivered by the machine is measured by an accurate flow sensor in the PAP device. As discussed, the total flow is then partitioned into two components (Figure 23–4): the PAP flow and the "bias" flow or leak. The PAP flow is sometimes called PAP device flow, PAP flow, CPAP flow, or Cflow. The PAP flow is used to score respiratory events. The PAP flow signal provides not only an estimate of the magnitude of flow but also information from the inspiratory flow contour. High upper airway resistance is manifested by a flattened inspiratory waveform.[164] The normal shape is a round one. A tracing in Figure 23–16 shows that the inspiratory portion PAP flow tracing is flat at a pressure of 7 cm H_2O, and snoring is noted. These findings suggest significant upper airway narrowing is still present. An increase in CPAP to 8 cm H_2O results in a round signal shape and elimination of snoring. PAP flow signals are usually either filtered or insufficiently sampled to show snoring. Snoring can be detected by a snoring sensor placed on the neck or from pressure vibrations in the mask (measured by a sensitive pressure transducer). Sleep-center PAP units also provide a "patient pressure" signal that can be recorded (sometime called Cpress or CPAP pressure). This is the pressure at the machine outlet and can differ slightly from the set pressure (value entered by technologist). Mask pressure can also be directly measured by connecting the mask to a pressure transducer. Actual mask pressure can then be recorded. The mask pressure may be somewhat lower during inhalation and sometimes slightly higher during exhalation than the pressure at the PAP device outlet due to pressure changes across the hose. The inspiratory mask pressure can be significantly lower than the pressure at the device outlet if there is a large pressure drop across the hose (due to high flow—often associated with high leak). PAP devices used at home for treatment have menu options to specify the mask type and the hose diameter. Some devices also allow a "resistance" setting based on mask type). This information is used to estimate the actual pressure at the mask.

Monitoring Leak During PAP Titrations

The trend in leak is more useful than the absolute number. If the patient has not moved and leak suddenly increases, this could provide a hint that mouth leak is occurring (assuming the patient is wearing a nasal mask). Sometimes, an **increase in leak** can occur with the **onset of REM sleep** (Figure 23–17). Relaxation in the facial musculature can sometime produce mask or mouth leaks. Observation using video (zooming in) can show an open mouth or fluttering of the lips during mouth leak (Video 23-1).

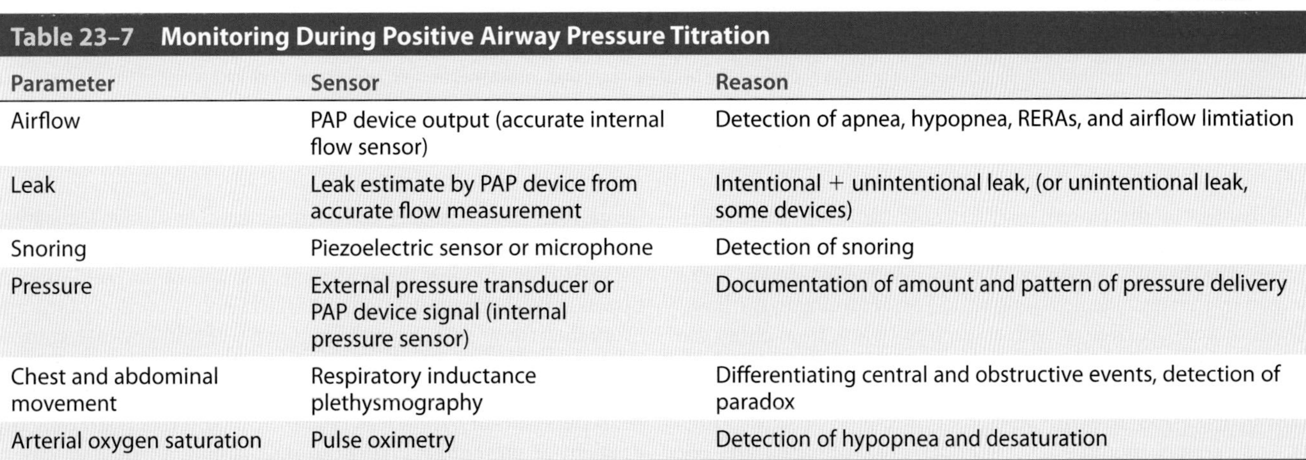

Table 23–7 Monitoring During Positive Airway Pressure Titration

Parameter	Sensor	Reason
Airflow	PAP device output (accurate internal flow sensor)	Detection of apnea, hypopnea, RERAs, and airflow limtiation
Leak	Leak estimate by PAP device from accurate flow measurement	Intentional + unintentional leak, (or unintentional leak, some devices)
Snoring	Piezoelectric sensor or microphone	Detection of snoring
Pressure	External pressure transducer or PAP device signal (internal pressure sensor)	Documentation of amount and pattern of pressure delivery
Chest and abdominal movement	Respiratory inductance plethysmography	Differentiating central and obstructive events, detection of paradox
Arterial oxygen saturation	Pulse oximetry	Detection of hypopnea and desaturation

PAP, Positive airway pressure; *RERA,* respiratory effort-related arousal.

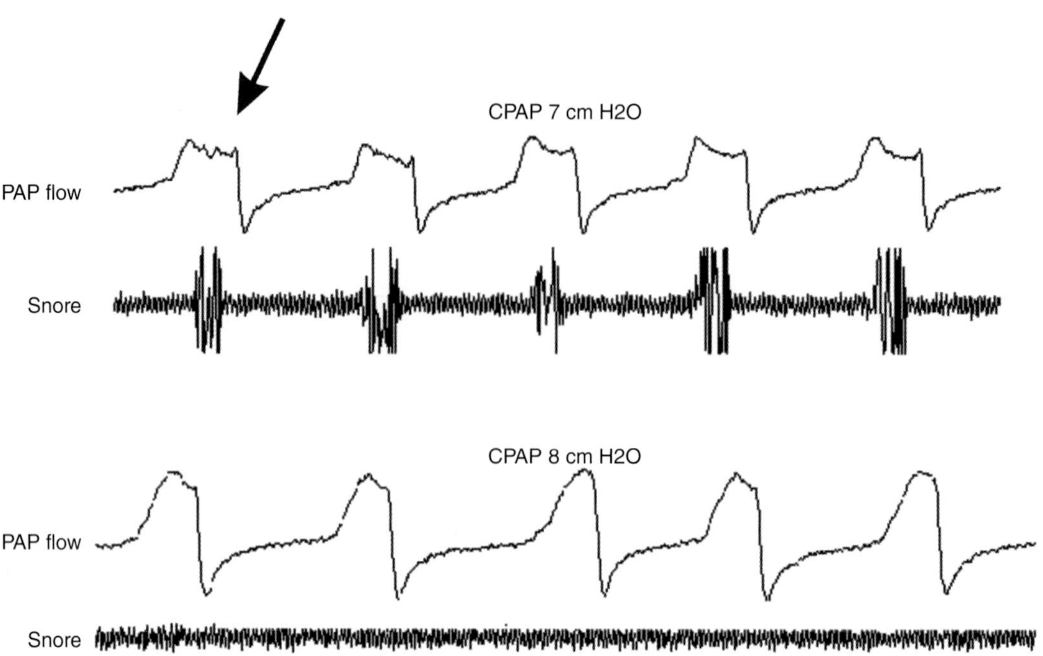

Figure 23–16 Example showing use of the inspiratory waveform shape of the positive airway pressure (PAP) flow signal. On continuous PAP (CPAP) of 7 cm H_2O, the shape is flat (arrow), consistent with airflow limitation (narrow upper airway), and snoring is also noted in the snore sensor data. After an increase of CPAP to 8 cm H_2O, the inspiratory shape is round, and snoring has resolved. (From Berry R. *Fundamentals of Sleep Medicine*. Elsevier; 2011:328.)

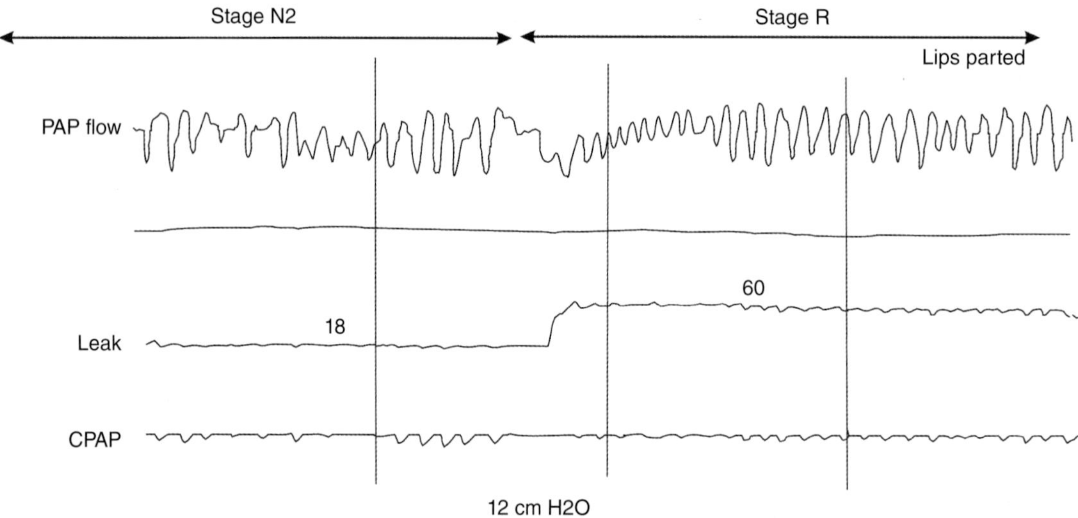

Figure 23–17 Example of increased leak associated with the transition from non-REM (NREM) to REM sleep. During REM sleep, muscle hypotonia can affect the facial muscles, and sometimes, mouth opening occurs. In this case, there is an abrupt increase in leak from 18 lpm to 60 lpm (the continuous positive airway pressure [CPAP] has not changed).

Changes in the pattern of PAP flow can also be useful in evaluating leak. If the flow signal becomes truncated during expiration, this means that part or all of flow during exhalation is not sensed by the machine flow sensor (no flow returning to the hose/device system), consistent with an expiratory leak from either the mask or the mouth. If the patient is wearing a nasal mask (which has not moved), the sudden appearance of truncated expiratory flow (often associated with vibration in the snoring sensor) suggests expiratory mouth leak (Figure 23–18). Azabarzin and coworkers[165] performed upper airway endoscopy simultaneously with PAP flow recording and documented that sudden truncation of expiratory airflow was associated with palatal prolapse, which shunts flow through the oral route. On the other hand, mouth opening without palatal prolapse shunts only a portion of expiratory flow through the mouth (Figure 23–19). In any case, truncation of expiratory flow is associated with oral venting during exhalation. The technician does not necessarily have to intervene for mild amounts of mouth leak unless the mouth leak is arousing the patient or preventing PAP from maintaining a patent airway. If mouth leak is a problem, a chin strap, an oronasal mask, or

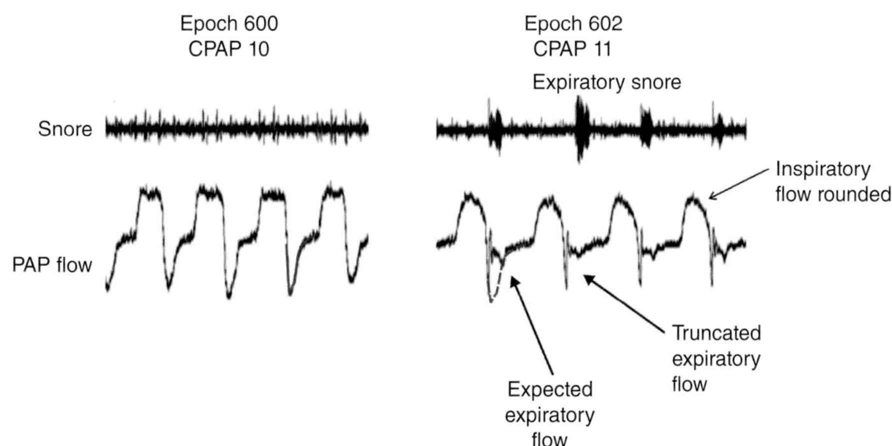

Figure 23–18 Truncation in the expiratory flow (inspiration is upward) associated with expiratory snore. In this patient, an open mouth and fluttering lips were noted on video. This pattern can be seen with expiratory venting via the mouth and can be associated with palatal prolapse (see Figure 23–19). On the right, the dashed line during exhalation on the first breath illustrates the expected shape during exhalation.

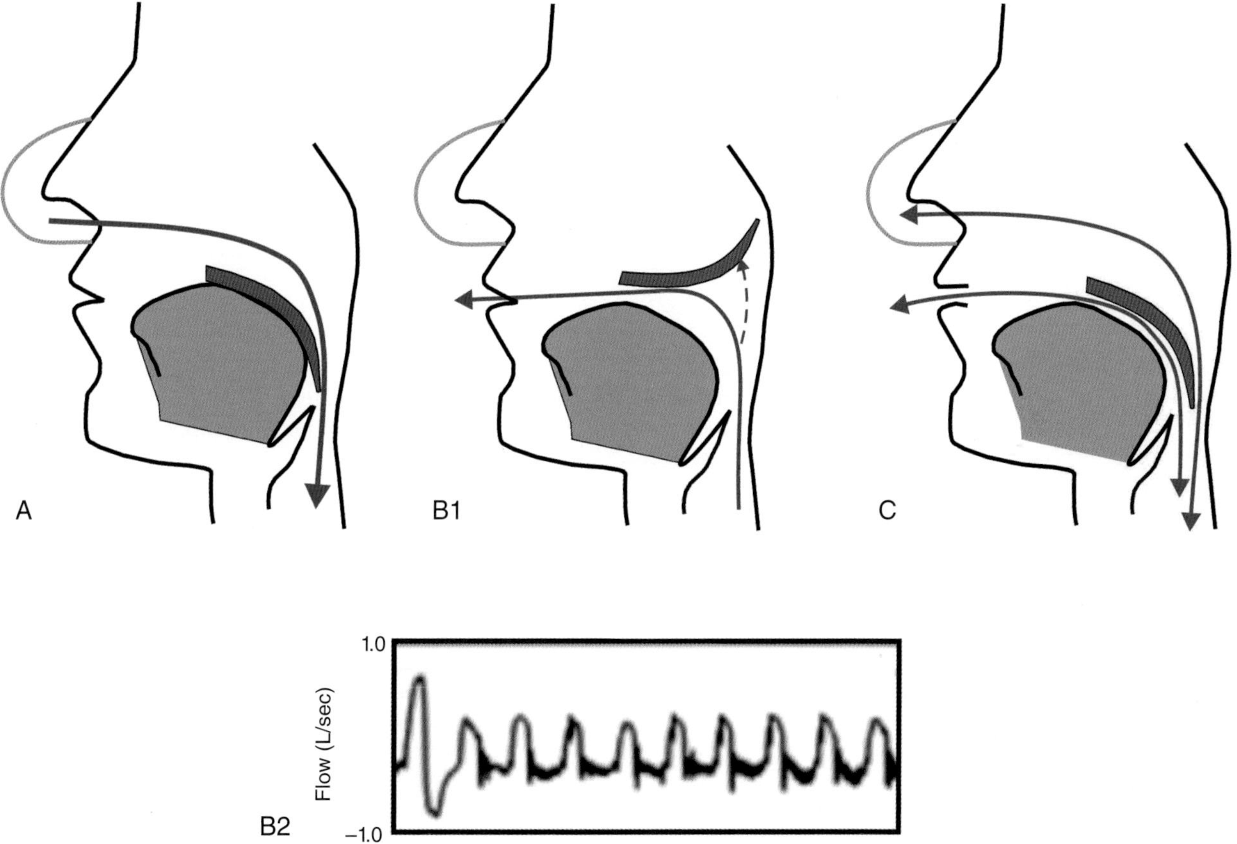

Figure 23–19 (A) The normal breathing route using nasal continuous positive airway pressure (CPAP) is illustrated. (B1) An example is shown of expiratory shunting of airflow through the mouth, associated with palatal prolapse, while using a nasal mask. The associated truncation in expiratory flow is shown on an actual tracing fragment below (B2). (C) The mouth is open, and both nasal and oral airflow is noted. See Figure 23-20 for an example of this pattern. (Reproduced with permission of the © ERS 2023: *Eur Respir J.* 2018;51(2):1701419; doi:10.1183/13993003.01419-2017 Published 14 February 2018.)

lowering the pressure could be considered. Using CPAP with EPR or BPAP might also reduce mouth leak, which typically occurs during exhalation (oral venting). There are also situations in which an increase in pressure can sometimes reduce leak during use of a nasal mask (especially at low or inadequate pressures).

Intermittent mouth leak when patients are using a nasal mask can also mimic respiratory events. Flow through the mouth is sensed as leak and does not contribute to deflections in flow sensed by the PAP device. Figurere 23–20 (left side) illustrates changes in PAP flow and leak during simulated

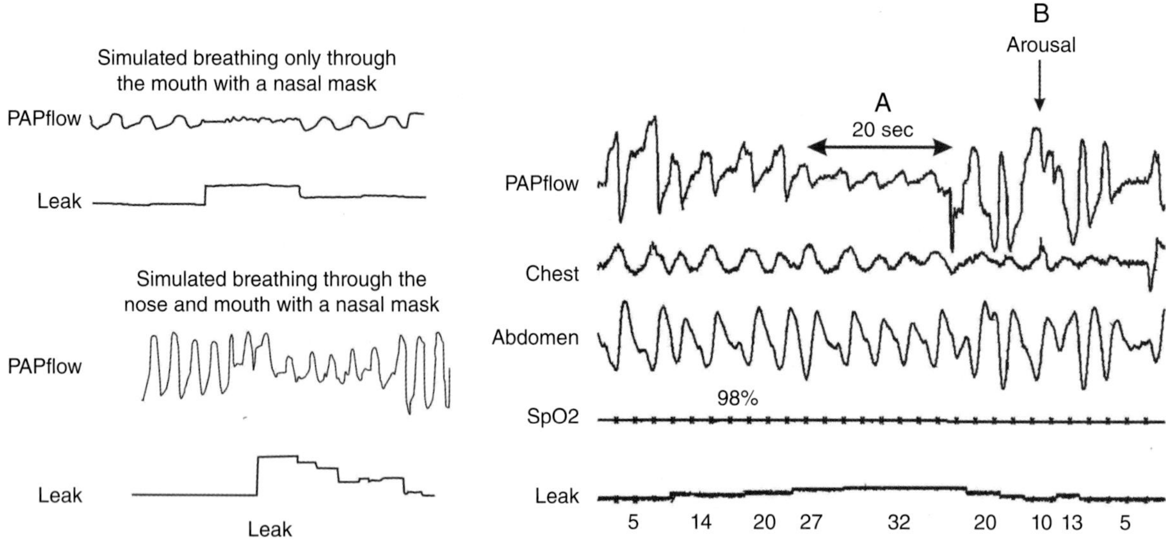

Figure 23–20 On the left are examples of recordings during simulated breathing via a nasal mask while on a low level of continuous positive airway pressure (CPAP). At the top there is an example of breathing only through the mouth. The PAP flow (PAP device flow signal) and leak signals suggest an apnea is present with increased leak. Changes in inspiratory and expiratory flow did not substantially change flow at the device sensor, which detects only flow through the nose (increase in oral flow interpreted as leak). On the bottom, simultaneous breathing through the nose and mouth while using a nasal mask is illustrated. The change in airflow resembles hypopnea. Note the rounded shape in the inspiratory waveform. In both examples, leak increases with mouth breathing while using a nasal mask. On the right is a 90-second tracing of a patient on CPAP of 9 cm H_2O. (A) There is a decrease in the positive airway pressure (PAP) flow signal, associated with a progressive increase in leak. (B) After an arousal, the leak suddenly decreased. On video, the lips were parted, and nasal and oral breathing were suspected. At arousal, the patient woke up and closed his mouth, immediately reducing leak. Multiple similar events, each causing an arousal, were noted. On 7 cm H_2O, this pattern was absent, and leak was not increased. The mouth opening (leak) was likely due to higher pressure. Placement of a chin strap resolved this pattern. (From Berry RB, Wagner MH. *Sleep Medicine Pearls*. 3rd ed. Elsevier; 2015:299.)

breathing through the nose and mouth or the mouth alone. In Figure 23–20 (right panel), an apparent event is shown during a period of increased leak. At arousal, the patient closed the mouth, resulting in a decrease in leak. This pattern may result in scoring a respiratory event (by technologist or PAP device). Rather than an intervention for mouth leak an increase in pressure occurs. However, as noted previously, there are also occasions when an increase in pressure can reduce the tendency for mouth leak, perhaps by opening the nasal airflow pathway and promoting movement of the palate against the posterior tongue sealing off the oral route of airflow.

If the patient is pressure intolerant or the arterial oxygen saturation remains low in the absence of discrete respiratory events, a switch to BPAP can be tried. BPAP not only eliminates upper airway obstruction but delivers PS (IPAP − EPAP). The PS can be adjusted to augment tidal volume. Typically, the starting IPAP − EPAP difference is 4 cm H_2O. IPAP can be increased to treat hypopnea, low tidal volume, or persistent hypoxemia from presumed hypoventilation. For example, patients with OHS may require BPAP for persistent hypoxemia or periods of low tidal volume (Figure 23–21). If the IPAP − EPAP difference is adjusted to augment tidal volume, displaying/recording the tidal volume signal from the PAP device can also be useful (Figure 23–6). The PAP device provides the tidal volume signal by integration of the flow. Tidal volume depends both on flow and inspiratory time. Therefore monitoring the flow signal alone may not provide an accurate estimate of ventilation. If arterial oxygen desaturation remains low in the absence of discrete respiratory events (apnea or hypopnea), the addition of supplemental oxygen is another option. An increase in pressure, change from CPAP to BPAP, or an increase in pressure support could be tried.

Titration Protocol

The recommended PAP titration protocols for adults and children[9] are summarized in Tables 23–8 (for CPAP) and 23–9 for (BPAP). The reader should consult the reference for additional information. CPAP is usually started at 4 or 5 cm H_2O (higher for a patient already on CPAP or for comfort in individuals with an elevated BMI), then increased for obstructive apneas, hypopneas, RERAs, and snoring. Usually, as pressure is increased, apneas → hypopneas → RERAs → snoring resolve in that order.[166] CPAP is increased in adults after two obstructive apneas, three hypopneas, or five RERAs and no more often than every 5 minutes. If events are controlled with ≥ 15 minutes in supine REM sleep on a given pressure, down titration in ≥ 1 cm H_2O increments every 10 min or more can be tried until events re-emerge. When titrating BPAP, starting IPAP/EPAP pressures of 8/4 cm H_2O are typically used. *Both IPAP and EPAP are increased together for obstructive apnea (no change in pressure support).* For obstructive hypopneas, RERAs, and snoring, the IPAP alone is increased. Clinical guidelines suggest that the IPAP − EPAP difference should be at least 4 cm H_2O but no greater than 10 cm H_2O. Note that, during noninvasive positive pressure ventilation (NPPV) titration, a wider IPAP − EPAP difference is used to augment tidal volume. *Higher PAP is needed for the supine position and during REM sleep.*[167] For this reason, an effective pressure during supine

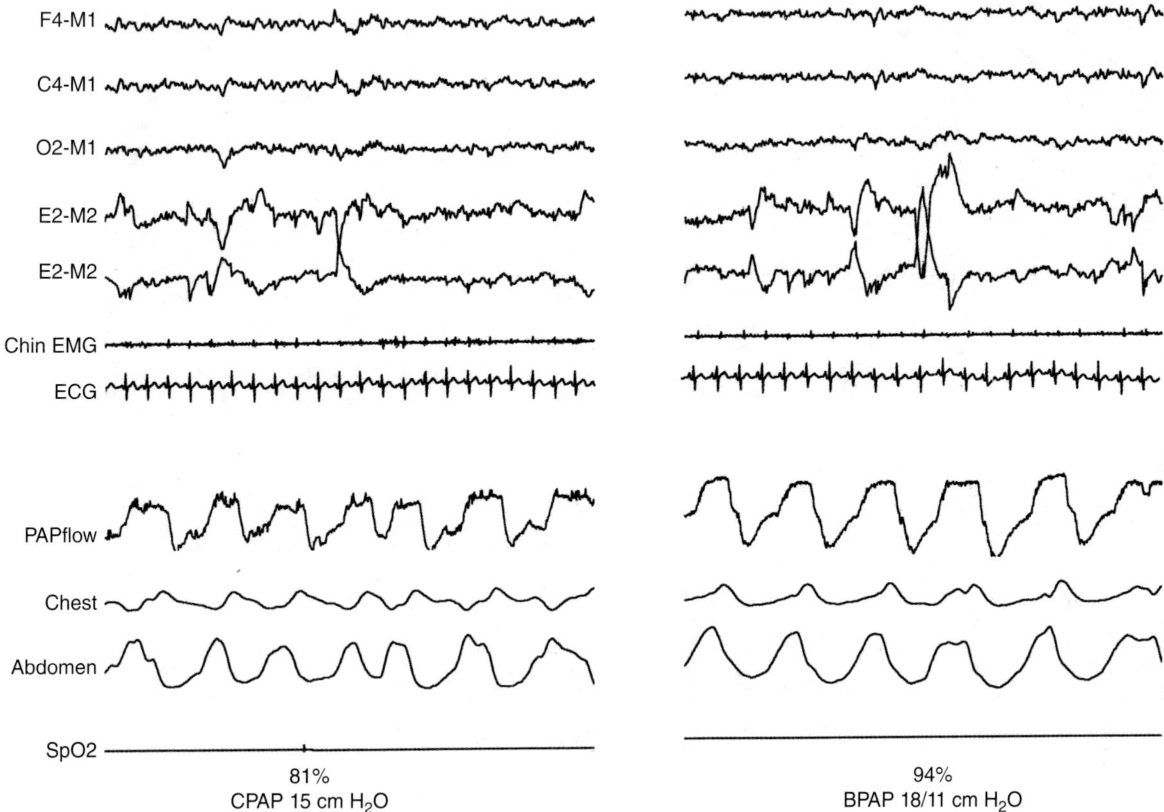

Figure 23–21 On the left, a tracing on continuous positive airway pressure (CPAP) of 15 cm H_2O is noted with what appears to be adequate airflow during REM sleep. However, the arterial oxygen saturation by oximetry (SpO_2) was decreased. The patient was changed to bilevel PAP (BPAP) 18/11 cm H_2O, which increased airflow and tidal volume (not shown) with normalization of the oxygen saturation. An increase in CPAP or change to BPAP can be tried for persistent desaturation without discrete events. If this had not worked, the addition of supplemental oxygen would have been needed. (From Berry RB, Wagner MH. *Sleep Medicine Pearls*. 3rd ed. Elsevier; 2015:287.)

Table 23–8 Positive Airway Pressure Titration Guidelines (CPAP)

	Adults and Children >12 Years	Children <12 Years
Beginning/minimum pressure (cm H_2O)	4 or 5*	4*
Maximum pressure (cm H_2O)	20	15
Increase CPAP in at least 1 cm H_2O increments, no more frequently than every 5 min	Increase pressure for ≥2 obstructive apneas ≥3 hypopneas ≥5 RERAs ≥3 min of loud or unambiguous snoring	Increase pressure for ≥1 obstructive apnea ≥1 hypopnea ≥3 RERAs ≥1 min of loud or unambiguous snoring
Pressure intolerance Switch to BPAP	Drop pressure enough to allow return to sleep Intolerant to CPAP Events still present on CPAP of 15 cm H_2O (option)	Same
(Optional) If control of breathing for at least 30 min including at least 15 min of supine REM Sleep	Drop pressure by ≥1 cm H_2O no more frequently than every 30 minutes. Stop if events return.	Same

BPAP, Bilevel positive airway pressure; *CPAP,* continuous positive airway pressure; *RERA,* respiratory effort-related arousal.
* Minimum. A higher CPAP setting may be selected if high BMI or for retitration studies.
Adapted from Kushida CA. Littner MR, Hirshkowitz M, et al: Practice parameters for the use of continuous and bilevel positive airway pressure devices to treat adult patients with sleep related breathing disorders. Sleep 2006; 29:375–380.

Table 23–9 Positive Airway Pressure Titration Guidelines (BPAP)

	Adults	Children <12 Years
Beginning pressure (cm H_2O) IPAP/EPAP	8/4*	8/4*
Maximum IPAP (cm H_2O)	30	20
Minimum PS (cm H_2O)	4	4
Maximum PS (cm H_2O)	10	10
Increase **both IPAP and EPAP** in at least 1 cm H_2O increments no more frequently than every 5 min	≥ 2 obstructive apneas	≥ 1 obstructive apnea
Increase **IPAP** in at least 1 cm H_2O increments no more frequently than every 5 min	Increase for ≥3 hypopneas ≥5 RERAs ≥3 min loud or unambiguous snoring	Increased for ≥1 hypopnea ≥3 RERAs ≥1 min of loud or unambiguous snoring
(Optional) If control of breathing for at least 30 min including at least 15 min of supine REM sleep	Drop IPAP by ≥1 cm H_2O no more frequently than every 30 minutes. Maintain PS≥PS min. Stop If events return.	Same
Pressure intolerance	Drop in pressure enough to allow return to sleep	Same

EPAP, Expiratory positive airway pressure; *IPAP,* inspiratory positive airway pressure; *PS,* pressure support (IPAP − EPAP); *RERA,* respiratory effort-related arousal.
* Minimum. A higher BPAP setting may be selected if high BMI or for retitration studies.
Adapted from Kushida CA. Littner MR, Hirshkowitz M, et al: Practice parameters for the use of continuous and bilevel positive airway pressure devices to treat adult patients with sleep related breathing disorders. Sleep 2006; 29:375–380.

REM sleep should be determined, if possible, during the titration.[9] If control of events is documented during supine REM sleep for ≥ 10 minutes on a given level of BPAP, down titration of IPAP in 1 cm H_2O increments every 10 minutes or can be tried until events are again noted. Note that the recommended maximum CPAP or IPAP and the number of events triggering pressure changes are lower in children. In both adults and children, the specified number of events is based on consensus; the goal is upward titration that is not too fast or too slow. If the patient awakens and complains of excessive pressure, the pressure should be lowered until a pressure is reached that the patient feels is comfortable enought to allow a return to sleep. If this does not work, a switch from CPAP to BPAP or use of flexible PAP may be tried. When switching from CPAP to BPAP, one approach is to use IPAP 2 cm H_2O higher than CPAP and EPAP 2 cm H_2O lower than CPAP. Thus for change from CPAP of 16, one would use BPAP 18/14 cm H_2O. Another approach is to use IPAP = CPAP and EPAP= IPAP − 4 cm H_2O and titrate pressure upward if needed. Of note, in pressure-intolerant patients, sleep in the lateral position or with the head elevated can be tried to reduce the required level of pressure.[168] If mouth leak is a problem, a chin strap can be tried, followed by an oronasal mask. In patients with allergic rhinitis or nasal congestion, *use of HH from the start of the study* is suggested. Although studies have not shown a benefit from using "prophylactic" HH in all patients, many sleep centers find this to be useful. Once the nose is congested, this problem is not easily reversed. If there is excessive mask leak, a readjustment of the mask or change in mask size or type is indicated. Overtightening of the mask straps is strongly discouraged. It is also worth mentioning again that some patients with very severe OSA and/or a large neck circumference may be more comfortable with a *higher initial pressure* (8–10 cm H_2O) than the usual starting pressure. This is also true of patients already using CPAP at home. If the patient is not able to fall asleep on PAP, the patient should be asked what is bothering him or her. The AASM PAP-CPG[9] also suggests that downward pressure titration could be tried during the study. If there is any doubt that the pressure was raised too rapidly, a lowering of pressure should be tried. As mentioned, one study found that, often, a lower pressure than used in the titration study may be effective.[98] It is also important to not increase pressure for brief events (often central) that occur after arousal. If increases in pressure do not eliminate respiratory events, the technologist should consider the effect of leak rather than sequential increases in pressure. If the leak is high, this should be addressed before increases in pressure (which will likely further increase the leak). The pressure recommended for treatment by the physician reading the titration sleep study should NOT be the final pressure used *if a lower pressure is clearly effective.*

Goals of Titration

The AASM PAP titration clinical guidelines provide recommendations for assessing the quality of a PAP titration[9] (Table 23–10). An optimal titration reduces the AHI < 5 events/hour for at least a 15-minute duration and should include supine REM sleep at the selected pressure. The SaO_2 should be ≥90%. A good titration reduces the AHI ≤ 10 events/hour or by 50% if the baseline AHI is <15 events/hour and should include supine REM sleep that is not continually interrupted by spontaneous arousals or awakenings at the selected pressure.[9] An adequate titration does not reduce the AHI ≤ 10 events/hour but reduces the AHI (or respiratory disturbance index if RERAs scored) by 75% from baseline (especially in patients with severe OSA). An adequate titration also includes the situation where the titration grading criteria for optimal or good are met with the exception that supine REM sleep did not occur at the selected pressure. An unacceptable titration does not meet criteria for optimal,

Table 23–10 Titration Quality and Goals

Treatment Pressure	Should reflect control of the patient's obstructive respiration with a low (preferably < 5/hr) AHI at the selected pressure, and a minimum sea level SpO_2 above 90% at the pressure and with a leak within acceptable parameters at the pressure.
Optimal	• AHI <5 events/hr for at least a 15-min duration • Supine REM sleep at the selected pressure that is not continually interrupted by spontaneous arousals or awakenings • The SaO_2 should be ≥90% at the selected pressure
Good	• AHI ≤ 10 events/hr (or 50% reduction in AHI from baseline if baseline AHI < 15 events/hr) • Should include supine REM sleep that is not continually interrupted by spontaneous arousals or awakenings at the selected pressure
Adequate	• AHI > 10 events/hr at the selected pressure but the AHI is reduced by 75% from baseline OR • Meets criteria for optimal or good except that no supine REM sleep at the selected pressure
Unacceptable	• Titration does not meet any of the above grades • A repeat PAP titration study should be considered if the initial titration does not achieve a grade of optimal or good and, if it is a split-night PSG study, it fails to meet the AASM criteria for a split study with ≥3 hrs for the titration

AHI, Apnea-hypopnea index; *AASM*, American Academy of Sleep Medicine; *PAP*, positive airway pressure; *PSG*, polysomnography; *REM*, rapid eye movement.
Adapted from reference 9.

good, or adequate titration. In most cases, a repeat PSG titration is indicated. If the optimal pressure is not identified and the patient or circumstances make a repeat titration difficult, one could use APAP with a pressure range based on information from the PSG titration. For example, if supine NREM sleep was noted on 10 cm H_2O with excellent control but minimal REM sleep was recorded, one might use APAP with a range of 8 to 12 (or 14) cm H_2O.

Treatment-Emergent Central Apneas

During a titration for OSA, central apneas may appear (or persist since the diagnostic study). In most patients, these are hypocapnic central apneas after arousal or due to an instability in the control of breathing. Hypocapnic central sleep apnea occurs when the arterial PCO_2 ($PaCO_2$) falls below the apneic threshold and ventilation ceases. It is important to note that, if the central apneas are of the Cheyne-Stokes type this usually indicates cardiac dysfunction. A common mistake is to intervene for central apneas with a change from CPAP to BPAP *without a backup rate*, which usually worsens central apnea.[169] There are three choices (wait, pressure down, pressure up). Often, if the patient reaches stage N3 or stable N2, the central apneas will resolve (wait). If the central apneas followed respiratory arousals from RERAs, one can try an increase in pressure (up). If the arousal was due to leak, intervene for leak. Some patients will respond to a drop in pressure (down). In any case, a relentless increase in pressure should be avoided. The best solution is to simply find a pressure that will eliminate upper airway obstruction. Treatment-emergent central apnea is further discussed in Chapters 24 and 30. Of note, a level of pressure that effectively reduces the AHI in REM sleep may not be as effective in NREM in patients with hypocapnic central apnea. Many sleep centers have a protocol for instituting a trial of some form of BPAP with a backup rate. However, to meet CMS criteria for complex sleep apnea, control of obstructive events must be documented with CPAP or BPAP without a backup rate *before change to a form of BPAP with a backup rate*.[170]

Supplemental Oxygen

The addition of supplemental oxygen during PAP titration is sometimes needed.[9] Some patients will exhibit significant arterial oxygen desaturation despite adequate airflow, especially during REM sleep. Persistent hypoxemia in these conditions may be caused by hypoventilation or ventilation-perfusion mismatch (often resulting from chronic lung disease). In some studies of titrations in patients with OHS, a substantial number of patients required the addition of supplemental oxygen. If, while awake and supine, the patient has an SaO_2 of 88% or lower or is already on supplemental oxygen to maintain an acceptable awake SaO_2, the addition of supplemental oxygen will be needed. Recall that even in healthy individuals, the arterial partial pressure of oxygen (PaO_2) falls on the order of 5 to 10 mm Hg during sleep. Before adding supplemental oxygen, one should attempt to adjust the PAP settings to prevent the need for this additional treatment. If the patient requires high oxygen flows, optimizing PAP may allow reduction in the required oxygen flow rate. First, an increase in CPAP can be tried to eliminate unrecognized high upper airway resistance. If this is not successful or not tolerated, CPAP can be changed to BPAP, which augments ventilation. PS ≥ 6 cm H_2O is often needed. In Figure 23–21, on CPAP of 15 cm H_2O, there are no discrete events, but there is persistent desaturation. A change to BPAP of 18/11 cm H_2O increased tidal volume (not shown) and normalized the SaO_2. If optimizing PAP does not relieve hypoxemia, the addition of oxygen is indicated at 1 to 2 lpm with upward titration to reach the goal of an SaO_2 > 90% to 92%. If the patient is on oxygen when awake, higher oxygen flow will usually be needed on PAP. The PAP flow dilutes the supplemental oxygen added to the system and reduces the effective fraction of inspiratory oxygen (FiO_2) (Figure 23–22).[171,172] Note that increases in PAP flow due to pressure increases or increases in mask or mouth leak will further dilute the added oxygen. Reduction in mask leak can raise the effective inhaled concentration of oxygen (FiO_2).

The CMS Local carrier determination L33718[23] has criteria for qualification for coverage of the addition of supplemental oxygen to PAP. The addition of supplemental oxygen to PAP is covered if a titration (PSG titration or titration portion of a split sleep study) is conducted over a minimum of 2 hours and during the titration the AHI is reduced to ≤ 10 events/hour (or if the initial AHI was less that 10 events per hour the titration demonstrated a further reduction in AHI), and while

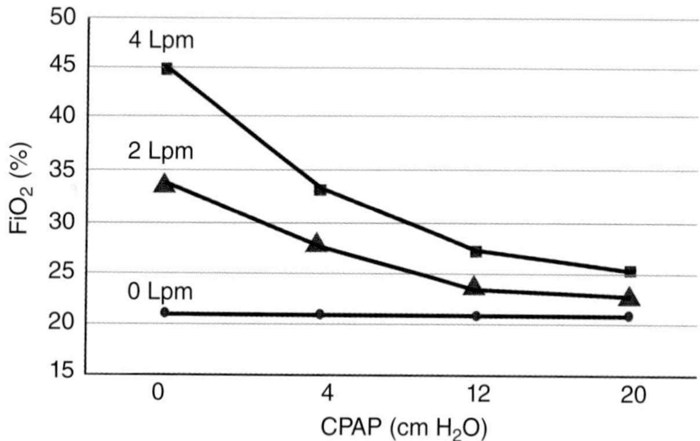

Figure 23–22 Reduction in the effective inspiratory fraction of oxygen (FiO_2) for a given supplemental oxygen flow into the positive airway pressure (PAP) system with increasing continuous PAP (CPAP). The effective FiO_2 falls as CPAP increases. This is due to the higher flow rate associated with high pressure, which dilutes the flow of oxygen. Increases in leak at a constant level of CPAP can also reduce the effective FiO_2. The data plotted are for illustration only as the actual FiO_2 will depend on the total PAP flow at each pressure which depends on unintentional as well as intentional leak. (Figure plotted from data in Yoder EA, Klann K, Strohl KP. Inspired oxygen concentrations during positive pressure therapy. *Sleep Breath.* 2004;8:1-5. Figure from Berry RB, Wagner MH. *Sleep Medicine Pearls.* 3rd ed. Elsevier; 2015:290.)

using the optimal setting oximetry during the PSG demonstrates oxygen saturation ≤ 88% for 5 minutes (need not to be continuous). Most private insurance companies follow CMS coverage requirements. The regulations change and the reader should consult the most recent version.

STARTING PAP TREATMENT WITHOUT A TITRATION

Several alternative options are available for starting PAP without a PSG titration after a diagnosis of OSA has been made using a PSG or HSAT (Figure 23–23). The titration alternatives can also be used for patients unwilling or unable to have a PSG PAP titration. A split sleep study or the combination of a diagnostic PSG followed by a PAP titration PSG are the traditional approaches, and they still have advantages, especially for complicated patients. Today, treating uncomplicated patients with APAP (titration not needed) after either a diagnostic PSG or HSAT is a commonly used approach. This may be required by insurance providers. Performing autotitration at home for several days to a week (optimally at least 3 days) to determine an effective level of CPAP (90% or 95% pressure over the autotitration period) and subsequent

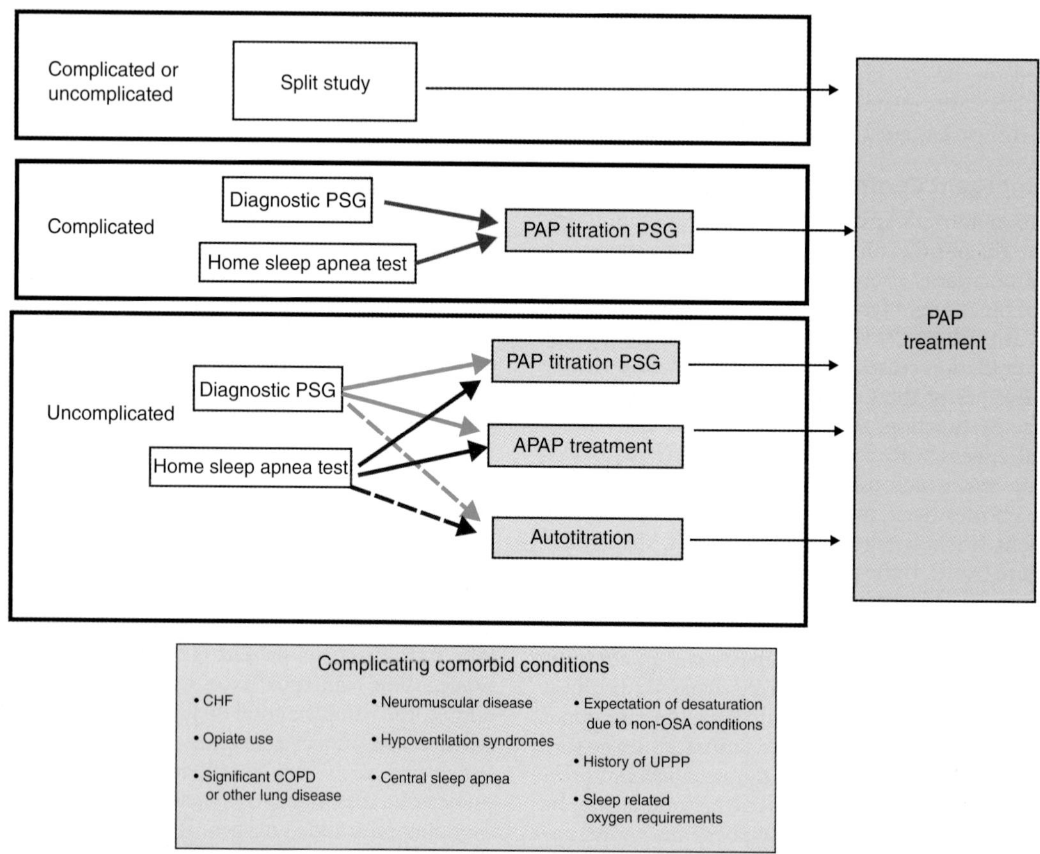

Figure 23–23 Clinical pathways for diagnosis of obstructive sleep apnea (OSA) and positive airway pressure (PAP) treatment. Complicated or uncomplicated patients can be diagnosed and treated using a split sleep study. Complicated patients diagnosed by polysomnography (PSG) or home sleep apnea testing (HSAT) should undergo a PAP titration with PSG. Such patients are not ideal candidates for HSAT, but sometimes this type of testing is mandated by insurance. In other cases, the "complicated" condition is only noted or suspected based on HSAT results. Uncomplicated patients diagnosed by PSG or HSAT can undergo a PAP titration, be started on AutoPAP (APAP) treatment, or undergo autotitration followed by CPAP treatment. The dashed arrows for this last option indicate that, currently, this option is rarely used unless the same device is used for autotitration and chronic treatment. Due to financial issues (APAP titration not reimbursed) and concerns about reuse of a device for autotitration between patients, this option is rarely used.

CPAP treatment with another device is an effective option. However, as noted, autotitration to determine an effective level of CPAP is rarely used because of issues with cleaning the autotitration device between patients, lack of reimbursement for autotitration, and a reduction in the price differential between CPAP and APAP devices. In any case, the viable alternatives really include a PSG titration or chronic treatment with an APAP device (without PSG titration). In fact, many practitioners even routinely treat patients undergoing a PAP PSG titration with APAP, adjusting the settings based on the PSG findings. This is especially true when documentation of an effective pressure during supine REM sleep does not occur during the titration. The APAP device provided to the patient for chronic treatment can also be used to determine an effective level of CPAP followed by treatment with that level of CPAP. That is, APAP devices can be used in the CPAP mode following an initial period of autotitraton.

Diagnosis by HSAT followed by APAP titration at home and CPAP treatment has been shown to produce outcomes similar to those of PSG for diagnosis and titration (either separate diagnostic and studies or a split study).[131,173-176] The adherence was either equal or better than traditional approaches using PSG. The approach of diagnosis by HSAT followed by APAP treatment (no intermediate autotitration) has also been validated.[48] However, these studies often *excluded a significant number of patients* and had a structured system with good patient education, mask fitting, and follow-up. The results may not apply when careful patient selection, education, and follow-up are not available. The AASM PAP-CPG recommends either initiation of PAP treatment using APAP at home or PAP after PSG titration in patients *without complicating* comorbidities (Table 23–1). Patients with complications listed at the bottom of Table 23–1 and Figure 23–23 are best treated after a PSG titration. A PSG titration allows detection and treatment of arterial oxygen desaturation present in the absence of respiratory events in patients with severe obesity, lung disease, or known or suspected hypoventilation. While unattended, APAP or autoBPAP devices can usually normalize the AHI; they do not respond to persistent desaturation or hypoventilation. The APAP and autoBPAP algorithms are designed to normalize the obstructive AHI and offer no interventions for central apneas, desaturation in the absence of respiratory events, or central apneas. Patients at risk for central apneas on PAP (congestive heart failure, opiate medication, or significant central apneas on the diagnostic sleep study) are also best treated using PSG titration. Individuals who may require very high pressures (high BMI or large neck circumference) benefit from PSG titration. High PAP pressure usually results in mask interface issues, and the availability of a sleep technologist to help with mask adjustment during PSG titrations is often crucial. Of note, APAP devices have a maximum pressure of 20 cm H_2O, whereas a sleep-center PAP device can provide up to 30 cm H_2O and has treatment modes with a backup rate. Supplemental oxygen can be added if needed. If insurance or clinical circumstances mandate use of APAP treatment without titration, patients at risk for significant residual oxygen desaturation often benefit from an oximetry at home on the final treatment settings. Although a low AHI on PAP download usually reflects good treatment (i.e., low actual AHI),[177] APAP devices do not assess oxygenation. One study evaluated the benefit of oximetry at home on PAP,[178] and oximetry was recommended when the baseline SaO_2 was <92% or the BMI was ≥30 kg/m^2. Nocturnal monitoring with oximetry at home should be considered for patients with an increased BMI, a borderline awake SaO_2, and any of the comorbid disorders listed in Figure 23–23 if they have not had a recent PSG titration. If significant desaturation is present on the current treatment at home, either adjustment of the APAP setting, or a positive pressure titration is indicated. It should also be appreciated that OHS should always be considered when OSA patients have significant obesity. The presence of OHS can change the treatment approach.[38]

General Consideration for PAP Treatment Without Titration

The indication and expectation for treatment outcomes needs to be discussed with the patient. This should be the job of the treating physician, not the DME company. Education on how to adjust the device (including use and adjustment of humidity and ramp), clean the device and mask, and change device filters is essential. In our experience, most patients require more than one educational encounter. We have patients bring the device and mask to every clinic visit for ongoing education. It is common for patients to state that they changed the pressure using the "big knob" (humidity control) or to find device filters that are black with dust. Mask selection and fitting are important. Testing mask seal under some pressure is essential to verify a reasonable mask seal. When starting PAP treatment without a titration, one useful technique is to have the patient put on the mask and turn on the device (a trial run) before leaving the DME office (if possible) with the PAP device for home treatment. The AASM PAP task force guidleine recommend educational; interventions and telemonitoring of adherence in all patients starting PAP.[5] Applications that allow patients to follow their adherence and/or internet sites sponsored by PAP device companies provide useful information to the patient and improve adherence.[120]

APAP Treatment

The ordering physician usually specifies the minimum and maximum APAP pressures and Flex (Aflex)/EPR settings. There are several approaches to setting pressure limits. One option is use of 4 to 20 cm H_2O ("wide open"). Another is choosing a lower pressure limit and pressure range set to match the patient's neck size and severity of sleep apnea. Information about previous determinations of an effective level of CPAP should be considered. The upper pressure limit is less crucial unless the patient has pressure intolerance (Flex or EPR should be used). The lower pressure should be high enough for comfortable breathing while awake but not so high that the patient cannot comfortably fall asleep. Larger patients may find falling asleep on 4 cm H_2O uncomfortable (not high enough). A pressure-intolerant patient may find starting on 8 cm H_2O difficult (too high). Empiric guidelines for choosing the minimum pressure are 6 cm H_2O for milder sleep apnea/small neck circumferences, 8 cm H_2O for moderately sized necks (16–17 in.), and 8 to 10 cm H_2O for larger neck sizes (≥18 in.). Another option would be resetting the lower pressure limit after a few days of treatment based on the 90th or 95th percentile pressure. PR devices have an "Opti-Start" option that, when enabled, starts at 90% pressure of the previous night of use. This option reduces the likelihood of events

Box 23–5 PAP FOLLOW-UP CHECKLIST AND REVIEW OF PAP DOWNLOAD

- What major PAP problems are you facing?
- How is your mask fitting?
- Do you have dryness? If so, do you know how to adjust your humidifier? (The download should provide information about humidifier settings or the device menus can be manually assessed.)
- Do you have hose or mask condensation?
- Are you cleaning your mask and hose regularly and changing filters?
- Are you changing your mask and cushion on a regular basis?
- How is the quality of your sleep?
- Does your bedpartner report that you snore while using PAP?
- Does your bedpartner report mask leak, noise, or air coming out your mouth?
- Do you feel refreshed in the morning?
- How many hours do you actually sleep? Do you keep PAP on the entire night? (This can be seen by looking at a detailed report showing pattern of use.)
- Are you still sleepy during the day (also review ESS).
- Do you use PAP if you take a nap?

Parameters on Download to Check

- Check adherence; look for patterns of nonuse (e.g., weekends).
- Is the average use similar to reported sleep duration? (Is the patient using PAP the entire night?)
- If using autoCPAP, is 90th or 95th percentile pressure close to the upper pressure limit? If the patient is doing well, an increase in the upper pressure limit may not be indicated.
- Check AHI; if elevated, what types of events? Is the number of clear airway apneas increased?
- Is the amount of periodic breathing on PR devices or Cheyne-Stokes breathing estimate on ResMed devices increased?
- Check for large leak.
- Check humidity settings.
- Check Flex or EPR setting, if applicable.
- Look at detailed reports of a few nights to determine patterns suggesting a need for interventions:
  - Are there are event clusters during periods of high leak?
  - Is pressure constrained by the upper pressure limit?
  - Are there clusters of events suggestive of insufficient pressure during REM sleep (clusters in the early morning hours)?

AHI, apnea-hypopnea index; *EPR,* expiratory pressure relief; *ESS,* Epworth Sleepiness Scale; *PAP,* positive airway pressure; *PR,* Philips Respironics; *REM,* rapid eye movement.

occurring while the device increases to an effective pressure from a low starting pressure. If information about an effective pressure (previous titration or 90th/95th percentile pressure on APAP) is known, one might use a range centered on this pressure. For example, if the 90% pressure is 12 cm H_2O, one could use 10 to 14 cm H_2O or 8 to 16 cm H_2O. On the other hand, a pressure-intolerant patient may prefer a lower starting pressure. APAP algorithms have difficulty with large and varying leak. Persistent REM-associated sleep apnea can occur on APAP if the device does not increase pressure rapidly enough after the transition from NREM to REM sleep. Increasing the lower pressure limit is one approach to this issue. Another is treatment with CPAP using a level of pressure effective during REM sleep.

FOLLOW-UP OF THE PAP PATIENT/USE OF DEVICE DATA

Key questions to ask patients during follow-up and important data to assess when reviewing download information are listed in Box 23–5. An example of a summary report is shown in Figure 23–24. Early telemonitoring of adherence can provide valuable information and allow early interventions. PAP usage information is essential to assure adequate treatment and to qualify for reimbursement for the PAP device. Typical adherence criteria for reimbursement were presented previously. However, treatment for 4 hours' duration is not adequate. The patient should be educated that using the PAP device all night is ideal. One strategy is to inform the patient that REM sleep occurs in the early morning hours, and that situation is often associated with the most severe OSA of the night.

Several types of reports of adherence and efficacy are available. These include summary reports, detailed single-night reports, and for PR PAP devices detailed waveform reports.

Premium PAP devices provide the clinician with detailed use and pressure information (PR, 90% pressure; ResMed, 95% pressure). CPAP, APAP, and BPAP devices manufactured by PR provide time or % of use time in large leak based on total leak. Recall that total leak is the intentional leak (mask nonrebreathing orifice) + unintentional leak. As noted previously, large leak in PR devices is defined as the total leak greater than two times the intentional leak at a given pressure expected from a typical mask. In PR devices, both blower hours and use (time at pressure) hours are provided. For example, if a patient left the device running while they were out of bed for 2 hours, the blower time might by 8 hours and use time 6 hours. Although often misunderstood, only **use hours** are used to determine time at large leak. Rarely a patient actually wearing CPAP has such a large leak that PAP device reports 2 hours of use while the patient vehemently insists the mask was worn for 6 hours. ResMed devices report an estimate of unintentional leak. One can specify the type of mask (nasal, nasal pillows, full) in the device menu of ResMed devices. An estimate of intentional leak is automatically subtracted from the total leak, and only unintentional leak is displayed. The maximum desired unintentional leak is 24 lpm. The impact of leak on patients is variable. A patient with an average of 1 hour of large leak may not complain of leak at all, whereas other patients will complain of smaller amounts of leak into the eyes or causing awakenings (sound or associated breathing event). For example, a patient using a nasal mask has repeated intermittent mouth leak. If the average leak is 1.5 times the expected leak, this could be associated with mouth dryness. The bedpartner can often provide useful information about mask seal and mouth leak.

PAP devices also provide an estimate of the residual AHI. Unfortunately, many clinicians forget the word "estimate" and assume the value is completely accurate. As previously noted, an ATS work group[146] recommended the term AHIflow be used to emphasize that only flow is used to detect respiratory events. Studies have compared automatic device event detection and classification with simultaneous PSG scoring.[177] Results have varied, but a machine AHI < 10 events/hour is usually associated with good treatment; a high device determined AHI acccurately detects an elevated residual AHI only

Usage days			
>= 4 hrs			30/30 days
< 4 hrs			19 days (63%)
Average use (total days)			11 days (37%)
Average use (days used)			5 hrs 2 min
Treatment			
Mode	APAP		
Min Pressure	6 cmH2O		
Max Pressure	14 cm H2O		
Pressure relief	2		
Therapy			
95% Pressure (cm H2O):	8.4		
Leak (L/min)	70.0 (95%)	40 (median)	Threshold 24
Events per hour	AI: 1.6	HI: 0.3	AHI: 1.9
Apnea Index	Central: 0.2	Obstructive: 1.0	Unknown: 0.2
Cheyne Stokes respiration (average duration per night)		0 min (0%)	

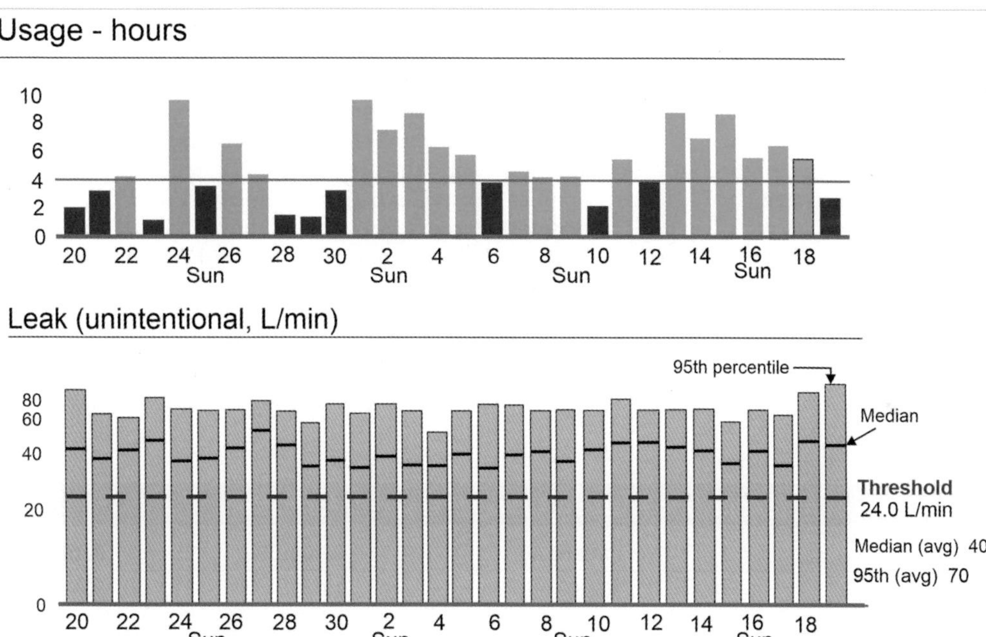

Figure 23–24 An example of download information for a patient on autoCPAP (APAP) with a format similar to that used for ResMed devices. Although the patient reliably uses the device every night, there are many nights when use is below 4 hours (dashed line). On the bottom graph the bars in red are the nights when use is below 4 hours. The overall adherence would not meet Medicare and other insurers criteria for continued reimbursement. The median and 95th percentile leak are above the 24 lpm threshold. The patient did not understand the 4-hour criteria and thought he was doing well because he was using the device every night. Nasal mask discomfort was the reason treatment was stopped on the short-use nights. The patient has adjusted the mask very tightly to prevent leak. A change of mask with careful fitting was provided.

about 60% of the time[177] (an appreciable number of falsely elevated values). A low machine AHI, good symptomatic response, and no report of snoring are consistent with good treatment. A high machine AHI should be viewed in the context of patient and bedpartner report. Basically, the same events that are detected and used for APAP devices to adjust pressure are reported. As arterial oxygen desaturation is not measured, the hypopnea index is the least accurate. Events are detected based on a moving average of flow. For example, for PR devices, an 80% reduction in flow compared with average airflow over several minutes previously for 10 seconds or longer (or no airflow for 10 seconds or longer) is considered an apnea. A 40% to 79% reduction in flow for 10 to 60 seconds is considered a hypopnea. As previously noted, apneas can be classified as central (clear-airway apnea) or obstructive (obstructed-airway apnea) events. However, as mentioned previously, one study found that a significant fraction of events classified as clear airway apneas were not classified as central apnea during a simultaneous PSG.[47] The physician reviewing download information, should understand the event definitions used by the manufacturer of the device.

It is important to remember that as CPAP is increased, first obstructive apneas are abolished, then hypopneas, and finally snoring. Therefore the apnea index should not exceed the hypopnea index. If the apnea index (AI) exceeds the hypopnea index (HI), this would raise concern about the accuracy of event detection or the presence of central apneas. If the device has the ability to classify apneas as obstructive (obstructed airway apnea) or central (clear airway apnea), finding an increase in clear airway apneas might explain the elevation in the apnea index. If apneas are predominantly classified as obstructed airway apneas, one possibility is that these are obstructed upper airway central apneas. The other possibility is the that the classification is not correct. A PAP titration may be needed to determine if the device determined AHI is accurate and if so, what is causing the high residual AHI. It is also important to assess the AHI in the context of the amount of leak and amount of adherence. If leak is elevated, mask intervention should be the first step rather than increasing pressure (or pressure limits on APAP). In Figure 23–7, a single night of APAP titration is shown. The residual AHI is elevated. One can see that events occurred when the pressure was constrained by the upper pressure limit. In this patient, an increase in the upper pressure limit is indicated. As the starting pressure is much lower than the pressure that is needed, an increase in the lower pressure limit would also be reasonable. In Table 23–11, some examples of download data are shown. Patient A has good adherence (although, ideally, average use should be 7 hours or longer), an AHI at goal, and minimal large leak. The 90th percentile pressure is within the pressure limit range (6–20 cm H_2O). However, the patient reports sleeping 7.5 hours/night and removing his mask for the last hour of sleep. Praise for good adherence but encouragement to use PAP all night is indicated. Patient B exhibits poor adherence, and although the AHI is above goal, the patient's use and large leak are the first issues to address. The reasons for poor adherence (possibly due to mask issues) should be addressed. The AHI may improve simply by improving mask fit. Patient C has good adherence, minimal large leak, but an elevated AHI. On the same treatment pressures, the previous AHI was less than 5 events/hour. A large proportion of events are clear airway apneas, and there has been a large increase in periodic breathing. The amount of periodic breathing (PR PAP devices) or Cheyne-Stokes breathing (ResMed devices) is available in download reports. Detailed waveform data showing airflow, pressure, event identification, and periods of large leak or periodic breathing is available for selected nights in PR PAP devices. In the case of patient C, observation of the detailed waveform data showed a pattern of Cheyne-Stokes breathing (Figure 23–25). The patient had known congestive heart failure with preserved ejection fraction. Given pedal edema on physical examination, cardiology was contacted. With diuresis and adjustment of his medications, the AHI improved, and periodic breathing was no longer present. Viewing single-night profiles showing overnight changes in pressure with event flags (device determined events) (Figure 23-7) and periods of increased leak (not shown in Figure 23-7) can be informative. If the single-night detail report reveals increased large leak at the time of increased respiratory events, addressing the leak before changing the pressure is indicated.

If a patient complains that PAP is not restorative and/or the device AHI is above the goal despite pressure changes or interventions for leak, a PAP titration is indicated. *The titration may find an unexpected cause of nonrestorative sleep, such as arousals from mouth leak.* The study can determine if an elevated machine-determined AHI is accurate and find an appropriate treatment.

Table 23–11 Examples of Autoadjusting Positive Airway Pressure Information

	Patient A	Patient B	Patient C
Days used/monitored	30/30	20/30	30/30
Average use (days used)	6 hrs 31 min	4 hrs 2 min	7 hrs 5 min
Average use (all days)	6 hrs 31 min	2 hrs 41 min	7 hrs 5 min
Percentage nights ≥4 hrs	100	5	100
Average time in large leak	5 min	2 hrs	12 min
AHI (events/hr)	4.0	12	17
90th percentile pressure (cm H_2O)	11.8	9.5	12.0
Clear airway apnea index	0	1.0	15
Obstructive airway apnea index	0	8.0	0
Hypopnea index	4	3.0	2
Periodic breathing	0	0	15%
Min pressure limit (cm H_2O)	6	4	8
Max pressure limit (cm H_2O)	20	20	20
Flex	3	3	3

Average use of all days (includes zero hours to compute average on days not used).
Large leak defined as twice the expected leak from an average mask at the given treatment pressure.
AHI, Apnea-hypopnea index; *Flex,* flexible pressure setting.

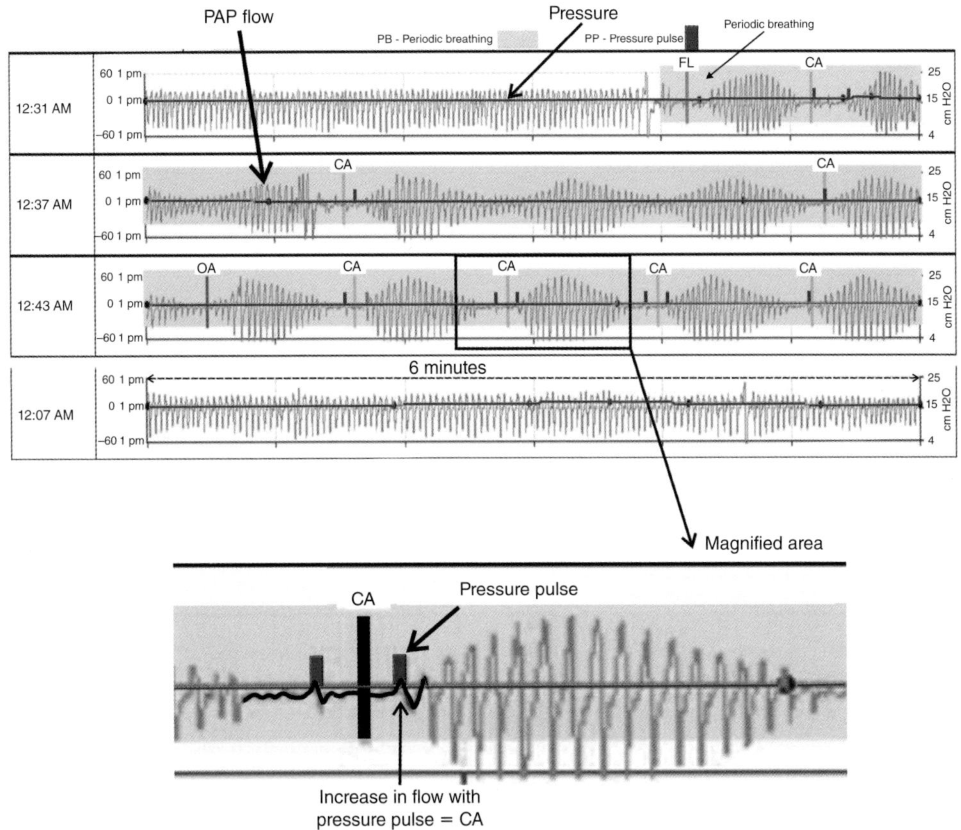

Figure 23–25 Detailed waveform data for the patient discussed in Table 23–11 (Patient C). Each line represents 6 minutes and the pattern of flow for each breath is shown. The concurrent level of pressure is also shown. **Periods of periodic breathing (gray background in the figure)** or large leak (not shown in this figure) are also identified. The download showed an increase in clear airway apneas and increased periodic breathing. Review of detailed waveform pattern during periods of periodic breathing indicates the presence of Cheyne-Stokes breathing. Clear airway apneas (CA) were classified by the device based on a pressure pulse that resulted in flow (see magnified area). The patient was using a DreamStation Auto CPAP device from Philips Respironics. Note that the second line shows Cheyne-Stokes breathing with two apneas and two hypopneas.

SUMMARY OF KEY POINTS

1. PAP is the treatment of choice for patients with moderate to severe OSA and is an option in symptomatic patients with mild OSA.
2. Although many variants of PAP have been developed, CPAP remains the treatment of choice for most patients with OSA. Guidelines suggest initial treatment with CPAP or autoCPAP (APAP) for uncomplicated patients.
3. BPAP devices deliver separately adjustable IPAP and EPAP, with IPAP > EPAP.
4. APAP devices provide the lowest effective pressure for a given sleeping position and sleep stage. High and variable leak can reduce the effectiveness of APAP algorithms and/or decrease the accuracy of event detection. Intervention for high leak rather than pressure changes is often effective in addressing a high device detected AHI. APAP algorithms may not always provide an optimal treatment pressure is some individuals.
5. BPAP, APAP, or flexible PAP devices have not significantly improved adherence to PAP treatment for unselected patients. However, individual patients may benefit from these treatment modes.
6. BPAP in the spontaneous mode is used for pressure-intolerant patients with OSA, to minimize bloating or mask leak (especially mouth leak if a nasal mask is being used), and to deliver pressure support (PS = IPAP − EPAP).
7. PAP treatment is effective at reversing or improving many manifestations of OSA, including daytime sleepiness and quality of life. However, acceptance and adherence are major problems.
8. There is a dose response to CPAP usage, with the ESS improving with as little as 4 hours of use; however, objective improvement in sleepiness and quality-of-life measures usually require longer nightly CPAP use (6 to 7 hours) for maximal benefit.
9. Objective monitoring of adherence is essential for successful PAP treatment. This should be performed early after treatment initiation and intermittently during chronic treatment. At a minimum, monitoring should be routine at clinic visits.
10. Documentation of adequate objective adherence is the first step to evaluate persistent sleepiness despite PAP treatment. Patients should extend PAP use to 7 hours/night if residual sleepiness is a complaint. Recurrent arousal from leak (including mouth leak) and inadequate pressure may also impair the restorative nature of sleep.
11. PSG PAP titration is the standard approach for choosing an effective pressure. For patients already on PAP it can be used to evaluate a high residual machine-estimated AHI,

persistent elevated leak, or absence of symptomatic improvement on PAP.

12. Higher CPAP is needed in the supine position and during REM sleep. Studies have shown that many patients can be treated with lower pressure than used in titration studies. However, other patients may require higher pressure for chronic treatment if an effective pressure for supine REM sleep was not documented during the PSG titration study.
13. Interventions to increase the efficacy of a given level of CPAP include weight loss, elevation of the head, sleep in the lateral position, and a change from an oronasal to a nasal interface.
14. Unattended APAP titration can be used to determine an effective level of CPAP (90th or 95th percentile pressure).
15. Chronic treatment with APAP devices in properly selected patients eliminates the need for a PSG titration. Treatment outcomes are similar to approaches using a PAP titration in uncomplicated patients.
16. Choosing a satisfactory mask interface is challenging despite many mask alternatives, including nasal pillow (prong) masks, nasal masks covering the nose, nasal masks with cradles under the nose, and oronasal masks. Oronasal masks are available either covering the nose and mouth or using cushions covering the mouth with the nose fitting down in a cradle at the top of the cushion.
17. Nasal masks are recommended rather than oronasal masks as the initial interface.
18. Oronasal masks may be useful in patients with nasal congestion or symptomatic mouth leak that does not respond to a chin strap. However, oronasal masks are associated with lower adherence, increased leak, and the requirement for higher pressure. Patients can often be converted to a nasal mask after appropriate treatment of nasal congestion or use of interventions to reduce mouth leak (lower pressure, BPAP, flexible PAP).
19. Telemonitoring of adherence, use of patient smartphone applications, and early CPAP coaching may improve adherence.
20. Device estimates of residual AHI can be useful if their limitations are recognized. If the device AHI is low, treatment is usually effective. If the device AHI is high, the result is not always correct. Technology to classify apnea as clear airway or obstructive airway or to detect periodic breathing/Cheyne Stokes breathing can be helpful, but the results are not always correct. Concerning device download information requires clinical correlation. A PAP titration may be needed to assess the accuracy of device determined information.
21. If both the device residual AHI and leak are elevated, the first intervention should be correction of leak.
22. Use of a heated tube may allow delivery of a high amount of moisture using heated humidity without mask and tubing condensation ("rain out").
23. In patients with OSA and COMISA, effective treatment of both OSA and insomnia is often needed for effective PAP therapy and improvement of insomnia.
24. Factors associated with good adherence include pretreatment daytime sleepiness with improvement sleepiness on PAP, and good early adherence. Factors associated with poor adherence include high mask leak, high residual AHI, high nasal resistance, use of an oronasal mask, and spouse referral. The mode of PAP, level of pressure, use of heated humidity, and type of mask (other than worse adherence with full face masks) do not affect adherence.

CLINICAL REVIEW QUESTIONS

1. Which of the following is most predictive of good PAP adherence?
A. ESS score 16
B. Treatment prescription CPAP = 8 cm H_2O vs. 16 cm H_2O
C. Spouse referral
D. Entire night for PAP titration

2. A patient with OSA undergoes an attended PAP titration. The CPAP treatment table is shown. What pressure do you recommend? Assume all sleep is in the supine position. *CA,* Central apnea; *HYP,* hypopnea; *MA,* mixed apnea; *OA,* obstructive apnea; *TST,* total sleep time.

CPAP (cmH_2O)	TST (min)	REM Sleep (min)	AHI (#/hr)	AHI REM (#/hr)	OA (#)	MA (#)	CA (#)	HYP (#)
7	30	0	20	0	10	0	0	0
8	30	10	10	30	0	0	0	5
9	30	20	4	6	0	0	0	2
10	30	10	10	0	0	0	5	0
11	30	10	20	0	0	0	10	0

A. 7
B. 8
C. 9
D. 10
E. 11

3. A patient with severe COPD requiring supplemental oxygen at 2 lpm during the day (SaO_2 awake on this flow rate is 94%) is found to have severe OSA with an AHI of 40 events/hour. BPAP of 16/12 cm H_2O is the optimal treatment pressure. The patient is started on the combination of BPAP and oxygen. Which of the following is likely true about the required oxygen flow on BPAP treatment?
A. 2.0 lpm should be adequate
B. Higher BPAP may require higher supplemental oxygen flow
C. The required supplemental oxygen flow would increase with high mouth or mask leak

D. A and B
E. B and C

4. Treatment with an oronasal mask (compared with use of a nasal mask) is associated with which of the following?
A. Lower leak
B. Lower effective pressure
C. Lower adherence
D. Less claustrophobia

5. A patient with OSA is undergoing a PAP titration. The tracing in Figure 23–26 shows BPAP (IPAP/EPAP) of 12/8 cm H_2O. At least three other similar events preceded the event shown. What change in pressure do you recommend?
A. IPAP 14 cm H_2O, EPAP 8 cm H_2O
B. IPAP 13 cm H_2O, EPAP 9 cm H_2O
C. IPAP 12 cm H_2O, EPAP 9 cm H_2O
D. IPAP 15 cm H_2O, EPAP 10 cm H_2O

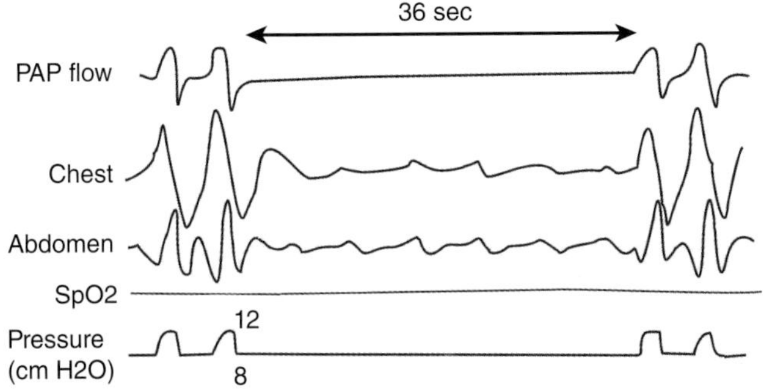

Figure 23–26 An event was noted on bilevel positive airway pressure (BPAP) of 12/8 cm H_2O. What change in pressure is indicated?

6. In Figure 23–27, an increase in CPAP has improved airflow but worsened the arterial oxygen saturation. What is the best explanation for worsening oxygen saturation?
A. The SpO_2 value is likely not correct.
B. This change is expected with higher pressure. Higher intentional leak is the cause of the worsening SpO_2.
C. Increased (unintentional and intentional) leak is the cause.

7. Which of the following factors is associated with good PAP adherence?
A. Improvement in daytime sleepiness with PAP
B. Spousal referral
C. Use of BPAP rather than CPAP
D. Use of CPAP of 10 cm H_2O rather than a CPAP of 15 cm H_2O

8. The following download information was obtained on a patient using APAP with a pressure range of 6 to 12 cm H_2O. **He reports mouth dryness and nonrestorative sleep.** What do you recommend?

Parameter	Result
Average usage	4 hours/night
Average large leak	2 hours/night
90% pressure (cm H_2O)	12
AHI (#/hr)	10
Flex (0–3)	1
Humidity setting	2 of 5
Large leak = total leak > 2 times the expected intentional leak based on mask type and treatment pressure.	

A. Change pressure range to 6 to 14 cm H_2O
B. Change pressure range to 4 to 10 cm H_2O
C. Intervention for leak
D. Increase Flex to 3 and Humidity to 5

9. A patient comes for a yearly follow-up appointment. He has always been very adherent to PAP treatment. He reports using his device every night for about 8 hours. The download from a PR PAP device shows average use of 2 hours and 44 minutes. A plot of the last 25 days is shown (Figure 23–28A). Note that the large leak is very low. The average duration of blower hours is much higher than use hours. What is the explanation for these findings? In Figure 23–28B, another 10 days are shown with a dramatic change after 6 days. What do you think happened?

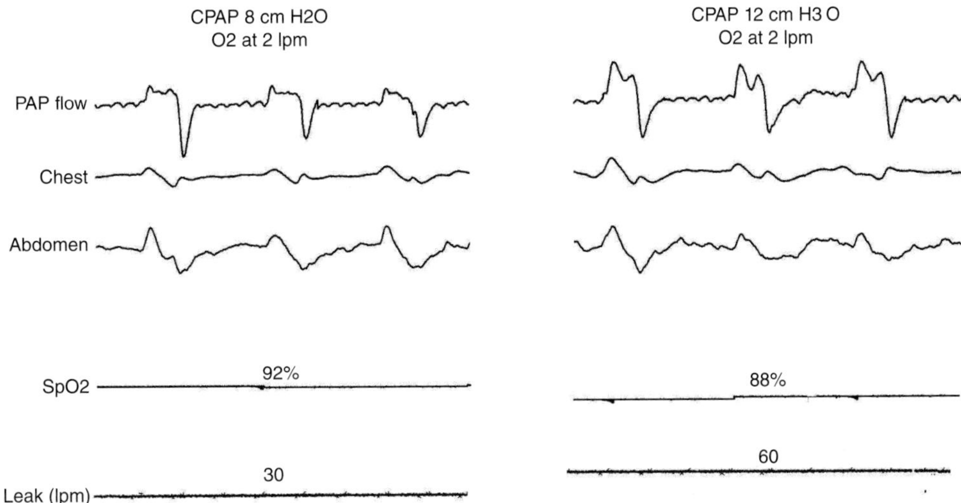

Figure 23–27 An increase in continuous positive airway pressure (CPAP) from 8 to 12 cm H_2O is associated with improved PAP flow but worsening arterial oxygen saturation on the same flow rate of supplemental oxygen. What has caused this finding? PAP flow is the device flow signal. The patient uses 2 lpm supplemental oxygen during the day. *Lpm*, Liters per minute.

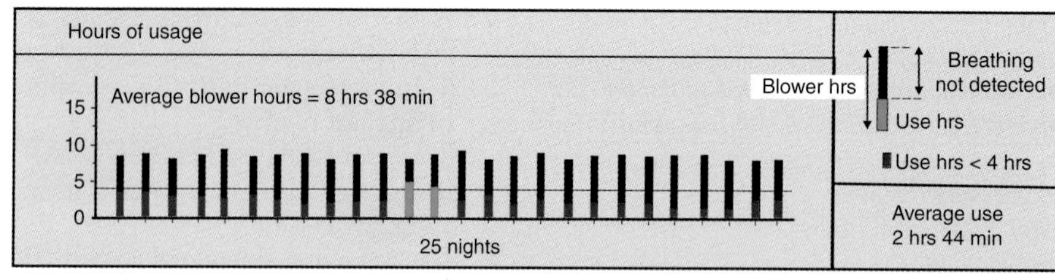

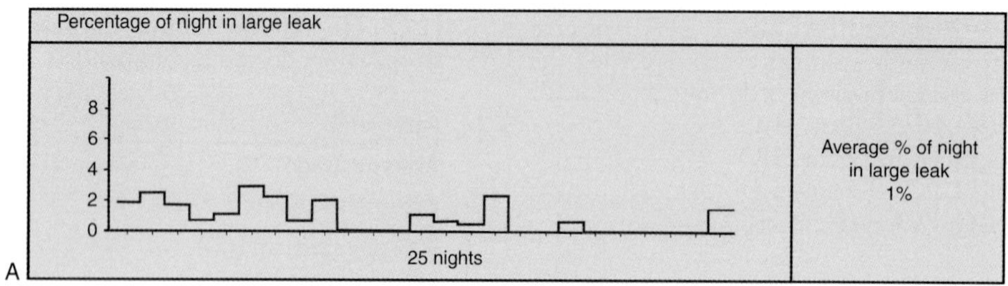

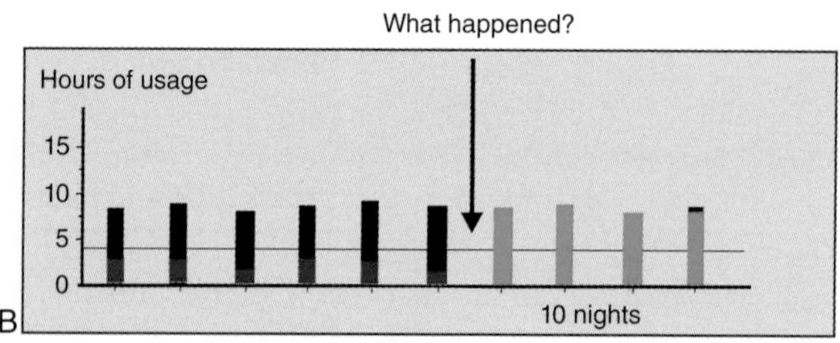

Figure 23–28 (A) A nightly average adherence report showing the duration of blower hours for each night and use hours (green if 4 hours or more or red if less than 4 hours). The black portion of the nightly use duration is the difference between blower hours and use hours. The average blower time was 8 hours and 38 minutes. The average use time was 2 hours and 44 min. (B) Hours of usage showing a sudden change in pattern.

ANSWERS

1. A. Improvement in sleepiness with PAP (or worse sleepiness at baseline) has been associated with better adherence. Spousal referral is associated with lower adherence, and the level of pressure or pressure mode does not seem to affect adherence.
2. C. On CPAP of 9 cm H_2O, the AHI was 4 events/hour, and supine REM sleep was recorded. Higher pressure was associated with central apneas. Of note, some clinicians might choose 10 cm H_2O, as this pressure was associated with a lower AHI REM.
3. E (B and C are correct). The patient likely requires fairly high BPAP; therefore, 2.0 lpm will likely not be adequate given that 2 lpm provides a daytime SaO_2 of only 94%. The required supplemental oxygen flow increases with increasing levels of PAP as a result of the higher delivered flow rate. The supplemental oxygen flow can be adjusted during a PSG PAP titration. However, checking nocturnal oximetry on treatment is suggested to determine oxygen requirements in the home setting.
4. C. Lower adherence. Oronasal masks are associated with higher mask leak and the need for higher PAP pressure. Patients with claustrophobia may find oronasal masks challenging. If necessary, oronasal mask featuring under the nose and over the mouth cushions may be better tolerated in patients with claustrophobia but a nasal or nasal pillows mask may be the best option.
5. B. The AASM titration guidelines recommend increasing both the IPAP and EPAP for obstructive apnea (the event shown). An increase of 1 cm H_2O in both the IPAP and EPAP is recommended after ≥3 obstructive apneas, no more frequently than every 5 minutes. Answers A, C, and D might all eliminate obstructive apnea, but an increase in EPAP, not pressure support, is recommended (A is not the best answer); maintaining the original pressure support is optimal (C is not the best answer); and although D may well work, a slow increase in pressure prevents over titration. Using a pressure support of less than 4 cm H_2O does not take advantage of BPAPs ability to maintain an open airway with lower EPAP. IPAP alone can be increased (increased pressure support) for hypopnea, RERA events, or snoring.
6. C. Higher flow has likely diluted the supplemental oxygen, reducing the effective FiO_2. The increase in pressure would be expected to increase total leak because of an increase in intentional leak (Figure 23–5). However, the total leak has doubled with a relatively small increase in CPAP. Therefore unintentional leak has increased. The first intervention would be adjustment of the mask (the same pressure can be delivered with lower total flow), and if the leak remains high and/or SpO_2 remains low, an increase in the oxygen flow rate would be indicated. Given that the patient required 2 lpm for a low normal awake SpO_2, it is not surprising that a higher flow rate will be needed during CPAP treatment.
7. A.
8. C. Intervention for leak. Although the AHI is above goal and the 90% pressure is at the upper pressure limit, the first intervention is reduction of leak. An increase in

humidity would not be wrong but is unlikely to be effective until the increased leak is addressed.

9. A mask change. When blower hours exceed the use hours, the difference is shown in black in PR CareOrchestrator download reports. This is the time when no breathing is detected. The mask could be off and the device simply running. However, if mask leak is high enough, the same pattern can occur while the patient is actually breathing on the device. Note that the large leak was very low. The time the device is blowing but no breathing is detected is NOT included in the time in large leak. When leak is large, machine detection of residual events is also impaired. The patient had not changed his mask for over one year. He was not aware of the high leak but did notice that the humidifier was dry in the morning (high flow in an attempt to maintain pressure). When the patient started using a new mask, nearly all blower hours were use hours.

SUGGESTED READING

Caples SM, Anderson WM, Calero K, Howell M, Hashmi SD. Use of polysomnography and home sleep apnea tests for the longitudinal management of obstructive sleep apnea in adults: an American Academy of Sleep Medicine clinical guidance statement. *J Clin Sleep Med.* 2021;17(6):1287-1293.

Patil SP, Ayappa IA, Caples SM, Kimoff RJ, Patel SR, Harrod CG. Treatment of adult obstructive sleep apnea with positive airway pressure: an American Academy of Sleep Medicine clinical practice guideline. *J Clin Sleep Med.* 2019;15(2):335-343.

REFERENCES

1. Sullivan CE, Issa FG, Berthon-Jones M, et al. Reversal of obstructive sleep apnoea by continuous positive airway pressure applied through the nares. *Lancet.* 1981;1:862-865.
2. Gay P, Weaver T, Loube D, et al. Evaluation of positive airway pressure treatment for sleep related breathing disorders in adults. *Sleep.* 2006;29:381-401.
3. Kushida CA. Littner MR, Hirshkowitz M, et al. Practice parameters for the use of continuous and bilevel positive airway pressure devices to treat adult patients with sleep related breathing disorders. *Sleep.* 2006;29:375-380.
4. Patil SP, Ayappa IA, Caples SM, Kimoff RJ, Patel SR, Harrod CG. Treatment of adult obstructive sleep apnea with positive airway pressure: an American Academy of Sleep Medicine systematic review, meta-analysis, and GRADE assessment. *J Clin Sleep Med.* 2019;15(2):301-334.
5. Patil SP, Ayappa IA, Caples SM, Kimoff RJ, Patel SR, Harrod CG. Treatment of adult obstructive sleep apnea with positive airway pressure: an American Academy of Sleep Medicine clinical practice guideline. *J Clin Sleep Med.* 2019;15(2):335-343.
6. Caples SM, Anderson WM, Calero K, Howell M, Hashmi SD. Use of polysomnography and home sleep apnea tests for the longitudinal management of obstructive sleep apnea in adults: an American Academy of Sleep Medicine clinical guidance statement. *J Clin Sleep Med.* 2021;17(6):1287-1293.
7. Chowdhuri S, Quan SF, Almeida F, et al. ATS Ad Hoc Committee on Mild Obstructive Sleep Apnea. An Official American Thoracic Society research statement: impact of mild obstructive sleep apnea in adults. *Am J Respir Crit Care Med.* 2016;193(9):e37-54.
8. Sanders MH, Kern N. Obstructive sleep apnea treated by independently adjusted inspiratory and expiratory positive airway pressures via nasal mask. *Chest.* 1990;98:317-324.
9. Kushida CA, Chediak A, Berry RB, et al; Positive Airway Pressure Titration Task Force; American Academy of Sleep Medicine. Clinical guidelines for the manual titration of positive airway pressure in patients with obstructive sleep apnea. *J Clin Sleep Med.* 2008;4(2):157-171.
10. Berry RB, Parish JM, Hartse KM. The use of auto-titrating continuous positive airway pressure for treatment of adult obstructive sleep apnea. An American Academy of Sleep Medicine review. *Sleep.* 2002;25(2):148-173.
11. Berry RB, Chediak A, Brown LK, et al. NPPV Titration Task Force of the American Academy of Sleep Medicine. Best clinical practices for the sleep center adjustment of noninvasive positive pressure ventilation (NPPV) in stable chronic alveolar hypoventilation syndromes. *J Clin Sleep Med.* 2010;6(5):491-509.
12. Weaver TE, Grunstein RR. Adherence to continuous positive airway pressure therapy: the challenge to effective treatment. *Proc Am Thorac Soc.* 2008;5:173-178.
13. Epstein LJ, Kristo D, Strollo PJ Jr., et al., Adult Obstructive Sleep Apnea Task Force of the American Academy of Sleep Medicine. Clinical guideline for the evaluation, management and long-term care of obstructive sleep apnea in adults. *J Clin Sleep Med.* 2009;5(3):263-276.
14. Kuna ST, Bedi DG, Ryckman C. Effect of nasal airway positive pressure on upper airway size and configuration. *Am Rev Respir Dis.* 1988;138:969-975.
15. Schwab RJ, Pack AI, Gupta KB, et al. Upper airway and soft tissue structural changes influences by CPAP in normal subjects. *Am J Respir Crit Care Med.* 1996;154:1106-1116.
16. Alex CG, Aronson RM, Onal E, Lopata M. Effects of continuous positive airway pressure on upper airway and respiratory muscle activity. *J Appl Physiol.* 1987;62:2026-2030.
17. Heinzer RC, Stanchina ML, Malhotra A, et al. Lung volume and continuous positive airway pressure requirements in obstructive sleep apnea. *Am J Respir Crit Care Med.* 2005;172:114-117.
18. Van de Graaff WB. Thoracic influences on upper airway patency. *J Appl Physiol.* 1988;65:2124-2131.
19. Koo BB, Wiggins R, Molina C. REM rebound and CPAP compliance. *Sleep Med.* 2012;13(7):864-868.
20. Cheng JX, Ren J, Qiu J, et al. Rapid eye movement sleep and slow wave sleep rebounded and related factors during positive airway pressure therapy. *Sci Rep.* 2021;11(1):7599.
21. Punjabi NM, Patil S, Crainiceanu C, Aurora RN. Variability and misclassification of sleep apnea severity based on multi-night testing. *Chest.* 2020;158(1):365-373.
22. American Academy of Sleep Medicine. *International Classification of Sleep Disorders.* 3rd ed, text revision. American Academy of Sleep Medicine; 2023.
23. *LCD—Positive Airway Pressure (PAP) Devices for the Treatment of Obstructive Sleep Apnea (L33718).* Available at: https://www.cms.gov/medicare-coverage-database/view/lcd.aspx?LCDId=33718. Accessed November 1, 2023.
24. Patil SP, Collop NA, Chediak AD, Olson EJ, Vohra KP, ONMAP Technical Expert Panel. Optimal NIV Medicare Access Promotion: Patients with OSA: A technical expert panel report from the American College of Chest Physicians, the American Association for Respiratory Care, the American Academy of Sleep Medicine, and the American Thoracic Society. *Chest.* 2021;160(5):e409-e417. Erratum in *Chest.* 2022;161(2):592.
25. American Academy of Sleep Medicine. *International Classification of Sleep Disorders.* 3rd ed. American Academy of Sleep Medicine; 2014.
26. Javaheri S, Barbe F, Campos-Rodriguez F, et al. Sleep apnea: types, mechanisms, and clinical cardiovascular consequences. *J Am Coll Cardiol.* 2017;69(7):841-858.
27. Pack AI, Magalang UJ, Singh B, Kuna ST, Keenan BT, Maislin G. Randomized clinical trials of cardiovascular disease in obstructive sleep apnea: understanding and overcoming bias. *Sleep.* 2021;44(2):zsaa229.
28. McEvoy RD, Sánchez-de-la-Torre M, Peker Y, Anderson CS, Redline S, Barbe F. Randomized clinical trials of cardiovascular disease in obstructive sleep apnea: understanding and overcoming bias. *Sleep.* 2021;44(4): zsab019.
29. Martínez-García MA, Capote F, Campos-Rodríguez F, et al; Spanish Sleep Network. Effect of CPAP on blood pressure in patients with obstructive sleep apnea and resistant hypertension: the HIPARCO randomized clinical trial. *JAMA.* 2013;310(22):2407-2415.
30. Reeves-Hoché MK, Hudgel DW, Meck R, et al. Continuous versus bilevel positive airway pressure for obstructive sleep apnea. *Am J Respir Crit Care Med.* 1995;151:443-449.
31. Smith I, Lasserson TJ. Pressure modification for improving usage of continuous positive airway pressure machines in adults with obstructive sleep apnoea. *Cochrane Database Syst Rev.* 2004;(4):CD003531.
32. Schafer H, Ewig S, Hasper E, et al. Failure of CPAP therapy in obstructive sleep apnea syndrome: predictive factors and treatment with bilevel positive airway pressure. *Respir Med.* 1998;92:208-215.
33. Schwartz SW, Rosas J, Iannacone MR, Foulis PR, Anderson WM. Correlates of a prescription for bilevel positive airway pressure for treatment of obstructive sleep apnea among veterans. *J Clin Sleep Med.* 2013;9(4): 327-335.
34. Ballard RD, Gay PC, Strollo PJ. Interventions to improve compliance in sleep apnea patients previously non-compliant with continuous positive airway pressure. *J Clin Sleep Med.* 2007;3:706-712.
35. Kushida CA, Berry RB, Blau A. Positive airway pressure initiation: a randomized controlled trial to assess the impact of therapy mode and titration process on efficacy, adherence, and outcomes. *Sleep.* 2011; 34(8):1083-1092.

36. Benjafield AV, Pépin JL, Valentine K, et al. Compliance after switching from CPAP to bilevel for patients with non-compliant OSA: big data analysis. *BMJ Open Respir Res*. 2019;6(1):e000380.
37. Piper AJ, Wang D, Yee BJ, et al. Randomized trial of CPAP vs. bilevel support in the treatment of obesity hypoventilation syndrome without severe nocturnal desaturation. *Thorax*. 2008;63:395-401.
38. Mokhlesi B, Masa JF, Brozek JL, et al. Evaluation and management of obesity hypoventilation syndrome. An official American Thoracic Society clinical practice guideline. *Am J Respir Crit Care Med*. 2019;200(3):e6-e24. Erratum in *Am J Respir Crit Care Med*. 2019;200(10):1326.
39. Gómez de Terreros FJ, Cooksey JA, Sunwoo BY, et al. Clinical practice guideline summary for clinicians: evaluation and management of obesity hypoventilation syndrome. *Ann Am Thorac Soc*. 2020;17(1):11-15.
40. Masa JF, Benítez I, Sánchez-Quiroga MÁ, et al; Spanish Sleep Network. Long-term noninvasive ventilation in obesity hypoventilation syndrome without severe OSA: the Pickwick Randomized Controlled Trial. *Chest*. 2020;158(3):1176-1186.
41. Littner M, Hirshkowitz M, Davila D, et al. Practice parameters for the use of auto-titrating continuous positive airway pressure devices for titrating pressures and treating adult patients with obstructive sleep apnea syndrome. An American Academy of Sleep Medicine report. *Sleep*. 2002;25:143-147.
42. Morgenthaler TI, Aurora RN, Brown T, et al; Standards of Practice Committee of the AASM: Practice parameters for the use of autotitrating continuous positive airway pressure devices for titrating pressures and treating adult patients with obstructive sleep apnea syndrome: an update for 2007. *Sleep*. 2008;31:141-147.
43. Randerath WJ, Schraeder O, Galetke W, et al. Autoadjusting CPAP therapy based on impedance efficacy, compliance and acceptance. *Am J Respir Crit Care Med*. 2001;163:652-657.
44. Isetta V, Navajas D, Montserrat JM, Farré R. Comparative assessment of several automatic CPAP devices' responses: a bench test study. *ERJ Open Res*. 2015;1(1):00031-2015.
45. McArdle N, King S, Shepherd K, et al. Study of a novel APAP algorithm for the treatment of obstructive sleep apnea in women. *Sleep*. 2015; 38(11):1775-1781.
46. Badr MS, Toiber F, Skatrud JB, et al. Pharyngeal narrowing/occlusion during central apnea. *J Appl Physiol*. 1995;78:1806-1815.
47. Li QY, Berry RB, Goetting MG, et al. Detection of upper airway status and respiratory events by a current generation positive airway pressure device. *Sleep*. 2015;38(4):597-605.
48. Berry RB, Sriram P. Auto-adjusting positive airway pressure treatment for sleep apnea diagnosed by home sleep testing. *J Clin Sleep Med*. 2014;10(12):1269-1275.
49. Fashanu OS, Quan SF. Factors associated with treatment outcomes after use of auto-titrating CPAP therapy in adults with obstructive sleep apnea. *Sleep Breath*. 2023;27(1):165-172.
50. Ayas NT, Patel SR, Malhotra A, et al. Auto-titrating versus standard continuous positive airway pressure for the treatment of obstructive sleep apnea: results of a meta-analysis. *Sleep*. 2004;27:249-253.
51. Kennedy B, Lasserson TJ, Wozniak DR, Smith I. Pressure modification or humidification for improving usage of continuous positive airway pressure machines in adults with obstructive sleep apnoea. *Cochrane Database Syst Rev*. 2019;12(12):CD003531.
52. Hukins C. Comparative study of autotitrating and fixed-pressure CPAP in the home: a randomized, single-blind crossover trial. *Sleep*. 2004; 27(8):1512-1517.
53. Lebret M, Rotty MC, Argento C, et al. Comparison of auto- and fixed-continuous positive airway pressure on air leak in patients with obstructive sleep apnea: data from a randomized controlled trial. *Can Respir J*. 2019;2019:6310956.
54. Shirlaw T, Hanssen K, Duce B, Hukins C. A randomized crossover trial comparing autotitrating and continuous positive airway pressure in subjects with symptoms of aerophagia: effects on compliance and subjective symptoms. *J Clin Sleep Med*. 2017;13(7):881-888.
55. Gentina T, Fortin F, Douay B, et al. Auto bi-level with pressure relief during exhalation as a rescue therapy for optimally treated obstructive sleep apnoea patients with poor compliance to continuous positive airways pressure therapy—a pilot study. *Sleep Breath*. 2011;15(1):21-27.
56. Powell ED, Gay PC, Ojile JM, Litinski M, Malhotra A. A pilot study assessing adherence to auto-bilevel following a poor initial encounter with CPAP. *J Clin Sleep Med*. 2012;8(1):43-47.
57. Carlucci A, Ceriana P, Mancini M, et al. Efficacy of bilevel-auto treatment in patients with obstructive sleep apnea not responsive to or intolerant of continuous positive airway pressure ventilation. *J Clin Sleep Med*. 2015;11(9):981-985.
58. Aloia MS, Stanchina M, Arnedt JT, et al. Treatment adherence and outcomes in flexible vs. standard continuous positive airway pressure therapy. *Chest*. 2005;172:2085-2093.
59. Bakker J, Campbell A, Neill A. Randomized controlled trial comparing flexible and continuous positive airway pressure delivery: effects on compliance, objective and subjective sleepiness and vigilance. *Sleep*. 2010;33:523-529.
60. Dolan DC, Okonkwo R, Gfullner F, et al. Longitudinal comparison study of pressure relief (C-Flex) vs. CPAP in OSA patients. *Sleep Breath*. 2009;13:73-77.
61. Marshall NS, Neill AM, Campbell AJ. Randomised trial of compliance with flexible (C-Flex) and standard continuous positive airway pressure for severe obstructive sleep apnea. *Sleep Breath*. 2008;12:393-396.
62. Pépin JL, Muir JF, Gentina T, et al. Pressure reduction during exhalation in sleep apnea patients treated by continuous positive airway pressure. *Chest*. 2009;136:490-497.
63. Nilius G, Happel A, Domanski U, Ruhle KH. Pressure-relief continuous positive airway pressure vs. constant continuous positive airway pressure: a comparison of efficacy and compliance. *Chest*. 2006;130:1018-1024.
64. Mulgrew AT, Cheema R, Fleetham J, et al. Efficacy and patient satisfaction with autoadjusting CPAP with variable expiratory pressure vs. standard CPAP: a two-night randomized crossover trial. *Sleep Breath*. 2007;11:31-37.
65. Martins de Araujo MT, Vieira SB, Vasquez EC, Fleury B. Heated humidification or face mask to prevent upper airway dryness during continuous positive airway pressure therapy. *Chest*. 2000;117:142-147.
66. Hayes MJ, McGregor FB, Roberts DN, et al. Continuous positive airway pressure with a mouth leak: effect on nasal mucosal blood flow and nasal geometry. *Thorax*. 1995;50:1179-1182.
67. Richards GN, Cistulli PA, Ungar RG, et al. Mouth leak with nasal continuous positive airway pressure increases nasal airway resistance. *Am J Respir Crit Care Med*. 1996;154:182-186.
68. Massie CA, Hart RW, Peralez K, Richards GN. Effects of humidification on nasal symptoms and compliance in sleep apnea patients using continuous positive airway pressure. *Chest*. 1999;116:403-408.
69. Ryan S, Doherty LS, Nolan GM, McNicholas WT. Effects of heated humidification and topical steroids on compliance, nasal symptoms, and quality of life in patients with obstructive sleep apnea syndrome using nasal continuous positive airway pressure. *J Clin Sleep Med*. 2009;5(5):422-427.
70. Nilius G, Domanski U, Franke KJ, Ruhle KH. Impact of a controlled heated breathing tube humidifier on sleep quality during CPAP therapy in a cool sleeping environment. *Eur Respir J*. 2008;31:830-836.
71. Duong M, Jayaram L, Camfferman D, et al. Use of heated humidification during nasal CPAP titration in obstructive sleep apnoea syndrome. *Eur Respir J*. 2005;26:679-685.
72. Dibra MN, Berry RB, Wagner MH. Treatment of obstructive sleep apnea: choosing the best interface. *Sleep Med Clin*. 2020;15(2):219-225.
73. Bachour A, Avellan-Hietanen H, Palotie T, Virkkula P. Practical aspects of interface application in CPAP treatment. *Can Respir J*. 2019;2019:7215258.
74. Genta PR, Kaminska M, Edwards BA, et al. The importance of mask selection on continuous positive airway pressure outcomes for obstructive sleep apnea. An official American Thoracic Society workshop report. *Ann Am Thorac Soc*. 2020;17(10):1177-1185.
75. Rowland S, Aiyappan V, Hennessy C, et al. Comparing the efficacy, mask leak, patient adherence, and patient preference of three different CPAP interfaces to treat moderate-severe obstructive sleep apnea. *J Clin Sleep Med*. 2018;14(1):101-108.
76. Westhoff M, Litterst P. Obstructive sleep apnoea and non-restorative sleep induced by the interface. *Sleep Breath*. 2015;19(4):1317-1325.
77. Ma Z, Hyde P, Drinnan M, Munguia J. Development of a smart-fit system for CPAP interface selection. *Proc Inst Mech Eng H*. 2021;235(1): 44-53.
78. Duong K, Glover J, Perry AC, et al. Feasibility of three-dimensional facial imaging and printing for producing customised nasal masks for continuous positive airway pressure. *ERJ Open Res*. 2021;7(1):00632-2020.
79. Zhu X, Wimms AJ, Benjafield AV. Assessment of the performance of nasal pillows at high CPAP pressures. *J Clin Sleep Med*. 2013;9(9):873-877.
80. Prosise GL, Berry RB. Oral-nasal continuous positive airway pressure as a treatment for obstructive sleep apnea. *Chest*. 1994;106:180-186.
81. Sanders MH, Kern NB, Stiller RA, et al. CPAP therapy via oronasal mask for obstructive sleep apnea. *Chest*. 1994;106:774-779.
82. Berry RB. Retrospective: when were oronasal masks first used to treat obstructive sleep apnea? *J Clin Sleep Med*. 2017;13(3):523-524.
83. Anderson FE, Kingshott RN, Taylor DR, et al. A randomized crossover efficacy trial of oral CPAP (Oracle) compared with nasal CPAP in the management of obstructive sleep apnea. *Sleep*. 2003;26:721-726.
84. Bachour A, Hurmerinta K, Maasilta P. Mouth closing device (chinstrap) reduces mouth leak during nasal CPAP. *Sleep Med*. 2004;5(3):261-267.

85. Foellner S, Guth P, Jorde I, et al. Prevention of leakage due to mouth opening through applying an oral shield device (Sominpax™) during nasal CPAP therapy of patients with obstructive sleep apnea. *Sleep Med.* 2020;66:168-173.
86. Kaminska M, Montpetit A, Mathieu A, Jobin V, Morisson F, Mayer P. Higher effective oronasal versus nasal continuous positive airway pressure in obstructive sleep apnea: effect of mandibular stabilization. *Can Respir J.* 2014;21(4):234-238.
87. Nascimento JA, de Santana Carvalho T, Moriya HT, et al. Body position may influence oronasal CPAP effectiveness to treat OSA. *J Clin Sleep Med.* 2016;12(3):447-448.
88. Teo M, Amis T, Lee S, Falland K, Lambert S, Wheatley J. Equivalence of nasal and oronasal masks during initial CPAP titration for obstructive sleep apnea syndrome. *Sleep.* 2011;34(7):951-955.
89. Andrade RGS, Viana FM, Nascimento JA, et al. Nasal vs. oronasal CPAP for OSA treatment: a meta-analysis. *Chest.* 2018;153:665-674.
90. Bakker JP, Neill AM, Campbell AJ. Nasal versus oronasal continuous positive airway pressure masks for obstructive sleep apnea: a pilot investigation of pressure requirement, residual disease, and leak. *Sleep Breath.* 2012;16(3):709-716.
91. Borel JC, Tamisier R, Dias-Domingos S, et al; Scientific Council of The Sleep Registry of the French Federation of Pneumology (OSFP). Type of mask may impact on continuous positive airway pressure adherence in apneic patients. *PLoS One.* 2013;8(5):e64382.
92. Ebben MR, Oyegbile T, Pollak CP. The efficacy of three different mask styles on a PAP titration night. *Sleep Med.* 2012;13(6):645-649.
93. Ebben MR, Milrad S, Dyke JP, Phillips CD, Krieger AC. Comparison of the upper airway dynamics of oronasal and nasal masks with positive airway pressure treatment using cine magnetic resonance imaging. *Sleep Breath.* 2016;20(1):79-85.
94. Edmonds JC, Yang H, King TS, et al. Claustrophobic tendencies and continuous positive airway pressure therapy non-adherence in adults with obstructive sleep apnea. *Heart Lung.* 2015;44(2):100-106.
95. Chasens ER, Pack AI, Maislin G, Dinges DF, Weaver TE. Claustrophobia and adherence to CPAP treatment. *West J Nurs Res.* 2005;27(3): 307-321.
96. Lebret M, Martinot JB, Arnol N, et al. Factors contributing to unintentional leak during CPAP treatment: a systematic review. *Chest.* 2017;151(3):707-719.
97. Lebret M, Arnol N, Martinot JB, et al. Determinants of unintentional leaks during CPAP treatment in OSA. *Chest.* 2018;153(4):834-842.
98. Fashanu OS, Budhiraja R, Batool-Anwar S, Quan SF. Titration studies overestimate continuous positive airway pressure requirements in uncomplicated obstructive sleep apnea. *J Clin Sleep Med.* 2021;17(9):1859-1863.
99. Chandrashekariah R, Shaman Z, Auckley D. Impact of upper airway surgery on CPAP compliance in difficult-to-manage obstructive sleep apnea. *Arch Otolaryngol Head Neck Surg.* 2008;134(9):926-930.
100. Egesi A, Davis MD. Irritant contact dermatitis due to the use of a continuous positive airway pressure nasal mask: 2 case reports and review of the literature. *Cutis.* 2012;90(3):125-128.
101. Benjafield AV, Oldstone LM, Willes LA, et al, on behalf of the medXcloud Group. Positive airway pressure therapy adherence with mask resupply: a propensity-matched analysis. *J Clin Med.* 2021;10(4):720.
102. Ely JR, Khorfan F. Unilateral periorbital swelling with nasal CPAP therapy. *J Clin Sleep Med.* 2006;2(3):330-331.
103. Dandekar F, Camacho M, Valerio J, Ruoff CM. Periorbital edema secondary to positive airway pressure therapy. *Case Rep Ophthalmol Med.* 2015;2015:126501.
104. Singh NP, Walker RJ, Cowan F, Davidson AC, Roberts DN. Retrograde air escape via the nasolacrimal system: a previously unrecognized complication of continuous positive airway pressure in the management of obstructive sleep apnea. *Ann Otol Rhinol Laryngol.* 2014;123(5):321-324.
105. Ryals S, Sharma S, Hadigal S, Wagner M, Berry R. An unusual case of PAP-related eye dryness. *J Clin Sleep Med.* 2020;16(9):1619-1621.
106. Bachour A, Maasilta P, Wares J, Uusitalo M. Bubbling test to recognize retrograde air escape via the nasolacrimal system during positive airway pressure therapy. *Sleep Med.* 2017;29:35-36.
107. Endara-Bravo A, Ahoubim D, Mezerhane E, Abreu RA. Alternobaric vertigo in a patient on positive airway pressure therapy. *J Clin Sleep Med.* 2013;9(12):1347-1348.
108. Chou DW, Huntley C, Rosen D. Tympanic membrane perforation as a complication of continuous positive airway pressure. *J Clin Sleep Med.* 2017;13(6):835-836.
109. Lobbezoo F, Li J, Koutris M, et al. Nasal CPAP therapy associated with masticatory muscle myalgia. *J Clin Sleep Med.* 2020;16(3):455-457.
110. Sanner BM, Fluerenbrock N, Kleiber-Imbeck A, Mueller JB, Zidek W. Effect of continuous positive airway pressure therapy on infectious complications in patients with obstructive sleep apnea syndrome. *Respiration.* 2001;68(5):483-487.
111. Ortolano GA, Schaffer J, McAlister MB, et al. Filters reduce the risk of bacterial transmission from contaminated heated humidifiers used with CPAP for obstructive sleep apnea. *J Clin Sleep Med.* 2007;3:700-705.
112. Mercieca L, Pullicino R, Camilleri K, et al. Continuous positive airway pressure: is it a route for infection in those with obstructive sleep apnoea? *Sleep Sci.* 2017;10(1):28-34.
113. Voelker R. Warning about cleaning CPAP devices with ozone gas, UV light. *JAMA.* 2020;323(13):1236.
114. Sunwoo BY, Light M, Malhotra A. Strategies to augment adherence in the management of sleep-disordered breathing. *Respirology.* 2020;25(4): 363-371.
115. Mehrtash M, Bakker JP, Ayas N. Predictors of continuous positive airway pressure adherence in patients with obstructive sleep apnea. *Lung.* 2019;197(2):115-121.
116. Weaver TE. Novel aspects of CPAP treatment and interventions to improve CPAP adherence. *J Clin Med.* 2019;8(12):2220.
117. Kribbs NB, Pack AI, Kline LR, et al. Objective measurement of patterns of nasal CPAP use by patients with obstructive sleep apnea. *Am Rev Respir Dis.* 1993;147(4):887-895.
118. Weaver TE, Kribbs NB, Pack AI, et al. Night-to-night variability in CPAP use over the first three months of treatment. *Sleep.* 1997; 20(4):278-283.
119. Budhiraja R, Parthasarathy S, Drake CL, et al. Early CPAP use identifies subsequent adherence to CPAP therapy. *Sleep.* 2007;30(3):320-324.
120. Malhotra A, Crocker ME, Willes L, Kelly C, Lynch S, Benjafield AV. Patient engagement using new technology to improve adherence to positive airway pressure therapy: a retrospective analysis. *Chest.* 2018; 153(4):843-850.
121. Naik S, Al-Halawani M, Kreinin I, Kryger M. Centers for Medicare and Medicaid Services positive airway pressure adherence criteria may limit treatment to many Medicare beneficiaries. *J Clin Sleep Med.* 2019;15(2):245-251.
122. Gaisl T, Rejmer P, Thiel S, et al. Effects of suboptimal adherence of CPAP therapy on symptoms of obstructive sleep apnoea: a randomised, double-blind, controlled trial. *Eur Respir J.* 2020;55(3):1901526.
123. Rotenberg BW, Murariu D, Pang KP. Trends in CPAP adherence over twenty years of data collection: a flattened curve. *J Otolaryngol Head Neck Surg.* 2016;45(1):43.
124. McArdle N, Devereux G, Heidarnejad H, Engleman HM, Mackay TW, Douglas NJ. Long-term use of CPAP therapy for sleep apnea/hypopnea syndrome. *Am J Respir Crit Care Med.* 1999;159(4 Pt 1):1108-1114.
125. Pépin JL, Krieger J, Rodenstein D, et al. Effective compliance during the first 3 months of continuous positive airway pressure. A European prospective study of 121 patients. *Am J Respir Crit Care Med.* 1999;160(4):1124-1129.
126. Sin DD, Mayers I, Man GC, Pawluk L. Long-term compliance rates to continuous positive airway pressure in obstructive sleep apnea: a population-based study. *Chest.* 2002;121(2):430-435.
127. Kohler M, Smith D, Tippett V, Stradling JR. Predictors of long-term compliance with continuous positive airway pressure. *Thorax.* 2010; 65(9):829-832.
128. Cistulli PA, Armitstead J, Pepin JL, et al. Short-term CPAP adherence in obstructive sleep apnea: a big data analysis using real world data. *Sleep Med.* 2019;59:114-116.
129. Platt AB, Field SH, Asch DA, et al. Neighborhood of residence is associated with daily adherence to CPAP therapy. *Sleep.* 2009;32: 799-806.
130. Brostrom A, Stromberg A, Martensson J, Ulander M, Harder L, Svanborg E. Association of type D personality to perceived side effects and adherence in CPAP-treated patients with OSAS. *J Sleep Res.* 2007;16:439-447.
131. Rosen CL, Auckley D, Benca R, et al. A multisite randomized trial of portable sleep studies and positive airway pressure autotitration versus laboratory-based polysomnography for the diagnosis and treatment of obstructive sleep apnea: the HomePAP study. *Sleep.* 2012;35(6):757-767.
132. Valentin A, Subramanian S, Quan SF, Berry RB, Parthasarathy S. Air leak is associated with poor adherence to autoPAP therapy. *Sleep.* 2011;34(6):801-806.
133. Sung C, Kim H, Kim J, et al. Patients with Epiglottic Collapse Are Less Adherent to Autotitrating Positive Airway Pressure Therapy for Obstructive Sleep Apnea. *Ann Am Thorac Soc.* 2022;19(11):1907-1912.
134. Ye L, Pack AI, Maislin G, et al. Predictors of continuous positive airway pressure use during the first week of treatment. *J Sleep Res.* 2012;21(4):419-426.
135. Hoy CJ, Vennelle M, Kingshott RN, Engleman HM, Douglas NJ. Can intensive support improve continuous positive airway pressure use in

patients with the sleep apnea/hypopnea syndrome? *Am J Respir Crit Care Med.* 1999;159(4 Pt 1):1096-1100.

136. Gentina T, Bailly S, Jounieaux F, et al. Marital quality, partner's engagement and continuous positive airway pressure adherence in obstructive sleep apnea. *Sleep Med.* 2019;55:56-61.
137. Weaver TE, Maislin G, Dinges DF, et al. Relationship between hours of CPAP use and achieving normal levels of sleepiness and daily functioning. *Sleep.* 2007;30(6):711-719.
138. Crook S, Sievi NA, Bloch KE, et al. Minimum important difference of the Epworth Sleepiness Scale in obstructive sleep apnoea: estimation from three randomised controlled trials. *Thorax.* 2019;74(4):390-396.
139. Campos-Rodriguez F, Pena-Grinan N, Reyes-Nunez N, et al. Mortality in obstructive sleep apnea-hypopnea patients treated with positive airway pressure. *Chest.* 2005;128:624-633.
140. Campos-Rodriguez F, Perez-Ronchel J, Grilo-Reina A, et al. Long-term effect of continuous positive airway pressure on BP in patients with hypertension and sleep apnea. *Chest.* 2007;132:1847-1852.
141. Askland K, Wright L, Wozniak DR, Emmanuel T, Caston J, Smith I. Educational, supportive and behavioural interventions to improve usage of continuous positive airway pressure machines in adults with obstructive sleep apnoea. *Cochrane Database Syst Rev.* 2020;4(4):CD007736.
142. Hwang D, Chang JW, Benjafield AV, et al. Effect of telemedicine education and telemonitoring on continuous positive airway pressure adherence. The Tele-OSA randomized trial. *Am J Respir Crit Care Med.* 2018;197(1):117-126.
143. Berry RB, Beck E, Jasko JG. Effect of cloud-based sleep coaches on positive airway pressure adherence. *J Clin Sleep Med.* 2020;16(4):553-562.
144. Richard D, Bartlett DJ, Wong K, et al. Increased adherence to CPAP with a group cognitive behavioral treatment intervention: a randomized trial. *Sleep.* 2007;30:635-640.
145. Aloia MS, Smith K, Arnedt JT, et al. Brief behavioral therapies reduce early positive airway pressure discontinuation rates in sleep apnea syndrome: preliminary findings. *Behav Sleep Med.* 2007;5:89-104.
146. Schwab RJ, Badr SM, Epstein LJ, et al; ATS Subcommittee on CPAP Adherence Tracking Systems. An official American Thoracic Society statement: continuous positive airway pressure adherence tracking systems. The optimal monitoring strategies and outcome measures in adults. *Am J Respir Crit Care Med.* 2013;188(5):613-620.
147. Fox N, Hirsch-Allen AJ, Goodfellow E, et al. The impact of a telemedicine monitoring system on positive airway pressure adherence in patients with obstructive sleep apnea: a randomized controlled trial. *Sleep.* 2012;35(4):477-481.
148. Labarca G, Schmidt A, Dreyse J, Jorquera J, Barbe F. Telemedicine interventions for CPAP adherence in obstructive sleep apnea patients: systematic review and meta-analysis. *Sleep Med Rev.* 2021;60:101543.
149. Luyster FS, Buysse DJ, Strollo Jr PJ. Comorbid insomnia and obstructive sleep apnea: challenges for clinical practice and research. *J Clin Sleep Med.* 2010;6(2):196-204.
150. Berry RB, Patel PB. Effect of zolpidem on the efficacy of continuous positive airway pressure as treatment for obstructive sleep apnea. *Sleep.* 2006;29:1052-1056.
151. Bradshaw DA, Ruff GA, Murphy DP. An oral hypnotic medication does not improve continuous positive airway pressure compliance in men with obstructive sleep apnea. *Chest.* 2006;130:1369-1376.
152. Lettieri CJ, Shah AA, Holley AB, et al. CPAP promotion and prognosis—the Army Sleep Apnea Program Trial. Effects of a short course of eszopiclone on continuous positive airway pressure adherence: a randomized trial. *Ann Intern Med.* 2009;151:696-702.
153. Lettieri CJ, Quast TN, Eliasson AH, Andrada T. Eszopiclone improves overnight polysomnography and continuous positive airway pressure titration: a prospective, randomized, placebo-controlled trial. *Sleep.* 2008;31:1310-1316.
154. Tang Y, Chen Y, Zhang S, et al. The effect of non-benzodiazepine sedative hypnotics on CPAP adherence in patients with OSA: a systematic review and meta-analysis. *Sleep.* 2021;44(8):zsab077.
155. Sweetman A, Lack L, Catcheside PG, et al. Cognitive and behavioral therapy for insomnia increases the use of continuous positive airway pressure therapy in obstructive sleep apnea participants with comorbid insomnia: a randomized clinical trial. *Sleep.* 2019;42(12):zsz178.
156. Alessi CA, Fung CH, Dzierzewski JM, et al. Randomized controlled trial of an integrated approach to treating insomnia and improving the use of positive airway pressure therapy in veterans with comorbid insomnia disorder and obstructive sleep apnea. *Sleep.* 2021;44(4):zsaa235.
157. Sweetman A, Lechat B, Catcheside PG, Smith S, Antic NA. Polysomnographic predictors of treatment response to cognitive behavioral therapy for insomnia in participants with co-morbid insomnia and sleep apnea: secondary analysis of a randomized controlled trial. *Front Psychol.* 2021;12:676763.
158. Ong JC, Crawford MR, Dawson SC, et al. A randomized controlled trial of CBT-I and PAP for obstructive sleep apnea and comorbid insomnia: main outcomes from the MATRICS study. *Sleep.* 2020; 43(9):zsaa041.
159. Rains JC. Treatment of obstructive sleep apnea in pediatric patients. Behavioral intervention for compliance with nasal continuous positive airway pressure. *Clin Pediatr (Phila).* 1995;34:535-541.
160. Marcus CL, Rosen G, Davidson-Ward S, et al. Adherence to and effectiveness of positive airway pressure therapy in children with obstructive sleep apnea. *Pediatrics.* 2006;117:e442-e451.
161. Koontz KL, Slifer KJ, Cataldo MD, Marcus CL. Improving pediatric compliance with positive airway pressure therapy: the impact of behavioral intervention. *Sleep.* 2003;26:1010-1015.
162. Khaytin I, Tapia IE, Xanthopoulos MS, et al. Auto-titrating CPAP for the treatment of obstructive sleep apnea in children. *J Clin Sleep Med.* 2020;16(6):871-878.
163. Kapur VK, Auckley DH, Chowdhuri S, et al. Clinical practice guideline for diagnostic testing for adult obstructive sleep apnea: an American Academy of Sleep Medicine clinical practice guideline. *J Clin Sleep Med.* 2017;13(3):479-504.
164. Condos R, Norman RG, Krishnasamy I, et al. Flow limitation as a noninvasive assessment of residual upper-airway resistance during continuous positive airway pressure therapy of obstructive sleep apnea. *Am J Respir Crit Care Med.* 1994;150:475-480.
165. Azarbarzin A, Sands SA, Marques M, Genta PR, Taranto-Montemurro L. Palatal prolapse as a signature of expiratory flow limitation and inspiratory palatal collapse in patients with obstructive sleep apnoea. *Eur Respir J.* 2018;51(2):1701419.
166. Montserrat JM, Ballester E, Olivi H, et al. Time-course of stepwise CPAP titration. Behavior of respiratory and neurological variables. *Am J Respir Crit Care Med.* 1995;152:1854-1859.
167. Oksenberg A, Silverberg DS, Arons E, Radwan H. The sleep supine position has a major effect on optimal nasal continuous positive airway pressure: relationship with rapid eye movements and non-rapid eye movements sleep, body mass index, respiratory disturbance index, and age. *Chest.* 1999;116(4):1000-1006.
168. Neill AM, Angus SM, Sajkov D, McEvoy RD. Effects of sleep posture on upper airway stability in patients with obstructive sleep apnea. *Am J Respir Crit Care Med.* 1997;155:199-204.
169. Johnson KG, Johnson DC. Bilevel positive airway pressure worsens central apneas during sleep. *Chest.* 2005;128(4):2141-2150.
170. *LCD L33800 Respiratory Assist Devices. Centers for Medicare and Medicaid Services.* Available at: https://www.cms.gov/medicare-coverage-database/view/lcd.aspx?lcdid=33800&ver=26&bc=CAAAAAAAAAAA. Accessed November 1, 2023.
171. Yoder EA, Klann K, Strohl KP. Inspired oxygen concentrations during positive pressure therapy. *Sleep Breath.* 2004;8:1-5.
172. Schwartz AR, Kacmarek RM, Hess DR. Factors affecting oxygen delivery with bilevel positive airway pressure. *Respir Care.* 2004;49: 270-275.
173. Berry RB, Hill G, Thompson L, McLaurin V. Portable monitoring and autotitration versus polysomnography for the diagnosis and treatment of sleep apnea. *Sleep.* 2008;31:1423-1431.
174. Antic NA, Buchan C, Esterman A, et al. A randomized controlled trial of nurse-led care for symptomatic moderate-severe obstructive sleep apnea. *Am J Respir Crit Care Med.* 2009;179:501-508.
175. Kuna ST, Gurubhagavatula I, Maislin G, et al. Noninferiority of functional outcome in ambulatory management of obstructive sleep apnea sleep apnea. *Am J Respir Crit Care Med.* 2011;183(9):1238-1244.
176. Skomro RP, Gjevre J, Reid J, et al. Outcomes of home-based diagnosis and treatment of obstructive sleep apnea. *Chest.* 2010;138(2): 257-263.
177. Berry RB, Kushida CA, Kryger MH, Soto-Calderon H, Staley B, Kuna ST. Respiratory event detection by a positive airway pressure device. *Sleep.* 2012;35(3):361-367.
178. Koivumäki V, Maasilta P, Bachour A. Oximetry monitoring recommended during PAP initiation for sleep apnea in patients with obesity or nocturnal hypoxemia. *J Clin Sleep Med.* 2018;14(11):1859-1863.

Advanced PAP Modes, NIV Titration, and Phrenic Nerve Stimulation

Chapter 24

INTRODUCTION TO ADVANCED PAP MODES

The modes of positive airway pressure (PAP) devices to be discussed in this chapter include bilevel positive airway pressure in the spontaneous mode (BPAP-S), the spontaneous-timed mode (BPAP-ST), and timed mode (BPAP-T); adaptive servoventilation (ASV); and volume-assured pressure support (VAPS) (Table 24–1). BPAP-S is primarily used for obstructive sleep apnea but can be used for some patients with hypoventilation disorders when these patients do not qualify for BPAP with a backup rate as the initial treatment due to insurance regulations. BPAP-ST, ASV, and VAPS devices are BPAP devices that have an available backup rate[1-5] and are all classified as E0471 respiratory assist devices (RADs) by the Centers for Medicare and Medicaid Services (CMS) and most insurance providers. BPAP without a backup rate (BPAP-S) is classified as an E0470 RAD device. BPAP devices deliver a higher inspiratory PAP (IPAP) and lower expiratory PAP (EPAP). The pressure support (PS) delivered by BPAP devices is the difference between IPAP and EPAP (IPAP – EPAP). In the spontaneous mode (BPAP-S), the patient **triggers** an *EPAP to IPAP transition* by generating inspiratory flow. The BPAP devices **cycle** from *IPAP to EPAP* based on proprietary algorithms when inspiratory flow falls below a threshold value, usually based on a fraction of the peak inspiratory flow (Figure 24–1). That is, changes in patient flow spontaneously trigger or cycle the device between IPAP and EPAP. The **rise time** is the time required for the transition from EPAP to IPAP. The EPAP prevents upper airway closure (prevents obstructive apnea) and results in a bias flow (intentional leak) via small orifices in the mask to wash out the exhaled CO_2, preventing rebreathing. The total leak is the sum of the intentional leak (non-rebreathing ports) and the unintentional leak (around the sides of the mask and mouth leak). The inspiratory time (Ti) as shown in Figure 24–1A is really the IPAPtime but Ti is the common nomenclature. As can be seen in Figure 24–1B inspiratory flow continues briefly as pressure transitions from IPAP to EPAP.

In the **BPAP-ST mode**, devices deliver a *fixed PS* with an available backup rate. Breaths can be triggered either spontaneously (S) or device triggered (T) if the patient fails to initiate a

Table 24–1 Advanced Modes of Positive Airway Pressure Devices

PAP Mode	Method	Use
No Backup Rate		
BPAP spontaneous mode (BPAP-S)	• All breaths spontaneously triggered • Fixed pressure support: PS= (IPAP-EPAP)	• OSA • OHS • Hypoventilation syndromes not requiring a backup rate
Backup Rate Available		
BPAP with backup rate (BPAP-ST)	Fixed PS Modes with backup rate • ST Spontaneous Timed • T Timed (some devices)	• NIV • Hypoventilation Syndromes • CSA Syndromes

Volume Assured Pressure Support (VAPS)
AVAPS, iVAPS
	• AVAPS – PS adjusted to deliver target tidal volume
	  • Used in ST, PC modes
	• iVAPS - PS adjusted to deliver target alveolar ventilation
	  • Used with intelligent backup rate (iBR)
		• NIV
		• Hypoventilation Syndromes
		• CSA Syndromes

Adaptive Servoventilation (ASV)	• PS varies to stabilize breathing
	• EPAP or autoEPAP to eliminate upper airway obstruction (obstructive apnea, hypopnea (PR), airflow limitation, snoring)
	• Backup rate for central apnea
		• Hypocapnic CSA
		  • Primary CSA
		  • CSA with CSB
		  • Treatment emergent CSA
		• CSA Due to a Medication

ASV, adaptive servoventilation; *BPAP*, bilevel positive airway pressure; *EPAP*, expiratory positive airway pressure; autoEPAP, device automatically adjusts the EPAP within pressure limits; *IPAP*, inspiratory positive airway pressure; *NPPV*, noninvasive positive pressure ventilation; *NIV*, noninvasive ventilation; *PAP*, positive airway pressure; *PS*, pressure support; *S mode*, spontaneous mode; *ST*, spontaneous timed; obesity hypoventilation syndrome, OHS; *CSA*, central sleep apnea; *CSB*, Cheyne-Stokes breathing; *AVAPS*, average volume assured pressure support; *iVAPS*, intelligent volume assured pressure support; *iBR*, intelligent backup rate. iVAPS ResMed, AVAPS Philips Respironics. The Centers for Medicare and Medicaid Services (CMS) classifies BPAP devices without a backup rate as E0470 and all types of BPAP devices with a backup rate as E0471. BPAP-S (BPAP spontaneous, no backup rate)

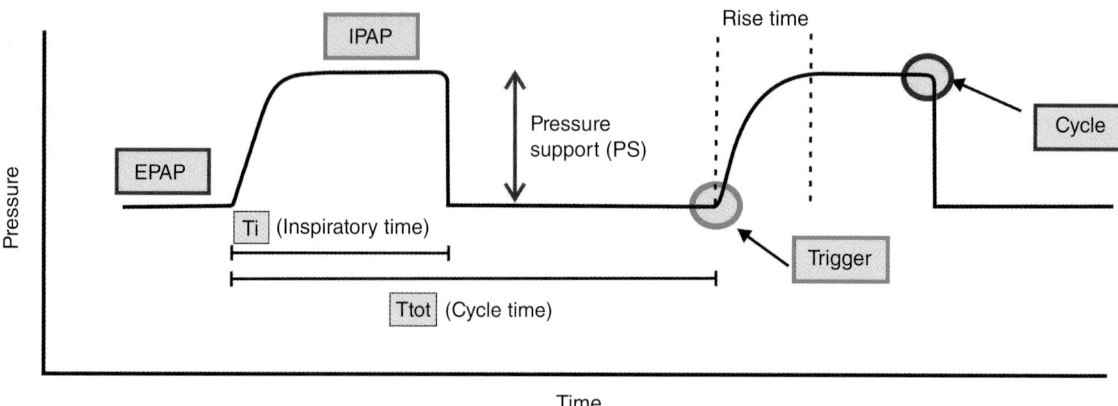

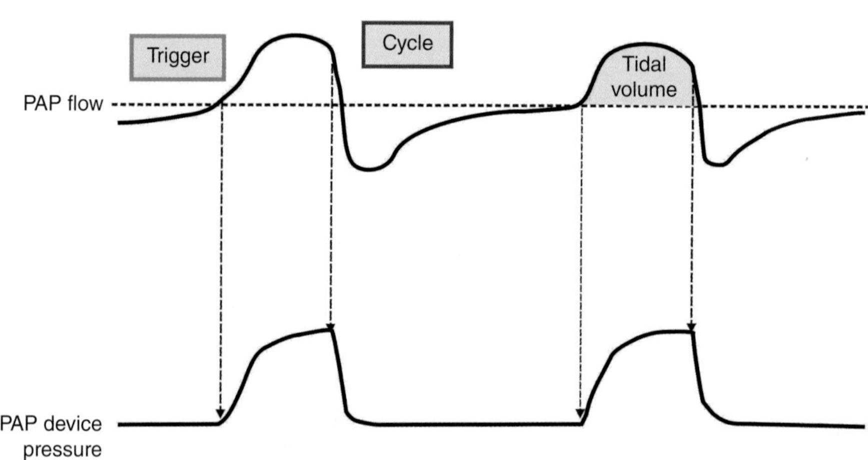

Figure 24–1 A Tracing of Pressure Versus Time for a Bilevel Positive Airway Pressure (BPAP) Device. (A) A schematic of pressure change using a BPAP device. Pressure support is the difference between inspiratory PAP (IPAP) and expiratory PAP (EPAP). The EPAP to IPAP transition is termed trigger (either spontaneous or device triggered), and the IPAP to EPAP transition is termed cycle (either spontaneous or device cycled). The inspiratory time (Ti) is the duration of the IPAP cycle (also called IPAP time). The total cycle time (Ttot) is the time from the start of a given pressure pulse until the start of the next breath (EPAP to IPAP transition). The rise time is the time from EPAP to IPAP once the transition has been triggered. (B) Tracings of PAP flow and PAP device pressure are shown, The PAP flow and PAP device pressure signals are provided by the sleep laboratory PAP device used for polysomnography PAP titrations). The area under the inspiratory portion of the flow curve is the tidal volume.

breath within a time window (seconds) set by the backup rate (60/backup rate). The backup rate is specified in breaths per minute (bpm). In **ASV**, the PS varies to stabilize peak flow (or minute ventilation). During periods of reduced peak flow or minute ventilation (below a target value), PS increases and when peak flow or minute ventilation increases (above a target value), PS decreases. The target is approximately 90-95% (depending on the device) of the average value (or time weighted average) over a preceding moving time window. The goal is to stabilize either the minute ventilation or peak flow depending on the brand of the device being used. A backup rate is available to treat central apnea. EPAP is available to treat obstructive apnea. An autoEPAP function is available on ASV devices to select an appropriate EPAP between EPAPmin and EPAPmax. In **VAPS** units, the PS varies to deliver a target tidal volume (or target alveolar ventilation), and a backup rate is available for central apneas and/or to ensure an adequate minute ventilation. In the United States, autoEPAP functionality is available only on home mechanical ventilators (HMVs) with VAPS capability. In ASV, the time window used to determine the target is 3 to 4 minutes based on the device, and PS changes from breath to breath or within a breath. In VAPS, there is a much shorter time window used to determine if the target tidal volume or alveolar ventilation is being delivered. The PS in VAPS varies at a much slower rate (VAPS rate), for example, an increase of 1 to 5 cm H_2O/min. The exact setup of the advanced devices varies among manufacturers. In this chapter, Philips Respironics (PR) and ResMed devices will be discussed (Table 24–2). At the time of writing PR will no longer sell PAP devices and HMVs in the USA. However, many patients continue to use refurbished (with replacement sound abatement foam) PR advanced PAP devices or HMVs (Trilogy-Evo not under recall). PR devices are still sold outside of the US.

BPAP-ST, BPAP-T, AND BPAP-PC MODES

BPAP in the ST mode and BPAP in the T mode are used to deliver noninvasive ventilation (NIV) in patients with central

Table 24–2 Current BPAP Devices

Device	Modes	Max pressure (cm H_2O)
PR BPAP Devices**		
DS BiPAP™ pro	CPAP, BPAP S	25
DS BiPAP™ S/T	CPAP, BPAP S, ST	30
DS BiPAP AVAPS™ (AVAPS)	CPAP, BPAP S, ST, T, PC, AVAPS™	30
DS BiPAP autoSV™ (ASV)	ASV	30
ResMed BPAP Devices		
AC S™	BPAP-S	25
AC ST™	CPAP, BPAP (S, ST, T)	25
AC ST-A™	CPAP, S, ST, T, PAC, iVAPS (with iBR)	30
AC ASV™	CPAP, ASV, ASVauto	25

BiPAP is a trademark of PR; AirCurve trademark of ResMed. Available devices and capabilities may change over time.
**At the time of writing PR will no longer sell PAP devices in the USA.
PR, Philips Respironics; *DS*, DreamStation; *AC*, AirCurve (at the time of writing AirCurve 10 for ResMed BPAP devices); *ASV*, adaptive servoventilation; *AVAPS*, average volume-assured pressure support; *iVAPS*, intelligent volume-assured pressure support; *S*, spontaneous; *ST*, spontaneous-timed; *T*, timed; *PC*, pressure control; *PAC*, pressure-assist control; *CPAP*, continuous positive airway pressure; *BPAP*, bilevel positive airway pressure; *iBR*, intelligent backup rate. Auto-SV PR brand name for BPAP with ASV capability, ST-A ResMed brand name for BPAP with iVAPS capability

sleep apnea (CSA) and chronic hypoventilation syndromes.[1-6] NIV is sometimes referred to as noninvasive positive pressure ventilation (NPPV). As noted above, BPAP devices in the ST mode deliver a combination of spontaneously triggered and device-triggered breaths. Breaths are cycled (IPAP to EPAP) either spontaneously (based on flow) or by the device (time cycled) depending on the manufacturer of the BPAP-ST device (PR versus ResMed). During polysomnography (PSG) titration studies, recording the PAP pressure as well as PAP flow signals is essential for the clinician to understand the pressure the BPAP device is delivering and if the breath is spontaneously or device triggered. Basic BPAP-ST devices include the DreamStation BiPAP S/T (PR) and AirCurve 10 ST (ResMed). These devices have a maximum pressure of 25 cm H_2O. More advanced ST devices that can also deliver VAPS include the DreamStation AVAPS (PR) and Aircurve 10 ST-A (ResMed) and have a maximum pressure of 30 cm H_2O. As noted above all BPAP devices with a backup rate are considered respiratory assist devices (RADs) by the Centers for Medicare and Medicaid Services (CMS) and other insurance providers. For CMS, any version of a BPAP device with a backup rate (BPAP ST, ASV, VAPS) is considered an E0471 device. In this chapter, when BPAP delivers an EPAP to IPAP (pressure pulse), this is considered a breath, even if no actual flow occurs. This situation usually occurs with device-triggered breaths when the upper airway is closed or very narrow.

In the ST mode, the clinician specifies the EPAP, IPAP, rise time, and backup rate. PAP devices operating in the BPAP-ST mode deliver a device-triggered breath if the patient does not trigger a spontaneous breath within a time window (device cycle time = 60/backup rate). PR PSG laboratory BPAP devices output a pressure signal (patient pressure) that adds a downward artifact in the signal for device-triggered breaths (Figure 24–2). In PR device spontaneously triggered breaths have variable inspiratory times, but **device-triggered breaths** all have a fixed duration (inspiratory time, Ti) specified by the clinician. For example, if the backup rate is 12 breaths/min, there is a 5-second window following the start of the last breath. As shown in Figure 24–2A, no spontaneous breath occurred in the 5-second window following the second breath (pressure pulse), and the BPAP device delivered a machine-triggered breath (T) identified by the artifact in the pressure tracing for the specified Ti. That is, the breath is device triggered based on the backup rate and device cycled based on the specified Ti. The first two breaths have different Ti values and are spontaneously triggered and spontaneously cycled. The Ttot (total cycle time) is the time from the start of a breath (pressure pulse) to the start of the next breath. The Ttot of a breath followed by a spontaneously triggered breath or the Ttot of a device triggered breath followed by a spontaneously triggered breath can vary (Figure 24-2B). The Ttot of a spontaneously triggered breath followed by a device triggered breath or the Ttot of a device triggered breath followed by another device triggered breath is always the same (device cycle time in seconds = 60/Backup rate in bpm). The Ttot=Ti +Te where Ti is the inspiratory time and Te is the expiratory time.

In ResMed devices operating in the ST mode, a backup rate and a *cycle time window* (rather than a fixed Ti) are specified.[3,7] Minimum and maximum Ti values are specified (TiMin, TiMax), and the device cycles between those time limits with a Ti based on decreasing inspiratory flow (Figure 24–3). The TiMin and TiMax are operative for both **spontaneous and device-triggered breaths**. Device-cycled breaths are also referred to as time-cycled breaths. For device cycled breaths, the Ti will be TiMin if decreases in inspiratory flow would otherwise cycle the device sooner then TiMin or TiMax if inspiratory flow would otherwise cycle the device later than TiMax. ResMed PSG laboratory devices provide a trigger signal that can be recorded during PSG that can identify device-triggered breaths as well as well a device-cycled breaths (Figure 24–3). In this figure, the first breath is spontaneously triggered and spontaneously cycled within the Ti cycle window. The second breath is spontaneously triggered but device cycled at TiMin. In this case, inspiratory flow (not shown) fell rapidly and would have resulted in a shorter Ti than TiMin. The third breath is device triggered, as no spontaneous breath was noted within the 5-second window (backup rate 12 breaths/min). The device was cycled at TiMax, as flow would have resulted in a longer Ti than TiMax. In summary, in the ST mode, a Ti is specified for device-triggered breaths in PR devices, and a Ti cycle window is specified for both spontaneously and device-triggered breaths in ResMed devices. Selection of Ti, TiMin, and TiMax will be discussed in more detail later in this chapter. For ResMed devices, one can essentially specify a desired Ti by setting the TiMin to the desired Ti and the TiMax to slightly longer than TiMin (narrow cycle window).

In the timed (T) mode, all breaths are device triggered and device cycled at the set Ti for both PR and ResMed devices (Figure 24–4). The T mode is not available on standard PR BPAP-ST units but is available on PR BPAP devices that

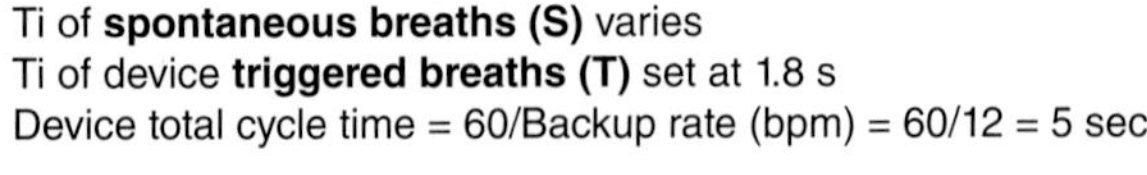

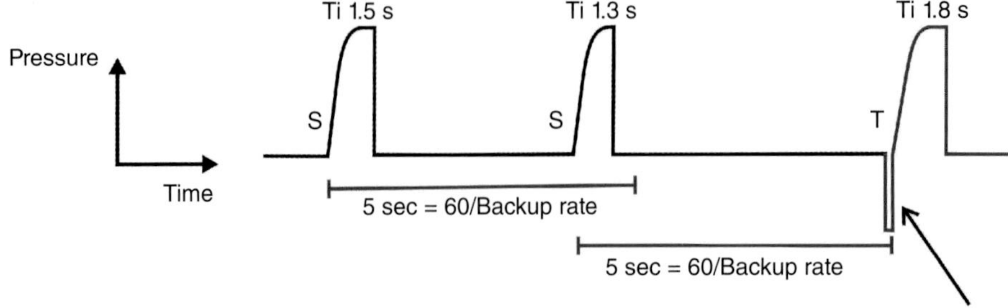

Artifact signifying a device triggered breath
(no S breath within 5 sec window)

A

Ttot = time from start of the current
breath to start of the next breath

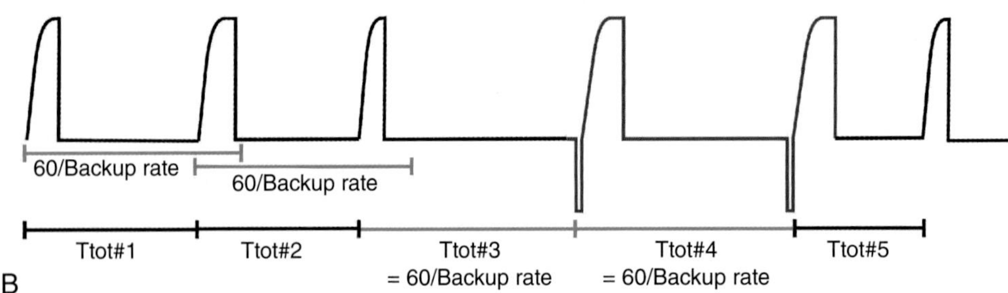

Ttot#1 Ttot#2 Ttot#3 = 60/Backup rate Ttot#4 = 60/Backup rate Ttot#5

B

Figure 24–2 (A) Pressure versus time tracing of the patient pressure signal From a laboratory Philips Respironics (PR) Bilevel Positive Airway Pressure (BPAP) Device operating in the Spontaneous-Timed (ST) Mode With an inspiratory Time (Ti) of 1.8 Seconds. Two spontaneously triggered and cycled breaths are shown followed by a device-triggered and device-cycled breath (pressure pulse). A downward artifact is added to the signal to designate a device-triggered breath. In this case, the backup rate was 12 breaths/min (device cycle time of 5 seconds). The spontaneously cycled breaths have different Ti values, but the device-triggered breaths have the specified Ti. (B) The Ttot (total cycle time) of a given breath is from the start of the breath to the start of the next breath (pressure pulse). The Ttot between two spontaneously triggered breaths (Ttot#1, Ttot#2) or between a device triggered breath and a spontanously triggered breath (Ttot#5) can vary. The Ttot of a spontaneously triggered breath followed by a device triggered breath (Ttot#3) or the Ttot of a device triggered breath followed by another device triggered breath (Ttot#4) is always the same (Ttot in seconds = 60/Backup rate in bpm).

have VAPS capability. ResMed BPAP-ST devices still have a timed mode option. In the timed mode, Ti rather than TiMin or TiMax is specified. This mode is rarely used, as most patients find it to be uncomfortable because they are unable to spontaneously trigger breaths.

Advanced BPAP devices made by PR and ResMed that have VAPS capability have an additional backup rate mode called *pressure control (PC)* for PR devices and *pressure assist control (PAC)* for ResMed devices. In this mode, *both spontaneous and device-triggered breaths* have the duration specified by Ti. This mode is especially useful for patients using PR devices, as it ensures an adequate Ti for spontaneous as well as device-triggered breaths. However, unlike the timed mode, the PC (or PAC) mode allows breaths to be *spontaneously triggered* and is better tolerated by patients. The three modes (ST, T, and PC) for a PR device are displayed in Figure 24–4.

As discussed, laboratory PAP devices can provide several useful signals that can be recorded during PSG. The PAP pressure signal was discussed previously. Other options include PAP flow, PAP leak (total or unintentional), and tidal volume (Figure 24–5). Device algorithms are able to separate the measured total flow into a leak component and a patient flow component (PAP flow). See Chapter 23 for a detailed discussion. The leak signal may be the total leak or the unintentional leak (estimated mask leak at the current pressure subtracted from total leak) depending on the device. *Estimates of the delivered tidal volume are determined by integrating the PAP flow* and value of the estimated tidal volume may be recorded. Complex algorithms are needed to segment total flow into PAP flow and leak, as the total leak may vary between breaths and during breaths. Devices determine an estimate of intentional leak based on the mask type and delivered pressure (see Chapter 23). The delivered tidal volume is useful in adjusting PS and Ti. As shown in Figure 24–5, *the tidal volume depends on both peak flow and Ti.* Knowing what PS the device is delivering, whether the backup rate has been activated, and the delivered Ti are very useful for the clinician. For example, looking at an ASV titration, one knows the set limits on EPAP and PS, but looking at the flow and pressure tracings (and trigger channel in ResMed devices) is the only method to see what treatment the device is actually delivering. In Figure 24–6, the **same** PS delivers entirely different flow

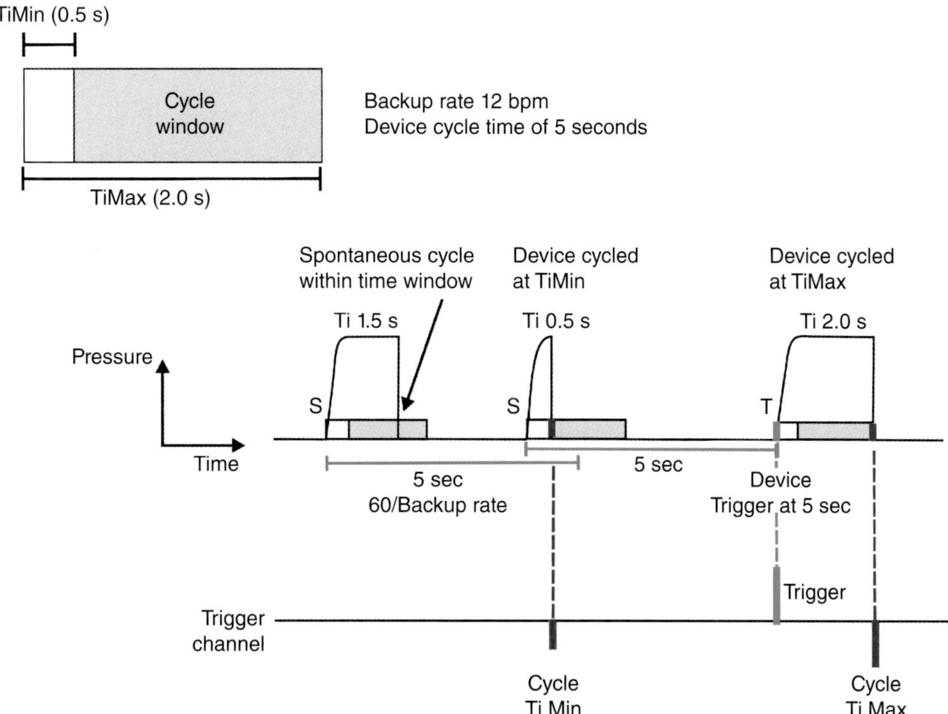

Figure 24–3 Pressure versus time tracing of the pressure and trigger signal from a laboratory ResMed Bi-level Positive Airway Pressure (BPAP) device operating in the Spontaneous-Timed (ST) Mode. Spontaneous breaths are cycled within a time window between inspiratory time TiMin and TiMax. Here, TiMin is 0.5 seconds (default value is 0.3 sec) and TiMax is 2 seconds (default value). The first breath is spontaneously triggered and cycled (based on flow). The second breath is spontaneously triggered but device cycled at TiMin (see downward deflection in Trigger channel). The third breath is device triggered (upward deflection in trigger channel) and device cycled at TiMax (larger downward deflection than for TiMin). Both spontaneous and device-triggered breaths are spontaneously cycled between TiMin and TiMax based on flow. Breaths are time cycled at TiMin if flow would have cycled the device before TiMin or time cycled at TiMax if flow would have cycled the device at a time later than TiMax.

depending on whether the breath is spontaneous or device triggered (different Ti). As will be discussed later in this chapter, lower PS is needed for spontaneously triggered breaths, as the patient is actively inhaling during these breaths. A higher PS is needed for device-triggered breaths, as inspiratory flow depends entirely on the PS and the resistance and compliance of the respiratory system (including the resistance and patency of the upper airway).

IMPORTANCE OF THE BACKUP RATE AND INSPIRATORY TIME

While it obvious that a backup rate is needed to treat patients with central sleep apnea (CSA) or abnormal ventilatory control, an available backup rate is also essential for optimal NIV treatment in patients with hypoventilation. Minute ventilation depends on both tidal volume and the respiratory rate. In some patients, a relatively high respiratory rate is needed due to limitations on delivering an optimal tidal volume. Use of a lower tidal volume may be needed in patients with a stiff chest wall (high PS required) or when the PS needed to deliver a target tidal volume is not tolerated. In such cases changing the Ti cn be very useful. *At the same PS, a larger tidal volume can be delivered with a longer Ti*, and a higher minute ventilation can be delivered with a higher respiratory rate. A method to ensure an adequate Ti is important in patients with neuromuscular weakness or a low respiratory system compliance. In these patients, the BPAP algorithm may cycle from IPAP to EPAP prematurely due to a rapid fall in inspiratory flow. With PR BPAP devices, one can specify Ti for device-triggered breaths in the BPAP-ST mode and for all breaths in the PC mode (VAPS units only). For ResMed devices, a TiMin can be specified for all breaths in the ST mode. A set Ti is specified for the PC mode (PR) and PAC mode (ResMed) for all breaths.

CHOOSING Ti AND UNDERSTANDING THE Ti/Ttot AND I:E RATIO PARAMETERS

The Ti is usually 1.0 to 1.6 seconds, depending on the backup rate (Table 24–3), but it can be longer for slower respiratory rates or shorter for faster respiratory rates. The total cycle time (Ttot) is the time from the start of a breath (EPAP to IPAP transition) until the start of the next EPAP to IPAP transition. In PR BPAP devices operating in the ST mode, *if all breaths are device triggered and cycled*, then Ttot = device cycle time = (60/backup rate), and Ti/Ttot for all breaths is the specified Ti divided by (60/backup rate). If there is a combination of spontaneously and device-triggered breaths, the Ti/Ttot can vary Figure 24–2B. However, expressing Ti as a fraction of Ttot is a useful method to choose Ti for a given backup rate. The Ti/Ttot conveys the relative time in inspiration and exhalation.

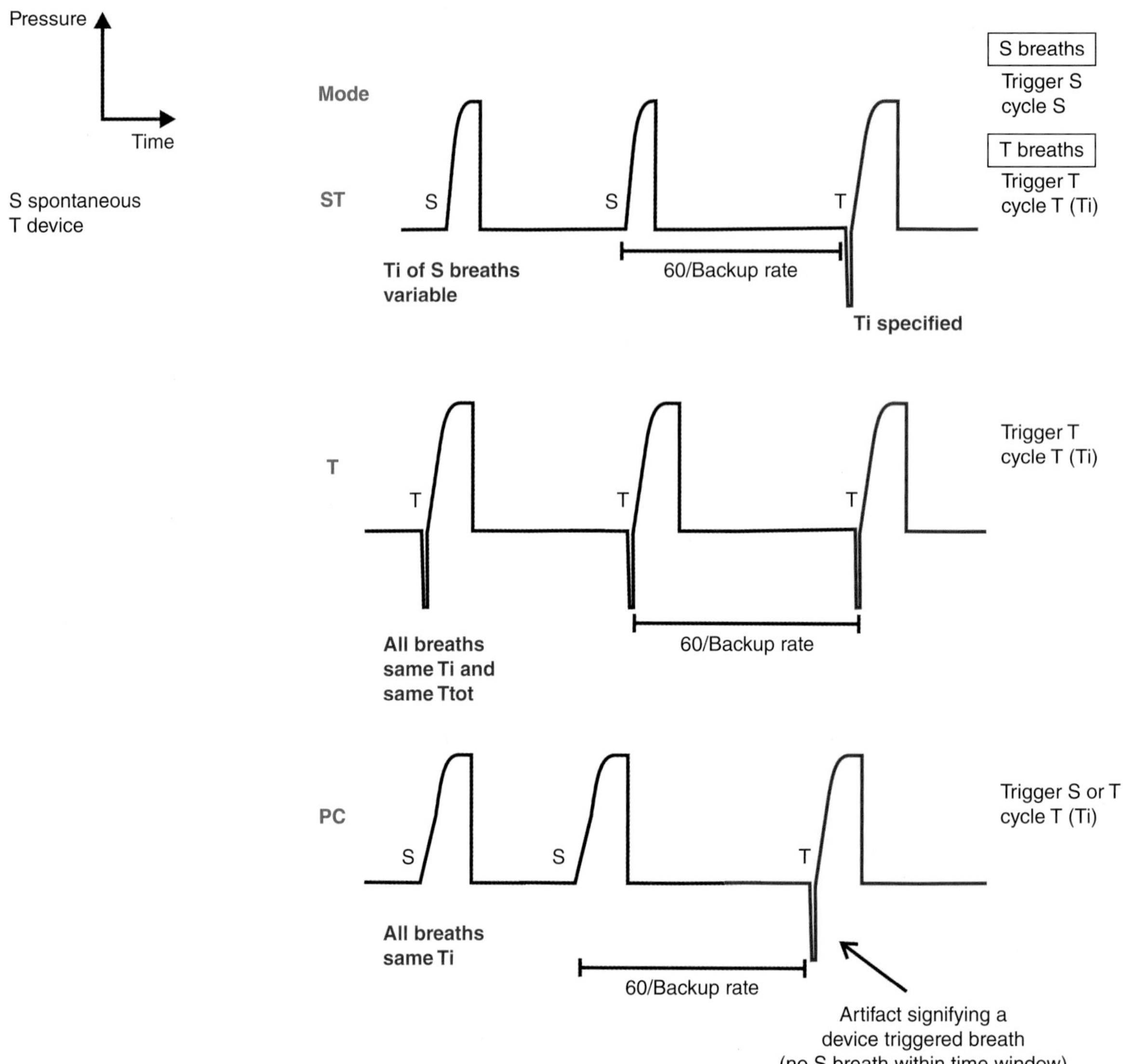

Figure 24–4 Pressure Versus Time Tracings of Different Bilevel Positive Airway Pressure (BPAP) Timed Modes Using a Philips Respironics (PR) Laboratory BPAP Device. *At the top,* spontaneous-timed (ST) mode: The first two S breaths are spontaneously triggered and cycled. The third breath is device triggered and cycled at the specified inspiratory time (Ti). In the timed (T) mode: all breaths are device triggered and device cycled. In the pressure-controlled (PC) mode: breaths can be spontaneous or device triggered, but all breaths are cycled by the device at the specified Ti. In the example of the PC mode the first two breaths are spontaneously triggered, but the third breath is device triggered. For ResMed devices, this mode is called pressure assist control (PAC). For ResMed devices functioning in the PAC mode, a Ti is specified for all breaths (no TiMin or TiMax).

In Table 24–3, a listing of Ti values as a fraction of Ttot for different respiratory rates is displayed. The Ti values are obtained by multiplying a chosen Ti/Ttot by the Ttot = device cycle time computed from the backup rate (60/backup rate). For example, using a Ti/Ttot = 0.3 and a backup rate of 15 breaths/min (device cycle time 4 seconds), the derived Ti would be 0.3 × 4 = 1.2 seconds. For ResMed devices, one can use the derived Ti as the TiMin (or as a guide to choose the TiMin). However, in the ST mode all breaths are cycled between TiMin and TiMax, the actual Ti can vary. ResMed recommendations for TiMin and TiMax are available (Table 24–4).[7]

Depending on the patient type, the Ti/Ttot is usually between 0.25 and 0.5. Patients with obstructive lung disease need a long exhalation time; therefore, a Ti/Ttot of 0.25 to 0.3 is recommended. Patients with restrictive lung disease may need a longer inhalation time; therefore, a Ti/Ttot of 0.3 to 0.4 is recommended. Summary download information usually provides an average Ti/Ttot (although providing an average Ti would be more useful).

The initial recommended setting for PR BPAP ST titrations is 1.5 seconds (assumes a backup rate of 12 breaths/min), and the backup rate is usually chosen one or two breaths below the spontaneous breathing rate. A longer Ti than 1.5 may be appropriate for rates lower than 12 bpm and a shorter Ti is appropriate for higher respiratory rartes. Another option is to match the patient's spontaneous Ti. Choosing TiMin and TiMax for ResMed devices will be discussed later in this chapter.

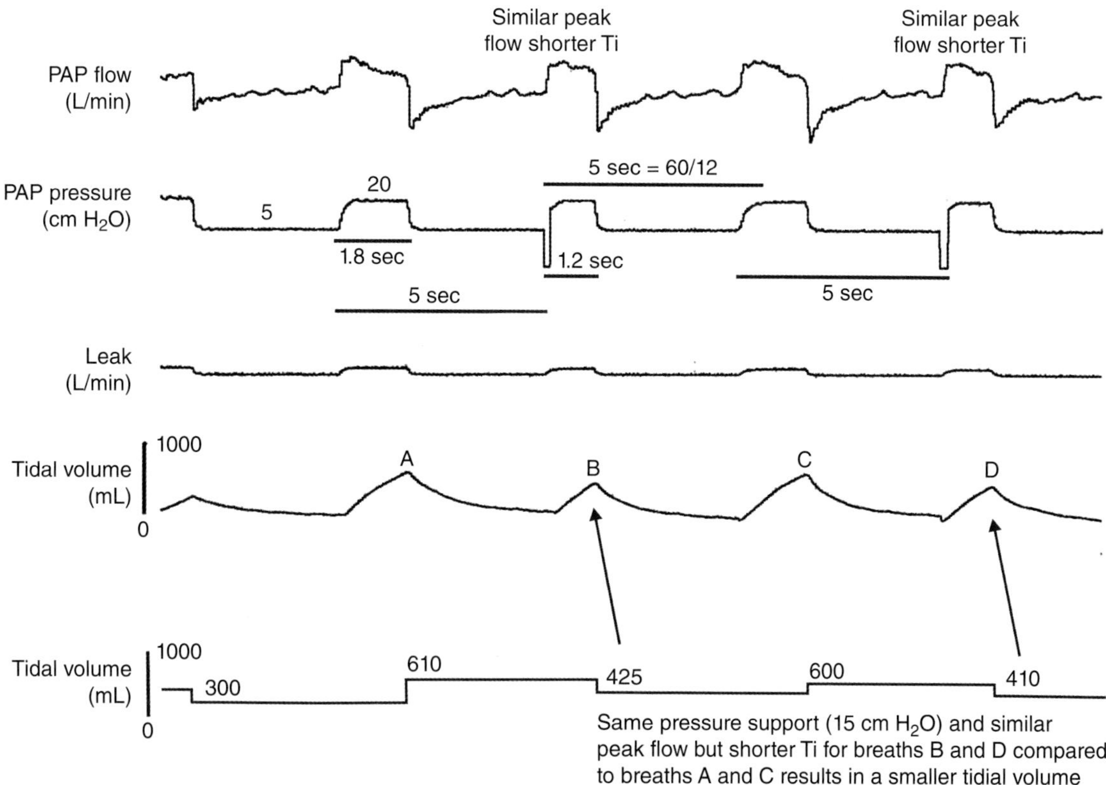

Figure 24–5 **Laboratory bilevel positive airway pressure (BPAP) device tracings (Philips Respironics) showing positive airway pressure (PAP) Flow, PAP device Pressure, Leak, and Tidal Volume.** Although breaths A, B, C, and D have the same pressure support and similar peak flow, the tidal volume is much smaller in breaths B and D due to a shorter inspiratory time (Ti). The delivered tidal volume depends both on value of the pressure support and the Ti.

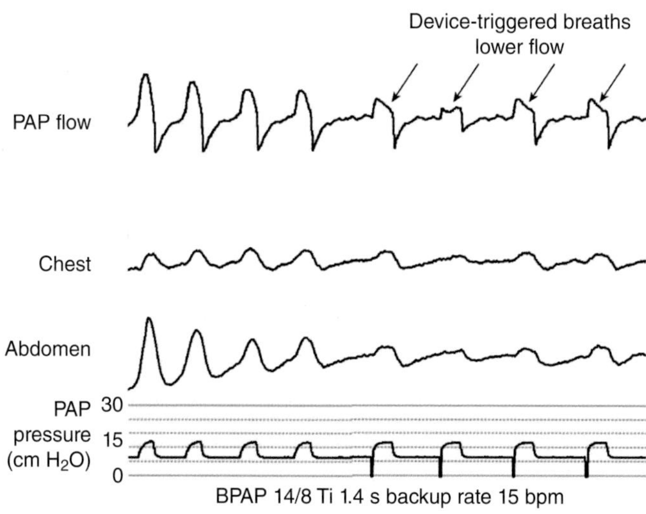

Figure 24–6 **This tracing shows actual flow and positive airway pressure (PAP) tracings from a patient on fixed bilevel positive airway pressure (BPAP, IPAP/EPAP) of 14/8 cm H_2O in the Spontaneous-Timed (ST) Mode.** The same pressure support (6 cm H_2O) during device-triggered breaths delivers lower flow with a different flow waveform. In spontaneous breaths, the driving pressure is PS + negative pressure generated by patient effort. The driving pressure is much lower during device-triggered breaths (in the figure 6 cm H_2O). In spontaneous breaths, upper airway muscles are activated, and this produces a different inspiratory flow profile.

While an adequate Ti is important, an adequate Te is also important and is of special concern for patients requiring a long exhalation time (chronic obstructive pulmonary disease [COPD], asthma). Another parameter expressing the relationship between inspiration and expiration is the ratio of Ti to Te, known as the "I:E" ratio. *By convention, the ratio is written so that the I is 1.* For example, if Ti = 1 second and Ttot = 3 seconds (Te = 2 seconds), the I:E ratio is 1:2. However, if the Ti = 1.5 seconds and Ttot = 6 seconds, then the Te is 4.5 seconds and the raw Ti/Te ratio is 1.5/4.5. Dividing the numerator and denominator by 1.5, the ratio is equal to 1/(4.5/1.5) or (1:3). Thus, the I:E ratio in the 1:X format uses X = [(1-a)/a] where a = (Ti/Ttot). For Ti/Ttot = 1/3 the X = ([2/3]/[1/3] = 2 and the I:E ratio is 1:2. For patients without a need for a long exhalation time, a I:E of 1:2 is adequate. Patients with COPD will benefit from an I:E of 1:3. This can be achieved by using a low Ti/Ttot. For example, for a respiratory rate of 15 breaths/min (Ttot = 4 s), using a Ti/Ttot of 0.25 corresponds to a Ti of 1 second. In this case, the Ti/Te is 1/3 or an I:E ratio of 1:3.

CHOOSING TiMin, TiMax, TRIGGER SENSITIVITY, AND CYCLE SENSITIVITY (ResMed DEVICES)

BPAP devices must determine the appropriate time to transition from EPAP to IPAP (trigger) and IPAP to EPAP (cycle).

Table 24–3 Inspiratory Time (Ti) for Different Respiratory Rates and Fractions of Total Cycle Time (Ti/Ttot)

Ti/Ttot	Backup Rate (bpm)	Device Total Cycle Time (Ttot)	Inspiratory Time (Ti)	I:E Ratio
0.25	10	6	1.5	1:3
	12	5	1.25	
	15	4	1.0	
	20	3	0.75	
0.30	10	6	1.8	1:2.33
	12	5	1.5	
	15	4	1.2	
	20	3	0.9	
0.33	10	6	2.0	1:2
	12	5	1.7	
	15	4	1.3	
	20	3	1.0	
0.40	10	6	2.4	1:1.5
	12	5	2.0	
	15	4	1.6	
	20	3	1.2	
0.5	10	6	3.0	1:1
	12	5	2.5	
	15	4	2.0	
	20	3	1.5	

In this table Ti is the inspiratory time, Ttot (the total cycle time) is equal to the device total cycle time in seconds based on the backup rate (60/backup rate in bpm); Ti = (Ti/Ttot) × Ttot; Ttot=Ti + Te where Te is the expiratory time
I:E ratio, inspiratory to expiratory time ratio; if A = Ti/Ttot, I:E = 1: ([1-A]/A).
For example, if Ti/Ttot = .40, I:E = 1:([1-.4]/.4) = 1:1.5.

The trigger decision is based on detection of inspiratory flow or inspiratory volume (for example, 6 mL percentage of peak flow) and other parameters using proprietary algorithms that must account for variable leak. ResMed devices allow adjustment of the sensitivity of BPAP devices for these transitions.[7] The **trigger sensitivity** determines the timing of the EPAP to IPAP transition (Figure 24–7). The settings are very high, high, medium, low, and very low. Medium is the default. Very high is quickest to trigger (low inspiratory flow triggers the transition) and very low the slowest to trigger. Weak patients might generate low inspiratory flow; therefore, a very high or high trigger sensitivity is appropriate (very little inspiratory flow needed). On the other hand, if the transition from EPAP to IPAP is too early, as when the device triggers a breath before the patient is ready (auto-triggering), a low trigger sensitivity might be useful. The **cycle** transition from IPAP to EPAP is determined by the **cycle sensitivity** (very high, high, medium, low, very low). The default cycle sensitivity is medium. A very high cycle sensitivity means an earlier transition from IPAP to EPAP. For example, for a very high cycle sensitivity when airflow is 50% of peak flow, a medium cycle sensitivity would be at 25% of peak flow, and a very low sensitivity would to 8% of peak flow (actual values may be different). If the patient feels the IPAP to EPAP transition is too early, a change in cycle sensitivity from medium to low (later transition) might improve patient synchrony. For patients with COPD who require a shorter Ti to provide adequate time for exhalation, use of a high cycle sensitivity setting might be appropriate (earlier transition and shorter Ti). The sensitivity terminology can be confusing but remember *high is early, low later transitions*.

If inspiratory flow drops quickly during the IPAP cycle due to a stiff chest wall, high resistance, or inspiratory muscle weakness, the device may cycle to EPAP prematurely (Figure 24–8). These patients would benefit from a longer Ti. On the other hand, patients who require a long exhalation time may benefit from a shorter Ti. For example, if flow continues during the

Table 24–4 Guidelines for TiMin and TiMax

Rate	Device Cycle Time (Ttot)	Ti with I:E = 1:2 (Ti/Ttot = 0.33)	Goal Sufficient Inhalation Time (can tolerate up to I:E = 1:1)		Ti With I:E = 1:3 or Ti/Ttot = 0.25	Goal; Secure Exhalation Time
		Reference (for comparison)	*TiMin (Restrictive)*	*TiMax (normal and Restrictive)*	*Reference (for comparison)*	*TiMax (COPD)*
10	6	2	1.0	2.0	1.5	1.5
12	5	1.7	1.0	2.0	1.25	1.25
15	4	1.3	1.0	2.0	1.0	1.0
20	3	1.0	0.8	1.5	0.75	0.8
25	2.4	0.8	0.7	1.2	0.6	0.8
30	2	0.7	0.6	1.0	0.5	0.7
			or set TiMin to desired Ti	or set TiMax slightly greater than the desired Ti=TiMin		or set TiMax to spontaneous wake Ti, and TiMin ≤ TiMax

In this table Ttot= device cycle time based on the backup rate (60/backup rate in bpm). Default values TiMin = 0.3 sec, TiMax = 2 sec
Alternate method: for restrictive or normal patients set TiMin to desired Ti (or Ti based on Ti/Tot = 0.3 or 0.33) and TiMax = TiMin + 0.5 sec. For COPD, set TiMax = awake Ti or set TiMin to Ti based on Ti/Ttot of 0.25 and TiMax = TiMin + 0.1 sec
For example, for restrictive patients using Ti/Ttot = 0.30 and Rate 15, TiMin = (.30 × 4) = 1.2 sec, TiMax = 1.7 sec.
For example, for COPD patients using Ti/Ttot of .25 and rate 15, TiMin = 1.0 sec and TiMax = 1..0 + .1 sec = 1.1 sec
Ti, inspiratory time; *Ttot*, total cycle time; *I:E*, inspiratory time to expiratory time.
Adapted from references 1 and 7

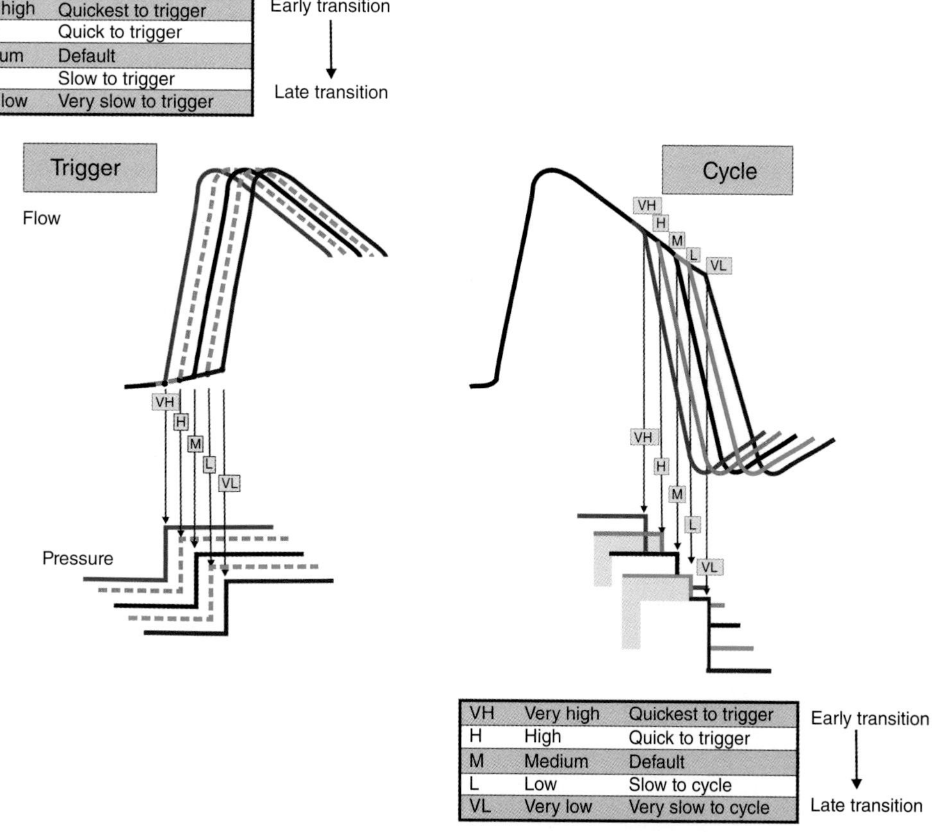

Figure 24–7 **This Figure Illustrates the Effects of Different Trigger and Cycle Sensitivity Settings Using a ResMed Bilevel Positive Airway Pressure (BPAP) Device.** Very high sensitivity in both cases means the earliest transition and very low sensitivity the latest transition. A very high trigger sensitivity means a very small amount of flow triggers an EPAP to IPAP transition. A very high cycle sensitivity means a smaller decrease in flow (compared to peak flow) triggers an IPAP to EPAP transition. When flow falls to 50% of peak flow (very high cycle sensitivity) or 8% of peak flow (very low sensitivity) an IPAP to EPAP transition occurs. The default setting for both cycle and trigger sensitivity is medium. Adapted from reference 7.

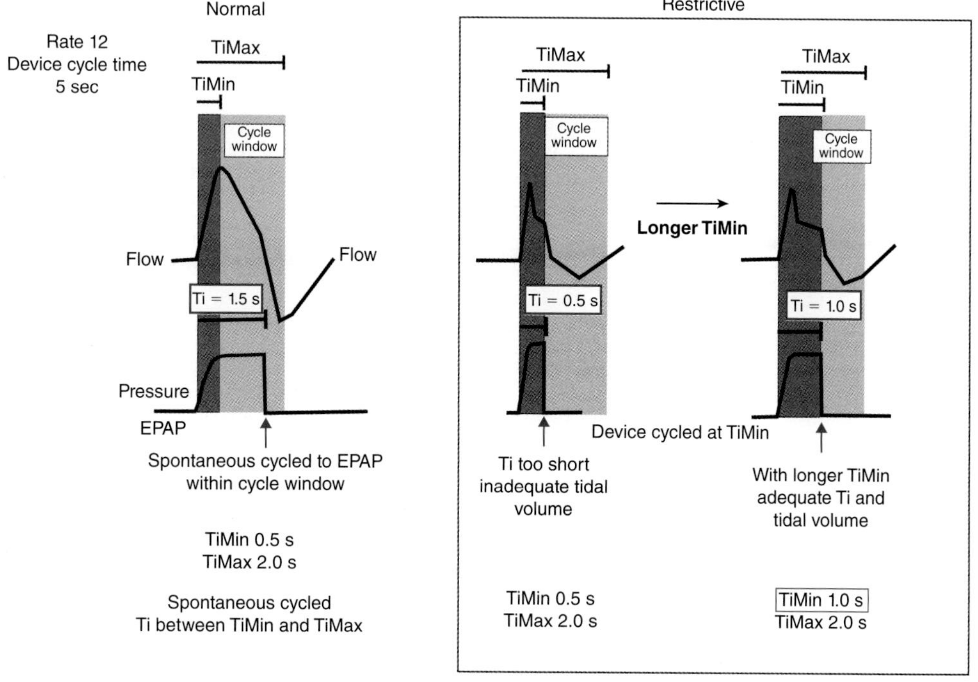

Figure 24–8 This schematic depicts the situation in which the inspiratory positive airway pressure (IPAP)/expiratory positive airway pressure (EPAP) transition is too early due to decreasing inspiratory flow associated with decreased respiratory system compliance or muscle weakness. Increasing the minimum inspiratory time (TiMin) will allow an adequate Ti and tidal volume.

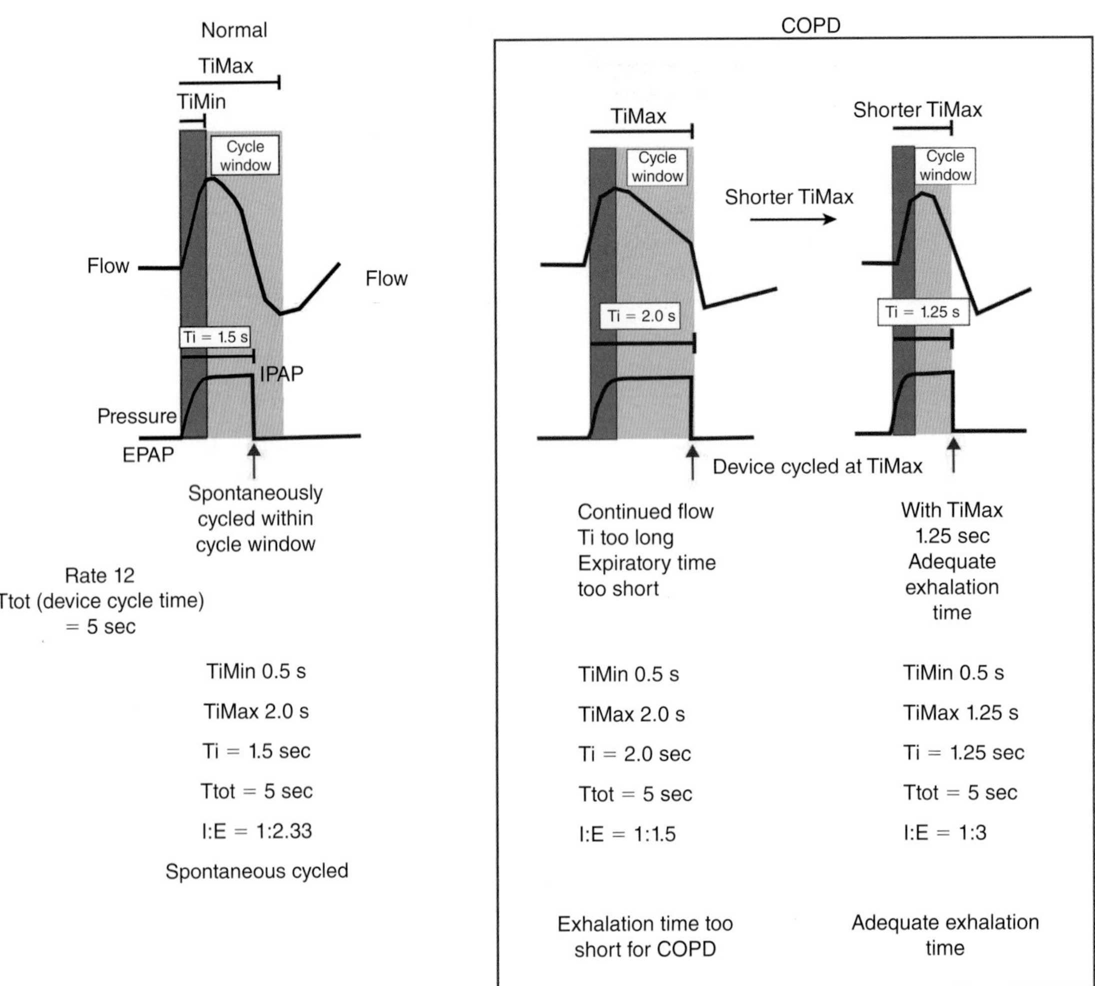

Figure 24–9 This schematic depicts the situation in which the inspiratory positive airway pressure (IPAP) to expiratory positive airway pressure (EPAP) transition is too late. This can occur with an increase in mask leak interpreted by the device as ongoing inspiratory flow. Decreasing the maximum inspiratory time (TiMax) can avoid a Ti that is too long to allow for an adequate expiratory time. *COPD*, chronic obstructive pulmonary disease.

IPAP cycle due to high leak, the Ti may be inappropriately long and will shorten the time for exhalation. Patients with chronic lung disease who require a long time for exhalation may benefit from a shorter Ti (Figure 24–9). As discussed previously, BPAP devices manufactured by ResMed allow setting the TiMin and TiMax durations rather than a fixed Ti for the ST mode. A fixed Ti is specified in the timed or PAC modes. The recommended TiMin and TiMax values depend on the respiratory rate and the type of patient being treated (Table 24–4). The default values are TiMin = 0.3 seconds and TiMax = 2 seconds. As previously discussed, the BPAP device cycles from IPAP to EPAP within the "cycle window" set by TiMin and TiMax based on flow. The default TiMin value of 0.3 seconds is well below the normal spontaneous Ti at even rapid respiratory rates. However, as noted above, patients with a restrictive chest wall disorder, low respiratory system compliance ("stiff chest wall"), or muscle weakness may exhibit an early fall in flow, and the BPAP device may cycle from IPAP to EPAP prematurely (short spontaneous Ti). To ensure an adequate Ti, the TiMin value is increased to the minimum acceptable Ti (depends on respiratory rate). At respiratory rates of 12 to 15 bpm a TiMin of approximately 1.2 to 1.5 seconds is appropriate. As the respiratory rate increases, the TiMin must decrease to allow adequate time for exhalation. The TiMax default value is 2 seconds and prevents excessively long spontaneous Ti value. The TiMax is set to provide sufficient time for exhalation and also depends on the respiratory rate. A TiMax shorter than the default 2-second value is useful to prevent excessive time in the IPAP cycle for patients with COPD who require a long exhalation time. One can use the recommended values in Table 24–4. However, a simple approach for normal or restrictive patients is to set TiMin to the desired Ti value (or slightly shorter) you would use based on an estimated respiratory rate and desired Ti/Ttot and the TiMax 0.3 to 0.5 seconds longer than TiMin). For a respiratory rate of 15 breaths/min (Ttot = 4 sec) and using a Ti/Ttot of 0.3 (I:E ratio 1:2.33), the Ti would be 1.2 seconds (0.3 × 4) and TiMax of 1.7 seconds (or use default of 2.0 seconds). For a patient with COPD, one could choose TiMax = awake Ti or use TiMin based on Ti/Ttot = 0.25 and TiMax = TiMin + 0.1 sec. For eample at a rate of 15 bpm choose TiMin = 1.0 seconds and TiMax = 1.1 seconds.

BACKUP RATE (BPAP-ST)

For PR and ResMed devices, the backup rate for the BPAP-ST mode is usually set 1 to 2 breaths below the patient's spontaneous breath rate (unless the rate is low). Usually, a rate of 10 breaths/min or higher is used. As will be discussed later in this chapter's section on titration, there are times the backup rate may be set higher than the spontaneous rate if an ideal tidal volume cannot be provided so that an adequate minute ventilation can be provided (minute ventilation [L/min] = respiratory rate [breaths/min] × tidal volume [in liters]). The parameters that must be specified for the BPAP-ST mode and BPAP-PC (PAC) mode are displayed in Table 24–5. The rise time is set for patient comfort. Usually longer for neuromuscular disease (NMD) and shorter for COPD.

ADAPTIVE SERVOVENTILATION (ASV)

ASV was developed for treatment of Cheyne-Stokes breathing (CSB) but can be used for any patient with ventilatory instability and/or hypocapnic CSA.[5,6] Recall that hypocapnic

Table 24–5 Parameters to Specify for BPAP-ST and BPAP in the PC or PAC Modes

	ST	PC and PAC
Parameters	• IPAP, EPAP • Backup rate • Ti (PR), TiMin and TiMax (ResMed) • Rise time • Trigger and cycle sensitivity (ResMed)	• IPAP, EPAP • Backup rate • Ti (PR) • Ti (ResMed) • Rise Time • Trigger and Cycle Sensitivity (ResMed)

PR, Philips Respironics; *Ti*, inspiratory time; *PC*, pressure control; *PAC*, pressure assist control; *IPAP*, inspiratory positive airway pressure; *EPAP*, expiratory positive airway pressure *BPAP*, bilevel positive airway pressure, *ST*, spontaneous timed.

CSA occurs when the $PaCO_2$ during sleep falls below the apneic threshold. This often occurs with a return to sleep after a period of increased ventilation.[8] This concept is discussed in more detail in Chapter 30. In ASV devices, the PS adapts to stabilize breathing, providing a higher PS when peak flow or minute ventilation are decreased below the target and a lower PS when peak flow or minute ventilation are increased above the target (Figure 24–10). ASV devices have a backup rate to address central apnea, but the goal is to stabilize the pattern of breathing so that device-triggered breaths are not needed. By preventing excessive ventilation and hypocapnia, central apnea is eliminated. Examples of disorders benefiting from ASV include CSA with CSB, primary CSA, and patients with complex sleep apnea (treatment-emergent CSA). It can also be used for patients with narcotic-induced CSA,[6,8] but a sufficient minimum PS must be used to deal with hypopnea or hypoventilation (if present). Two brands of ASV devices that are being used in the United States. They work differently, and the setups are slightly different (Tables 24–6 and 24–7).[4,5] The PR ASV device is called the DreamStation BiPAP AutoSV and automatically adjusts the EPAP between the EPAPmin and EPAPmax to eliminate upper airway obstruction (APAP algorithm). The APAP algorithm responds to apnea, hypopnea, airflow limitation, and airway vibration. An apnea is defined by a ≥ 80% reduction in flow and a hypopnea by a ≥ 40% reduction in flow. The PS is adjusted by the device between the minimum and maximum PS settings (between PSmin and PSmax) to stabilize ventilation by delivering a target **peak inspiratory flow** rate based on the average peak flow of preceding breaths determined over a 4 minute moving time window. The target is ≈ 90-95% of the average peak flow. If respiratory events are occurring, this can change the PS algorithm. The PS is adjusted within each breath based on the early flow rate to reach the peak flow target. A fixed backup rate (4 to 30 breaths/min) can be specified and the Ti can be set based on

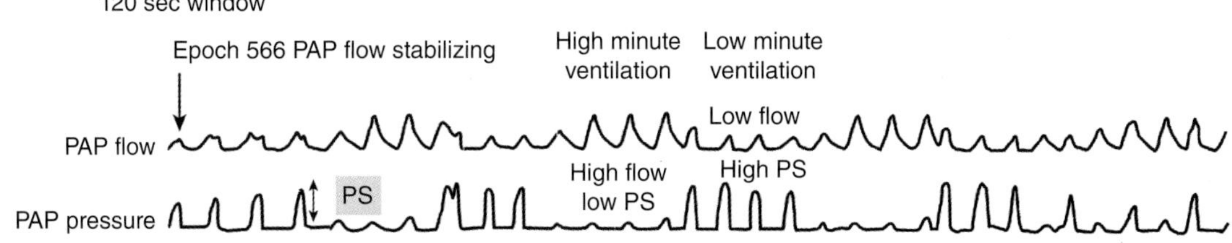

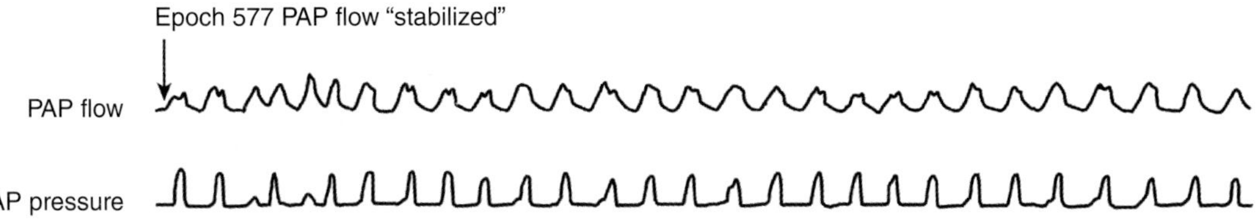

Figure 24–10 A tracing positive airway pressure (PAP) flow and pressure for a patient being treated with a ResMed adaptive servoventilation device. The pressure support (PS) varies to stabilize breathing (minute ventilation), delivering higher PS when flow (minute ventilation) is low (below target) and lower PS when flow (minute ventilation) is high (above target). Over time, the ventilation stabilized. PAP pressure is the PAP device delivered presssure.

Table 24–6 Adaptive Servoventilation Characteristics

	ResMed AirCurve ASV	Philips Respironics DreamSation BiPAP AutoSV
Target	90% of previous average minute ventilation (MV) over a weighted 3 minute moving time window, most recent MV given greater weight	90-95% average peak flow over a 4 minute moving time window Target higher if respiratory events
EPAP	• **ASV mode** EPAP set manually (4-15 cm H_2O) • **ASVAuto mode** EPAP automatically adjusted between EPAPmin and EPAPmax (EPAP range 4-15 cm H_2O) EPAPmax ≥ EPAPmin Responds to apnea, airflow limitation, snoring	• EPAP automatically adjusted between EPAPmin and EPAPmax to prevent upper airway obstruction • Responds to apnea, hypopnea, airflow limitation, snoring (EPAP will also increase if flow does not respond to higher PS)
PS	• PS varies between PSmin and PSmax to meet MV target • Pmax 25 cm H_2O (not adjustable) • PSmin 0 to 6 cm H_2O • PSmax 5 - 20 cm H_2O (PSmax constrained by EPAP (EPAPmin), PSmin, and Pmax)	• PS varies between PSmin and PSmax to meet peak flow target • Pmax up to 30 cm H_2O (usually 25 or 30 cm H_2O) • PSmin range 0 to (Pmax - EPAPmax), ≤ PSmax • PSmax range PSmin to (Pmax-EPAPmin), ≥ PSmin
Backup rate	Based on recent patient rate (default 15 bpm), Ti set automatically, backup rate cannot be set manually	• Breaths/min: off, auto, 4-30 bpm • **Manual rate:** 4 to 30 bpm, set Ti = 1.5 sec or based on rate • **Auto rate:** Fixed rate option 2: 4–30 fixed rate (if fixed rate must specify Ti) If fixed rate Ti = 1 .5 seconds recommended, lower higher rates
Typical settings	**ASV mode:** • EPAP = 5 cm H_2O **ASVAuto mode:** • EPAPmin = 5 cm H_2O • EPAPmax = 10 cm H_2O • PSmin = 3 cm H_2O • PSmax 15 to 20 cmH_2O	• EPAPmin = 4 cm H_2O If previous CPAP >10 cm H_2O use EPAPmin = 6 - 8 cm H_2O or patient comfort • EPAPmax =15 cm H_2O • PSmin = 0 or higher if hypopnea persists • PSmax = 20 cm H_2O (assumes Pmax -EPAPmin ≥ 20 cmH_2O) • Rate: Auto

BiPAP, bilevel positive airway pressure; *EPAP*, expiratory positive airway pressure; *IPAP,* inspiratory positive airway pressure; *PS*, pressure support; *ASV*, adaptive servo-ventilation; *Ti,* inspiratory time, *MV*, minute ventilation.

Adapted from Javaheri S, Brown LK, Randerath WJ. Positive airway pressure therapy with adaptive servoventilation: part 1: operational algorithms. *Chest.* 2014;146(2):514-523.

Table 24–7 Adaptive Servoventilation Setting Range and Defaults

DreamStation BiPAP AutoSV	Range	Typical settings
Pmax (cm H_2O)	Up to 30	25 or 30
PS (cm H_2O)	PSmin 0–20 Constrained by EPAP and Pmax (0 to [Pmax-EPAPmax]) PSmax 0–20 Constrained by EPAP and Pmax (PSmin to Pmax – EPAPmin)	PSmin = 0 PSmax = 20 Set PSmin >4 if many residual hypopneas
EPAPmin (cm H_2O)	4 to lesser of 20 or Pmax	4 (6–8, if known CPAP ≥10)
EPAPmax (cm H_2O)	EPAPmin to lesser of 20 or Pmax	15
Rate and inspiratory time (Ti) (bpm, sec)	Rate: off, auto, 4–30 Ti Range 0.5–3.0 sec Auto-rate (Ti automatic)	Rate: Auto If rate specified use, Ti = 1.5 sec or based on rate
Rise time (can be specified if Flex = none and PSmax ≠ 0)	1–6 (100–600 msec)	2 to 3 or patient comfort

Table 24-7 Adaptive Servoventilation Setting Range and Defaults—cont'd

AirCurve 10 ASV	Range	Typical settings
Pmax (cm H_2O)***	Up to 25 cm H_20	25 cm H_20
PSmin (cm H_2O)	0–6	3
PSmax (cm H_2O)	5–20 (constrained by EPAP and Pmax)	15 or 20
EPAP manual* (cm H_2O)	4–15	5, adjusted manually
EPAPmin** (cm H_2O)	4–15	4
EPAPmax** (cm H_2O)	4–15	15
Rise time, Rate (bpm), Ti (sec)	Automatic	15 per minute (default)

Pressures in cm H_2O, time in seconds
P, pressure; *PS*, pressure support; *EPAP*, expiratory positive airway pressure; *Ti*, inspiratory time.
*ASV mode
** ASVauto mode
***cannot be adjusted

the respiratory rate. An auto option (auto-rate) can be used. In the auto-rate mode, both the backup rate and Ti are automatically determined. *The auto rate option is recommended for most patients.* The rate and Ti are determined by a proprietary algorithm based on the preceding average respiratory rate (12 breath window) and the time since the last breath was delivered. The PSmin and PSmax settings are constrained by the EPAP settings and the maximum pressure setting (Pmax, usually 25 or 30 cm H_2O). For example, if EPAPmin is 5 cm H_2O and Pmax is 25 cm H_2O, the highest allowed value of PSmax is 20 cm H_2O. That is, EPAPmin + PSmax = Pmax. PSmin can vary between 0 and (Pmax – EPAPmax, assuming PSmin ≤ PSmax). For example if the EPAPmax = 15 cmH_2O and Pmax 25 cm H_2O, the upper limit of PSmin would be 10 cm H_2O (PSmin ≤ PSmax). The rise time can also be adjusted (setting 1–6, meaning approximately 100–600 milliseconds) based on comfort. If the flex option is is enabled the rise time cannot be manually set. As noted patients with restrictive disorders usually benefit from a longer rise time, and those with COPD usually benefit from a shorter rise time. The flex option can be selected allowing an early expiratory drop in pressure (similar to Biflex - see chapter 23). There is a ramp option where EPAP increases in a linear manner with PS = 0 over the ramp time.

The AirCurve 10 ASV (formerly VPAP Adapt SV) by ResMed delivers PS and a backup rate to achieve a target **minute ventilation** (MV), computed as an average MV over a 3 minute moving time window (target ≈ 90% of weighted average minute ventilation). In the weighted average the, most recent breaths contribute the most to the average. The device automatically adjusts the backup rate and Ti. In the **ASV mode,** the EPAP must be specified, but in **ASVAuto** mode, EPAP varies automatically between EPAPmin and EPAPmax. The algorithm that adjusts the EPAP responds to apnea, airflow limitation, and airway vibration (but not hypopnea). The algorithm adjusting the Ti and backup rate in the ResMed ASV device is proprietary but has a baseline default of 15 breaths/min. However, the Ti at any time depends on the average Te of preceding breaths, the time since the last breath, and the recent respiratory rate.

When using ASV for treatment, it is important to consider the possibility of closed airway central apneas.[9] During central apnea, the upper airway may close. For example, during a mixed apnea, the airway closes during the central portion. If a closed airway central apnea occurs, the device-triggered PS will not effectively deliver flow (or tidal volume). In this case, higher EPAP is needed (Figure 24–11). In the past, this depended on the sleep technologist recognizing that closed airway central apnea was occurring and increasing the EPAP. With automatic adjustment of EPAP, this may be less of an issue. The exact algorithms for EPAP adjustment are proprietary, and the monitored parameters depend on the specific device. However, EPAP may increase in the absence of closed airway apnea if increases in PS are not effective in increasing flow/tidal volume (narrowed but not closed upper airway) (Figures 24–12 and 24–13). As noted, the PR autoEPAP algorithm responds to apnea, hypopnea, snoring, airway vibration (snoring), and airflow limitation (inspiratory flattening). The ResMed autoEPAP algorithms respond to apnea, airway vibration, and airflow limitation. Hypopneas are addressed by increasing PS.

The default PSmin is 0 cm H_2O in PR ASV devices and 3 cm H_2O for the ResMed ASV devices. However, current ResMed ASV devices do allow a PSmin of 0 cm H_2O. For patients with ventilatory instability due to high loop gain, delivering CPAP (PSmin = 0 cm H_2O) during periods of stable ventilation is desired to avoid overshoots in ventilation following arousals. However, a PSmin >0 cm H_2O is desired in several situations. A pressure-intolerant patient may benefit from EPAP of 10 cm H_2O and PSmin of 4 cm H_2O (equivalent to BPAP 14/10) versus EPAP of 12 cm H_2O with a PSmin of 0 cm H_2O. ASV devices were not specifically designed for patients with nocturnal hypoventilation. However, some patients with complex sleep apnea associated with opioid use have some degree of hypoventilation as well as instability in both breathing rate and tidal volume (ataxic breathing). A higher PSmin (≥6 to 8 cm H_2O) may be needed if the arterial oxygen saturation (SaO_2) remains low but breathing is regular (e.g., in patients with hypoventilation) or if persistent hypopneas are noted.[5,10] An occasional patient with a very low spontaneous respiratory rate may be better treated with ASV using a fixed backup rate (fixed rate option available on PR ASV devices). One study comparing BPAP-ST and ASV for treatment of opioid-related CSA found ASV to be more successful based on a single night of PSG (BPAP-ST or ASV, in random order).[11] It is important to

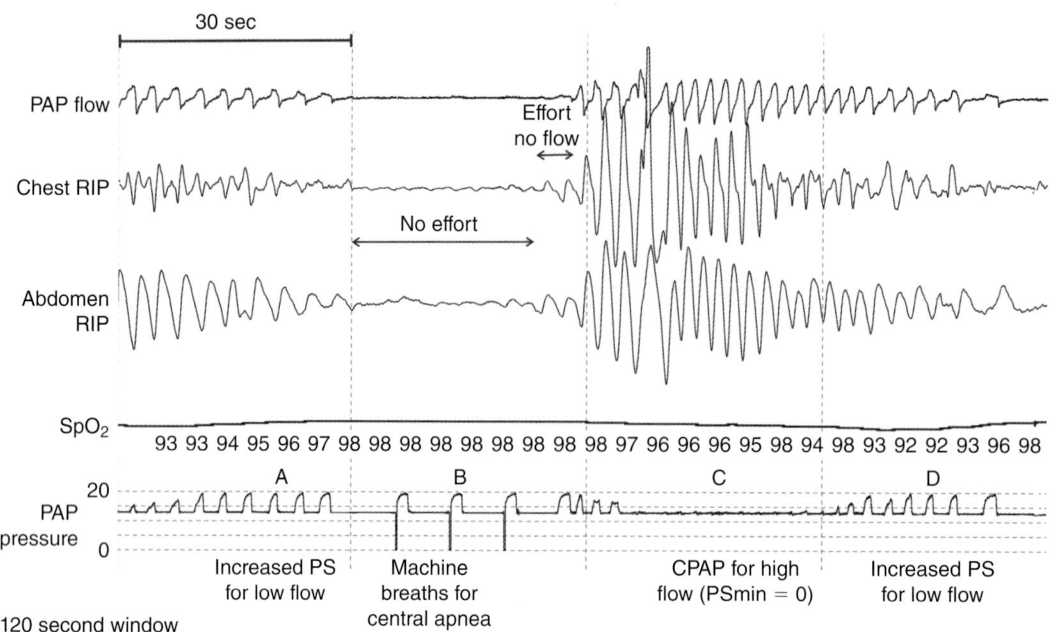

Figure 24–11 A tracing of a patient being treated with adaptive servoventilation (Philips Respironics device with **fixed** expiratory positive airway pressure [EPAP]) and PSmin = 0 cm H_2O. (A) Pressure support increases for low flow (B) A mixed apnea with a long central portion is shown. During the central apnea portion device-triggered pressure pulses (pressure support) do not produce airflow (closed airway central apnea). At the end of the apnea there is an obstructive portion (respiratory effort but no airflow). An increase in EPAP is needed.(C) For high flow continuous positive airway pressure (CPAP) is provided (PSmin = 0). (D) Increased pressure support for low flow.

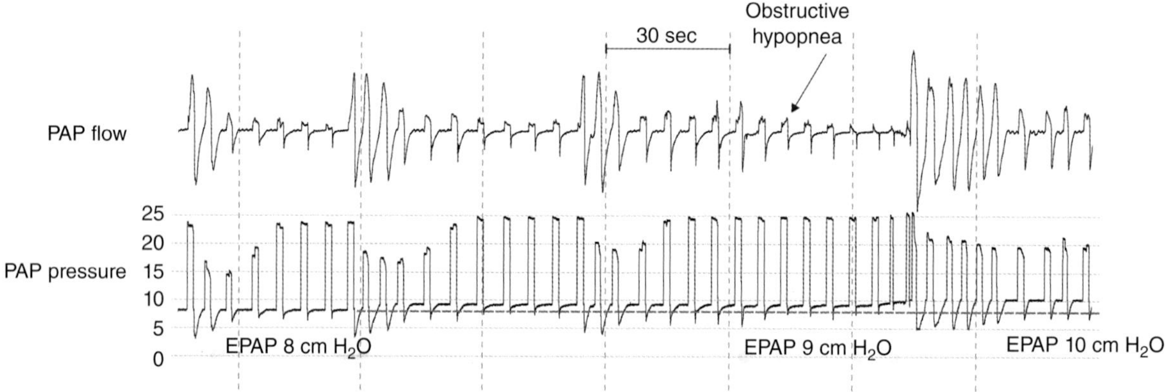

Figure 24–12 A tracing of a patient being treated with Philips Respironics (PR) adaptive servoventilation (ASV) device. High pressure support over several respiratory events does not produce adequate flow. A gradual increase in expiratory positive airway pressure (EPAP) finally restores adequate flow. The EPAP algorithm responds to apnea, hypopnea, airflow limitation, and airflow vibration (snoring).

note that, for ASV devices to work well, accurate estimates of flow and ventilation are needed. *High and variable leak may reduce the efficacy of ASV device titration algorithms.* For PR ASV devices a rise time setting is only available if Biflex is set to None. The rise time setting are integers 1 to 6. For ResMed ASV device a rise time of 100-600 msec can be set. Of note both PR and ResMed ASV devices have optional alarms and depending on the device, turning the device off requires pressing the off button for several seconds.

Of note, BPAP-ST with a fixed PS can also be used to treat hypocapnic CSA. However, this usually requires a fairly high PS to deliver an adequate tidal volume during device-triggered breaths. For example, in a given patient, a BPAP (IPAP/EPAP) of 12/8 cm H_2O maintains an open airway and adequate tidal volume on spontaneous breaths. However, for device-triggered breaths, 18/8 cm H_2O is needed. As IPAP and EPAP are fixed, the device must deliver 18/8 cm H_2O on all breaths to deliver effective flow on device-triggered breaths. In Figure 24–6, spontaneously triggered breaths at a given PS (BPAP setting) result in much higher flow than during device-triggered breaths. ASV devices treat hypocapnic CSA with a higher percentage of *patient-triggered* breaths and usually much lower average pressure. On the other hand, some patients may be more effectively treated with BPAP-ST than ASV, especially if a high PS is needed or there is a significant component of hypoventilation. In Figure 24–14, tracings from

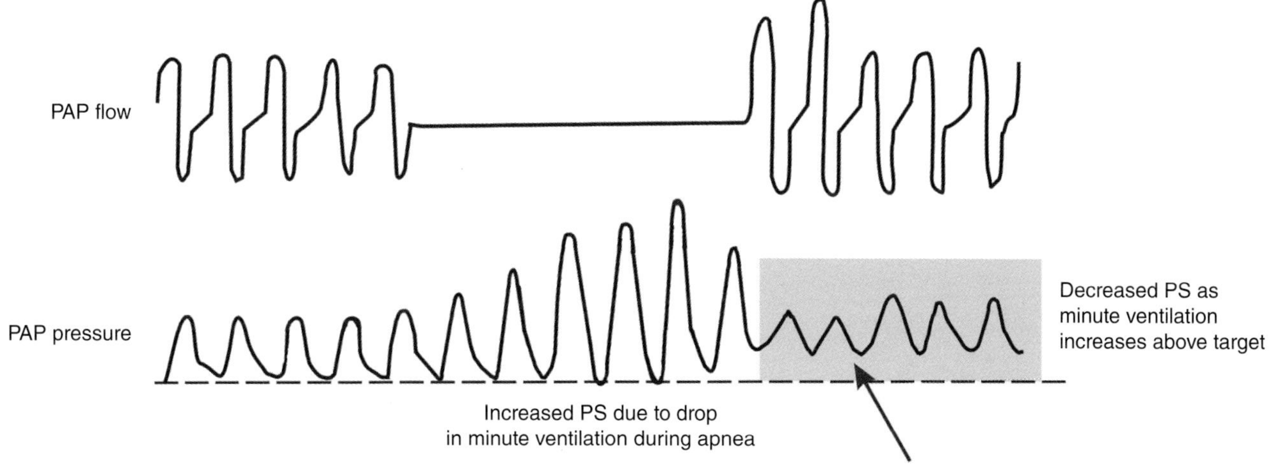

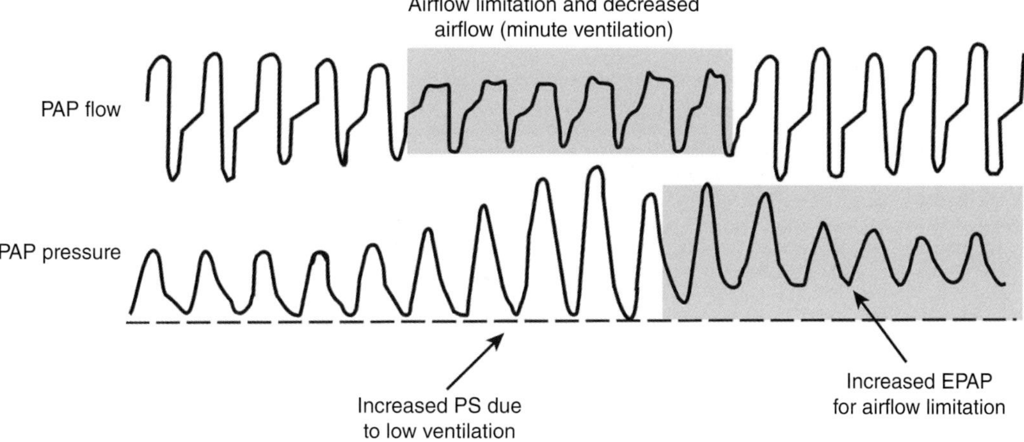

Figure 24–13 A schematic tracing illustrating the response of a ResMed adaptive servoventilation (ASV) device to obstructive apnea (*top*) and obstructive hypopnea (*bottom*). For the obstructive apnea, expiratory positive airway pressure (EPAP) increases. For the obstructive hypopnea, the EPAP increases due to airflow limitation. Pressure support (PS) increases for reduced ventilation rather than a hypopnea itself. ResMed ASV devices use an EPAP algorithm responding to airflow limitation, apnea, and airflow vibration (snoring), but not hypopnea.

a patient with a high body mass index (BMI) and central apnea due to methadone are displayed. This patient required high EPAP, high PS, and a high backup rate for adequate control of respiratory events. Table 24–7 lists the settings for ASV, including ranges and typical settings.

VOLUME ASSURED PRESSURE SUPPORT

The PS required for an adequate tidal volume may vary in a patient over time secondary to disease progression (changes in muscle strength and system compliance). Often, there is a need to start a patient on NIV based on empiric settings before a PSG titration is possible (or practical). To meet this challenge, VAPS devices were developed to automatically assure an adequate PS (Figure 24–15A).[12-21] At the time of this writing, the two VAPS technologies being used in the USA (Tables 24–8 and 24–9) are Average Volume-Assured PS (AVAPS) by PR and Intelligent Volume-Assured PS (iVAPS) by ResMed. The corresponding devices are DreamStation AVAPS and AirCurve 10 ST-A. These are RADs (respiratory assist devices), in contrast to home mechnical ventilators (HMVs) made by the same companies that can also operate in the VAPS mode (Trilogy, Trilogy-Evo for PR, Astral for ResMed). The DreamStation AVAPS and AirCurve 10 ST-A can be used in the S, ST, PC (PAC), or T modes. As noted previously Philips Resironics will no longer sell PAP devices in the USA. The HMVs have an automatic EPAP functionality (EPAPmin and EPAPmax must be specified) but the RAD devices sold in the US do not have an autoEPAP option. Therefore an EPAP must be specified for both AVAPS and iVAPs RAD devices.

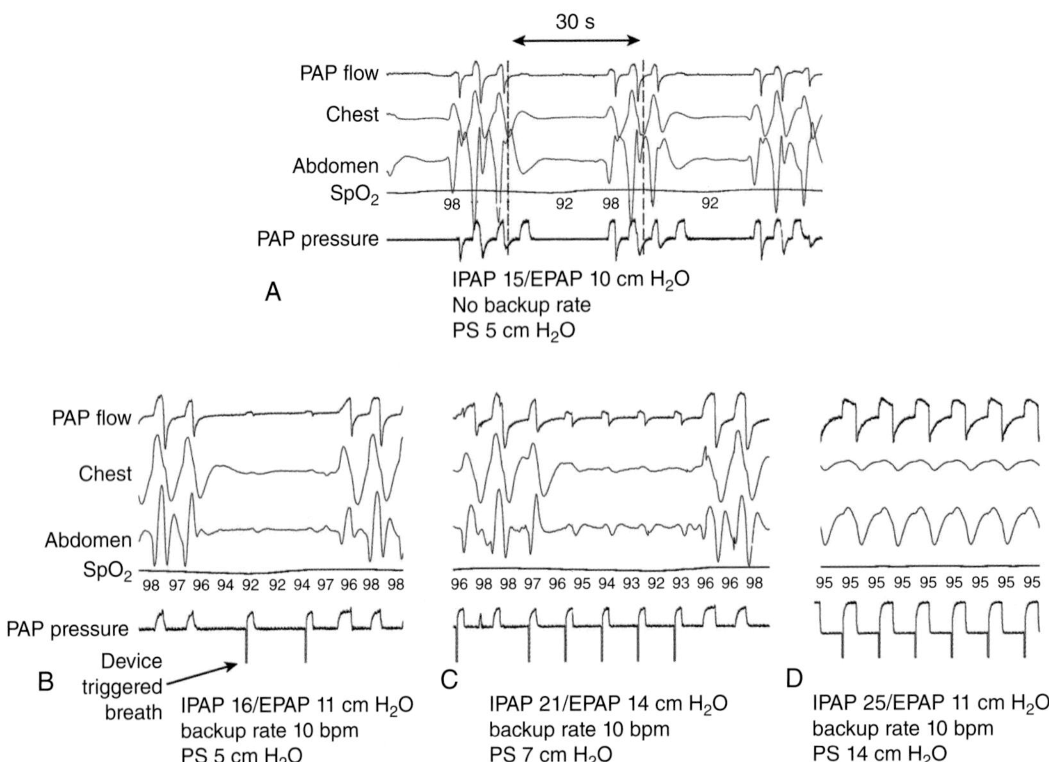

Figure 24–14 Several tracings in a patient with Central Sleep Apnea and Hypoventilation due to Methadone. (A) Central apneas are noted on bilevel positive airway pressure (BPAP) in the spontaneous (S) mode. (B) In the BPAP spontaneous-timed (ST) mode, device-triggered breaths do not deliver airflow (closed airway central apnea). The small deflections at A are due to slight movement due to the pressure pulses and are not patient effort. (C) Higher EPAP opened the upper airway and higher pressure support improved flow, but a hypopnea is still present. (D) Higher pressure support delivered adequate flow. Using a higher PS maintained an open airway, although the EPAP is the same as associated with a closed airway at B. A lower EPAP was used to avoid use of an inspiratory positive airway pressure (IPAP) greater than 25 cm H_2O. A pressure of 25 cm H_2O is the maximum pressure available on basic BPAP-ST devices (VAPS not available). Note that because the spontaneous respiratory rate was low (about 8 bpm), a backup rate of 10 breaths/min resulted in all device triggered breaths. However, the patient tolerated this treatment very well.

AVAPS is usually used in the ST or PC mode. In the ST mode a Ti is specified but only applies to device triggered breaths. In the PC mode, a Ti must also be specified but applies to both spontaneous and device-triggered breaths. In both the ST and PC modes a backup rate is specified for device triggered breaths (usually 1 or 2 breaths lower than the spontaneous rate). IPAPmin and IPAPmax are specified along with an EPAP level. Therefore the PSmin is IPAPmin-EPAP and PSmax is IPAPmax-EPAP. If Pmax is the maximum pressure setting (usually 30 cm H_2O), the possible IPAPmax values can range from EPAP to Pmax and the IPAPmin range from EPAP to IPAPmax. The range of pressure support is 0 to (Pmax-EPAP).

The ResMed iVAPS devices are usually used in the iVAPS mode, although S, ST, T, and PAC modes are options. In the iVAPS mode the intelligent backup rate (iBR) is provided by default. In the IVAPs/iBR mode a target backup rate is specified (as the patients's actual rate) (Figure 24–15B). The Ti cycle time window for both spontaneous and device triggered breaths is determined by specifying TiMin and TiMax. In the PAC mode a Ti and target backup rate are specified for all breaths (iBR not available). In the iVAPS mode Pmax is automatically set at 30 cm H_2O. PSmin and PSmax must be specified. The PSmax and PSmin values are constrained by the Pmax=30 cm H_2O and EPAP. That is PSmin varies from 0 to PSmax, and the PSmax varies from 0 to Pmax-EPAP.

AVAPS devices vary PS to reach a tidal volume target (usually 8 mL/kg of ideal body weight [IBW]). A chart of height, IBW, and tidal volume at 8 mL/kg IBW is supplied in Table 24–10. ResMed devices functioning in the iVAPS mode vary both PS and the respiratory rate (when iBR is active) to reach a target alveolar ventilation. The alveolar ventilation is calculated as the minute ventilation minus the dead space ventilation. The anatomic dead space (V_D) is estimated based on the patient's height (which must be specified), and the dead space ventilation is equal to $V_D \times$ respiratory rate. At setup the respiratory rate is the target rate. One enters the patient height and target respiratory rate (usually 15 breaths/min), then scrolls through alveolar ventilation target values—each showing the associated **computed** minute ventilation, tidal volume, and tidal volume as mL/Kg IBW (Figure 24–16). These are calculated based on the estimated dead space (based on height) and the target respiratory rate. A value of alveolar ventilation is chosen as the target based on the associated desired tidal volume (absolute value or as mL/kg of IBW). A common tidal volume target is 8 mL/Kg of IBW (based on

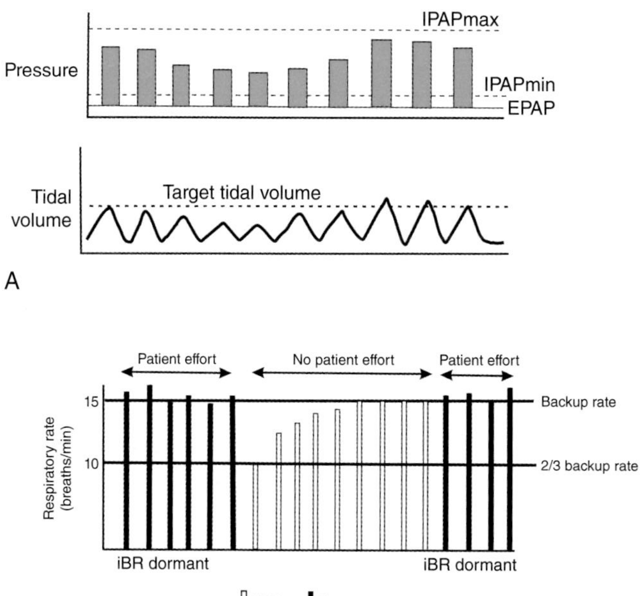

Figure 24–15 The top tracing is a schematic illustrating the change in pressure support to deliver the target tidal volume in an average Volume-Assured Pressure Support (AVAPS) device (PR). The bottom tracing illustrates the intelligent backup rate (iBR) function in the intelligent volume-assured pressure support (iVAPS) mode (ResMed). When no spontaneous breath occurs within a time window based on 2/3 of the backup rate, device-triggered breaths are delivered starting at a rate of *two-thirds the target rate*. The respiratory rate increases with subsequent breaths until either the target backup rate is reached or spontaneous breathing resumes. If a spontaneous breath with a rate > 2/3 the target rate occurs, iBR becomes dormant. This approach ensures an adequate respiratory rate but allows resumption of spontaneous breathing, if possible. When the iBR is active, both PS and rate vary to deliver the target alveolar ventilation. The iBR does not exceed the target backup rate. Once the target backup rate is reached the PS increases to address alveolar ventilation below target.

height). A PS range must be specified on iVAPS devices. Typically, PSmin = 4 and PSmax = 20 or up to (Pmax − EPAP) with Pmax = 30 cm H_2O.

The backup rates on the PR and ResMed VAPS devices are different as noted above. In the PR AVAPS device, the backup rate is fixed and usually set one or two breaths below the spontaneous breathing rate. The Ti is chosen as previously discussed.

In the iVAPS device, the target backup should be the patient's acutal breathing rate (and not less than 15 bpm). When the iBR is active it varies between 2/3 the target rate and the target rate[3,7]. When no patient effort is noted based on a time window set at two-thirds of the target respiratory rate, the iBR begins to deliver breaths at a rate that is **two-thirds of the set backup rate** (Figure 24–15B). This rate progressively increases up to the set target backup rate to deliver adequate alveolar ventilation. The speed with which the iBR increases toward the set target backup rate following apnea depends on the ventilation (faster if ventilation is low), but usually this occurs within the duration of 4 to 5 breaths. The PS also increases when the iBR is active to reach the target alveolar ventilation. It is important to note that, while the alveolar ventilation target is chosen with a target tidal volume/Kg IBW in mind, the **PS responds to target alveolar ventilation and not a target tidal volume.** The iBR is dormant if the spontaneous patient respiratory rate is above two-thirds the target respiratory rate and does not exceed the target respiratory rate. For example with a target rate of 15 bpm, 2/3 of 15 is 10 bpm (or a device cycle time of 6 seconds). If **no** spontaneous breath is noted within 6 seconds of the last breath iBR is activated and increases toward 15 bpm. Suppose iBR reaches 13 bpm but a spontaneous breath occurs 4.3 seconds after the last breath (60/4.3 = 14 bpm) then iBR becomes dormant. Figure 24–17 illustrates that both the PS and the iBR increase to meet the alveolar ventilation goal until a spontaneous breath in the time window set by two-thirds the target rate to the target rate occurs. As noted, the iBR can vary from 2/3 the target rate to the target rate (but no higher). The TiMin, TiMax, and rise time are also set. Typical values would be TiMin = 1 to 1.5 seconds, TiMax = 2 seconds, and rise time = 300 milliseconds. At a backup rate of 15 breaths/min (cycle time 4 seconds), the Ti for a Ti/Ttot of 0.3 is 1.2 seconds and for a Ti/Ttot of 0.4 is 1.6 seconds. The rise time on the PR AVAPS devices can be specified as 1 to 6 (approximately 100 to 600 msec) and for the ResMed iVAPS devices (150, 200 to 600 msec in 50 msec increments).

In setting the respiratory rate, it is important to recall that, if the tidal volume increases with higher PS, the spontaneous respiratory rate may decrease. In patients with decreased respiratory-system compliance, the combination of a lower tidal volume and higher respiratory rate is sometimes used to avoid excessive pressure, keeping in mind that this pattern increases dead space ventilation. In patients with neuromuscular weakness, a more aggressive backup rate may be needed to provide muscle rest. *A greater percentage of device-triggered breaths will provide greater respiratory muscle rest (reducing muscle effort needed to trigger breaths)*. One treatment issue with AVAPS devices in the ST mode is that the specified Ti applies only to device-triggered breaths. One has no control over the Ti of spontaneous breaths. In this situation, use of the PC mode allows setting the Ti for all breaths. In ResMed devices a TiMin can be set for all breaths. ResMed iVAPS devices also allow setting trigger and cycle sensitivity. As discussed previously, a high or very high trigger sensitivity is useful in patients with muscle weakness. The TiMin should also be set to provide an adequate Ti. For patients with COPD, a high cycle sensitivity or a shorter TiMax may prevent an excessively long Ti and allow sufficient time for exhalation. A comparison summary of the VAPS settings for AVAPS and iVAPS is provided in Table 24–11.

VAPS, Automatic EPAP, Home Mechanical Ventilators

AVAPS and iVAPS are available for HMVs (Trilogy or Trilogy Evo by PR, Astral by ResMed) (Tables 24–12 and 24–13). The Trilogy is under recall but will be discussed as some patients are using the device. In addition Philips Respironics has decided not to continue sale of home ventilators is the US. However, many patients will continue to use these for several years. Routine RAD devices (PR and ResMed) sold in the US do not have an autoEPAP capability. HMV devices have an autoEPAP function (AE option, but the physician must specify EPAP limits).[20,21] The AE function is especially useful when treatment must be started without titration. The AE function may not work well when there is high mask leak. The PR ventilators use a forced oscillation technique to assess upper airway narrowing.[3] In AVAPS-AE (AE for autoEPAP) the mode is ST (specify respiratory rate and Ti), or there is an option to choose an auto-rate (breathing rate and Ti chosen

Table 24–8 Average Volume Assured Pressure Support (AVAPS) (Philips Respironics)

Parameter	Typical Settings (AVAPS on)
Target tidal volume	6-8 mL/kg IBW
Pmax (cm H_2O)	25 or 30 (use 30 if high PS needed)
EPAP (cm H_2O)	Manual 4–15 cm H_2O, to prevent obstructive apnea
IPAPmin (cm H_2O)	EPAP + 4 to 6 cm H_2O (PSmin = IPAPmin - EPAP)
IPAPmax (cm H_2O)	25 (30) cm H_2O (PSmin = IPAPmin - EPAP)
Backup Rate (bpm)	One or two breaths below spontaneous or at least 8 to 10 bpm
AVAPS	On
Mode:	ST, PC (S, T available, rarely used)
Inspiratory time (Ti) (sec)	Based on backup rate and Ti/Ttot, usually Ti = 1.2–1.5 seconds
Rise time	(1–6 by integers, ≈ 100–600 msec) adjust for comfort
Disease Specific Considerations	• Target tidal volume: 10 mL/kg IBW in OHS, If high intensity NIV for COPD may need 8–10 mL/kg IBW to reach PCO_2 goal • EPAP 4 cm H_2O In NMD 4–6 cm H_2O, COPD 6–8 cm H_2O, OHS, consider BMI and previous CPAP treatment • Adjust IPAPmin for long term treatment so it is closer to average IPAP • Ti based on Ti/Ttot and rate In NMD Ti/Tot 0.3 to 0.4, consider PC mode, COPD Ti/Ttot 0.25,
Titration	• Start with EPAP 4–8 cm H_2O see disease considerations, increase for obstructive apnea **maintaining the same PS** • IPAPmin = 8 cm H_2O (EPAP + 4 cm H_2O), increase for hypopnea, snoring, or airflow limitation • IPAP max = 25(or 30)cm H_2O, Target tidal volume 6 to 8 mL/kg IBW • Backup rate = 1 to 2 breaths below spontaneous breath rate, increase for central apnea or PCO_2 or SaO_2 not at goal when tidal volume optimized • Ti based on backup rate and desired Ti/Ttot • If many spontaneous breaths with low Ti consider PC mode

For AVAPS with autoEPAP (Trilogy or Evo home ventilators use PSmin, PSmax rather than IPAPmin, IPAPmax).
S, spontaneous; *ST*, spontaneous-timed; *PC*, pressure control; *P*, pressure; *T*, timed; *OHS*, obesity hypoventilation syndrome; *COPD*, chronic obstructive pulmonary disease; *OSA*, obstructive sleep apnea; *IPAP*, inspiratory positive airway pressure; *EPAP*, expiratory positive airway pressure; *AVAPS*, average volume-assured pressure support; *NMD*, neuromuscular disease; *IBW*, ideal body weight.

Table 24–9 Intelligent Volume-Assured Pressure Support (iVAPS) – (ResMed)

Parameter	Typical Settings (iVAPs mode)**
Target Alveolar Ventilation (Va) (L/min)	• Enter patient height and target rate • Adjust Va until tidal volume is 8 mL/kg of ideal body weight (or 6 mL/kg for adaptation)
EPAP (cm H_2O)	Manual, adjust set to eliminate obstructive apnea Default: 5 cm H_2O
Height (in)	Used to estimate dead space (V_D), Default 70 in Alveolar ventilation = minute ventilation – (V_D x RR)
Target Backup Rate (breaths/min)	Fixed, (using iBR), usually at least 15 bpm, use actual patient spontaneous respiratory rate
PSmin (cm H_2O)	4 cm H_2O
PSmax	20 cm H_2O (or sufficiently high to reach target Va), constrained by Pmax and EPAP
Mode	• iVAPS, iBR (ST with iBR)
Ti	• TiMin, TiMax • NMD adequate TiMin • COPD shorter TiMax
Rise Time	Default 200 msec, Range 150–650 msec in 50 msec increments, constrained by Ti or TiMax • NMD 300 msec (especially with bulbar disease) • COPD 100–200 msec
Trigger Setting (TS)	Default: medium • Auto-triggering, breath starts too early – use low TS • Difficulty initiating a breath – use high TS • NMD – use high TS (quicker, easier trigger) • COPD – use medium TS

Table 24-9 Intelligent Volume-Assured Pressure Support (iVAPS) - (ResMed)—cont'd

Parameter	Typical Settings (iVAPs mode)**
Cycle Setting (CS)	Default: medium • NMD – use low CS (later cycle) • COPD – use high CS (earlier cycle to allow sufficient exhalation time)
Disease Specific Considerations	• In obesity hypoventilation syndrome – use up to 10 mL/kg IBW for tidal volume (start 6-8 mL/kg IBW) • In chest wall disorders – use tidal volume of 6–8 mL/kg IBW • In NMD, use tidal volume 6–8 mL/kg IBW • In COPD, start 6-8 mL/kg higher than 8 mL/kg IBW may be needed (as Va increased to normalize SpO_2 and CO_2). In high intensity NIV IPAP >18 cm H_2O, up to 10 mL/kg has been used. • During start of titration or treatment, can use 6 mL/kg IBW (to allow adaptation to pressure) • See rise time, trigger, cycle settings, TiMin, TiMax settings
Titration	• Increase EPAP for obstructive apnea, increase PSmin for hypopnea, airflow limitation, snoring • Increase rate if central apneas persist (one to two breaths/min every 20 min) • For persistent SaO_2 <90% or high PCO_2, increase target Va by 0.3 L/min every >5 min until resolved

iBR, intelligent backup rate; *IBW*, ideal body weight; *NMD*, neuromuscular disease; *COPD*, chronic obstructive pulmonary disease; *Va*, alveolar ventilation; *EPAP*, expiratory positive airway pressure; *PS*, pressure support; *ST*, spontaneous-timed; *Ti*, inspiratory time.
High sensitivity means early trigger or cycle; low sensitivity means later trigger or cycle.
** iVAPS settings for AirCurve ST-A RAD device. For iVAPS settings for Astral Home Ventilator see Table 24-13

Table 24-10 Sample Target Tidal Volume Based on Ideal Body Weight

Height (in)	Ideal Body Weight (Kg)**	Target Tidal Volume (8 mL/kg of IBW)*
59	51.7	410
61	55.2	440
63	59.0	470
65	62.7	500
67	66.5	530
69	70.5	560
71	74.5	600
73	78.5	630
75	83.0	660

*Values are rounded.
**Ideal body weight assumed to be the weight associated with a body mass index (BMI) of 23 kg/m^2.

automatically) based on the spontaneous breathing rate. While the auto-rate may be useful at initiation of treatment, a set backup rate may be more effective (especially in patients with muscle weakness or in those not reliably triggering an EPAP-to-IPAP transition). Rather than specifying IPAPmin and IPAPmax, when using AVAPS on an HMV, PSmin and PSmax are specified, as the actual EPAP can vary. The **AVAPS rate** refers to how fast the IPAP is increased to meet tidal volume goals (1-5 cm H_2O/min). Here, choosing 3 means the IPAP can increase up to 3 cm H_2O per minute to meet the target tidal volume goal. In the older Trilogy devices, one can choose the PC mode and then select the AVAPS option. However, AVAPS-AE is not available with the PC mode. In the new Trilogy-Evo models, one can choose the A/C-PC mode, then the AVAPS-AE option is chosen. Then, one can select the PCbreath-off (ST mode) or PCbreath-on (PC mode) options. If one wants to replicate the T mode, then triggering is turned off. In addition, in advanced options, TiMin and TiMax can now be specified for spontaneous breaths. The triggering options are Auto-Trak, Auto-Trak sensitive, and flow triggering (used for weaker patients, often 0.5-1 L/min). The device has Bluetooth connectivity to communicate with the cloud-based adherence/monitoring program Care Orchestrator via a separate wireless hub.

In ResMed Astral units, AE is an option, or EPAP must be specified. The trigger and cycle sensitivities as well as TiMin and TiMax can be set as in the nonventilator iVAPS units. There are more options available such as pressure or flow triggering. The reader should refer to Astral manuals for details. The other settings are chosen as for nonventilator iVAPS.

Studies Comparing BPAP-ST and VAPS

Several studies have compared BPAP-ST and VAPS in patients with obesity hypoventilation syndrome (OHS),[12,13,15,16] neuromuscular and chest wall disorders,[14,19] and COPD.[22] In these studies, BPAP-ST was adjusted per protocol. In some studies, the use of autoEPAP was also evaluated.[20,21] As reviewed by Shaughnessy et al.,[18] there was no clear advantage for VAPS with respect to sleep quality or $PaCO_2$. Thus, a clear advantage of VAPS compared to BPAP-ST has not been demonstrated. On the other hand, VAPS was not inferior to BPAP-ST. It should also be appreciated that *studies comparing VAPS and BPAP-ST were performed with careful adjustment of BPAP-ST settings using standard protocols and the results may not reflect what happens in actual clinical practice.* In a retrospective study of NIV treatment of ALS,[19] which likely represents real-world experience, VAPS was associated with a greater probability of reaching an effective tidal volume. The advantage of VAPS is that it can adapt to changes in patient status, avoiding the need for periodic titration, and it is useful when NIV is started with empirical settings without an NIV titration. When VAPS is used, major purposes of a PSG PAP titration include selecting a level of EPAP that eliminates

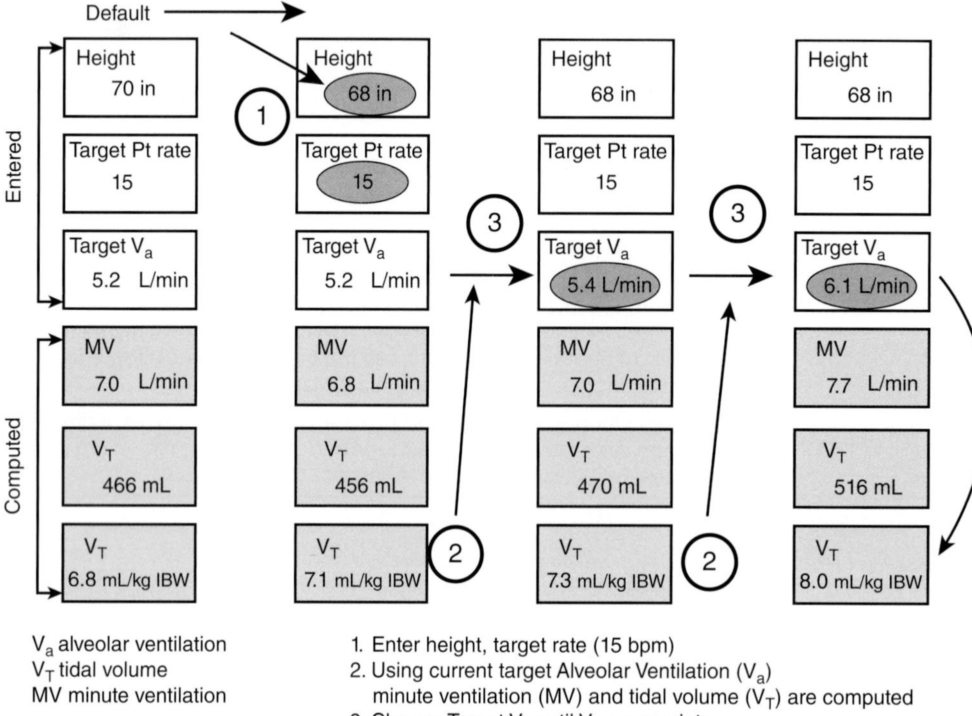

Figure 24–16 This schematic shows an approach to setting a ResMed iVAPS device using a target alveolar ventilation (V_a). (1) The patient height and backup rate are set (actual target rate). Based on these settings and the current target alveolar ventilation, a tidal volume given as mL/kg of ideal body weight is computed. If this is not satisfactory, the alveolar ventilation target is increased or decreased until a desired computed tidal volume is reached. The dead space ventilation is computed from the respiratory rate and the height (using a nomogram giving dead space volume versus height). The alveolar ventilation = minute ventilation – (respiratory rate × *dead space). Note that the required alveolar ventilation associated with an appropriate tidal volume may be inadequate in patients* with lung disease, as the actual dead space usually exceeds the predicted value. That is, the target alveolar ventilation will need to be increased if the arterial PCO_2 goal is not met.

obstructive events (obstructive apnea and hypopnea), determine an optimal mask interface, and documenting that the device does deliver adequate tidal volumes. As previously noted, in the United States, an autoEPAP function is not available on VAPS devices other than HMVs (AVAPS-AE for AVAPS-autoEPAP). In the future, less expensive nonhome ventilator VAPS devices will hopefully offer an autoEPAP setting. VAPS RADs communicate information to cloud-based programs that can provide the physician with useful information (CareOrchestrator PR, AirView ResMed). In the past, HMV VAPS units only had data card download capability, but newer devices can also communicate with cloud-based programs. The HMVs communicate with a hub via Bluetooth, and the hub communicates with cloud-based programs (wireless modem).

CHOOSING THE ADVANCED PAP MODE (VAPS VERSUS ASV VERSUS BPAP-ST)

There is some overlap in the patient populations that may benefit from these devices. However, ASV devices use a relatively **long time window** to determine a target (minute ventilation or peak flow), and PS varies breath to breath with the goal of stabilizing ventilation. In contrast, VAPS devices respond with a slow increase or decrease in PS (the AVAPS rate, usually 1–5 cm/H_2O/minute), using a short time window to determine if the *tidal volume or alveloar ventilation meets the target.* VAPS is appropriate for hypoventilation disorders but not ideal for hypocapnic CSA. Treatment of patients with CSA is discussed in Chapter 30, but limited information will be presented here for completeness.

Hypocapnic CSA

Some patients with hypocapnic CSA (primary CSA, CSA with CSB, treatment-emergent CSA) and CSA due to medication will respond to CPAP alone either acutely or with chronic treatment. Although most insurance providers do not consider CSA an indication for CPAP (even if effective),[23,24] many of these patients also have enough OSA to make the diagnosis of both CSA and OSA and qualify them for CPAP. BPAP **without** a backup rate tends to worsen hypocapnic CSA. If CPAP is not effective, patients with hypocapnic CSA are candidates for ASV treatment, which is usually very effective. Patients with narcotic-induced CSA and mild hypoventilation may respond to BPAP-ST or ASV. As previously noted, if ASV is used, a PSmin of 6 to 8 cm H_2O or higher may be needed. If ASV is not effective, patients can be treated with BPAP-ST. An occasional patient with CSA due to a medication with a very low respiratory rate will respond better to ASV using a fixed backup rate (only available on PR ASV devices) than ASV using the auto-rate option. Those patients with more significant hypoventilation can be treated with

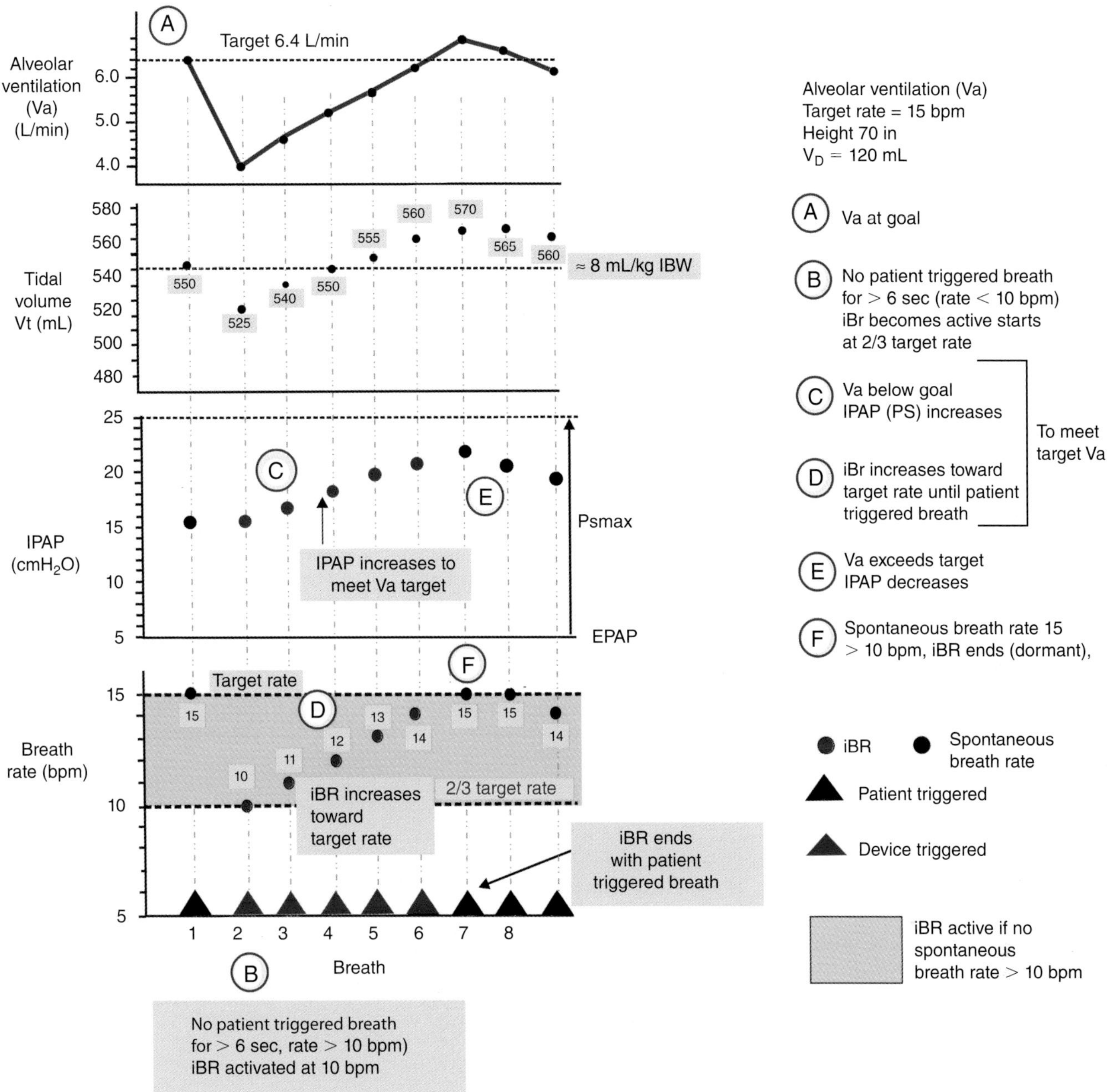

Figure 24–17 This figure illustrates the responses of intelligent Volume-Assured Pressure Support (iVAPS) and Intelligent Backup Rate (iBR) to Provide the target alveolar ventilation. Although the tidal volume is illustrated, the pressure support (PS) varies in response to the alveolar ventilation (Va) target. When the spontaneous rate falls below two-thirds of the target rate, the iBR is activated and increases toward the target rate until a spontaneous breath occurs. A fixed expiratory positive airway pressure (EPAP) of 5 cm H_2O and a PSmax of 20 cmH_2O) are illustrated. When the iBR is active it increases toward the target rate to help meet the Va target along with increases in PS. However, the iBR does not exceed the target rate and is not operative during spontaneous breathing at a rate above two-thirds the target rate. The calculation of the Va uses the estimated dead space volume based on height from a ResMed nomorgram.

BPAP-ST (or VAPS). *Of note, the major intervention should be reduction in opioid dose (or weaning and cessation).*[25] As previously mentioned, if BPAP in the ST mode is used for treatment of hypocapnic CSA or CSA due to medication, this tends to require more machine-triggered breaths and higher average PS than does ASV. ASV is the preferred treatment for most patients with hypocapnic CSA requiring an advanced PAP mode, as ventilation can be stabilized with fewer device-triggered breaths and lower average PS. ASV may be better tolerated than BPAP-ST with a fixed PS. ASV units also have the ability to auto-titrate the EPAP and can be used to treat both OSA and CSA. The American Academy of Sleep Medicine (AASM) published practice parameters for treatment of the CSA syndromes (CSAS).[26] A recommendation for the use of PAP for treatment of primary CSA was made without specifying a definite mode. A recommendation

Table 24–11 Comparison of Required Settings for AVAPS and iVAPS

AVAPS (Philips Respironics)	iVAPS (ResMed)
Target **tidal volume** mL	Target **alveolar ventilation** (L/min)
EPAP (cm H_2O)	EPAP (cm H_2O)
Pmax (maximum allowed IPAP), usually 30 cm H_2O	No setting, assumed to be 30 cm H_2O
IPAPmin (cm H_2O) (EPAP + 4 cm H_2O) (PSmin = IPAPmin – EPAP)	PSmin (4 cm H_2O, range 0 to PSmax)
IPAPmax (cm H_2O) (PSmax = IPAPmax – EPAP)	PSmax (20 cm H_2O, range 0 to [30-EPAP])
Respiratory rate (one to two breaths below spontaneous)	Target respiratory rate (actual desired respiratory rate), default 15 bpm)
Mode: ST or PC Specify Ti inspiratory time based on rate and desired Ti/Ttot	Mode: iBR (intelligent backup rate) Specify TiMin (default 0.3 sec), TiMax (default 2.0 sec), set based on desired Ti/Ttot and target respiratory rate
Rise time (1–6, 100–600 msec) (set for comfort)	Rise time (150–900 msec in 50-msec increments) (typical setting 300 or 150 for COPD)
—	Cycle sensitivity (default medium) Trigger sensitivity (default medium)

ST, spontaneous-timed; *PC*, pressure control; *PS*, pressure support; *AVAPS*, average volume-assured pressure support; *iVAPS*, intelligent volume-assured pressure support; *EPAP*, expiratory positive airway pressure; *IPAP*, inspiratory positive airway pressure; *Ti*, inspiratory time; *iBR*, intelligent backup rate.

Shaughnessy GF, Gay PC, Olson EJ, Morgenthaler TI Noninvasive volume-assured pressure support for chronic respiratory failure: a review. Curr Opin Pulm Med. 2019;25(6):570–577.

Table 24–12 AVAPS Home Ventilators – Philips Respironics (Trilogy, Evo)

AVAPS-AE	
Parameter	Typical settings:
Pmax	30 cm H_2O
Target tidal volume	8 mL/kg IBW
Automatic EPAP (AE) • Range EPAPmin to EPAPmax	EPAPmin 4 or 5 cm H_2O EPAPmax 15 cm H_2O
PS varies to meet tidal volume goal • Range PSmin to PSmax	PSmin 4 to 5 cm H_2O PSmax 20 cm H_2O (constrained by EPAPmin and Pmax)
Mode: ST (can use PC) Specify backup rate and Ti	Backup rate: 10–12 breaths/min or one to two breaths/min below spontaneous rate Ti = 1.5 seconds or based on backup rate
Mode: ST	Use in NMD, specify rate and Ti
Mode: ST with automatic rate	Automatic rate and automatic Ti Useful for initial setup, but not in severe NMD or unreliable triggering
AVAPS rate How fast PS changes in cm H_2O/min	Range (1–5 cm H_2O/min) Use 3 or 4
Trigger	Auto-Trak, Auto-Trak sensitive, Flow trigger In NMD use, Auto-Trak sensitive or Flow trigger (0.5 L/min)
PC Mode Option	
Trilogy	
Specify: PC mode AVAPS but not AVAPS-AE available	AVAPS on Specify EPAP and Target tidal volume Specify backup rate and Ti
Evo	
AVAPS-AE available with PC mode ON option	Specify AVAPS-AE Specify PC Breath ON (if PC mode desired) Specify target tidal volume, EPAPmin, and EPAPmax Specify backup rate, and Ti

NMD, neuromuscular disease; *IBW*, ideal body weight; *AVAPS*, average volume-assured pressure support; *EPAP*, expiratory positive airway pressure; *AE*, automatic EPAP; *PS*, pressure support; *ST*, spontaneous-timed; *PC*, pressure control; *Ti*, inspiratory time.

Table 24–13 Astral Home Ventilator – ResMed *iVAPS with iBR*

Parameter	Typical settings:
Pmax	30 cm H_2O
Height	Used to calculate dead space and alveolar ventilation
Backup rate (BR)	Use iBR Set actual respiratory rate goal (usually 15 breaths/min)
Ti	Specify TiMin, TiMax
Alveolar ventilation target (Va)	Adjust alveolar ventilation target until calculated tidal volume reaches target tidal volume or until (8 mL/kg IBW)
Automatic EPAP not enabled	Set EPAP 5 cm H_2O or higher
Enable: automatic EPAP – Range EPAPmin to EPAPmax	EPAPmin 5 cm H_2O EPAPmax 15 cm H_2O
Set PSmin, PSmax	PSmin 4, PSmax 20 Set sufficient PSmax so alveolar ventilation target can be met PSmax constrained by EPAPmin and Pmax

iVAPS, intelligent volume-assured pressure support; *iBR*, intelligent backup rate; *P*, pressure; *Ti*, inspiratory time; *Va*, ventilation target; *EPAP*, expiratory positive airway pressure; *PS*, pressure support; *IBW*, ideal body weight.

for CPAP therapy targeted to normalize the apnea-hypopnea index (AHI) was recommended as the initial treatment of CSAS related to congestive heart failure (CHF). As discussed in Chapter 30, about 50% of patients with CSA with CSB secondary to heart failure with a low ejection fraction respond to CPAP, although the AHI may not be reduced to as low a level as with ASV. ASV targeted to normalize the AHI was recommended for the treatment of CSA related to CHF. BPAP therapy in an ST mode targeted to normalize the AHI was recommended for the treatment of CSAS related to CHF only if there is no response to adequate trials of CPAP, ASV, and oxygen therapies. Of note, the AASM practice parameters did not make recommendations concerning treatment-emergent CSA or CSA associated with a medication. In 2015, a study of ASV for **CSA** due to CHF using a ResMed ASV device by Cowie et al.[27] found increased mortality in a group with low ejection fraction (EF <45%). This resulted in the AASM publishing an updated recommendation for treatment of CSAS.[28] Given the data from the study by Cowie et al., there was a recommendation (at the standard level) against use of ASV to treat CHF-associated CSAS in patients with a left ventricular EF (LVEF) of ≤45% and moderate or severe CSAS. There was a recommendation at the option level for the use of ASV in the treatment CHF-associated CSAS in patients with an LVEF >45% or mild CHF-related CSAS. ASV is not currently recommended in patients with moderate-to-severe CSA with CSB due to heart failure with a low EF (<45%).

The ADVENT-HF study compared treatment with a PR ASV device (peak flow target) to optimal medical therapy using a randomized parallel-group, open-label controlled design of patients with heart failure and a low ejection fraction (≤45%) and moderate to severe sleep disordered breathing (AHI ≥15/hour). The study included both patients with predominately OSA and patients with predominately CSA. The results of the study found no improvement with ASV on a composite outcome including all cause mortality compared to optimal medical treatment. However, ASV effectively eliminated sleep-disordered breathing safely.[29] More details of the study results are presented in chapter 30. The effect of the study results on clinical practice remains to be determined.

Non-hypocapnic CSA and Hypoventilation Disorders

Patients with hypoventilation syndromes include those with OHS, neuromuscular weakness, chest wall disease, or disorders of the central control of ventilation.[6] In these disorders, a backup rate is needed to ensure adequate ventilation. BPAP-ST (fixed PS) or VAPS devices in the ST mode are used to augment tidal volume and ensure an adequate respiratory rate. An exception is the group of stable patients with OHS and severe OSA. In this group, treatment with CPAP or BPAP-S may be sufficient.[30,31] Volume-assured PS is useful for patients in whom the amount of PS needed may vary and often increases with disease progression. Comparison of BPAP-ST and VAPS was previously discussed.[18] In general, VAPS more reliably reduces the $PaCO_2$ and attains the target tidal volume. In actual practice, one typically starts with a lower target tidal volume to allow adaptation (6 mL/kg IBW). It is important to emphasize that a much larger PS is needed to treat hypoventilation (8–20 cm H_2O) than the usual 4 cm H2O used to treat OSA. The lowest EPAP possible allows an effective PS without the need for an excessively large IPAP, which may produce pressure intolerance and mask leak issues. On the other hand, higher EPAP levels are needed in some patients with a high BMI and severe OSA. An increase in the EPAP can also improve oxygenation in some patients.

NIV (NPPV) TITRATION AND TREATMENT

The AASM recommends a PSG titration when starting NIV in stable patients.[1] The titration allows selection of NIV settings (IPAP, EPAP, backup rate, Ti) that will eliminate obstructive apnea/hypopnea and deliver an optimal PS and backup rate. Some patients will also require the addition of supplemental oxygen. An alternative is initiating treatment at home, in clinic, or at a durable medical equipment (DME) provider office based on empiric settings or with the use of devices that automatically adjust the device settings.[3] For example, NIV can be started on an outpatient basis at low pressure (IPAP/EPAP 8/4–13/6 cm H_2O and backup rate based on the spontaneous rate—a few breaths lower) and increased as tolerated based on patient symptoms and oximetry, daytime $P_{ET}CO_2$ measurements, or daytime arterial blood gas measurements. Use of VAPS devices allow setting a target tidal volume or target alveolar ventilation. However, unless an HMV is used, EPAP must be set empirically. An advantage of the NIV titration is determination of an appropriate EPAP and a trial of multiple mask interfaces. In addition, an NIV titration may provide information about the efficacy of a minute ventilation target, especially if transcutaneous PCO_2 is measured (for example, a minute ventilation of 6 L/min associated with a $PaCO_2$ of 55 mmHg requires a higher minute ventilation). Patients with lung diesase often require a greater than normal minute ventilation to deliver an adequate alveolar ventilation. Whether treatment is started empirically or with a PSG titration, careful outpatient follow-up is needed with optimization of mask and device settings based on machine download information, oximetry, and home PCO_2 monitoring.

Goals of NIV Titration and Treatment

The titration of NIV focuses on providing ventilatory support in addition to maintaining an open airway. The goals of NIV treatment vary among patients but generally include[1]: (1) improving sleep quality and preventing nocturnal dyspnea, (2) prevention of nocturnal hypoventilation (or worsening of hypoventilation during sleep if daytime hypoventilation is present), and (3) providing respiratory muscle rest. For patients with daytime hypoventilation, use of NIV can improve the quality of life and delay the development of respiratory failure. The nocturnal $PaCO_2$ goal is a value equal to or less than the daytime $PaCO_2$. However, sufficient PS may not be tolerated initially. If using a VAPS device, a lower tidal volume target may be needed to allow adaptation to pressure. As the patient improves and the daytime $PaCO_2$ decreases, a lower nocturnal $PaCO_2$ goal would also be appropriate. Improvement in the daytime $PaCO_2$ depends on adherence,[30] and some studies suggest "high intensity" treatment (with a goal of normalizing or substantially improving nocturnal hypercapnia) may improve outcomes in patients with hypercapnic COPD.[32,33,34]

NIV Titration Protocol

If NIV (NPPV) is titrated in the sleep center, recording of pressure, flow, tidal volume, and leak signals from the laboratory PAP device is recommended (Figure 24–5). Recording the PAP pressure allows the clinician to determine the delivered pressure on each breath and, depending on the laboratory PAP device, whether the breath was spontaneous or device triggered. While this discussion targets hypoventilation, recording of PAP pressure is also very useful for the clinician reviewing ASV titration studies.

As adequate minute ventilation is a goal, recording the tidal volume is helpful as the tidal volume depends on both the PS and the Ti. Although the programs used to control PAP devices in the sleep lab can also display the tidal volume on a breath-to-breath basis (can be included as a comment by the sleep technologist), having the information recorded on the PSG tracing is of great help to the clinician reading the study. Monitoring transcutaneous PCO_2 is also useful, if validated (requires calibration). In the morning, a simultaneous capillary arterial blood gas test (ABG) can be used to verify the accuracy of transcutaneous PCO_2 readings (requires a respiratory therapist to draw a sample and transportation of the sample to a clinical laboratory). The PCO_2 by capillary ABG is usually within a few mmHg of the $PaCO_2$.[35]

A best clinical practice NPPV titration protocol was published by the AASM and is a useful guide for NIV titration.[1] However, the general recommendations need to be altered to meet the needs of special patient populations. Some sleep centers are not equipped to handle patients with severe neuromuscular disorders. Sometimes, daytime titration in the home or clinic by a skilled respiratory therapist may be a better option.[36] Titration recommendations are summarized in Table 24–14. A schematic of NIV titration is shown in Figure 24–18.

Table 24–14 Recommendations for Adjustment of Pressure Support during Noninvasive Positive Pressure Ventilation Titration

Pressure Change	Trigger	Duration Between Changes	Goal
IPAP/ and EPAP increased by 1 to 2 cm H_2O (maintaining current PS)	Eliminate obstructive apnea	≥5 min	Prevent obstructive apnea.
IPAP increased (1-2 cm H_2O)	Eliminate hypopnea, RERAs, and snoring	≥ 5 min	Prevent hypopneas, RERAs, and snoring.
PS increased 1–2 cm H_2O	Low tidal volume (<6–8 mL/kg IBW)	≥5 min	Adequate tidal volume.
PS increased 1–2 cm H_2O	$PaCO_2$ >10 mm Hg above goal	≥10 min	Adequate ventilation and $PaCO_2$.
PS increased 1–2 cm H_2O	Respiratory muscle rest not achieved	≥10 min	Adequate respiratory muscle rest. Reduction of respiratory rate with higher tidal volumes and/or reduction in inspiratory EMG activity.
PS increased 1–2 cm H_2O	SaO_2 <90% with tidal volume <8 mL/kg (assumes discrete apnea, hypopnea, RERAs not present)	≥5 min	Adequate oxygenation. Tidal volume up to 10 mL/kg IBW maybe needed in some patients.

EMG, electromyogram; *IPAP*, inspiratory positive airway pressure; *EPAP*, expiratory positive airway pressure; *IBW*, ideal body weight; *$PaCO_2$*, arterial carbon dioxide pressure; *PS*, pressure support; *RERA*, respiratory effort-related arousal; *SaO_2*, arterial oxygen saturation. Adapted from reference 1.

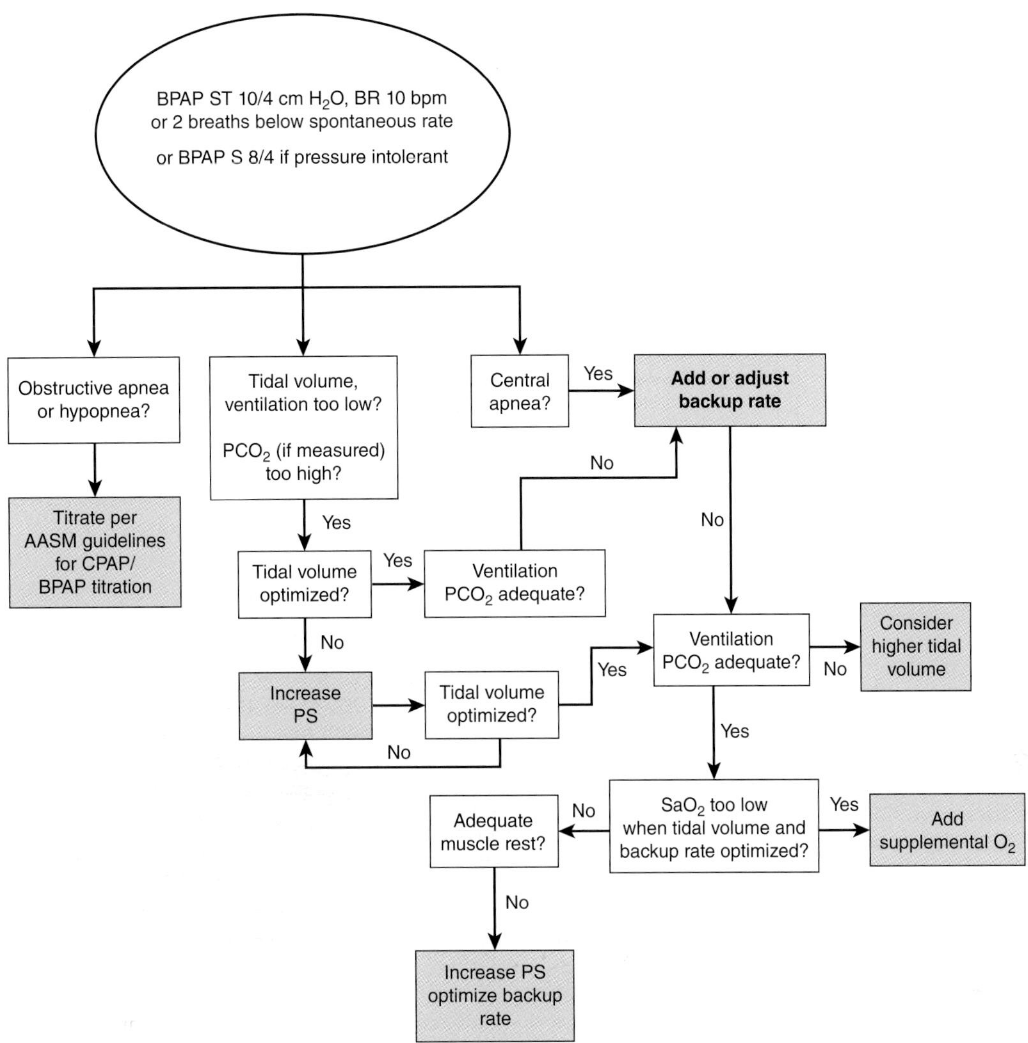

Figure 24–18 A schematic algorithm for titration of noninvasive Ventilation (NIV) in the sleep center. In this approach, a backup rate is utilized from the start (or added if not used initially). Pressure support is increased based on a target tidal volume. Expiratory positive airway pressure (EPAP) is increased to prevent obstructive apnea. An increase in respiratory rate or inspiratory time is needed if the delivered minute ventilation does not result in adequate control of the SaO_2 or transcutaneous PCO_2 or deliver adequate muscle rest. Of note, if this is the first night on NIV, the patient may not tolerate optimal settings. These can be gradually adjusted on an outpatient basis. Schematic adapted from reference 1.

Some of the basics of PAP titration in general were covered in the chapter on PAP treatment, Chapter 23. Both the IPAP and EPAP are increased maintaining the same pressure suppport to eliminate obstructive apnea. For example an increase in IPAP/EPAP from 8/4 to 10/6 cm H_2O. The IPAP is increased as per the protocol discussed in chapter 23 to eliminate hypopneas, respiratory effort-related arousals (RERAs), and snoring. In addition, IPAP is increased during an NIV titration to augment tidal volume. In general, a starting BPAP (IPAP/EPAP) of 8/4 cm H_2O to 10/6 cmH_2O is used. Higher pressure can be used for patient comfort. The effectiveness of ventilatory support can be assessed by monitoring the SaO_2, delivered flow and tidal volume, and transcutaneous PCO_2 ($TcPCO_2$). A goal of delivering a tidal volume of 6 to 8 mL/kg IBW is recommended. While one may start at 6 mL/Kg IBW for adaptation, really 8 mL/kg or higher is the usual tidal volume goal. The PS is incrementally increased if the tidal volume is not reached or the PCO_2 remains above goal. If there is continued desaturation, a higher tidal volume goal or EPAP may be needed. The backup rate is usually set 1 to 2 breaths below the sleeping spontaneous breathing rate (8 to 10 breaths/min minimum). Information on choosing the Ti is provided previously in this chapter. For ResMed devices, the TiMin can be set at the desired Ti, although the actual Ti may be slightly longer but within the TiMin-to-TiMax window based on patient flow. Adjustment of both the PS and backup rate (as well as the Ti) has the goal of achieving an adequate minute ventilation, appropriate PCO_2 (if measurement available), and oxygen saturation. A tidal volume goal higher than 8 cc/kg IBW and a backup rate of 15 to 20 breaths/min may be needed. In patients with muscle weakness, providing muscle rest is also an important goal. In Figure 24–19, an example of reduced diaphragmatic electromyogram (EMG) activity with higher PS is illustrated. Of note, the spontaneous rate also decreased with higher flow (and tidal volume) associated with higher PS.

If further increases in ventilation are desired but the patient does not tolerate a higher PS, use of a higher backup

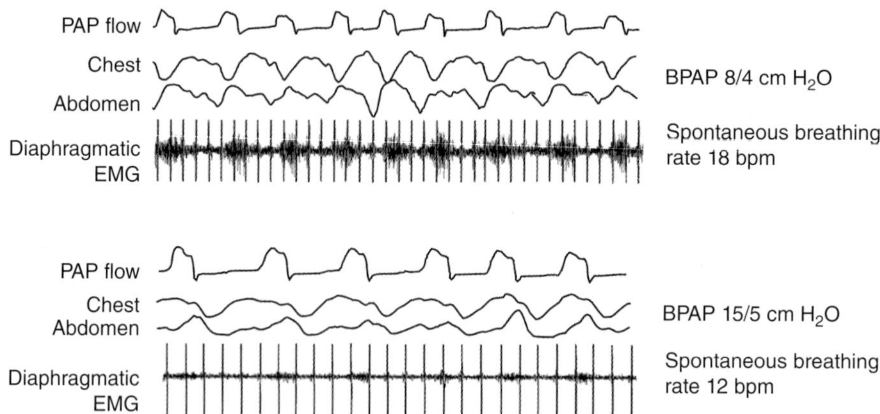

Figure 24–19 This figure shows the effect of increasing pressure support on surface diaphragmatic electromyography (EMG). The reduction in EMG activity suggests that muscle rest is occurring secondary to the increased ventilatory support. Note the increase in positive airway pressure (PAP) flow and decrease in spontaneous respiratory rate. Optimal ventilation occurs with a higher tidal volume (associated with higher PAP flow) and a lower respiratory rate.

rate can be tried. Typical initial pressures for a thin patient with neuromuscular disease (NMD) might be IPAP/EPAP of 12/4 or 13/5 cm H_2O for initial treatment with adjustment up to as high as 25/4 cm H_2O. *The goal in NIV is to use as low an EPAP as possible so that adequate PS can be delivered without excessive IPAP.* Patients with neuromuscular disorders, thoracic cage disorders, or disorders of inadequate ventilatory control may not be obese and may not require as high an EPAP as patients with OSA or OHS. Higher EPAP is needed for patients with a high BMI and a significant component of OSA. Typical pressures for OHS patients might be IPAP/EPAP of (16 to 20)/8 or (20-25)/12 cm H_2O. Note that tidal volume can be increased by increasing the Ti, but that only applies to device-triggered breaths in PR devices. For PR devices, if the Ti is too short, the backup rate can be increased so more breaths are device-triggered breaths. In PR BPAP devices with AVAPS capability the PC mode can be chosen. Then both spontaneous and device triggered breaths have the specified Ti. For ResMed devices, the TiMin can be increased, as noted, and will affect both spontaneous and machine-triggered breaths.

The AASM titration guidelines[1] state that a backup rate should be used in all patients with central hypoventilation, those with a significant number of central apneas or an inappropriately low respiratory rate, and those who unreliably trigger IPAP/EPAP cycles due to muscle weakness. However, currently use of a backup rate is recommended for all patients requiring NIV for CSA and hypoventilation syndromes (especially neuromuscular disorders). Stable obesity hypoventilation syndrome patients with severe OSA are an exception.[30,31] However, as will be discussed, obtaining insurance coverage for a device with a backup rate may be difficult in some disorders.

If the NIV titration is using VAPS in the ST mode, the appropriate target tidal volume, backup rate, Ti, and EPAP are set. For thinner patients, an EPAP of 4 or 5 cm H_2O is typically used; for more obese patients, 8 to 10 cm H_2O is used. IPAPmin is usually set at 4 cm H_2O above the current EPAP, and IPAPmax is usually set at 20 to 25 cm H_2O (constrained by EPAP and the maximum pressure). If there is information from a prior titration, that should be utilized.

Specifying treatment parameters for the ResMed iVAPS device was previously discussed. Important differences are that the patient height, a target alveolar ventilation, and a target respiratory rate must be specified. Recall that the intelligent backup rate uses the actual patient respiratory rate (default 15 breaths/min) rather than the backup rate used in PR AVAPS devices (slightly lower than the spontaneous breathing rate). It may be appropriate to use an alveolar ventilation target associated with a tidal volume of 6 mL/kg IBW to allow the patient to adapt to pressure. Typical values are EPAP = 5 cm H_2O, PSmin = 4 cm H_2O, PSmax = 20 cm H_2O, and a target respiratory rate of 15 bpm. *If the SaO_2 is <90% in the absence of respiratory events, an increase in the target alveolar ventilation by 0.3 L/min every ≥5 minutes is recommended.*[7] If there are persistent central apneas, the target respiratory rate can be increased. *It is important to note that, in iVAPS devices, the alveolar ventilation is calculated using a dead space based on height in* ***normal individuals***. In patients with lung disease, *the dead space is increased,* and a higher minute ventilation is needed to provide a given alveolar ventilation target. This implies that a higher alveolar ventilation target than one based on a tidal volume of 8 mL/kg IBW) may be needed. Of interest a study of severe COPD patients with hypercapnia that compared high intensity NIV delivered with BPAP-ST (mean IPAP about 18 cm H_2O) versus iVAPS (mean IPAP of 20 cm H_2O found that an iVAPS target alveolar ventilation of approximately 7.7 L/min was needed to reach a sleeping PCO_2 goal around 50 mmHg[22]. For comparison, using computations in iVAPs software an alveolar ventilation target of 6.1 L/min is associated with a 68 inch height. a tidal volume of 8 cc/kg IBW, and a target respiratory rate of 15 bpm. For these parameters a target alveoalr entilation of 8 L/min correspond to the tidal volume of about 10 mL/kg IBW.

Supplemental oxygen can be added if desaturation persists despite optimization of NIV. However, if tolerated, a higher EPAP, tidal volume, or respiratory rate may be a better choice. *In a study of outcomes in patients with OHS,*[15] *use of a target tidal volume of 10 mL/kg of ideal body weight was associated with better improvement in daytime $PaCO_2$, and in another study by Priou et al.,*[37] *use of supplemental oxygen as well as NIV in patients with*

OHS was associated with worse survival. While the need for supplemental oxygen may simply have been a marker for greater disease severity, *optimization of NIV before addition of oxygen* is an important goal. On **chronic** treatment with NIV, some patients with hypoventilation will have lower daytime and nocturnal $PaCO_2$ and may no longer need supplemental oxygen. On the other hand, patients with hypercapnic COPD may require supplemental oxygen 24 hours per day. Some special considerations for NIV treatment in hypercapnic COPD will be discussed.

Initiating NIV Without Titration

Studies have shown that NIV can be effectively initiated at home or in a clinic if sufficiently trained personnel, and facilities are available.[2,3,36] Mask fitting and education are essential. Frequent follow-up in the home by respiratory therapists and/or in the clinic is needed at the start of treatment. Usually, lower pressure settings or target tidal volume are used initially to allow adaptation. Information from the devices is available from cloud-based programs, and most devices can communicate via wireless connections. The current status and response to interventions can be quickly noted.[38]

Disease-Specific Recommendations for Chronic Treatment

Some disease-specific recommendations for NIV titration or chronic NIV treatment are listed in Table 24–15. As noted above, for patients with OHS requiring NIV, a target tidal volume of 10 mL/kg IBW is recommended rather than 8 mL/kg IBW,[3,15] as the higher goal was associated with optimal reduction in daytime $PaCO_2$. However, the degree of adherence is the most important factor determining the decrease in daytime $PaCO_2$ during chronic treatment of OHS, so a lower tidal volume target may have to be accepted if there is pressure intolerance or inability to find a good mask seal. In the Pickwick study of the use of NIV in OHS *without* severe sleep apnea, *the highly adherent group had reduced mortality* and delay to the first hospital admission.[39] However, adherence is not generally worse in studies using an aggressive tidal volume. As noted, it is preferable to use NIV with a higher tidal volume (higher minute ventilation) for treatment of OHS rather than NIV and supplemental oxygen.[37] Unless transcutaneous PCO_2 is measured, supplemental oxygen may obscure the fact that significant residual hypoventilation is still present. That is, supplemental oxygen can normalize the SaO_2, even though significant hypoventilation is still present. However, in some patients, use of supplemental oxygen cannot be avoided. If supplemental oxygen is needed with NIV at the start of treatment, with clinical improvement (lower daytime $PaCO_2$), oxygen may no longer be needed. Patients with OHS may require relatively high EPAP (8 to 12 cm H_2O) compared to patients with NMD or COPD. However, with higher pressure support a lower than expected EPAP may be effective. For example, in Figure 24–14 when IPAP/EPAP

Table 24–15 Noninvasive Ventilation – Disease Specific Considerations

	OHS	NMD	Restrictive Thoracic	COPD
Rise Time	• Medium • PR setting 3 • ResMed 300 msec	• Longer • at least 300 msec • (esp bulbar dysfunction)	Same as NMD	• Shorter • PR setting 1 to 2 • ResMed 150 msec (100-200 msec) • Goal adequate exhalation time
EPAP	• Higher, 7 to 8 cm H_2O • 10–12 if high BMI	• 4–5 cm H_2O • Low as possible	Same as NMD	6–8 cm H_2O
Tidal volume Target	• 8–10 mL/kg IBW • start lower for adaptation • Use adequate Ti • Avoid supplemental oxygen if possible	• 6–8 mL/kg IBW • PS 10 to 20 cm H_2O	Same as NMD	• 6–8 mL/kg IBW • May need 8-10 mL/kg IBW to meet PCO_2, SpO_2 goals • High intensity IPAP >18 cmH_2O
Mode	• CPAP, BPAP-S if stable, severe OSA • If NIV indicated BPAP-ST, adequate Ti • Can use VAPS	• BPAP-ST, adequate Ti • set TiMin= Desired Ti (1-1.5 sec depending on Backup Rate) • Consider PC or PAC mode • Can use VAPS	Same as NMD	• BPAP-ST • Can use VAPS
Trigger/Cycle Sensitivity High= early Low= late	• Trigger Medium • Cycle Medium	• Trigger - High(early) • Cycle - Low (late) • Goal - less effort to trigger and avoid cycle too early	Same as NMD	• Trigger Low to Medium • Cycle Low (early) • Goal: Adequate exhalation time
TiMin, TiMax	• Can set TiMin = desired Ti (Ti/Ttot = .3 to 0.4) • TiMax = 2.0 sec	• TiMin = adequate Ti (1 to 1.5 sec) • TiMax 2.0 sec	Same as NMD	• TiMin use Ti/Ttot = .25 • TiMax shorter than 2 sec slightly longer than TiMin • Goal: avoid long Ti, I:E 1:3

IBW, ideal body weight; *OHS*, obesity hypoventilation syndrome; *NMD*, neuromuscular disease, *COPD*, chronic obstructive pulmonary disease, *PR*, Philips Respironics; *VAPS*, volume-assured pressure support; IPAP, inspiratory positive airway pressure; BMI, body mass index; *S*, spontaneous; *BPAP*, bilevel positive airway pressure; *PC*, pressure control; *EPAP*, expiratory positive airway pressure; *ST*, spontaneous timed; *CPAP*, continuous positive airway pressure, *Ti*, inspiratory time.

was changed from 21/14 to 25/11 cm H_2O no obstructuve events were noted,

For patients with neuromuscular disorders, setting the trigger sensitivity to high or very high (easily triggered) and using flow triggering (HMVs), if available, is recommended, as weak patients may have difficulty triggering the device. A retrospective study of NIV in a large group of patients with ALS[19] found that, overall, more than 80% of breaths were spontaneously triggered, but a much lower percentage were spontaneously cycled. The study used a ResMed device, and TiMin and TiMax were set. The trigger sensitivity was set to high and the cycle sensitivity to low. A low cycle senstivity (later transition) avoids early termination of IPAP. In this study a device-cycled breath was Ti=TiMin, and a spontaneously cycled breath was one cycled between TiMin and TiMax. The high percentage of device-cycled breaths means the patients could not spontaneously maintain inspiratory flow for a Ti longer than TiMin. In summary, if using a high trigger sensitivity, patients with muscle weakness were better able to trigger a breath than maintain inspiratory flow greater than TiMin. Ensuring an adequate Ti is important in patients with neuromuscular weakness or thoracic cage abnormalities. *Increasing the Ti also provides a method of increasing the tidal volume in situations in which higher PS is not tolerated.* Rise time is usually adjusted for patient comfort but is longer in NMD (especially in those with bulbar dysfunction) and chest wall disorders and shorter in COPD (shorter Ti, longer time for exhalation).

In some NIV studies, a higher backup rate was associated with better reduction in the $PaCO_2$. For patients with chest wall disorders, a lower tidal volume and higher respiratory rate may be needed. However, Budweiser et al.[40] used both a high tidal volume target and a high respiratory rate in a group with thoracic cage disorders.

For delivery of chronic NIV treatment in patients with hypercapnic COPD, a few issues are worth noting. For patients with hypercapnic COPD, high intensity NIV (with IPAP of 18 to 25 cm H_2O and a high backup rate, 14-15 bpm) has been recommended, as this has been associated with improved outcomes and does not reduce adherence.[32,33] However, an earlier study found that the component of high intensity ventilation that matters is the use of high IPAP (high PS and high target tidal volume) rather than a high respiratory rate.[33] Of note, the patients in these studies of high intensity NIV had very severe COPD with FEV_1 values 23-30% of predicted and mean awake $PaCO_2$ levels of approximately 57 to 60 mm Hg. In some studies of high intensity NIV tidal volumes up to 10 mL/kg ideal body weight were used. On the other hand there is a concern about barotrauma in patients with COPD. The American Thoracic Society has published a clinical practice guideline for NIV (NPPV) in patients with chronic stable hypercapnic COPD.[34] In contrast to patients with OHS admitted with hypercapnic respiratory failure, waiting for stabilization of respiratory acidosis in patients with COPD after discharge is recommended rather than discharging COPD patients on NIV. **Stable** COPD patients with residual hypercapnia are more likely to benefit and comply with treatment.

The recommendations for treatment of hypercapnic COPD[34] are as follows: "1) We suggest the use of nocturnal NIV in addition to usual care for patients with chronic stable hypercapnic COPD (conditional recommendation, moderate certainty); 2) We suggest that patients with chronic stable hypercapnic COPD undergo screening for OSA before initiation of long-term NIV (conditional recommendation, very low certainty); 3) We suggest not initiating long-term NIV during an admission for acute-on-chronic hypercapnic respiratory failure, favoring instead reassessment for NIV at 2 to 4 weeks after resolution (conditional recommendation, low certainty); 4) We suggest not using in-laboratory overnight PSG to titrate NIV in patients with chronic stable hypercapnic COPD who are initiating NIV (conditional recommendation, very low certainty); and 5) We suggest NIV with ***targeted normalization of $PaCO_2$*** in patients with hypercapnic COPD on long-term NIV (conditional recommendation, low certainty)." Normalization of PCO_2 requires high levels of IPAP in most patients (high intensity NIV). Starting NIV as an outpatient requires an appropriate setting, well trained respiratory therapists with experience in NIV, and specific protocols. In many locales, starting NIV using a titration in the sleep center may be a better option. However, not all sleep centers have experience with NIV titrations. It should be noted that in the studies of "high intensity" NIV the level of EPAP was 4 or 5 cm H_2O. With high levels of pressure support lower EPAP was able to maintain an open upper airway. Low EPAP allows delivery of a high pressure support (for example 15 cm H_2O) while using a lower level of IPAP. EPAP of 5 or 6 cm H_2O is recommended by some clinicians to address auto PEEP in COPD patients. As noted, using AVAPS or iVAPS for COPD patients higher than 8 mL/kg IBW may be needed to significantly improve the $PaCO_2$ as these patients need a higher minute ventilation due to an increased dead space ventilation. As previously noted, for iVAPS the recommendation is to increase the Alveolar ventilation target by .3 L/min every 5 minutes if the SpO_2 and PCO_2 (transcutaneous PCO_2) is not at goal[7]. It is important to allow patients to adapt and an ideal $PaCO_2$ goal may not be reached during the initial titration.

Supplemental Oxygen – Special Considerations

The supplemental oxygen flow rate used for treatment (added to NIV circuit -"bleed in") is usually based on an NIV titration, if available, or adjusted based on oximetry at home while the patient uses NIV with the current flow rate of supplemental oxygen. It is important to realize that the required liter flow rate of supplemental oxygen is usually higher than the flow rate used with nasal cannula during the day due to dilution of the oxygen flow by the device flow. The total device flow increases with leak, so the effective FIO_2 can decrease if leak increases.[41] As patients improve, the requirement for supplemental oxygen may decrease. As previouly mentioned, adjustment of NIV settings to optimize nocturnal PCO_2 is an important goal, and use of supplemental oxygen may prevent the recognition of inadequate ventilatory support if depending on the SpO_2 to guide treatment. That is, as noted, supplemental oxygen can normalize the SaO_2, even though significant hypoventilation is still present.

Leak

Most physicians find interpretation of leak data challenging due to the fact that data presentation varies between PR and ResMed devices and between certain PR devices. Total leak is the combination of intentional leak and unintentional leak. Traditionally, PR reports for CPAP and APAP presented total leak and determined the amount of large leak, defined as a leak greater than two times the expected intentional leak based on mask type and pressure. Intentional leak is higher with higher delivered pressure and higher in full face than nasal masks. Mask type can be specified in the device menu so the device can make a more accurate intentional leak estimate. Unintentional leak is determined (total leak minus intentional leak) and displayed in some advanced PR devices. ResMed devices allow specification of mask type in the menu and present *unintentional leak* with a value of 24 L/min representing the highest optimal unintentional leak. Leak is presented as a median and 95th percentile values. Trends in leak are often more important than absolute values. A trend of increasing leak could represent failure to change the mask cushion in a timely manner or indicate the mask straps were wearing out. Frequent variation in leak (visualized on detailed download information) can occur with intermittent mouth leak. One sign of variable leak is a complaint of varying amounts of water used in the humidifier chamber even though the humidity setting is unchanged. PAP devices are leak tolerant, which means higher flow is delivered to compensate for leak. High flow across the water removes more water from the chamber.

LONG-TERM FOLLOW-UP

NIV device information can be obtained via card download or cloud-based portals (wireless modem).[38] This includes important adherence and effectiveness information. Close follow-up is needed, as the given level of PS, target tidal volume, backup rate, or delivered Ti may prove inadequate if respiratory muscles weaken. Table 24–16 lists some important considerations in reviewing an NIV device download. Some patients do not tolerate an adequate PS or target tidal volume initially, but these can be slowly increased with adaptation. Device download information provides estimates of tidal volume, average respiratory rate, the percentage of patient triggered breaths, and average Ti/Ttot (some devices). *A low delivered tidal volume or high respiratory rate are clues that the amount of support is not adequate.* The *rapid shallow breathing index* (RSBI = respiratory rate/tidal volume in liters) should be less than 40. For example, with a respiratory rate of 20 breaths/min and a tidal volume of 400 mL, the RSBI is 50. In patients with NMD, a high percentage of device-triggered breaths may provide more respiratory muscle rest, and a relatively high backup rate may be needed. A change from the ST to PC mode could be needed to ensure an adequate Ti (depending on device type). In VAPS devices, unless pressure intolerance is an issue, using a starting IPAPmin (or PSmin) closer to what is needed to deliver an adequate tidal volume prevents delay in reaching the goal. Patients with severe neuromuscular weakness rarely tolerate a ramp period. Although download information is important, questioning patients is equally important. Mask issues, dryness issues, and pressure issues (intolerance, bloating, starting pressure too low or too high) are important and can affect adherence. There are specific questions that allow adjustment for patient and device synchrony (Table 24–17).[2,3,38]

Table 24–16 Using NIV Device Download Information

Adherence	• Nightly use too short, needs troubleshooting (mask, dryness, pressure) • 10–12 hours suggests need for daytime mouthpiece ventilation in NMD patients
AHI	• Too high, check EPAP, PS, backup rate, leak

Respiratory parameters	• Look at trends
	  • Progressive increase in leak - a mask intervention is needed. Is the mask cushion being changed on a regular basis?
	  • Progressive decrease in tidal volume – weakness? high leak? need for more PS?

Leak	• Too high (unintentional leak >30 L/min), mask intervention, ? adequate mask resupply
Respiratory rate	• >20 breaths/min or rapid shallow breathing index >40 suggests inadequate tidal volume and PS
Tidal volume, or Alveolar Ventilaton	• Tidal volume above target – breathing exceeds ventilatory support (needs higher tidal volume or alveolar ventilation target). Higher PSmax or IPAPmax setting may be needed if delivered PS is constrained by IPAPmax or PS max. • Below target tidal volume or target minute/alveolar ventilation (need higher PS, longer Ti or TiMin, higher respiratory rate, or switch to PC mode) • Trends are important
PS	• Is IPAPmax (PSmax) too low? If average IPAP ≈ maximum possible IPAP • Is IPAPmin (PSmin) too low? Should be near average delivered IPAP unless there is pressure intolerance
Average percentage patient triggered breaths	• For NMD goal is <20% to provide rest but <10% consider difficulty triggering device • >90% with high spontaneous rate, tidal volume may be too low–high spontaneous rate to compensate (need to increase PS, target tidal volume, backup rate ?)
Actual Ti	• Average, median not available on all devices • Actual mean Ti << set Ti for device-triggered breaths suggests early cycling on spontaneous breaths, use lower cycling sensitivity (later cycling), increase TiMin, consider PC mode
Ti/Ttot	• Compare average Ti/Ttot to Ti/Ttot determined using Ti on device triggered breaths and Ttot = (60/ actual average respiratory rate) • Ti/Ttot too low (need longer TiMin, PC mode, higher backup rate in PR devices). • Ti/Ttot too high (consider decrease in TiMax, decrease Ti use, higher cycle sensitivity (earlier cycle)

Trigger and cycle sensitivity – high (earlier) and low (later) transition

PS, pressure support; *Ti*, inspiratory time; *Ttot*, total cycle time; *PC*, pressure control; *TiMin*, minimum Ti; *TiMax*, maximum Ti; *NMD* neuromuscular disease; *AHI*, apnea-hypopnea index; *EPAP*, expiratory positive airway pressure; *IPAP*, inspiratory positive airway pressure; *NIV*, noninvasive ventilation; *PR*, Philips Respironics.

Table 24–17 Adjustment for Comfort and Synchrony

Question	Settings to Adjust
Is pressure too high?	**Pressure Adjustment** Reduce IPAPmax or PSmax, use longer rise time Use smaller tidal volume or maintain tidal volume with lower pressure support but longer Ti
Does machine easily trigger a breath every time you want one?	**Trigger Adjustment** If no – adjust trigger to higher sensitivity (from medium to high), triggering earlier with less effort On Trilogy/Evo, use Auto-Trak sensitive or flow triggering (0.5 L/min)
Does machine sometimes trigger a breath before you want one?	**Trigger Adjustment** If yes – adjust (lower trigger sensitivity, change from medium to low), **triggering later**
Does the machine **END** a breath too soon, too late, or at the right time?	Too soon – increase Ti or TiMin, lower cycle sensitivity (change medium to low cycle sensitivity – later cycling) Too late – decrease TiMax, higher cycle sensitivity (change medium to high cycle sensitivity – earlier cycle)
After you start a breath, how does air flow in? Too slow? Too fast? About right?	**Rise Time Adjustment** Too slow (decrease rise time) Too fast (increase rise time) About right (current setting)
Are breaths too small, too big, or about right?	Adjust tidal volume target, PS, or cycle sensitivity

For trigger and cycle sensitivity, see Figure 24–7. Higher sensitivity, earlier transition; lower sensitivity, later transition.
PS, pressure support; *Ti*, inspiration time; *IPAP*, inspiratory positive airway pressure.
Adapted from Ackrivo J, Elman L, Hansen-Flaschen J. Telemonitoring for home-assisted ventilation: a narrative review. *Ann Am Thorac Soc.* 2021;18(11):1761-1772.

Adjustment in clinic while the patient breathes on the device or by a respiratory therapist in the patient's home are ways to quickly determine whether changes in settings achieve the desired result.

REIMBURSEMENT FOR NIV DEVICES

A noted previously Bilevel PAP devices are called respiratory assist devices (RADs) by the CMS[24] and classified based on the ability to deliver a backup rate. BPAP without a backup rate is E0470 device and BPAP with a backup rate [BPAP ST, ASV, VAPS] is an E0741 device. RADs have specific criteria for reimbursement depending on the type of patient. The different categories include NMD/chest wall disorders, hypoventilation, CSA/complex sleep apnea, and severe COPD. The criteria are listed in Tables 24–18 to 24–22. General requirements are listed in Table 24–18. The FIO_2 is the fractional concentration of oxygen delivered to the beneficiary for inspiration. The beneficiary's prescribed FIO_2 refers to the oxygen concentration the beneficiary normally breathes when not undergoing testing to qualify for coverage of a RAD. That is, if the beneficiary does not normally use supplemental oxygen, their prescribed FIO_2 is that found on room air (0.21). Obtaining a BPAP device with a backup rate is relatively easy for restrictive thoracic disease (including neuromuscular weakness and thoracic cage disorders) and in patients with CSA/Complex Sleep Apnea syndromes. However, for hypoventilation and hypercapnic COPD, a BPAP without a backup rate must be used first and found to be ineffective. The RAD criteria are flawed for a number of reasons, including the fact that patients often have more than one disorder (i.e., OSA and COPD). A tri-society task force reviewed the entire range of CMS PAP criteria and submitted suggestions for improvement.[23,42-45] A major concern was that, for the hypoventilation syndrome and severe COPD categories, an E0470 device must be tried for up to 61 days in some qualification categories before an E0471 device can be obtained. However, most of these patients are best treated with an E0471. It should be noted that, *while the time window for a provider adherence visit for CPAP (E0601)/BPAP(E0470) treatment of OSA is day 31 to 90, for a patient qualifying for a device under RAD criteria, the visit must be on day 61 or later after starting treatment with the device* (Table 24–18). The treating physician must document benefit and adequate adherence (average of 4 hours or more per day). The difficulty in qualifying patients under the RAD criteria, especially if they are acutely ill and ready to be discharged from the hospital, has resulted in prescription for a home mechancial ventilator (HMV) using a diagnosis of acute and chronic or chronic respiratory failure) in an increasing number of patients.[46,47] These devices are appropriate for patients who are likely to have a steady downhill course and will need some degree of daytime ventilatory support (mouthpiece ventilation) as well as a battery backup (for uninterrupted ventilatory support). However, other patients can be treated with a less expensive RAD device.

The criteria for restrictive thoracic disease[24] allow the physician to choose either E0470 or E0471 (Table 24–19). *However, in these patients, an E0471 device is definitely needed.* Note that the reimbursement of BPAP-ST, ASV, and VAPS devices (all classified as E0471) is the same, though the prices vary considerably. *A sleep study is not required to obtain an RAD for these patients,* and treatment can be started with daytime adjustment of the device at home, in the clinic, or at the DME supplier office. However, a titration sleep study is useful for ensuring an adequate EPAP and optimizing mask selection and pressure settings. This is especially true if a significant component of OSA is present. Routine RAD devices do not have autoEPAP capability (HMVs do).

For the CSA/complex sleep apnea category, *an E0470 or E0471 can be obtained* if a patient meets the criteria

Table 24–18 Respiratory Assistance Devices – General Requirements

- Medical records include documentation of a face-to-face encounter between the beneficiary and the ordering practitioner that occurred *within 6 months prior to completion of the detailed written order.*
- The medical record fully documents symptoms characteristic of sleep-associated hypoventilation (daytime hypersomnolence, excessive fatigue, morning headache, cognitive dysfunction, dyspnea, etc.).
- Medical records support that the beneficiary has one of the following clinical disorders (see Tables 24-19, 24-20, 24-21, 24-22) and meets all coverage criteria for that clinical disorder.

FIO_2 is the fractional concentration of oxygen delivered to the beneficiary for inspiration. The beneficiary's prescribed FIO_2 refers to the oxygen concentration the beneficiary normally breathes when not undergoing testing to qualify for coverage of a respiratory assist device (RAD). That is, if the beneficiary does not normally use supplemental oxygen, their prescribed FIO_2 is that found in room air.

Continued Coverage (Beyond the first 3 months of therapy)

The medical record contains a re-evaluation on or after the 61st day of therapy. The re-evaluation records the progress of relevant symptoms; **and**

- The re-evaluation documents beneficiary usage of the device up to that time.
- The supplier's file includes a signed and dated statement completed by the treating physician no sooner than 61 days after initiating use of the device.
- The statement declares that the beneficiary compliantly uses the device (an average of 4 hours per 24-hour period); and
- The statement confirms that the beneficiary is benefiting from its use.

LCD: L33800[24]

Table 24–19 Respiratory Assistance Devices – Restrictive Thoracic Disorder

(E0470 or E0471) covered

- The beneficiary's medical record documents a neuromuscular disease (for example, amyotrophic lateral sclerosis) or a severe thoracic cage abnormality (for example, postthoracoplasty for tuberculosis);
  AND
- The medical record documents **ONE** of the following:
  - An arterial blood gas $PaCO_2$, done while the beneficiary is awake and breathing the prescribed FIO_2, is **≥45 mm Hg**;
  OR
  - Sleep oximetry demonstrates oxygen saturation ≤88% for ≥5 minutes of nocturnal recording time (minimum recording time of 2 hours), done while breathing the beneficiary's prescribed recommended FIO_2;
  OR
  - For neuromuscular disease only,
    - The maximal inspiratory pressure is less than 60 cm H_2O or
    - Forced vital capacity is less than 50% of predicted
- The medical record supports that chronic obstructive pulmonary disease (COPD) does not contribute significantly to the beneficiary's pulmonary limitation.

LCD: L33800[24]

(Table 24–20).[24] However, use of an E0471 device is essential. *A facility-based sleep study is required,* and one must document "significant improvement of the *sleep-associated hypoventilation* with the use of the device on the settings prescribed for initial use at home, while breathing the beneficiary's prescribed FIO_2." It is not enough for a sleep study to meet diagnostic criteria for CSA or complex sleep apnea; improvement on the E0470 or E0471 device must be documented. Of note, the criteria wording is obviously flawed, as one of the criterion in this category is that *hypoventilation is not present,* while another states that *there must be improvement in the sleep-associated hypoventilation.*[23,24] The intent is that the CSA/complex sleep apnea has improved on the E0471 device. The other issue with the complex sleep apnea criteria is that the obstructive AHI must be less than 5 events/hour. This is not always possible. In addition, the length of time the complex sleep apnea definition must be met is not specified. Unfortunately, *interpretation* of the RAD criteria varies among durable medical administration contractors (DMACs) who administer Medicare payments for DME.

For the hypoventilation group[24] (Table 24–21), which includes OHS and hypoventilation due to medication, qualifying for a *BPAP without a backup rate (E0470)* requires an awake ABG showing a $PaCO_2$ ≥45 mm Hg, spirometry showing no evidence of COPD, and a *facility-based PSG or home sleep test (HST) demonstrating* ≥5 minutes with an SaO_2 ≤88% not caused by OSA. An alternative to the PSG/HST is demonstration of a $PaCO_2$ during sleep or upon awakening that is 7 mm Hg higher than the awake $PaCO_2$ used to meet the first criterion. That is, if the awake $PaCO_2$ is 47 mm Hg, the sleeping or awakening $PaCO_2$ is ≥54 mm Hg. *BPAP with a backup rate (E0471)* can be obtained only after treatment with BPAP without a backup rate fails. Failure of treatment with an E0470 is documented by an ABG $PaCO_2$, done while awake and breathing the beneficiary's prescribed FIO_2, showing that the beneficiary's $PaCO_2$ worsens ≥7 mm HG compared to the ABG result performed to qualify the beneficiary for the E0470 device; or a **facility-based PSG or HST** demonstrating oxygen saturation ≤88% for ≥5 minutes of nocturnal recording time (minimum recording time of 2 hours) that is not caused by

Table 24–20 Respiratory Assistance Devices – CSA or Complex Sleep Apnea

(E0470 or E0471 covered if criteri A-D met)

An E0470 or E0471 are covered when prior to initiating therapy, a **complete facility-based, attended polysomnogram** was performed documenting the following (A and B).

A. The diagnosis of central sleep apnea (CSA) or complex sleep apnea; **and**

B. Significant improvement of the **sleep-associated hypoventilation** with the use of the device on the settings prescribed for initial use at home, while breathing the beneficiary's prescribed FIO_2

(Note this means both diagnosis of CSA/complex sleep apnea AND effectiveness of the device is documented by polysomnography)

Definitions:

CSA Definition

1. An apnea-hypopnea index (AHI) >5, **and**
2. The sum total of central apneas plus central hypopneas is greater than 50% of the total apneas and hypopneas, **and**
3. A central apnea-central hypopnea index (CAHI) is ≥5 per hour, **and**
4. The presence of at least one of the following:
   - Sleepiness
   - Awakening short of breath
   - Difficulty initiating or maintaining sleep
   - Snoring frequent awakenings or nonrestorative sleep
   - Witnessed apneas
5. There is no evidence of daytime or nocturnal hypoventilation

Complex Sleep Apnea definition:

Complex sleep apnea is a form of central apnea specifically identified by all of the following:

1. With use of a positive airway pressure device without a backup rate (E0601 or E0470), the polysomnogram shows a pattern of apneas and hypopneas that demonstrates the persistence or emergence of central apneas or central hypopneas upon exposure to continuous positive airway pressure (CPAP) (E0601) or a bi-level device without backup rate (E0470) **when titrated to the point where obstructive events have been effectively treated (obstructive AHI <5 per hour).**
2. After resolution of the obstructive events, the sum total of central apneas plus central hypopneas is greater than 50% of the total apneas and hypopneas; and
3. After resolution of the obstructive events, a CAHI ≥5 per hour.

LCD: L33800[24]

Table 24–21 Respiratory Assist Devices – Hypoventilation Syndrome

E0470 is covered if:

A. An initial arterial blood gas (ABG) $PaCO_2$, done while awake and breathing the beneficiary's prescribed FIO_2, is ≥45 mm Hg;
and

B. Spirometry shows an FEV1/FVC ≥70% and an FEV_1 ≥50% of predicted. (Refer to SEVERE COPD section for information about device coverage for beneficiaries with FEV1/FVC <70% or FEV1 <50% of predicted);
and

Beneficiary's condition also meets one of the following:

C. An ABG $PaCO_2$, done during sleep or immediately upon awakening and breathing the beneficiary's prescribed FIO_2, shows the beneficiary's $PaCO_2$ worsened ≥7 mm HG compared to the original result in criterion A;
or

D. **Facility-based polysomnography (PSG) or a home sleep apnea test (HST)** demonstrates oxygen saturation ≤88% for ≥5 minutes of nocturnal recording time (minimum recording time of 2 hours) that is not caused by obstructive upper airway events – i.e., apnea-hypopnea index (AHI) <5. (Refer to Positive Airway Pressure Devices LCD for information about E0470 coverage for obstructive sleep apnea).

E0471 is covered if:

A. A covered E0470 is being used;
and

B. Spirometry shows an FEV1/FVC ≥70% and an FEV1 ≥50% of predicted (otherwise, refer to COPD coverage);
and

One of the following criteria are being met:

C. An ABG $PaCO_2$, done while awake and breathing the beneficiary's prescribed FIO_2, shows that the beneficiary's $PaCO_2$ **worsens ≥7 mm HG** compared to the ABG result performed to qualify the beneficiary for the E0470 device;
or

D. A **facility-based PSG or HST** demonstrates oxygen saturation ≤88% for ≥5 minutes of nocturnal recording time (minimum recording time of 2 hours) that is not caused by obstructive upper airway events – i.e., AHI <5 **while using an E0470 device**.

Table 24–22 Respiratory Assist Devices - Severe COPD

E0470

E0470 is covered if A-C met:

A. An arterial blood gas $PaCO_2$, done while the beneficiary is awake and breathing the prescribed FIO_2, **is ≥52 mm Hg**; and
B. **Sleep oximetry** demonstrates oxygen saturation ≤88% for greater than or equal to a cumulative 5 minutes of nocturnal recording time (minimum recording time of 2 hours), done **while breathing oxygen at 2 LPM or the beneficiary's prescribed FIO_2 (whichever is higher)**; and
C. The medical record shows that, prior to initiating therapy, obstructive sleep apnea (OSA) and treatment with continuous positive airway pressure (CPAP) has been considered and ruled out. Note: Formal sleep testing is not required if there is sufficient information in the medical record to demonstrate that the beneficiary does not suffer from some form of sleep apnea (OSA, central sleep apnea [CSA], and/or complex sleep apnea) as the **predominant cause of awake hypercapnia** or nocturnal arterial oxygen desaturation.

E0471

An E0471 device will be covered for a beneficiary with COPD in either ot the two situations below, depending on the testing performed to demonstrate the need.

Situation 1

For severe COPD beneficiaries who qualifed for an E0470 device, an E0471 **started any time after a period of initial use of an E0470 device** is covered if both criteria A and B are met.

A. An arterial blood gas (ABG) $PaCO_2$, done while **awake** and breathing the beneficiary's prescribed FIO_2, shows that the beneficiary's **PaCO2 worsens ≥7 mm Hg** compared to the ABG result performed to qualify the beneficiary for the E0470 device; and
B. **Facility-based polysomnography (PSG)** demonstrates oxygen saturation ≤88% for greater than or equal to a cumulative 5 minutes of nocturnal recording time (minimum recording time of 2 hours) while using an E0470 device that is not caused by obstructive upper airway events – i.e., apnea-hypopnea index (AHI) <5.

Situation 2

For severe COPD beneficiaries who qualified for an E0470 device, an E0471 device will be covered if, at a time no sooner than 61 days after initial use of the E0470 device, both of the following criteria A and B are met:

A. An ABG $PaCO_2$, done while awake and breathing the beneficiary's prescribed FIO_2, still remains ≥52 mm Hg.
B. **Sleep oximetry** while **breathing with the E0470 device** demonstrates oxygen saturation ≤88% for ≥5 minutes of nocturnal recording time (minimum recording time of 2 hours), done *while breathing oxygen at 2 LPM or the beneficiary's prescribed FIO_2 (whichever is higher)*.

LCD: L33800[24]

obstructive upper airway events-i.e., AHI less than 5 events/hour **while using an E0470 device.**

In the severe COPD group (Table 24–22), *pulmonary function testing is actually not required.* To qualify for a E0470 device an awake $PaCO_2$ while breathing the prescribed FIO_2 (or oxygen flow rate) is ≥52 mm Hg *and* sleep oximetry (sleep study not necessary) demonstrates ≥5 minutes with a SaO_2 ≤88% ***while breathing either oxygen at 2 LPM*** (or prescribed oxygen, if at a higher flow rate) are both required. The medical record must show that OSA and treatment with CPAP were considered but ruled out (formal sleep study not needed). Obtaining coverage of a BPAP with a backup rate is more complicated. Coverage of BPAP with a backup rate (E0471) requires demonstration of failure of treatment with a BPAP without a backup rate (E0470) at any time after starting the E0470 (situation 1) or no sooner than 61 days after initial issue of the E0470 (situation 2). In situation 1, demonstration of an increase in $PaCO_2$ while awake and breathing the prescribed FIO_2 shows a ≥7 mm Hg increase in the $PaCO_2$ compared to the value qualifying for an E0470 device, and a **facility-based PSG** shows significant desaturation (SaO_2 ≤88% for ≥5 minutes) while using the E0470 that is not caused by obstructive airway events. In situation 2, there must be an awake $PaCO_2$ ≥52 mm Hg while using the prescribed FIO_2, **and** *sleep oximetry* (sleep study not needed) while using the E0470 device demonstrates an SaO_2 ≤88% for ≥5 minutes while breathing oxygen at 2 LPM or the beneficiary's prescribed FIO_2 (whichever is higher) (minimum recording time of 2 hours). Basically situation 1 documents hypoventilation is worse and requires a PSG and situation 2 documents that hypoventilation has not improved and requires sleep oximetry.

HOME MECHANICAL VENTILATORS

HMVs can deliver BPAP-ST and VAPS (Tables 24–12 and 24–13). Some details of providing VAPS using these devices were provided in a previous section. HMVs differ from the usual devices used for RADs in several ways (Table 24–23). First, they are approved by the U.S. Food and Drug Administration (FDA) for invasive (via tracheostomy, E0465) or noninvasive ventilation (mask, E0466). They can provide pressure control or volume ventilation. Some devices (Trilogy, Trilogy-Evo by PR) provide an option to automatically titrate EPAP (AVAPS-AE option) and have an automatic backup rate option (Ti automatically set). The Astral (RedMed)

Table 24–23 Considerations of Home Mechanical Ventilator (HMV) versus Respiratory Assist Device (RAD)

Pro HMV versus RAD Devices	Con HMV versus RAD Devices
• Automatic EPAP • Can be used with tracheostomy or mask • Can provide mouth-piece ventilation, breath stacking to prevent atelectasis • Battery backup • Complex alarms • FSS provided (respiratory therapist home visits routine for equipment maintenance and adjustment)	• Expensive, monthly payment often ≥$1000 without a cap (= monthly payments as long as the HMV is being used). (no separate charges for ongoing mask, hose, and other supplies allowed) • No integrated humidification • RAD units are less expensive, payment for only 13 months • Until recently, HMVs not assessed by wireless modems

HMV, home ventilator; *FSS*, frequent and substantial servicing payment category; *RAD*, respiratory assist device; *EPAP*, expiratory positive airway pressure.

provides iVAPS and also has extended capability, including the ability to titrate EPAP. HMVs can be used with a battery, which allows emergency treatment if power fails or the device is to be used in an ambulatory mode (attached to a wheelchair). HMVs also have a "sip and puff" (mouth ventilation mode) option, allowing for intermittent oral ventilation, which permits a patient to be free from a mask for limited periods. HMVs have extensive alarms, as interruption of delivery of ventilation could be fatal to some patients. In general, the devices *do not contain integrated humidifiers*. An external humidifier can be supplied. *If an external humidifier is added, higher pressure settings may be needed to compensate for any pressure drop across the humidifier.* HMVs are covered under the *Frequently & Substantially Serviced* (FSS) payment category, which means respiratory therapist visits, masks, hoses, and humidifiers are bundled into the ventilator reimbursement (monthly rental for the duration of documented need) and are not separately billable.[24,46] While RAD reimbursement is capped at 13 months, monthly reimbursement for HMVs is over $1000/month on a **continual basis as long as the device is being used**. The FSS reimbursement does provide an increased level of DME care, including home visits. At the time of this writing, newer HMVs have the capability to communicate with cloud-based programs, though older devices require a data card download. Philips Respironics has decided to no longer provide home ventilators for sale in the US. However, a large number of the Philips devices are currently used by patients and will likely still be used for many years. At the time or writing the Trilogy but not the Trilogy Evo devices are under recall.

HMVs are indicated for many of the same conditions as typical RADs (home ventilators are covered by Medicare for the treatment of NMD, thoracic restrictive disease, and chronic respiratory failure consequent to chronic obstructive pulmonary disease),[46,47] but if prescribed, the medical record must document the reason the HMV was prescribed instead of a typical RAD device (Table 24–24).[24,47] While qualifications for RAD devices are documented in local carrier determinations (LCDs), the qualification for HMVs is under a national carrier determination (NCD). The NCD is difficult to find on the CMS website[46] and is embedded in LCDs for RAD devices[24] or in other documents published by DMACs.[48] The history of HMV qualifications is well summarized in an Office of the Inspector General (OIG) report evaluating the large increase in utilization of these devices.[47] The HMV is considered reasonable and necessary only when the "beneficiary has a severe condition in which the interruption of respiratory support could lead to serious harm." Usually, describing the need for daytime ventilation, a backup battery to address power outages and extensive alarms will suffice. Documentation of awake hypercapnia and multiple admissions for respiratory failure are often used to support use of an HMV. The diagnoses used to support the need for an HMV include J96.20 (acute or chronic respiratory failure/acute-on-chronic respiratory failure,

Table 24–24 Qualification for a Home Ventilator

Excerpt from L33800 LCD for Respiratory Assist Devices[24]:

Ventilators

The Centers for Medicare & Medicaid Services (CMS) National Coverage Determinations Manual (CMS Pub. 100-03) in Chapter 1, Part 4, Section 280.1[46] stipulates that ventilators (E0465, E0466, and E0467)* are covered for the following conditions:

"Neuromuscular diseases, thoracic restrictive, and chronic respiratory failure consequent to chronic obstructive pulmonary disease."

Each of these disease categories are comprised of conditions that can vary from severe and life-threatening to less serious forms. These ventilator-related disease groups overlap conditions described in this Respiratory Assist Devices LCD** used to determine coverage for bi-level positive airway pressure (PAP) devices. Each of these disease categories are conditions where the specific presentation of the disease can vary from beneficiary to beneficiary. For conditions such as these, the specific treatment plan for any individual beneficiary will vary as well. Choice of an appropriate treatment plan, including the determination to use a ventilator versus a bi-level PAP device, is made based upon the specifics of each individual beneficiary's medical condition. *In the event of a claim review, there must be sufficient detailed information in the medical record to justify the treatment selected.*

Sample documentation (requirements may vary):

- Beneficiary has a severe condition in which the interruption of respiratory support could lead to serious harm
- Need for battery backup and ability for daytime ventilation
- Severe daytime hypoventilation
- Frequent hospitalizations for hypercapnic respiratory failure

*Note: E0465 Home ventilator, invasive (with tracheostomy), E0466 Home Ventilator, Noninvasive, E0467 multifunction ventilator
**LCD (local carrier determination): L33800

unspecified as to associated hypoxia or hypercapnia), J96.10 (chronic respiratory failure, unspecified as to associated hypoxia or hypercapnia), or J96.12 (chronic respiratory failure with hypercapnia). Note that qualification for an HMV on the basis of respiratory failure is usually restricted to those with a NMD, thoracic cage disorder, or COPD.

When patients are admitted with respiratory failure, it is often impossible to qualify them for a typical RAD device quickly enough for discharge on the needed device. In this case, the HMV is often prescribed based on a diagnosis of respiratory failure. For some patients, a less-expensive RAD device may work, although at the time of this writing, RAD VAPS devices do not offer automatic titration of EPAP.

TRANSVENOUS PHRENIC NERVE STIMULATION

Although phrenic pacing for central sleep apnea is not an advanced PAP mode, it is a new advanced treatment for CSA and is briefly mentioned here as an advanced treatment mode for CSA including CSA due to medications. Transvenous phrenic nerve stimulation is an FDA-approved treatment for moderate-to-severe CSA (AHI ≥15/hour).[49-51] This indication does not specify the exact proportion of respiratory events that are central versus obstructive, but the pivotal trial required that the obstructive apnea index was ≤20% of the total AHI, central apneas were at least 50% of the total number of apneas and there were at least 30 central apnea events during the night. A central apnea index ≥5/hour and greater than the obstructive apnea index with a total AHI ≥15/hour would reasonable minimal requirements. The device is not routinely covered by Medicare or most insurance providers. However, coverage for the device can usually be obtained under "special circumstances" (pass-through payments). Transitional pass-through payments provide additional payment for new devices, drugs, and biologicals that met eligibility criteria for a period of at least two years but not more than three years while CMS gathers additional data on the cost of those items. The device (remedē system Zoll) is implanted by a cardiac electrophysiologist and consists of a pulse generator implanted below the clavicle, usually on the right, and a stimulation lead placed either in the left pericardiophrenic or right brachiocephalic vein near the phrenic nerve. Originally, a sensing lead was placed in the azygos vein, but now, sensing is performed via the stimulation lead. The device turns on automatically at night when the patient assumes a recumbent posture and is not moving. Stimulation of the phrenic nerve activates the diaphragm, eliminating central apnea. Use of the system in patients with a concomitant cardiac device is safe but requires special testing to document that the devices are not interacting. The need for magnetic resonance imaging (MRI) is a relative contraindication but the use of an MRI is conditionally approved (the reader should check the current criteria). In a pivotal randomized controlled trial, 51% of the patients with active stimulation had a 50% reduction in the AHI (compared to 11% in the control group (device implantated but not activated) with improvement in Epworth sleepiness scale value and quality of life in the active treatment group. The arousal index and the amount of REM sleep were improved with active pacing. The device usually functions in the asynchronous mode, with the rate of stimulation slightly below the patient's respiratory rate and automatic increase in stimulation amplitude, if needed. A different stimulation strength is often needed in the supine, left lateral, and right lateral positions. The 5-year outcomes show the near elimination of central apneas (central apnea index, CAI) but persistently increased AHI and oxygen desaturation index (ODI4), although they were significantly reduced from baseline. A study documented the efficacy of pacing in primary CSA,[51] and another potential group might be those patients with CSA associated with heart failure who cannot be treated with adaptive servoventilation. A tracing of breathing before and after stimulation is shown in Figure 24–20. While a

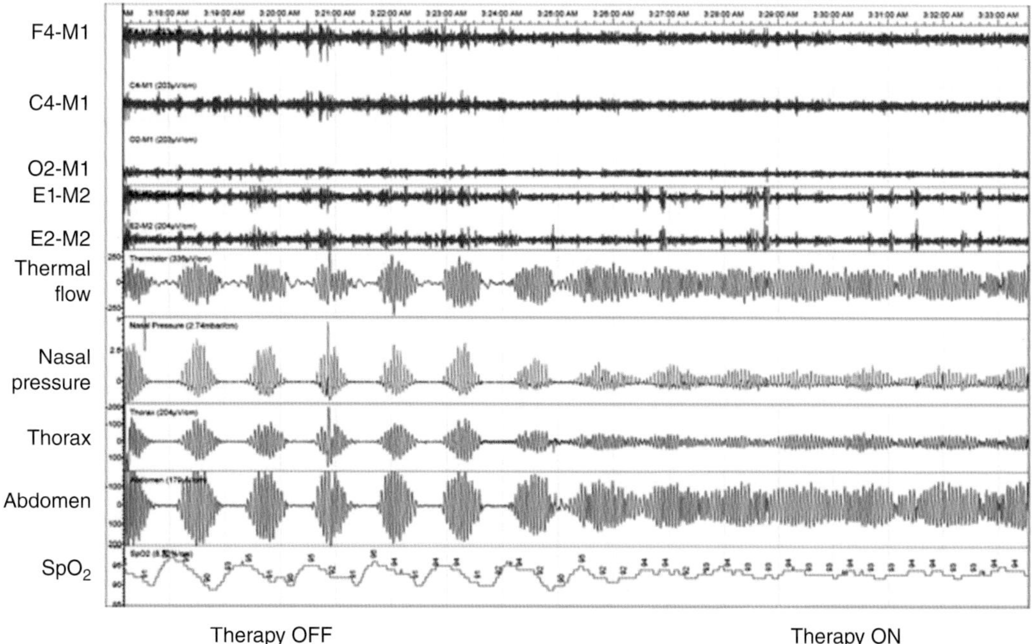

Figure 24–20 This figure illustrates the elimination of central apnea with pacing using Transvenous Phrenic Nerve Stimulation. Thermal flow is an oronasal thermal flow sensor. (From Abraham WT, Jagielski D, Oldenburg O, et al. Phrenic nerve stimulation for the treatment of central sleep apnea. *JACC Heart Fail*. 2015;3[5]:360-369.)

substantial amount of obstructive events can persist on pacing, additional treatment of the obstructive events can be combined with pacing. More information on the use of transvenous phrenic nerve stimulation to treat central sleep apnea is presented in chapter 30.

SUMMARY OF KEY POINTS

1. BPAP devices deliver a higher pressure in inspiration (IPAP) and lower pressure during exhalation (EPAP). The delivered pressure support [PS (IPAP – EPAP)] can be used to maintain an open airway or to augment tidal volume. The device is **triggered** (EPAP to IPAP) or **cycled** (IPAP to EPAP) either spontaneously, based on patient airflow, or by the device, based on specified criteria. For example, spontaneously cycled when the inspiratory flow has decreased to 25% of peak inspiratory flow.
2. BPAP in the spontaneous-timed mode (BPAP-ST), adaptive servoventilation (ASV), and devices with the ability to provide volume-assured PS (VAPS) are all advanced PAP devices. These (BPAP) devices have in common the ability to provide a backup rate that can be used to address central apnea or assist in treatment of hypoventilation. However, the goal and method of PS delivery differs among the devices.
3. The following summarizes PS in the various devices. The PS is fixed in BPAP-ST devices (specified with the goal of providing an adequate tidal volume). In ASV devices, the PS varies to stabilize breathing based on a target peak flow or minute ventilation determined as approximately 90-95% of the average peak flow or minute ventilation determined over a 3- or 4-minute moving time window, depending on the device. The PS is higher when peak flow (minute ventilation) is low compared to the target, and the PS is lower when peak flow (minute ventilation) is high compared to the target. ASV devices have a backup rate to address central apnea, but the goal is to stabilize ventilation without the need for the backup rate being triggered. An automatic EPAP option is available to address obstructive events. The PS in VAPS devices varies to provide the PS needed to maintain a target tidal volume (or target alveolar ventilation in ResMed VAPS devices) determined over a short moving time window. The PR VAPS device is called AVAPS (average volume-assured PS), and the ResMed VAPS device mode is called iVAPS (intelligent volume-assured PS).
4. BPAP-ST or VAPS devices in the spontaneous-timed mode consist of spontaneously triggered and cycled breaths and timed breaths (device triggered and cycled) based on the set backup rate and a specified inspiratory time (Ti) for PR devices or a cycle time window (inspiratory time range TiMin to TiMax) for ResMed devices). If no breath is spontaneously triggered in a time widow of 60/backup rate, a breath is triggered by the device. The duration of the breath is specified as a single value (Ti = inspiratory time) in PR devices and applies only to device triggered breaths. In ResMed devices the a cycle time window (TiMin to TiMax) applies to both spontaneous and device triggered breaths. In ResMed devices, the TiMin can be set to the desired Ti, with TiMax slightly longer. The backup rate is usually set one or two breaths less than the spontaneous rate for PR devices and ResMed BPAP-ST devices. ResMed iVAPs use an intelligent backup rate (iBR) and the target rate is the actual spontanous respiratory rate.
5. In ResMed devices, the device cycles within the TiMin to TiMax time window based on inspiratory flow. Within the cycle time window the device can be spontanteously cycled based on falling flow. However, the Ti = TiMin if the device would spontaneously cycle with a Ti shorter than TiMin or Ti = TiMax if the device fails to spontaneously cycle before TiMax.
6. BPAP-ST devices can be used to treat central apnea of all types as well as hypoventilation syndromes. These include disorders of control of ventilation, thoracic cage disorders, neuromuscular disorders, and some patients with the obesity hypoventilation syndrome. The EPAP is set to maintain an open airway (prevent obstructive apnea), and IPAP is set to prevent hypopnea and provide the needed PS for an adequate tidal volume. PS of 4 to 6 cm H_2O is typically used with BPAP devices in the spontaneous mode to treat OSA, but much higher PS is needed to allow device-triggered breaths to provide adequate flow and tidal volume (often 10 to 20 cm H_2O). The backup rate prevents central apnea and and a rate higher than the spontaneous respiratory rate can increase the delivered minute ventilation when PS has been optimized but minute ventilation is below goal.
7. ASV devices are used for hypocapnic CSA, including primary CSA, CSA with CSB (usually due to congestive heart failure), and treatment-emergent CSA. ASV can also be used to treat CSA due to medications (usually potent narcotics).
8. Volume-assured PS (VAPS) is used for hypoventilation syndromes. It functions similar to BPAP-ST, but the PS varies to provide a target tidal volume (or alveolar ventilation). VAPS devices address changes in the patient condition that might require higher PS. Therefore, VAPS devices are useful for empiric treatment of hypoventilation without a PAP titration study. Overall, studies have not documented an advantage in efficacy, adherence, or patient comfort compared to *carefully adjusted BPAP-ST*. However, in the real world where BPAP-ST may not be well adjusted, the VAPS devices have a useful role. The ResMed VAPS device (iVAPS) varies PS to meet a target alveolar ventilation. The intelligent backup rate (iBR) is triggered when the respiratory rate falls below two-thirds of the target respiratory rate and increases toward the target rate until a spontaneous breath occurs. The more the alveolar ventilation is below the target, the faster the iBR increases. While active, the iBR increases along with PS to meet the alveolar ventilation goal. However, the iBR does not exceed the target tidal volume.
9. *The delivery of an adequate tidal volume depends on both an adequate PS and an adequate Ti.* In patients with neuromuscular weakness or chest wall disease, flow may fall quickly during inspiration, prompting an earlier-than-desired device cycling from IPAP to EPAP. An *inadequate* Ti will prevent delivery of an adequate tidal volume. In ResMed BPAP-ST and iVAPS devices, one may specify the TiMin, which ensures an adequate Ti for all breaths. In PR devices, the specified Ti does not affect spontaneous breaths. However, the pressure-controlled (PC) mode is available on PR VAPS devices. In the PC mode the set Ti applies to all breaths. In the PC mode, breaths may still be spontaneous or device triggered. In ResMed VAPS devices the PAC mode allows specification of a fixed Ti for all breaths.
10. Treatment with BPAP-ST, ASV, or VAPS is best initiated in the sleep center with an NIV (NPPV) titration that allows selection of a good mask interface and adjustment of EPAP, PS, the backup rate, the rise time and Ti (or TiMin and TiMax). PS is increased to reach a target tidal volume of 8 mL/kg IBW. However, a lower goal (6 mL/kg IBW or lower) may be needed to allow adaptation to pressure. If minute ventilation is not optimized at the current settings (based on the SaO_2, transcutaneous PCO_2, or muscle rest assessment), increases

in the PS and/or backup rate can be tried. Patients with hypercapnia associated with OHS may benefit from tidal volumes up to 10 mL/kg IBW.

11. NIV (NPPV) treatment of hypoventilation disorders in stable patients can be initiated effectively in the clinic, hospital, or home if experienced respiratory therapists and well-structured protocols are in place. *This may be preferred in some patients with neuromuscular disorders or if the sleep center is not proficient at NIV titrations.*
12. BPAP devices are considered respiratory assist devices (RADs), E0470 without a backup rate and E0471 with a backup rate. RADs are used to treat hypoventilation or central sleep apnea disorders. Home mechanical ventilators (HMVs) can treat the same hypoventilation disorders as RADS but have more extensive capabilities. HMVs can deliver VAPS and also have an auto-adjusting EPAP option and battery backup. Daytime ventilation modes via a mouthpiece are also available. However, HMVs do not have an integrated humidifier. Use of HMVs is indicated with patients with neuromuscular disorders, thoracic cage disorders, and respiratory failure due to COPD when a RAD device is not adequate. The physician must indicate that, if an HMV is not provided, there may be a significant unfavorable impact on the patient's health.
13. It is important to understand the RAD criteria for reimbursement for BPAP with and without a backup rate. The criteria differ between patient types and are detailed. For some disorders, an awake ABG or sleep oximetry rather than a sleep study can qualify patients. In other disorders such as CSA/complex sleep apnea, efficacy of a BPAP device with backup rate must be demonstrated by PSG.
14. Detailed machine download information is available in cloud-based programs that allow the physician to follow adherence and the effectiveness of treatment with BPAP devices with a backup rate. Interventions for excessive leak are a first priority, as device algorithms may not work well with high and variable leak.

CLINICAL REVIEW QUESTIONS

1. A thin patient with an neuromuscular disorder (NMD) and a weight of 70 kg complains of nocturnal dyspnea. Pulmonary function testing reveals a forced vital capacity (FVC) less than 50% of predicted. Which of the following statements is true?
   A. Diagnostic PSG is not needed to qualify the patient for PAP treatment.
   B. BPAP **without** a backup rate must be used for initial treatment.
   C. An appropriate long-term tidal volume goal is 480 mL.
   D. Setting an adequate Ti for use in the BPAP-ST mode using a PR device ensures an adequate Ti.
2. A patient is being treated with ASV with an EPAP range (EPAPmin to EPAPmax) of 5 to 15 cm H_2O, and PS range of 0 to 20 cm H_2O, auto-rate, and Pmax 25. The table below shows download results. What intervention is most appropriate?

Average use (days used)	7 hours 10 min
Pmax	25 cm H_2O
90% EPAP	10 cm H_2O
90% PS	10 cm H_2O
% patient triggered breaths	85%
AHI	20 events/hour
Obstructed apnea index	1 event/hour
Clear airway apnea index	4 events/hour
Hypopnea index	16 events/hour
Average large leak	2 hours 10 minutes

90% PS and EPAP means the value is exceeded only 10% of the time.

   A. Change the EPAP range to 5 to 15 and PS range 10 to 25 cm H_2O.
   B. Change the PS range to 10 to 20 cm H_2O; maintain the same EPAP setting.
   C. Intervention for large leak
   D. Change EPAPmin to 10 cm H_2O; same PS setting.
3. A thin patient weighing 70 kg with NMD is using BPAP with a PR device delivering AVAPS in the ST mode. The table shows settings and results of a recent download. The IPAPmax was *reduced to 15 cm H_2O due to pressure intolerance*. What intervention do you recommend?

Parameter	Value
Mode	ST
EPAP	5 cm H_2O
Actual average tidal volume	450 mL
Target tidal volume	560 mL
IPAPmin/IPAPmax	10/15 cm H_2O
Average IPAP	14.9 cm H_2O
Ti	1.2 seconds
Backup rate	15 bpm
Respiratory rate (average)	18 bpm
% patient triggered breaths	80%
Ti/Ttot (average)	0.24

   A. Increase the backup rate.
   B. Increase IPAPmax back to 20 cm H_2O.
   C. Increase Ti to 1.5 seconds.
   D. Change from ST to PC mode.
4. What is the rapid shallow breathing index in question 3 before changes were made in ventilation?
5. A 30-year-old male patient has primary CSA and an AHI of 30 events/hour with 70% central apneas. CPAP was not effective. What treatment mode do you suggest?
   A. ASV with autoEPAP
   B. ASV with fixed EPAP
   C. BPAP-ST
   D. AVAPS
6. A patient is undergoing a PAP titration after a diagnostic study revealed moderate OSA with no central apneas. On CPAP of 10 cm H_2O, he has no more obstructive events but frequent central apneas. The technologist changes to BPAP of 12/8 cm H2O with a backup rate of 12 breaths/min and a Ti of 1.5 seconds. The central apneas resolve, but instead, hypopneas occur when the backup rate is triggered. Obstructive apnea was not present on these settings. What is the most likely problem?
   A. The EPAP is too low.
   B. The PS is too low.
   C. The backup rate is too low.
   D. The Ti is too short.

7. A 40-year-old male patient is being treated for OHS. He had evidence of severe hypercapnia, but his AHI was only 20 events/hour. He was begun on AVAPS in the ST mode. Below are settings and download parameters. The patient originally complained of pressure intolerance, and machine settings were adjusted for adaptation. Now the patient states that the pressure was too low. Based on this data, what would you do?

Settings	
Mode	AVAPS, ST
8 mL/kg IBW = 625 mL	
Pmax	30 cm H_2O
EPAP	10 cm H_2O
IPAPmax	25 cm H_2O
IPAPmin	14 cm H_2O
Backup rate	12 breaths/min
Ti	1.5 seconds
Target tidal volume	500 mL
Download Information	
Average nightly use	4.5 hours
Average tidal volume	600 mL
% patient triggered breaths	90%
Average IPAP	18.6 cm H_2O
Average respiratory rate	14 breaths/min

A. Increase the Ti.
B. Increase the IPAPmax.
C. Increase the EPAP.
D. Increase the target tidal volume.
E. Increase the backup rate.

8. Which of the following are potential causes of a low tidal volume in a patient on a VAPS device?
A. High leak
B. Inadequate PS
C. Ti is too short.
D. PS limits inappropriate
E. All of the above

9. You are setting an iVAPS device for a patient with a height of 72 inches using a target respiratory rate of 15 breaths/min. As you scroll through the target alveolar ventilation (Va) values and view the computed values, which alveolar ventilation target do you pick (Options A–F)? Note that the actual Target Va options are incremented by 0.1, and all the options are not shown for convenience.

iVAPS Menu Options

Option	A	B	C	D	E	F
Height (inches)	72	72	72	72	72	72
Target rate (bpm)	15	15	15	15	15	15
Target Va (L/min)	5.2	5.7	6.1	6.5	6.9	7.3
MV (L/min)	7.1	7.6	8.0	8.4	8.8	9.2
VT (mL)	476	510	536	563	590	616
Vt/kg (mL/Kg IBW)	6.5	6.9	7.3	7.7	8.0	8.4

Vt//kg tidal volume is in mL per kg of ideal body weight (based on height). *Target rate,* target respiratory rate in breaths/min; *VT,* tidal volume (mL); *Va,* alveolar ventilation (L/min), *MV,* minute ventilation (L/min).

ANSWERS

1. A. The patient qualifies for a BPAP device with a backup rate on the basis of having an NMD and a FVC less than 50% of predicted under the RAD criteria. A **PSG for titration** of BPAP with a backup rate would be useful. Although BPAP without a backup rate is covered under RAD criteria, BPAP with a backup rate is also covered and should be used. An appropriate tidal volume goal would be 8 mL Kg/IBW × 70 kg = 560 mL. A lower target tidal volume goal might be needed for initial adaptation to positive airway pressure. In PR BPAP-ST devices, the Ti only specifies the Ti of device-triggered breaths. In ResMed devices, TiMin and TiMax are specified and affect both spontaneous and machine-triggered breaths. Setting an adequate TiMin (usually 1–1.2 seconds, depending on the respiratory rate) can ensure an adequate Ti.
2. C. ASV algorithms depend on accurate measurements of flow and ventilation. They function poorly in the setting of a large leak. Answer A is incorrect, as an EPAPmin of 5 cm H_2O + a PSmax of 25cm H_2O = 30 cm H_2O exceeds the Pmax of 25 cm H_2O (the device would not permit this setting). Answer B is a valid setting, and one could argue that a higher PSmin is needed for hypopneas. However, the first intervention should be correction of large leak. Answer D is incorrect, as this would not address the high leak, and higher EPAP addresses apnea but not hypopnea.
3. D. Change to PC mode. The average IPAP is essentially equal to IPAPmax, so the maximum PS allowed (10 cm H_2O is being delivered). Changing to the PC mode would mean all breaths have a Ti of 1.2 seconds. Although the set Ti is appropriate for the backup rate of 15 breaths/min (0.3 × 60/15 = 1.2), the actual respiratory rate is higher than the backup rate, and 80% of the breaths are NOT device triggered. Therefore, only 20% of breaths have a guaranteed Ti of 1.2 seconds. The overall average Ti/Ttot is 0.24, and average Ttot = 60/18 = 3.3 seconds (using the actual respiratory rate). If 100% of the breaths were device triggered, the average Ti/Ttot would be 1.2/3.3 = 0.36. Thus the spontaneous Ti must be much less than 1.2 seconds. The actual average Ti is approximately equal to the average (Ti/Ttot) × average (Ttot) = 0.24 × 3.3 = 0.79 seconds. This means the **spontaneous** Ti is much less than 1.2 seconds. Increasing the IPAP is incorrect because the patient has pressure intolerance. Increasing the Ti is not unreasonable, but this would affect only machine-triggered breaths (20% of breaths). Increasing the backup rate is not the best option, as the average rate is already high. While it might increase the percentage of machine-triggered breaths and the average Ti, it would be better to switch to the PC mode and deliver a higher tidal volume with a lower respiratory rate. However, if the PC mode were not available, that might be the only option. If the device allowed setting the TiMin for all breaths, then TiMin could be set to the desired Ti, and continuing the ST mode would be an option. The results from changing to the PC mode are shown below:

Effect of Changing Mode on Ventilation

Mode	ST	PC
EPAP	5	5
Target tidal volume	560 mL	536 mL
IPAPmin/IPAPmax	10/15	same
Ti	1.2 seconds	1.2

Effect of Changing Mode on Ventilation

Mode	ST	PC
Backup rate	15	15
Average respiratory rate (bpm)	18	14
Average tidal volume	**440 mL**	**540**
Average IPAP (cm H_2O)	14.9	14.9
% patient triggered breaths	80%	50%
Ti/Ttot (average)	0.24	**0.28**

4. The RSBI = 18/.45 = 40. The ideal RSBI is less than 40.
5. Answer: A. (ASV with autoEPAP). ASV will be the most comfortable treatment, and if breathing is stabilized, few machine-triggered breaths will be needed. Patients with primary CSA have hypocapnic CSA, and central apnea occurs when the $PaCO_2$ is below the apneic threshold (see Chapter 30). The patient had nearly 30% non-central events, and the autoEPAP option will handle these. BPAP-ST would be effective but would likely require more device-triggered breaths and higher fixed PS. AVAPS is not the most appropriate treatment, as the patient does not have hypoventilation. The goal is to stabilize breathing and prevent central apneas due to hypocapnia.
6. B. The PS is too low. PS of 4 cm H_2O would not be expected to deliver an adequate tidal volume or flow during device-triggered breaths in most individuals. Apnea is not present, and an EPAP of 8 cm H_2O is only slightly below the CPAP of 10 cm H_2O, which eliminated obstructive events. The Ti of 1.5 seconds is appropriate for a rate of 12 breaths/min (0.3 × 5 seconds = 1.5 seconds). Increasing the Ti would only affect device triggered breaths. Increasing the backup rate will not increase airflow and tidal volume during device-triggered breaths.
7. D. Increase the target tidal volume. *The actual tidal volume exceeds the target volume.* The patient is spontaneously breathing at a higher tidal volume. There is room to deliver higher IPAP, as the IPAPmax is 25 cm H_2O and the average delivered IPAP is only 18.6 cm H_2O (PS 8.6 cm H_2O). Increasing the backup rate will not be helpful, as the respiratory rate is already adequate.
8. E. All of the above. If download information shows a low tidal volume, all of the factors A–D should be considered. For example, in an AVAPS device, if the actual average IPAP is 19.6 and the IPAPmax is 20 cm H_2O, the device cannot increase PS. However, if the PS seems adequate, a low average Ti can reduce the delivered tidal volume. *One method is to compute an ideal Ti/Ttot as if all breaths were device triggered using set Ti and average Ttot = 60/actual respiratory rate.* If the actual average Ti/Ttot is much lower, this suggests the spontaneous Ti is lower than the specified Ti. High leak can decrease the ability of the device to determine tidal volume as well as decrease the effective mask pressure.
9. Option E (Va=6.9 L/min). This corresponds to an ideal tidal volume of 8 mL/kg of IBW. Of course, one would choose another value depending on the target tidal volume/kg IBW. One should remember that the computations to determine the Va assume a normal dead space (estimated based on the patient height). A higher Va target could be needed to deliver an appropriate actual Va. The ResMed titration guidelines recommend an increase in the target Va of .3 L/min every 5 minutes if significant desaturation or hypoventilation (based on the transcutaneous PCO_2) is still present on the current iVAPS settings.

REFERENCES

1. Berry RB, Chediak A, Brown LK, et al. Best clinical practices for the sleep center adjustment of noninvasive positive pressure ventilation (NPPV) in stable chronic alveolar hypoventilation syndromes. *J Clin Sleep Med.* 2010;6(5):491-509.
2. Selim B, Ramar K. Sleep-related breathing disorders: when CPAP is not enough. *Neurotherapeutics.* 2021;18(1):81-90.
3. Selim BJ, Wolfe L, Coleman JM III, Dewan NA. Initiation of noninvasive ventilation for sleep related hypoventilation disorders: advanced modes and devices. *Chest.* 2018;153(1):251-265.
4. Javaheri S, Brown LK, Randerath WJ. Positive airway pressure therapy with adaptive servoventilation: part 1: operational algorithms. *Chest.* 2014;146(2):514-523.
5. Javaheri S, Brown LK, Randerath WJ. Clinical applications of adaptive servoventilation devices: part 2. *Chest.* 2014;146(3):858-868.
6. American Academy of Sleep Medicine. *International Classification of Sleep Disorders,* 3rd ed. Darien, IL: American Academy of Sleep Medicine; 2014.
7. ResMed. *Sleep Lab Titration Guide.* 2022. Available at: https://document.resmed.com/en-us/documents/products/titration/s9-vpap-tx/user-guide/1013904_Sleep_Lab_Titration_Guide_amer_eng.pdf. Accessed August 28, 2022.
8. Javaheri S, Badr MS. Central sleep apnea: pathophysiologic classification. *Sleep.* 2023 9;46(3):zsac113. doi: 10.1093/sleep/zsac113.
9. Badr MS, Toiber F, Skatrud JB, Dempsey J. Pharyngeal narrowing/occlusion during central sleep apnea. *J Appl Physiol (1985).* 1995;78(5):1806-1815.
10. Javaheri S, Harris N, Howard J, Chung E. Adaptive servoventilation for treatment of opioid-associated central sleep apnea. *J Clin Sleep Med.* 2014;10(6):637-643.
11. Cao M, Cardell C-Y, Willes L, Mendoza J, Benjafield A, Kushida C. A novel adaptive servoventilation (ASVAuto) for the treatment of central sleep apnea associated with chronic use of opioids. *J Clin Sleep Med.* 2014;10(8):855-861.
12. Storre JH, Seuthe B, Fiechter R, et al. Average volume-assured pressure support in obesity hypoventilation: a randomized crossover trial. *Chest.* 2006;130(3):815-821.
13. Janssens J-P, Metzger M, Sforza E. Impact of volume targeting on efficacy of bi-level non-invasive ventilation and sleep in obesity-hypoventilation. *Respir Med.* 2009;103(2):165-172.
14. Jaye J, Chatwin M, Dayer M, Morrell MJ, Simonds AK. Autotitrating versus standard noninvasive ventilation: a randomised crossover trial. *Eur Respir J.* 2009;33(3):566-571.
15. Murphy PB, Davidson C, Hind MD, et al. Volume targeted versus pressure support non-invasive ventilation in patients with super obesity and chronic respiratory failure: a randomised controlled trial. *Thorax.* 2012;67(8):727-734.
16. Royer CP, Schweiger C, Manica D, Rabaioli L, Guerra V, Sbruzzi G. Efficacy of bilevel ventilatory support in the treatment of stable patients with obesity hypoventilation syndrome: systematic review and meta-analysis. *Sleep Med.* 2019;53:153-164.
17. Huang XA, Du YP, Li LX, et al. Comparing the effects and compliance between volume-assured and pressure support non-invasive ventilation in patients with chronic respiratory failure. *Clin Respir J.* 2019;13(5):289-298.
18. Shaughnessy GF, Gay PC, Olson EJ, Morgenthaler TI. Noninvasive volume-assured pressure support for chronic respiratory failure: a review. *Curr Opin Pulm Med.* 2019;25(6):570-577.
19. Nicholson TT, Smith SB, Siddique T, et al. Respiratory pattern and tidal volumes differ for pressure support and volume-assured pressure support in amyotrophic lateral sclerosis. *Ann Am Thorac Soc.* 2017;14(7):1139-1146.
20. Kelly JL, Jaye J, Pickersgill RE, Chatwin M, Morrell MJ, Simonds AK. Randomized trial of 'intelligent' autotitrating ventilation versus standard pressure support non-invasive ventilation: impact on adherence and physiological outcomes. *Respirology.* 2014;19(4):596-603.
21. Orr JE, Coleman J, Criner GJ, et al. Automatic EPAP intelligent volume-assured pressure support is effective in patients with chronic respiratory failure: a randomized trial. *Respirology.* 2019;24(12):1204-1211.
22. Nilius G, Katmadzi N, Domanski, et al. Non-invasive ventilation with intelligent volume-assured pressure support versus pressure-controlled ventilation: effects on the respiratory event rate and sleep quality in COPD with chronic hypercapnia. Int J Chron Obstruct Pulmon Dis. 2017;12:1039–1045.
23. Morgenthaler TI, Malhotra A, Berry RB, Johnson KG, Raphaelson M. Optimal NIV Medicare access promotion: patients with central sleep apnea: a technical expert panel report from the American College of Chest Physicians, the American Association for Respiratory Care,

the American Academy of Sleep Medicine, and the American Thoracic Society. *Chest*. 2021;160(5):e419-e425.
24. Centers for Medicare and Medicaid Services (CMS). *LCD L33800 Respiratory Assist Devices*. Available at: https://www.cms.gov/medicare-coverage-database/view/lcd.aspx?lcdid=33800&ver=26&bc=CAAAAAAAAAAA. Accessed December 23, 2021.
25. Javaheri S, Patel S. Opioids cause central and complex sleep apnea in humans and reversal with discontinuation: a plea for detoxification. *J Clin Sleep Med*. 2017;13(6):829-833.
26. Aurora RN, Chowdhuri S, Ramar K, et al. The treatment of central sleep apnea syndromes in adults: practice parameters with an evidence-based literature review and meta-analyses. *Sleep*. 2012;35(1):17-40.
27. Cowie MR, Woehrle H, Wegscheider K, et al. Adaptive servo-ventilation for central sleep apnea in systolic heart failure. *N Engl J Med*. 2015;373(12):1095-1105.
28. Aurora RN, Bista SR, Casey KR, et al. Updated adaptive servo-ventilation recommendations for the 2012 AASM Guideline: "The treatment of central sleep apnea syndromes in adults: practice parameters with an evidence-based literature review and meta-analyses." *J Clin Sleep Med*. 2016;12(5):757-761.
29. Bradley TD, Logan AG, Lorenzi Filho G, et al. ADVENT-HF Investigators. Adaptive servo-ventilation for sleep-disordered breathing in patients with heart failure with reduced ejection fraction (ADVENT-HF): a multicentre, multinational, parallel-group, open-label, phase 3 randomised controlled trial. *Lancet Respir Med*. 2024 Feb;12(2):153-166.
30. Mokhlesi B, Masa JF, Brozek JL, et al. Evaluation and management of obesity hypoventilation syndrome. An official American Thoracic Society Clinical Practice Guideline. *Am J Respir Crit Care Med*. 2019;200(3):e6-e24.
31. Gómez de Terreros FJ, Cooksey JA, Sunwoo BY, et al. Clinical practice guideline summary for clinicians: evaluation and management of obesity hypoventilation syndrome. *Ann Am Thorac Soc*. 2020;17(1):11-15.
32. Coleman JM, Wolfe LF, Kalhan R Noninvasive Ventilation in Chronic Obstructive Pulmonary Disease. Annals ATS. 2019;16(9):1091–1098.
33. Murphy PB, Brignall K, Moxham J, Polkey MI, Davidson AC, Hart N. High pressure versus high intensity noninvasive ventilation in stable hypercapnic chronic obstructive pulmonary disease: a randomized cross-over trial. *Int J Chron Obstruct Pulmon Dis*. 2012;7:811-818.
34. Macrea M, Oczkowski S, Rochwerg B, et al. Long-term noninvasive ventilation in chronic stable hypercapnic chronic obstructive pulmonary disease. An official American Thoracic Society Clinical Practice Guideline. *Am J Respir Crit Care Med*. 2020;202(4):e74-e87.
35. Hollier CA, Maxwell LJ, Harmer AR, et al. Validity of arterialised-venous P CO_2, pH and bicarbonate in obesity hypoventilation syndrome. *Respir Physiol Neurobiol*. 2013;188(2):165-171.
36. Volpato E, Vitacca M, Ptacinsky L, et al. Home-based adaptation to night-time non-invasive ventilation in patients with amyotrophic lateral sclerosis: a randomized controlled trial. *J Clin Med*. 2022;11(11):3178.
37. Priou P, Hamel JF, Person C, et al. Long-term outcome of noninvasive positive pressure ventilation for obesity hypoventilation syndrome. *Chest*. 2010;138(1):84-90.
38. Ackrivo J, Elman L, Hansen-Flaschen J. Telemonitoring for home-assisted ventilation: a narrative review. *Ann Am Thorac Soc*. 2021;18(11):1761-1772.
39. Masa JF, Benítez I, Sánchez-Quiroga M, et al. Long-term noninvasive ventilation in obesity hypoventilation syndrome without severe OSA: the Pickwick randomized controlled trial. *Chest*. 2020;158(3):1176-1186.
40. Budweiser S, Heinemann F, Fischer W, Dobroschke J, Wild PJ, Pfeifer M. Impact of ventilation parameters and duration of ventilator use on non-invasive home ventilation in restrictive thoracic disorders. *Respiration*. 2006;73(4):488-494.
41. Yoder EA, Klann K, Strohl KP. Inspired oxygen concentrations during positive pressure therapy. *Sleep Breath*. 2004;8(1):1-5.
42. Mokhlesi B, Won CH, Make BJ, Selim BJ, Sunwoo BY. Optimal NIV Medicare access promotion: patients with hypoventilation syndromes: A technical expert panel report from the American College of Chest Physicians, the American Association for Respiratory Care, the American Academy of Sleep Medicine, and the American Thoracic Society. *Chest*. 2021;160(5):e377-e387.
43. Patil SP, Collop NA, Chediak AD, Olson EJ, Vohra KP. Optimal NIV Medicare access promotion: patients with OSA: a technical expert panel report from the American College of Chest Physicians, the American Association for Respiratory Care, the American Academy of Sleep Medicine, and the American Thoracic Society. *Chest*. 2021;160(5):e409-e417.
44. Wolfe LF, Benditt JO, Aboussouan L, Hess DR, Coleman JM III. Optimal NIV Medicare access promotion: patients with thoracic restrictive disorders: a technical expert panel report from the American College of Chest Physicians, the American Association for Respiratory Care, the American Academy of Sleep Medicine, and the American Thoracic Society. *Chest*. 2021;160(5):e399-e408.
45. Hill NS, Criner GJ, Branson RD, Celli BR, MacIntyre NR, Sergew A. Optimal NIV Medicare access promotion: patients with COPD: a technical expert panel report from the American College of Chest Physicians, the American Association for Respiratory Care, the American Academy of Sleep Medicine, and the American Thoracic Society. *Chest*. 2021;160(5):e389-e397.
46. Centers for Medicare & Medicaid Services. *CMS Home Ventilator Requirements*. Available at: https://www.cms.gov/medicare-coverage-database/view/technology-assessments.aspx? Accessed January 22, 2023.
47. Office of Inspector General. *Escalating Medicare Billing for Ventilators Raises Concerns*. Available at: https://oig.hhs.gov/oei/reports/oei-12-15-00370.pdf. Accessed January 22, 2023.
48. Palmetto GBA. *Correct Coding and Coverage of Ventilators-Revised*. Available at: https://oig.hhs.gov/oei/reports/oei-12-15-00370.pdf. Accessed February 22, 2023.
49. Costanzo MR, Ponikowski P, Javaheri S, et al. Transvenous neurostimulation for central sleep apnoea: a randomised controlled trial. *Lancet*. 2016;388(10048):974-982.
50. Costanzo MR, Javaheri S, Ponikowski P, et al. Transvenous phrenic nerve stimulation for treatment of central sleep apnea: five-year safety and efficacy outcomes. *Nat Sci Sleep*. 2021;13:515-526.
51. Javaheri S, McKane S. Transvenous phrenic nerve stimulation to treat idiopathic central sleep apnea. *J Clin Sleep Med*. 2020;16(12):2099-2107.

Oral Appliance Treatment for Obstructive Sleep Apnea

Chapter 25

ORAL APPLIANCES

An oral appliance (OA) can be defined as a device inserted into the mouth for treatment of snoring or obstructive sleep apnea (OSA).[1-5] There are two main types: the tongue retaining/stabilizing devices (TRD/TSDs)[1-5,6] (Fig. 25–1) and the mandibular advancement devices (MADs) (Fig. 25–2). Other names for MADs include mandibular advancement splints (MASs), mandibular repositioning devices (MRDs), mandibular repositioning splints (MRSs) or mandibular repositioning appliances (MRAs). Treatment with OAs is abbreviated OAT in the literature. The TSD/TRDs hold the tongue in a forward position by retaining the tongue in a suction bulb. The MADs are attached to the dental arches and provide variable degrees of bite opening and mandibular advancement. A picture of the Herbst MAD is shown in Figure 25–3, and side views of a patient with and without the MAD in place are shown in Figure 25–4.

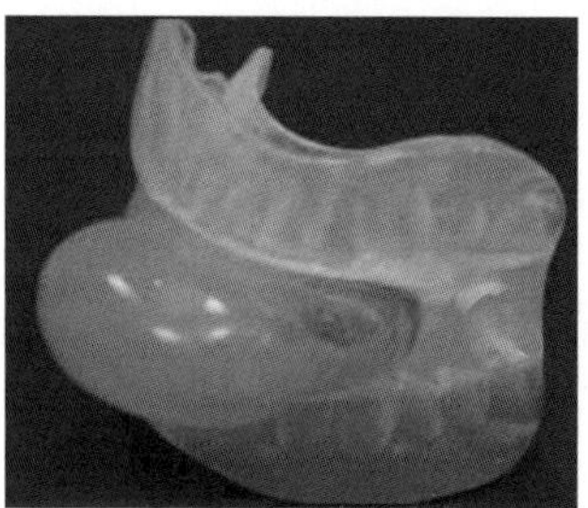
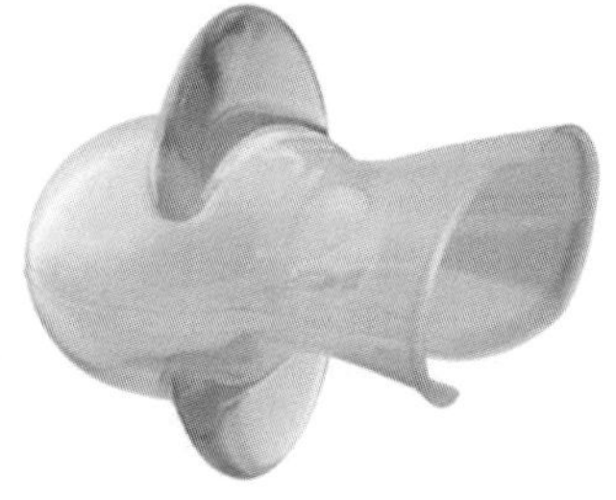

Figure 25–1 *Left,* Tongue retaining device (TRD). *Right,* Tongue stabilizing device (TSD). The TRD is fabricated for each patient, whereas the TSD comes in three standard sizes (small, medium, large). (From Berry RB. Fundamentals of Sleep Medicine. Philadelphia: Elsevier; 2012:350.)

INDICATIONS FOR ORAL APPLIANCES

An American Academy of Sleep Medicine (AASM) review of the evidence for the use of OAs was published in 2006.[1] The same year, the AASM published an update of practice parameters for use of OAs in the treatment of OSA.[2] Since that time, OAs have improved, and scientific literature supporting the use of OAs has grown considerably. An updated review of the use of OAs to treat OSA was published in 2014.[3] In 2015, the results of a meta-analysis and AASM clinical practice guidelines for the use of OA therapy for treatment of OSA and snoring were published.[4] While the guidelines were meant to update the 2006 guidelines, the 2006 guidelines are more extensive. Therefore, both will be summarized. The 2006 guidelines (Table 25–1) state that OAs are indicated for treatment of snoring and mild-to-moderate OSA. Patients with severe OSA should have an initial trial of CPAP. Surgery may precede OAs in patients for whom surgery is predicted to be highly effective. To ensure adequate treatment of OSA, polysomnography (PSG) or home sleep apnea testing (HSAT) should be performed after the OA is optimally adjusted. A dental specialist (usually the individual providing the OA) should follow-up with the patients every 6 months in the first year, then yearly. The purpose of follow-up is to monitor patient adherence, evaluate device deterioration

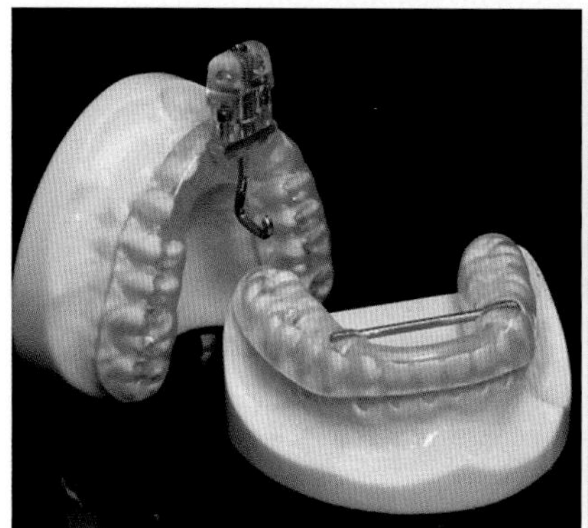
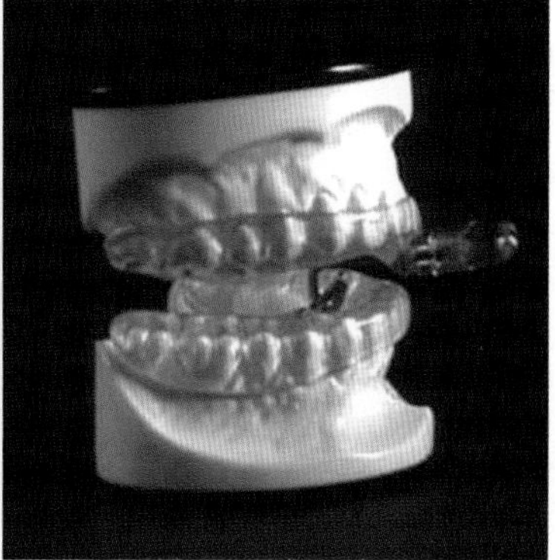
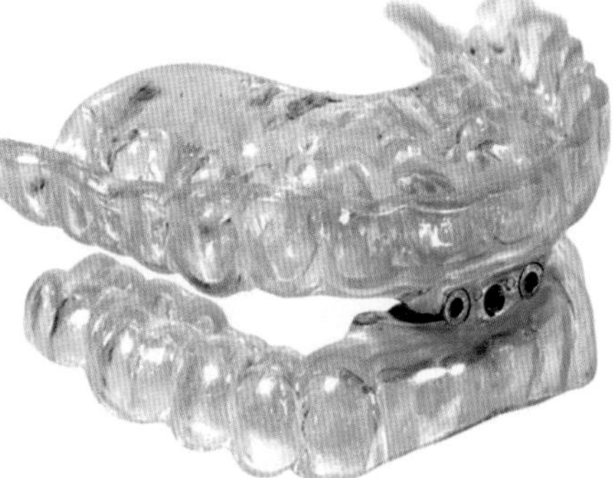

Figure 25–2 Versions of the Thornton anterior positioner (TAP) oral appliance, which consists of two separate arches connected by an advancing mechanism. *Left two panels,* The adjustment apparatus extends outward from the maxillary arch. This is turned to change the amount of protrusion of the mandible by moving the hook, which pulls the bar forward. *Right,* In the TAP-3 appliance, a key is used to advance the mandibular arch. (From Berry RB. *Fundamentals of Sleep Medicine*. Philadelphia: Elsevier; 2012:351.)

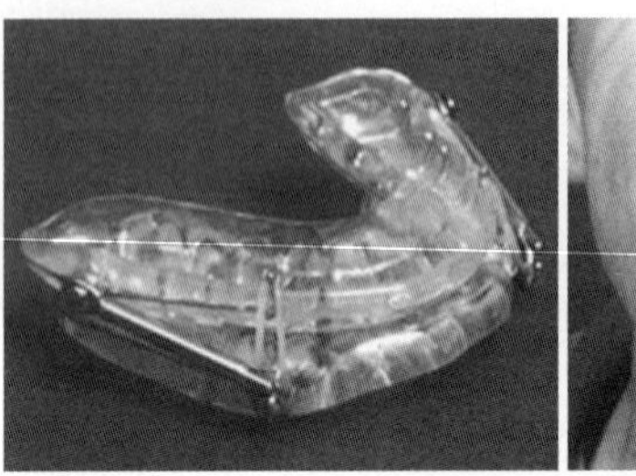
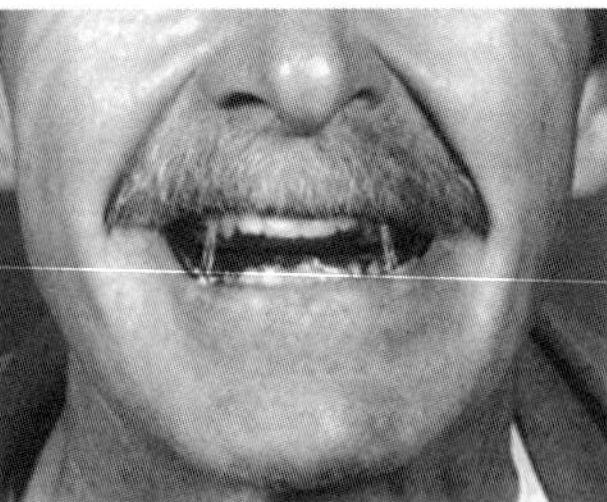

Herbst appliance

Figure 25–3 A Herbst Appliance. The side arms allow adjustment of the amount of mandibular protrusion. (From Berry RB. *Sleep Medicine Pearls*, 2nd edition. Philadelphia: Hanley & Belfus; 2003:175.)

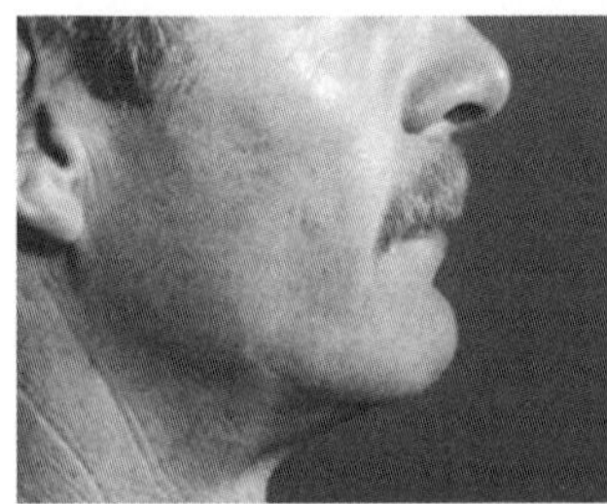
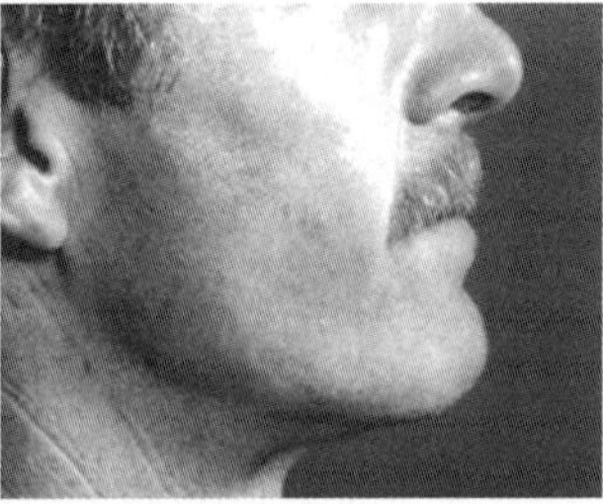

Before Herbst appliance

Figure 25–4 Side view of a patient with and without the Herbst oral appliance in place, showing the advancement of the mandible. (From Berry RB. *Sleep Medicine Pearls*, 2nd edition. Philadelphia: Hanley & Belfus; 2003:175.)

Table 25–1 Oral Appliance Treatment Guidelines (2006)

1. **Initial diagnosis:** Presence or absence of obstructive sleep apnea (OSA) must be determined before oral appliance (OA) treatment **for snoring or OSA**.
2. **Appliance fitting:** OA treatment should be managed by dental practitioners with training in sleep medicine and sleep-related breathing disorders.
3. **Cephalometrics** are not always needed, but if used, qualified professionals should perform and evaluate.
4. **Primary snoring:** The goal of OA treatment is to reduce snoring to a subjectively acceptable level.
5. **OSA:** Goals of treatment include resolution of clinical signs and symptoms of OSA, normalization of the apnea-hypopnea index (AHI), and oxyhemoglobin saturation.
6. OAs are indicated for treatment of **primary snoring** in patients who do not respond to or are not appropriate candidates for weight loss or sleep-position change.
7. OA treatment is indicated for **mild-to-moderate OSA**.
   a. OA is not as efficacious (reducing the AHI) as continuous positive airway pressure (CPAP) but is preferred by some patients.
   b. OA is indicated in cases of CPAP failure.
   c. OA treatment is indicated when there is failure of weight loss or side sleep position treatments.
8. OAs are not indicated for initial treatment of **severe OSA**. Upper-airway surgery may also supersede use of OA treatment in patients for whom surgery is predicted to be highly effective.

Adapted from Kushida CA, Morgenthaler TI, Littner MR, et al.; American Academy of Sleep Medicine. Practice parameters for the treatment of snoring and obstructive sleep apnea with oral appliances: an update for 2005. *Sleep*. 2006;29:240-243.

or maladjustment, evaluate the health of the oral structures and integrity of the occlusion, and assess the patient for signs and symptoms of worsening OSA. Intolerance and improper use of the device are potential problems. OAs can aggravate temporomandibular joint disease and cause dental misalignment and discomfort. A physician (usually the individual who referred the patient for an OA) should follow up with the patient to assess device adherence and the ongoing adequacy of the OAT for OSA. The 2015 clinical guidelines for OAT (Table 25–2) recommend OAT for snoring as well as for adult patients with OSA *(without regard to severity)* rather than no treatment. It was recommended that a qualified dentist use a custom titratable appliance over a non-custom

Table 25–2 2015 Clinical Practice Guideline for Treatment of OSA and Snoring with Oral Appliances

1. We recommend that sleep physicians prescribe oral appliances, rather than no therapy, for adult patients who request treatment of primary snoring (without obstructive sleep apnea). (Standard)
2. When oral appliance (OA) therapy is prescribed by a sleep physician for an adult patient with obstructive sleep apnea, we suggest that a qualified dentist use **a custom, titratable appliance over non-custom oral devices.** (Guideline)
3. We recommend that sleep physicians consider prescription of OAs, rather than no treatment, for adult patients with obstructive sleep apnea who are intolerant of continuous positive airway pressure (CPAP) therapy or prefer alternate therapy. (Standard)
4. We suggest that qualified dentists provide oversight—rather than no follow-up—of OA therapy in adult patients with obstructive sleep apnea to survey for dental-related side effects or occlusal changes and reduce their incidence. (Guideline)
5. We suggest that sleep physicians conduct follow-up sleep testing to improve or confirm treatment efficacy, rather than conduct follow-up without sleep testing, for patients fitted with OAs. (Guideline)
6. We suggest that sleep physicians and qualified dentists instruct adult patients treated with OAs for obstructive sleep apnea to return for periodic office visits—as opposed to no follow-up—with a qualified dentist and a sleep physician. (Guideline)

Meta-analysis findings:

- OAs were effective for treatment of snoring.
- OAs reduced the apnea-hypopnea index (AHI).
- CPAP reduced the AHI more than OAs.
- OAs (all types analyzed) improved the minimum SpO_2 and reduced the oxygen desaturation index (ODI)—most evidence was for custom titratable OAs.
- OAs were not shown to improve sleep architecture (% REM) but did decrease the arousal index.
- OAs reduced daytime sleepiness (subjective).
- OAs improved quality-of-life measures.
- Custom OA treatment was associated with the most improvement in blood pressure.

From Ramar K, Dort LC, Katz SG, et al. Clinical practice guideline for the treatment of obstructive sleep apnea and snoring with oral appliance therapy: an update for 2015. *J Clin Sleep Med*. 2015;11(7):773-827.

device. In general, custom OAs are more effective and better tolerated than non-adjustable monobloc OAs.[7-9] As per the 2006 guidelines, follow-up testing to document OA efficacy and follow-up with both dental and medical providers are recommended. The 2015 guidelines recognize that some patients with severe OSA who do not tolerate positive airway pressure (PAP) and do not want surgery (or are surgical failures) may benefit significantly from OAT, even if the apnea-hypopnea index (AHI) is not normalized by OAT. The AASM practice parameters for surgical modifications of the upper airway recommend that patients with severe OSA should initially be offered PAP therapy, while those with moderate OSA should initially be offered either PAP therapy or OA therapy.[10] That is, the AASM practice parameters for upper-airway surgery suggest that OAs be considered before upper-airway surgery for moderate OSA (although some patients will prefer surgery). OAs can also be used in patients with OSA who have failed uvulopalatopharyngoplasty (UPPP).[11] For severe OSA, the treatment of choice is PAP, second is complex upper-airway surgery, and last is OA therapy. OAs may substantially reduce the AHI in severe OSA,[12] and in one study, they normalized the AHI in about 25% of patients.[5] As noted, the *2015 guidelines recommend OAs be prescribed for patients with OSA (all severities) who are intolerant to CPAP or prefer alternative treatment (rather than no treatment)*. As will be discussed, though OAs rarely lower the AHI as well as CPAP in patients with OSA of all severities, they may improve daytime sleepiness and other indices of successful treatment equal to CPAP likely because of superior adherence to OAT.[5,13]

MECHANISM OF ACTION

One might assume that the mechanism of action of OAs is to increase the retroglossal space. However, the improvement is actually in the velopharyngeal (retropalatal) area in most studies. Airway imaging and nasal endoscopy have shown anteroposterior (AP) mandibular protrusion predominantly increases the caliber of the airway at the retropalatal area via lateral expansion and displacement of parapharyngeal fat pads,[14-16] while the tongue and tongue-base muscles shift forward. The lateral widening from AP movement was attributed to stretching of soft tissue connections between the tongue, soft palate, and lateral pharyngeal walls. Isono studied patients under general anesthesia and found that anterior movement of the mandible widened the *retropalatal airway as well as at the base of the tongue* in the passive pharynx of patients with OSA.[15] Using dynamic magnetic resonance imaging (MRI), Brown et al. found that mandibular advancement had two mechanisms of action that increased airway size. The first mechanism of upper airway enlargement by mandibular advancement (most relevant to patients with a low AHI) was due to forward movement of the tongue. The second mechanism of increased airway size with mandibular advancement was lateral airway expansion via a direct connection between the lateral walls and the lateral mandible (ramus of the mandible). The connection is postulated to be the pterygomandibular raphe. In the majority of patients the anterior portion of the tongue moved forward (tongue elongation).[14] Another MRI study showed TSDs actually increased airway size more than an MRA.[16] These devices directly move the tongue forward. However, difficulty with device retention during sleep and adherence limit this potential benefit. The retropalatal location of the greatest effect of OA on airway size is surprising given the finding from other studies that patients with airway collapse in the oropharyngeal area are more likely to respond to OAT.[17,18] Marques et al. found that a posteriorly placed tongue and less upper-airway collapsibility was associated with the best response to OA therapy.[18] It is apparent that both airway shape and size AND upper-airway collapsibility determine the effects of the OA. The effect of an OA on upper-airway muscle activity remains uncertain.[5] Awake studies have shown an increase in genioglossus activity in normal individuals wearing a TRD but a decrease in OSA patients wearing a TRD. Studies during sleep have shown a decrease in genioglossus activity with progressive mandibular advancement. Another study on CPAP showed no change in muscle activity with progressive mandibular advancement. If the passive upper airway is kept patent by an OA, one would not expect an increase in muscle activity simply due to the MAD. There is more discussion of the mechanisms by which OA improves upper airway patency in the next section and the section on patient evaluation.

EVALUATION OF THE PATIENT AND PREDICTION OF SUCCESS OF OA TREATMENT

Each candidate for an OA should be examined by a qualified dentist to determine whether an OA is feasible and safe from a dental standpoint (Table 25–3). The dental examination should focus on the temporomandibular joint (TMJ), evidence or history of bruxism, quality of dental occlusion, the presence of significant periodontal disease, overall dental health, and protrusive ability. The patient must also be able to open their mouth sufficiently (no trismus). A minimum number of stable teeth in each arch (usually eight) is required for stabilization and retention of the OA.[19,20] During evaluation for the suitability of OAT, cephalometric or dental radiographs may be indicated.[21] The patient's occlusion type should be noted. Three classes (types) of skeletal occlusions are illustrated in Figure 25–5. Cone beam computed tomography (CT) is increasingly used in dental medicine, as it requires less

Table 25–3 Dental Evaluation for OSA and Device Adjustment

Pre-OA evaluation

- PSG or HSAT in all patients (even if only snoring expected)
- Dental evaluation
    - Condition of teeth and gums (minimum 8–10 teeth in each arch)*
    - Edentulous patients can use a tongue-stabilizing device
    - Type of occlusion (class III not a good candidate)
    - TMJ (moderate-to-severe problems are a contraindication)
    - Bruxism (complicates treatment, may improve with OA treatment, requires a "hardy" OA)
    - Ability to open mouth and protrude mandible at least 3 mm

Titration

- Progressive adjustment (protrusion) based on symptoms, bed partner report of snoring, HSAT, oximetry, or PSG
- During PSG, some devices may be titrated

OSA, obstructive sleep apnea; *OA*, oral appliance; *PSG*, polysomnography; *HSAT*, home sleep apnea testing; *TMJ*, temporomandibular joint.
*Some dentists recommend minimum of 6 teeth in the upper and 6 teeth in the lower jaw with at least 2 teeth in each quadrant

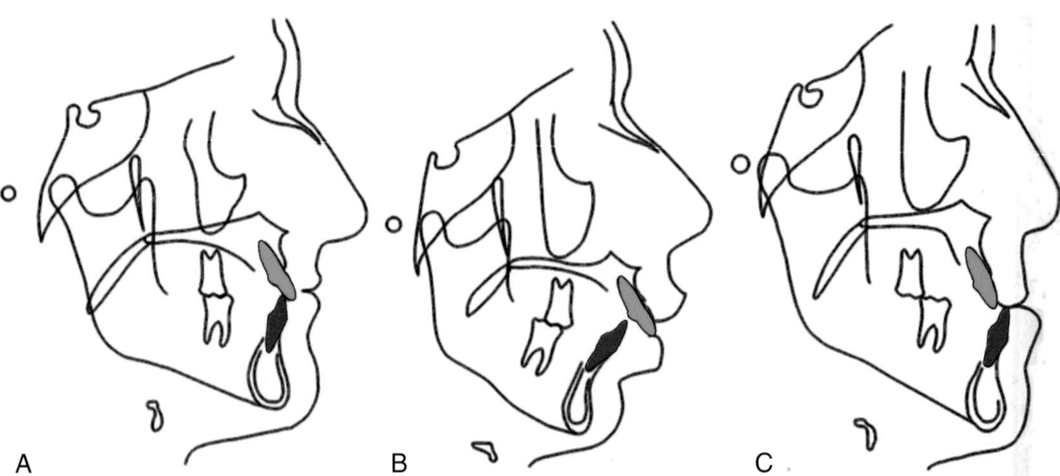

Figure 25–5 Lateral Cephalometric Views of Three Distinct Skeletal Occlusions. **A**, A skeletal class I occlusion. There is a nearly ideal skeletal and dental balance. **B**, A skeletal class II malocclusion (overjet or retrognathia). There is mandibular deficiency. Note the everted lower lip and distance between the upper and lower incisors. **C**, A skeletal class III occlusion with mandibular hyperplasia and maxillary hypoplasia (or prognathia). The upper incisor is behind the lower incisor. (From Conely RS. Orthodontic considerations related to sleep disordered breathing. *Sleep Med Clin.* 2009;5:71-89.)

radiation than conventional CT and also provides volumetric information.[22] One might expect that patients with mandibular deficiency (retrognathia) would benefit the most from an OA, but the amount of improvement is somewhat unpredictable. The tongue position and nature of upper-airway collapsibility are also important. It also should be noted that dental imaging in the upright position or imaging during wakefulness may not reflect upper-airway anatomy during sleep. As noted, some studies suggest that patients with collapse mainly in the retroglossal area rather than the retropalatal area might be expected to improve the most with an MAD (although awake studies have shown the major change in upper-airway size with MADs in the retropalatal area). Awake nasal endoscopy in the supine position may eliminate concerns about positional effects, and drug-induced sleep endoscopy (DISE) may better reflect what happens during supine sleep. DISE was found to help predict OAT success.[23,24] Patients showing increased airway dimensions at the level of the velum and/or oropharynx with a jaw thrust may benefit the most from OAT. However, at this point, DISE should be considered investigational unless the patient is being considered for other treatment such as hypoglossal nerve stimulation or upper-airway surgery. The use of PSG airflow was used to predict a response to OAT.[25] Several studies found that positional OSA[26,27] and OSA responding to lower levels of CPAP[28] may respond better to OAT. On the other hand, Sutherland and coworkers[29] did not find patients with positional OSA responded better to OAT. This difference in findings could be due to the fact that the amount of time an individual with positional OSA spends in the supine position can significantly alter the effect of an OA on the overall AHI. Determination of endotypes using advanced analysis of PSG found that *less ventilatory instability (low loop gain)*,[30,31] *mild-to-moderate upper-airway collapsibility, and a higher arousal threshold* were associated with a better response to OAT.[31] Dutta and coworkers[32] used routine polysomnography and clinical characteristics to predict a good response to OAT using machine learning techniques. Sophisticated functional imaging, by means of 3D models obtained from low-dose CT scans of the upper airway coupled with computational fluid dynamics (CFD) simulations,[33] gives information about the upper-airway volume, upper-airway resistance, and several cephalometric measurements. Using this technique, a study concluded that MADs act by increasing the total upper-airway volume, predominantly from an increase in the velopharyngeal volume. Responders showed a significant increase in the total upper-airway volume with MAD treatment, while there was no significant increase in non-responders. However, such a technique is unlikely to be used as a routine clinical evaluation. As summarized by Sutherland,[5] no technique that is practical for routine clinical use accurately predicts a good response to OAT.

Overall, the following factors have been associated with improvement with MADs: *younger age, female sex, supine-dependent OSA, a lower body mass index (BMI), lower AHI, lower CPAP pressure, a posteriorly placed tongue, lower loop gain, mild-to-moderate upper-airway collapsibility, and a high arousal threshold.* As noted, there is some disagreement in the literature about some of these factors. In any case, these associations only partially predict MAD treatment efficacy, and a significant fraction of patients (up to one-third) may not have improvement with MAD treatment.

EXCLUSIONS AND CONTRAINDICATIONS

A patient with Class III occlusion (prognathia) would not be a candidate for an MAD. Patients must have a minimum of eight healthy teeth in each arch (some references say at least six teeth each of the upper and lower jaw with at least 2 teeth in each quadrant).[1,19,20] Edentulous patients may be treated with a TRD/TSD. Treatment with dental implants can permit future MRA treatment in patients with insufficient dentition at the time of evaluation for an OA. Patients must be able to *open the mouth adequately and be able to voluntarily protrude the mandible at least 3 mm for OA insertion* and must have the ability to voluntarily protrude the mandible. Moderate-to-severe TMJ disease or inadequate protrusive ability are contraindications. Mild TMJ dysfunction may improve with the jaw positioned anteriorly during sleep. Bruxism is not a contraindication, as bruxism may improve in some patients with OAT. However, bruxism during sleep can damage some types of OAs, and a history of bruxism may alter the choice of the type of OA (a "hardy" device is needed). An experienced dental practitioner should evaluate patients with bruxism for suitability for an OA.

TONGUE STABILIZING/RETAINING DEVICES

TSD/TRDs hold the tongue in a forward position by retaining the tongue in a suction bulb. TRDs are a monobloc device *customized to each patient*, while TSDs are manufactured in three prefabricated sizes (small, medium, and large). The patient inserts the tongue into the device and gently pumps the bulb to apply suction. Once the tongue is inserted, the bulb is released, and the tongue is held forward by suction. A study by Deane et al.[6] found TSDs to significantly reduce the AHI, although not quite as well as MRAs. In addition, the TSD had a lower compliance rate and was more likely to come out during the night. Dort et al.[34] made a TSD-like device themselves and performed a randomized crossover trial of a suction and non-suction (NS) device. The suction device produced a significant decrease in the AHI compared to the NS device (15.5 [±17.6] to 8.9 [±7.6]). A similar device is commercially available. Lazard and coworkers[35] performed a retrospective review of patients treated with a TRD and found a complete or partial response in 71% of patients with a decrease in the mean AHI from 38 to 14/hour ($p < 0.001$). There were 33 users (52%) and 30 nonusers (48%) after a mean follow-up period of 5 years. While not as well tolerated as customizable TRDs, the TSDs (Fig. 25–1) may be an affordable alternative for some patients. Two currently available TSDs are the AVEOtsd® and the Good Morning Snore Solution (by MPowrx). The AVEOtsd® is cleared by the U.S. Food and Drug Administration (FDA) as an anti-snoring device, made from Dow Corning silicone, and has been available since 1999. Purchase of the device no longer requires a prescription (cost about $90). Many other TSD knockoffs are available at lower prices, but quality is questionable. The Good Morning Snore Solution is FDA cleared as an anti-snore device and costs about $90 to $100 and does not require a prescription. The AVEOtsd® rests on the lips while the Good Morning Snore Solution rests on the gums. TSDs are marketed as antisnore devices but are effective for mild to moderate OSA in some patients.

MANDIBULAR ADVANCEMENT DEVICES

MADs can have a monobloc (boil and bite) fixed configuration or are custom-fitted appliances (requiring impressions) that can be adjusted to change the amount of mandibular protrusion (advancement). There are also OAs that do not require impressions but do allow adjustment of protrusion. In the 2015 AASM meta-analysis of OAT,[4] devices were classified as *custom titratable, custom non-titratable, non-custom titratable, and non-custom non-titratable.* This classification shows the wide variety of OAs that are available. Characteristics of an ideal MAD are listed in Table 25–4. The ideal device has coverage of both arches (for good retention) and is adjustable (protrusion can be changed). One study compared a custom-made OA with a thermoplastic OA for the treatment of mild OSA. The custom-made device was more effective.[7] A later randomized trial of readymade versus custom-made OAs found custom devices resulted in better efficacy and adherence.[8,9] However, custom-made devices are typically much more expensive. The 2015 clinical guidelines for OAT state, "When oral appliance therapy is prescribed by a sleep physician for an adult patient with obstructive sleep apnea, we suggest that a qualified dentist use a *custom, titratable appliance* over non-custom oral devices." OAs are now viewed by the FDA as class II medical devices and, as such, must adhere to more detailed standards with special controls.[36] Oral devices for both snoring and mild OSA are now considered to be in the same category. "FDA cleared" refers to a device the FDA has allowed to be marketed through the 510(k) process based on substantial equivalence to a legally marketed predicate device. It does not sound as glamorous as "FDA approved," but clearance is a critical step on the path to market for many devices. An FDA approved device (class III medical device) has undergone rigorous review and an approval process.

Table 25–4 Characteristics of an Ideal Oral Appliance

Titratable	Ability to adjust both vertical opening and amount of mandibular advancement
Full tooth coverage	Makes certain the upper and lower teeth are fully engaged in the appliance to prevent undesirable tooth movement and for adequate retention of the device
Posterior support	The upper and lower components should have contact in the posterior aspect for stabilization of the temporomandibular joint
Mandibular mobility	Allows free movement of mandible during sleep and may be beneficial if bruxism is present
Ability to breathe through the mouth (adequate mouth opening)	Improves breathing
Adequate tongue space	Assists in preventing tongue from collapsing into the oropharyngeal airway

From Baily D. Oral appliance therapy in sleep medicine. In: Bailey DR, ed. *Dentistry's Role in Sleep Medicine.* Sleep Medicine Clinics; 2010;5(1):91-98.

MEDICARE AND INSURANCE COVERAGE OF OA(MADS)

The Centers for Medicare and Medicaid Services (CMS) has published specific guidelines for coverage of OA devices.[37] There are four durable medical equipment (DME) medical area contractors (MACs), but they all use the same local coverage determination (LCD; L33611) (Table 25–5). Only E0486 devices, as defined herein, are deemed medically necessary (Table 25–6). Most private insurance providers follow CMS guidelines (or have slight variations). Custom-made OAs for OSA are categorized as DME under Medicare. DME includes a broad range of items used by a patient in a home

Table 25–5 Local Coverage Determination (LCD): Oral Appliances for Obstructive Sleep Apnea (L33611)[37]

A custom fabricated mandibular advancement oral appliance (E0486) used to treat obstructive sleep apnea (OSA) is covered if criteria A-D are met:

A. The beneficiary has a face-to-face clinical evaluation by the treating practitioner prior to the sleep test to assess the beneficiary for OSA testing.

B. The beneficiary has a Medicare-covered sleep test that meets one of the following criteria (1–3):

1. The apnea-hypopnea index (AHI) or respiratory disturbance index (RDI) is greater than or equal to 15 events/hour with a minimum of 30 events; or,
2. The AHI or RDI is greater than or equal to 5 and less than or equal to 14 events/hour with a minimum of 10 events and documentation of:
   a. Excessive daytime sleepiness, impaired cognition, mood disorders, or insomnia; or,
   b. Hypertension, ischemic heart disease, or history of stroke; or,
3. If the AHI is >30 or the RDI is >30 and meets either of the following (a or b):
   a. The beneficiary is not able to tolerate a positive airway pressure (PAP) device; or,
   b. The treating practitioner determines that the use of a PAP device is contraindicated.

C. The device is ordered by the treating practitioner following a review of the report of the sleep test. (The practitioner who provides the order for the oral appliance could be different from the one who performed the clinical evaluation in criterion A.)

D. The device is provided and billed for by a licensed dentist (DDS or DMD).

If all of these criteria (A–D) are not met, the custom fabricated oral appliance (E0486) will be denied as not reasonable and necessary.

RDI is the AHI determined by home sleep testing (HST).
L33611 approved for CGS Administrators LLC, Noridian Health Care Solutions LLC which are DME MACs (durable medical equipment [DME] medical area contractors [MAC] or DMACs)

setting to serve a medical purpose, such as wheelchairs, PAP devices, canes, and more. To bill Medicare for DME items, a practice (or company) must enroll as a DME supplier (participating or non-participating). The current Medicare payment depends on the jurisdiction, but in general, it is about 80% of the allowable cost (about 1100-$2000 allowable cost). A participating supplier is one that agrees to accept assignment for all services furnished to Medicare beneficiaries during a 12-month period, beginning January 1 of each year. By completing the CMS-460 Participating Physician or Supplier Agreement Form each year, the supplier accepts the Medicare allowed amount as payment in full. Medicare will pay 80% of that amount to the supplier/provider. The supplier can collect the 20% coinsurance, any unmet deductible, and payment for statutorily non-covered services from the beneficiary at the time of service. By accepting assignment, the reimbursement is sent to the supplier. For example, the provider would normally charge $2000 for the service. However, the Medicare allowable charge is $1600. If the provider/supplier is participating, Medicare will pay the provider/supplier $1280 directly and the patient (or coinsurance) will pay $320 to the provider/supplier.

Table 25–6 Requirements for an E0486 Device

To be coded as E0486, custom fabricated mandibular advancement devices must meet all of the following criteria:

- Have a fixed mechanical hinge at the sides, front, or palate
  A fixed hinge is defined as a mechanical joint containing an inseparable pivot point. Interlocking flanges, tongue-and-groove mechanisms, hook-and-loop or hook-and-eye clasps, elastic straps or bands, monoblock articulation, traction-based articulation, compression-based articulation, etc. (not all-inclusive), do not meet this requirement.
- Able to protrude the individual beneficiary's mandible beyond the front teeth when adjusted to maximum protrusion
- Incorporate a mechanism that allows the mandible to be easily advanced by the beneficiary in increments of 1 millimeter or less
- Retain the adjustment setting when removed from the mouth
- Maintain the adjusted mouth position during sleep
- Remain fixed in place during sleep so as to prevent dislodging the device
- Require no return dental visits beyond the initial 90-day fitting and adjustment period to perform ongoing modification and adjustments to maintain effectiveness

TITRATION/ADJUSTMENT OF OAS

After OAs are fabricated, they are usually adjusted by the dentist caring for the patient for fit and comfort. A number of titration protocols are utilized.[38] The maximal protrusion is determined using a George gauge (top portion abuts anterior incisors of the maxilla and the lower part the anterior incisors of the mandible, lower portion can slide forward as the mandible is protruded allowing measurement of the amount of protrusion). In general, the initial protrusion setting is at or less than 70% of maximal protrusion. Starting at a more conservative protrusion with slow advancement is more likely to be tolerated. In one approach, patients are instructed to slowly increase mandibular protrusion until symptoms improve (cessation of snoring and improvement in sleep quality) or until either the maximum protrusion is reached or further advances are not tolerated. At that time, PSG or HSAT is ordered to determine whether the device is effective. Unfortunately, a large percentage of patients have a higher than desired AHI on OA based on this approach. This is likely due in part to reliance on patient titration at home. If the device is not effective, further adjustment could be performed by the patient or dentist with repeat PSG or HSAT. However, use of multiple nights of PSG is an expensive option. Other OA titration approaches include home advancement followed by further titration during PSG[39,40]; remote-controlled mandibular protrusion during PSG[41-43]; endoscopy to evaluate changes in airway anatomy with an MAD in place[44]; titration of a temporary appliance, with either one or multiple nights of PSG/HSAT study[38,40]; adjustment based on HSAT[38]; and home titration based on a combination of patient symptoms and oximetry.[45,46]

Titration during PSG is one method to improve the effectiveness of OAT. The sleep technologist or patient has the "key" to advance the mandible until OSA is controlled. A remotely controlled MAD has been used and the mandible advanced until respiratory events were controlled or until further advances were not tolerated.[41-43] The results of the remotely controlled OA PSG titration (with a temporary OA/dentral tray) were highly predictive of the effectiveness of chronic OAT with a permanent device. In another study, a combination of home adjustment and PSG OA titration was used. First, patients were directed to adjust their devices at home.[40] Then, during a subsequent PSG with the OA in place, further adjustment was allowed per protocol (increased protrusion in 1-mm increments). Of the patients completing the protocol, 55% were successfully treated (AHI <10 events/hour) after home titration. A total of 64.9% of patients were successfully treated overall. Thus, some patients will likely need further adjustments either during or after PSG documenting the efficacy of OAT.

Fleury et al.[45] used a combination of patient symptoms and the arterial oxygen desaturation index by pulse oximetry to adjust the OA with a subsequent PSG on the adjusted OA. They found that 25% of advancements were for an elevated oxygen desaturation index (ODI) despite resolution of symptoms, 20% were motivated by persistent symptoms with normal ODI, and 50% were motivated by symptoms and increased ODI. The use of high resolution oximetry was able to achieve success in 63% of patients using a Herbst device.[46] In summary, the most practical approach appears to be home titration assisted with some form of objective home monitoring, such as oximetry. Today, a number of consumer smartphone applications (with a separate oximetry device) are available, and some have the ability to monitor oxygen saturation.

ADHERENCE TO OA TREATMENT

Studies of adherence to OAT have almost always relied on patient report.[47] The option of thermal sensors to determine objective adherence is available.[48-50] However, this currently remains an option for research studies due to the added expense. One study did show that there was relatively little difference between objective and reported adherence, but these individuals were likely motivated.[51] The initial adherence to OAT is usually around 80%. However, OA adherence rates tend to decrease with the duration of use.[47] An analysis by Sutherland et al.[47] of adherence in several long-term studies[52-59] is shown in Figure 25–6. A study comparing outcomes of an OA versus UPPP found a 4-year adherence rate of 62%.[60] In a questionnaire study of OA patients 5 years after starting treatment, 64% of respondents (46% returned the questionnaire) were using the OA. Of these, 93% were using the OA more than 4 nights/week. Of those stopping OAT, the causes were discomfort (44%), little or no effect (34%), and the patient changing to CPAP treatment (23%).[61] A meta-analysis of treatment usage in trials comparing OA and PAP therapies[62] indicated that PAP was used 1.1 hours per night less than OAs over the trial period. Greater OA usage could contribute to the equivalent health effects observed, despite the presence of higher residual OSA (OAT compared to CPAP). However, a limitation of this analysis was that, while PAP usage was *objective, OA usage was determined by patient report.* Sutherland et al.[47] reviewed five short-term treatment studies and two longer-term follow-up studies (about 1 year), all using **objective monitoring** with thermal sensors. The average short-term use was 6.5 hours, and average long-term use was 6.7 hours. Defining adherence as a percentage of patients using the device for more than 4 hours, the adherence ranged from 33% to 96%. A long-awaited 12-month objective adherence study (OA vs. CPAP) with objective adherence available in both treatments was performed.[63] Objective adherence with MADs and CPAP was comparable and consistent over time, although *self-reported adherence to OAT was higher.* Self-reported adherence was higher with MADs than objective adherence, while subjective PAP use tended to underestimate objective adherence. The adherence with OAT and PAP were similar, giving rise to an interesting discrepancy between objective and self-reported adherence between OAT and CPAP. The findings of this study need to be confirmed, but they show the importance of objective adherence monitoring. There are a number of factors associated with poor adherence. A meta-analysis of studies on factors influencing adherence found that nonadherent patients reported more side effects with OAT than users and tended to discontinue the treatment within the first 3 months.[64] The most common self-reported reason for discontinuing treatment was a lack of treatment effect or discomfort or pain. Custom-made OAs were preferred, and increased adherence with custom-made OAs was reported in comparison to ready-made appliances. In summary, objective adherence to OAT appears to be good in the short term (at least up to 1 year) but declines considerably over time. Like CPAP treatment, OAT adherence would likely benefit from regular physician-patient interaction. Studies comparing adherence in OAT and CPAP have tended to show better adherence with OAT than PAP, *but a reliable comparison awaits more studies with objective adherence in* ***both*** *treatments.*

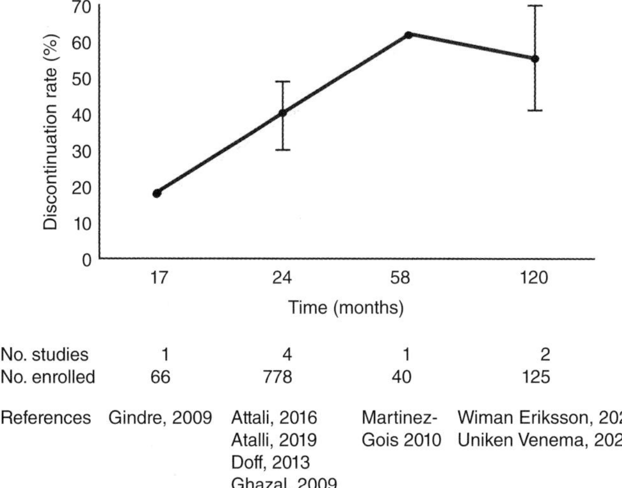

Figure 25–6 A plot of the discontinuation rate of oral appliance use over time based on eight studies. (From Sutherland K, Dalci O, Cistulli PA. What do we know about adherence to oral appliances? *Sleep Med Clin.* 2021;16[1]:145-154.)

SIDE EFFECTS AND COMPLICATIONS

Common OAT side effects included TMJ pain, myofascial pain, tooth pain, excessive salivation, TMJ sounds, dry mouth, gum irritation, and morning-after occlusal changes (Box 25–1). These phenomena were observed in a wide range of frequencies from 6% to 86% of patients.[1] Patients undergoing TRD/TSD treatment may report a sore tongue or difficulty with the device slipping off during the night. Hammond et al.[65] found that the most commonly reported OA (MAD) side effects found that

Box 25–1 SIDE EFFECTS OF ORAL APPLIANCES

1. Minor and temporary
   A. Excessive salivation
   B. Tooth pain
   C. TMJ tenderness
   D. Tongue pain (TRD/TSD)
2. Chronic and more severe
   a. Tooth movement (decreased overjet and overbite in most patients)
   b. TMJ dysfunction or pain
   c. Gum disease
   d. Dry mouth

TMJ, temporomandibular joint; *TRD/TSD,* tongue retaining/stabilizing devices. Based on Marklund M. Subjective versus objective dental side effects from oral sleep apnea appliances. *Sleep Breath.* 2020;24[1]:111-117.

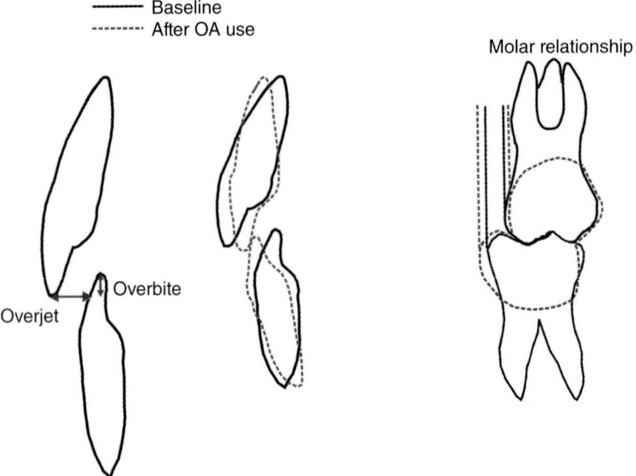

Figure 25–7 Changes in Overbite and Overjet with oral appliance treatment. These are often actually beneficial changes, as many patients have a large overjet at baseline. The molar changes are also noted. In most studies, the patients were not aware of these changes. However, forward movement of the teeth with respect to the mandible tends to decrease mandibular protrusion and could reduce device efficacy. (From Marklund M. Subjective versus objective dental side effects from oral sleep apnea appliances. *Sleep Breath.* 2020;24[1]:111-117.)

the most commonly reported were jaw discomfort, tooth tenderness, excessive salivation, and dry mouth. Several studies have found long-term changes in dental occlusion, but the results vary between studies. The changes are relatively mild in most patients. A study by Rose and coworkers[66] found the anteroposterior position of the molars and the inclination of upper and lower incisors changed with OAT (mean follow-up of 30 months). No skeletal changes in mandibular position were noted. In another study, only 4% noted long-term bite changes, while 41% noted temporary bite changes. In this study, 25% had objective evidence of bite change.[67] Marklund and coworkers[68] used plaster casts before and after OAT for over 3 years and found occlusal changes in most patients. Overjet and overbite decreased, the lower molars repositioned anteriorly in relation to the upper molars, and irregularity of the lower front teeth increased (Fig. 25–7). The changes in overbite and overjet were beneficial to most patients. Most patients did not notice these changes. However, the *forward shift in teeth tends to decrease the amount of mandibular protrusion and can reduce the efficacy of OAT.* Some studies have found that patients tend to notice early "temporary changes" but not long-term changes. Hamoda et al.[69] confirmed that bite changes progressed in their patients with an average of 12 years of OA use. Pliska and coworkers[70] found similar results. In the morning after removal of the OA, patients may experience TMJ discomfort or muscle tenderness. *Many dentists/physicians have patients wear a bite splint (repositioning splint) in the morning to help minimize changes in TMJ positioning and muscle tenderness.* An alternative is to have patients perform jaw exercises.[71,72]

EFFECTIVENESS OF ORAL APPLIANCES AND COMPARISON WITH CPAP

The effectiveness of OAs has been evaluated in many studies and depends on the severity of sleep apnea and type of OA. Sutherland et al.[29] reported on 425 patients treated with an OA (Fig. 25–8) and found that about two-thirds of all patients had a >50% decrease in the AHI and about one-third had normalization of the AHI. The improvement did differ across severities of OSA. *Of interest, almost 25% of patients with severe OSA had normalization of the AHI.* The 2015 clinical practice guidelines for OAT[4] were based on a meta-analysis of a large number of studies to determine the effect of OAT on a number of parameters. The results showed that OAT reduced the AHI by 13.6 events/hour, the oxygen desaturation index by 12.8 events/hour, and the arousal index by 10.8 events/hour. The minimum oxygen saturation was 3.1% higher (improved) on OAT. The Epworth sleepiness scale decreased by 3.81. Compared to CPAP, the AHI on OAT was 6.3 events/hour higher. For some parameters of interest, the analysis for overall OAs versus custom titratable versus custom non-titratable OAs found differing results. The reader should consult the reference for details.[4] A meta-analysis of the studies comparing CPAP and an OAT by Schwartz and coworkers[62] found that, as expected, CPAP reduced the AHI more than OAs but that improvement in daytime sleepiness was similar; *reported* adherence was higher with OAT.

Given the difficulties with CPAP adherence, a number of studies of the effect of OAT on cardiovascular or quality-of-life outcomes have been performed.[4] A few selected studies will be discussed here. A randomized controlled crossover trial of the effect of OAT on blood pressure compared active OAT and control OAT (no mandibular advance) in patients with an AHI ≥10 events/hour, with each treatment arm of 4 weeks duration.[73] Treatment with active OA was associated with a 50% reduction in the mean AHI; the mean 24-hour diastolic blood pressure dropped by 1.8 mm Hg, and awake systolic blood pressure dropped by 3.3 mm Hg compared to the control. These values are similar to the results of studies on the effect of CPAP treatment on blood pressure. Bratton and coworkers[74] found that, among patients with OSA, both CPAP and MADs were associated with reductions in blood pressure. A network meta-analysis did not identify a statistically significant difference between the blood pressure outcomes associated with these therapies. Phillips et al.[75] compared cardiovascular outcomes (24-hour blood pressure, arterial stiffness), neurobehavioral outcomes (subjective sleepiness, driving simulator performance), and quality-of-life outcomes (Functional Outcomes of Sleep Questionnaire, Short Form-36) between 1 month of OAT or CPAP treatment in patients with moderate-to-severe OSA using a crossover design (patients had both treatments). CPAP was more efficacious than

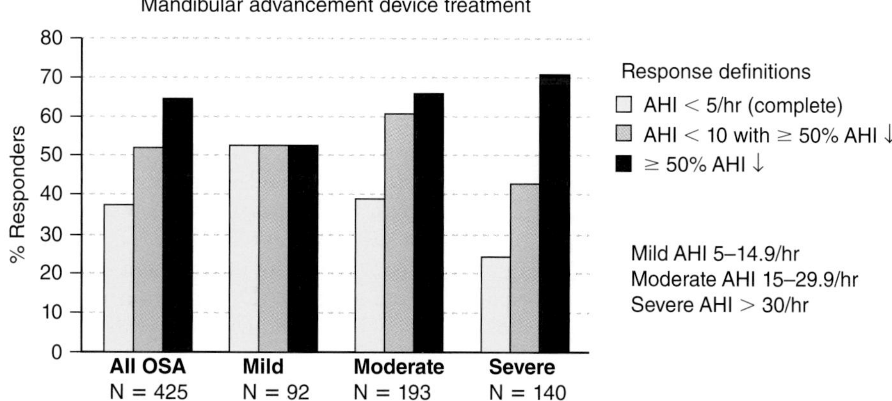

Figure 25–8 The percentage of responders to oral appliance treatment (see response definitions) in mild, moderate, and severe obstructive sleep apnea (OSA). Results of the study showed that about one-third of all patients with OSA and 25% with severe OSA had normalization of the AHI. Overall, about two-thirds had a ≥50% drop in the AHI. (From Sutherland K, Takaya H, Qian J, Petocz P, Ng AT, Cistulli PA. Oral appliance treatment response and polysomnographic phenotypes of obstructive sleep apnea. *J Clin Sleep Med.* 2015;11[8]:861-868.)

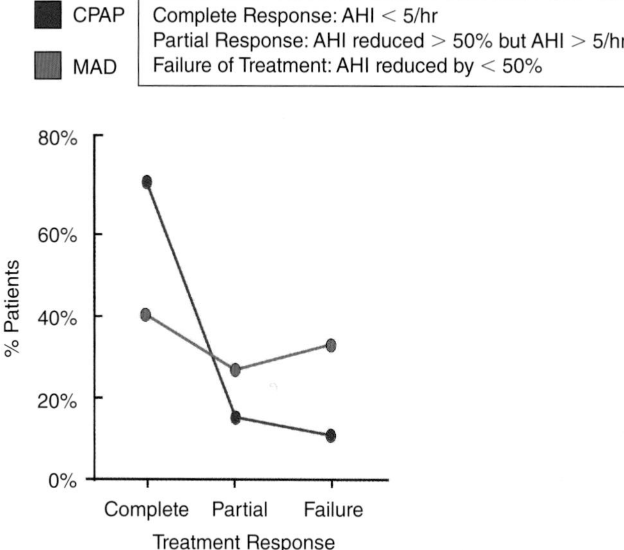

Figure 25–9 The results of treatment with continuous positive airway pressure (CPAP) and a mandibular advancing device (MAD) in a group of patients with moderate-to-severe obstructive sleep apnea (OSA; apnea-hypopnea index [AHI] 25.6 event/hour). The average AHI was 4.6 events/hour on CPAP and 11.1 events/hour on an MAD. (Plotted using data from Phillips CL, Grunstein RR, Darendeliler MA, et al. Health outcomes of continuous positive airway pressure versus oral appliance treatment for obstructive sleep apnea: a randomized controlled trial. *Am J Respir Crit Care Med.* 2013;187[8]:879-887.)

MADs in reducing AHI (CPAP AHI, 4.5 events/hour vs. MAD AHI, 11.1 events/hour) (Fig. 25–9), but **reported** compliance was higher on MAD treatment (MAD, 6.50 hours vs. CPAP, 5.2 hours). Neither treatment improved 24-hour blood pressure, but daytime sleepiness, driving simulator performance, and disease-specific quality of life *improved on both treatments by similar amounts.* However, MAD treatment was superior to CPAP for improving four general quality-of-life domains. More participants chose to use OAT than CPAP at the end of the study. This study shows that OAT and CPAP have similar outcomes with slightly better control of the AHI with CPAP and better adherence with OAT (OAT adherence self-reported). This result is typical of a number of studies comparing OAT and CPAP.

A study comparing OAT and CPAP in a group of veterans with post-traumatic stress disorder (PTSD). These individuals often have difficulty with CPAP due to claustrophobia. The study found equal improvement in PTSD measures and quality of life with both treatments.[76] CPAP was more effective at reducing the AHI, but reported adherence was better on OAT. Successful reduction in cardiac septal thickness (reversal of ventricular hypertrophic remodeling)[77] with successful MAD treatment for 6 months was demonstrated with maintenance of blood pressure similar to that pretreatment. In those NOT successfully treated with an MAD, no improvement in the AHI was noted. More studies on the effects of MAD treatment on cardiovascular outcomes are anticipated.

COMBINATIONS OF OAT AND OTHER TREATMENTS

OAT can be combined with other treatments for OSA. For example, OAT can be used for residual OSA after surgery. Use of OAT in patients with persistent sleep apnea after UPPP was reported by Millman and coworkers[11] in 18 patients. The post-UPPP AHI was 37.2 events/hour, and the arterial oxygen saturation (SaO_2) nadir was 84%. With OAT, the AHI fell to 15.3 events/hour, and the SaO_2 nadir was 87.9%. With the addition of a Herbst device, 10 of the patients had a fall in the AHI to less than 10 events/hour. OAs can be used with CPAP; some are specially designed for this purpose. The required level of CPAP may decrease. A small pilot study of patients with residual OSA on OAT used a combination of autoCPAP and OAT. The treatment pressure was reduced by about 2 cm H_2O.[78] Another small pilot study found that hybrid treatment with an OA and low levels of CPAP was well tolerated.[79] The use of CPAP and an OA was utilized in individuals intolerant to CPAP but in whom the AHI remained elevated on monobloc OAT.[80] Combined treatment lowered the required level of CPAP and reduced the AHI when compared to MAD treatment alone. Combined treatment has potential, but the ability to comfortably use both treatments at the same time is a challenge. One area of possible improvement is the design of an OA that is not associated with mouth leak if using a nasal CPAP interface. Tong et al. used a novel one-way valve to address this issue.[81] In this study, the combination of CPAP and a novel OA (addition of a covering with a one-way valve [inhalation but not exhalation]) reduced the epiglottic pressure swings (less upper airway resistance) with a lower level of delivered CPAP. Combined CPAP and OAT reduced the therapeutic CPAP requirements by 35% to 45% and minimized epiglottic pressure swings. The authors concluded that the combination of CPAP and an OA may be a therapeutic alternative for patients with incomplete responses to OAT alone and those who cannot tolerate high CPAP levels.

FOLLOW-UP

The success of OAT depends on ongoing involvement of both the dentist constructing the OA and the physician treating the patient for OSA (Table 25–7). The 2006 practice parameters do not mandate repeat sleep testing while using an OA for treatment of **snoring**. The most recent guidelines recommend repeat sleep testing for all severities of OSA with the patient wearing the OA to document effectiveness.[4] HSAT and PSG are acceptable methods. During PSG, some devices can be titrated using a protocol determined by the treating dentist and sleep physician. The 2015 AASM clinical guidelines for OAT state, "We suggest that sleep physicians conduct follow-up sleep testing to improve or confirm treatment efficacy, rather than conduct follow-up without sleep testing, for patients fitted with oral appliances." If significant sleep apnea persists on OAT, several options are possible. These include increased protrusion, weight loss (if obese), or the addition of positional treatment (if patients have positional OSA on the OA). There are patients who will elect another trial of CPAP treatment or request referral for evaluation for surgery (including hypoglossal nerve stimuation). The 2006 practice parameters recommend follow-up visits with the dentist who fabricated the OA device every 6 months, then yearly. This is to ensure side effects are not significant and the amount of protrusion is optimized. The 2015 OAT guidelines state, "We suggest that qualified dentists provide oversight rather than no follow-up of OA therapy in adult patients with obstructive sleep apnea, to survey for dental-related side effects or occlusal changes and reduce their incidence."

Table 25–7 Follow-up After Oral Appliance Treatment

1. Follow-up sleep testing is not indicated after OA treatment of primary snoring.
2. Follow-up sleep testing with OA in place IS indicated after OA treatment of OSA after final adjustments of fit have been performed for all OSA severities. (PSG or HST acceptable)
3. Follow-up visits with dental specialist until optimal fit and efficacy is demonstrated.
4. Follow-up dental visits every 6 months for first year and annually thereafter to detect change in occlusion.
5. Regular visits with clinician supervising treatment of OSA.
6. Repeat sleep study with OA in place if signs or symptoms of OSA worsen or recur.

HST, home sleep test; *OA*, oral appliance; *OSA*, obstructive sleep apnea; *PSG*, polysomnography.

Follow-up with the clinician directing sleep-apnea treatment is also indicated to assure that OSA symptoms are controlled and do not recur. The 2015 clinical practice guidelines for OAT of OSA state, "We suggest that sleep physicians and qualified dentists instruct adult patients treated with OAs for obstructive sleep apnea to return for periodic office visits—as opposed to no follow-up—with a qualified dentist and a sleep physician." *If symptoms return on OAT, repeat sleep testing with the OA in place is indicated. The average lifespan of most OAs is 3 to 5 years.* The involvement of the dentist is needed to be certain the MAD is in good repair. A new OA device will likely be needed in 3 to 5 years.

SUMMARY OF KEY POINTS

1. The presence or absence of OSA must be determined before OAT for snoring or suspected OSA. It is important to determine whether OSA or snoring is being treated. If OSA is present, the severity has implications for treatment selection and the probability of success with OAT.
2. The OA should be fitted by a qualified dental professional. Use of a custom titratable device is recommended.
3. OAs are indicated for treatment of primary snoring and mild-to-moderate OSA. CPAP may be more effective at reducing the AHI in mild to moderate OSA but patients may prefer OAT. Reported OA adherence was better than objective CPAP adherence in some studies comparing OA and CPAP treatment and treatment outcomes did not differ.
4. CPAP rather than OAT should be the first treatment for severe OSA. If CPAP is not accepted, upper airway surgery or an OA should be considered. OA treatment of severe OSA is much better than no treatment at all. Up to 25% of patients with severe OSA may have normalization of the AHI, and significant improvement in the AHI on OAT is common in a significant fraction of these patients.
5. PSG or HSAT (with the patient wearing the OA) is needed to document the effectiveness of the OA (after adjustment) for treatment of OSA.
6. OAs are believed to work by enlarging the retropalatal upper airway in the lateral dimension and by movement of the tongue base forward in some patients. A connection between the lateral pharyngeal wall and mandible is believed to be the reason mandibular advancement increases lateral airway dimensions.
7. Titration of OAs is possible with PSG (some devices) and may improve the efficacy. Other options are to use oximetry or HSAT to titrate the OA.
8. Follow-up of OAT should include both visits with a dentist to address OAT side effects and any changes in dentition or occlusion (as well as the condition of the OA) and a physician visits to assess if symptoms of OSA are well controlled and to verify continued adherence to treatment.
9. A significant number of patients stop using the OA within 3 years (40% to 50%), and there is some change in occlusion in a majority of patients. In some cases, the change in occlusion is beneficial. In most cases, the patient does not notice the changes in occlusion.
10. Thermal sensitive sensors are available to monitor objective adherence with OAT. Some studies of research protocols have documented very good initial adherence with OAT.

11. Cross-over studies comparing OA and CPAP usually show better adherence with OAT (patient-reported) and better control of the AHI with CPAP, and equivalent improvements in outcomes including daytime sleepiness and quality of life measures. However, adherence to OAT is by self-report in nearly all studies. The explanation for equivalent benefits is that better adherence overcomes less control of the AHI; this results in similar outcomes.

12. Medicare and many insurance providers will pay for an OA if criteria are met. However, the amount provided is much less than the cost of many custom devices. For Medicare to pay for an OA, the device must meet criteria for a custom titratable device.

13. There is currently no method to reliably predict a good response to OAT. A lower baseline AHI, lower BMI, female gender, supine-dependent OSA, lower loop gain, mild-to-moderate upper-airway collapsibility, lower required CPAP, and high arousal threshold are associated with a good response to OAT.

CLINICAL REVIEW QUESTIONS

1. Of the following, which is predictive of a good response to OAT?
   A. Higher BMI
   B. Higher CPAP needed
   C. Positional OSA
   D. Higher AHI
2. Which type of OA is most effective at opening the upper airway?
   A. TSD/TRD
   B. MAD
3. What is the minimum number of teeth required in each arch for an OA?
   A. 3
   B. 4
   C. 8
   D. 11
4. In studies comparing the effectiveness of OAT with that of CPAP, which of the following is **NOT** true?
   A. CPAP was more effective at reducing the AHI.
   B. Reported OAT adherence was greater than objective CPAP adherence.
   C. Outcome measures such as improvement of daytime sleepiness were better with CPAP.
   D. Patient satisfaction with treatment was often greater with OAT.
5. Which of the following statements about side effects of OAT is **NOT** true?
   A. Early discontinuation is often due to discomfort or lack of benefit.
   B. Movement of teeth is almost universal (if followed objectively) and continues with longer duration of treatment.
   C. Reductions in overbite and overjet (usually beneficial) are common.
   D. Change in occlusion is almost always noticed by the patient.
   E. Anterior movement of teeth tends to decrease the efficacy of OAT.

ANSWERS

1. C. Positional OSA was associated with better OAT outcomes in many (but not all) studies. A lower CPAP pressure, BMI, and AHI were associated with better OAT outcomes in most studies.
2. A. An MRI study suggested that TSD/TRDs produced a greater enlargement of the upper airway. However, adherence was much lower with TSD/TRDs than with MADs.
3. C. The literature varies, but eight teeth in each arch is the most commonly mentioned number. Some references state as low as six teeth, others as high as 10 teeth.
4. C. Outcome measures are similar with OAT and CPAP.
5. D. Only a minority of patients are aware of changes in occlusion.

REFERENCES

1. Ferguson KA, Cartwright R, Rogers R, et al. Oral appliances for snoring and obstructive sleep apnea: a review. *Sleep*. 2006;29:244-262.
2. Kushida CA, Morgenthaler TI, Littner MR, et al.; American Academy of Sleep Medicine. Practice parameters for the treatment of snoring and obstructive sleep apnea with oral appliances: an update for 2005. *Sleep*. 2006;29:240-243.
3. Sutherland K, Vanderveken OM, Tsuda H, et al. Oral appliance treatment for obstructive sleep apnea: an update. *J Clin Sleep Med*. 2014; 10(2):215-227.
4. Ramar K, Dort LC, Katz SG, et al. Clinical practice guideline for the treatment of obstructive sleep apnea and snoring with oral appliance therapy: an update for 2015. *J Clin Sleep Med*. 2015;11(7):773-827.
5. Sutherland K, Cistulli PA. Oral appliance therapy for obstructive sleep apnoea: state of the art. *J Clin Med*. 2019;8(12):2121.
6. Deane SA, Cistulli PA, Ng AT, Zeng B, Petocz P, Darendeliler MA. Comparison of mandibular advancement splint and tongue stabilizing device in obstructive sleep apnea: a randomized controlled trial. *Sleep*. 2009;32(5):648-653. Erratum in: *Sleep*. 2009;32(8):table of contents.
7. Vanderveken OM, Devolder A, Marklund M, et al. Comparison of a custom-made and a thermoplastic oral appliance for the treatment of mild sleep apnea. *Am J Respir Crit Care Med*. 2008;178(2):197-202.
8. Johal A, Haria P, Manek S, Joury E, Riha R. Ready-made versus custom-made mandibular repositioning devices in sleep apnea: a randomized clinical trial. *J Clin Sleep Med*. 2017;13(2):175-182.
9. Johal A, Agha B. Ready-made versus custom-made mandibular advancement appliances in obstructive sleep apnea: a systematic review and meta-analysis. *J Sleep Res*. 2018;27(6):e12660.
10. Aurora RN, Casey KR, Kristo D, et al.; American Academy of Sleep Medicine. Practice parameters for the surgical modifications of the upper airway for obstructive sleep apnea in adults. *Sleep*. 2010;33(10): 1408-1413.
11. Millman RP, Rosenberg CL, Carlisle CC, et al. The efficacy of oral appliances in the treatment of persistent sleep apnea after uvulopalatopharyngoplasty. *Chest*. 1998;113:992-999.
12. Henke KG, Fratnz DE, Kuna ST. An oral mandibular advancement device for obstructive sleep apnea. *Am J Respir Crit Care Med*. 2000; 161:420-425.
13. Marklund M, Braem MJA, Verbraecken J. Update on oral appliance therapy. *Eur Respir Rev*. 2019;28(153):190083.
14. Brown EC, Cheng S, McKenzie DK, et al. Tongue and lateral upper airway movement with mandibular advancement. *Sleep*. 2013;36(3): 397-404.
15. Isono S, Tanaka A, Sho Y, et al. Advancement of the mandible improves velopharyngeal airway patency. *J Appl Physiol (1985)*. 1995;79(6): 2132-2138.
16. Sutherland K, Deane SA, Chan AS, et al. Comparative effects of two oral appliances on upper airway structure in obstructive sleep apnea. *Sleep*. 2011;34(4):469-477.
17. Ng AT, Qian J, Cistulli PA. Oropharyngeal collapse predicts treatment response with oral appliance therapy in obstructive sleep apnea. *Sleep*. 2006;29(5):666-671.
18. Marques M, Genta PR, Azarbarzin A, et al. Structure and severity of pharyngeal obstruction determine oral appliance efficacy in sleep apnoea. *J Physiol*. 2019;597(22):5399-5410.

19. Bailey DR, Hoekema A. Oral appliance therapy in sleep medicine. *Sleep Med Clin*. 2010;5:91-98.
20. Hamoda MM, Kohzuka Y, Almeida FR. Oral appliances for the management of OSA: an updated review of the literature. *Chest*. 2018; 153(2):544-553.
21. Conely RS. Orthodontic considerations related to sleep disordered breathing. *Sleep Med Clin*. 2009;5:71-89.
22. Marcussen L, Henriksen JE, Thygesen T. Do mandibular advancement devices influence patients' snoring and obstructive sleep apnea? A cone-beam computed tomography analysis of the upper airway volume. *J Oral Maxillofac Surg*. 2015;73(9):1816-1826.
23. Huntley C, Cooper J, Stiles M, Grewal R, Boon M. Predicting success of oral appliance therapy in treating obstructive sleep apnea using drug-induced sleep endoscopy. *J Clin Sleep Med*. 2018;14(8):1333-1337.
24. Vroegop AV, Vanderveken OM, Verbraecken JA. Drug-induced sleep endoscopy: evaluation of a selection tool for treatment modalities for obstructive sleep apnea. *Respiration*. 2020;99(5):451-457.
25. Vena D, Azarbarzin A, Marques M, et al. Predicting sleep apnea responses to oral appliance therapy using polysomnographic airflow. *Sleep*. 2020;43(7):zsaa004.
26. Chung JW, Enciso R, Levendowski DJ, et al. Treatment outcomes of mandibular advancement devices in positional and nonpositional OSA patients. *Oral Surg Oral Med Oral Pathol Oral Radiol Endod*. 2010;109: 724-731.
27. Dieltjens M, Braem MJ, Van de Heyning PH, Wouters K, Vanderveken OM. Prevalence and clinical significance of supine-dependent obstructive sleep apnea in patients using oral appliance therapy. *J Clin Sleep Med*. 2014;10(9):959-964.
28. Sutherland K, Phillips CL, Davies A, et al. CPAP pressure for prediction of oral appliance treatment response in obstructive sleep apnea. *J Clin Sleep Med*. 2014;10(9):943-949.
29. Sutherland K, Takaya H, Qian J, Petocz P, Ng AT, Cistulli PA. Oral appliance treatment response and polysomnographic phenotypes of obstructive sleep apnea. *J Clin Sleep Med*. 2015;11(8):861-868.
30. Op de Beeck S, Dieltjens M, Azarbarzin A, et al. Mandibular advancement device treatment efficacy is associated with polysomnographic endotypes. *Ann Am Thorac Soc*. 2021;18(3):511-518.
31. Bamagoos AA, Cistulli PA, Sutherland K, et al. Polysomnographic endotyping to select patients with obstructive sleep apnea for oral appliances. *Ann Am Thorac Soc*. 2019;16(11):1422-1431.
32. Dutta R, Tong BK, Eckert DJ. Development of a physiological-based model that uses standard polysomnography and clinical data to predict oral appliance treatment outcomes in obstructive sleep apnea. *J Clin Sleep Med*. 2022;18(3):861-870.
33. Van Gaver H, Op de Beeck S, Dieltjens M, et al. Functional imaging improves patient selection for mandibular advancement device treatment outcome in sleep-disordered breathing: a prospective study. *J Clin Sleep Med*. 2022;18(3):739-750.
34. Dort L, Brant R. A randomized, controlled, crossover study of a noncustomized tongue retaining device for sleep disordered breathing. *Sleep Breath*. 2008;12:369-373.
35. Lazard DS, Blumen M, Lévy P, et al. The tongue-retaining device: efficacy and side effects in obstructive sleep apnea syndrome. *J Clin Sleep Med*. 2009;5(5):431-438.
36. Center for Devices and Radiologic Health, U.S. Food and Drug Administration. Intraoral devices for snoring and/or obstructive sleep apnea—Class II Special Controls Guidance Document for Industry and *FDA*. November 12, 2002. Available at: https://www.fda.gov/medical-devices/guidance-documents-medical-devices-and-radiation-emitting-products/intraoral-devices-snoring-andor-obstructive-sleep-apnea-class-ii-special-controls-guidance-document. Accessed 8/13/2022.
37. *Oral Appliances for OSA. LCD L33611*. Available at: www.cms.gov/medicare-coverage-database/details/lcd-details.aspx?LCDId=33611&ContrId=389. Accessed August 28, 2021.
38. Dieltjens M, Vanderveken OM, Van de Heyning PH, Braem MJ. Current opinions and clinical practice in the titration of oral appliances in the treatment of sleep-disordered breathing. *Sleep Med Rev*. 2012;16:177-185.
39. Almeida FR, Parker JA, Hodges JS, Lowe AA, Ferguson KA. Effect of a titration polysomnogram on treatment success with a mandibular repositioning appliance. *J Clin Sleep Med*. 2009;5:198-204.
40. Krishnan V, Collop N, Scherr S. An evaluation of a titration strategy for prescription of an oral appliance for obstructive sleep apnea. *Chest*. 2008;133:1135-1141.
41. Remmers JE, Topor Z, Grosse J, et al. A feedback-controlled mandibular positioner identifies individuals with sleep apnea who will respond to oral appliance therapy. *J Clin Sleep Med*. 2017;13:871-880.
42. Tsai WH, Vazquez J, Oshima T, et al. Remotely controlled mandibular positioner predicts efficacy of an oral appliance in sleep apnea. *Am J Respir Crit Care Med*. 2004;170:366-370.
43. Sutherland K, Ngiam J, Cistulli PA. Performance of remotely controlled mandibular protrusion sleep studies for prediction of oral appliance treatment response. *J Clin Sleep Med*. 2017;13(3):411-417.
44. Okuno K, Ikai K, Matsumura-Ai E, Araie T. Titration technique using endoscopy for an oral appliance treatment of obstructive sleep apnea. *J Prosth Dent*. 2018;119:350-353.
45. Fleury B, Rakotonanahary D, Petelle B, et al. Mandibular advancement titration for obstructive sleep apnea: optimization of the procedure by combining clinical and oximetric parameters. *Chest*. 2004;125(5):1761-1767.
46. Metz JE, Attarian HP, Harrison MC, et al. High-resolution pulse oximetry and titration of a mandibular advancement device for obstructive sleep apnea. *Front Neurol*. 2019;10:757.
47. Sutherland K, Dalci O, Cistulli PA. What do we know about adherence to oral appliances? *Sleep Med Clin*. 2021;16(1):145-154.
48. Kirshenblatt S, Chen H, Dieltjens M, Pliska B, Almeida FR. Accuracy of thermosensitive microsensors intended to monitor patient use of removable oral appliances. *J Can Dent Assoc*. 2018;84:i2.
49. Vanderveken OM, Dieltjens M, Wouters K, De Backer WA, Van de Heyning PH, Braem MJ. Objective measurement of compliance during oral appliance therapy for sleep-disordered breathing. *Thorax*. 2013; 68(1):91-96.
50. Gjerde K, Lehmann S, Naterstad IF, Berge ME, Johansson A. Reliability of an adherence monitoring sensor embedded in an oral appliance used for treatment of obstructive sleep apnoea. *J Oral Rehabil*. 2018;45(2): 110-115.
51. Dieltjens M, Braem MJ, Vroegop AVMT, et al. Objectively measured vs self-reported compliance during oral appliance therapy for sleep-disordered breathing. *Chest*. 2013;144(5):1495-1502.
52. Martínez-Gomis J, Willaert E, Nogues L, Pascual M, Somoza M, Monasterio C. Five years of sleep apnea treatment with a mandibular advancement device. Side effects and technical complications. *Angle Orthod*. 2010;80(1):30-36.
53. Wiman Eriksson E, Leissner L, Isacsson G, Fransson A. A prospective 10-year follow-up polygraphic study of patients treated with a mandibular protruding device. *Sleep Breath*. 2015;19(1):393-401.
54. Ghazal A, Sorichter S, Jonas I, Rose EC. A randomized prospective long-term study of two oral appliances for sleep apnoea treatment. *J Sleep Res*. 2009;18(3):321-328.
55. Attali V, Chaumereuil C, Arnulf I, et al. Predictors of long-term effectiveness to mandibular repositioning device treatment in obstructive sleep apnea patients after 1000 days. *Sleep Med*. 2016;27-28:107-114.
56. Attali V, Vecchierini M-F, Collet J-M, et al.; ORCADES investigators. Efficacy and tolerability of a custom-made Narval mandibular repositioning device for the treatment of obstructive sleep apnea: ORCADES study 2-year follow-up data. *Sleep Med*. 2019;63:64-74.
57. Doff MH, Veldhuis SK, Hoekema A, et al. Long-term oral appliance therapy in obstructive sleep apnea syndrome: a controlled study on temporomandibular side effects. *Clin Oral Investig*. 2012;16(3):689-697.
58. Gindre L, Gagnadoux F, Meslier N, Gustin J-M, Racineux J-L. Mandibular advancement for obstructive sleep apnea: dose effect on apnea, long-term use and tolerance. *Respiration*. 2008;76(4):386-392.
59. Uniken Venema JAM, Doff MHJ, Joffe-Sokolova D, et al. Long-term obstructive sleep apnea therapy: a 10-year follow-up of mandibular advancement device and continuous positive airway pressure. *J Clin Sleep Med*. 2020;16(3):353-359.
60. Walker-Engström M-L, Tegelberg Å, Wilhelmsson B, Ringqvist I. 4-year follow-up of treatment with dental appliance or uvulopalatopharyngoplasty in patients with obstructive sleep apnea: a randomized study. *Chest*. 2002;121:739-746.
61. de Almeida FR, Lowe AA, Tsuiki S, et al. Long-term compliance and side effects of oral appliances used for the treatment of snoring and obstructive sleep apnea syndrome. *J Clin Sleep Med*. 2005;1:143-152.
62. Schwartz M, Acosta L, Hung YL, et al. Effects of CPAP and mandibular advancement device treatment in obstructive sleep apnea patients: a systematic review and meta-analysis. *Sleep Breath*. 2018;22(3):555-568.
63. de Vries GE, Hoekema A, Claessen JQPJ, et al. Long-term objective adherence to mandibular advancement device therapy versus continuous positive airway pressure in patients with moderate obstructive sleep apnea. *J Clin Sleep Med*. 2019;15(11):1655-1663.
64. Tallamraju H, Newton JT, Fleming PS, Johal A. Factors influencing adherence to oral appliance therapy in adults with obstructive sleep apnea: a systematic review and meta-analysis. *J Clin Sleep Med*. 2021; 17(7):1485-1498.

65. Hammond RJ, Gotsopoulos H, Shen G, Petocz P, Cistulli PA, Darendeliler MA. A follow-up study of dental and skeletal changes associated with mandibular advancement splint use in obstructive sleep apnea. *Am J Orthod Dentofacial Orthop.* 2007;132(6):806-814.
66. Rose E, Statts R, Virchow C, Jonas IE. Occlusal and skeletal effects of an oral appliance in treatment of obstructive sleep apnea. *Chest.* 2002; 122:871-877.
67. Marklund M, Franklin KA, Persson M. Orthodontic side-effects of mandibular advancement devices during treatment of snoring and sleep apnoea. *Eur J Orthod.* 2001;23(2):135-144.
68. Marklund M. Subjective versus objective dental side effects from oral sleep apnea appliances. *Sleep Breath.* 2020;24(1):111-117.
69. Hamoda MM, Almeida FR, Pliska BT. Long-term side effects of sleep apnea treatment with oral appliances: nature, magnitude and predictors of long-term changes. *Sleep Med.* 2019;56:184-191.
70. Pliska BT, Nam H, Chen H, Lowe AA, Almeida FR. Obstructive sleep apnea and mandibular advancement splints: occlusal effects and progression of changes associated with a decade of treatment. *J Clin Sleep Med.* 2014;10(12):1285-1291.
71. Ishiyama H, Inukai S, Nishiyama A, et al. Effect of jaw-opening exercise on prevention of temporomandibular disorders pain associated with oral appliance therapy in obstructive sleep apnea patients: a randomized, double-blind, placebo-controlled trial. *J Prosthodont Res.* 2017;61(3): 259-267.
72. Ueda H, Almeida FR, Chen H, Lowe AA. Effect of 2 jaw exercises on occlusal function in patients with obstructive sleep apnea during oral appliance therapy: a randomized controlled trial. *Am J Orthod Dentofacial Orthop.* 2009;135(4):430.e1-e7; discussion 430-431.
73. Gotsopoulos H, Kelly JJ, Cistulli PA. Oral appliance therapy reduces blood pressure in obstructive sleep apnea: a randomized, controlled trial. *Sleep.* 2004;27(5):934-941.
74. Bratton DJ, Gaisl T, Wons AM, Kohler M. CPAP vs. mandibular advancement devices and blood pressure in patients with obstructive sleep apnea: a systematic review and meta-analysis. *JAMA.* 2015;314(21): 2280-2293.
75. Phillips CL, Grunstein RR, Darendeliler MA, et al. Health outcomes of continuous positive airway pressure versus oral appliance treatment for obstructive sleep apnea: a randomized controlled trial. *Am J Respir Crit Care Med.* 2013;187(8):879-887.
76. El-Solh AA, Homish GG, Ditursi G, et al. A randomized crossover trial evaluating continuous positive airway pressure versus mandibular advancement device on health outcomes in veterans with posttraumatic stress disorder. *J Clin Sleep Med.* 2017;13(11):1327-1335.
77. Dieltjens M, Vanderveken OM, Shivalkar B, et al. Mandibular advancement device treatment and reverse left ventricular hypertrophic remodeling in patients with obstructive sleep apnea. *J Clin Sleep Med.* 2022;18(3):903-909.
78. El-Solh AA, Moitheennazima B, Akinnusi ME, Churder PM, Lafornara AM. Combined oral appliance and positive airway pressure therapy for obstructive sleep apnea: a pilot study. *Sleep Breath.* 2011;15(2):203-208.
79. De Vries GE, Do MH, Hoekema A, Kerstjens HA, Wijkstra PJ. Continuous positive airway pressure and oral appliance hybrid therapy in obstructive sleep apnea: Patient comfort, compliance and preference: a pilot study. *J Dent Sleep Med.* 2016;3:5-10.
80. Liu HW, Chen YJ, Lai YC, et al. Combining MAD and CPAP as an effective strategy for treating patients with severe sleep apnea intolerant to high-pressure PAP and unresponsive to MAD. *PLoS One.* 2017;12(10):e0187032. Erratum in: *PLoS One.* 2018;13(4):e0196319.
81. Tong BK, Tran C, Ricciardiello A, et al. CPAP combined with oral appliance therapy reduces CPAP requirements and pharyngeal pressure swings in obstructive sleep apnea. *J Appl Physiol (1985).* 2020;129(5): 1085-1091.

Chapter 26

Surgical Treatment for Obstructive Sleep Apnea

INTRODUCTION

Tracheostomy was the first treatment (and first surgical treatment) available for obstructive sleep apnea (OSA). Now, many surgical procedures are available to treat adults with OSA.[1-7] The newer procedures are more acceptable to patients and have less morbidity. However, none of the newer procedures are more effective than tracheostomy. The major surgical options are listed in Table 26–1. Each of the major procedures is discussed briefly below. Surgery for nasal obstruction is considered adjunctive treatment; laser-assisted uvuloplasty (LAUP) and palatal implants are recommended mainly for snoring. The use of tonsillectomy and adenoidectomy to treat pediatric OSA is discussed in Chapter 27. Hypoglossal nerve stimulation for treatment of OSA will also be discussed in this chapter.

INDICATIONS FOR SURGICAL TREATMENT

An update of the American Academy of Sleep Medicine (AASM) practice parameters for surgical treatment of OSA and the accompanying review were published in 2010 (Table 26–2).[1,2] In 2021 a clinical practice guideline for referral of adults with OSA for surgical consultation was published along with a review of surgical treatment of OSA.[4,5] These guidelines will be discussed, as well as an overview of surgical options. The 2010 guidelines used levels of recommendation: standard > guideline > option. The practice parameters state that the presence and severity of OSA must be determined before initiating surgical therapy. The patient should be advised about the success of surgical procedures and side effects as well as the success rate of alternative treatments. The practice parameters state that positive airway pressure (PAP) should first be offered to patients with severe OSA, and either PAP or an oral appliance (OA) should first be offered to patients with moderate OSA. In cases potentially requiring the stepped surgical procedure approach, patients should be informed that multiple surgical procedures may be needed. These guidelines preceded the option of hypoglossal nerve stimulation. The more recent guidelines by Kent et al.[5] recommend that clinicians discuss referral to a sleep surgeon for adults with OSA and a body mass index (BMI) <40 kg/m^2 who are intolerant or unaccepting of PAP as part of a patient-oriented discussion of alternative treatment options. Another recommendation suggests that clinicians discuss referral to a sleep surgeon with adults with OSA, a BMI <40 kg/m^2, and persistent inadequate PAP adherence due to pressure-related side effects as part of a patient-oriented discussion of adjunctive or alternative treatment options. Sometimes, surgical procedures, if not curative, may allow PAP treatment at lower pressures.

Table 26–1 Surgical Options for Treatment of Adult OSA

Adjunctive Nasal Surgery
- Turbinate reduction
- Repair of nasal valve collapse
- Repair of septal deviation

Snoring procedures
- Pillar procedure
- LAUP

Bypasses All Obstruction
- Tracheostomy

Selectively Improves Upper Airway Obstruction
- Palatal Surgery
  1. Uvulopalatopharyngoplasty (UPPP) – retropalatal area
  2. Non-ablative palatal surgery (Expansion Sphincter Pharyngopalatoplasty and others)
- Genioglossus advancement (GA) – retroglossal area
- Hyoid advancement (HA) – retroglossal area
- Maxillomandibular advancement (MMA) – retroglossal > retropalatal areas
- Temperature-controlled radiofrequency and robotic tongue base reduction – retroglossal areas
- Tongue base suspension surgery

Hypoglossal Nerve Stimulation

EVALUATION FOR POSSIBLE SURGICAL TREATMENT

The AASM practice parameters for surgical treatment of OSA mandate that all patients scheduled for surgery **to correct snoring or OSA** undergo polysomnography (PSG) for diagnosis and to assess severity.[1,2] If a surgery is planned for snoring, a PSG may reveal significant OSA and mandate a different surgical approach. Additional evaluation of patients with snoring or OSA for possible upper airway surgery includes fiberoptic examination of the nose, pharynx, and hypopharynx to evaluate the anatomy for abnormalities and the location of narrowing/obstruction. During fiberoptic examination, the patient performs a Müller maneuver (inspiration with the nose occluded). This maneuver is performed to help identify the most prominent site of collapse (retropalatal or retroglossal/hypopharyngeal area).[8] A jaw thrust during endoscopy might also give information regarding stabilization of the upper airway affected by forward movement of the mandible. A limitation of nasopharyngeal endoscopy, which is typically performed during wakefulness and often in an upright posture, is that the results may not correspond to what happens during supine sleep. Lateral

Table 26–2 Summary of the 2010 AASM Surgical Treatment of OSA Practice Parameter Recommendations

Procedure	Indications/Conditions:
Tracheostomy	• Other options do not exist or have failed. • Clinical urgency (e.g., repeated bouts of hypercapnic respiratory failure)
MMA	• Severe OSA • Unwilling or unable to tolerate PAP • OA considered and undesirable or ineffective
UPPP	• Snoring, mild OSA • Moderate OSA – only after offering PAP treatment and oral appliances
Palatal implants	• "May be effective in some patients with mild OSA" • Indicated for OSA treatment IF patients cannot tolerate/adhere to PAP therapy and OA treatment is considered and found ineffective and undesirable.
GA or HA	• No specific recommendations • Used for patients with hypopharyngeal narrowing
Maxilloman-dibular advance-ment (MMA)	• Moderate to severe OSA in whom CPAP treatment is not accepted or effective • Substantial and consistent reductions in AHI, highest rate of success (other than tracheostomy) • Addresses upper airway narrowing at multiple sites
Multilevel or step-wise surgery	• Upper airway narrowing at multiple sites • Have failed UPPP as sole treatment

General Recommendations:

1. The presence and severity of OSA must be determined before initiating surgical therapy.
2. The patient should be advised of potential surgical success rates and complications as well as the availability of other treatment options and the success rates of these options.
3. Desired treatment outcomes include resolution of the signs and symptoms of OSA and normalization of sleep quality, the AHI, and oxygen saturation levels.
4. Post-operatively (after healing) the patient should undergo objective testing to determine the presence and severity of sleep disordered breathing and drops in oxygen saturation as well as and clinical assessment of residual symptoms. Patient follow-up over time is needed to detect recurrence of disease.

OA, oral appliance; *OSA*, obstructive sleep apnea; *UPPP*, uvulopalatopharyngoplasty; *GA*, genioglossus advancement; *HA*, hyoid advancement; *MMA*, maxillomandibular advancement; *CPAP*, continuous positive airway pressure; *PAP*, positive airway pressure; *AHI*, apnea-hypopnea index.

Adapted from Caples SM, Rowley JA, Prinsell JR, et al: Surgical modifications of the upper airway for obstructive sleep apnea in adults: a systematic review and meta-analysis. *Sleep*. 2010;33:1396–1407.

cephalometric radiographs are also standard and can help visualize bony abnormalities and the posterior airspace. Patients with OSA tend to have long soft palates, small posterior air spaces (<10 mm behind the tongue), mandibular deficiency, and a long distance to the hyoid[9] (Figure 26–1).

Friedman et al. proposed a classification for preoperative evaluation based on palate position, tonsil size, and BMI (Table 26–3).[10] Stage I patients are the most likely to benefit from a palatal procedure alone. Stage II and stage III patients will need multilevel surgery, and stage IV patients are not good candidates for palate surgery. In a group of stage I patients UPPP was associated with a success rate of 80% (reduction in the AHI of 50% or more with a reduction in AHI to < 20 events/hour).[10]

Drug-induced sleep endoscopy (DISE) is a relatively new approach that allows dynamic, three-dimensional evaluation of the patterns of vibration and collapse of the upper airway of patients with sleep disordered breathing.[11-16] Several classification systems have been introduced to characterize DISE findings. The VOTE classification system, which examines the Velum, Oropharyngeal (lateral walls), Tongue, and Epiglottis, is widely used for DISE scoring (Table 26–4). The most common finding from DISE is multilevel collapse, despite heterogeneity among studies. The patterns of complete concentric collapse (CCC), multilevel collapse, and tongue-base collapse are associated with a higher apnea-hypopnea index (AHI). CCC has been associated with poor surgical outcomes in multilevel surgery and upper airway stimulation (UAS) but is well addressed by maxillomandibular advancement (MMA), to be discussed in detail below.

DISE may change the initial surgical planning in a high percentage of cases. However, a universally accepted and methodologically standardized DISE procedure is still not available. The procedure requires an anesthesiologist skilled in the approach so that an adequate (but not excessive) amount of sedation is given the patient. Medications that have been used include propofol, midazolam, and dexmedetomidine. The ideal sedation depth is essential, consisting of a stable pattern of light sedation, defined as the transition from consciousness to unconsciousness (loss of response to verbal stimulation: modified Ramsay score of 5).

A multicenter cohort study by Green et al.[13] reported that any DISE findings of lateral oropharyngeal wall obstruction and complete tongue obstruction pattern may lead to a higher risk of surgical failure. Certal et al.[14] published a systematic review comparing upper airway awake examination versus DISE as diagnostic tools for surgical decision making. A total of eight studies with 535 patients were included in the review. Surgical treatment was changed after DISE in about 50% of cases. The change in surgical planning was mainly due to the presence of hypopharyngeal or laryngeal dynamic collapse that is only seen on DISE. However, the change in surgical planning did not lead to a significantly higher success rate. A clinical guideline publication by Aljassim et al.[15] summarized evidence on the role of DISE in planning for upper airway surgery. The authors found that, in a majority of studies, DISE was found to change the overall surgical plan based on the findings seen in the airway while the patient was under sedation. The guideline included the following statements: "However, the available evidence suggests that DISE findings, and the subsequent alteration of surgical plan, do not strongly correlate with improved overall surgical success. Therefore, this article recommends that when DISE is offered to patients, it should be clear that the purpose of the procedure is diagnostic alone, and that the findings may not necessarily change the final outcome if subsequent surgery is to be offered. An exception may be *when DISE identifies epiglottis*

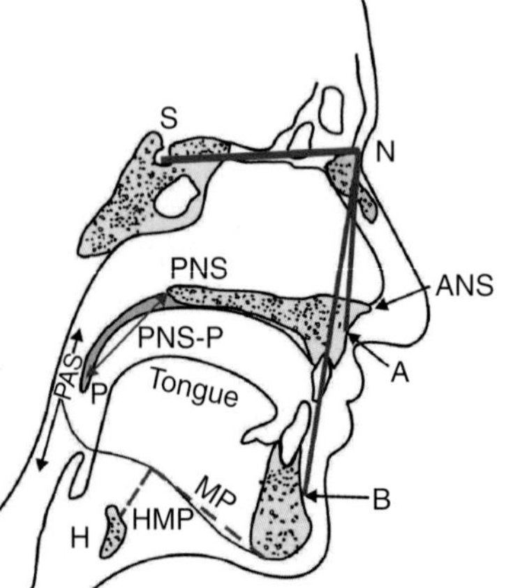

Figure 26–1 Cephalometric parameters are illustrated. Patients with OSA have a longer distance from the hyoid to the mandibular plane (HMP), a longer palate, a small posterior d to the mandibular plane (HMP), a longer palate, a small posterior airspace (PAS), and a larger angle reflecting the relationship of the maxilla and mandible (ANB). (Figure adapted from Li KK, Powell NB, Riley RW. Surgical Management of Obstructive Sleep Apnea. In: Lee-Chiong TL, Sateia MJ, Carskadon MA, eds. *Sleep Medicine*. Philadelphia: Hanly & Belfus; 2002:437.)

Table 26–3 Friedman Staging Systems

Stage	Palate position	Tonsil size	Body mass index (kg/m²)
1	1		<40
	2		<40
2	1, 2	1, 2	<40
	3, 4	3, 4	<40
3	3	0, 1, 2	<40
	4	0, 1, 2	<40
4	1, 2, 3, 4, All patients with significant craniofacial or other anatomic deformities	0, 1, 2	>40

Tonsil size is graded from 0 to 4.

- 0 denotes surgically removed tonsils.
- 1 implies tonsils hidden within the pillars.
- 2 implies the tonsils extending to the pillars.
- 3 tonsils are beyond the pillars but not to the midline.
- 4 implies tonsils extend to the midline.

The Friedman palate position is based on visualization of structures in the mouth with the mouth open widely without protrusion of the tongue.

Palate grade I allows the observer to visualize the entire uvula and tonsils.

Grade II allows visualization of the uvula but not the tonsils.

Grade III allows visualization of the soft palate but not the uvula.

Grade IV allows visualization of the hard palate only.

Adapted from Friedman M, Ibrahim H, Joseph NJ. Staging of obstructive sleep apnea/hypopnea syndrome: a guide to appropriate treatment. *Laryngoscope*. 200;114(3):454-459. PMID: 15091218.

Table 26–4 VOTE Classification

Structure	Degree of obstruction*	Configuration (if obstructed)
Velum	0 / 1 / 2 / X	( ) A-P ( ) Lateral ( ) Concentric
Oropharynx (lateral walls)	0 / 1 / 2 /X	Lateral
Tongue Base	0 / 1 / 2/ X	A-P
Epiglottis	0 / 1/ 2 / X	( ) A-P ( ) Lateral
	0 / 1/ 2/ X	

*Degree of obstruction: 0 none (no vibration), 1 partial obstruction (vibration), 2 complete obstruction (collapse), X not visualized

From Eric J, Kezirian EJ, Hohenhorst W, de Vries N. Drug-induced sleep endoscopy: the VOTE classification. *Eur Arch Otorhinolaryngol*. 2011;268:1233-1236.

collapse as a source of OSA; this is often not visible under awake circumstances, and this particular finding may have a direct bearing on surgical outcomes." The European Position Consensus Meeting on DISE[16] reached consensus for indications, required preliminary examinations, where to perform DISE, technical equipment required, staffing, local anaesthesia, nasal decongestion, other medications, patient positioning, basic and special diagnostic manoeuvres, drugs, and observation windows. However, no consensus could be reached on scoring and classification. As will be discussed in the section on hypoglossal nerve stimulation (HNS), DISE is an essential part of the evaluation of a patient being considered for HNS. A circumferential versus anterior-posterior pattern of collapse is associated with poor HNS treatment outcomes.[17] DISE can document epiglottic collapse, but at least one study suggested that if the tongue-base obstruction is addressed, separate surgery for epiglottic collapse may not be necessary.[18]

SURGERY FOR NASAL OBSTRUCTION AND SNORING

Surgery for Nasal Obstruction and Maxillary Expansion

Nasal obstruction can lead to mouth breathing during sleep. This causes rotation of the mandible and retrodisplacement of the tongue base back into the pharynx. Patients with chronic nasal obstruction often have a laterally narrow maxilla and high arched palate (adenoid facies). The major areas of surgical focus for nasal obstruction include the nasal valve/alar cartilage area, nasal septum, and turbinates (mostly inferior turbinates). Radiofrequency ablation (RFA) of turbinate hypertrophy can improve nasal continuous PAP (CPAP) adherence in selected patients.[19] A meta-analysis of surgery for nasal obstruction in patients being treated with CPAP concluded that isolated nasal surgery in patients with OSA and nasal obstruction reduces therapeutic CPAP device pressures, and the currently published literature's objective and subjective data consistently suggest that it also increases CPAP use in select patients.[20] One limitation of the analysis of the effect of nasal surgery on CPAP adherence was differences in inclusion criteria among the studies analyzed (for example, the degree of difficulty with CPAP treatment). With improved nasal breathing, patients can sometimes be changed from a full face mask to a nasal mask, which may reduce leak and improve comfort in some patients. It should be noted that the benefits from nasal surgery may not be apparent until after healing, which can take up to 6 weeks. Long-term studies with more precise inclusion criteria are needed to better define the indications for this procedure. A number of approaches to reduce inferior turbinate size include coblation (radiofrequency energy applied using a bipolar electrode with a conductive solution such as saline), electrocautery, and microdebrider technology.[21] Both RFA and coblation have been used for palatal surgery. Of note, coblation (a word derived from "controlled ablation") involves using low-temperature radiofrequency and a saline solution to remove the problematic tissues gently and precisely. The risk of injury to surrounding tissue is much lower than that with cautery.

A randomized, controlled trial of nasal surgery (vs. placebo surgery) found that surgery resulted in improvement in the amount of nasal breathing during sleep (less mouth breathing) *but minimal effects on the AHI.* The surgeries included resection of the deviated nasal septum and submucous resection of the inferior turbinates.[22] In summary, although nasal surgery can improve the quality of life for some patients, it is considered an adjunctive rather than primary treatment for OSA. It has the potential to improve satisfaction with PAP treatment (or even adherence).

Although not traditional nasal surgery, nasal floor expansion using distraction osteogenesis maxillary expansion (DOME) can be useful for patients with a narrow and high arched maxilla.[23] The procedure is similar to one used in children before the maxilla have fused in the midline. In adults, minimally invasive osteotomies can be made at the Le Fort I level via an intranasal incision. Then, an expander is anchored to the roof of the maxilla intraorally. The patient turns the expander each day, and this method usually expands the maxilla by 8 to 10 mm in a month. Orthodontic treatment is needed to restore occlusion. Liu et al. recommended that nasal surgery be considered as part of multilevel surgery for OSA.[6]

Surgery for Snoring

In the text below procedures that target snoring but that can be used for very mild OSA are discussed. Most insurance providers do not cover the cost of procedures for snoring.

Palatal Implants

The Pillar procedure involves surgically placing small polyester rods in the soft palate. Each implant measures 18 mm in length—slightly less than an inch—and 1.5 mm in diameter. The subsequent healing of tissue around the implants stiffens the soft palate, thereby reducing relaxation and vibration of the tissue (reduced snoring). The procedure can be performed in the office or outpatient surgery center. The success is variable, and sometimes additional strip insertion is needed.[24] Although the evidence that palatal implant surgery is effective in patients with OSA is very marginal, the 2010 AASM surgical practice parameters state, "Palatal implants may be effective in some patients with mild OSA who cannot tolerate or are unwilling to adhere to PAP therapy or in whom oral appliances have been considered and found ineffective or undesirable (Option)."[2] Palatal implant surgery is often not reimbursed by insurance, as it is mainly for snoring. The best results are in individuals with small tonsils who are not obese.

Laser-Assisted Uvuloplasty

Laser-assisted palatoplasty or uvuloplasty (LAP or LAUP) was introduced as a treatment for snoring.[24,25] In this procedure, only a small portion of the uvula/soft palate is removed (Figure 26–2). Usually, two trenches on either side of the uvula are cut. Some surgeons also remove the end of the uvula. With time and scarring, the palate stiffens and elevates. This procedure can be done on an outpatient basis using local anesthesia. It is generally considered a treatment for snoring but has been used for very mild sleep apnea when suitable upper airway anatomy exists. The long-term efficacy of LAP remains to be established. The 2010 AASM practice parameters for surgical treatment of OSA[2] state, "LAUP is NOT routinely recommended as a treatment for OSA syndrome (Standard)." A recent systematic review by Camacho et al. reported that LAUP can increase the AHI in about 44% of patients and recommended the procedure be performed with caution or not at all.[25]

SURGERY FOR OBSTRUCTIVE SLEEP APNEA

Tracheostomy

This procedure bypasses all upper airway obstruction and is uniformly effective at preventing upper airway obstruction.[26-28] However, it is cosmetically unacceptable to most patients. The indications for tracheostomy in one large series

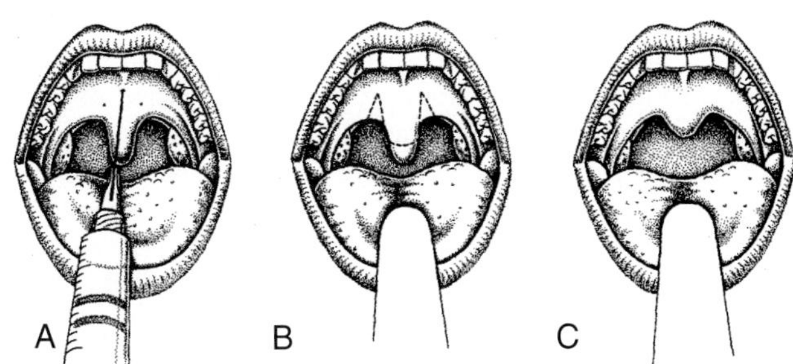

Figure 26–2 Laser uvulopalatoplasty. (A) Local anesthetic is injected. (B) The CO_2 laser is used to excise vertical trenches of the soft palate on either aspect of the uvula up to the muscular sling. Thirty percent to 90% of the uvula is excised or vaporized. (C) The postoperative result necessitates 4 to 5 weeks for complete healing and scarring to produce traction forces to improve airway patency. (A–C from Li KK, Powell NB, Riley RW. Surgical Management of OSA. In: Lee-Chiong TL, Sateia MJ, Carskadon MA, eds. *Sleep Medicine.* Philadelphia: Hanley & Belfus; 2002:439, reproduced with permission.)

included: (1) disabling sleepiness with severe consequences, (2) cardiac arrhythmias with sleep apnea, (3) cor pulmonale, (4) AHI >40 events/hour, (5) frequent desaturations below 40%, and (6) no improvement after other therapy. The main use of tracheostomy is for patients who have life-threatening OSA (often the obesity hypoventilation syndrome with recurrent hypercapnic respiratory failure) and who are poorly adherent to PAP treatment. Another use is as a temporary measure while patients recover from other upper airway surgery.[29] For example, in very severe OSA cases, tracheostomy could be performed with MMA and later closed if MMA surgery is successful. The 2010 AASM practice parameters state that tracheostomy has been found to be an effective single intervention.[2] However, this "operation should be considered only when other options do not exist, have failed, are refused, or when this operation is deemed necessary by clinical urgency." There are a number of potential adverse effects of tracheostomy for OSA.[26-28] Postoperative complications include stomal infection/granulation tissue, accidental decannulation, obstruction of the tube when the head is turned or hyperextended, recurrent purulent bronchitis, and psychosocial difficulties (depression). Non-cuffed, size 6 French tubes usually suffice. A longer-than-usual tracheostomy tube may be needed for very obese patients with thick necks. The end of the tracheostomy tube is typically plugged during the day, and because of its small size, air entering the nose and mouth can flow around the tube into the lungs. During sleep, the tracheostomy tube is unplugged to bypass the upper airway obstruction. However, one must not forget that very obese patients can still occlude the tracheostomy opening with "triple chins."

Palatal Surgery

Options for palatal surgery have increased significantly in an effort to improve effectiveness and reduce impairment of palatal function. While some are office procedures, most require general anesthesia and have considerable discomfort in the postoperative period. Some side effects and impairment of palatal function are temporary, but others remain a long-term issue.

Radiofrequency Ablation and Palatal Stiffening Procedures

RFA (also known as radiofrequency volumetric tissue reduction [RFVTR]) has been used in the upper airway, usually with temperature control of the probe tip. A probe is inserted into the area of interest, and tissue is heated to create cellular damage. With time, the tissue shrinks. RFA has been used for treatment of the soft palate, base of the tongue, and at multiple levels.[30] Somnoplasty (a variant of RFA) is a method of palatoplasty for treatment of snoring, appears to be well tolerated (possibly less pain) but is not more effective than traditional uvulopalatopharyngoplasty (UPPP). It can be performed as an outpatient procedure. Repeated treatments may be needed. The same technique can be used for turbinate reduction. Several other procedures that utilize coblation, cautery (cautery assisted palatal stiffening operation, CAPSO), or injection of sclerotic agents to stiffen the palate have also been used.[31] The 2010 AASM practice parameters for surgical treatment of OSA state, "RFA can be considered as a treatment in patients with mild to moderate OSA who cannot tolerate or who are unwilling to adhere to PAP or in whom oral appliances have been considered and have been found ineffective or undesirable (Option)." However, today, procedures that do not reduce palatal function are preferred. For certain patients with snoring or mild OSA who do not wish to undergo more extensive surgery, the above procedures are an option.

Uvulopalatopharyngoplasty

Traditional UPPP is the most frequently performed sleep upper airway surgery worldwide. The original technique introduced by Fujita involved removal of the uvula and a portion of the soft palate.[32,33] The UPPP was the first procedure used to treat OSA other than tracheostomy. This surgery includes removal of residual tonsillar tissue, the uvula and a portion of the soft palate, and redundant tissue from the pharyngeal area, as well as sewing together the cut edges of the remaining portion of the soft palate and sides of the throat (Figure 26–3). Compared to other palatal OSA surgeries, UPPP typically involves more tissue removal from the soft palate.

UPPP Limitations and Side Effects. Disadvantages of UPPP include the need for general anesthesia and considerable postoperative pain. The most frequent complication is velopharyngeal insufficiency, which is manifested as some degree of nasal reflux when drinking fluids. This usually resolves within a month of surgery. Other potential complications include voice change, postoperative bleeding, nasopharyngeal stenosis (secondary to scarring), or a persistent globus sensation. However, the major problem with UPPP is less-than-perfect efficacy as a treatment for OSA.[34] UPPP does not address airway narrowing behind the tongue or in the hypopharynx; therefore, it is not universally effective in preventing sleep apnea. UPPP is generally reasonably effective in decreasing the incidence or loudness of snoring (vibration of the soft palate). In general, 40% to 50% of all patients undergoing UPPP have about a 50% decrease in their AHI, to less than 20 events/hour, or about a 30% chance of the postoperative AHI dropping below 10 events/hour.[1,35] The results will, of course, depend on the pre-surgery AHI and the location of upper airway obstruction. Frequently, the relative amount of apneas decreases and hypopneas increases after UPPP. That is, before surgery apneas compose 40% of the total number of respiratory events and hypopneas 60%. Then post UPPP apneas compose 20% of the respiratory events and hypopneas 80%. The 2010 AASM practice parameters for surgical treatment of OSA state, "UPPP as a sole procedure, with or without tonsillectomy, does not reliably normalize the AHI when treating moderate to severe OSA. Therefore, patients with severe OSA should initially be

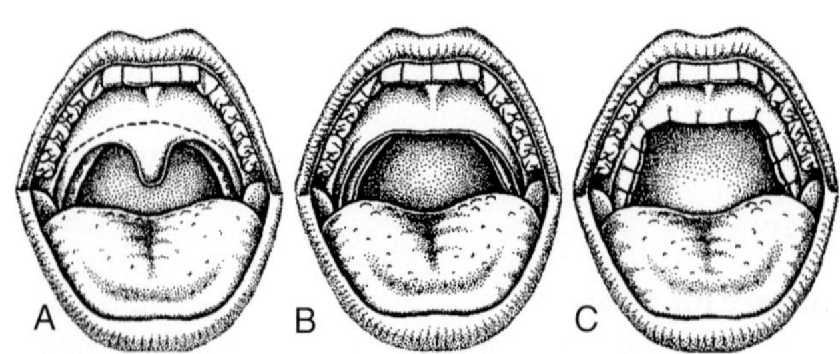

Figure 26–3 Technique of uvulopalatopharyngoplasty. (A) Redundant soft palate and tonsillar pillar mucosa are outlined. (B) Tonsils, tonsil pillar mucosa, and posterior soft palate are excised. (C) Mucosal flaps of the lateral pharyngeal wall and nasal palatal muscle are advanced to the anterior pillar and/or mucosa of the soft palate. (A–C from Li KK, Powell NB, Riley RW. Surgical Management of OSA. In: Lee-Chiong TL, Sateia MJ, Carskadon MA, eds. *Sleep Medicine.* Philadelphia: Hanley & Belfus; 2002:439, reproduced with permission.)

offered positive airway pressure therapy, while those with moderate OSA should initially be offered either PAP therapy or oral appliances (Option)."[2] Improved success of UPPP occurs when patients are properly selected for the procedure (Friedman class 1). Newer advanced palatal techniques offer the possibility of targeting specific types of palatal collapse with less morbidity.

New Palatal Procedures

Today there are several non-ablative palatal procedures available for treatment of sleep apnea. In general, removal of muscle or scarring of tissue is avoided. With the increasing use of DISE, it has become apparent that *different types of palatal collapse may benefit from different approaches*. Velopharyngeal obstruction can be divided into lateral, anterior-posterior (A-P), and concentric collapse under observation during DISE in VOTE classification. Different procedures target different patterns of collapse. For example, lateral pharyngoplasty, expansion sphincter pharyngoplasty, or similar procedures can be applied to lateral pharyngeal collapse, while suspension palatoplasty or transpalatal advancement pharyngoplasty can be utilized in anteroposterior narrowing of the palate.[36,37] What follows is a brief summary of some types of palatal surgery. Only an overview of the general surgical approach will be provided. More details about the procedures can be found in the individual sections to follow.[36-42]

Uvulopalatal Flap. This surgery is a modification of the UPPP and, in many centers, has replaced the traditional UPPP.[3,39] Uvulopalatal flap (Figure 26–4) is a treatment that preserves the palatal musculature and can be performed in patients with thin, soft palates. The procedure involves almost no removal of muscle of the soft palate. Instead, the lining of the oral surface (mucosa) found on a portion of the soft palate and the uvula are removed to allow a folding of the soft palate muscle onto itself. Effectively, it makes the soft palate shorter without removing muscle. Muscle removal is avoided because it can likely affect swallowing in these patients. The tonsillar pillars may be sutured together, and the tonsils are removed in this procedure, if indicated. The advantages are less postoperative pain and perhaps less nasopharyngeal reflux. The results are similar to those of UPPP. The procedure **cannot** be done if the palate is very long or bulky.[3]

Modified UPPP. The meaning of the term "modified UPPP" can vary among clinicians. As originally described by Li et al.,[40] this was an extended form of the uvulopalatal flap. It includes tonsillectomy, removal of adipose tissue of the soft palate and tonsils, and suturing together of the anterior and posterior tonsillar pillars. Only the tip of the uvula is removed; the other palatal muscles are left intact. Other variations are also performed. The goal is to expand the velopharyngeal inlet in the anteroposterior dimension as well as the lateral dimension while preserving the palatal musculature. Sometimes, the term is used to describe variants of palatal surgeries that do not remove palatal muscles.

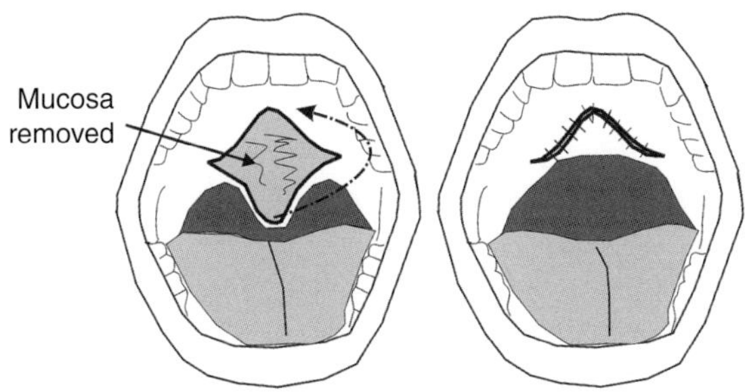

Figure 26–4 The uvulopalatal flap procedure is illustrated. The procedure involves the shortening of the soft palate by folding the distal soft palate with uvula forward upon itself. The intervening mucosal surfaces of the folded palate are removed, and the palate is sutured in its new position in two layers with interrupted sutures.

Expansion Sphincter Pharyngoplasty (ESP). ESP involves tissue repositioning and little or no tissue removal.[41-43] The muscle that is directly behind the posterior tonsillar arch (palatopharyngeus muscle) is freed from the side of the throat and moved forward (Figure 26–5). Because it is still attached to the soft palate, it pulls the soft palate forward to open the area behind the soft palate for breathing. The surgery targets those with *lateral pharyngeal wall collapse*. Pang and Woodson[41] randomized a group with OSA and small tonsils to ESP or traditional UPPP. The mean BMI was 28.7 kg/m^2. The mean AHI improved from 44.2 to 12.0 events/hour ($P < 0.005$) after ESP and from 38.1 to 19.6 after UPPP ($P < 0.005$). Selecting the threshold of a 50% reduction in AHI and an AHI less than 20, success was 82.6% in the ESP and 68.1% in the uvulopalatopharyngoplasty group ($P < 0.05$).

Lateral Pharyngoplasty. This surgery for sleep apnea involves extensive repositioning of tissue of the soft palate and the lateral pharyngeal tissues (side of the throat). Only some tissue removal is required. The technique is complicated.

Palatal Advancement Pharyngoplasty. This surgery for sleep apnea treats the palate by removing some of the bone toward the back of the roof of the mouth (hard palate).[43,44] After removal of the bone, the soft palate is pulled forward and sewn into place. This opens the space behind the soft palate for breathing. It may be useful for anterior-posterior collapse.

Z-palatoplasty. This surgery for sleep apnea requires dividing part of the soft palate in the middle and pulling each half forward and laterally. This can be most effective for patients with scarring on the sides of the throat that can occur after a tonsillectomy or other previous soft palate procedures.[45] Z-palatoplasty tends to be associated with more difficulty swallowing post-surgery compared to other palate procedures.

Relocation Pharyngoplasty (Barbed Reposition Pharyngoplasty). Relocation pharyngoplasty includes sewing together the muscles on the side of the throat to open the space for breathing.[46] "Barbed" refers to the use of knotless bidirectional absorbable sutures. Reposition/relocation means a displacement of the posterior tonsillar pillar (palatopharyngeal muscle) in a more lateral and anterior position to enlarge the oropharyngeal inlet as well as the retropalatal space. In addition, there is a suspension of the posterior pillar to the pterygomandibular raphe.

Complications of New Palatal Procedures. A study of long-term (mean, 41 weeks)[47] complications in 217 patients undergoing various types of new palatal surgery found the following complications that were either constant or occurred twice a

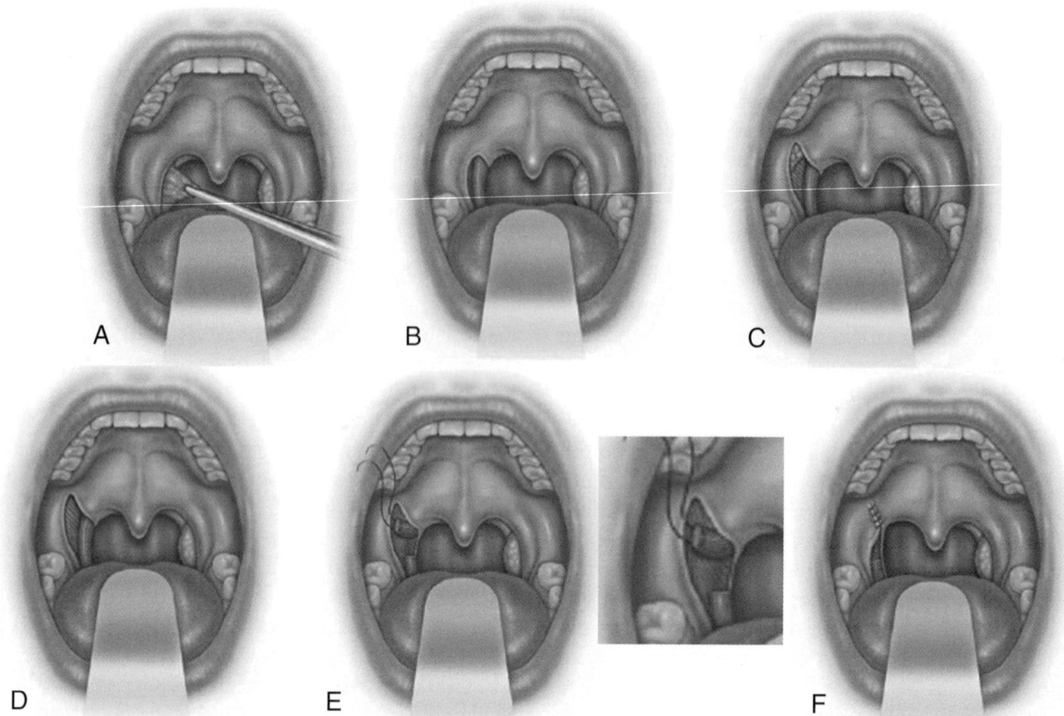

Figure 26–5 Expansion sphincter pharyngoplasty (or expansion sphincteroplasty) technique is illustrated. (A) Tonsillectomy. (B) Exposure of palatopharyngeus and superior constrictor muscles within the tonsillar fossa. (C) Lateral palatal incision over lateral palatal space with exposure of supratonsillar fat. (D) Removal of fat and fibers of palatoglossus provides exposure to superior constrictor and arching fibers of palatopharyngeus muscles. (E) Palatopharyngeus muscle incised 1.5 cm inferior to the fulcrum of rotation, and the pedicle is sutured to pterygomandibular raphe or fibrous tissue lateral to the hamulus. (F) Mucosal closure.(From Olszewska E, Woodson BT. Palatal anatomy for sleep apnea surgery. *Laryngoscope Investig Otolaryngol.* 2019;4(1):181-187. PMID: 30828637.)

week: dry throat (7.8%), throat lump feeling (11.5%), throat phlegm (10.1%), throat scar feeling (3.7%), and difficulty swallowing (0.5%). With the many variants of palatal surgery, it is difficult to compare side effects among the surgeries. In this study, the lowest number of symptom complaints was after expansion sphincter palatoplasty, and the highest numbers were after modified UPPP, relocation palatoplasty, and suspension palatoplasty.

Hypopharyngeal Surgery

Surgical approaches to obstruction at the retroglossal/hypopharyngeal level include genioglossus advancement and hyoid suspension, maxillomandibular advancement (treatment for multilevel obstruction), and tongue-base procedures.

Genioglossus Advancement/Hyoid Advancement

In genioglossus advancement (GA) (Figure 26–6), the attachment of the genioglossus at the glenoid tubercle of the mandible is advanced by making a limited rectangular mandibular osteotomy to include the genial tubercle (site of attachment of genioglossus and geniohyoid on the mandible).[48-50] The rectangular piece of bone with muscular attachments is advanced and rotated to prevent retraction of the piece of bone back into the mandible. A screw is then placed for stabilization. The major issues with the surgery have included damage to the roots of the lower incisors or nerves. With wide availability of computed tomography (CT) scans or other types of imaging, virtual surgical planning and osteotomy guides allow contemporary GA to be considerably more precise and less likely to damage the roots of teeth. Cutting templates are constructed to help with the osteotomy, and various hardware has been developed to securely hold the advanced segment of the mandible in place. Other methods of genial tubercle advancement include a "mortised" rather than rectangular piece of bone or an anterior visor osteotomy to move the genial tubercle forward.[49]

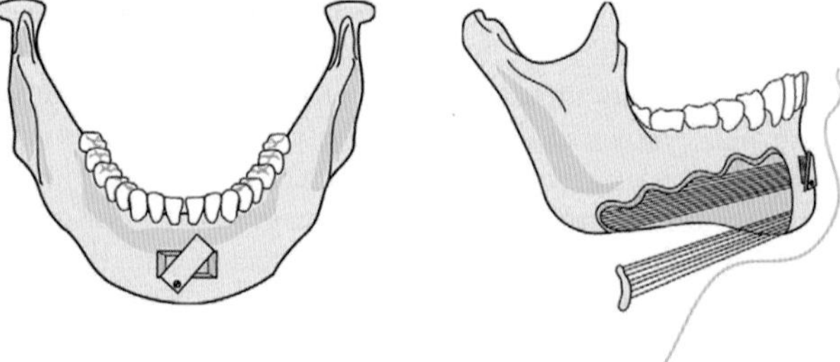

Figure 26–6 Technique of genioglossus advancement (GA). A rectangular window of symphyseal bone consisting of the genial tubercle is advanced anteriorly, rotated to allow body overlap, and immobilized with a titanium screw. *Left*, Anterior view. *Right*, Lateral view. Currently, there are many variations of this technique, including different types of mandibular osteotomy and stabilization hardware. (From Li KK. Hypoglossal airway surgery. *Otolaryngol Clin North Am.* 2007;40:845-853.)

When initially introduced, the second component of the surgery, hyoid advancement (HA) (Figure 26–7), was called "hyoid myotomy with suspension (HMS)." The original

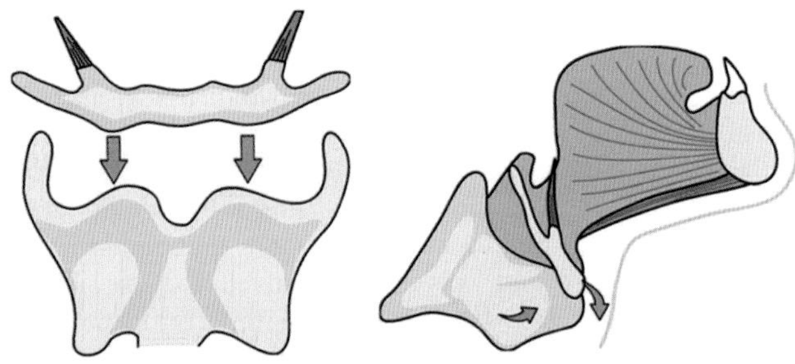

Figure 26–7 Technique of hyoid advancement (HA). The hyoid bone is isolated, the inferior body is dissected clean, and the majority of the suprahyoid musculature remains intact. The hyoid is advanced over the thyroid lamina and immobilized with sutures placed through the superior aspect of the thyroid cartilage. *Left*, Anterior view. *Right*, Lateral view. (From Li KK. Hypoglossal airway surgery. *Otolaryngol Clin North Am*. 2007;40:845-853.)

surgery consisted of release of the hyoid from its inferior muscular attachments and suspension from the anterior mandible with suture or ligament. Today, the hyoid is often attached to the superior border of the thyroid cartilage. Some surgeons perform only the GA at the first surgery, with the HA performed only if needed in a subsequent operation. GAHA does not require any change in dental occlusion. Complications of GAHA include transient anesthesia of the lower anterior teeth (all) and, rarely, tooth injury. Indications for GAHA include a small posterior airspace by lateral cephalometric assessment (<10 mm), an increased mandible-to-thyroid distance (>20 mm) by cephalometrics, mandibular deficiency, tongue-base prominence on nasopharyngoscopy, or macroglossia.[49,50]

The 2010 AASM practice parameters for surgical treatment of OSA[2] did not provide a specific statement about the GA or HA procedures. The practice parameters state, "multilevel or stepwise surgery (MLS), as a combined procedure or stepwise operations, is acceptable in patients with narrowing of multiple sites in the upper airway, particularly if they have failed UPPP as a sole treatment (Option)."

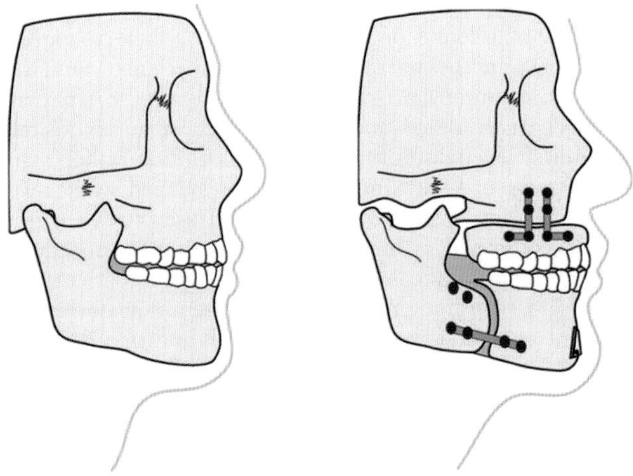

Figure 26–8 Technique of maxillomandibular advancement osteotomy procedure (*lateral view*). Le Fort I maxillary osteotomy with rigid plate fixation and a bilateral sagittal split mandibular osteotomy with bicortical screw fixation. The advancement is at least 10 mm. (From Li KK. Hypoglossal airway surgery. *Otolaryngol Clin North Am*. 2007;40:845-853.)

Box 26–1 INDICATIONS FOR MAXILLARY MANDIBULAR ADVANCEMENT

First Surgical Option

- Severe obstructive sleep apnea (OSA) (especially with minimally redundant palate)
- Retrognathia or facial skeletal deficiency
- Morbid obesity
- Drug-induced sleep apnea (DISE): concentric collapse, collapse of lateral pharyngeal walls
- Adequate health to undergo surgery

Second Surgery

- Failed previous surgical procedures (oral appliance unacceptable or likely ineffective, intolerant of positive airway pressure)

Maxillomandibular Advancement (MMA)

MMA is the most complex upper airway surgery, but excluding tracheostomy, this procedure has the best record of success as a treatment for OSA[51-53] (Figure 26–8). MMA is also called maxillomandibular osteotomy and advancement (MMO). The procedure is a treatment alternative for patients who have failed UPPP with or without GA and HA. Some surgeons would recommend MMA as the first surgical procedure in a patient with severe OSA who has retrognathia or in whom multiple surgeries are not acceptable. Indications for MMA are listed in Box 26–1. For patients with retroglossal upper airway obstruction, tongue-base reduction surgery is another option.[54-57] The maxilla and mandible are advanced together, and both upper and lower teeth are moved to maintain adequate occlusion. An orthodontic dentist is usually part of the surgical team and may optimize occlusion before MMA surgery. The MMA procedure increases the retrolingual and, to a lesser extent, retropalatal segments of the upper airway. The maxilla is moved by a Le Fort I osteotomy and the mandible by a sagittal split osteotomy. MMA enlarges the pharyngeal and hypopharyngeal areas by moving the skeletal framework and tensions the suprahyoid and velopharyngeal musculature. While patients with retrognathia may be especially good candidates, this procedure does not require that a patient has this problem.

A noted, in some institutions, MMA is performed only after UPPP and GAHA. However, for patients with severe OSA and/or mandibular deficiency, MMA can also be offered as the initial surgery. If the palate is long, doing a UPPP at the same time as the MMA is also an option. However, *some surgeons prefer a UPPP NOT to* ***precede*** *MMA, as any associated scaring can make moving the mandible forward more difficult.* Numbness of the chin and cheek areas is an expected complication that resolves in 6 to 12 months in most patients. The response rates from MMA vary from 50% to 80% or higher depending on the definition of surgical success. Li and coworkers[51] reported a 95% "cure" rate defined as an AHI < 20 events/hour and at least a 50% reduction. In a group of 36 to 40 patients who were responders, the AHI dropped from 69.6 events/hour preoperatively to 7.7 events/hour postoperatively. A meta-analysis by Elshaug et al. found MMA to reduce the AHI to less than 20 events/hour in 80% to 90%.[35] This procedure is usually offered only at large tertiary hospitals by experienced maxillofacial surgeons. The AASM practice parameters for surgical treatment of OSA state, "MMA is indicated for surgical treatment of severe OSA in patients who cannot tolerate or are unwilling to adhere to positive airway pressure therapy or in whom oral appliances, which are often more appropriate in mild and moderate OSA patients, have been considered and found ineffective or undesirable (Option)."[2] The reason for the grade of Option rather than a higher grade of Guideline is that the published studies were considered "low quality of evidence" because they were small and not controlled. Other than tracheostomy, the procedure is most likely to significantly improve the AHI in patients with severe OSA, although the AHI is often not normalized. A recent meta-analysis compared MMA and multilevel surgery for OSA. Although both were fairly effective, the MMA approach had better outcomes but a slightly higher rate of complications.[53]

Tongue Procedures

To avoid surgery involving the mandible or maxilla, procedures directed at the tongue have also been developed. Tongue-base reduction surgery aims to increase the retroglossal airway by removing tongue tissue. Surgical resection, laser resection, and temperature-controlled radiofrequency (TCRF) tongue-base reduction have all been tried with variable success.[54-57]

Coblation of the tongue (multiple channels with wand) can be performed as an outpatient surgery, although many surgeons admit patients overnight for observation, at least after the first surgery. Location of the channels helps surgeons avoid important neurovascular tongue structures. The use of robotic surgery has allowed better access to the tongue (transoral robotic surgery, TORS).[56] A number of side effects, including postoperative bleeding, odynophagia, tongue abscess, swallowing difficulty, and alterations in speech, are possible.

Tongue-Base Suspension Suture. A suspension suture is looped from the anchor screw on the inner surface of the mandible to the base of the tongue. The suture is tensioned, bringing the tongue forward. The procedure can be performed in less than half an hour and has few side effects (infection, injury to tooth roots, and detachment of screw). The success rates are variable.[58-61] In the United States, the Airvance®(formerly Repose®) system (Medtronics) and the AirLift procedure/Encore™ system (Siesta Medical) are available. The Airvance is a minimally invasive procedure that involves stabilizing the tongue base using a triangular suture configuration anchored to a titanium screw embedded in the mandibular cortex and was first approved for use in the United States in 1998. The Airlift is a similar procedure but creates a suture loop within the tongue without having to create penetrations through the mucosal surface of the tongue.[60] Only a small surgical incision a few centimeters below the mandible is needed. A similar system can be used for hyoid stabilization/elevation. The Airlift procedure is often performed with a UPPP or another procedure. The transoral tongue suspension procedure for tongue stabilization (TOTS) has also been developed.[61]

Overall Surgical Approach

The overall surgical approach depends on OSA severity, upper airway anatomy, prior treatment failures, and patient preference. A traditional approach was to classify patients as type 1 to 3. Obstruction can be classified as type 1 to 3 based on the predominant level of upper airway obstruction.[62] A type 1 obstruction is at the retropalatal area. Type 3 obstruction is at the hypopharyngeal area (behind the tongue or lower), and type 2 is a combined obstruction (palate + hypopharynx). Type 1 patients are considered favorable candidates for palatal procedures (UPPP). Type 3 are candidates for procedures addressing the retroglossal space (GA, with or without HA). Type 2 patients are candidates for UPPP + GAHA, UPPP + tongue-base reduction, or MMA. A systematic stepped surgical approach has been used at Stanford. A postoperative PSG is performed 6 months post-surgery, and treatment failures can then be offered MMA (Figure 26–9). Because an occasional patient with type 2 obstruction will improve with UPPP, in some centers, a retrolingual procedure is added only after UPPP fails. In some other centers, patients with severe OSA, severe mandibular deficiency, or very small posterior air spaces are offered MMA

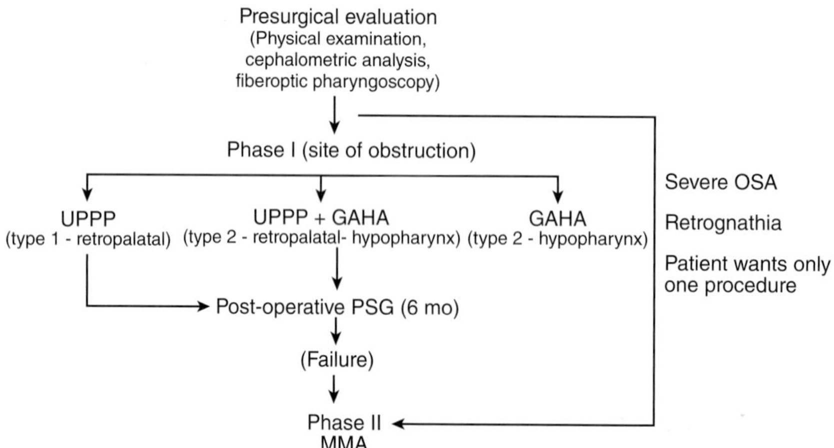

Figure 26–9 Original Stanford algorithm for upper airway surgery for treatment of sleep apnea. Stepped surgical approach to treatment of obstructive sleep apnea (OSA) based on the site of upper airway obstruction. *GAHA*, genioglossal advancement/hyoid advancement; *MMA*; maxillomandibular advancement; *PSG*; polysomnography; *UPPP*, uvulopalatopharyngoplasty. (Adapted from Li KK, Powell NB, Riley RW. Surgical Management Of Obstructive Sleep Apnea. In: Lee-Chiong TL, Sateia MJ, Caraskadon MA, eds. *Sleep Medicine.* Philadelphia: Hanley & Belfus; 2002:435-446.)

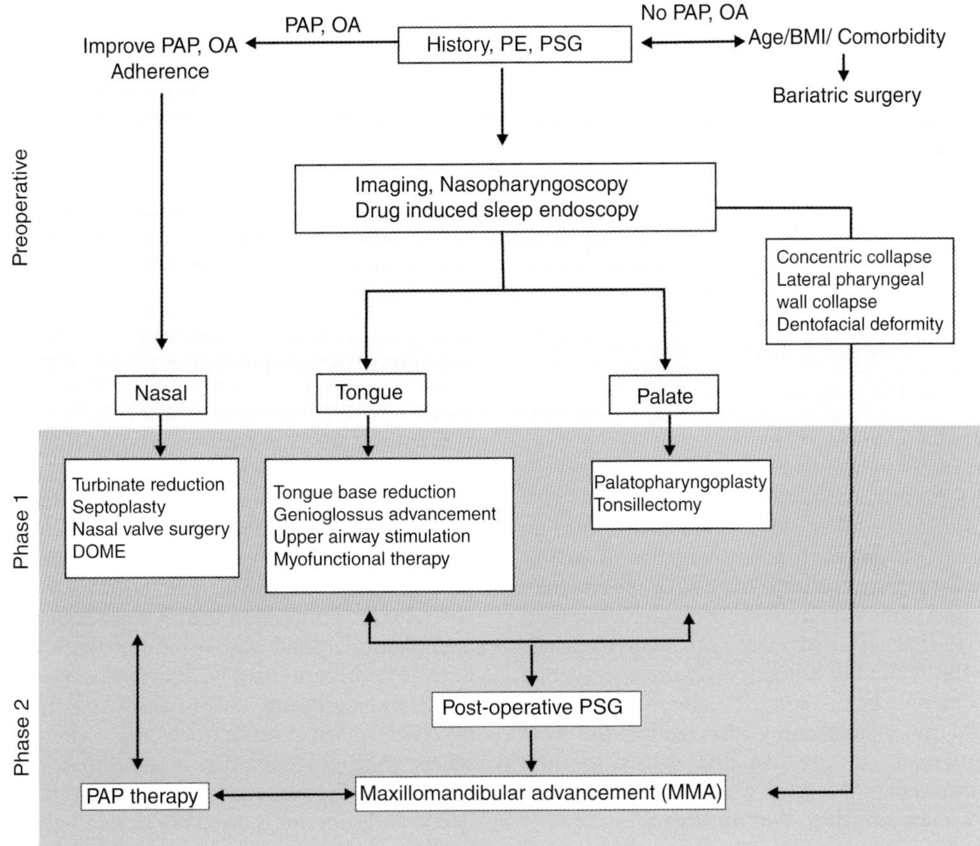

Figure 26–10 Updated algorithm for upper airway surgery for treatment of obstructive sleep apnea (OSA). Patients with severe OSA, concentric or lateral wall collapse, or skeletal deformity (mandibular deficiency) should undergo maxillomandibular advancement (MMA) without other intermediate surgical interventions. Otherwise, interventions are targeted at one or more sites of obstruction. Nasal surgery can be used to improve tolerance and adherence with of positive airway pressure (PAP) or oral appliance (OA) treatment. In very obese individuals with comorbidity associated with obesity, bariatric surgery should be considered. (From: Liu SY, Awad M, Riley R, Y, Capasso R. The role of the revised Stanford protocol in today's precision medicine. *Sleep Med Clinics*. 2019:14:99-107.

with or without UPPP as the first procedure. Some patients also want to *avoid* multiple procedures, and this more aggressive approach may be more acceptable to them.

Given the widespread use of DISE before surgery, a modified Stanford algorithm has been created. If there is concentric collapse of the palate, inward collapse of the lateral walls, or narrowing behind the base of the tongue these findings suggest that an aggressive approach targeting all areas of concern is needed to avoid multiple procedures and result in a better outcome (modified surgical algorithm).[6] The approach is illustrated in Figure 26–10. The approach emphasizes the use of nasal surgery to improve CPAP effectiveness and the importance of DISE to guide surgical management. The early use of MMA is recommended if DISE findings suggest an aggressive approach is needed to avoid the need for multiple procedures.

Table 26–5 Meta-Analysis Results for Upper Airway Surgery (% success rates)

Criteria	50% Reduction in AHI to ≤20 events/hour	AHI <10 events/hour	AHI <5 events/hour
Phase I*	55%	31.5%	13%
Phase II†	86%	45 %	43%

*Phase I (UPPP, GA, HA, or combination).
†Phase II (MMA).
AHI, apnea-hypopnea index; *GA*, genioglossus advancement; *HA*, hyoid advancement; *MMA*, maxillomandibular advancement; *UPPP*, uvulopalatopharyngoplasty.
Data from Elshaug AG, Moss JR, Southcott A, et al. Redefining success in airway surgery for obstructive sleep apnea: a meta-analysis and synthesis of the evidence. *Sleep*. 2007;30:461-467.

Success of Upper Airway Surgery

Because of the proliferation of upper airway surgical approaches, it is difficult to define the probability of success. Meta-analysis has often reviewed the results of fairly specific approaches. A meta-analysis and synthesis of evidence for success in upper airway surgery was reported by Elshaug and colleagues in 2007[35] (Table 26–5). A traditional metric of success has been a 50% reduction in the AHI and/or decrease to 20 events/hour or less. These authors suggested a more rigorous approach, with reduction to less than 10 or 5 events/hour the goal of success. Phase I surgery included palatal surgery without or without other procedures such as GA or GAHA. Phase II surgery was MMA with or without additional procedures. Of course, the percentage termed successful will depend on the initial severity and the definition of success. An updated meta-analysis of multilevel upper airway surgery[63] defined success as a reduction in AHI (events/hour) of 50% or more and an AHI of less than 20 events/hour found a success rate of 60.2%. A study by Mackay et al.[64] evaluated the results of multilevel surgery versus medical management (weight loss and avoidance of supine sleep) in a group of patients with OSA who had failed other approaches, including CPAP. The surgical approach included modified UPPP and tongue-base ablation. While the AHI was significantly reduced (47.9 to 20.8 events/hour), the AHI remained in the moderate or higher range in a significant proportion of treated patients at 6 months.

New Viewpoints of Surgical Success

Historically, analysis of surgical success has considered mainly the AHI. For most procedures, the AHI is not reduced as well as it is with CPAP. On the other hand, "adherence" is not an issue with surgical treatment except for avoidance of weight gain. Given the fact that many patients use CPAP for less than half of the night, the nightly average AHI is much higher than the AHI on CPAP. That is, CPAP may have greater efficacy (ability to reduce the AHI) but much less effectiveness when adherence is considered. For example, surgery reduces the AHI from 40 to 20 events/hour, and CPAP reduces the AHI from 40 to 5 events/hour. However, if CPAP is used for 50% of the night the on average the AHI would by (5+40)/2 or 22.5 events/hour, a value similar to that of surgery.

A large meta-analysis of "rescue surgery" focused on outcomes.[4] The results were as follows:

1. Surgery as a rescue therapy resulted in a clinically significant reduction in excessive sleepiness, snoring, blood pressure (BP), AHI, respiratory disturbance index (RDI), and oxygen desaturation index (ODI); an increase in lowest oxygen saturation (LSAT) and sleep quality; and an improvement in quality of life in adults with OSA who are intolerant or unaccepting of PAP therapy.

2. Surgery as an adjunctive therapy resulted in a clinically significant reduction in optimal PAP pressure and improvement in PAP adherence in adults with OSA who are intolerant or unaccepting of PAP due to side effects associated with high pressure requirements.

3. Surgery as an initial treatment resulted in a clinically significant reduction in AHI/RDI, sleepiness, snoring, BP, and ODI and an increase in the lowest oxygen saturation in adults with OSA and major anatomical obstruction.

An example of a different viewpoint of success is the previously mentioned study by MacKay et al.[64] The authors performed a parallel group open-label randomized trial to determine if combined palatal and tongue surgery (modified UPPP and minimally invasive tongue volume reduction to enlarge or stabilize the upper airway) is an effective treatment when compared to medical therapy alone in patients in whom conventional device treatment has failed. Rather than a comparison to CPAP, a better analysis is to compare surgery with standard medical care (weight loss, side sleep position). This recognizes the reality that *patients failing CPAP often get no treatment beyond standard medical care.* The mean AHI was 47.9 events/hour at baseline and 20.8 events/hour after 6 months (vs. 45.3 to 34.5 events/hour in the medical group). The mean Epworth sleepiness scale decreased from 12.4 to 5.3 (versus 11.1 to 10.5 in the medical group). The improvements with surgery were statistically better (and clinically significant) compared to medical therapy alone. Therefore, if CPAP fails, surgical treatment (compared to standard medical treatment or, often, no treatment at all) is much more effective with respect to improvement in subjective daytime sleepiness.

HYPOGLOSSAL NERVE STIMULATION (HNS)

HNS is a relatively new treatment for OSA that is a good alternative for many patients who do not tolerate PAP treatments and who meet the criteria for HNS treatment.[65-81] Stimulation of the hypoglossal nerve results in forward tongue movement, opening the retroglossal and, to a lesser extent, the retropalatal airway. A stimulator (impulse generator, IPG) is placed in a subcutaneous pocket, usually on the right upper chest, and a stimulation lead is tunneled up through the neck and placed around the median branch of the hypoglossal nerve[65,66] (Figure 26–11). Previously, another lead was tunneled, and a pressure sensor was placed in the fourth intercostal space to sense respiratory effort. The pressure/respiratory sensor permits stimulation to coordinate with respiratory effort. Currently, the sensor to detect respiratory effort is placed lateral and superior to the IPG device, below a layer of muscle in the same "pocket." At implantation of the device, the main trunk of the hypoglossal nerve (XII) is exposed by means of a horizontal incision in the upper neck at the inferior border of the submandibular gland. The hypoglossal nerve is followed anteromedially until it branchs into a lateral and a medial (m-XII) division. The stimulation lead cuff is placed around the m-XII branch. The cuff section of the stimulation lead includes three electrodes that can be arranged in a variety of unipolar or bipolar configurations for stimulation of the upper airway. Appropriate placement of the stimulation lead is confirmed by observing tongue protrusion during stimulation and by electromyographic monitoring during surgery. A tablet programmer is used to test stimulation cuff placement during surgery. The controller communicates with the implanted stimulator via an external antennae (wand) placed over the device. Specific training is needed for certification to be able to implant the device. Usually, implantation is performed by an ear, nose, and throat (ENT) surgeon. Tongue movement is tested before stabilization of the stimulation electrodes. The goal is to stimulate the tongue protruders and not the retractors.[66] The presence of a pacemaker is not an absolute contraindication but requires the assistance of a cardiologist at implantation to make adjustments so the two devices do not interfere with each other. The stimulator has a battery life of 7 to 10 years. The newer IPG model (made after 2018) has recently been cleared for magnetic resonance imaging (MRI) of most body areas (cannot be performed with the previous model). This full-body MRI approval expands the labeling that previously allowed only head, neck, and extremity MRI scans. Most importantly, this approval is retroactive, applying to all patients with the Inspire IV neurostimulator device introduced in 2018 already in place. However, approval is **conditional** for certain areas of the body and depends on the

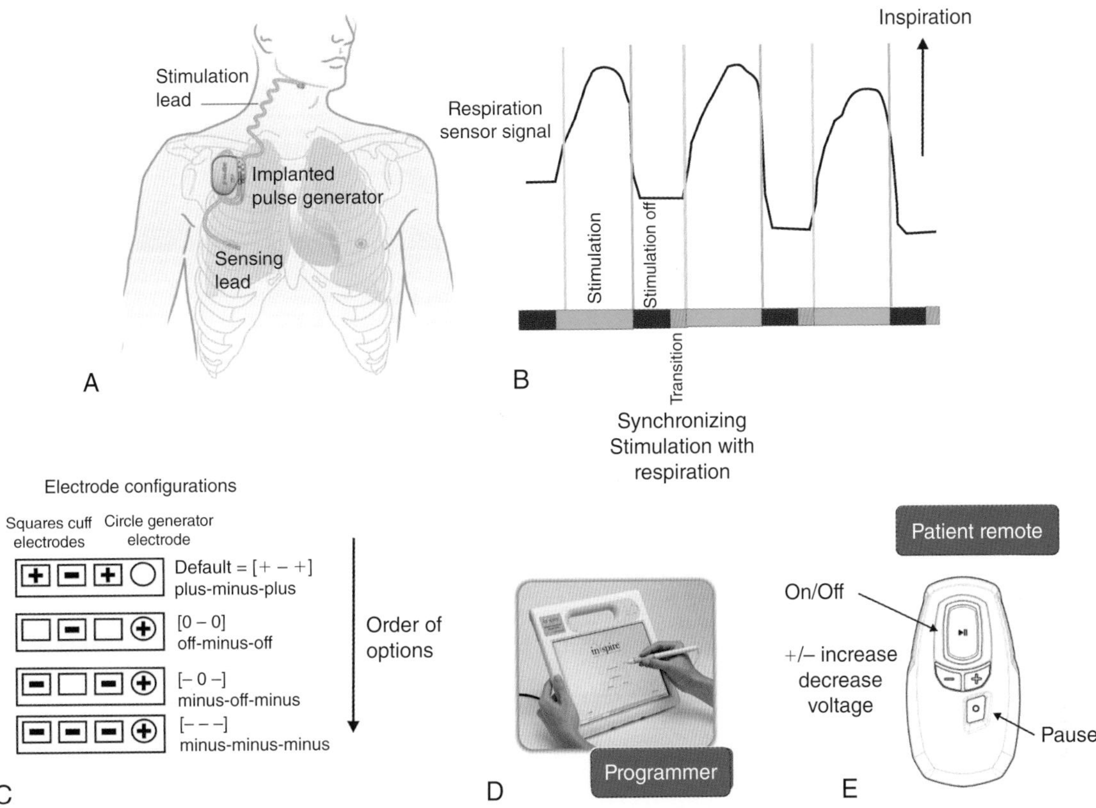

Figure 26–11 (A) The Inspire hypoglossal nerve stimulation system and positioning. The system includes the hypoglossal nerve stimulation device (impulse generator, IPG), a stimulation lead, and respiratory sensor (sensing lead). As illustrated, the position of the respiratory sensor is in the 4th intercostal space. Currently, the sensor is placed in the same pocket at the IPG, somewhat laterally and upward toward the right clavicle. The neurostimulator delivers electrical stimulating pulses to the hypoglossal nerve through the stimulation lead; the stimulating pulses are synchronized with ventilation detected by the sensing lead (B). Different electrode stimulation configurations are possible (C). A physician programmer can communicate with the IPG to obtain stored data or make changes (D). A patient remote allows the patient to turn the device on or off, pause the device, or change the stimulation voltage (E). The remote is held near the IPG to communicate with the stimulator. (From de Vries N, Maurer JT. Upper airway stimulation for obstructive sleep apnea. *Oper Tech Otolaryngol Head Neck Surg.* 2015;26(4):216-220; *Right,* © Inspire Medical Systems, Inc.)

MRI device being used. The reader should consult the most recent guidelines.[67]

A handheld controller unit (patient remote) that is placed over the stimulator by the patient is used to turn the device on and off, pause the device, and adjust the voltage output. Typical criteria for qualification for HNS treatment are listed in Table 26–6. The criteria have been modified several times, so the reader should look for updates. Criteria may vary among insurance providers. The U.S. Food and Drug Administration (FDA) widened its approved indications for HNS to an AHI of 15 to ≤100 events/hour (formerly 15 to ≤65 events/hour) and a BMI up to ≤40 kg/m^2. However, at the time of writing Medicare uses a maximum AHI of 65 events/hour and a BMI of 35 kg/m^2. A DISE procedure is performed to exclude the presence of circumferential airway collapse (an exclusion criteria for HNS). A schematic of A-P collapse and concentric collapse is shown in Figure 26–12.

Effectiveness of HNS

The pivotal STAR trial of HNS in the United States by Strollo et al. found that HNS demonstrated good effectiveness in carefully selected patients.[65] The initial part of the study did not have a control group. In the final portion of the study, those patients who responded were randomized to active or inactive treatment. The inclusion criteria were the presence of moderate to severe OSA (AHI 15 to 65 events/hour with less than 25% of respiratory events being central or mixed apneas). Exclusions were a BMI >32 kg/m^2, tonsil size (3 or 4), concentric collapse on DISE, neuromuscular disease, hypoglossal nerve palsy, severe restrictive or obstructive pulmonary disease, moderate to severe pulmonary hypertension, severe valvular heart disease, recent myocardial infarction, severe persistent uncontrolled hypertension despite medication use, active psychiatric disease, and coexisting non-respiratory sleep disorders that would confound functional sleep assessment. The co-primary outcomes were a reduction in the AHI by 50% to an AHI <20 events/hour and a reduction in the oxygen desaturation index by 25% from baseline.

The mean age of the study group was 54.5 years, and the mean BMI was 28.4 kg/m^2. The median screening AHI was 32 events/hour. The results for the co-primary outcomes at 12 months of treatment included 66% of individuals meeting the AHI outcome criteria and 75% meeting the ODI criteria. This means that a substantial fraction had a significant residual AHI. Some of the outcomes of interest are illustrated in Figure 26–13. In the second part of the study 46 consecutive individuals with a response to treatment were randomized to continued treatment or withdrawal of treatment (for at least

Table 26–6 Qualifying Criteria for Hypoglossal Nerve Stimulation (HNS)

Qualifying Criteria

- Age >22 years
- CPAP not accepted or tolerated (or effective)
- Apnea-hypopnea index (AHI) 15 to 65 events/hour on polysomnography within 24 months of first consultation for HNS
- Body mass index <35 kg/m^2
- *Less than 25% of events are central or mixed apneas*
- Absence of circumferential collapse on drug-induced sleep endoscopy (DISE)
- Absence of other upper airway abnormalities (tonsil size 3 or 4)

Exclusions

- Beneficiaries who require magnetic resonance imaging (MRI) (model 3024)
- Neuromuscular disease
- Recent myocardial ischemia or severe cardiac arrhythmias within 6 months
- New York Heart Classification class 3 or 4 heart failure
- Severe restrictive or obstructive pulmonary disease
- Adverse interaction with other implanted device
- Unable to operate remote

Adapted from LCD L38398 (Hypoglossal Nerve Simulation for Obstructive Sleep Apnea). Note the qualifying criteria and regulations pertaining to the use of MRI are frequently changing. The most recent information should be reviewed. A higher upper limit of AHI and BMI are acceptable for some insurance providers.[68]

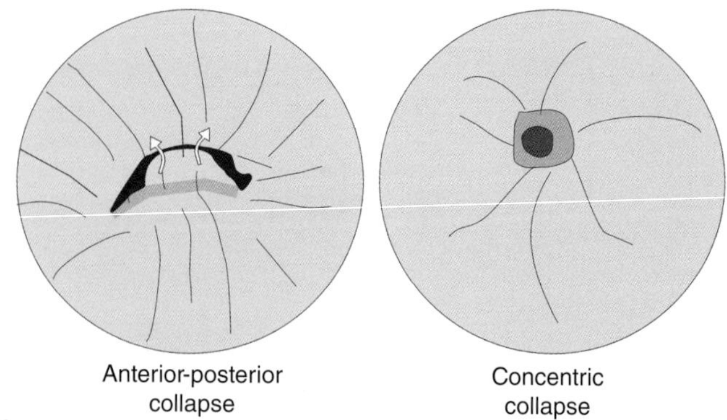

Figure 26–12 A schematic illustrating the appearance of anterior-posterior versus concentric upper airway collapse as seen during drug-induced sleep endoscopy.

5 nights, N=23 both groups) and another PSG was performed on HNS treatment. The change (decrease) in AHI from baseline in the continuation group was significantly greater than in the withdrawal group (Figure 26–13).

Other studies have documented the effectiveness of HNS treatment and its reasonable maintenance effectiveness over time.[69-71] An analysis by Kent et al.[70] did find an increase in the mean AHI of 3.24 events/hour from 6 to 12 months. A larger reduction in the AHI was seen with a higher preoperative

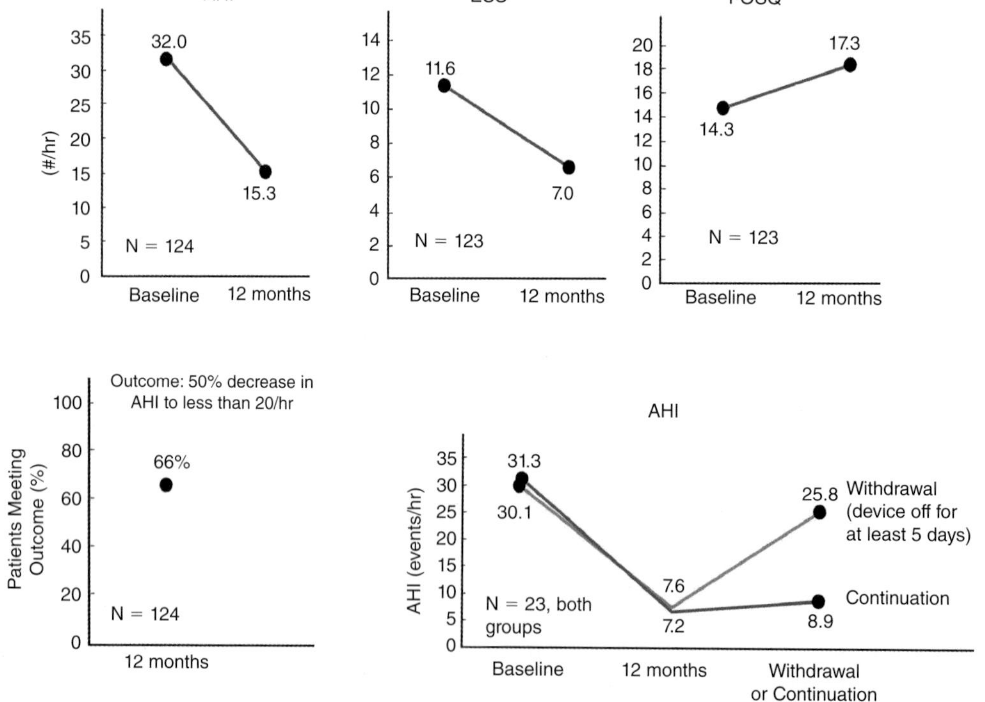

Figure 26–13 A summary of the results of the STAR trial. Compared to baseline at 12 months, there as a significant decrease in the apnea-hypopnea index (AHI), and Epworth sleepiness scale and an increase in the Functional Outcomes of Sleep Questionnaire (FOSQ), a quality of life measure. The 12 month data for ESS (lower better) and FOSQ (higher better) were missing for one individual. A change of 2 or more in the FOSQ is felt to be clinically significant with a lower bound of 17.9 for individuals with normal sleep. Median values are shown. The changes were all statistically significant (p <0.001). Overall, 66% of patients had a reduction in the AHI of 50% or greater to less than 20 events/hour. In the second part of the study, a consecutive group of 46 individuals who responded were randomized to continuation or withdrawal of treatment for at least 5 days. Mean values are shown for continuation (number of individuals N =23) or withdrawal of treatment (N =23). The difference in the change in AHI from baseline to 12 months was higher in those who continued treatment (16.4/hr), (p <0.001). (Data plotted from Strollo PJ Jr, Soose RJ, Maurer JT, et al. Upper-airway stimulation for obstructive sleep apnea. *N Engl J Med.* 2014;370[2]:139-149.)

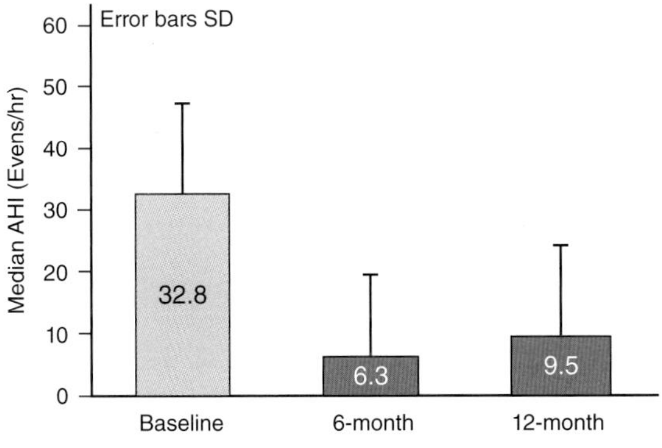

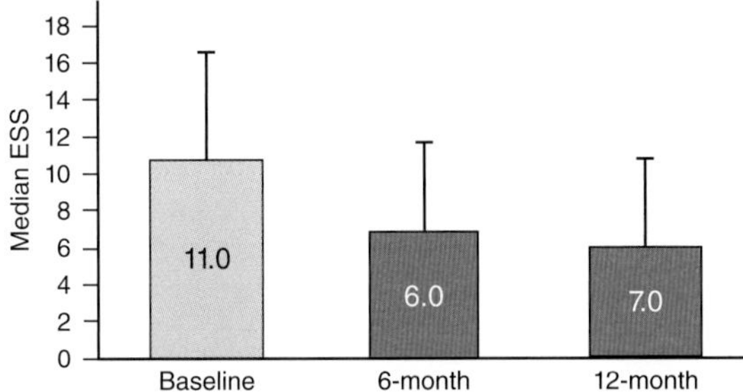

Figure 26–14 The median Epworth sleepiness scale (lower better) and the apnea-hypopnea index (AHI) at baseline, 6 months and 12 months post-surgery from the ADHERE registry (error bars are the standard deviation). Improvements in subjective sleepiness and the AHI were maintained at 12 months. The median adherence was 5.7 hours per night. (Adapted from Thaler E, Schwab R, Maurer J, et al. Results of the ADHERE upper airway stimulation registry and predictors of therapy efficacy. *Laryngoscope*. 2020;130(5):1333-1338. PMID: 31520484.)

AHI, older age, and lower BMI. The ADHERE Registry is a multicenter prospective observational study following outcomes of UAS therapy in patients who have failed CPAP therapy for OSA.[71] The aim of this registry and purpose of the article was to examine the longer term outcomes of patients receiving HNS for treatment of OSA. In this study, improvements in daytime sleepiness and reduction in the AHI were well maintained (Figure 26–14), and the mean usage was 5.6 hours per night after 12 months. Adherence to HNS can be objectively determined, as the IPG records usage that may be assessed during patient visits. The IPG can provide treatment information using a bluetooth enabled remote that communicates with both the IPG and via a Bluetooth connection with the patient's smart phone Inspire App. The patient activates an option in the app and information is sent from the remote to the app. This allows the patient to track their objective adherence. The app also sends more detailed data to a cloud based platform (Sleep Synch) that allows the physician to track adherence and the current stimulation voltage. The Sleep Synch platform shows detailed information including the current pulse width, stimulation frequency, and electrode configuration. Information about where the patient currently is in the clinical pathway (implantation, activation etc.) is also displayed and visible to the patient's care team.

The main side effect reported by patients using HNS is discomfort associated with the stimulation. As with all treatments, there are some patients who may find using HNS uncomfortable or who are unable to tolerate a voltage sufficient to keep the upper airway open in all body positions and

Table 26–7 Steps in Hypoglossal Nerve Stimulation Treatment

- Evaluation for inclusion, exclusion criteria
- DISE (rule out concentric collapse)
- Implantation
- Healing for at least 1 month
- Activation and training (determine sensation and functional thresholds)
- Adaptation, patient increases voltage at home
- Check-in visit (telephone or clinic) 4 to 6 weeks after activation
- Second clinic visit* 4 to 6 weeks after check-in visit to determine adherence, current voltage, intervene for issues
- Sleep study to fine-tune voltage (no sooner than 3 months after activation)
- Post fine-tune visit – setting voltage range (to include therapeutic voltage)
- Routine follow-up (Green pathway)

or

- Follow-up for poor adherence, high AHI, side effects (yellow pathway)

*Clinic visits: check adherence, current voltage, symptoms, make adjustments as needed

DISE, drug-induced sleep endoscopy; *AHI*, apnea-hypopnea index.

Adapted from Soose RJ, Faber K, Greenberg H, et al. Post-implant care pathway: lessons learned and recommendations after 5 years of clinical implementation of hypoglossal nerve stimulation therapy. *Sleep*. 2021;44(Supplement_1):S4-S10.

sleep stages. However, overall, there is a high rate of patient satisfaction. Algorithms have been developed to adjust stimulation parameters to improve both the residual AHI and comfort.[72,73,74] These interventions will be discussed in the next section of the chapter.

HNS Treatment Details

The steps in evaluation and treatment are listed in Table 26–7. After implantation, there is a period of surgical healing (at least 1 month). After healing, the patient returns to sleep clinic for device activation. The surgical site is inspected and appearance of the tongue is observed to rule out neuropraxia (traumatic nerve injury). Stimulation is started at a low voltage and slowly increased. The voltage threshold for sensation (patient can detect stimulation) and for tongue movement (functional threshold) are documented. In addition, the direction of tongue movement with stimulation is documented. About 40% of patients will have stimulation of the contralateral as well as ipsilateral tongue muscles with unilateral hypoglossal nerve stimulation.[75] The pattern of response does not affect the ability of stimulation to move the tongue or treat sleep apnea.[74] The output of the respiration sensor is visualized to determine if detection of respiration and synchronization of stimulation with breathing is working adequately. A voltage range is set (usually starting at 0.2 volts below the functional threshold, with a total range of 10 levels, each level .1 volt higher than the previous level). For example, if level 3 is 2.0 volts, levels 1–10 are 1.8, 1.9, 2.0, 2.1, 2.2, 2.3, 2.4, 2.5, 2.6, and 2.7 volts, respectively. At this point, the patient learns how to turn on the device at night and adjust the voltage. The controller has an on and off button, a pause button, and + and − buttons to increase or decrease the stimulation voltage. Typically, there is a set "Start Delay" period to allow the patient to fall asleep, and voltage may be decreased or paused during the night (pause time duration is specified). A duration of treatment is also programmed

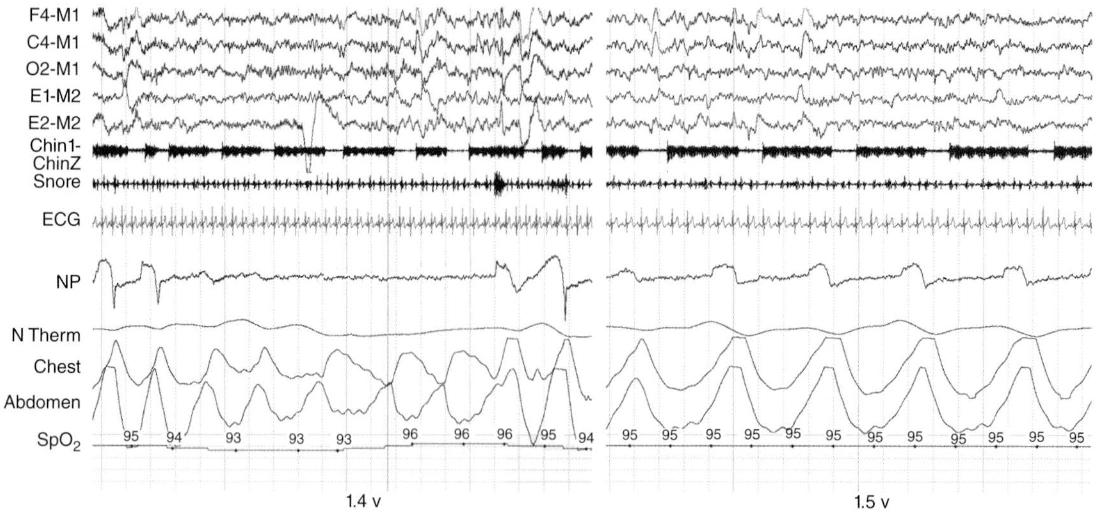

Figure 26–15 Tracings from a patient undergoing a hypoglossal nerve stimulation titration (Fine Tune) study. An increase in voltage was associated with an improvement in airflow. *NP,* Nasal pressure; *N Therm,* nasal oral thermal flow sensor. Note the stimulation artifact in the chin EMG.

(usually 8 hours). The patient has the ability to stop stimulation but a duration is set to avoid stimulation stopping while the patient is asleep. The patient returns home with the instruction to slowly increase the voltage as tolerated. Formerly, an HNS titration fine tune study occurred at about 6 weeks, but now the time from activation until the titration study is typically 12 weeks or longer. About 4–6 weeks after activation, the patient is seen in the office (or via telephone check) to determine whether the device is working, assess subjective benefit and objective adherence as well as documenting pliance the current stimulation voltage the patient is using. If necessary, the stimulation voltage range can be changed to allow the patient to continue to advance to higher levels in pursuit of a more therapeutic voltage/subjective benefit. After another 4 to 6 weeks of voltage adaptation and adjustment, the patient is seen in clinic to check for adherence and efficacy. If treatment is thought to be optimized, a PSG titration fine tune study is subsequently performed to document a "therapeutic voltage". The incoming voltage is the setting the patient has been using at home prior to the sleep study. The voltage may be changed remotely during the sleep study with a tablet programmer that can communicate with the device. The stimulation voltage is increased slowly to reduce or eliminate respiratory events. If the patient cannot tolerate a given voltage level the stimulation voltage is decreased. Of note, respiratory inductance plethysmography effort belts cannot be used as they interfere with communication between the programmer and the IPG. After the study, the outgoing voltage range and stimulation level are reset to the incoming values. The patient is seen at a post-tune study visit and the current settings and therapeutic voltage are reviewed with the patient If the therapeutic voltage is at or below the incoming voltage, the outgoing voltage (from the clinic) is set to the therapeutic voltage with a range of 2 levels below and 2 levels above the outgoing treatment level. If the therapeutic voltage is higher than the incoming voltage the patient is requested to return home and try to slowly increased the voltage 0.1 volts every 1 week with a goal of reaching the optimal voltage. If the patient cannot tolerate higher voltage then setting are manipulated as discussed below. Of note there are times where the patient is actually using a voltage that is higher than needed ("over patient titration" and the treatment voltage is reduced. In Figure 26–15, a small increase in voltage amplitude improved patient low.

In some patients, the maximum tolerated voltage is not effective. Clinical pathways have been established: green for patients doing well and yellow for those having issues with adherence, comfort, or a high residual AHI. These patients return for a clinic visit and one or more changes of the stimulation pattern (pulse width and stimulation frequency) for comfort and electrode configuration (for ability to reduce the AHI with a lower stimulation voltage if possible) are performed with a reduction in functional (and treatment) voltage, if possible[72-74] In cases where adherence is a problem, there are algorithms for adjustment in pulse rate and width to improve patient comfort. The standard pulse width and rate (stimulation frequency) is 90 microseconds/33 Hz. If the pulse width is increased a lower voltage amplitude may provide similar results, for example (120 microseconds/33 Hz). The standard electrode stimulation configuration is (+,−,+) (Figure 26–11) but other configurations may provide equivalent tongue protrusion with a lower stimulation voltage. There are detailed recommended protocols for changing electrode configuration and pulse rate and width. Note that,algorithms for adjustment in pulse rate and width to improve patient comfort Figure 26–11 are visualized to verify the functioning of the sensor. In some cases, a repeat in-lab or home sleep study may be ordered to determine the efficacy of the new settings. For the occasional patient not doing well despite pulse rate/stimulation frequency and electrode adjustments, an office titration with simultaneous endoscopy can be performed to optimize treatment. Another alternative is an "advanced" titration. If adequate treatment is still not being provided, combination treatment (HNS + CPAP, HNS+positional treatment) can be considered. The steps in the current clinical pathway may be different from those described here and the reader should consult the most recent information.

Lee et al. analyzed the ability of the required level of CPAP to predict a therapeutic response to HNS.[76] Patients with CPAP <8 cm H_2O had a greater drop in the AHI (36.7 versus 18.4 events/hour) and a greater response (defined as an AHI

<40 events/hour and a >50% reduction in the AHI) of 92% versus 44%. Of note, body weight did not differ (in part due to maximum of 32 kg/m^2 as a qualification for HNS). The authors noted that neither pre-AHI nor BMI has been successful at predicting HNS response. A two-center study by Huntley et al. compared outcomes between 113 patients with a BMI <32 kg/m^2 and 40 patients with a BMI >32 kg/m^2. There were no significant differences in postoperative AHI, Epworth sleepiness scale, or surgical success between the low and high BMI groups.[77] As noted, the FDA has increased the upper BMI limit to ≤40 kg/m^2. Many insurance providers allow a BMI of up to 35 kg/m^2. There are also some insurance carriers who do not have an upper AHI limit. The reader should consult the latest qualifications for Inspire treatment as well as the most current MRI guidelines. It is possible that upper airway surgery might address concentric collapse so that previously ineligible patients can now be treated with HNS for residual apnea after upper airway surgery.[78] A pivotal study found that hypoglossal nerve stimulation was effective in children with Down syndrome.[79] The FDA has expanded the approval of Inspire therapy to include pediatric patients 13 years of age and older with Down syndrome who have OSA with an AHI between 10 and 50 events/hour and who do not have the ability to benefit from CPAP.[80] There are ongoing efforts to improve the effectiveness of HNS.[81]

SUMMARY OF KEY POINTS

1. The presence and severity of OSA must be determined before initiating any type of surgical treatment (including treatment for "presumed primary snoring").
2. Before undergoing surgery, patients should be advised of potential success rates and complications, as well as treatment alternatives.
3. Tracheostomy is the only surgery uniformly effective for severe OSA, although some series suggest MMA may approach 80% to 90% success depending on how surgical success is defined. Tracheostomy is rarely indicated except in patients with recurrent severe hypercapnic respiratory failure who do not adhere to PAP treatment.
4. DISE can localize areas of upper airway obstruction and may change the surgical treatment. DISE has NOT been demonstrated to improve outcomes but may be especially useful in documenting epiglottic collapse and qualifying patients for (HNS).
5. UPPP does not reliably normalize the AHI in patients with moderate to severe OSA. Patients with severe OSA should be offered PAP treatment before proceeding with surgical options. Patients with moderate OSA should initially be offered PAP therapy or an oral appliance. HNS in a patient meeting the inclusion criteria for treatment is another option for patients with moderate to severe OSA not tolerating PAP.
6. Modifications of traditional UPPP are less ablative and more effectively address specific types of palatal collapse. There are many options. Palatal surgery is most effective in Friedman class 1 patients. Other patients will need multilevel surgery for optimal results.
7. Multilevel surgery consisting of a combination of a modified/non-ablative UPPP and either GA and HA or tongue surgery may improve the results in patients with multilevel obstruction.
8. MMA is indicated for initial treatment of severe OSA in patients who cannot tolerate or are unwilling to adhere to PAP therapy and in whom oral appliance treatment has been considered and found ineffective or undesirable.
9. MMA should be considered *as the initial surgery* in patients with severe OSA and in those with concentric collapse, collapse of the lateral pharyngeal walls, or skeletal deformities. Some patients will prefer MMA to avoid the need for multiple surgeries.
10. HNS is an effective treatment for patients meeting qualifying criteria who do not tolerate CPAP. Studies have demonstrated maintenance of efficacy and good adherence. However, only 66% of patients in the STAR trial had a >50% decrease in AHI to less than 20 events/hour. Significant residual AHI may still be present in up to one-third of individuals on HNS. However, these individuals may still experience symptomatic improvement. Good adherence and lasting efficacy for at least 5 years have been demonstrated.
11. Difficulty with HNS adherence (interventions for comfort) and effectiveness (AHI reduction) can be addressed by changes in the stimulation pulse duration and frequency and/or stimulating electrode configuration. These changes may result in improved effectiveness at a lower stimulation amplitude or improved comfort at the same voltage level.
12. HNS devices can track adherence, which has generally been excellent in most studies.
13. The effectiveness of PAP versus upper airway surgery depends on the amount of PAP adherence. If adherence with PAP is suboptimal, the actual nightly AHI is much higher than the "residual AHI" on PAP and may be similar to results from surgery (adherence not an issue).
14. The benefits of upper airway surgery cannot be judged by AHI alone but on the basis of other outcome measures such improvements in sleepiness and quality of life. A recent large meta-analysis determined that "rescue" upper airway surgery resulted in clinically significant improvements in daytime sleepiness, quality of life, the AHI, and oxygen desaturation indices in OSA patients who did not accept or who had poor adherence to PAP treatment.

CLINICAL REVIEW QUESTIONS

1. A 40-year-old man has severe daytime sleepiness and an AHI of 50 events/hour with moderate arterial oxygen desaturation. The patient's only medical problems are obesity (BMI 45 kg/m^2) and hypertension. Multiple attempts at PAP treatment have been unsuccessful. Which treatment alternatives do you recommend?
A. UPPP
B. UPPP + GAHA
C. MMA
D. HNS

2. In the original STAR trial of HNS, which of the following percentages is close to the actual proportion of patients who had a decrease in the AHI of ≥50% to an AHI <20 events/hour?
A. 40%
B. 60%
C. 80%
D. 89%

3. Which of the following is not a criteria for qualification for HNS?
A. Inability to accept or adhere to CPAP
B. Age less than 65 years
C. BMI <32 kg/m^2 (35 or 40 kg/m^2 for some insurance providers)
D. AHI 15 to 65 events/hour (15 to 100 events/hour for some health insurance providers)
E. Absence of concentric collapse on DISE

4. A patient with mild obstructive sleep apnea complains of severe nasal congestion that has not responded to medical treatment and, on examination, has inferior turbinate hypertrophy and nasal septal deviation. Which of the following does **NOT** describe the role of nasal surgery?
A. May improve quality of life
B. May reduce mouth breathing
C. May improve tolerance to PAP treatment
D. Reduces the AHI (sole treatment)

5. A patient with an AHI of 15 events/hour and a BMI of 27 kg/m^2 cannot tolerate CPAP. His teeth are in poor repair (not a good candidate for an oral appliance), and he is referred for surgical options. Nasopharyngoscopy reveals collapse at the palate and retroglossal areas. Which of the following surgical procedures is most appropriate for this patient?
A. UPPP
B. Modified UPPP (non-ablative palate surgery)
C. Modified UPPP and GA
D. MMA

ANSWERS

1. C. MMA is most likely to be effective in this individual with severe sleep apnea and a high BMI. His BMI is above that acceptable for HNS. UPPP and GAHA might be an alternative but is less likely to be effective. Of note, the maximum BMI approved for HNS has increased from 32 to 35 kg/m^2 for some providers. The FDA raised the BMI level to $\leq$ 40 kg/m^2.

2. B. The actual number is 66%.

3. B. There is currently no upper age limit on qualification for HNS.

4. D. Nasal surgery may improve symptoms and, in selected individuals, may improve adherence to PAP (depending on the cause of poor adherence). However, nasal surgery does not reliably decrease the AHI.

5. C. This patient needs surgery that will address two sites of obstruction. While MMA is likely to be effective, it is usually reserved for more severe sleep apnea. Modified UPPP and GA would address both sites of obstruction. The AHI barely meets criteria for hypoglossal nerve stimulation but that would be another reasonable option.

SELECTED READING

Kent D, Stanley J, Aurora RN, et al. Referral of adults with obstructive sleep apnea for surgical consultation: an American Academy of Sleep Medicine systematic review, meta-analysis, and GRADE assessment. *J Clin Sleep Med.* 2021;17(12):2507-2531.

Kent D, Stanley J, Aurora RN, et al. Referral of adults with obstructive sleep apnea for surgical consultation: an American Academy of Sleep Medicine clinical practice guideline. *J Clin Sleep Med.* 2021;17(12):2499-2505.

Liu SY, Riley RW, Yu MS. Surgical algorithm for obstructive sleep apnea: an update. *Clin Exp Otorhinolaryngol.* 2020;13(3):215-224.

Strollo Jr PJ, Soose RJ, Maurer JT, et al. Upper-airway stimulation for obstructive sleep apnea. *N Engl J Med.* 2014;370(2):139-149.

REFERENCES

1. Caples SM, Rowley JA, Prinsell JR, et al. Surgical modifications of the upper airway for obstructive sleep apnea in adults: a systematic review and meta-analysis. *Sleep.* 2010;33:1396-1407.
2. Aurora RN, Casey KR, Kristo D, et al. Practice parameters for the surgical modifications of the upper airway for obstructive sleep apnea in adults. *Sleep.* 2010;33:1408-1413.
3. Won CHJ, Li KK, Guilleminault C. Surgical treatment of obstructive sleep apnea. *Proc Am Thorac Soc.* 2008;5:193-199.
4. Kent D, Stanley J, Aurora RN, et al. Referral of adults with obstructive sleep apnea for surgical consultation: an American Academy of Sleep Medicine systematic review, meta-analysis, and GRADE assessment. *J Clin Sleep Med.* 2021;17(12):2507-2531.
5. Kent D, Stanley J, Aurora RN, et al. Referral of adults with obstructive sleep apnea for surgical consultation: an American Academy of Sleep Medicine clinical practice guideline. *J Clin Sleep Med.* 2021;17(12): 2499-2505.
6. Liu SY, Riley RW, Yu MS. Surgical algorithm for obstructive sleep apnea: an update. *Clin Exp Otorhinolaryngol.* 2020;13(3):215-224.
7. MacKay SG, Lewis R, McEvoy D, Joosten S, Holt NR. Surgical management of obstructive sleep apnoea: a position statement of the Australasian Sleep Association. *Respirology.* 2020;25(12):1292-1308.
8. Sher AE, Thorpy MJ, Spielman AJ, et al. Predictive values of Müller maneuver in selection of patients for uvulopalatopharyngoplasty. *Laryngoscope.* 1985;95:1483-1487.
9. Sforza E, Bacon W, Weiss T, Thibault A, Petiau C, Krieger J. Upper airway collapsibility and cephalometric variables in patients with obstructive sleep apnea. *Am J Respir Crit Care Med.* 2000;161(2 Pt 1):347-352.
10. Friedman M, Ibrahim H, Joseph NJ. Staging of obstructive sleep apnea/hypopnea syndrome: a guide to appropriate treatment. *Laryngoscope.* 2004;114(3):454-459.
11. Zhao C, Viana Jr A, Ma Y, Capasso R. Insights into Friedman stage II and III OSA patients through drug-induced sleep endoscopy. *J Thorac Dis.* 2020;12(7):3663-3672.
12. Kezirian EJ, Hohenhorst W, de Vries N. Drug-induced sleep endoscopy: the VOTE classification. *Eur Arch Otorhinolaryngol.* 2011;268(8): 1233-1236.
13. Green KK, Kent DT, D'Agostino MA, et al. Drug-induced sleep endoscopy and surgical outcomes: a multicenter cohort study. *Laryngoscope.* 2019;129(3):761-770.
14. Certal VF, Pratas R, Guimarães L, et al. Awake examination versus DISE for surgical decision making in patients with OSA: a systematic review. *Laryngoscope.* 2016;126(3):768-774.
15. Aljassim A, Pang KP, Rotenberg BW. Does drug-induced sleep endoscopy improve sleep surgery outcomes? *Laryngoscope.* 2020;130(11): 2518-2519.
16. De Vito A, Carrasco Llatas M, Ravesloot MJ, et al. European position paper on drug-induced sleep endoscopy: 2017 update. *Clin Otolaryngol.* 2018;43(6):1541-1552.
17. Vanderveken OM, Maurer JT, Hohenhorst W, et al. Evaluation of drug-induced sleep endoscopy as a patient selection tool for implanted upper airway stimulation for obstructive sleep apnea. *J Clin Sleep Med.* 2013;9(5):433-438.
18. Kwon OE, Jung SY, Al-Dilaijan K, Min JY, Lee KH, Kim SW. Is epiglottis surgery necessary for obstructive sleep apnea patients with epiglottis obstruction? *Laryngoscope.* 2019;129(11):2658-2662.
19. Powell NB, Zonato AI, Weaver EM, et al. Radiofrequency treatment of turbinate hypertrophy in subjects using continuous positive airway pressure: a randomized, double-blind, placebo-controlled clinical pilot trial. *Laryngoscope.* 2001;111:1783-1790.
20. Camacho M, Riaz M, Capasso R, et al. The effect of nasal surgery on continuous positive airway pressure device use and therapeutic treatment pressures: a systematic review and meta-analysis. *Sleep.* 2015;38(2): 279-286.
21. Abdullah B, Singh S. Surgical interventions for inferior turbinate hypertrophy: a comprehensive review of current techniques and technologies. *Int J Environ Res Public Health.* 2021;18(7):3441.
22. Koutsourelakis I, Georgoulopoulos G, Perraki E, et al. Randomized trial of nasal surgery for fixed nasal obstruction in obstructive sleep apnea. *Eur Respir J.* 2008;31:110-117.

23. Liu SY, Guilleminault C, Huon LK, Yoon A. Distraction osteogenesis maxillary expansion (DOME) for adult obstructive sleep apnea patients with high arched palate. *Otolaryngol Head Neck Surg.* 2017;157(2): 345-348.
24. Friedman M, Schalch P. Surgery of the palate and oropharynx. *Otolaryngol Clin North Am.* 2007;40:829-843.
25. Camacho M, Nesbitt NB, Lambert E, et al. Laser-assisted uvulopalatoplasty for obstructive sleep apnea: a systematic review and meta-analysis. *Sleep.* 2017;40(3).
26. Guilleminault C, Simmons B, Motta J, et al. Obstructive sleep apnea syndrome and tracheostomy. *Arch Intern Med.* 1981;141:985-988.
27. Conway WA, Victor L, Magilligan DJ, et al. Adverse effects of tracheostomy for sleep apnea. *JAMA.* 1981;246:347-350.
28. Camacho M, Certal V, Brietzke SE, Holty JE, Guilleminault C, Capasso R. Tracheostomy as treatment for adult obstructive sleep apnea: a systematic review and meta-analysis. *Laryngoscope.* 2014;124(3):803-811.
29. Camacho M, Teixeira J, Abdullatif J, et al. Maxillomandibular advancement and tracheostomy for morbidly obese obstructive sleep apnea: a systematic review and meta-analysis. *Otolaryngol Head Neck Surg.* 2015;152(4):619-630.
30. Powell NB, Riley RW, Troell RJ, et al. Radiofrequency volumetric tissue reduction of the palate in subjects with sleep-disordered breathing. *Chest.* 1998;113:1163-1174.
31. Llewellyn CM, Noller MW, Camacho M. Cautery-assisted palatal stiffening operation for obstructive sleep apnea: a systematic review and meta-analysis. *World J Otorhinolaryngol Head Neck Surg.* 2018;5(1): 49-56.
32. Fujita S, Conway W, Zorick F, Roth T. Surgical correction of anatomic abnormalities in obstructive sleep apnea: uvulopalatopharyngoplasty. *Otolaryngol Head Neck Surg.* 1981;89:923-934.
33. Larsson LH, Carlsson-Norlander B, Svanborg E. Four year follow-up after uvulopalatopharyngoplasty in 50 unselected patients with obstructive sleep apnea syndrome. *Laryngoscope.* 1994;104:1362-1368.
34. Fairbanks DNF. Uvulopalatopharyngoplasty complications and avoidance strategies. *Otolaryngol Head Neck Surg.* 1990;102:239-245.
35. Elshaug AG, Moss JR, Southcott A, et al. Redefining success in airway surgery for obstructive sleep apnea: a meta-analysis and synthesis of the evidence. *Sleep.* 2007;30:461-467.
36. Li HY. Palatal surgery for obstructive sleep apnea: from ablation to reconstruction. *Sleep Med Clin.* 2019;14(1):51-58.
37. Alcaraz M, Bosco G, Pérez-Martín N, et al. Advanced palate surgery: what works? *Curr Otorhinolaryngol Rep.* 2021;9:271-284.
38. Puccia R, Woodson BT. Palatopharyngoplasty and palatal anatomy and phenotypes for treatment of sleep apnea in the twenty-first century. *Otolaryngol Clin North Am.* 2020;53(3):421-429.
39. Neruntarat C. Uvulopalatal flap for obstructive sleep apnea: short-term and long-term results. *Laryngoscope.* 2011;121(3):683-687.
40. Li HY, Li KK, Chen NH, Wang PC. Modified uvulopalatopharyngoplasty: the extended uvulopalatal flap. *Am J Otolaryngol.* 2003;24(5):311-316.
41. Pang KP, Woodson BT. Expansion sphincter pharyngoplasty: a new technique for the treatment of obstructive sleep apnea. *Otolaryngol Head Neck Surg.* 2007;137(1):110-114.
42. Hong SN, Kim HG, Han SY, et al. Indications for and outcomes of expansion sphincter pharyngoplasty to treat lateral pharyngeal collapse in patients with obstructive sleep apnea. *JAMA Otolaryngol Head Neck Surg.* 2019;145(5):405-412.
43. Woodson BT, Sitton M, Jacobowitz O. Expansion sphincter pharyngoplasty and palatal advancement pharyngoplasty: airway evaluation and surgical techniques. *Oper Tech Otolaryngol Head Neck Surg.* 2012;23:3-10.
44. Askar SM, El-Bary MEA, Elshora ME, et al. Anterolateral advancement palatoplasty with tonsillectomy for retropalatal obstruction in selected cases of obstructive sleep apnea. *Eur Arch Otorhinolaryngol.* 2022;279(5):2679-2687.
45. Eesa M, Hendawy E, El-Anwar MW. Modified Z-palatoplasty for correction of acquired nasopharyngeal stenosis following palatal surgery: a case series. *Cleft Palate Craniofac J.* 2022;59(6):774-778.
46. Oh H, Kim HG, Pyo S, et al. The clinical efficacy of relocation pharyngoplasty to improve retropalatal circumferential narrowing in obstructive sleep apnea patients. *Sci Rep.* 2020;10(1):2101.
47. Pang KP, Vicini C, Montevecchi F, et al. Long-term complications of palate surgery: a multicenter study of 217 patients. *Laryngoscope.* 2020; 130(9):2281-2284.
48. Goh YH, Abdullah V, Kim SW. Genioglossus advancement and hyoid surgery. *Sleep Med Clin.* 2019;14(1):73-81.
49. Hendler B, Silverstein K, Giannakopoulos H, Costello BJ. Mortised genioplasty in the treatment of obstructive sleep apnea: an historical perspective and modification of design. *Sleep Breath.* 2001;5(4):173-180.
50. Li KK. Hypopharyngeal airway surgery. *Otolaryngol Clin North Am.* 2007;40(4):845-853.
51. Li KK, Powell NB, Riley RW, Troell RJ, Guilleminault C. Long-term results of maxillomandibular advancement surgery. *Sleep Breath.* 2000; 4(3):137-140.
52. Awad M, Capasso R. Skeletal surgery for obstructive sleep apnea. *Otolaryngol Clin North Am.* 2020;53(3):459-468.
53. Zhou N, Ho JTF, Huang Z, et al. Maxillomandibular advancement versus multilevel surgery for treatment of obstructive sleep apnea: a systematic review and meta-analysis. *Sleep Med Rev.* 2021;57:101471.
54. Li K, Powell NB, Riley RW, Guilleminault C. Temperature controlled radiofrequency tongue base reduction for sleep disordered breathing: long term outcomes. *Otolaryngol Head Neck Surg.* 2002;127:230-234.
55. Woodson BT, Nelson L, Mickelson S, Huntley T, Sher A. A multi-institutional study of radiofrequency volumetric tissue reduction for OSAS. *Otolaryngol Head Neck Surg.* 2001;125(4):303-311.
56. Friedman M, Hamilton C, Samuelson CG, et al. Transoral robotic glossectomy for the treatment of obstructive sleep apnea-hypopnea syndrome. *Otolaryngol Head Neck Surg.* 2012;146(5):854-862.
57. Miller SC, Nguyen SA, Ong AA, Gillespie MB. Transoral robotic base of tongue reduction for obstructive sleep apnea: a systematic review and meta-analysis. *Laryngoscope.* 2017;127(1):258-265.
58. Lee JA, Byun YJ, Nguyen SA, Lentsch EJ, Gillespie MB. Transoral robotic surgery versus plasma ablation for tongue base reduction in obstructive sleep apnea: meta-analysis. *Otolaryngol Head Neck Surg.* 2020;162(6):839-852.
59. Handler E, Hamans E, Goldberg AN, Mickelson S. Tongue suspension: an evidence-based review and comparison to hypopharyngeal surgery for OSA. *Laryngoscope.* 2014;124(1):329-336.
60. Ong AA, Buttram J, Nguyen SA, Platter D, Abidin MR, Gillespie MB. Hyoid myotomy and suspension without simultaneous palate or tongue base surgery for obstructive sleep apnea. *World J Otorhinolaryngol Head Neck Surg.* 2017;3(2):110-114.
61. Hsi LJ, Lee YC, Lin WN, et al. Transoral tongue suspension for obstructive sleep apnea a preliminary study. *J Clin Med.* 2022;11:4960.
62. Li KK, Powell NB, Riley RW. Surgical management of obstructive sleep apnea. In: Lee-Chiong TL, Sateia MJ, Caraskadon MA, eds. *Sleep Medicine.* Philadelphia: Hanley & Belfus; 2002:435-446.
63. Su YY, Lin PW, Lin HC, et al. Systematic review and updated meta-analysis of multi-level surgery for patients with OSA. *Auris Nasus Larynx.* 2022;49(3):421-430.
64. MacKay S, Carney AS, Catcheside PG, et al. Effect of multilevel upper airway surgery vs medical management on the apnea-hypopnea index and patient-reported daytime sleepiness among patients with moderate or severe obstructive sleep apnea: the SAMS randomized clinical trial. *JAMA.* 2020;324(12):1168-1179.
65. Strollo Jr PJ, Soose RJ, Maurer JT, et al. Upper-airway stimulation for obstructive sleep apnea. *N Engl J Med.* 2014;370(2):139-149.
66. Heiser C, Thaler E, Soose RJ, Woodson BT, Boon M. Technical tips during implantation of selective upper airway stimulation. *Laryngoscope.* 2018;128(3):756-762.
67. *Inspire Sleep Apnea Innovation.* Available at: https://manuals.inspiresleep.com (see Inspire MRI Guidelines for Inspire Therapy). Accessed January 14, 2023.
68. U.S Food and Drug Administration. *Inspire Upper Airway Stimulation – P130008/S090.* Available at: https://www.fda.gov/medical-devices/recently-approved-devices/inspire-upper-airway-stimulation-p130008s090. Accessed July 27, 2023.
69. Woodson BT, Strohl KP, Soose RJ, et al. Upper airway stimulation for obstructive sleep apnea: 5-year outcomes. *Otolaryngol Head Neck Surg.* 2018;159(1):194-202.
70. Kent DT, Carden KA, Wang L, Lindsell CJ, Ishman SL. Evaluation of hypoglossal nerve stimulation treatment in obstructive sleep apnea. *JAMA Otolaryngol Head Neck Surg.* 2019;145(11):1044-1052.
71. Thaler E, Schwab R, Maurer J, et al. Results of the ADHERE upper airway stimulation registry and predictors of therapy efficacy. *Laryngoscope.* 2020;130(5):1333-1338.
72. Soose RJ, Faber K, Greenberg H, et al. Post-implant care pathway: lessons learned and recommendations after 5 years of clinical implementation of hypoglossal nerve stimulation therapy. *Sleep.* 2021;44(suppl 1):S4-S10.
73. Steffen A, Jeschke S, Soose RJ, Hasselbacher K, König IR. Impulse configuration in hypoglossal nerve stimulation in obstructive sleep apnea: the effect of modifying pulse width and frequency. *Neuromodulation.* 2022;25(8):1312-1316.
74. Pawlak D, Bohorquez D, König IR, Steffen A, Thaler ER. Effect of electrode configuration and impulse strength on airway patency in

neurostimulation for obstructive sleep apnea. *Laryngoscope*. 2021;131(9):2148-2153.

75. Sturm JJ, Modik O, Koutsourelakis I, Suurna MV. Contralateral tongue muscle activation during hypoglossal nerve stimulation. *Otolaryngol Head Neck Surg*. 2020;162(6):985-992.
76. Lee CH, Seay EG, Walters BK, Scalzitti NJ, Dedhia RC. Therapeutic positive airway pressure level predicts response to hypoglossal nerve stimulation for obstructive sleep apnea. *J Clin Sleep Med.* 2019;15(8):1165-1172.
77. Huntley C, Steffen A, Doghramji K, Hofauer B, Heiser C, Boon M. Upper airway stimulation in patients with obstructive sleep apnea and an elevated body mass index: a multi-institutional review. *Laryngoscope*. 2018;128(10):2425-2428.
78. Liu SY, Hutz MJ, Poomkonsarn S, Chang CP, Awad M, Capasso R. Palatopharyngoplasty resolves concentric collapse in patients ineligible for upper airway stimulation. *Laryngoscope*. 2020;130(12):E958-E962.
79. Yu PK, Stenerson M, Ishman SL, et al. Evaluation of upper airway stimulation for adolescents with Down syndrome and obstructive sleep apnea. *JAMA Otolaryngol Head Neck Surg*. 2022;148(6):522-528.
80. *Inspire Medical Systems, Inc. announces FDA approval for pediatric patients with Down Syndrome*. News release. Inspire Medical Systems, Inc. Available at: https://www.globenewswire.com/news-release/2023/03/21/2631228/0/en/Inspire-Medical-Systems-Inc-Announces-FDA-Approval-for-Pediatric-Patients-with-Down-Syndrome.html. Accessed March 21, 2023.
81. Suurna MV, Jacobowitz O, Chang J, et al. Improving outcomes of hypoglossal nerve stimulation therapy: current practice, future directions and research gaps. Proceedings of the 2019 International Sleep Surgery Society Research Forum. *J Clin Sleep Med*. 2021;17(12):2477-2487.

Pediatric Obstructive Sleep Apnea—Diagnosis and Treatment

Chapter 27

INTRODUCTION

There are significant differences in the diagnosis and management of obstructive sleep apnea (OSA) in pediatric patients compared to adults.[1-5] The American Academy of Sleep Medicine (AASM) scoring manual[6] definitions for respiratory events in children are discussed in detail in Chapter 12. The major differences in the presentation and characteristics of OSA between children and adults are listed in Table 27–1. Although very obese children or those with structural upper airway abnormalities can present with symptoms similar to those of adults, the typical history in childhood OSA may include inattentiveness, aggressive behavior, and/or impulsiveness[1-4] combined with abnormal sleep behaviors observed by the parents. These nocturnal behaviors include snoring, labored breathing, diaphoresis, paradoxical chest movement, or frequent movements during sleep. Less commonly, children can present with failure to thrive. A systematic review and associated recommendations for the evaluation and treatment of pediatric OSA are available.[1,2]

EPIDEMIOLOGY

The age range with the highest prevalence of patients with OSA is typically from 4 to 6 years (some authors state 2 to 8 years), when hypertrophy of the tonsils occurs.[1-5,7] A 2008 review of breathing in children concluded that the prevalence of "always" snoring ranged from 1.5% to 6% and that of *"habitual snoring" ranged from 5% to 12%.*[7] The prevalence of parent-reported apneic events ranged from 0.2% to 4%. Using questionnaires completed by parents, the prevalence of OSA has been estimated to be 4% to 11%. *The prevalence of OSA in children by diagnostic studies has been estimated to be 1% to 4%* (reported range 0.1%–13%). Evidence suggests that pediatric OSA is more common among heavier children. Studies of younger children (<13 years) have generally found an *equal prevalence of OSA in boys and girls.* In the majority of studies including older children, a male predominance was found.[5] There may be a higher prevalence of pediatric OSA among African Americans than among Whites.

Consequences of Childhood OSA

Many of the consequences of untreated pediatric OSA[5-8] are listed in Table 27–2. The consequences are divided into neurobehavioral, metabolic, and cardiovascular groups.

Neuro-Behavioral Consequences

Studies have suggested that both habitual snoring and childhood OSA are associated with behavioral problems, particularly impulsiveness, aggressiveness, and inattentive behaviors.[4] These may improve after effective treatment (usually tonsillectomy and adenoidectomy, TNA). Sometimes, a diagnosis of attention-deficit/hyperactive disorder (ADHD) is made when a child actually has OSA. However, one should not assume every child with ADHD has OSA. Children with OSA often have poor school performance and impaired performance on intelligence tests that improve with treatment. Both hypoxia and sleep fragmentation may cause neurocognitive issues. While studies suggest impairment is reversible with treatment, it is still unknown if an irreversible component of central nervous system (CNS) damage occurs with untreated OSA.

One study[9] of 3- to 12-year-old children compared a group with snoring and a mean apnea hypopnea index (AHI) of 0.5 events/hr with a group with OSA and a mean AHI of 5.2 events/hour. The children with snoring had more abnormal executive function scores than the children with OSA. There were also elevated Conners scores for inattention and hyperactivity in the snoring group. The authors concluded that young, snoring children with only minimally elevated apnea-hypopnea levels may still be at risk for deficits in executive function and attention. The CHAT study[10] compared watchful waiting versus TNA for OSA in school-aged children and found that surgery did reduce symptoms and improve outcomes of behavior, quality of life, and polysomnography (PSG) findings. The study did not a find a significant improvement in inattention or executive function as measured by neuropsychological testing. As in adults, individuals with similar AHIs may have variable benefits from treatment. It is also difficult to show an improvement in individuals without symptoms at baseline.

Although excessive daytime sleepiness is less prominent in childhood OSA than in adult OSA, it does occur and may be unrecognized. Using the multiple sleep latency test, daytime sleepiness is thought to occur in between 13% and 40% of children with OSA.[11,12] *Daytime sleepiness is often more prominent in obese children with pediatric OSA or in older children.* Given the obesity epidemic, more obese children are being evaluated in sleep clinics.

Metabolic and Inflammatory Consequences

Untreated pediatric OSA has been associated with a failure to thrive[7]. The possible origin is a reduction in insulin-like growth factor (IGF) and growth hormone secretion. IGF binding protein levels (IGF-3) correlate with growth hormone secretion and are decreased in some children with OSA. These changes are reversible, and catch-up growth occurs with adequate treatment. With the obesity epidemic, obesity is more often noted than failure to thrive. *Up to half of pediatric patients with OSA are obese.* Leptin, an adipocyte secreted hormone, is increased in children with OSA and decreases after treatment.[13,14]

Leukotrienes and their receptors are increased in adenotonsillar tissue and in exhaled condensates of children with OSA.[15,16] The combination of nasal inhaled steroid and leukotriene inhibitors (montelukast) was found to have benefit in a study of patients with residual sleepiness after tonsillectomy and adenoidectomy.[17] However, long-term success with anti-inflammatory therapy has not been established.[18] Of note, the

Table 27-1 Differences Between Children and Adults With Obstructive Sleep Apnea

	Children	Adults
Clinical Findings		
Peak age	Preschool (4–6 years)	60–70 years
Sex ratio	M = F age < 13 years M > F if older children included	M > F
Etiology	Adenotonsillar hypertrophy	Obesity/upper airway structural shape
Weight	Failure to thrive to obese, many normal in size	Obese
Excessive daytime sleepiness	Less common	Common
Neurobehavioral	Impulsiveness, aggression, inattention	Impaired vigilance
Polysomnography		
Study type	Diagnostic, PAP titration, no split studies	Diagnostic, titration, split night PSG Home sleep apnea testing
Definition of abnormal	Obstructive apnea index > 1 event/hour OAHI > 1.0–1.4 events/hour	AHI ≥ 5/hr
Definition of severity	OAHI 1 to < 5 events/hour mild, 5 to 10 events/hour moderate, >10 events/hour severe	AHI 5 to <15 events/hour mild, 15–30 events/hour moderate, >30 events/hour severe
Pattern of obstruction	Obstructive hypoventilation Apnea and hypopnea during REM sleep	Obstructive apnea/hypopnea in NREM and REM sleep Higher AHI in REM sleep
Sleep architecture	Normal	Reduced stage N3 and REM sleep
Sleep stage with OSA	REM (stage R)	REM > NREM
Cortical arousal	Low rates <50% of apneas	High rates 60%–80% of apneas/hypopneas

AHI, apnea-hypopnea index; *NREM*, non-rapid eye movement; *OAHI*, obstructive apnea-hypopnea index (OA+MA+H) × 60/total sleep time (TST) min; *OSA*, obstructive sleep apnea; *PSG*, polysomnography; *REM*, rapid eye movement; *RDI*, respiratory disturbance index; *RERA*, respiratory effort related arousal.

Table 27-2 Sequelae of Pediatric Obstructive Sleep Apnea

Neurocognitive
Decreased quality of life
Aggressive behavior
Poor school performance
Depression
Attention deficit
Hyperactivity
Moodiness
Metabolic
Elevated C-reactive protein
Insulin resistance
Hypercholesterolemia
Elevated transaminases
Decreased insulin like growth factor (IGF)
Decreased/altered growth hormone secretion
Increased leptin
Cardiovascular
Autonomic dysfunction
Systemic hypertension
Absent blood pressure "dipping" during sleep
Left ventricular dysfunction
Pulmonary hypertension
Abnormal heart rate variability
Elevated vascular endothelial growth factor

Adapted from Katz ES, D'Ambrosio CM. Pediatric obstructive sleep apnea syndrome. *Clin Chest Med.* 2010;31(2):221-234.

labeling approved by the U.S. Food and Drug Administration (FDA) for montelukast includes a black box warning that serious neuropsychiatric events that may include suicidal thoughts or actions have been reported in patients taking this medication.[19]

Children with OSA may also have elevated serum levels of tumor necrosis factor alpha (TNF-α), C-reactive protein, interleukin (IL) 6 and 8, and interferon gamma.[5] These changes can occur independent of obesity.

Cardiovascular Consequences

Children with OSA have cardiovascular consequences similar to those of adults, but changes occur at much lower AHI values typical in children.[5] Children with "severe" OSA (AHI > 10 events/hour) may have a lack of nocturnal blood pressure dipping and high morning blood pressure. In severe cases, right and left ventricular hypertrophy have been described.

DIAGNOSIS

PSG is the test indicated for the diagnosis of OSA in children.[20] A position statement by the AASM does not recommend home sleep apnea testing (HSAT) in children.[21] This recommendation followed a review of the literature. However, it is likely HSAT will be increasingly used in the future (especially in older children). A study of a neural network-based automated analyses of nocturnal oximetry recordings was found to provide accurate identification of OSA severity among habitually snoring children with a **high pretest probability of OSA.**[22] Thus, nocturnal oximetry may enable a simple and effective diagnostic alternative to nocturnal PSG, leading to more timely interventions and potentially improved outcomes when traditional sleep testing is not available or delayed. The recommended sensors for monitoring respiratory events during PSG and the event definitions are included in the AASM scoring manual[4] and discussed in Chapters 10 and 12.

The *International Classification of Sleep Disorders*, 3rd edition, text revision (ICSD-3-TR) diagnostic criteria for pediatric OSA[23] includes the following (criteria A–C must be met):

A. The presence of *one or more* of the following:
- Snoring
- Labored, paradoxical, or obstructed breathing during the child's sleep.
- Sleepiness, hyperactivity, behavioral problems, or learning and other cognitive problems.

B. PSG demonstrates *one or more* of the following:
1. One or more obstructive or mixed apneas, or hypopneas, per hour of sleep (OAHI)
2. A pattern of obstructive hypoventilation, defined as at least 25% of total sleep time with hypercapnia ($PaCO_2$ > 50 mm Hg), arterial oxygen desaturation, or combined hypercapnia and desaturation, in association with *one or more* of the following:
   - snoring
   - flattening of the inspiratory nasal pressure waveform
   - paradoxical thoracoabdominal motion

C. The symptoms are not better explained by another current sleep disorder, medical disorder, medication, or substance use.

Note that respiratory effort-related arousals (RERAs) are not included, as their physiological consequences are unknown. In addition, given the inclusive pediatric hypopnea definition using an associated ≥3% desaturation or arousal, there are very few RERAs. Some pediatric sleep centers report not only the AHI but the obstructive apnea and hypopnea index (obstructive and mixed apneas + hypopneas per hour of sleep, OAHI) and a central apnea index (CAI). The values of respiratory indices considered to be diagnostic of pediatric OSA vary, but typically, an OAHI of >1 or >1 to 2 events/hour is used as a criteria for diagnosis.[24] Some clinicians use an OAHI of ≥1.4 events/hour as the cutoff for diagnosis of OSA. The decision to treat is based on symptoms as well as PSG findings (OAHI). No widely accepted severity ranges are available, but many centers treat patients with an OAHI of 2 to 5 events/hour. An AHI of 5 to 10 events/hour is considered *moderate OSA*, and an AHI of >10 events/hour is considered severe in children.[24] As noted, a diagnosis of OSA can also be made based on obstructive hypoventilation, defined as the presence of hypoventilation PCO_2 >50 mm Hg for >25% of the total sleep time, arterial oxygen desaturation, or a combination of hypoventilation and desaturation associated with snoring, flattening of the inspiratory nasal pressure waveform, or paradoxical thoracoabdominal motion. The requirement of the associated findings differentiates between OSA and disorders of hypoventilation due to abnormal ventilatory control or muscle weakness in the absence of upper airway abnormality.[23]

Physical Examination

General examination of children with OSA may reveal mouth breathing, adenoidal facies, or findings of craniofacial abnormality. The voice may have a hyponasal quality (adenoidal obstruction). Tonsils are often (but not always) enlarged. The child's weight with respect to norms is important, as obesity is a major factor, especially in older children. The head and neck examination should focus on findings of retrognathia, micrognathia, nasal obstruction, macroglossia, and midfacial hypoplasia. A higher Mallampati score is associated with a greater risk of OSA but examination is not always possible.

Polysomnography in Pediatric OSA

Children with OSA may exhibit cyclic obstructive apneas, as in adults, or a pattern of hypopneas and long periods of upper airway narrowing termed *obstructive hypoventilation. Most obstructive apneas and hypopneas in pediatric patients occurs during REM sleep* (Fig. 27–1). Obstructive events can also occur in stage N2 but are uncommon in stage N3. Hypopneas are more common than apneas. Of note, even short apneas can be associated with severe arterial oxygen desaturation, especially in younger children who have a small functional residual capacity or reduced oxygen stores. Obstructive hypoventilation is characterized by long periods of airflow limitation, increased inspiratory effort, increased end-tidal partial pressure of carbon dioxide ($P_{ET}CO_2$), and variable amounts of arterial oxygen desaturation (Fig. 27–2). Traditional monitoring using oronasal thermistor flow often demonstrates few changes, but nasal pressure monitoring shows airflow limitation (flattening) and reduced but stable flow. There is an elevation in $P_{ET}CO_2$, perhaps associated with mild drops in the SaO_2. Paradoxical motion of the chest and abdomen may be noted (chest moving inward during inspiration). This common pattern is the reason that $P_{ET}CO_2$ monitoring is an integral part of pediatric sleep studies. Note paradoxical chest wall motion can be normal during REM sleep in children 1 to 3 years of age due to immaturity of the chest wall structures. As noted, typical severity ranges for pediatric OSA are mild (OAHI ≥1–5 events/hour), moderate (>5–10 events/hour), and severe (>10 events/hour).

The AASM scoring manual[4] states that sleep-related hypoventilation in children should be scored when greater than 25% of the total sleep time is spent with a PCO_2 >50 mm Hg using transcutaneous carbon dioxide ($TcPCO_2$) monitoring or measurement of $P_{ET}CO_2$. However, other definitions for what constitute abnormal CO_2 values have been suggested (peak CO_2 >49 torr, mean CO_2 >50 torr, 2% of total sleep time with $TcCO_2$ above 50 torr).[25,26] A study analyzed data from the CHAT study[10] with respect to the relationship of end-tidal PCO_2 findings and the AHI.[25] In this study, the mean $P_{ET}CO_2$ increased an average of 3 mm Hg from wakefulness to sleep. The average awake value was 41.7 mm Hg. This knowledge is useful for interpreting the results of $P_{ET}CO_2$ monitoring. Only 13% of 876 children screened for OSA had $P_{ET}CO_2$ findings that met AASM criteria for hypoventilation. A plot of the percentage of screening sleep studies meeting criteria for hypoventilation in each AHI category is shown in Figure 27–3. On average, the percentage of studies meeting criteria for hypoventilation increased as the AHI increased. *However, the correlation between the AHI and the percentage of total sleep time (TST) with $P_{ET}CO_2$ >50 mm Hg was low* ($r = 0.33$, $P < 0.0001$). Thus, the AHI and measurements of end-tidal PCO_2 appear to provide different information. Some clinicians believe the AASM definition of hypoventilation may be too strict and that each patient must be considered individually.[26] For example, a patient with 20%

100%
95%
90%
SaO2
85%
80%
75%
70%
Hypopnea
Ob Apnea
Wake
REM
Stage
N1
N2
N3
60 120 180 240 300 360 420 480 540 600 660 720 780 840 900 960
21:50:31 23 00 01 02 03 04 05 06:02:44

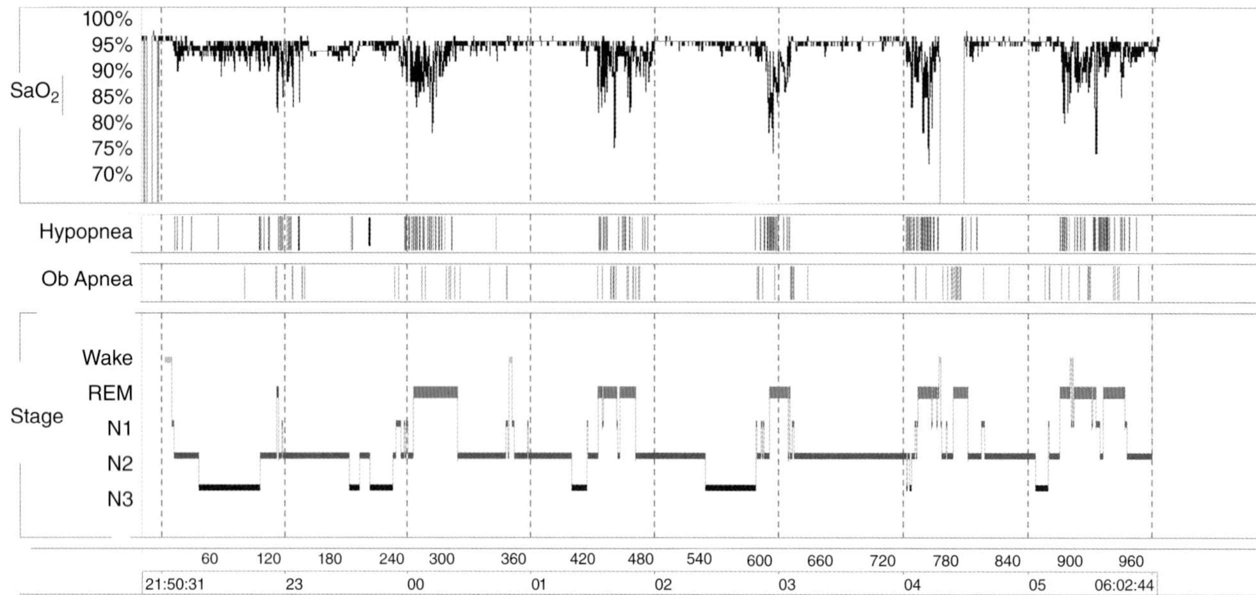

Figure 27–1 All-night summary of polysomnography (PSG) in 3-year-old girl with very loud snoring and disturbed sleep. Note that most of the respiratory events were noted during REM sleep. The overall AHI was 26.2/hour with 74 obstructive apneas, 4 central apneas, and 128 hypopneas. The AHI during REM sleep was 72.4/hour. *AHI,* Apnea-hypopnea index; *Ob Apnea,* Obstructive apnea.

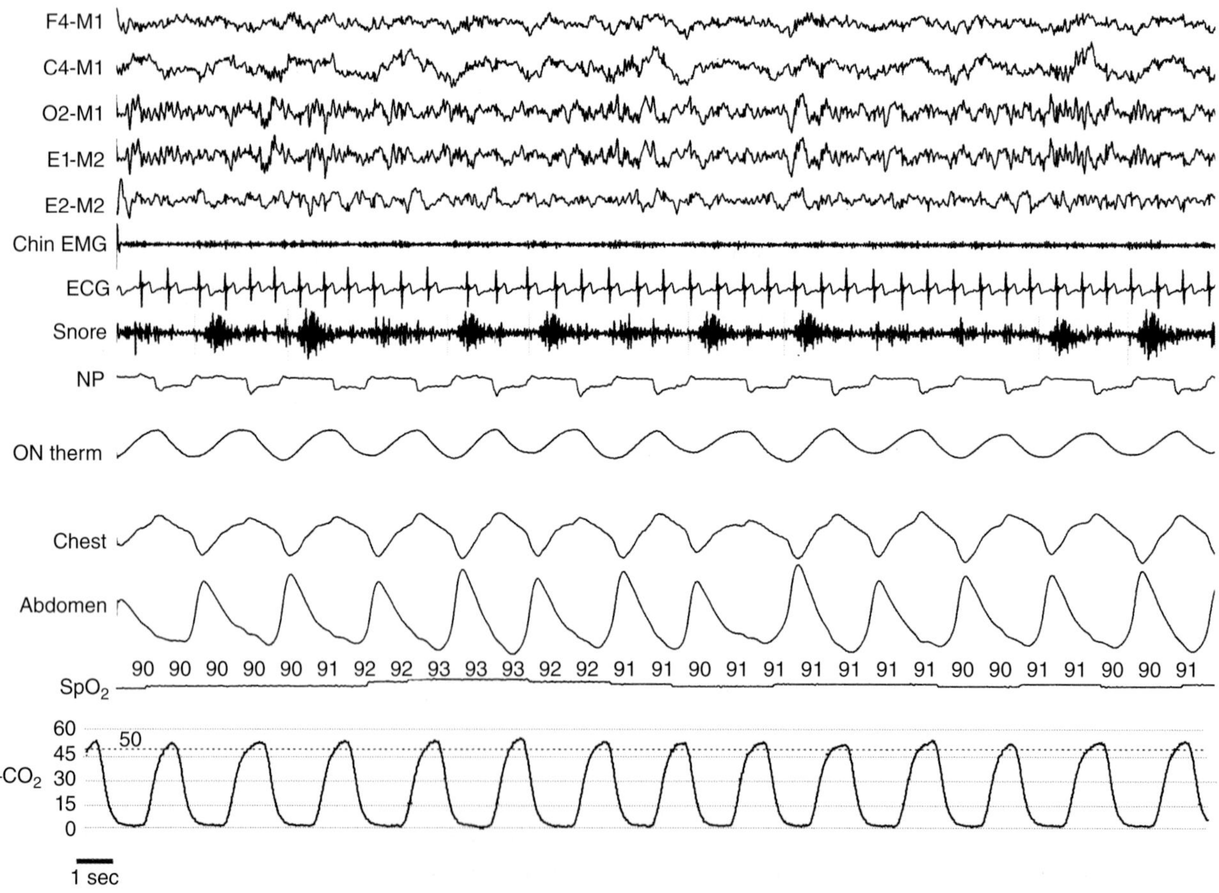

F4-M1
C4-M1
O2-M1
E1-M2
E2-M2
Chin EMG
ECG
Snore
NP
ON therm
Chest
Abdomen
90 90 90 90 90 91 92 92 93 93 93 92 92 91 91 90 91 91 91 91 91 91 90 90 91 91 90 90 91
SpO2
60
50
45
PETCO2 30
15
0
1 sec

Figure 27–2 **Obstructive Hypoventilation in a Pediatric Patient With OSA (30-second tracing).** The end-tidal partial pressure of CO_2 (PCO_2) is greater than 50 mm Hg, and there is evidence of flattening of the nasal pressure (airflow limitation). Paradoxical breathing (chest and abdomen out of phase), snoring, and a very mild drop in the arterial oxygen saturation (SpO_2) are noted. Inspiration is in an upward direction.

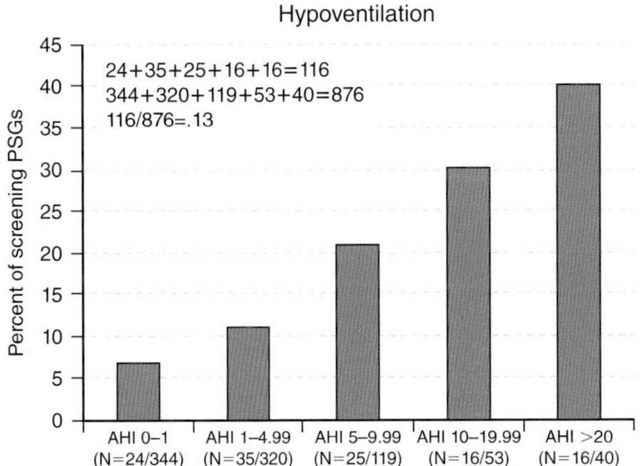

Figure 27–3 The relationship between the apnea-hypopnea index (AHI) and percentage of studies in each AHI category meeting criteria for hypoventilation (surrogate of $PaCO_2$ >50 mm Hg for >25% of total sleep time) based on end-tidal PCO_2 ($P_{ET}CO_2$) measurements. Note that, on average, the percentage meeting hypoventilation criteria increases with AHI severity. Only 13% of 876 children screened for obstructive sleep apnea (OSA) had a $P_{ET}CO_2$ meeting the American Academy of Sleep Medicine (AASM) criteria for hypoventilation. (From Paruthi S, Rosen CL, Wang R, et al. End-tidal carbon dioxide measurement during pediatric polysomnography: signal quality, association with apnea severity, and prediction of neurobehavioral outcomes. *Sleep.* 2015;38[11]:1719-1726.)

TST with a PCO_2 >50 mm Hg should not be considered "normal." Measurement of hypercapnia and AHI provide valuable but different information.[25] Of note, the CHAT study[10,25] demonstrated that hypercapnia improved after TNA but less so than the AHI and did the finding of hypercapnia was not predictive of neurocognitive improvement after TNA.[3] However, the presurgery AHI *also did not predict neurocognitive improvements* following TNA.

The sleep architecture may be relatively preserved in pediatric OSA,[3] as fewer arousals may be noted following obstructive events (high arousal threshold). In addition, the long periods of obstructive hypoventilation do not result in frequent arousals. The infrequent arousals may explain why sleep architecture is often fairly normal in pediatric patients with OSA.

TREATMENT OF PEDIATRIC OSA

The major treatment options for pediatric OSA are listed in Box 27–1. Because the majority of pediatric OSA is associated with adenotonsillar hypertrophy, the initial treatment is TNA[1,2] (unless tonsillar hypertrophy is not present). It is important to note, however, that *the presence or severity of OSA does not correlate with tonsillar size.* Other factors such as upper airway structure or obesity contribute to the effect of tonsillar hypertrophy on breathing during sleep. The epidemic of childhood obesity has tremendous implications for treatment and treatment outcomes. OSA in obese children is more similar to adult OSA. However, the current recommendations continue to be TNA (even in obese children) if tonsillar hypertrophy is present. A 2012 systematic review[2] concluded: "Although OSA improved postoperatively, the proportion of patients who had residual OSA ranged from 13% to 29% in low-risk populations to 73% when obese children were included and stricter polysomnographic criteria were used. Nevertheless, OSA may improve after TNA even in obese children, thus supporting surgery as a reasonable initial treatment."[1,2] Certainly, patients with residual symptoms or with a pretreatment

Box 27–1 TREATMENT FOR PEDIATRIC OBSTRUCTIVE SLEEP APNEA

Treatment options
- TNA – first line treatment unless tonsillar tissue absent
- Distraction osteogenesis (in special populations)
- Rapid maxillary expansion (if maxillary constriction present)
- Maxillomandibular advancement – severe cases of intractable OSA
- PAP
- Medical treatments:
  - Weight loss
  - Nasal medications (intranasal steroids)

Mild OSA
- Watchful waiting (6 months)
- Weight Loss
- Nasal medications
- TNA

Moderate OSA
- Specialist referral
- TNA*
- Weight loss, if indicated
- If residual OSA:
  - Weight loss
  - Nasal medications
  - CPAP
  - Dental and surgical options

Severe OSA
- Specialist referral
- Cardiology evaluation, if indicated
- TNA with additional monitoring post-surgery*
- If residual OSA:
  - Weight loss
  - Nasal medications
  - CPAP
  - Dental and surgical options

Severe Structural Upper Airway Abnormality
- Combined sleep specialist, surgical evaluation
- Airway and/or craniofacial surgery
- High level of monitoring after surgical procedures

OSA, obstructive sleep apnea; *TNA,* tonsillectomy and adenoidectomy; *PAP,* positive airway pressure; *CPAP,* continuous PAP.
*Follow-up polysomnography recommended after TNA.

OAHI in the moderate-to-severe range should be restudied. If a significant residual OAHI is present after TNA, possible treatments include weight loss, positive airway pressure, dental procedures such as rapid maxillary expansion, or medications to reduce upper airway/swelling obstruction.

Medical Treatment of OSA in Pediatric Patients

In obese children, weight management should be instituted even if TNA is planned. Some studies suggest a role for anti-inflammatory therapy in management of adenotonsillar hypertrophy. Such treatments may suffice in patients with mild OSA or when surgery is delayed or not possible. As noted, the combination of nasal inhaled steroid and leukotriene inhibitors (montelukast) was found to have benefit in a study of patients with residual sleepiness after TNA.[17] A Cochran review concluded that leukotriene inhibitors worked for milder OSA but did not find evidence for use of nasal steroids alone.[18] However, use of montelukast should be considered carefully due to reports of neuropsychiatric side effects of this medication.[19]

Tonsillectomy and Adenoidectomy

TNA has been the standard treatment for OSA in pediatric patients for many years (Fig. 27–4). There are over 400,000 such surgeries performed per year. It is estimated that PSG is performed in only about 10% of patients undergoing TNA.[27-29] Studies have shown that history and physical examination are not accurate in predicting the presence or absence of OSA. Tonsil size is not predictive of OSA. However, the need for routine PSG before TNA for childhood sleep apnea is still debated.[27,28]

Guidelines published by the American Academy of Pediatrics[2] include:

- All children/adolescents should be screened for snoring.
- PSG should be performed in children/adolescents with snoring and symptoms/signs of OSA; if PSG is not available, then alternative diagnostic tests or referral to a specialist for more extensive evaluation may be considered.
- Adenotonsillectomy is recommended as the first-line treatment for patients with OSA and adenotonsillar hypertrophy.
- High-risk patients should be postoperatively monitored as inpatients.
- Patients should be reevaluated postoperatively to determine whether further treatment is required. Objective testing should be performed in patients who are high risk or have persistent symptoms/signs of OSA after therapy.
- Continuous positive airway pressure (CPAP) is recommended as treatment if adenotonsillectomy is not performed or if OSA persists postoperatively.
- Weight loss is recommended in addition to other therapy in patients who are overweight or obese.
- Intranasal corticosteroids are an option for children with mild OSA in whom adenotonsillectomy is contraindicated or for mild postoperative OSA.

Performing PSG before TNA has a number of advantages: (1) accurate diagnosis and avoiding unnecessary surgery, (2) PSG results provide parents with an estimate of chance of surgical success (patients with an elevated AHI may require additional treatment beyond TNA), and (3) the PSG and clinical evaluation may reveal factors indicating increased risk for postoperative complications.

The American Academy of Otolaryngology-Head and Neck Surgery[29] suggests considering TNA in children with tonsillar hypertrophy and comorbid conditions that may improve after surgery, including growth failure, poor academic performance, behavioral issues, enuresis, and asthma. They also suggest PSG in certain populations (aged <2 years, Trisomy 21, craniofacial abnormalities, mucopolysaccharidoses, neuromuscular dysfunction, and sickle cell anemia) in which potential symptoms may be difficult to discern.

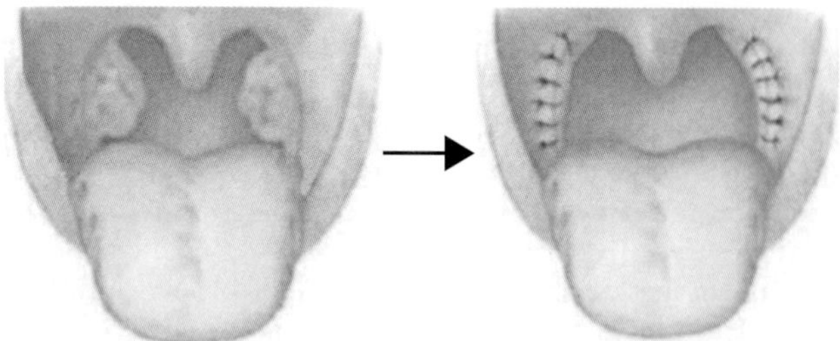

Figure 27–4 Tonsillectomy and Adenoidectomy (TNA). The adenoid and tonsillar tissues are removed, and the lateral pharyngeal walls are sutured to prevent collapse.

Studies before the obesity epidemic found that TNA successfully eliminated OSA in 75% to 100% of patients. More recent prospective studies using postoperative PSG have found lower cure rates (depending on the definition of success).[30-32] Treatment success has been defined over an AHI range of 1 to 5 events/hour. A meta-analysis by Brietzke et al.[30] found 82% of patients to be successfully treated for OSA by TNA. Another meta-analysis of the efficacy of TNA by Friedman and associates[31] found that a “cure,” defined as an AHI <1 event/hour, occurred in about 60% of patients. Most patients undergoing TNA do improve, but frequently, significant residual OSA is still present. A meta-analysis published in 2017 of 11 studies[32] found that, relative to watchful waiting, most studies reported better sleep-related outcomes in children who had tonsillectomies. A meta-analysis of three of the eleven studies showed a 4.8-point improvement in the AHI in children who underwent tonsillectomy compared to that of children with no surgery. Sleep-related quality of life and negative behaviors (e.g., anxiety and emotional lability) also improved more among children who had a tonsillectomy. Changes in executive function were not significantly different between TNA and watchful waiting.

The CHAT study randomized 464 children who met entry criteria to early TNA (eTNA) or watchful waiting care (WWC).[10] Follow-up data were available for 86% with 397 having attention and executive function tested at 7 months. The entry criteria were OAHI ≥2 events/hour or an obstructive apnea index (OAI ≥1 event/hour). Children with an AHI score of more than 30 events/hour, an OAI score of more than 20 events/hour, or arterial oxyhemoglobin saturation of less than 90% for 2% or more of TST were excluded. Recurrent tonsillitis, medication for ADHD or significantly increased body weight were other exclusions. Health outcomes were assessed at 7 months. The median AHI in the eTNA group was 4.8 events/hour and in the WWC group was 4.5 events/hour. Children randomized to TNA did NOT have greater improvement in attention or executive function. On the other hand, both groups had improved scores, suggesting WWC is a reasonable approach in properly selected children. The eTNA group did have greater improvement in behavioral, quality of life, and PSG findings. Normalization of PSG findings was greater in the eTNA group than in the WWC group (79% vs. 46%). Normalization was defined by a reduction in both the OAHI score to fewer than 2 events/hour and the OAI score to fewer than 1 event/hour. The study did document benefit from TNA but also showed that WWC did not adversely affect attention or executive function (at least in 7 months). Of interest, while the percentage of children with normalized AHI with TNA was higher in non-obese children (85%), *65% of obese children still had normalization.* This study did not show a correlation between the severity of OSA, as measured by PSG, and neurobehavioral outcomes—a finding similar to those in other studies. The normalization of the AHI in the WWC group was of interest, and the etiology of improvement is unknown. A limitation of the study was that it did not include children younger than 5 years of age, those with severe obesity, or those with significant desaturation.

Given the finding that TNA normalized the AHI in 65% of obese children, TNA is still considered the initial treatment of choice in pediatric patients with OSA and tonsillar hypertrophy,[2] even if obesity is present.

Complications from TNA

Complications of TNA include bleeding, pain, infection, and weight loss. Classic tonsillectomy dissects the tonsillar capsule off the pharyngeal constrictor muscles using "cold" dissection. Alternatives to conventional cold dissection include electrosurgery (mono- or bi-polar) and plasma-mediated ablation (coblation). Partial tonsillectomy, a modified procedure in which the majority of tonsillar tissue is removed but the tonsillar capsule remains in place, is increasingly being utilized to treat OSA in children.[33] Complication rates of partial tonsillectomy (also known as tonsillotomy and intracapsular tonsillectomy) are lower than those of standard tonsillectomy; however, few studies have examined its therapeutic effect.[33] The subset of children with both obesity and asthma are more likely to experience resolution of OSA following traditional tonsillectomy compared to partial tonsillectomy.[34]

A list of proposed risk factors for TNA requiring overnight hospitalization or more long-term recovery-room monitoring is listed in Table 27–3.[29,35] Nasal CPAP can be used to manage postoperative complications in very severely affected individuals. The need for routine **postoperative** PSG in patients who have undergone TNA (after surgical healing) is also a subject of controversy. The American Academy of Pediatric guidelines[2] recommend "Patients should be reevaluated postoperatively to determine whether further treatment is required. Objective testing should be performed in patients who are high risk or have persistent symptoms/signs of OSA after therapy." High-risk patients include those with moderate or severe OSA (AHI of 5–10 or >10 events/hour, respectively) presurgery as well as those with failure to thrive, craniofacial abnormalities, pulmonary hypertension, or significant obesity (Table 27–4). Nasal CPAP and weight loss (if applicable) can be used to treat significant residual OSA after TNA.

Table 27–3 Criteria for Increased Risk of Tonsillectomy and Adenoidectomy (overnight hospitalization indicated post-operatively)

Clinical Criteria

- Age <3 years
- Craniofacial abnormalities affecting the pharyngeal airway (especially midface hypoplasia or micrognathia/retrognathia)
- Failure to thrive
- Hypotonia
- Obesity
- Neuromuscular disorders
- Cardiac complications of OSA (right ventricular hypertrophy, cor pulmonale)
- Previous upper airway trauma
- Undergoing a UPPP in addition to TNA

PSG Criteria

- Severe OSA on PSG
- SaO_2 nadir less than 80%

OSA, obstructive sleep apnea; *UPPP*, uvulopalatopharyngoplasty; *TNA*, tonsillectomy and adenoidectomy; *PSG*, polysomnography. Adapted from references 29 and 35.

Table 27–4 Indications for Repeat PSG after TNA

- Persistent symptoms or return of symptoms
- AHI moderate-to-severe OSA (AHI of 5–10 events/hour, or >10 events/hour, respectively)
- Failure to thrive
- Craniofacial abnormalities
- Pulmonary hypertension
- Severe obesity

TNA, tonsillectomy and adenoidectomy; *PSG*, polysomnography; *AHI*, apnea-hypopnea index; *OSA*, obstructive sleep apnea.

Rapid Maxillary Expansion and Distraction Osteogenesis

Rapid maxillary expansion (RME) in conjunction with TNA has been shown to be successful in treating children with OSA and maxillary contraction (high arched palate and unilateral or bilateral crossbite).[36-38] RME requires an orthodontic device (Fig. 27–5) anchored to two upper molars on each side of the jaw that applies daily pressure, causing each half of the maxilla to grow apart. This technique aims to expand the hard palate laterally, raise the soft palate, and widen the nasal passages. RME needs to occur before cartilage becomes bone (5–16 years of age). Of interest, one publication found that RME can decrease the size of tonsils and adenoids.[39] Distraction osteogenesis is defined as the mechanical induction of new bone between two bony surfaces that are gradually distracted (separated). If RME is not successful or deemed insufficient, mandibular distraction osteogenesis is surgically performed.[40] In this procedure, osteotomies are created in the mandible, then either an internal or external device is used to distract the bones. Mandibular distraction osteogenesis is often used to treat sleep apnea in patients with severe congenital abnormalities of the mandible (mandibular retrognathia), as in Treacher Collins syndrome or Pierre Robin syndrome.

Positive Airway Pressure Treatment in Pediatric Patients

Positive airway pressure (PAP) titrations in children require special considerations.[41-47] The AASM has published guidelines for titration of PAP that include recommendations for children.[41] However, a number of issues are worth mentioning. First, split studies are not recommended for children. If a child without previous mask desensitization undergoes a split-night study, during the PAP titration portion, the child may be frightened, making subsequent CPAP use unlikely. Children are often given a mask to play with and try on during the day for a period of time before attempting a titration study. The child should be desensitized to the mask during the day by wearing it for increasing periods of time while engaging in a fun activity (e.g., watching a favorite video). Pediatric-sized masks should be used. In patients with neuromuscular disorders or ventilatory control disorders, wearing a mask for long hours can result in midface hypoplasia. Therefore, awareness of this potential problem, alternating treatment with different types of mask, and avoiding overtightening of the mask are important considerations. Durable medical equipment providers and sleep technologists skilled and willing to provide care for pediatric patients should be utilized. Studies have shown that structured behavioral interventions help with compliance (graduated exposure, positive reinforcement, dealing with escape and avoidance behavior), and

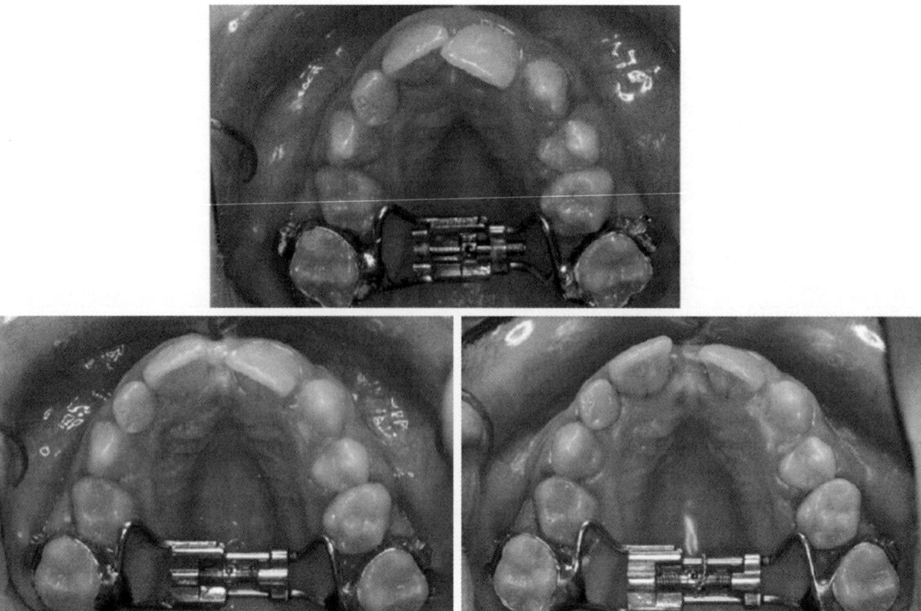

Figure 27–5 Occlusal sequence of treatment with rapid maxillary expansion from crowding in the upper central incisors (top) to a wide space (bottom). Note how the palatal vault has changed. (From Pirelli P, Saponara M, Gulleminault C. Rapid maxillary expansion in children with obstructive sleep apnea syndrome. *Sleep.* 2004;27:764.)

praising and distracting activities that allowed the child to wear a mask.[43-44] As in adults, objective monitoring of adherence in children and adolescents is essential to guide treatment. Since the sleep duration in children is longer than in adults, no widely accepted values for adequate adherence exists. Many studies of CPAP in children have documented average usage in the 3-to-4 hour range, a duration that is clearly inadequate. Studies of PAP adherence and discussion of possible interventions for improvement are summarized by Parmar et al. in a review of PAP treatment for OSA in children.[45]

A prospective study of PAP adherence in children and adolescents found that adherence is related primarily to family and demographic factors rather than severity of apnea or measures of psychosocial functioning.[46] The authors concluded that further research is needed to determine the relative contributions of maternal education, socioeconomic status, and cultural beliefs to PAP adherence in children and to develop better adherence programs. The involvement of psychologists and social workers skilled in behavioral interventions in children should be an integral part of CPAP programs for children. A questionnaire has been developed to identify barriers to CPAP use.[47]

Special Populations

OSA is very common in Down syndrome (Trisomy 21), which is associated with obesity and macroglossia. The American Academy of Pediatrics (AAP) recommends that all Down syndrome children have a PSG between the ages of 3 and 4 years[48]. Referral to a pediatric sleep specialist is also recommended to assist with treatment of OSA. The initial treatment in most Down children with OSA is TNA (unless minimal tonsillar tissue is present). A significant fraction will continue to have residual OSA following surgery. The AAP recommends a PSG after TNA (after surgical healing). While some patients do surprisingly well with CPAP, many others do not accept or adhere to PAP treatment. Recently, use of hypoglossal nerve stimulation has been shown to be a reasonable alternative if CPAP treatment is not possible.[49] The FDA has approved hypoglossal nerve stimulation treatment of OSA in patients with Down syndrome 13 years of age or older with an AHI between 10 and 50 events/hour who do not have the ability to benefit from CPAP.[50]

The care of patients with OSA and craniofacial abnormalities requires a team approach, including pediatric pulmonologists; dentists; ear, nose, and throat specialists; and maxillofacial surgeons. Physicians should also be aware that use of nasal CPAP can produce midfacial and dental changes, especially in children with craniofacial conditions.[51]

Most of the information in this chapter concerns children older than one year of age. Reference PSG values for healthy newborns have been published and the results differ from older children.[52] A group with a conceptual age between 37 and 42 weeks were tested before 30 days of age. The mean AHI was 14.9/hour with central, obstructive, mixed apnea indices of 5.4, 2.3, and 1.2 events/hour, respectively. Only 6.2% of the time was spent with an end-tidal PCO_2 above 45 mmHg. All events were brief and no event lasted longer that 20 seconds.[52] Other studies have shown lower AHI values at 3 months (4.9/hour)[53]. As PSG is more frequently performed in very young infants this information may be useful to clinicians.

SUMMARY OF KEY POINTS

1. The presentation of pediatric OSA differs from that of adult OSA. Frequently, behavioral issues and disturbed sleep rather than daytime sleepiness prompt evaluation.
2. Criteria vary, but an OAHI ≥1 to 2 events/hour and an OAI ≥1 event/hour are typical diagnostic criteria for pediatric OSA. Levels of severity for the OAHI are mild (2 to <5 events/hour), moderate (5–10 events/hour), and severe (>10 events/hour). PSG findings in children are

characterized by obstructive apneas and hypopneas during REM sleep and long periods of obstructive hypoventilation during NREM sleep (see next Key Point). Hypopneas can occur during stage N2 but much more frequently occur during REM sleep. Overall hypopneas are more common than apneas. Arousals following respiratory events are much less common in children than in adults, and sleep architecture often remains normal. Of note, severe arterial oxygen desaturation can occur with short respiratory events given the lower oxygen stores or small functional residual capacity in children.

3. According to the ICSD-3-TR, a diagnosis of pediatric OSA can be made based on the following:
   1. The presence of *one or more* of the following:
      - Snoring
      - Labored, paradoxical or obstructed breathing during the child's sleep
      - Sleepiness, hyperactivity, behavioral problems, or learning and other cognitive problems
   2. PSG demonstrates *one or more* of the following:
      One or more obstructive or mixed apneas, or hypopneas, per hour of sleep (OAHI)
      OR
      A pattern of obstructive hypoventilation is defined as at least 25% TST with hypercapnia ($PaCO_2$ >50 mm Hg), arterial oxygen desaturation, or combined hypercapnia and desaturation in association with *one or more* of the following:
      - Snoring
      - Flattening of the inspiratory nasal pressure waveform
      - Paradoxical thoracoabdominal motion
4. The treatment of choice for pediatric patients with OSA and tonsillar hypertrophy is TNA, even if obesity is present.
5. Residual sleep apnea is present in a significant proportion of children following TNA. Those with persistent symptoms or risk factors for failure of TNA (obesity, OAHI in the moderate to severe range, facial abnormalities) should have a post-operative PSG to evaluate for residual OSA.
6. Watchful waiting is reasonable in children who are not symptomatic with PSG findings in the mild-to-moderate range. However, close follow-up is essential.
7. Hypoglossal nerve stimulation is a new treatment for patients with Down syndrome 13 years of age or older with an AHI between 10 and 50 events/hour and who do not have the ability to benefit from CPAP.

CLINICAL REVIEW QUESTIONS

1. Which of the following is NOT true for OSA in children:
   A. The prevalence of OSA in **prepubertal** children is equal in boys and girls.
   B. The AHI for the diagnosis of OSA in children is higher than in adults.
   C. Obstructive hypoventilation is a common pattern noted on a PSG in children with OSA.
   D. Sleep architecture may be normal in children with OSA.
   E. Obstructive apneas are less common than hypopneas and often confined to REM sleep.
2. Adenotonsillectomy is the first line of treatment for OSA in children with tonsillar hypertrophy, even if they are obese. True or false.
3. Which of the following results are standard diagnostic criteria for OSA in a child?
   A. AHI ≥5 events/hour
   B. OAHI >5 events/hour, OAI >3 events/hour
   C. OAHI >1 to 2 events/hour, OAI >1 event/hour
   D. OAHI >2 events/hour
4. Which of the following is **NOT** true concerning $P_{ET}CO_2$ measurements in children?
   A. Values are highly correlated with AHI.
   B. Values are weakly correlated with AHI.
   C. About 10% to 15% of pediatric sleep studies meet criteria for hypoventilation.
   D. Hypoventilation is more likely if the AHI is higher.

ANSWERS

1. All answers are correct except for B. Obstructive apnea is less common than hypopneas, and both are less common in children than in adults. Long periods of obstructive hypoventilation are commonly found. The AHI that is considered abnormal is much lower in children. All other statements are correct.
2. This statement is true, as most children will benefit even if there is a significant residual AHI. A high residual AHI is more common with a higher presurgery AHI, obesity, craniofacial abnormality, and cardiovascular consequences of OSA.
3. C. Answer A refers to adult criteria, and the AHI criteria considered abnormal in children is much lower. B and D are also incorrect. Most clinicians would include the OAI in the criteria since obstructive apnea is less common than hypopnea in children.
4. A. The statement is false. The average $P_{ET}CO_2$ is weakly correlated with the AHI, although a higher AHI is associated with a greater percentage of children meeting the criteria for hypoventilation. In a study of 876 children 13% had hypoventilation.[25]

SUGGESTED READING

Mitchell RB, Archer SM, Ishman SL, et al. Clinical practice guideline: tonsillectomy in children (update)-executive summary. *Otolaryngol Head Neck Surg*. 2019;160(2):187-205.

Marcus CL, Brooks LJ, Draper KA, et al.; American Academy of Pediatrics. Diagnosis and management of childhood obstructive sleep apnea syndrome. *Pediatrics*. 2012;130(3):576-584.

REFERENCES

1. Marcus CL, Brooks LJ, Draper KA, et al.; American Academy of Pediatrics. Diagnosis and management of childhood obstructive sleep apnea syndrome. *Pediatrics*. 2012;130(3):576-584.
2. Marcus CL, Brooks LJ, Draper KA, et al.; American Academy of Pediatrics. Diagnosis and management of childhood obstructive sleep apnea syndrome. *Pediatrics*. 2012;130(3):e714-e755.
3. Marcus CL. Sleep-disordered breathing in children. *Am J Respir Crit Care Med*. 2001;164(1):16-30.
4. Chervin RD, Archbold KH, Dillon JE, et al. Inattention, hyperactivity, and symptoms of sleep-disordered breathing. *Pediatrics*. 2002;109(3):449-456.
5. Katz ES, D'Ambrosio CM. Pediatric obstructive sleep apnea syndrome. *Clin Chest Med*. 2010;31(2):221-234.
6. Troester MM, Quan SF, Berry RB, et al. American Academy of Sleep Medicine. *The AASM Manual for the Scoring of Sleep and Associated Events: Rules, Terminology and Technical Specifications*. Version 3. Darien, IL: American Academy of Sleep Medicine; 2023.
7. Lumeng JC, Chervin RD. Epidemiology of pediatric obstructive sleep apnea. *Proc Am Thorac Soc*. 2008;5(2):242-252.

8. Bitners AC, Arens R. Evaluation and management of children with obstructive sleep apnea syndrome. *Lung*. 2020;198(2):257-270.
9. Yu PK, Radcliffe J, Gerry Taylor H, et al. Neurobehavioral morbidity of pediatric mild sleep-disordered breathing and obstructive sleep apnea. *Sleep*. 2022;45(5):zsac035.
10. Marcus CL, Moore RH, Rosen CL, et al. Childhood Adenotonsillectomy Trial (CHAT). A randomized trial of adenotonsillectomy for childhood sleep apnea. *N Engl J Med*. 2013;368(25):2366-2376.
11. Chervin RD, Weatherly RA, Ruzicka DL, et al. Subjective sleepiness and polysomnographic correlates in children scheduled for adenotonsillectomy vs other surgical care. *Sleep*. 2006;29(4):495-503.
12. Gozal D, Kheirandish-Gozal L. Obesity and excessive daytime sleepiness in prepubertal children with obstructive sleep apnea. *Pediatrics*. 2009;123(1):13-18.
13. Tauman R, Serpero LD, Capdevila OS, et al. Adipokines in children with sleep disordered breathing. *Sleep*. 2007;30:443-449.
14. Nakra N, Bhargava S, Dzuira J, Caprio S, Bazzy-Asaad A. Sleep-disordered breathing in children with metabolic syndrome: the role of leptin and sympathetic nervous system activity and the effect of continuous positive airway pressure. *Pediatrics*. 2008;122(3):e634-e642.
15. Goldbart AD, Goldman JL, Li RC, et al. Differential expression of cysteinyl leukotriene receptors 1 and 2 in tonsils of children with obstructive sleep apnea syndrome or recurrent infection. *Chest*. 2004;126:13-18.
16. Goldbart AD, Krishna J, Li RC, et al. Inflammatory mediators in exhaled condensate of children with obstructive sleep apnea syndrome. *Chest*. 2006;130:143-148.
17. Kheirandish L, Goldbart AD, Gozal D. Intranasal steroids and oral leukotriene modifier therapy in residual sleep-disordered breathing after tonsillectomy and adenoidectomy in children. *Pediatrics*. 2006;117(1):e61-e66.
18. Kuhle S, Hoffmann DU, Mitra S, Urschitz MS. Anti-inflammatory medications for obstructive sleep apnoea in children. *Cochrane Database Syst Rev*. 2020;1(1):CD007074.
19. Aschenbrenner DS. New boxed warning for Singulair. *Am J Nurs*. 2020; 120(7):27.
20. Aurora RN, Zak RS, Karippot A, et al.; American Academy of Sleep Medicine. Practice parameters for the respiratory indications for polysomnography in children. *Sleep*. 2011;34(3):379-388.
21. Kirk V, Baughn J, D'Andrea L, et al. American Academy of Sleep Medicine position paper for the use of a home sleep apnea test for the diagnosis of OSA in children. *J Clin Sleep Med*. 2017;13(10):1199-1203.
22. Hornero R, Kheirandish-Gozal L, Gutiérrez-Tobal GC, et al. Nocturnal oximetry-based evaluation of habitually snoring children. *Am J Respir Crit Care Med*. 2017;196(12):1591-1598.
23. American Academy of Sleep Medicine. *International Classification of Sleep Disorders*. 3rd ed., text revision. Darien IL: American Academy of Sleep Medicine; 2023.
24. Katz E, Marcus C. Diagnosis of obstructive sleep apnea. In: Sheldon S, Ferber R, Kryger M, Gozal D, eds. *Principles and Practice of Pediatric Sleep Medicine*. 2nd ed. New York: Elsevier Saunders; 2014:221-230.
25. Paruthi S, Rosen CL, Wang R, et al. End-tidal carbon dioxide measurement during pediatric polysomnography: signal quality, association with apnea severity, and prediction of neurobehavioral outcomes. *Sleep*. 2015; 38(11):1719-1726.
26. Amaddeo A, Fauroux B. Oxygen and carbon dioxide monitoring during sleep. *Paediatr Respir Rev*. 2016;20:42-44.
27. Hoban TF. Polysomnography should be required both before and after adenotonsillectomy for childhood sleep disordered breathing. *J Clin Sleep Med*. 2007;3(7):675-677.
28. Friedman NR. Polysomnography should not be required both before and after adenotonsillectomy for childhood sleep disordered breathing. *J Clin Sleep Med*. 2007;3(7):678-680.
29. Mitchell RB, Archer SM, Ishman SL, et al. Clinical practice guideline: tonsillectomy in children (update)-executive summary. *Otolaryngol Head Neck Surg*. 2019;160(2):187-205.
30. Brietzke SE, Gallagher D. The effectiveness of tonsillectomy and adenoidectomy in the treatment of pediatric obstructive sleep apnea/hypopnea syndrome: a meta-analysis. *Otolaryngol Head Neck Surg*. 2006;134(6):979-984.
31. Friedman M, Wilson M, Lin HC, Chang HW. Updated systematic review of tonsillectomy and adenoidectomy for treatment of pediatric obstructive sleep apnea/hypopnea syndrome. *Otolaryngol Head Neck Surg*. 2009;140(6):800-808.
32. Chinnadurai S, Jordan AK, Sathe NA, et al. Tonsillectomy for obstructive sleep-disordered breathing: a meta-analysis. *Pediatrics*. 2017;139(2): e20163491.
33. Parikh SR, Archer S, Ishman SL, Mitchell RB. Why is there no statement regarding partial intracapsular tonsillectomy (tonsillotomy) in the new guidelines? *Otolaryngol Head Neck Surg*. 2019;160(2):213-214.
34. Mukhatiyar P, Nandalike K, Cohen HW, et al. Intracapsular and extracapsular tonsillectomy and adenoidectomy in pediatric obstructive sleep apnea. *JAMA Otolaryngol Head Neck Surg*. 2016;142(1):25-31.
35. Rosen GM, Muckle RP, Mahowald MW, Goding GS, Ullevig C. Postoperative respiratory compromise in children with obstructive sleep apnea syndrome: can it be anticipated? *Pediatrics*. 1994;93(5):784-788.
36. Pirelli P, Saponara M, Guilleminault C. Rapid maxillary expansion in children with obstructive sleep apnea syndrome. *Sleep*. 2004;27(4):761-766.
37. Cistulli PA, Palmisano RG, Poole MD. Treatment of obstructive sleep apnea syndrome by rapid maxillary expansion. *Sleep*. 1998;21(8):831-835.
38. Villa MP, Malagola C, Pagani J, et al. Rapid maxillary expansion in children with obstructive sleep apnea syndrome: 12-month follow-up. *Sleep Med*. 2007;8(2):128-134.
39. Yoon A, Abdelwahab M, Bockow R, et al. Impact of rapid palatal expansion on the size of adenoids and tonsils in children. *Sleep Med*. 2022;92:96-102.
40. Cohen SR, Simms C, Burstein F. Mandibular distraction osteogenesis in the treatment of upper airway obstruction in children with craniofacial deformities. *Plast Reconstr Surg*. 1998;101:312-318.
41. Kushida CA, Chediak A, Berry RB, et al. Positive Airway Pressure Titration Task Force; American Academy of Sleep Medicine. Clinical guidelines for the manual titration of positive airway pressure in patients with obstructive sleep apnea. *J Clin Sleep Med*. 2008;4(2):157-171.
42. Marcus CL, Rosen G, Ward SL, et al. Adherence to and effectiveness of positive airway pressure therapy in children with obstructive sleep apnea. *Pediatrics*. 2006;117(3):e442-e451.
43. Koontz KL, Slifer KJ, Cataldo MD, Marcus CL. Improving pediatric compliance with positive airway pressure therapy: the impact of behavioral intervention. *Sleep*. 2003;26:1010-1015.
44. Rains JC. Treatment of obstructive sleep apnea in pediatric patients. Behavioral intervention for compliance with nasal continuous positive airway pressure. *Clin Pediatr (Phila)*. 1995;34:535-541.
45. Parmar A, Baker A, Narang I. Positive airway pressure in pediatric obstructive sleep apnea. *Paediatr Respir Rev*. 2019;31:43-51.
46. DiFeo N, Meltzer LJ, Beck SE, et al. Predictors of positive airway pressure therapy adherence in children: a prospective study. *J Clin Sleep Med*. 2012;8(3):279-286.
47. Simon SL, Duncan CL, Janicke DM, Wagner MH. Barriers to treatment of paediatric obstructive sleep apnoea: development of the adherence barriers to continuous positive airway pressure (CPAP) questionnaire. *Sleep Med*. 2012;13(2):172-177.
48. Bull MJ, Trotter T, Christensen C, et al. Health Supervision for Children and Adolescents With Down Syndrome. *Pediatrics*. 2022;149(5): e2022057010. doi:10.1542/peds.2022-057010.
49. Yu PK, Stenerson M, Ishman SL, et al. Evaluation of upper airway stimulation for adolescents with Down syndrome and obstructive sleep apnea. *JAMA Otolaryngol Head Neck Surg*. 2022;148(6):522-528.
50. *Inspire Medical Systems, Inc. Announces FDA Approval for Pediatric Patients with Down Syndrome*. News release. Inspire Medical Systems, Inc.; 2023. Available at: https://www.globenewswire.com/news-release/2023/03/21/2631228/0/en/Inspire-Medical-Systems-Inc-Announces-FDA-Approval-for-Pediatric-Patients-with-Down-Syndrome.html. Accessed March 21.
51. Roberts SD, Kapadia H, Greenlee G, Chen ML. Midfacial and dental changes associated with nasal positive airway pressure in children with obstructive sleep apnea and craniofacial conditions. *J Clin Sleep Med*. 2016;12(4):469-475.
52. Daftary A, Jalou H, Shivley L, et al. Polysomnography Reference Values in Healthy Newborns. *J Clin Sleep Med*. 2019;15(3):437-443.
53. Brockman P, Poets A, Poets C Reference values for respiratory events in overnight polygraphy from infants aged 1and 3 months. *Sleep Med*. 2013;14(12):1323-1327.

Chapter 28

Sleep and Cardiovascular Disease

INTRODUCTION

The consequences of untreated obstructive sleep apnea (OSA) on cardiovascular disease and benefits from treatment are discussed in Chapter 20. In this chapter, more general information about the effects of sleep and sleep apnea on the autonomic nervous system and the effects of both OSA and central sleep apnea (CSA) on the cardiovascular system will be discussed. Additional information concerning heart failure and sleep apnea will be presented, as many patients have a *combination* of CSA and OSA. Some of the changes in physiology during the night could be due to circadian influences as well as the influences of sleep. However, in many cases, the relative roles of sleep and circadian influences have not been determined.

NORMAL SLEEP-RELATED CHANGES IN AUTONOMIC ACTIVITY

Hemodynamic changes during sleep depend on the sympathetic-parasympathetic balance.[1-4] Activity of the autonomic nervous system has been assessed by measurements of sympathetic nerve activity (SNA) using microneurography,[5,6] which provides direct measurements of efferent SNA related to muscle blood vessels (muscle SNA, MSNA), blood and urine catecholamine levels, and power spectral analysis of heart rate variability.[4,7]

During NREM sleep, there is an increase in parasympathetic nervous system activity (PSNA) and a decrease in sympathetic activity (SNA) (Box 28–1).[1,2] In normal individuals, blood pressure and heart rate decrease with sleep onset, reflecting a predominance of the parasympathetic nervous system during NREM sleep. Stroke volume, cardiac output, and systemic vascular resistance also decrease. The decrease in heart rate is due to increased parasympathetic activity (PSNA), and the reduction in systemic vascular resistance is due to the decrease in muscle sympathetic tone. MSNA, as measured by needle electrodes,[5] progressively decreases from wakefulness to stage N3 sleep (Fig. 28–1).[2,8,9] However, it should be recognized that MSNA may not reflect the amount of sympathetic output to all areas of the body (cardiac, gastrointestinal, or renal). In Figure 28–2, the changes in heart rate, blood pressure, sympathetic burst frequency, and amplitude during different sleep stages are shown. During NREM sleep the heart rate and blood pressure are lower than during wakefulness. The heart rate and blood pressure values during REM sleep are similar to those during wakefulness. The SNA is lower during NREM sleep compared to REM sleep. The SNA during REM sleep is higher than during wakefulness in most studies (Fig. 28–1) while in other studies the SNA during REM sleep was similar to that in wakefulness.[8,9] Of note, during REM sleep, episodic large bursts of SNA are often noted. Thus, the SNA during REM sleep is variable, which may explain some differences in results between studies. The reduction in SNA during NREM sleep is associated with **a decrease in ventricular premature beats.** Respiration affects the heart rate and is mediated by vagal efferent activity to the heart. Vagal afferent input to the brainstem from slowly adapting pulmonary stretch receptors communicate *changes in lung volume to the brainstem, and this information, as well as the activity of respiratory motor neurons, changes vagal activity.*[3] During NREM sleep, *respiratory sinus arrhythmia* is often noted, characterized by a speeding of the heart rate during inspiration and a slowing of the heart rate during expiration.[3] Lung inflation reduces vagal activity and the heart rate increases during inspiration. However, in general, the pulse rate during NREM sleep is very regular. *Of note, lung inflation evokes a decrease in measured sympathetic nerve activity.*[10] *During obstructive apnea, sympathetic tone increases due to hypoxia and hypercapnia and is unopposed by the usual sympathetic-inhibitory lung inflation reflexes.* At apnea termination, there is evidence of sympathetic excitation and vagal withdrawal (increased heart rate and blood pressure).[11] However, at apnea termination, there is an abrupt decrease in MSNA (Fig. 28–3). Decreased MSNA is caused in part by restoration of the inhibitory effects of lung inflation. However, the manifestations of previous increased sympathetic activity continue to be present for some time after apnea termination because of previously secreted norepinephrine, such that *increases in the heart rate and blood pressure continue for several seconds after apnea termination; evidence of vasoconstriction in peripheral arterial blood vessels also continues for several seconds after apnea termination. In addition*

Box 28–1 KEY POINTS ABOUT SLEEP AND THE AUTONOMIC NERVOUS SYSTEM

NREM Sleep

- Parasympathetic predominance
- Lower blood pressure and heart rate compared to wakefulness
- Decreased low frequency/high frequency ratio index of heart rate variability
- High baroreceptor sensitivity (helps maintain steady blood pressure)
- Progressively lower muscle sympathetic nerve activity in transitions from wakefulness to N2 to N3

REM Sleep

- Sympathetic and parasympathetic surges
- Overall irregular heart rate, mean heart rate higher than in NREM sleep
- Parasympathetics surges associated with bradycardia, heart block, asystole
- Increased low frequency/high frequency ratio index of heart rate variability

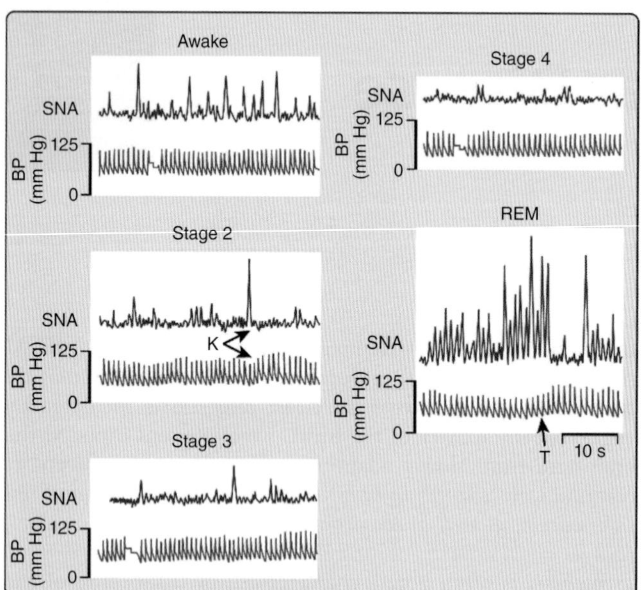

Figure 28–1 Recordings of muscle sympathetic nerve activity (here labeled as SNA) and mean blood pressure (BP) in a single subject while awake and while in stages 2, 3, 4, and REM sleep. SNA and BP gradually decrease with the deepening of non-REM sleep. Heart rate, BP, and BP variability increase during REM sleep, together with a profound increase in the frequency and amplitude in SNA. K marks the appearance of a K complex in the electroencephalogram (EEG; not shown). There was a frequent association between REM twitches (momentary periods of restoration of muscle tone (not shown), denoted by T in the tracing) and abrupt inhibition of sympathetic-nerve discharge and increases in blood pressure. As noted in the text the effects of increased SNA on blood pressure may lag changes in muscle SNA due to the effects of secreted norepinephrine. (Somers VK, Dyken ME, Mark AL, Abboud FM. Sympathetic-nerve activity during sleep in normal subjects. *N Engl J Med.* 1993;328[5]:303-307, with permission of the publisher.)

while sinus node activity responds quickly to increases and decreases in vagal activity the response of the sinus node to a sympathetic activity increase is slower and the increase in heart rate is more prolonged after sympathetic activity decreases.[3]

During REM sleep, breathing is not completely under metabolic control and breathing changes with the phasic events of REM sleep. *During REM sleep, there are also bursts of both SNA and PSNA.* These changes in activity are associated with periods of increased and decreased heart rate. Overall, the mean heart rate is often higher in REM sleep than in NREM sleep (Fig. 28–4) and similar to that in wakefulness. There is also a profound increase in muscle and skin SNA during REM sleep (in both frequency and amplitude)[5] (Fig. 28–2). In untreated OSA, SNA is increased at night and is associated with the respiratory events, but increased SNA *continues to be present during the day* (Fig. 28–5).[11] Surges of PSNA during REM sleep can be associated with profound bradycardia (including asystole) or atrioventricular (AV) block due to increased vagal activity[12-15] (Fig. 28–6).

Heart rate variability (variability in the RR interval) has been used to assess the sympathetic-parasympathetic (vagal) balance.[7,16] While widely used the accuracy in reflecting the true sympathetic -r parasympathetic balance of cardiac nerve activty has been questioned. However, the analysis is widely used and has reasonable clinical correlates. The analysis of the changes in heart rate over time can be in the time domain (RR interval, and indices derived from the RR interval) or in the frequency domain. In the frequency domain, the low-frequency (LF) band (0.04–0.15 Hz) is comprised of rhythms with periods between 7 and 25 seconds and is affected by breathing from ~3 to 9 breaths/min. Within a 5 minute sample, there are 12 to 45 complete periods of oscillation. The LF band is felt to represent both PSNA and SNA. The high frequency or *respiratory band*

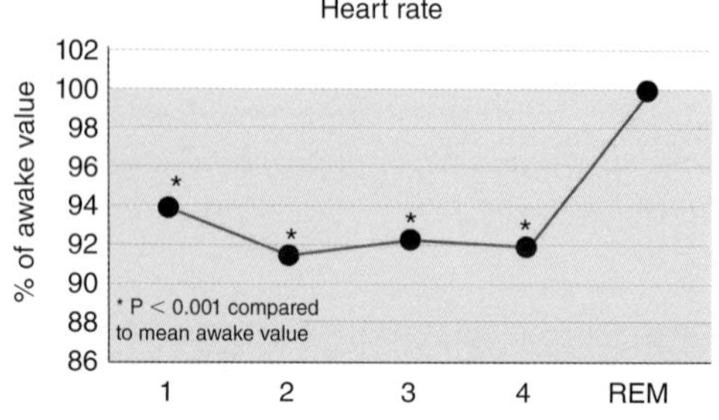

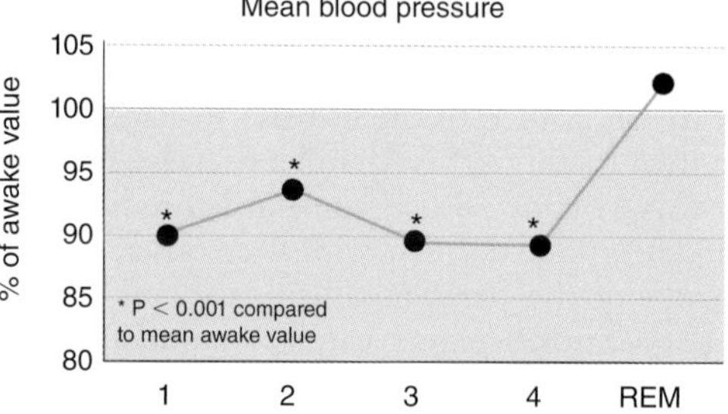

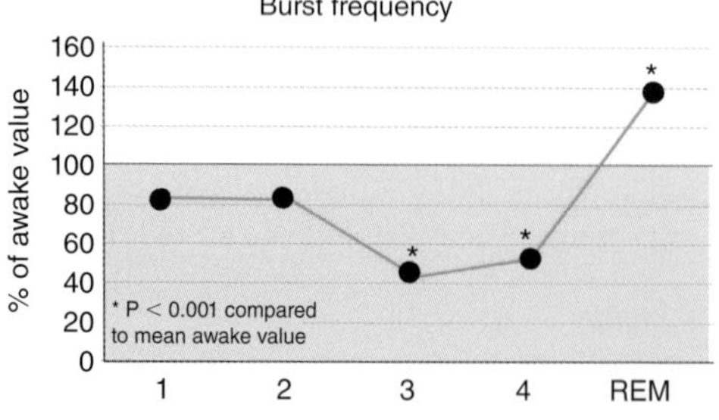

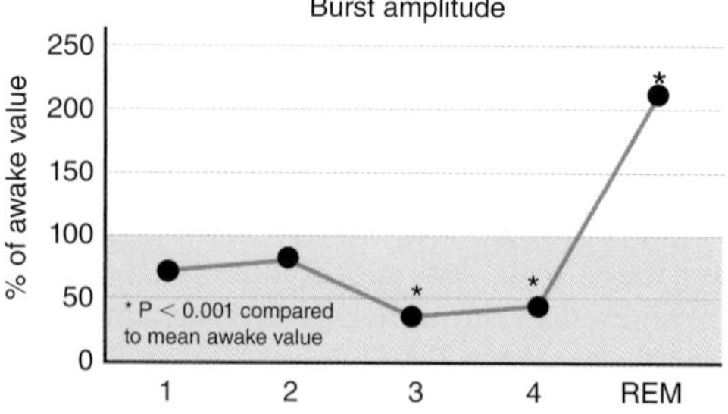

Figure 28–2 Mean heart rate, blood pressure, sympathetic nerve burst frequency, and amplitude ***expressed as a percentage of the mean values during wakefulness*** are shown in a group of normal individuals. Heart rate and blood pressure are lower during NREM sleep than wakefulness but similar during REM sleep and wakefulness (for example REM heart rate about 100% of mean awake value). Muscle sympathetic activity is lower than that of wakefulness during deep sleep (stages 3 and 4) and higher than that of wakefulness during REM sleep (both burst frequency and burst amplitude). (Graphs plotted using data from Somers VK, Dyken ME, Mark AL, Abboud FM. Sympathetic-nerve activity during sleep in normal subjects. *N Engl J Med.* 1993;328[5]:303-307.)

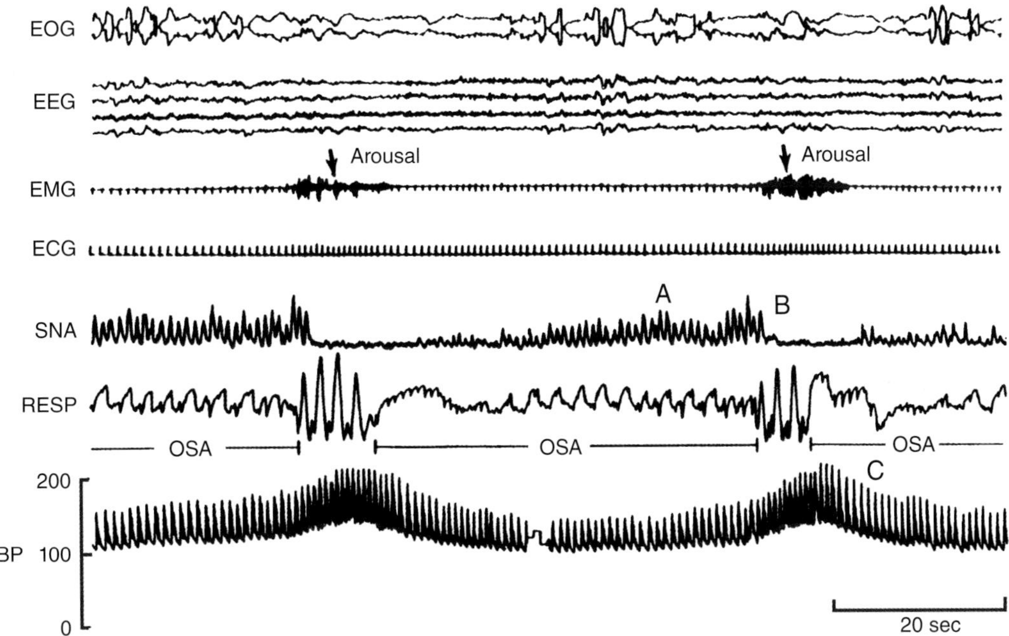

Figure 28–3 **(A) During Obstructive Sleep Apnea, Muscle Sympathetic Activity (SNA) Increases. (B)** At apnea termination, muscle sympathetic activity decreases (inhibition of activity by lung inflation). However, the effects of sympathetic activation, including increased blood pressure and heart rate, continue for several seconds (C) because of increased synaptic norepinephrine and persistent effects of sympathetic stimulation. (From Somers VK, Dyken ME, Clary MP, Abboud FM. Sympathetic neural mechanisms in obstructive sleep apnea. *J Clin Invest.* 1995;96[4]:1897-1904.)

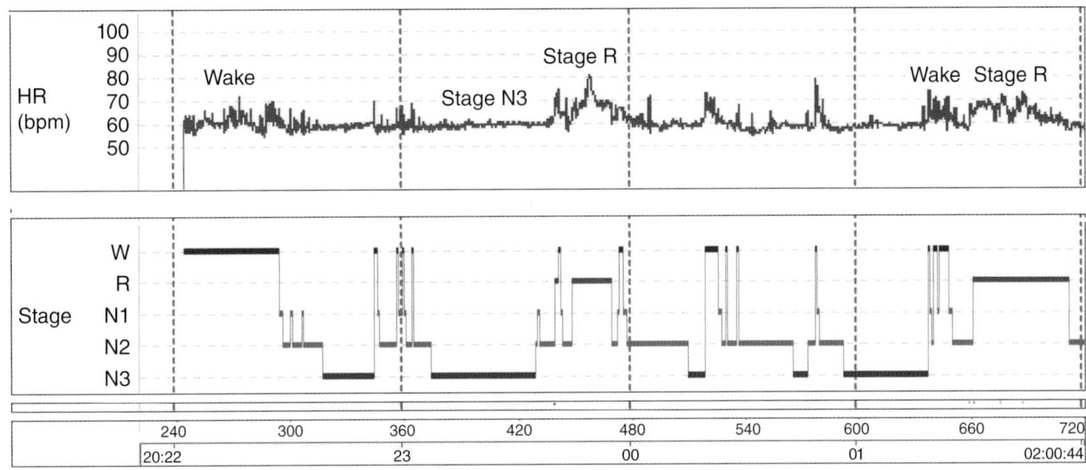

Figure 28–4 **Hypnogram (Sleep Stages) and Heart Rate.** Note the heart rate is lower and regular during NREM sleep compared to wakefulness. During REM sleep (stage R), the heart rate is higher than that in NREM sleep and irregular and similar to that in wakefulness. This hypnogram is from a individual without sleep apnea.

(0.15–0.40 Hz) is influenced by breathing from 9 to 24 breaths/min and is felt to represent PSNA. For example, breathing at a rate of 12 breaths/min is a frequency of 12/60 or 0.2 Hz. The ratio of low frequency power (LF) divided by the high frequency power (HF) written as (LF/HF) is used to estimate the sympathetic/parasympathetic balance. A conceptual method of thinking about the LF/HF ratio is consider the LF/HF ≈ [PSNA+SNA]/[PSNA]). Thus the L/H ratio depends on BOTH PSNA and SNA. An **increase** in the LF/HF ratio is thought to represent a *relative increase in SNA.*[16] A decrease in the LF/HF ration is thought to represent a relative increase in PSNA. In Figure 28–7, an example of measurements of the LF ratio during wakefulness, NREM sleep, and REM sleep for normal patients and patients after a recent myocardial infarction is shown. In normal individuals, the LF/high frequency ratio was lowest during NREM sleep (parasympathetic predominance), higher during REM sleep than NREM sleep, and highest during wakefulness. Although in some studies the L/H ratio is similar between relaxed wakefulness (or during wake after sleep onset) and REM sleep. In this study after myocardial infarction, there was an increase in the LH/HF ratio (higher SNA during sleep.[17] In summary, the LF/high frequency ratio is decreased during NREM sleep, reflecting parasympathetic predominance, and increased during REM sleep (relative to that during NREM sleep), reflecting overall sympathetic predominance with respect to the heart. However, bursts of PSNA also

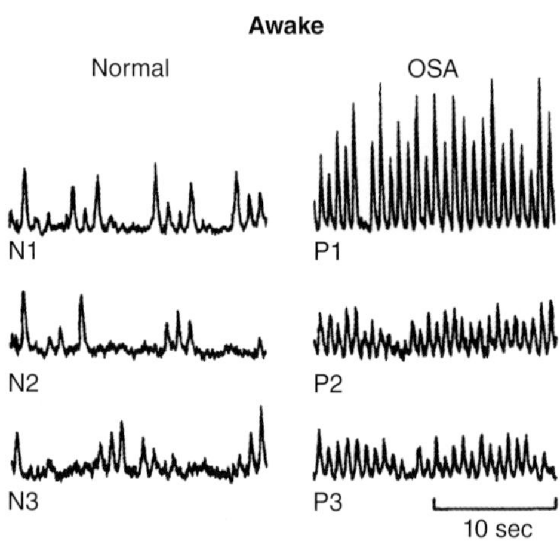

Figure 28–5 Recordings of muscle sympathetic nerve activity (here labeled as SNA) during wakefulness in patients with obstructive sleep apnea (OSA) and matched controls, showing high levels of SNA in patients with sleep apnea. (Somers VK, Dyken ME, Clary MP, Abboud FM. Sympathetic neural mechanisms in obstructive sleep apnea. *J Clin Invest.* 1995;96[4]:1897-1904.)

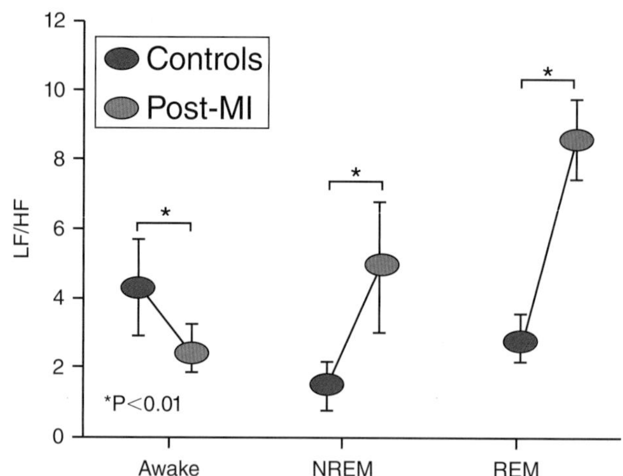

Figure 28–7 Mean low frequency to high frequency (LF/HF) ratio an index of heart rate variability during the awake state (*left*), during NREM sleep (*middle*), and during REM sleep (*right*) in healthy subjects and in patients post–myocardial infarction (MI) (P < 0.01 when comparing control subjects and patients post-MI). Values are means ± standard error of the mean. Asterisks indicate statistically significant differences. (Data from Vanoli E, Adamson PB, Ba-Lin, et al. Heart rate variability during specific sleep stages: a comparison of healthy subjects with patients after myocardial infarction. *Circulation.* 1995;91:1918-1922.)

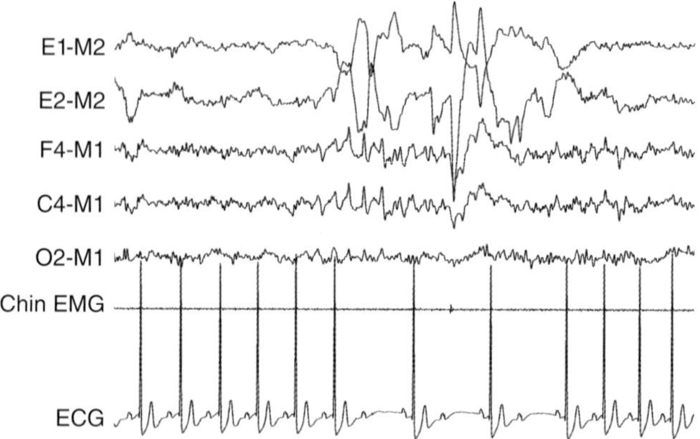

Figure 28–6 Second-degree atrioventricular (AV) block (Mobitz type II) during REM sleep (stage R). Block is noted during a burst of rapid eye movements during phasic REM sleep.

occur during REM sleep and can have important consequences, as noted. Given the increased sympathetic tone during the day in many patients with sleep apnea, it is not surprising that measures of heart rate variability are abnormal but can be improved with continuous positive airway pressure (CPAP) treatment with good adherence.[18] The baroreflex sensitivity = (decrease in heart rate [commonly determined as an increase in the RR interval]/increase in blood pressure) opposes the increase in heart rate after apnea given the increase in blood pressure. However, baroreflex sensitivity is reduced in patients with OSA[3].

HEART RATE AND BLOOD PRESSURE DURING SLEEP

Resting awake heart rate has prognostic significance, as does absence of heart rate dipping during sleep (normally about 10%). In a study by Ben-Dov et al.,[19] the authors found that a blunted heart rate dip during sleep was associated with an increase in all-cause mortality. Blood pressure is reduced during sleep by 10-15% (dipping), then starts to rise slightly before awakening with a peak soon after awakening in the morning. After this morning "surge" blood pressure falls slightly and then slowly increases showing a peak around mid-day and then falls in the afternoon and evening. Studies have found that nighttime blood pressure is, in general, a better predictor of outcome than daytime pressure in hypertensive patients, and the night/day blood pressure ratio predicts mortality. Non-dipping is associated with increased mortality.[20] There is also an increased risk of complex ventricular arrhythmia,[21] myocardial ischemia,[22] stroke,[23] and cardiac hypertrophy.[24] A study of a group of patients with OSA found non-dipping blood pressure was a significant and independent risk factor for *incident cardiovascular events*, even when adjusted for OSA severity and CPAP use.[25]

The increase in blood pressure from the minimum during sleep until the maximum soon after awakening is termed the *morning surge in blood pressure* (Fig. 28–8).[26] The normal morning BP surge is a normal physiological phenomenon. However, studies have demonstrated that an excessive morning surge in BP is a risk factor for cardiovascular disease, including stroke.[27]

NIGHTTIME ACUTE CARDIAC EVENTS

About 20% of all myocardial infarctions, 15% of sudden deaths, and 15% of automated implantable cardioverter defibrillator (AICD) discharges happen between midnight and 6:00 AM.[28] When looking at the details, there is a non-uniform distribution. The peak incidence of myocardial infarction was from midnight to 1:00 AM, and peak incidence of sudden cardiac death was from 1:00 AM to 1:59 AM. This finding is consistent with the hypothesis that sleep-state dependent fluctuations in autonomic nervous system activity may trigger the onset of major cardiovascular events. However, both NREM and REM sleep are associated with factors that can potentially worsen ischemia. The effects of NREM and REM sleep on ischemia will be discussed below.

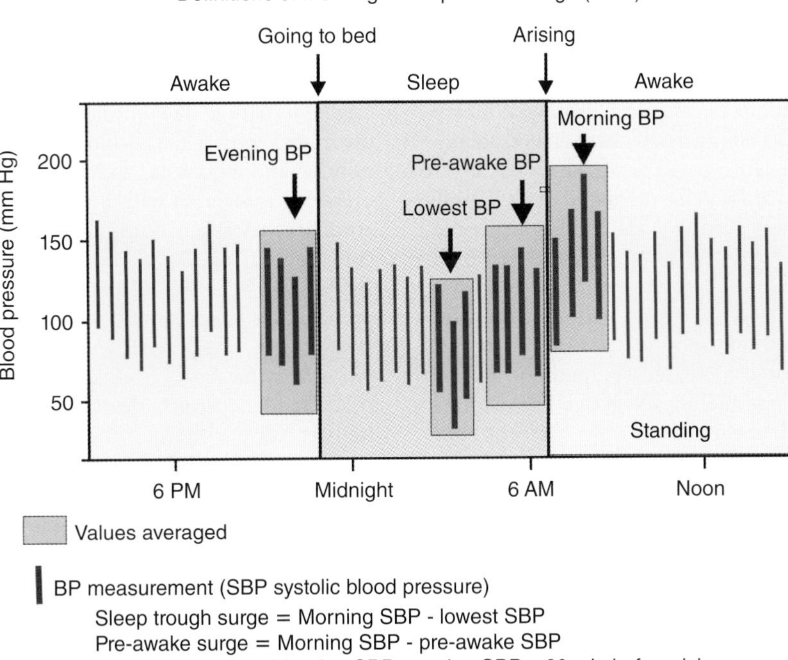

Figure 28–8 Definition of morning surge in blood pressure (BP) characterizing time-dependent measures, that is, sleep-trough surge, pre-waking surge, and rising BP surge. The *vertical lines* represent BP measurement by cuff (usually every 30 minutes during the night). The *blue boxes* are the values averaged for each definition (for example, four values for evening BP). Clinical relevance is underscored by increased stroke incidence in those with exaggerated morning BP surges relative to that in those without this exaggerated morning surge. *BP*, blood pressure; *ME*, morning-evening; *SBP*, systolic blood pressure. (Adapted from Kario K. Morning surge in blood pressure and cardiovascular risk: evidence and perspectives. *Hypertension*. 2010;56:765-773, with permission from the American Heart Association.)

PREMATURE VENTRICULAR COMPLEXES AND VENTRICULAR ARRHYTHMIAS

Surges in cardiac SNA during REM sleep have been implicated in nocturnal arrythmias. Several electrocardiogram (ECG) parameters have been studied to determine risk factors for ventricular arrhythmias and sudden cardiac death. The corrected QT interval (QTc) represents ventricular depolarization-repolarization, including the vulnerable period for induction of reentry tachycardia. Research has concentrated on patients with OSA. Studies have found QT prolongation during apnea events (vagal activity) and abrupt QT shortening post apnea due to increased sympathetic tone and vagal withdrawal.[29] The interval from the peak to the end of the T wave (TpTe) on the 12-lead ECG is a measure of transmural dispersion of repolarization in the left ventricle and is a possible marker of ventricular arrhythmogenesis. The TpTe/QT or TpTe/(corrected QT) [also known as the corrected Tp/Te ratio] have also been used to assess risk of ventricular arrhythmias, but studies have found some conflicting results. In a 6-month observational study of patients newly diagnosed with OSA who had heart failure (HF) and an ICD in place, the effect of CPAP was determined. CPAP treatment did reduce the frequency of premature ventricular contractions (PVCs) and the Tpeak to T-end/corrected ratio.[30] A systematic review of OSA and ventricular arrythmias was unable to draw conclusions because of heterogeneity of the data.[31] An early study of PVCs and OSA found the greatest risk of PVCs was in patients with OSA with desaturation to below 60%.[32] Ryan and coworkers[33] found that CPAP did reduce PVCs in a group of patients with HF and OSA. A case report showed reduction of PVCs in a patient with OSA and a very large PVC burden using CPAP.[34] It is possible that the presence of OSA can worsen the severity of ventricular arrhythmias in patients with underlying heart disease but may not increase the risk for the *presence of arrhythmias*. Analysis of the sleep heart health cohort[35] found that, while the absolute arrhythmia rate was low, the relative risk of paroxysmal atrial fibrillation (AF) and non-sustained ventricular tachycardia during sleep was *markedly increased shortly after a respiratory disturbance. Of interest a normal decline in PVC frequency with sleep predicts success of beta blockers in suppressing PVCs during the daytime.*[3]

ATRIAL FIBRILLATION

AF is the most common sustained arrhythmia and is increasing in prevalence and incidence. Some studies have found a nocturnal peak in the total duration of paroxysmal AF in patients younger than 60 years of age.[97] In the foundational study by Gami et al., obesity and the magnitude of nocturnal desaturation were independent risk factors for **incident AF** in individuals <65 years of age.[36] The incidence of AF was more closely associated with nocturnal hypoxemia than with the apnea-hypopnea index (AHI). The incidence of AF was higher with a higher AHI but this was better explained by the association with the severity of desaturation. In another study, there was a strong association between OSA and AF, such that OSA was strikingly more prevalent in patients with AF than in high-risk patients with multiple other cardiovascular diseases.[37] Lin et al.[38] found an association between *physician-reported OSA and incident AF* in a multiethnic study of atherosclerosis. As noted, analysis of the Sleep Heart Health cohort found the relative risk of paroxysmal AF to be higher after respiratory events. These results support a direct temporal link between sleep disordered breathing (SDB) events and the development of these arrhythmias.

It has been shown that 10% to 25% of AF episodes are facilitated by vagal influence (vagally mediated AF).[39] Since parasympathetic tone is high during NREM sleep, this may predispose to this type of AF. Some characteristics of vagally versus adrenergic mediated AF are shown in Table 28–1. Obstructive apnea is associated with coactivation of the parasympathetic and sympathetic autonomic nervous system, and this may trigger AF. Chronic increased sympathetic tone in OSA may result in atrial remodeling. Negative intrathoracic pressures could also stretch the atrial walls. In a recent study in patients investigated for OSA, nocturnal hypoxemia and measures of pulse-rate variability (PRV) derived from oximetry (not ECG) were independent predictors of AF incidence.[41] Oximetry may be used to identify patients with OSA at greatest risk of developing AF. As discussed in Chapter 20, untreated OSA is associated with an increased risk of recurrence after cardioversion or ablation.[42] To date, observational but not randomized trials suggest CPAP treatment can reduce the risk of recurrence of AF.[43]

Table 28–1 Vagally and Adrenergic Mediated Atrial Fibrillation

Vagally Mediated AF	Adrenergic Mediated AF
More common in middle-aged men	More common in older population
Structurally normal hearts	Abnormal heart of known cardiovascular disease
Occurs with vagal stimuli such as sleep, alcohol consumption, postprandial, or post exercise	Provoked by physical or emotional stress
Presence mainly at night	Presence mainly during day
Preceded by bradycardia	Preceded by tachycardia
Worsened by beta-blockers	Improved by beta-blockers
Less likely to progress to permanent atrial fibrillation	More likely to be permanent

Rattanawong P, Kewcharoen J, S Srivathsan K, Shen WK. Drug therapy for vagally-mediated atrial fibrillation and sympatho-vagal balance in the genesis of atrial fibrillation: a review of the current literature. *J Atr Fibrillation.* 2020;13(1):2410.

Box 28–2 SLEEP AND MYOCARDIAL ISCHEMIA

- Both the *elevated heart rate and blood pressure* of REM sleep and the *hypotension* of NREM sleep can promote myocardial ischemia.
- Twenty percent of myocardial infarctions and 15% of sudden cardiac deaths occur at night.
- Conditions predisposing to nocturnal myocardial infarction
  - Nadir in fibrinolytic activity
  - Diabetes (endothelial dysfunction)
  - Hypotension during NREM sleep
  - Increased sympathetic activity (REM sleep)

MYOCARDIAL ISCHEMIA AND INFARCTION

About 20% of all myocardial infarction events occur at night. Important facts about the interaction between sleep and myocardial ischemia are summarized in Box 28–2. NREM sleep is associated with a fall in blood pressure, and this can result in nondemand nocturnal ischemic episodes (reduced perfusion pressure) associated with a critical underlying coronary lesion, coronary vasospasm, and transient coronary stenosis. This risk could potentially be worsened by antihypertensive treatment. REM sleep is associated with increased SA and surges in blood pressure, also predisposing to periods of ischemia. *Myocardial infarction is more likely in the morning, with a threefold increased risk within the first 3 hours of awakening that peaks around 9:00 AM.* Sudden cardiac death and ischemic episodes have the highest risk during morning hours (6:00 to 9:00 AM). As discussed in chapter 20, the greatest risk of sudden death in OSA patients is midnight to 6AM. Fibrinolytic activity in the blood showed a sinusoidal variation with a period of 24 hours; it increased several fold during the day, reaching a peak at 6:00 PM, then dropping to trough levels at 3:00 to 4:00 AM.[44] This could predispose to nocturnal myocardial infarction. Specific patient groups experience an increased incidence of nighttime myocardial infarctions, particularly those with poor ventricular function, advanced age, or diabetes mellitus.[45,46] Although OSA via sympathetic nerve surges and intermittent hypoxia is a risk factor for coronary heart disease and myocardial infarction, it has been proposed that ischemic preconditioning as a result of intermittent hypoxia may confer cardioprotection.[47]

CONGESTIVE HEART FAILURE

The two types of congestive HF (CHF) include HF with a *preserved* ejection fraction (HFpEF, diastolic HF) and HF with a *reduced* ejection fraction (HFrEF, systolic HF). Here, the ejection fraction refers to the left ventricle (LVEF). Introduction of beta blockers in the therapeutic armamentarium of HF has had no impact on the prevalence of sleep apnea in HF. The incidence of moderate-to-severe sleep apnea (AHI ≥15 events/hour, CSA, OSA, or both) is about 50% in both HFpEF and HFrEF[48,49] (Fig. 28–9). Many patients have components of both OSA and CSA, and the predominant component is used to make the diagnosis. Oldenberg and coworkers[50] published an observational study of 700 patients *with systolic HF (LVEF <40%)* that showed sleep apnea (AHI ≥15 events/hour) was present in 53% of the patients, including *33% with CSA and 20% with OSA.* Using a cut off of AHI ≥5 events/hour, the corresponding numbers were 76%, 40%, and 36%. Bitter et al.[51] prospectively evaluated 244 consecutive patients (87 women) with preserved ejection fraction (HFpEF). Forty-seven percent had an AHI of 15 or more events/hour; of these, 23% had CSA and 24% had OSA. The designation of OSA or CSA was made according to the majority of events. Other studies of HFpEF have found a higher percentage of OSA than of CSA.[52] Studies have also found a very high percentage of sleep apnea (47% OSA, 31% CSA in one study) in patients admitted with decompensated HF.[53,54] As the prevalence of either OSA, CSA with Cheyne-Stokes respiration (CSA-CSB), or both is high in patients with significant systolic or diastolic HF, one should not assume that complaints of disturbed nocturnal sleep are simply secondary to HF.

The relative proportions of OSA and CSA can vary within a given patient over time and even within the same night.

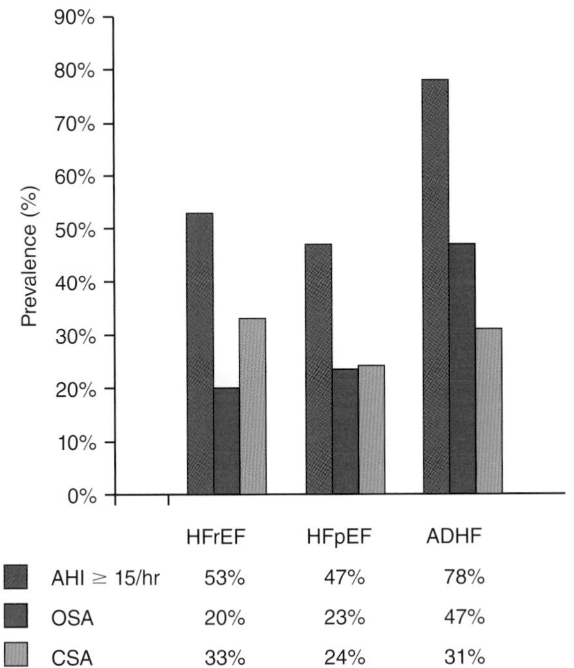

	HFrEF	HFpEF	ADHF
AHI ≥ 15/hr	53%	47%	78%
OSA	20%	23%	47%
CSA	33%	24%	31%

Figure 28–9 Prevalence (%) of moderate-to-severe sleep apnea (apnea-hypopnea index [AHI] ≥15) in heart failure with preserved ejection fraction (HFpEF) or heart failure with reduced ejection fraction (HFrEF) AND acutely decompensated heart failure (ADHF). *AHI*, apnea-hypopnea index; *CSA*, central sleep apnea; *OSA*, obstructive sleep apnea. (Modified from Javaheri S, Barbe F, Campos-Rodriguez F, et al. Sleep apnea: types, mechanisms, and clinical cardiovascular consequences. *J Am Coll Cardiol*. 2017;69[7]:841-858.)

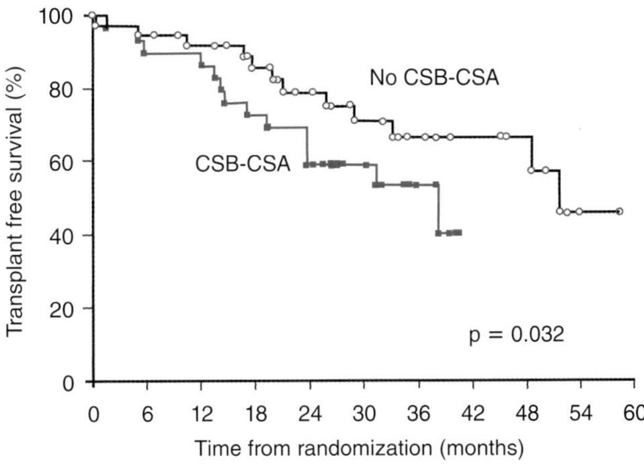

Figure 28–10 Transplant-free survival in patients with congestive heart failure (low ejection fraction) with Cheyne-Stokes respiration (CSB-CSA) was significantly worse than in those without CSB-CSA independent of the use of CPAP. (From Sin DD, Logan AG, Fitzgerald FS, Liu PP, Bradley TD. Effects of continuous positive airway pressure on cardiovascular outcomes in heart failure patients with and without Cheyne-Stokes respiration. *Circulation*. 2000;102:61-66.)

A study by Tcakova et al.[55] found an increase in the percentage of central events from the first quarter to the last quarter of the night that was associated with a reduction in the transcutaneous PCO_2. During the night, there is redistribution of fluid into the lungs (higher wedge pressure). Pulmonary congestion stimulates J receptors, and this increases ventilatory drive and lowers the PCO_2 (increasing the tendency for central apnea). Central apnea in HF patients usually meets criteria for CSB, with a crescendo-decrescendo pattern of ventilation between central apneas or hypopneas and a cycle length of at least 40 seconds. CSA-CSB is common in both systolic and diastolic HF but has a shorter cycle time in diastolic HF.[56]

The presence of either OSA or CSA in a patient with HF implies a worse prognosis.[57] Javaheri et al. examined retrospectively analyzed data concerning Medicare beneficiaries (30,719 patients) with newly diagnosed HF and determined that sleep apnea was underdiagnosed. Patients who were tested, diagnosed, and treated for sleep apnea with positive airway pressure (PAP) therapy, supplemental oxygen, or both had a better 2-year overall survival than patients who were tested and diagnosed with sleep apnea but not treated.[57] The presence of OSA in patients with HFrEF (LVEF ≤45%) was associated with an increased risk of death independent of confounding factors in a retrospective study performed by Wang and coworkers.[58] In a study of HFrEF by Sin et al. of patients *with and without CSA-CSB*, the presence of CSA-CSB was associated with a worse prognosis (Fig. 28–10).[59]

Another study retrospectively evaluated 450 patients with *significant left ventricular (LV) failure* referred to the sleep laboratory and found that risk factors for OSA included an increased body mass index (BMI) for men and increased age for women. Risk factors for CSA included AF, male gender, age >60 years, and hypocapnia.[60] In patients with CHF and OSA, negative intrathoracic pressure, hypoxemia, and increased sympathetic tone are associated with apneas and are believed to negatively affect ventricular function. Patients with HF and CSA have a higher pulmonary capillary wedge pressure than do patients with HF with predominantly OSA or those without any type of apnea.[61] In another study, in patients with HF,[62] a lower awake PCO_2 was associated with a higher pulmonary capillary wedge pressure. Thus, a higher pulmonary capillary wedge pressure is associated with both CSA and a lower $PaCO_2$ in patients with HF. The factors determining the relative amounts of obstructive and central apneas are illustrated in Figure 28–11.

Sleep Apnea With Heart Failure and Preserved EF

HFpEF is not a benign condition and *is the most common type of heart failure in the elderly population*, especially in women.[63] The exact cutoff used to define HFpEF has varied from an EF ≥40% to an EF ≥55%. Symptoms **do not differ** from those associated with systolic HF and include decreased exercise tolerance, orthopnea, paroxysmal nocturnal dyspnea, and edema. The largest prospective study of HFpEF to date by Bitter et al.[64] evaluated 244 consecutive patients (87 women) with an LVEF ≥55%. The two major causes of HFpEF were *systemic hypertension and coronary artery disease.* As noted, 47% of the patients had an AHI of 15 or more events/hour, of whom 23% had CSA and 24% had OSA. Patients with *CSA had a lower $PaCO_2$ but higher pulmonary capillary wedge pressure.* Pulmonary congestion is important for development of CSA because of increased hypercapnic ventilatory response (associated with a small PCO_2 difference between the eupnea and the apneic threshold).

Some, but not all, studies have found a similar mortality between HFpEF and HFrEF (lower mortality with normal EF in some studies), but all have found similar impacts from HFpEF and HFrEF on outcomes including similar hospitalization rates, hospital stay duration, and patient quality of life.[63,65] Studies in community-based cohorts suggest that HFpEF accounts for approximately 40% to 50% of incident HF and 50% to 60% prevalent HF overall.[63]

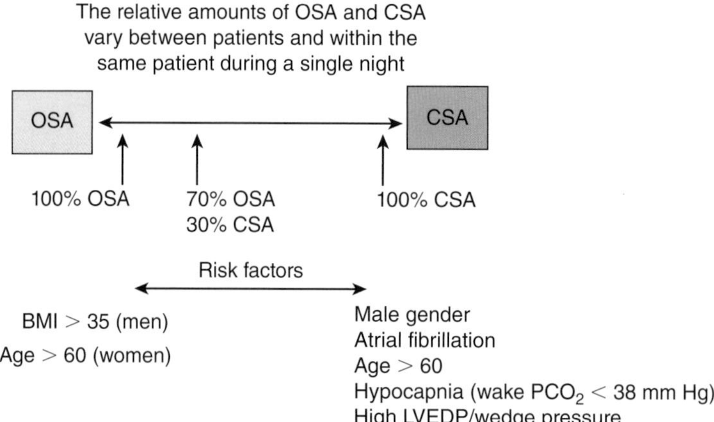

Figure 28–11 Factors Determining the Relative Risk of Obstructive Sleep Apnea (OSA) Versus Central Sleep Apnea (CSA) in Patients With Heart Failure. An example of a patient with 70% OSA and 30% CSA is shown. (From Berry RB, Wagner MH. *Sleep Medicine Pearls.* Elsevier; 2015:364.)

The pathophysiologic consequence of LV diastolic dysfunction relates to a hypertrophied or a noncompliant left ventricle shifting the pressure volume curve upward and to the left. Therefore, for a given LV volume, LV end-diastolic pressure increases, resulting in elevated left atrial and pulmonary capillary pressures, pulmonary congestion, and edema. Similar to asymptomatic LV systolic dysfunction, which with time leads to HFrEF, asymptomatic LV diastolic dysfunction is also independently associated with incident HFpEF.

Heart Failure in Patients With OSA

As noted, a retrospective analysis found the presence of OSA in patients with HF (LVEF ≤45%) to be associated with an increased risk of death, independent of confounding factors.[58] Patients with mild or no sleep apnea were compared to those with moderate-to-severe OSA. A subgroup of patients was treated with CPAP, and in these patients, no deaths were reported. However, the increase in survival (compared to that among patients with untreated moderate-to-severe OSA) did not quite reach statistical significance. The effect of 3 months of CPAP treatment in patients with OSA and HF (LVEF <55%) was evaluated by Mansfield et al.[66] using a randomized controlled design. Compared to the control group, CPAP treatment was associated with improvements in the LVEF, reductions in overnight urinary norepinephrine excretion, and improvements in quality of life. A previous study by Kaneko and coworkers[67] showed benefit of 1 month of CPAP treatment of OSA in idiopathic and ischemic cardiomyopathy (improvement in the LVEF and reduced daytime systolic blood pressure) using a randomized controlled trial. The effect of CPAP appears to occur because of a reduction in sympathetic tone and a decrease in ventricular afterload. In a prospective observational study, Kasai et al.[68] studied patients with *predominant moderate-to-severe OSA,* stable symptomatic HF, and LVEF less than 50%. All patients were offered CPAP treatment. Outcomes (death and hospitalizations) in the group using CPAP were compared to those in the group not using CPAP. The subgroups of CPAP users who were more adherent or less adherent were also compared. During a mean follow-up period of 25 months, 44.3% of the patients died or were hospitalized. Multivariant analysis showed that the risk of death and hospitalization was increased in the untreated group and in the group with poor adherence to CPAP treatment. The median time of CPAP use in the treated group was 4.9 hours. A randomized controlled trial conducted by Arias and coworkers[69] in patients with newly diagnosed OSA but without overt CHF demonstrated a benefit of CPAP on diastolic function. This provides support for the idea that treatment of OSA may reduce the risk of development of HFpEF. Analysis of a large Medicare cohort also suggested that treatment of OSA will benefit patients with HF.[57] A task force of the American Academy of Sleep Medicine (AASM) performed a meta-analysis concerning use of PAP.[70] The meta-analysis found that, while there was a statistically significant improvement in LVEF with CPAP treatment in patients with HF, the difference was small and NOT clinically significant. The meta-analysis also found survival benefit with CPAP treatment for patients with cardiovascular disorders in non-randomized trials but not in randomized trials and concluded there is no convincing evidence of a survival benefit with CPAP treatment. In particular, the large SAVE trial[71] found no benefit in composite cardiovascular outcomes (including HF) in patients with known cardiovascular disease with CPAP treatment. However, CPAP adherence was low in this study, and sleepy patients were excluded. Overall, the AASM CPAP task force made no recommendation concerning CPAP treatment with respect to OSA and cardiovascular disorders.[70] In summary, the presence of OSA in patients with systolic CHF worsens the prognosis, and retrospective and observational studies have shown modest improvement in cardiac function with CPAP treatment of OSA as well improved short-term cardiovascular outcomes. However, there is no convincing evidence of benefit from CPAP treatment in patients with OSA and HF from randomized controlled trials. As noted, the trials included only non-sleepy patients, and CPAP adherence was not optimal. The ADVENT-HF trial,[96] studied the effects of treatment of patients with HFrEF and either predominant OSA or CSA with a modern adaptive servoventilation device with the ability to treat OSA and CSA.[73-75] The results were published in 2024. The study found no benefit with respect to mortality or hospitalization in either the OSA-predominant or CSA-predominate groups. Treatment adherence was adequate, and the AHI was effectively decreased. *The OSA patients had to be non-sleepy*. Therefore, sleepy patients could conceivably benefit, but this would need to be studied.

There is additional discussion of the Advent-HF trial with respect to patients with HF with predominant CSA later in this chapter.

Given this information, what treatment can be recommended for patients with HF and predominant OSA? *The first line of treatment of patients with HF and OSA is to optimize treatment of the HF.*[48,76,77] In the past, many physicians would treat moderate-to-severe OSA in patients with HF with CPAP, even if they had no symptoms[76]. Based on the current information, this practice could change in the future. On the other hand, if daytime sleepiness is present this symptom could improve with CPAP treatment. However, the majority of patients with OSA and HF do not report symptoms such as daytime sleepiness.[76,78] Many complain of insomnia. Of interest, a study found that insomnia complaints are associated with incident HF.[79] In a study by Mehra et al.[78] of 26 patients with stable HF, only 4 of 26 had an Epworth sleepiness scale (ESS) greater than 10. However, there was *evidence of objective sleepiness, with a mean sleep latency of 7 minutes.* There was no correlation between the ESS and mean sleep latency on the multiple sleep latency test. The authors concluded that there was a dissociation between objective and subjective sleepiness in patients with HF. In conclusion, based on the current evidence, the most convincing reason for treatment of a patient with CHF and predominant OSA is to improve daytime sleepiness or perhaps other nocturnal symptoms such as frequent awakenings that might improve with treatment. This sleepy group may be a minority of the patients with HF and OSA in a cardiology clinic but will likely be more common in patients evaluated in sleep clinic.

Heart Failure in Patients With CSB-CSA

As noted, the presence of CSA (usually with CSB) in patients with systolic CHF is associated with a worse prognosis.[59] In a randomized controlled study of 3 months duration and a median of 2.2 years of follow up by Sin et al., patients with systolic HF with and without CSA-CSB were randomized to medical care or CPAP groups.[59] The group with CSA-CSB had a worse prognosis independent of the presence or absence of CPAP treatment (Fig. 28–10). The patients with CHF and CSA-CSB treated with CPAP had an improved LVEF at 3 month and a reduction in transplant-free mortality over a median of 2.2 years of follow up. The group with HF without CSA-CSB showed neither benefit.

A study by Naughton and coworkers[80] randomized patients with stable *systolic HF* (LVEF ≤45%) and CSA-CSB to 3 months of CPAP or routine care. The AHI was reduced by 28.5 events/hour in the CPAP group (significantly greater than in the control group) and the CPAP group had a greater improvement in ejection fraction. Another study showed that CSA-CSB treatment with CPAP in patients with systolic CHF can reduce markers of increased sympathetic tone.[81] These findings led to a large, randomized trial of patients with systolic CHF and moderate-to-severe predominantly CSA (CANPAP trial).[82] However, this study did not find an improvement in mortality compared to that of standard care and was terminated when preliminary analysis showed a higher short-term mortality in the CPAP group. However, only 50% of patients had an improved AHI, with CPAP (AHI <15 events/hour). The titration of CPAP in this study differed from the approach used in OSA patients. CPAP was increased to around 10 to 12 cm H_2O,

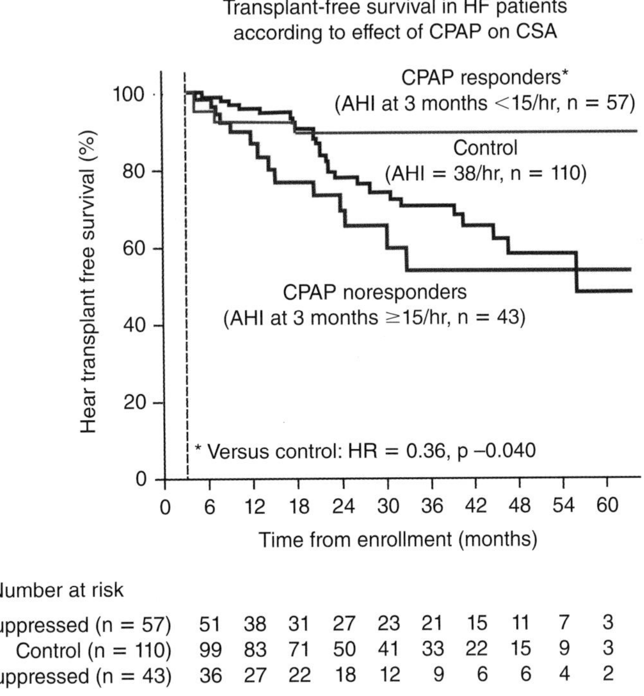

Number at risk

CPAP-CSA-suppressed (n = 57)	51	38	31	27	23	21	15	11	7	3
Control (n = 110)	99	83	71	50	41	33	22	15	9	3
CPAP-CSA-unsuppressed (n = 43)	36	27	22	18	12	9	6	6	4	2

Figure 28–12 Kaplan-Meier survival plots demonstrating that, compared with the control group, the continuous positive airway pressure (CPAP)-central sleep apnea (CSA)-suppressed group had significantly improved heart transplant-free survival (*unadjusted P = 0.043), whereas the CPAP-unsuppressed group did not (unadjusted P=0.260). (From Arzt M, Floras JS, Logan AG, et al. Suppression of central sleep apnea by continuous positive airway pressure for patients with central sleep apnea and transplant-free survival in heart failure: a post hoc analysis of the Canadian Suppression of Central Sleep Apnea by Continuous Positive Airway Pressure and Heart Failure Trial (CANPAP). *Circulation*. 2007;115:3173-3180.)

as tolerated (and sufficiently high to eliminate obstructive events). This level of pressure had been shown effective in several previous studies. A subsequent analysis of the subroup of *CPAP responders* showed improvements in ejection fraction and mortality (Fig. 28–12)[83]. That is, the group responding to CPAP might benefit from this treatment. Post-hoc analysis of studies showing a benefit is generally thought to be weaker evidence.

However, because only about 50% of patients with CSA-CSB and systolic heart failure respond to CPAP, adaptive servoventilation (ASV) was developed. This mode of PAP (Chapter 24) is a type of anticyclic bilevel PAP in which higher pressure support is provided during periods of reduced ventilation or flow and lower pressure support during periods of higher ventilation or flow.[73-75] A backup rate is available to treat central apneas. This form of PAP was shown to be very effective at reducing the AHI commonly to levels less than 5 to 10 events/hour in most patients with CSA-CSB in several studies.[73-75,84-86] These promising results led to a large randomized controlled trial of ASV versus guideline-based medical care in patients with **systolic HF** and moderate-to-severe sleep apnea with a predominance of central events (CSA-CSB; SERVE-HF study).[87] Inclusion criteria were an EF ≤45%, >50% central events (apneas or hypopneas) with a central AHI ≥10 events/hour. The patients had an average AHI around 30 events/hour and central apnea-central hypopnea index around 80% of the total AHI (both groups). The primary end points in the time-to-event analysis were the first event of death from any cause, lifesaving cardiovascular intervention (cardiac transplantation, implantation of a ventricular assist device, resuscitation after sudden cardiac arrest, or appropriate lifesaving shock), or unplanned hospitalization for worsening HF. In the ASV group, the AHI at 12 months was 6.6 events/hour, *but the primary end point results were not different between the ASV and control groups*. However, the all-cause mortality and cardiovascular mortality were higher in the ASV group, and the study was terminated.

Given the results of this trial, a physician task force of the AASM performed a meta-analysis of trials of ASV for treatment of CSA due to HF.[88] The meta-analysis demonstrated an improvement in LVEF and a normalization of AHI. However, the analysis also demonstrated an increased risk of cardiac mortality in patients with an LVEF of ≤45% and moderate or severe CSA-predominant sleep-disordered breathing. The task force concluded "these data support a standard level recommendation against the use of ASV to treat CHF-associated CSAs in patients with an LVEF of ≤45% and moderate or severe CSA, and an option level recommendation for the use of ASV in the treatment of CHF-associated CSA in patients with an LVEF >45% or mild CHF-related CSA."[88] Therefore, use of ASV was not recommended for patients with LVEF ≤45% in patients with moderate-to-severe CSA but could be used with a normal EF and moderate-to-severe CSA or in patients with mild CHF-related CSA.

The SERVE-HF trial was criticized for use of an ASV device that did not automatically titrate the expiratory PAP (EPAP) and use of an algorithm delivering high levels of PAP. As briefly mentioned, a trial using a modern ASV device in patients with HFrEF with moderate-to-severe sleep apnea and variable proportions of central and obstructive events[96] has been completed without evidence of harm in these patients (ADVENT-HF trial). However, results show no improvement in the primary outcomes (cardiovascular hospitalization, death from any cause, new onset AF, and ICD discharges). There was also no improvement in overall mortality. The device was very effective at reducing central and obstructive apnea. ASV treatment was also effective in with respect to a reduction in the arousal frequency, and improvement in indices of sleep quality and quality of life. Due to publicity concerning the SERVE-HF trial, the recall of Philips PAP devices, and the COVID-19 pandemic, the study did not meet the patient recruitment goals and relatively few patients with predominantly CSA completed the study (control N=06, ASV N=92). The impact of the study results on the treatment approach to patients with predominant CSA and a reduced ejection fraction remains to be determined. The entire history of attempts at treating sleep apnea associated with CHF is well summarized by Lorenzi-Filho and coworkers.[89]

In summary, use of a modern ASV device showed no improvement in cardiovascular outcomes in groups with both predominant OSA (non-sleepy) and predominant CSA and HFrEF. Treatment with the modern ASV device appears to be safe in HFrEF and could potentially be used in **sleepy** OSA or CSA with symptoms associated with disturbed sleep. This would require patient consent and education on potential risks. In the future, treatment of patients with OSA or CSA and HF will likely target symptoms rather than cardiovascular outcomes.

Treatment Alternatives for Heart Failure and CSA-CSB

The first treatment for CSA-CSB in patients with CHF is optimization of cardiac function. ASV is effective at reducing the AHI in patients **with HFpEF** and CSB.[90] However, the benefit of this treatment on long-term cardiovascular outcomes remains uncertain. At the time of this writing, use of ASV in patients with a low LVEF is not recommended. Time will tell if the results of the ADVENT-HF trial showing no harm with a modern ASV device will change medical practice. CPAP will work in about 50% of patients with CSA-CSB, and this treatment could be used in those *who do respond*. In summary, modern ASV devices with automatically adjusting EPAP are usually effective at reducing the AHI in CSA-CSB with or without co-existent OSA in both patients with HFpEF and HFrEF. Use of modern ASV devices in patients with CSA-CSB and HFrEF appears to do no harm. However, long-term benefits with respect to cardiovascular outcomes have not been demonstrated. *At this point, improvement in symptoms is the most reasonable goal of treatment of any type of sleep apnea in a patient with HF.* The patients with HF most likely to benefit from ASV treatment are sleepy patients or those with prominent nocturnal symptoms improved with this treatment.

Supplemental oxygen does reduce the AHI[48,76] in patients with HF and CSA-CSB, but long-term benefit has not been demonstrated, and the treatment is not currently reimbursed by most insurance providers. As discussed in Chapter 24, transvenous phrenic pacing has been shown to be an effective treatment in patients with moderate-to-severe central sleep apnea, although some obstructive events remain in many patients.[91] Studies using transvenous phrenic nerve pacing to treat CSA have found improvement in sleep quality and quality of life,[91] so one could make a case for this treatment, even if the effect on long-term HF survival was neutral. Combined treatment with pacing and CPAP or an oral appliance to address obstructive events is another possibility.

INSOMNIA, DAYTIME SLEEPINESS, AND CARDIOVASCULAR DISEASE

Insomnia associated with **objectively documented short sleep duration** is associated with unfavorable cardiovascular outcomes, including an increased risk of incident hypertension (several studies) or HF and all-cause mortality (in some studies).[79,92-95] A meta-analysis of 13 prospective studies found that insomnia was associated with an increased risk of developing and/or dying from cardiovascular disease.[94] While many patients with insomnia complain of short sleep, in some, a short sleep duration cannot be documented objectively. Therefore, the phenotype *of insomnia complaints and objectively documented short sleep* may be an important group. For example, Bertisch and coworkers found that *objectively measured short sleep duration* increased the odds of reporting hypertension more than threefold after adjusting for potential confounders. This relationship was *not significant for subjectively measured sleep duration*.[93] Daytime sleepiness in older adults has also been shown to predict mortality and cardiovascular disease.[95] There is certainly overlap between insomnia and daytime sleepiness, so future studies need to address the relative importance of short sleep duration versus the presence and type of symptoms. Many patients with insomnia do not report daytime sleepiness.

SUMMARY OF KEY POINTS

1. NREM sleep is associated with parasympathetic predominance and a decrease in blood pressure and heart rate compared to wakefulness. Regular heart rate and respiratory rate are noted in normal individuals. There is a decrease in low frequency to high frequency ratio (LF/HF), an index of heart rate variability, from wakefulness to NREM sleep consistent with parasympathetic predominance. Muscle sympathetic nerve activity (MSNA) progressively decreases from wakefulness to stage N3 sleep.
2. REM sleep is associated with autonomic instability and surges in both PSNA and SNA. The heart rate is variable (increases and decreases), but the mean heart rate is usually higher than during NREM sleep (and often similar to wakefulness). Parasympathetic surges can be associated with bradycardia, heart block, or asystole. The LF/HF ratio, a heart rate variability index, is increased in REM compared to NREM sleep and similar to wakefulness. In some studies the LF/HF ratio was higher during wakefulness compared to REM sleep although the LF/HF ratio during wakefulness was similar to that during REM sleep if the LF/HF was determined during wake after sleep onset. MSNA is increased during REM sleep compared to that in NREM sleep and, in most studies, compared to that in wakefulness. Sympathetic tone is not homogenous during REM sleep, with periods of profound increase. It is important to remember that MSNA may not represent global SNA.
3. In untreated OSA, the MSNA is high during NREM sleep and even higher during REM sleep. *Elevated SNA is still present during the day in many patients. Acute treatment with CPAP can reduce the elevated SNA during REM sleep. Chronic treatment with CPAP can reduce daytime sympathetic activity and improve heart rate variability (if CPAP adherence is adequate).*
4. Sleep is associated with a 10% to 15% drop in blood pressure ("dipping"). A non-dipping pattern is associated with an increased risk or mortality, arrhythmias, stroke, and LV hypertrophy. There is a normal increase in blood pressure on awakening, but this is exaggerated in some patients with hypertension and OSA. An abnormal increase in blood pressure on awakening in the AM is also associated with a worse prognosis. *About 70% of patients with resistant hypertension have OSA.* Evaluation for OSA in patients with resistant hypertension is recommended.
5. The heart rate also decreases from wakefulness to sleep, and a **non-dipping pattern in heart rate** is also associated with worsening cardiovascular outcomes.
6. About 50% of patients with HF with either a reduced ejection fraction (HFrEF) or a preserved ejection fraction (HFpEF) have moderate-to-severe OSA with variable amounts of CSA and OSA. A very high percentage of patients (70–80%) admitted with decompensated HF have moderate-to-severe OSA. The presence of sleep apnea (OSA or CSA) in a patient with HF is associated with a worse prognosis. Patients with HFrEF tend to have more CSA than OSA. Patients with HFpEF tend to have fairly equal amounts of CSA and OSA.
7. Both HFpEF and HFrEF are associated with increased mortality, impaired quality of life, and increased hospital admissions. HFpEF is the most common form of HF in older patients
8. A high percentage of patients with AF have moderate-to-severe OSA. The presence of OSA is associated with an increased risk of incident AF and recurrent AF after cardioversion or ablation. Observational studies suggest CPAP can reduce the risk of AF recurrence, but to date, a randomized controlled trial has not confirmed this benefit.
9. About 15% of AF is "vagally mediated" and is more common at night and in younger patients without structural heart disease. For community populations age $<$ 65 years, incident AF is associated with *obesity and nocturnal arterial oxygen desaturation.*
10. CSA-CSB can occur *in both HFrEF and HFpEF (although with a shorter cycle time with a normal EF).* The presence of CSA-CSB is associated with a poor prognosis in HF (increased mortality).
11. Observational studies suggest CPAP treatment of (predominant) OSA in patients with HF can improve the EF and reduce sympathetic nervous system activation. No randomized controlled trial has documented a benefit with respect to mortality or cardiovascular adverse events. Based on current knowledge, the best reason to treat a patient with HF and OSA is improvement in symptoms. However, a significant percentage of the group with HF and OSA do not report symptoms.
12. About 50% of patients with HF and predominant CSA-CSB will respond to CPAP, and post-hoc analysis of a large trial (CANPAP) found benefit in this group with an increase in EF and reduction in mortality. In this group, CPAP treatment could be considered. In those who do not respond, most physicians would not recommend this treatment, as CPAP was associated with a worse survival in non-responders. However, modern ASV devices more reliably reduce the AHI and can be used to treat both OSA and CSA (if indicated and safe).
13. ASV can effectively reduce the AHI in patients with CSA-CSB with both HFpEF and HFrEF. Newer ASV devices with automatically adjusting EPAP can effectively treat both OSA and CSA. A large, randomized trial showed that ASV treatment with an older generation device increased mortality in patients with a low EF ($\leq$45%) and use of ASV in moderate-to-severe CSA in patients with a low EF is currently not recommended. Recent findings of a trial of a modern ASV device with the ability to treat OSA and CSA in patients with HFrEF (groups with predominant OSA and predominant CSA) found no evidence of harm and an effective reduction in the AHI. However, the study found no benefit with respect

to cardiovascular outcomes. *Only non-sleepy patients with OSA were studied.* Treatment with ASV was associated with improved sleep quality and quality of life measures. Improvement in symptoms (daytime sleepiness or disturbed sleep) is likely the most valid reason for treatment of patients with sleep apnea and HF with an appropriate PAP device.

14. Insomnia with **an objectively documented short sleep time** is associated with an increased risk of hypertension and other cardiovascular morbidity.

CLINICAL REVIEW QUESTIONS

1. Which of the following factors may **increase** nocturnal ischemia?
   A. Hypotension during NREM sleep
   B. Hypotension during REM sleep
   C. Increased fibrinolytic activity during sleep
2. Which of the following is **NOT** associated with REM sleep?
   A. Increased and variable heart rate compared to NREM sleep
   B. Surges of SNA and PSA
   C. Decreased LF/HF an index of heart rate variability
   D. Period of bradycardia or heart block can occur
3. Which of the following statements about the presence of moderate to severe sleep apnea is true?
   A. Present in 50% of HFrEF but 20% of HFpEF
   B. Present in 50% HFpEF but 70% of HFrEF
   C. Present in about 50% of patients with both HFrEF and HFpEF
   D. Present in about 30% of patients with both HFrEF and HFpEF
4. Which of the following is **NOT true** about atrial fibrillation and sleep apnea?
   A. Sleep apnea increases the risk of incident atrial fibrillation.
   B. After cardioversion, the presence of untreated sleep apnea increases the risk of recurrence.
   C. Randomized controlled trials have demonstrated that CPAP reduces the risk of recurrence of AF after cardioversion or ablation.
   D. About 15% of AF is vagally mediated and especially likely to occur at night.
5. Which of the following is **NOT a true statement**?
   A. Non-dipping in blood pressure is associated with increased mortality.
   B. The termination of obstructive apnea is associated with sympathetic activation and parasympathetic (vagal) withdrawal.
   C. About 40% of myocardial infarctions occur at night.
   D. There is a progressive decrease in MSNA on transitions from wakefulness to stage N1 to stage N2 to stage N3.

ANSWERS

1. A. During NREM sleep, hypotension can occur (especially in patients taking antihypertensive medication), which can lead to reduced coronary perfusion pressure and ischemia, particularly in a severely stenosed coronary circulation. During REM sleep, arterial blood pressure is either unchanged compared to wakefulness or transiently elevated; therefore, reduced coronary perfusion pressure is generally not a factor in myocardial ischemia during this stage of sleep. Decreased rather than increased fibrinolytic activity would predispose to nocturnal ischemia. Fibrinolytic activity in blood shows a sinusoidal variation with a period of 24 hours; it increased severalfold during the day, reaching a peak at 6:00 PM, and then dropped to trough levels at 3:00 to 4:00 AM.[44]
2. C. The LF/HF ratio an index of heart rate variability is **increased** during REM sleep imply sympathetic predominance.
3. C. Sleep apnea is present in about 50% of patients with both HFrEF and HFpEF. The relative amounts of predominantly CSA and OSA are relatively equal in HFpEF but predominantly CSA is higher in patients with HFrEF
4. C. Observational studies but not randomized trials have demonstrated that CPAP treatment of OSA reduces the risk of recurrence of AF after cardioversion or ablation.
5. C. About 20% of myocardial infarctions occur at night. The peak occurrence is shortly after awakening in the early morning. Apnea termination is associated with vagal withdrawal and sympathetic activation. However, SNA abruptly decreases with restoration of the inhibitory influences of lung inflation. Sympathetic activation persists for 5-10 seconds or more due to the actions of previously secreted norepinephrine and the prolonged residual response of vascular smooth muscle and the heart following a decrease in SNA.

REFERENCES

1. Fink AM, Bronas UG, Calik MW. Autonomic regulation during sleep and wakefulness: a review with implications for defining the pathophysiology of neurological disorders. *Clin Auton Res.* 2018;28(6):509-518.
2. Lurie A. Hemodynamic and autonomic changes in adults with obstructive sleep apnea. In: Borer JS, ed. *Advances in Cardiology.* Karger; 2011:171-195. doi:10.1159/000325109.
3. Leung RS. Sleep-disordered breathing: autonomic mechanisms and arrhythmias. *Prog Cardiovasc Dis.* 2009;51(4):324-338.
4. Coy TV, Dimsdale JE, Ancoli-Israel S, Clausen J. Sleep apnoea and sympathetic nervous system activity: a review. *J Sleep Res.* 1996;5(1):42-50.
5. Carter JR. Microneurography and sympathetic nerve activity: a decade-by-decade journey across 50 years. *J Neurophysiol.* 2019;121(4):1183-1194.
6. Greenlund IM, Carter JR. Sympathetic neural responses to sleep disorders and insufficiencies. *Am J Physiol Heart Circ Physiol.* 2022;322(3):H337-H349. doi:10.1152/ajpheart.00590.2021.
7. Malik M. Heart rate variability: standards of measurement, physiological interpretation and clinical use. Task Force of the European Society of Cardiology and the North American Society of Pacing and Electrophysiology. *Circulation.* 1996;93:1043-1065.
8. Okada H, Iwase S, Mano T, Sugiyama Y, Watanabe T. Changes in muscle sympathetic nerve activity during sleep in humans. *Neurology.* 1991;41(12):1961-1966. doi:10.1212/wnl.41.12.1961.
9. Somers VK, Dyken ME, Mark AL, Abboud FM. Sympathetic-nerve activity during sleep in normal subjects. *N Engl J Med.* 1993;328(5):303-307.
10. Somers VK, Abboud FM. Chemoreflexes—responses, interactions and implications for sleep apnea. *Sleep.* 1993;16(suppl 8):S30-S33; discussion S33-S34.
11. Somers VK, Dyken ME, Clary MP, Abboud FM. Sympathetic neural mechanisms in obstructive sleep apnea. *J Clin Invest.* 1995;96(4):1897-1904.
12. Janssens W, Willems R, Pevernagie D, Buyse B. REM sleep-related brady-arrhythmia syndrome. *Sleep Breath.* 2007;11(3):195-199.
13. Guilleminault C, Pool P, Motta J, Gillis AM. Sinus arrest during REM sleep in young adults. *N Engl J Med.* 1984;311(16):1006-1010.
14. Biswas A, Berry RB, Sriram PS, Prasad A. A man with sleep-associated symptomatic bradycardia. *Ann Am Thorac Soc.* 2017;14(4):597-600.
15. Holty JE, Guilleminault C. REM-related bradyarrhythmia syndrome. *Sleep Med Rev.* 2011;15(3):143-151.
16. Shaffer F, Ginsberg JP. An overview of heart rate variability metrics and norms. *Front Public Health.* 2017;5:258.

17. Vanoli E, Adamson PB, Ba-Lin, Pinna GD, Lazzara R, Orr WC. Heart rate variability during specific sleep stages. A comparison of healthy subjects with patients after myocardial infarction. *Circulation.* 1995; 91(7):1918-1922. doi:10.1161/01.cir.91.7.1918.
18. Khoo MC, Belozeroff V, Berry RB, Sassoon CS. Cardiac autonomic control in obstructive sleep apnea: effects of long-term CPAP therapy. *Am J Respir Crit Care Med.* 2001;164(5):807-812.
19. Ben-Dov IZ, Kark JD, Ben-Ishay D, Mekler J, Ben-Arie L, Bursztyn M. Blunted heart rate dip during sleep and all-cause mortality. *Arch Intern Med.* 2007;167(19):2116-2121.
20. Fagard RH, Celis H, Thijs L, et al. Daytime and nighttime blood pressure as predictors of death and cause-specific cardiovascular events in hypertension. *Hypertension.* 2008;51(1):55-61.
21. Schillaci G, Verdecchia P, Borgioni C, et al. Association between persistent pressure overload and ventricular arrhythmias in essential hypertension. *Hypertension.* 1996;28:284-289.
22. Pierdomenico SD, Bucci A, Costantini F, et al. Circadian blood pressure changes and myocardial ischemia in hypertensive patients with coronary artery disease. *J Am Coll Cardiol.* 1998;31:1627-1634.
23. Schwartz GL, Bailey KR, Mosley T, et al. Association of ambulatory blood pressure with ischemic brain injury. *Hypertension.* 2007;49:1228-1234.
24. Verdecchia P, Schillaci G, Guerrieri M, et al. Circadian blood pressure changes and left ventricular hypertrophy in essential hypertension. *Circulation.* 1990;91:523-536.
25. Sasaki N, Ozono R, Edahiro Y, et al. Impact of non-dipping on cardiovascular outcomes in patients with obstructive sleep apnea syndrome. *Clin Exp Hypertens.* 2015;37(6):449-453.
26. Kario K. Morning surge in blood pressure and cardiovascular risk: evidence and perspectives. *Hypertension.* 2010;56(5):765-773.
27. Yano Y, Kario K. Nocturnal blood pressure, morning blood pressure surge, and cerebrovascular events. *Curr Hypertens Rep.* 2012;14(3):219-227.
28. Lavery CE, Mittleman MA, Cohen MC, Muller JE, Verrier RL. Nonuniform nighttime distribution of acute cardiac events: a possible effect of sleep states. *Circulation.* 1997;96(10):3321-3327.
29. Gillis AM, Stoohs R, Guilleminault C. Changes in the QT interval during obstructive sleep apnea. *Sleep.* 1991;14(4):346-350.
30. Seyis S, Usalan AK, Rencuzogullari I, Kurmuş Ö, Gungen AC. The effects of continuous positive airway pressure on premature ventricular contractions and ventricular wall stress in patients with heart failure and sleep apnea. *Can Respir J.* 2018;2018:2027061.
31. Raghuram A, Clay R, Kumbam A, Tereshchenko LG, Khan A. A systematic review of the association between obstructive sleep apnea and ventricular arrhythmias. *J Clin Sleep Med.* 2014;10(10):1155-1160.
32. Shepard JW Jr, Garrison MW, Grither DA, Dolan GF. Relationship of ventricular ectopy to oxyhemoglobin desaturation in patients with obstructive sleep apnea. *Chest.* 1985;88(3):335-340.
33. Ryan CM, Usui K, Floras JS, Bradley TD. Effect of continuous positive airway pressure on ventricular ectopy in heart failure patients with obstructive sleep apnoea. *Thorax.* 2005;60(9):781-785.
34. Sakai T, Takemoto M, Koga T, Tsuchihashi T. A case report of an improvement in premature ventricular complex-induced cardiomyopathy following continuous positive airway pressure therapy in a patient with severe obstructive sleep apnoea. *Eur Heart J Case Rep.* 2022;6(9):ytac349.
35. Monahan K, Storfer-Isser A, Mehra R, et al. Triggering of nocturnal arrhythmias by sleep-disordered breathing events. *J Am Coll Cardiol.* 2009;54(19):1797-1804.
36. Gami AS, Hodge DO, Herges RM, et al. Obstructive sleep apnea, obesity, and the risk of incident atrial fibrillation. *J Am Coll Cardiol.* 2007;49(5):565-571.
37. Gami AS, Pressman G, Caples SM, et al. Association of atrial fibrillation and obstructive sleep apnea. *Circulation.* 2004;110(4):364-367.
38. Lin GM, Colangelo LA, Lloyd-Jones DM, et al. Association of sleep apnea and snoring with incident atrial fibrillation in the Multi-Ethnic Study of Atherosclerosis. *Am J Epidemiol.* 2015;182(1):49-57.
39. Huang B, Liu H, Scherlag BJ, et al. Atrial fibrillation in obstructive sleep apnea: neural mechanisms and emerging therapies. *Trends Cardiovasc Med.* 2021;31(2):127-132.
40. [deleted in review]
41. Blanchard M, Gervès-Pinquié C, Feuilloy M, et al. Association of nocturnal hypoxemia and pulse rate variability with incident atrial fibrillation in patients investigated for obstructive sleep apnea. *Ann Am Thorac Soc.* 2021;18(6):1043-1051.
42. Linz D, McEvoy RD, Cowie MR, et al. Associations of obstructive sleep apnea with atrial fibrillation and continuous positive airway pressure treatment: a review. *JAMA Cardiol.* 2018;3(6):532-540.
43. Traaen GM, Aakerøy L, Hunt TE, et al. Effect of continuous positive airway pressure on arrhythmia in atrial fibrillation and sleep apnea: a randomized controlled trial. *Am J Respir Crit Care Med.* 2021;204(5):573-582.
44. Andreotti F, Kluft C. Circadian variation of fibrinolytic activity in blood. *Chronobiol Int.* 1991;8(5):336-351.
45. Hjalmarson A, Gilpin EA, Nicod P, et al. Differing circadian patterns of symptom onset in subgroups of patients with acute myocardial infarction. *Circulation.* 1989;90:267-275.
46. Rana JS, Mukamal KJ, Morgan JP, et al. Circadian variation in the onset of myocardial infarction: effect of duration of diabetes. *Diabetes.* 2003;52:1464-1468.
47. Shah N, Redline S, Yaggi HK, et al. Obstructive sleep apnea and acute myocardial infarction severity: ischemic preconditioning? *Sleep Breath.* 2013;17(2):819-826. Erratum in: *Sleep Breath.* 2013;17(3):1119.
48. Javaheri S, Barbe F, Campos-Rodriguez F, et al. Sleep apnea: types, mechanisms, and clinical cardiovascular consequences. *J Am Coll Cardiol.* 2017;69(7):841-858.
49. Javaheri S, Parker TJ, Wexler L, et al. Occult sleep-disordered breathing in stable congestion heart failure. *Ann Intern Med.* 1995;122:487-492.
50. Oldenburg O, Lamp B, Faber L, et al. Sleep-disordered breathing in patients with symptomatic heart failure: a contemporary study of prevalence in and characteristics of 700 patients. *Eur J Heart Fail.* 2007;9:251-257.
51. Bitter T, Faber L, Hering D, Langer C, Horstkotte D, Oldenburg O. Sleep-disordered breathing in heart failure with normal left ventricular ejection fraction. *Eur J Heart Fail.* 2009;11(6):602-608.
52. Herrscher TE, Akre H, Øverland B, Sandvik L, Westheim AS. High prevalence of sleep apnea in heart failure outpatients: even in patients with preserved systolic function. *J Card Fail.* 2011;17(5):420-425.
53. Khayat R, Jarjoura D, Porter K, et al. Sleep disordered breathing and post-discharge mortality in patients with acute heart failure. *Eur Heart J.* 2015;36(23):1463-1469.
54. Khayat RN, Jarjoura D, Patt B, et al. In-hospital testing for sleep disordered breathing in hospitalized patients with decompensated heart failure-report of prevalence and patient characteristics. *J Card Fail.* 2009; 15(9):739-746.
55. Tkacova R, Niroumand M, Lorenzi-Filho G, Bradley TD. Overnight shift from obstructive to central apneas in patients with heart failure: role of PCO2 and circulatory delay. *Circulation.* 2001;103:238-243.
56. Wedewardt J, Bitter T, Prinz C, Faber L, Horstkotte D, Oldenburg O. Cheyne-Stokes respiration in heart failure: cycle length is dependent on left ventricular ejection fraction. *Sleep Med.* 2010;11(2): 137-142.
57. Javaheri S, Caref EB, Chen E, Tong KB, Abraham WT. Sleep apnea testing and outcomes in a large cohort of Medicare beneficiaries with newly diagnosed heart failure. *Am J Respir Crit Care Med.* 2011;183(4):539-546.
58. Wang H, Parker JD, Newton GE, et al. Influence of obstructive sleep apnea on mortality in patients with heart failure. *J Am Coll Cardiol.* 2007;49(15):1625-1631.
59. Sin DD, Logan AG, Fitzgerald FS, Liu PP, Bradley TD. Effects of continuous positive airway pressure on cardiovascular outcomes in heart failure patients with and without Cheyne-Stokes respiration. *Circulation.* 2000;102(1):61-66.
60. Sin DD, Fitzgerald F, Parker JD, Newton G, Floras JS, Bradley TD. Risk factors for central and obstructive sleep apnea in 450 men and women with congestive heart failure. *Am J Respir Crit Care Med.* 1999;160(4): 1101-1106.
61. Solin P, Bergin P, Richardson M, Kaye DM, Walters EH, Naughton MT. Influence of pulmonary capillary wedge pressure on central apnea in heart failure. *Circulation.* 1999;99(12):1574-1579.
62. Lorenzi-Filho G, Azevedo ER, Parker JD, Bradley TD. Relationship of carbon dioxide tension in arterial blood to pulmonary wedge pressure in heart failure. *Eur Respir J.* 2002;19(1):37-40.
63. Pfeffer MA, Shah AM, Borlaug BA. Heart failure with preserved ejection fraction in perspective. *Circ Res.* 2019;124(11):1598-1617.
64. Ahmed A, Perry GJ, Fleg JL, Love TE, Goff DC Jr, Kitzman DW. Outcomes in ambulatory chronic systolic and diastolic heart failure: a propensity score analysis. *Am Heart J.* 2006;152(5):956-966. doi:10.1016/j.ahj.2006.06.020.
65. Bitter T, Faber L, Hering D, Langer C, Horstkotte D, Oldenburg O. Sleep-disordered breathing in heart failure with normal left ventricular ejection fraction. *Eur J Heart Fail.* 2009;11(6):602-608.
66. Mansfield DR, Gollogly NC, Kaye DM, Richardson M, Bergin P, Naughton MT. Controlled trial of continuous positive airway pressure in obstructive sleep apnea and heart failure. *Am J Respir Crit Care Med.* 2004;169(3):361-366.

67. Kaneko Y, Floras JS, Usui K, et al. Cardiovascular effects of continuous positive airway pressure in patients with heart failure and obstructive sleep apnea. *N Engl J Med.* 2003;348:1233-1241.
68. Kasai T, Narui K, Dohi T, et al. Prognosis of patients with heart failure and obstructive sleep apnea treated with continuous positive airway pressure. *Chest.* 2008;133(3):690-696.
69. Arias MA, García-Río F, Alonso-Fernández A, et al. Obstructive sleep apnea syndrome affects left ventricular diastolic function: effects of nasal continuous positive airway pressure in men. *Circulation.* 2005;112(3): 375-383.
70. Patil SP, Ayappa IA, Caples SM, Kimoff RJ, Patel SR, Harrod CG. Treatment of adult obstructive sleep apnea with positive airway pressure: an American Academy of Sleep Medicine systematic review, meta-analysis, and GRADE assessment. *J Clin Sleep Med.* 2019;15(2):301-334.
71. McEvoy RD, Antic NA, Heeley E, et al. SAVE Investigators and Coordinators. CPAP for prevention of cardiovascular events in obstructive sleep apnea. *N Engl J Med.* 2016;375(10):919-931.
72. [deleted in review]
73. Randerath WJ, Nothofer G, Priegnitz C, et al. Long-term auto-servoventilation or constant positive pressure in heart failure and coexisting central with obstructive sleep apnea. *Chest.* 2012;142(2):440-447.
74. Kasai T, Usui Y, Yoshioka T, et al. JASV Investigators. Effect of flow-triggered adaptive servo-ventilation compared with continuous positive airway pressure in patients with chronic heart failure with coexisting obstructive sleep apnea and Cheyne-Stokes respiration. *Circ Heart Fail.* 2010;3(1):140-148.
75. Galetke W, Ghassemi BM, Priegnitz C, et al. Anticyclic modulated ventilation versus continuous positive airway pressure in patients with coexisting obstructive sleep apnea and Cheyne-Stokes respiration: a randomized crossover trial. *Sleep Med.* 2014;15(8):874-879.
76. Javaheri S, Brown LK, Abraham WT, Khayat R. Apneas of heart failure and phenotype-guided treatments: part one: OSA. *Chest.* 2020;157(2):394-402.
77. Khattak HK, Hayat F, Pamboukian SV, et al. Obstructive sleep apnea in heart failure: review of prevalence, treatment with continuous positive airway pressure, and prognosis. *Tex Heart Inst J.* 2018;45(3):151-161.
78. Mehra R, Wang L, Andrews N, et al. Dissociation of objective and subjective daytime sleepiness and biomarkers of systemic inflammation in sleep-disordered breathing and systolic heart failure. *J Clin Sleep Med.* 2017;13(12):1411-1422.
79. Laugsand LE, Strand LB, Platou C, Vatten LJ, Janszky I. Insomnia and the risk of incident heart failure: a population study. *Eur Heart J.* 2014;35(21):1382-1393.
80. Naughton MT, Liu PP, Bernard DC, Goldstein RS, Bradley TD. Treatment of congestive heart failure and Cheyne-Stokes respiration during sleep by continuous positive airway pressure. *Am J Respir Crit Care Med.* 1995;151(1):92-97.
81. Naughton MT, Benard DC, Liu PP, Rutherford R, Rankin F, Bradley TD. Effects of nasal CPAP on sympathetic activity in patients with heart failure and central sleep apnea. *Am J Respir Crit Care Med.* 1995; 152(2):473-479.
82. Bradley TD, Logan AG, Kimoff RJ, et al. CANPAP Investigators. Continuous positive airway pressure for central sleep apnea and heart failure. *N Engl J Med.* 2005;353(19):2025-2033.
83. Arzt M, Floras JS, Logan AG, et al. Suppression of central sleep apnea by continuous positive airway pressure and transplant-free survival in heart failure: a post hoc analysis of the Canadian Continuous Positive Airway Pressure for Patients with Central Sleep Apnea and Heart Failure Trial (CANPAP). *Circulation.* 2007;115:3173-3180.
84. Teschler H, Döhring J, Wang YM, Berthon-Jones M. Adaptive pressure support servoventilation: a novel treatment for Cheyne-Stokes respiration in heart failure. *Am J Respir Crit Care Med.* 2001;164:614-619.
85. Oldenburg O, Schmidt A, Lamp B, et al. Adaptive servoventilation improves cardiac function in patients with chronic heart failure and Cheyne-Stokes respiration. *Eur J Heart Fail.* 2008;10:581-586.
86. Pepperell JC, Maskell NA, Jones DR, et al. A randomized controlled trial of adaptive ventilation for Cheyne-Stokes breathing in heart failure. *Am J Respir Crit Care Med.* 2008;168:1109-1114.
87. Cowie MR, Woehrle H, Wegscheider K, et al. Adaptive servo-ventilation for central sleep apnea in systolic heart failure. *N Engl J Med.* 2015; 373(12):1095-1105.
88. Aurora RN, Bista SR, Casey KR, et al. Updated adaptive servo-ventilation recommendations for the 2012 AASM Guideline: "the treatment of central sleep apnea syndromes in adults: practice parameters with an evidence-based literature review and meta-analyses". *J Clin Sleep Med.* 2016;12(5):757-761.
89. Lorenzi-Filho G, Drager LF, Bradley TD. Adaptive servo-ventilation for central sleep apnea: what are the lessons learned? *Pulmonology.* 2023; 29(2):105-107.
90. Bitter T, Westerheide N, Faber L, et al. Adaptive servoventilation in diastolic heart failure and Cheyne-Stokes respiration. *Eur Respir J.* 2010; 36(2):385-392.
91. Schwartz AR, Goldberg LR, McKane S, Morgenthaler TI. Transvenous phrenic nerve stimulation improves central sleep apnea, sleep quality, and quality of life regardless of prior positive airway pressure treatment. *Sleep Breath.* 2021;25(4):2053-2063.
92. Bathgate CJ, Edinger JD, Wyatt JK, Krystal AD. Objective but not subjective short sleep duration associated with increased risk for hypertension in individuals with insomnia. *Sleep.* 2016;39(5):1037-1045.
93. Bertisch SM, Pollock BD, Mittleman MA, et al. Insomnia with objective short sleep duration and risk of incident cardiovascular disease and all-cause mortality: Sleep Heart Health Study. *Sleep.* 2018;41(6):zsy047.
94. Sofi F, Cesari F, Casini A, Macchi C, Abbate R, Gensini GF. Insomnia and risk of cardiovascular disease: a meta-analysis. *Eur J Prev Cardiol.* 2014;21(1):57-64.
95. Newman AB, Spiekerman CF, Enright P, et al. Daytime sleepiness predicts mortality and cardiovascular disease in older adults: the Cardiovascular Health Study Research Group. *J Am Geriatr Soc.* 2000;48:115-123.
96. Bradley TD, Logan AG, Lorenzi Filho G, et al. Adaptive servo-ventilation for sleep-disordered breathing in patients with heart failure with reduced ejection fraction (ADVENT-HF): a multicentre, multinational, parallel-group, open-label, phase 3 randomised controlled trial. *Lancet Respir Med.* 2024;12(2):153-156. doi:10.1016/S2213-2600(23)00374-0.
97. Mehra F, Mittleman M, Verrier RL. Cardiac Arrhythmogenesis during Sleep. In: Kryger M, Goldstein CA, Roth T, Dement WC, eds. *Princpiles and Practice of Sleep Medicine.* Philadelphia PA: Elsevier; 2022: 1421-1429.

Sleep and Lung Disease

Chapter 29

INTRODUCTION

Patients with lung disease may have both impaired nocturnal gas exchange and poor sleep quality. The combination of lung disease and obstructive sleep apnea (OSA) is common, but one of the components is often not recognized. Sleep physicians may concentrate on the OSA and pulmonary physicians the lung disease. However, optimal treatment requires addressing both disorders. Pulmonary function testing is discussed in Chapter 13 but will be briefly reviewed in this chapter as well. When taking a history for evaluation of a patient suspected of having a sleep disorder, attention to the presence and severity of lung disease and current medications used for treatment is important. One should not assume that the patient's lung disease is adequately diagnosed or treated. A detailed discussion of lung disease is beyond the scope of this chapter, but a broad overview will be provided.

OBSTRUCTIVE VENTILATORY DEFECT AND ASSOCIATED DISORDERS

An obstructive ventilatory defect (OVD) describes a pattern of pulmonary dysfunction characterized by a reduced ratio of the forced expiratory volume in 1 second (FEV_1) to the forced vital capacity (FVC) on spirometry. In addition to the reduced FEV_1/FVC ratio, there is a reduction in flow manifested by a reduction in the FEV_1 (Figure 29–1).[1-31] Patients with very mild OVD may have a normal FEV_1 but a reduced FEV_1/FVC ratio. For convenience, the lower limit of normal for the FEV_1 and FVC is often assumed to be 80% of predicted, and the lower limit of normal for the FEV_1/FVC ratio is assumed to be 0.70. However, using a slightly higher value of the FEV_1/FVC ratio for the lower limit of normal is appropriate in younger patients. For example, using 90% of predicted as the lower limit of normal for the FEV_1/FVC ratio may be more sensitive for identification of OVDs.[3] The recommended method to determine the lower limit of normal for the FEV_1 is to define the 5% percentile value (95% of the normal population have a greater value).[1-4] However, the Global Initiative for Chronic Obstructive Lung Disease (GOLD) defines chronic obstructive pulmonary disease (COPD) based on a **post-bronchodilator** FEV1/FVC ratio <0.70 in combination with symptoms (exertional dyspnea, cough, sputum production).[5-9] A discussion of methods to define a normal range and grade the severity of lung disease is presented in chapter 13.

Patients with an OVD have normal or increased lung volumes, including the residual volume (RV), function residual capacity (FRC), and total lung capacity (TLC) (Figure 29–2). The first lung volume to be affected is the RV. Most patients with an OVD have an elevated RV due to air-trapping from small airway narrowing and closure. With more severe disease, the FRC and then the TLC may also be increased (hyperinflation). However, the relative increase in the RV is greater than any increase in the FRC or TLC. In moderate to severe OVD, the increase in RV is large enough (compared with any increase in the TLC) to cause a reduction in the FVC (Figure 29–2). The increase in the FRC and TLC is due to loss of lung elastic recoil (emphysema) and/or airway disease (asthma, chronic bronchitis).

A significant acute response to inhaled bronchodilator has been defined by a 12% or greater increase in the FEV_1 or FVC, with a minimum of 200 mL absolute increase. However more recent guidlines use >10% improvement in the FEV_1 or FVC as significant (see chapter 13).[4] Lack of an acute bronchodilator response does not rule out a benefit from chronic bronchodilator therapy. Some patients with lung disease require a course of steroids to exhibit an improvement in the FEV_1 and FVC. If the patient is currently using bronchodilators, these should be withheld for an appropriate period prior to testing. Patients with asthma often have a 25% or greater increase in the FEV_1, while patients with COPD may demonstrate some degree of bronchospasm and have increases in the 10% to 15% range. The single breath diffusing capacity for carbon monoxide (DLCO) is used to detect abnormalities in the diffusion of gases from alveoli to the pulmonary capillaries. In this test, the patient inspires a mixture of carbon monoxide and helium from RV to TLC, holds the breath for 10 seconds, then exhales. After discarding dead space gas, the exhaled concentration of CO and a marker gas for lung volume (usually helium or methane) are measured. The lung volume at breath-hold and the amount of CO transferred can be computed. The units of the DLCO are ml/min/mm Hg. Individuals with asthma and chronic bronchitis (airway disease) usually have a normal DLCO, while the diffusing capacity is reduced in patients with a significant component of emphysema.[1,2,10]

Common OVD disorders are listed in Table 29–1. These include asthma (bronchospasm = reversible airway obstruction), chronic bronchitis (productive cough/sputum production and evidence of OVD), and emphysema (destruction of alveoli and increased size of terminal airspaces). Patients often have a mixture of these manifestations and are said to have COPD. Patients with asthma may have normal pulmonary function between exacerbations that can occur due to upper respiratory tract infections, exposure to allergens, or exercise. They typically demonstrate a large improvement in the FEV_1 or FVC after administration of an inhaled bronchodilator. Asthmatics have bronchial hyperresponsiveness to methacholine challenge (>20% fall in FEV_1 after inhaling low concentrations), allergens, or exercise challenges (>20% fall in FEV_1 after exercise). A diagnosis of asthma can be made in a patient with normal pulmonary function by demonstration of bronchial hyperresponsiveness. Some patients with asthma have

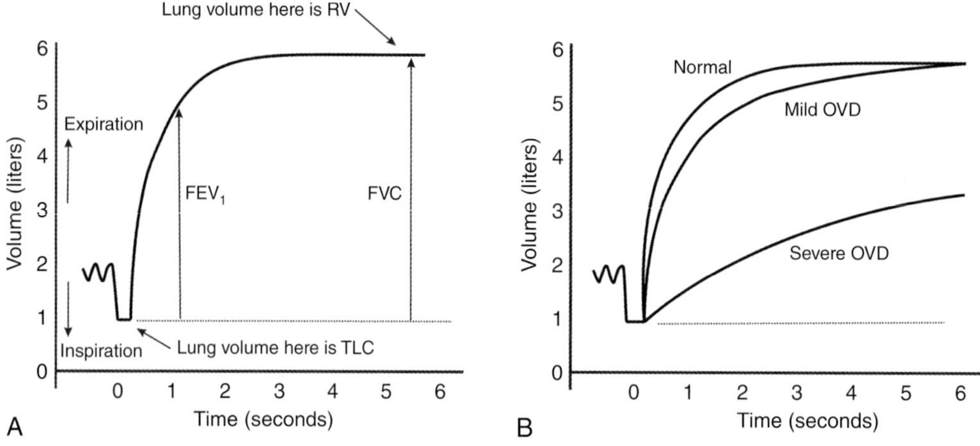

Figure 29–1 A, Spirometry measures the exhaled volume versus time. The individual being tested inhales to total lung capacity and forcibly exhales to residual volume. The forced exhaled volume in 1 second (FEV_1) and forced vital capacity (FVC) are shown. B, Patterns of patients with mild and severe obstructive ventilatory dysfunction (OVD). The hallmark of obstruction is a reduced FEV1/FVC ratio. *RV*, residual volume; *TLC*, total lung capacity.

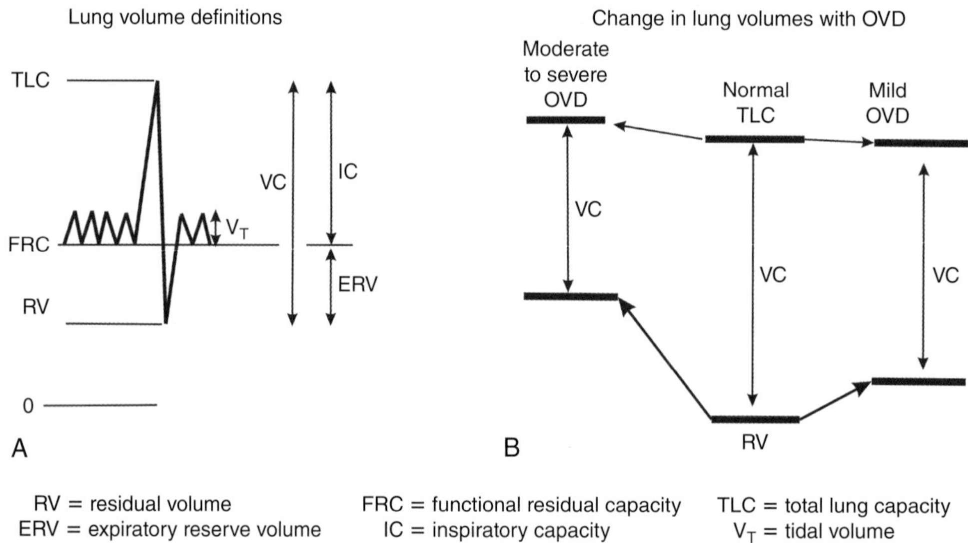

Figure 29–2 A, A slow vital capacity maneuver. Lung volumes, including the total lung capacity (TLC), functional residual capacity (FRC), and residual volume (RV), are shown. The vital capacity (VC) is TLC-RV. The expiratory reserve volume = FRC − RV. The inspiratory capacity (IC) = TLC-FRC. B, In obstructive ventilatory dysfunction (OVD), the RV increases more than the FRC and TLC. In moderate to severe OVD, the RV increase may be enough to decrease the vital capacity (VC).

persistent airflow obstruction and require inhaled or even oral corticosteroids for improvement. Patients with severe asthma can have hyperinflation and hypercapnic respiratory failure with severe exacerbations. Those individuals with COPD and predominantly chronic bronchitis typically have recurrent exacerbations and tend to have lower arterial partial pressure of oxygen (PaO_2) values earlier in the disease course. Some may develop hypercapnia and cor pulmonale (blue bloaters). Other patients with OVD have predominantly emphysema with severe hyperinflation (due to loss of lung elastic recoil) and relative preservation of PaO_2 levels until late in the disease course. They present with dyspnea and, because of the relatively spared PaO_2, are called "pink puffers." Patients with a combination of COPD and OSA are said to have overlap syndrome (OLS) and can have especially severe drops in the arterial oxygen saturation (SaO_2) associated with apneas and hypopneas. The importance of an overlap between asthma and COPD has also been appreciated.

CHRONIC OBSTRUCTIVE PULMONARY DISEASE

The 2023 GOLD[9] definition of COPD is "a heterogeneous lung condition characterized by chronic respiratory symptoms (dyspnea, cough, expectoration, and/or exacerbations) due to abnormalities of the airways (bronchitis, bronchiolitis) and/or alveoli (emphysema) that cause persistent, often progressive, airflow obstruction." *COPD is the fourth leading cause of death in the United States.*[11,12] Patients with COPD may die from respiratory failure, lung cancer, or from comorbid conditions. Significant comorbidities may have an impact on morbidity and mortality. The major cause of COPD is cigarette smoking (about 80%), but inhalation of toxic gases, including industrial

Table 29–1 Spectrum of Obstructive Ventilatory Dysfunction

	Diagnosis	Diffusing Capacity	Bronchodilator Response	Airtrapping and Hyperinflation
Asthma	Reversible airflow obstruction (physiological diagnosis)	Normal	Yes >12% increase, often 25%	High RV can occur High FRC, TLC can occur in severe disease
Chronic Bronchitis	Productive sputum for ≥3 months for more than 2 consecutive years (clinical diagnosis)	Normal	Sometimes 10–15% increase	High RV
Emphysema	Destruction of gas exchanging units and enlargement of terminal airspaces (pathological diagnosis)	Decreased	Rarely	High (RV, FRC) or High (TLC, FRC, and RV)
Mixed Chronic-Bronchitis and Emphysema (COPD)	Combination	Decreased	None or small increase	High RV or High (RV, FRC) or High (TLC, FRC, and RV)

COPD, chronic obstructive pulmonary disease; *RV*, residual volume; *TLC*, total lung capacity, *FRC*, functional residual capacity.
Airtrapping: increased RV
Hyperinflation: increased FRC and TLC.

pollution, causes the remainder.[11,12] Alpha-1-antitrypsin (AAT) deficiency is an inherited cause of about 3% of COPD cases and is characterized by the development of panlobular emphysema, often at a young age, and can be diagnosed by testing of blood for the level of AAT and genetic type. The nomenclature for COPD varies among clinicians. Chronic bronchitis is defined based on symptoms as a chronic productive cough for at least 3 months in each of 2 successive years in a patient in whom other causes of chronic cough (e.g., bronchiectasis) have been excluded. It may precede or follow development of airflow limitation. These patients tend to have frequent exacerbations. Patients with chronic bronchitis without evidence of an OVD are not classified as having COPD in the GOLD classification of the disease.[6-8] The GOLD diagnostic criteria and treatment recommendations undergo frequent updates, and the reader is referred to the GOLD website for the most recent version (www.goldcopd.org). Emphysema is a pathological term, and this subtype of COPD has abnormal and permanent enlargement of the distal airspaces distal to terminal bronchioles and is accompanied by destruction of the airspace walls. Patients with asthma that is incompletely reversible are considered to have a form of COPD, and those with a bronchodilator response (but not completely reversible) and chronic bronchitis are sometimes referred to as having "asthmatic bronchitis."

Although individuals with COPD typically present to physicians with complaints of bronchitis (cough and sputum production) or dyspnea, they also frequently complain of poor sleep quality. The GOLD criteria for the severity of airflow limitation is based on the **post-bronchodilator** FEV_1 as a percentage of predicted *(≥80% mild, 50–79% moderate, 30–49% severe, and <30% very severe)*.[9] The importance of symptoms and risk of exacerbations also plays a critical role in classifying severity in patients The 2023 scheme first considers exacerbation history and separates this from symptoms. The former ABCD scheme is replaced by E, A, and B. The E group has either ≥2 exacerbations per year or ≥1 leading to hospitalization. The A and B groups have 0 or 1 moderate exacerbations per year (not leading to hospitalization). The A and B groups are differentiated based on the fact that the B group has more severe symptoms as assessed by the modified Medical Research Council (mMRC) dyspnea score[13,14] or COPD assessment test (CAT)[15] than those of the A group (A: mMRC 0–1, CAT <10; B: mMRC ≥2, CAT ≥10). A higher score in both the mMRC and CAT scales is more severe. The mMRC scale is as follows: 1 = breathless with strenuous exercise, 2 = short of breath when hurrying on the leve or walking up a slight hill, 3 = walking slower than people of the same stage of the level or stopping for breath while walking at own pace on the level, 4 = stopping for breath after walking 100 meters, and 5 = too breathless to leave the house or breathless while dressing.

The ABE scheme places greater emphasis on the history of exacerbations in assessing the severity of disease. *The greatest risk factor for future exacerbations is the history of prior exacerbations.*[16] The ABE scheme is used in the GOLD guidelines to make treatment recommendations. Changes in the GOLD reports with respect to treatment recommendations have included more emphasis on the number of exacerbations and symptoms to guide treatment choices, a greater emphasis on longer acting bronchodilators, and limitation of inhaled steroids to target the patients most likely to benefit from steroid treatment.[17]

Although the FEV_1 remains an important predictor of mortality, the predictive value is limited when the FEV_1 is greater than 50% of predicted. Other factors such as exercise capacity, pulmonary artery size, and indices of dyspnea have been used to quantify disease severity and mortality risk. The importance of comorbid conditions, including heart disease, have also been noted. In general, an FEV_1 less than 30% to 40% of predicted or 1.0 L for a normal-sized individual indicates very severe disease. Daytime hypercapnia is usually associated with an FEV_1 of 30% to 40% or less of predicted (usually an FEV_1 <1.0 L). Patients with the overlap syndrome (OLS) defined as a combination of COPD and OSA can develop hypercapnia with a higher FEV_1 (milder reduction) value than patients with COPD without associated OSA.

Sleep in COPD

Sleep in patients with COPD is often impaired in both duration and quality.[18,19] Omachi et al.[19] analyzed a group of patients with COPD and found that sleep disturbance was associated with

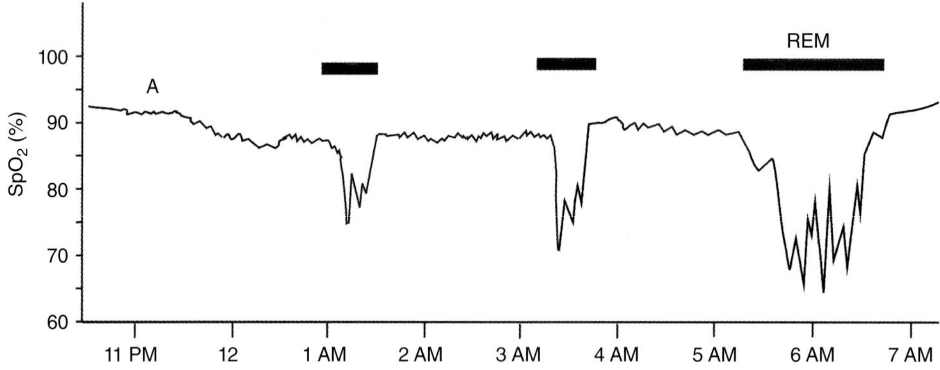

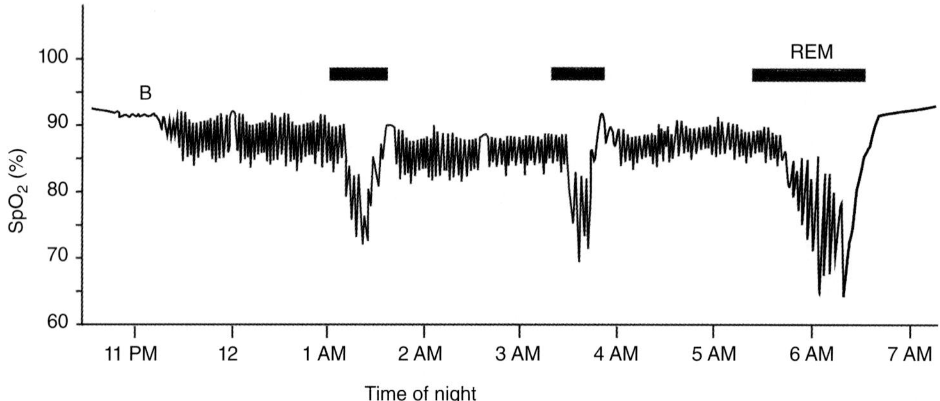

Figure 29–3 In the upper schematic tracing, there is an example of typical nocturnal oximetry in a patient with COPD. There is a mild decrease in the awake SaO_2 (92%), which decreases slightly in NREM (87–88%) sleep but has a more significant decrease during REM sleep. The bottom schematic tracing displays an example of an individual with both COPD and obstructive sleep apnea (OSA) showing a saw-tooth pattern. The worst period of desaturation was noted in the early morning hours.

Table 29–2 Medicare Criteria for Oxygen Treatment (NCD 240.2 and L33797)

Required qualifying PaO_2 or oximetry studies must be performed at the time of need.

Patients exhibiting hypoxemia:

Group 1

- $PaO_2 \leq 55$ mm Hg or $SaO_2 \leq 88\%$, taken at rest (awake), breathing room air; or
- $PaO_2 \leq 55$ mm Hg or $SaO_2 \leq 88\%$, taken during **sleep** for a patient who demonstrates a $PaO_2 \geq 56$ mm Hg or $SaO_2 \geq 89\%$ while awake; or a greater than normal fall in oxygen during **sleep** (a decrease in $PaO_2 > 10$ mm Hg or decrease in $SaO_2 > 5\%$) associated with symptoms or signs reasonably attributable to hypoxemia (e.g., impairment of cognitive processes and nocturnal restlessness or insomnia. In either of the cases, coverage is provided only for use of oxygen during **sleep**, and only one unit will be covered). Portable oxygen, therefore, would not be covered in this situation.
- $PaO_2 \leq 55$ mg Hg or $SaO_2 \leq 88\%$, taken during **exercise** (defined as either the functional performance of the patient or a formal exercise test) for a patient who demonstrated a $PaO_2 \geq 56$ mm Hg or $SaO_2 \geq 89\%$ during the day while at rest. In this case, supplemental oxygen is provided during **exercise** if the oxygen improves the hypoxemia that was demonstrated during **exercise** when the patient was breathing room air.

Group 2

Coverage is available for patients whose PaO_2 is 56–59 mm Hg or whose SaO_2 is 89% if there is:

- Dependent edema suggesting congestive heart failure, or
- Pulmonary hypertension or cor pulmonale, determined by measurement of pulmonary artery pressure, gated blood pool scan, echocardiogram (ECG), or "P" pulmonale on ECG (P wave greater than 3 mm in standard leads II, III, or aVF); or,
- Erythrocythemia with a hematocrit greater than 56%

Note: *PaO_2,* arterial PO_2; *SaO_2,* arterial oxygen saturation.
Implementation Date: 1/3/2023
Oxygen and Oxygen Equipment Local Coverage Determination (LCD) L33797 and Related Policy Article (PA) A52514 Update

Table 29–3 Studies of Effects of Supplemental Oxygen on Sleep Quality in Chronic Obstructive Pulmonary Disease

	Calverly ($N = 6$)	Fleetham ($N = 15$)
Total sleep time	Increased	No change
Stage N3	Increased	No change
REM sleep	Increased	No change
Arousals	Decreased	No change

REM, rapid eye movement.

Calverley PM, Brezinova V, Douglas NJ, et al. The effect of oxygenation on sleep quality in chronic bronchitis and emphysema. *Am Rev Respir Dis.* 1982;126:206-210. PMID: 7103244.

Fleetham J, West P, Mezon B, et al. Sleep, arousals, and oxygen desaturation in chronic obstructive pulmonary disease: the effect of oxygen therapy. *Am Rev Respir Dis.* 1982;126:429-433. PMID: 7125332.

increased cough, dyspnea, and a COPD severity score (incorporating COPD symptoms, requirement for COPD medications and oxygen, and hospital-based utilization) *but not the FEV1. Sleep disturbance predicted incident COPD exacerbations and predicted poorer survival.* These findings may simply document the fact that patients with more severely symptomatic COPD have worse sleep quality. Many patients with COPD also have significant hypercapnia and hypoxemia at night. Ten percent to 15% of patients may also have concomitant OSA that worsens nocturnal gas exchange (OLS). A schematic of a typical pattern of **nocturnal oxygen desaturation** (NOD) in a patient with COPD is shown in Figure 29–3 (*top panel*). The arterial oxygen saturation (SaO_2), which is mildly reduced when awake at 92% and falls 2% to 4% during non–rapid eye movement (NREM) sleep with minor fluctuations until much larger drops are noted during rapid eye movement (REM; stage R) sleep.[20,21] In contrast, typical nocturnal oximetry of a patient with OLS is shown in Figure 29–3 (*lower panel*). There is a low baseline sleeping SaO_2 and a sawtooth pattern consistent with repeated discrete events. Whereas central sleep apnea could cause a saw-tooth pattern, this is most likely representative of OSA. Polysomnography (PSG) is indicated to document the presence and severity of the sleep apnea. In Figure 29–4, changes in the arterial oxygen saturation and transcutaneous PCO_2 are shown. During NREM sleep, there is a mild decrease in the SpO_2 without discrete apnea or hypopneas, and during REM sleep, there is a further decrease in the SpO_2 and increase in the transcutaneous PCO_2.

Etiology of Abnormal Nocturnal Gas Exchange

Patients with COPD often experience exaggerations of normal sleep-related changes in ventilation. The most severe desaturation occurs during REM sleep.[21-25] The major mechanisms of nocturnal arterial oxygen desaturation are listed in Box 29–1. The relative importance of hypoventilation and ventilation-perfusion ($\dot{V}/\dot{Q}$) mismatch is still debated. If the baseline sleeping SaO_2 is on the steep portion of the hemoglobin saturation curve, small drops in PaO_2 result in larger drops in the SaO_2 (Figure 29–5). To understand sleep-associated changes in breathing in COPD, a brief review of normal changes in breathing during sleep is informative.

Normal Individuals

During NREM sleep, CO_2 production falls, but alveolar ventilation falls proportionately more, and arterial pressure of carbon dioxide ($PaCO_2$) increases slightly (Figure 29–6). Recall that $PaCO_2$ = constant × (CO_2 production)/(alveolar ventilation) (see Chapter 13). The fall in ventilation is due to a loss of the wakefulness stimulus to breathe, decreased

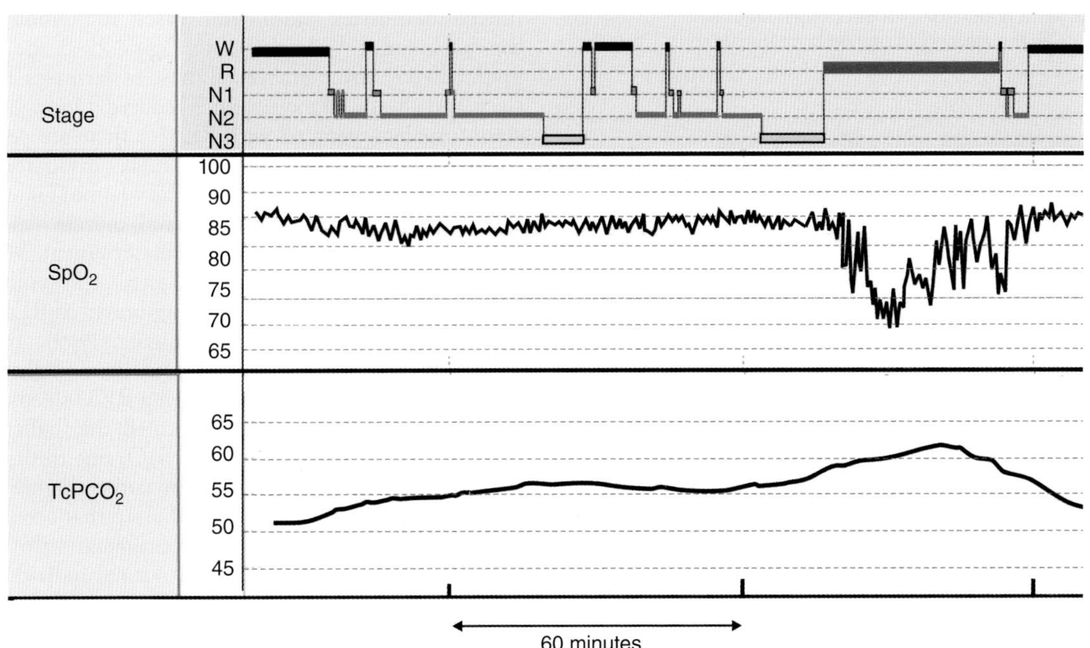

Figure 29–4 An example of arterial oxygen desaturation in a patient with moderate COPD. With sleep onset, the arterial oxygen saturation by oximetry (SpO_2) falls slightly, with a more significant fall during REM sleep. The transcutaneous PCO_2 ($TcPCO_2$) shows a small increase from wakefulness to NREM sleep and a further increase during REM sleep. There is a delay in changes in the transcutaneous PCO_2 due to a longer response time.

Box 29–1 MAJOR MECHANISMS OF NOCTURNAL OXYGEN DESATURATION IN CHRONIC OBSTRUCTIVE PULMONARY DISEASE

- Hypoventilation
  - Decreased chemosensitivity (REM < NREM < Wakefulness)
  - Reliance on accessory respiratory muscles and loss of this assistance during REM atonia
  - Increased upper airway resistance
  - Lower alveolar ventilation per minute ventilation (high dead space-to-tidal volume ratio—due to high dead space and low tidal volume)
- Ventilation-perfusion mismatching (drop in PaO_2 exceeds increase in $PaCO_2$)
  - High closing volume and decreases in FRC—especially during REM-associated hypopnea
  - V/Q mismatch in lungs
- Co-existing sleep apnea (12–15%)—especially blue bloaters
- Low awake SaO_2—starting on the steep portion of the oxygen-hemoglobin dissociation curve (larger fall in SaO_2 for a given fall in PaO_2)

FRC, functional residual capacity; *$PaCO_2$*, arterial partial pressure of carbon dioxide; *PaO_2*, arterial partial pressure of oxygen; *REM*, rapid eye movement.

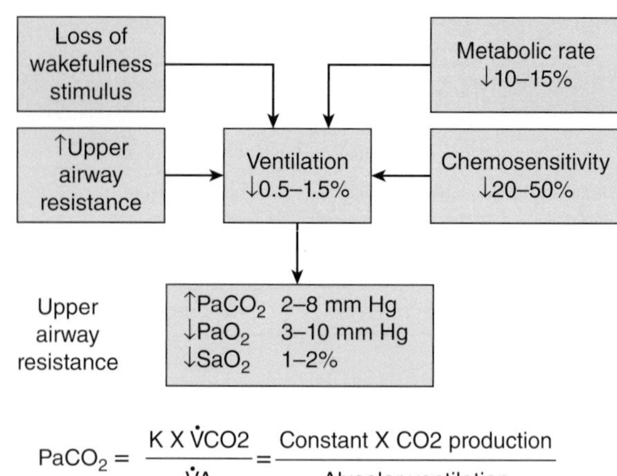

Figure 29–6 Normal changes in gas exchange during sleep. Although the metabolic rate falls from wakefulness to sleep, the ventilation fall is greater, such that the PCO_2 is mildly increased during sleep and the PaO_2 mildly decreased. *$PaCO_2$*, arterial partial pressure of carbon dioxide; *PaO_2*, arterial partial pressure of oxygen; *SaO_2*, arterial oxygen saturation. (Adapted from Mohsenin V. Sleep in chronic obstructive pulmonary disease. *Semin Respir Crit Care Med.* 2005;26:109-115.)

ventilatory responses (chemosensitivity) to hypoxia and hypercapnia, and increased upper-airway resistance.[22-25] The increase in $PaCO_2$ results in a mild decrease in the PaO_2. However, because the awake PaO_2 value is on the flat portion of the oxygen-hemoglobin saturation curve (Figure 29–5), minimal drops in the SaO_2 are noted (e.g., from 97% to 95%). The FRC decreases slightly from wakefulness to NREM sleep.[26,27] In the study by Ballard et al.,[27] the FRC values

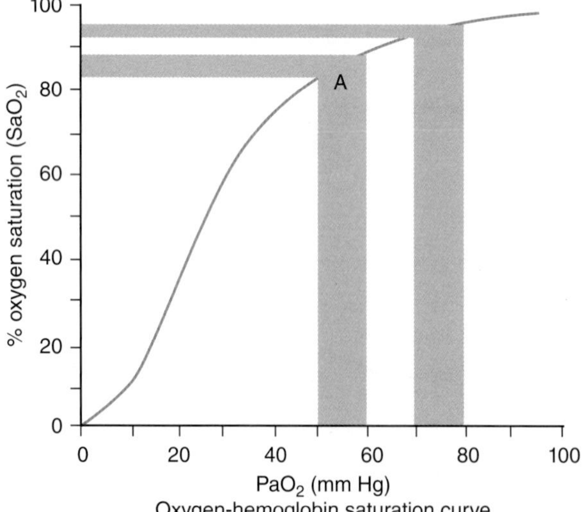

Figure 29–5 The same drop in the arterial partial pressure of oxygen (PaO_2) is associated with a greater drop in the arterial oxygen saturation (SaO_2) when the initial partial pressure of oxygen (PO_2) is 60 (A) on the steep portion of the hemoglobin oxygen dissociation curve rather than 80 mm Hg on the flat part of the curve.

during NREM and REM sleep were similar in normal individuals (Figure 29–7), and in the study by Hudgel et al.,[26] the FRC values in stage N3 and REM sleep were similar. Using magnetometers, Mueller and coworkers concluded that the FRC does decrease during REM sleep.[28] REM sleep is not homogeneous, and a fall in FRC could occur during "phasic" REM sleep associated with bursts of rapid eye movements.[29]

During REM sleep in normal individuals, ventilation is irregular, and periods of reduced tidal volume occur, often during bursts of REMs.[30] Ventilatory drive is lower during REM sleep than during NREM sleep.[31] Skeletal muscle hypotonia reduces the contribution from the accessory respiratory muscles and intercostal muscles, and for this reason, respiration depends on the diaphragm.[28,32] As shown in Figure 29–8, the electromyogram (EMG) of the intercostal muscles decreases during REM sleep, and chest wall movement is reduced. During phasic REM sleep (usually associated with REMs), there are periods of decreased chest wall and diaphragm EMG inspiratory bursts associated with decreased flow and tidal volume (Figure 29–8).[28,32] Thus, both tonic and phasic chest wall muscle hypotonia is associated with a decrease in chest wall movement.[28,32] The EMG of the diaphragm does not show a decrease in tonic activity but has an irregular pattern, and during bursts of REMs, reduced phasic activity is often noted (Figure 29–9). These REM-associated physiologic changes result in a slight increase in $PaCO_2$ and a decrease in PaO_2 during REM sleep compared to that during NREM sleep. But as noted, the slight fall in PaO_2 results in minimal changes in the SaO_2 due to the position of the oxygen-hemoglobin saturation curve (Figure 29–5). The changes in breathing during REM sleep that occur in patients with COPD are believed to be an "exaggeration" of the changes during REM sleep that occur in normal individuals. An example of periods of reduced and irregular airflow as well as an example of reduced chest wall movement during REM sleep is shown in Figure 29–10. During this period, hypoventilation occurs (increase in the transcutaneous PCO_2). The mechanisms of hypopneic breathing during REM sleep are summarized in schematic form in Figure 29–11.

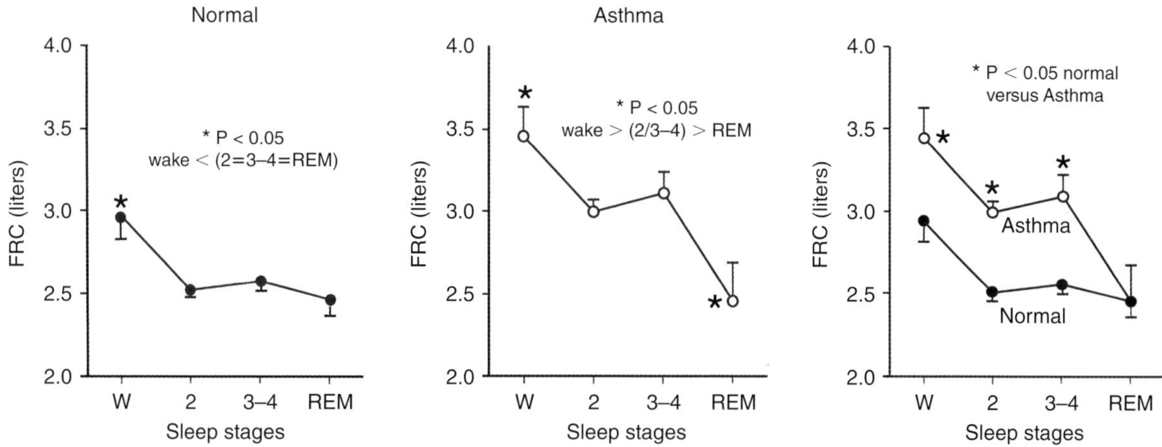

Figure 29–7 In normal individuals, the functional residual capacity (FRC) falls from wakefulness to sleep with no significant change between the sleep stages. In asthma, the FRC is lower during NREM sleep than during wakefulness and lower during REM sleep than during NREM sleep. Overall, the FRC values during wakefulness and NREM sleep were greater in asthmatics than in normal individuals. (From Ballard RD, Irvin CG, Martin RJ, et al. Influence of sleep on lung volume in asthmatic patients and normal subjects. *J Appl Physiol.* 1990;68:2034-2041. PMID: 2361905)

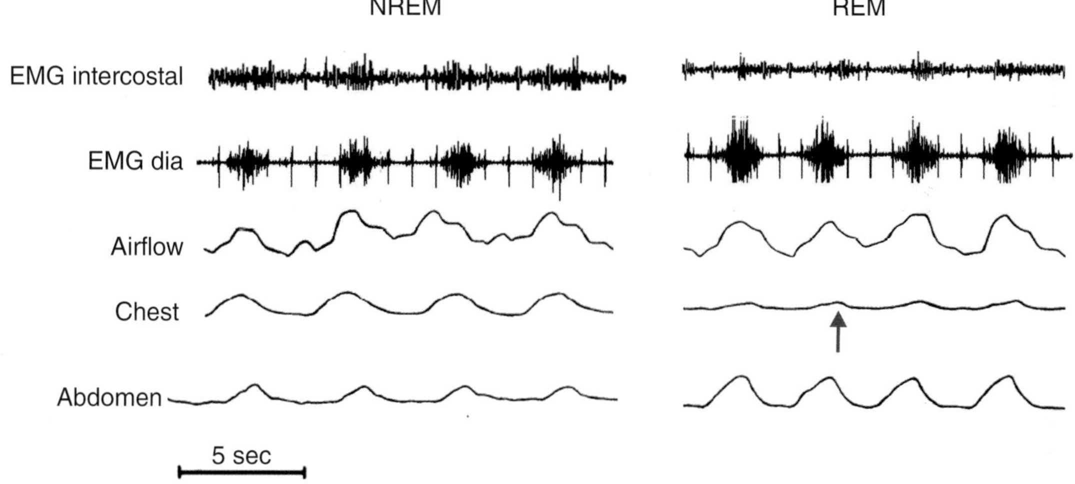

Figure 29–8 Changes in respiration between NREM and REM sleep in a normal individual. On transition from NREM to REM sleep, intercostal muscle activity decreases as does chest wall movement (*red arrow*). To compensate the diaphragm, increases contraction (increased EMGdia activity) resulting in increased abdominal movement. EMG Dia is the diaphragmatic EMG, V_T is tidal volume.

Sleep-Related Changes in Respiration in COPD

Koo and colleagues[33] studied 15 patients with severe COPD (mean FEV_1 of 0.96 L) with a mean daytime PaO_2 of approximately 60 mm Hg. They found a mean decrease in PaO_2 of 13.5 mm Hg and a mean increase in $PaCO_2$ of 8.3 mm Hg from wakefulness to sleep (average of measurements in all sleep stages) (Figure 29–12). In some individuals, the decrease in PaO_2 could be explained by alveolar hypoventilation, and in others, the decrease in PaO_2 exceeded that expected from an increase in $PaCO_2$ (suggesting the presence of ventilation perfusion mismatch). There was no relationship between the fall in PaO_2 during sleep and the severity of awake airway obstruction or the awake PaO_2. Although patients with daytime hypercapnia or a low awake PaO_2 or SaO_2 are likely to have worse gas exchange during sleep, in one study, *about 25% of patients with COPD exhibited REM-related NOD, despite having an average daytime PaO_2 ≥60 mm Hg.*[34]

Non–Rapid Eye Movement Sleep. During supine wakefulness, patients with COPD often start with low-normal or slightly decreased SaO_2 values. Therefore, even the normal fall in PaO_2 with sleep will cause a greater decrease in the SaO_2. Koo and colleagues[33] documented stage-specific changes in arterial blood gases in eight patients with severe COPD and found a fall in PaO_2 of approximately 8 mm Hg from wakefulness to NREM sleep and an increase in $PaCO_2$ of about 5 mm Hg in patients with COPD. In patients with COPD, the onset of NREM sleep is often associated with mild falls in the SaO_2 (4–8%) and mild $PaCO_2$ increases.[34] If obstructive apneas or hypopneas are present, the degree of desaturation is worsened. Due to hyperinflation, the diaphragm is at a mechanical disadvantage,[35] and there is more dependence on the accessory muscles. In a study by Becker and coworkers[36] of a group of **hypercapnic** patients with COPD, the minute ventilation fell by 16% from wakefulness to NREM sleep, mainly due to a *decrease in tidal volume.*

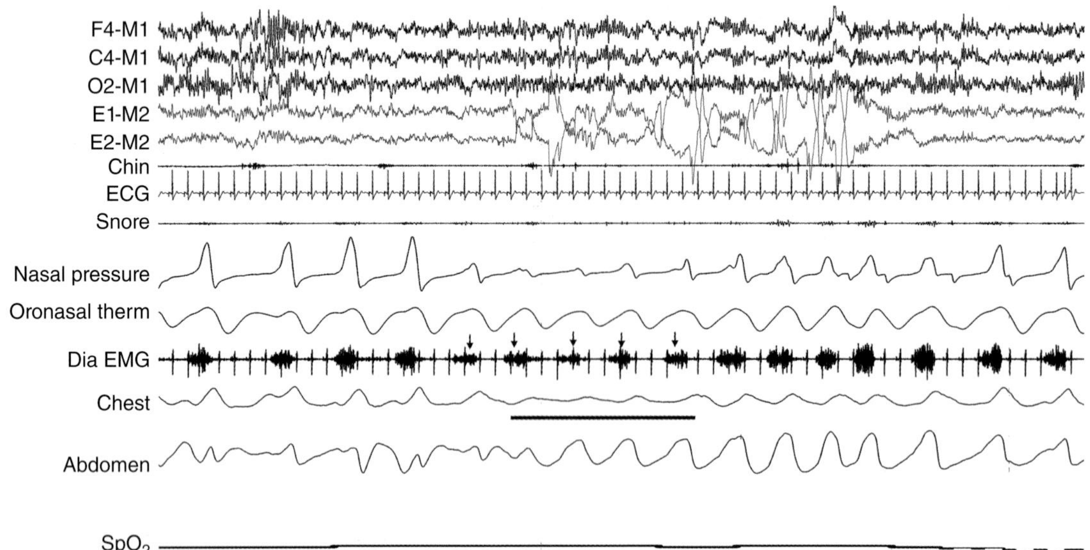

Figure 29–9 Decreased airflow and chest and abdominal movement associated with a burst of rapid eye movements (REMs) during REM sleep in a patient with chronic obstructive pulmonary disease (COPD). The surface diaphragm electromyogram (EMG) activity (EMG Dia) is inhibited (decreased) during the rapid eye movements (*down arrows*), reflecting inhibition of phrenic motor neurons during phasic REM sleep. Note the decrease in chest wall movement during the period of hypopneic breathing (*dark line*). The baseline oxygen saturation by oximetry (SpO_2) is reduced.

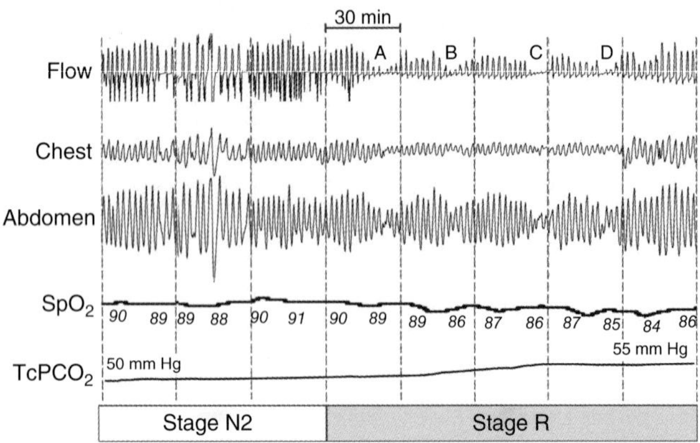

Figure 29–10 A 240-second tracing shows changes in airflow as well as chest and abdominal movement during transition from NREM to REM sleep in a patient with severe chronic obstructive pulmonary disease (COPD). Note the greater decrease in chest movement. Some periods of very significantly decreased airflow and chest and abdominal movements were noted at A, B, C, and D. These were associated with burst of eye movements (not shown). There was a progressive increase in the transcutaneous PCO_2 ($TcPCO_2$) and decrease in the arterial oxygen saturation (SpO_2) during this episode of REM sleep.

Rapid Eye Movement Sleep. During REM sleep, there are more profound periods of arterial oxygen desaturation than during NREM sleep in patients with COPD. These episodes of desaturation are characterized by long periods of irregular breathing and reduced tidal volume (Figures 29–9 and 29–10). *This pattern is sometimes called non-apneic desaturation or hypopneic breathing.* In contrast to obstructive hypopnea in patients with OSA, the onset and termination of these non-apneic periods of REM desaturation are less well defined, and the duration can be longer than with hypopneas typically seen in patients with OSA. As noted, it is believed that REM-associated hypotonia reduces the contribution from the intercostal muscles so that ventilation depends on the diaphragm. However, as also noted, hyperinflation in patients with COPD reduces the effectiveness of the diaphragm.[35] In EMG nomenclature, tonic activity refers to background activity and phasic activity to the increases in activity during inspiration. As in normal individuals, REM sleep is associated with hypotonia of the non-diaphragm respiratory muscles and a reduction in tonic activity. During bursts of REMs, there is also a further fall in the *phasic activity* of intercostal muscles associated with decreased chest movement (Figure 29–11). At the same time, there are periods of diaphragmatic inhibition associated with the phasic changes during REM sleep usually associated with the presence of REMs (Figures 29–9 and 29–11)[28,32]; the airflow, tidal volume, and minute ventilation often decrease dramatically (Figure 29–9 and Figure 29–10). In a study by Becker et al. of a group of hypercapnic patients with COPD, the minute ventilation fell by 32% from wakefulness to REM sleep (compared with 16% from wakefulness to NREM).[36] Studies have documented increases in $PaCO_2$ during these episodes (Figure 29–10).[37,38]

$\dot{V}/\dot{Q}$ Mismatch. Does the hypoventilation that occurs during periods of non-apneic desaturation (hypopneic breathing) explain the changes in PaO_2 and SaO_2? Catterall and associates[38,39] directly measured arterial blood gases and found the PaO_2 dropped more than the $PaCO_2$ increased (Figure 29–13). Therefore, increased ($\dot{V}/\dot{Q}$) mismatch could play a role in REM-associated desaturation (in addition to hypoventilation).[21,22] However, as Catterall and associates[38,39] and others have pointed out, the usual blood gas analysis of the relationship between PaO_2 and $PaCO_2$ depends on an assumption of steady state. This condition does not exist during the transient periods of hypopneic breathing. *Because oxygen stores in the body are much smaller than carbon dioxide stores, a change in ventilation may affect PaO_2 more than $PaCO_2$.*

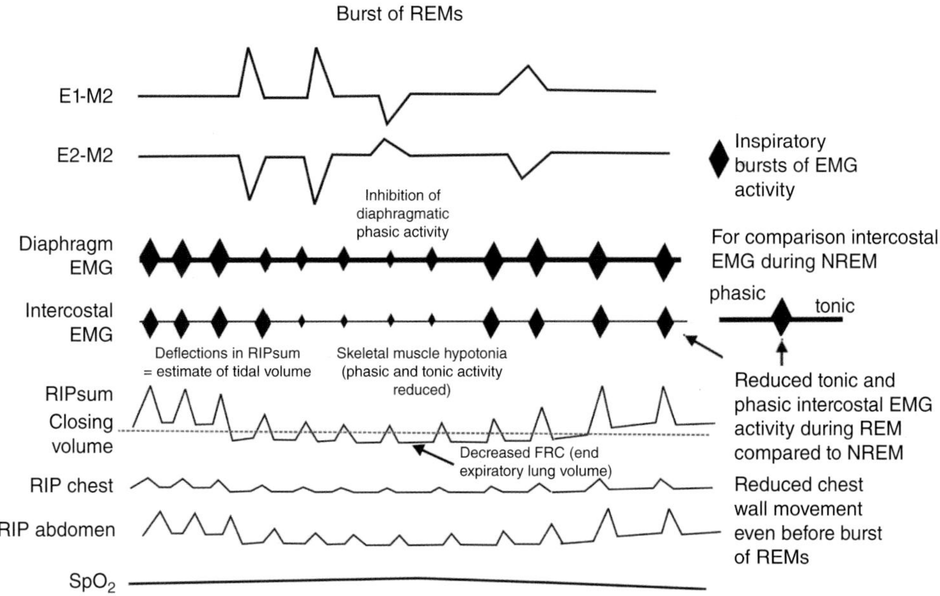

Figure 29–11 A schematic illustration of the physiology of hypopneic breathing during rapid-eye movement (REM) sleep. REM-associated hypotonia reduces tonic intercostal electromyogram (EMG) (activity of accessory muscles of respiration). This phenomenon occurs during tonic REM sleep. During bursts of REMs, the phasic (inspiratory) intercostal activity also decreases and is associated with reduced chest wall excursions. There is also inhibition of inspiratory diaphragmatic activity associated with bursts of REMs (phasic REM sleep). In this schematic, the end-expiratory lung volume falls during the period of hypopneic breathing. Respiratory inductance plethysmography, RIP; RIPsum is the sum of RIP chest and RIP abdomen effort belt signals. Deflections in the RIPsum signal are estimates of tidal volume. Here RIPsum is acquired as a DC signal and reduction of the signal during exhalation is assumed to reflect a reduction in the end expiratory lung volume 26 (see Figure 29-14).

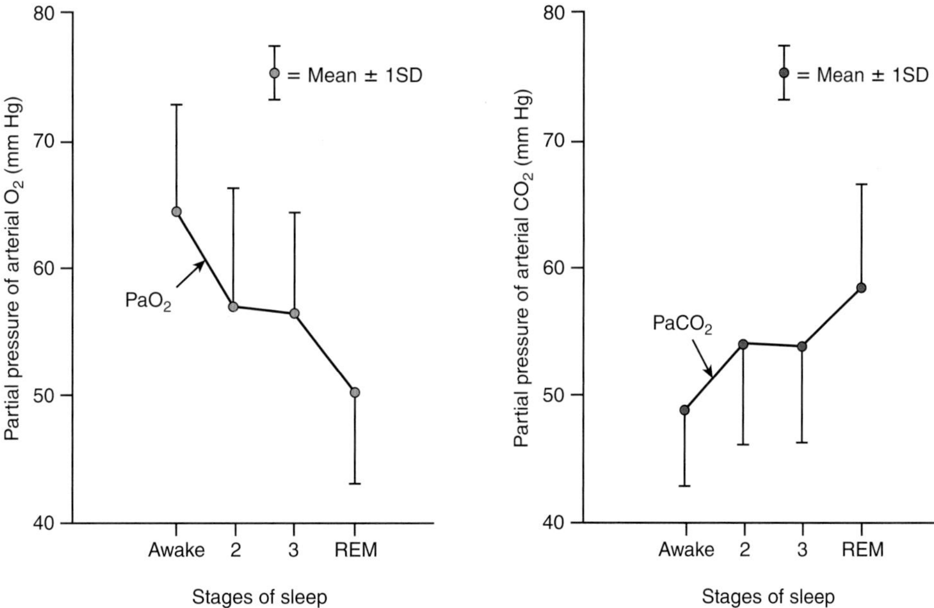

Figure 29–12 Changes in the arterial partial pressure of carbon dioxide (PaO_2) and the arterial partial pressure of oxygen ($PaCO_2$) during sleep in a group of patients with severe COPD. *REM*, rapid eye movement; *SD*, standard deviation. (From Koo KW, Sax DS, Snider GL. Arterial blood gases and pH during sleep in chronic obstructive pulmonary disease. *Am J Med.* 1975;58:663-670.)

What are the reasons for the increase in ($\dot{V}/\dot{Q}$) mismatch during hypopneic breathing during REM sleep? Many patients with COPD have an increase in FRC in the upright position (hyperinflation). In the supine position, the FRC may be slightly lower than during wakefulness, and the change may also be affected by the degree of obesity. Ballard and coworkers[40] found similar FRC values during wakefulness, NREM, and REM sleep in patients with emphysema. However, in another study in asthmatics, the group found that the FRC does decrease from wakefulness to NREM sleep and from NREM to REM sleep (Figure 29–7).[27] Therefore, patients with COPD with a significant component of airway

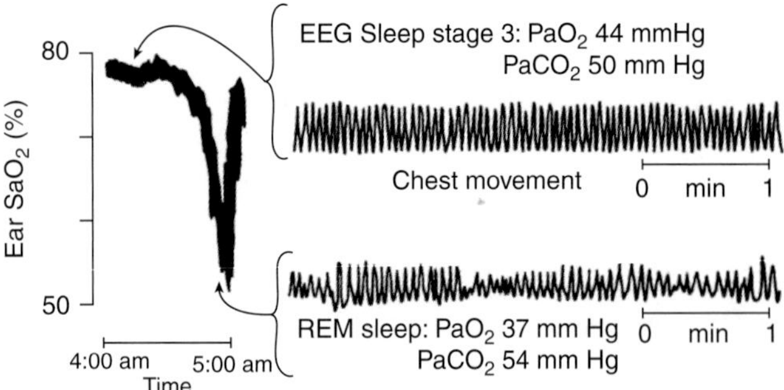

Figure 29–13 An episode of rapid eye movement (REM)–associated nonapneic desaturation in a patient with chronic obstructive pulmonary disease (COPD). On transition from stage 3 (N3) sleep to REM sleep, the $PaCO_2$ increased by 4 mm Hg, but the PO_2 decreased by 7 mm Hg. Maintaining a constant alveolar-to-arterial gradient, the ideal gas equation (R = 0.8) predicts that the PaO_2 should be 39.0 mm Hg, not 37.5 mm Hg. That is, the decrease in arterial partial pressure of oxygen (PaO_2) was slightly greater than predicted based entirely on an increase in the $PaCO_2$. The assumes R=0.8 in both NREM and REM sleep and the alveolar-arterial PaO_2 gradient is the same. $PaCO_2$, arterial partial pressure of carbon dioxide; PaO_2; arterial partial pressure of oxygen; R, gas-exchange ratio; EEG, electroencephalogram; SaO_2, arterial oxygen saturation. (From Catterall JR, Calverley PMA, MacNee W, et al. Mechanism of transient nocturnal hypoxemia in hypoxic chronic bronchitis and emphysema. *J Appl Physiol.* 1985;59:1698-1703.)

disease could also experience a fall in FRC from NREM to REM sleep. Furthermore, assigning a single FRC value to stage R sleep is problematic because breathing during REM sleep is very inhomogeneous. Hudgel and coworkers[29] found *no decrease in FRC* during transition from stage N2 to stage R sleep in a group of five patients with COPD. However, during episodes of hypopneic breathing in REM sleep, there was a fall in FRC (Figure 29–14). The same study found that those patients with COPD who desaturated during REM *sleep had longer periods of hypopneic breathing*. Thus, it seems likely that the FRC **during hypopneic breathing** in REM sleep in COPD is lower than that during NREM sleep. Whether the absolute value is below normal may vary among patients. A fall in the FRC during hypopneic breathing in patients with COPD may have greater consequences than in normal individuals. In COPD, the closing volume (CV), the volume at which small airway closure is significant, is closer to the FRC than in normal individuals. During the hypopneic breathing of REM sleep, the FRC falls below the CV (Figure 29–15).[41,42] This means that, during tidal breathing, more alveoli are either not ventilated or under-ventilated. This results in worsening of ($\dot{V}/\dot{Q}$) mismatch (already abnormal awake) and worsening hypoxemia.

What are the relative roles of hypoventilation and ($\dot{V}/\dot{Q}$) mismatch? Hudgel and coworkers[29] concluded that hypoventilation and, to a lesser extent, ($\dot{V}/\dot{Q}$) mismatch cause REM-associated desaturation. Fletcher and associates[37] found an increase in venous admixture during REM hypopnea episodes and concluded that ($\dot{V}/\dot{Q}$) mismatch was a significant cause of hypoxemia. The relative roles of hypoventilation and ($\dot{V}/\dot{Q}$) mismatch in inducing nocturnal desaturation during hypopneic breathing in REM sleep are still debated. As noted, the analysis is complicated by the non–steady-state condition of transient hypopneic breathing and, because oxygen stores in the body are much smaller than carbon dioxide stores, a change in ventilation may affect PaO_2 more than $PaCO_2$.

Time of Night and Circadian Variation in Lung Function

REM episodes in the early morning have the greatest REM density (number of REMs per minute) and the greatest variation in ventilation, even in normal individuals.[43] These REM periods are also typically longer. In the early morning hours, the lower airway resistance is *greater* due to circadian changes in bronchomotor tone that are exaggerated in patients with asthma and many patients with COPD and significant airway disease.[44] Ballard and colleagues[40] found an *increase in upper airway resistance* but not lower airway resistance during the night in a group of patients with emphysema. Conversely, lower airway resistance does increase during the night in asthmatics[45] and, likely, in some patients with COPD with a significant component of airway disease. These factors help *explain why the most severe and longest REM-associated desaturation typically occurs in the early morning hours.*

COPD Types and Respiration During Sleep

Several studies have tried to find factors predicting more severe desaturation during sleep in COPD. As might be expected, a lower awake PaO_2 and higher $PaCO_2$ predict more dramatic changes in gas exchange during sleep. One study compared blue bloaters and pink puffers and found the former were more likely to desaturate during sleep[46] Analysis of the Sleep Heart Health data suggested the odds of desaturation more than 5% of total sleep time was minimally increased until the FEV_1/FVC ratio was less than 60%.[47] Connaughton and coworkers found that patients with lower **awake** SaO_2 or PaO_2 values tended to have lower values at night.[48] However, there is considerable variability, and oximetry or PSG is needed to reliably exclude nocturnal oxygen desaturation (NOD). A study by Lewis et al.[49] did not find that patients with COPD and isolated nocturnal desaturation had worse quality of life or sleep quality. Connaughton et al.[48] did not recommend routine evaluation of nocturnal oxygenation in patients with COPD. However, use of nocturnal oximetry (or PSG, if sleep apnea is suspected) is indicated in patients with prominent nocturnal complaints, daytime hypercapnia, or evidence of cor pulmonale. If OSA is suspected, polysomnography rather than oximetry is indicated.

Sleep Quality in COPD. Sleep quality is impaired with reductions in total sleep time, stage N3 sleep, and REM sleep. In contrast, wakefulness after sleep onset (WASO) and stage N1 sleep are increased consistent with impaired sleep quality. The total arousal index is also increased.[18,19] Patients often complain of insomnia but can also complain of daytime sleepiness if OSA is also present. A study of NOD in patients with COPD *not on 24-hour oxygen* found *no difference in quality of life, subjective sleepiness, or subjective sleep quality* in patients with COPD who had NOD when compared with those of patients who did not.[48] It is likely that other factors such as cough, nocturnal dyspnea, and medication side effects have greater effect than transient hypoxemia on sleep quality. In many patients, the NOD is less than 15 minutes and confined to the last few REM periods of the night. Insomnia is a frequent complaint in patients with COPD. A survey conducted by Budihraja et al.[50] of 183 patients with COPD found complaints of chronic sleep disturbance with impaired daytime function in 27%. Of interest, current tobacco users or those with frequent mood complaints were at high risk,

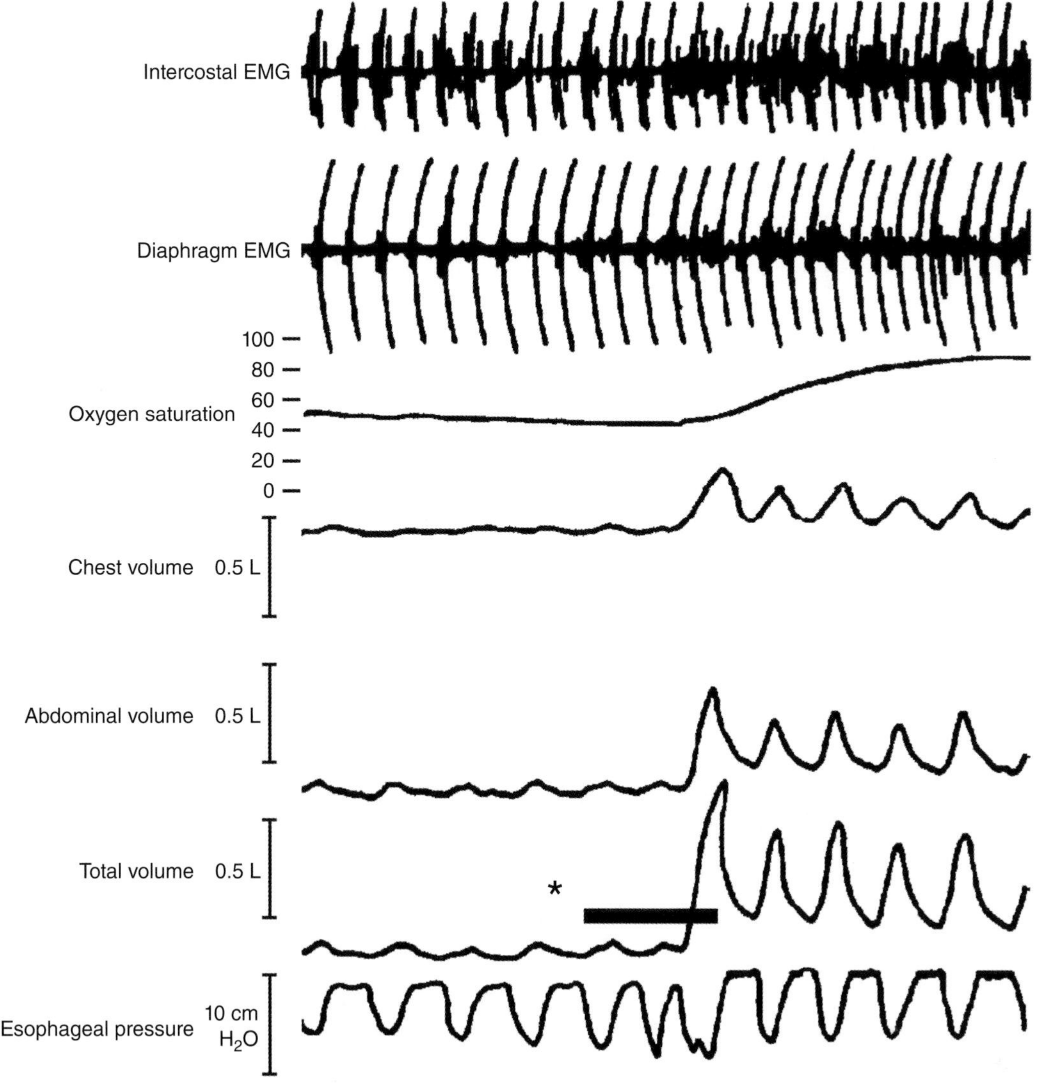

Figure 29–14 Hypopnea and hyperpnea during REM sleep of a patient with chronic obstructive pulmonary disease (COPD). Raw intercostal and diaphragmatic electromyogram (EMG) activity, esophageal pressure, and arterial oxygen saturation (SaO_2) are shown. This is the end of an episode of REM hypopneic breathing. Note the increase in end-expiratory volume (*) at the end of the episode. The solid bar shows that the end-expiratory volume after the hypopnea ends is higher than that during the hypopneic breathing. Also note the decreased intercostal EMG phasic (inspiratory activity) and greater reduction in chest wall movement due the period of hypopneic breathing. (From Hudgel DW, Martin RJ, Capehart M, et al. Contribution of hypoventilation to sleep oxygen desaturation in chronic obstructive pulmonary disease. *J Appl Physiol.* 1983;55:669-677.)

while those using oxygen were at a lower risk. **Potential** interventions to improve sleep are reduction in nocturnal symptoms of cough and dyspnea with bronchodilators, supplemental oxygen in those with nocturnal hypoxemia, and possibly, hypnotics. These possible interventions are discussed in following sections of the chapter, but all have significant limitations. Smoking cessation is also an important intervention. Impaired sleep quality in COPD patients can also be due to the presence of comorbid depression, chronic pain syndromes, or congestive heart failure.

Treatment of Sleep-Related Hypoxemia in COPD. Studies have shown that long-term oxygen therapy (LTOT) improves survival in patients with COPD with **daytime** hypoxemia.[51-53] The studies showing benefit used oxygen for 12 hours or more per day. The standard indication for 24-hour supplemental oxygen is a daytime $PaO_2 \leq 55$ mm Hg at rest breathing room air (or $SaO_2 \leq 88\%$) when the patient is in a stable condition. PaO_2 values from 56 to 59 mm Hg are also an indication of a need for oxygen therapy if signs of dysfunction (right heart failure, increase hematocrit) are present.[54] The national carrier determination for oxygen NCD 240.2 has been revised and the local carrier determinations L33797 revised to conform to the new guidelines.[55,56] The major change is that the *duration of low oxygen during sleep* has been eliminated (Table 29–2). The criteria may vary among regions (Local Carrier Determinations). Patients qualifying for 24-hour supplemental oxygen will obviously be using nocturnal oxygen. One study found that at least 50% of patients on LTOT needed increased oxygen flow during sleep.[57] Medicare and most insurance providers do provide

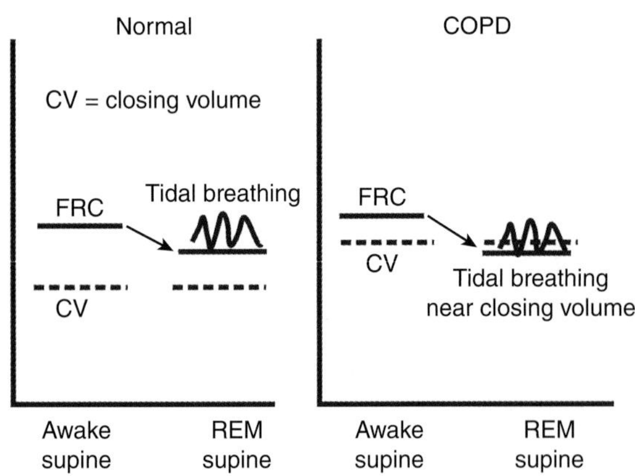

Figure 29–15 A possible explanation for increased ventilation perfusion mismatch during hypopneic breathing episodes in patients with chronic obstructive pulmonary disease (COPD). The closing volume (CV) is the volume at which small airway closure begins. In a normal individual, any drops in function residual capacity (FRC) during REM sleep result in tidal breathing above the closing volume. In COPD, the closing volume is elevated, and any drops in the FRC are associated with tidal breathing below the closing volume, resulting in ventilation perfusion mismatch. Although the average FRC may not be lower during REM sleep, periods of hypopneic shallow breathing are likely associated with lower end-expiratory lung volume. See Figure 29–13.

nocturnal oxygen (for sleep only) for patients with NOD who do not meet requirements for daytime oxygen if a sleeping SaO_2 ≤88% is documented for supplemental oxygen during sleep. Previously, the qualifying saturation had to be present for ≥5 minutes (need not be continuous).

Qualification can also occur if there is a greater than normal fall in oxygen during sleep (a decrease in PaO_2 >10 mm Hg or decrease in SaO_2 >5 %). One study found an improvement in sleep quality with supplemental oxygen,[58] and another did not.[59] Both studies evaluated a relatively small number of patients, and this question remains to be answered (Table 29–3). A randomized trial of supplemental oxygen in patients with isolated NOD (daytime PaO_2 >60 mm Hg) did not find a survival benefit (although there were only a small number of deaths), but nocturnal oxygen did improve the pulmonary artery pressure.[60] Chaouat and coworkers[61] also performed a randomized trial of nocturnal oxygen in a similar patient group. They found no benefit of oxygen treatment with respect to mortality, the pulmonary artery pressure, or the subsequent need for daytime oxygen. The INOX study[62] was a multicenter randomized controlled trial to determine if supplemental oxygen in patients with COPD with only nocturnal desaturation was of benefit. Unfortunately, the study was stopped due to low recruitment and was underpowered. However, based on the available data, there was no indication of benefit. As noted, studies have not found evidence that patients with a worse NOD than expected based on daytime gas exchange had a worse prognosis[48,49] and have argued against the use of routine sleep studies or nocturnal oximetry in patients with COPD. On the other hand, nocturnal oximetry is indicated if the patient complains of nocturnal symptoms or symptoms of OSA or has evidence of cor pulmonale. The results of oximetry may suggest the presence of OSA (saw-tooth oximetry pattern) and the need for PSG. In summary, the benefit of treating *isolated* NOD (daytime PaO_2 >60 mm Hg) is unproven. However, many clinicians would treat patients who have a nocturnal SaO_2 less than 88% for a substantial period of time, especially if there was evidence of cor pulmonale. Of interest, *treatment with bronchodilators can improve nocturnal oxygenation in some patients*. In the NOTT trial,[51] 21% of individuals initially qualifying for the study were excluded when oxygenation improved after a period of intense bronchodilator treatment and they no longer met inclusion criteria (a standard part of the protocol).

In acute respiratory failure, administration of high-flow oxygen can significantly worsen hypercapnia, but low-flow supplemental oxygen produces only mild to moderate increases in nocturnal $PaCO_2$ during sleep in stable patients with COPD. Goldstein and coworkers[20] studied a group of 15 stable patients with severe COPD and both hypoxemia and hypercapnia during wakefulness. One night the patient breathed room air, and one night supplemental oxygen was added at 1 to 2 lpm, sufficient to bring the SaO_2 during sleep to ≥90%. Transcutaneous PCO_2 was measured and increased about 4 mm Hg from wakefulness to sleep (highest during REM sleep) while breathing room air. The administration of supplemental oxygen increased the PCO_2 about 6 mm Hg during sleep when compared to room air. However, three patients with both COPD and OSA (the overlap syndrome) had a much larger increase in PCO_2 on oxygen. For example, in one patient, the sleeping PCO_2 increased from about 60 mm Hg to 85 to 90 mm Hg. In both room air and oxygen breathing conditions, the PCO_2 during REM sleep was about 3 to 4 mm Hg higher than during NREM sleep. A schematic illustrating the findings of the study is shown in Figure 29–16.[20] Another study found that increasing the nocturnal oxygen flow rate by even 1 LPM resulted in a lower pH and higher $PaCO_2$ in the morning.[63] It seems prudent to use the lowest oxygen flow required to maintain adequate nocturnal oxygenation, especially in hypercapnic patients.

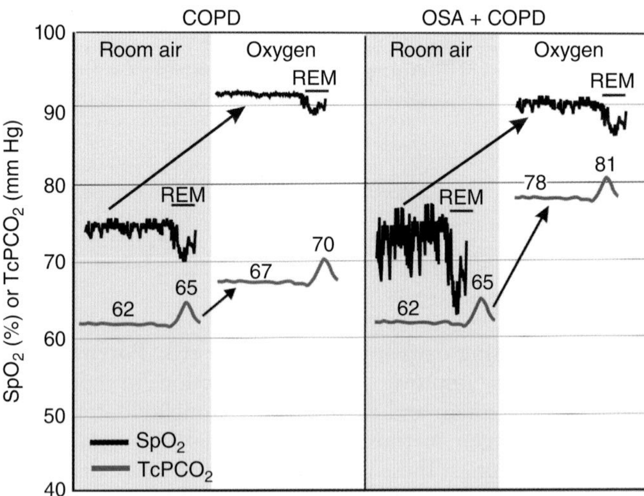

Figure 29–16 Schematic showing nocturnal oximetry (SpO_2) and transcutaneous PCO_2 monitoring ($TcPCO_2$) in a patient with chronic obstructive pulmonary disease (COPD) on the left and one with COPD + obstructive sleep apnea (OSA) on the right. Supplemental oxygen improves but does not completely eliminate oxygen desaturation. In the patient with COPD, the increase in the transcutaneous PCO_2 with the addition of supplemental oxygen is modest. In the patient with COPD and OSA, the increase in the transcutaneous PCO_2 is much larger. (Schematic based on Goldstein RS, Ramcharan V, Bowes G, et al. Effect of supplemental nocturnal oxygen on gas exchange in patients with severe obstructive lung disease. *N Engl J Med*. 1984;310:425-429. PMID: 6420700.)

Bronchodilators

With the exception of smoking cessation and 24-hour LTOT in qualifying patients, no treatment has been shown to reduce the decline in lung function or improve mortality in patients with COPD. However, bronchodilator therapy can provide symptomatic improvement, reduce the number of exacerbations, and improve exercise capacity. Treatment with bronchodilators, especially long-acting inhaled bronchodilators, does improve nocturnal oxygenation in patients with COPD.[64-70] However, only a few studies of the effects of bronchodilators on sleep have not shown objective improvement in **sleep quality**.[65,68,69] Conversely, sleep quality was not worsened, and subjective sleep quality improved in some patients. One study compared the combination of sustained-action theophylline and a short-acting inhaled beta-agonist bronchodilator at bedtime versus a short-acting inhaled bronchodilator + placebo.[64] The addition of theophylline did not worsen sleep quality but improved the morning FEV_1 and SaO_2 during NREM sleep. Martin and associates[65] found that inhaled ipratropium bromide (a short-acting anticholinergic) given by nebulizer improved subjective sleep quality, NOD, and the amount of REM sleep. This study used 4 nights of sleep monitoring, allowing patients to acclimate to the monitoring equipment. McNicholas and coworkers[66] found that tiotropium (a long-acting inhaled anticholinergic bronchodilator) given either in the morning or in the evening improved the SaO_2 during REM sleep compared with placebo but did not improve objective sleep quality. Ryan and colleagues[67] found that salmeterol, a long-acting inhaled beta agonist, improved nocturnal oxygenation without impairing sleep quality. Donahue and associates[68] compared fluticasone propionate/salmeterol with ipratropium bromide/albuterol during an 8-week period. Both fluticasone propionate/salmeterol and ipratropium bromide/albuterol improved lung function and symptoms and reduced supplemental albuterol use compared with baseline. Fluticasone propionate/salmeterol was more effective than ipratropium bromide/albuterol for improvement in morning pre-dose FEV_1, daytime symptom score, nighttime awakenings, sleep symptoms, and albuterol-free nights ($p \leq 0.013$). These results are not surprising given the shorter duration of activity with ipratropium. Bouloukaki et al.[69] compared the effects of tiotropium applied via the Respimat soft mist inhaler and HandiHaler in a group with COPD. Medication increased total sleep time and the amount of REM sleep as well as the time spent with a $SaO_2 \leq 90\%$. However, there was no placebo control arm, and sleep may have improved on the second night due to first-night effects of monitoring. There was a small advantage with the Respimat versus HandiHaler. Krachman and coworkers[70] evaluated the change in lung function, sleep quality, and oxygenation from baseline to treatment with tiotropium-placebo versus triple treatment with Budesonide-Formoterol-Tiotropium. Only the triple treatment improved the FEV_1, but *neither treatment* improved sleep quality or oxygenation. However, sleep quality was not worsened by either treatment. In summary, long-acting bronchodilator therapy improves morning spirometry and oxygenation (some studies) overnight without consistent improvement in sleep quality. The sleep of individual patients complaining of nocturnal cough or dyspnea may improve from bronchodilator treatment at night.

A detailed discussion of bronchodilator treatment of COPD is beyond the scope of this chapter. Table 29–4 lists some commonly used bronchodilators. A simplified graphic of a treatment approach in stable patients (Figure 29–17) is presented

Table 29–4 Bronchodilator Treatment: Overview of Bronchodilator Options

Terminology	Abbreviation	Examples and FDA approved indications
Short-acting beta agonist	SABA	Albuterol
Long-acting beta agonist	LABA	Formoterol (bid) Perforomist (nebulization) – COPD Salmeterol (bid) Serevent Diskus – asthma and COPD Olodaterol (qd) (Striverdi Respimat) – COPD Vilanterol – not available as single agent in USA
Short-acting muscarinic agonist	SAMA	Ipratropium
Long-acting muscarinic agonist	LAMA	Tiotropium (Spiriva) (Spiriva Respimat – asthma and COPD, Spiriva HandiHaler – COPD) Aclidinium (Tudorza Pressair) – COPD Glycopyrrolate (Lonhala Magnair, solution and nebulizer) – COPD Umeclidinium (Incruse Ellipta) – COPD
Combinations		
	ICS+LABA+ LAMA	beclomethasone/formoterol/glycopyrronium, (Trimbow) – COPD fluticasone /vilanterol/umeclidinium (Trelegy Ellipta) – asthma, COPD budesonide/formoterol/glycopyrrolate (Breztri Aerosphere) – asthma
	LAMA + LABA	Tiotropium-olodaterol (Stiolto Respimat) – COPD
	ICS + LABA	Budesonide-formoterol (Symbicort) – asthma and COPD Fluticasone-Salmeterol (Advair) – Asthma and COPD Mometasone-Formoterol (Dulera) – Asthma Fluticasone – vilanterol (Breo Ellipta) – COPD
	SABA + SAMA	Albuterol-Ipratropium (Combivent Respimat)

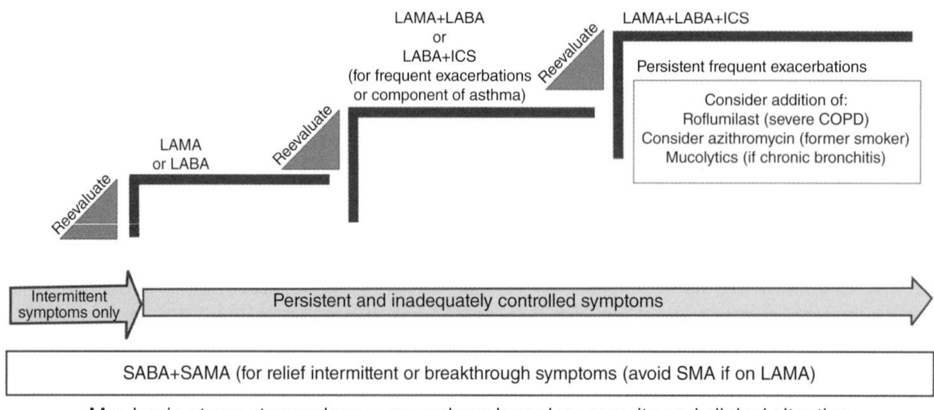

Figure 29–17 A step approach to treatment of chronic obstructive pulmonary disease (COPD). *LABA*, long-acting beta agonist; *LAMA*, long-acting muscarinic agonist; *SABA*, short-acting beta agonist; *SAMA*, short-acting muscarinic agonist. (Adapted from Mirza S, Clay RD, Koslow MA, Scanlon PD. COPD guidelines: a review of the 2018 GOLD report. *Mayo Clin Proc.* 2018;93(10):1488-1502. PMID: 30286833.)

(treatment of exacerbations will not be addressed).[7,9] Short-acting beta2 agonists (SABAs; for example, albuterol) or a short-acting muscarinic agonists (SAMAs; for example, ipratropium) are used for patients with intermittent symptoms or as treatment of breakthrough symptoms in patients on long-acting medications. A SAMA should not be used if a patient is on a long-acting muscarinic agonist (LAMA). For persistent or inadequately controlled symptoms, a step approach can be used. Step 1 would be a long-acting beta2 agonist (LABA; for example, formoterol) or an LAMA (for example, tiotropium). Step 2 would include using a LAMA+ LABA (two different inhalers or a single combined formulation) or combination of an LABA and an inhaled corticosteroid (LABA+ICS). In general, use of an ICS is recommended only for patients with a significant asthmatic component, higher eosinophil levels, and frequent exacerbations. Continued use of an ICS is NOT recommended if the addition of an ICS does not provide improvement or if frequent bouts of pneumonia are noted. Step 3 would be use of "triple therapy" with LABA+LAMA+ICS. A few triple medication inhalers exist. The addition of roflumilast (a PDE4 inhibitor that reduces intracellular inflammation by inhibiting the breakdown of cyclic AMP, no bronchodilator action) for patients with severe airflow limitation/chronic bronchitis/frequent exacerbations is another option. The addition of a mucolytic could be considered for patients with chronic/bronchitis/frequent exacerbation. Azithromycin (a macrolide antibiotic) could be added for former smokers or those older than 65 years with frequent exacerbations). The use of inhaled corticosteroids does not improve mortality, but in some studies it improved the quality of life, reduced exacerbations, and improved lung function when added to a long-acting bronchodilator. Based on the previously mentioned studies, most clinicians would use a long-acting anticholinergic or long-acting beta2 agonist (or both) in patients with significant COPD who complain of nocturnal dyspnea, cough, or poor sleep quality. Inhaled corticosteroids are also a reasonable addition, especially if the patient has repeated COPD exacerbations, a significant component of bronchospasm, a high blood eosinophil count, or does not respond to other treatments. However, if the addition of an ICS does not improve COPD manifestations, the ICS should be stopped, given the side effects. The GOLD guidelines[9] have recommendations for initial treatment based on the ABE classification. LABA+LAMA is recommended for group E ($\geq$2 moderate exacerbation or $\geq$1 leading to hospitalization). Addition of an ICS could be considered if the blood eosinophil count is increased (>300 cells/μL). For Group B (0 to 1 moderate exacerbation [not leading to hospitalization] and more severe symptoms), use of a LABA+LAMA is also suggested. For group A (same exacerbations as B but less severe symptoms), a bronchodilator is recommended. Options could include an as-needed SABA, SAMA, LAMA, or LABA. Further guidelines for addressing dyspnea and exacerbations are also presented. The reader should consult the most recent GOLD guidelines for additional information.

Treatment of Insomnia in COPD – Hypnotics and Cognitive Behavioral Treatment of Insomnia

Nighttime cough, dyspnea, and insomnia are frequent complaints in patients with COPD.[18,19,50] In general, patients with COPD have a decreased total sleep time and amount of REM sleep compared to normal individuals of the same age. A number of interventions have been proposed, including bronchodilators, hypnotics, and supplemental oxygen. Treatment of nocturnal cough and dyspnea is a recommended intervention that might improve sleep quality. As discussed, studies have documented improvement in airflow and gas exchange with bronchodilators, but improvement in sleep quality has been demonstrated in only a few studies. Hypnotics have been used with some caution in patients with COPD. In general, in non-hypercapnic patients, clinically significant worsening of gas exchange does not occur with benzodiazepine receptor agonists,[71] although benzodiazepine receptor agonist (BZRA) use is a risk factor for respiratory failure.[72] The non-benzodiazepine BZRAs including zolpidem, zaleplon, and eszopiclone are believed to be safer than traditional benzodiazepine BZRAs. Girault and coworkers[73] studied 10 patients with severe COPD before and after 10 days of zolpidem 10 mg and could find no worsening in performance or gas exchange. Of interest, the only objective improvement in sleep was an increase in stage N2 sleep. Subjective sleep quality was also improved (not placebo-controlled). Another study found no detrimental effects from temazepam 10 mg (a dose lower than typically used).[74] Steens and colleagues[75] studied the effects of zolpidem and triazolam in mild to moderate COPD. Total sleep time was increased as well as sleep efficiency without an adverse effect on gas exchange.[75] This was a single dose, randomized cross-over, double-blind, and placebo-controlled study. A double-blind, placebo-controlled crossover study of patients with moderate to severe COPD evaluated the effects of 8 mg of ramelteon, a melatonin receptor agonist with no respiratory depressant properties. This study found no worsening of nocturnal gas exchange.[76] However, there was an improvement in total sleep time, sleep efficiency, and the latency to persistent sleep on ramelteon compared to those on placebo. This medication has a short duration of action and is generally used for sleep-onset insomnia. However, the duration of action may vary among individuals. A meta-analysis of hypnotics in COPD[77] was limited by the small number of published studies but concluded that BZRAs improved objective sleep and did not decrease oxygenation. However, there was evidence of an increase in the maximum nocturnal transcutaneous PCO_2 in one study. In summary, the BZRAs are probably safe in non-hypercapnic non-hypoxemic patients. Use of a non-benzodiazepine BZRA is preferred. However, caution is still required. Ramelteon is a safe hypnotic (a melatonin receptor agonist) that may be effective in some patients with COPD. The drug is most effective for sleep-onset insomnia. A study of suvorexant[78] (dual hypocretin receptor antagonist [DORA]) using a randomized, placebo-controlled, double-blind format found no adverse effects on breathing in a group of patients with mild to moderate COPD (a history of insomnia not required). There was no significant change in the SpO_2 for total sleep time or apnea-hypopnea index (AHI) on suvorexant compared to those on placebo, but there was an increase in total sleep time and the amount of REM sleep. The authors concluded that the data do not suggest an overt respiratory depressant effect with 30 to 40 mg daily doses of suvorexant, up to twice the maximum dose recommended for treatment of insomnia in the United States. A study found that daridorexant (another DORA) improved objective sleep parameters (i.e., prolonged total sleep time, increased sleep efficiency, and decreased wakefulness after sleep onset), reached expected plasma concentrations, and was safe and well tolerated in a group with moderate COPD.[79] This medication (brand name Quviviq) was recently approved by the U.S. Food and Drug Administration (FDA) for treatment of insomnia. DORAs may prove useful for treatment of insomnia in COPD, but they are relatively expensive. Many clinicians use sedating antidepressants as hypnotics (e.g., trazodone), believing this treatment option is safer. However, a benefit of the use of sedating antidepressants to improve sleep quality in COPD patients has never been documented.

As noted, data on the ability of supplemental oxygen to improve sleep quality are conflicting. Some patients who meet criteria for supplemental oxygen do report improvement in sleep. Cognitive behavioral treatment of insomnia is felt to be the treatment of choice for both primary insomnia and insomnia comorbid with mental and medical disorders. Limited data suggest this approach may work in patients with COPD.[80,81]

Nocturnal Noninvasive Ventilation (NIV) for Patients With COPD and Chronic Hypercapnia

One can divide patients with COPD into 3 groups with respect to hypoventilation, although there may be some overlap between the groups. Group 1 comprises COPD patients without OSA who may develop hypoventilation during a COPD exacerbation but otherwise have a normal awake $PaCO_2$. They can be treated with bronchodilators and oxygen if needed. Group 2 consists of patients with the overlap syndrome who may exhibit mild to moderate daytime hypoventilation when stable that may improve with CPAP treatment of the OSA. They usually have mild to moderate COPD. Optimal treatment includes interventions for both OSA (CPAP) and COPD. Group 3 consists of patients with moderate to severe COPD who manifest significant daytime and nocturnal hypercapnia even when clinically stable (daytime $PaCO_2$ 50 to 60 mmHg). Severe COPD rather than OSA is the main etiology of the hypercapnia in these patients. The presence of daytime hypercapnia is associated with increased hospital admissions and mortality. NIV can improve the outcomes in the group 3 patients.

For patients with COPD who present to the hospital with acute hypercapnic respiratory failure, noninvasive ventilation (NIV), also known as noninvasive positive-pressure ventilation (NPPV), has proven to be an effective treatment, often avoiding the need for intubation and mechanical ventilation. NIV usually consists of bilevel positive airway pressure (BPAP) with a backup rate using sufficient pressure support to augment ventilation. Should long-term NIV be used in stable patients with COPD and chronic daytime hypercapnia? COPD represents the third most common cause of hospital readmissions among Medicare beneficiaries (22.6%).[82,83] Thus, treatment to prevent readmissions is of great interest. A noted above, *chronic hypercapnia is a risk factor for mortality*. Patients with COPD most likely to benefit from chronic NIV are individuals with *substantial chronic daytime CO_2 retention* and NOD who are highly motivated. In 1999, a consensus conference recommended the following indications for NIV in patients with COPD[84]: (1) symptom criteria (e.g., fatigue, dyspnea, morning headache); (2) physiologic criteria daytime $PaCO_2$ >55 or 50 to 54 mm Hg with NOD; or (3) awake $PaCO_2$ 50 to 54 mm Hg with recurrent hospitalization related to episodes of hypercapnic respiratory failure. Patients with severe swallowing dysfunction or those who cannot protect their airway were thought not to be ideal candidates for NIV. However, considerable research evidence supporting use of NIV has been published since those recommendations. Both the European Respiratory Society and American Thoracic Society have published guidelines for treatment with long-term NIV for chronic hypercapnia in stable patients with COPD.[85,86] The results of studies of NIV in stable hypercapnic COPD are well outlined in the review by Coleman et al.[87] Early studies failed to show benefit. However, studies in Europe using high-intensity NIV (high inspiratory positive airway pressure [IPAP] >18 cm H_2O and use of a high mandatory backup rate [for example, 2 breaths/min below awake respiratory rate]) showed significant improvement in **daytime PCO_2** and reduced hospital readmissions. Struik et al.[88] randomized COPD patients with a prior admission for respiratory failure to NIV or standard care. The NIV group had improvements in gas exchange, but there was no difference in readmission rates. Köhnlein and coworkers[89] found that the addition of long-term NIV to standard treatment improved survival of patients with hypercapnic, stable COPD when *NIV was targeted to significantly reduce hypercapnia*. In this study, the mean IPAP was 21.6 cm H_2O, the mean expiratory PAP (EPAP) was 4.5 cm H_2O, and the mean backup rate was 16 breaths/min. *The goal was a 20% decrease in the $PaCO_2$ or a value less than 48 mm Hg*. Another study compared high-intensity ventilation (high pressure and high backup rate) and high pressure alone and found that the addition of a high backup rate did not improve outcomes.[90]

However, very high IPAP was used, and using a lower pressure support and a higher backup rate may be appropriate for some patients with pressure intolerance or intractable mask leak. Murphy and coworkers[91] randomized patients with persistent hypercapnia ($PaCO_2$ >53 mm Hg) at 2 to 4 weeks after resolution of respiratory acidemia to supplemental oxygen alone or supplemental oxygen and NIV. Patients underwent daytime *NIV acclimatization*, followed by nocturnal titration with oxygen entrained at the daytime prescription rate. The aim was to achieve control of nocturnal hypoventilation with a high-pressure ventilation strategy. *The median IPAP was 24 cm H_2O, the median EPAP was 4 cm H_2O,* and the median backup rate was 14 breaths/min. Median ventilator use was 4.7 hours per night at 6 months but increased to 7.6 hours at 12 months. The authors found that, among patients with persistent hypercapnia following an acute exacerbation of COPD, adding home NIV to home oxygen therapy prolonged the time to readmission or death within 12 months of follow-up. Dreher et al. found that high ventilatory support was actually better tolerated than low levels of support.[92] The American Thoracic Society recommendations for NIV in stable hypercapnic COPD[87] include: (1) nocturnal NIV in addition to usual care for patients with chronic stable hypercapnic COPD (conditional recommendation, moderate certainty); (2) patients with chronic stable hypercapnic COPD undergo screening for OSA before initiation of long-term NIV (conditional recommendation, very low certainty); (3) not *initiating* **long-term** NIV prior to discharge after an admission for acute-on-chronic hypercapnic respiratory failure, favoring instead reassessment for NIV at 2 to 4 weeks after resolution (conditional recommendation, low certainty); (4) not using an in-laboratory overnight PSG to titrate NIV in patients with chronic stable hypercapnic COPD who are initiating NIV (conditional recommendation, very low certainty); and (5) NIV with *targeted normalization of $PaCO_2$ in patients with hypercapnic COPD* on long-term NIV (conditional recommendation, low certainty). It is not necessary to initiate NIV in the sleep center, as it can be done in the clinic or at home. However, adequate facilities and skilled respiratory therapists are not available in many locales, and this expertise may only be available in sleep centers with experience with NIV. NIV titration during PSG[93] allows titration of EPAP (autoEPAP is not available in bilevel PAP [BPAP] devices with a backup rate in the United States [except in home ventilators]). Mask fitting and changes/interventions for mask leak are possible, and the patient can be allowed to adapt to pressure. It is not necessary to achieve the final settings on the initial titration. In addition, monitoring of transcutaneous PCO_2 and oxygenation can guide the titration and the amount of supplemental oxygen (if needed). The American Academy of Sleep Medicine guidelines suggest the sleep center for titration of NIV in chronic stable patients with hypoventilation.[93] BPAP devices used for hypoventilation and central sleep apnea are known as respiratory assist devices (RAD), and Medicare and other insurance providers have specific qualifications for reimbursement for these devices[94] (E0470 BPAP without a backup rate, E0471 with backup rate)

Table 29–5 CMS LCD 33800 Criteria for Coverage of a RAD Device for Severe Chronic Obstructive Pulmonary Disease (COPD)

An **E0470** device is covered if criteria A–C are met.

A. An arterial blood gas $PaCO_2$, done while awake and breathing the beneficiary's prescribed fraction of inspired oxygen (FIO_2), is greater than or equal to 52 mm Hg.
B. Sleep oximetry demonstrates oxygen saturation less than or equal to 88% for greater than or equal to a cumulative 5 minutes of nocturnal recording time (minimum recording time of 2 hours), done **while breathing oxygen at 2 LPM** or the beneficiary's prescribed FIO_2 (whichever is higher).
C. Prior to initiating therapy, sleep apnea and treatment with a continuous positive airway pressure (CPAP) device has been considered and ruled out. (Note: Formal sleep testing is not required if there is sufficient information in the medical record to demonstrate that the beneficiary does not suffer from some form of sleep apnea (obstructive sleep apnea [OSA], central sleep apnea [CSA] and/or complex sleep apnea [CompSA]) as the **predominant cause of awake hypercapnia** or nocturnal arterial oxygen desaturation.

If all of the above criteria for beneficiaries with COPD are met, an E0470 device will be covered for the first 3 months of therapy.

An **E0471** device will be covered for a beneficiary with COPD in either of the two situations below, depending on the testing performed to demonstrate the need.

Situation 1. For severe COPD beneficiaries who qualified for an E0470 device, an E0471 started **any time after a period of initial use of an E0470 device** is covered if **both** criteria A and B are met.

A. An arterial blood gas $PaCO_2$, done while awake and breathing the beneficiary's prescribed FIO_2, shows that the **beneficiary's $PaCO_2$ worsens greater than or equal to 7 mm Hg compared to the original result from criterion A,** (above).**
B. **Facility-based polysomnography (PSG)** demonstrates oxygen saturation less than or equal to 88% for greater than or equal to a cumulative 5 minutes of nocturnal recording time (minimum recording time of 2 hours) **while using an E0470 device that is not caused by obstructive upper airway events** – i.e., apnea-hypopnea index (AHI) less than 5 events/hour. (Refer to Positive Airway Pressure (PAP) Devices for the Treatment of Obstructive Sleep Apnea LCD for information about E0470 coverage for OSA).

Situation 2. For severe COPD beneficiaries who qualified for an E0470 device, an E0471 device will be covered if, **at a time no sooner than 61 days after initial issue of the E0470 device**, **both** of the following criteria A and B are met:

A. An arterial blood gas $PaCO_2$, done while awake and breathing the beneficiary's prescribed FIO_2, still remains greater than or equal to 52 mm Hg.
B. **Sleep oximetry** while breathing with the E0470 device demonstrates oxygen saturation less than or equal to 88% for greater than or equal to a cumulative 5 minutes of nocturnal recording time (minimum recording time of 2 hours), done while breathing oxygen at 2 LPM or the beneficiary's prescribed FIO_2 (whichever is higher).

**Criteria A in qualifying for E0470, E0470 BPAP, E0471 BPAP with a backup rate

From https://www.cms.gov/medicare-coverage-database/view/lcd.aspx?LCDId=33800 Accessed 8/24/022.

Box 29–2 KEY POINTS: OVERLAP SYNDROME (OLS)

- Coexistence of OSA and COPD defines the overlap syndrome
- Prevalence of OSA in COPD patients is the same as in the general population
- The presence of COPD predisposes patients with OSA to more severe arterial oxygen desaturation
- Hypercapnia may occur in patients with OLS with a less severe reduction in the FEV_1 than is typical for hypercapnia in patients with COPD alone.
- Optimal Treatment of OLS
  - PAP (CPAP or BPAP), BPAP may be better tolerated
  - Supplemental oxygen, if needed (low awake or baseline sleeping SpO_2 not responding to PAP)
  - Bronchodilator treatment and smoking cessation
- Treatment of OLS patients with nocturnal supplemental oxygen alone is not adequate treatment, may be associated with significant hypercapnia during sleep and worse outcomes
- An observational study found that CPAP treatment was associated with higher survival in patients with moderate to severe OSA and hypoxemic COPD on long term oxygen treatment (LTOT) compared to a a similar group who did not use CPAP.*
- An observational study found that OLS patients not on CPAP had greater all cause mortality and a higher risk of hospitalization for a COPD exacerbation compared to OLS patients on CPAP.**

OSA, obstructive sleep apnea; *COPD*, chronic obstructive pulmonary disease; *OLS*, overlap syndrome; *FEV_1*, forced expiratory volume in 1 second; *PAP*, positive airway pressure, *CPAP*, continuous PAP; *BPAP*, bilevel PAP.

* Machado MCL, Vollmer WM, Togeiro SM, et al. CPAP and survival in moderate to severe obstructive sleep apnea syndrome and hypoxemic COPD. *Eur Respir J.* 2010;35:132-137.

** Marin JM, Soriano JB, Carrizo SJ, et al. Outcomes in patients with chronic obstructive pulmonary disease and obstructive sleep apnea. *Am J Respir Crit Care Med.* 2010;182:325-331.

(Table 29–5). There are four categories of RAD qualifications, and the pertinent one is labeled *"severe COPD" (although no spirometry criteria* are listed and spirometry is not required, see Table 29–5). The ordering physician would need to state that COPD rather than OSA is the predominant cause of the awake hypercapnia or nocturnal arterial oxygen desaturation. Note that oximetry *and not formal sleep testing* is required.

While most experts recommend a BPAP device with a backup rate for treatment of hypoventilation in patients with COPD, the Medicare RAD criteria make it difficult to obtain such a device initially[94] (Table 29-5). Rather than a RAD device, many clinicians have opted for a home ventilator (has a backup rate), which can be obtained under a diagnosis of chronic respiratory failure associated with COPD[94] with medical documentation supporting the need for the home ventilator (frequent admissions, need for battery backup). Thus, patients are discharged from the hospital on a home ventilator (and oxygen, if needed) after an acute or chronic episode of hypercapnic respiratory failure. Studies suggest that the optimal time to start outpatient NIV is not at discharge following hospitalization for hypercapnic respiratory failure, but several weeks after discharge when the patient has stabilized. This allows targeting of patients with stable chronic hypercapnia who are more likely to tolerate and adhere to treatment. Home ventilators are more expensive than RAD BPAP devicesdevices. Both a RAD E0471 BPAP device and a HMV can provide BPAP with a backup rate. Treatment with the RAD device will suffice for many individuals. However, use of a E0470 device is required before the patient can qualify for a device with a backup rate (E0471).[94] The difficulty qualifying patients with hypercapnic COPD for the correct device has been outlined in a publication with recommendations for changing the existing RAD criteria.[95] See Chapter 24 for more discussion about home ventilators and the use of RAD devices to treat patients with COPD and chronic hypoventilation. If NIV is used, studies suggest aggressive treatment with a goal of significantly improving (or normalizing) the nocturnal $PaCO_2$. However, many patients initially need lower pressure for adaptation. Detailed information regarding NIV treatment of the severe COPD group with chronic hypoventilation is provided in chapter 24. Of interest a low level of EPAP 4–6 cm H_2O is typically sufficient but a high level of IPAP is needed to provide the pressure support of 15 to 20 cm H_2O necessary to normalize or significantly improve hypercapnia. If OSA is also present higher EPAP may be needed.

OVERLAP SYNDROME

The Overlap Syndrome (OLS) consists of patients with both OSA and COPD (Box 29–2). One study found that OSA is no more frequent in COPD patients than in the general population.[47] That is, the prevalence of OSA in patients with COPD is the same as in the general population. However, because both are common, the combination is also fairly common. The two groups of patients with OSA with daytime hypercapnia include patients with the obesity hypoventilation syndrome and some patients with OLS.[96-101] Patients with OLS tend to have severe NOD, even if they do not have daytime hypercapnia. Usually, patients with COPD become hypercapnic when the FEV_1 is around 1.0 L (or 40% of predicted). Patients with OLS can be hypercapnic with milder reductions in the FEV_1 (Table 29–6). For example, Resta et al.[102] found a group of patients with COPD had an awake mean $PaCO_2$ of 40 mm Hg with a mean FEV_1 of 47% of predicted, while a group with OLS had a mean $PaCO_2$ of 45 mm Hg with a mean FEV_1 of 63% of predicted. However, patients with OLS can also maintain a normal daytime PCO_2, even when their FEV_1 is quite reduced.[101] Of interest, the OLS group compared to a pure OSA group had a higher $PaCO_2$ and greater time with a $SaO_2 \leq 88\%$ although the AHI was similar in the two groups (Table 29–6). In clinical practice, one often treats patients with a combination of COPD, OSA, and severe obesity who have significant hypoventilation. It is difficult to know how to label them because they likely have components of both the obesity hypoventilation syndrome and OLS. The amount of CO_2 retention in patients with OLS does **not** necessarily correlate with the AHI. One study comparing hypercapnic and non-hypercapnic patients with OLS found *no difference in the FEV1 and AHI between the two groups.*[101] The hypercapnic

Table 29–6 Characteristics of COPD, Overlap Syndrome, and OSA Only

	Groups			Comparisons	
	COPD Group (n = 32)	Overlap Group (n = 29)	Pure OSA Group (n = 152)	COPD vs. Overlap Group	Overlap Group vs. Pure OSA
Age (y)	60.1 (10.4)	57.2 (9.5)	48.9 (12.9)	NS	$P < 0.01$
Weight (kg)	87.6 (17.5)	**102.2** (20.6)	106.8 (28.8)	NS	NS
BMI (kg/m^2)	31 (7)	**36 (6)**	39 (10)	$P < 0.05$	NS
FVC (% predicted)	60 (19)	**72 (17)**	87 (20)	$P < 0.05$	*
FEV1 (% predicted)	47 (16)	**63 (16)**	89 (20)	$P < 0.005$	*
FEV1/FVC (%)	59 (9)	67(5)	87 (9)	$P < 0.005$	*
PaO_2 (mm Hg)	69 (10.4)	70 (11)	79 (12)	NS	$P<0.01$
PCO_2 (mm Hg)	40 (5)	**45 (5)**	39 (4)	$P < 0.005$	$P<0.01$
AHI (events/h)	6.1 (5)	40 (20)	42 (23)	$P < 0.005$	NS
% Time SpO_2 <90%	16 (28)	**48 (28)**	30(28)	$P < 0.001$	$P < 0.05$

*no statistical comparison as by definition pure OSA group has normal pulmonary function; *NS*, not significant. Data from reference[102]
Data are means (standard deviation); overlap is OSA + COPD.
COPD, chronic obstructive pulmonary disease; *OSA*, obstructive sleep apnea; *BMI*, body mass index; *FVC*, forced vital capacity; *FEV_1*, forced expiratory volume in 1 second; *AHI*, apnea-hypopnea index.
Resta O, Foschino Barbaro MP, Brindicci C, et al. Hypercapnia in overlap syndrome: possible determinant factors. *Sleep Breath.* 2002;6(1):11-18 PMID: 11917259.

group was heavier and had a history of heavy ethanol use. The authors hypothesized that the hypercapnic patients had depressed respiratory drives possibly secondary to the effects of alcohol. As effective treatment of OSA in patients with OLS can result in a reduction of daytime PCO_2, nocturnal CO_2 retention secondary to untreated apnea probably contributes to the development of daytime hypercapnia in patients with OLS.

TREATMENT OF OVERLAP SYNDROME

As discussed, treatment of patients with OLS with supplemental oxygen **alone** can result in significant increases in nocturnal $PaCO_2$.[20] Alford and colleagues[103] administered 4 LPM supplemental oxygen to 20 men with both OSA and COPD. While nocturnal oxygenation improved, the duration of obstructive events increased from 25.7 seconds to 31.4 seconds, resulting in an end-apneic PCO_2 increase from 52.8 mm Hg to 62.3 mm Hg, with corresponding decreases in pH. Fletcher and associates[104] followed patients with chronic lung disease and OSA, including a group treated with oxygen but no effective treatment for sleep apnea. They found that patients who did not have adequate treatment for OSA had no improvement in their pulmonary hemodynamics, whereas those who had effective treatment improved. One should recall that hypoxemia and acidosis result in pulmonary arterial vasoconstriction and pulmonary hypertension. This can lead to the development of in cor pulmonale.

An observational study by Machado and coworkers of patients with OSA and hypoxemic COPD receiving LTOT found that those who accepted and adhered to continuous PAP (CPAP) treatment in addition to oxygen had a better long-term survival (71% vs. 26%) than those who did not.[105] Another observational study by Marin et al.[106] of patients with OLS (including patients who did or did not use CPAP) found an increased risk of death and hospitalization due to COPD exacerbations in those not treated with CPAP. CPAP treatment was associated with improved survival and decreased hospitalizations (Figure 29–18). The amount of CPAP adherence needed for improved outcomes is unknown. Stanchina et al.[107] performed a post-hoc analysis of 10,272 patients identified from an outpatient database. Of these, 227 patients were identified as having OLS. Multivariant analysis revealed that greater time on CPAP was associated with reduced mortality; although age did not correlate with CPAP use ($p = 0.2$), the mean age of those with CPAP use <2 hours per night was significantly higher than that of those using CPAP >2 hours per night. Another study of adults suspected of having OSA in addition to COPD found the co-occurrence of nocturnal hypoxemia and COPD was associated with an increased hazard of cardiovascular events and mortality with a synergistic effect found only in women. This study suggests the worsening of hypoxemia by the addition of COPD to OSA rather than the AHI itself is the reason the co-occurrence of OSA and COPD caries a higher risk.[108]

The optimal treatment for patients with OLS includes treatment of COPD (smoking cessation and bronchodilators)

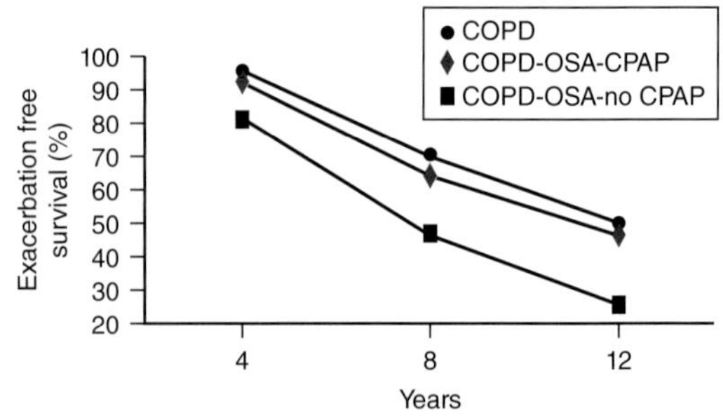

Figure 29–18 Data points from Kaplan Meier survival curves of exacerbation-free survival among patients with chronic obstructive pulmonary disease (COPD) without OSA, COPD with OSA on CPAP, and COPD with OSA not on CPAP. The curves from COPD only and COPD with OSA treated with CPAP differ significantly from those from COPD and untreated OSA ($P < 0.001$). (Figure plotted using data from Marin JM, Soriano JB, Carrizo SJ, et al. Outcomes in patients with chronic obstructive pulmonary disease and obstructive sleep apnea. *Am J Respir Crit Care Med.* 2010;182:325-331.)

and OSA (CPAP or BPAP with supplemental oxygen, if needed).[109,110] If significant CO_2 retention is present, most clinicians would use BPAP. Some patients with COPD have difficulty exhaling on CPAP and may be more adherent to treatment with BPAP. Patients with OLS who have a low awake PaO_2 (and SaO_2) value will likely need both oxygen and PAP to prevent nocturnal oxygen desaturation. However, the PAP levels should be optimized, even if supplemental oxygen is used for chronic treatment. When the upper airway obstruction of patients with hypercapnic OLS is adequately treated, the daytime PCO_2 frequently improves. If there is persistent significant CO_2 retention after treatment of COPD and OSA, NIV treatment could be considered (see section on hypercapnic COPD). As previously discussed the optimal use of BPAP to deliver NIV requires a different approach than simply treating OSA. That is, studies suggest that aggressive use of high-pressure support using a backup rate with a goal of normalizing the PCO_2 may be the best approach. However, the treatment approach needs to be individualized.[86,110]

ASTHMA

The definition of asthma endorsed by the Global Initiative for Asthma (GINA)[111,112] is as follows: "Asthma is a heterogeneous disease, usually characterized by chronic airway inflammation. It is defined by the history of respiratory symptoms such as wheeze, shortness of breath, chest tightness, and cough that vary over time and in intensity, together with variable expiratory airflow limitation." Airflow limitation may later become persistent. Asthma is associated with airway hyperresponsiveness and airway inflammation, but these are not necessary or sufficient to make a diagnosis. The airflow limitation may or may not be reversible by inhaled bronchodilators or corticosteroids. The National Asthma Education and Prevention Program 2020 (NAEPP 2020) expert panel also published asthma severity classification and treatment recommendations.[113] Separate guidelines for management of severe asthma have also been published.[114] *The estimated prevalence of asthma across all ages is about 8%.*[115] Women, African Americans, and individuals with lower socioeconomic status are at increased risk for asthma.[115-122] Asthma severity is defined by both *the symptoms and the level of treatment needed to control* the disease. Nighttime asthma symptoms are one of the factors to consider in assessing asthma control.[110-115] Some important manifestations of nocturnal asthma are listed in Box 29–3. Braido et al.[121] surveyed a large group of asthmatics and found that 58% had impaired sleep quality. *After analyzing a number of factors, they found that asthma control was the best predictor of sleep quality and health-related quality of life.* Levin and coworkers[122] found an increased risk of significant nocturnal asthma in African Americans compared to patients of European descent.

Box 29–3 MANIFESTATIONS OF NOCTURNAL ASTHMA

- Morning drop in FEV_1 >15% (often 15–50%)
- Increased circadian variation in FEV_1
- Decreased response to bronchodilators during early morning
- Increased bronchial hyperresponsiveness to methacholine in early morning
- Nocturnal awakenings with symptoms of asthma (cough, dyspnea)
- Impaired sleep quality
- Presence of nocturnal asthma symptoms used to determine asthma severity

FEV_1, forced expiratory volume in 1 second.

Nocturnal asthma is usually defined as asthma occurring in patients with a 15–20% or greater drop in the peak flow (or FEV_1) between bedtime and morning awakening.[44,123,124] Even normal persons have a circadian variation in lung function with the best function around 4:00 PM and the worst at 4:00 AM (usually 5–10% drop at 4:00 AM). However, the variation is much greater in patients with asthma.[118,124,127] Asthmatic patients can experience a 20% to 50% drop in the FEV_1 from bedtime to morning ("morning dippers") (Figure 29–19). Of note, the same patient will see greater circadian variation in airflow during exacerbations or after antigen challenge.[125] The overnight drop in lung function is also associated with increased airway hyperresponsiveness, increasing airway inflammation, and a decreased response to inhaled bronchodilators.[126,127] Important considerations for the diagnosis and treatment of nocturnal asthma are listed in Box 22–4. Of note, *sleep has an important impact on nocturnal asthma independent of circadian factors.*

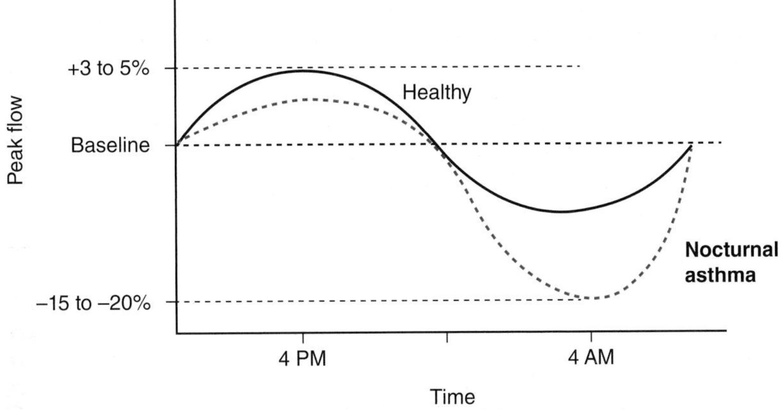

Figure 29–19 Both healthy individuals (*solid line*) and subjects with nocturnal asthma (*dotted line*) have circadian alterations in lung function with nadirs occurring at approximately 4:00 AM. The circadian variation in lung function is increased in subjects with nocturnal asthma and might exceed 20% over the course of the 24-hour period. (From Sutherland ER. Nocturnal asthma. *J Allergy Clin Immunol.* 2005;116:1179-1186.)

Epidemiology

Turner-Warwick[128] surveyed 7729 asthmatics to determine the prevalence of nocturnal asthma. According to the report, 74% revealed they woke up at least once each week with asthma symptoms and *65% woke up with symptoms at least three times per week*. In those who considered their asthma "mild," 26% woke up every night with symptoms of asthma. The majority of respiratory arrests or sudden death in asthmatic patients occurred from midnight to 8:00 AM.[129,130] Asthma control has two dimensions: (1) symptoms and (2) risk of future adverse events. *Poor asthma control is characterized by frequent symptoms or reliever inhaler use, activity limited by asthma, and night-waking due to asthma.*[116,123,131]

Etiology of Nocturnal Asthma

The etiology of the circadian variation in asthma severity is likely multifactorial with a number of proposed mechanisms (Box 29–4). These include circadian changes in the amounts of circulating steroids, catecholamines, and inflammatory mediators in the lungs, as well as a nocturnal increase in cholinergic tone associated with sleep.[132-137] Studies of infusions of epinephrine[134] or administration of high-dose steroids[135] were not able to eliminate the circadian variation in bronchomotor tone. The relative role of circadian rhythms and sleep in causing nocturnal worsening of asthma has been controversial. Sleep appears to have an adverse effect on asthma, independent of other factors. Clark et al. found a dip in peak flow during sleep **during the day** in shift workers moved to the daytime sleep period.[136] The *increase in parasympathetic activity* during sleep is associated within increased vagally mediated bronchoconstriction that can be improved with atropine.[137] Ballard and colleagues[45] found that sleep increased lower airway resistance by comparing nighttime changes between asthmatics and normal individuals who either slept in the supine position or were kept awake while supine. In asthmatics, there was a progressive increase in lower airway resistance over the night (in both wakefulness and sleep), but the increase in resistance was greater during sleep (Figure 29–20). This suggest sleep has an important adverse effect on airway function independent of circadian factors. In another study, Ballard and associates[27] found that, despite elevated lung volumes during wakefulness, the FRC of asthmatics had a larger than normal drop during sleep, with the lowest levels during REM sleep. The FRC was lower during REM sleep than that during NREM sleep (Figure 29–7). Lower lung volume tends to increase lower airway resistance.

Box 29–4 POSSIBLE CAUSES OF CIRCADIAN VARIATION IN ASTHMA

- Increased nocturnal parasympathetic (vagal) tone
- Decreased circulating cortisol and epinephrine
- Influx of inflammatory cells into the lung
- Nocturnal gastroesophageal reflux
- Allergen exposure (bed mites, dust)
- Obstructive sleep apnea (snoring)
- Adverse effect of sleep (controlling for time of day and body position)

Airway Inflammation and Response to Steroids or Beta2 Agonists

Kraft and coworkers[138] found the biopsy of the small airway at 4:00 AM showed differences in the number of eosinophils per unit volume in asthmatics with nocturnal asthma compared with patients with non-nocturnal asthma. No differences in eosinophils were found in the large airways. In patients with nocturnal asthma, there were more alveolar eosinophils at 4:00 AM than at 4:00 PM. A later study by the same group[139] found that CD4+ lymphocytes (important for eosinophil recruitment) were increased in alveolar tissue at night in patients with nocturnal asthma but not in asthmatic patients without nocturnal asthma. Kelly and colleagues[140] investigated circadian changes in airway inflammation in patients with mild atopic asthma (mean FEV_1 93% of predicted). In this patient population, bronchoalveolar lavage (BAL) fluid contained increased numbers of macrophages, neutrophils, and CD4+ T lymphocytes at 4:00 AM versus 4:00 PM. In addition, the percentage of CD4+ T lymphocytes in the 4:00 AM lavage fluid was inversely correlated with the 4:00 AM FEV_1. Kraft et al. found that nocturnal asthma was associated with reduced glucocorticoid receptor binding affinity and decreased steroid responsiveness at night.[141]

Szefler and coworkers found that a significant change in beta-adrenergic receptor density and function occured at night in patients with nocturnal asthma. Only patients with nocturnal asthma had a significant 33% decrease in mononuclear and polymorphonuclear leukocyte beta-adrenergic

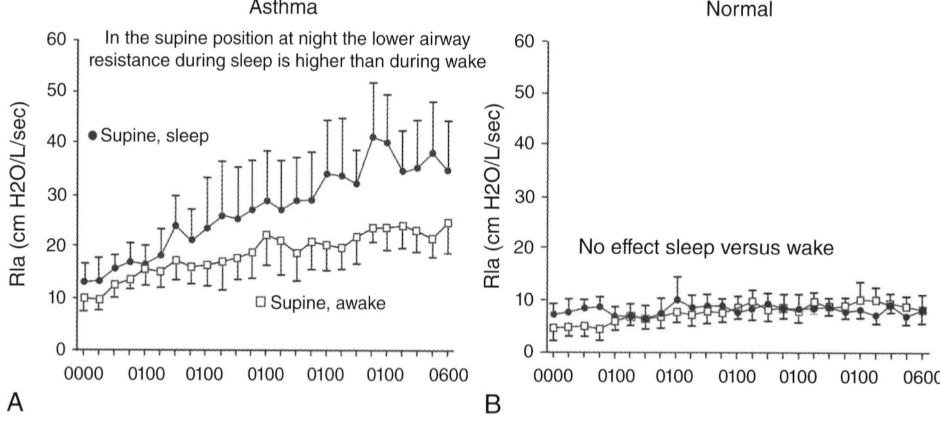

Figure 29–20 A, Lower airway resistance (R_{la}) increased overnight during supine wakefulness and supine sleep in asthmatics. However, during sleep, the increase was greater. B, In normal subjects, there was minimal change overnight and no difference between wakefulness and sleep. (From Ballard RD, Saathoff MC, Patel DK, et al. Effect of sleep on nocturnal bronchoconstriction and ventilatory patterns in asthmatics. *J Appl Physiol.* 1989;67:243-249.)

receptor density, with no difference in binding (compared to controls and asthmatics without nocturnal asthma).[142]

Melatonin

Melatonin, a hormone secreted by the pineal gland at night (in darkness), has proinflammatory effects. The addition of melatonin to zymosan stimulation of peripheral blood monocytes increased the production of interleukin-1 (IL-1), IL-6, and tumor necrosis factor-alpha (TNF-alpha) when compared with zymosan stimulation alone in normal controls and asthmatic patients.[143,3] The cytokine production was higher in patients with asthma than in normal subjects. Another study found that melatonin levels were higher in patients with nocturnal asthma than in both asthmatic patients without nocturnal asthma and healthy controls.[144] In subjects with nocturnal asthma, there was an inverse correlation between melatonin level and overnight decrease in lung function. The clinical importance of the effects of melatonin on asthma remains to be determined.

Factors Worsening Nocturnal Asthma

Allergens in the Bedroom

The importance of allergens in the bedroom is still under evaluation. Woodcock and associates[145] were not able to find a benefit from having patients use allergen-impermeable bed covers. It still seems prudent to minimize exposure to allergens, if possible. Reduction in allergen exposure is still a component of many treatment programs.

Gastroesophageal Reflux

Several studies have supported the idea that gastroesophageal reflux (GER) may worsen asthma. Studies have shown that GER, as defined by abnormal esophageal pH monitoring, can occur in 62% of patients without GER symptoms.[146] Harding and coworkers[147] treated 22 patients with both asthma and GER (documented by 24-hour pH monitoring) for 3 months, with doses of omeprazole documented to normalize 24-hour pH monitoring. Seventy-three percent of the patients had improvement in either asthma symptoms (67%) or peak expiratory flow (20%). Cuttitta and colleagues[148] investigated the relationship between reduced esophageal pH (evidence of GER) and lower airway resistance. The most important predictor of an increase in lower airway resistance was the duration of esophageal acid contact. However, studies have not conclusively shown that treatment of GER will improve asthma. A systematic review published in 2001 concluded that treatment of GER does not improve asthma.[149] A parallel-group, randomized, double-blind study of esomeprazole for treatment of poorly controlled asthma (patients did not complain of GER) found no difference in episodes of asthma exacerbations between placebo and esomeprazole groups.[150] GER was found in 40% of patients using pH monitoring (asymptomatic). No subgroup of patients could be identified in which treatment of GER improved asthma. The investigators concluded that GER is unlikely to be a major factor in uncontrolled asthma. However, this group of patients *did not have GER symptoms*. A randomized trial studying the effects of esomeprazole once or twice daily on asthma found only a small improvement in pulmonary function and symptoms, but the improvement was thought to be clinically insignificant.[151] The current recommendation is to treat asthmatic patients with GER symptoms (for improvement of GER symptoms) but with the realization that this may help asthma in individual patients. However, there is no evidence that treatment of GER in patients with intractable asthma without symptomatic GER is of benefit.

Asthma Overlap (Asthma + OSA)/Obesity

If OSA is present in a patient with asthma, this is considered a type of OLS.[98,152] However, more commonly the term *asthma overlap* is used for the combination of asthma and COPD. OSA appears to be more common in asthmatics than in non-asthmatics. A study by Julien et al. showed OSA was significantly more prevalent among patients with severe asthma than in those with moderate asthma and more prevalent in both asthma groups than in controls without asthma.[153] These observations suggest potential pathophysiologic interactions between OSA-hypopnea and asthma severity and control. Treatment with nasal CPAP in patients with OSA and asthma can improve the comorbid asthma. A number of observational studies have been performed, but many lacked a control group or objective assessment of CPAP use. Chan and associates[154] treated patients with both OSA and asthma and found that the peak expiratory flow rate improved in the morning and night after 2 weeks of treatment. Serrano-Pariente studied the effect of CPAP treatment in patients with asthma and moderate to severe OSA over a 6 month period. CPAP improved asthma control and quality of life.[155] The biggest improvement was in those with the *moderate to severe asthma and severe OSA*. Kauppi and coworkers[156] used questionnaires to determine the impact of CPAP on asthma and found evidence of improved asthma control. On the other hand, Ng et al.[157] randomized patients with asthma and OSA to 3 months of CPAP or a control group. Asthma control based on symptom assessment did not improve. However, the AHI was in the moderate range. The benefit from CPAP treatment may be confined to those with asthma and severe OSA. More studies on this topic are needed. Treatment of asthma can also affect OSA. For example, weight gain associated with oral corticosteroids can worsen OSA. A study of **inhaled** fluticasone[158] in a group of mildly asthmatic individuals never treated with inhaled steroids found an improvement in the critical pressure for upper airway closure (P_{crit}, more negative) in most patients. The etiology of this effect is unknown, but reduced inflammation in the upper airway may reduce edema and improve airway patency. There was an increase in tongue fat as assessed by magnetic resonance imaging (MRI) but no associated deterioration in P_{crit}. The study does suggest that treatment of asthma with inhaled steroids could affect the function of the upper airway. Obesity is believed to worsen asthma. In another study, weight loss in a group of obese asthmatics improved pulmonary function.[159]

Diagnosis of Nocturnal Asthma

The easiest way to objectively diagnose a severe nocturnal worsening of asthma is to have the patient record peak flow measurements at bedtime and upon awakening. Although there is not a widely accepted criteria, a fall in the peak flow of greater than 15% (evening to awakening) supports the diagnosis of nocturnal asthma. Of note, only taking measurements at two times in the day can underestimate the circadian variability of asthma.

Chronotherapy

Chronotherapy is the design of treatment to respond to circadian changes in disease. Theophylline is rarely used today due to the need to closely monitor serum levels to avoid severe side effects, but at one time, it was the only long-acting bronchodilator available. Illustrating the importance of adjusting treatment to circadian changes in disease, dosing theophylline so that peak levels will occur in the early morning might improve effectiveness in nocturnal asthma. Martin and coworkers[160] compared twice-daily sustained-release theophylline and once-daily sustained-release theophylline in subjects with nocturnal asthma and demonstrated that administration of the once-daily preparation at 7:00 PM resulted in a higher serum theophylline concentration at night than did an equivalent dose of the twice-daily preparation given at 7:00 PM and 7:00 AM. The FEV_1 at 7:00 AM was higher in subjects who received the once-daily preparation. While theophylline is rarely used today, the study highlights the importance of targeting treatment for the times of day asthma is worse.

The effectiveness of oral or inhaled steroids also appears to be affected by the time of day of dosing. The dosing of oral steroids[161] from 3:00 to 4:00 PM appears to have a greater effect on nocturnal asthma. A double-blind, placebo-controlled study evaluated the effects of a 50-mg oral dose of prednisone given at 8:00 AM, 3:00 PM, or 8:00 PM on overnight spirometry, blood eosinophil counts, and BAL cytology in seven individuals with asthma. A single prednisone dose at 3:00 PM resulted in a reduction in the overnight percentage decrease in FEV_1 and improvement in the FEV_1 measured at 4:00 AM. In contrast, neither the 8:00 AM nor the 8:00 PM prednisone dose resulted in overnight spirometric improvement. Using a 3:00 PM prednisone dose, blood eosinophil counts were also significantly reduced at both 8:00 PM and 4:00 AM. In a later study, Pincus and coworkers[162] found the optimal timing of once-a-day inhaled steroids was 5:30 PM. These findings have not altered the usual clinical practice of administering oral steroids in the morning or inhaled steroids in the morning and at bedtime.

Treatment of Nocturnal Asthma

Important treatment considerations for nocturnal asthma are listed in Box 29–5. Reducing the burden of allergen exposure by keeping the bedroom free of dust may help. A detailed discussion of asthma treatment with medications is beyond the scope of this chapter. The reader is referred to the references on this topic.[112,113,1,2] However, a very general overview will be provided here. Treatment inhalers are often divided into reliever medications (immediate relief) and maintenance/controller medications (chronic treatment of disease). The groups of medications used to treat asthma include inhaled corticosteroids (ICS) alone or as combined treatment, short and long acting beta agonists (SABA and LABA, respectively) and long acting anticholinergic medications (LAMAs). The use of SABAs alone as reliever medications in intermittent asthma has been criticized, as patients with intermittent asthma can have severe exacerbations, and bronchodilators without an inhaled steroid component do not address the inflammatory nature of asthma. Traditionally, a SABA such as albuterol has been used as a symptom reliever (quick onset of action but short duration). However, one or two inhalations of a low-dose inhaled corticosteroid (ICS) combined with a *rapid onset* LABA such as budesonide-formoterol is recommended for immediate relief (up to 12 inhalations daily by some guidelines).[112,113] This is called SMART therapy (Single Maintenance And Reliever Therapy) and is recommended for patients 4 years of age or older with moderate to severe asthma by several guidelines.[112,113,163-165] However, this is an off-label use, as the FDA-approved dosing for ICS-formoterol medications

Box 29–5 KEY POINTS: DIAGNOSIS AND TREATMENT OF NOCTURNAL ASTHMA

1. The degree of diurnal variation in airflow can most easily be documented by peak flow measurements at bedtime and on awakening.
2. Inhaled corticosteroids are essential treatment for nocturnal asthma.
3. The addition of a long-acting bronchodilator is indicated if patients with nocturnal asthma do not respond to inhaled steroids or if the required dose of inhaled steroids is higher than desired.
4. When OSA is present in asthmatic patients, adequate treatment of OSA may improve the asthma.
5. Long-acting inhaled beta agonists taken at bedtime have been shown to improve morning flow rates as well as (if not better than) theophylline and may improve perceptions of sleep quality more than theophylline in some patients.
6. Today, theophylline is rarely used given other options. If theophylline is used, dosing should be such that the highest levels are during the night or the early morning hours.
7. If nocturnal asthma symptoms persist on treatment with ICS and LABA, options include increasing the dose of ICS or addition of a long-acting anticholinergic medication (tiotropium).
8. Treatment of gastroesophageal reflux does not appear to improve asthma in patients who do not complain of GER symptoms. Treatment of GER is indicated in symptomatic patients (those who complain of GER symptoms).

OSA, obstructive sleep apnea; *LABA*, long-acting beta agonist; *ICS*, inhaled corticosteroids; *GER*, gastroesophageal reflux.

for asthma is for maintenance twice daily. When used daily for maintenance, most ICS-LABA inhalers are used twice daily (fluticasone-salmeterol [ADVAIR HFA] – *two inhalations* twice daily; mometasone-formoterol [Dulera] – two inhalations twice daily; budesonide-formoterol [Symbicort] – *two inhalations* twice daily; fluticasone-salmeterol [Advair Diskus] – *one inhalation* twice daily). Of note a formulation (Spiriva Respimat) of the LAMA tiotropium has been approved for treatment of asthma in adults and children 6 years and older as well as COPD in adults. Treatment recommendations use a step approach based on the severity of asthma (off-label use of inhaled budesonide-formoterol as a reliever in the United States). The following is adapted from portions of several guidelines[112,113]:

- Intermittent asthma: daytime symptoms ≤2 days/week, nocturnal awakenings ≤2 time per month, normal FEV_1, ≤1 exacerbation per year
  - SABA (e.g., albuterol), as needed
  - Low-dose ICS with SABA, as needed
  - Low-dose ICS and rapid-onset LABA, as needed (off-label in the United States)

- Mild persistent asthma: daytime symptoms >2 but <7 per week, nocturnal awakenings >1 per week, daily need for SABA, ≥2 exacerbations per year.
  - Daily low-dose ICS + SABA, as needed

  or
  - Low-dose ICS-formoterol, as needed

- **Moderate persistent asthma**: daily symptoms, nocturnal awakenings ≥1 week, FEV1 60% to 80% predicted , ≥2 exacerbations per year

- Low-dose ICS-formoterol (maintenance bid daily and as a reliever)
- Low-dose ICS-LABA daily (maintenance bid daily) + SABA (as reliever), as needed (LABA not formoterol)

- **Severe persistent asthma**: symptoms all day, need for SABA several times per day, FEV_1 <60% predicted, nocturnal awakenings nightly, extreme limitation of activity, ≥2 exacerbations per year.
  - Medium-dose ICS-formoterol (daily bid as maintenance and as reliever)
  - Daily medium dose ICS-LABA daily bid, + SABA, as needed (LABA not formoterol)
  - Add LAMA or use ICS-LABA-LAMA
  - Add biological treatments (anti–IL-5, anti-IgE if high eosinophils count or increased exhaled nitric oxide, trial of chronic macrolide therapy for recurrent exacerbations)

Most patients with significant nocturnal asthma fall into the moderate to severe persistent asthma group, although mild persistent asthma also includes patients with less frequent nocturnal asthma. The foundation of treatment of chronic persistent asthma is inhaled corticosteroids. Weersink and colleagues[166] studied a group with nocturnal asthma, and patients were treated with inhaled fluticasone, salmeterol (a LABA), or the combination. The three treatments all reduced the circadian variation in peak flow to less than 12%, improved the bronchial hyperresponsiveness to methacholine both day and night, and improved cognitive performance during daytime testing. Therefore, use of inhaled steroids alone may be effective in many patients with nocturnal asthma. A common practice is to start with inhaled steroids and add a long-acting inhaled beta agonist if symptoms persist. Both inhaled long-acting beta agonists and sustained-action theophylline preparations have been effective in treatment of nocturnal asthma.[166-169] Selby and associates[168] found only a slight advantage of salmeterol compared with theophylline for sleep quality (fewer arousals). The falls in morning flow rates were similar, but awakenings were less frequent on salmeterol. Weigand and coworkers[169] found salmeterol to be more effective than theophylline at preventing the morning drop in flow rate. The drugs did not differ in PSG findings, but patients perceived better sleep with salmeterol than with theophylline. In any case, the long-acting beta agonists require less attention to dosing than theophylline (rarely used today). Whereas asthmatics generally have a greater response to beta agonists than to anticholinergic medications, *vagal tone is increased during sleep*. Therefore, one might expect that inhaled anticholinergics might be helpful. There is evidence that the *addition of an inhaled anticholinergic* to standard treatment may be helpful in some patients with moderate to severe asthma. An important study[170] documented the effectiveness of the addition of tiotropium (long-acting anticholinergic) to patients still not well controlled with an inhaled steroid. In a three-way, double-blind crossover trial involving 210 patients, the addition of tiotropium bromide to an inhaled glucocorticoid was compared with a doubling of the dose of the inhaled glucocorticoid (primary superiority comparison) or the addition of the long-acting beta agonist salmeterol (secondary noninferiority comparison). The tiotropium combination was superior to doubling the corticosteroid dose and equivalent to the addition of salmeterol to the inhaled steroid. If a low dose inhaled steroid combined with a LABA does not control nocturnal asthma, the addition of a long acting antimuscarinic medication (LAMA, eg tiotropium) provides an alternative to using a higher dose of inhaled steroid with a LABA. A similar study of tiotropium in "real world asthma" documented the effectiveness of add-on tiotropium (to a corticosteroid).[171] A formulation of tiotropium (Spiriva Respimat) is the only anticholinergic approved for maintenance treatment of asthma in children and adults. The benefits may take up to 4 to 8 weeks.

In summary, inhaled corticosteroids are the foundation of treatment for most patients with nocturnal asthma. The addition of a long-acting beta agonist may help nocturnal symptoms. If symptoms persist, increasing the dose of the inhaled steroid is the next step. Addition of an anticholinergic medication is another option. The reader is referred to GINA treatment guidelines[165] for more details. If there are symptoms of nocturnal GER, treatment with a proton pump inhibitor may improve asthma in some patients. The evening proton pump inhibitor should be given before the evening meal rather than at bedtime. Finally, if sleep apnea is present, treatment with CPAP may improve asthma in some patients.

SUMMARY OF KEY POINTS

1. Patients with COPD may experience nocturnal oxygen desaturation (NOD) without discrete apneas and hypopneas.
2. In COPD, the NOD is worse during REM sleep. Hypopneic breathing during REM sleep is characterized by long periods of irregular but reduced tidal volume.
3. A saw-tooth pattern on a nocturnal oximetry tracing in a patient with COPD suggests the possibility of coexisting sleep apnea (OLS).
4. If the awake SaO_2 is low, even the normal fall in PaO_2 with sleep will result in greater desaturation (drop in SaO_2) due to the initial position on the steep portion of the oxyhemoglobin dissociation curve.
5. Mechanisms of NOD in patients with COPD include a low baseline SaO_2, hypoventilation during phasic REM sleep characterized by low tidal volume, and a reduction in FRC during hypopneic episodes (greater ventilation-perfusion mismatch).
6. Long-term oxygen treatment (ideally 24 hours/day) improves survival in patients with COPD and **daytime hypoxemia** (PaO_2 <55 mm Hg, SaO_2 ≤88%) OR PaO_2 55 to 59 mm Hg and certain symptoms/manifestations (Table 29–2). The benefit of supplemental oxygen in patients with isolated nocturnal desaturation (**daytime** PaO_2 ≥60 mm Hg) is unproven (although often administered if the patient meets criteria; Table 29–2).
7. *Nocturnal* oxygen supplementation has NOT been proven to improve sleep quality or quality of life measures in patients with COPD and NOD without daytime hypoxemia (PaO_2 ≥ 60 mm Hg). Treatment with long-acting bronchodilators can improve nocturnal oxygenation in some patients.
8. The national carrier determination for qualification for oxygen has changed and no longer specifies a duration of nocturnal desaturation. If a sleeping SaO_2 of ≤88% is documented, the patient qualifies (in the absence of OSA). However, many clinicians would consider the actual duration of nocturnal desaturation and the clinical status of the patient before adding supplemental oxygen in this situation.
9. Poor sleep quality in patients with COPD is believed to be a result of medication side effects, nocturnal cough, and

dyspnea. Many patients also have significant comorbid disorders impacting sleep.

10. Bronchodilator therapy improves nocturnal gas exchange in COPD, but only a few studies have documented an improvement in sleep quality. If bronchodilators are used, medications with a long duration of action are preferred.
11. Benzodiazepine receptor agonists can be used with caution to treat insomnia in stable patients with COPD without hypercapnic respiratory failure. A melatonin receptor agonist (ramelteon) did not worsen gas exchange and did improve sleep quality in one study. The medication is approved for sleep-onset insomnia. Sedating antidepressants are another option, but their efficacy as a hypnotic in patients with COPD is unproven. Recently dual orexin antagonists have been used in patients with COPD and do not appear to worsen nocturnal gas exchange and may improve sleep quality. More studies with these medications and patients with COPD are needed. Cognitive behavioral treatment of insomnia is considered the treatment of choice for insomnia and may be effective in patients with COPD and insomnia.
12. Patients with a combination of COPD and OSA (OLS) often require treatment with a combination of PAP and supplemental oxygen. Bronchodilator therapy may improve nocturnal gas exchange, and smoking cessation should be encouraged. BPAP may be better tolerated than CPAP in some patients with COPD and OSA.
13. Nocturnal oxygen therapy in hypercapnic patients with COPD **without OSA** generally results in only mild increases in the $PaCO_2$. A much greater increase in nocturnal $PaCO_2$ may occur in patients with a combination of OSA and COPD when supplemental oxygen is administered.
14. Patients with OLS have a worse prognosis than those with equivalent amounts of COPD and no concomitant OSA. Observational studies suggest that prognosis improves if the OSA component is adequately treated with PAP.
15. The use of high-intensity NIV in patients with moderate to severe COPD with stable hypercapnia has been shown to improve outcomes (mortality, intubations, and hospitalizations) if patients are adherent to treatment. High-intensity NIV has a goal of significantly decreasing or normalizing the nocturnal $PaCO_2$ and may require high levels of IPAP and a backup rate. Usually only low levels of EPAP are needed.
16. Patients with nocturnal asthma experience a larger than normal fall in the FEV_1 (morning dippers). This can be documented by peak flow or spirometry.
17. Nocturnal asthma is one of the defining characteristics of moderate to severe asthma. The presence of nocturnal asthma symptoms means asthma is suboptimally treated.
18. Inhaled corticosteroids are the first step in treating patients with nocturnal asthma. The next option is the addition of a long-acting beta agonist. If this is not successful, a higher dose of inhaled corticosteroids or the addition of a long-acting anticholinergic medication are options.

CLINICAL REVIEW QUESTIONS

1. A 50-year-old man with moderate COPD has a room air blood gas showing a PaO_2 of 60 mm Hg. He undergoes nocturnal oximetry that reveals 200 minutes with an SaO_2 less than 88%. There are long periods in which the average SaO_2 is around 85%. A sawtooth pattern is seen in about half of the tracing. The patient reports snoring but no daytime sleepiness. What do you recommend?
   A. Treatment with supplemental oxygen at 2 LPM.
   B. Treatment with supplemental oxygen at 2 LPM and repeat the oximetry.
   C. Polysomnography.
   D. Addition of an inhaled long-acting beta agonist and repeat the oximetry.
2. Which of the following is (are) mechanisms of nonapneic (hypopneic) NOD during REM sleep?
   A. Low baseline SaO_2.
   B. Intercostal muscle hypotonia.
   C. Hypoventilation.
   D. $\dot{V}/\dot{Q}$ mismatch.
   E. All of the above.
3. Which of the following is thought to play a role in the morning fall in FEV_1 in patients with asthma?
   A. High cortisol levels at night.
   B. High circulating catecholamines.
   C. Increased inflammatory cells in the lung.
   D. Low parasympathetic tone.
4. Which of the following are predictive of significant arterial oxygen desaturation during sleep in a patient with COPD?
   A. Daytime $PaCO_2$ = 52 mm Hg.
   B. Pink puffer COPD type.
   C. Blue bloater clinical type.
   D. Daytime PaO_2 = 70 mm Hg.
   E. A and C.
   F. B and D.
5. In spirometry, which of the following is used to assess the severity of COPD (GOLD criteria)?
   A. FEV_1 (% predicted).
   B. FVC (% predicted).
   C. FEV_1/FVC (% predicted).
   D. Postbronchodilator FEV_1 (% predicted).
   E. Postbronchodilator FVC (% predicted).
6. A 30-year-old patient with known intermittent asthma has begun to develop awakenings with dyspnea and cough twice weekly. The evening peak flow is 450 LPM, and that on awakening in the morning is 300 LPM. The patient has been using a short-acting beta agonist intermittently. What do you recommend for the initial treatment?
   A. Short-acting beta agonist at bedtime.
   B. Long-acting beta agonist at bedtime.
   C. Inhaled corticosteroids.
   D. Inhaled corticosteroids and long-acting beta agonist at bedtime.
7. A patient with stable moderate COPD on appropriate bronchodilator treatment has an awake $PaCO_2$ of 55 mm Hg and PaO_2 of 51 mm Hg. In the past, he has been hospitalized for an acute exacerbation of chronic hypercapnic respiratory failure. Nocturnal oximetry does not reveal a sawtooth pattern. What do you suggest?
   A. 24-hour supplemental oxygen at 2 LPM.
   B. Daytime oxygen and nocturnal NIV with a goal of "high-intensity" settings (IPAP up to 20–25 cm H_2O) adjusted for significant improvement in nocturnal $PaCO_2$, with oxygen added to the NIV, as needed.
   C. Daytime supplemental oxygen and nocturnal NIV with a goal of comfort, and an acceptable tidal volume, and normal oxygenation (IPAP up to 15–20 cm H_2O) and oxygen, as needed.

ANSWERS

1. C. Although the patient may well require supplemental oxygen as a component of therapy, the presence or absence of OSA must be determined. The sawtooth pattern suggests sleep apnea is present and that the patient has the OLS. Optimal therapy includes treatment of both OSA and COPD.
2. E. All of the above is the correct answer as all choices are factors resulting in NOD. Hypoventilation is likely the main cause of the decrease in PaO_2. The drop in SaO_2 is greater for a given decrease in the PaO_2 if the awake or sleeping PaO_2 is positioned on the steep portion of the oxygen hemoglobin saturation curve. Hypopneic breathing during REM sleep is often associated with bursts or rapid eye movements and is characterized by low and variable tidal volume.
3. C. Increased inflammatory cells appear to enter the airways and lungs at night. Cortisol and circulating catecholamine levels are lower during the night, and *parasympathetic tone is higher during sleep. Although circadian factors are important, sleep has an independent adverse effect on lower airway function in asthmatics.*
4. E. Worse nocturnal SaO_2 is predicted by a lower daytime SaO_2/PaO_2, hypercapnia, and the blue bloater clinical type. Of note, nocturnal oximetry is needed if there is a suspicion for nocturnal desaturation.
5. D. The GOLD criteria are based on the post-bronchodilator FEV_1.
6. C. The patient has nocturnal asthma, evidenced by a 22% fall in the peak flow as well as symptoms. The treatment of choice is inhaled corticosteroids. If this is not effective, the addition of a long-acting beta agonist is the next step. However, the patient may improve with inhaled corticosteroids alone.
7. B. High-intensity NIV with a goal of normalizing or significantly improving the nocturnal $PaCO_2$ (transcutaneous PCO_2) has been shown to improve outcomes. Very high pressures may not be tolerated initially. Use of a backup rate (if available) for chronic treatment is ideal.

SUGGESTED READING

Agusti A, Celli B, Criner GJ, et al. Global Initiative for Chronic Obstructive Lung Disease 2023 report: GOLD executive summary. Am J Respir Crit Care Med. 2023;207:819-837.

Celli BR, Wedzicha JA. Update on clinical aspects of chronic obstructive pulmonary disease. N Engl J Med. 2019;381(13):1257-1266.

Dempsey TM, Scanlon PD. Pulmonary function tests for the generalist: a brief review. Mayo Clin Proc. 2018;93(6):763-771.

Hill NS, Criner GJ, Branson RD, et al. ONMAP Technical Expert Panel. Optimal NIV Medicare access promotion: patients with COPD: a technical expert panel report from the American College of Chest Physicians, the American Association for Respiratory Care, the American Academy of Sleep Medicine, and the American Thoracic Society. Chest. 2021;160(5):e389-e397.

Macrea M, Oczkowski S, Rochwerg B, et al. Long-term noninvasive ventilation in chronic stable hypercapnic chronic obstructive pulmonary disease. An official American Thoracic Society clinical practice guideline. Am J Respir Crit Care Med. 2020;202(4):e74-e87.

Mauer Y, Taliercio RM. Managing adult asthma: the 2019 GINA guidelines. Cleve Clin J Med. 2020;87(9):569-575.

Reddel HK, Bateman ED, Schatz M, Krishnan JA, Cloutier MM. A practical guide to implementing SMART in asthma management. J Allergy Clin Immunol Pract. 2022;10(1S):S31-S38.

REFERENCES

1. Pellegrino R, Viegi G, Brusasco V, et al. Interpretative strategies for lung function tests. *Eur Respir J.* 2005;26:948-968.
2. Dempsey TM, Scanlon PD. Pulmonary function tests for the generalist: a brief review. *Mayo Clin Proc.* 2018;93(6):763-771.
3. Pennock BE, Cottrell JJ, Rogers RM. Pulmonary function testing. What is 'normal'? *Arch Intern Med.* 1983;143(11):2123-2127.
4. Stanojevic S, Kaminsky DA, Miller MR, et al. ERS/ATS technical standard on interpretive strategies for routine lung function tests. *Eur Resp J.* 2022;60:2101499. doi:10.1183/13993003.01499-2021.
5. Vestbo J, Hurd SS, Agustí AG, et al. Global strategy for the diagnosis, management, and prevention of chronic obstructive pulmonary disease: GOLD executive summary. *Am J Respir Crit Care Med.* 2013;187(4):347-365.
6. Martinez CH, Curtis JL. Implications of the GOLD COPD classification and guidelines. *Fed Pract.* 2015;32(suppl 10):14S-18S.
7. Mirza S, Clay RD, Koslow MA, Scanlon PD. COPD guidelines: a review of the 2018 GOLD report. *Mayo Clin Proc.* 2018;93(10):1488-1502.
8. Singh D, Agusti A, Anzueto A, et al. Global strategy for the diagnosis, management, and prevention of chronic obstructive lung disease: the GOLD science committee report 2019. *Eur Respir J.* 2019;53(5):1900164.
9. Agusti A, Celli B, Criner GJ, et al. Global initiative for chronic obstructive lung disease 2023 report: GOLD executive summary. *Am J Respir Crit Care Med.* 2023;207:819-837.
10. DeCato TW, Hegewald MJ. Breathing red: physiology of an elevated single-breath diffusing capacity of carbon monoxide. *Ann Am Thorac Soc.* 2016;13(11):2087-2092.
11. Agustí A, Hogg JC. Update on the pathogenesis of chronic obstructive pulmonary disease. *N Engl J Med.* 2019;381(13):1248-1256.
12. Celli BR, Wedzicha JA. Update on clinical aspects of chronic obstructive pulmonary disease. *N Engl J Med.* 2019;381(13):1257-1266.
13. Bestall JC, Paul EA, Garrod R, Garnham R, Jones PW, Wedzicha JA. Usefulness of the Medical Research Council (MRC) dyspnoea scale as a measure of disability in patients with chronic obstructive pulmonary disease. *Thorax.* 1999;54(7):581-586.
14. Paladini L, Hodder R, Cecchini I, Bellia V, Incalzi RA. The MRC dyspnoea scale by telephone interview to monitor health status in elderly COPD patients. *Respir Med.* 2010;104(7):1027-1034.
15. Jones PW, Harding G, Berry P, Wiklund I, Chen WH, Kline Leidy N. Development and first validation of the COPD assessment test. *Eur Respir J.* 2009;34(3):648-654.
16. Hurst JR, Vestbo J, Anzueto A, et al. Evaluation of COPD Longitudinally to Identify Predictive Surrogate Endpoints (ECLIPSE) investigators: susceptibility to exacerbation in chronic obstructive pulmonary disease. *N Engl J Med.* 2010;363(12):1128-1138.
17. Brożek GM, Nowak M, Zejda JE, Jankowski M, Lawson J, Pierzchała W. Consequences of changing the GOLD reports (2007-2011-2017) on the treatment regimen of patients with COPD. *COPD.* 2019;16(2):126-132.
18. Agusti A, Hedner J, Marin JM, Barbé F, Cazzola M, Rennard S. Night-time symptoms: a forgotten dimension of COPD. *Eur Respir Rev.* 2011;20(121):183-194.
19. Omachi TA, Blanc PD, Claman DM, et al. Disturbed sleep among COPD patients is longitudinally associated with mortality and adverse COPD outcomes. *Sleep Med.* 2012;13(5):476-483.
20. Goldstein RS, Ramcharan V, Bowes G, et al. Effect of supplemental nocturnal oxygen on gas exchange in patients with severe obstructive lung disease. *N Engl J Med.* 1984;310:425-429.
21. Phillipson EA, Goldstein RS. Breathing during sleep in chronic obstructive pulmonary disease. State of the art. *Chest.* 1984;85(suppl 6):24S-30S.
22. Collop N. Sleep and sleep disorders in chronic obstructive pulmonary disease. *Respiration.* 2010;80:78-86.
23. Shah NM, Murphy PB. Chronic obstructive pulmonary disease and sleep: an update on relevance, prevalence and management. *Curr Opin Pulm Med.* 2018;24(6):561-568.
24. D'Cruz RF, Murphy PB, Kaltsakas G. Sleep disordered breathing and chronic obstructive pulmonary disease: a narrative review on classification, pathophysiology and clinical outcomes. *J Thorac Dis.* 2020;12(suppl 2): S202-S216. doi: 10.21037/jtd-cus-2020-006.
25. Mohsenin V. Sleep in chronic obstructive pulmonary disease. *Semin Respir Crit Care Med.* 2005;26(1):109-116. doi:10.1055/s-2005-864204.
26. Hudgel DW, Devodatta P. Decrease in functional residual capacity during sleep in normal humans. *J Appl Physiol.* 1984;57:1319-1325.
27. Ballard RD, Irvin CG, Martin RJ, et al. Influence of sleep on lung volume in asthmatic patients and normal subjects. *J Appl Physiol.* 1990;68:2034-2041.
28. Muller NL, Francis PW, Gurwitz D, Levison H, Bryan AC. Mechanism of hemoglobin desaturation during rapid-eye-movement sleep in normal

subjects and in patients with cystic fibrosis. *Am Rev Respir Dis*. 1980;121(3):463-469.

29. Hudgel DW, Martin RJ, Capehart M, et al. Contribution of hypoventilation to sleep oxygen desaturation in chronic obstructive pulmonary disease. *J Appl Physiol*. 1983;55:669-677.
30. Gould GA, Gugger M, Molloy J, et al. Breathing pattern and eye movement density during REM sleep in humans. *Am Rev Respir Dis*. 1988;138:874-877.
31. Douglas NJ, White DP, Weil JV, Pickett CK, Zwillich CW. Hypercapnic ventilatory response in sleeping adults. *Am Rev Respir Dis*. 1982;126(5):758-762.
32. Tabachnik E, Muller NL, Bryan C, et al. Changes in ventilation and chest wall mechanics during sleep in normal adolescents. *J Appl Physiol*. 1981;51:557-564.
33. Koo KW, Sax DS, Snider GL. Arterial blood gases and pH during sleep in chronic obstructive pulmonary disease. *Am J Med*. 1975;58:663-670.
34. Fletcher EC, Miller J, Divine GW, et al. Nocturnal oxyhemoglobin desaturation in COPD patients with arterial oxygen tensions above 60 mm Hg. *Chest*. 1987;92:604-608.
35. De Troyer A. Effect of hyperinflation on the diaphragm. *Eur Respir J*. 1997;10(3):708-713.
36. Becker HF, Piper AJ, Flynn WE, et al. Breathing during sleep in patients with nocturnal desaturation. *Am J Respir Crit Care Med*. 1999;159:112-118.
37. Fletcher EC, Gray BA, Levin DC. Nonapneic mechanisms of arterial oxygen desaturation during rapid-eye-movement sleep. *J Appl Physiol*. 1983;54:632-639.
38. Catterall JR, Calverley PMA, MacNee W, et al. Mechanism of transient nocturnal hypoxemia in hypoxic chronic bronchitis and emphysema. *J Appl Physiol*. 1985;59:1698-1703.
39. Catterall JR, Douglas NJ, Calverley PM, et al. Transient hypoxemia during sleep in chronic obstructive pulmonary disease is not a sleep apnea syndrome. *Am Rev Respir Dis*. 1983;128:24-29.
40. Ballard RD, Clover CW, Suh BY. Influence of sleep on respiratory function in emphysema. *Am J Respir Crit Care Med*. 1995;151:945-951.
41. Craig DB, Wahba WM, Don HF, Couture JG, Becklake MR. "Closing volume" and its relationship to gas exchange in seated and supine positions. *J Appl Physiol*. 1971;31(5):717-721.
42. Milic-Emili J, Torchio R, D'Angelo E. Closing volume: a reappraisal (1967-2007). *Eur J Appl Physiol*. 2007;99(6):567-583.
43. Neilly JB, Gaipa EA, Maislin G, Pack AI. Ventilation during early and late rapid-eye-movement sleep in normal humans. *J Appl Physiol (1985)*. 1991;71(4):1201-1215.
44. Martin RJ. Nocturnal asthma: circadian rhythms and therapeutic interventions. *Am Rev Respir Dis*. 1993;147(6 Pt 2):S25-S28.
45. Ballard RD, Saathoff MC, Patel DK, et al. Effect of sleep on nocturnal bronchoconstriction and ventilatory patterns in asthmatics. *J Appl Physiol*. 1989;67:243-249.
46. DeMarco Jr FJ, Wynne JW, Block AJ, et al. Oxygen desaturation during sleep as a determinant of the "blue and bloated" syndrome. *Chest*. 1981;79:621-625.
47. Sanders MH, Newman AB, Haggerty CL, et al. Sleep and sleep-disordered breathing in adults with predominantly mild obstructive airway disease. *Am J Respir Crit Care Med*. 2003;167:7-14.
48. Connaughton JJ, Catterall JR, Elton RA, et al. Do sleep studies contribute to the management of patients with severe chronic obstructive pulmonary disease? *Am Rev Respir Dis*. 1988;138:341-344.
49. Lewis CA, Fergusson W, Eaton T, et al. Isolated nocturnal desaturation in COPD: prevalence and impact on quality of life and sleep. *Thorax*. 2009;64:133-138.
50. Budhiraja R, Parthasarathy S, Budhiraja P, Habib MP, Wendel C, Quan SF. Insomnia in patients with COPD. *Sleep*. 2012;35(3):369-375. doi:10.5665/sleep.1698.
51. Nocturnal Oxygen Therapy Trial Group. Continuous or nocturnal oxygen therapy in hypoxemic chronic obstructive lung disease. *Ann Intern Med*. 1980;93:391-398.
52. Medical Research Council Working Party. Long-term domiciliary oxygen therapy in chronic hypoxic cor pulmonale complicating chronic bronchitis and emphysema: report of the Medical Research Council Working Party. *Lancet*. 1981;1:681-686.
53. Kim V, Benditt JO, Wise RA, Sharafkhaneh A. Oxygen therapy in chronic obstructive pulmonary disease [review]. *Proc Am Thorac Soc*. 2008;5:513-518.
54. Jacobs SS, Krishnan JA, Lederer DJ, et al. Home oxygen therapy for adults with chronic lung disease: an official American Thoracic Society clinical practice guideline. *Am J Respir Crit Care Med*. 2020;202(10):e121-e141. Erratum in: *Am J Respir Crit Care Med*. 2021;203(8):1045-1046.
55. *National Carrier Determination 240.2*. Available at: https://www.cms.gov/medicare-coverage-database/view/ncd.aspx?NCDId=169. Accessed July 31, 2023.
56. *Local Coverage Determination for Oxygen L33797*. Available at: https://www.cms.gov/medicare-coverage-database/view/lcd.aspx?lcdid=33797&ver=28&keywordtype=starts&keyword=oxygen&bc=0lcd.aspx?LCDId=33797. Accessed July 31, 2023.
57. Plywaczewski R, Sliwinski P, Nowinski A, et al. Incidence of nocturnal desaturation while breathing oxygen in COPD patients undergoing long-term oxygen therapy. *Chest*. 2000;117:679-683.
58. Calverley PM, Brezinova V, Douglas NJ, et al. The effect of oxygenation on sleep quality in chronic bronchitis and emphysema. *Am Rev Respir Dis*. 1982;126:206-210.
59. Fleetham J, West P, Mezon B, et al. Sleep, arousals, and oxygen desaturation in chronic obstructive pulmonary disease: the effect of oxygen therapy. *Am Rev Respir Dis*. 1982;126:429-433.
60. Fletcher EC, Luckett RA, Goodnight-White S, et al. A double-blind trial of nocturnal supplemental oxygen for sleep desaturation in patients with chronic obstructive pulmonary disease and a daytime PO_2 above 60 mm Hg. *Am Rev Respir Dis*. 1992;145:1070-1076.
61. Chaouat A, Weitzenblum E, Kessler R, et al. A randomized trial of oxygen therapy in chronic obstructive pulmonary disease. *Eur Respir J*. 1999;14:1002-1008.
62. Lacasse Y, Sériès F, Corbeil F, et al. INOX Trial Group. Randomized trial of nocturnal oxygen in chronic obstructive pulmonary disease. *N Engl J Med*. 2020;383(12):1129-1138.
63. Samolski D, Tárrega J, Antón A, et al. Sleep hypoventilation due to increased nocturnal oxygen flow in hypercapnic COPD patients. *Respirology*. 2010;15:283-288.
64. Berry RB, Desa MM, Branum JP, et al. Effect of theophylline on sleep and sleep-disordered breathing in patients with chronic obstructive pulmonary disease. *Am Rev Respir Dis*. 1991;143:245-250.
65. Martin RJ, Bartelson BL, Smith P, et al. Effect of ipratropium bromide treatment on oxygen saturation and sleep quality in COPD. *Chest*. 1999;115:1338-1345.
66. McNicholas WT, Calverly PMA, Edward JC. Long-acting inhaled anticholinergic therapy improves sleeping oxygen saturation in COPD. *Eur Respir J*. 2004;23:825-831.
67. Ryan S, Doherty LS, Rock C, et al. Effects of salmeterol on sleeping oxygen saturation in chronic obstructive pulmonary disease. *Respiration*. 2010;79:475-481.
68. Donohue JF, Kalberg C, Emmett A, et al. A short-term comparison of fluticasone propionate/salmeterol with ipratropium bromide/albuterol for the treatment of COPD. *Treat Respir Med*. 2004;3:173-181.
69. Bouloukaki I, Tzanakis N, Mermigkis C, et al. Tiotropium Respimat Soft Mist Inhaler versus HandiHaler to improve sleeping oxygen saturation and sleep quality in COPD. *Sleep Breath*. 2016;20(2):605-612. doi:10.1007/s11325-015-1259-y.
70. Krachman SL, Vega ME, Yu D, et al. Effect of triple therapy with budesonide-formoterol-tiotropium versus placebo-tiotropium on sleep quality in patients with chronic obstructive pulmonary disease. *Chronic Obstr Pulm Dis*. 2021;8(2):219-229.
71. Roth T. Hypnotic use for insomnia management in chronic obstructive pulmonary disease. *Sleep Med*. 2009;10:19-25.
72. Chen SJ, Yeh CM, Chao TF, et al. The use of benzodiazepine receptor agonists and risk of respiratory failure in patients with chronic obstructive pulmonary disease: a nationwide population-based case-control study. *Sleep*. 2015;38(7):1045-1050.
73. Girault C, Muir JF, Mihaltan F, et al. Effects of repeated administration of zolpidem on sleep, diurnal and nocturnal respiratory function, vigilance, and physical performance in patients with COPD. *Chest*. 1996;110:1203-1211.
74. Stege G, Heijdra YF, van den Elshout FJ, et al. Temazepam 10 mg does not affect breathing and gas exchange in patients with severe normocapnic COPD. *Respir Med*. 2010;104:518-524.
75. Steens RD, Pouliot Z, Millar TW, et al. Effects of zolpidem and triazolam on sleep and respiration in mild to moderate chronic obstructive pulmonary disease. *Sleep*. 1993;16:318-326.
76. Kryger M, Roth T, Wang-Weigand S, et al. The effects of ramelteon on respiration during sleep in subjects with moderate to severe chronic obstructive pulmonary disease. *Sleep Breath*. 2009;13:79-84.
77. Lu XM, Zhu JP, Zhou XM. The effect of benzodiazepines on insomnia in patients with chronic obstructive pulmonary disease: a meta-analysis of treatment efficacy and safety. *Int J Chron Obstruct Pulmon Dis*. 2016;11:675-685.
78. Sun H, Palcza J, Rosenberg R, et al. Effects of suvorexant, an orexin receptor antagonist, on breathing during sleep in patients with chronic obstructive pulmonary disease. *Respir Med*. 2015;109(3):416-426.

79. Boof ML, Dingemanse J, Brunke M, et al. Effect of the novel dual orexin receptor antagonist daridorexant on night-time respiratory function and sleep in patients with moderate chronic obstructive pulmonary disease. *J Sleep Res*. 2021;30(4):e13248.
80. Kapella MC, Herdegen JJ, Perlis ML, et al. Cognitive behavioral therapy for insomnia comorbid with COPD is feasible with preliminary evidence of positive sleep and fatigue effects. *Int J Chron Obstruct Pulmon Dis*. 2011;6:625-635.
81. Kapella M, Steffen A, Prasad B, et al. Therapy for insomnia with chronic obstructive pulmonary disease: a randomized trial of components. *J Clin Sleep Med*. 2022;18(12):2763-2774.
82. Jencks SF, Williams MV, Coleman EA. Rehospitalizations among patients in the Medicare fee-for-service program. *N Engl J Med*. 2009; 360:1418-1428.
83. Sharif R, Parekh TM, Pierson KS, Kuo YF, Sharma G. Predictors of early readmission among patients 40 to 64 years of age hospitalized for chronic obstructive pulmonary disease. *Ann Am Thorac Soc*. 2014;11:685-694.
84. Clinical indications for noninvasive positive pressure ventilation in chronic respiratory failure due to restrictive lung disease, COPD, and nocturnal hypoventilation a consensus conference report. *Chest*. 1999;116:521-534.
85. Ergan B, Oczkowski S, Rochwerg B, et al. European Respiratory Society guidelines on long-term home non-invasive ventilation for management of COPD. *Eur Respir J*. 2019;54(3):1901003.
86. Macrea M, Oczkowski S, Rochwerg B, et al. Long-term noninvasive ventilation in chronic stable hypercapnic chronic obstructive pulmonary disease: an official American Thoracic Society clinical practice guideline. *Am J Respir Crit Care Med*. 2020;202(4):e74-e87.
87. Coleman JM III, Wolfe LF, Kalhan R. Noninvasive ventilation in chronic obstructive pulmonary disease. *Ann Am Thorac Soc*. 2019;16(9): 1091-1098.
88. Struik FM, Sprooten RT, Kerstjens HA, et al. Nocturnal non-invasive ventilation in COPD patients with prolonged hypercapnia after ventilatory support for acute respiratory failure: a randomised, controlled, parallel-group study. *Thorax*. 2014;69(9):826-834.
89. Köhnlein T, Windisch W, Köhler D, et al. Non-invasive positive pressure ventilation for the treatment of severe stable chronic obstructive pulmonary disease: a prospective, multicentre, randomised, controlled clinical trial. *Lancet Respir Med*. 2014;2(9):698-705.
90. Murphy PB, Brignall K, Moxham J, Polkey MI, Davidson AC, Hart N. High pressure versus high intensity noninvasive ventilation in stable hypercapnic chronic obstructive pulmonary disease: a randomized crossover trial. *Int J Chron Obstruct Pulmon Dis*. 2012;7:811-818.
91. Murphy PB, Rehal S, Arbane G, et al. Effect of home noninvasive ventilation with oxygen therapy vs oxygen therapy alone on hospital readmission or death after an acute COPD exacerbation: a randomized clinical trial. *JAMA*. 2017;317(21):2177-2186.
92. Dreher M, Storre JH, Schmoor C, Windisch W. High-intensity versus low-intensity non-invasive ventilation in patients with stable hypercapnic COPD: a randomised crossover trial. *Thorax*. 2010;65(4):303-308.
93. Berry RB, Chediak A, Brown LK, et al. NPPV Titration Task Force of the American Academy of Sleep Medicine. Best clinical practices for the sleep center adjustment of noninvasive positive pressure ventilation (NPPV) in stable chronic alveolar hypoventilation syndromes. *J Clin Sleep Med*. 2010;6(5):491-509.
94. *LCD L33800 Respiratory Assist Devices*. CMS.gov website. Available at: https://www.cms.gov/medicare-coverage-database/view/lcd.aspx?lcdid=33800&ver=26&bc=CAAAAAAAAAAA. Accessed December 23, 2021.
95. Hill NS, Criner GJ, Branson RD, et al. Optimal NIV Medicare access promotion: patients with COPD: a technical expert panel report from the American College of Chest Physicians, the American Association for Respiratory Care, the American Academy of Sleep Medicine, and the American Thoracic Society. *Chest*. 2021;160(5):e389-e397.
96. Weitzenblum E, Chaouat A, Kessler R, Canuet M. Overlap syndrome. Obstructive sleep apnea syndrome in patients with chronic obstructive pulmonary disease. *Proc Thorac Soc*. 2008;5:237-241.
97. McNicholas WT. COPD-OSA overlap syndrome: evolving evidence regarding epidemiology, clinical consequences, and management. *Chest*. 2017;152(6):1318-1326.
98. Owens RL, Macrea MM, Teodorescu M. The overlaps of asthma or COPD with OSA: a focused review. *Respirology*. 2017;22(6):1073-1083. doi:10.1111/resp.13107.
99. Kessler R, Chaouat A, Schinkewitch PH, et al. The obesity-hypoventilation syndrome revisited: a prospective study of 34 consecutive cases. *Chest*. 2001;120:369-376.
100. Bradley TD, Rutherford R, Lue F, et al. Role of diffuse airway obstruction in the hypercapnia of obstructive sleep apnea. *Am Rev Respir Dis*. 1986;134:920-924.
101. Chan CS, Grunstein RR, Bye PTP, et al. Obstructive sleep apnea with chronic airflow limitation: comparison of hypercapnic and eucapnic patients. *Am Rev Respir Dis*. 1989;140:1274-1278.
102. Resta O, Foschino Barbaro MP, Brindicci C, et al. Hypercapnia in overlap syndrome: possible determinant factors. *Sleep Breath*. 2002;6(1):11-18.
103. Alford NJ, Fletcher EC, Nickeson D. Acute oxygen in patients with sleep apnea and COPD. *Chest*. 1986;89(1):30-38.
104. Fletcher EC, Schaaf JW, Miller J, Fletcher JG. Long-term cardiopulmonary sequelae in patients with sleep apnea and chronic lung disease. *Am Rev Respir Dis*. 1987;135:525-533.
105. Machado MCL, Vollmer WM, Togeiro SM, et al. CPAP and survival in moderate to severe obstructive sleep apnea syndrome and hypoxemic COPD. *Eur Respir J*. 2010;35:132-137.
106. Marin JM, Soriano JB, Carrizo SJ, et al. Outcomes in patients with chronic obstructive pulmonary disease and obstructive sleep apnea. *Am J Respir Crit Care Med*. 2010;182:325-331.
107. Stanchina ML, Welicky LM, Donat W, Lee D, Corrao W, Malhotra A. Impact of CPAP use and age on mortality in patients with combined COPD and obstructive sleep apnea: the overlap syndrome. *J Clin Sleep Med*. 2013;9(8):767-772.
108. Kendzerska T, Leung RS, Aaron SD, Ayas N, Sandoz JS, Gershon AS. Cardiovascular outcomes and all-cause mortality in patients with obstructive sleep apnea and chronic obstructive pulmonary disease (overlap syndrome). *Ann Am Thorac Soc*. 2019;16(1):71-81.
109. Sampol G, Sagalés MT, Roca A, de la Calzada MD, Bofill JM, Morell F. Nasal continuous positive airway pressure with supplemental oxygen in coexistent sleep apnoea-hypopnoea syndrome and severe chronic obstructive pulmonary disease. *Eur Respir J*. 1996;9(1):111-116.
110. Suri TM, Suri JC. A review of therapies for the overlap syndrome of obstructive sleep apnea and chronic obstructive pulmonary disease. *FASEB Bioadv*. 2021;3(9):683-693.
111. Boulet LP, Reddel HK, Bateman E, Pedersen S, FitzGerald JM, O'Byrne PM. The Global Initiative for Asthma (GINA): 25 years later. *Eur Respir J*. 2019;54(2):1900598.
112. *GINA-Main Report 2023*. Available at: https://ginasthma.org/wp-content/uploads/2023/07/GINA-2023-Full-report-23_07_06-WMS.pdf. Accessed August 30, 2023.
113. Expert Panel Working Group of the National Heart, Lung, and Blood Institute (NHLBI) administered and coordinated National Asthma Education and Prevention Program Coordinating Committee (NAEPPCC), Cloutier MM, Baptist AP, Blake KV, et al. 2020 focused updates to the asthma management guidelines: a report from the National Asthma Education and Prevention Program Coordinating Committee Expert Panel Working Group. J Allergy Clin Immunol. 2020;146(6):1217-1270. doi:10.1016/j.jaci.2020.10.003. Erratum in: *J Allergy Clin Immunol*. 2021;147(4):1528-1530.
114. Holguin F, Cardet JC, Chung KF, et al. Management of severe asthma: a European Respiratory Society/American Thoracic Society guideline. *Eur Respir J*. 2020;55(1):1900588.
115. Akinbami LJ, Moorman JE, Liu X. Asthma prevalence, health care use, and mortality: United States, 2005-2009. *Natl Health Stat Report*. 2011;(32):1-14.
116. Atanasov ST, Calhoun WJ. The relationship between sleep and asthma. *Sleep Med Clin*. 2007;2:9-18.
117. Khan WH, Mohsenin V, D'Ambrosio CM. Sleep in asthma. *Clin Chest Med*. 2014;35(3):483-493.
118. Sutherland ER. Nocturnal asthma. *J Allergy Clin Immunol*. 2005; 116:1179-1186.
119. Pinyochotiwong C, Chirakalwasan N, Collop N. Nocturnal asthma. *Asian Pac J Allergy Immunol*. 2021;39(2):78-88.
120. Kavanagh J, Jackson DJ, Kent BD. Sleep and asthma. *Curr Opin Pulm Med*. 2018;24(6):569-573.
121. Braido F, Baiardini I, Ferrando M, et al. The prevalence of sleep impairments and predictors of sleep quality among patients with asthma. *J Asthma*. 2021;58(4):481-487.
122. Levin AM, Wang Y, Wells KE, et al. Nocturnal asthma and the importance of race/ethnicity and genetic ancestry. *Am J Respir Crit Care Med*. 2014;190(3):266-273.
123. Clark TJ, Hetzel MR. Diurnal variation of asthma. *Br J Dis Chest*. 1977;71:87-92.
124. Hetzel MR, Clark TJ. Comparison of normal and asthmatic circadian rhythms in peak expiratory flow rate. *Thorax*. 1980;35(10):732-738. doi:10.1136/thx.35.10.732.

125. Wang R, Murray CS, Fowler SJ, Simpson A, Durrington HJ. Asthma diagnosis: into the fourth dimension. *Thorax*. 2021;76(6):624-631.
126. Hendeles L, Beaty R, Ahrens R, et al. Response to inhaled albuterol during nocturnal asthma. *J Allergy Clin Immunol*. 2004;113:1058-1062.
127. Martin RJ, Cicutto LC, Ballard RD. Factors related to the nocturnal worsening of asthma. *Am Rev Respir Dis*. 1990;141:33-38.
128. Turner-Warwick M. Epidemiology of nocturnal asthma. *Am J Med*. 1988;85(1B):6-8.
129. Cochrane GM, Clark JH. A survey of asthma mortality in patients between ages 35 and 64 in the Greater London hospitals in 1971. *Thorax*. 1975;30:300-305.
130. Hetzel MR, Clark TJ, Branthwaite MA. Asthma: analysis of sudden deaths and ventilatory arrests in hospital. *Br Med J*. 1977;1(6064):808-811. doi:10.1136/bmj.1.6064.808.
131. Mauer Y, Taliercio RM. Managing adult asthma: the 2019 GINA guidelines. *Cleve Clin J Med*. 2020;87(9):569-575.
132. Martin RJ, Banks-Schlegel S. Chronobiology of asthma. *Am J Respir Crit Care Med*. 1998;158:1002-1007.
133. Hetzel MR, Clark TJ. Does sleep cause nocturnal asthma? *Thorax*. 1979;34:749-754.
134. Morrison JF, Teale C, Pearson SB, et al. Adrenaline and nocturnal asthma. *BMJ*. 1990;301:473-476.
135. Soutar CA, Costello J, Ijaduola O, Turner-Warwick M. Nocturnal and morning asthma: relationship to plasma corticosteroids and response to cortisol infusion. *Thorax*. 1975;30(4):436-440. doi:10.1136/thx.30.4.436.
136. Clark TJ, Hetzel MR. Diurnal variation of asthma. *Br J Dis Chest*. 1977;71(2):87-92.
137. Morrison JF, Pearson SB, Dean HG. Parasympathetic nervous system in nocturnal asthma. *Br Med J (Clin Res Ed)*. 1988;296(6634):1427-1429.
138. Kraft M, Djukanovic R, Wilson S, et al. Alveolar tissue inflammation in asthma. *Am J Respir Crit Care Med*. 1996;154:1505-1510.
139. Kraft M, Martin RJ, Wilson S, et al. Lymphocyte and eosinophil influx into alveolar tissue in nocturnal asthma. *Am J Respir Crit Care Med*. 1999;159:228-234.
140. Kelly EA, Houtman JJ, Jarjour NN. Inflammatory changes associated with circadian variation in pulmonary function in subjects with mild asthma. *Clin Exp Allergy*. 2004;34:227-233.
141. Kraft M, Vianna E, Martin RJ, Leung DY. Nocturnal asthma is associated with reduced glucocorticoid receptor binding affinity and decreased steroid responsiveness at night. *J Allergy Clin Immunol*. 1999;103(1 Pt 1):66-71.
142. Szefler SJ, Ando R, Cicutto LC, Surs W, Hill MR, Martin RJ. Plasma histamine, epinephrine, cortisol, and leukocyte beta-adrenergic receptors in nocturnal asthma. *Clin Pharmacol Ther*. 1991;49(1):59-68. doi:10.1038/clpt.1991.11.
143. Sutherland ER, Martin RJ, Ellison MC, et al. Immunomodulatory effects of melatonin in asthma. *Am J Respir Crit Care Med*. 2002;166:1055-1061.
144. Sutherland ER, Ellison MC, Kraft M, et al. Elevated serum melatonin is associated with the nocturnal worsening of asthma. *J Allergy Clin Immunol*. 2003;112:513-517.
145. Woodcock A, Forster L, Matthews E, et al. Control of exposure to mite allergen and allergen impermeable bed covers for adults with asthma. *N Engl J Med*. 2003;349:225-257.
146. Harding SM, Guzzo MR, Richter JE. The prevalence of gastroesophageal reflux in asthma patients without reflux symptoms. *Am J Respir Crit Care Med*. 2000;162(1):34-39.
147. Harding SM, Richter JE, Guzzo MR, Schan CA, Alexander RW, Bradley LA. Asthma and gastroesophageal reflux: acid suppressive therapy improves asthma outcome. *Am J Med*. 1996;100(4):395-405.
148. Cuttitta G, Cibella F, Visconti A, et al. Spontaneous gastroesophageal reflux and airway patency during the night in adult asthmatics. *Am J Respir Crit Care Med*. 2000;161:177-181.
149. Coughlan JL, Gibson PG, Henry RL. Medical treatment for reflux oesophagitis does not consistently improve asthma control: a systematic review. *Thorax*. 2001;56:198-204.
150. ALA Asthma Clinical Research Centers: efficacy of esomeprazole for treatment of poorly controlled asthma. *N Engl J Med*. 2009;360:1487-1499.
151. Kiljander TO, Junghard O, Beckman O, Lind T. Effect of esomeprazole 40 mg once or twice daily on asthma: a randomized, placebo-controlled study. *Am J Respir Crit Care Med*. 2010;181(10):1042-1048.
152. Prasad B, Nyenhuis SM, Imayama I, et al. Asthma and Obstructive Sleep Apnea Overlap: What Has the Evidence Taught Us. *Am J Respir Crit Care Med*. 2020;201(11):1345-1357.
153. Julien JY, Martin JG, Ernst P, et al. Prevalence of obstructive sleep apnea-hypopnea in severe versus moderate asthma. *J Allergy Clin Immunol*. 2009;124(2):371-376.
154. Chan CS, Woolcock AJ, Sullivan CE. Nocturnal asthma: role of snoring and obstructive sleep apnea. *Am Rev Respir Dis*. 1988;137(6):1502-1504.
155. Serrano-Pariente J, Plaza V, Soriano JB, et al. Asthma outcomes improve with continuous positive airway pressure for obstructive sleep apnea. *Allergy*. 2017;72:802-812.
156. Kauppi P, Bachour P, Maasilta P, Bachour A. Long-term CPAP treatment improves asthma control in patients with asthma and obstructive sleep apnoea. *Sleep Breath*. 2016;20(4):1217-1224.
157. Ng SSS, Chan TO, To KW, et al. Continuous positive airway pressure for obstructive sleep apnoea does not improve asthma control. *Respirology*. 2018;23(11):1055-1062.
158. Teodorescu M, Xie A, Sorkness CA, et al. Effects of inhaled fluticasone on upper airway during sleep and wakefulness in asthma: a pilot study. *J Clin Sleep Med*. 2014;10:183-193.
159. Hakala K, Stenius-Aarniala B, Sovijarvi A. Effects of weight loss on peak flow variability, airways obstruction, and lung volumes in obese patients with asthma. *Chest*. 2000;118:1315-1321.
160. Martin RJ, Cicutto LC, Ballard RD, et al. Circadian variations in theophylline concentrations and the treatment of nocturnal asthma. *Am Rev Respir Dis*. 1989;139:475-478.
161. Beam WR, Weiner DE, Martin RJ. Timing of prednisone and alterations of airways inflammation in nocturnal asthma. *Am Rev Respir Dis*. 1992;146:1524-1530.
162. Pincus DJ, Humeston TR, Martin RJ. Further studies on the chronotherapy of asthma with inhaled steroids: the effect of dosage timing on drug efficacy. *J Allergy Clin Immunol*. 1997;100:771-777.
163. Krings JG, Gerald JK, Blake KV, et al. A call for the United States to accelerate the implementation of reliever combination inhaled corticosteroid-formoterol inhalers in asthma. *Am J Respir Crit Care Med*. 2023;207(4):390-405.
164. Reddel HK, Bateman ED, Schatz M, Krishnan JA, Cloutier MM. A practical guide to implementing SMART in asthma management. *J Allergy Clin Immunol Pract*. 2022;10(1S):S31-S38.
165. Mauer Y, Taliercio RM. Managing adult asthma: the 2019 GINA guidelines. *Cleve Clin J Med*. 2020;87(9):569-575.
166. Weersink EJM, Douma RR, Postma DS, et al. Fluticasone propionate, salmeterol xinafoate, and their combination in the treatment of nocturnal asthma. *Am J Resp Crit Care Med*. 1997;155:1241-1246.
167. Kraft M, Wenzel SE, Bettinger CM, et al. The effect of salmeterol on nocturnal symptoms, airway function, and inflammation in asthma. *Chest*. 1997;111:1249-1254.
168. Selby C, Engleman HM, Fitzpatrick MF, et al. Inhaled salmeterol or oral theophylline in nocturnal asthma? *Am J Respir Crit Care Med*. 1997;155:104-108.
169. Weigand L, Mende CN, Zaidel G, et al. Salmeterol vs theophylline. Sleep and efficacy outcomes in patients with nocturnal asthma. *Chest*. 1999;115:1525-1532.
170. Peters SP, Kunselman SJ, Icitovic N, et al. National Heart, Lung, and Blood Institute Asthma Clinical Research Network. Tiotropium bromide step-up therapy for adults with uncontrolled asthma. *N Engl J Med*. 2010;363:1715-1726.
171. Chipps B, Mosnaim G, Mathur SK, et al. Add-on tiotropium versus step-up inhaled corticosteroid plus long-acting beta-2-agonist in real-world patients with asthma. *Allergy Asthma Proc*. 2020;41(4):248-255.

Central Sleep Apnea and Sleep-Related Hypoventilation Disorders

Chapter 30

INTRODUCTION

This chapter discusses the diagnosis and treatment of central sleep apnea (CSA) and sleep-related hypoventilation disorders. The CSA syndromes include a diverse group of disorders[1-9] associated with the presence of central apnea during sleep. In many CSA disorders, the daytime arterial partial pressure of carbon dioxide ($PaCO_2$) is normal or low. In the sleep-related hypoventilation syndromes the $PaCO_2$ is elevated during sleep or during both sleep and wakefulness. Many of the patients with nocturnal hypoventilation have an inadequate tidal volume and/or respiratory rate with relatively few discrete central apneas. However, discussion of patients with central apnea and hypoventilation syndromes together is useful because they have many similar aspects of pathophysiology and treatment. The obesity hypoventilation syndrome (OHS) is discussed with obstructive sleep apnea (OSA) in Chapters 18 and 21. Scoring rules for central apneas, Cheyne-Stokes breathing (CSB), and hypoventilation for both adults and children[10] are discussed in Chapters 11 and 12. Traditionally, patients with CSA have accounted for 5% to 15% of patients with sleep apnea evaluated at most sleep centers. However, two factors have increased the number of patients with CSA being evaluated. First, there has been an increased recognition of sleep-disordered breathing in congestive heart failure (CHF), and a substantial number of patients with systolic or diastolic heart failure have CSA with CSB (CSA-CSB) (Chapter 28). Second, there has been more aggressive use of opioids to control pain. As discussed below, many patients develop central apnea as a result of the use of potent narcotics (oxycodone, methadone). Central apnea may occur in patients with CSA-CSB or those on potent opioid treatment *either at baseline or once the patients are exposed to positive airway pressure (PAP) treatment.*

The International Classification of Sleep Disorders, 3rd edition, text revision (ICSD-3-TR)[1] provides diagnostic criteria for CSA and sleep-related hypoventilation disorders and refers to the American Academy of Sleep Medicine (AASM) scoring manual for respiratory definitions.[10]

The following is a list of CSA disorders to be discussed in this chapter:

1. Primary CSA
2. CSA with CSB
3. CSA Due a Medication or Substance
4. CSA Due to High-Altitude Periodic Breathing
5. Treatment-Emergent CSA
6. CSA Due to a Medical Disorder without Cheyne-Stokes Breathing
7. Primary CSA of Infancy
8. Primary CSA of Prematurity

Daytime hypoventilation is usually defined as a $PaCO_2 \geq 45$ mmHg (some references use >45 mmHg). As noted, some patients with primarily hypoventilation may have some central apneas, but the predominant pattern is a reduced tidal volume. *It should be noted that many patients have a combination of obstructive and central apneas and may qualify for a diagnosis of both OSA and a CSA disorder.* Often, patients are diagnosed with the predominant disorder. For some of the CSA syndromes, *diagnostic criteria may be met based on a PAP titration study*. For example, a patient may have obstructive apneas and hypopneas during the diagnostic portion of a split sleep study but develop CSA-CSB during the PAP titration portion of the study, once obstructive events are eliminated or reduced. Central apnea predisposes to closure of the upper airway from decreased caudal traction associated with the absence of an increase in respiratory system volume with inspiration and decreased ventilatory drive to both upper airway and respiratory pump muscles.[11,12] Thus, closed airway central apneas can occur. Mixed apneas are an example of this phenomenon, there is a central apnea portion followed by an obstructive apnea portion. The diagnostic criteria for CSA disorders require that central apneas or central hypopneas compose more than 50% of the respiratory events.

Hypoventilation disorders include:

1. Obesity Hypoventilation Syndrome (discussed in detail in Chapters 18, 21, and 24)
2. Congenital Central Alveolar Hypoventilation Syndrome
3. Late-Onset Central Hypoventilation with Hypothalamic Dysfunction
4. Idiopathic Central Alveolar Hypoventilation
5. Sleep-Related Hypoventilation Due to a Medication or Substance
6. Sleep-Related Hypoventilation Due to a Medical Disorder

Some patients with a sleep-related hypoventilation disorder have hypoventilation only during sleep. Others have hypoventilation during wakefulness that worsens during sleep. OHS is the only disorder with *daytime hypoventilation* as a diagnostic criteria. There is some overlap between CSA and hypoventilation disorders. For example, a patient taking opioid medications might have both CSA and hypoventilation.

To understand the pathophysiology of CSA, one can divide the CSA disorders into hypocapnic and non-hypocapnic (sometimes classified as hypercapnic) groups. The physiology of both groups will be discussed below, as well as relevant aspects of normal physiology.

PATHOPHYSIOLOGY OF CENTRAL SLEEP APNEA

Effects of Normal Physiological Changes on Ventilation During Sleep

In normal individuals, there is a 2 to 8 mmHg rise in the $PaCO_2$ during non–rapid eye movement (NREM) sleep compared to wakefulness. This is thought to be caused by loss of the wakefulness drive, reduction of the hypercapnic and hypoxic ventilatory drives, and increased upper airway resistance (Table 30-1).[3,13] The wakefulness drive is a poorly understood generalized augmentation of ventilation associated with the wakefulness state. During NREM sleep, ventilation is totally under metabolic control (chemoreceptors). Ventilatory control centers respond to information from the peripheral chemoreceptors, including the carotid body (arterial partial pressure of oxygen [PaO_2] and the $PaCO_2$) and medullary chemoreceptors (changes in the hydrogen on concentration (H^+) associated with of changes in the $PaCO_2$).[4,5] During NREM sleep, an **apneic threshold (AT)** is present, and central apnea occurs when the $PaCO_2$ is below this value.[4,5] In Figure 30-1, three central apneas are noted (no airflow and no inspiratory effort) in a patient with primary CSA. The arousals following each apnea are associated with increased ventilation that reduces the $PaCO_2$ to a level below the AT, resulting in a subsequent central apnea. The AT and primary CSA will be discussed in detail below.

During rapid eye movement (REM) sleep, ventilation is irregular, and nonmetabolic factors also affect ventilation. The hypercapnic and hypoxic ventilatory drives are lower during REM sleep than those during NREM sleep. An apneic threshold cannot be defined during REM sleep.[14] Central apnea occurring predominantly during REM sleep is *uncommon in adults* but has been reported.[15] The cause is unknown. If occasional central apneas occur, they may represent a more extreme manifestation of hypopneas occurring during REM sleep associated with inhibition of respiratory control centers or respiratory muscle motor neurons associated with the phasic events of REM sleep.[16] It is of interest that some patients with hypocapnic CSA syndromes may have better oxygen saturation and fewer central apneas *during REM sleep than during NREM sleep. For example, central apneas do not occur during REM sleep in primary CSA, CSA-CSB, and treatment emergents CSA.*

Table 30-1 Effect of Sleep on Ventilatory Control

	Wakefulness	NREM	REM sleep
Wakefulness Drive	Present	Absent	Absent
Chemoreceptors/Ventilatory Drive	Intact	Reduced	Reduced more
Upper Airway Resistance	Normal	Increased	Increased/Variable
Apneic Threshold	Not present	Present	Not present
Behavioral and Non-Respiratory Influences on Respiratory Motor Neurons (such as during phasic REM sleep)	Present	Absent	• Present • Periods of reduced tidal volume during phasic REM sleep often associated with bursts of rapid eye movements (REMs)

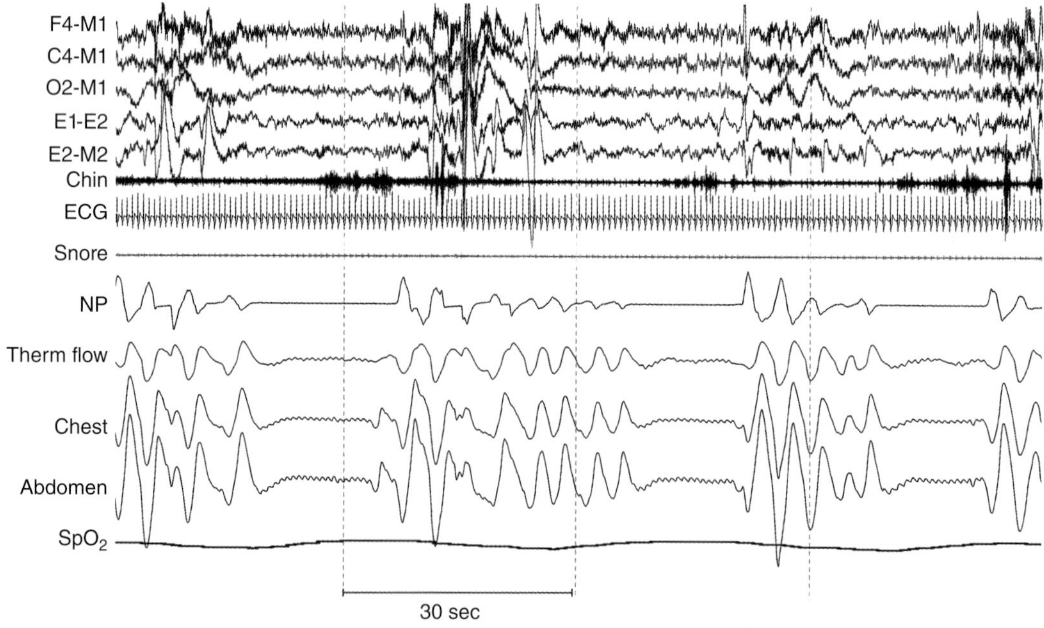

Figure 30-1 Three central apneas in a patient with primary central sleep apnea. The arousals before each apnea are associated with increased ventilation that reduces the arterial partial pressure of carbon dioxide ($PaCO_2$) below the apneic threshold, resulting in a central apnea after return to sleep. The small deflections in the chest and abdominal effort belt tracings are cardioballistic artifact.

In addition, during REM sleep, there is generalized skeletal muscle hypotonia.[16,17] The contribution of accessory muscles of ventilation is either reduced or absent, and ventilation depends entirely on the diaphragm. The loss of accessory inspiratory muscles can compromise the ability to maintain adequate ventilation, especially in patients with muscle weakness or a high work of breathing. During the phasic changes of REM sleep (associated with bursts of eye movements), there is often additional inhibition of upper airway muscles and diaphragmatic activity resulting in episodes of reduced tidal volume (rarely central apnea) (Figure 30-2).[16,17] Patients with non-hypocapnic/hypercapnic CSA/hypoventilation disorders usually have the worst oxygenation and the highest $PaCO_2$ during REM sleep. However, in the Central Congenital Hypoventilation Syndrome breathing is worse during NREM sleep. Note that, while CSA during REM sleep is uncommon in adults, in central sleep apnea of prematurity and infancy, the *associated central apneas usually occur during REM sleep* (stage R, Active sleep).[1]

Apneic Threshold and Loop Gain

As noted previously, during NREM sleep, an AT for the $PaCO_2$ is present, and when the $PaCO_2$ falls below this level, a central apnea occurs. For most individuals, the *AT is at or 1 to 2 mmHg below the awake $PaCO_2$* or approximately 3 to 6 mmHg below the sleeping $PaCO_2$ during stable NREM sleep.[3-5] The $PaCO_2$ in normal individuals increases from 2 to 8 mmHg on transition from wakefulness to sleep. Most patients in stable sleep have $PaCO_2$ levels around 4 to 5 mmHg higher than the wakefulness values (e.g., an awake $PaCO_2$ of 40 mmHg, an NREM sleep $PaCO_2$ of 45 mmHg, and an AT $PaCO_2$ of 38 to 40 mmHg). During central apnea, the $PaCO_2$ rises but must reach a level 1 to 4 mmHg higher than the AT for ventilation to resume ("system inertia"). The higher $PaCO_2$ at apnea termination results in an increased chemoreceptor stimulus and contributes to ventilatory control instability. Hyperventilation during wakefulness does not cause central apnea, because of the presence of the wakefulness stimulus—a poorly defined but important component of ventilatory drive that is lost during sleep—and centrally mediated short-term potentiation of ventilatory output that lingers after the increase in ventilation. During NREM sleep, ventilation depends on metabolic control. If the PCO_2 falls below the AT for any reason (even in normal individuals), central apnea is the result. The AT can be determined by passive increases in ventilation during sleep with a bilevel PAP (BPAP) device with lowering of the $PaCO_2$ followed by a sudden termination of ventilatory support.[18] If the $PaCO_2$ is below the AT, a central apnea occurs (Figure 30-3).

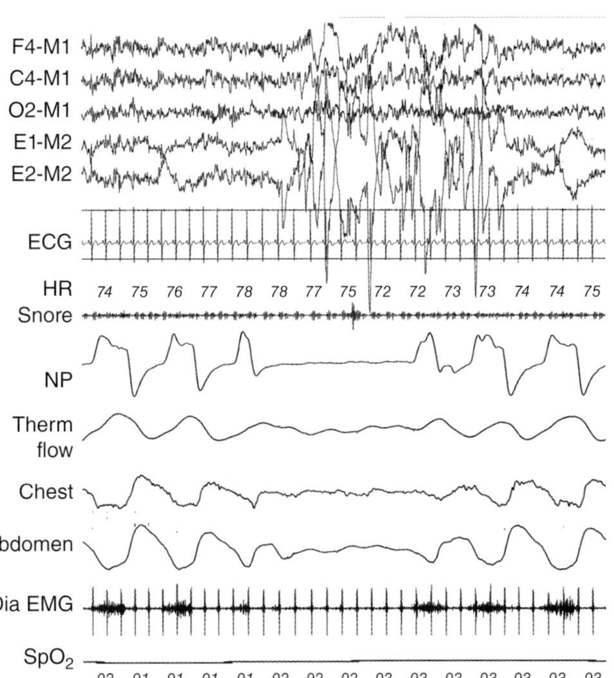

Figure 30-2 An example of a central apnea during REM sleep associated with a burst of rapid eye movements (REMs) in an adult patient. A hypopnea rather than an apnea is more commonly noted. The baseline sleeping arterial oxygen saturation by oximetry (SpO_2) is mildly decreased in this tracing. Inspiration is upward. *NP,* nasal pressure; *Therm flow,* an oronasal thermal airflow sensor; *Dia EMG,* the surface electromyography monitored with electrodes in the right 8th intercostal space near the anterior axillary line.

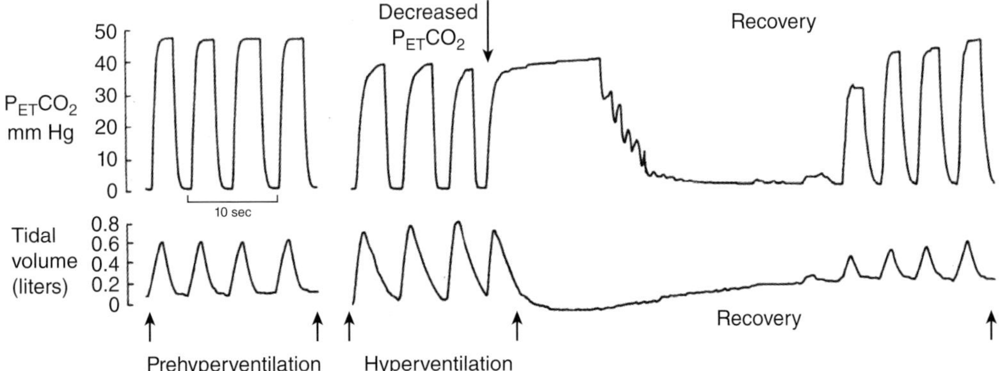

Figure 30-3 Determination of the apneic threshold (AT). The individual being tested undergoes increasing levels of positive-pressure ventilation until the end-tidal partial pressure of carbon dioxide ($P_{ET}CO_2$) drops below baseline and the passive ventilation is discontinued. In the figure, prehyperventilation is baseline stable sleep, hyperventilation is increased ventilation resulting in an increase in tidal volume and reduction in the $P_{ET}CO_2$. The ventilatory support is suddenly terminated, and if the $P_{ET}CO_2$ is below the AT, central apnea ensues. This procedure is performed with various drops in the $P_{ET}CO_2$ to define the AT. For example, if the baseline sleeping value is 45 mmHg, the procedure is repeated with $P_{ET}CO_2$ targets of 43, 41, 40, 39, and 38 mmHg. If central apnea is first noted at 38 mmHg, this is the AT. (From Skatrud JB, Dempsey JA. Interaction of sleep state and chemical stimuli in sustaining rhythmic ventilation*J Appl Physiol.* 1983;55:813-822.)

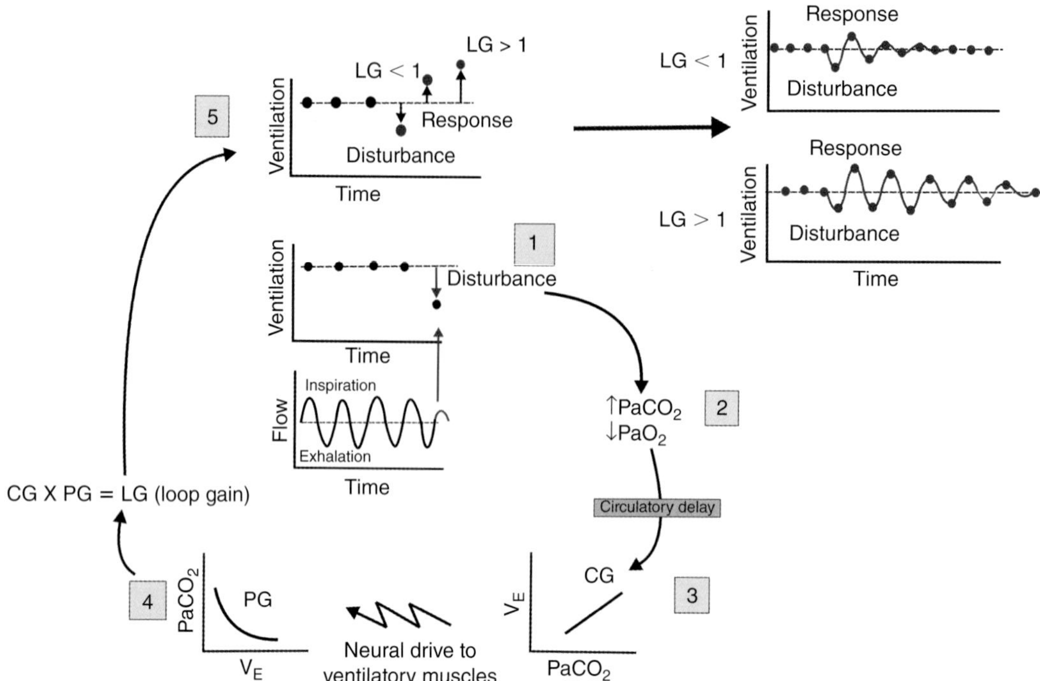

Figure 30-4 Schematic of ventilatory loop gain. (1) A disturbance to breathing causes a reduction in ventilation below eupnea (*red arrow*). (2) Reduced ventilation (V_E) increases arterial PCO_2 ($PaCO_2$) and reduces arterial PO_2 (PaO_2). (3) Controller gain (CG) reflects the sensitivity of the peripheral and central chemoreceptors to blood gases and dictates the magnitude of neural drive to ventilatory muscles ($\Delta V_E/\Delta PaCO_2$). (4) Plant gain (PG) represents the effectiveness of the lungs to change blood gases ($\Delta PaCO_2/\Delta V_E$). (5) The product of controller and plant gain determines overall loop gain (LG). If loop gain is less than 1 (LG < 1), the fluctuations in ventilation will dampen out, and breathing will stabilize. If loop gain is greater than 1 (LG > 1), the response in ventilation will exceed the amplitude of the disturbance (5), and instability will be self-perpetuating. For simplicity, the effect of delay of the information concerning changes in the PCO_2 and PO_2 from reaching the chemoreceptors is shown but not included in the LG formula. (Adapted from Deacon-Diaz N, Malhotra A. Inherent vs. induced loop gain abnormalities in obstructive sleep apnea. *Front Neurol.* 2018;9:896.)

The stability of ventilatory control depends on the loop gain of the system, which reflects the response of the ventilatory control system to a disturbance (such as apnea or an increase in ventilation associated with an arousal). With high loop gain, the disturbance results in an oscillation between apnea and hyperpnea; with low loop gain, the system quickly returns to baseline (Figure 30-4).[6,9,19] The loop gain is equal to the controller gain × plant gain × circulatory delay. The circulatory delay is the delay in changes in $PaCO_2$ and PaO_2 reaching the ventilatory control centers (sometime called the "mixing gain"). The controller gain can be represented by the hypercapnic ventilatory response (change in ventilation/change in $PaCO_2$), which depends on the $PaCO_2$ but is also increased by hypoxia. The plant gain is the change in $PaCO_2$ for a given change in ventilation. As will be discussed, plant gain is increased by a low lung volume (supine position) and hypercapnia and decreased by hypocapnia (a low steady state $PaCO_2$) during sleep. Patients with hypocapnic CSA are thought to have high loop gain caused by an increase in controller gain (high hypercapnic ventilatory response) even if plant gain is reduced. That is, the effect of increased controller gain is predominant. In patients with systolic CHF, there is also a long circulation time and a delay in the current $PaCO_2$ and PO_2 reaching ventilatory control centers, predisposing to an overshoot in ventilation.

High ventilatory drive increases both loop gain and the likelihood of reaching the AT.[4-6] Schematic illustration of the physiology determining the AT and the change in $PaCO_2$ and ventilation to reach the AT from the stable NREM sleeping $PaCO_2$ is illustrated in Figures 30-5 to 30-7. As illustrated in Figure 30-5, the AT (the $PaCO_2$ at which ventilation is zero) and the change in the $PaCO_2$ to reach the AT ($PaCO_2$ reserve) depend on the hypercapnic ventilatory response (steepness of the slope) above and below eupnea and the eupneic (steady state) position on the isometabolic hyperbola that defines the relationship between the alveolar ventilation ($\dot{V}_A$) and the $PaCO_2$ (Figure 30-5). A high hypercapnic ventilatory response results in a small difference between the eupneic $PaCO_2$ and the $PaCO_2$ at the AT (small $PaCO_2$ reserve), predisposing to central apnea, as only a small increase in ventilation is needed to reach the AT. Plant gain also affects loop gain and is defined as the change in $PaCO_2$ per change in ventilation. Decreased plant gain occurs when the baseline NREM eupneic $PaCO_2$ is lower than normal because of the position (leftward shift) to the steeper portion of the isometabolic hyperbola (Figures 30-5 and 30-6). However, the effects of high ventilatory drive predominate in patients with hypocapnic CSA (even if plant gain is decreased), and a smaller change in ventilation is needed to reach the AT. Changes in plant gain are illustrated in Figure 30-6. A lower $PaCO_2$ at baseline is associated with a lower plant gain and a higher baseline ventilation, which increases the $PaCO_2$ reserve even with normal ventilatory drive. In Figure 30-7, examples of the effects of increased and decreased chemosensitivity are shown. The fact that the $PaCO_2$

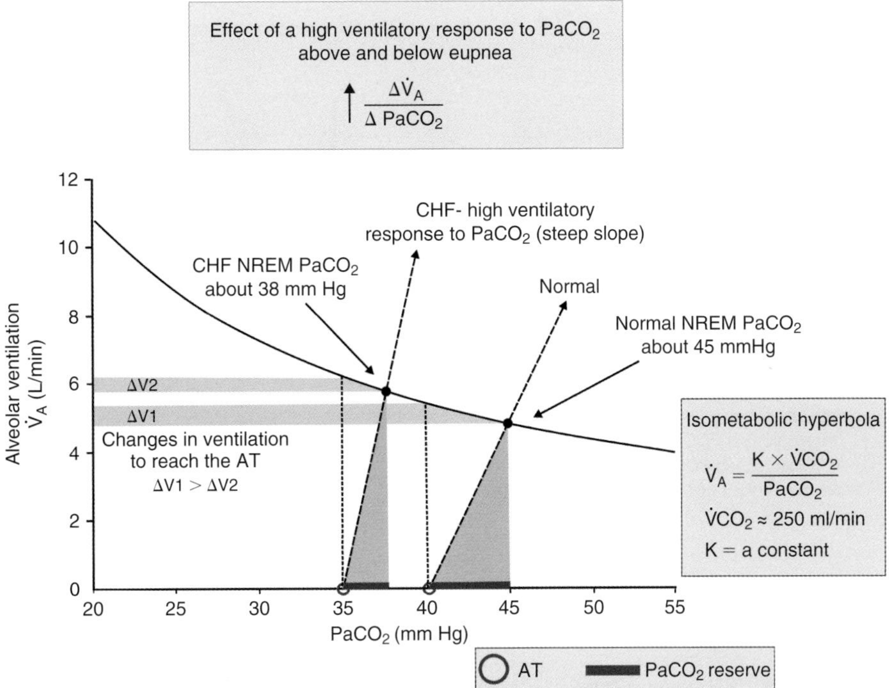

Figure 30-5 Examples showing the associated physiology determining the apneic threshold in a normal individual and a patient with heart failure and increased ventilatory drive. The relationship between the $PaCO_2$ and alveolar ventilation ($\dot{V}_A$) is defined by the isometabolic hyperbola. All possible combinations of the $PaCO_2$ and alveolar ventilation lie along this line. The *straight dashed lines* represent the relationship between the ventilation and $PaCO_2$ above and below eucapnia. When ventilation increases, the $PaCO_2$ falls until reaching the apneic threshold (AT = $PaCO_2$, at which ventilation is zero). In the patient with high ventilatory drive (steeper slope), the PCO_2 reserve (the change in $PaCO_2$ needed to reach the AT) is much smaller. The plant gain (change in $PaCO_2$/change in ventilation) is smaller in the individual with high ventilatory drive because the baseline sleeping $PaCO_2$ is lower and on the steeper portion of the hyperbola (more change in ventilation for a given change in $PaCO_2$, which is the reciprocal of the plant gain; see Figure 30-6). However, the effect of increasing ventilatory drive predominates, loop gain is increased, and the change in ventilation to reach the AT is much smaller (ΔV2 < ΔV1).

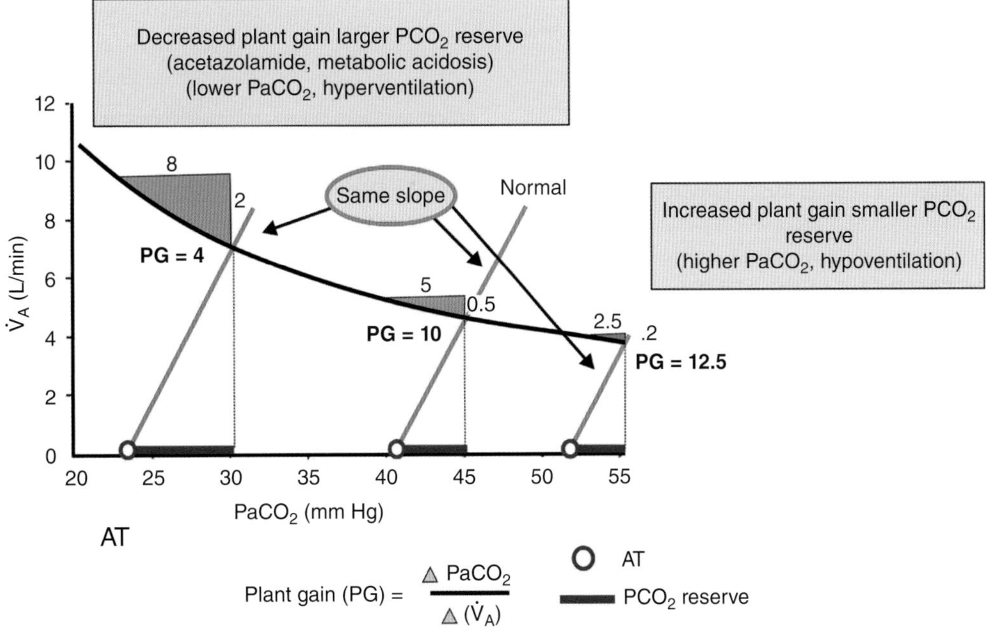

Figure 30-6 This figure shows the effect of varying the baseline (eupneic) sleeping $PaCO_2$ with the same amount of chemosensitivity (same slope). A lower than normal sleeping $PaCO_2$ is associated with a lower plant gain (steeper portion of the isometabolic parabola) and a larger PCO_2 reserve. Acidosis and acetazolamide are causes of a decreased plant gain. A higher than normal $PaCO_2$ (hypoventilation) is associated with a larger plant gain and a smaller $PaCO_2$ reserve. A lower plant gain reduces the loop gain and increases the required ventilation to reach the apneic threshold (AT). A higher plant gain increases loop gain and decreases the required ventilation to reach the AT.

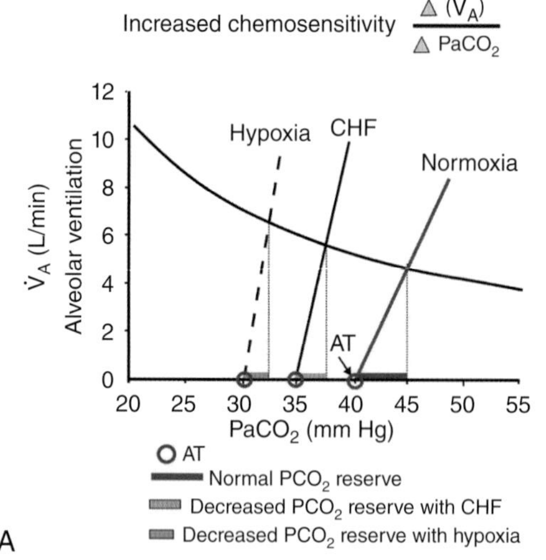

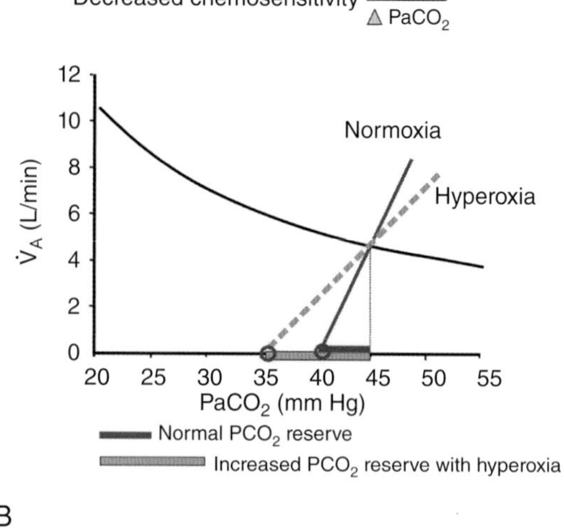

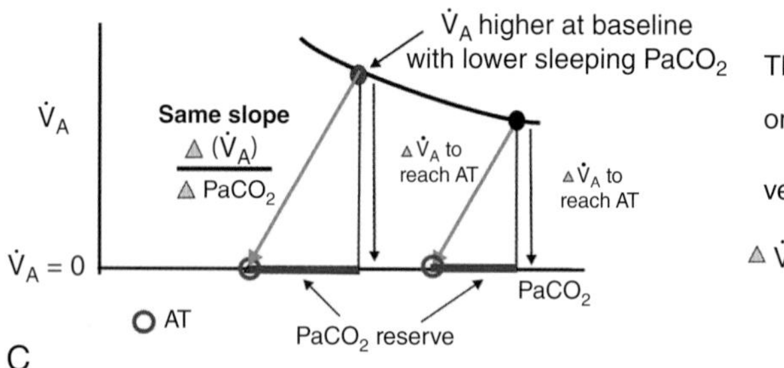

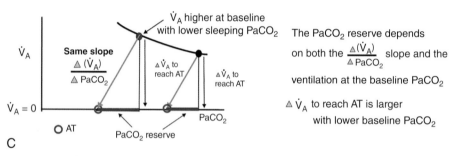

Figure 30-7 Changes in the apneic threshold (AT) and PCO_2 reserve with lower and higher chemosensitivity. Both the slope (chemosensitivity) and the baseline sleeping $PaCO_2$ determine the AT and the $PaCO_2$ reserve. In general, a higher chemosensitivity is also associated with a lower sleeping $PaCO_2$. **A**, Hypoxia and CHF are associated with increased chemosensitivity and are associated with a small $PaCO_2$ reserve. **B**, Supplemental oxygen has been used to lower loop gain and treat central sleep apnea associated with a high chemosensitivity. Hyperoxia decreases the chemosensitivity and increases the PCO_2 reserve. **C**, The ventilation at baseline also influences the AT and PCO_2 reserve. The ventilation is greater with a lower eucapnic $PaCO_2$.

reserve depends on both the slope (chemosensitivity) and ventilation at baseline (determined by the baseline sleeping $PaCO_2$ and position on the isometabolic hyperbola) is also illustrated.

HYPOCAPNIC CENTRAL SLEEP APNEA

The hypocapnic CSA group (Table 30-2) includes patients with an **awake** $PaCO_2$ that is normal or decreased. CSA during sleep occurs because the $PaCO_2$ decreases to a level below the hypocapnic AT.[3-9] Hypocapnic CSA is believed to be caused by a high hypercapnic ventilatory response above and below eupnea during sleep that results in a small difference between the $PaCO_2$ during sleep and the AT (**decreased $PaCO_2$ reserve**), as well as increased loop gain.[3-6] As noted, a high loop gain is associated with an instability in ventilatory control. Any disturbance in ventilation (a decrease or an increase from baseline) results in an over correction (overshoot or undershoot, respectively) in ventilation, and the system oscillates between apnea and hyperpnea. Often, a central apnea occurs following an arousal, and the arousal initiates a series (run) of central apneas caused by high loop gain (ventilatory instability). Patients with hypocapnic CSA tend to have

Table 30-2 Characteristics of Hypocapnic CSA

Awake $PaCO_2$	Normal or decreased
Sleep-related hypoventilation	No
Pathophysiology	• CSA due to sleeping $PaCO_2$ below the AT • High ventilatory drive (increased hypercapnic ventilatory response) • Small difference between AT and the sleeping $PaCO_2$ • Unstable sleep, frequent arousals • Circulatory delay (Cheyne-Stokes Breathing) – delay in SaO_2 nadir also noted • **AHI NREM > AHI REM sleep**
Disorders	• Primary Central Sleep Apnea • CSA with Cheyne-Stokes Breathing • CSA due to High Altitude Periodic Breathing • Treatment Emergent Central Sleep Apnea

AT, Apnea threshold; *AHI*, apnea-hypopnea index; *CSA*, central sleep apnea.

low awake and sleeping $PaCO_2$ values. As noted, this results in a decrease in plant gain, which tends to increase the change in ventilation needed to reach the AT and decrease loop gain. However, the effect of the increased hypercapnic ventilatory response (controller gain) is predominant and causes a low $PaCO_2$ reserve and an increase in loop gain. *The lower baseline sleeping $PaCO_2$ is a* ***marker of high ventilatory drive*** *and does* ***not*** *itself reduce the $PaCO_2$ reserve (a high controller gain/high hypercapnic ventilatory response does)*. As noted, a lower $PaCO_2$ actually reduces plant gain.

As ventilatory drive is lower during REM sleep than during NREM sleep and ventilation is irregular and not completely under metabolic control, hypocapnic CSA is unlikely during REM sleep; it is not possible to define an AT during REM sleep.[14] Thus, in patients with hypocapnic CSA, the apnea-hypopnea index (AHI) during REM sleep is often lower than that during NREM sleep (a pattern opposite to that typical of OSA). As discussed, central apneas can occur during REM sleep and are often associated with bursts of eye movements,[15] but these central apneas are likely an extreme manifestation of the periods of decreased ventilatory drive (and tidal volume) that occur during phasic REM sleep (REMs present).[16] The characteristics of hypocapnic CSA syndromes are listed in Table 30-2.

NON-HYPOCAPNIC CSA AND HYPOVENTILATION DISORDERS

The non-hypocapnic CSA group (Table 30-3) includes patients with a normal or increased awake $PaCO_2$ and CSA. In some references, this group is referred to as hypercapnic CSA, although some awake $PaCO_2$ values in this group may be normal or at the upper limit of normal. Some of patients in this group also have sleep-related hypoventilation. In the hypoventilation syndromes, some central apnea may also be present, but hypoventilation with a reduced tidal volume is the prominent feature. Patients with hypoventilation (high baseline $PaCO_2$) are predisposed to central apnea caused by an increase in plant gain (Figure 30-6), although controller gain is usually low. Hypoventilation during wakefulness may also be present in patients with sleep-related hypoventilation. If hypoventilation is present during wakefulness, it always worsens during sleep (lower ventilatory drive during sleep).

OSA, CSA, AND COMPLEX SLEEP APNEA

In sleep apnea, it is common to have a mixture of obstructive and central events. Many patients with predominantly obstructive apneas and hypopneas on a diagnostic study will have a few mixed and central apneas. Typically, treatment with CPAP eliminates all types of events. On the other hand, most patients with predominantly central apneas will have some obstructive apneas. For example, a patient may have central apneas during NREM sleep and obstructive apneas during REM sleep. As noted, the ICSD-3-TR diagnostic criteria allow for the diagnosis of OSA in addition to a CSA disorder if the criteria for both are met. For example, a patient may have an overall AHI of 30 events/hour, a central AHI (central apneas and/or central hypopneas) of 20 events/hour, and an obstructive AHI (obstructive apneas, mixed apneas, obstructive hypopneas) of 10 events/hour with symptoms (daytime sleepiness). In this case, the obstructive AHI is ≥5 events/hour with symptoms meeting the criteria for OSA[1]. As more than 50% of the events are central and the central AHI is ≥5 events/hour with symptoms, a diagnosis of one of the CSA disorders can also be made. Note that, if hypopneas are not classified as obstructive or central, they are assumed to be obstructive.

Using ICSD-3-TR criteria,[1] a diagnosis of CSA can also be made *based on findings during a PAP titration sleep study*. Often, a patient will exhibit mainly obstructive events during a diagnostic study, but a significant number of central apneas will *emerge or persist* on PAP once obstructive events are no longer present or constitute a minority of the residual events. This pattern is often called complex sleep apnea (CompSA). The terms *CompSA and treatment emergent CSA (TECSA)* are often used as synonyms, but according to the ICSD-3-TR, TECSA is restricted to disorders in which the CSA that emerges or persists on PAP *is not better explained by another entity*. The designation CompSA is defined by the Centers for Medicare and Medicaid Services (CMS)[20] and is **not** an ICSD-3-TR term. The term *CompSA* refers to a **pattern** of primarily obstructive events on a diagnostic study with primarily central events (persistent or emergent) on PAP after obstructive events have been significantly reduced. This is illustrated in (Figure 30-8). Here obstructive apnea is noted during the diagnostic portion of a

Table 30-3 Non-Hypocapnic CSA/Hypoventilation Syndromes

Awake $PaCO_2$	Normal or increased
Sleep-related hypoventilation	Yes, in hypoventilation disorders
Pathophysiology	• Abnormal ventilatory control due to structural or functional abnormality of ventilatory control centers • Drug or substance suppressing ventilation • Immature ventilatory control centers • Disorders of structures innervating respiratory muscles, myopathy, disorders of the neuromuscular junction • Chest wall disorders • Pulmonary disorders (airways, parenchyma, pulmonary vasculature)
Non-Hypocapnic CSA Disorders	• CSA due to a Medical Disorder without CSB • CSA due to a Medication or Substance • Primary Central Sleep Apnea of Infancy • Primary Central Sleep Apnea of Prematurity
Sleep-Related Hypoventilation Disorders	• Obesity hypoventilation syndrome • Congenital Central Alveolar Hypoventilation syndrome • Late-Onset Central Hypoventilation with Hypothalamic Dysfunction • Idiopathic Central Alveolar Hypoventilation • Sleep-Related Hypoventilation Due to a Medication or Substance • Sleep-Related Hypoventilation Due to a Medical Disorder

CSB, Cheyne-Stokes breathing; *CSA*, central sleep apnea.

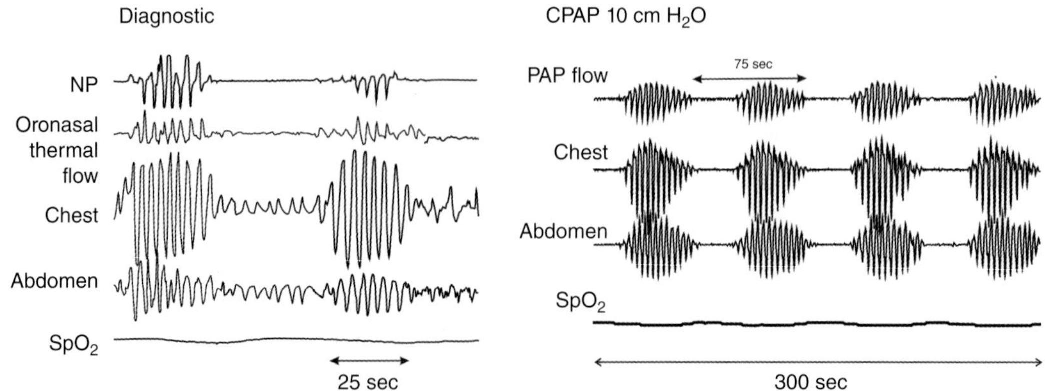

Figure 30-8 An example of a patient with obstructive sleep apnea during the diagnostic portion of a split sleep study who developed central sleep apnea of the Cheyne-Stokes type on CPAP. This is a type of complex sleep apnea. The diagnosis is obstructive sleep apnea and central sleep apnea with Cheyne-Stokes Breathing. One might suspect that CSB would be noted on CPAP given the crescendo-decrescendo pattern of respiration between obstructive apneas. (From Berry RB, Wagner MH. *Sleep Medicine Pearls*, 3rd edition. Elsevier Health Sciences; 410.)

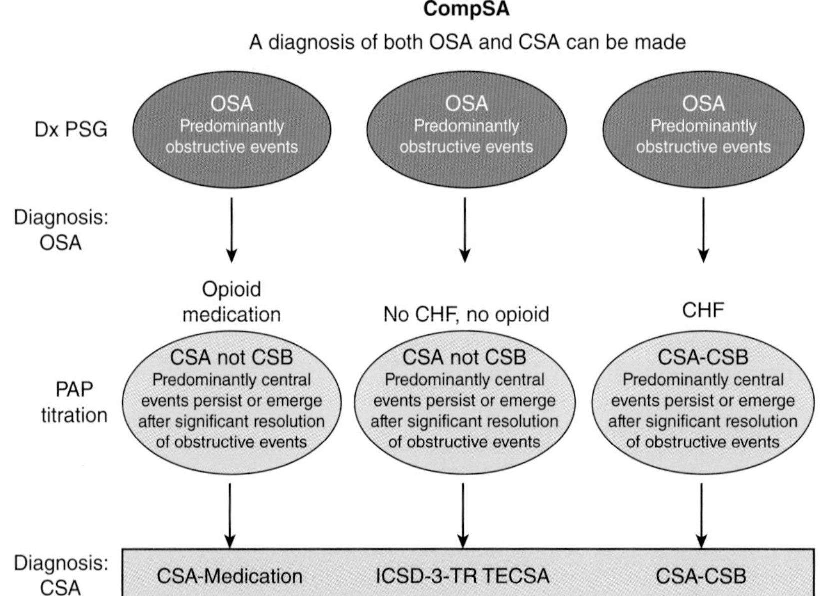

Figure 30-9 A schematic of the forms of complex sleep apnea. (1) A patient on opioids has obstructive sleep apnea (OSA) on the diagnostic polysomnography (PSG) but develops CSA during the positive airway pressure (PAP) titration. In this case, the diagnosis is OSA and CSA due to a Medication or Substance. (2) This patient has no known risk factors for CSA, has OSA on a diagnostic PSG, and has CSA on PAP. The diagnosis is OSA and treatment-emergent CSA (TECSA) using ICSD-3-TR criteria. This assumes symptoms or signs are present with residual CSA. (3) This patient has CHF and OSA on a diagnostic PSG but CSA with Cheyne-Stokes breathing (CSB) on the PAP titration. The diagnosis is OSA and CSA-CSB (due to congestive heart failure).

split sleep study. However, CSA-CSB events are predominant after obstructive events are reduced on CPAP. Using ICSD-3-TR criteria, the diagnosis would NOT be TECSA but instead OSA and CSA associated with CSB. However, many clinicians apply the term *TECSA* to central apneas meeting the CompSA definition rather than the more restrictive definition in the ICSD-3-TR. A schematic illustrating CompSA and TECSA according to the ICSD-3-TR is shown in Figure 30-9. The precise definitions of CSA and CompSA used by the CMS[20] to determine qualification for a BPAP device with a backup rate for treatment of central apnea/CompSA (one of the four categories of respiratory assist device [RAD] criteria) is shown in Table 30-4. Definitions of both CSA and CompSA are listed. Note that, currently, a decrease in the **obstructive AHI** to less than 5 events/hour is required on PAP to meet the definition of CompSA. This degree of effectiveness is not always attainable during the PAP titration. Patients with CHF and those taking opioid medications may *predominantly exhibit CSA during a* ***diagnostic study*** *that meets the CMS definition of CSA.* On the other hand, these patient groups may have primarily OSA during a diagnostic study but exhibit CSA on PAP once obstructive events have resolved (CompSA). A number of scenarios are possible (Table 30-5). For example, if a patient with CHF has primarily obstructive events on a diagnostic study but exhibits a significant number of central apneas of the CSB type on PAP after obstructive apneas resolve, a diagnosis

Table 30-4 Definition of CSA and Complex Sleep Apnea (Centers of Medicare and Medicaid Services)*

Central sleep apnea (CSA) is defined by all of the following:
1. An apnea-hypopnea index (AHI) greater than or equal to 5; **and**
2. The sum total of central apneas plus central hypopneas is greater than 50% of the total apneas and hypopneas; **and**
3. A central apnea-central hypopnea index (CAHI) is greater than or equal to 5 events/hour; **and**
4. The presence of at least one of the following:
   - Sleepiness
   - Difficulty initiating or maintaining sleep, frequent awakenings, or non-restorative sleep
   - Awakening short of breath
   - Snoring
   - Witnessed apneas
5. **There is no evidence of daytime or nocturnal hypoventilation.****

Complex sleep apnea (CompSA) is a form of central apnea specifically identified by all of the following:
1. With use of a *positive airway pressure (PAP) device without a backup rate (E0601 or E0470)*, the polysomnogram (PSG) shows a pattern of apneas and hypopneas that demonstrates the persistence or emergence of central apneas or central hypopneas upon exposure to continuous PAP (CPAP) (E0601) or a bilevel device without backup rate (E0470) *when titrated to the point where obstructive events have been effectively treated (obstructive AHI less than 5 events/hour).*
2. After resolution of the obstructive events, the sum total of central apneas and central hypopneas is greater than 50% of the total apneas and hypopneas; and
3. After resolution of the obstructive events, a central apnea-central hypopnea index (CAHI) greater than or equal to 5 events/hour.

Qualification for RAD devices (LCD L33800)

Central sleep apnea or complex sleep apnea

An E0470 or E0471 device is covered when, prior to initiating therapy, **a complete facility-based, attended PSG is performed** documenting the following:
1. The diagnosis of CSA or CompSA; and
2. Significant improvement of the sleep-associated hypoventilation** (*this really means CSA*) with the use of an E0470 or E0471 device on the settings that will be prescribed for initial use at home while breathing the beneficiary's prescribed FiO_2.

If all of the above criteria are met, either an E0470 or an E0471 device (based on the judgment of the treating practitioner) will be covered for beneficiaries with documented CSA or CompSA for the first 3 months of therapy.

*Used to determine qualification for bilevel PAP (BPAP) with or without a backup rate using RAD criteria. However, BPAP with a backup rate is clinically indicated.
**Criteria are inconsistent.
E0601, CPAP; *E0470*, BPAP without a backup rate; *E0471*, BPAP with a backup rate; *RAD*, respiratory assist device.
Adapted from Centers for Medicare and Medicaid Services. Local Coverage Determination Respiratory Assist Devices (L33800). Updated 08/08/ 2021. Accessed September 16, 2022.

Table 30-5 Examples of Complex Sleep Apnea and the Appropriate Diagnosis Using the ICSD-3-TR Diagnostic Criteria

Example	Diagnostic PSG	PAP PSG	Diagnosis ICSD-3-TR	CMS Terminology*
1. CHF present	Predominantly OSA	Obstructive events resolve CSA-CSB events emerge/persist	OSA CSA-CSB	Complex Sleep Apnea (CompSA RAD category)*
2. CHF present	Predominantly CSA-CSB Obstructive AHI ≥ 5/hr +symptoms	CSA-CSB resolves or persists	CSA-CSB OSA	Central Sleep Apnea (CSA RAD category)*
3. On potent opioids	Predominantly OSA	Obstructive events resolve CSA - not CSB noted	OSA CSA Due to Medication or Substance	Complex Sleep Apnea (CompSA RAD Category)*
4. On potent opioids	Predominantly CSA	CSA not CSB resolves or persists	CSA Due to a Medication or Substance	Central Sleep Apnea (CSA RAD category)*
5. No CHF or narcotics	Predominantly OSA	Obstructive events resolve CSA not CSB emerges/persists	OSA TECSA	Complex Sleep Apnea (Complex SA RAD category)*

*RAD category definition used to determine qualification for a bilevel positive airway pressure (BPAP) device with a backup rate.
CSA, central sleep apnea; *TECSA*, treatment-emergent CSA; *CMS*, Centers for Medicare and Medicaid Services; *CSB*, Cheyne-Stokes breathing; *CHF*, congestive heart failure; *RAD*, respiratory assist device; *CompSA*, complex sleep apnea. The diagnostic PSG and PAP PSG can occur on the same night during a split sleep study.

of both OSA and CSA-CSB can be made according to ICSD-3-TR criteria but using CMS terminology this is a patient with OSA and Complex SA. On the other hand, if a patient with CHF has mainly CSA-CSB on a diagnostic study but the pattern persists on CPAP or BPAP without a backup rate, this *CSA*[20] *as defined by CMS and NOT CompSA.* The patient would qualify for BPAP with a backup rate using the CMS criteria for CSA if this treatment is shown to be effective during polysomnography (PSG). There are occasions when a patient shows primarily CSA on a diagnostic study but has resolution of events on CPAP.[21-23] According to CMS criteria, they would not qualify for CPAP (treatment reimbursed for OSA but not

CSA). However, often sufficient obstructive events are present on the diagnostic study to make a diagnosis of OSA and qualify the patient for CPAP. If CSA does not respond to CPAP, use of BPAP with a backup rate is needed (BPAP spontaneous timed [BPAP-ST] or adaptive servoventilation [ASV]). These devices are classified as RADs and have specific criteria for reimbursement qualification.[20] Several difficulties in qualifying patients with CSA for PAP treatment, including issues with the local carrier determinations (LCD) for RAD devices, have been identified (including the need for the obstructive AHI to be ≤ 5 events/hour and the requirement that "significant improvement in sleep-related hypoventilation" using BPAP with a backup rate is documented when CSA rather than hypoventilation is really what is being treated) and recommendations made to the CMS.[23] Notable problems with the CMS criteria include the need for the obstructive AHI to be < 5/hour and the requirement that "significant improvement in sleep-related hypoventilation" using BPAP with a backup rate is documented. Improvement in CSA not hypoventilation is the relevant outcome.

HYPOCAPNIC CENTRAL SLEEP APNEA DISORDERS

Primary Central Sleep Apnea

Primary CSA (idiopathic CSA) is an uncommon syndrome (5–10% of patients with sleep apnea) of **unknown etiology (idiopathic)** characterized by recurrent central apneas.[1] Some studies suggest the syndrome is **more common in men,** but others do not confirm this finding. The major ICSD-3-TR diagnostic criteria for primary CSA are listed here. See the ICSD-3-TR for a complete discussion of the diagnostic criteria.

Primary CSA diagnostic criteria (Criteria A-D must be met):

A. The presence of at least one of the following (in children, daytime symptoms may not be evident):
   1. Sleepiness
   2. Difficulty initiating or maintaining sleep, frequent awakenings, or non-restorative sleep
   3. Awakening short of breath
   4. Witnessed apneas

B. PSG demonstrates all of the following:
   - Five or more central apneas or central hypopneas per hour of sleep
   - The total number of central apneas and/or central hypopneas is >50% of the total number of apneas and hypopneas.
   - Absence of CSB.

C. There is no evidence of daytime or nocturnal hypoventilation.

D. The disorder is not better explained by another current sleep disorder, medical disorder, medication, or substance use.

PSG findings **alone** are not sufficient for a diagnosis of primary CSA. Symptoms must be present (one or more of the following: *sleepiness, insomnia, awakening short of breath, or witnessed apnea*). PSG reveals five or more central apneas or central hypopneas per hour of sleep with >50% of the total number of apneas and hypopneas being central in nature. **CSB is absent.** The morphology of the central apneas is different from that associated with CSB. There is no evidence of hypoventilation. The disorder is not better explained by another current sleep disorder, medical or neurologic disorder, medication use, or substance use disorder. Patients with a known medical or neurological disorder that is believed to cause central apneas are classified elsewhere. Key points concerning primary CSA are listed in Box 30-1. Of note, formerly snoring was included as a symptom in the diagnostic criteria but is not included in ICSD-3-TR. However, snoring can be present and often OSA rather than CSA is expected.

Patients with primary CSA tend to be thinner than those with OSA and are more likely to complain of insomnia. However, in one series, a complaint of daytime sleepiness was the most common symptom.[24] Complaints of snoring and choking during sleep are common, and PSG is often ordered because a diagnosis of OSA is suspected. The finding of predominant CSA on a sleep study is often an unexpected. The awake $PaCO_2$ is normal or low (less than 40 mmHg). The central apneas do not have the Cheyne-Stokes morphology (Figures 30-1 and 30-10) and have a short cycle time (less than 40 seconds).[1,10,25] In some studies, the central apnea index was much higher (or greater than zero) in the supine position.[21,22] The differential diagnosis of primary CSA includes other causes of CSA without CSB, including CSA due to a medical disorder without CSB and CSA due to a Medication or Substance. That is, primary CSA is a diagnosis of exclusion. One should consider the possibility of CSA caused by Chiari syndrome[1] before making a diagnosis of primary CSA. Often, the only complaint different from the usual CSA complaints in Chiari syndrome is frequent headaches.

Box 30-1 KEY POINTS: PRIMARY CENTRAL SLEEP APNEA (CSA)

- A type of hypocapnic central apnea with a normal or low awake $PaCO_2$
- No obvious associated disease (neurologic disorder or congestive heart failure) and patients are not being treated with respiratory depressant medications (narcotics).
- A diagnosis of primary CSA is a diagnosis of exclusion
- High ventilatory drive (controller gain) and unstable sleep (arousals) are the etiology
- Arousal from sleep may trigger several large breaths with a subsequent central apnea
- The morphology of the central apneas differs from those with Cheyne-Stokes breathing (short cycle time, lack of crescendo-decrescendo ventilatory pattern between events).
- Central apnea occurs when the sleeping $PaCO_2$ is less than the apneic threshold in NREM. NREM AHI > REM AHI. Central apnea more frequent in supine position.
- Most patients with primary CSA complain of excessive daytime sleepiness and have a history of snoring; some complain primarily of insomnia (frequent awakenings)
- Primary CSA is uncommon, less than 5% of patients with sleep apnea
- Treatment options for primary CSA:*
  - PAP treatment,* (CPAP, BPAP-ST, ASV)
  - Acetazolamide*
  - Zolpidem, triazolam* (if no underlying risk factors for respiratory depression)
  - Transvenous phrenic nerve stimulation
  - Oxygen

*Recommended for treatment of primary CSA at the option level[35]; for PAP treatment, type of PAP not specified

CSA, central sleep apnea; *PAP*, positive airway pressure; *CPAP*, continuous PAP; *BPAP*, bilevel PAP; *ST*, spontaneous timed; *ASV*, Adaptive servoventilation.

*Aurora RN, Chowdhuri S, Ramar K, et al. The treatment of central sleep apnea syndromes in adults: practice parameters with an evidence-based literature review and meta-analyses. *Sleep.* 2012;35(1):17-40.

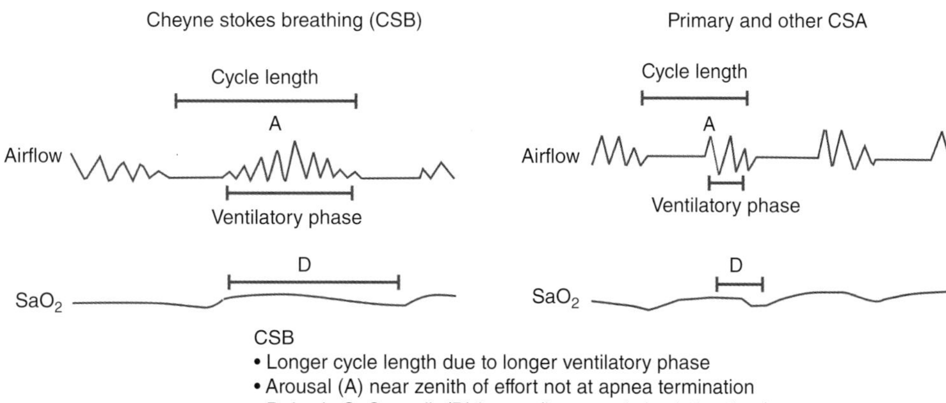

Figure 30-10 Schematic representation of differences between morphology of central apneas in primary central sleep apnea (CSA) and central apnea associated with Cheyne-Stokes breathing (CSB) with heart failure. The cycle length of CSA-CSB is ≥40 seconds, and the ventilation between apneas has a crescendo-decrescendo pattern. A longer length of the ventilatory phase in CSA-CSB is associated with a lower ejection fraction. A longer ventilatory phase is associated with a longer cycle length.

Patients with primary CSA are believed to have an *increased hypercapnic ventilatory response*, a normal to decreased awake $PaCO_2$, and a small difference between the AT and the sleeping $PaCO_2$ level (decreased $PaCO_2$ reserve).[3,26-28] Central apneas often follow periods of increased ventilation from any cause, such as an arousal[28] (Figure 30-1), or associated with sleep onset (transitional central apnea). If central apneas are isolated events and are only associated with wakefulness to sleep transitions, the *transitional central apneas* are felt to be normal. In contrast, in primary CSA, a transition from wakefulness to sleep can be associated with a series of central apneas. Periods of increased ventilation triggering central apneas in patients with primary CSA are often associated with a preceding arousal.[28] Arousal may trigger a transient increase in ventilation and a fall in $PaCO_2$. This transient fall in $PaCO_2$ is then associated with a central apnea as the patient returns to sleep ($PaCO_2$ below the AT). Thus, arousal may initiate or predispose to continuation of central apnea. Sleep studies may show frequent isolated central apneas. However, usually, the central apneas occur in groups with continued oscillations between apnea and hyperpnea (a form of periodic breathing) caused by a high loop gain. A run of central apneas may follow arousal from a non-respiratory stimulus. As noted, the events do NOT have CSB morphology. For CSB, the cycle length is ≥40 seconds,[10] with ventilatory periods having a crescendo-decrescendo pattern. Differences in central apnea morphology in primary CSA and CSB are illustrated in Figure 30-10. The central apneas in patients with primary CSA occur *during stages N1 and N2* and are uncommon during stage N3 sleep and REM sleep. The central apneas may also be more common in the supine position,[21,22] and often the *AHI-NREM is higher than the AHI-REM* in patients with primary CSA. A diagnosis of Primary CSA does not rule out a simultaneous diagnosis of OSA if the obstructive AHI is ≥ 5/hour and symptoms are present.

Treatment of Primary CSA

In research studies, the addition of *dead space or inhalation of CO_2* with the goal of increasing and/or stabilizing the $PaCO_2$ has been shown to reduce central apnea in patients with primary CSA.[29] However, these interventions have not been tried for long-term treatment, nor are they practical.

There are no controlled studies of treatments for primary CSA. Treatments have included PAP (CPAP, BPAP with a backup rate, and ASV), respiratory stimulants (acetazolamide), benzodiazepine receptor agonists, and supplemental oxygen.[21,22,30-35] Transvenous phrenic nerve stimulation has also been used to treat primary CSA and is effective, though invasive (Figure 30-11).[36] The addition of supplemental oxygen is believe to decrease ventilatory drive, thereby stabilizing ventilation (decreased loop gain).[34] Benzodiazepine receptor agonists may reduce arousals, which can precipitate runs of central apneas. Acetazolamide decreases loop gain by decreasing plant gain.[4,5,30] The medication reduces the baseline sleeping $PaCO_2$ and plant gain and increases the PCO_2 reserve (Figure 30-6). The net effect is that a greater increase in ventilation is needed to reach the AT. Plant gain is reduced because of the position of the baseline sleeping $PaCO_2$ on the steep portion of the isometabolic hyperbola.

Treatment options for primary CSA are listed in Box 30-1, including those recommended in the 2012 AASM practice parameters[35] (at the option level because of limited data). Later, updated guidelines for use of ASV in CHF were published.[37] Treatment with PAP (type not specified) and acetazolamide are listed as options for treatment of primary CSA. Zolpidem and triazolam are listed as a treatment option only if the patient does not have underlying risk factors for respiratory depression.[35] A study by Quadri et al.[31] found that zolpidem decreased the central AHI in patients with primary CSA and improved sleep continuity and decreased subjective daytime sleepiness without a worsening of oxygenation or obstructive events in the majority of patients. Caution is still advised. Of note, PAP (rather than a specific type of PAP) was recommended in the 2012 treatment guidelines, although the discussion in the publication lists CPAP, BPAP-ST, and ASV.[35] Use of oxygen for primary CSA was not recommended. Supplemental oxygen was recommended for CSA associated with CHF. At the time of this writing, oxygen treatment for any type of CSA is not covered by insurance.

A retrospective analysis of patients identified as having some form of sleep apnea found primary CSA in 3.8%, with male predominance. PAP was prescribed in 23%, and 78% were adherent.[24] PAP treatments included CPAP and ASV. At first follow-up, a majority were adherent, and the AHI was <15 events/hour in most patients.

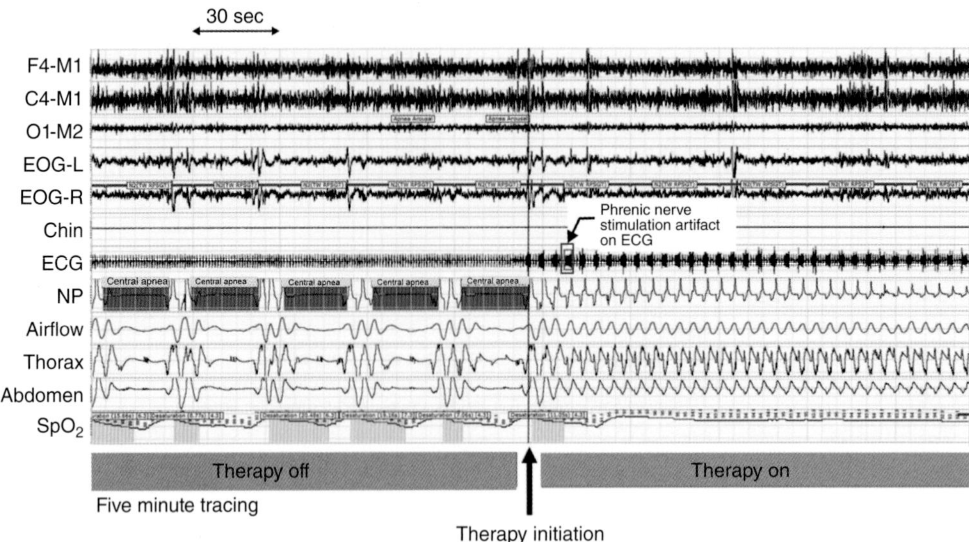

Figure 30-11 A tracing showing use of transvenous phrenic nerve pacing for treatment of primary central sleep apnea. On the left is the baseline (treatment turned off), and on the right is after treatment was turned on. (From: Javaheri S, McKane S. Transvenous phrenic nerve stimulation to treat idiopathic central sleep apnea. *J Clin Sleep Med.* 2020;16(12):2099–2107.)

It is interesting that CPAP is effective in some patients with primary CSA.[21,22] This is probably the treatment of choice if patients also have significant OSA as well as CSA. The reason CPAP works in patients with primary CSA is unknown, but CPAP may result in a slight increase in $PaCO_2$ or prevent triggering of arousal by episodes of high upper airway resistance. High upper airway resistance may trigger an arousal, resulting in subsequent central apnea in patients with instability in ventilatory control caused by high ventilatory drive and a low arousal threshold. One study found that central apnea was present mainly in the supine position.[21] A reduction in resting lung volume during supine sleep could increase plant gain. In contrast, PAP could increase resting lung volume and decrease plant gain. As noted, CPAP is not currently covered by insurance for treatment of central sleep apnea. Fortunately, most patients have enough obstructive events to qualify for CPAP reimbursement with diagnoses of both OSA and CSA. If CPAP does not work as a treatment for primary CSA, treatment with spontaneously timed BPAP (BPAP-ST) or ASV should be effective. ASV has an advantage, as the automated expiratory PAP (autoEPAP) option treats both central and obstructive events. Case series report effective treatment with ASV for a wide variety of hypocapnic CSA syndromes. Although BPAP-ST should be effective for primary CSA, ASV may require fewer device-triggered breaths to treat central apnea, as ventilation is stabilized. Overall, a lower level of PAP is usually needed, and ASV may be better tolerated than BPAP-ST. Transvenous phrenic nerve stimulation is a new treatment option in patients with primary CSA (Figure 30-11).[36] More details about this treatment are presented in this chapter's section on treatment of CSA-CSB.

CSA With Cheyne-Stokes Breathing (CSA-CSB)

CSA-CSB is characterized by recurrent central apneas or central hypopneas alternating with a respiratory phase exhibiting a crescendo-decrescendo pattern of flow (or tidal volume).[10] The longer cycle length (≥40 seconds and typically 45 to 60 seconds) and the crescendo-decrescendo pattern of breathing distinguishes CSB from other CSA types (Figures 30-10 and 30-12). Central hypopneas, rather than

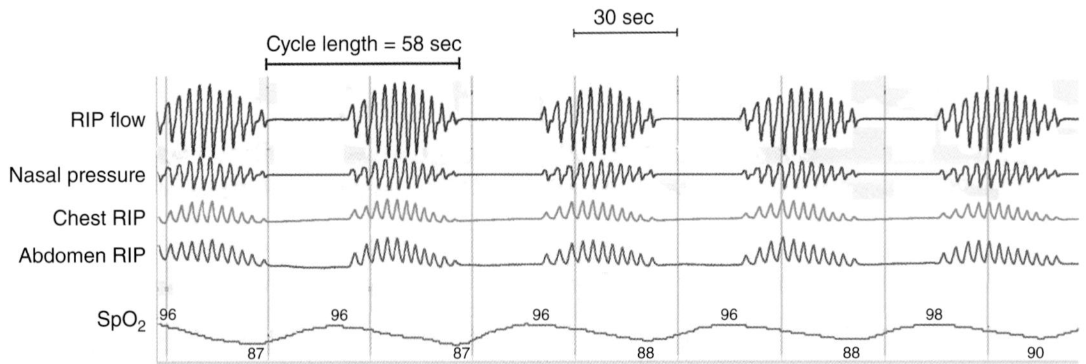

Figure 30-12 A tracing illustrating central sleep apnea with Cheyne-Stokes breathing (CSA-CSB). Note the crescendo-decrescendo breathing pattern between central apneas, the cycle length ≥40 seconds, and the delay in the SpO_2 nadir after the central apneas. RIPflow is the first time derivative of the RIPsum of the chest and abdomen and RIP deflections are an estimate of airflow. *RIP*, respiratory inductance plethysmography. (From Berry RB, Wagner MH. *Sleep Medicine Pearls*, 3rd edition. Philadelphia, PA: Elsevier; 419.)

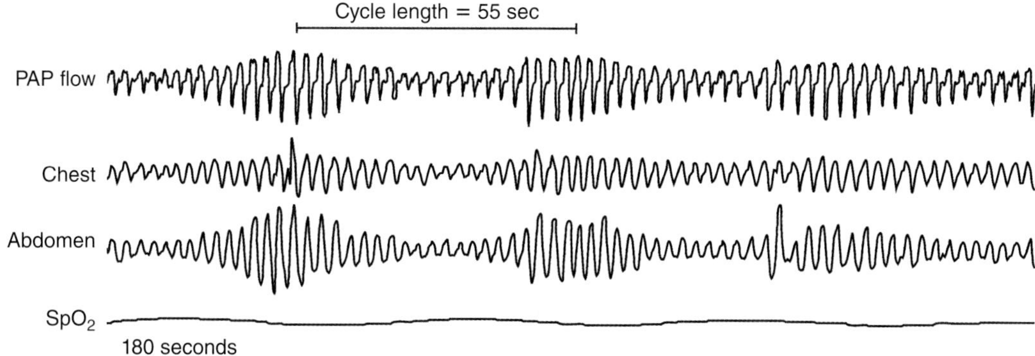

Figure 30-13 An example of Cheyne-Stokes breathing with hypopneas at the nadir of respiration (central hypopnea) on positive airway pressure (CPAP of 12 cm H_2O). PAP flow is the flow signal from the PAP device. In the diagnostic portion the patient had predominantly obstructive apneas. In this case the cycle length is measured from the peak ventilation of one cycle to the peak ventilation in the next cycle. From Berry RB, Wagner MH. *Sleep Medicine Pearls*, 3rd edition, Philadelphia, PA: Elsevier; 410.

central apneas, can occur at the nadir in effort (Figure 30-13). Not all sleep centers differentiate between central and obstructive hypopneas. The latest edition of the AASM scoring manual allows undifferentiated hypopneas to be included to determine the amount of CSB if the flow shows a crescendo-decrescendo pattern:

Score a respiratory event as CSB if BOTH of the following are met:[10]

- There are episodes of ≥3 consecutive central apneas and/or hypopneas separated by a crescendo and decrescendo change in breathing amplitude with a cycle length of ≥40 seconds. *To be included, the hypopneas must have a symmetrical crescendo-decrescendo pattern of tidal volume or flow.*
- There are ≥5 central apneas and/or hypopneas per hour of sleep associated with the crescendo-decrescendo breathing pattern recorded over ≥2 hours of monitoring.

The majority of patients with CSA with CSB (CSA-CSB) have either systolic or diastolic heart failure. Systolic heart failure is associated with a reduced ejection fraction (HFrEF) and diastolic heart failure with a preserved ejection fraction (HFpEF). In one study of stable patients with CHF with *reduced ejection fraction* treated with beta blockers, about 61% had moderate to severe sleep apnea (AHI ≥15 events/hour), 31% had predominantly central apnea with CSB, and 30% had predominantly OSA.[38] Other studies have found a higher percentage of predominant CSA (33%) versus predominant OSA (20%) in patients with HFrEF who have moderate to severe sleep apnea (AHI ≥ 15/hr, see Chapter 28).[39] CSA-CSB can also occur in patient with HFpEF (diastolic heart failure). About 47% of these patients have an AHI ≥ 15/hr and of these 47% predominant OSA was present in 23% and predominant CSA was present in 24%. Risk factors for the presence of CSA-CSB in CHF include the presence of *atrial fibrillation, male gender, age >60 years, hypocapnia, an increased left ventricular end diastolic pressure, and an increased left atrial size.*[40] Many patients with both HFrEF and HFpEF have a mixture of obstructive and central apneas. More discussion of sleep apnea and CHF is found in Chapters 20 and 28. CSA-CSB can also be noted in patients with atrial fibrillation, although most of these patients has some form of heart failure. Patients may also manifest CSA-CSB after a cerebrovascular accident (CVA) or associated with other neurological disorders.[41,42] In a meta-analysis of stroke and sleep apnea, about 38% had an AHI ≥20 events/hour, and 7% of the syndromes were primarily CSA.[42] That is, *OSA is the most common type of sleep apnea after stroke*. CSA is believed to be more common *early after stroke* and often resolves or converts to OSA. CSA-CSB in stroke could be caused by underlying CHF (including HFpEF/diastolic dysfunction). A study by Kim and coworkers[41] found CSB to frequently occur in strokes involving large arteries or those caused by cardioembolism, regardless of the location or severity of the stroke. Predisposing conditions such as preexisting neurologic disability, low left ventricular ejection fraction (LVEF), and left atrial enlargement were associated with CSB in acute stroke. CSA-CSB has been reported in patients with *renal disease* and could be a manifestation of fluid overload.[43] Idiopathic CSA-CSB has also been reported.[44]

In summary CSA-CSB is commonly noted in patients with HFpEF and HFrEF but can occur following stroke, as an idiopathic form, or associated with renal failure. The ICSD-3-TR diagnostic criteria for CSA with CSB include the following. Criteria (A **or** B) + (C–E) must be met[1]:

A. The presence of one or more of the following:
   1. Sleepiness.
   2. Difficulty initiating or maintaining sleep, frequent awakenings, or non-restorative sleep.
   3. Awakening short of breath
   4. Witnessed apneas
B. The presence of atrial fibrillation/flutter, CHF, or a neurological disorder
C. PSG (during ***diagnostic or PAP titration***) shows all of the following:
   1. Five or more central respiratory events (central apneas or central hypopneas) per hour of sleep
   2. The total number of central apneas plus central hypopneas is >50% of the total number of apneas and hypopneas
D. The pattern of ventilation meets criteria for CSB
E. The syndrome is not better explained by another current sleep disorder, medication use (e.g. opioids), or substance use

The diagnosis of CSA with CSB requires either symptoms (sleepiness, insomnia, awakening short of breath, or witnessed apnea) **or comorbidity** (atrial fibrillation/flutter, CHF, or a neurological disorder). In the absence of symptoms or comorbidities, one can simply say that CSA with a CSB pattern is present (a PSG finding). The comorbidity option was added, as many patients with CSA-CSB associated with heart failure do not report sleep issues or daytime sleepiness. PSG must show five or more central apneas or hypopneas per hour of sleep, and the total number of central events must be >50% of the total number of apneas and hypopneas. The pattern of ventilation must meet criteria for CSB according to the AASM scoring manual.[10] Note that the ICSD-3-TR specifies the PSG findings can occur *either during diagnostic or PAP titration sleep study*. A diagnosis of CSA-CSB ***during a PAP titration*** requires that respiratory events be predominantly central apneas and central hypopneas, at least during a portion of the night. For patients with a mixture of OSA and CSA-CSB, *the central apneas may appear only after elimination of obstruction on PAP (a type of CompSA)* (Figures 30-8 and 30-9). This scenario is often seen in patients with CHF who also have OSA.[45] CSA-CSB is uncommon during REM sleep, and in patients with CSA-CSB, a level of CPAP that is **not** effective during NREM sleep (continued CSA) may be effective during REM sleep (stage R) (Figure 30-14). The lateral sleeping position appears to reduce the severity of CSA-CSB.[46-48] Some key features of CSA-CSB are listed in Box 30-2. Note that, if CSA-CSB events are not sufficiently frequent to meet criteria, the presence of the events may simply be mentioned. As specified in the ICSD-3-TR, *a diagnosis of CSA with CSB does not preclude a simultaneous diagnosis of OSA. For example, if a patient meets diagnostic criteria for OSA during the diagnostic portion of a split sleep study but meets criteria for CSB-CSA during the titration portion of the study.*

CSA-CSB and Heart Failure

Many patients with heart failure have a mixture of obstructive, mixed, and central apneas.[38] The exact proportion of OSA and CSA in a given case can vary over time or during a single night. Patients with CSA-CSB caused by CHF have a low awake $PaCO_2$, an *increased* hypercapnic ventilatory response above and below eupnea, and a decreased $PaCO_2$ reserve. That is, the gap between the eupneic NREM $PaCO_2$ and the AT is reduced. The lower sleeping $PaCO_2$ reduces the plant gain, but the increase in ventilatory response to $PaCO_2$ results in a **net increase in loop gain** and a decrease in the gap between the AT and the baseline NREM $PaCO_2$, predisposing to central apnea (Figure 30-5). In addition, the long circulation time delays chemoreceptor measurement of the current $PaCO_2$, resulting in ventilatory overshoot (and undershoot) and giving the classic CSB crescendo-decrescendo breathing pattern between apneas. A study by Xie et al. compared patients with CHF with and without periodic breathing. Both groups had *similar awake $PaCO_2$ and AT values*. However, the *group with periodic breathing had a smaller increase in the $PaCO_2$ with sleep*, and this reduced the gap between the sleeping $PaCO_2$ and the AT (Figure 30-15).[49]

The increased ventilatory drive in patients with CSB during sleep is thought to be secondary to redistribution of fluid to the lungs, which results in interstitial edema and stimulates J receptors, which increase ventilatory drive via vagal afferents. The higher the pulmonary capillary pressure, the lower the

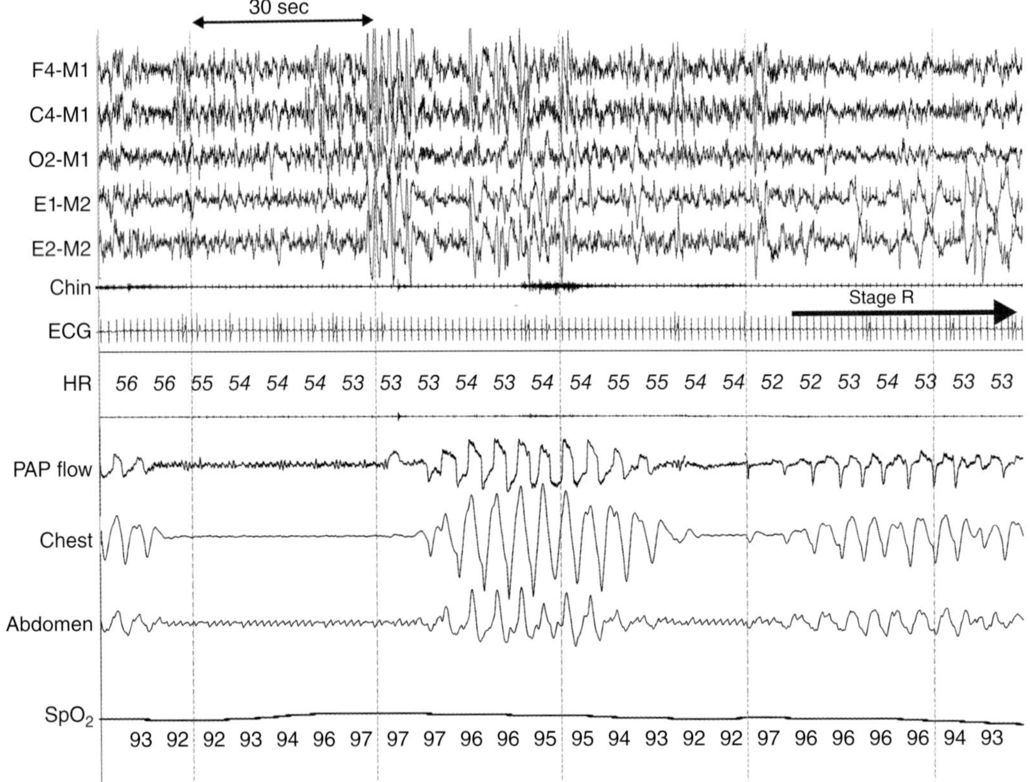

Figure 30-14 This tracing shows Cheyne-Stokes breathing on continuous positive airway pressure (CPAP) (PAP flow is flow from the laboratory PAP device) that suddenly resolves without any pressure change with the onset of REM sleep.

Box 30-2 KEY FEATURES OF CSA-CSB IN CHF

- Common in both HFrEF and HFpEF,
- Patients may have both OSA and CSA-CSB and CSA-CSB may be first noted during a PAP titration (a form of Complex Sleep Apnea)
- Common in stages N1, N2
- Uncommon in REM sleep (stage R)
- Worse in the supine position
- Longer cycle length is correlated with lower ejection fraction
- Low or normal daytime PCO_2
- High hypercapnic ventilatory response
- Small difference between sleeping $PaCO_2$ and the apneic threshold
- Relative amount of central versus obstructive apnea can increase during the night with redistribution of fluid to the lungs increasing pulmonary congestion and ventilatory drive. A decreasing $PaCO_2$ is a manifestation of the increased ventilatory drive

$PaCO_2$ (awake and asleep)[50] and the greater the amount of central apnea[51] (Figure 30-16). Note that there is often a shift from obstructive to central respiratory events over the night, with a progressive reduction in $PaCO_2$ caused by an increase in filling pressure.[52] The amount of CSA-CSB is greater in the second half of the night[53] and is likely caused by redistribution of fluid to the lungs with an increase in ventilatory drive contributing to ventilatory instability.

In patients with CSA-CSB caused by CHF, the cycle length depends on the ejection fraction (Table 30-6).[54] Patients with HFpEF tend to have shorter cycle lengths of 40 to 55 seconds,[54] and those with systolic CHF and lower ejection fractions have longer cycle lengths mainly *caused by a longer ventilatory phase*. Typically, there is also a delay in the nadir of desaturations following the events (longer circulation time). The crescendo-decrescendo pattern is caused by circulatory delay with a greater delay (longer ventilatory phase) associated with worse cardiac function. In patients with CSA-CSB, arousal from sleep tends to occur between apnea termination and the zenith of respiratory effort between contiguous central apneas or hypopneas (Figure 30-10). In contrast, in OSA, arousal typically occurs just before, at, or soon after event termination. *It is important to note that a normal ejection fraction does not rule out CSA-CSB.* In one study of heart failure with a normal ejection fraction, about 30% of a group with a normal ejection fraction had CSA-CSB.[55]

It has been estimated that CSA with CSB is present in approximately 25% to 40% of patients with heart failure (HF), including both HrEF and HpEF, and exposes the failing heart to hypoxia, arousals from sleep, sympathetic nervous system activation, and ventricular arrhythmias.[56] The presence of CSA-CSB in CHF implies a worse prognosis than that of patients without CSA-CSB.[57] There is ongoing debate about whether CSA contributes to mortality independently of other risk factors. That is, CSA-CSB may simply be a manifestation of poor cardiac function. In fact, it has been argued that CSB is a compensatory mechanism in patients with CHF.[58] On the other hand, CSB is associated with hypoxia, arousals, and sympathetic activation. For these reasons, treatment of CSA-CSB in CHF is considered desirable.[56]

Treatment of CSA-CSB

Treatment options for CSA-CSB are displayed in Table 30-7. The first treatment for CSA-CSB in patients with CHF is to *optimize treatment of heart failure*. Improvement or resolution of CSA-CSB can occur with medical treatment,[59] transplant,[60] or effective treatment of atrial fibrillation[61] and other

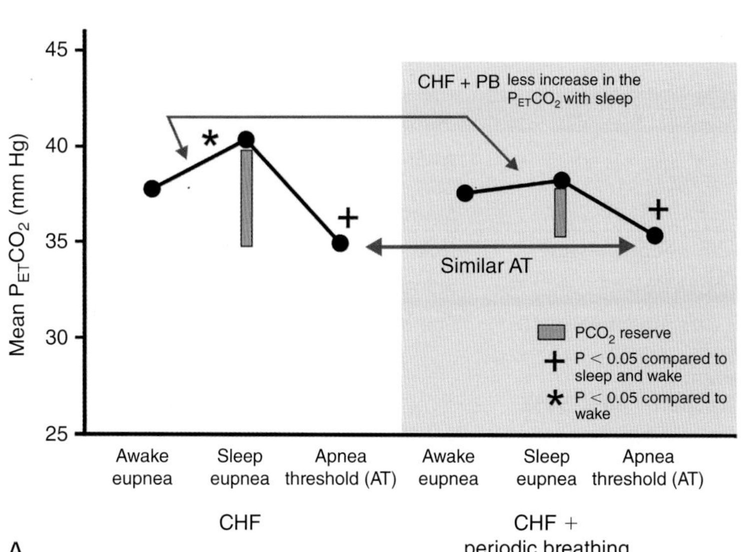

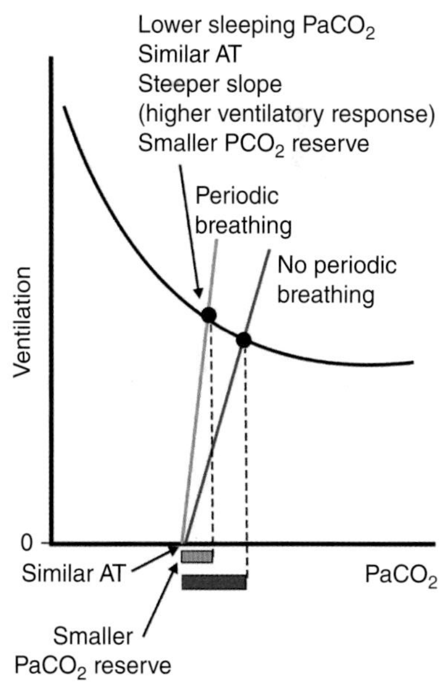

Figure 30-15 **A**, The awake eupnea end-tidal partial pressure of carbon dioxide ($PaCO_2$), sleeping $P_{ET}CO_2$, and apneic threshold (AT) for patients with congestive heart failure (CHF) with and without periodic breathing. The patients with periodic breathing had a small sleeping $P_{ET}CO_2$-AT difference. Although the AT values are similar between the two groups, there was a smaller increase in the PE_TCO_2 with sleep onset in the group with periodic breathing. **B**, Schematic illustrating findings of similar AT but lower sleeping $PaCO_2$. The slope (ventilatory drive above and below eucapnic) is higher in the group with periodic breathing. (Plotted using data from Xie A, Skatrud JG, Puelo DS, et al. Apnea-hypopnea threshold for CO_2 in patients with congestive heart failure. *Am Respir Crit Care Med.* 2002;165:1245-1250.)

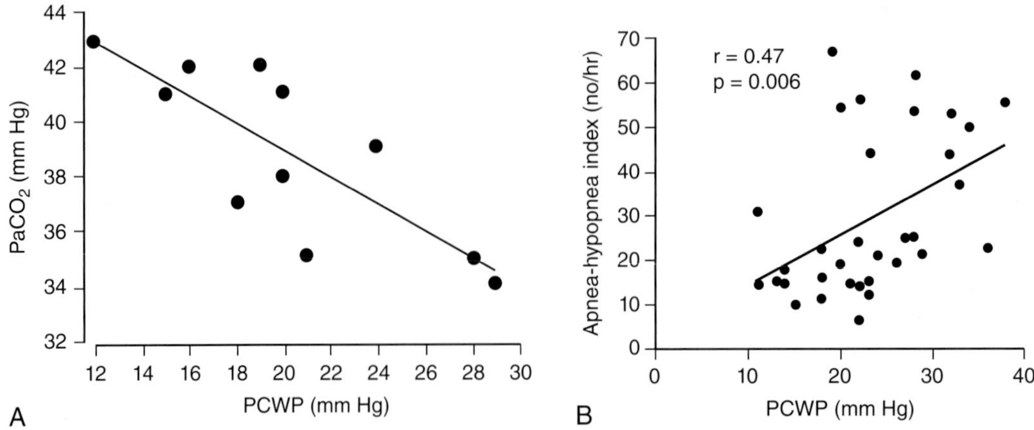

Figure 30-16 **A**, The higher the pulmonary capillary wedge pressure (PCWP), the lower the daytime arterial partial pressure of carbon dioxide ($PaCO_2$) in a group of patients with congestive heart failure. **B**, The relationship between the PCWP and the apnea-hypopnea index in patients with congestive heart failure in a group of patients with predominantly central apnea (>85% of respiratory events were central apneas or hypopneas). A higher PCWP is associated with a higher apnea-hypopnea index. Higher filling pressure and pulmonary congestion (interstitial edema) is believed to stimulate J receptors in the lung, which increase ventilatory drive via vagal afferents, as reflected in a lower awake $PaCO_2$ and during sleep and a higher apnea-hypopnea index due to increased central apneas. (A, Reproduced with permission of the © ERS 2023: *Euro Respir J.* 2002;19(1):37-40. doi:10.1183/09031936.02.00214502. B, From Solin P, Bergin P, Richardson M, et al. Influence of pulmonary capillary wedge pressure on central apnea in heart failure. *Circulation.* 1999;99:1574-1579.)

Table 30-6 Cheyne-Stokes Breathing (CSB) Cycle Length and Ejection Fraction (EF)

EF group	>50%	40%–49%	30%–39%	20%–29%	<20%
	Preserved EF	*Mildly impaired EF*	*Moderately impaired EF*	*Severely Impaired EF*	*Highly impaired*
EF mean (%)	61	43	33	24	15
Cycle length (sec)	49	59	60	74	85
Ventilatory Phase Duration (sec)	28	35	38	47.3	54.5
Apnea length (sec)	20.6	23.6	22.2	26.8	31.1

EF, left ventricular ejection fraction. The ventilatory phase occurs between central apneas (see Figure 30-10)
Wedewaredt J, Bitter T, Prinz C, et al. Cheyne-Stokes respiration in heart failure: cycle length is dependent of left ventricular ejection fraction. *Sleep Medicine.* 2010;11:137-142.

Table 30-7 Treatment Options for CSA-CSB Caused by CHF

Treatment of CSA-CSB	Comments	AASM Practice Parameters for Treatment of CSA due to CHF[37,39] (level of recommendation)-Standard>Guideline>Option
Optimize treatment of CHF	Central AHI correlated with wedge pressure	N/A
CPAP	Effective in about 50% of CSA-CSB	Standard
Adaptive servoventilation	Effective in most patients, treatment AHI <10 events/hour is common Also treats obstructive events **Do not use if ejection fraction <40%–50%**	Standard
Oxygen	Prevents desaturation, may reduce central apnea Can be used with CPAP (CPAP for obstructive events) Not covered by most insurance plans for CHF	Standard
BPAP-ST	If CPAP, ASV, oxygen are not effective	Option
Theophylline	Consider if PAP therapy not successful; can worsen ventricular arrhythmias	Limited evidence (option), rarely used
Acetazolamide	Consider if PAP therapy not successful	Limited evidence (option)
Transvenous phrenic nerve pacing	Effective for CSA but effects on mortality unknown	New treatment (not in guidelines)

CSA, central sleep apnea; *CSB*, Cheyne-Stokes breathing; *CHF*, congestive heart failure; PAP, positive airway pressure; *CPAP*, continuous PAP; *BPAP*, bilevel PAP; *ASV*, adaptive servoventilation; *AHI*, apnea-hypopnea index.

arrythmias. The use of beta blockers, afterload reduction, resynchronization, or left ventricular assist devices (LVADS) may improve CSA if the ejection fraction improves. A number of treatments can reduce CSA-CSB, at least in the short term. These include CPAP,[57,62,63] ASV,[64-67] oxygen,[68-71] BPAP with a backup rate,[65] acetazolamide,[72] theophylline,[73] and transvenous phrenic nerve pacing.[74,75] Avoidance of the supine position may also reduce CSA-CSB.[46-48] Benzodiazepines may reduce arousal in CSA-CSB.[76] While some observational studies show short-term benefit of PAP treatment, to date, no randomized controlled PAP study has shown mortality benefit in CHF with CSA-CSB. The 2012 AASM practice parameters for treatment of CSA[35,37] recommend the following for treatment of CSA associated with CHF: CPAP, nocturnal oxygen, ASV, and BPAP-ST (if oxygen, CPAP, and ASV are not effective). Options mentioned included theophylline and acetazolamide (limited evidence). The guidelines were updated to **not** recommend the use of ASV in patients with a low ejection fraction but did give ASV as an option in patients with better cardiac function or milder CSA-CSB.[37] A comparison of four treatments for CSA-CSB is shown in Figure 30-17.

A large trial of CPAP treatment in patients with CHF, a low ejection fraction, a moderate to severe AHI and predominantly CSA (CANPAP trial) randomized patients to CPAP (usually 8 to 9 cm H_2O) or a control arm. The titration was started at a CPAP of 5 cm H_2O and increased to 10 cm H_2O if tolerated. The study was stopped because of an increase in mortality in the treatment arm.[62] In this study, CPAP suppressed CSA (AHI <15 events/hour) in about 50% of individuals randomized to this treatment arm. Post-hoc analysis of CPAP **responders** found improvements in transplant-free survival and LVEF at 3 months compared to control.[63] Post-hoc findings are less convincing but suggest benefit from CPAP if there is a response in CSA-CSB. ASV was developed to treat periodic breathing, and several observational studies showed a benefit in patients with CSA-CSB.[65,64] For example, a study by Tescheler et al.[65] found that treatment with CPAP, BPAP with a backup rate, and oxygen treatment lowered the central AHI, but ASV was the most effective (Figure 30-17). However, a large trial (SERVE-HF) of ASV in patients with CHF (ejection fraction ≤ 45%, AHI ≥ 15/hour, and predominantly central events) was stopped because of increased all-cause and cardiovascular mortality in the treatment arm.[66] This led to the AASM recommendation to not use ASV in this group (EF ≤ 45%) but instead (option level) to use ASV in patients with a better ejection fraction or mild CSA-CSB.[37] There were a number of issues with the SERVE-HF study, including use of an older generation ASV that did not have the ability to adjust EPAP for obstructive events and an algorithm delivering relatively high pressure.[56,77] Another trial of a modern ASV device (Philips BiPAP AutoSV Advanced System One), also known as the ADVENT-HF[67] trial, was completed without a safety signal (the trial was not stopped for evidence of an adverse outcome with ASV) but the findings showed no improvement in cardiovascular outcomes including mortality with ASV treatment. ASV did improve dayime sleepiness and a quality of life measure and effectively lowered the AHI. The device used in this study automatically adjusts the EPAP and has the ability to deliver low pressure support. As many patients have a combination of OSA and CSA, this device can treat both issues. The study group had a low ejection fraction (<45%) and an AHI ≥15 events/hour and was divided into groups with predominant OSA (>50% of events obstructive) and predominant CSA (>50% of events central). The main study endpoints were survival and hospitalizations.[67] The effect of the ADVENT-HF study results on clinical practice remains to be determined. One option would be treatment with ASV in HFrEF patient with the goal of improving symptoms (if the patient consents in view of the possible risks). BPAP-ST could be tried rather than ASV, but most clinicians feel this is also contraindicated and will certainly deliver significant amounts of PAP to the chest. The group with CSA-CSB and a low ejection fraction could be treated with transvenous phrenic nerve pacing. Benefits with respect to sleep and quality of life have been demonstrated, but a mortality benefit remains undocumented at the time of this writing.[74,75]

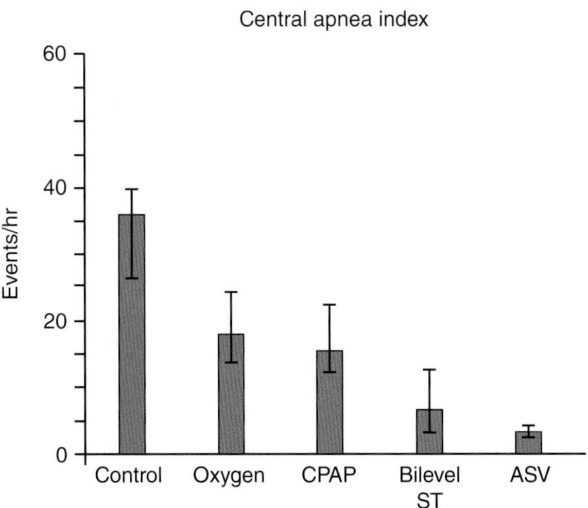

Figure 30-17 Median values (*bars are interquartile limits*) of the central apnea index at baseline and on treatment in patients with central apnea with Cheyne-Stokes breathing and heart failure. The patients all had systolic heart failure but were stable. Four treatments (oxygen, continuous positive airway pressure [CPAP], bilevel positive airway pressure [BPAP] with a backup rate, and adaptive servoventilation [ASV]) all reduced the central apnea index. All four treatments resulted in a central apnea index significantly lower than that of the controls (P <0.001). The greatest reduction was with ASV, but the difference was significantly different only when compared to CPAP and oxygen. The effects of ASV and spontaneous timed BPAP were similar. (Figure plotted using data from Teschler H, Döhring J, Wang YM, Berthon-Jones M. Adaptive pressure support servo-ventilation: a novel treatment for Cheyne-Stokes respiration in heart failure. *Am J Respir Crit Care Med.* 2001;164:614-619. PMID: 11520725.)

The AASM practice parameters recommend oxygen for CSA in patients with heart failure.[35] The recommendation is based on studies showing a benefit from treatment with supplemental oxygen.[65,68-71] For example, a study by Javaheri et al. found a reduction in the central AHI from 28 to 13 events/hour.[69] Using low flow oxygen will avoid the toxicity associated with higher oxygen concentrations. However, oxygen treatment for CSA in currently not covered by insurance. Not all patients respond to oxygen, which is believed to work by reducing loop gain (reduction in controller gain). One study found that those with the lowest awake $PaCO_2$ values (a maker for high ventilatory drive) were least likely to respond (a somewhat counterintuitive finding).[70] However, though oxygen may lower the loop gain in non-responders, the absolute value of loop gain may still remain elevated because of a higher baseline loop gain. Another group found a higher awake end-tidal PCO_2 (possibly associated with a lower controller gain) predicted a response to oxygen.[71] The group responding to oxygen in the study by Javaheri et al. also had a higher $PaCO_2$.[69] A combination of PAP and oxygen can also be used to treat CSA.[78]

Acetazolamide produces metabolic acidosis and increases the difference between the prevailing $PaCO_2$ and the AT $PaCO_2$ (the $PaCO_2$ reserve). This effect is thought to be the result of a reduction in plant gain. In a randomized, double-blind, placebo-controlled crossover study of 12 patients with HFrEF and severe CSA-CSB, acetazolamide administered before bedtime significantly decreased the central apnea index (CAI) from 57 to 34 per hour of sleep.[79] Patients reported improved sleep quality and reduced fatigue and daytime sleepiness. However, not all patients responded to this treatment.

Transvenous phrenic nerve stimulation is another potential treatment for CSA-CSB when other treatments are not effective or not appropriate. The device is approved by the U.S. Food and Drug Administration (FDA) for the treatment of moderate to severe CSA.[74,75] The indications are broad (moderate to severe CSA), without specific requirements for the exact allowable percentage of obstructive events. The device is implanted by an interventional cardiologist in a position to stimulate one phrenic nerve (left pericardiophrenic or right brachiocephalic vein). The potential use of magnetic resonance imaging (MRI) is a concern. There is conditional MRI clearance, depending on the body area and the strength of the MRI device. The pivotal trial (prospective observational study) had inclusion criteria that required an AHI >20 events/hour with *no more than 20% obstructive events*. The study found a >50% reduction in the AHI in the treatment group but only 11% in the control group (device implanted but not turned on). The median AHI in the treatment group decreased from 49.7 to 25.9 events/hour in the treatment group over 6 months and remained unchanged in the control group (43 to 45 events/hour). There was a significant improvement in the Epworth sleepiness scale, quality-of-life measures, and arousal index. Roughly 50% of the patients had CHF. Five year safety and efficacy outcomes documented continued efficacy in reduction of CSA and improvements in sleep architecture and daytime sleepiness. Of note, the device turns on automatically at night when the patient is in a supine position and not moving. The firing rate is usually set one or two breaths below the native respiratory rate, and stimulation strength (milliamps) can be set for different body positions (right, left, supine). The stimulator records adherence and efficacy information. The settings can be adjusted for improved efficacy. The role of this treatment in patients with CSA remains to be seen but seems promising. One issue to be resolved is how to approach the residual obstructive events. However, the concern that the device might increase obstructive events is not an issue. Combined treatment with CPAP (or an oral appliance) and pacing is one option. The treatment has a billing code. A few payors have published coverage policies for this treatment for eligible patients who meet certain criteria (usually moderate CSA). Other insurance providers, including Medicare, may cover the pacing treatment on a case-by-case basis, with evidence of medical necessity. Medicare has granted the device a pass through status (awarded by the US Department of Health and Human Services on a case-by-case basis for newly FDA-approved drug and device products). A useful publication discusses billing issues and methods to establish a pacing program.[80]

In summary, for patients with a normal ejection fraction and CSA-CSB that persists after optimization of cardiac function, one could start with CPAP. The effect of CPAP in this group with a normal EF has not been well studied but about 50% of patients with a low EF and CSA responsed to CPAP in the CANPAP trial.[62] Treatment with ASV in this population with a preserved EF is effective[64] at reducing the AHI and may provide symptomatic improvement (cardiovascular outcome benefit has not be proven by a randomized controlled trial). In those patients with CSA-CSB and a low ejection fraction, use of ASV is currently felt to be contraindicated. About 50% will respond to CPAP alone[63] and that treatment could be considered. Given the results of the ADVENT-HF study the medical community may someday be comfortable with use of modern ASV devices in patients with CSA-CSB and a low EF. Even if safe ASV has not been proven to improve cardiovascular outcomes. ASV treatment may improve symptoms. Those CHF patients with a low ejection fraction or not tolerating ASV could be candidates for phrenic nerve pacing. Transvenous phrenic nerve pacing might be beneficial but the effects on mortality are unknown. Supplemental oxygen, acetazolamide and position treatment could be tried. To date large randomized trials have not documented efficacy. It should be noted that neither supplemental oxygen nor CPAP treatment for CSA is covered by insurance. Many patients with CSA have some degree of obstructive apnea. If the obstructive AHI is ≥5 events/hour, CPAP treatment can be reimbursed for that indication.

Central Sleep Apnea Due to High-Altitude Periodic Breathing (CSA-HAPB)

High-altitude periodic breathing (HAPB) is characterized by alternating periods of central apnea and hyperpnea associated with a recent ascent to high altitude.[1,81-83]

The ICSD-3-TR[1] diagnostic criteria include (Criteria A-D must be met):

A. The breathing disturbance occurs at high altitude
B. The presence of one or more of the following:
   1. Sleepiness
   2. Difficulty initiating or maintaining sleep, frequent awakenings, or non-restorative sleep
   3. Awakening short of breath or morning headache
C. Witnessed periodic breathing or PSG performed at altitude demonstrates recurrent central apneas or central hypopneas with a central AHI ≥5 events/hour.
D. The syndrome is not better explained by another current sleep disorder, medical disorder, medication (e.g., narcotics), or substance use.

Key points concerning CSA-HAPB are listed in Box 30-3. Hypobaric hypoxia occurs at high altitude (fraction of inspired oxygen [FiO_2] = 0.21, but barometric pressure is lower than at sea level). CSA-HAPB should not be confused with altitude sickness, which is usually divided into three syndromes: acute mountain sickness, high-altitude cerebral edema, and high-altitude pulmonary edema. A discussion of these is beyond the scope of this chapter, and the subject is reviewed elsewhere.[84,85] The percentage of individuals exhibiting periodic breathing during sleep increases at higher altitudes. Approximately 25% exhibit periodic breathing at 2500 meters (8202 feet) and virtually 100% demonstrate periodic breathing at 4000 m (13,123 feet). Periodic breathing has been described at altitudes as low as 1500 meters (4900 feet)[1] As periodic breathing is a common response to altitude; *associated symptoms are required to make the diagnosis of a disorder*. There is no level of the central AHI separating a normal and abnormal response to high altitude. The cycle length of

Box 30-3 KEY POINTS: CSA DUE TO HIGH-ALTITUDE PERIODIC BREATHING (HAPB)

- Above 2500 to 3000 ft, most healthy subjects develop high-altitude periodic breathing, during NREM sleep. HAPB can occur at altitudes as low as 1500 m (4200 feet). About 25% have HAPB at 2500m (about 8200 feet) and and 100% have HAPB above 4000 m (about 13,000 feet)
- Underlying etiology is hypobaric hypoxia due to reduced partial pressure of inhaled oxygen (FiO_2 normal, Pb reduced)
- A hypoxia-induced increase in chemoreceptor sensitivity to changes in PCO_2 – both above and below eupnea – leads to periods of apnea and hyperpnea
- Hypoxic and hypercapnic ventilatory responses increase with altitude but the amount varies considerably between individuals (variation in basal individual responses to hypoxia)
- Central apnea caused by sleeping PCO_2 less than apneic threshold
- Cycle length shorter than Cheyne-Stokes breathing, as there is no circulatory delay. Quoted cycle lengths vary (shorter with higher altitude) but less than 40 seconds.
- Sleep architecture slowly improves after acclimatization to altitude with increased NREM and REM sleep **despite persistence of periodic breathing**
- The hypoxic ventilatory response continues to increase for several weeks in some individuals
- CSA due to HAPB is more common in men (higher ventilatory drive)
- Total sleep time and amount of REM sleep fairly preserved, increased stage N1, decreased stage N3, CSA usually in stage N1 and N2.

the periodic breathing is commonly less than 40 seconds and often as short as 12 to 20 seconds (some references say 12–34 seconds, and others report a cycle time of 12 to 20 or 30 to 45 seconds) (Figure 30-18). The variability in cycle time is likely caused by different experimental methods and the fact that studies were performed at different altitudes (cycle length decreases at higher altitude). Unlike in CSA-CSB, there is no circulatory delay. Differences in ventilatory time constants and circulation time between lung and chemoreceptors result in phase offset, thereby producing a cyclical pattern of breathing. The etiology of the periodic breathing during sleep at altitude depends on the removal of the "wakefulness drive" and the presence of an AT, usually a few mmHg below the waking levels of eupneic PCO_2 and the associated propensity for overshoot and undershoot in ventilation. Hypoxic stimulation of chemoreceptors (hypobaric hypoxia) in the carotid

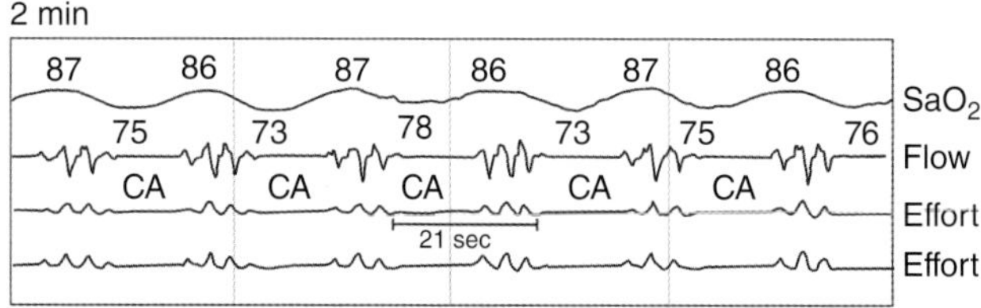

Figure 30-18 A 2-minute tracing of central sleep apnea occurring at high altitude (5050 meters). Note the relatively short central apneas and the cycle time. Even during the hyperpnea phases, the arterial oxygen saturation remains low due to hypobaric hypoxia. Flow was measured by a nasal cannula connected to a pressure transducer. (Adapted from Ainslie PN, Lucas SJ, Burgess KR. Breathing and sleep at high altitude. *Respir Physiol Neurobiol.* 2013;188(3):233-256. PMID: 23722066.)

body increases both the hypoxic and hypercapnic ventilatory responses. The resulting hyperventilation and lowering of the $PaCO_2$ tends to decrease loop gain by decreasing plant gain (sleeping $PaCO_2$ on the steep portion of the ventilation versus $PaCO_2$ isometablic hyperbola). However, the potential benefit is overwhelmed by the hypoxia-induced increase in the hypercapnic ventilatory response (overall loop gain increases). The increase in hypercapnic ventilatory drive above and below eupnea causes a decrease in the difference between the AT and the $PaCO_2$ (the PCO_2 reserve), predisposing to apnea following any decrease in the $PaCO_2$. The system oscillates between hypocapnic-induced apnea and apnea-induced hyperventilation. During the breathing clusters, the most obvious aspect of the periodicity is the oscillation of tidal volume with a less obvious change in breathing frequency. Like periodic breathing at sea level, resultant periodic breathing at **altitude** is often initiated by a movement, an arousal, or a deeper breath associated with a subsequent fall in the $PaCO_2$.

The amount of periodic breathing varies from night to night and among individuals and is usually most prominent in stages N1 and N2. The periodic breathing may persist even after sleep architecture improves with increases in stage N3 and stage R. That is, with acclimatization, sleep quality tends to improve, even though the amount of periodic breathing persists (may actually increase in some individuals). With acclimatization, one might expect that the increase in PaO_2 and cerebral blood flow (CBF) would mitigate the CSA. However, over time, both the hypoxic and hypercapnic ventilatory responses increase, causing an increase in loop gain, which is a counteracting force. The pattern of longtime residents at high altitude is periodic breathing and a normal sleep architecture.

Treatments for periodic breathing are listed in Table 30-8. Treatment for HAPB was not discussed in the AASM CSA treatment guidelines.[37] Descent is the most effective treatment and reverses the hypoxia that drives the process. Slow ascent, at a rate of 500 meters (1640 ft) per day above 2500 meters (8200 ft) elevation may help minimize HAPB. Acetazolamide improves both the mean level and stability of oxygenation during sleep at altitude and reduces the proportion of periodic breathing during sleep. The medication causes metabolic acidosis by increasing renal excretion of bicarbonate. This acts as a respiratory stimulant and lowers the baseline sleeping $PaCO_2$, thereby decreasing plant gain. Supplemental oxygen is also effective in reducing periodic breathing (as well as high altitude pulmonary edema). Several studies suggest the safety and potential utility of benzodiazepines for the treatment of sleep disturbance of high altitude.[86] Studies have evaluated the effects of temazepam, zaleplon, and zolpidem on sleep at altitude. In general, sleep quality improves (fewer arousals) without an effect on breathing. One study of BPAP with a backup rate found improved oxygenation during sleep.[87] Orr et al. compared supplemental oxygen and ASV and found oxygen but not ASV to be effective.[88] The standard ASV algorithms may not be effective with the pattern of breathing and shorter cycle length of HAPB. Another study found that stabilizing breathing (ASV) or increasing oxygenation (supplemental oxygen) during sleep can reduce feelings of fatigue and confusion, but that daytime hypoxia may play a larger role in other cognitive impairments reported at high altitude. Furthermore, this study provides evidence that some aspects of cognition (executive control, risk inhibition, sustained attention) improve with acclimatization.[89]

Table 30-8 Treatments of CSA Due to High-Altitude Periodic Breathing	
Descent to lower altitude	Reduces hypoxia stimulation of ventilatory control
Acetazolamide	Improves sleep and periodic breathing by inducing a metabolic acidosis and induced hyperventilation, decreasing plant gain, and widening the PCO_2 reserve. The increased PCO_2 reserve reduces the development of central apneas during sleep (PCO_2 reserve = eucapnic PCO_2 – AT) An effective prophylactic dose of acetazolamide is 125 mg twice daily, to be taken a day before ascent and continued for 2 days after the highest sleeping altitude
Supplemental oxygen	Reduces hypoxia and hypercapnic ventilatory drives
Benzodiazepine receptor agonists (BZ and Z drugs)	Improve sleep without affecting breathing pattern or cognitive function
Addition of dead space, positive pressure ventilation	Possible benefit, more studies needed. ASV algorithm may need adjustment

BZ, benzodiazepine; *Z drugs*, zaleplon, zolpidem, eszopiclone; *CSA*, central sleep apnea; *ASV*, adaptive servoventilation; *AT*, apneic threshold.

Treatment-Emergent Central Sleep Apnea

As discussed, the terms *CompSA* (used by the CMS and other insurance providers) and *TECSA* are often used to designate the same condition, but the ICSD-3-TR diagnostic criteria specify that the CSA in TECSA is not better explained by another CSA syndrome (e.g., CSA with CSB due to CHF or CSA due to a medication or substance). *The ICSD-3-TR added another requirement for the diagnosis of TECSA, mainly that symptoms or signs must be attributable to with the finding of residual central apneas.* That is, one cannot make a diagnosis at the time of a PAP titration. Strictly speaking, only if central events persist and *are associated with symptoms* can a diagnosis of TECSA be made using ICSD-3-TR criteria.

The ICSD-3-TR diagnostic criteria include (Criteria A-D) must be met:

A. Diagnostic PSG or home sleep apnea testing (HSAT) demonstrates five or more predominantly obstructive respiratory events (obstructive and mixed apneas, hypopneas, or respiratory effort-related arousals [RERAs] per hour of sleep (PSG) or per hour of monitoring (HSAT). (RERAs cannot be scored using most HSAT devices)

B. PSG during use of CPAP shows significant resolution of obstructive events and emergence or persistence of central apnea or central hypopnea with all of the following:
   1. Five or more central respiratory events (central apneas or central hypopneas) per hour of sleep
   2. The total number of central apneas plus central hypopneas is >50% of the total number of apneas and hypopneas

C. The presence of at least one of the following symptoms or signs thought to be attributable to the central events:
   1. Sleepiness
   2. Difficulty initiating or maintaining sleep, frequent awakenings, or nonrestorative sleep
   3. Awakening short of breath
   4. Witnessed apneas

D. The CSA is not better explained by another CSA disorder (e.g., CSA with CSB or CSA due to a medication or substance)

The ICSD-3-TR also states that the diagnosis should not be made solely on the treatment device report to detect clinically significant new or residual central events. It should be recognized that the CAI of a device download is often not accurate (see Chapter 23).[113] Repeat PSG should be considered to document the central nature of respiratory events, if clinically indicated.

There is ongoing discussion about how to define CompSA/TECSA.[90] Many studies of TECSA discussed herein included a few patients on opioids and with CHF, who can exhibit a CompSA pattern. This discussion focuses primarily on TECSA as defined in the ICSD-3-TR. *It should be emphasized that a diagnosis of both OSA and TECSA can be made.* Many studies of the natural history of TECSA required a CAI ≥ 5 events/hour on PAP to qualify for this diagnosis, while others required a CAI ≥10 events/hour. The finding of a shift from obstructive to central apnea after treatment of OSA is not new and was noted after tracheostomy for OSA.[91,92] The central apneas usually resolved with time. It has also been noted that some patients had frequent central events during NREM sleep on the same pressure that was effective during REM sleep.[93] TECSA shares the same propensity for central events to occur during NREM sleep but not during REM sleep, as with the other causes of hypocapnic CSA (Figure 30-19).

Patients with TECSA are thought to have instability in ventilatory control (high loop gain) or a sleep-state instability.[6,93] The increased loop gain is due to a high controller gain. The underling instability is believed to be exacerbated ("uncovered") by CPAP or BPAP without a backup rate which eliminate high upper airway resistance and increase ventilation for a given amount of ventilatory drive (increased effective plant gain). CPAP also increases lung volume, and this would decrease plant gain, but the effect of high controller gain is predominant. Patients with OSA exhibit a higher propensity to induced central apnea and higher loop gain than healthy matched adults.[94,95] PAP therapy for 4 weeks is associated with decreased controller gain and widening of the CO_2 reserve (difference between the sleeping $PaCO_2$ and the $PaCO_2$ at the AT).[95] This may explain the resolution of TECSA with chronic CPAP treatment in the majority of patients. Hypoxia reduces PCO_2 reserve (Figure 30-7) and increases the propensity for central apnea.[96] Resolution of hypoxia on CPAP could reduce the chance of central apnea. Intermittent hypoxia has been shown to increase peripheral chemoreceptor activity and is associated with increased propensity for central apnea.[97] Patients with TECSA tend to have small difference between the sleeping PCO_2 and the AT and difficulty reaching stable sleep (frequent arousals). Arousal results in a lower PCO_2 on

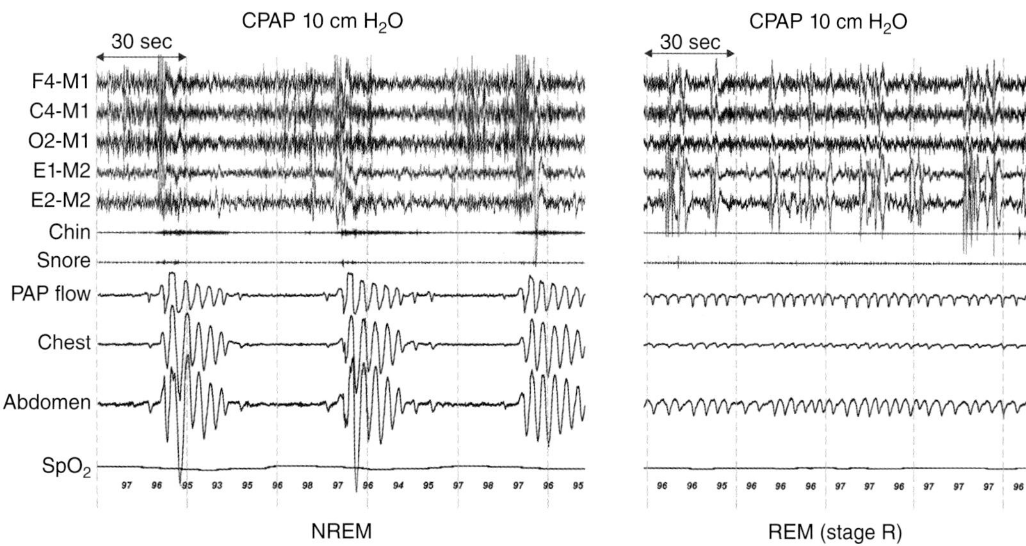

Figure 30-19 Effect of REM sleep on central apnea. During the diagnostic portion of a split sleep study, this patient had obstructive apneas and hypopneas. When placed on CPAP, he developed central apneas during NREM sleep, but during REM sleep on the same pressure, ventilation was stable. This patient had no history of heart failure (normal echocardiogram) or opioid medication intake. The respiration between central apneas shows a peak flow on the second breath followed by a decrescendo pattern (not a CSB pattern). This is an example of central apnea meeting the ICSD-3-TR definition of treatment-emergent central sleep apnea. Hypocapnic central sleep apnea usually resolves during REM sleep. Note that the ICSD-3-TR requires that the residual central apneas be associated with symptoms or signs.

return to sleep and increases the risk for CSA. If central apneas appear on CPAP, a switch to BPAP **without a backup rate** is likely **to increase** the amount of central apnea,[98,99] as this augments ventilation (increasing plant gain). *It should be noted that the AT and CO_2 reserve can vary in a given individual over time and can be altered by a number of conditions.*[19] For example, TECSA is much more common at high altitude. Identified risk factors for TECSA have varied among studies (Box 30-4) but include NREM > REM, men > women, residence at high altitude, high levels of CPAP or BPAP without a backup rate, high mask leak, high AHI, presence of central apneas on the diagnostic study or diagnostic portion of a split study, supine > non-supine position, and use of a split sleep study.[100-104] As noted, *a change from CPAP to BPAP without a backup rate in response to central apneas is not indicated.* BPAP will increase the chance of ventilatory overshoot and may increase the frequency of central apneas. Measurement of loop gain may predict those patients with TECSA that may respond to chronic CPAP treatment.[104] Higher loop gain is associated

Box 30-4 RISK FACTORS FOR TREATMENT EMERGENT CENTRAL SLEEP APNEA**

- NREM (stages N1, N2) > Stage R
- Men > women
- Supine position > non-supine position
- High AHI in diagnostic study
- Central apneas during the diagnostic study
- Split study > a separate night for PSG titration
- High CPAP (over-titration), use of BPAP without a backup rate
- High altitude, oral breathing
- Mask leak

**Opioids and congestive heart failure are additional risk factors for/CompSA.
AHI, apnea-hypopnea index; *PSG*, polysomnography; *CPAP*, continuous positive airway pressure; *BPAP*, bilevel positive airway pressure.

with persistent CSA on PAP. Tracings from a CPAP titration of a patient with TECSA who had no central apneas during the diagnostic study are shown in Figure 30-19. *On the same level of CPAP, there is good control of respiratory event during REM sleep but central apneas during NREM sleep.*[93]

In reviewing the literature on TECSA, it is important to note that the goal of many studies was to determine how many patients *undergoing a CPAP study* had TECSA on the PAP titration. *An entirely different question to be answered* is, how many patients with TECSA on an initial PAP titration study have persistent TECSA on chronic PAP treatment? The overall incidence of TECSA (of patients with a PAP titration) varies among studies but is believed to be about 8% with a wide range (3.5–20%), with TECSA defined as a CAI >5 events/hour on CPAP.[100,101] The outcome of patients with TECSA treated with chronic CPAP has been investigated by several observational studies[102-110] and one randomized trial.[111] The percentage of patients with sustained CSA after chronic treatment varied from 14% to 46%, with an average of around 25% to 30%.[100,101] In some of these studies, a good percentage of patients with TECSA on an initial study did not complete a second titration and possibly stopped using PAP. Therefore, the percentage with **sustained CSA** on CPAP may be underestimated. A meta-analysis by Nigram et al. found 0.9% to 3.2% of ***patients with OSA undergoing PAP treatment*** *had persistent CSA on long-term treatment.*[100] This should not be confused with the percentage of those with TECSA/CompSA on the CPAP titration *with persistent CSA on chronic CPAP treatment.* Of interest, a small percentage of patients *without* TECSA on the initial study will have CSA on a later titration study – the so called "delayed emergent group."[109] A large study using telemonitoring found 3.5% of patients treated with PAP had CSA on CPAP at either week 1 or week 3 of treatment. A CAI ≥5 events/hour was required to define CSA on CPAP. Three trajectories were noted (Figure 30-20) over

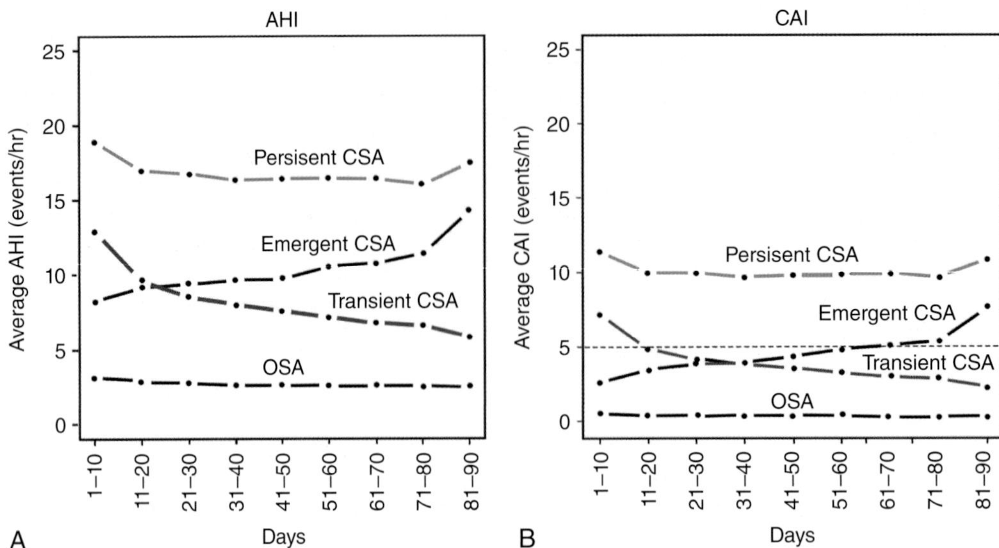

Figure 30-20 The trajectory of patients with obstructive sleep apnea treated with CPAP studies during a titration and at a later time. The graphs show the values of the apnea-hypopnea index (AHI) (**A**) and the central apnea index (CAI) (**B**). There was a group with resolution of central sleep apnea (CSA) (transient CSA), a group having CSA only on the follow-up study (emergent CSA), and a group with persistent CSA on CPAP. (From Liu D, Armitstead J, Benjafield A, et al. Trajectories of emergent central sleep apnea during CPAP therapy. *Chest*. 2017;152(4):751-760. PMID: 28629918.)

90 days of treatment: transient CSA (central apnea resolved on treatment in about 55%), persistent CSA (central apnea did not resolve on CPAP in about 25%), and delayed emergent CSA (CSA was not present at the first titration or on early treatment but appeared on treatment in 19.7%).[112] Patients with TECSA were at higher risk of therapy termination than those who did not develop CSA. Those patients with TESCA that do not experience resolution of central apneas on chronic PAP treatment are found to have a high number of residual events on PAP machine interrogation in clinic follow-up. Nocturnal oximetry at home on PAP treatment may show persistent arterial oxygen desaturation. Sleep fragmentation and daytime sleepiness may persist if a significant number of central apneas remain. This may explain the potential for poor adherence and decreased acceptance of PAP treatment in those with persistent CSA. It should be noted that the PAP device classification of residual events as clear airway (central) is often not accurate,[113] and the residual AHI estimate based on flow may not be accurate if there is high leak. Therefore, one should not assume that device data showing residual central apneas on PAP is always accurate. The other question to consider is, *does a residual CAI of 5 events/hour have clinical significance*? The symptomatic response of the patient to treatment is an important consideration when evaluating the clinical significance of residual central apnea on CPAP. The ICSD-3-TR diagnostic criteria would not classify a patient without symptoms or complaints as having TECSA-solely on the basis of residual central apneas.

TECSA After Non-PAP Treatment

TESCA has been reported after non-PAP treatments for OSA,[114-118] including mandibular advancement devices (MADs),[115] upper airway surgery (including tracheostomy, uvulopalatopharyngoplasty [UPPP], and mandibular maxillary advancement),[116] and hypoglossal nerve stimulation (HNS).[117] TECSA has also been reported followin nasal surgery.[118]

Treatment of TECSA/CompSA

There are really two approaches to treatment of TECSA on CPAP: a trial of CPAP for several months or an immediate move to titration with BPAP with a backup rate (BPAP-ST or ASV). While treatment with CPAP alone may be an effective treatment approach in many patients, several studies have documented the effectiveness of ASV[111,119-121] or noninvasive positive pressure ventilation (NPPV; BPAP-ST).[119,121] Two randomized trials comparing BPAP-ST with ASV (one trial included a mixture of TECSA and other CSAs) found both treatments to effectively reduce the AHI, but ASV was more effective.[119,121] A randomized trial of *CPAP versus ASV* for treatment of TECSA[111] required a CAI ≥10 events/hour on CPAP for entry. On long-term CPAP, treatment about one-third in the CPAP group had a residual AHI >10 events/hour and about two-thirds had an AHI > 5 events/hour. The mean residual AHI was lower on ASV (4.4 vs. 9.9 events/hour, $p = 0.0024$) and a higher percentage achieved the goal of a residual AHI <10 events/hour (90% in the ASV group and 65% in the CPAP group, $p = 0.0214$). *However, neither the adherence, improvement in sleepiness (Epworth sleepiness scale) or change in quality of life differed between the CPAP and ASV groups.* Thus, though ASV was better at reducing the residual AHI, other outcomes were similar with CPAP. Though ASV is almost uniformly effective, using ASV on every patients with TECSA would result in use of a $4000 device in many patients when an $800 device would suffice. On the other hand, the "CPAP failures" are at risk for treatment failure (high residual AHI, low adherence, or cessation of PAP treatment). A telemonitoring study by Pepin et al.[122] compared three groups of patients with TECSA: those using only CPAP, those using only ASV, and those who switched from CPAP to ASV. The adherence rates for CPAP only (73.8%) and ASV only (73.2%) were similar, but the initial adherence in the switch group was 62.7% initially on CPAP, improving to 76.6% on ASV. This suggests that overall adherence in patients with TECSA is slightly better with ASV but that switching a patient with lower adherence on CPAP to ASV may improve adherence.

Approach to Treatment of TECSA (CompSA)

The best treatment approach for patients with CompSA/TECSA is still controversial. The AASM practice parameters for CSA do not address treatment for TECSA. If central apneas appear during a titration observation is indicated as they may resolve if the patient transitions to stable sleep. High leak should be addressed as frequent arousals from leak or ineffective mask pressure due to high leak could be preventing stable sleep. Otherwise one could try lower or higher levels of CPAP. Over titration can cause central apneas. If the patient was doing well on a lower pressure a reduction in pressure is definitely indicated. BPAP without a backup rate should not be used as this can cause worsening of CSA. It is important to demonstrate that a level CPAP has effectively reduced obstructive events. The ICSD-3-TR says "a significant resolution off obstructive events". CMS requires an obstructive AHI < 5/hour to qualify a patient for BPAP with a backup rate. To obtain a BPAP with a backup rate under CMS RAD criteria three findings must be demonstrated (Table 30-4). First, there has been a resolution of obstructive events with CPAP (obstructive AHI < 5/hr). Second, the emergence or persistence of a sufficient number of central apneas to meet criteria for CompSA once there is significant improvement or resolution of obstructive events. Third, one must demonstrate effective treatment of central events with BPAP with a backup rate.

A clinical pathway for treatment of CompSA/TECSA is shown in (Figure 30-21). In patients with a CompSA pattern associated with CSA-CSB or CSA due to a medication or substance many clinicians would immediately proceed with ASV treatment if the **central AHI** is high (>5 to 10 events/hour) and/or sleep was poor on the initial CPAP titration. In these patient CSA rarely resolves with chronic CPAP treatment. Some sleep centers have a protocol for addressing CompSA during the titration portion of a split sleep study. However, this is often difficult due to a time constraint. In most cases a subsequent PAP titration study is needed. An entire night for the titration is available either as a repeat titration following a split sleep study or as the initial titration following a diagnostic PSG. The titration must demonstrate the three finidings previously discussed to qualify the patient for either a E0470 or E0471. However, E0471 (BPAP with a backup rate should be used. It is not enough to simply demonstrate a pattern of CompSA (Table 30-4).

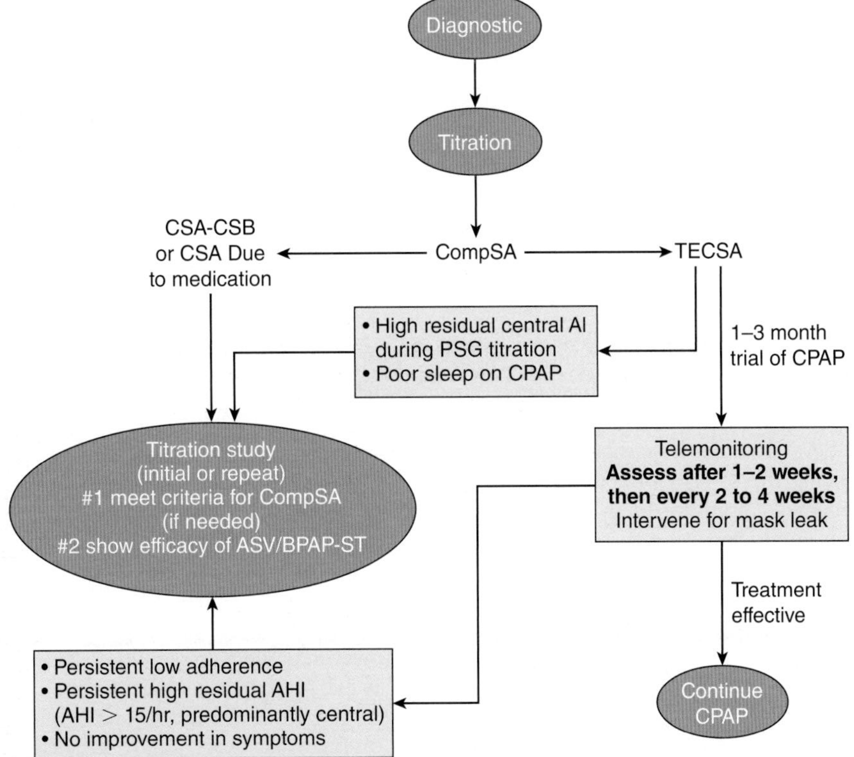

Figure 30-21 An approach to complex sleep apnea (CompSA), including treatment-emergent central sleep apnea (TECSA) (using the ICSD-3-TR definition) is shown. If patients with central sleep apnea (CSA) with Cheyne-Stokes breathing (CSB) or CSA due to a medication or substance exhibit persistent or emergent central apnea during the continuous positive airway pressure (CPAP) titration, the central apnea usually does not resolve with chronic CPAP treatment and initial treatment with BPAP with a backup rate is indicated. Effective treatment of CSA with BPAP with a backup rate must be demonstrated by PSG. This assumes ASV is not contraindicated due to a low ejection fraction. If no explanation is apparent for the emergence/persistence of central apneas on PAP, the diagnosis is TECSA, and there are two approaches. #1. A trial of chronic treatment with CPAP will result in resolution of CSA in about two-thirds of patients (higher in some studies) and is less expensive. The risks are low adherence, cessation of treatment because of lack of symptomatic benefit, and ineffective treatment. These issues can be noted with close follow-up. Lack of improvement would result in a titration with ASV (or BPAP-ST). #2. The other approach is to proceed with titration and treatment with a BPAP device with a backup rate rather than chronic CPAP treatment. This approach is expensive but reasonable in patients with a high residual central apnea-hypopnea index or poor sleep on CPAP during the initial titration. These patients are likely at a higher risk of failure of CPAP treatment.

If CSA-CSB is present and the ejection fraction is <45%, at this point in our knowledge, treatment with ASV is contraindicated. For those with TECSA (as defined by the ICSD-3-TR), it appears that roughly 60% of patients will respond to chronic CPAP, depending on the definition of success. A CPAP level for treatment at home is chosen that will eliminate most obstructive events (avoiding high pressures associated with frequent central apneas). However, those with a high residual central AHI (> 10/hr) or poor sleep on the initial exposure CPAP may benefit from immediate ASV treatment. If CPAP is used for patients with TECSA, close follow-up in the first few weeks after the initiation of treatment is essential (typically with telemonitoring and interventions for mask leak and pressure issues). If the AHI remains elevated, symptoms have not improved, or adherence remains poor, an ASV/BPAP-ST titration should be ordered (initial documentation of CSA on CPAP and resolution on ASV/BPAP-ST). Fortunately, now that telemonitoring is possible, one can easily follow the course of the residual AHI and adherence. *The main challenge is to review the data in a timely manner.* BPAP- ST can also be used for TECSA. Overall, ASV is more efficacious than CPAP or BPAP-ST in eliminating respiratory events in patients with TECSA.[121] An alternative treatment for TECSA is a combination of oxygen and CPAP.[78] However, currently CSA is not an approved indication for oxygen therapy for most insurance providers. Oxygen therapy has been proven to reduce the CAI even in the absence of associated nocturnal hypoxemia. Hyperoxia works by lowering carotid-body chemosensitivity, therefore buffering oscillations in ventilatory control. The addition of oxygen to CPAP may result in better control of TECSA via reduction of the respiratory drive. One study of Veterans Affairs patients showed use of CPAP and oxygen was effective at reducing central apnea in those not responding to CPAP alone.[78] Acetazolamide is a carbonic anhydrase inhibitor or mild diuretic that increases bicarbonate excretion causing a mild metabolic acidosis. The induced acidosis is associated with shift in the hypercapnic ventilatory response to the left without a change in the slope (Figure 30-6). The results is a mild decrease in the baseline sleeping $PaCO_2$ and an increase in the PCO_2 reserve decreasing the chance of reaching the AT and the associated central apnea. Several studies have shown the efficacy of acetazolamide in reducing the severity of central apnea,[72,79] and a case report documented improvement in TECSA with acetazolamide.[4,123] There is empiric evidence that administration of acetazolamide is associated with widening of the PCO_2 reserve, in part attributed to decreased plant gain. Some patients with TECSA will have more central events in the supine position, and positional treatment was useful in one case of TECSA that developed on hypoglossal nerve stimulation.[124,5] Several other studies have noted increased central apnea frequency in the supine position in other CSA conditions.[46-48] This finding is likely attributed to the association of the supine position with passive upper airway collapse during CSA, lower lung volumes (increased plant gain), and worsened pulmonary vascular congestion and the associated increase in ventilatory drive. *Therefore, positional treatment could be a possible therapy for TECSA* (on CPAP or other treatments for OSA).

NON-HYPOCAPNIC CSA DISORDERS

Central Sleep Apnea Due to a Medication or Substance

In this disorder, the central apneas are believed to be caused by a potent long-acting opioid or other respiratory suppressant medication. *The most common offending drug is methadone.* However, the condition has also been described in patients taking long-acting forms of morphine or oxycodone and in individuals being treated with fentanyl patches or constant narcotic infusions.[125,127-130] Suboxone (a combination of buprenorphine and naloxone) is often used for treatment of patients with narcotic dependence and pain but can also cause drug-induced central apnea. The description of the population with CSA Due to a Medication or Substance is complicated by the fact that many of the patients are on several drugs (both prescribed and illicit) that may affect sleep and breathing. It is also worth noting that the dose of methadone used for treatment of opioid dependance is much lower than typically used for pain. At lower doses, daytime sleepiness or breathing abnormalities are less common. Central apnea has also been reported to be associated with ticagrelor (an antiplatelet medication used in acute coronary syndrome),[131] baclofen (a muscle relaxant and $GABA_B$ agonist),[132] and sodium oxybate (also a $GABA_B$ agonist).[133]

An adaptation of the ICSD-3-TR diagnostic criteria for CSA Due to a Medication or Substance include the following (criteria A-D must be met):

A. The patient is taking an opioid, ticagrelor, or other medication known to impact respiratory control.
B. The presence of one or more of the following:
   1. Sleepiness
   2. Difficulty initiating or maintaining sleep, frequent awakenings, or non-restorative sleep
   3. Awakening short of breath
   4. Witnessed snoring
C. PSG (**diagnostic or on PAP**) shows all of the following:
   1. Five or more central respiratory events (central apneas or central hypopneas) per hour of sleep (PSG)
   2. The total number of central apneas plus central hypopneas is >50% of the total number of apneas and hypopneas
D. The disorder is not better explained by another current sleep disorder or medical disorder.

Abnormal breathing patterns in this disorder include ataxic breathing (irregular variations in respiratory cycle time and tidal volume), Biot's breathing (irregular tidal volume), cluster breathing, or Cheyne-Stokes breathing. In the ICSD-3[125] the absence of CSB was a diagnostic criteria. This criterion was removed in the ICSD-TR given some reports of a pattern of CSB in patients on respiratory suppressing medications. However, while a crescendo decrescendo pattern of breathing may be present secondary to medications,true CSB with a cycle length of at least 40 seconds is usually not seen unless a component of heart failure is present. The typical breathing pattern in CSA due to a medication is NOT consistent with CSB. Nocturnal or daytime hypoventilation may be present but is not required.An additional diagnosis of Sleep-Related Hypoventilation Due to Medication or Substance can be made if criteria are met. In the ICSD-3[125] diagnostic criteria included a statement that the PSG findings could be present on either a diagnostic or PAP titration sleep study. *This is not included in the ICSD-3-TR but is included here as a pattern of CompSA can occur as will be discussed below.*

As noted, patients commonly have both CSA and additional abnormalities of respiration, including a low respiratory rate, severe OSA, and ataxic breathing (variation in rate and magnitude of flow) Figure 30-22. A diagnosis of CSA due to

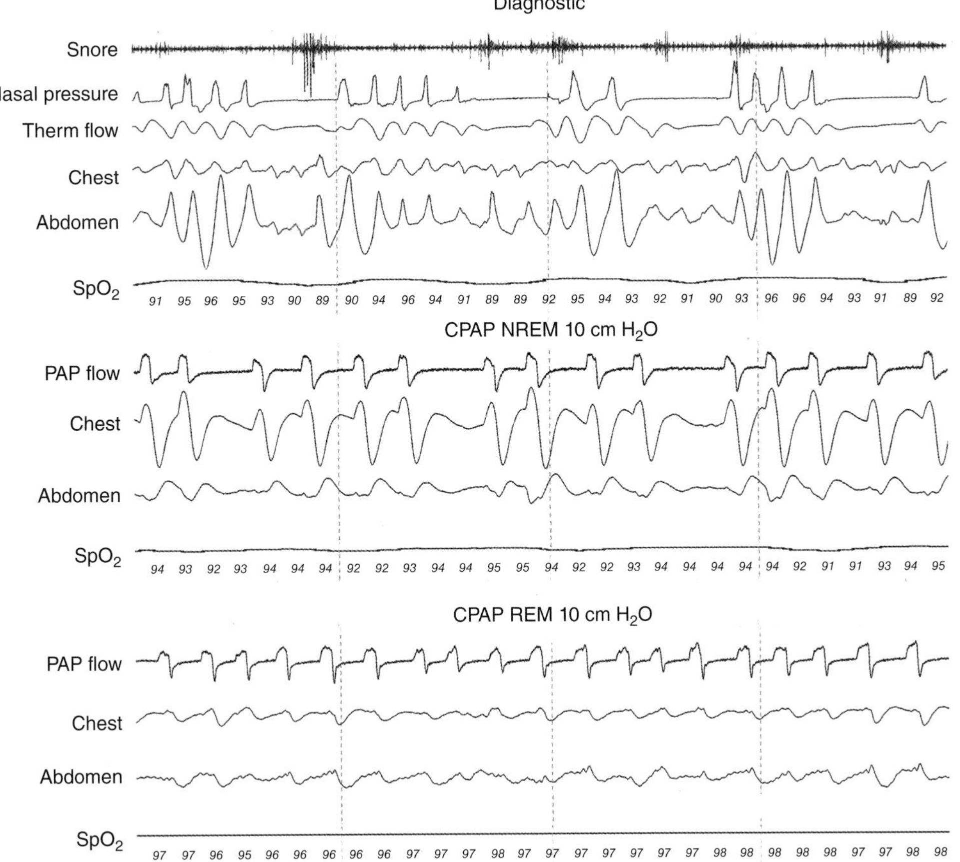

Figure 30-22 Three 120-second tracings of a patient taking methadone. The top tracing is the diagnostic study showing obstructive sleep apnea (OSA) and an irregular pattern of breathing. This is an example of ataxic breathing. The second is on continuous positive airway pressure (CPAP) of 10 cm H_2O during NREM sleep, showing central apneas also with an irregular pattern of breathing (ataxic breathing). The third is on CPAP of 10 cm H_2O during REM sleep. This pattern of better control on CPAP during REM sleep compared to NREM sleep is similar to that noted in patients with CSA-CSB on CPAP and with TECSA on CPAP. Unlike TECSA (ICSD-3-TR definition), CSA in patients on opioids usually does not improve with chronic CPAP treatment, and most need treatment with some type of BPAP with a backup rate (e.g., adaptive servoventilation). Although usually not possible, weaning and discontinuation of the responsible medication is the best treatment.

Box 30-5 KEY POINTS: CENTRAL SLEEP APNEA DUE TO A MEDICATION OR SUBSTANCE

Opioid-Induced Sleep-Related Breathing Disorders

- Low respiratory rate
- Ataxic breathing – variations in cycle length and airflow magnitude
- Obstructive sleep apnea (OSA) – long events, OSA is the most common form of breathing disorder in patients taking narcotics
- Central sleep apnea – intermittent events or as a form of periodic breathing. More common during NREM than REM sleep
- Complex sleep apnea pattern can occur
- Sleep-related hypoventilation (with or without awake hypoventilation) can be present
- Excessive daytime sleepiness – even with effective treatment
- CSA due to effects of opioid on Mu receptors in the Pre-Botzinger Complex (ventral respiratory group in the medulla)

Medications Associated With CSA Due to a Medication or Substance

Opioids

- Methadone – medication most frequently associated with CSA Due to a Medication or Substance
- Oxycodone
- Fentanyl
- Suboxone (buprenorphine and naloxone)
- Morphine sulfate
- Hydromorphone

Other Respiratory Suppressant Medications

- Ticagrelor
- Sodium oxybate ($GABA_B$ receptor agonist)
- Baclofen ($GABA_B$ receptor agonist)

a medication or substance does not exclude a diagnosis of OSA (if obstructive AHI ≥ 5 events/hour). *The central apneas may appear only after the patient has been started on PAP (a form of CompSA).*[130,134] Patients may be completely unaware that significant hypoventilation is present, as the opioid medications decrease dyspnea.

Important facts concerning CSA Due to a Medication or Substance are listed in (Box 30-5). Webster et al.[128] evaluated a group of patients on narcotics for pain and found an AHI ≥5 events/hour in 75% of patients (39% had OSA, 4% had sleep apnea of indeterminate type, 24% had CSA, and 8% had both CSA and OSA). They found a direct relationship between the AHI and the daily dosage of methadone ($p = 0.002$).

The etiology of opioid-induced sleep-related breathing disorders is believed to be depression of central drive by opioid mediations (specifically, *action on the Mu opioid receptors on respiratory pattern generating neurons of the pre-Bötzinger area of the ventral respiratory group in the medulla).* Upper-airway muscle activity is also reduced by these opioid medications. Although opioid-induced CSA is typically placed in the non-hypercapnic/hypercapnic CSA group, patients often have either normal or only mildly increased awake $PaCO_2$ values (45–50 mmHg). During sleep, patients may develop sleep-related hypoventilation even if the awake $PaCO_2$ is normal. Patients with awake hypoventilation experience a further increase in $PaCO_2$ during sleep. As noted, a high level of suspicion for hypoventilation is needed, as patients often report no sensation of dyspnea. Of interest in some patients with opioid-induced sleep-related breathing disorders with CSA is that the AHI NREM is greater than the AHI REM. That is, central apneas are more common in NREM sleep than in REM sleep (Figure 30-22). A level of CPAP effective during stage R may not be effective in NREM sleep (high number of residual central apneas, a CompSA pattern).[134]

Some patients taking potent opioids may have *relatively few arousals and an increase in stage N3 sleep.* However, other studies have reported impaired sleep quality, including a reduction in REM sleep, increased arousals, and decreased stage N3. In any case, patients often complain of severe sleepiness that may not improve with chronic PAP treatment.

This is likely because of a sedative medication effect. Note that, in studies of patients on methadone maintenance, sleepiness is not a common complaint. However, the dose of medication used for methadone maintenance is typically much lower than that used for pain.

Treatment of CSA Caused by Drug or Substance Use

Treatment options for CSA caused by drug or substance use are displayed in Box 30-6. Some patients will improve with a reduction in narcotic dose or weaning and discontinuation,[130] but this is rarely acceptable to the patient. However, complete reversal of central apnea has been reported following withdrawal of an opioid.[130] Patients with mainly obstructive events may respond to CPAP. Patients who have predominantly central apneas on a diagnostic study sometimes respond to CPAP alone. However, BPAP with a backup rate or ASV[134-137] is usually needed. If very severe hypoventilation is present, volume-assured pressure support may be a good option. CPAP treatment of CSA is not covered by insurance, but most patients have enough obstructive apneas and hypopneas on the diagnostic study to qualify for CPAP reimbursement. On the other hand, as mentioned patients on opioids may have mainly obstructive events during a diagnostic study but develop central apneas (persistent or emergent) on CPAP (a form of CompSA). Treatment with either BPAP with a backup rate (BPAP-ST) or ASV is usually successful for narcotic-induced CompSA. Unlike TESCA without an apparent cause, opioid-associated persistent/emergent central apneas *rarely resolve on chronic CPAP treatment.*[134] Farney and coworkers[136] reported that ASV was not effective in opioid-induced central apneas, but the study likely used an insufficient EPAP. Javaheri and associates found ASV to be a very effective treatment for both central and obstructive apneas in patients on narcotics, including those with opioid-associated Co mpSA.[134,135,137] Current ASV devices can address both the obstructive and central components of opioid-induced sleep apnea (auto-EPAP feature). Adaptive servoventilation is effective, but if frequent machine-triggered breaths occur or if hypopneas persist, patients may require a higher minimum pressure support ($PS = 6$ to 8 cm H_2O). This is especially true in patients with a component of hypoventilation. Glidewell et al.[138] combined acetazolamide with CPAP for successful treatment of CSA due to a medication or substance.

Box 30-6 TREATMENT OPTIONS FOR CSA CAUSED BY DRUG OR SUBSTANCE USE

- Stop or reduce dose of causative agent
- CPAP works in some especially if significant OSA is also present
- BPAP-ST (with backup rate), especially if significant hypoventilation
- Adaptive servoventilation (automatic EPAP can also treat OSA)

CPAP, continuous positive airway pressure; *OSA*, obstructive sleep apnea; *EPAP*, expiratory positive airway pressure; *ST*, spontaneous timed.

Central Sleep Apnea Due to a Medical Disorder Without Cheyne-Stokes Breathing

The nomenclature "medical disorder" is meant to include neurological disorders. In this group of disorders, CSA is attributed to a medical or neurological condition (and does not have the pattern of CSB). The majority of these patients have brainstem lesions of developmental, vascular, neoplastic, degenerative, demyelinating, or traumatic origin. For example, multiple system atrophy (an atypical Parkinson syndrome) can present as a CSA syndrome or with hypoventilation.[139-141] Patients generally present with sleep fragmentation, excessive daytime sleepiness, or insomnia. Other signs and symptoms that are often, but not invariably, present include snoring, witnessed apnea, and awakening with shortness of breath. The presentation varies with the cause of central apnea and may include neurological findings.

The inclusion of Chiari malformation (CM) in this group of patients with CSA is important to note. Patients with this syndrome may be relatively asymptomatic and without abnormal neurological findings. The finding of CSA on a sleep study is often the only clue that the syndrome is present. If clinically indicated, surgical treatment can resolve the CSA as well as the associated symptoms, if present.

The ICSD-3-TR diagnostic criteria for CSA Due to a Medical Disorder without CSB includes the following criteria (A-C must be met)[1]:

A. The presence of one or more of the following (in infants and small children, symptoms are supportive but not required):
    1. Sleepiness
    2. Difficulty initiating or maintaining sleep, frequent awakenings, or nonrestorative sleep
    3. Awakening short of breath
    4. Witnessed apnea
B. PSG shows all of the following:
    1. Five or more central respiratory events (central apneas or central hypopneas) per hour of sleep
    2. The total number of central apneas plus central hypopneas is >50% of the total number of apneas and hypopneas
    3. Absence of CSB

C. The disorder occurs as a consequence of a *medical or neurological* disorder and is not better explained by medication/substance use.

Note that the central apneas must be attributed to a medical or neurological condition. A pattern of CSB is not present by definition. *A mixture of obstructive and central apnea may be present, and a simultaneous diagnosis of OSA is not excluded.* Sleep-related *hypoventilation may or may not be present.* If present, a diagnosis of both CSA and Sleep-Related Hypoventilation due to a Medical Disorder can be made. Common syndromes associated with CSA Due to a Medical Disorder without CSB are listed in Box 30-7.

Arnold Chiari Malformation

CSA caused by a Chiari malformation (CM) is included in the category of central sleep apnea Due to a Medical Disorder without CSB.[142-148] With the increased use of MRI, cases are often detected before symptoms begin. CM-I is defined as herniation of the cerebellar tonsils through the foramen magnum. CM-II includes caudal displacement of the vermis and is usually associated with myelodysplasia and meningomyelocele. *In CM-I, obstructive apneas, central apneas, or a combination can occur.* A tracing from a sleep study of a patient with CM is shown in Figure 30-23. Nocturnal hypoventilation without discrete apneas can also occur. A *minority* of patients with CM-I have daytime hypercapnia. Presenting symptoms of CM with CSA include snoring, breathing pauses, headaches, neck pain, ataxia, oculomotor disturbances, scoliosis, and lower cranial nerve palsies. Although CM-I can present in infancy and childhood, the most common presentation is in adulthood (**20 to 40 years of age**). In many cases of CM, the neurological examination is completely normal, an*d often the only symptom is unexplained headaches, especially with exertion*. Important facts to note about CSA caused by CM are listed in Box 30-8.

In CM, the CSA is believed to be caused by pressure on the medullary structures controlling ventilation and upper-airway muscles. Surgical decompression (posterior fossa decompression,

Box 30-7 CAUSES OF CSA DUE TO A MEDICAL DISORDER WITHOUT CSB

- Brainstem Abnormality
  - Tumor
  - CVA
  - Chiari Malformation
  - Trauma
  - Vasculitis (infection)
- Demyelinating disorders
- Neurodegenerative disorders – multiple system atrophy

CSB, Cheyne-Stokes breathing; *CVA*, cerebrovascular accident.

Box 30-8 CENTRAL SLEEP APNEA IN CHIARI MALFORMATION AND STROKE

Chiari Malformation

- Consider a diagnosis of Chiari malformation (CM) in patients with unexplained central sleep apnea or a *combination of obstructive and central sleep apneas*
- *Headache (especially worsened with exertion) in young to middle aged adults should alert the clinician to the possibility of CM*
- Neurological examination is frequently normal
- Central Sleep apnea in patients with CM often resolves after surgical decompression

Stroke (Cerebrovascular event)

- Obstructive sleep apnea is the most commonly observed type of sleep apnea after stroke. However, central sleep apnea with Cheyne-Stokes breathing can be present in up to 30% of patients after stroke. Central apneas tend to resolve with time.

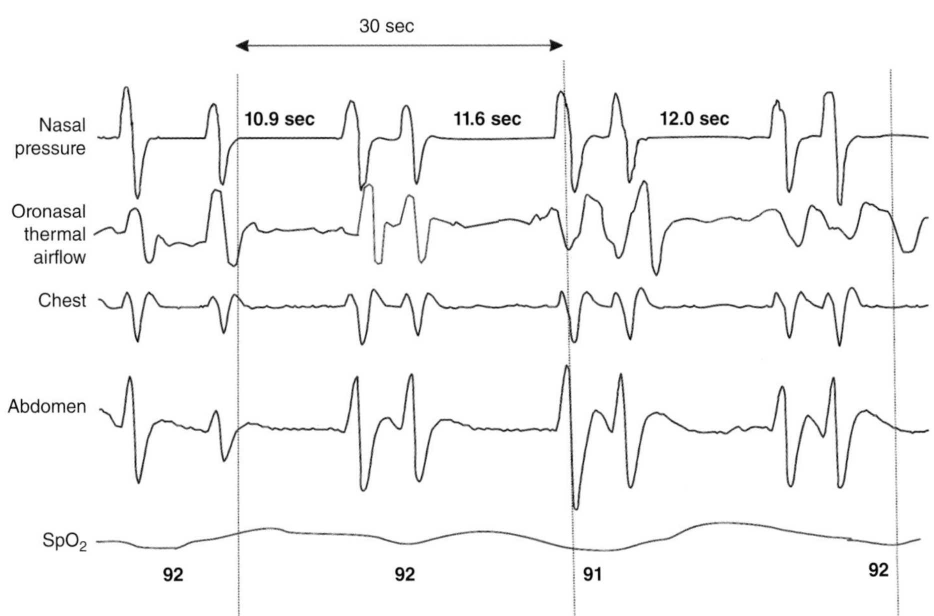

Figure 30-23 A tracing from a patient with central sleep apnea (CSA) associated with arnold chiari malformation. Inspiration is upward. The patient was evaluated for snoring and apnea. He complained only of headaches (worse with exertion). Frequent central apneas are noted. The cycle length is too short from Cheyne-Stokes Breathing. (From Berry RB, Wagner MH. *Sleep Medicine Pearls*, 3rd edition. Philadelphia, PA: Elsevier; 431.)

duraplasty, and cervical laminectomy) often improves the degree of sleep apnea,[148] although significant apnea can be present in the postoperative period. There have been reports of patients treated for obstructive hydrocephalus with shunts who experienced an acute worsening of sleep apnea as the only manifestation of shunt failure.

Central sleep apnea can occur associated with a cerebrovascular event. Obstructive sleep apnea is more common after stroke (Box 30-8). Central sleep apnea tends to occur early in the course after a stroke and may resolve.

Extensive discussion regarding sleep apnea and stroke is presented in Chapter 40.

PRIMARY CENTRAL SLEEP APNEA OF INFANCY

Primary CSA of infancy (PCSAOI) is characterized by prolonged central, mixed, or obstructive apneas or hypopneas associated with physiological compromise (hypoxemia, bradycardia, or the need for intervention such as stimulation or resuscitation).[1,149-152]

The ICSD-3-TR diagnostic criteria for this syndrome include (criteria A-D must be met)[1]:

A. Apnea or cyanosis is noted by an observer, or an episode of sleep-related central apnea or desaturation is detected by monitoring in the postnatal period.

B. The infant has a **conceptional age** (gestational age + chronological age) **of at least (≥) 37 weeks.**

C. PSG or alternative monitoring such as portable apnea monitoring shows one of the following:
  1. Recurrent, prolonged (>20 seconds duration) central apneas
  2. Recurrent central apneas of shorter duration associated with bradycardia or oxygen desaturation
  3. Periodic breathing for ≥5% of total sleep time after a chronological age of 3 months

D. The disorder is not better explained by another sleep disorder, medical, disorder or medication.

The predominant feature is central apnea. Less than 0.5% of term infants have symptomatic central apnea. Note that normative data concerning the number of prolonged central apneas per hour is not well established.[149] Short (<20 seconds) central apneas associated with significant desaturation are more likely to be a sign of decreased pulmonary reserve than of central nervous system pathology. Definitive determination of the central nature of apneas requires simultaneous monitoring of airflow and respiratory effort, ideally by PSG. Obstructive and mixed apneas may also be present, but *central apneas are predominant.* Awake or sleeping hypoventilation may or may not be present. Central apneas are more common during REM sleep.

PCSAOI is a syndrome of abnormal respiratory control that can be either a developmental problem associated with immaturity of the brainstem respiratory centers[149,150] or secondary to other medical conditions that produce direct depression of central respiratory control or lung function. Apnea in the neonate or infant may be exacerbated or precipitated by a variety of medical conditions that must be recognized and treated to stabilize the apnea, such as *anemia, infection, hypoxemia, or metabolic abnormality.* A study by Ginsburg et al.[151] found that the three most common etiologies of PCSAOI were gastroesophageal reflux disease (GERD), upper-airway abnormalities/obstruction, and neurological disease. In this study, infants underwent full PSG, and an infant was diagnosed as having PCSAOI if the AHI was greater than 1 event/hour.

The terms *sudden infant death syndrome (SIDS)* and *apparent life-threatening event (ALTE)* should **not** be used. If another medical condition appears to be the cause rather than an exacerbating factor of CSA, then the condition should be classified as CSA caused by a medical disorder or CSA due to a medication or substance. Despite the heterogeneity of infant risk groups and underlying pathophysiology, most studies report a progressive decrease in frequency of apneas and risk of symptomatic apnea secondary to other medical conditions after the early weeks of life.[1,151]

ALTE, SIDS, and BRUE

The American Academy of Pediatrics (AAP) published a clinical guideline[152] that recommends dropping the previously used term apparent life threaening event (*ALTE*) and replacing it with *brief resolved unexplained event (BRUE).*

BRUE is defined as:
1. An event occurring in an **infant <12 months of age**
2. Brief, <1 minute episode of apnea or cyanosis that resolves spontaneously
3. Association with a reassuring history and normal physical examination
4. The patient is **afebrile**, and there is no history of choking or gagging to suggest GERD

Nocturnal PSG, EEG, and neuroimaging tests are not required in patients with uncomplicated events. Higher risk patients in whom more detailed evaluation may be necessary include those with: possible *child abuse, family history of sudden death, with need to exclude a cardiac arrhythmia, fever and concerns for infection, choking and spitting up suggestive of GERD.* AASM guidelines for use of PSG in children state that PSG is indicated when there is clinical evidence of a sleep related breathing disorder in infants who have experienced an apparent life-threatening event.

The Sudden Infant Death Syndrome (SIDS) is the sudden, unexplained death of a baby younger than 1 year of age that doesn't have a known cause even after a complete investigation. This investigation includes performing a complete autopsy, examining the death scene, and reviewing the clinical history. Interventions to decrease the risk of SIDS include: sleep on the back, firm mattress, no loose bedding/soft stuffed animals/crib bumpers, no incline, no over dressing, no co-sleeping, and avoidance of exposure to cigarette smoke (ABC-alone on back in crib). Baby monitors have **not** been shown to reduce the risk of SIDS. Primary Central Sleep Apnea of infancy has not be established as a risk factor for SIDS.

A summary of important facts about primary CSA of Infancy: 1. Age ≥ 37 weeks conceptional age, 2. Diagnostic criteria include observation of apnea or cyanosis, PSG/other monitoring reveals central apnea > 20 seconds, central apnea of any length associated with bradycardia or desaturation, or periodic breathing ≥ 5% of total sleep time after a chronological age of 3 months, 3. Apneas are most common during REM sleep.

PRIMARY CENTRAL SLEEP APNEA OF PREMATURITY

Apnea is very common in preterm infants, and the prevalence varies inversely with gestational age.[1,153] The syndrome caused by abnormality of respiratory control affects 70% to 90% of premature infants weighing less than 1500 g at birth or less than 28 weeks' gestation. It is characterized by prolonged apneas of 20 or more seconds or shorter respiratory pauses that are accompanied by decreases in oxyhemoglobin saturation and/or bradycardia (heart rate less than 60 beats per minute [BPM] for 15 seconds for age less than 1 year[10]). In the preterm infant, sleep apnea can be anticipated, is primarily related to immaturity, may require supportive ventilatory and pharmacologic treatment, and will improve with maturation unless extenuating conditions, such as hypoxemia caused by chronic lung disease or gastroesophageal reflux, are present. *Apneas may be central, mixed, or obstructive* or hypopneas associated with physiological compromise (hypoxemia, bradycardia) or the need for interventions such as stimulation or resuscitation, although the predominant feature is central apnea. There may be recurrent episodes of *periodic breathing, oxygen desaturation, and bradycardia.*[153] In periodic breathing, between 5-second and 10-second periods of apnea alternate with regular breathing.

The ICSD-3-TR diagnostic criteria include the following (criteria A-D must be met)[1]:

A. **Apnea** or **cyanosis** is noted by an observer, or and an episode of sleep-related central apnea, desaturation, or bradycardia is detected by hospital monitoring in the postnatal period.

B. The infant has a conceptional age (gestational age + chronological age) **less than 37 weeks' at the time of onset of symptoms**

C. PSG or alternative monitoring such as hospital or home apnea monitoring shows either:
   1. Recurrent prolonged (>20 seconds duration) central apneas
   2. Recurrent central apneas of shorter duration associated with bradycardia or oxgen desaturation

D. The syndrome is not better explained by another current sleep, medical, or neurological disorder or medication.

In preterm infants apnea on day 1 of life is rare. The most common period of onset is between the second and seventh day of life. Presentation on day 1 suggests other etiologies. Males and females are equally affected. Their is a higher incidence with lower birth weight and lower gestational age (incidence inversely proportional to birth weight and gestational age) Obstructive and mixed apneas may also be present, but central apneas are predominant. Normative data concerning the number of prolonged central apneas per hour are not well established. Apnea in the preterm infant is *commonly associated with bradycardia. Primary CSA of prematurity is state dependent, and the frequency of respiratory events* ***increases during stage R (REM or active) sleep.*** Paradoxical chest-wall movements are common during active sleep in neonates and may cause a fall in arterial oxygen saturation as a result of ventilation or perfusion defects associated with a *decrease in functional residual capacity*. Periodic breathing is common in premature infants. Underlying comorbidities (for example, chronic lung disease or abnormal neurological status) can predispose the infant to having a more severe or prolonged course for apnea. Apnea of prematurity is complex and multifactorial and reflects immaturity of respiratory control. Passive collapse of the hypotonic upper airway of premature infants predisposes them to obstructive apnea. Furthermore, preterm infants of 30 to 32 weeks' conceptional age spend close to 80% of their total sleep time in active (REM) sleep and thus have an increased likelihood of hypotonic collapse of the upper airway when asleep. Their central control of ventilation is immature, characterized by a blunted central ventilatory response to the accumulation of carbon dioxide. There is also immaturity of the excitatory N-methyl-D-aspartate (NMDA) receptors located in the nucleus of the tractus solitarius in the medulla. These receptors increase ventilation in response to recurrent hypoxia. *An important causative factor in apnea of prematurity is that preterm infants respond by* decreasing *ventilation when challenged with hypoxia*. This is most likely a consequence of suppression of the central ventilatory drive by hypoxia. Adenosine probably plays a role in mediating this inhibition. Caffeine, the most widely used psychoactive compound, is an adenosine receptor antagonist. It promotes wakefulness by blocking adenosine A2A receptors and is a standard treatment for apnea of prematurity.[154] Paradoxical chest and abdominal wall motion is common during the active sleep of premature infants, and this may further exacerbate inefficient breathing. Yet another contributing factor might be immaturity of the Hering-Breuer reflex—small increases in lung volume may thus trigger apnea. The neurologic mechanism behind the Hering Breuer reflex is complex[155] and is a prime example of an inhibitory feedback loop. In human adults, the reflex begins with a prolonged inspiration well exceeding the usual eupneic tidal volume. This thoracic expansion subsequently and gradually activates, slowly adapting pulmonary stretch receptors. These receptors relay a signal through the vagus nerve (on a breath-by-breath basis) to "pump cells" located within the ventrolateral nucleus of the solitary tract. The pump cells receive these vagal inputs and project the information to the medullary post-inspiratory neurons. These neurons subsequently project inhibitory signals back to the inspiratory neurons along the lateral portion of the respiratory column, thereby terminating inspiration and beginning a prolonged expiration. As adults demonstrate reduced ability to illustrate the Hering Breuer reflex (require volumes greater than typical tidal volume), it is much more prominent among preterm infants and newborns. GERD is a factor in some patients. Although "cardiorespiratory events" and GERD are common in preterm infants, they are not causally related. Perhaps they are dual manifestations of central autonomic nervous system immaturity. The influence of *inherited factors* in the pathogenesis of apnea of prematurity has also been recognized recently.

Treatment options for apnea of prematurity include supportive care, caffeine therapy, nasal CPAP via nasal prongs, and high flow via nasal cannula (Box 30-9). Supportive care is very important and is focused on prevention of factors that increase apnea. This care includes tactile stimulation (if necessary), a stable thermal environment, treatment of anemia, maintaining nasal patency, and avoiding extreme neck flexion or extension. Caffeine treatment has been associated with improved long-term outcomes with respect to cognitive and motor function.[156,157] Caffeine citrate is preferred, as it has a longer half-life. Apneic events subside spontaneously and resolve after 46 to 48 weeks' conceptional age. The benefits of home apnea monitoring are uncertain, but monitoring can be provided to cover the risk period.

A summary of major points: 1. apnea on day 1 of life is rare and suggests other etiologies. The most common time of onset of apnea is the second through seventh day of life, 2. apnea is more common during REM sleep, 3. apnea, cyanosis, bradycardia, and paradoxical chest motion are typically observed,

Box 30-9 TREATMENT OF APNEA OF PREMATURITY

- Supportive care—Focused on eliminating factors that increase the risk of apnea, including maintenance of a stable thermal environment, transfusion for significant anemia, tactile stimulation, as needed, maintaining nasal patency (vigorous nasal suctioning), avoidance of extreme neck flexion, and extension (narrow the upper airway)
- Caffeine therapy—Caffeine citrate is the preferred agent because of its longer half-life and wider safety margin. The recommended dose is a 20-mg/kg intravenous or oral loading dose, followed by 5 mg/kg per day by mouth or the intravenous route, and may be increased to 10 mg/kg per day for persistent apnea. Improved long-term outcomes from the standpoint of cognitive and motor function have also been reported with the use of caffeine in the newborn period.
- Supplemental oxygen
- Nasal continuous positive airway pressure (CPAP), in general provided via prongs or use of high flow via nasal cannula
- Noninvasive ventilation if other methods fails.

Obstructive and mixed apneas can also occur but central apneas predominate. Periodic breathing is very common. 4. Persistent of apnea beyond 43 weeks conceptional age (suggests other etiologies, 4. Use of caffeine is a mainstay of treatment.

SLEEP-RELATED HYPOVENTILATION DISORDERS

Sleep-related hypoventilation syndromes meet the criteria for hypoventilation as defined in the AASM scoring manual.[10]

The major sleep related hypoventilation syndromes include[1]:

1. Obesity Hypoventilation Syndrome (OHS)
2. Congenital Central Alveolar Hypoventilation Syndrome
3. Late-Onset Central Hypoventilation with Hypothalamic Dysfunction
4. Idiopathic Central Alveolar Hypoventilation
5. Sleep-Related Hypoventilation Due to a Medication or Substance
6. Sleep-Related Hypoventilation Due to a Medical Disorder

Hypoventilation during sleep meeting the AASM scoring manual criteria for hypoventilation during sleep is required for a diagnosis of sleep-related hypoventilation[10]. Arterial oxygen desaturation is usually present but is not required for the diagnosis. Daytime hypoventilation may or may not be present. In fact, daytime hypoventilation ($PaCO_2$ ≥45 mmHg) is a requirement only for the OHS. OHS is discussed in Chapters 18 and 21. In Figure 30-24, many of the **causes** of sleep-related hypoventilation and associated syndromes are illustrated. Diagnostic criteria for the Sleep-Related Hypoxemia, Disorder are included in a separate category in the sleep-related breathing disorders section in the ICSD-3-TR, These are included here for completeness.

The ICSD-3-TR diagnostic criteria for sleep-related hypoxemia syndrome include (A and B must be met)[1]:

A. PSG, HSAT, or nocturnal oximetry shows an arterial SpO_2 ≤88% in adults or ≤90% in children for ≥5 minutes (cumulative).

B. The desaturation is not fully explained by *sleep-related hypoventilation*, OSA, or other sleep-related breathing disorders.

The diagnosis should not be used if sleep-related hypoventilation has been confirmed (instead, classify the disorder as sleep-related hypoventilation). If evaluation to exclude sleep-related hypoventilation (end-tidal PCO_2 or transcutaneous PCO_2 monitoring) *has not been performed the hypoxemia should be noted as a test result and a diagnosis of sleep-related hypoxemia disorder should NOT be made*[1].

Evaluation of Patients With Suspected Hypoventilation

The ICSD-3-TR general criteria for sleep-related hypoventilation require demonstration of a $PaCO_2$ (or surrogate) meeting the AASM criteria for hypoventilation during sleep (see Chapters 11 and 12). Surrogates of the $PaCO_2$ include end-tidal PCO_2 testing (diagnostic sleep studies) or transcutaneous PCO_2 ($TcPCO_2$) (diagnostic and PAP titration sleep studies). The diagnosis of hypoventilation (daytime or nocturnal) should be considered in all patients with the syndromes listed in Table 30-9 or Figure 30-24 who complain of nocturnal symptoms including insomnia, dyspnea, disturbed sleep, or frequent awakenings. However, lack of symptoms does not rule out hypoventilation. The development of right heart failure should also trigger suspicion but is often a late sign (Figure 30-25). A reduced daytime SaO_2 (≤92%) or an elevated serum HCO^-_3 (possible compensation for chronic respiratory acidosis) should also increase suspicion of hypoventilation. In patients with normal lungs (normal alveolar-arterial [A-a] gradient), significant hypoventilation can be present, and the SaO_2 can still remain in the low normal range. For example, a patient with presumed "chronic obstructive pulmonary disease (COPD)" may have arterial blood gas results breathing room air showing a PCO_2 of 60 mmHg and a PO_2 of 65 mmHg. The A-a gradient (see Chapter 13) can be computed as the ideal or alveolar value (PaO_2) minus the measured PaO_2. Breathing room air the PAO_2 is 150 – 60/0.8 = 75 mmHg. The A-a gradient is only 10 mmHg, which is normal. Lung disease severe enough to cause hypoventilation has an increased A-a gradient typically 25 mmHg or higher (see Chapter 13 for more information on the A-a gradient). Thus, this patient has hypoventilation not caused by lung disease and a disorder of ventilatory control, or more likely, neuromuscular weakness is present. Arterial blood gas results showing a $PaCO_2$ ≥45 mmHg during the day is the most definite method to diagnose daytime hypoventilation. The ICSD-3-TR diagnostic criteria for the OHS include an awake arterial $PaCO_2$, end-tidal PCO_2, or transcutaneous PCO_2 ≥ 45 mmHg[1]. An elevated awake end-tidal PCO_2 result can identify unsuspected daytime hypoventilation. While the presence of lung disease increases the gradient between the $P_{ET}CO_2$ and the $PaCO_2$, an elevated $P_{ET}CO_2$ is still useful, even though the value underestimates the $PaCO_2$. A capillary arterial blood gas test is also a fairly accurate means of detecting an elevated $PaCO_2$, and the $PcapCO_2$ is usually within ± 2 to 3 mmHg of the $PaCO_2$.[158] A venous arterial blood gas test can also be useful, but the PCO_2 in the venous blood ($PvCO_2$) is higher than the $PaCO_2$ by 4 to 5 mmHg (central venous) or 3 to 8 mmHg (peripheral venous).[159,160] On average, the $PvCO_2$ is about 6 mmHg higher than the

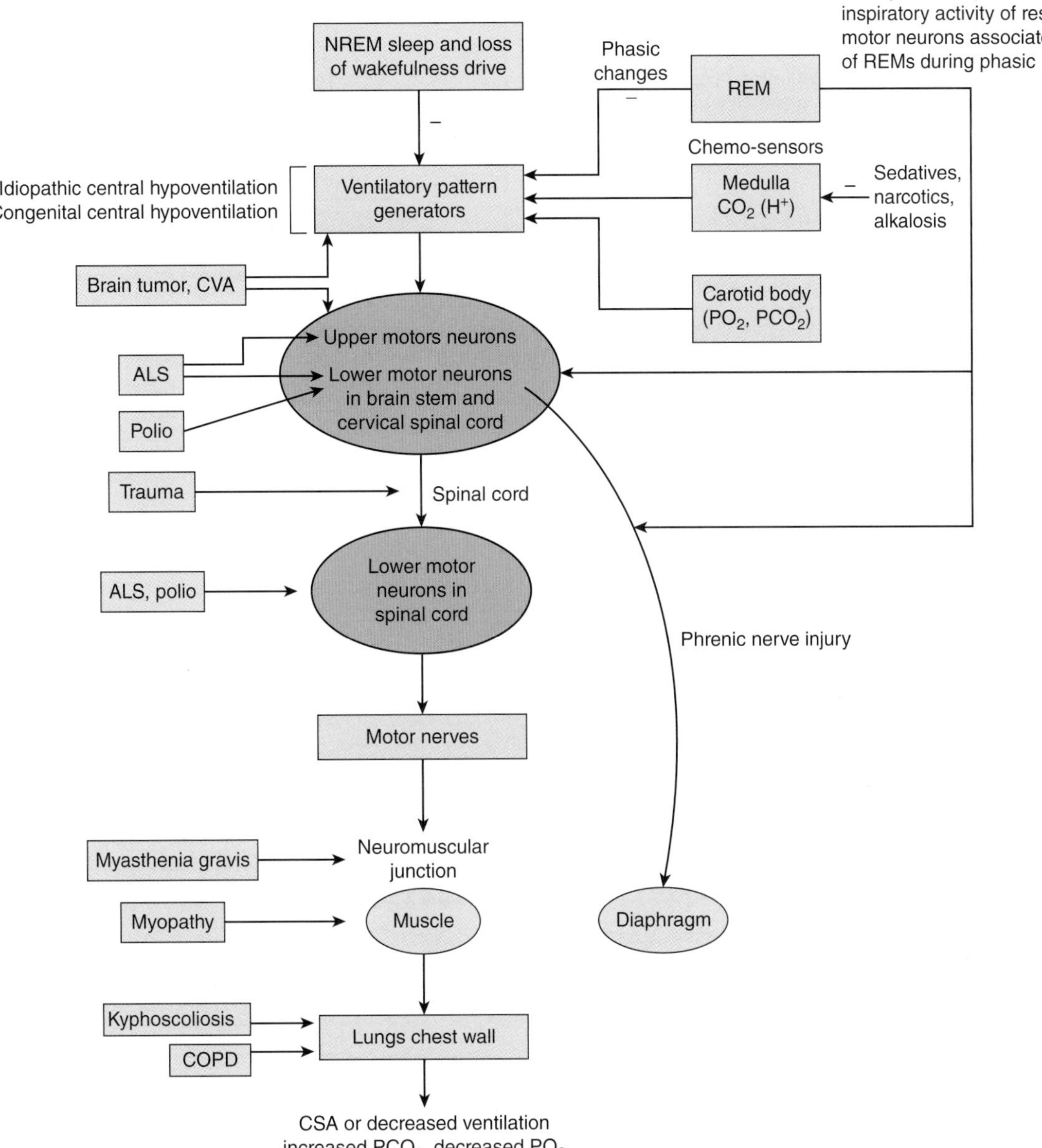

Figure 30-24 Schematic illustration of various causes of sleep-related hypoventilation. Some of these patients may have daytime hypoventilation as well. (Adapted from Malhotra A, Berry RB, White DP. Central Sleep Apnea. In: Carney P, Berry RB, Geyer JW, editors. *Clinical Sleep Medicine*. Philadelphia: Lippincott Williams & Wilkins; 2005:338.)

$PaCO_2$. The upper limit of normal for the $PvCO_2$ is approximately 51-52 mm Hg.

Depending on the clinical setting, a careful neurologic examination, pulmonary function testing, chest radiography, central nervous system imaging (ventilatory control dysfunction suspected), genetic testing, and PSG may be useful. Early in the disease course, some patients have only nocturnal hypoventilation (Figure 30-25). An arterial blood gas test drawn immediately on awakening can confirm nocturnal hypoventilation. As noted, noninvasive methods such as $P_{ET}CO_2$ monitoring or $TcPCO_2$ monitoring can be used during sleep studies if their accuracy can be documented. Figure 30-26 shows a tracing from a patient with muscular dystrophy with hypoventilation documented by $P_{ET}CO_2$. Nocturnal oximetry in patients with suspected hypoventilation may detect unexpected arterial oxygen desaturation. Whereas this *does not document nocturnal hypoventilation*, it would indicate the need for further diagnostic and therapeutic interventions. Further comments on diagnostic evaluation are included below in sections on the specific syndromes.

Congenital Central Alveolar Hypoventilation (Congenital Central Hypoventilation Syndrome, CCHS)

Central congenital hypoventilation syndrome (CCHS) is a rare syndrome affecting approximately one per 200,000 live births,[161-163] Although the condition is termed *congenital*, some patients with a *PHOX2B* genotype may present phenotypically

Table 30-9 Medical Disorders Associated With Sleep-Related Hypoventilation

1. Central respiratory control disturbances
   - Brainstem neoplasms or lesions (astrocytoma, CVA, Chiari malformation)
   - Congenital central alveolar hypoventilation syndrome
   - Hypoventilation caused by drug or substance use
2. Obesity Hypoventilation Syndrome (OSA)
3. Inherited disorders associated with OSA – Prader Willi Syndrome
4. Phrenic nerve disorders
   - Idiopathic
   - Parsonage Turner Syndrome
   - Remote Radiation therapy for Hodgkins or other tumors
   - Devic's syndrome (neuromyelitis optica)
   - Damage from surgical procedures
   - Spinal cord injury (trauma)
5. Restrictive cage disorders (RTCD) – Kyphoscoliosis, Ankylosing Spondylitis
6. Neuromuscular disorders
   - Neuromuscular junction – Myasthenia Gravis
   - Upper/lower motor neuron disease – polio, amyotrophic lateral sclerosis (ALS)
   - Myopathy – Duchenne muscular dystrophy, Myotonic Dystrophy
7. Chronic lung disease (chronic obstructive pulmonary disease [COPD], interstitial lung disease)

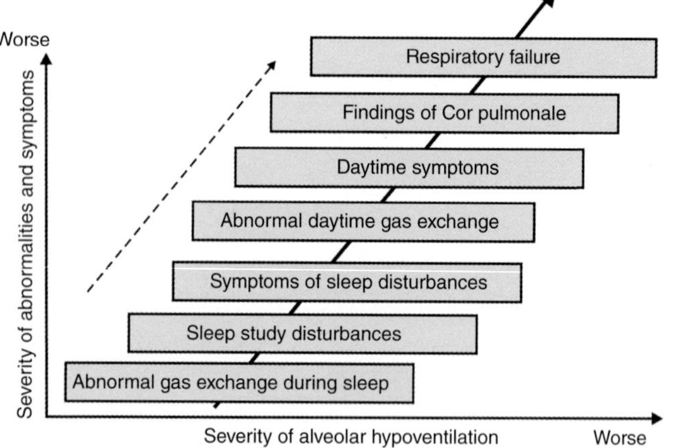

Figure 30-25 The progression of manifestations of disease in a patient with hypoventilation during sleep. With time, abnormal gas exchange during the day develops, and eventually, respiratory failure develops if hypoventilation is not addressed. In some individuals, treatment of nocturnal hypoventilation will delay, prevent, or improve daytime hypoventilation. The goal is early intervention to prevent the progression of disease. (From American College of Chest Physicians. Clinical indications for noninvasive positive pressure ventilation in chronic respiratory failure due to restrictive lung disease, COPD, and nocturnal hypoventilation—a consensus conference report. *Chest*. 1999;116(2):521-534. PMID: 10453883.)

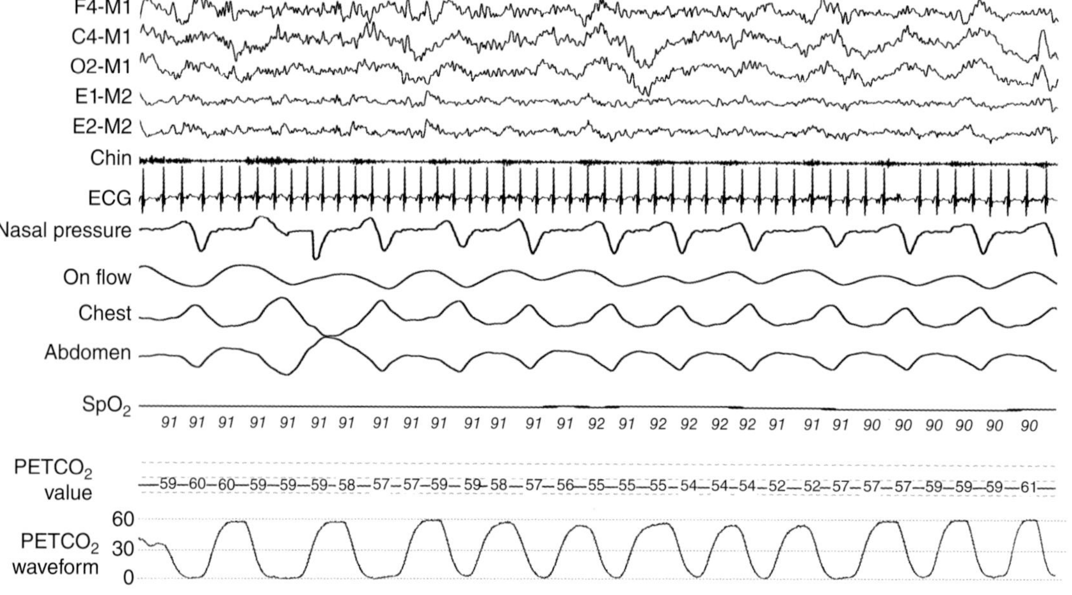

Figure 30-26 A 30-second tracing in a patient with muscular dystrophy and nocturnal hypoventilation. Although the arterial oxygen saturation by oximetry (SpO_2) is only mildly reduced, there is evidence of very significant hypoventilation using end-tidal PCO_2 ($P_{ET}CO_2$) monitoring. $P_{ET}CO_2$ value is the recent maximum value, and $P_{ET}CO_2$ waveform is the PCO_2 versus time tracing.

later in life[164] (and even in adulthood) following the presence of a stressor such as general anesthesia or a severe respiratory illness.[161-164] However, most cases of CCHS are present from birth and characterized by alveolar hypoventilation without evidence of lung, neuromuscular, or structural brainstem abnormalities.

Recall that the definition of hypoventilation in children is an elevation in the $PaCO_2$ (or surrogate) >50 mmHg for >25% of the total sleep time.

The ICSD-3-TR diagnostic criteria (A-C must be met) for CCHS are:

A. Sleep-related hypoventilation is present.
B. Central nervous system autonomic dysfunction is present, most often caused by a mutation of the *PHOX2B* gene.
C. The syndrome is not better explained by another sleep disorder, medical disorder, medication use, or substance use.

The central nervous system dysfunction typically is manifested by an abnormal ventilatory response to hypercapnia with significant hypercapnia and hypoxia during sleep. awake hypoventilation may or may not be present, but the $PaCO_2$ is elevated during sleep. PSG monitoring demonstrates severe hypercapnia and arterial oxygen desaturation. Some central apneas may occur, but the *predominant pattern is reduced flow/tidal volume*. Note that the previous ICSD-3 version required a mutation of the *PHOX2B* gene, but the latest version states, " most often due to a mutation of the *PHOX2B* gene." Mutations of the genes *MYO1H* and *LBX1* have been reported to cause CCHS.[1]

A typical presentation is an infant who is noted to have cyanosis, feeding difficulties, hypotonia, or occasionally, central apnea. The infant may require intubation and mechanical ventilation, but the chest radiograph is normal. During wakefulness, many patients with CCHS have normal ventilation (~15% manifest hypoventilation during wakefulness), but all patients with the syndrome manifest hypoventilation during sleep. Those with hypoventilation during wakefulness have worsening of hypoventilation during sleep and require continuous ventilatory support. Ventilatory responses to hypercapnia or hypoxemia by the rebreathing method are absent or blunted, and a *perception of dyspnea is absent*.[1,161] As noted, the patients most severely affected by CCHS also have hypoventilation during wakefulness. Those patients with normal awake ventilation do have peripheral chemoreceptor responses to hypoxemia or hypercapnia.[165] It has been hypothesized that the central integration of chemoreceptor information rather than the chemoreceptors themselves is abnormal in patients with CCHS. One study found that those with CCHS did have intact arousal responses to hypercapnia.[166] However, such arousals do not reliably result in an appropriate ventilatory response and rapid reversal of hypoxemia.

During sleep, all patients with CCHS have worsening of ventilation with profound hypoxemia and hypercapnia on PSG. Central apneas may occur, but hypoventilation exhibited by diminished tidal volume and normal or decreased respiratory rates is the predominant pattern[161] (Figure 30-27). In contrast to most types of sleep-disordered breathing in children, **abnormalities may be more severe during NREM sleep than during REM sleep**. Patients may not arouse from sleep despite severe gas exchange abnormalities.

Because CCHS is a generalized syndrome of the autonomic nervous system (ANS), affected patients may manifest features of ANS dysfunction, such as severe bradycardia or asystole that may require implantation of a cardiac pacemaker, Hirschsprung disease (HD), and risk for developing a neural crest tumor (NCT) such as neuroblastoma, ganglioneuroma, and ganglioneuroblastoma. Hirschsprung disease (present in about 20%) usually presents with constipation, esophageal dysmotility, and associated with feeding difficulty. Cardiac manifestations of CCHS in addition to bradycardia or periods of asystole include decreased heart rate variability and a decreased heart rate response to exercise. Other manifestions of autonomic dysfunction include a decreased papillary light response, intermittent profuse sweating, and dysregulation of body temperature with a decreased baseline body temperature. *Patients with CCHS are at risk for adverse outcomes from respiratory infections because they may not exhibit a* fever or complain of dyspnea *even if severely hypoxemic.*

The diagnosis of CCHS should be considered in early infancy when apneic or cyanotic spells are noted, especially during sleep. The most severe cases occur in patients who do not breathe during wakefulness after birth and require immediate ventilatory support. In others, the abnormalities are noted when the infants sleep. Milder cases may present later, with

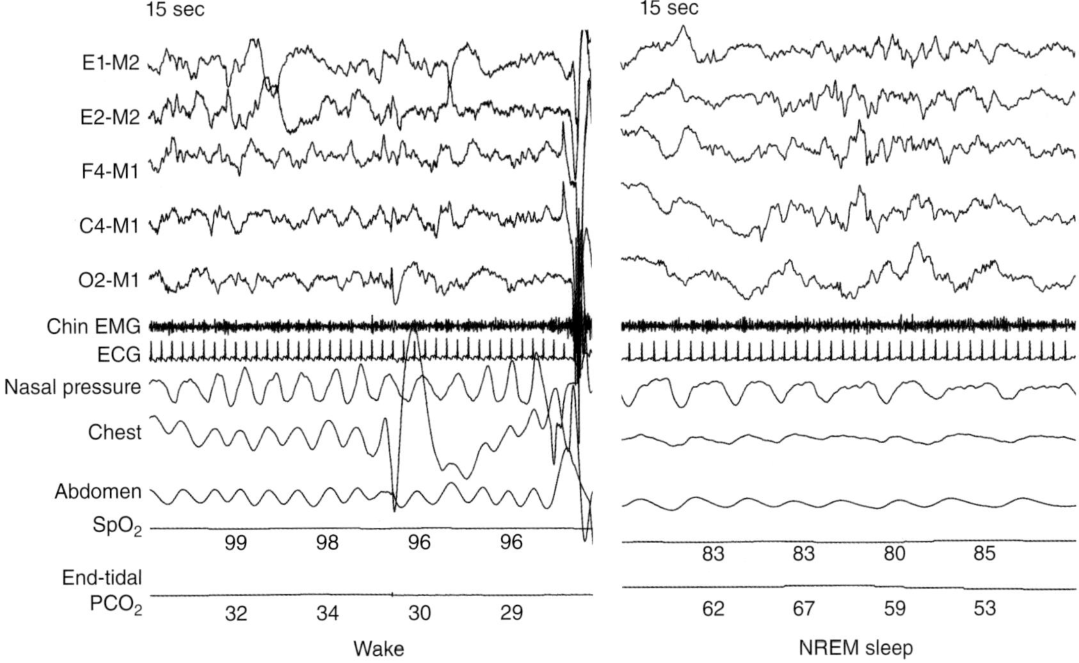

Figure 30-27 Tracings (15 seconds each) from a patient with congenital central hypoventilation during wake and NREM sleep. With sleep onset, there is a profound increase in the end-tidal PCO_2 and severe arterial oxygen desaturation. Note that ventilation and respiratory effort are decreased, and hypoxemia is NOT associated with a change in heart rate (autonomic dysfunction). The end-tidal PCO_2 tracing is tracking the most recent end-tidal PCO_2 values. (From Berry RB, Wagner MH. *Sleep Medicine Pearls*, 3rd edition. Philadelphia, PA: Elsevier; 2015:429.)

signs of cor pulmonale or hypoxic damage to central nervous system structures. Some cases may not present until late childhood and can present in adulthood.[164] The diagnosis of CCHS depends on genetic testing. While waiting for results, exclusion of other causes of hypoventilation such as brainstem malformation, inborn errors of metabolism, myopathy, diaphragmatic paralysis, and lung or respiratory pump abnormalities may be needed. PSG with $P_{ET}CO_2$ monitoring usually reveals high $P_{ET}CO_2$ and low tidal volume (Figure 30-27).

Most patients with CCHS are **heterozygous** for a de novo *polyalanine repeat expansion mutations* (PARM) in exon 3 of *PHOX2B*. **Ninety percent are spontaneous mutations**. The *PHOX2B* gene is located on **chromosome 4p12** and encodes a transcription factor that is important for the development of the autonomic nervous system. The *PHOX2B* gene normally contains a repeat sequence of 20 alanines in exon 3. The majority (90%) of patients with CCHS have increased polyalanine repeats in exon 3 of the *PHOX2B* gene (25–33 repeats). *Those with **more** polyalanine repeats are more likely to have severe disease, including awake hypoventilation.* Approximately 10% of patients are heterozygous for a non-polyalanine repeat mutation [non-PARM (**NPARM**)] in the *PHOX2B* gene that include *frameshift, nonsense, and missense mutations*, whereas less than 1% have *PHOX2B* exon or whole gene deletion.[167] The majority of patients with **NPARM are reported to have severe phenotypes** with need for continuous assisted ventilation, Hirschsprung disease, and increased NCT risk. A previously noted, the NCTs include neuroblastoma, ganglioneuroma, and ganglioneuroblastoma. Most mutations occur de novo, but in *families with CCHS, it is inherited* as an ***autosomal dominant trait.*** Research suggests that severity of illness is related to the type of mutation present. However, there is tremendous variability in the manifestations. Patients with NPARM have been described with relatively mild manifestations not discovered until adulthood.

Treatment includes lifelong ventilatory support for all patients during sleep.[168] As noted, more severely affected patients require ventilatory support while awake as well. Ventilatory support for severe cases is usually provided by a volume-cycled ventilator via a tracheostomy. In older patients and those with milder symptoms, noninvasive mask ventilation may suffice. Diaphragmatic pacing has also been used during the day. Diaphragmatic pacing at night usually requires the presence of a tracheostomy because obstructive events often occur when the upper-airway muscles do not contract in synchrony with the diaphragm. Infants with CCHS must be closely monitored because they are at risk for hypoventilation or apnea at sleep onset. These children are also at increased risk during chest infections due to their abnormal temperature control, lack of perception of dyspnea, and nonappearance of respiratory distress. Noninvasive positive-pressure ventilation (NPPV) with BPAP with a back-up rate has been successfully used in infants when parents have refused tracheostomy.[169] Appropriate alarms are essential. Older children initially treated with tracheostomy may be transitioned to NPPV via mask if their symptoms are milder, and they are adherent to treatment.

Late Onset Central Hypoventilation With Hypothalamic Dysfunction

Late onset central hypoventilation with hypothalamic dysfunction is a syndrome of central control of ventilation. The syndrome is also known as the Rapid Onset Obesity with Hypothalamic Dysfunction, and Autonomic Dysregulation (ROHHAD) syndrome.

The ICSD-3-TR diagnostic criteria[1] are the following:
A. Sleep-related hypoventilation is present
B. Symptoms are absent during the first few years of life
C. The patient has at least two of the following
  1. Obesity
  2. Endocrine abnormalities of hypothalamic origin
  3. Severe emotional or behavioral disturbances
  4. Tumor of neural origin
D. Mutation of the PHOX2B gene is **not present.**
E. The disorder is not better explained by another sleep disorder, medical disorder, medication, or substance use.

Patients ROHHAD are usually healthy until early childhood (often 2-3 years of age) when they develop hyperphagia and severe obesity, followed by central hypoventilation,[170-174] which often presents as respiratory failure. *Hypoventilation often develops several years afrer the rapid onset of obesity and endocrine manifestations.* The ROHHAD phenotype evolves with advancing age and is characterized by rapid-onset obesity in the first 7–10 years of life, followed by hypothalamic dysfunction, onset of symptoms of autonomic dysregulation and later onset of alveolar hypoventilation. Children with ROHHAD typically have an absent or attenuated response to hypoxia and hypercapnia. Respiratory failure may be precipitated by a mild respiratory illness or anesthesia. Patients require ventilatory support during sleep; most patients breathe adequately during wakefulness but some need ventilatory support during both wakefulness and sleep. The hypoventilation persists even if the patients lose weight, differentiating the condition from OHS. There are manifestations of hypothalamic endocrine dysfunction characterized by increased or decreased hormone levels, which may include one or more of the following: diabetes insipidus, inappropriate antidiuretic hormone hypersecretion, *precocious puberty*, hypogonadism, hyperprolactinemia, hypothyroidism, and decreased growth hormone secretion. Other symptoms of hypothalamic dysfunction, such as temperature dysregulation, have been reported. However, Hirschsprung's disease is NOT associated with ROHHAD. Mood and behavior abnormalities, sometimes severe, have been reported frequently. There is a wide variation in the interval between the onset of hypothalamic dysfunction, autonomic dysregulation and hypoventilation, and the severity of the phenotype evolves with advancing age.

Hypoxemia and hypercapnia are present on PSG during sleep. *Central apneas may be present, but hypoventilation associated with decreased tidal volume and respiratory rate is more common.* Patients have flat hypoxic and hypercapnic responses. Arterial blood gases may be normal during wakefulness but will be abnormal if obtained from an arterial line during sleep. In patients with chronically untreated or poorly controlled hypoventilation, a compensated respiratory acidosis may be present, with elevated serum bicarbonate levels. In these patients, polycythemia may be present. Serum tests may show evidence of endocrine abnormalities; *hypernatremia is common* (diabetes inspidus). Computed tomography and magnetic resonance imaging scans of the head are normal.

Early recognition is important as there is a high prevalence of cardio-respiratory arrest. **This is a rare syndrome with only about 100 cases reported.** Forty percent of the cases are associated with ganglioneuroma or ganglioneuroblastoma. At present, treatment for ROHHAD is symptom based. The primary goal is to optimize the neurocognitive potential of these children.

Idiopathic Central Alveolar Hypoventilation

This is a diagnosis of exclusion. Sleep-related hypoventilation must be present and known causes should be excluded.[1]

Diagnostic criteria in the ICSD-3-TR include (A and B must be met):

A. Sleep-related hypoventilation is present.
B. Hypoventilation is not primarily caused by lung parenchymal or airway disease, pulmonary vascular pathology, chest wall disorder, medication use, neurologic disorder, muscle weakness, obesity, or congenital hypoventilation syndromes.

Arterial oxygen desaturation is often present but is not required for the diagnosis. Although OSA may be present, it is not believed to be the major cause of hypoventilation and the predominant respiratory pattern is one of reduced tidal volume or ataxic breathing and associated arterial oxygen desaturation; in such cases, a diagnosis of both OSA and idiopathic central alveolar hypoventilation may be made.

Known causes of hypoventilation should be excluded. These include pulmonary vascular pathology, a chest wall disorder, medication use, neurological disorders (including those causing muscle weakness) and the obesity hypoventilation syndrome. Daytime and nocturnal hypoventilation is believed to occur because of blunted chemoresponsivenss to CO_2 and O_2. Only a few cases have been reported. Symptoms include morning headache, neurocognitive dysfunction, and sleep disturbance. Some cases could be asymptomatic. PSG reveals episodes of shallow breathing (reduced tidal volume and ataxic breathing). Imaging of the central nervous system is usually unremarkable. The differential diagnosis includes other causes of hypoventilation.

Sleep-Related Hypoventilation Due to Medication or Substance

Most of the medications that can cause CSA Due to a Medication or Substance can also cause sleep-related hypoventilation and in some cases daytime hypoventilation. By far the most common group of medications suppressing respiration are the potent opioids. As the medications decrease dyspnea the patient or for that matter many of their physicians may not detect daytime hypoventilation.

The ICSD-3-TR diagnostic criteria[1] for Sleep Related Hypoventilation Due to Medication or Substance are as follows (Criteria A-C must be met):

A. Sleep-related hypoventilation is present.
B. A medication or substance known to inhibit respiration and/or ventilatory drive is believed to be the primary cause of sleep-related hypoventilation.
C. Hypoventilation is not primarily caused by lung parenchymal or airway disease, pulmonary vascular pathology, chest wall disorder, neurologic disorder, muscle weakness, OHS, or a known congenital or idiopathic central alveolar hypoventilation syndrome.

Often more than one factor is causing nocturnal hypoxemia and hypoventilation. For example a patient with severe OSA and use of a potent opioid. The best treatment is a reduction in the pain medication dose or weaning and stopping the offending medication. Usually BPAP treatment is needed and a backup rate is essential. If the patient has CSA they can be qualified for a backup rate under RAD criteria for central sleep apnea/complex apnea. It is unusual for a patient to have sleep-related hypoventilation caused by an opioid without some degree of central apnea. If central apneas are not present during a diagnostic study, sometimes they appear when a patient is placed on CPAP or BPAP without a backup rate. If sufficient central apneas are present the patient may meet criteria for CompSA and qualify for a BPAP device with a backup rate (if effectiveness of BPAP with a backkup rate is demonstrated). In cases of very severe hypoventilation, an advanced PAP device may be needed with volume assured pressure support or even a home ventilator if the patient can qualify.

Sleep-Related Hypoventilation Due to a Medical Disorder

A diverse number of syndromes are included in this group and various classifications have been used.

ICSD-3-TR diagnostic criteria are as follows (Criteria A-C must be met):

A. Sleep-related hypoventilation is present.
B. A lung parenchymal or airway disease, chest wall disorder, neurologic disorder, or muscle weakness is believed to be the primary cause of hypoventilation.
C. Hypoventilation is NOT primarily due to the OHS, medication use, or a known congenital central alveolar hypoventilation syndrome.

Although OHS is certainly a medical disorder it is classified separately. Daytime hypoventilation may be present but is not required for the diagnosis. If is possible for a given patient to meet criteria for OSA, CSA Due to a Medical Disorder, and Sleep-Related Hypoventilation Due to Medical Disorder (if all criteria are met). While central apneas may be present the usual pattern for most patients with this disorder is a reduction in tidal volume. A summary of common disorders associated with sleep-related hypoventilation caused by a medical disorder is shown in Table 30-9. The Centers for Medicare and Medicaid uses the terminology restrictive thoracic disorders to include restrictive thoracic cage disorders and disorders associated with neuromuscular weakness[20] (Table 30-10). Noninvasive ventilation (NIV) is the treatment of choice in these disorders, whether started in the sleep center, at home, or in the clinic.[175,176] Recommendations for the delivery of NIV are discussed in Chapter 24. A difficult but very important decision in most cases is when to start NIV.

Restrictive Thoracic Cage Disorders

Disorders causing restriction of the thoracic cage caused by disease of the spine, chest wall, or pleura can result in hypoventilation. Causes include thoracoplasty, fibrothorax, kyphoscoliosis, and ankylosing spondylitis. In general, isolated nocturnal hypoventilation precedes daytime hypoventilation. These disorders result in extrinsic restrictive ventilatory dysfunction[177] with a reduced total lung capacity and a normal or mildly reduced diffusing capacity (see Chapter 13). Typical lung volume findings in thoracic cage disorders are shown in Figure 13-25. In patients with chest wall disease, the total lung capacity is decreased, and the functional residual capacity is either normal to increased

Table 30-10 Respiratory Assistance Device (RAD) Criteria: Restrictive Thoracic Disorders: Neuromuscular Diseases or Severe Thoracic Cage Abnormalities

For an E0470 or an E0471 RAD to be covered, the treating practitioner must fully document in the beneficiary's medical record symptoms characteristic of sleep-associated hypoventilation, such as daytime hypersomnolence, excessive fatigue, morning headache, cognitive dysfunction, and dyspnea.

An E0470 or E0471 device is covered when criteria A–C are met.

A. There is **documentation in the beneficiary's medical record** of a neuromuscular disease (for example, amyotrophic lateral sclerosis) or a severe thoracic cage abnormality (for example, post-thoracoplasty for tuberculosis).

B. One of the following:
   a. An arterial blood gas $PaCO_2$, done while **awake** and breathing the beneficiary's prescribed FiO_2 is **greater than or equal** to 45 mmHg, **OR**
   b. Sleep oximetry demonstrates oxygen saturation ≤88% for ≥5 minutes of nocturnal recording time (minimum recording time of 2 hours), done while breathing the beneficiary's prescribed recommended FiO_2, **OR**
   c. For a neuromuscular disease (only), either i or ii:
      i. Maximal inspiratory pressure is less than 60 cm H_20, or
      ii. Forced vital capacity is less than 50% predicted

C. Chronic obstructive pulmonary disease does not contribute significantly to the beneficiary's pulmonary limitation.

E0470, bilevel PAP; *E0471*, bilevel PAP with backup rate; *FiO2*, fraction of oxygen in inspired air. Although the criteria qualify a patient for either E0470 or E0471, a E0471 should be used.
LCD 33800[16]

(ankylosing spondylitis) or decreased (kyphoscoliosis). The residual volume is typically normal. An increased residual volume can occur in patients with expiratory muscle weakness (for example, spinal cord injury). In thoracic cage disorders, the chest wall has decreased compliance, so there is an increased work of breathing. Patients tend to take rapid, shallow breaths. The severity of impairment may be roughly gauged by the forced vital capacity (FVC). An FVC less than 50% of predicted is considered severe.[178] However, patients with thoracic cage disorders or neuromuscular disorders who have an FVC higher than 50% of predicted may have hypoventilation and desaturation at night (Figure 30-28). Symptoms of morning headache or nonrestorative sleep **are not sensitive** for detection of nocturnal hypoventilation. Nocturnal oximetry is a useful tool in this setting. The CMS RAD criteria for restrictive thoracic disorder[20] are shown in Table 30-10. Only patients with neuromuscular disease (NMD) can qualify on the basis of a reduced FVC (<50% of predicted) or inspiratory pressure (< 60 cm H_2O). Note that, while evidence of daytime hypoventilation ($PaCO_2$ ≥45 mmHg) will qualify the patient for treatment with BPAP with or without a backup rate (a backup rate should always be used), nocturnal oximetry documenting ≥5 minutes with an SaO_2 ≤88% (on the beneficiary's usual FiO_2) will also meet the criteria. Note that COPD should not contribute significantly to the limitation, *although pulmonary function testing is not required.* The criteria do not mention sleep apnea. While PSG is the most sensitive test to determine nocturnal hypoventilation and rule out coexistent OSA, *a sleep study is NOT needed to qualify a patient with a neuromuscular disorder or thoracic cage disorder under RAD criteria if the nocturnal oximetry meets the criteria.* The best use of a sleep study is for a BPAP titration to optimize BPAP-ST settings.[176,179] Of course, there are occasions when the cause of hypoventilation is uncertain and a diagnostic PSG with CO_2 monitoring can be helpful. Monitoring of $TcPCO_2$ can also be performed during the titration studies, which will address sleep apnea if present and determine an appropriate level of ventilatory support. The most severe desaturation in patients with thoracic cage disease or a neuromuscular disorders usually occurs during REM sleep (Figure 30-29). If $TcPCO_2$ is monitored, this usually shows an increase from wakefulness to NREM sleep and a further increase during REM sleep. If a diagnostic sleep study is performed to demonstrate nocturnal hypoventilation, $TcPCO_2$ is preferred, as a patient with restrictive ventilatory dysfunction often has a small tidal volume and the $P_{ET}CO_2$ may not accurately reflect the alveolar PCO_2. The technique of delivering noninvasive ventilation is discussed in Chapter 24.

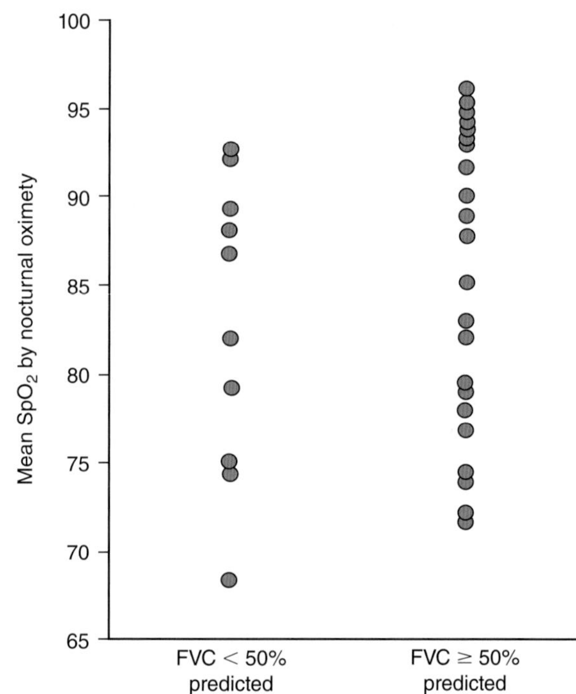

Figure 30-28 The mean arterial oxygen saturation (SpO_2) determined by nocturnal oximetry in individual patients with amyotrophic lateral sclerosis (ALS) is shown for a group with a forced vital capacity (FVC) <50% predicted and a group with an FVC ≥50% predicted. Many patients in the higher FVC group showed significant arterial oxygen desaturation. (Figure plotted using data from Morgan RK, McNally S, Alexander M, Conroy R, Hardiman O, Costello RW. Use of Sniff nasal-inspiratory force to predict survival in amyotrophic lateral sclerosis. *Am J Respir Crit Care Med.* 2005;171(3):269-274. PMID: 15516537.)

Treatment of Restrictive Thoracic Cage Disorders. Early intervention with NIV to provide respiratory muscle rest and prevent nocturnal hypoventilation in patients with restrictive thoracic cage disorders may improve sleep quality, prevent the

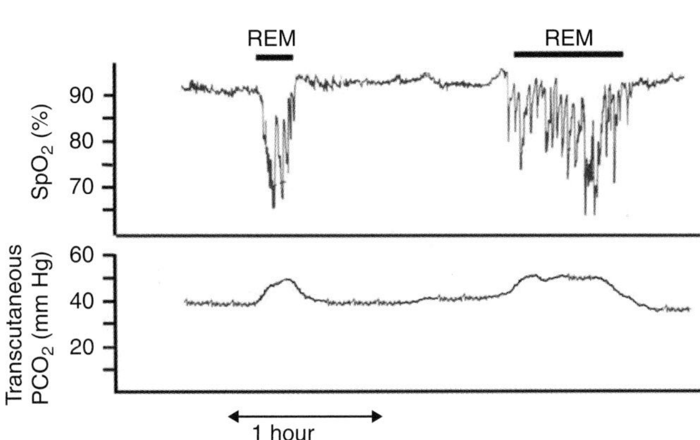

Figure 30-29 Trends in the SpO_2 and transcutaneous partial pressure of carbon dioxide ($TcPCO_2$) during the night in a patient with neuromuscular disease. Note the simultaneous increase in $TcPCO_2$ and decrease in the SpO_2 during episodes of REM sleep. *REM,* rapid eye movement; *PCO_2,* partial pressure of carbon dioxide; *SpO_2,* pulse oximetry.

onset of cor pulmonale, and prevent or delay daytime hypoventilation.[180] With NIV at night, the quality of life is improved, and survival ≥25 years has been reported in a significant proportion of patients.[180] Most clinicians would start treatment after documentation of nocturnal desaturation or hypoventilation. Nocturnal ventilatory support rather than supplemental oxygen is the treatment of choice. An FVC <50% of predicted could be used to determine when to initiate NIV, but many patients with a *higher FVC (70%–80% of predicted)* have significant desaturation at night. NIV is usually provided using BPAP-ST with a mask interface. As discussed in Chapter 24, using volume-assured pressure support allows the BPAP device to change the amount of pressure support to obtain a target tidal volume or alveolar ventilation. NIV can be started effectively on an outpatient basis, but a NIV titration with PSG is the ideal method to select appropriate treatment in many clinical settings. Because of the low compliance of the respiratory system, high pressure support (IPAP-EPAP) up to 20 cm H_2O may be needed to deliver an adequate tidal volume. Some patients may be ventilated with lower pressure support and a backup rate that is higher than spontaneous respiratory rates. A patient may not tolerate an effective amount of pressure support on the first night. A tidal volume goal less than 8 ml/Kg ideal body weight (for example, 6 ml/Kg ideal body weight) and prevention of a significant increase in PCO_2 rather than normalization of the nocturnal PCO_2 would be reasonable initial goals. BPAP devices may cycle from IPAP to EPAP prematurely in patients with a stiff chest wall, and it is important to ensure an adequate inspiratory time (see Chapter 24). If patients are not obese, using as low an EPAP as possible will allow an adequate pressure support without an excessive IPAP (e.g., an IPAP/EPAP of 15/5 rather than 20/10 cm H_2O).

Neuromuscular Disorders (NMD)

Hypoventilation can occur with disorders that impair function at any point from premotor neuron to respiratory muscle. These sites include disorders of the premotor neurons, neural pathways to lower motor neurons, the motor neurons, peripheral nerve disorders (phrenic nerve damage), disorders of the neuromuscular junction (myasthenia gravis), or myopathies (muscular dystrophy).

These disorders result in extrinsic restrictive ventilatory dysfunction (reduction in the total lung capacity (TLC) and vital capacity with relatively normal diffusing capacity for carbon monoxide). For more details on pulmonary function testing, see Chapter 13. Later in the disease course of patients with NMD, abnormalities of the chest wall and lung can also occur, and a reduced functional residual capacity (FRC) and diffusing capacity may be observed.[177,181] In patients with diaphragmatic weakness, spirometry or maximal inspiratory pressure testing in the supine position may be more sensitive (in the supine position, respiration depends more on the diaphragm).[182] *Severe orthopnea and or chest/abdominal paradox while supine may also alert the clinician to the presence of diaphragmatic weakness.* Although it is often said that testing respiratory muscle strength (maximum inspiratory force, expiratory force) is the most sensitive method to detect respiratory weakness, these tests require special expertise to avoid erroneous measurements, and normative values for strength vary considerably.[183,184] The FVC is a very useful measurement in NMD. Studies have shown that the FVC is reduced more than predicted for a given muscle strength (using a normal respiratory system compliance) (Figure 30-30).[185] This implies a decreased compliance of the chest wall and/or lung is present in patients with chronic muscle weakness. The American College of Chest Physicians (ACCP) consensus guidelines[178] recommended an FVC less than 50% of predicted or a maximal inspiratory pressure less than 60 cm H_2O as indications for NPPV treatment. However, a patient with a high FVC can still have significant nocturnal desaturation[186] (Figure 30-28). Therefore, nocturnal oximetry or PSG is recommended if the patient complains of poor sleep quality, frequent awakenings, or nocturnal dyspnea. A discussed below, unless OSA is suspected nocturnal oximetry may be sufficient. Of interest, some patients with NMD cannot make a good mouth seal to allow for an estimate of inspiratory force. One study found using nasal "sniff" inspiratory pressure was useful in assessing prognosis.[187] Patients with a neuromuscular disorder do NOT need a sleep study to qualify them for BPAP with a backup rate if

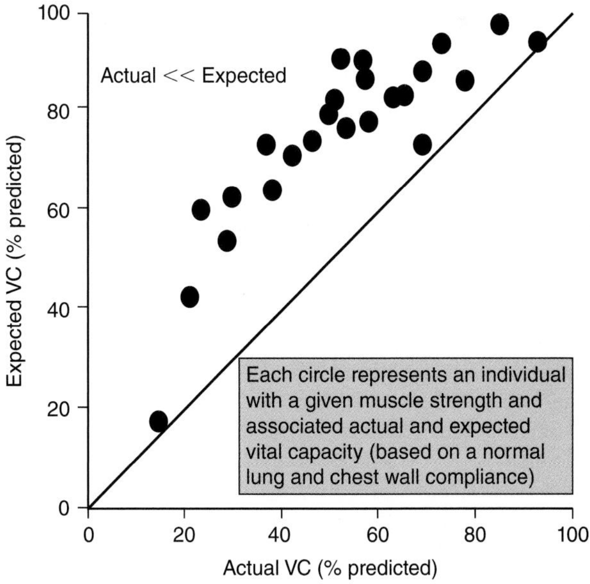

Figure 30-30 A plot of the actual forced vital capacity (FVC) versus the FVC predicted based on the patient's muscle strength and normal respiratory system compliance. The actual FVC is lower than predicted as a result of chronic changes in the chest wall or lungs decreasing respiratory system compliance. (Plotted with data from De Troyer A, Borenstein S, Cordier R. Analysis of lung volume restriction in patients with respiratory muscle weakness. *Thorax.* 1980;35:603-610.)

they meet RAD criteria. A daytime $PaCO_2 \geq 45$ mmHg or nocturnal oximetry showing ≥5 minutes with an $SaO_2 \leq 88\%$, an FVC <50% of predicted, or a maximum inspiratory force of <60 cm H_2O will all qualify a patient with NMD for a RAD device (Table 30-10). If PSG is performed, the results can be used to find effective NIV settings. Similar to most patients with hypoventilation, patients with NMD typically have the lowest oxygen saturation and highest $PaCO_2$ during REM sleep.[188] It is important to realize that hypopneas during REM sleep can be caused by diaphragmatic weakness as much as upper-airway narrowing (so called "pseudo-obstructive apnea").[188] While thoracoabdominal paradox is suggestive of an obstructive hypopnea, it can also occur with a weak diaphragm (inward/upward motion during inspiration).

Treatment of Nocturnal Hypoventilation Caused by NMD. In the past, volume ventilation via a tracheostomy was the usual mode of ventilatory support in patients with NMD. Today, NIV using BPAP with a backup rate (BPAP-ST and other modes) with a mask interface is the most widely used treatment. However, some patients may require tracheostomy if they cannot protect their upper airway. The decision for or against tracheostomy in end-of-life care is always challenging. NIV can be started without a sleep study in the clinic or at home with low levels of pressure support to allow adaptation and adjusted for comfort. Later adjustments can be made based on nocturnal oximetry, daytime $PaCO_2$ measurements, or symptoms[176] (e.g., using BPAP-ST at 12/4 cm H_2O with a backup rate of 1 to 2 breaths/min below the spontaneous rate). If the patient is thin, a low EPAP may be sufficient and allow a greater pressure support without an excessive IPAP. NIV with volume-assured pressure support (see Chapter 24) allows setting a target tidal volume (or alveolar ventilation), and the device will adjust the pressure support within limits set by the physician to achieve the goal. While the ultimate goal is 8 ml/kg ideal body weight (or higher), a lower target can be chosen initially to allow adaptation. At the time of this writing, the only devices that can provide VAPS with automatic EPAP adjustment in the USA are home ventilators. A more precise approach to finding optimal settings for a routine RAD device (not home ventilator) is an NIV titration with PSG. The PSG titration can utilize $TcPCO_2$ monitoring and allow for a trial of multiple mask interfaces. Not all patients will tolerate an optimal degree of pressure support on the first night of treatment. BPAP with a backup rate is recommended because patients may not consistently trigger IPAP-EPAP cycles because of muscle weakness. NIV treatment initiation is discussed in more detail in Chapter 24.

The goals of NIV treatment should be individualized but include improved sleep quality and quality of life, prevention of worsening of hypoventilation, avoiding cor pulmonale, and providing respiratory muscle rest. Delivery of NIV with a home ventilator has advantages in chronic progressive disorders such as amyotrophic lateral sclerosis (ALS), including availability of a battery backup and the ability to deliver daytime mouth-piece ventilation. While the ST mode is commonly used, the pressure control (PC) or pressure assist control (PAC) modes assure an adequate inspiratory time (Ti) for every breath (both machine triggered and patient triggered). Details on adjustment of NIV settings, including the use of a home ventilator, are discussed in Chapter 24.

An initial randomized study of patients with ALS found increased survival with NIV in the group of patients with less severe bulbar dysfunction.[189] The average IPAP and EPAP settings were 15 and 6 cm H_2O, respectively. This and other studies reported improvement in quality of life with NIV. Patients with bulbar involvement may have more difficulty tolerating NPPV and mask ventilation. These patients may also have a greater risk of aspiration than those without upper-airway dysfunction. However, an analysis of NIV and ALS by Berlowitz et al.[190] found the greatest survival benefit with NIV to be in those with bulbar ALS. Ackrivo and coworkers[191] examined whether the amount of NIV use matters in patients with ALS. After adjustment for body mass index and age at diagnosis, the authors showed that ≥4 hours per day of use was associated with a 33% reduction in the rate of death (median, unadjusted survival of 10.7 months if use >4 hours/day vs. 5.9 months with use <4 hours/day). In an editorial discussing this study, Berlowitz and Sheers pointed out the important benefits of NIV in ALS but noted that increasing adherence is important and will take a team effort involving the patient, family, physicians, and respiratory therapists.[192] Home initiation of NIV can result in treatment that is as effective as that following a PSG NPPV titration.[193] However, this requires a home care system and respiratory therapy team experienced in taking care of patients with NMD. Patient ventilatory asynchrony and other issues may reduce the benefit of NIV. A single-site, randomized controlled trial determined that careful alignment of NIV settings to patient effort using an overnight sleep study can increase adherence with NIV in ALS.[194] Adherence was improved only in participants who initially used NIV for <4 hours/day, and optimizing NIV increased adherence by 118 minutes compared with controls. Home ventilators have the option of mouthpiece ventilation (sip and puff) and allow ventilatory support during the day without the need for a mask. Providing NIV to severely ill neuromuscular patients requires an emphasis on respiratory muscle rest, increased triggering sensitivity (triggering with a small amount of inspiratory flow), and assuring adequate inspiratory time. These may not be familiar to some physicians used to using BPAP for sleep apnea or NIV for COPD. For chronic progressive disorders, the best care is provided by a dedicated clinic and multidisciplinary team to address the total integrated treatment of the NMD, including NIV, nutrition, cough assist, and psychological support for the patient and family. Guidelines for the respiratory management of patients with neuromuscular weakness were published in 2023 and address airway clearance techniques as well as mouth piece ventilation and treatment of sialorrhea.[196]

Chronic Lung Disease

Severe lung disease of many different etiologies is often associated with hypoventilation as well as hypoxemia. Initially, only nocturnal hypoventilation may be present. Chapter 29 discusses sleep and lung disease and treatment of hypoventilation associated with COPD. Patients with overlap syndrome (OSA + COPD) may exhibit hypoventilation even with an FEV_1 in the mild to moderate range. Treatment of OSA may improve hypoventilation. Aggressive NIV treatment of patients with severe COPD and stable hypoventilation may also improve their prognosis. "High intensity" NIV aims to normalize or significantly improve the degree of hypoventilation at night. Treatment of hypercapnic COPD patient is discussed in chapter 29.

Nocturnal oxygen desaturation is common in patients with interstitial lung disease and may not be recognized until evaluation for pulmonary hypertension is initiated. Some studies suggest a poor prognosis in patients with interstitial lung disease and nocturnal oxygen desaturation.[196] There is little information concerning sleep-related hypoventilation in interstitial lung disease.

SUMMARY OF KEY POINTS

1. Hypocapnic CSA occurs because the arterial PCO_2 falls below the apneic threshold (AT) during NREM sleep. The propensity for this type of central apnea to occur is increased when there is a small difference between the $PaCO_2$ during sleep and the AT (small $PaCO_2$ reserve) because of high ventilatory drive. The AT is usually at or slightly below the awake $PaCO_2$.
2. Hypocapnic CSA syndromes include Primary CSA (idiopathic CSA), CSA with CSB, High Altitude Periodic Breathing, and Treatment-Emergent CSA (TECSA).
3. Primary CSA is an uncommon form of hypocapnic central apnea characterized by symptoms of snoring, daytime sleepiness, and/or insomnia; a normal or low awake $PaCO_2$; an *elevated hypercapnic ventilatory response*; and central apneas with a short cycle time, not having a Cheyne-Stokes morphology, without an obvious associated disease (neurologic disorder or heart failure), and not being treated with a respiratory depressant medication (opioid).
4. CSA-CSB is characterized by a cycle time of ≥40 seconds and a crescendo-decrescendo pattern of ventilation between central apneas or hypopneas and is most commonly caused by CHF—both with and without a reduced ejection fraction. Many patients have a combination of OSA and CSA-CSB. If OSA is present on a diagnostic study, CSA-CSB may emerge on PAP treatment (a form of CompSA). CSA-CSB can also be the predominant diagnostic study finding, and about 50% of patients with HFrEF and CSB-CSA will respond to CPAP. Adaptive servoventilation is very effective at reducing the AHI in CSB-CSA. However, this treatment is currently contraindicated in patients with a low ejection fraction (<40%–45%). A study using a modern ASV device found the treatment to be safe in HFrEF patients with CSA-CSB although cardiovascular outcomes were not improved. ASV is also effective in patients with CSA-CSB and HFpEF. CSA-CSB can also occur after stroke, although OSA is more common.
5. CompSA is a **pattern** consisting of primarily obstructive events on a diagnostic study but predominantly central apneas or hypopnea that are persistent or emerge on PAP (CPAP or BPAP without a backup rate) after obstructive events are eliminated or substantially reduced. The ICSD-3-TR reserves the diagnosis of TECSA for when a pattern of CompSA is not explained by another central apnea syndrome (usually CSA-CSB or a medication-associated CSA). In the ICSD-3-TR *symptoms caused by the persistent central apneas on CPAP treatment are required for a diagnosis*.
6. The percentage of patients with persistent central apnea (compared to the total number undergoing a PAP titration or treatment) is believed to be small (3%–8%). The percentage of patients with significant CSA during an initial PAP titration after obstructive events have resolved who have persistent central apnea on chronic PAP treatment is 25% to 40%. Though the majority of patients with OSA with initial CSA on PAP have resolution of CSA (transient CSA), a significant number will continue to experience CSA. These patients are at risk for continued symptoms, low adherence, and cessation of treatment. Careful objective follow-up and changing from CPAP to ASV, if indicated, may improve outcomes. Patients with CompSA associated with CHF or narcotics that does not respond to CPAP are unlikely to have a resolution of central apnea on chronic CPAP and are best initially treated with some form of BPAP with a backup rate (if not contraindicated). It is important to treat the patient and not the AHI, as the persistence of a low central AHI may have little impact on symptoms in many patients. Risk factors for development of TECSA include male gender, a high diagnostic AHI, central apnea during the diagnostic study, use of a split night protocol, supine > nonsupine position, NREM > REM, high altitude, oral breathing, high levels of CPAP (overtitration), use of BPAP without a backup rate, and high mask leak.
7. Primary CSA and CSA-CSB are associated with instability in ventilatory control. The instability is caused by increased hypercapnic ventilatory response (high controller gain), unstable sleep (frequent arousals), increased circulation time (CSA-CSB), and a small sleeping $PaCO_2$ – AT difference.
8. Hypocapnic CSA is often absent *during REM sleep*, as this sleep stage is associated with lower ventilatory responses to PCO_2 and PO_2, and ventilation varies because of the phasic changes associated with this stage of sleep. The results is that an AT does not exist. Some patients with hypocapnic CSA will respond better to CPAP during REM sleep than during NREM sleep.
9. CSA caused by high altitude periodic breathing is a result of hypobaric hypoxia, which increases ventilatory drive. The fraction of patients developing this issue increases with higher altitude. In many individuals remaining at a high altitude (depending on the altitude), the ventilatory drive continues to increase; as compensation for chronic hypoxia, periodic breathing persists, but sleep quality improves. Acetazolamide started prior to assent and taken a few days at altitude can be helpful.
10. CCHS is a rare disorder usually present from birth and is characterized by alveolar hypoventilation without evidence of lung, neuromuscular, or structural brainstem abnormalities. The syndrome is usually caused by de novo mutations in the *PHOX2B* gene on chromosome 4 (very rarely other gene abnormalities). Most patients with CCHS are heterozygous for phenylalanine repeat mutations (PARM) in exon 3 of *PHOX2B*. Longer polyalanine repeat expansions and NPARM defects in the *PHOX2B* gene are associated with more severe phenotypes (including daytime hypoventilation). The majority of patients with NPARM are reported to have severe phenotypes with need for continuous assisted ventilation and are more likely to have Hirschsprung disease or a neural crest tumor (NCT). Most mutations occur de novo, but in families with CCHS, it is inherited as an autosomal dominant trait. Late-onset (teenage years) or even adult-onset CCHS has been described. Some patients need 24-hour ventilatory support, but others can be treated with nocturnal ventilatory support. In CCHS hypoventilation is usually worse during NREM than REM sleep.
11. Opioid (narcotic)-associated sleep disordered breathing can be manifested by long obstructive apneas, ataxic breathing, a low respiratory rate during sleep, CSA, CompSA, and nocturnal hypoventilation. Some patients also manifest daytime hypoventilation, which can be severe but is usually mild. When central apnea persists or emerges on PAP (a form of CompSA), most patients have better control of respiratory events during REM sleep. The best treatment is weaning and cessation of the offending medication. Medications associated with CSA include methadone, oxycodone, morphine, hydromorphone, fentanyl, baclofen, ticagrelor, and sodium oxybate.
12. OHS is the only sleep-related hypoventilation syndrome that requires the presence of daytime hypoventilation ($PaCO_2$ ≥45 mmHg).

13. Patients with thoracic cage disorder or NMD may manifest daytime hypoventilation that worsens during sleep or exhibit hypoventilation only during sleep. Although sometime classified under the hypercapnic CSA subgroup, most patients have relatively few discrete central apneas but have abnormal decreases in tidal volume during sleep. In these patients, nocturnal gas exchange is usually more abnormal during REM sleep.

14. NIV (BPAP with a backup rate) is the treatment of choice for most patients with sleep-related hypoventilation. With early intervention, sleep quality can be improved, and the development of daytime hypoventilation delayed or, if present, the severity improved. The respiratory assist device (RAD) criteria specify the qualifications for a BPAP device with a backup rate. This chapter discussed the first two of the four categories: restrictive thoracic disorder and CSA/CompSA. The other two categories include hypoventilation syndromes and severe COPD. Except for stable patients with OHS and severe OSA, all patients with hypoventilation should be treated with a BPAP device with a backup rate. See Chapter 24 for more details.

15. In restrictive chest-wall disorders, a daytime $PaCO_2$ $\geq$45 mmHg OR nocturnal oximetry showing $\geq$5 minutes with an SaO_2 $\leq$88% meets RAD criteria for BPAP with a backup rate and is considered an indication for nocturnal NIV. This assumes COPD does not contribute (but pulmonary function testing is not required). A sleep study is not needed to qualify these patients under RAD criteria. However, a sleep study is useful for adjustment of NIV settings. Patients with restrictive chest-wall disorders may require relatively high pressure support and/or an increased respiratory rate.

16. Patients with an FVC less than 50% of predicted are considered to have severe restrictive ventilatory dysfunction. However, patients with much milder pulmonary impairment may experience significant arterial oxygen desaturation. Nocturnal oximetry is useful to detect a nocturnal gas exchange abnormality. If sleep apnea is suspected, PSG is indicated. However, if patients already qualify for a BPAP with a backup rate under RAD criteria, a PAP titration sleep study is useful for optimizing NIV settings (and treating OSA, if present).

17. In patients with NMD: One of the following qualify a patient for a BPAP device with a backup rate under RAD criteria: 1) a daytime $PaCO_2$ $\geq$45 mmHg; 2) sleep oximetry showing $\geq$5 minutes with an SaO_2 $\leq$88%); OR 3) an FVC <50% of predicted or a maximal inspiratory force less than 60 cm H_2O. PSG is not needed to qualify these patients for a RAD device with a backup rate. Many patients benefit from early intervention even if the FVC is greater than 50% of predicted. Aggressive NIV has been shown to improve outcomes in many NMD disorders. Many NMD patients can be treated with a RAD device-BPAP using a backup rate (BPAP-ST or volume assured pressure support). Patients with severe progressive disease will benefit from a home ventilator at some point in their disease course (battery backup, mouthpiece ventilation). The use of home mechanical ventilators is discussed in Chapter 24.

CLINICAL REVIEW QUESTIONS

1. All of the following are true about central congenital hypoventilation syndrome **EXCEPT**?
   A. Associated with Hirschsprung disease
   B. Caused by mutations in the *PHOX2B* gene in most cases
   C. Hypoventilation manifested by low tidal volume
   D. Patients have dyspnea when hypoxic
   E. May require 24-hour ventilatory support from birth
2. Which of the following does not predispose a patient to hypocapnic central sleep apnea?
   A. Large PCO_2 – AT gradient
   B. Increased hypercapnic ventilatory drive
   C. Frequent arousals
   D. NREM > REM sleep
   E. Supine > non-supine sleep
3. Which of the following patients with Cheyne-Stokes central sleep apnea likely has the lowest cardiac output and the longest delay in the SaO_2 nadir?

	Cycle length in seconds*	Apnea length
A	40	20
B	75	25
C	50	25
D	50	20

*Start of one central apnea until the next

4. A patient with suspected sleep apnea and CHF **with a preserved ejection fraction** undergoes a split sleep study. During the diagnostic portion, the AHI is 50 events/hour with 40 obstructive apneas, 10 mixed apneas, 0 central apneas, and 30 hypopneas. During the CPAP titration on CPAP of 10 cm H_2O, obstructive apneas are abolished but frequent **central apneas of the Cheyne-Stokes type are noted.** The AHI on 10 cm H_2O is 40 events/hour, all residual events are CSA-CSB. Higher pressure is not more effective. What do you recommend?
   A. Optimize cardiac function
   B. Treatment with CPAP of 10 cm H_2O
   C. Titration with ASV
   D. A and B
   E. A and C
5. Which of the following is likely present in a patient with CSB central apnea associated with heart failure?
   A. High wedge pressure (left ventricular end diastolic pressure)
   B. Low hypercapnic ventilatory response
   C. Daytime $PaCO_2$ = 44 mmHg
   D. Normal left atrial size
   E. Sinus rhythm
6. A 50-year-old male undergoes a split sleep study. The results are shown below. The central apneas were **not** of the Cheyne-Stokes type. He does not have CHF and is not taking opioid medications. What do you recommend?

	Diagnostic	Titration
Total sleep time (min)	120	150
REM sleep (min)	10	40
AHI (events/hr)	50	22
Obstructive apneas (No.)	40	15
Central apneas (No.)	5	30
Mixed apneas (No.)	5	0
Hypopneas (No.)	40	10

CPAP Treatment Table

CPAP (cm H_2O)	TST (min)	REM sleep (min)	AHI (events/hr)	AHI REM (events/hr)	OA (No.)	MA (No.)	CA (No.)	Hypopnea (No.)
6	15	0	40	0	10	0	0	0
7	15	0	40	0	5	0	0	5
8	30	10	10	30	0	0	0	5
9	30	20	0	0	0	0	0	0
10	30	10	10	0	0	0	5	0
11	30	10	40	0	0	0	20	0

A. Treatment with CPAP of 8 cm H_2O
B. Treatment with CPAP of 9 cm H_2O
C. Treatment with CPAP of 10 cm H_2O
D. ASV titration
E. BPAP ST titration

7. A patient with a progressive NMD reports moderate snoring and has a daytime $PaCO_2$ of 42 mmHg. However, nocturnal oximetry reveals 15 minutes with an SaO2 ≤88%. The FVC is 60% of predicted, and the maximum inspiratory force is 70 cm H_2O. What do you recommend?
   A. Nocturnal supplemental oxygen
   B. Diagnostic PSG and PSG for titration with CPAP
   C. Diagnostic PSG and PSG for titration with BPAP
   D. PSG for titration with BPAP-ST
   E. Empiric treatment with BPAP ST 12/4 cm H_2O and backup rate of 12 BPM
8. Which of the following would **NOT** be consistent with PSG showing CSA in a thin male using high-dose methadone? The overall AHI was 30 events/hour with 85% of the respiratory events being central apneas.
   A. Periods of ataxic breathing
   B. Lower AHI in NREM than REM sleep
   C. Low respiratory rate
   D. Repetitive central apneas with a cycle time of 35 seconds.

ANSWERS

1. D. Patients with CCHS do not experience dyspnea when hypoxemic and are at risk of death from respiratory infections.
2. A. A small $PaCO_2$-AT gradient predisposes to hypocapnic central sleep apnea
3. B. A longer ventilatory phase between events is associated with a longer circulation time, a lower cardiac output, and a longer delay in the SaO_2 nadir. The ventilatory phase = cycle length − apnea duration = A (20 sec), B (50 sec), C (25 sec), D (30 sec)
4. E. (A and C). CSB may improve with optimization of cardiac function. Even if the patient has a normal ejection fraction treatment may reduce left atrial and pulmonary venous pressures. The patient may receive some benefit from CPAP, which did eliminate OSA, but the residual AHI caused by central apnea is quite high. ASV can often reduce the AHI to less than 5 events/hour. Because this patient has both OSA and CSA-CSB and a normal ejection fraction, an ASV with an autoEPAP function is the best approach. However, to date, no improvement in long-term outcomes has been demonstrated with ASV treatment in this type of patient.
5. A. Patients with CSA-CSB are more likely to have a large left atrium, atrial fibrillation, a low daytime PCO_2, and an elevated wedge pressure.
6. B. The patient has TECSA. CPAP of 9 cm H_2O was effective at eliminating obstructive events, even during REM sleep. Higher pressure was associated with central apneas. In other patients, TECSA may occur on pressures needed to prevent obstructive apneas during REM sleep. TECSA may resolve with chronic CPAP treatment (especially if the patient does not have CHF and is not taking potent opioids). However, close follow-up is needed, as central apneas may persist in 25%–40% of patients (about one-third).
7. D. The patient has NMD and qualifies for a BPAP with a backup rate under RAD criteria; as such, treatment would definitely be indicated, no matter what a diagnostic PSG showed. Only one of the following three is required: 1. awake $PaCO_2$ ≥45mmHg; 2. sleep oximetry ≥5 min with SaO_2 ≤88%; or 3. FVC <50% of predicted or maximal inspiratory pressure <60 cm H_2O. This patient meets the second of the three criteria (Table 30-10). A diagnostic PSG may provide useful information, but the best use of a sleep study is to find an appropriate mask and pressure to begin NPPV treatment. The empiric approach might work with very close follow-up and adjustment of settings but is not practical in most settings. NIV rather than supplemental oxygen is indicated for treatment or prevention of nocturnal hypoventilation. A titration with NIV (BPAP-ST) can eliminate OSA events, (document an effective EPAP), treat nocturnal hypoventilation, and provide respiratory muscle rest. BPAP with a backup rate is recommended for patients with neuromuscular disorders, as they may not trigger IPAP/EPAP cycles caused by weak muscles (especially during REM sleep). A backup rate will also provide intervention for central apneas
8. B. Central apneas caused by drug or substance use are more common during NREM sleep, and often the AHI in REM sleep is low (unless severe OSA is also present). On CPAP, this patient might have continued central apneas during NREM but good control during REM sleep.

SUGGESTED READING

1. American Academy of Sleep Medicine. *International Classification of Sleep Disorders*. 3rd ed. Darien, IL: American Academy of Sleep Medicine; 2014.
2. Dempsey JA. Central sleep apnea: misunderstood and mistreated! *F1000Res*. 2019;8:F1000 Faculty Rev-981.
3. Orr JE, Malhotra A, Sands SA. Pathogenesis of central and complex sleep apnoea. *Respirology*. 2017;22(1):43-52.
4. Badr MS, Dingell JD, Javaheri S. Central sleep apnea: a brief review. *Curr Pulmonol Rep*. 2019;8(1):14-21. doi:10.1007/s13665-019-0221-z.

5. Selim BJ, Wolfe L, Coleman JM III, Dewan NA. Initiation of noninvasive ventilation for sleep related hypoventilation disorders: advanced modes and devices. *Chest.* 2018;153(1):251-265.
6. Javaheri S, Dempsey JA. Central sleep apnea. *Compr Physiol.* 2013; 3(1):141-163.
7. Morgenthaler TI, Malhotra A, Berry RB, Johnson KG, Raphaelson M. Optimal NIV Medicare access promotion: patients with central sleep apnea: a technical expert panel report from the American College of Chest Physicians, the American Association for Respiratory Care, the American Academy of Sleep Medicine, and the American Thoracic Society. *Chest.* 2021;160(5):e419-e425.

REFERENCES

1. American Academy of Sleep Medicine. *International Classification of Sleep Disorders.* 3rd ed., text revision. Darien, IL: American Academy of Sleep Medicine; 2023.
2. Bradley TD, McNicholas WT, Rutherford R, Popkin J, Zamel N, Phillipson EA. Clinical and physiologic heterogeneity of the central sleep apnea syndrome. *Am Rev Respir Dis.* 1986;134(2):217-221.
3. Eckert DJ, Jordan AS, Merchia P, Malhotra A. Central sleep apnea: pathophysiology and treatment. *Chest.* 2007;131(2):595-607.
4. Dempsey JA. Central sleep apnea: misunderstood and mistreated! *F1000Res.* 2019;8:F1000 Faculty Rev-981.
5. Javaheri S, Dempsey JA. Central sleep apnea. *Compr Physiol.* 2013; 3(1):141-163.
6. Orr JE, Malhotra A, Sands SA. Pathogenesis of central and complex sleep apnoea. *Respirology.* 2017;22(1):43-52.
7. Roberts EG, Raphelson JR, Orr JE, et al. The pathogenesis of central and complex sleep apnea. *Curr Neurol Neurosci Rep.* 2022;22(7):405-412.
8. Hernandez AB, Patil SP. Pathophysiology of central sleep apneas. *Sleep Breath.* 2016;20(2):467-482.
9. Badr MS, Dingell JD, Javaheri S. Central sleep apnea: a brief review. *Curr Pulmonol Rep.* 2019;8(1):14-21.
10. Troester MM, Quan SF, Berry RB, et al.; for the American Academy of Sleep Medicine. *The AASM Manual for the Scoring of Sleep and Associated Events: Rules, Terminology and Technical Specifications.* Version 3. Darien, IL: American Academy of Sleep Medicine; 2023.
11. Badr MS, Toiber F, Skatrud JB, Dempsey J. Pharyngeal narrowing/occlusion during central sleep apnea. *J Appl Physiol (1985).* 1995;78(5):1806-1815.
12. Sankri-Tarbichi AG, Rowley JA, Badr MS. Expiratory pharyngeal narrowing during central hypocapnic hypopnea. *Am J Respir Crit Care Med.* 2009;179(4):313-319.
13. Mohsenin V. Sleep in chronic obstructive pulmonary disease. *Semin Respir Crit Care Med.* 2005;26(1):109-116. doi:10.1055/s-2005-864204.
14. Xi L, Smith CA, Saupe KW, Henderson KS, Dempsey JA. Effects of rapid-eye-movement sleep on the AT in dogs. *J Appl Physiol (1985).* 1993;75(3):1129-1139.
15. Jouett NP, Smith ML, Watenpaugh DE, Siddiqui M, Ahmad M, Siddiqui F. Rapid-eye-movement sleep-predominant central sleep apnea relieved by positive airway pressure: a case report. *Physiol Rep.* 2017; 5(9):e13254. doi:10.14814/phy2.13254.
16. Wiegand L, Zwillich CW, Wiegand D, White DP. Changes in upper airway muscle activation and ventilation during phasic REM sleep in normal men. *J Appl Physiol (1985).* 1991;71(2):488-497.
17. Tabachnik E, Muller NL, Bryan AC, Levison H. Changes in ventilation and chest wall mechanics during sleep in normal adolescents. *J Appl Physiol Respir Environ Exerc Physiol.* 1981;51(3):557-564.
18. Skatrud JB, Dempsey JA. Interaction of sleep state and chemical stimuli in sustaining rhythmic ventilation. *J Appl Physiol Respir Environ Exerc Physiol.* 1983;55(3):813-822.
19. Deacon-Diaz N, Malhotra A. Inherent vs. induced loop gain abnormalities in obstructive sleep apnea. *Front Neurol.* 2018;9:896. doi:10.3389/fneur.2018.00896.
20. Centers for Medicare and Medicaid Services. *Local Coverage Determination Respiratory Assist Devices (L33800).* Last Update August 8, 2021. Available at: https://www.cms.gov/medicare-coverage-database/view/lcd.aspx?LCDId=33800. Accessed Sept 16, 2012.
21. Issa FG, Sullivan CE. Reversal of central sleep apnea using nasal CPAP. *Chest.* 1986;90(2):165-171.
22. Hoffstein V, Slutsky AS. Central sleep apnea reversed by continuous positive airway pressure. *Am Rev Respir Dis.* 1987;135(5):1210-1212.
23. Morgenthaler TI, Malhotra A, Berry RB, Johnson KG, Raphaelson M. Optimal NIV Medicare access promotion: patients with central sleep apnea: a technical expert panel report from the American College of Chest Physicians, the American Association for Respiratory Care, the American Academy of Sleep Medicine, and the American Thoracic Society. *Chest.* 2021;160(5):e419-e425.
24. Kouri I, Kolla BP, Morgenthaler TI, Mansukhani MP. Frequency and outcomes of primary central sleep apnea in a population-based study. *Sleep Med.* 2020;68:177-183.
25. Hall MJ, Xie A, Rutherford R, Ando S, Floras JS, Bradley TD. Cycle length of periodic breathing in patients with and without heart failure. *Am J Respir Crit Care Med.* 1996;154(2 Pt 1):376-381.
26. Xie A, Rutherford R, Rankin F, Wong B, Bradley TD. Hypocapnia and increased ventilatory responsiveness in patients with idiopathic central sleep apnea. *Am J Respir Crit Care Med.* 1995;152(6 Pt 1):1950-1955.
27. Nakayama H, Smith CA, Rodman JR, Skatrud JB, Dempsey JA. Effect of ventilatory drive on carbon dioxide sensitivity below eupnea during sleep. *Am J Respir Crit Care Med.* 2002;165(9):1251-1260.
28. Xie A, Wong B, Phillipson EA, Slutsky AS, Bradley TD. Interaction of hyperventilation and arousal in the pathogenesis of idiopathic central sleep apnea. *Am J Respir Crit Care Med.* 1994;150(2):489-495.
29. Xie A, Rankin F, Rutherford R, Bradley TD. Effects of inhaled CO2 and added dead space on idiopathic central sleep apnea. *J Appl Physiol (1985).* 1997;82(3):918-926.
30. DeBacker WA, Verbraecken J, Willemen M, Wittesaele W, DeCock W, Van deHeyning P. Central apnea index decreases after prolonged treatment with acetazolamide. *Am J Respir Crit Care Med.* 1995;151(1):87-91.
31. Quadri S, Drake C, Hudgel DW. Improvement of idiopathic central sleep apnea with zolpidem. *J Clin Sleep Med.* 2009;5(2):122-129.
32. Grimaldi D, Provini F, Vetrugno R, et al. Idiopathic central sleep apnoea syndrome treated with zolpidem. *Neurol Sci.* 2008;29(5):355-357.
33. Bonnet MH, Dexter JR, Arand DL. The effect of triazolam on arousal and respiration in central sleep apnea patients. *Sleep.* 1990;13(1):31-41.
34. Franklin KA, Eriksson P, Sahlin C, Lundgren R. Reversal of central sleep apnea with oxygen. *Chest.* 1997;111(1):163-169.
35. Aurora RN, Chowdhuri S, Ramar K, et al. The treatment of central sleep apnea syndromes in adults: practice parameters with an evidence-based literature review and meta-analyses. *Sleep.* 2012;35(1):17-40.
36. Javaheri S, McKane S. Transvenous phrenic nerve stimulation to treat idiopathic central sleep apnea. *J Clin Sleep Med.* 2020;16(12): 2099-2107.
37. Aurora RN, Bista SR, Casey KR, et al. Updated adaptive servo-ventilation recommendations for the 2012 AASM Guideline: "The Treatment of Central Sleep Apnea Syndromes in Adults: Practice Parameters with an Evidence-Based Literature Review and Meta-Analyses". *J Clin Sleep Med.* 2016;12(5):757-761.
38. MacDonald M, Fang J, Pittman SD, White DP, Malhotra A. The current prevalence of sleep disordered breathing in congestive heart failure patients treated with beta-blockers. *J Clin Sleep Med.* 2008;4(1):38-42.
39. Javaheri S, Barbe F, Campos-Rodriguez F, et al. Sleep apnea: types, mechanisms, and clinical cardiovascular consequences. *J Am Coll Cardiol.* 2017;69(7):841-858.
40. Sin DD, Fitzgerald F, Parker JD, Newton G, Floras JS, Bradley TD. Risk factors for central and obstructive sleep apnea in 450 men and women with congestive heart failure. *Am J Respir Crit Care Med.* 1999; 160(4):1101-1106.
41. Kim Y, Kim S, Ryu DR, Lee SY, Im KB. Factors associated with Cheyne-Stokes respiration in acute ischemic stroke. *J Clin Neurol.* 2018;14(4):542-548.
42. Johnson KG, Johnson DC. Frequency of sleep apnea in stroke and TIA patients: a meta-analysis. *J Clin Sleep Med.* 2010;6(2):131-137.
43. Nigam G, Pathak C, Riaz M. A systematic review of central sleep apnea in adult patients with chronic kidney disease. *Sleep Breath.* 2016; 20(3):957-964.
44. Banno K, Okamura K, Kryger MH. Adaptive servo-ventilation in patients with idiopathic Cheyne-Stokes breathing. *J Clin Sleep Med.* 2006;2(2):181-186.
45. Bitter T, Westerheide N, Hossain MS, et al. Complex sleep apnoea in congestive heart failure. *Thorax.* 2011;66(5):402-407.
46. Sahlin C, Svanborg E, Stenlund H, Franklin KA. Cheyne-Stokes respiration and supine dependency. *Eur Respir J.* 2005;25(5):829-833.
47. Szollosi I, Roebuck T, Thompson B, Naughton MT. Lateral sleeping position reduces severity of central sleep apnea / Cheyne-Stokes respiration. *Sleep.* 2006;29(8):1045-1051.
48. Joho S, Oda Y, Hirai T, Inoue H. Impact of sleeping position on central sleep apnea/Cheyne-Stokes respiration in patients with heart failure. *Sleep Med.* 2010;11(2):143-148.

49. Xie A, Skatrud JB, Puleo DS, Rahko PS, Dempsey JA. Apnea-hypopnea threshold for CO2 in patients with congestive heart failure. *Am J Respir Crit Care Med.* 2002;165(9):1245-1250.
50. Lorenzi-Filho G, Azevedo ER, Parker JD, Bradley TD. Relationship of carbon dioxide tension in arterial blood to pulmonary wedge pressure in heart failure. *Eur Respir J.* 2002;19(1):37-40.
51. Solin P, Bergin P, Richardson M, Kaye DM, Walters EH, Naughton MT. Influence of pulmonary capillary wedge pressure on central apnea in heart failure. *Circulation.* 1999;99(12):1574-1579.
52. Tkacova R, Niroumand M, Lorenzi-Filho G, Bradley TD. Overnight shift from obstructive to central apneas in patients with heart failure: role of PCO2 and circulatory delay. *Circulation.* 2001;103(2):238-243.
53. Javaheri S, McKane SW, Cameron N, Germany RE, Malhotra A. In patients with heart failure the burden of central sleep apnea increases in the late sleep hours. *Sleep.* 2019;42(1):zsy195. doi:10.1093/sleep/zsy195.
54. Wedewardt J, Bitter T, Prinz C, Faber L, Horstkotte D, Oldenburg O. Cheyne-Stokes respiration in heart failure: cycle length is dependent on left ventricular ejection fraction. *Sleep Med.* 2010;11(2):137-142.
55. Bitter T, Faber L, Hering D, Langer C, Horstkotte D, Oldenburg O. Sleep-disordered breathing in heart failure with normal left ventricular ejection fraction. *Eur J Heart Fail.* 2009;11(6):602-608.
56. Javaheri S, Brown LK, Khayat R. CON: persistent central sleep apnea/Hunter-Cheyne-Stokes breathing, despite best guideline-based therapy of heart failure with reduced ejection fraction, is not a compensatory mechanism and should be suppressed. *J Clin Sleep Med.* 2018;14(6):915-921.
57. Sin DD, Logan AG, Fitzgerald FS, Liu PP, Bradley TD. Effects of continuous positive airway pressure on cardiovascular outcomes in heart failure patients with and without Cheyne-Stokes respiration. *Circulation.* 2000;102(1):61-66.
58. Naughton MT. PRO: persistent central sleep apnea/Hunter-Cheyne-Stokes breathing, despite best guideline-based therapy of heart failure with reduced ejection fraction, is a compensatory mechanism and should not be suppressed. *J Clin Sleep Med.* 2018;14(6):909-914.
59. Dark DS, Pingleton SK, Kerby GR, et al. Breathing pattern abnormalities and arterial oxygen desaturation during sleep in the congestive heart failure syndrome. Improvement following medical therapy. *Chest.* 1987;91(6):833-836.
60. Braver HM, Brandes WC, Kubiet MA, Limacher MC, Mills Jr RM, Block AJ. Effect of cardiac transplantation on Cheyne-Stokes respiration occurring during sleep. *Am J Cardiol.* 1995;76(8):632-634.
61. Hadigal S, Sharma S, Wagner MH, Ryals S, Berry RB. Sudden improvement in PAP download indices without treatment change. *J Clin Sleep Med.* 2019;15(5):791-793.
62. Bradley TD, Logan AG, Kimoff RJ, et al. Continuous positive airway pressure for central sleep apnea and heart failure. *N Engl J Med.* 2005;353(19):2025-2033.
63. Arzt M, Floras JS, Logan AG, et al. Suppression of central sleep apnea by continuous positive airway pressure and transplant-free survival in heart failure: a post hoc analysis of the Canadian Continuous Positive Airway Pressure for Patients with Central Sleep Apnea and Heart Failure Trial (CANPAP). *Circulation.* 2007;115(25):3173-3180.
64. Bitter T, Westerheide N, Faber L. Adaptive servoventilation in diastolic heart failure and Cheyne–Stokes respiration. *Eur Resp J.* 2010;36:385-392.
65. Teschler H, Döhring J, Wang YM, Berthon-Jones M. Adaptive pressure support servo-ventilation: a novel treatment for Cheyne-Stokes respiration in heart failure. *Am J Respir Crit Care Med.* 2001;164(4):614-619.
66. Cowie MR, Woehrle H, Wegscheider K, et al. Adaptive servo-ventilation for central sleep apnea in systolic heart failure. *N Engl J Med.* 2015;373(12):1095-1105.
67. Bradley TD, Logan AG, Lorenzi Filho G, et al. Adaptive servo-ventilation for sleep-disordered breathing in patients with heart failure with reduced ejection fraction (ADVENT-HF): a multicentre, multinational, parallel-group, open-label, phase 3 randomised controlled trial. *Lancet Respir Med.* 2024;12(2):153-166.
68. Krachman SL, Nugent T, Crocetti J, D'Alonzo GE, Chatila W. Effects of oxygen therapy on left ventricular function in patients with Cheyne-Stokes respiration and congestive heart failure. *J Clin Sleep Med.* 2005;1(3):271-276.
69. Javaheri S, Ahmed M, Parker TJ, Brown CR. Effects of nasal O2 on sleep-related disordered breathing in ambulatory patients with stable heart failure. *Sleep.* 1999;22(8):1101-1106.
70. Sakakibara M, Sakata Y, Usui K, et al. Effectiveness of short-term treatment with nocturnal oxygen therapy for central sleep apnea in patients with congestive heart failure. *J Cardiol.* 2005;46(2):53-61.
71. Sugimura K, Shinozaki T, Fukui S, Ogawa H, Shimokawa H. End-tidal CO2 tension is predictive of effective nocturnal oxygen therapy in patients with chronic heart failure and central sleep apnea. *Tohoku J Exp Med.* 2016;239(1):39-45.
72. Javaheri S. Acetazolamide improves central sleep apnea in heart failure: a double-blind, prospective study. *Am J Respir Crit Care Med.* 2006;173(2):234-237.
73. Javaheri S, Parker TJ, Wexler L, Liming JD, Lindower P, Roselle GA. Effect of theophylline on sleep-disordered breathing in heart failure. *N Engl J Med.* 1996;335(8):562-567.
74. Costanzo MR, Ponikowski P, Javaheri S, et al. Transvenous neurostimulation for central sleep apnoea: a randomised controlled trial. *Lancet.* 2016;388(10048):974-982.
75. Voigt J, Emani S, Gupta S, Germany R, Khayat R. Meta-analysis comparing outcomes of therapies for patients with central sleep apnea and heart failure with reduced ejection fraction. *Am J Cardiol.* 2020;127:73-83. doi:10.1016/j.amjcard.2020.04.011. Erratum in: *Am J Cardiol.* 2020;134:162.
76. Biberdorf DJ, Steens R, Millar TW, Kryger MH. Benzodiazepines in congestive heart failure: effects of temazepam on arousability and Cheyne-Stokes respiration. *Sleep.* 1993;16(6):529-538.
77. Javaheri S, Brown LK, Khayat RN. Update on apneas of heart failure with reduced ejection fraction: emphasis on the physiology of treatment: part 2: central sleep apnea. *Chest.* 2020;157(6):1637-1646.
78. Chowdhuri S, Ghabsha A, Sinha P, Kadri M, Narula S, Badr MS. Treatment of central sleep apnea in U.S. veterans. *J Clin Sleep Med.* 2012;8(5):555-563.
79. Javaheri S, Sands SA, Edwards BA. Acetazolamide attenuates Hunter-Cheyne-Stokes breathing but augments the hypercapnic ventilatory response in patients with heart failure. *Ann Am Thorac Soc.* 2014;11(1):80-86.
80. Teckchandani PH, Truong KK, Zezoff D, Healy WJ, Khayat RN. Transvenous phrenic nerve stimulation for central sleep apnea: clinical and billing review. *Chest.* 2022;161(5):1330-1337.
81. Ainslie PN, Lucas SJ, Burgess KR. Breathing and sleep at high altitude. *Respir Physiol Neurobiol.* 2013;188(3):233-256.
82. Burgess KR, Ainslie PN. Central sleep apnea at high altitude. *Adv Exp Med Biol.* 2016;903:275-283.
83. Mohsenin V. Common high altitudes illnesses a primer for healthcare provider. *Br J Med Med Res.* 2015;7(12):1017-1025.
84. Hackett PH, Roach RC. High-altitude illness. *N Engl J Med.* 2001;345(2):107-114.
85. Luks AM, McIntosh SE, Grissom CK, et al. Medical Society consensus guidelines for the prevention and treatment of acute altitude illness. *Wilderness Environ Med.* 2010;21(2):146-155.
86. Beaumont M, Batéjat D, Piérard C, et al. Zaleplon and zolpidem objectively alleviate sleep disturbances in mountaineers at a 3,613 meter altitude. *Sleep.* 2007;30(11):1527-1533.
87. Johnson PL, Popa DA, Prisk GK, Edwards N, Sullivan CE. Non-invasive positive pressure ventilation during sleep at 3800 m: relationship to acute mountain sickness and sleeping oxyhaemoglobin saturation. *Respirology.* 2010;15(2):277-282.
88. Orr JE, Heinrich EC, Djokic M, et al. Adaptive servoventilation as treatment for central sleep apnea due to high-altitude periodic breathing in nonacclimatized healthy individuals. *High Alt Med Biol.* 2018;19(2):178-184.
89. Heinrich EC, Djokic MA, Gilbertson D, et al. Cognitive function and mood at high altitude following acclimatization and use of supplemental oxygen and adaptive servoventilation sleep treatments. *PloS One.* 2019;14(6):e0217089.
90. Randerath W, Verbraecken J, Andreas S, et al. Definition, discrimination, diagnosis and treatment of central breathing disturbances during sleep. *Eur Respir J.* 2017;49(1):1600959.
91. Guilleminault C, Cummiskey J. Progressive improvement of apnea index and ventilatory response to CO2 after tracheostomy in obstructive sleep apnea syndrome. *Am Rev Respir Dis.* 1982;126(1):14-20.
92. Fletcher EC. Recurrence of sleep apnea syndrome following tracheostomy. A shift from obstructive to central apnea. *Chest.* 1989;96(1):205-209.
93. Thomas RJ, Terzano MG, Parrino L, Weiss JW. Obstructive sleep-disordered breathing with a dominant cyclic alternating pattern: a recognizable polysomnographic variant with practical clinical implications. *Sleep.* 2004;27(2):229-234.
94. Zeineddine S, Badr MS. Treatment-emergent central apnea: physiologic mechanisms informing clinical practice. *Chest.* 2021;159(6):2449-2457.

95. Salloum A, Rowley JA, Mateika JH, Chowdhuri S, Omran Q, Badr MS. Increased propensity for central apnea in patients with obstructive sleep apnea: effect of nasal continuous positive airway pressure. *Am J Respir Crit Care Med.* 2010;181(2):189-193.
96. Xie A, Skatrud JB, Puleo DS, Dempsey JA. Influence of arterial O2 on the susceptibility to posthyperventilation apnea during sleep. *J Appl Physiol (1985).* 2006;100(1):171-177.
97. Chowdhuri S, Shanidze I, Pierchala L, Belen D, Mateika JH, Badr MS. Effect of episodic hypoxia on the susceptibility to hypocapnic central apnea during NREM sleep. *J Appl Physiol (1985).* 2010;108(2):369-377.
98. Hommura F, Nishimura M, Oguri M, et al. Continuous versus bilevel positive airway pressure in a patient with idiopathic central sleep apnea. *Am J Respir Crit Care Med.* 1997;155(4):1482-1485.
99. Johnson KG, Johnson DC. Bilevel positive airway pressure worsens central apneas during sleep. *Chest.* 2005;128(4):2141-2150.
100. Nigam G, Riaz M, Chang ET, Camacho M. Natural history of treatment-emergent central sleep apnea on positive airway pressure: a systematic review. *Ann Thorac Med.* 2018;13(2):86-91.
101. Nigam G, Pathak C, Riaz M. A systematic review on prevalence and risk factors associated with treatment-emergent central sleep apnea. *Ann Thorac Med.* 2016;11(3):202-210.
102. Pusalavidyasagar SS, Olson EJ, Gay PC, Morgenthaler TI. Treatment of complex sleep apnea syndrome: a retrospective comparative review. *Sleep Med.* 2006;7(6):474-479.
103. Montesi SB, Bakker JP, Macdonald M, et al. Air leak during CPAP titration as a risk factor for central apnea. *J Clin Sleep Med.* 2013; 9(11):1187-1191.
104. Stanchina M, Robinson K, Corrao W, Donat W, Sands S, Malhotra A. Clinical use of loop gain measures to determine continuous positive airway pressure efficacy in patients with complex sleep apnea. A pilot study. *Ann Am Thorac Soc.* 2015;12(9):1351-1357.
105. Kuzniar TJ, Pusalavidyasagar S, Gay PC, Morgenthaler TI. Natural course of complex sleep apnea—a retrospective study. *Sleep Breath.* 2008;12(2):135-139.
106. Javaheri S, Smith J, Chung E. The prevalence and natural history of complex sleep apnea. *J Clin Sleep Med.* 2009;5(3):205-211.
107. Dernaika T, Tawk M, Nazir S, Younis W, Kinasewitz GT. The significance and outcome of continuous positive airway pressure-related central sleep apnea during split-night sleep studies. *Chest.* 2007; 132(1):81-87.
108. Lehman S, Antic NA, Thompson C, Catcheside PG, Mercer J, McEvoy RD. Central sleep apnea on commencement of continuous positive airway pressure in patients with a primary diagnosis of obstructive sleep apnea-hypopnea. *J Clin Sleep Med.* 2007;3(5): 462-466.
109. Cassel W, Canisius S, Becker HF, et al. A prospective polysomnographic study on the evolution of complex sleep apnoea. *Eur Respir J.* 2011;38(2):329-337.
110. Westhoff M, Arzt M, Litterst P. Prevalence and treatment of central sleep apnoea emerging after initiation of continuous positive airway pressure in patients with obstructive sleep apnoea without evidence of heart failure. *Sleep Breath.* 2012;16(1):71-78.
111. Morgenthaler TI, Kuzniar TJ, Wolfe LF, Willes L, McLain WC III, Goldberg R. The complex sleep apnea resolution study: a prospective randomized controlled trial of continuous positive airway pressure versus adaptive servoventilation therapy. *Sleep.* 2014;37(5):927-934.
112. Liu D, Armitstead J, Benjafield A, et al. Trajectories of emergent central sleep apnea during CPAP therapy. *Chest.* 2017;152(4): 751-760.
113. Li QY, Berry RB, Goetting MG, et al. Detection of upper airway status and respiratory events by a current generation positive airway pressure device. *Sleep.* 2015;38(4):597-605. doi:10.5665/sleep.4578.
114. Berger M, Solelhac G, Horvath C, Heinzer R, Brill AK. Treatment-emergent central sleep apnea associated with non-positive airway pressure therapies in obstructive sleep apnea patients: a systematic review. *Sleep Med Rev.* 2021;58:101513.
115. Kuźniar TJ, Kovačević-Ristanović R, Freedom T. Complex sleep apnea unmasked by the use of a mandibular advancement device. *Sleep Breath.* 2011;15(2):249-252.
116. Goodday RH, Fay MB. Emergence of central sleep apnea events after maxillomandibular advancement surgery for obstructive sleep apnea. *J Oral Maxillofac Surg.* 2019;77(11):2303-2307.
117. Patel J, Daniels K, Bogdan L, Huntley C, Boon M. Elevated central and mixed apnea index after upper airway stimulation. *Otolaryngol Head Neck Surg.* 2020;162(5):767-772.
118. Goldstein C, Kuzniar TJ. The emergence of central sleep apnea after surgical relief of nasal obstruction in obstructive sleep apnea. *J Clin Sleep Med.* 2012;8(3):321-322.
119. Morgenthaler TI, Gay PC, Gordon N, Brown LK. Adaptive servoventilation versus noninvasive positive pressure ventilation for central, mixed, and complex sleep apnea syndromes. *Sleep.* 2007;30(4):468-475.
120. Allam JS, Olson EJ, Gay PC, Morgenthaler TI. Efficacy of adaptive servoventilation in treatment of complex and central sleep apnea syndromes. *Chest.* 2007;132(6):1839-1846.
121. Dellweg D, Kerl J, Hoehn E, Wenzel M, Koehler D. Randomized controlled trial of noninvasive positive pressure ventilation (NPPV) versus servoventilation in patients with CPAP-induced central sleep apnea (complex sleep apnea). *Sleep.* 2013;36(8):1163-1171.
122. Pépin JL, Woehrle H, Liu D, et al. Adherence to positive airway therapy after switching from CPAP to ASV: a big data analysis. *J Clin Sleep Med.* 2018;14(1):57-63.
123. Kwok CT, Wong KC, Kwok CL, Lee SH, Yee KS. Treatment-emergent central sleep apnoea managed by CPAP with adjunctive acetazolamide: a case report. *Respirol Case Rep.* 2022;10(4):e0916.
124. Palmer W, Jaziri M, Tovar A. Positional therapy in a patient with refractory treatment-emergent central sleep apnea. *J Sleep Med.* 2021;18(3):182-185.
125. American Academy of Sleep Medicine. *International Classification of Sleep Disorders.* 3rd ed. Darien, IL: American Academy of Sleep Medicine; 2014.
126. Correa D, Farney RJ, Chung F, Prasad A, Lam D, Wong J. Chronic opioid use and central sleep apnea: a review of the prevalence, mechanisms, and perioperative considerations. *Anesth Analg.* 2015; 120(6):1273-1285.
127. Wang D, Teichtahl H, Drummer O, et al. Central sleep apnea in stable methadone maintenance treatment patients. *Chest.* 2005; 128(3):1348-1356.
128. Webster LR, Choi Y, Desai H, Webster L, Grant BJ. Sleep-disordered breathing and chronic opioid therapy. *Pain Med.* 2008; 9(4):425-432.
129. Chowdhuri S, Javaheri S. Sleep disordered breathing caused by chronic opioid use: diverse manifestations and their management. *Sleep Med Clin.* 2017;12(4):573-586.
130. Javaheri S, Patel S. Opioids cause central and complex sleep apnea in humans and reversal with discontinuation: a plea for detoxification. *J Clin Sleep Med.* 2017;13(6):829-833.
131. Lamberts V, Baele P, Kahn D, Liistro G. Dyspnea or Cheyne-Stokes respiration associated with Ticagrelor? *Sleep Med.* 2018;43:4-6.
132. Olivier PY, Joyeux-Faure M, Gentina T, et al. Severe central sleep apnea associated with chronic baclofen therapy: a case series. *Chest.* 2016;149(5):e127-e131.
133. Frase L, Schupp J, Sorichter S, Randelshofer W, Riemann D, Nissen C. Sodium oxybate-induced central sleep apneas. *Sleep Med.* 2013;14(9):922-924.
134. Javaheri S, Harris N, Howard J, Chung E. Adaptive servoventilation for treatment of opioid-associated central sleep apnea. *J Clin Sleep Med.* 2014;10(6):637-643.
135. Javaheri S, Malik A, Smith J, Chung E. Adaptive pressure support servoventilation: a novel treatment for sleep apnea associated with use of opioids. *J Clin Sleep Med.* 2008;4(4):305-310.
136. Farney RJ, Walker JM, Boyle KM, Cloward TV, Shilling KC. Adaptive servoventilation (ASV) in patients with sleep disordered breathing associated with chronic opioid medications for non-malignant pain. *J Clin Sleep Med.* 2008;4(4):311-319.
137. Morgenthaler TI. The quest for stability in an unstable world: adaptive servoventilation in opioid induced complex sleep apnea syndrome. *J Clin Sleep Med.* 2008;4(4):321-323.
138. Glidewell RN, Orr WC, Imes N. Acetazolamide as an adjunct to CPAP treatment: a case of complex sleep apnea in a patient on long-acting opioid therapy. *J Clin Sleep Med.* 2009;5(1):63-64.
139. Cormican LJ, Higgins S, Davidson AC, Howard R, Williams AJ. Multiple system atrophy presenting as central sleep apnoea. *Eur Respir J.* 2004;24(2):323-325.
140. Ralls F, Cutchen L. Respiratory and sleep-related complications of multiple system atrophy. *Curr Opin Pulm Med.* 2020;26(6):615-622.
141. Glass GA, Josephs KA, Ahlskog JE. Respiratory insufficiency as the primary presenting symptom of multiple-system atrophy. *Arch Neurol.* 2006;63(7):978-981.
142. Lam B, Ryan CF. Arnold-Chiari malformation presenting as sleep apnea syndrome. *Sleep Med.* 2000;1(2):139-144.

143. Leu RM. Sleep-related breathing disorders and the Chiari 1 malformation. *Chest*. 2015;148(5):1346-1352.
144. Abel F, Tahir MZ. Role of sleep study in children with Chiari malformation and sleep disordered breathing. *Childs Nerv Syst*. 2019; 35(10):1763-1768.
145. Dauvilliers Y, Stal V, Abril B, et al. Chiari malformation and sleep related breathing disorders. *J Neurol Neurosurg Psychiatry*. 2007;78(12):1344-1348.
146. Hershberger ML, Chidekel A. Arnold-Chiari malformation type I and sleep-disordered breathing: an uncommon manifestation of an important pediatric problem. *J Pediatr Health Care*. 2003;17(4):190-197.
147. Zolty P, Sanders MH, Pollack IF. Chiari malformation and sleep-disordered breathing: a review of diagnostic and management issues. *Sleep*. 2000;23(5):637-643.
148. Gagnadoux F, Meslier N, Svab I, Menei P, Racineux JL. Sleep-disordered breathing in patients with Chiari malformation: improvement after surgery. *Neurology*. 2006;66(1):136-138.
149. Levin JC, Jang J, Rhein LM. Apnea in the otherwise healthy, term newborn: national prevalence and utilization during the birth hospitalization. *J Pediatr*. 2017;181:67-73.e61.
150. MacLean JE, Fitzgerald DA, Waters KA. Developmental changes in sleep and breathing across infancy and childhood. *Paediatr Respir Rev*. 2015;16(4):276-284.
151. Ginsburg D, Maken K, Deming D, et al. Etiologies of apnea of infancy. *Pediatr Pulmonol*. 2020;55(6):1495-1502.
152. Tieder JS, Bonkowsky JL, Etzel RA, et al. Clinical practice guideline: brief resolved unexplained events (formerly apparent life-threatening events) and evaluation of lower-risk infants: executive summary. Pediatrics. 2016:137(5):e20160591. *Pediatrics*. 2016;138(2):e20161488.
153. Eichenwald EC, Committee on Fetus and Newborn, American Academy of Pediatrics. Apnea of prematurity. *Pediatrics*. 2016;137(1).
154. Schmidt B, Roberts RS, Davis P, et al. Long-term effects of caffeine therapy for apnea of prematurity. *N Engl J Med*. 2007;357(19): 1893-1902.
155. Vadhan J, Tadi P. *Physiology, Herring Breuer Reflex*. Treasure Island, FL: StatPearls Publishing; 2022.
156. Long JY, Guo HL, He X, et al. Caffeine for the pharmacological treatment of apnea of prematurity in the NICU: dose selection conundrum, therapeutic drug monitoring and genetic factors. *Front Pharmacol*. 2021;12:681842.
157. Salemi LA, Sahlstrom AL, Lim SY, Johnson PN, Dannaway D, Miller JL. Evaluation of the use of caffeine citrate maintenance doses >5 mg/kg/day in preterm neonates for apnea of prematurity. *J Pediatr Pharmacol Ther*. 2021;26(6):608-614.
158. Hollier CA, Maxwell LJ, Harmer AR, et al. Validity of arterialised-venous P CO2, pH and bicarbonate in obesity hypoventilation syndrome. *Respir Physiol Neurobiol*. 2013;188(2):165-171.
159. Malatesha G, Singh NK, Bharija A, Rehani B, Goel A. Comparison of arterial and venous pH, bicarbonate, PCO2 and PO2 in initial emergency department assessment. *Emerg Med J*. 2007;24(8):569-571.
160. Theodore AC. *Venous Blood Gases and Other Alternatives to Arterial Blood Gases*. Available at: https://www.uptodate.com/contents/venous-blood-gases-and-other-alternatives-to-arterial-blood-gases?search=venous%20abg§ionRank=2&usage_type=default&anchor=H1942934&source=machineLearning&selectedTitle=1,150&display_rank=1#H1942934. Accessed September 8, 2023.
161. Weese-Mayer DE, Berry-Kravis EM, Ceccherini I, Keens TG, Loghmanee DA, Trang H. An official ATS clinical policy statement: congenital central hypoventilation syndrome: genetic basis, diagnosis, and management. *Am J Respir Crit Care Med*. 2010;181(6):626-644.
162. Berry-Kravis EM, Zhou L, Rand CM, Weese-Mayer DE. Congenital central hypoventilation syndrome: PHOX2B mutations and phenotype. *Am J Respir Crit Care Med*. 2006;174(10):1139-1144.
163. Trang H, Samuels M, Ceccherini I, et al. Guidelines for diagnosis and management of congenital central hypoventilation syndrome. *Orphanet J Rare Dis*. 2020;15(1):252.
164. Weese-Mayer DE, Berry-Kravis EM, Zhou L. Adult identified with congenital central hypoventilation syndrome—mutation in PHOX2b gene and late-onset CHS. *Am J Respir Crit Care Med*. 2005;171(1):88.
165. Gozal D, Marcus CL, Shoseyov D, Keens TG. Peripheral chemoreceptor function in children with the congenital central hypoventilation syndrome. *J Appl Physiol (1985)*. 1993;74(1):379-387.
166. Marcus CL, Bautista DB, Amihyia A, Ward SL, Keens TG. Hypercapneic arousal responses in children with congenital central hypoventilation syndrome. *Pediatrics*. 1991;88(5):993-998.
167. Kasi AS, Li H, Jurgensen TJ, Guglani L, Keens TG, Perez IA. Variable phenotypes in congenital central hypoventilation syndrome with PHOX2B nonpolyalanine repeat mutations. *J Clin Sleep Med*. 2021;17(10):2049-2055.
168. American Thoracic Society. Idiopathic congenital central hypoventilation syndrome: diagnosis and management. American Thoracic Society. *Am J Respir Crit Care Med*. 1999;160(1):368-373.
169. Ramesh P, Boit P, Samuels M. Mask ventilation in the early management of congenital central hypoventilation syndrome. *Arch Dis Child Fetal Neonatal Ed*. 2008;93(6):F400-F403.
170. Katz ES, McGrath S, Marcus CL. Late-onset central hypoventilation with hypothalamic dysfunction: a distinct clinical syndrome. *Pediatr Pulmonol*. 2000;29(1):62-68.
171. Ize-Ludlow D, Gray JA, Sperling MA, et al. Rapid-onset obesity with hypothalamic dysfunction, hypoventilation, and autonomic dysregulation presenting in childhood. *Pediatrics*. 2007;120(1): e179-e188.
172. Goldbart AD, Arazi A, Golan-Tripto I, Levinsky Y, Scheuerman O, Tarasiuk A. Altered slow-wave sleep activity in children with rapid-onset obesity with hypothalamic dysregulation, hypoventilation, and autonomic dysregulation syndrome. *J Clin Sleep Med*. 2020; 16(10):1731-1735.
173. Lazea C, Sur L, Florea M. ROHHAD (rapid-onset obesity with hypoventilation, hypothalamic dysfunction, autonomic dysregulation) syndrome-what every pediatrician should know about the etiopathogenesis, diagnosis and treatment: a review. *Int J Gen Med*. 2021;14:319-326.
174. Harvengt J, Gernay C, Mastouri M, et al. ROHHAD(NET) syndrome: systematic review of the clinical timeline and recommendations for diagnosis and prognosis. *J Clin Endocrinol Metab*. 2020;105(7):dgaa247.
175. Berry RB, Chediak A, Brown LK, et al. Best clinical practices for the sleep center adjustment of noninvasive positive pressure ventilation (NPPV) in stable chronic alveolar hypoventilation syndromes. *J Clin Sleep Med*. 2010;6(5):491-509.
176. Selim BJ, Wolfe L, Coleman JM III, Dewan NA. Initiation of noninvasive ventilation for sleep related hypoventilation disorders: advanced modes and devices. *Chest*. 2018;153(1):251-265.
177. Bergofsky EH. Respiratory failure in disorders of the thoracic cage. *Am Rev Respir Dis*. 1979;119(4):643-669.
178. American College of Chest Physicians. Clinical indications for noninvasive positive pressure ventilation in chronic respiratory failure due to restrictive lung disease, COPD, and nocturnal hypoventilation—a consensus conference report. *Chest*. 1999;116(2): 521-534.
179. Wolfe LF, Benditt JO, Aboussouan L, Hess DR, Coleman JM III, ONMAP Technical Expert Panel. Optimal NIV Medicare access promotion: patients with thoracic restrictive disorders: a technical expert panel report from the American College of Chest Physicians, the American Association for Respiratory Care, the American Academy of Sleep Medicine, and the American Thoracic Society. *Chest*. 2021;160(5):e399-e408.
180. Kinnear W, Watson L, Smith P, et al. Long-term survival on noninvasive ventilation in adults with thoracic scoliosis. *Respir Care*. 2021; 66(6):972-975.
181. Gartman EJ. Pulmonary function testing in neuromuscular and chest wall disorders. *Clin Chest Med*. 2018;39(2):325-334.
182. Lechtzin N, Wiener CM, Shade DM, Clawson L, Diette GB. Spirometry in the supine position improves the detection of diaphragmatic weakness in patients with amyotrophic lateral sclerosis. *Chest*. 2002;121(2):436-442.
183. Laveneziana P, Albuquerque A, Aliverti A, et al. ERS statement on respiratory muscle testing at rest and during exercise. *Eur Respir J*. 2019;53(6):1801214.
184. Evans JA, Whitelaw WA. The assessment of maximal respiratory mouth pressures in adults. *Respir Care*. 2009;54(10):1348-1359.
185. De Troyer A, Borenstein S, Cordier R. Analysis of lung volume restriction in patients with respiratory muscle weakness. *Thorax*. 1980;35(8):603-610.
186. Morgan RK, McNally S, Alexander M, Conroy R, Hardiman O, Costello RW. Use of sniff nasal-inspiratory force to predict survival in amyotrophic lateral sclerosis. *Am J Respir Crit Care Med*. 2005; 171(3):269-274.
187. American Thoracic Society ERS. ATS/ERS Statement on respiratory muscle testing. *Am J Respir Crit Care Med*. 2002;166(4):518-624.

188. Aboussouan LS. Sleep-disordered breathing in neuromuscular disease. *Am J Respir Crit Care Med.* 2015;191(9):979-989.
189. Bourke SC, Tomlinson M, Williams TL, Bullock RE, Shaw PJ, Gibson GJ. Effects of non-invasive ventilation on survival and quality of life in patients with amyotrophic lateral sclerosis: a randomised controlled trial. *Lancet Neurol.* 2006;5(2):140-147.
190. Berlowitz DJ, Howard ME, Fiore Jr JF, et al. Identifying who will benefit from non-invasive ventilation in amyotrophic lateral sclerosis/motor neurone disease in a clinical cohort. *J Neurol Neurosurg Psychiatry.* 2016;87(3):280-286.
191. Ackrivo J, Hsu JY, Hansen-Flaschen J, Elman L, Kawut SM. Noninvasive ventilation use is associated with better survival in amyotrophic lateral sclerosis. *Ann Am Thorac Soc.* 2021;18(3):486-494.
192. Berlowitz DJ, Sheers N. Not only about the drugs: improved survival with noninvasive ventilation in amyotrophic lateral sclerosis. *Ann Am Thorac Soc.* 2021;18(3):419-420.
193. Van den Biggelaar RJM, Hazenberg A, Cobben NAM, Gaytant MA, Vermeulen KM, Wijkstra PJ. A randomized trial of initiation of chronic noninvasive mechanical ventilation at home vs in-hospital in patients with neuromuscular disease and thoracic cage disorder: the Dutch Homerun trial. *Chest.* 2020;158(6):2493-2501.
194. Hannan LM, Rautela L, Berlowitz DJ, et al. Randomised controlled trial of polysomnographic titration of noninvasive ventilation. *Eur Respir J.* 2019;53(5):1802118.
195. Khor YH, Ng Y, Sweeney D, Ryerson CJ. Nocturnal hypoxaemia in interstitial lung disease: a systematic review. *Thorax.* 2021;76(12):1200-1208. doi:10.1136/thoraxjnl-2020-216749.
196. Khan A, Frazer-Green L, Amin R. Respiratory management of patients with neuromuscular weakness. *Chest.* 2023;164(2):394-413.

Chapter 31

Restless Legs Syndrome (Willis-Ekbom Disease), Periodic Limb Movements in Sleep, and Periodic Limb Movement Disorder

INTRODUCTION

Restless legs syndrome (RLS), periodic limb movements in sleep (PLMS), and the periodic limb movement disorder (PLMD) are three distinct but related entities[1-16] (Table 31-1). A diagnosis of RLS is based on clinical history. PLMS is a finding on polysomnography (PSG) that may or may not be clinically important. PLMD is diagnosed via PSG in patients with PLMS who have a sleep complaint (sleep-onset or maintenance insomnia or, less commonly, daytime sleepiness) not better explained by another sleep disorder. A **diagnosis of RLS excludes a diagnosis of PLMD**. PLMS is a very common finding, especially in older patients (Figure 31-1), and is often asymptomatic.[5] The PLMS index (PLMSI) is the number of periodic limb movements per hour of sleep. Approximately 80% to 90% of patients with RLS will have findings of PLMS (PLMSI >5/hour) on PSG, especially if monitored for two nights.[1] The percentage of patients with PLMS who have RLS has not been well defined but is estimated to be about 25% to 30% (depending on the population studied and the criteria used to diagnose RLS). In a multi-ethnic atherosclerosis study, 433 individuals had PLMS (PLMSI >15/hour) and no RLS and 137 had PLMS with RLS; therefore, about 24% (137 × 100)/(137+433) of those with PLMS had RLS.[17] While the majority of patients with PLMS do not have RLS, the presence of PLMS does increase the risk of concomitant RLS and should always trigger an assessment for the presence of RLS symptoms.

PLMS has been associated with narcolepsy, rapid eye movement (REM) sleep behavior disorder (RBD), and obstructive sleep apnea (OSA). PLMS is very common, RLS is common, and PLMD is thought to be rare[10]. Using a population survey based on telephone interviews, Ohyaon et al. estimated RLS to occur in 5.5% of the population and PLMD in 3.9%.[6] However, as this study used telephone interviews, the diagnosis of PLMD may not be reliable given the diagnosis requires exclusion of other causes of symptoms such as sleep apnea. Therefore, the true incidence of PLMD is likely lower. Chapter 15 outlines the criteria for scoring PLMS with illustrative tracings. This chapter emphasizes the clinical significance of PLMS and discusses RLS and PLMD.

RESTLESS LEGS SYNDROME

RLS is also known as Willis-Ekbom disease, and sometimes the amalgamated terminology (RLS/WED) is used. There are five essential diagnostic criteria for RLS established through consensus in 2014 by the *International Restless Legs Syndrome Study Group* (IRLSSG).[2] A useful pneumonic is URGES: **U**rge to move, **R**est induced, **G**ets better with activity, worse during the **E**vening and night, and not **S**olely due to another entity. The consensus document states, "RLS/WED, a neurologic sensorimotor disease, is diagnosed by ascertaining symptom patterns that meet the five essential criteria, adding clinical specifiers where appropriate."

RLS Diagnostic Criteria (IRLSSG)[2] (all criteria must be met)

1. An **Urge** to move the legs *usually, but not always,* accompanied or felt to be caused by uncomfortable and unpleasant sensations in the legs.
2. The urge to move the legs and any accompanying unpleasant sensations **begin or worsen** during periods of **Rest** or inactivity such as lying down or sitting.
3. The urge to move the legs and any accompanying unpleasant sensations are partially or totally relieved by movement **(Gets better)**, such as walking or stretching, *at least as long as the activity continues.*
4. The urge to move the legs and any accompanying unpleasant sensations during rest or inactivity *only occur or are worse* in the **Evening** or night than during the day.
5. The occurrence of the above features is not **Solely** accounted for as symptoms primary to another medical or a behavioral condition (e.g., myalgia, venous stasis, leg edema, arthritis, leg cramps, positional discomfort, habitual foot tapping).

The addition of the fifth diagnostic criteria ("Solely") was based in part on a study by Hening et al.[18] that found 16% of RLS "mimics" could satisfy all four RLS diagnostic criteria. There were a number of notes accompanying the diagnostic criteria providing clarification. The urge to move the legs can be present *without the uncomfortable sensations,* and sometimes the *arms or other parts of the body are involved* in addition to the legs. For children, the description of symptoms should be in the child's own words. When symptoms are very severe, relief by activity may not be noticeable but must have been previously present. In addition, when symptoms are very severe, the worsening in the evening or night may not be noticeable but must have been previously present.

Box 31-1 lists some conditions that are commonly confused with RLS. RLS/WED may also occur with any of these conditions, but the RLS/WED symptoms will differ from those usually expected with the other condition with

Table 31-1 Different Leg Movement Conditions

	RLS	PLMS	PLMD
Diagnosis	History	PSG	PSG + History
Prevalence	Common	Very common • Asymptomatic individuals • Narcolepsy • REM sleep behavior disorder • OSA	Rare
PSG findings	~80% have PLMS	PLMSI ≥15/hour is commonly noted in asymptomatic elderly patients	PLMD PLMSI criteria: >5/hour children >15/hour adults
Relationship with other leg movement conditions	A diagnosis of RLS excludes a diagnosis of PLMD	A PSG finding not a disorder Usually asymptomatic or symptoms are not due to PLMS ~25% with PLMSI >15/hour have RLS	Not diagnosed if RLS is present Must exclude other causes of insomnia or daytime sleepiness

OSA, obstructive sleep apnea; *PLMD*, periodic limb movement disorder; *PLMS*, periodic limb movements during sleep; *PLMSI*, PLMS index; *PSG*, polysomnography; *REM*, rapid eye movement; *RLS*, restless legs syndrome.

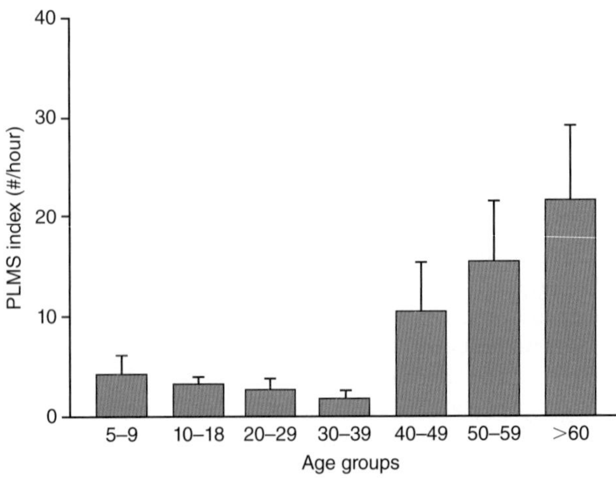

Figure 31-1 Mean periodic limb movements during sleep (PLMS) index (hour of sleep) at different ages for normal healthy individuals. The error bars are the standard error of the mean. The average PLMS index increases in older individuals. (From Pennestri M, Whittom S, Adam B, et al. PLMS and PLMW in healthy subjects as a function of age: prevalence and interval distribution. *Sleep*. 2006;29:1183-1187.)

Box 31-1 DIFFERENTIAL DIAGNOSES OF RLS/WED

Common Conditions	Less Common Conditions
• Leg cramps* • Positional discomfort* • Peripheral neuropathy* • Radiculopathy* • Local leg injury • Arthritis • Leg edema • Venous stasis • Habitual foot tapping/leg rocking • Anxiety • Myalgia • Drug-induced akathisia	• Myelopathy • Myopathy • Vascular or neurogenic claudication • Hypotensive akathisia • Orthostatic tremor • Painful legs and moving toes

* Especially likely to meet or nearly meet RLS diagnostic criteria 1–4.
RLS, restless legs syndrome; *WED*, Willis-Ekbom disease.
Adapted from Allen RP, Picchietti DL, Garcia-Borreguero D, et al. International Restless Legs Syndrome Study Group. Restless legs syndrome/Willis-Ekbom disease diagnostic criteria: updated International Restless Legs Syndrome Study Group (IRLSSG) consensus criteria–history, rationale, description, and significance. *Sleep Med*. 2014;15(8):860-873.

respect to severity, character, or circumstances associated with the onset of the other condition or interventions that improve the other condition. For example, positional discomfort can be associated with abnormal sensations and an urge to move as well as being worse at night. However, positional discomfort is improved simply by a change in position. Improvement of RLS requires prolonged stretching, walking, rubbing the legs etc to provide temporary improvement in symptoms. Box 31-2 lists common descriptions of the undesirable sensations usually (but not always) associated with the urge to move the legs.

Box 31-2 COMMON DESCRIPTIONS OF ABNORMAL SENSATIONS IN THE RESTLESS LEGS SYNDROME

- Creepy, crawly.
- Ants crawling under the skin.
- Worms crawling in the veins.
- Pepsi-Cola in the veins.
- Nervous feet, "gotta move."
- Itching under the skin, itchy bones.
- Crazy legs/Elvis legs.
- Tooth ache feeling—cannot leave it alone.
- Excited nerves, electric-like shocks.
- Painful sensation in 20–50%
- Sensation involves arms in 50%

Specifiers for Clinical Course of RLS/WED

A. Chronic-persistent RLS/WED: symptoms, when not treated, occured on average at least twice weekly for the past year.
B. Intermittent RLS/WED: symptoms, when not treated, occured on average less than twice weekly for the past year, with at least five lifetime events.

Specifier for Clinical Significance of RLS/WED

The symptoms of RLS/WED cause significant distress or impairment in social, occupational, educational, or other important areas of functioning as a result of their impact on sleep, energy/vitality, daily activities, behavior, cognition, or mood.

The clinical significance specifier is important, as if there are no associated impairments, these are isolated symptoms and usually do not need treatment. As discussed below, the International Classification of Sleep Disorders, 3rd edition Text Revision (ICSD-3-TR) RLS diagnostic criteria[10] specify that some impairment **must be present** and therefore differs from the IRLSSG definition.

Patients with RLS symptoms twice weekly tend to have significant symptoms.[13,14] Population-based surveys, however, indicate that many have RLS/WED symptoms only intermittently. The REST general population survey found that, of those reporting RLS/WED symptoms during the past year, 30% had symptoms less than once a week and 12.5% had symptoms about once a week.[14] Of the remaining 57.5% with symptoms occurring twice a week or more, the majority (66%) also reported the symptoms as moderate to severely disturbing. This group was called the "RLS sufferers" group. The prevalence of symptoms increased with age (Figure 31-2). The frequency of different complaints in the "RLS sufferers" group is shown in Figure 31-3. Commonly reported RLS-associated sensations (Box 31-2) were reported to be painful by about 20% of the patients. Of note, there may be an urge to move (akathisia) without accompanying sensations, or *there may be involuntary leg movement without a noticeable urge to move ("the legs just move on their own")*. Involvement of parts of the body other than the legs (such as the arms) occurs in 30% to 50% of patients. However, the *legs should also be involved*. While the unpleasant sensations (dysesthesia) can be painful, pain alone (no urge to move) does not meet diagnostic criteria for RLS. There are RLS variants that involve ONLY other body areas (arms, genitalia) but are not included in this classification.[19,20] Although RLS symptoms are usually bilateral, *they can occur mainly in one extremity*. As noted, in severe RLS, there may not be noticeable relief with activity (but relief with activity should have been present previously). Immobility and decreased mental activity can worsen RLS. Rubbing the legs or taking hot or cold baths may improve symptoms in some patients. Of note, increased mental activity or eating can improve the symptoms ("popcorn therapy" while watching a movie). As also noted, in very severe RLS, there may no longer be worsening in the evening or with immobility, but this should have been present at disease onset.

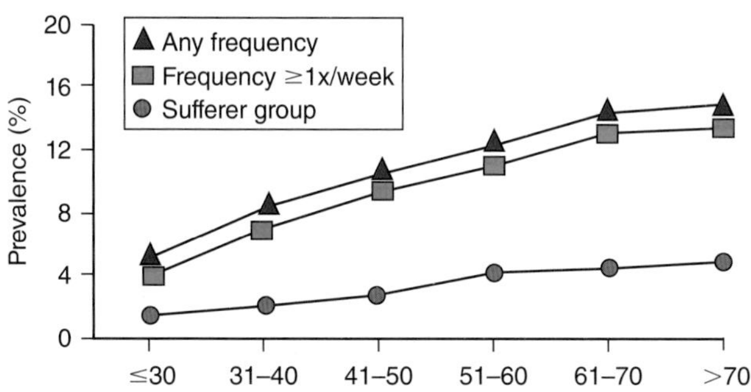

Figure 31-2 Prevalence of restless legs syndrome (RLS) at different age groups in patients reporting any frequency of RLS symptoms, reporting frequency greater than once per week, and "sufferers" (reporting RLS symptoms at least twice per week and some impact from the symptoms when they occurred). (Data from Hening WA, Buchfuhrer MJ, Lee HB. *Clinical Management of RLS.* West Islip, NY: Professional Communications, 2008; and Hening W, Walters AS, Allen RP, Montplaisir J, Myers A, Ferini-Strambi L. Impact, diagnosis and management of RLS in a primary care population: the REST [RLS Epidemiology, Symptoms, and Treatment] Primary Care Study. *Sleep Med.* 2004;5:237-246.)

The important points of the diagnostic criteria (A-C must be met) for RLS in the ICSD-3-TR[10] are (see the ICSD-3-TR for the complete criteria):

A. An urge to move the legs, usually but not always accompanied by or felt to be caused by uncomfortable and unpleasant sensations in the legs. These symptoms must:
   1. Begin or worsen during periods of rest or inactivity such as lying down or sitting;
   2. Be partially or totally relieved by movement, such as walking or stretching, at least as long as the activity continues; and
   3. Occur exclusively or predominantly in the evening or night rather than during the day.
B. These features are *not solely accounted for* as symptoms primary to another medical or behavioral condition (e.g., leg cramps, positional discomfort, myalgia, venous stasis, leg edema, arthritis, habitual foot tapping).
C. The symptoms of RLS cause concern, distress, sleep disturbance, or impairment in mental, physical, social, occupational, educational, behavioral, or other important areas of functioning.

These criteria are similar to the IRLSSG criteria with the additional requirement of criterion C.

Differentiating RLS From "Mimics"

It is not always easy to distinguish RLS from mimics (Table 31-2). It is important to note that *both RLS mimics and true RLS* can occur together.[18,21] For example, there may be a patient with diabetic neuropathy who also has RLS. Most RLS mimics are not usually associated with an urge to move. However, patients with neuroleptic akathisia do have an urge to move (but symptoms are *less likely* to worsen with rest or in the evening, and the urge to move is a generalized inner sensation)[2.1,22] The major clue to distinguish between RLS and neuroleptic akathisia is the history of the patient taking a dopamine antagonist medication (phenothiazines, atypical antipsychotic, metoclopramide) currently or previously. Often, RLS mimics are not worse at night, and symptoms are not temporarily improved by movement. If patients describe their symptoms entirely associated with leg cramps, this is not RLS. If symptoms are present only in **certain body positions** such as with crossed legs, this is more likely to be positional discomfort and less likely to be RLS. In such cases, a *change in body position* (rather than movement) brings relief. If patients describe symptoms as painful and associated with a localized problem area (painful joint, leg edema) or painful in a pattern consistent with radiculopathy or neuropathy (numbness in a specific area), this is less likely to be RLS. However, both neuropathy and RLS can be present. Individuals with RLS are very aware of leg movements. If individuals report pronounced or frequent unconscious foot or leg movements (e.g., hypnic jerks, habitual foot taping, leg shaking, general nervous movements), this is likely not RLS. RLS symptoms are more likely to be described as **irresistible** or a cause of sleep disturbance. Peripheral neuropathy can be worse at night, but symptoms are also present during the day. Patients with RLS do

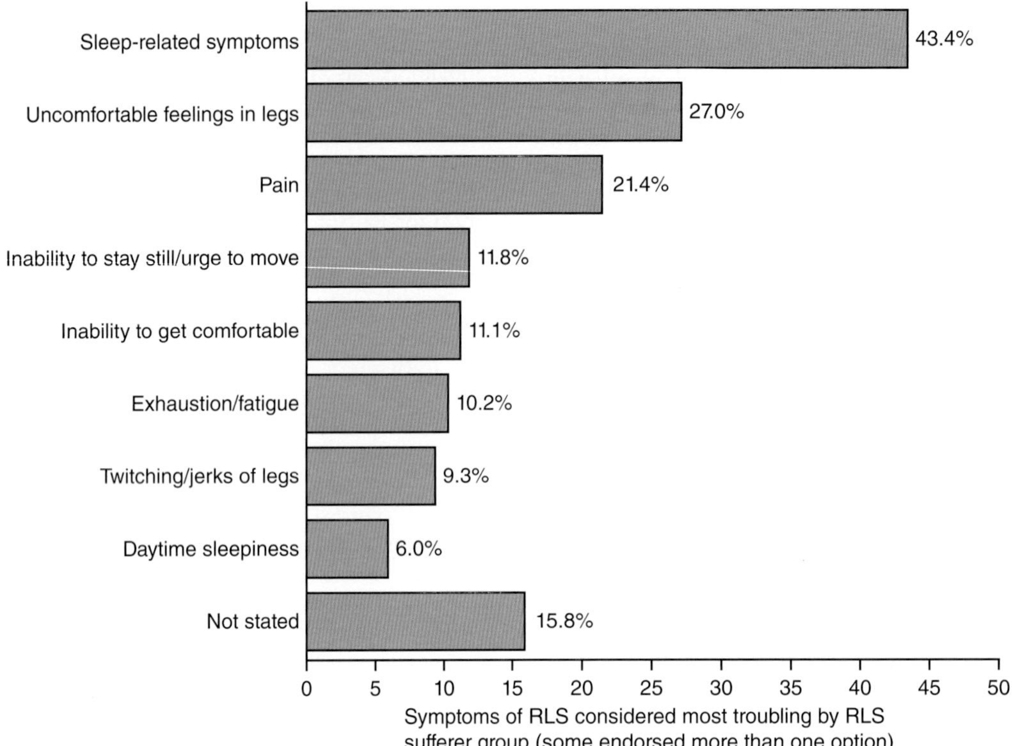

Figure 31-3 Symptoms reported in the restless legs syndrome (RLS) "sufferer" group (symptoms at least twice weekly with moderate to severe symptoms). Note that *daytime sleepiness is infrequent.* The most commonly reported symptoms are sleep related symptoms (impairment) and uncomfortable feeling in the legs. (From Hening W, Walters AS, Allen RP, Montplaisir J, Myers A, Ferini-Strambi L. Impact, diagnosis and management of RLS in a primary care population: the REST [RLS Epidemiology, Symptoms, and Treatment] Primary Care Study. *Sleep Med.* 2004;5:237-246.)

not tolerate confinement (e.g., long airplane trips). Occasionally, some RLS mimics as well as true RLS are reported to improve with walking. The painful legs and moving toes syndrome[23] consists of pain in the legs and involuntary movement in the toes (often "fanning out"). The etiology is varied and includes nerve root lesions, peripheral trauma, neuropathy (e.g., polyneuropathy from alcoholism, hypertrophic mononeuritis, or tarsal tunnel syndrome), Wilson disease, herpes zoster myelitis, human immunodeficiency virus (HIV), neuroleptics, and chemotherapeutic agents.

Supportive Clinical Features

Supportive clinical features of RLS (Box 31-3) may help resolve diagnostic uncertainty but are not required for a diagnosis.[2] These features include: (1) a family history of RLS, (2) a response to dopaminergic treatment, (3) the presence of PLMS, (4) a low ferritin level, and (5) associated sleep disturbance. A familial history is reported in 50% to 60% of RLS cases and is supportive of the diagnosis. Improvement with a trial of dopaminergic treatment is also evidence that symptoms represent RLS. However, placebo-controlled studies in RLS report considerable improvement in symptoms with inactive medication. It is difficult to define normal periodic limb movements in terms of a sleep index (PLMSI). In the past, some sleep centers considered a PLMSI >5/hour to be abnormal. However, many asymptomatic individuals have a much higher PLMSI value.[5,7] One study using a PLMSI cutoff of 5/hours reported 80.2% of patients with RLS had PLMS (87% if two nights were monitored).[1] Other studies in adults have used a PLMSI ≥15/hour to identify a significant PLMSI. However, older normal individuals can have a similar PLMSI (Figure 32-1). Patients with RLS often report repetitive involuntary leg movements during wake when at rest, especially at night. This is a manifestation of periodic limb movements during wake (PLMW).

Causes of RLS

RLS is often divided into primary RLS (independent of other disorders, cause unknown, idiopathic) and secondary RLS (from an identifiable cause such as a medical disorder, condition, or medication). Familial RLS (genetic factors) play a contributory role in about 50% of RLS cases. The common causes of secondary RLS are listed in Box 31-4. RLS associated with renal failure is *not helped by dialysis but is usually cured by kidney transplantation.* Return of RLS symptoms can be an early indictor of transplant failure. RLS symptoms can make tolerating dialysis very difficult. RLS in pregnancy is common (19%) is worse in the third trimester and but usually vanishes or improves with delivery (>90–96% if no RLS was present pre-pregnancy).[24] RLS in pregnancy may respond to iron supplementation if the serum ferritin is ≤ 50 μg/L. If the onset of RLS can be linked to the start of a given medication, a switch to an alternate medication can be tried. Medications commonly associated with worsening RLS have been specified by Hoque and coworkers.[25] RLS can occur within a few days of starting antidepressants.[26] In one study, mirtazapine was by far

Table 31-2 Characteristics of Common Mimics of RLS/PLMS

Mimic	Description	Abnormal Sensations	Urge to Move	Relief by Movement	Timing
Hypnic jerk	Single, whole-body jerk at sleep onset, involuntary	**No**	**No**	N/A	At sleep onset
Positional discomfort	Need to move to relieve discomfort from pressure on nerves, blood vessels, or stretched tissue.	**Usually**	**Yes**	Change in position (not movement) brings relief	Worse at night
Nocturnal leg cramps	Muscle hardening and pain localized to specific muscle groups; tenderness and sensitivity remain after cramping subsides	**Pain**	**No**	Relieved with stretching	Night
Peripheral neuropathy	Sensory symptoms of numbness or burning and pain	**Can be** painful	**No**	**Usually no** Typically, not improved with walking or sustained movement	Day and night (Symptoms night > day typical)
Neuroleptic induced akathisia	Involuntary movement of face, extremities **History of neuroleptic (dopamine antagonist**)**	Whole body sensation rather than centered only on the limbs	Yes, but whole-body inner restlessness	Not usually	Not usually
Volitional movements (foot tapping, leg rocking)	Anxiety or boredom, fidgety patient	**No**	**No**	**n/a**	Boring, stressful activities
Painful toes, moving leg syndrome	Pain in lower limbs with spontaneous movements of toes and feet	**Pain**	**No**	**No**	**Not usually**

**Neuroleptic (dopamine blocker) – phenothiazines (Haldol), can occur with atypical antipsychotics, metoclopramide
RLS, restless legs syndrome; *PLMS*, periodic limb movements during sleep.

Box 31-3 SUPPORTIVE CLINICAL FEATURES FOR RLS

- Family history (50%)
- Response to dopaminergic treatment (at least initially, placebo effect can be large)
- PLMS (present in 80–90% but not required), PLMW
- Low ferritin level
- Associated sleep disturbance but lack of profound sleepiness

RLS, restless legs syndrome; *PLMS*, periodic limb movements in sleep; *PLMW*, periodic limb movements during wake.
Allen RP, Picchietti DL, Garcia-Borreguero D, et al. International Restless Legs Syndrome Study Group. Restless legs syndrome/Willis-Ekbom disease diagnostic criteria: updated International Restless Legs Syndrome Study Group (IRLSSG) consensus criteria–history, rationale, description, and significance. *Sleep Med.* 2014;15(8):860-873. PMID: 25023924.

Box 31-4 CAUSES OF RESTLESS LEGS SYNDROME

Primary RLS (idiopathic, often familial)
Secondary RLS
- Iron deficiency
- Pregnancy
- Neuropathy—diabetic and others
- Multiple sclerosis
- Renal failure
- Parkinson disease
- Medications
  - First-generation (sedating) antihistamines (e.g., diphenhydramine)
  - Antinausea medication—prochlorperazine
  - Dopamine receptor blockers—metoclopramide
  - Antidepressants (SSRIs, SNRIs)—exception is bupropion

RLS, restless legs syndrome, *SNRI*, serotonin-norepinephrine reuptake inhibitor; *SSRI*, selective serotonin reuptake inhibitor.

the antidepressant most frequently associated with new-onset RLS (28%), with other commonly used medications (sertraline, paroxetine, escitalopram, fluoxetine, venlafaxine, and duloxetine) in the 5% to 10% range.[26] If a selective serotonin reuptake inhibitor (SSRI) is believed to worsen RLS, one might consider switching to bupropion, an antidepressant that does not worsen RLS.[27] Of interest, first-generation antihistamines such as diphenhydramine, triprolidine, chlorpheniramine, and doxylamine that are contained in many over-the-counter (OTC) sleep aids or cough syrups can worsen RLS. Patients may not report their use of OTC medications. Medications with *dopamine antagonist* activity can also worsen RLS (phenothiazines, atypical antipsychotics, metoclopramide, prochlorperazine [a phenothiazine antiemetic]). RLS occurs in about 35% of patients with iron deficiency anemia and at only a slightly lower rate in patients with iron deficiency without anemia. RLS occurs commonly in patients with Parkinson disease but appears NOT to be increased in untreated Parkinson disease and may be associated with treatment with dopaminergic medications.

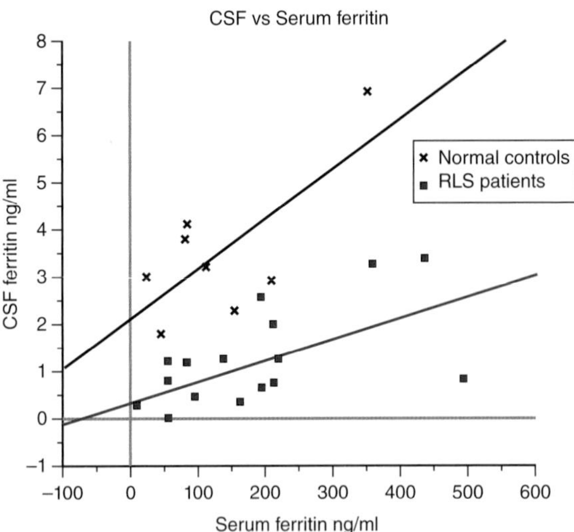

Figure 31-4 Cerebrospinal fluid (CSF) versus serum ferritin in normal controls and patients with restless legs syndrome (RLS). The patients with RLS tend to have lower CSF ferritin for a given serum ferritin than normal controls. In addition, one can see that it is possible to have a high serum ferritin and low CSF ferritin. (From Earley CJ, Connor JR, Beard JL, Malecki EA, Epstein DK, Allen RP. Abnormalities in CSF concentrations of ferritin and transferrin in restless legs syndrome. *Neurology.* 2000;54(8):1698-700. PMID: 10762522.)

As will be discussed, brain iron deficiency is felt to be a major cause of RLS.[28,29] The cerebrospinal fluid (CSF) iron levels are roughly correlated with serum iron but may be low, even if peripheral iron stores are normal. Patients with RLS tend to have a lower CSF ferritin for the same serum ferritin than normal controls (Figure 31-4). Heritable factors may influence cerebral iron transport and storage in some patients with RLS. It should be appreciated that conditions associated with secondary RLS can worsen primary RLS.

Epidemiology of RLS

The prevalence of RLS in adults has been estimated at approximately 5% to 10%.[6] RLS is approximately **1.5 to 2 times more common in women than in men**. It is believed that most of the increased incidence is due to the increase in RLS during pregnancy. *RLS appears to be more common in Caucasian than in Asian populations.* Therefore, RLS is more common in Europe, Canada, and the United States than in Asia. The prevalence of RLS in Africa has not been adequately studied. Defining the prevalence of RLS depends on the criteria (severity of symptoms) required for the presence of RLS. If one requires *symptoms at least twice weekly and causing at least moderate distress*, the population prevalence is approximately 1.5% to 2.7%.[15,16]

Age of Onset

RLS can begin at any age, and the clinical course is variable. Some clinicians find it useful to classify RLS on the basis of the age at onset (Box 31-5). Early-onset RLS (<45–50 years of age) has an insidious onset, is slowly progressive, usually familial, usually primary, and tends to be less severe. Late-onset RLS (>45–50 years of age) tends to have a rapid onset, be rapidly progressive, sporadic, more likely secondary, and with more severe symptoms. Patients with late-onset RLS also tend to have lower ferritin levels than those of patients with early onset RLS.

Box 31-5 CHARACTERISTIC OF RLS BY AGE

Early Onset*	Late Onset*
Age ≤45 years	Age >45 years
Slowly progressive	Rapidly progressive
Familial	Sporadic
Primary (idiopathic)	Secondary > primary
Less severe	More severe

*Some use 50 years as the dividing age between early and late onset.

Genetics of RLS

RLS is a genetically complex disorder.[30-32] Epigenetic factors appear to be important. As noted, about 50% to 60% of individuals with RLS have a family history of the disorder. Monozygotic twin concordance of 54% to 83% has been reported. Linkage studies identified susceptibility loci—predominantly with an autosomal dominant inheritance pattern (but recessive patterns can occur). The disorder is not monogenetic (more than one gene is involved). Genome-wide association studies (GWAS) have identified risk loci: *MEIS1, BTBD9, MAP2K5/SKORI, PTPRD, TOX3, SEMA6D, SETBP1*, and *MYTI*. However, these regions of interest appear to account for only a small amount of heritability. Most variants of interest are associated with neural development and iron pathways. *Alteration in MEIS1 is believed to be the strongest risk factor for RLS*, and *MEIS1* appears to play an important role in brain iron metabolism. The most common variant of *MEIS1* associated with RLS results in decreased expression of MEIS1 in embryonic areas, leading to development of the basal ganglia (important for control of movement). The reader is referred to sources that review the current knowledge on genetics and RLS for more detailed information.[30,32]

Pathophysiology of RLS

Our understanding of the pathophysiology of RLS is complex and undergoing rapid expansion. The previous hypothesis was that dopamine signaling was low. Evidence for this hypothesis was the rapid response to dopaminergic medications. At the time of this writing, it is believed that the major factors causing RLS include: (1) brain iron deficiency (BID), (2) dopamine dysfunction (hyperdopaminergic state), (3) hyperglutamatergic activity, and (4) alterations in adenosine signaling (Figure 31-5).[12,33-35] Histopathology and MRI studies have shown decreased iron stores in areas of the brain important for control of movement in patients with RLS. Brain iron deficiency alters glutaminergic transmission, resulting in cortico-striatal hypersensitivity. The striatum is part of the basal ganglia—clusters of neurons deep in the center of the brain including the ventral striatum (the nucleus accumbens and the olfactory tubercle) and the dorsal striatum (the caudate nucleus and the putamen). A white matter tract (the internal capsule) in the dorsal striatum separates the caudate nucleus and the putamen. The term *striatum* describes its striped (striated) appearance of grey-and-white matter. The striatum is a critical component of the motor and reward systems; it receives glutamatergic and dopaminergic inputs from different sources and serves as the primary input to the rest of the basal ganglia.

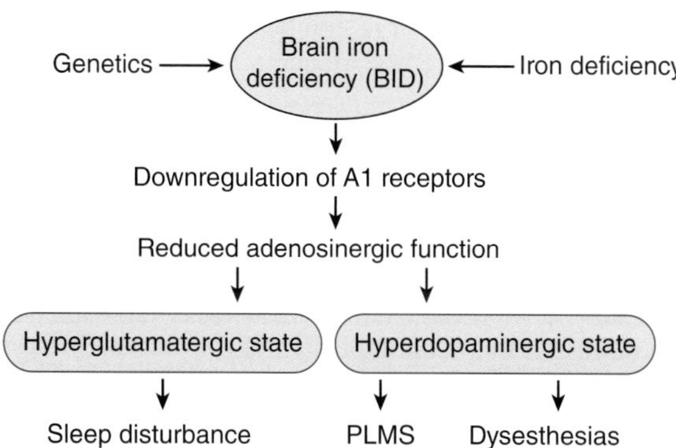

Figure 31-5 Schematic of pathogenesis of restless legs syndrome (RLS). Brain iron deficiency results in downregulation of adenosine A1 receptors and increased activity of A2A receptors associated with reduced adenosine function resulting in an increase in glutamatergic and hyperdopaminergic activity. Genetics influences the brain handling of iron, and some individuals may be predisposed to low brain iron, which is exacerbated by iron deficiency.

Alpha-2-delta (voltage gated calcium channels) and dopamine presynaptic receptors on glutaminergic neurons, when stimulated, reduce transmission. Ligands acting at these receptors inhibit glutamatergic neurons, reducing glutamatergic transmission, and may explain the therapeutic action of alpha-2-delta ligands and dopaminergic medications in RLS. Adenosine A1 and A2A receptors form a complex and modulate glutamatergic and dopamine activity in the striatum. Low adenosine concentrations **activate A1 receptors** and reduces glutamate transmission, and high concentrations **activate A2A receptors** and increase glutamate release. Brain iron deficiency decreases (downregulates) A1 more than A2A receptors, resulting in a **hypo**-adenosinergic state and promoting a hyperglutamatergic state, which in turn results in a hyperdopaminergic state. Thus, RLS is believed to be caused by a hyperglutamatergic and hyperdopaminergic state resulting in part from decreased adenosine signaling (associated with brain iron deficiency).[35] An increase in glutamate signaling causes arousal, and the increase in dopamine signaling causes PLMS (Figure 31-5). The adenosine system is also believed to have inhibitory influences in the spinal cord. Of interest, dipyridamole, a medication known to inhibit the nucleoside transporter (ENT1) responsible for terminating the actions of adenosine (enhancing the effects of endogenous adenosine), improved RLS symptoms in a preliminary study[36] and then a randomized crossover trial.[37] Equilibrative nucleoside transporters (ENTs) are polytopic integral membrane proteins that mediate the transport of nucleosides, nucleobases, and therapeutic analogs.

Sleep Disturbance, Depression, and Suicide Risk Associated With RLS

The two most common complaints that lead patients with RLS to seek medical attention are the **uncomfortable leg sensations** and the **disturbance of sleep** (Figure 31-3). Beyond the significant discomfort caused by RLS symptoms, the disorder can cause difficulty with sleep initiation and maintenance. In a group of patients with RLS with symptoms on at least two nights a week, sleep-related symptoms (prolonged sleep latency or awakenings) were present in 43.4%, but *only 6% complained of daytime sleepiness.*[15] It is not surprising that RLS symptoms can prolong sleep latency. However, RLS can also potentially reduce total sleep time. If the patient awakens, the return to sleep may also be delayed by RLS symptoms. Because the majority of patients with RLS have PLMS, it might be assumed that patients with a higher PLMSI or PLMS arousal index (PLMSAI) have more sleep disturbance. However, the PLMSI has not been correlated with any measure of sleep disturbance in most studies of RLS patients. In a study of two groups of unmedicated patients with RLS, Hornyak and coworkers[38] analyzed the relationship between RLS severity and the PLMSI and PLMSAI. In the first group, the RLS symptom severity correlated with the PLMSAI but not the PLMSI. However, the relationship between RLS severity and the PLMSAI was very weak ($r = 0.22$, $P = 0.03$). In the second group, neither the PLMSI or PLMSAI correlated with RLS symptom severity. Entry criteria for the first group was a PLMSAI > 5/hour, but this was not required for the second group. Overall, sleep disturbance from PLMS associated with RLS did not seem to significantly contribute to RLS-induced sleep disturbance. Of note, many patients with RLS have a low PLMSI, and there is considerable night-to-night variability in the PLMSI,[39] while RLS symptoms are often more consistent.

Untreated RLS via sleep disturbance can have significant morbidity beyond disturbed sleep. RLS is associated with both *depression and increased suicidal risk.*[40,41] In one study, treatment of RLS improved depression but not suicidal/self-harm risk.[41]

Medical Evaluation in RLS

The diagnostic evaluation (Box 31-6) should include a history to elicit the essential and associated features of RLS. A detailed medication history including OTC medications is very important, as sedating antihistamines worsen RLS. Behaviors during sleep should be assessed (question the bed partner about body movement and kicking). Patients with a high PLMSI often leave the bedcovers in disarray. As OSA and RBD are commonly associated with PLMS, symptoms of those disorders should also be assessed. Physical examination should look for signs of neuropathy. Laboratory studies should check renal and thyroid function. A serum iron level, total iron binding capacity (TIBC), percentage of iron saturation, and

Box 31-6 ESSENTIAL ELEMENTS FOR EVALUATION OF A PATIENT WITH RLS

History

- Presence of essential RLS criteria?
- RLS in family members?
- Neuroleptic use?
- Detailed medication history (including OTC medications, antihistamines, neuroleptics).

Physical Examination

- Neurologic examination—look for signs of neuropathy

Laboratory

- Fasting ferritin, TIBC, % iron saturation
- Renal function

OTC, over the counter; *RLS*, restless legs syndrome; *TIBC*, total iron-binding capacity.

ferritin levels should be checked. The ferritin is the most useful single test. However, ferritin can be elevated by inflammatory processes, and ordering tests for both the ferritin level and percentage of iron saturation (also known as transferrin saturation) is recommended.[42,43] If the ferritin level is ≤75 μg/L (ng/ml) or the iron saturation is less than 20%, iron supplementation may improve symptoms.[44] Iron treatment for RLS will be discussed in following sections of the chapter. *PSG is NOT required in most cases of RLS unless sleep apnea or another sleep disorder is suspected* (Box 31-7). Of note, abnormal movements during sleep, including leg kicks, can occur with OSA, epilepsy, sleep-related rhythmic movement disorder, and RBD. If there is a suspicion of other causes of abnormal nocturnal movements, a sleep study is indicated. As noted, *daytime sleepiness is NOT a common symptom of RLS,* and the presence of this symptom should prompt consideration of disorders other than RLS. A combination of sleep disorders, for example, RLS and sleep apnea, is common. If RLS symptoms are very mild but sleep disruption occurs nightly or is significant or if sleep disturbance continues despite apparently adequate RLS treatment, a PSG should be considered. *PSG is needed for the diagnosis of PLMD,* both to document significant PLMS and to eliminate other obvious causes of symptoms. As PLMD is not common, the main use of PSG is to exclude other causes of sleep disruption, such as OSA. If PSG reveals an increased PLMSI and there is no other explanation for sleep complaints, a diagnosis of PLMD should be considered. Diagnostic criteria for PLMD will be discussed in a section on PLMD.

Box 31-7 WHEN TO CONSIDER ORDERING POLYSOMNOGRAPHY FOR PATIENT WITH RLS

- Daytime sleepiness a prominent feature
- Sleep apnea or PLMD suspected (uncertain RLS)
- RLS symptoms minimal/intermittent but sleep disruption significant/nightly
- Sleep disturbance present despite apparently effective RLS treatment

RLS, restless legs syndrome; *PLMD*, periodic limb movement disorder.

The International Restless Legs Syndrome Study Group (IRLSSG) developed a rating scale for RLS symptoms (Box 31-8) called the *International Restless Legs Scale* (***IRLS***).[45,46] A slight revision of the validated scale[46] was published as an appendix to an editorial. The IRLS is useful to quantify RLS symptom severity and the effects of treatment. The scale is validated under conditions of a face-to-face interview with the patient in which clarifications regarding the questions can be made to the patient. The IRLS consists of 10 questions, and each question has a four-point scale from no RLS (score = 0) to very severe RLS (score = 4); the total score range is from 0 to 40.

The scale is used in research studies but also has clinical utility in following patients on treatment. Most research studies use an IRLS score >5 to 20 to define symptomatic RLS. The self-administered form of IRLS has also been validated.[47] The IRLS does not examine all aspects of RLS. For example, the scale does not examine the number of involved limbs or the rapidity with which symptoms develop when a patient first sits or lies down.

Box 31-8 INTERNATIONAL RESTLESS LEGS SCALE (IRLS) – VERSION 2.1

In the past week:

1. Overall, how would you rate the RLS discomfort in your legs or arms?
   4) Very severe (3) Severe (2) Moderate (1) Mild (0) None
2. Overall, how would you rate the need to move around because of your RLS symptoms?
   (4) Very severe (3) Severe (2) Moderate (1) Mild (0) None
3. Overall, how much relief of your RLS arm or leg discomfort did you get from moving around?
   (4) No relief (3) Slight relief (2) Moderate relief (1) Either complete or almost complete relief (0) No RLS symptoms to be relieved
4. Overall, how severe was your **sleep disturbance** due to your RLS symptoms?
   (4) Very severe (3) Severe (2) Moderate (1) Mild (0) None
5. How severe was your **tiredness or sleepiness** due to your RLS symptoms?
   (4) Very severe (3) Severe (2) Moderate (1) Mild (0) None
6. How severe was your RLS as a whole?
   (4) Very severe (3) Severe (2) Moderate (1) Mild (0) None
7. How often did you get RLS symptoms?
   (4) Very often [6–7 days/week] (3) Often [4–5 days/wk] (2) Sometimes [2–3 days/week] (1) Occasionally [≤1 day/week] (0) Never
8. When you had RLS symptoms, how severe were they on average?
   (4) Very severe [≥8 hours/24 hours] (3) Severe [3–8 hours/24 hours] (2) Moderate [1–3 hours/24 hours] (1) Mild [<1 hour/24 hours] (0) None
9. Overall, how severe was the impact of your RLS symptoms on your ability to carry out your daily affairs—for example, carrying out a satisfactory family, home, social, or work life?
   (4) Very severe (3) Severe (2) Moderate (1) Mild (0) None
10. How severe was your mood disturbance due to your RLS symptoms—for example, angry, depressed, sad, anxious, or irritable?
    (4) Very severe (3) Severe (2) Moderate (1) Mild (0) None

RLS, restless legs syndrome. Most studies use a score > 5 to 20 to define symptomatic RLS
From International Restless Legs Syndrome Study Group. Validation of the International Restless Legs Syndrome Rating Scale for the restless legs syndrome. *Sleep Med.* 2003;4:121-122.

PSG Findings in Patients With RLS

In a study of 133 patients with RLS, it was found that the PLMSI was greater than 5/hour in 80.2% of patients.[1] The **PLMSI did increase with RLS severity**. There was also a significant correlation between the PLMSI and the PLMW index (PLMWI). However, there was no correlation between PLMSI and measures of sleep disturbance such as sleep efficiency and nocturnal awakenings. As mentioned, another study found a weak correlation between the PLMSAI and RLS severity in only one of two groups of unmedicated patients with RLS.[38] Therefore, PLMS does not appear to be a major cause of sleep disturbance in most patients with RLS. *The major importance of an elevated PLMSI is to alert the clinician to the possibility of RLS.*

Diagnosis of RLS in Children

RLS can be difficult to diagnose in children.[2,3,48,49] Some children complain of typical RLS symptoms, while others complain of "growing pains" or simply have difficulty "sitting still." The Peds REST study found criteria for definite RLS in 1.9% of children aged 8 to 11 years and in 2% of adolescents aged 12 to 17 years.[49] Of note, PLMS is less common in children, and a PLMSI of greater than 5 /hour is considered abnormal. Some children with attention deficit hyperactivity disorder (ADHD) have PLMS and possible RLS (and vice versa).[50] The relationship between RLS and ADHD remains to be determined. The IRLSSG published separate revised criteria for diagnosis of RLS in children in 2013.[3] The 2014 IRLSSG diagnostic criteria for RLS combined adult and pediatric criteria[2] based on the study group's 2013 recommendations. The 2014 diagnostic criteria publication states that symptoms should be recorded "in the child's own words." Rather than urge to move children often state their legs "need to move", "have to move" or "legs want to kick". Sensations are often described as "bugs in my legs" or legs feeling "wiggly or shaky". Another interesting difference is that children are much less likely to report symptoms being worse at night. This is likely due to the long periods when they are sitting (at rest) during school. Because of the difficulty in establishing a diagnosis of RLS based on history in children, often a diagnosis of PLMD is made initially but changed to RLS when the child matures and can better provide a description of symptoms.

PERIODIC LIMB MOVEMENTS IN SLEEP

The manifestations of PLMS have been studied in several cohorts.[16,51-55] A common finding is that the PLMSI increases with age. In early descriptions of PLMS, the phenomenon was referred to as "nocturnal myoclonus," but this terminology is no longer used. The criteria for scoring PLMS are presented in Chapter 15. The ICSD 1st edition[56] lists the following grading of the PLMS severity: PLMSI <5 normal, 5–24 mild, 25–49 moderate, and ≥50 severe/hour. However, these cutoffs are entirely arbitrary and are not based on any outcome data. Given the high prevalence of PLMS in asymptomatic individuals, there is unlikely to be a value separating asymptomatic from symptomatic populations. In the ICSD-3-TR,[10] PLMSIs **greater than** 15/hour in adults and **greater than** 5/hour in children are part of the diagnostic criteria for PLMD. However, as noted, asymptomatic individuals can have quite high PLMSI values. There may be information in the periodicity of periodic limb movements (PLMs) that can identify those patients with RLS. Ferri et al. found that normal individuals displayed a unimodal distribution of PLMS periodicity, while those with RLS had a bimodal pattern with a larger second peak (Figure 31-6); for this reason, the minimum PLM inter-movement (period) used in the World Association of Sleep Medicine diagnostic criteria for a candidate leg movement to be included in a PLMS series changed from 5 to 10 seconds (Chapter 15).[57,58]

PLMs occur most commonly in stage N1 and N2 but can also occur in stage N3 or, less commonly, in stage R sleep.[59] *The PLMSI is often higher during the first part of the night.* Culpepper and colleagues[60] described two patterns of PLMS. In one pattern, PLMS was much more common in the first part of the night. In the second pattern, PLMS was more evenly distributed across the night. The interval between individual PLMs increases from stage N1 to stage N3. PLMs are less likely to cause arousal in stage N3 sleep. *Frequent PLMs during REM sleep have been noted in patients with RBD and narcolepsy.*[61-63]

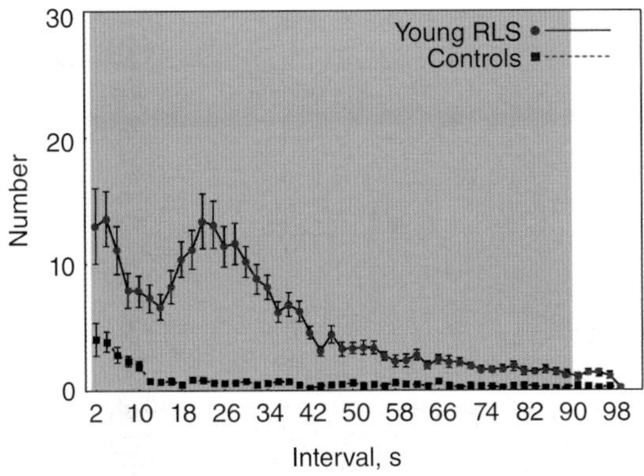

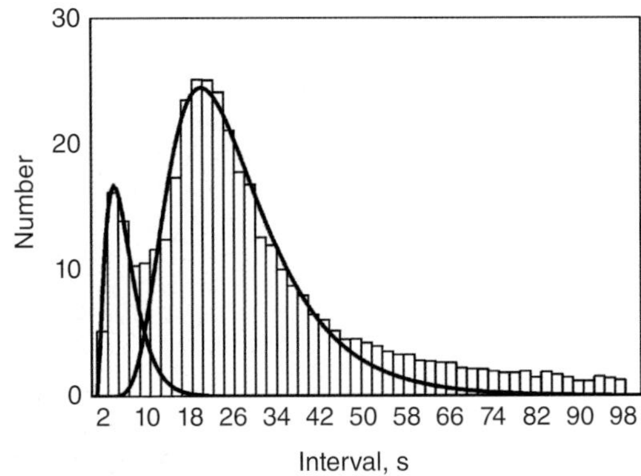

Figure 31-6 (*Left panel*) Intermovement intervals for leg movements (LMs) in young patients with restless legs syndrome (RLS) and controls. The control group did not have the second peak at 18-26 seconds. (*Right panel*) Bimodal distribution for intermovement intervals in patients with RLS. An interval of 10 seconds separates the first and second groups of LMs. The dark grey background in the left figure stops at 90 seconds as the maximum intermovement interval for a LM to be included in a PLMS series is 90 seconds. (From Ferri R, Zucconi M, Manconi M, Plazzi G, Bruni O, Ferini-Strambi L. New approaches to the study of periodic leg movements during sleep in restless legs syndrome. *Sleep*. 2006;29(6):759-769. PMID: 16796214.)

The individual leg movements in PLMS consist of dorsiflexion of the foot and often flexion at the knee or hip. Although the movements are often relatively small and involve one leg at a time, they can be quite *large, violent, bilateral, and involve the arms*. Bed partners may complain of being kicked. In cases in which the movements are violent, PSG may be needed to rule out other pathology such as RBD. Gaig and coworkers described patients with PLMS mimicking RBD.[64] On the other hand, patients with narcolepsy and RBD are most likely to have PLMS during REM sleep.[61-64]

PLMS and Arousals

An individual leg movement (LM) that is a member of a PLMS series is considered to be associated with an arousal if it occurs simultaneously, if it overlaps, or if there is 0.5 second or less from the end of one event to the onset of another, regardless of which is first.[11] See Chapter 15 for examples. The PLMSAI is the number of PLMS arousals per hour of sleep. The ICSD-1[56] lists a PLMSAI of 25 arousals/hour or more as severe. However, there is no widely accepted method to grade the severity of the PLMSAI. One study looking at the association of PLMs and arousals found that 49% of electroencephalogram (EEG) arousals occurred before PLMs, 30.6% simultaneously, and 23.2% occurred just after the LMs.[65] Approximately 30% of PLMS are associated with cortical arousal, whereas more than 60% are associated with K-complexes or bursts of delta waves that do not meet criterial for cortical arousal. Of note, autonomic changes (increases in heart rate or blood pressure)[66] commonly occur in association with PLMs, with and without cortical arousals (Figure 31-7). At least in some individuals, the changes may have clinical significance.

Differential Diagnosis of PLMS

The differential of other periodic movements includes hypnagogic foot tremor (HFT), alternating leg movement activation (ALMAs), excessive fragmentary myoclonus, and the rhythmic movement disorder. The reader is referred to Chapter 15 for more details on these entities. Leg kicks can be a manifestation of RBD. Hypnic jerks are usually single, whole-body jerks that occur at sleep onset and are not periodic.

Clinical Significance of the PLMSI and PLMSAI

The clinical significance of PLMS and the utility of monitoring LMs have been the subject of controversy.[67-70] The utility of counting PLMS arousals has also been questioned because the index does not appear to correlate with subjective measures of disturbed sleep, daytime sleepiness, or the sense of nonrestorative sleep. Claman and associates[7] studied 455 older community-dwelling women and found that 66% had a PLMSI greater than 5/hour and 52% greater than 15/hour. The associations between the PLMSI and the PLMSAI and measures of sleep quality were determined. The associations were adjusted for age, body mass index (BMI), apnea-hypopnea index, and antidepressant medication use. An increased PLMSI was associated with a statistically significant higher total arousal index but not impairment of other indices of sleep quality. A higher PLMSAI was associated with lower total sleep time, less stage N3, and a higher total arousal index. However, neither a higher PLMSI nor a higher PLMSAI was associated with worse subjective daytime sleepiness by the Epworth Sleepiness Scale. When Leary and coworkers analyzed the Wisconsin cohort to compare groups with PLMSIs of <15/hour and ≥15/hour, there was no difference in objective or subjective sleepiness between the groups.[52] *Looking at those with RLS*, those with a PLMSI ≥15/hour were sleepier. Thus, the PLMSAI might have significance if RLS is present. However, this may simply mean that RLS is more severe. It remains unknown whether determination of the PLMSAI really adds anything of clinical significance to other measures of sleep quality. The study results suggest that those with *both PLMS and RLS* often have more impaired sleep quality and worse symptoms than those with PLMS alone. For example,

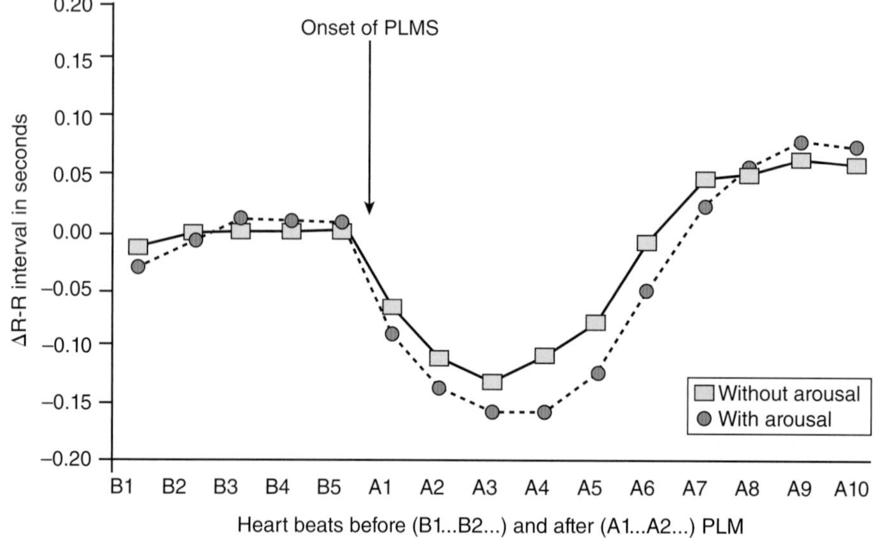

Figure 31-7 Change in heart rate after periodic limb movements during sleep (PLMS). The heart rate increased (respiratory rate [R-R] decreases) whether or not the PLM is associated with a cortical arousal. The heart rate is higher for a few beats after the periodic leg movement (PLM) if an arousal is present. (From Sforza E, Nicolas A, Lavigne G, et al, EEG and cardiac activation during periodic leg movements in sleep. *Neurology*. 1999;52:786-792. PMID: 10078729.)

an awakening with an LM might result in a longer time to return to sleep if RLS is present. The relative importance of RLS and PLMS is also informed by the fact that many patients with RLS have impaired sleep and a PLMSI <15/hour. There is often considerable night-to-night variability in the PLMSI, without similar variability in RLS symptoms. As mentioned, the finding of PLMS should always trigger determination of the presence and severity of RLS.

PLMS and Other Disorders

PLMS is common in a number of disorders (Box 31-9) other than RLS, including narcolepsy, RBD, neuropathy of diverse etiology, and OSA.[61-63,71-75] An increase in the PLMSI on continuous positive airway pressure (CPAP) compared with baseline was noted in a study of patients with OSA by Fry et al.[71] Common patterns are persistent PLMS on diagnostic and PAP titration studies, emergence of PLMS on CPAP, and resolution of PLMS on CPAP. With respect to split night studies, it is important to note that the PLMSI decreases in the second part of the night in many individuals. Lee and coworkers[72] evaluated PLMS on a diagnostic night and a subsequent CPAP titration night. The proportions of participants with PLMS on both PSGs (persistent PLMS), those with CPAP-emergent PLMS, and those with CPAP-resolved PLMS were 12.9%, 9.2%, and 3.9%, respectively. Compared with individuals in the non-PLMS group, those in the persistent group were more likely to be men of older age and have a higher BMI and worse symptoms of RLS. Patients in the CPAP-emergent group were also older and more likely to have RLS, as well as more severe apnea. Patients in the CPAP-resolved group were more likely to be women of older age and have a higher BMI but less severe apnea. Chervin and colleagues[73] evaluated 1124 patients with suspected or confirmed OSA and found that *24% of the patients with OSA had a PLMSI greater than 5/hour*. Of interest, the presence of PLMS was associated with *less sleepiness*. The presence of PLMS can be associated with very mild sleep apnea (upper airway resistance syndrome).[74] A retrospective analysis of data from the Apnea Positive Pressure Long-Term Efficacy Study[75] was performed to analyze the PLMS frequency. A total of 1105 patients with OSA underwent a PSG investigation at baseline, another for CPAP titration, and another 6 months after randomization to either active CPAP or sham CPAP groups. Of all participants, 14.8% had a PLMI ≥15/hour, and 7.5% had a PLMSI ≥30/hour. The odds of having a PLMI ≥10/hour were higher in older participants, men, those using antidepressants, and those with higher caffeine use. After controlling for OSA and depression, PLMS was associated with increased sleep latency, reduced sleep efficiency, and reduced total sleep time. *No significant relationships were noted between PLMS frequency and subjective sleepiness (Epworth Sleepiness Scale score) or objective sleepiness (Maintenance of Wakefulness Test)*. There was no differential effect of CPAP in comparison to sham CPAP on PLMS after 6 months of therapy. It was concluded that *PLMS is common in patients with OSA and is associated with a significant reduction in sleep quality over and above that conferred by OSA*. Treatment with CPAP did not affect the severity of PLMS. An important limitation of this study was lack of information on the presence or absence of RLS. That is, PLMS could simply be a marker of RLS, and treatment of RLS may improve sleep quality. Future studies should evaluate the impact of treating both OSA and PLMS (no RLS) with respect to adherence and improvement in daytime sleepiness. In summary, the finding of PLMS and OSA should trigger the physician to evaluate and treat RLS, if present. It is possible that a patient with OSA could have PLMD, so this possibility should be considered in patients with persistent sleepiness on CPAP.

Box 31-9 SYNDROMES IN WHICH PERIODIC LIMB MOVEMENTS IN SLEEP IS COMMON

Disorder	Prevalence
RLS	80–90% with PLMSI > 5/hour
Narcolepsy	~45–65%[6,62,63]
OSA	~24%[6]

Disorders Associated With PLMS During Stage R

- Narcolepsy[63]
- REM sleep behavior disorder[61]

OSA, obstructive sleep apnea; *PLMS*, periodic limb movements in sleep; *PLMSI*, PLMS index; *REM*, rapid eye movement; *RLS*, restless legs syndrome.

PLMS and Cardiovascular Risk

PLMS causes repetitive sympathetic activation and may be associated with increased cardiovascular risk. Khoo et al. evaluated 2911 men in the observational Outcomes of Sleep Disorders in Older Men (MrOS) Sleep Study cohort who underwent in-home PSG with PLMS measurement.[76] At a 4-year follow-up, they were evaluated for **incident** coronary heart disease, cerebrovascular disease, peripheral arterial disease, and all-cause cardiovascular disease, which included coronary heart disease, cerebrovascular disease, and peripheral arterial disease. The investigators found an association between an increased PLMSI (>30/hour) and incident cardiovascular disease compared to the group with a PLMSI <5/hour.[76] Because RLS and PLMS could have differential effects, the same cohort was analyzed with respect to both RLS and the finding of PLMS.[77] Physician-diagnosed RLS was reported by 2.2%, and a PLMI ≥15/hour was found in 59.6% of men. RLS was not associated with composite cardiovascular disease but was significantly associated with incident myocardial infarction (MI), even after adjustment for multiple covariates. Results were only modestly attenuated when PLMI was added to the model. An increased PLMI was also found to predict incident MI and was materially unchanged after addition of RLS. Therefore, the presence of PLMS and RLS appear to independently increase risk of some cardiovascular disorders. However, other studies have not documented increased cardiovascular risk with RLS.[78] Kendzerska and coworkers[79] performed a systematic review of studies of the associations among RLS, PLMS, and incident cardiovascular events (CVE) or all-cause mortality and concluded the results are limited and inconclusive. The data suggest PLMS may be a prognostic factor for incident CVE and mortality. A major issue is that using the PLMSI from a single night is problematic, given the night-to-night variability. For RLS observational analyses, most prior studies have used limited question sets to make the diagnosis of RLS, and no efforts were made to assess severity or duration. The association between RLS and PLMS with incident CVE remains controversial, and as with all association studies, it is the ability to influence outcomes with treatment that is the most important issue.

PERIODIC LIMB MOVEMENT DISORDER

In PLMD, the presence of PLMS results in clinical sleep disturbance (sleep onset or maintenance insomnia, non-restorative sleep), daytime sleepiness, or fatigue. Of note, excessive daytime sleepiness is NOT a common complaint in patients with RLS. The clinical symptoms are not better explained by another primary sleep disorder. Thus, the diagnosis depends on PSG to demonstrate PLMS and exclusion of other causes of the symptoms by a clinical history and PSG. *It is important to note that a diagnosis of RLS excludes a diagnosis of PLMD.*

The major elements of ICSD-3-TR diagnostic criteria for PLMD are[10]:

A. PSG demonstrates PLMS (as described in the American Academy of Sleep Medicine [AASM] Manual for the scoring of sleep and associated events).
B. The frequency (PLMSI) is >5/hour in children or >15/hour in adults.
C. The PLMS cause clinically significant sleep disturbance or impairment in mental, physical, occupational, behavioral, or other important areas of functioning
D. The PLMS symptoms are not better explained by another current sleep disorder, medical disorder, or mental disorder (e.g., PLMS occurring with apnea, hypopnea, and respiratory arousals should not be scored[11]).

There are a number of important notes in the ICSD-3-TR diagnostic criteria for PLMD. The reader is referred to the reference for a complete listing of the notes. The most important aspects will be mentioned here. PLMD cannot be diagnosed in the presence of RLS, narcolepsy, untreated OSA, or the REM sleep behavior disorder. PLMS commonly occur with these disorders and PLMD is not diagnosed if the PLMS finding and symptoms are better explained by these disorders. PLMD also should not be diagnosed on the basis of the presence of insomnia or hypersomnolence without ruling out other more common causes of insomnia such as anxiety or more common causes of excessive sleepiness such as OSA or narcolepsy. PLMD is thought to be rare in adults. It is often difficult to document a causal relationship between the PLMS and symptoms. There is a significant overlap in the PLMSIs of normal and symptomatic individuals. The ICSD-3-TR mentions that *certain elements can suggest a cause-and-effect relationship between PLMS and symptoms*: (1) improvement in symptoms with a suppression of PLMS with medication, (2) a positive correlation between symptoms and PLMS over several nights (recall there is considerable night-to-night variability in PLMS), and (3) a strong correlation between PLMS and cortical arousals (and possibly autonomic activation). A high PLMSAI would suggest PLMs are important.

Prevalence and Manifestations of PLMD

Although PLMS is common, PLMD is thought to be less common. In fact PLMD is said to be rare in the ICSD-3-TR[10]. The exact prevalence of the PLMD is unknown,[7] although one population study estimated a prevalence of 3.9% based on telephone interview questions. The prevalence of PLMS in adults depends on age, and the defining PLMSI has been estimated to be present in 4% to 11% but is likely much higher in older populations. The population prevalence of a PLMSI > 15/hour has been estimated at 7.6% in ages 18 to 65 years, 28% in ages 35-75 years, and up to 60% in those older than 65 years.[10] In a multiethnic study of atherosclerosis using a PLMSI of >15/hour, about 28% of the participants had PLMS (mean age 68.4 years). However, given the difficulty of making the diagnosis, the true incidence of PLMD in adults is unknown. Patients are rarely aware that they have PLMS until informed by their bed partner. Disturbance of the bed partner's sleep is thought to be more common in PLMS than in PLMD. Some of the patients previously thought to have PLMD on the basis of sleep studies that monitored airflow with a thermal device rather than nasal pressure may have actually had respiratory effort-related arousals (RERAs) or hypopnea-associated PLMS. In these patients, the symptoms of daytime sleepiness may be caused by mild OSA rather than PLMD.[74] Other patients diagnosed with PLMD may have actually had somewhat atypical RLS without prominent sensations. The finding of PLMS in children can be especially helpful because RLS symptoms are often difficult to elicit. It has also been proposed that, in children, PLMD (PLMS with sleep disturbance) may precede the development of RLS symptoms.

PSG Findings in PLMD

The PLMSIs of asymptomatic patients and patients with PLMD overlap. The ICSD-3-TR criteria for PLMD include the requirement of a PLMSI of >15/hour in adults and >5/hour in children. However, as noted, many asymptomatic individuals have a PLMSI greater than 15 movements. Mendelson[70] evaluated a group of 67 patients considered to have PLMD. The patients had both a PSG and a multiple sleep latency test (MSLT). The overall sleep latency was around 10 minutes (near normal). There was no significant correlation between the PLMSAI and sleep latency (a measure of objective sleepiness). In a study of PLMS and OSA, Chervin and coworkers found that patients with a higher PLMSI were actually less sleepy.[73] Eisensehr et al. compared the sleep of patients with PLMD with that of patients with RLS and found the PLMSI and PLMSAI to be higher in PLMD than in RLS.[80] Patients with RLS had a higher overall arousal index and more wake after sleep onset, while patients with PLMD had more stage N1 sleep. However, another study comparing patients with "isolated PLMD" and patients with RLS found minimal differences.[81] Given PLMD is a diagnosis of exclusion, one approach is a therapeutic trial of treatment of PLMS with a dopaminergic medication to see if symptoms improve. There is a large placebo effect in RLS, so this may also be present in patients with suspected PLMD. Simply studying changes in the PLMS symptoms after medication treatment might be helpful, but there is the issue of night-to-night variability.

Clinical Example

A 70-year-old man was evaluated for complaints of nonrestorative sleep and daytime sleepiness (Epworth Sleepiness Scale: 14). There was no history of cataplexy or snoring, and sleep duration was more than 7.5 hours nightly. The patient's wife did report that he kicked at night. He denied depression and was on no regular medications. A PSG was only remarkable for a PLMSI of 80/hour and a PLMSAI of 15 arousals/hour (overall arousal index 25/hour). An MSLT documented a short sleep latency of 7 minutes with no sleep-onset REM periods. An empiric trial of ropinirole resulted in dramatic improvement in subjective sleep quality and, after an increase in dose, there was resolution of daytime sleepiness (Epworth Sleepiness Scale: 3). Ropinirole was used, as the patient declined use of gabapentin because of previous side effects. The patient's wife reported that she rarely noted the patient kicking during sleep. Iron stores were checked and revealed low ferritin, and iron supplementation was initiated. A repeat PSG was considered to determine if the PLMSI was lower, but the patient declined. A diagnosis of PLMD was made.

TREATMENT OF RLS AND PLMD

Overview

Over the years, a number of guidelines for treatment of RLS/PLMD have been published.[82-88] More recently, recognition of issues with the long-term effectiveness of dopaminergic drugs has resulted in significant changes. The majority of treatment studies have focused on RLS symptoms, with limited data concerning changes in the PLMSI. While dopaminergic medications were once considered first-line treatment of RLS, recommendations have shifted toward use of alpha-2-delta ligands (gabapentin, pregabalin) when possible. An overall summary of treatment options is listed in Table 31-3. The treatments for RLS are also effective for PLMS/PLMD, with the exception of opioids, which have not been well studied for treatment of PLMS/PLMD.

Nonpharmacologic Treatments for RLS

In mild and intermittent RLS, nonpharmacologic treatments may be useful. These include stretching, heating, or cooling of the extremities (warm bath) and avoidance of alcohol and caffeine. Antidepressant treatment can sometimes be associated with initiation or worsening of RLS.[25,26] However, if treatment with a given antidepressant is deemed necessary (only effective medication after trying many different drugs), RLS treatment can be attempted without stopping the antidepressant. Concerns about RLS should not limit effective treatment of depression. Studies have suggested that bupropion either improves or does not worsen PLMS and RLS,[27,89] so use of this medication could be considered. Physical devices have also been tried as RLS treatment.[90-98] These include compression stockings,[91] heating and vibrating pads,[92,93] and foot pressure wraps.[94,95] None of these are approved by the U.S. Food and Drug Administration (FDA) for treatment of RLS. The Relaxis, a vibrating pad that improved RLS sleep loss but not RLS severity, has been discontinued by the manufacturer (the FDA ruled that devices that vibrate are considered pleasure devices). The Restiffic,[95] a device consisting of a compressive foot wrap, is currently available. The Nidra Tonic Motor Activation System (Noctrix Health) is a device cleared by the FDA for treatment of moderate to severe RLS refractory to drug

Table 31-3 Treatments for RLS, PLMD

Class	Interventions	Comments
Nonpharmacologic	• Exercise, stretching, warm baths • Avoid caffeine • Avoid first-generation antihistamines • Avoid medications worsening RLS • Iron supplementation (po or IV) if Ferritin ≤75 μg/L (ng/ml)	• Low iron stores increase the risk for DA augmentation • Oral iron: (65 mg elemental iron; for example, 325 mg $FeSO_4$ daily with 100–200 mg vitamin C daily or every other day)
Dopaminergic medications (DA)	Carbidopa/levodopa—intermittent RLS DA—daily RLS • Pramipexole (Mirapex)* • Ropinirole (Requip)* • Rotigotine patch (NeuPro*)	• Generic forms of pramipexole, ropinirole available

Anticonvulsants (alpha-2-delta ligands)	• Gabapentin (Neurontin)
	• Gabapentin enacarbil (Horizant)*
	• Pregabalin (Lyrica)
		• RLS with pain, anxiety, insomnia
		• Combination with DA
		• Generic formulations of gabapentin and pregabalin are available
		• Intolerance of DA
		• Situations where DA may be preferred over alpha-2-delta ligand
		  • Depression
		  • Obesity
		  • Gait instability
		  • History of drug abuse/dependence
		  • Severe respiratory disorders, at risk for respiratory failure

Narcotics	• Tramadol • Hydrocodone/APAP • Oxycodone • Methadone	• Intractable RLS • Augmentation with DA, alpha-2-delta meds not effective • Cannot tolerate DA or alpha-2-delta ligands • Opioids contraindicated if history of substance abuse/dependence
Hypnotics	Adjunctive or mild RLS May not reduce the PLMS index	Clonazepam most studied

*FDA approved for RLS; all except narcotics have been used to treat PLMD; generic forms of ropinirole, pramipexole, gabapentin, and pregabalin are available., Hydrocodone/APAP is a combination of hydrocodone and acetaminophen; *DA*, dopamine agonists; *PLMD*, periodic limb movement disorder; *PLMS*, periodic limb movements during sleep; *RLS*, restless legs syndrome.

treatment.[97,98] The device consists of bilateral bands around each upper calf that stimulates the peroneal nerve, causing tonic contraction of leg muscles that mimic the effects of stretching the legs (known to temporarily reduce RLS sensation in many patients). The device is available on a prescription basis only and not available at the time of this writing.

Medication Treatment for RLS

The major medication groups (Table 31-3) for treatment of RLS include dopaminergic medications (dopamine precursor levodopa [LD] and dopamine agonists [DAs]), opioids, anticonvulsant medications (alpha-2-delta receptor ligands), and sedative-hypnotic medications (usually benzodiazepine receptor agonists [BZRAs]).[82-88] Similar medications have been used to treat PLMD, with the exception of opiates, which have not been well studied for this indication. Of note, three DAs (ropinirole, pramipexole, rotigotine patch) and gabapentin enacarbil extended release are the only medications that are FDA approved for RLS treatment (in adults). Few studies have been published concerning treatment of PLMD and RLS in children.[99] Of the alpha-2-delta ligands, only gabapentin enacarbil (Horizant) is FDA approved for treatment of adult RLS. Although no alpha-2-delta ligand is FDA approved for RLS in children, treatment guidelines suggest these drugs should be used as first-line treatment if nonpharmacologic interventions and iron supplementation (if indicated) are not effective.[87] Dopaminergic medications have also been used.[99] No opioid is FDA approved for treatment of RLS in the United States. The medication groups will be discussed in chapter sections below, followed by algorithms for treatment.

Alpha-2-Delta Calcium Channel Ligands

Although this group is often listed under the class "anticonvulsants," the drugs are rarely used for this indication. Alpha-2-delta ligands bind receptors on voltage-gated calcium channels.[100] Three alpha-2-delta receptor ligands have been shown to be effective for use in **RLS** (Table 31-4). Because of issues with DA treatment of RLS, these agents are considered the first-line treatment for chronic persistent RLS (daily moderate to severe RLS) unless there are contraindications or they are not effective. There is no augmentation associated with use of these drugs. They can also be used in combination with DAs or opioids to reduce the dose of the DA or opioid medications. The alpha-2-delta ligand medications are especially useful for painful RLS or patients with RLS and insomnia.[85-87] DAs are generally preferred in patients with significant or uncontrolled depression, unstable gait, severe obesity, a history of drug abuse, or a severe respiratory disorder predisposing the patient to hypoventilation, as alpha-2-delta ligands can worsen these conditions.[87] Gabapentin is an analog of GABA but binds to the alpha-2-delta subunit of voltage-gated calcium channels in the central nervous system (CNS). It is FDA approved for treatment of the pain of herpetic neuralgia and as an adjunct for patients with partial seizures. It has also been used for diabetic neuropathy but is not FDA approved for this indication. It is excreted unchanged in the urine, with a ***half-life of 5 to 7 hours***. The dose must be reduced in patients with decreased renal function. The efficacy of gabapentin treatment for RLS has been demonstrated by a number of trials.[101-104] One of these studies also reported a decrease in the PLMSI compared with placebo.[102] In this study, patients reporting the symptoms of pain received the most benefit from gabapentin. In Figure 31-8, one can see a progressive improvement in RLS symptoms (lower IRLS value) with an increase in the daily gabapentin dose. Of note, a dose above 1500 mg was required for significant improvement. The failure of gabapentin treatment of RLS is often the result of an insufficient dose. However, patients may not

Table 31-4 Alpha-2-Delta Ligand Medications for Treatment of the Restless Legs Syndrome

Medication	Dose forms	Bioavailability (Time to Max Blood level)	Elimination (Half life)	Initial Daily Dose**	Usual Effective dose** (Max Dose)	Side Effects
Gabapentin (Neurontin and Generics)	100, 300, 400 mg capsules; 600, 800 mg tablets	Unpredictable Saturable absorption (2 hrs)	Renal (5–7 hrs)	300 mg (100 mg elderly) Q 1–2 hrs before bedtime	900–1200 mg (Max Dose 2400 mg to 3600 mg multiple doses) Can give additional earlier than PM dose if early symptoms	Dizziness/ ataxia Somnolence Tremor Headache Weight gain Dry mouth
Gabapentin Enacarbil* (Horizant)	300, 600 mg ER tablets (do not cut or chew	Extended release Predictable Active transport in GI tract (Hydrolyzed in GI tract cells to gabapentin (7–9 hrs))	Renal (6 hrs) (Stable levels 18–24 hrs)	600 mg at 5 PM **with food**	600–1200 mg FDA max 600 mg Up to 1200 mg used in some studies	Same
Pregabalin (Lyrica and Generics)	25, 50, 75, 100, 150, 200, 225, 300 mg capsules)	Predictable (1.5 hrs)	Renal (6 hrs)	75 mg (50 mg in elderly) q to 1 to 2 hrs before bedtime	150–450 mg Max Dose (450 mg PM dose, 600 mg multiple doses)	Same

Gabapentin, pregabalin structural analogs of GABA, bind alpha-2-delta receptors
*Only Horizant is FDA approved for treatment of RLS
**Reduced dosage in renal insufficiency (initial dose 100 mg gabapentin, 300 mg Horizant, 50 mg pregabalin)
Adapted from reference 87

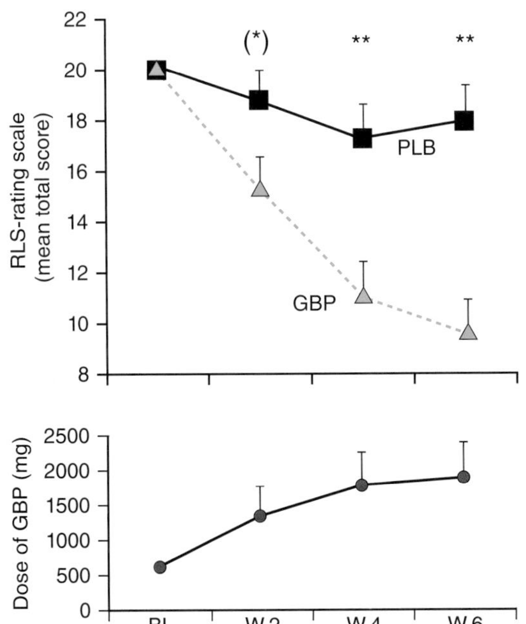

Figure 31-8 Change in restless legs syndrome (RLS) symptoms (RLS rating scale) on gabapentin (GBP) and placebo (PLB) during dose escalation. (*)p = NS; ** $p < .05$ GBP vs. PLB. Note that fairly high doses of GBP were needed to be effective (over 1200 to 1500 mg). *BL*, baseline. (From Garcia-Borreguero D, Larrosa O, de la Llave Y, et al. Treatment of restless legs syndrome with gabapentin. *Neurology*. 2002;59:1573-1579.)

tolerate an effective dose, and the dosage should be gradually increased to improve tolerance. A study by Saletu et al.[103] comparing gabapentin and ropinirole found that both improved RLS, but gabapentin improved sleep quality more while ropinirole decreased the PLMs to a greater degree.

The usual starting dose of gabapentin is 300 mg administered at night 1 to 2 hour before symptoms (100 to 200 mg in the elderly), with progressive gradual increases in dosage if needed (or tolerated). The average effective dose is quite high (900–1200 mg) (Figure 31-8). Some patients will benefit from a lower dose, and some need a higher dose. A slow upward titration has been used in studies of gabapentin with an increase of 300 to 600 mg every 1 to 2 weeks. This may improve tolerance to relatively high doses of gabapentin. One should not assume the medication does not work unless a reasonable dose has been reached. Common side effects include sedation, fatigue, ataxia, nausea, peripheral edema, and weight gain. Serious reactions include leukopenia, thrombocytopenia, and **depression**. Associated with depression there is an increase in suicidal ideation. While the dose of gabapentin must be reduced in patients with renal failure, it can be used in a low dose in patients on dialysis. For a creatinine clearance treatment with 100–300 mg daily or with supplemental doses after hemodialysis has been suggested. A controlled crossover study demonstrated that gabapentin was effective treatment of RLS in patients with renal failure on hemodialysis.[104] In this study, a dose of 200 to 300 mg was given after each dialysis session. Gabapentin toxicity in renal failure consists of sedation, falls, and severe myoclonic twitching of the face and arms.

While many physicians have tried gabapentin only after problems have been encountered with dopaminergic medications, *a study found a reduced response to gabapentin enacarbil after previous long-term RLS treatment with DAs.*[105] This fact is another reason to consider alpha-2-delta ligands as first-line treatment for RLS.

Administration with antacids reduces absorption of gabapentin, while some medications (methadone, morphine, hydrocodone) increase the plasma levels of gabapentin. On the other hand, gabapentin lowers the levels of hydrocodone. A major problem with the use of gabapentin is that it has a dose-dependent bioavailability (as the dose increases, the proportion absorbed medication decreases). This is a manifestation of saturable absorption in the upper intestine. In addition, the ability to absorb gabapentin varies among individuals. Because gabapentin is mildly sedating, it also tends to improve sleep quality and can increase stage N3 sleep. Unlike with DAs, augmentation has not been described.

Gabapentin enacarbil (GBPen; Horizant) is the first non-dopamine FDA-approved treatment for moderate to severe RLS.[106,107] GBPen is **an extended-release** preparation using a prodrug of gabapentin that is rapidly absorbed throughout the gastrointestinal (GI) tract via high-capacity active rapid intestinal transporters and, once absorbed, is converted to gabapentin (hydrolysis) in the GI enterocytes. This extended release form of gabapentin delays the time to peak gabapentin plasma levels and provides dose-proportional exposure. That is, this formulation of gabapentin has reliable absorption. The preparation is extended release to provide an effective level for the entire night. Side effects are similar to gabapentin, e.g., headaches, dizziness, somnolence. There are no significant drug interactions. The medication is given as a single dose at 5 PM and *should not be chewed or cut*. Of note, while 600 mg is the FDA-approved dose (300 mg in the elderly), a dose of 1200 mg in many studies was found to be most effective,[108] especially for improving sleep quality. The usual dose is 600 mg at 5:00 PM. As there is no generic formulation, the medication is more expensive than gabapentin. On the other hand, one can avoid the dose titration needed with gabapentin. The efficacy of GBPen for RLS treatment has been documented by double-blind placebo-controlled studies.[106,107]

Pregabalin (Lyrica) is a structural analog to GABA that binds to the alpha-2-delta subunit of the voltage-dependent calcium channels in the CNS. Pregabalin was developed as an anticonvulsant but is FDA approved for treatment of fibromyalgia, postherpetic neuralgia, neuropathic pain associated with spinal cord injury or diabetic neuropathy, and as an adjunct for partial-onset seizures in patients 4 years of age and older. It has primarily renal elimination with a *half-life of about 6.3 hours in adults and 3-6 hrs in children. The dose must be reduced in renal failure.* No significant drug interactions are noted with pregabalin. The usual starting dose is 75 mg (50 mg in the elderly) one to two hours before bedtime (or symptoms). The dose can be increased by 75 to 150 mg weekly as needed with a usual effective dose of 150–450 mg with a maximum dose of 450 mg for a PM dose (or 600 mg if multiple doses). If the creatinine clearance is <15 ml/min one approach is 75 mg daily or 75–100 mg after each hemodialysis. A double-blind placebo-controlled study found that pregabalin at a **mean dose of 333 mg** was an effective treatment for RLS.[109] Treatment was started at 150 mg and increased as needed. In contrast, a dose ranging study found 90% effectiveness at a daily dose of 123.9 mg (although higher doses were most effective).[110] Pregabalin was also effective as an "add-on" to other treatments.[111] Treatment with pregabalin was found to be as effective as pramipexole in another study (compared to placebo), and augmentation rates were significantly lower with pregabalin than with 0.5 mg pramipexole.[112] Side effects of pregabalin include dizziness, drowsiness, blurred vision, and ataxia. In 2019, the FDA approved generic forms of pregabalin that are less expensive. An advantage of pregabalin over generic gabapentin is that the absorption of pregabalin is reliable.[113] Given the availability of generic pregabalin, it is an attractive alternative to generic gabapentin. Of note, pregabalin is a schedule V medication (schedule V includes cough medications with a low dose of codeine) and is considered to have some abuse potential but lower than schedule IV medications (e.g., tramadol). Gabapentin has also been classified as a schedule V medication in some states. *In 2019, the FDA issued a warning that gabapentinoids (gabapentin, gabapentin enacarbil, pregabalin) may be associated with respiratory depression in patients with breathing disorders, especially when combined with opioid medications or benzodiazepines.*[114]

Dopaminergic Medications

Levodopa (LD) is a precursor that is converted to dopamine by dopa decarboxylase (DDC). Carbidopa (CD) does not penetrate the blood-brain barrier but acts as an inhibitor of DDC outside the CNS. Therefore, there is less peripheral conversion of LD to dopamine. This results in fewer side effects (nausea) and an increased amount of LD reaching the brain. Since LD competes with certain amino acids for transport across the gut wall, the absorption of LD may be impaired in some patients on a high-protein diet. LD may activate melanoma and should not be used in a patient with known or suspected melanoma. LD should not be used in patients with narrow-angle glaucoma or in patients taking a nonselective monoamine oxidase (MAO) inhibitor.

The combination of CD and LD (CD/LD) is very effective in RLS and has a quick onset of action (but a short duration of action). The onset of CD/LD is 30 to 50 minutes after ingestion, and the half-life of the CD/LD combination is about 1.5 hours. The starting dose is half to one pill of the CD/LD 25/100 mg preparation with a usual effective dose range of 100 to 200 mg of LD (max 200 mg LD). There are two problems with use of CD/LD in treating RLS. First, the drug has a short duration of action, and there may be a rebound in symptoms in the early morning hours. The patient can take another dose at that time. There are longer-acting forms of CD/LD but they have a slower onset of action. The second problem is that continued use of CD/LD, especially at high doses (LD >200 mg/day), commonly results in augmentation (a change in the effectiveness of dopaminergic medications). In some studies, up to 80% of patients taking CD/LD for RLS develop augmentation.[115] For this reason, CD/LD is rarely used except in cases of intermittent RLS. The immediate-release form is rapid acting and will suffice if a short duration of effect is needed; otherwise, controlled-release preparations are used (or repeated dosing with the immediate-acting formulation).

The non-ergotamine DAs pramipexole, ropinirole, and rotigotine (patch) are all FDA-approved treatments for RLS (Table 31-5). Randomized, controlled studies have documented the efficacy of these medications for treating RLS and PLMD. They have a sufficiently long duration of action, such that rebound does usually not occur. The half-life of pramipexole is longer than ropinirole. Dopagmine agonists were once considered first-line medications for treatment of daily moderate to severe RLS.[116-124]

Augmentation and side effects of DAs can be minimized by starting at a low dose (0.125 mg for pramipexole and 0.25 mg for ropinirole), with a slow upward titration as needed (Table 31-5). It is important to note that both drugs have a long time of onset and should be taken several hours before symptoms are expected (2 to 3 hours for pramipexole, 1 to 2 hours for ropinirole). If patients have symptoms in the morning, one can try treatment with dosing twice or three times a day. Of note, some patients will respond better to pramipexole than to ropinirole, and vice versa. Some patients will tolerate one medication better than the other (less nausea). Studies have suggested that the equivalent dose of ropinirole is about four times the dose of pramipexole. In the manufacturers' drug prescribing information, the **maximum recommended doses for RLS treatment are 0.5 mg of pramipexole and 4 mg of ropinirole**. The drug labeling states pramipexole doses up to 0.75 mg have been used in studies, but there was little additional benefit from doses above 0.5 mg. However, most physicians would accept a 0.75-mg dose as the upper limit for treatment of RLS. The rotigotine transdermal patch is potentially useful for patients with daytime RLS symptoms or augmentation. The risk of augmentation may be lower with the rotigotine patch. Switching from ropinirole or pramipexole to rotigotine is a possible intervention for mild augmentation[123] or daytime symptoms. Methods of switching from oral DAs to the rotigotine patch have been published.[124,125]

Dopaminergic Side Effects

All dopaminergic medications share similar side effects (Table 31-6). All DAs are category C and not recommended for use during pregnancy. Although the A-X classification is no longer officially used by the FDA, it can still be informative. *Nausea is the most common side effect of DA medications*, but headache, light-headedness, somnolence, peripheral edema, and nasal congestion can occur. Severe side effects include severe hypersomnia (including sudden sleep attacks), nightmares, augmentation, and dopamine dysregulation syndrome/impulse control disorders. As noted, long-term studies of patients using DAs have shown that a significant proportion (up to 50%) of patients stop taking the medications because of lack of efficacy, augmentation, or side effects.[126,127] The **dopamine dysregulation syndrome** is a dysfunction of the reward system in patients taking dopamine treatment. The most common symptom is craving for dopaminergic medication, sometimes associated with taking extra doses even in the absence of symptoms that indicate the need for additional medication. DAs can also be associated with **defects in impulse control** (compulsive gambling, hypersexuality, punding, or compulsive shopping).[128,129] Punding is characterized by compulsive fascination with and performance of repetitive, mechanical tasks, such as assembling and disassembling, collecting, or sorting household objects. Although impulse control disorders are more common during DA treatment of Parkinson's disease than during that of RLS, the problem is increasingly reported as a complication of DA treatment of RLS. It is important to ask about abnormal behaviors **during every clinical visit** in patients on a DA and to warn patients about this potential side effect (they may note the problem but not associate it with the medication and often do not spontaneously report these issues to the treating physician).

Table 31-5 Dopamine Precursor and Agonists Used for RLS Treatment

	Dopamine Precursor	Dopamine Agonists		
Medication	Carbidopa/levodopa (CD/LD)	Pramipexole	Ropinirole	Rotigotine
	L-DOPA dopamine precursor Carbidopa does not penetrate blood-brain barrier, inhibits dopa decarboxylase, less peripheral conversion to dopamine, less side effects, more L-DOPA reaches CNS	Non-ergotamine DA	Non-ergotamine DA	Non-ergotamine DA
Brand/generic	Sinemet/generic (Sinemet CR no longer available except as generic) IR CD/LD: 10 mg/100 mg, 25 mg/100 mg, 25 mg/250 mg ER 25 mg/100 mg, 50 mg/200 mg	Mirapex, generic available	Requip, generic available	NeuPro, no generic
Time to max blood level	Time to effect (delayed by high protein foods) IR 20–50 min CR 50 min	2 hours	1–1.5 hours	Transdermal Patch
Elimination half life	IR 0.75-1.5h IR effect lasts about 2–3 hours ER effects last 4–6 hours	8–12 hours	6 hours	N/A
Metabolism and excretion	Converted to dopamine by dopa decarboxylase Renal excretion (80%) as dopamine, norepinephrine, and homovanillic acid	Renal excretion	Hepatic metabolism, renal excretion, dose adjustment in severe renal impairment (maximum dose 3 mg)	Hepatic metabolism; renal excretion (no dose adjustment for rean insufficiency)
Starting dose/ titration	½–1 tablet of 25/100 mg qhs (max 200 mg levodopa) to avoid high risk of augmentation	• 0.125 mg • 2–3 hours before bedtime step 1: 0.125 mg step 2: 0.25 mg step 3: 0.5 mg Increase to next step every 4–7 days Max dose 0.5–0.75 mg	• 0.25 mg • 1–2 hours before bedtime • Increase by 0.5 mg weekly if needed • Max dose 4 mg	• 1 mg/24 hours • Increase by 1 mg/24 hours to max of 3 mg/24 hours

CD/LD, carbidopa/levodopa; *CNS*, central nervous system; *CR*, continuous release; *DA*, dopamine agonists; *ER*, extended release; *IR*, immediate release.

Table 31-6 Dopamine Agonist Side Effects

Acute	Subacute/Severe	Parkinson Disorders

• Nausea, vomiting (less common)
• Light-headedness, syncope (rare)
• Headache
• Somnolence
• Insomnia
• Local site reactions (Rotigotine)
Less common
• Peripheral edema
• Nasal congestion
• Constipation
	• Augmentation
	• Hypersomnia—including sleep attacks
	• Dopamine dysregulation syndrome
	• Impulse control disorders
	  • Hypersexuality
	  • Pathologic gambling
	  • Excessive shopping
	  • Punding
	• Rotigotine patch—allergic reactions
		(Higher doses)
		• Dyskinesias
		• Hallucinations
		• Psychosis

When the DAs are used to treat Parkinson's disease in much higher doses than those used to treat RLS, they can be associated with dyskinesias, hallucinations, or psychosis. Patients with RLS who develop impulse control disorder should be switched to an alternative class of medications.

The rotigotine patch is associated with a significant number of local site reactions. The location of patch placement should be changed with each application. The rotigotine patch contains sodium metabisulfite, a substance that may cause allergic-type reactions, including anaphylactic symptoms and life-threatening or less severe asthmatic episodes in certain susceptible people. Sulfite sensitivity is seen more frequently in asthmatic individuals than in non-asthmatics individuals. Of note, allergy to metabisulfites is not the same as allergy to sulfa.

Pramipexole is renally excreted, whereas ropinirole and rotigotine undergo hepatic metabolism and are preferred for patients with renal insufficiency. A maximum dose of 3 mg of ropinorole is recommended of end stage renal disease on hemodialysis. There is no renal impairment dose adjustment for rotigotine.

Augmentation

Augmentation is defined as a change in the efficacy of RLS treatment with dopaminergic medications[130-135] (Box 31-10). It is characterized by one or more of the following: (1) worse symptoms before dose administration than before initially starting DA treatment, (2) greater severity of symptoms at the same dose (assuming prior response to the dose), (3) earlier symptom onset and longer delay in medication effect after taking the medication, (4) paradoxical response to treatment: RLS symptom severity increases after a dose increase (not immediately) and improves after a dose decrease (not always, and can be delayed), (5) reduced latency to onset of symptoms with rest, and (6) spread of symptoms to involve new body parts (arms as well as legs). The paradoxical response is difficult to determine, as worsening after an increase in DA dosage may be delayed. If the dosage is reduced, improvement in symptoms may also be delayed. Decreasing the CD/LD dosage can be associated with improvement in symptoms over 72 hours. However, improvement after a decrease in the dosage of a DA may take several weeks to months. Thus, the paradoxical response is not very helpful in clinical practice.[86,130] There are mimics of augmentation (Table 31-7). An end-of-dose rebound (wearing off) effect can occur with early morning symptoms. However, symptoms **do not occur earlier** and are not **more intense than before** starting DA treatment. Using a longer- duration DA, giving another dose of DA at bedtime (assuming total dose within guidelines), or giving an early-morning dose of a DA are options. Tolerance is a reduced effect of a given dose of medication. This is usually manifested by breakthrough in middle-of-the-night or early-morning symptoms. With tolerance, *symptoms do not occur earlier, are not more intense than before starting treatment, and are not present in the arms.* A higher dose of DA medication is usually needed, but another option is adding an alpha-2-delta ligand. Natural progression of the disease is very difficult to differentiate from augmentation, as symptoms can appear earlier, be more intense, and involve the arms. In progression of disease, there is no paradoxical response to DAs, but this is difficult to document. Certainly, *if more than one dosage escalation of a DA is needed in a patient who has been on a stable dose*, this is suggestive of augmentation. Exacerbating factors can also mimic augmentation, but there is no paradoxical response. Such factors include low iron stores, addition of an exacerbating medication (first-generation antihistamines, antidepressant medications), and increased immobility. **Iron deficiency increases the risk of augmentation.**[135]

The prevalence of augmentation is difficult to evaluate, as it depends on dose, schedule, and duration of follow-up. *The risk of augmentation increases with treatment duration.* An analysis of the literature found the prevalence of augmentation to be 80% with CD/LD (especially with LD over 200 mg)[131] and with DAs to be 10% to 12% at 1 year, 30%

Box 31-10 IMPORTANT AUGMENTATION CHARACTERISTICS

- Unmedicated symptoms worse than before starting dopamine agonist treatment
- Greater severity of symptoms at a given dosage (assumes a better prior response to the dosage)
- RLS symptom onset earlier in the day
- Symptoms in the arms
- Shorter latency to symptoms when at rest (delayed)
- Longer latency after dose ingetion to onset of medication effiacy
- Symptoms better following DA dose decrease (improvement can be quite delayed with dopamine agonists) or symptoms worse after DA dose increase

Questions to ask the patient:

1. Do RLS symptoms appear earlier than when the drug was first started?
2. Are higher doses of the drug now needed, or do you need to take the medicine earlier, to control the RLS symptoms compared with the original effective dose?
3. Has the intensity of symptoms worsened since starting the medication?
4. Have symptoms spread to other parts of the body (e.g., the arms) since starting the medication?

Adapted from García-Borreguero D, Allen RP, Kohnen R, et al. International Restless Legs Syndrome Study Group. Diagnostic standards for dopaminergic augmentation of restless legs syndrome: report from a World Association of Sleep Medicine-International Restless Legs Syndrome Study Group consensus conference at the Max Planck Institute. *Sleep Med.* 2007;8(5):520-530. Erratum in: *Sleep Med.* 2007;8(7-8):788. Earley CJ [added].

Table 31-7 Differential Diagnosis of Augmentation

	Augmentation	End-of-Dose Rebound	Tolerance	Natural Progression	Exacerbating Factors**
Worse than before DA treatment started	Yes	Yes, in early AM	No	Yes	Yes
Earlier onset	Yes	Yes, in early AM	No	Yes	Yes
Spread to arms	Yes	No	No	Yes	Yes
Breakthrough at night	Yes	Yes, but in early AM	Yes	Yes	Yes
Worse with increased dose	Yes, but not immediately	No	No	No	No
Improved with decreased dose	Yes, but not always*	No	No	No	No

* After decreased dose, may take weeks to months with DA (72 hours with CD/LD)
**Low ferritin, immobility, addition of exacerbating medications
CD/LD, carbidopa/levodopa; *DA*, dopamine agonists.
From García-Borreguero D, Allen RP, Kohnen R, et al. International Restless Legs Syndrome Study Group. Diagnostic standards for dopaminergic augmentation of restless legs syndrome: report from a World Association of Sleep Medicine-International Restless Legs Syndrome Study Group consensus conference at the Max Planck Institute. *Sleep Med.* 2007;8(5):520-530. Erratum in: *Sleep Med.* 2007;8(7-8):788. Earley CJ [added]. PMID: 17544323.

over 2 to 3 years, and 42% to 68% over long-term studies (10 years or more).[86,130] The progression of augmentation in a community sample is shown in Figure 31-9. All dopaminergic medications and tramadol can result in augmentation. The risk is greater for CD/LD than for DAs and less for longer-acting DAs (rotigotine patch) than for pramipexole or ropinirole. There are extended-release forms of pramipexole and ropinirole, but these have not been well studied. Newer studies suggest augmentation with DAs is more of a problem than realized, and a substantial percentage of patients stop DA treatment as a result of augmentation (or lack of efficacy) when followed over 5 to 10 years.[126-129] One study analyzed follow up with DA and opioid treatments and found that stopping DA medication was common, while discontinuing opioid treatment for RLS was rare (Figure 31-10).[126] Assessment of augmentation in community samples shows that the

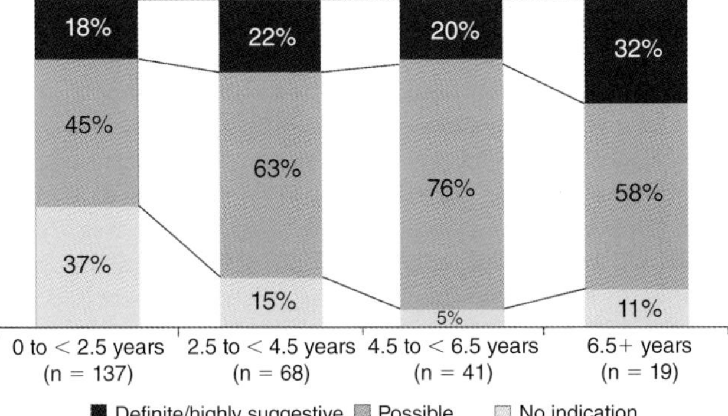

Figure 31-9 A progressive increase in the amount of augmentation with a longer duration of treatment in a community sample. Note that possible augmentation was over 50% at 2.5 years or longer. (From Allen RP, Ondo WG, Ball E, et al. Restless legs syndrome (RLS) augmentation associated with dopamine agonist and levodopa usage in a community sample. *Sleep Med.* 2011;12(5):431-439. PMID: 21493132.)

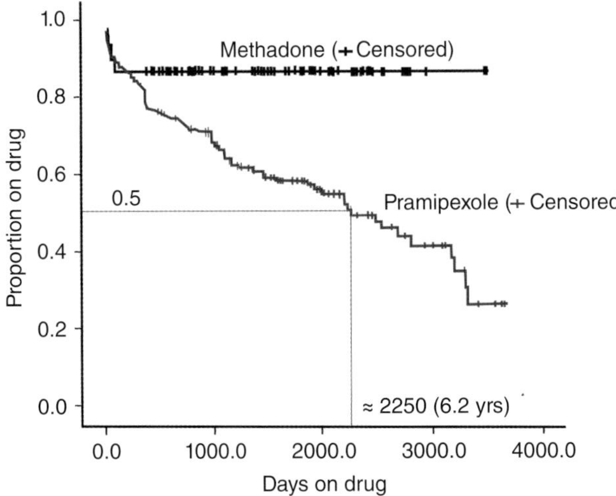

Figure 31-10 Long-term follow-up of patients treated with pramipexole or methadone. The vertical lines are the time at which follow-up was censored (the last observation made at that time). After a slight decrease in patients on methadone, most continued the medication. In contrast with pramipexole, there was a large decrease in the number of patients still on the medication over time. Patients stopped because of lack of efficacy or development of augmentation. (From Silver N, Allen RP, Senerth J, Earley CJ. A 10-year, longitudinal assessment of dopamine agonists and methadone in the treatment of restless legs syndrome. *Sleep Med.* 2011;12(5):440-444.)

risk increases with a higher DA dosage and longer duration of treatment.[133] One reason for the high prevalence of augmentation is that physicians have been *prescribing DAs at doses much higher than those recommended for RLS.*[134] When using a DA, it is imperative to be certain the patient is taking the DA *early enough* **before** increasing the dose. Using the lowest effective dose of DA is prudent to minimize the risk of augmentation. Many patients have an occasional bad night, and *taking an additional dose at those times rather than a chronic increase in DA dose is preferred.*

Treatment of Augmentation

The best approach is to **avoid augmentation** by using an alpha-2-delta ligand as first-line treatment and, if using a DA, to keep the dose as low as possible and below the recommended maximum doses (ropinirole 4 mg, pramipexole 0.5 to 0.75 mg). Patients must take the medications early enough (2 hours before bedtime), as the delay in effect might result in an increase in dosage that is really not needed. Low iron stores appear to increase the frequency or severity of augmentation, so ferritin should be checked[135] if augmentation is present and should actually be checked routinely in all patients with RLS. If a patient is being treated with a DA but control of RLS is not adequate, rather than increase the DA dosage, another option is the addition of an alpha-2-delta ligand or low-dose opioid (if alpha-2-delta ligands are not tolerated) to keep the DA dose as low as possible.

Once augmentation is suspected, multiple interventions are possible, depending on the current dopaminergic medication and the severity of symptoms[86,87] (Box 31-11 and Figure 31-11). If the patient is on CD/LD, the first approach would be to change to an alpha-2-delta ligand. If the patient is on a DA and symptoms occur earlier in the evening, the medication dose could be split or another dose added earlier (e.g., pramipexole 0.125 mg at 6:00 PM and 9:00 PM). If the problem is morning symptoms, a morning dose could be added (bid to tid dosing). Usually, a midday dose is not needed because of the "RLS protected time period" in the middle of the day. Switching to the rotigotine patch is an option to address daytime symptoms. This long-acting preparation may reduce the risk of augmentation. Switching to another DA (e.g., from ropinirole to pramipexole) is reasonable at the *initiation* of DA treatment if the current DA is not tolerated or effective (sometimes patients respond to or tolerate treatment with an alternative DA). However, switching between pramipexole and ropinirole *if augmentation is suspected* is usually not recommended. For moderate augmentation, starting an alpha-2-delta ligand and weaning the DA is often effective (cross-titration). Reaching an effective dose of the alpha-2-delta ligand before reducing the DA dosage may make the switch more tolerable (but some temporary worsening of symptoms may occur, and patient education is important). For severe augmentation, starting a high-potency opioid and then weaning the DA medication is usually necessary. There are variable opinions regarding how rapidly a DA is weaned. This depends on patient preference (ability to tolerate withdrawal worsening of symptoms) and effectiveness of the replacement medication.

In general, *higher dosages of DAs should never be discontinued abruptly*, as serious withdrawal effects can occur, characterized by severe RLS, sleep disturbance, and depression. Rates of reduction should not exceed 0.25 mg (pramipexole) or 0.5 mg (ropinirole)

Box 31-11 APPROACHES TO AUGMENTATION

Avoid Augmentation

- Use alpha-2-delta ligand as first-line treatment.
- Avoid CD/LD in daily RLS; avoid LD dose >200 mg.
- If using DA agonists, use pramipexole dose ≤0.5 mg (0.75 mg) and ropinirole ≤4 mg.
- Document proper timing of administration (early enough) to avoid unneeded dose increase.
- Use combination treatment rather than increase DA agonist dosage (alpha-2-delta ligand or opioid).
- Intervene for low iron stores or exacerbating factors.

Mild Augmentation (earlier symptoms, no recent increase in dosage above what was previously effective)

- If on CD/LD, stop and change to a DA or alpha-2-delta ligand.
- If on a DA and earlier symptom onset is the problem, split the dose and give half of the dose earlier.
  - Or, if not effective, add an earlier dose (increased total dosage should be within guidelines).
- Breakthrough symptoms – increase nighttime dose (or give part of current dose later).
- If morning symptoms are a problem, try evening and morning doses of medication or use a rotigotine patch.
- Change to a longer acting DA medication (rotigotine patch).

Moderate to Severe Augmentation

- Switch to a longer acting DA such as the rotigitine patch (mild to moderate augmentation).
- Wean DA over 10 to 14 days (if tolerated); if treatment is needed, use an alpha-2-delta ligand or opioid.**
- Cross-titration: Add an alpha-2-delta ligand and wean the DA; try to ultimately stop the DA (or continue at a low dose).
- Cross-titration (Severe augmentation or alpha-2-delta ligand not tolerated/effective): Add a potent opioid and wean off DA.
- If opioid started, attempt long-term conversion to alpha-2-delta ligand, if possible (assuming medications are effective/tolerated). Many patients will require long-term opioid medication.
- If serum ferritin below goal and oral iron is not working, consider IV iron.

** Most patients have severe symptoms if a DA is weaned without cross-titration with another medication. If cross-titration with an alpha-2-delta ligand is planned, an adequate dosage should be reach before DA is completely eliminated.
CD/LD, carbidopa/levodopa; *DA*, dopamine agonist; *RLS*, restless legs syndrome.

every 3 days. Some favor an approach of weaning the DA before starting a new drug. However, this is usually poorly tolerated, as RLS symptoms are usually severe. The cross-titration method in which the DA is weaned, the new medication started, and the dosage increased as needed is better tolerated by patients.

Opioids/Opioid agonists

Opioids and opioid receptor agonists (tramadol) can be effective treatments for RLS (Table 31-8).[136-144] They are rapid acting and can be used either singly or in combination with other medication groups such as DAs. While most studies of opioids in RLS have been small or uncontrolled,[137-142] a double-blind, randomized placebo-controlled study of long-acting oxycodone-naloxone (not available in the United States) documented efficacy of opioid medication for RLS.[143] Except for tramadol, augmentation has not been described with opioid treatment of RLS. Milder RLS may respond to low-potency opiates (codeine) or an opioid agonist (tramadol). Moderate to severe RLS may respond to high-potency opiates (hydrocodone, oxycodone, methadone). Hydrocodone is available in the United States in combination with acetaminophen (APAP). One must be cautious not to prescribe an excessive dose of APAP. For example, it is preferable to use hydrocodone/APAP of 10/325 mg rather than two tablets of 5/325 mg. A maximum of 2 g of APAP per day can be used, although lower doses can be harmful if liver disease is present. Side effects of opiates include nausea, itching, and constipation. These medications should not be used with alcohol and should be used with caution in patients with OSA, central sleep apnea, or hypoventilation. Advantages and disadvantages of opioid treatment of RLS are listed in Box 31-12. Because of the potential of abuse and dependence, opioids are not the drugs of choice for daily RLS. However, studies and clinical experience suggest dependence is not a problem if patients do not have a history of opioid dependence and take the medication only at night. A detailed discussion of the appropriate use of opioids in RLS is contained in the reference by Silber et al.[136] Screening for opioid abuse risk, an opioid contract of patient expectations, monitoring, and controlled substance prescription websites (required in many states) are appropriate interventions to minimize risk. A national registry for opioid treatment in RLS was started, and findings to date show that the dosage is rarely increased over time (and if so, only a mild increase).[144]

Typical doses of opiates/opioid agonists include tramadol 50 to 100 mg, hydrocodone 5 to 15 mg, oxycodone 5 to 15 mg, and methadone 5 to 15 mg. Many physicians find methadone to be especially effective in very severe augmentation/intractable RLS. Methadone has a long duration of action and can be used when patients have significant RLS symptoms during the day. The medication is excreted by the kidneys (dosage adjustment for renal insufficiency) and *can increase the QT interval* (usually at higher doses). Therefore, it is prudent to perform an electrocardiogram (ECG) before and after starting the medication. Of note, narcotics are not FDA approved for treatment of RLS. There is limited information about the treatment of PLMD with narcotics.

Sedative Hypnotics

The BZRAs, including both benzodiazepines (triazolam, temazepam, clonazepam) and nonbenzodiazepines (zolpidem, zaleplon, eszopiclone), can be used for treatment of RLS or PLMD.[145-149] The BZRAs work mainly by reducing sleep latency, increasing sleep efficiency, and possibly reducing arousals resulting from PLMS. Most studies have NOT found a decrease in the PLMSI. Studies found clonazepam was effective, but this medication can cause profound morning grogginess because of its long half-life. The BZRAs with a short duration of action (triazolam,[147,148] zaleplon, zolpidem) or intermediate duration of action (zolpidem-CR, eszopiclone, temazepam) are likely to be as effective and better tolerated. In patients with early morning awakening, a change from the shorter-acting to the medium-duration medications may be helpful. This class of medications should be used with caution in patients with OSA or severe lung disease. The BZRAs are generally used as *adjunctive treatment* unless RLS is mild and/or insomnia is an independent problem only worsened by RLS. In general the combined use of a BZRA and opioid is problematic and increases the risk of respiratory

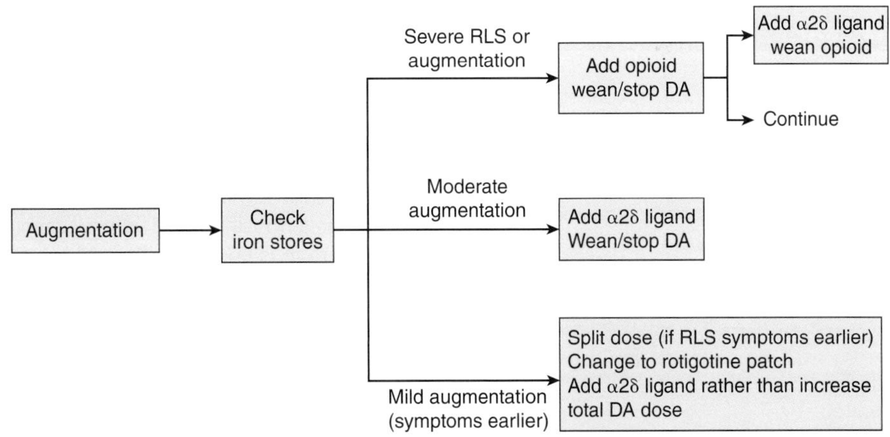

Figure 31-11 Approach to Treatment of Augmentation. The approach depends on the severity of restless legs syndrome (RLS) and symptoms. In milder cases, the dopamine agonist (DA) dose can be split into an earlier dose for early symptoms and a dose nearer bedtime for nocturnal symptoms. A change to the rotigotine patch is another option. One could also add an alpha-2-delta ligand and reduce the DA dosage or wean and stop the DA, if possible. For moderate RLS, a switch to an alpha-2-delta agonist and weaning the DA is an option. In severe RLS, most patients need an opioid at an effective dose followed by weaning of the DA (stopping, if possible). Before the DA is weaned, reasonable control with the other medication being substituted is ideal to minimize symptoms. Some patients can then be weaned from the opioid after starting an alpha-2-delta ligand (cross-titration).

Table 31-8 Opioid Treatment of the Restless Legs Syndrome

Medication	Dose Forms	Initial Dose	Usual Effective Dose	Max Dose (24 hours)	Time of onset	Half – life (Elimination)
Tramadol* IR or ER	IR 50,100 mg ER 100, 200 mg Tablets	50 mg IR 100 mg ER	100–200 mg	400 mg If high dose Wean	1 hour onset 2–3 hours peak level	6–7 hours
Codeine (COD)/ APAP	15/300 mg, 30/300 mg, 60/300 mg	30 mg codeine	60–180 mg COD	300 mg COD	Onset 30–45 min, Peak 1–2 hours	COD 2.9 hrs APAP 2 to 3 hrs
Hydrocodone (HC)/APAP (Lortab, Vicoden)	5/325 mg, 7.5/325 mg, 10/325 mg	5/325 mg	5–20 mg HC	20–30 mg/day 2 or 3 divided doses	1–30 min onset 1.3 hours peak level	3–4 hours
Oxycodone	5, 10, 15 mg	5 mg qhs	5–20 mg	5–15 q4h for acute paint	10–15 min onset 30–60 min peak level	3–6 hours
Oxycodone/APAP (Percocet)	5/325 mg 7.5/326 mg 10/325 mg	5/325 mg	5 to 20 mg of oxycodone	Same, Avoid excessive APAP	Same	Same
Methadone	5, 10 mg tablets	2.5 to 5 mg Bid dosing	5–20 mg per day	20 mg For RLS	30–60 min	8–59 hours

*Augmentation, seizure risk reported
APAP, acetaminophen.
Adapted from reference 87

Box 31-12 OPIOIDS FOR RLS

Advantages	Disadvantages/Side Effects

• Rapid action
• Quick titration of dose
• No augmentation (except tramadol)
• No evidence of decreased effect with time
	• Abuse potential
	• Dependence potential
	• Most states allow only 30-day prescriptions
	• Side effects:
	  • Drowsiness
	  • Exacerbates OSA/CSA
	  • Itch
	  • Nausea
	  • Constipation
	  • Prolonged QT (methadone)

CSA, central sleep apnea; *OSA*, obstructive sleep apnea; *RLS*, restless legs syndrome.

depression. The same caution applies to the combination of an alpha2-delta ligand and a BZRA. Like many adverse effects the lowest dose possible and slow increases in doses may reduce the risk. These combinations are especially problematic in older patients and those with lung disease.

Iron and RLS

Iron deficiency can cause or worsen RLS. The IRLSSG published consensus guidelines for iron treatment in RLS.[44] Some general guidelines are listed in Box 31-13. Checking the fasting ferritin level[42-44] is recommended in patients with RLS, because this disorder may be the only indication that low iron stores are present. Note that, while low serum ferritin means CSF ferritin is low, *normal serum ferritin can also be associated with low CSF ferritin*. The ferritin level can be elevated in patients with

Box 31-13 IRON THERAPY

- Determine iron status in all patients with restless legs syndrome (RLS) with an early morning fasting iron panel [serum ferritin, iron total binding capacity (TIBC), and percentage transferrin saturation (%TIBC)].
- If serum ferritin concentration ≤75 μg/L in adults and transferrin saturation <45%, administer an oral iron preparation (elemental iron 65 mg) with 100 to 200 mg vitamin C every 1 or 2 days on empty stomach (taken with food if better tolerated). Repeat the iron panel after 3 months.
- Consider intravenous iron if transferrin saturation is <45% and
  (1) Serum ferritin <100 μg/L and a more rapid response needed than with oral iron.
  (2) Oral iron not tolerated.
  (3) Oral iron is not absorbed due to disorders of the gastrointestinal tract, bariatric surgery, or chronic inflammatory conditions.
  (4) RLS symptoms do not improve despite an adequate (3-month) trial of oral iron.
  (5) Moderate daily RLS that is uncontrolled or with refractory RLS in whom a rapid response is needed.

Notes:

1. In the presence of inflammation or malignant disease, serum ferritin concentration may be misleadingly high, and thus transferrin saturation <20% may be a more accurate measure of iron deficiency.
2. In children, iron supplementation indicated if ferritin <50 μg/L.
3. For IV iron, 100 μg/L is used rather than 75 μg/L because IV iron does improve iron stores when ferritin levels are 76 to 100 μg/L. In contrast, oral iron absorption is minimal when ferritin levels are >75 μg/L.

Adapted from Allen RP, Picchietti DL, Auerbach M, et al. International Restless Legs Syndrome Study Group (IRSG). Evidence-based and consensus clinical practice guidelines for the iron treatment of restless legs syndrome/Willis-Ekbom disease in adults and children: an IRLSSG task force report. *Sleep Med.* 2018;41:27-44. PMID: 29425576.

inflammation; therefore, TIBC and iron saturation should also be tested.[43,44] Most clinicians recommend that a ferritin level above >75 μg/L be achieved in patients with RLS.[44] Wang et al. demonstrated that oral iron supplementation in patients with serum ferritin levels of 15 to 75 μg/L improved RLS symptoms in a randomized, double-blind placebo-controlled study.[150] Patients with low iron stores should also be evaluated for occult GI blood loss, if clinically indicated. Typical iron supplementation is 65 mg of elemental iron daily (324 mg of ferrous sulfate) with the addition of 100 to 200 mg of ascorbic acid with each dose (to improve absorption). Studies have suggest that giving iron supplements more than once a day increases side effects without increasing iron absorption. Another approach is taking an iron supplement every other day. Taking oral iron when the ferritin is >75 μg/L is not effective at increasing iron stores (hence the recommendation of using 75 μg/L as a threshold). Preparations using iron bound to a polysaccharide may be better tolerated in some patients and often contain 150 mg of elemental iron. Iron absorption is best achieved on an empty stomach, but it may need to be taken with food to avoid severe GI upset. Monitoring of ferritin levels is recommended to ensure adequate replenishment of iron stores and to avoid inducing iron overload. *In children, a ferritin level <50 μg/L is considered an indication for oral iron,*[44,151] *which can decrease symptoms and PLMS. The usual dosage is 3 mg/kg/day.* Guidelines suggest[24] pregnant women with ferritin levels <30 μg/L will likely benefit from iron supplementation and may benefit if the ferritin is <75 μg/L.

In patients in whom oral iron supplementation is not successful, intravenous (IV) iron can be very effective at improving iron stores. Consensus guidelines state: Consider IV administration of iron if transferrin saturation is <45% and (1) serum ferritin concentration is <100 μg/L and a more rapid response is desired than is possible with oral iron; (2) oral iron cannot be adequately absorbed because of disorders of the GI system, bariatric surgery, or chronic inflammatory conditions; (3) oral iron is not tolerated; and (4) restless legs symptoms do not improve despite an adequate (3-month) trial of oral intake of iron.[87] The main indication for IV iron is in patients who cannot tolerate oral iron or who demonstrate iron malabsorption. Patients with significant ongoing GI blood loss or those who require a quick response to iron are also candidates. IV iron is also recommended in patients with moderate daily RLS that is uncontrolled or with refractory RLS in whom a rapid response is needed. The use of 100 rather than 75 μg/L is because absorption of oral iron is not effective when ferritin levels are > 75 μg/L. In contrast IV iron does improve iron stores when ferritin levels are 76 to 100 μg/L. The best evidence is for ferritin < 100 μg/L, although benefit from use of IV iron with ferritin in the 100 to 300 μg/L range may occur in some patients (IV iron could be considered) as long as the iron saturation is less than 45%. **Of note it may take 6 to 8 weeks for symptoms to improve after IV iron administration.** Current recommendations are to limit IV iron to those with ferritin levels <100 μg/L and iron saturation levels less than 45%. Referral to a hematologist for direction of IV iron administration is prudent, as they are familiar with the preparations and side effects. Several newer IV iron preparations are less likely to result in anaphylaxis. During iron infusions, significant side effects other than anaphylaxis may occur. Use of IV iron gluconate, iron sucrose, low-molecular-weight (LMW) iron dextran,[44,152] or ferric carboxymaltose is recommended, as use of high-molecular-weight iron dextran (no longer available) is associated with a high frequency of allergic reactions. Ferric carboxymaltose or LMW iron dextran are generally used. *The best evidence from randomized controlled studies is for ferric carboxymaltose.*[153] When ferritin levels exceed the goal, iron supplementation can be stopped. It is important to note that iron supplementation alone does not always improve RLS. However, many patients will have better results on treatment with standard RLS medications. Transcranial sonography of the substantia nigra has been used to assess brain iron deficiency and changes after iron supplementation[154]; this might be a method to assess CNS iron stores and improve selection of candidates for IV iron. A recent Cochrane database systematic review of iron treatment in RLS[155] concluded, "Iron therapy probably improves restlessness and RLS severity in comparison to placebo. Iron therapy may not increase the risk of side effects in comparison to placebo. We are uncertain whether iron therapy improves quality of life in comparison to placebo." More studies are needed, but without more data, most physicians will follow published treatment guidelines concerning iron supplementation.

RLS Treatment Algorithm

In choosing treatment, it is useful to classify the patient using the approach of Silber and coworkers[87] into the following groups: (1) mild/intermittent RLS symptoms, (2) daily RLS/chronic persistent symptoms, and (3) severe/refractory RLS

Box 31-14 RESTLESS LEGS SYNDROME TREATMENT OVERVIEW

General Considerations:

- Assess systemic iron status and consider appropriate iron replacement if needed, especially in patients with refractory RLS.
- Consider and manage any coexisting sleep disorders.
- Consider the role of medications in causing or exacerbating RLS.

Intermittent RLS:

- Use nonpharmacologic strategies, including mental alerting and a trial of abstinence from caffeine and alcohol.
- Consider intermittent use of carbidopa/levodopa, low-potency opioids, or benzodiazepine receptor agonists.

Chronic Persistent RLS:

- Use alpha-2-delta calcium channel ligands unless contraindications exist. Possible benefits with comorbid pain or insomnia.
- Use a dopamine agonist (pramipexole, ropinirole, rotigotine patch) if alpha-2-delta calcium channel ligands are contraindicated or ineffective.
- Use of dopamine agonist would be preferred with history of severe depression, obesity, gait instability, or very severe RLS.
- If dopamine agonists are used, administer the lowest dose possible, do not exceed recommended doses for RLS, consider combination treatment, monitor for augmentation and impulse control disorders, and modify treatment accordingly.

Refractory RLS:

- Consider combination therapy with alpha-2-delta calcium channel ligands, opioids, dopamine agonists, or benzodiazepines.
- Consider opioid monotherapy (low to medium dose opioid therapy with appropriate precautions).

RLS, restless legs syndrome.
Adapted from Silber MH, Buchfuhrer MJ, Earley CJ, Koo BB, Manconi M, Winkelman JW; Scientific and Medical Advisory Board of the Restless Legs Syndrome Foundation. The management of restless legs syndrome: an updated algorithm. *Mayo Clin Proc.* 2021;96(7):1921-1937. PMID: 34218864.

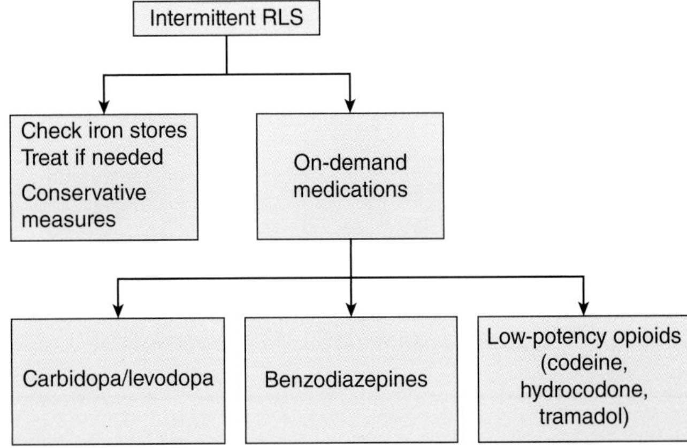

Figure 31-12 An algorithm for the treatment of intermittent/mild restless legs syndrome (RLS). (Adapted from Silber MH, Buchfuhrer MJ, Earley CJ, Koo BB, Manconi M, Winkelman JW; Scientific and Medical Advisory Board of the Restless Legs Syndrome Foundation. The management of restless legs syndrome: an updated algorithm. *Mayo Clin Proc.* 2021;96(7):1921-1937. PMID: 34218864.)

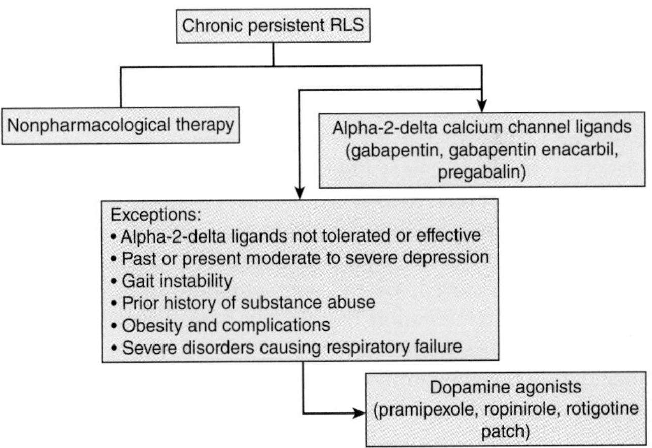

Figure 31-13. An algorithm for treatment of daily/persistent restless legs syndrome (RLS). (Adapted from Silber MH, Buchfuhrer MJ, Earley CJ, Koo BB, Manconi M, Winkelman JW; Scientific and Medical Advisory Board of the Restless Legs Syndrome Foundation. The management of restless legs syndrome: an updated algorithm. *Mayo Clin Proc.* 2021;96(7):1921-1937. PMID: 34218864.)

symptoms. A general overview is provided in Box 31-14. Algorithms for treatment of intermittent RLS, chronic persistent RLS, and refractory RLS are shown in Figures 31-12, 31-13, and 31-14, respectively. Treatment of RLS in children is discussed in a separate section.

The mild/intermittent group may be treated with conservative measures such as avoiding precipitating medications (sedating antihistamines) and substances (alcohol, caffeine), warm baths, and iron supplementation if they have low irons stores (Figure 31-12). If an RLS medication is used, it should be rapid acting, because the patient can often not predict that symptoms will occur. CD/LD in the short-acting form is active within half an hour and, therefore, is a good choice for treatment of intermittent RLS (occurrence of RLS episodes not predictable). A DA is effective, although the time to onset is delayed for 1 to 3 hours. Ropinirole has a more rapid effect than pramipexole. Other choices are low-potency opiates such as propoxyphene or codeine. Sedative-hypnotics may also be effective in patients with mild/intermittent RLS but should be used with caution.

Daily RLS of moderate severity requires a different approach. Guidelines recommend using an alpha-2-delta ligand as the initial treatment (Figure 31-13). As gabapentin often requires a slow upward titration, reaching an effective dose may take some time. Pregabalin and gabapentin enacarbil have more reliable absorption, and one of these would be preferred if a quick response is needed. This class of medications would **not** be the initial choice in patients with significant depression, obesity, or impaired gait. Alpha-2-delta ligands can worsen these issues. In this situation, DAs are preferred. If DAs are used, the goal is to use a low dosage and stay within treatment guidelines. Some patients benefit from alpha-2-delta ligands but do not tolerate a fully effective dosage. The addition of a low-potency opioid or low dosage of a DA is an option. If the DA treatment is started but a dose increase is needed after initial stabilization, the addition of another class of medication is preferable to repeated increases in the DA dose. Rotigotine may have an advantage in patients with daytime symptoms and may have less risk of

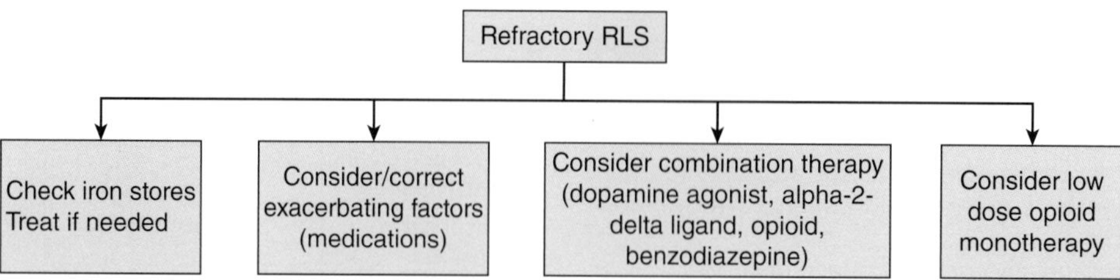

Figure 31-14 An algorithm for treatment of severe/refractory restless legs syndrome (RLS). (Adapted from Silber MH, Buchfuhrer MJ, Earley CJ, Koo BB, Manconi M, Winkelman JW; Scientific and Medical Advisory Board of the Restless Legs Syndrome Foundation. the management of restless legs syndrome: an updated algorithm. *Mayo Clin Proc.* 2021;96(7):1921-1937. PMID: 34218864.)

augmentation than ropinirole or pramipexole. There is no generic rotigotine, and skin reactions to the patch are problematic. If daytime symptoms are a problem, use of rotigotine should be considered. If comorbid pain, anxiety, or insomnia is present, use of an alpha-2-delta ligand has advantages over DAs. If one medication in a class is not effective or tolerated, one could try an alternative medication in the same class. For example, if a patient has severe nausea on pramipexole, they might tolerate ropinirole. If the clinical response to a DA is inadequate or side effects prevent the use of the DA, a low- to moderate-potency opiate, gabapentin, or a sedative-hypnotic should be tried. If side effects are noted at higher dosages of a DA, one might also combine a lower dosage of DA with a medication from another class (e.g., lower dosage of DA with gabapentin).

Refractory/severe RLS is defined as: (1) inadequate initial response despite adequate dose (and timing of dose), (2) response has become inadequate over time, (3) intolerable side effects have occurred, or (4) augmentation is present. The approach to augmentation has already been discussed. Treatment approaches to refractory/severe RLS (Figure 31-14) include: (1) checking iron stores and treating if needed, (2) correcting exacerbating factors, (3) combination treatment, and (4) consider low-dose opioid monotherapy. For example, if the patient is on a DA, add an alpha-2-delta ligand or opioid. In this case, if augmentation is a concern, the dopamine dosage should be reduced or the medication weaned and stopped. If the patient is on an alpha-2-delta ligand, adding a low-dose DA (without a subsequent increase) or low-potency opioid is an option. In cases of severe augmentation or intractable RLS, low-dose, high-potency opioid monotherapy can be effective. For example, a patient on a DA with severe augmentation may not tolerate gabapentin or pregabalin. Use of methadone might be effective at lower doses than typically used for pain. Because of the difficulty in treating severe augmentation, it is best to avoid very high doses of DAs, if possible. If combination treatment is used in a patient with mild augmentation, a reduction in the DA dosage should be considered. If combination treatment for moderate to severe augmentation is used, withdrawal (weaning) of the DA is recommended after the other agent (usually an opioid) has been titrated to an effective dose. In general, at the start of treatment, if one medication in a class does not work or is not tolerated, trial of another medication in the same class should be considered. For example, if pramipexole is not effective or not tolerated, one could try ropinirole. However, switching between pramipexole and ropinirole *for augmentation* is generally not recommended. One could try a switch to rotigotine if augmentation is mild to moderate. Weaning and discontinuing DAs in response to moderate to severe augmentation is likely the best approach. If one opioid is not effective or tolerated, another medication can be tried. For example, if oxycodone is not tolerated or effective, methadone could be tried. In using combination treatment, one must be mindful of the potential for worsening side effects (e.g., respiratory depression with the combination of an alpha-2-delta ligand and opioid in a patient at risk for hypoventilation).

Treatment of RLS in Children

Nonpharmacologic approaches such as elimination of caffeine and avoiding sleep deprivation may help some patients. The mainstay of RLS treatment in children is iron replacement. *Iron supplementation is recommended if serum ferritin is <50 μg/L.*[44,87] Iron stores are lower in adolescents than in adults because of an increase in red cell mass during growth periods and, in women, the onset of menstruation. Thus, serum ferritin concentration is usually lower in children than in adults. Although optimal levels are uncertain, iron supplementation should be considered if the serum ferritin concentration is <50 μg/L.[44,87] Oral ferrous sulfate 3 to 5 mg/kg in either tablet or liquid form should be administered once daily before breakfast. As in adults, constipation or abdominal discomfort are frequent side effects. Rechecking serum ferritin after 3 months is suggested. There are no large, controlled trials of medications to treat RLS in children. No medication is approved for treatment of PLMD or RLS in children. However, it appears that dopaminergic therapy is an effective treatment for PLMD or RLS in children.[98,156-159] A recent RLS treatment algorithm[87] made the following recommendations based on anecdotal experience and case series. Alpha-2-delta ligands were recommended as first-line agents in adults. However, many clinicians have limited experience using them in children. Gabapentin (5–15 mg/kg) and pregabalin (2–3 mg/kg) are first-line agents if iron is not needed or is ineffective. Second-line agents include clonazepam (0.1–1 mg), with sedation and paradoxical hyperactivity as possible adverse effects. DAs used in children include pramipexole (0.0625–0.25 mg), ropinirole (0.25–0.5 mg), and the rotigotine patch (1–3 mg), but they should preferably be avoided in adolescents because of the risk of precipitating schizophrenia in predisposed patients.[87] If long-term therapy is contemplated, there is a significant risk for augmentation, and monitoring for impulse control disorders is important. Clonidine, an alpha-2-adrenergic agonist, can be considered in children (0.05–0.4 mg) who also have an anxiety disorder or ADHD. Its use may be limited by adverse effects including sedation, irritability, depression, and orthostatic hypotension. Treatment with IV iron has also been reported in pediatric patients (ferric carboxymaltose).[160]

RLS and Renal Failure

As previously noted, RLS is common in patients with renal insufficiency, especially in those on hemodialysis. Treatment with hemodialysis requires the patient remain at rest for long periods. RLS symptoms can be severe and sometimes require discontinuation of a dialysis session. Management of iron stores is essential. Ropinirole and rotigotine have hepatic metabolism and can be used with caution. Gabapentin and pregabalin are effective, but the dose must be reduced as previously discussed. Use of gabapentin 200 to 300 mg after dialysis is one approach. Careful monitoring is needed to minimize falls and mental confusion.[161] One study found that supplementation with vitamins E and C improved symptoms.[162] As noted, RLS often improves or resolves with kidney transplantation.

RLS and Pregnancy and Lactation

RLS symptoms are common in pregnancy. About 20% of pregnant women in the United States and Europe experience RLS in pregnancy, but the prevalence is **lower in Asia** (but higher than in non-pregnant women). Most RLS in pregnancy is new onset, but up to one-third of women with RLS during pregnancy report a previous history of RLS. If RLS is present before pregnancy, it may worsen during pregnancy. The prevalence and severity of RLS/WED has been found to progressively increase over the course of pregnancy in most studies, with a *peak around the 7th to 8th month* and stability or a slight decrease in the last month of pregnancy. There is a clear and large drop in RLS/WED symptoms around delivery, with complete resolution of symptoms for approximately 70% of affected women and a significant decrease in severity for the remainder.[24,163] For women with new-onset RLS/WED during pregnancy, the resolution rate appears to exceed 90%.[164] However, for women who experience the transient form of RLS/WED during pregnancy, there is a significant fourfold increased rate of subsequently developing RLS/WED independent of pregnancy.[2,163] *Risk factors for RLS during pregnancy include prior RLS, RLS in prior pregnancy, low hemoglobin, and a family history of RLS.*

Consensus guideline for the diagnosis and treatment of RLS in pregnancy were published in 2015,[24] and additional recommendations were made in a treatment guidelines update.[87] Most physicians first try nonpharmacologic treatment (stretching, warm baths) and/or iron supplementation, if indicated. Using the older classification of pregnancy risk, DAs and gabapentin were category C (animal reproduction studies have shown an adverse effect on the fetus, and there are no adequate and well-controlled studies in humans), and clonazepam was category D (there is positive evidence of human fetal risk based on adverse reaction data from investigational or marketing experience or studies in humans). However, later studies did not confirm the high risk with clonazepam, and anecdotal experience suggests it is reasonably safe in the second and third trimesters. Oxycodone was category B (animal reproduction studies have failed to demonstrate a risk to the fetus, and there are no adequate and well-controlled studies in pregnant women). As noted, the A-X classification is no longer used by the FDA but is presented here for perspective.

For the first trimester, iron and nonpharmacologic treatments are recommended. Consensus guidelines[24,87,163] recommend the following approach for drug treatment in the second and third trimesters, if needed: Clonazepam 0.25 mg to 0.5 mg can be considered in the second and third trimesters. Use is not recommended with anticonvulsants or antihistamines during pregnancy. Low-dose CD/LD can be considered. L dopa should not be used with benserazide (used with LD instead of CD in Canada and much of Europe) because this medication increased the risk of congenital malformations. Oxycodone 5 to 10 mg at bedtime can be considered in the second and third trimesters. The infant should be monitored for signs of opioid withdrawal after birth.

During lactation, nonpharmacologic approaches can be tried. Clonazepam 0.25 to 0.5 mg and gabapentin 50 to 100 mg can be considered.[24] Of interest, LD and DAs inhibit prolactin secretion and should not be used during lactation. If RLS is very severe and an opioid must be used, tramadol 50 to 100 mg is recommended.

If oral iron supplementation is not adequate, IV iron has been used prior to or during pregnancy.[164-166] Consensus guidelines[24] recommend, “IV iron may be considered for the treatment of refractory RLS/WED during the second or third trimester of pregnancy and postpartum period *if there is failure of oral iron and serum* ***ferritin is*** <30 ***μg/L***.” Because of the demands of pregnancy, it may be difficult to attain mid-normal iron stores with oral iron.

Administration of IV Iron During Pregnancy

IV iron should be considered only after the first trimester to allow sufficient time for a response to oral iron and other nonpharmacologic interventions and to avoid administration during embryogenesis. Open-label studies using IV sucrose[164,165] and IV ferric carboxymaltose[167] have been published. Overall, IV iron has been shown to be safe during pregnancy, but because of possible anaphylaxis, it should be administered at facilities with staff who are familiar with appropriate infusion rates and management of adverse reactions. Iron transports very poorly to breast milk, and limited data indicate that breast milk iron levels are not increased after IV iron infusion.

Other RLS Treatment Options and the Restless Sleep Disorder (RSD)

While magnesium supplementation has been recommended for RLS, to date there is no convincing evidence of benefit.[168] Vitamin C and E preparations were useful for RLS in patients undergoing hemodialysis.[162] Botulinum toxin injections have been tried with conflicting results.[169,170] Cannabis and cannabinoids have also been tried. No controlled clinical trials have evaluated the use of cannabis for RLS. A case series suggests the possibility of some benefit,[171] but the formulation, dosage, and mode of administration that may be beneficial are unclear. Anecdotal experience suggests that ingested cannabis (brownies, cookies, or other edibles) is ineffective, whereas inhaled cannabis maybe be effective in some patients. A review[172] emphasized the potentially harmful interactions between cannabis and many medications. Although legalized for medical use in a few states, its use is still illegal under federal law.

The restless sleep disorder (RSD) has been proposed as a new sleep disorder in children ag 6–18 years and is charaterized by restless sleep and large body movements during sleep. Video-PSG documents ≥ 5 body movements per hour of sleep. An urge to move is not present. The movements may respond to iron supplementation.[173]

SUMMARY OF KEY POINTS

1. A diagnosis of RLS is based on clinical history, not PSG. Use "URGES" to make the diagnosis of RLS (**U**rge to move**, R**est induced, **G**ets better with activity, worse during the **E**vening and night, and not **S**olely due to another entity). Patients with leg cramps, unconscious foot tapping, positional discomfort, and pain cause by identifiable conditions (e.g., arthritis, leg edema) should not be diagnosed as RLS.
2. Abnormal RLS sensations may be **absent** (only an urge to move legs can be present). The abnormal sensations may be painful and involve the arms. In severe RLS, *worsening of symptoms in the evening or improvement with movement* may not be present but should have been present at the start of RLS.
3. PSG is needed in a patient with RLS only if another sleep disorder such as OSA or a parasomnia is suspected (both can cause leg during sleep). If RLS is not present, PSG findings are needed to diagnose PLMD (PLMSI >5/hour in children and >15/hour in adults) and confirm the absence of other causes of sleep complaints. **A diagnosis of RLS excludes a diagnosis of PLMD**.
4. RLS is more common in women and worsened by first-generation antihistamines and many antidepressants (especially mirtazapine). Bupropion is an antidepressant that does not worsen RLS. RLS is less common in Asian compared to Caucasian individuals. A family history of RLS is an important risk factor for developing early onset RLS.
5. PLMS is a common finding in sleep studies, and the average PLMSI increases with age. No definite PLMSI value separates asymptomatic from symptomatic patients.
6. Daytime sleepiness is an uncommon complaint in patients with RLS alone compared to complaints about sleep or uncomfortable sensations in the legs (Figure 31-3). The **presence** of prominent daytime sleepiness should prompt consideration of other disorders such as OSA or narcolepsy.
7. An elevated PLMSI on a sleep study should prompt evaluation for RLS (by history).
8. PLMS (PLMSI >5/hour) is present in 80% to 90% of patients with RLS. There is considerable night-to-night variability in PLMSI.
9. An elevated PLMSI in children (>5/hour) should prompt consideration of a diagnosis of PLMD. Children may not report RLS symptoms.
10. Brain iron deficiency impairs adenosine regulation of glutamate and dopamine signaling in brain areas important for control of movement. A hyperdopaminergic and hyperglutamatergic state causes RLS. DAs and alpha-2-delta ligands reduce glutamate signaling, and this likely explains their efficacy for RLS treatment.
11. An early-morning fasting blood sample to test for ferritin, TIBC, and iron saturation is recommended for patients with RLS and should be repeated at intervals if a patient begins iron supplementation. Repeat testing determines if oral iron supplementation has been effective and should be continued and helps avoid excessive iron supplementation (ferritin >300 μg/L).
12. Treatment options for RLS include nonpharmacologic interventions (avoiding medications that worsen RLS), normalization of iron stores, CD/LD for mild intermittent RLS, alpha-2-delta ligands (gabapentin, pregabalin, gabapentin enacarbil), DAs (pramipexole, ropinirole, rotigotine patch), opioids, and hypnotics (in selected cases).
13. The alpha-2-delta ligands (gabapentin, gabapentin enacarbil, pregabalin) are effective for daily RLS/PLMD. **They are now considered first-line agents for treatment of moderate to severe/daily RLS** and are especially useful if there is comorbid insomnia, anxiety, or pain. If there is known moderate to severe depression, obesity, gait issues, a significant disorder predisposing a patient to hypoventilation, or a history of drug/substance abuse, a DA is generally preferred.
14. The DAs ropinirole, pramipexole, and rotigotine patch are FDA approved for treatment of RLS in adults and are effective in the short term, but loss of efficacy over time or development of augmentation are major issues.
15. Impulse control is an important DA side effect that a patient may not recognize as a serious complication of DA treatment. Questions to assess the presence of this issue should be asked at each clinical visit.
16. Pramipexole and ropinirole must be taken about 2 hours before symptoms to be most effective and avoid excessive dose increases. The rotigotine transdermal patch is useful for patients with daytime RLS symptoms and/or augmentation associated with other DAs.
17. Gabapentin enacarbil (no generic available) and pregabalin (generic available) have more reliable absorption than gabapentin. For gabapentin, a slow upward titration of the dose starting at 300 mg (100–200 mg in elderly patients) may improve tolerance. The effective dose range is 900 to 1200 mg in many patients. Pregabalin is usually started at 75 mg about 1 to 2 hours before bedtime or symptoms. In studies, an average dose of about 300 mg was needed. Slow upward titration using the lowest effective dose is recommended. Pregabalin is a schedule V medication.
18. Opioids are an effective treatment for RLS. They may be especially useful in patients who develop severe augmentation or who do not tolerate DAs. If given only at bedtime, they usually do not result in dependence (unless there is a history or prior medication dependence/abuse). There are usually no progressive increases in dosage once an effective dosage is reached. For milder cases, codeine or tramadol may be effective. For moderate RLS, hydrocodone (combined with acetaminophen in the United States) or oxycodone are often used. For severe RLS, low dosages of oxycodone or methadone have been used with success. Methadone is particularly effective and has a fairly long duration of action but can increase the QT interval.
19. Benzodiazepine hypnotics may be useful in milder RLS associated with insomnia or can be combined with DAs. Over-sedation when combined with an alpha-2-delta ligand or respiratory depression when combined with an opioid are important considerations. The combination of a hypnotic and an opioid should be avoided.
20. Combination treatment avoids the need for high dosages of each agent and is a good approach to avoid augmentation (lower DA dosages) or treatment of augmentation while DAs are being weaned. Alpha-2-delta ligands or opioids can be used with DAs during weaning of a DA (cross-titration). In general DAs should be weaned rather abruptly stopped to avoid severe withdrawal symptoms. Some clinicians advocate complete weaning of the DA before starting another medication. This approach is poorly tolerated by most patients.
21. Augmentation describes a complication of dopamine treatment that can be very severe and is characterized by one or more of the following: (1) earlier symptom onset in the afternoon/evening, (2) greater severity of symptoms at

the same dosage or escalating dosage or greater symptoms before medication administration than before treatment began, (3) reduced latency to onset of symptoms with rest, and (4) spread of symptoms to involve new body parts (arms as well as legs).

22. Low serum ferritin is a risk factor for development of augmentation.

23. Patients with RLS with a ferritin level ≤75 μg/L and an iron saturation is less than 45% may improve with oral iron supplementation. The usual dosage is 65 mg of elemental iron (ferrous sulfate 325 mg) daily combined with 100 mg of ascorbic acid to improve absorption. Once daily (or every other day) is an adequate schedule. More frequent administration increases side effects and is not more effective. Patients with augmentation may improve with iron supplementation. If oral iron supplementation is not effective and the ferritin is <100 μg/L and iron saturation is <45%, IV iron is a reasonable option. Safer IV iron preparations are available, but a physician and clinic experienced in administration of IV iron are recommended. For children, oral iron is recommended for a ferritin level <50 μg/L. During pregnancy, ferritin <30 μg/L is an indication for oral iron, although some use ≤75 μg/L if RLS symptoms are significant.

24. RLS is very frequent in pregnancy (about 20% and worse in the third trimester) but usually resolves after delivery *if RLS was not present before pregnancy*. Treatment is usually iron supplementation and nonpharmacologic treatments (especially in the first trimester). RLS prior to pregnancy or RLS in past pregnancies are risk factors for developing RLS in future pregnancies. Patients with new onset RLS during pregnancy are at increased risk for developing RLS later in life.

25. Moderate to severe augmentation is treated by "cross-titration." The DA is weaned at the same time the new medication (alpha-2-delta ligand, an opioid, or a combination of both) is started, and the dosage of the new medication is increased as needed. In patients with very severe augmentation, weaning of the DA may not be tolerated until there is reasonable control of the RLS with the new medication.

26. Brain iron deficiency results in hypoadenosinergic, hyperdopaminergic, and hyperglutaminergic states, and is thought to be the etiology of RLS. Dopamine agonists and alpha-2-sodium channel ligands act on glutaminergic neurons reducing their activity. This is thought to be the reason these medications are effective in RLS.

CLINICAL REVIEW QUESTIONS

1. You are starting treatment for moderate to severe daily RLS. Which of the following patients is most suitable for treatment with an alpha-2-delta agonist?
A. 30-year-old man with a BMI of 35 kg/m^2
B. 40-year-old woman with painful RLS symptoms
C. 30-year-old man with a history of moderate to severe depression
D. 70-year-old woman with a history of falls

2. A 30-year-old pregnant woman in her second trimester is experiencing bothersome RLS symptoms. She has no history of the RLS prior to becoming pregnant. Which of the following statements is true?
A. She is not at risk for developing RLS in the future.
B. Her RLS will get better in the third trimester.
C. Her RLS will likely continue after delivery.
D. Her iron stores should be checked.

3. Which of the following is true about treatment of RLS with methadone?
A. High dosages >20 mg per day will be needed.
B. Methadone can increase the QT interval.
C. Dosage does not have to be reduced in renal failure.
D. Augmentation is a risk.
E. Progressive increases in dosage are likely needed.

4. Which of the following is not a factor in the development of RLS?
A. Family history
B. Brain iron deficiency
C. Upregulation of adenosine A1 receptors
D. Hyperglutamatergic cortical striatal signaling

5. A 40-year-old woman currently on ropinirole for RLS, which is under good control, complains of difficulty in her relationship with her husband (arguments about excessive spending). What do you recommend?
A. Referral for marriage counseling
B. Starting bupropion for depression
C. Stop ropinirole and start gabapentin
D. Start zolpidem

6. Which of the following patients with RLS would benefit from iron supplementation (more than one answer may be correct)?
A. Ferritin 125 μg/L, iron saturation 15%
B. Ferritin 100 μg/L, iron saturation 25%
C. Ferritin 80 μg/L, iron saturation 30%
D. Ferritin 200 μg/L, iron saturation 15%

7. A 40-year-old woman has nightly restless legs symptoms that delay her sleep onset. She was started on pramipexole 0.125 mg, taken at bedtime, and this was increased to 0.25 mg without much benefit. What do you recommend?
A. Change to ropinirole.
B. Increase pramipexole dosage to 0.5 mg.
C. Add tramadol 50 mg.
D. Administer current dose of pramipexole earlier.

8. A 30-year-old woman has intermittent RLS that occurs only on long car trips. Although these episodes occur infrequently, they are quite distressing. She has to stop and walk around every 100 miles, or the symptoms become intolerable. A recent ferritin level was 100 μg/L and iron saturation 25%. What do you recommend?
A. Pramipexole 0.125 mg on long car trips when symptoms begin
B. CD/LD 25/100 mg before long car trips (repeat dose if needed)
C. Iron supplementation
D. Gabapentin 300 mg before long car trips

9. A 40-year-old man has developed severe RLS symptoms nearly every night. He was started on CD/LD 25/100 mg at bedtime with good initial response. When RLS symptoms returned, the dosage was progressively increased to four (25/100 mg) tablets. After several months of taking this dosage, RLS symptoms were noted in both the arms and the legs, and the symptoms started at 6:00 PM rather than 10:00 PM nightly. What do you recommend?
A. Increase CD/LD dosage.
B. Take an earlier dose of CD/LD.
C. Add oxycodone 5 mg at 5:00 PM with another dose 1 hour before bedtime if needed and wean the CD/LD.
D. Start gabapentin 300 mg at 5:00 PM with another dose 1 hour before bedtime and wean/stop CD/LD.

10. A 25-year-old woman with daily RLS symptoms was started on pramipexole 0.125 mg, and this was increased to 0.75 mg over several weeks. The patient feels that her RLS symptoms have improved but continue at a significant level. Her ferritin level is 100 μg/L. What do you recommend?
    A. Increase pramipexole to 1.0 mg.
    B. Switch to ropinirole 0.75 mg.
    C. Add oxycodone 5 to 10 mg.
    D. Add gabapentin 300 mg.
11. A patient with diabetic neuropathy reports RLS symptoms that are quite painful and distressing. There is a history of alcohol and valium dependence in the past. What do you recommend for initial treatment?
    A. Gabapentin 300 mg in the evening (1 hour before symptoms)
    B. Ropinirole 0.25 mg in the evening (2 hours before symptoms)
    C. Oxycodone 10 mg in the evening (1 hour before symptoms)
    D. Clonazepam 0.25 mg at bedtime (1/2 to 1 hour before bedtime)
12. A 50-year-old woman is currently taking pramipexole 0.75 mg at 9:00 PM and zolpidem 10 mg at 10:30 PM (bedtime 11:00 PM) for severe symptoms of RLS. The symptoms were under fair control but are now present much earlier than when she started treatment. Initially, her symptoms began around 10:30 PM but now are noted as early as 9 PM. Her normal bedtime is midnight. What do you recommend?
    A. Change pramipexole dosing to 0.25 mg at 7:00 PM and 0.5 mg at 9:00 PM.
    B. Change from pramipexole to ropinirole.
    C. Add gabapentin 300 mg at 7:00 pm.
    D. Change pramipexole dosing to 0.5 mg at 7:00 PM and 0.5 mg 9:00 PM.
13. A 50-year-old man with a history of snoring undergoes a split-night sleep study. The diagnostic portion shows an apnea-hypopnea index (AHI) of 50 events/hour with a PLMSI of 5/hour. The CPAP titration portion of the study shows that on CPAP of 10 cm H_2O, the AHI is 5 events/hour. The PLMSI on treatment is 50/hour during the titration portion of the study. The patient does **not** report symptoms of RLS. The patient's wife does report that he kicks during sleep. What treatment do you recommend?
    A. CPAP of 10 cm H_2O and pramipexole
    B. CPAP of 10 cm H_2O
    C. CPAP of 10 cm H_2O and gabapentin
    D. CPAP of 10 cm H_2O and iron supplementation
14. Which of the following disorders has been associated with PLMS?
    A. Narcolepsy
    B. REM Sleep Behavior Disorder
    C. OSA
    D. All of the above
15. A 12-year-old boy has difficulty staying awake. He does NOT report an urge to move the legs or unusual sensations. His parents have noted that the patient is a restless sleeper, moves around in bed a lot, and sometimes snores. The patient is "fidgety" in school and has problems concentrating. A PSG is ordered to rule out OSA. The sleep study shows mild snoring, no apneas and hypopneas, and no elevation in end-tidal partial pressure of CO_2. The PLMSI is 15 events/hour. What is your diagnosis?
    A. RLS
    B. Snoring
    C. PLMD
    D. ADHD

ANSWERS

1. B. Alpha-2-delta agonists are helpful in painful RLS. Obesity, depression, and gait instability favor choice of a DA.
2. D. Her iron stores should be checked. RLS during pregnancy is a risk factor for future RLS (answer A is incorrect). Symptoms worsen in the third trimester (answer B is incorrect). RLS developing during pregnancy will usually resolve at or soon after delivery if RLS was not present prepregnancy (answer C is incorrect). Iron stores should be checked, but the threshold for iron supplementation is lower than in non-pregnant women or in men.
3. B. Methadone can increase the QT interval. Dosages lower than 20 mg are often effective; dosage escalation is usually not needed once an effective dose is reached. Augmentation does not occur with opioids (tramadol is an exception). The dosage of methadone should be reduced in patients with significant renal failure.
4. C. Adenosine **A1 receptors are downregulated (***A2 receptors upregulated***).**
5. C. Stop ropinirole and start treatment with a different class of medications. An impulse control disorder has developed on the DA.
6. A and D. If the ferritin is ≤75 μg/L or the iron saturation is less than 20% iron, supplementation is needed (A and D). The ferritin can be increased as a result of inflammation (D). If the iron saturation is low, iron stores are low. Most clinicians recommended checking the iron saturation in the fasting state.
7. D. Ropinirole and pramipexole should be given about 2 hours before bedtime (or evening symptom onset). These medications have a slow onset of action. A higher dosage of pramipexole could be needed, but the first intervention is to have the patient take the medication earlier. Ropinirole may have a more rapid onset than pramipexole.
8. B. CD/LD is a useful medication for intermittent RLS owing to the rapid onset of action. However, the duration of action is short, and augmentation frequently occurs with daily use. The medication could be used on a long car trip, but repeated dosing may be needed. DAs (pramipexole or ropinirole) have a longer duration of action **but must be taken 2 hours before symptoms**. An effective option would be taking one of these medication 2 hours before starting on a long car trip. Iron supplementation is recommended for patients with RLS with a ferritin level ≤75 μg/L, but restoration of iron stores takes time and may not completely resolve symptoms. Gabapentin might be effective but can result in sedation. In some patients, this might be an option if they are not driving and an effective dose is known.
9. D. This patient has significant augmentation on CD/LD. The patient should be started on gabapentin and CD/LD weaned and stopped. A higher dosage of gabapentin could be needed. Using oxycodone instead would work but

would not be the first choice for long-term treatment. One could start with oxycodone 5 mg, but a higher dose will usually be needed with severe augmentation. Low iron stores should also be ruled out.

10. D. The patient is on a fairly high dosage of pramipexole for RLS treatment. The maximum dosage recommended by drug labeling is 0.5 mg, although many physicians would consider 0.75 mg acceptable. She is tolerating the medication, but significant symptoms persist. It is possible that an increase to 1 mg pramipexole will be effective but could increase the risk of augmentation. A change to a different DA is another option. The equivalent dose of ropinirole is around four times that of pramipexole, so 0.75 mg would be too low. Ropinirole at a dosage of 0.5 mg is **not** equivalent to pramipexole 0.75 mg. To avoid the risk of augmentation, most clinicians avoid high dosages of DAs. The addition of oxycodone 5 to 10 mg might be an effective option, but alpha-2-delta ligands should be tried first. If the combination of gabapentin and pramipexole is effective, one could try to wean the pramipexole (or reduce the dosage) and increase the dosage of gabapentin (if tolerated). If gabapentin is not effective, pregabalin could be tried.

11. A versus B. The patient has a history of drug dependence; therefore, benzodiazepines and narcotics should be avoided. Some clinicians might also avoid alpha-2-ligands in this situation. Pregabalin is a schedule V medication (in some states, gabapentin is a schedule V medication). However, schedule II medications (oxycodone) or schedule IV medications (benzodiazepines) have a higher risk of abuse. DAs could be used in this situation. On the other hand, augmentation and impulse control disorder are concerns. Ropinirole might not improve the painful aspects of RLS. Gabapentin is recommended when RLS symptoms are painful, and an alpha-2-delta ligand is recommended for initial treatment of RLS. Of note, gabapentin at a dosage of 300 mg may not be effective. A dosage of 900 to 1500 mg is often needed. Slow upward titration may reduce side effects. A combination of lower dosages of a DA and gabapentin would be another option.

12. A. The earlier onset of symptoms is a mild form of augmentation. Because pramipexole was fairly effective and well tolerated, the first intervention should be use of a split dose, with a portion of the medication given earlier in the evening. The patient is already on the maximal dosage of pramipexole for RLS (prescribing information says 0.5 mg), so the first intervention would be splitting the current dose (D is not the best choice). The patient is already on a high dosage of pramipexole; therefore, a further increase in dosage in the setting of augmentation is probably not indicated. C would be a reasonable intervention, but before adding another medication, a split dose of the current medication without a dose increase could be tried. If augmentation continues to worsen, gabapentin could be added with a reduction in pramipexole (or weaning this medication). While it is true that a patient may respond to (or tolerate) ropinirole better than pramipexole, or vice versa, this would not be the best option in this situation; however, it could be tried during initiation of therapy when one of the medications does not appear to be effective or well tolerated. Use of a rotigotine patch might be another consideration.

13. B. The patient has **no** RLS symptoms. PLMS is frequently associated with OSA, may worsen during a CPAP titration, and usually does not require treatment. Treatment with CPAP of 10 cm H_2O should be started. If frequent LMs persist and are significantly impairing sleep quality, treatment could then be considered. Iron supplementation should not be started without demonstration of low iron stores.

14. D. PLMS have been associated with narcolepsy, RBD, and OSA.

15. C. PLMD. In pediatric patients, PLMD sometimes precedes symptoms of RLS. A PLMSI of 15/hour might be of borderline significance in an adult but for a child is significantly elevated. There has been an association between ADHD and RLS/PLMD, but PSG findings and symptoms suggest PLMD is the issue. The patient's sleep will likely improve with effective treatment of PLMD. Normalization of iron stores

SUGGESTED READING

Allen RP, Picchietti DL, Auerbach M, et al. International Restless Legs Syndrome Study Group (IRLSSG). Evidence-based and consensus clinical practice guidelines for the iron treatment of restless legs syndrome/Willis-Ekbom disease in adults and children: an IRLSSG task force report. *Sleep Med.* 2018;41:27-44.

Allen RP, Picchietti DL, Garcia-Borreguero D, et al. International Restless Legs Syndrome Study Group. Restless legs syndrome/Willis-Ekbom disease diagnostic criteria: updated International Restless Legs Syndrome Study Group (IRLSSG) consensus criteria—history, rationale, description, and significance. *Sleep Med.* 2014;15(8):860-873.

Garcia-Borreguero D, Silber MH, Winkelman JW, et al. Guidelines for the first-line treatment of restless legs syndrome/Willis-Ekbom disease, prevention and treatment of dopaminergic augmentation: a combined task force of the IRLSSG, EURLSSG, and the RLS-foundation. *Sleep Med.* 2016;21:1-11.

Picchietti DL, Hensley JG, Bainbridge JL, et al. International Restless Legs Syndrome Study Group (IRLSSG). Consensus clinical practice guidelines for the diagnosis and treatment of restless legs syndrome/Willis-Ekbom disease during pregnancy and lactation. *Sleep Med Rev.* 2015; 22:64-77.

Silber MH, Becker PM, Buchfuhrer MJ, et al.; Scientific and Medical Advisory Board, Restless Legs Syndrome Foundation. The appropriate use of opioids in the treatment of refractory restless legs syndrome. *Mayo Clin Proc.* 2018;93(1):59-67.

Silber MH, Buchfuhrer MJ, Earley CJ, et al. The management of restless legs syndrome: an updated algorithm. *Mayo Clin Proc.* 2021;96(7):1921-1937.

REFERENCES

1. Montplaisir J, Boucher S, Poirier G, Lavigne G, Lapierre O, Lespérance P. Clinical, polysomnographic, and genetic characteristics of restless legs syndrome: a study of 133 patients diagnosed with new standard criteria. *Mov Disord.* 1997;12(1):61-65.
2. Allen RP, Picchietti DL, Garcia-Borreguero D, et al. International Restless Legs Syndrome Study Group. Restless legs syndrome/Willis-Ekbom disease diagnostic criteria: updated International Restless Legs Syndrome Study Group (IRLSSG) consensus criteria—history, rationale, description, and significance. *Sleep Med.* 2014;15(8):860-873.
3. Picchietti DL, Bruni O, de Weerd A, et al.; International Restless Legs Syndrome Study Group (IRLSSG). Pediatric restless legs syndrome diagnostic criteria: an update by the International Restless Legs Syndrome Study Group. *Sleep Med.* 2013;14(12):1253-1259.
4. Ferri R, Fulda S, Allen RP, et al. International and European Restless Legs Syndrome Study Groups (IRLSSG and EURLSSG). World Association of Sleep Medicine (WASM) 2016 standards for recording and scoring leg movements in polysomnograms developed by a joint task force from the International and the European Restless Legs Syndrome Study Groups (IRLSSG and EURLSSG). *Sleep Med.* 2016;26:86-95.

5. Pennestri M, Whittom S, Adam B, et al. PLMS and PLMW in healthy subjects as a function of age: prevalence and interval distribution. *Sleep*. 2006;29:1183-1187.
6. Ohayon MM, Roth T. Prevalence of restless legs syndrome and periodic limb movement disorder in the general population. *J Psychosom Res*. 2002;53(1):547-554.
7. Claman DM, Redline S, Blackwell T, Study of Osteoporotic Fractures Research Group. Prevalence and correlates of periodic limb movements in older women. *J Clin Sleep Med*. 2006;2(4):438-445.
8. Hornyak M, Feige B, Riemann D, Voderholzer U. Periodic leg movements in sleep and periodic limb movement disorder: prevalence, clinical significance, and treatment. *Sleep Med Rev*. 2006;10(3):169-177.
9. American Academy of Sleep Medicine. *ICSD-2 International Classification of Sleep Disorders. Diagnostic and Coding Manual*. 2nd ed. Westchester, IL: American Academy of Sleep Medicine; 2005.
10. American Academy of Sleep Medicine. *ICSD-3 International Classification of Sleep Disorders*. 3rd ed., text revision edition. Darien, IL: American Academy of Sleep Medicine; 2023.
11. Troester MM, Quan SF, Berry RB, et al.; for the American Academy of Sleep Medicine. *The AASM Manual for the Scoring of Sleep and Associated Events: Rules, Terminology and Technical Specifications*. Version 3. Darien, IL: American Academy of Sleep Medicine; 2023.
12. Romero-Peralta S, Cano-Pumarega I, García-Borreguero D. Emerging concepts of the pathophysiology and adverse outcomes of restless legs syndrome. *Chest*. 2020;158(3):1218-1229.
13. Allen RP, Walters AS, Montplaisir J, et al. Restless legs syndrome prevalence and impact: REST general population study. *Arch Intern Med*. 2005;165(11):1286-1292.
14. Hening W, Walters AS, Allen RP, Montplaisir J, Myers A, Ferini-Strambi L. Impact, diagnosis and treatment of restless legs syndrome (RLS) in a primary care population: the REST (RLS epidemiology, symptoms, and treatment) primary care study. *Sleep Med*. 2004;5(3):237-246.
15. Allen RP, Bharmal M, Calloway M. Prevalence and disease burden of primary restless legs syndrome: results of a general population survey in the United States. *Mov Disord*. 2011;26(1):114-120.
16. Allen RP, Stillman P, Myers AJ. Physician-diagnosed restless legs syndrome in a large sample of primary medical care patients in western Europe: prevalence and characteristics. *Sleep Med*. 2010;11(1):31-37.
17. Doan TT, Koo BB, Ogilvie RP, Redline S, Lutsey PL. Restless legs syndrome and periodic limb movements during sleep in the Multi-Ethnic Study of Atherosclerosis. *Sleep*. 2018;41(8):zsy106.
18. Hening WA, Allen RP, Washburn M, Lesage SR, Earley CJ. The four diagnostic criteria for Restless Legs Syndrome are unable to exclude confounding conditions ("mimics"). *Sleep Med*. 2009;10(9):976-981.
19. Ruppert E. Restless arms syndrome: prevalence, impact, and management strategies. *Neuropsychiatr Dis Treat*. 2019;15:1737-1750.
20. Sforza E, Hupin D, Roche F. Restless genital syndrome: differential diagnosis and treatment with pramipexole. *J Clin Sleep Med*. 2017;13(9): 1109-1110.
21. Benes H, Walters AS, Allen RP, Hening WA, Kohnen R. Definition of restless legs syndrome, how to diagnose it, and how to differentiate it from RLS mimics. *Mov Disord*. 2007;22(suppl 18):S401-S408. Erratum in: *Mov Disord*. 2008;23(8):1200-1202.
22. Walters AS, Hening W, Rubinstein M, Chokroverty S. A clinical and polysomnographic comparison of neuroleptic-induced akathisia and the idiopathic restless legs syndrome. *Sleep*. 1991;14(4):339-345.
23. Alvarez MV, Driver-Dunckley EE, Caviness JN, Adler CH, Evidente VG. Case series of painful legs and moving toes: clinical and electrophysiologic observations. *Mov Disord*. 2008;23(14):2062-2066.
24. Picchietti DL, Hensley JG, Bainbridge JL, et al. International Restless Legs Syndrome Study Group (IRLSSG). Consensus clinical practice guidelines for the diagnosis and treatment of restless legs syndrome/ Willis-Ekbom disease during pregnancy and lactation. *Sleep Med Rev*. 2015;22:64-77.
25. Hoque R, Chesson Jr AL. Pharmacologically induced/exacerbated restless legs syndrome, periodic limb movements of sleep, and REM behavior disorder/REM sleep without atonia: literature review, qualitative scoring, and comparative analysis. *J Clin Sleep Med*. 2010;6(1):79-83.
26. Rottach KG, Schaner BM, Kirch MH, et al. Restless legs syndrome as side effect of second generation antidepressants. *J Psychiatr Res*. 2008; 43(1):70-75.
27. Nofzinger EA, Fasiczka A, Berman S, Thase ME. Bupropion SR reduces periodic limb movements associated with arousal from sleep in depressed patients with period limb movement disorder. *J Clin Psychiatry*. 2000; 61:858-862.
28. Earley CJ, Connor J, Garcia-Borreguero D, et al. Altered brain iron homeostasis and dopaminergic function in restless legs syndrome (Willis-Ekbom disease). *Sleep Med*. 2014;15(11):1288-1301.
29. Earley CJ, Connor JR, Beard JL, Malecki EA, Epstein DK, Allen RP. Abnormalities in CSF concentrations of ferritin and transferrin in restless legs syndrome. *Neurology*. 2000;54(8):1698-1700.
30. Jiménez-Jiménez FJ, Alonso-Navarro H, García-Martín E, Agúndez JAG. Genetics of restless legs syndrome: an update. *Sleep Med Rev*. 2018;39:108-121.
31. Trotti LM. Restless legs syndrome and sleep-related movement disorders. *Continuum (Minneap Minn)*. 2017;23(4, Sleep Neurology):1005-1016.
32. Winkelmann J, Schormair B, Xiong L, Dion PA, Rye DB, Rouleau GA. Genetics of restless legs syndrome. *Sleep Med*. 2017;31:18-22.
33. Ferré S, García-Borreguero D, Allen RP, Earley CJ. New insights into the neurobiology of restless legs syndrome. *Neuroscientist*. 2019;25(2):113-125.
34. Ferré S, Quiroz C, Guitart X, et al. Pivotal role of adenosine neurotransmission in restless legs syndrome. *Front Neurosci*. 2018;11:722.
35. Quiroz C, Gulyani S, Ruiqian W, et al. Adenosine receptors as markers of brain iron deficiency: implications for restless legs syndrome. *Neuropharmacology*. 2016;111:160-168.
36. Garcia-Borreguero D, Guitart X, Garcia Malo C, Cano-Pumarega I, Granizo JJ, Ferré S. Treatment of restless legs syndrome/Willis-Ekbom disease with the non-selective ENT1/ENT2 inhibitor dipyridamole: testing the adenosine hypothesis. *Sleep Med*. 2018;45:94-97.
37. Garcia-Borreguero D, Garcia-Malo C, Granizo JJ, Ferré S. A randomized, placebo-controlled crossover study with dipyridamole for restless legs syndrome. *Mov Disord*. 2021;36(10):2387-2392.
38. Hornyak M, Hundemer HP, Quail D, Riemann D, Voderholzer U, Trenkwalder C. Relationship of periodic leg movements and severity of restless legs syndrome: a study in unmedicated and medicated patients. *Clin Neurophysiol*. 2007;118(7):1532-1537.
39. Trotti LM, Bliwise DL, Greer SA, et al. Correlates of PLMs variability over multiple nights and impact upon RLS diagnosis. *Sleep Med*. 2009;10(6):668-671.
40. Zhuang S, Na M, Winkelman JW, et al. Association of restless legs syndrome with risk of suicide and self-harm. *JAMA Netw Open*. 2019;2(8):e199966.
41. Chenini S, Barateau L, Guiraud L, et al. Depressive symptoms and suicidal thoughts in restless legs syndrome. *Mov Disord*. 2022;37(4):812-825.
42. Sun ER, Chen CA, Ho G, Earley CJ, Allen RP. Iron and the restless legs syndrome. *Sleep*. 1998;21(4):371-377.
43. Mackie S, Winkelman JW. Normal ferritin in a patient with iron deficiency and RLS. *J Clin Sleep Med*. 2013;9(5):511-513.
44. Allen RP, Picchietti DL, Auerbach M, et al. International Restless Legs Syndrome Study Group (IRSG). Evidence-based and consensus clinical practice guidelines for the iron treatment of restless legs syndrome/ Willis-Ekbom disease in adults and children: an IRLSSG task force report. *Sleep Med*. 2018;41:27-44.
45. Walters AS, LeBrocq C, Dhar A, et al.; International Restless Legs Syndrome Study Group. Validation of the International Restless Legs Syndrome Study Group rating scale for restless legs syndrome. *Sleep Med*. 2003;4(2):121-134.
46. Hening WA, Allen RP. Restless legs syndrome (RLS): the continuing development of diagnostic standards and severity measures. *Sleep Med*. 2003;4(2):95-97.
47. Sharon D, Allen RP, Martinez-Martin P, et al. International RLS Study Group. Validation of the self-administered version of the International Restless Legs Syndrome Study Group severity rating scale - the sIRLS. *Sleep Med*. 2019;54:94-100.
48. Picchietti MA, Picchietti DL. Advances in pediatric restless legs syndrome: Iron, genetics, diagnosis and treatment. *Sleep Med*. 2010;11(7): 643-651.
49. Picchietti D, Allen RP, Walters AS, et al. Restless legs syndrome: prevalence and impact in children and adolescents—the Peds REST Study. *Pediatrics*. 2007;120:253-266.
50. Cortese S, Lecendreux M, Arnulf I, et al. Restless legs syndrome and attention-deficit/hyperactivity disorder: a review of the literature. *Sleep*. 2005;28:1007-1013.
51. Scofield H, Roth T, Drake C. Periodic limb movements during sleep: population prevalence, clinical correlates, and racial differences. *Sleep*. 2008;31(9):1221-1227.
52. Leary EB, Moore HE IV, Schneider LD, Finn LA, Peppard PE, Mignot E. Periodic limb movements in sleep: prevalence and associated sleepiness in the Wisconsin Sleep Cohort. *Clin Neurophysiol*. 2018;129(11): 2306-2314.

53. Haba-Rubio J, Marti-Soler H, Marques-Vidal P, et al. Prevalence and determinants of periodic limb movements in the general population. *Ann Neurol*. 2016;79(3):464-474.
54. Drakatos P, Olaithe M, Verma D, et al. Periodic limb movements during sleep: a narrative review. *J Thorac Dis*. 2021;13(11):6476-6494.
55. Ferri R, Fulda S, Manconi M, et al. Night-to-night variability of periodic leg movements during sleep in restless legs syndrome and periodic limb movement disorder: comparison between the periodicity index and the PLMS index. *Sleep Med*. 2013;14(3):293-296.
56. American Sleep Disorders Association. *International Classification of Sleep Disorders*. 1st ed. Rochester, MN: American Sleep Disorders Association; 1990.
57. Ferri R, Zucconi M, Manconi M, Plazzi G, Bruni O, Ferini-Strambi L. New approaches to the study of periodic leg movements during sleep in restless legs syndrome. *Sleep*. 2006;29(6):759-769.
58. Ferri R, Koo BB, Picchietti DL, Fulda S. Periodic leg movements during sleep: phenotype, neurophysiology, and clinical significance. *Sleep Med*. 2017;31:29-38.
59. Pollmacher T, Schulz H. Periodic leg movements: their relationship to sleep stages. *Sleep*. 1993;16:572-577.
60. Culpepper WJ, Badia P, Shaffer JI. Time-of-night patterns in PLMS activity. *Sleep*. 1992;15(4):306-311.
61. Fantini ML, Michaud M, Gosselin N, Lavigne G, Montplaisir J. Periodic leg movements in REM sleep behavior disorder and related autonomic and EEG activation. *Neurology*. 2002;59(12):1889-1894.
62. Dauvilliers Y, Pennestri MH, Petit D, Dang-Vu T, Lavigne G, Montplaisir J. Periodic leg movements during sleep and wakefulness in narcolepsy. *J Sleep Res*. 2007;16(3):333-339.
63. Pizza F, Tartarotti S, Poryazova R, Baumann CR, Bassetti CL. Sleep-disordered breathing and periodic limb movements in narcolepsy with cataplexy: a systematic analysis of 35 consecutive patients. *Eur Neurol*. 2013;70(1-2):22-26.
64. Gaig C, Iranzo A, Pujol M, Perez H, Santamaria J. Periodic limb movements during sleep mimicking rem sleep behavior disorder: a new form of periodic limb movement disorder. *Sleep*. 2017;40(3).
65. Karadeniz D, Ondze B, Besset A, Billiard M. EEG arousals and awakenings in relation with periodic leg movements during sleep. *J Sleep Res*. 2000;9(3):273-277.
66. Sforza E, Nicolas A, Lavigne G, et al. EEG and cardiac activation during periodic leg movements in sleep. *Neurology*. 1999;52:786-792.
67. Mahowald MW. Periodic limb movements are not associated with disturbed sleep. *Con J Clin Sleep Med*. 2007;3(1):15-17.
68. Högl B. Periodic limb movements are associated with disturbed sleep. *Pro J Clin Sleep Med*. 2007;3(1):12-14.
69. Montplasir J, Michaud M, Denesle R, Gosseline A. Periodic leg movements are not more prevalent in insomnia of hypersomnia but are specifically associated with sleep disorders involving a dopaminergic impairment. *Sleep Med*. 2000;1:163-167.
70. Mendelson WB. Are periodic leg movements associated with clinical sleep disturbance? *Sleep*. 1996;19(3):219-223.
71. Fry JM, DiPhillipo MA, Pressman MR. Periodic leg movements in sleep following treatment of obstructive sleep apnea with nasal continuous positive airway pressure. *Chest*. 1989;96(1):89-91.
72. Lee SA, Kim SJ, Lee SY, Kim HJ. Clinical characteristics of periodic limb movements during sleep categorized by continuous positive airway pressure titration polysomnography in patients with obstructive sleep apnea. *Sleep Breath*. 2022;26(1):251-257.
73. Chervin RD. Periodic leg movements and sleepiness in patients evaluated for sleep-disordered breathing. *Am J Respir Crit Care Med*. 2001;164(8 Pt 1):1454-1458.
74. Exner EN, Collop NA. The association of upper airway resistance with periodic limb movements. *Sleep*. 2000;24:188-192.
75. Budhiraja R, Javaheri S, Pavlova MK, Epstein LJ, Omobomi O, Quan SF. Prevalence and correlates of periodic limb movements in OSA and the effect of CPAP therapy. *Neurology*. 2020;94(17):e1820-e1827.
76. Koo BB, Blackwell T, Ancoli-Israel S, et al. Association of incident cardiovascular disease with periodic limb movements during sleep in older men: outcomes of sleep disorders in older men (MrOS) study. *Circulation*. 2011;124(11):1223-1231.
77. Winkelman JW, Blackwell T, Stone K, Ancoli-Israel S, Redline S. Associations of incident cardiovascular events with restless legs syndrome and periodic leg movements of sleep in older men, for the Outcomes of Sleep Disorders in Older Men Study (MrOS Sleep Study). *Sleep*. 2017;40(4):zsx023.
78. Szentkirályi A, Völzke H, Hoffmann W, Happe S, Berger K. A time sequence analysis of the relationship between cardiovascular risk factors, vascular diseases and restless legs syndrome in the general population. *J Sleep Res*. 2013;22(4):434-442.
79. Kendzerska T, Kamra M, Murray BJ, Boulos MI. Incident cardiovascular events and death in individuals with restless legs syndrome or periodic limb movements in sleep: a systematic review. *Sleep*. 2017;40(3).
80. Eisensehr I, Ehrenberg BL, Noachtar S. Different sleep characteristics in restless legs syndrome and periodic limb movement disorder. *Sleep Med*. 2003;4(2):147-152.
81. Hardy De Buisseret FX, Mairesse O, Newell J, Verbanck P, Neu D. While isolated periodic limb movement disorder significantly impacts sleep depth and efficiency, co-morbid restless legs syndrome mainly exacerbates perceived sleep quality. *Eur Neurol*. 2017;77(5-6):272-280.
82. Littner MR, Kushida C, Anderson WM, et al. Practice parameters for the dopaminergic treatment of restless legs syndrome and periodic limb movement disorder. *Sleep*. 2004;27:557-559.
83. Silber MH, Ehrenberg BL, Allen RP, et al.; Medical Advisory Board of the Restless Legs Syndrome Foundation. An algorithm for the management of restless legs syndrome. *Mayo Clin Proc*. 2004;79(7):916-922. Erratum in: *Mayo Clin Proc*. 2004;79(10):1341.
84. Aurora RN, Kristo DA, Bista SR, et al. The treatment of restless legs syndrome and periodic limb movement disorder in adults-an update for 2012: practice parameters with an evidence-based systematic review and meta-analyses: an American Academy of Sleep Medicine Clinical Practice Guideline. *Sleep*. 2012;35(8):1039-1062.
85. Winkelman JW, Armstrong MJ, Allen RP, et al. Practice guideline summary: treatment of restless legs syndrome in adults: report of the Guideline Development, Dissemination, and Implementation Subcommittee of the American Academy of Neurology. *Neurology*. 2016;87(24): 2585-2593.
86. Garcia-Borreguero D, Silber MH, Winkelman JW, et al. Guidelines for the first-line treatment of restless legs syndrome/Willis-Ekbom disease, prevention and treatment of dopaminergic augmentation: a combined task force of the IRLSSG, EURLSSG, and the RLS-foundation. *Sleep Med*. 2016;21:1-11.
87. Silber MH, Buchfuhrer MJ, Earley CJ, et al. The management of restless legs syndrome: an updated algorithm. *Mayo Clin Proc*. 2021;96(7): 1921-1937.
88. Gossard TR, Trotti LM, Videnovic A, St Louis EK. Restless legs syndrome: contemporary diagnosis and treatment. *Neurotherapeutics*. 2021; 18(1):140-155.
89. Bayard M, Bailey B, Acharya D, et al. Bupropion and restless legs syndrome: a randomized controlled trial. *J Am Board Fam Med*. 2011;24(4): 422-428.
90. Harrison EG, Keating JL, Morgan PE. Non-pharmacological interventions for restless legs syndrome: a systematic review of randomised controlled trials. *Disabil Rehabil*. 2019;41(17):2006-2014.
91. Lettieri CJ, Eliasson AH. Pneumatic compression devices are an effective therapy for restless legs syndrome: a prospective, randomized, double-blinded, sham-controlled trial. *Chest*. 2009;135:74-80.
92. Burbank F, Buchfuhrer MJ, Kopjar B. Sleep improvement for restless legs syndrome patients. Part I: pooled analysis of two prospective, double-blind, sham-controlled, multi-center, randomized clinical studies of the effects of vibrating pads on RLS symptoms. *J Parkinsonism Restless Legs Syndr*. 2013;3:1-10.
93. Burbank F, Buchfuhrer M, Kopjar B. Improving sleep for patients with restless legs syndrome. Part II: meta-analysis of vibration therapy and drugs approved by the FDA for treatment of restless legs syndrome. *J Parkinsonism Restless Legs Syndr*. 2013;3:11-22.
94. Park A, Ambrogi K, Hade EM. Randomized pilot trial for the efficacy of the MMF07 foot massager and heat therapy for restless legs syndrome. *PLoS One*. 2020;15(4):e0230951.
95. Kuhn PJ, Olson DJ, Sullivan JP. Targeted pressure on abductor hallucis and flexor hallucis brevis muscles to manage moderate to severe primary restless legs syndrome. *J Am Osteopath Assoc*. 2016;116(7): 440-450.
96. Rozeman AD, Ottolini T, Grootendorst DC, Vogels OJ, Rijsman RM. Effect of sensory stimuli on restless legs syndrome: a randomized crossover study. *J Clin Sleep Med*. 2014;10(8):893-896.
97. Buchfuhrer MJ, Baker FC, Singh H, et al. Noninvasive neuromodulation reduces symptoms of restless legs syndrome. *J Clin Sleep Med*. 2021;17(8):1685-1694.
98. Charlesworth JD, Adlou B, Singh H, Buchfuhrer MJ. Bilateral high-frequency noninvasive peroneal nerve stimulation evokes tonic leg muscle activation for sleep-compatible reduction of restless legs syndrome symptoms. *J Clin Sleep Med*. 2023;19(7):1199-1209.

99. Walters AS, Mandelbaum DE, Lewin DS, Kugler S, England SJ, Miller M. Dopaminergic therapy in children with restless legs/periodic limb movements in sleep and ADHD. Dopaminergic Therapy Study Group. *Pediatr Neurol.* 2000;22(3):182-186.
100. Stahl SM. Mechanism of action of alpha2delta ligands: voltage sensitive calcium channel (VSCC) modulators. *J Clin Psychiatry.* 2004;65(8): 1033-1034.
101. Happe S, Sauter C, Klösch G, Saletu B, Zeitlhofer J. Gabapentin versus ropinirole in the treatment of idiopathic restless legs syndrome. *Neuropsychobiology.* 2003;48(2):82-86.
102. Garcia-Borreguero D, Larrosa O, de la Llave Y, Verger K, Masramon X, Hernandez G. Treatment of restless legs syndrome with gabapentin: a double-blind, cross-over study. *Neurology.* 2002;59(10):1573-1579.
103. Saletu M, Anderer P, Saletu-Zyhlarz GM, et al. Comparative placebo-controlled polysomnographic and psychometric studies on the acute effects of gabapentin versus ropinirole in restless legs syndrome. *J Neural Transm (Vienna).* 2010;117(4):463-473.
104. Thorp ML, Morris CD, Bagby SP. A crossover study of gabapentin in treatment of restless legs syndrome among hemodialysis patients. *Am J Kidney Dis.* 2001;38(1):104-108.
105. Garcia-Borreguero D, Cano-Pumarega I, Garcia Malo C, Cruz Velarde JA, Granizo JJ, Wanner V. Reduced response to gabapentin enacarbil in restless legs syndrome following long-term dopaminergic treatment. *Sleep Med.* 2019;55:74-80.
106. Kushida CA, Becker PM, Ellengoben AL, et al. Randomized, double-blind, placebo-controlled study of XP135412/GSK1838262 in patients with RLS. *Neurology.* 2009;72:439-446.
107. Lee DO, Ziman RB, Perkins AT, et al. A randomized, double-blind, placebo-controlled study to assess the efficacy and tolerability of gabapentin enacarbil in subjects with restless legs syndrome. *J Clin Sleep Med.* 2011;7(3):282-292.
108. Kume A. Gabapentin enacarbil for the treatment of moderate to severe primary restless legs syndrome (Willis-Ekbom disease): 600 or 1,200 mg dose? *Neuropsychiatr Dis Treat.* 2014;10:249-262.
109. Garcia-Borreguero D, Larrosa O, Williams AM, et al. Treatment of restless legs syndrome with pregabalin: a double-blind, placebo-controlled study. *Neurology.* 2010;74:1897-1904.
110. Allen R, Chen C, Soaita A, et al. A randomized, double-blind, 6-week, dose-ranging study of pregabalin in patients with restless legs syndrome. *Sleep Med.* 2010;11(6):512-519.
111. Bae H, Cho YW, Kim KT, Allen RP, Earley CJ. The safety and efficacy of pregabalin add-on therapy in restless legs syndrome patients. *Front Neurol.* 2021;12:786408.
112. Allen RP, Chen C, Garcia-Borreguero D, et al. Comparison of pregabalin with pramipexole for restless legs syndrome. *N Engl J Med.* 2014;370(7):621-631.
113. Calandre EP, Rico-Villademoros F, Slim M. Alpha-2-delta ligands, gabapentin, pregabalin and mirogabalin: a review of their clinical pharmacology and therapeutic use. *Expert Rev Neurother.* 2016;16(11): 1263-1277. Erratum in: *Expert Rev Neurother.* 2016;16(11):iii.
114. *FDA Warns about Serious Breathing Problems with Seizure and Nerve Pain Medicines Gabapentin (Neurontin, Gralise, Horizant) and Pregabalin (Lyrica, Lyrica CR) When used with CNS Depressants or in Patients with Lung Problems.* Available at: https://www.fda.gov/drugs/drug-safety-and-availability/fda-warns-about-serious-breathing-problems-seizure-and-nerve-pain-medicines-gabapentin-neurontin#:,:text=The%20 U.S.%20Food%20and%20Drug,who%20have%20respiratory%20 risk%20factors. Accessed April 30, 2022.
115. Earley CJ, Allen RP. Pergolide and carbidopa/levodopa periodic leg movements in sleep in a consecutive series of patients. *Sleep.* 1996;19: 801-810.
116. Montplaisir J, Nicolas A, Denesle R, et al. Restless legs syndrome improved by pramipexole: a double-blind randomized trial. *Neurology.* 1999;52:938-943.
117. Montplaisir J, Denesle R, Petit D. Pramipexole in the treatment of restless legs syndrome: a follow-up study. *Eur J Neurol.* 2000;1:27-31.
118. Adler CH, Hauser RA, Sethi K, et al. Ropinirole for restless legs syndrome. *Neurology.* 2004;62:1405-1407.
119. Allen R, Becker PM, Bogan R, et al. Ropinirole decreases periodic leg movements and improves sleep parameters in patients with restless legs syndrome. *Sleep.* 2004;27:907-914.
120. Saletu M, Anderer P, Saletu B, et al. Sleep laboratory studies in periodic limb movement disorder (PLMD) patients as compared to normals and acute effects of ropinirole. *Hum Psychopharm.* 2001;16:177-187.
121. Inoue Y, Hirata K, Hayashida K, et al. Efficacy, safety and risk of augmentation of rotigotine for treating restless legs syndrome. *Prog Neuropsychopharmacol Biol Psychiatry.* 2013;40:326-333.
122. Hening WA, Allen RP, Ondo WG, et al.; SP792 Study Group. Rotigotine improves restless legs syndrome: a 6-month randomized, double-blind, placebo-controlled trial in the United States. *Mov Disord.* 2010; 25(11):1675-1683.
123. Trenkwalder C, Canelo M, Lang M, et al. Management of augmentation of restless legs syndrome with rotigotine: a 1-year observational study. *Sleep Med.* 2017;30:257-265.
124. Chung SJ, Asgharnejad M, Bauer L, et al. Switching from an oral dopamine receptor agonist to rotigotine transdermal patch: a review of clinical data with a focus on patient perspective. *Expert Rev Neurother.* 2017;17(7):737-749.
125. Winkelman JW, Mackie SE, Mei LA, Platt S, Schoerning L. A method to switch from oral dopamine agonists to rotigotine in patients with restless legs syndrome and mild augmentation. *Sleep Med.* 2016;24: 18-23.
126. Silver N, Allen RP, Senerth J, Earley CJ. A 10-year, longitudinal assessment of dopamine agonists and methadone in the treatment of restless legs syndrome. *Sleep Med.* 2011;12(5):440-444.
127. Lipford MC, Silber MH. Long-term use of pramipexole in the management of restless legs syndrome. *Sleep Med.* 2012;13(10):1280-1285.
128. Cornelius JR, Tippmann-Peikert M, Slocumb NL, Frerichs CF, Silber MH. Impulse control disorders with the use of dopaminergic agents in restless legs syndrome: a case-control study. *Sleep.* 2010;33:81-87.
129. Voon V, Schoerling A, Wenzel S, et al. Frequency of impulse control behaviours associated with dopaminergic therapy in restless legs syndrome. *BMC Neurol.* 2011;11:117.
130. García-Borreguero D, Allen RP, Kohnen R, et al. International Restless Legs Syndrome Study Group. Diagnostic standards for dopaminergic augmentation of restless legs syndrome: report from a World Association of Sleep Medicine-International Restless Legs Syndrome Study Group consensus conference at the Max Planck Institute. *Sleep Med.* 2007;8(5):520-530. Erratum in: *Sleep Med.* 2007;8(7-8):788.
131. Allen RP, Earley CJ. Augmentation of the restless legs syndrome with carbidopa/levodopa. *Sleep.* 1996;19:205-213.
132. Winkleman JW, Johnson L. Augmentation and tolerance with long-term pramipexole treatment of restless legs syndrome. *Sleep Med.* 2004;5:9-14.
133. Allen RP, Ondo WG, Ball E, et al. Restless legs syndrome (RLS) augmentation associated with dopamine agonist and levodopa usage in a community sample. *Sleep Med.* 2011;12(5):431-439.
134. Winkelman JW. High national rates of high-dose dopamine agonist prescribing for restless legs syndrome. *Sleep.* 2022;45(2):zsab212.
135. Trenkwalder C, Hogl B, Benes H, et al. Augmentation in restless legs syndrome is associated with low ferritin. *Sleep Med.* 2008;9:572-574.
136. Silber MH, Becker PM, Buchfuhrer MJ, et al.; Scientific and Medical Advisory Board, Restless Legs Syndrome Foundation. The appropriate use of opioids in the treatment of refractory restless legs syndrome. *Mayo Clin Proc.* 2018;93(1):59-67.
137. Walters AS, Wagner ML, Hening WA, et al. Successful treatment of the idiopathic restless legs syndrome in a randomized double-blind trial of oxycodone versus placebo. *Sleep.* 1993;16:327-332.
138. Kaplan PW, Allen RP, Bucholz DW, Walters JK. A double-blind, placebo-controlled study of the treatment of periodic limb movements in sleep using carbidopa/levodopa and propoxyphene. *Sleep.* 1993;16: 717-723.
139. Walters AS, Winkelmann J, Trenkwalder C, et al. Long-term follow-up on restless legs syndrome patients treated with opioids. *Mov Disord.* 2001;16(6):1105-1109.
140. Ondo WG. Methadone for refractory restless legs syndrome. *Mov Disord.* 2005;20(3):345-348.
141. Walters AS. Review of receptor agonist and antagonist studies relevant to the opiate system in restless legs syndrome. *Sleep Med.* 2002;3(4): 301-304.
142. de Biase S, Valente M, Gigli GL. Intractable restless legs syndrome: role of prolonged-release oxycodone-naloxone. *Neuropsychiatr Dis Treat.* 2016;12:417-425.
143. Trenkwalder C, Beneš H, Grote L, et al.; RELOXYN Study Group. Prolonged release oxycodone-naloxone for treatment of severe restless legs syndrome after failure of previous treatment: a double-blind, randomised, placebo-controlled trial with an open-label extension. *Lancet Neurol.* 2013;12(12):1141-1150. Erratum in: *Lancet Neurol.* 2013;12(12):1133.

144. Winkelman JW, Purks J, Wipper B. Baseline and 1-year longitudinal data from the National Restless Legs Syndrome Opioid Registry. *Sleep*. 2021;44(2):zsaa183.
145. Mitler MM, Browman CP, Menn SJ, et al. Nocturnal myoclonus: treatment efficacy of clonazepam and temazepam. *Sleep*. 1986;9:385-392.
146. Peled R, Lavie P. Double-blind evaluation of clonazepam on periodic leg movements in sleep. *J Neurol Neurosurg Psychiatry*. 1987;50: 1679-1681.
147. Bonnet MH, Arand DL. The use of triazolam in older patients with periodic leg movements, fragmented sleep, and daytime sleepiness. *J Gerontol*. 1990;45:M139-M144.
148. Doghramji K, Browman CP, Gaddy JR, et al. Triazolam diminishes daytime sleepiness and sleep fragmentation in patients with periodic leg movements in sleep. *J Clin Psychopharmacol*. 1991;11:284-290.
149. Saletu M, Anderer P, Saletu-Zyhalrz G, et al. Restless legs syndrome (RLS) and periodic limb movement disorder (PLMD): acute placebo-controlled sleep laboratory study with clonazepam. *Eur Neuropsychopharmacol*. 2001;11:153-161.
150. Wang J, O'Reilly B, Venkataraman R, Mysliwiec V, Mysliwiec A. Efficacy of oral iron in patients with restless legs syndrome and a low-normal ferritin: a randomized, double-blind, placebo-controlled study. *Sleep Med*. 2009;10(9):973-975.
151. Dye TJ, Jain SV, Simakajornboon N. Outcomes of long-term iron supplementation in pediatric restless legs syndrome/periodic limb movement disorder (RLS/PLMD). *Sleep Med*. 2017;32:213-219.
152. Cho YW, Allen RP, Earley CJ. Lower molecular weight intravenous iron dextran for restless legs syndrome. *Sleep Med*. 2013;14(3):274-277.
153. Cho YW, Allen RP, Earley CJ. Clinical efficacy of ferric carboxymaltose treatment in patients with restless legs syndrome. *Sleep Med*. 2016; 25:16-23.
154. Garcia-Malo C, Wanner V, Miranda C, et al. Quantitative transcranial sonography of the substantia nigra as a predictor of therapeutic response to intravenous iron therapy in restless legs syndrome. *Sleep Med*. 2020; 66:123-129.
155. Trotti LM, Becker LA. Iron for the treatment of restless legs syndrome. *Cochrane Database Syst Rev*. 2019;1(1):CD007834. doi:10.1002/14651858.CD007834.pub3.
156. DelRosso L, Bruni O. Treatment of pediatric restless legs syndrome. *Adv Pharmacol*. 2019;84:237-253.
157. Kotagal S, Silber MH. Childhood-onset restless legs syndrome. *Ann Neurol*. 2004;56(6):803-807.
158. Simakajornboon N, Kheirandish-Gozal L, Gozal D. Diagnosis and management of restless legs syndrome in children. *Sleep Med Rev*. 2009; 13(2):149-156.
159. Rulong G, Dye T, Simakajornboon N. Pharmacological management of restless legs syndrome and periodic limb movement disorder in children. *Paediatr Drugs*. 2018;20(1):9-17.
160. DelRosso LM, Ferri R, Chen ML, et al. Clinical efficacy and safety of intravenous ferric carboxymaltose treatment of pediatric restless legs syndrome and periodic limb movement disorder. *Sleep Med*. 2021;87:114-118.
161. Zand L, McKian KP, Qian Q. Gabapentin toxicity in patients with chronic kidney disease: a preventable cause of morbidity. *Am J Med*. 2010;123(4):367-373.
162. Sagheb MM, Dormanesh B, Fallahzadeh MK, et al. Efficacy of vitamins C, E, and their combination for treatment of restless legs syndrome in hemodialysis patients: a randomized, double-blind, placebo-controlled trial. *Sleep Med*. 2012;13(5):542-545.
163. Jahani Kondori M, Kolla BP, Moore KM, Mansukhani MP. Management of restless legs syndrome in pregnancy and lactation. *J Prim Care Community Health*. 2020;11:2150132720905950.
164. Uglane MT, Westad S, Backe B. Restless legs syndrome in pregnancy is a frequent disorder with a good prognosis. *Acta Obstet Gynecol Scand*. 2011;90(9):1046-1048.
165. Picchietti DL, Wang VC, Picchietti MA. Intravenous iron given prior to pregnancy for restless legs syndrome is associated with remission of symptoms. *J Clin Sleep Med*. 2012;8(5):585-586.
166. Vadasz D, Ries V, Oertel WH. Intravenous iron sucrose for restless legs syndrome in pregnant women with low serum ferritin. *Sleep Med*. 2013;14(11):1214-1216.
167. Schneider J, Krafft A, Manconi M, et al. Open-label study of the efficacy and safety of intravenous ferric carboxymaltose in pregnant women with restless legs syndrome. *Sleep Med*. 2015;16(11):1342-1347.
168. Marshall NS, Serinel Y, Killick R, et al. Magnesium supplementation for the treatment of restless legs syndrome and periodic limb movement disorder: a systematic review. *Sleep Med Rev*. 2019;48:101218.
169. Nahab FB, Peckham EL, Hallett M. Double-blind, placebo-controlled, pilot trial of botulinum toxin A in restless legs syndrome. *Neurology*. 2008;71(12):950-951.
170. Mittal SO, Machado D, Richardson D, Dubey D, Jabbari B. Botulinum toxin in restless legs syndrome: a randomized double-blind placebo-controlled crossover study. *Toxins (Basel)*. 2018;10(10):401.
171. Ghorayeb I. More evidence of cannabis efficacy in restless legs syndrome. *Sleep Breath*. 2020;24(1):277-279.
172. Antoniou T, Bodkin J, Ho JM. Drug interactions with cannabinoids. *CMAJ*. 2020;192(9):E206.
173. DelRosso LM, Ferri R, Allen R, et al. International Restless Legs Syndrome Study Group: Consensus diagnostic criteria for a newly defined pediatric sleep disorder (RSD). Sleep Med. 2020;75:335–340.

Chapter

32 Central Disorders of Hypersomnolence

INTRODUCTION

The disorders of hypersomnolence of central origin (Table 32-1) are an important part of the differential diagnosis of patients presenting with excessive daytime sleepiness.[1-3] The term *hypersomnolence* is preferred over *hypersomnia*, which actually means a long sleep duration. Of these disorders, insufficient sleep syndrome is likely the most common. In the International Classification of Sleep Disorders (ICSD-2),[1] narcolepsy was divided into narcolepsy with and without cataplexy (N+C, N–C). Cataplexy (emotionally induced weakness) is the only symptom virtually specific for narcolepsy. In the ICSD-3, narcolepsy is classified based on a low or absent cerebrospinal fluid (CSF) hypocretin-1 level (type 1, NT1) or a normal CSF hypocretin-1 level (type 2, NT2).[1] Most, but not all, NT1 patients have cataplexy (N+C), and most, but not all, N–C patients have a normal hypocretin level. Neither classification (N+C, N–C nor NT1, NT2) is completely satisfactory because, currently, hypocretin deficiency can be documented only by determination of the CSF hypocretin-1 level. However, a CSF hypocretin-1 level is not available for most patients. On the other hand, determining whether cataplexy is truly present is often challenging, and there is a delay between the onset of daytime sleepiness and cataplexy in some patients.[3-6] In the ICSD-3-TR,[3] the diagnostic criteria for NT1 were changed, and a sleep-onset rapid eye movement (REM) period (SOREMP) on the polysomnogram (PSG) preceding a multiple sleep patency test (MSLT) can be used as a standalone PSG/MSLT finding to diagnose narcolepsy. In the ICSD-2, idiopathic hypersomnia (IH) was divided into patients with and without long sleep time (< or > 10 hours). In the ICSD-3 and ICSD-3-TR, patients with IH are no longer classified according to sleep time. However, IH with long sleep time can be considered a subtype of IH.

Table 32-1 Hypersomnolence of Central Origin

1. Narcolepsy Type I (NT1, hypocretin deficiency) – usually with cataplexy*
2. Narcolepsy Type II (NT2, normal hypocretin levels) – usually without cataplexy*
3. Idiopathic Hypersomnia (IH)
4. Kleine-Levin Syndrome (KLS)
5. Hypersomnia Due to a Medical Disorder (HDMD)
6. Hypersomnia Due to a Medication or Substance (HDMS)
7. Hypersomnia Associated with a Mental Disorder (HAMD)
8. Insufficient Sleep Syndrome
9. Normal Variant – Long Sleeper

*A CSF hypocretin-1 level is often not available. Some patients without cataplexy are later found to have a low hypocretin level and are classified as NT1.

NARCOLEPSY

Narcolepsy is a disorder characterized by excessive daytime sleepiness and symptoms related to the abnormal regulation of wakefulness and sleep.[4-7] A short REM latency and intrusion of REM sleep features into wakefulness are characteristic of the disorder. The cause of NT1 (N+C) is loss of hypocretin-secreting neurons in the lateral hypothalamus and loss of the stabilizing effects the hypocretins have on wakefulness and sleep. Hypocretin 1 (orexin 1) and hypocretin 2 (orexin 2) were described in 1998,[8,9] and the association of hypocretin deficiency with narcolepsy (N+C) was described only a short time later.[10] Hypocretin deficiency is documented by determining the level of hypocretin-1 in the CSF. Loss of hypocretin is the result of destruction of the hypocretin-producing cells in the lateral hypothalamus. The destruction is thought to be autoimmune mediated. However, to date, this etiology has not been proven by experimental evidence.[6,7] A low CSF hypocretin level has rarely been found in other neurological disorders, but the combination of sleepiness, a low CSF hypocretin-1 level, and a normal neurological examination firmly establishes a diagnosis of NT1. In patients with or without cataplexy and an unknown hypocretin level, the diagnosis of narcolepsy is based on the presence or absence of cataplexy and findings from PSG followed by a daytime MSLT using standard procedures (see Chapter 17).[11,12]

The diagnostic criteria for NT1 include[3]:

A. The patient has daily periods of irrepressible need to sleep or daytime lapses into drowsiness or sleep.

B. The presence of **one or both** of the following:
   1. Cataplexy (typical) and either a or b:
      a. Mean sleep latency of ≤8 minutes and two or more SOREMPs on an MSLT performed in accordance with current recommended protocols
      b. An SOREMP within 15 minutes of sleep onset on nocturnal PSG
   2. CSF hypocretin-1 concentrations measured by immunoreactivity either ≤110 pg/ml (using a Stanford reference sample) or <1/3 of mean values obtained in normal subjects with the same standard assay

C. The symptoms and signs are not better explained by chronic insufficient sleep, a circadian rhythm sleep-wakefulness disorder or another current sleep disorder, mental disorder, or medication/substance use or withdrawal.

The standard MSLT protocol is discussed in Chapter 17. The ICSD-3-TR states that a sleep log for at least 1 week, accompanied whenever possible by actigraphy, prior to in-laboratory sleep testing is **required** to evaluate for insufficient sleep and circadian rhythm disturbances. Ideally, this should be for a period of 2 weeks, including a weekend, but a minimum of 1 week. Note that diagnostic criteria require daily symptoms, but the *duration of the symptoms is no longer specified* (previously at least a 3-month duration).[123] The characteristics of typical cataplexy will be discussed below. The new criteria specify that daytime sleepiness + a SOREMP on the PSG + a history of typical cataplexy can be used to diagnose narcolepsy (assuming criteria C is met). A history of daytime sleepiness + typical cataplexy and MSLT findings of a short mean sleep latency (≤8 minutes) and two or more SOREMPs on the MSLT can also be used to diagnose NT1 (assuming criteria C is met). Finally, a low CSF hypocretin-1 level can be used to diagnose NT1 if daily symptoms are present *with or without a history of cataplexy*. This is true even if PSG and MSLT findings are not supportive or if other untreated sleep disorders are present. Some patients diagnosed with NT1 based on a low hypocretin-1 level may not have exhibited cataplexy (usually present within 1 or 2 years of the onset of sleepiness).

The ICSD-3-TR diagnostic criteria for NT2 have not substantially changed from those of the ICSD-3 and include[3]:

A. The patient has daily periods of irrepressible need to sleep or daytime lapses into drowsiness or sleep occurring for at **least 3 months.**

B. A mean sleep latency of ≤8 minutes and two or more SOREMPs are found on an MSLT performed according to standard techniques. An SOREMP (within 15 minutes of sleep onset) on the preceding nocturnal PSG may replace one of the SOREMPs on the MSLT.

C. Cataplexy is absent.

D. *If* the CSF hypocretin-1 level is measured by radioimmunoassay, it is either >**110 pg/ml** (when using a Stanford reference standard) **or** >**1/3** of mean values obtained in normal subjects with the standard assay.

E. The symptoms and signs are not better explained by chronic insufficient sleep, a circadian rhythm sleep-wakefulness disorder or another current sleep disorder, mental disorder, or medication/substance use or withdrawal.

Using the MSLT, the finding of two or more SOREMPs is specific for the presence of narcolepsy in the absence of other explanations for this findings (PSG and history).[11,12] As noted, an SOREMP is defined as the onset of REM sleep within 15 minutes of sleep onset. The finding of SOREMPs is much more specific than the finding of a mean sleep latency ≤ 8 minutes. Unfortunately, the MSLT is not absolutely sensitive (70–90%, depending on the population studied). False positives and false negatives do occur (see Chapter 17). In both the ICSD-3 and ICSD-3-TR, a history of sleepiness and cataplexy is *not sufficient* to make a diagnosis of NT1. Other evidence must be present, including a low CSF hypocretin-1 level, a PSG SOREMP, or an MSLT with a mean sleep latency ≤8 minutes and two or more SOREMPs. As false negatives do occur, repeat testing is indicated when the history of cataplexy is felt to be reliable. As nearly all patients with NT1 and hypocretin deficiency are positive for HLA-DQB1*06:02, a negative antigen test would mean that true cataplexy was likely not present. However, a positive antigen test is not helpful, as it can occur in normal individuals.

The finding of a nocturnal SOREMP on PSG preceding an MSLT was found to be highly specific (few false positives) for diagnosis of NT1 in a study by Andlauer et al.[13] In this study, a diagnosis of narcolepsy (NT1) was defined as the finding of cataplexy plus HLA-DQB1*06:02 positivity (no CSF hypocretin-1 results available) or the finding of a low (≤110 pg/mL) CSF hypocretin-1 level. This study supports the use of a PSG SOREMP as a standalone PSG/MSLT finding to diagnose NT1, assuming other criteria are met. The use of a PSG SOREMP as one of the two or more required MSLT SOREMPs for **diagnosis of NT2** is retained in the ICSD-3-TR.

If a patient initially classified as NT2 (no cataplexy, no CSF available) later develops cataplexy (or a low CSF hypocretin-1 level is documented), the patient is reclassified as NT1. As noted, if CSF hypocretin-1 is low, a patient is classified as NT1 even if cataplexy is absent. Many of these patients will develop cataplexy in the following years. In this discussion, the terminology NT1 is used instead of N+C with the understanding that most (but not all) patients with NT1 have cataplexy and that the majority of patients diagnosed clinically with N+C in the past or included in more recent clinical studies did not (do not) have a known CSF hypocretin-1 level. If the notations NT1 (N+C) or NT2 (N–C) are used, this is to emphasize that the particular study classified patients with narcolepsy based on the presence or absence of cataplexy rather than a hypocretin level. Of note, there exists a small group of patients (5–10%) *otherwise meeting criteria for NT1 who are found to have normal hypocretin levels.*[3] The etiology of the narcolepsy in these patients is unknown. They are still classified as NT1.[3]

Core Symptoms of Narcolepsy

The core symptoms of narcolepsy are listed in Table 32-2. All of the symptoms may not be present is a given patient with narcolepsy. The only symptom virtually specific for narcolepsy is cataplexy.

1. **Excessive sleepiness** is present in virtually 100% of patients (duration ≥3 months required in NT2) and is defined as an irrepressible need for sleep or unintended lapses into drowsiness or sleep. Sleepiness may vary in severity and is more likely if the individual is at rest or in monotonous situations. The sudden onset of sleepiness without a prodromal warning can occur (sleep attacks). Sleepiness is usually the first initial symptom of narcolepsy (Figure 32-1). Rarely, cataplexy can be the first symptom.[3,4,14-16] In one study, cataplexy was the initial symptom in 9% of children[16]; it can be the most prominent symptom in children.
2. **Cataplexy** is the only symptom virtually specific for narcolepsy, but it is present in only 60% to 70% of patients, defined by excessive sleepiness and a + PSG-MSLT without other causes of sleepiness.[4,14-18] Typical cataplexy is characterized by brief periods (<2 minutes) of muscle weakness triggered by emotion (excitedly laughing, telling a joke) with preserved consciousness (Figure 32-2). The severity can vary from frequent episodes of collapse to infrequent partial weakness. Cataplexy usually appears within a few

Table 32-2 Core Symptoms of Narcolepsy

Symptom	Comments	Specific for Narcolepsy
Excessive daytime sleepiness	• Continuous daytime sleepiness, with exacerbations (sleep attacks) • Usually the first symptom • Present in virtually 100% of patients with narcolepsy	No
Cataplexy	• Muscle weakness triggered by emotion • Most common triggers: hearing or telling a joke • Usually occurs within a few years of onset of sleepiness • Duration: Seconds to minutes • Consciousness preserved at least at beginning of episodes • Present in 60% to 70% of patients with narcolepsy	Yes
Hypnagogic (sleep onset) Hypnopompic (on awakening) Hallucinations	• Vivid dreamlike images that occur at sleep-wakefulness transitions • Duration: Several minutes • Can be associated with sleep paralysis	No
Sleep Paralysis (SP)	• A partial or complete paralysis of the skeletal muscles that occurs at sleep onset or sleep offset. Most commonly on awakening (hypnopompic) • Can be associated with sleep hallucination; the patient is awake but cannot move • Can be associated with dyspnea, although the diaphragm is not affected • Duration: A few seconds to several minutes	No
Disturbed nocturnal sleep	• Increased stage N1 • Frequent awakenings • 20% to 30% have short nocturnal REM latency (<15 min) • PLMS is common, PLMS can occur in REM	No
Automatic behavior	• Semi-purposeful activity with amnesia	No
REM sleep behavior disorder	• Dream enactment—often violent • REM sleep without atonia	No
PLMS	• Common • Can be present during Stage R	No
Weight gain	Common at onset in NT1	

PLMS, periodic limb movement disorder; *REM*, rapid eye movement.

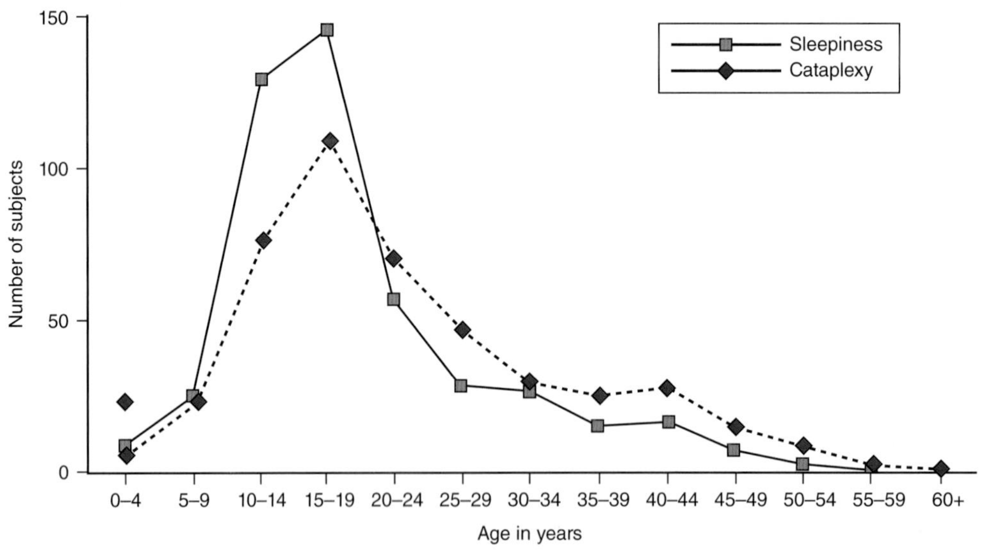

Figure 32-1 The number of subjects diagnosed with narcolepsy versus age in years. Data for the onset of sleepiness and cataplexy are shown. Sleepiness slightly precedes cataplexy. In this group, the peak age of diagnosis was around 15 years. (Adapted from Okun ML, Lin L, Pelin Z, Hong S, Mignot E. Clinical aspects of narcolepsy-cataplexy across ethnic groups. *Sleep*. 2002;25(1):27-35. PMID: 11833858.)

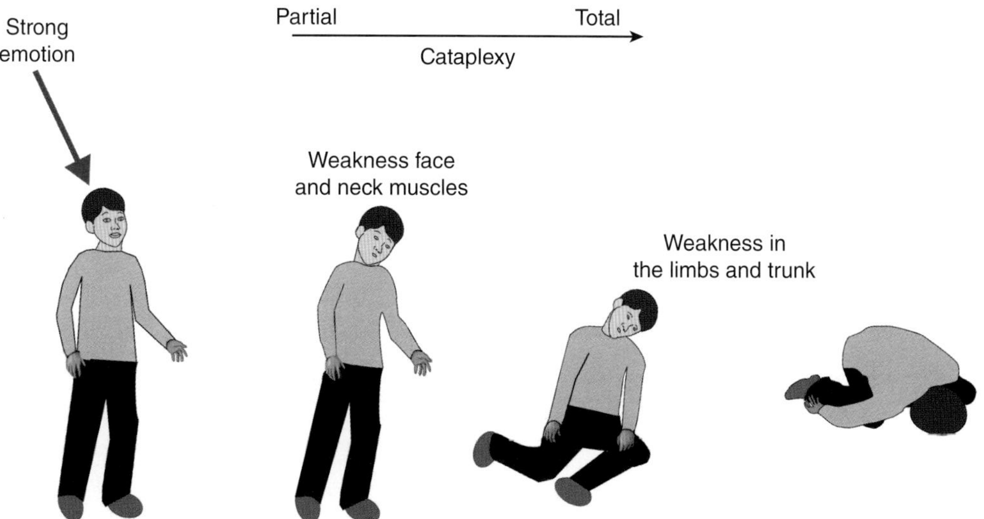

Figure 32-2 Cartoon illustration of cataplexy. Following a strong emotional trigger there can be partial or complete cataplexy. Partial cataplexy can include weakness in the muscles of the face and neck with jaw drop or head bobbing and progress to weakness of the limbs and trunk.

years of the onset of sleepiness (Figure 32-1).[14] Typical cataplexy is bilateral and usually precipitated by positive emotion. However, cataplexy can be asymmetrical, can involve the muscles of the neck (head bobbing) and face (jaw drop), and dysarthria may be noted. The onset of muscle weakness is usually not instantaneous but evolves over a few seconds. Muscle twitching, especially in the face, can also be observed. In children, cataplexy may often be more dramatic, with total loss of postural muscle strength. In children, cataplexy can be the first symptoms of narcolepsy and is not always associated with an emotional trigger. *During cataplexy, deep tendon reflexes (DTRs) are absent.* Sudden withdrawal of a medication that suppresses cataplexy can result in nearly continual bouts of cataplexy (status cataplecticus). Overeem and coworkers[17] performed a survey of symptoms triggering cataplexy (Box 32-1) and found that not just laughing, but excitedly laughing was the most common precipitating emotion. Anic-Labat and coworkers[18] found that cataplexy was best differentiated from other types of muscle weakness when triggered by only three typical situations: "when hearing and telling a joke," "while laughing," or "when angry." The Swiss Narcolepsy Scale and other questionnaires have been used to help clinicians identify patients with narcolepsy.[19] Features of typical, atypical, and unlikely cataplexy are listed in Table 32-3. Typical cataplexy is used to confidently make a diagnosis of NT1 (if other criteria are met and a CSF hypocretin-1 level is not available).

3. **Sleep-related hallucinations**[3-5] are vivid, often bizarre, dreamlike images associated with sleep onset (hypnagogic) or awakening (hypnopompic). The patient often is aware that the images are not real but is still frightened by them. A commonly described vision is an animal or stranger in the room. The hallucinations can be associated with sleep paralysis (SP). Sleep-related hallucinations can also occur in normal individuals and patients with idiopathic hypersomnia. Sleep-related hallucinations can have visual and auditory components.

Box 32-1 CATAPLEXY CHARACTERISTICS

- Emotional trigger (but not always)
- Brief seconds to minutes (15% last longer than 2 minutes)
- Preserved consciousness
- Bilateral > unilateral
- Weakness in legs, sagging to the floor, or falls
- Neck muscle weakness – head bobbing, jaw drop, eye-lid droop
- "Partial attacks" (30%) more common in jaw and face
- "Partial" and "complete" attacks in 45%
- 60% report some spontaneous attacks (no emotion trigger more common in children)
- Children – "cataplectic facies" (repetitive mouth opening, tongue protrusion, and ptosis).
- Complete return of muscle strength after event
- Absent deep tendon reflexes during the event

Triggers (Descending Order of Frequency)

1. Laughing excitedly
2. Making a sharp minded remark
3. Telling a joke
4. Before reaching punch line of a joke
5. Being tickled
6. Hearing a joke
7. Angry
8. Unexpectedly meeting someone well known
9. Being startled
10. Tickling someone
11. Laughing
12. Chuckling
13. Experiencing an orgasm
14. Being the center of attention
15. Expectedly meeting someone well known
16. Unexpectedly meeting an acquaintance
17. Feeling stressed
18. Feeling ashamed
19. Hearing an unexpected sound
20. Spontaneously
21. In the waiting room at the doctor
22. Hearing an expected sound
23. While eating
24. In pain

Adapted from Overeem S, van Nues SJ, van der Zande WL, Donjacour CE, van Mierlo P, Lammers GJ. The clinical features of cataplexy: a questionnaire study in narcolepsy patients with and without hypocretin-1 deficiency. *Sleep Med.* 2011;12(1):12-18. PMID: 21145280.

Table 32-3 Typical, Atypical, and Doubtful Cataplexy

Factor	Typical Cataplexy	Atypical Cataplexy	Doubtful Cataplexy
Inciting emotion	Most attacks precipitated by an emotion Most often positive emotion	Absence of clear precipitants or always negative emotion Never precipitated by a positive emotion (laughing, mirth, joking)	Almost never with precipitating emotion (but common in young children)
Consciousness	Present at least at the start (can lapse into sleep)	Uncertain level of conscious ness	Unconscious from the start of the episode
Duration of episodes	Seconds to <2 minutes	>3 minutes duration in adults	>10 minutes unless continued precipitant
HLA-DBQ1*602	Present	Not present or unknown	Not present
Bilateral weakness	Usually bilateral, can be asymmetrical	Always unilateral	Fatigue, impaired mood, drained
Cataplexy severity	Partial and total	Most always total	Total but vague manifestations
Onset	Slow build up Total episodes usually start in the neck and build up over several seconds	Hyperacute generalized weakness	Prolonged build up
Recovery time	Quick	Prolonged	Hours
Warning sensation	None	Usually none	Aura, nausea

4. **Sleep paralysis** (SP)[3-5] can be either partial or complete and usually is noted on awakening. The affected individual is awake but cannot move. SP can occur with sleep-related hallucinations. The diaphragm and extraocular muscles are not paralyzed. However, a patient may experience dyspnea. SP is experienced on at least one or two occasions in a large fraction of the normal population, and recurrent SP can occur in the absence of narcolepsy (isolated recurrent SP). SP is also reported in patients with idiopathic hypersomnia.
5. **Other symptoms**: Other manifestation frequently associated with narcolepsy include poor nocturnal sleep (increased stage N1), automatic behavior (performing a seemingly purposeful task without memory of having preformed the activity), periodic limb movement syndrome (PLMS) (both non-REM [NREM] and REM sleep),[20] and the REM sleep behavior disorder.[21] PLMS during REM sleep is rare in most individuals but common in patients with narcolepsy.[20] REM sleep behavior disorder can be present in patients with narcolepsy[21] but is not thought to be associated with risk of a future neurodegenerative disorder. Obesity and weight gain around the time of symptom onset is seen in NT1.[4,5]

History of Narcolepsy

The key symptoms of narcolepsy were described by Westphal in 1877.[22] The term *narcolepsy*, meaning "to seize with drowsiness," was coined by Gelinau.[22] Aidie termed the loss of muscle tone as "cataplexy" in the early 20th century.[23,24] Yoss and Daly[25] described the classic tetrad of daytime sleepiness, cataplexy, hypnogogic hallucinations, and SP. In 1960, Vogel[26] reported that SOREMPs were associated with narcolepsy. Initially, the association of narcolepsy with the human leukocyte antigen (HLA) DR2 antigen was described in Japanese patients.[27] In 1997, HLA-DQB1*602 was found to be strongly associated with narcolepsy in white and African American populations.[28] In 1998, two groups simultaneously reported the existence of hypocretin (orexin) peptides in the lateral and posterior hypothalamus.[8,9] In 2000, the association of narcolepsy with cataplexy and low or undetectable levels of CSF hypocretin-1 was first described.[10]

Epidemiology

Narcolepsy is present in about 1/2000 persons. Approximately 60% to 70% of patients with narcolepsy have cataplexy[4,5,14,29,30] *Men and women are affected equally*. The average age of onset in most studies is between 20 and 30 years. However, narcolepsy can begin at any age. Dauvilliers and coworkers[30] found two peaks in the age of onset, with one around 15 years of age and the other around 35 years of age. Okun et al.[14] found a single peak at about 15 years of age. Daytime sleepiness usually appears before cataplexy. Cataplexy typically follows within 3 years of the onset of daytime sleepiness.

Genetics

Familial canine narcolepsy is transmitted as a single autosomal recessive gene (canarc-1) with complete penetrance.[31] This form of narcolepsy is caused by an abnormal hypocretin-2 receptor. However, the human form of narcolepsy is not a simple genetic disease. Although the majority of cases of human narcolepsy are sporadic, there have been numerous reports of familial narcolepsy in the literature.[31,32] Studies of families of patients with narcolepsy revealed that the risk of a first-degree relative of a narcoleptic developing NT1 is 1% to 2%, a 10 to 40 times higher risk than in the general population.[31] However, studies of identical twins show a high degree of discordance for NT1. That is, if one twin has narcolepsy, the other twin will have or develop narcolepsy only about 25% to 31% of the time[31] (Table 32-4). Thus, factors other than genetics are important for the development of human narcolepsy. Polymorphisms in the vicinity of the hypocretin/orexin gene are not associated with narcolepsy.[33] Genetic variants for T-cell receptors have been found and would be consistent with an autoimmune etiology of narcolepsy.[34] In summary, the development of hypocretin-deficient narcolepsy is believed to be associated with autoimmune and genetic predisposition;

Table 32-4 Narcolepsy Facts

Incidence of Narcolepsy	
General Population	1/2000
Identical twin has narcolepsy with cataplexy.	Other twin has narcolepsy 25–31% of the time.
First-degree relative has narcolepsy.	1–2% (10–40 × higher risk).
HLA - DQB1*0602 Positive	
General population	12–38% Caucasian (25%), Asian (12%), Black (38%)
NT1	90% (≥10% negative).
NT2	40–60%
CSF Hypocretin-1	
NT1 (N+C)	Absent or low 90–100%
NT2 (N–C)	80-85% normal levels, 15-20% reduced levels*,**
Unusual Testing Circumstances	
Diagnosis NT2 then patient develops Cataplexy	Change diagnosis to NT1
Diagnosis NT2 then CSF Hypocretin-1 measured and is low (most positive for DQB1*0602	Change diagnosis to NT1
• Diagnosis NT1 (Typical cataplexy plus PSG/ MSLT meets criteria) • CSF Hypocretin-1 level measured and NOT low	Keep diagnosis of NT1***

*If low CSF-Hypocretin-1 level is known, diagnosis changed to NT1.
**(most + for DQB1*0602)
***Still considered of NT1 in ICSD-3-TR[3]
CSF, cerebrospinal fluid; *HLA*, human leukocyte antigen; *N+C* = narcolepsy with cataplexy; *N–C* = narcolepsy without cataplexy.

this, coupled with an antigen challenge (infection or vaccine), may trigger an immune response and damage to the cells in the hypothalamus that make hypocretin.

Human Leukocyte Antigen Typing

NT1 is strongly linked to specific HLAs. Approximately 90% to 95% of patients with NT1 have the DQB1*0602 allele, regardless of race[28] (Table 32-4). Nearly all patients with typical cataplexy and a low CSF hypocretin-1 level are positive for HLA-DQB1*0602. A low CSF hypocretin-1 in an HLA-negative patient is rare (1/500 cases). However, *the presence of this antigen is not diagnostic for narcolepsy*. This allele is present in about 12% of Japanese, 25% of whites, and 38% of African Americans without narcolepsy. In this discussion, HLA+ and HLA– refer to patients with and without the presence of the DQB1*0602 antigen, respectively. The percentage of NT2 patients positive for DQB1*0602 is lower (40–60%). In general, patients with narcolepsy who are DQB1*0602 positive have more severe symptoms.[4,5] A positive test for DQB1*0602 is not very helpful given that the allele is present in a significant proportion of the normal population. The results of HLA typing are useful when a spinal tap is contemplated to assess hypocretin-1 values. If the patient is DQB1*0602 negative, hypocretin-1 levels are most likely normal (procedure not indicated). Of note, patients with a low CSF hypocretin-1 level but without cataplexy are usually positive for the DQB1*0602 antigen.

Hypocretin Levels

Hypocretin-1 levels of the CSF can be assayed at a few centers. In patients with NT1 (N+C), over 90% have very low or undetectable hypocretin-1 levels (Figure 32-3). In one study of patients with many neurologic diseases, only patients with NT1 (N+C) and a few patients with Guillain-Barré syndrome had undetectable hypocretin levels.[35-40] Patients with a number of neurologic diseases had levels that were lower than normal but still detectable. There is small subset of patients with cataplexy and a PSG/MSLT meeting criteria for NT1 who are found to have a normal hypocretin level. They are still classified as NT1.[3] As noted patients with NT2 (no cataplexy) usually have a normal CSF hypocretin-1 level. However, CSF hypocretin-1 levels have not been measured in most patients with NT2. Some patient without cataplexy are found to have low CSF hypocretin-1 levels but the exact percentage of NT2 patients that are hypocretin deficient is unknown. It is estimated that 15-20% of NT2 patients have a low CSF hypocretin-1 level. However, estimates are based on research studies of selected populations and the percentage is likely lower than 15% in routine clinical populations. If low CSF hypocretin-1 is found in a patient with a diagnosis of NT2, the diagnosis is changed to NT1. Most of these patients with a low CSF hypocretin-1 without cataplexy are positive for the HLA-DBQ1*0602.[35-40]

IMPORTANCE OF HYPOCRETIN NEURONS

Orexin-A (hypocretin-1) signals through both types of orexin receptors (OX1R and OX2R), whereas orexin-B signals mainly through OX2R.[41] Hypocretin neurons located in the lateral hypothalamus project widely in the CNS (Figure 32-4). They augment the activity of brain areas active during wakefulness, including the tuberomammillary nucleus (histamine), the locus coeruleus (norepinephrine), and the dorsal raphe (serotonin).[41-43] The activity of hypocretin neurons is believed to stabilize the sleep-wakefulness system to prevent abrupt transitions between sleep and wakefulness. For example, histaminergic neurons are located exclusively in the tuberomammillary nucleus (TMN) of the posterior hypothalamus and project to various brain regions associated with regulation of sleep-wakefulness cycles. Activity of these histaminergic neurons is believed to help promote wakefulness. Hypocretin neurons project to the TMN and stimulate the TMN neurons via hypocretin-2 receptors.[44] For further discussion of the neurobiology of wakefulness and sleep, please see Chapter 8.

Pathophysiology of Narcolepsy

NT1 Group

Canine narcolepsy with cataplexy is usually secondary to a defect in the receptor for hypocretin-2. Human NT1 is associated with absent or very low CSF levels of hypocretin-1 (90–100% of patients).[35-40] The brains of patients with NT1 have reduced staining for hypocretin in the hypothalamus consistent with loss of hypocretin secreting neurons.[45-47] NT1 is associated with loss of approximately 90% of hypocretin neurons (Figure 32-5). Melanin-concentrating hormone neurons, which are

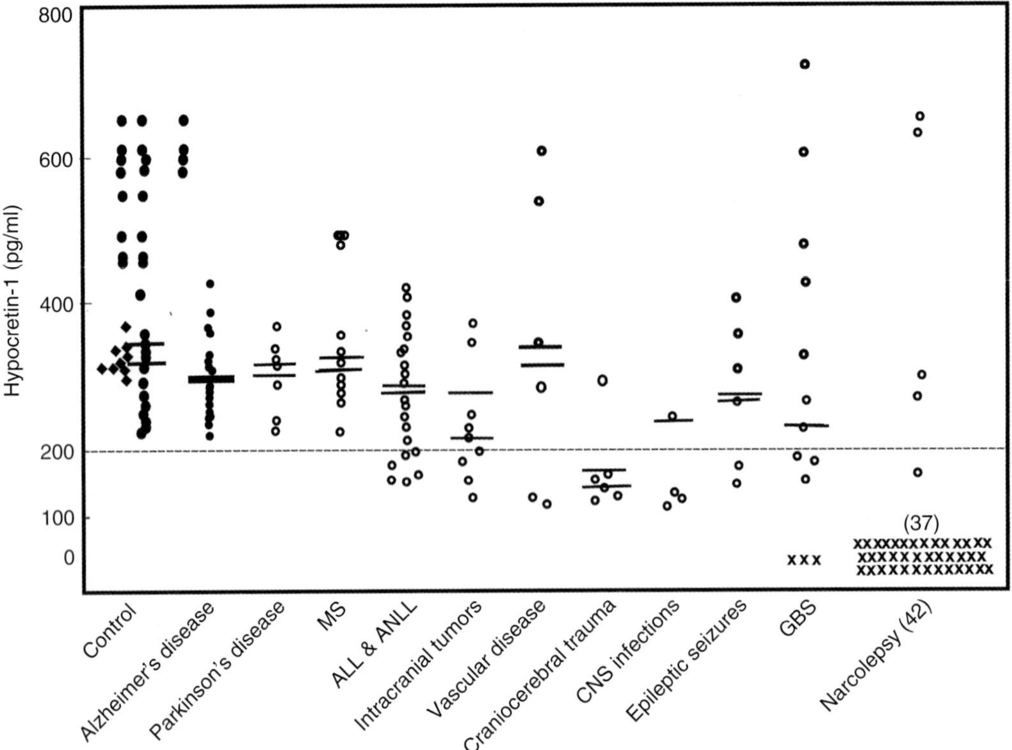

Figure 32-3 CSF hypocretin levels for patients with various diseases and narcolepsy. The ICSD-3-TR criteria for reduced hypocretin levels are a value ≤110 pg/ml or a value less than one-third of the mean values obtained in normal subjects with the same standardized assay. Thick bars represent mean values and thin bars represent median values. *MS*, multiple sclerosis; *ALL/ANLL*, acute lymphocytic leukemia and non-lymphocytic leukemia; *GBS*, Guillain-Barre syndrome. Control subjects that were tapped at night (6:00 PM to 2:00 AM) are indicated with diamonds. The dashed line is the hypocretin-1 cutoff level for abnormally low levels in this study. Here "x" means hypocretin-1 level less than 100 pg/ml considered non-detectable. In the individuals with narcolepsy 37/42 (88%) had undetectable levels and one individual had a a low level. (Adapted from Ripley BN, Overeem S, Fujiki N, et al. CSF hypocretin/orexin levels in narcolepsy and other neurological conditions. *Neurology*. 2001;57:2253-2258. PMID: 11756606.)

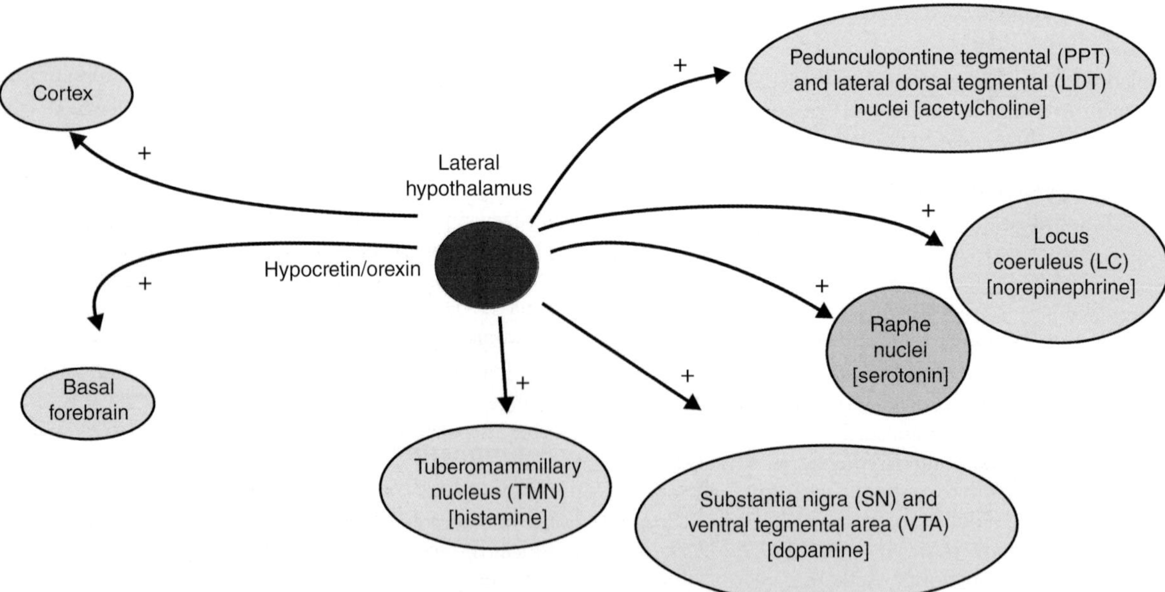

Figure 32-4 A summary of brain areas receiving stimulation by hypocretin/orexin neurons. Hypocretin-secreting neurons in the lateral hypothalamus innervate and excite multiple brain areas important for arousal and maintenance of wakefulness. Areas important for maintaining wakefulness receive facilitation. These included the tuberomammillary nucleus (TMN), the locus coeruleus (LC), dorsal raphe (DR), basal forebrain (BF), pedunculopontine tegmentum and lateral dorsal tegmentum (PPT/LDT), and substantia nigra/ventral tegmental area (SN/VTA).

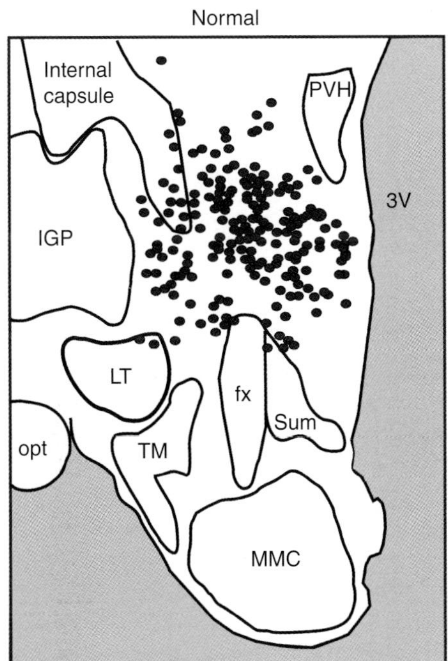

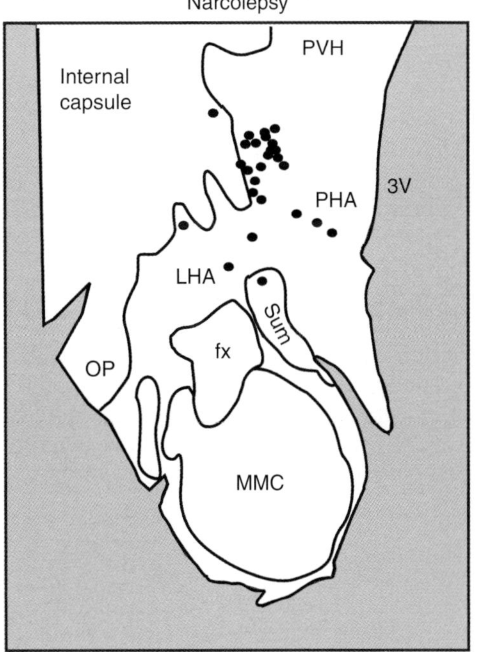

Figure 32-5 Sections of the hypothalamus in a normal individual and a patient with narcolepsy. Hypocretin staining cells on the left are numerous. In the patient with narcolepsy, most hypocretin cells have been destroyed. This is believed to be mediated by an autoimmune process. *3V*, third ventricle; *fx*, fornix; *IGP*, internal globus pallidus; *LHA* and *PHA*, lateral and posterior hypothalamic areas; *LT*, lateral tubercle nucleus; *MMC*, mamillary nucleus; *opt*, optic tract; *PVH*, paraventricular hypothalamus; *SUM*, supramammillary nucleus; *TM*, tuberomammillary nucleus. (Adapted from Crocker A, España RA, Papadopoulou M, et al. Concomitant loss of dynorphin, NARP, and orexin in narcolepsy. *Neurology*. 2005;65(8):1184-1188. PMID: 16247044.)

intermixed with hypocretin cells in the normal brain, are not reduced in number, indicating cell loss is relatively specific for hypocretin neurons. It is believed that hypothalamic hypocretin cells are destroyed before disease onset. Mutations in hypocretin genes do not appear to be the cause of most human narcolepsy.[33] *As mentioned, up to 10% of patients with NT1 have normal CSF hypocretin-1 levels although otherwise meeting diagnostic criteria for NT1.*[35-40] Thus, other abnormalities of the hypocretin system or other mechanisms must be the cause of the syndrome in these patients. Of note, these patients would not strictly meet criteria for NT1 (reduced hypocretin, if known) or NT2 (requires absent cataplexy). *However, they are classified as a variant of NT1.*[3] This issue illustrates the ambiguity in the current system for classifying narcolepsy.

The cause of the loss of hypocretin cells in patients with narcolepsy with cataplexy is unknown. Because of the association of narcolepsy with specific HLA antigens, an autoimmune mechanism has been hypothesized but difficult to document.[7,48-50] For example, the recent onset of NT1 was associated with elevated antistreptococcal antibodies.[51] A detailed discussion of the evidence for an autoimmune cause of narcolepsy is beyond the scope of this chapter but is discussed in detail in the reference by Mahonney et al.[7] The most direct evidence that NT1 can be caused by an autoimmune process occurred with the H1N1 influenza pandemic in the winter of 2009–2010. Clinicians noticed a surge in individuals developing NT1 after vaccination with Pandemrix, a brand of flu vaccine mainly used in northern Europe. Pandemrix inoculation was associated with an 8- to 12-fold increase in new cases of NT1 in children and adolescents and a 3- to 5-fold increase in adults.[52,53] Importantly, all these affected individuals carried the HLA allele DQB1*0602 and developed NT1 a few weeks to months after vaccination. Another study found that narcolepsy was also associated with a polymorphism in the T-cell receptor alpha gene.[54] Several studies have found that some patients with narcolepsy have elevated levels of antibodies against a protein known as Tribbles homolog 2 (TRIB2).[7] However, this protein is not unique to hypocretin-producing cells. Currently, autoimmune destruction of the hypocretin cells is believed to be mediated by killer T cells, and the antigen triggering the attack may be hypocretin itself, as the antigen differentiating these cells from others is the presence of the hypocretin proteins. Genetic polymorphisms in T-cell receptors may predispose an individual to react abnormally. The autoimmune attack can be triggered by bacterial or viral infections or immunization.

Recall that histamine neurons in the tuberomammillary nucleus are active during wakefulness. Destruction of histamine-producing areas does not eliminate wakefulness in animals. However, maintaining wakefulness during motivational states appears to require histamine.[44] The number of histamine-secreting neurons maybe increased in narcolepsy with cataplexy (NT1),[55] but CNS levels of histamine in patients with narcolepsy[44] appear to be normal. Initial studies found CSF histamine to be low in patients with narcolepsy and others with hypersomnia,[56,57] but this was ***not*** confirmed by later studies of large groups with a sensitive assay.[58] Although cataplexy and the atonia of REM sleep share some common pathways, there are differences. In contrast to REM sleep, during attacks of cataplexy, *TMN neurons have a high firing rate associated with preservation of consciousness.*[59] The pathophysiology of cataplexy will be discussed later in this chapter.

NT2 Group

The pathophysiology of NT2 is not well understood. A small percentage (15 to 20%) of patients with NT2 have reduced CSF hypocretin levels (most are positive for HLA-DQB1*0602). These patients would be classified as NT1. Patients with NT2 who are negative for HLA-DQB1*0602 almost always have normal CSF hypocretin-1 levels.[35-40] The etiology of NT2 is currently unknown but may represent a dysfunction of the hypocretin system without total loss of hypocretin-producing cells. Thannickal and coworkers examined portions of two brains of patients with NT2 and found a 33% reduction in hypocretin cells, with the loss confined to the posterior hypothalamus.[60] Thus, partial loss of hypocretin neurons and other alterations in the hypocretin system without a reduction in CSF hypocretin could be the etiology of excessive sleepiness in NT2. Loss of hypocretin secreting cells has also been described in Parkinson's Disease.

Mechanisms of Cataplexy

The mechanisms inducing cataplexy are still under investigation.[7,42,61] The atonia of REM sleep is thought to be caused by inhibition of the spinal alpha motor neurons of the anterior horn cells by glycine and gamma-aminobutyric acid (GABA) secreted by spinal interneurons or premotor neurons in the ventromedial medulla (Figure 32-6). The interneurons are activated directly by projections from areas in the pons responsible for atonia or via an intermediate relay area in the ventral medulla. Glutamate is believed to activate the spinal interneurons that produce GABA and glycine. In some references, the term *premotor neuron* is used instead of interneuron. The atonia neurons of the pontine reticular formation are located ventral to the locus coeruleus and are often called the subcoeruleus (SubC) or sublaterodorsal nucleus (SLD). The neurons are believed to be glutaminergic. During REM sleep, there also appears to be inhibition of pathways normally promoting alpha motor neuron activity (e.g., from the locus coeruleus).

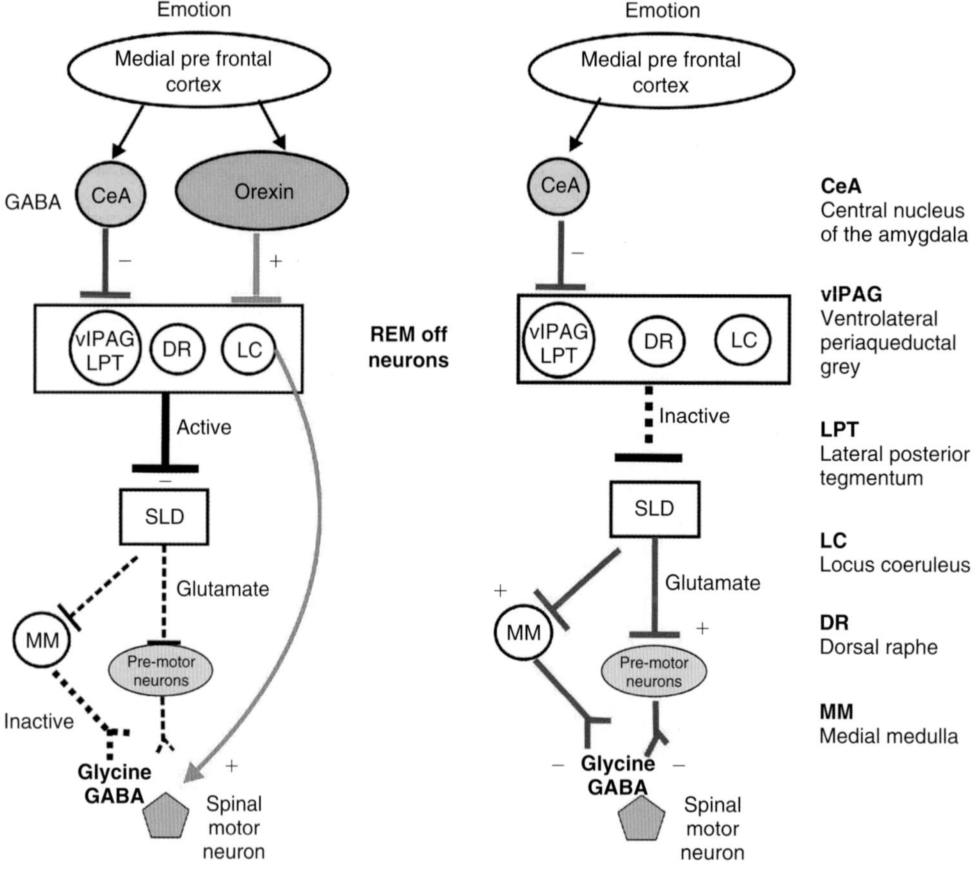

Figure 32-6 Proposed mechanism of cataplexy. Strong emotion excites both neurons in the central nucleus of the amygdala (CeA) and orexin neurons. Innervation from the CeA inhibits brain areas important for wakefulness, including the locus coeruleus (LC), dorsal raphe (DR), and REM-off neurons in the ventrolateral periaqueductal grey (vlPAG) and lateral pontine tegmentum (LPT). These neurons inhibit the atonia-producing neurons in the pons (sublateral dorsal nucleus, SLD). However, this inhibition is balanced by stimulation from orexin neurons. In narcolepsy, the balancing influence of orexin is absent, and atonia-producing neurons are activated by emotion, resulting in depolarization of motor neurons by GABA and glycine. The pathways are either direct from the SLD to premotor (interneurons) or indirectly through medial medulla neurons (MM). (Based on information and figures from Mahoney CE, Cogswell A, Koralnik IJ, Scammell TE. The neurobiological basis of narcolepsy. *Nat Rev Neurosci.* 2019;20(2):83-93. PMID: 30546103.)

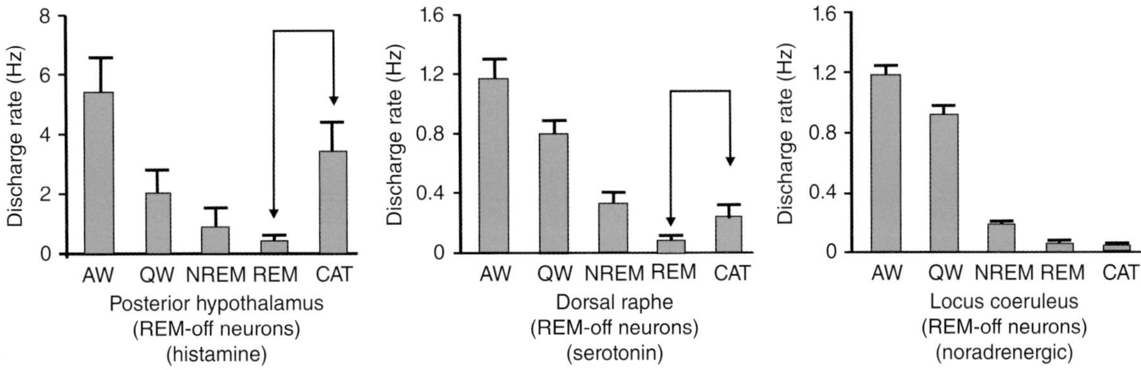

Figure 32-7 This figure shows activity of several important brain areas during active wakefulness (AW), quiet wakefulness (QW), NREM sleep, REM sleep, and episodes of cataplexy (CAT). The pattern during CAT is different from that during REM sleep. Histamine neurons in the tuberomammillary nucleus in the posterior hypothalamus remain active during cataplexy compared to those during REM sleep and help preserve consciousness during cataplexy attacks. (From John J, Wu MF, Boehmer LN, Siegel JM. Cataplexy-active neurons in the hypothalamus: implications for the role of histamine in sleep and waking behavior. *Neuron*. 2004;42(4):619-634. PMID: 15157423.)

Although cataplexy is often considered a manifestation of atonia associated with REM sleep, as mentioned, there are important differences. John and colleagues[59] reported that histaminergic neurons in the ventral posterior lateral hypothalamus remain active during cataplexy as opposed to REM sleep (Figure 32-7). Because histamine is associated with wakefulness, this may at least partially explain why patients remain conscious during cataplexy but not during REM sleep. Signaling from the dorsal raphe serotonin nucleus area is reduced in cataplexy but not to the same degree as during REM sleep. The other important difference between REM-associated atonia and cataplexy is the triggering emotional stimulus for cataplexy. The current theory[7,42,61] is that, during wakefulness, orexin stimulation of the REM-off neurons in the ventrolateral periaqueductal grey (vlPAG), lateral posterior tegmental area (LPT), locus coeruleus (norepinephrine), and dorsal raphe (serotonin) results in inhibition of the atonia-producing SLD area. Emotion acting through the medial prefrontal cortex and GABA neurons in the central nucleus of the amygdala inhibits the REM-off neurons. However, because of orexin stimulation, this inhibition is balanced, and no atonia is generated. In patients with narcolepsy lacking orexin, the sudden inhibition of REM-off areas allows the SLD neurons to be active and generate atonia. Other mechanisms may also be important for causing attacks of cataplexy. Of note, medications that increase serotonin and norepinephrine signaling have anticataleptic activity. The reason sodium oxybate reduces cataplexy is unknown. However, reductions in cataplexy take weeks to reach peak effect, so chronic changes induced by the medication are likely needed.

Diagnosis of Narcolepsy

History

Patients being evaluated for daytime sleepiness should be questioned about the severity and nature of their sleepiness, the age of onset, their normal sleep duration, medications, and the presence of cataplexy, sleep hallucinations, and SP. Concerning possible cataplexy, the patient should be questioned about typical triggers, the nature of muscle weakness, and the duration of the episodes. Daytime naps are often refreshing in patients with narcolepsy. In contrast, naps are not commonly refreshing in many patients with idiopathic hypersomnia.[3]

Polysomnography in Narcolepsy

The nocturnal sleep study is used to rule out other significant sleep disorders (sleep apnea) that might explain daytime sleepiness. Nocturnal PSG often reveals a short sleep latency and impaired sleep quality with increased stage N1 sleep and decreased stage N3 sleep. The total sleep time may be reduced, but the amount of REM sleep is usually normal.[4,5,62,63] Patients with narcolepsy usually have a near normal or slightly increased amount of 24-hour sleep, but their sleep is spread over 24 hours and is characterized by multiple transitions between wakefulness, sleep, and REM sleep (Figure 32-8).

On average, patients with NT1 have lower sleep efficiency, lower amounts of stage N3 sleep, more stage N1 sleep, and more awakenings than those with NT2.[4,5] Periodic limb movements in sleep (PLMS) is common in patients with narcolepsy.[20] However, the occurrence of PLMS is less common during REM sleep in most patients. Patients with narcolepsy may have a significant amount of periodic limb movements during REM sleep.[20] Aldrich and colleagues[64] found that 33% of patients with NT1 (N+C), 24% of patients with NT2 (N–C), and 1% of patients with sleep-related breathing disorder (SRBD) had a SOREMP on nocturnal PSG. Of interest, the finding of a nocturnal SOREMP + nocturnal sleep latency less than 10 minutes had a specificity of 98.9% and a positive predictive value of 73% (true positive/total number of positives) for the diagnosis of narcolepsy. Therefore, although a minority of patients with narcolepsy have a nocturnal SOREMP on a given PSG, the finding is highly suggestive of narcolepsy. This is especially true if no other factor is present to explain the short REM latency such as depression, obstructive sleep apnea (OSA), recent withdrawal of REM-suppressing medication, or sleep deprivation. Andlauer et al.,[13] using NT1 confirmed with a low CSF hypocretin level or a history of typical cataplexy + the presence of HLA-DBQ1*602, found that about 50% of patients with narcolepsy had a nocturnal SOREMP, and the presence of a nocturnal SOREMP had a high positive predictive value for NT1 narcolepsy. The higher percentage of nocturnal SOREMPs than in the study by Aldrich et al. is likely a result of more stringent diagnostic criteria for identification of patients with NT1. The presence of a PSG SOREMP in a patient with OSA is extremely unlikely if narcolepsy is not present. After treatment of OSA, evaluation for

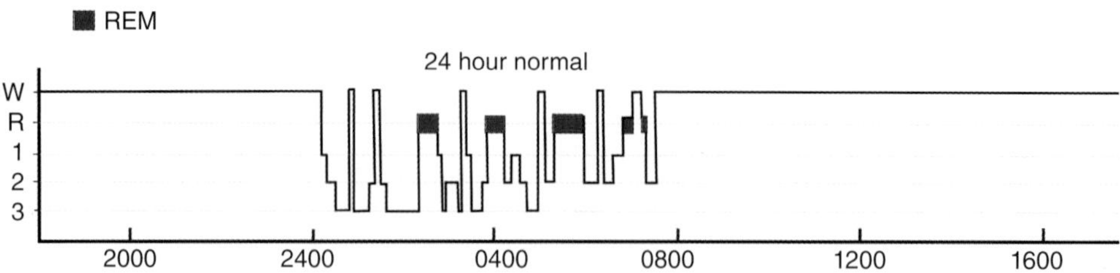

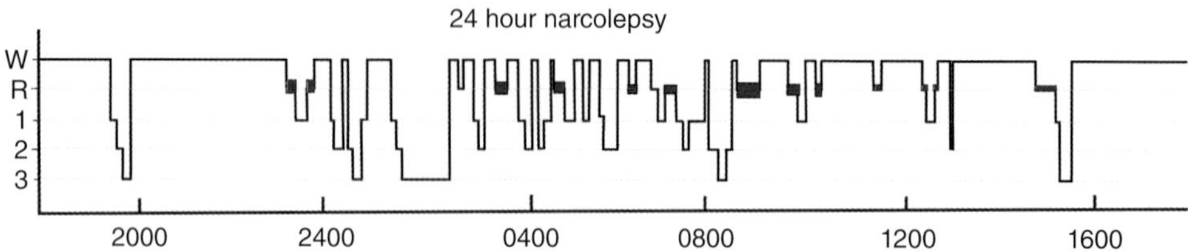

Figure 32-8 Hypnograms (plots of sleep stage vs. time) of a normal individual top and a patient with narcolepsy on the bottom. The patient with narcolepsy has frequent transitions between wakefulness, NREM sleep, and REM sleep that occur during the entire 24-hour period. (Adapted from Rogers AE, Aldrich MS, Caruso CC. Patterns of sleep and wakefulness in treated narcolepsy subjects. *Sleep.* 1994;17:590-597. PMID: 7846456.)

narcolepsy should be performed if daytime sleepiness is persistent or if typical cataplexy is present. As noted in the study by Aldrich et al.,[64] only 1% of patients with sleep-disordered breathing had a nocturnal SOREMP.

PSG/MSLT Criteria for Diagnosis of Narcolepsy

Use of the MSLT for diagnosis of narcolepsy is discussed in detail in Chapter 17. For proper interpretation, the MSLT is preceded by PSG that does not demonstrate another sleep disorder believed to cause abnormal MSLT findings. A *minimum of 360 minutes of sleep* should be recorded (preferably more). Medications that can affect sleep (including REM sleep) and alertness should be withdrawn for 2 weeks (or 5 half-life intervals) prior to testing. In the 2 weeks prior to the MSLT, the patient should have a normal sleep schedule and adequate sleep (>7 hours per night), ideally documented by actigraphy (or sleep log if actigraphy is not available). The criteria for a *positive PSG/MSLT for NT1* require either a PSG SOREMP or a mean sleep latency ≤8 minutes and two or more SOREMPs on the MSLT. The criteria for a positive MSLT for the diagnosis of NT2 are a mean sleep latency ≤8 minutes and two or more SOREMPs on an MSLT. A SOREMP on PSG (nocturnal REM latency ≤15 minutes) can be used as one of the two SOREMPs for the diagnosis of NT2. The MSLT is not 100% sensitive[11] for narcolepsy, and false negatives can occur 10% to 30% of the time, depending on the population studied and the criteria used as the gold standard for diagnosis of narcolepsy. A repeat MSLT may be needed if there is high clinical suspicion of narcolepsy and initial testing does not meet diagnostic criteria.[65] However, studies have shown that MSLT results are repeatable in NT1 but not NT2.[66,67]

Specific Information About NT1

The manifestations of NT1 generally begin between the ages of 15 and 30 years.[4,14-16] However, this form of narcolepsy can be present in the pediatric age group or in patients older than 60 years. Excessive daytime sleepiness alone or in combination with sleep hallucination and/or SP is the presenting symptom in approximately 90% of patients.[13,14] Cataplexy may develop several years after symptoms begin. However, most patients with NT1 develop cataplexy within 3 to 5 years of the onset of daytime sleepiness. As noted, cataplexy can rarely precede daytime sleepiness in adults. Presentation of cataplexy before sleepiness is more common in pediatric narcolepsy.[16]

Nearly all NT1 patients will have symptoms of cataplexy and are positive for HLA- DQB1*0602. A rare exception is a patient with a low CSF hypocretin-1 level and absent cataplexy (still classified as NT1 if other criteria are met). In clinical practice, this is a very rare occurrence, as most patients will not have a CSF hypocretin-1 level available. As noted, in the ICSD-3-TR, *the presence of sleepiness and a history of cataplexy alone are not sufficient for a diagnosis of NT1.* The rationale is avoiding over diagnosis given the uncertainly of determining whether true cataplexy is present. If the PSG/MSLT does not meet criteria for narcolepsy, the studies could be repeated.[3,65] If a patient is negative for the DQB1*0602 antigen, a history of cataplexy should be considered doubtful given the fact that virtually 100% of patients with a low CSF hypocretin level and cataplexy are positive for this antigen. If a patient has atypical cataplexy and a negative MSLT, determining the CSF hypocretin-1 level is an option. However, obtaining a CSF sample in a patient negative for HLA-DQB1*0602 is not indicated, as the CSF hypocretin-1 level will almost always be normal. In cases where withdrawal of REM suppressing medications is problematic and an initial PSG/MSLT does not meet diagnostic criteria, obtaining a CSF hypocretin 1 level if the patient is positive for HLA-DQB1*0602 is an option. Patients with NT1 tend to have lower mean sleep latency and more SOREMPs than patients with NT2. The PSG will often show increased stage N1, and there is a tendency of obesity. In some series, SP and hypnagogic hallucinations were more common in NT1 than in NT2.[4,5]

There are two variants of NT1 listed in the ICSD-3-TR.[3] The first is NT1 due to a Medical Condition (NT1-DMC). The medical conditions thought to cause NT1 include tumors or lesions (vascular, inflammatory, or infectious) of the hypothalamic area, autoimmune disorders, and anti-Ma2 antibodies. The second variant is NT1 based on excessive *daytime sleepiness and a low CSF hypocretin-1 level but no cataplexy.* It is assumed that cataplexy may occur in the future. Although not listed as a variant, about *5% to 10% of patients diagnosed with NT1 based on cataplexy and a PSG/MSLT meeting criteria for narcolepsy have a normal hypopcretin-1 level in the CSF. A diagnosis of NT1 is made even if the hypocretin-1 CSF level is not low. There is no known explanation for this finding.* It is possible that other causes of narcolepsy with cataplexy besides hypocretin deficiency exist.

Specific Information About NT2

Patients with NT2 (N–C) exhibit daytime sleepiness in the absence of cataplexy. They can also manifest the other core symptoms of narcolepsy. The diagnosis of NT2 is based on the symptom of *daytime sleepiness* ***for at least 3 months****, absent cataplexy, the presence of PSG/MSLT criteria for narcolepsy,* CSF hypocretin-1 levels are unavailable or normal, and *hypersomnia and MSLT findings not better explained by insufficient sleep, OSA, delayed sleep-wake phase disorder, or the use of medications or substances (or their withdrawal).* One study by Andlauer and coworkers found that 24% of a sample of patients with with N–C that were HLA-DBQ1*602 positive had low CSF hypocretin levels.[68] However, this was a selected population seen at a research center, and most studies suggest that only 15% to 20% of patients with N–C have low hypocretin. Nearly all patients with N–C with low CSF hypocretin-1 are DQB1*0602 positive. It is presumed that some of these patients will develop cataplexy in the following years. The study by Andlauer and coworkers[68] compared patients with NT2 (N–C) and normal CSF hypocretin-1 levels with NT2 patients with low levels. Those with low CSF hypocretin-1 levels had higher HLA-DQB1*0602 frequencies, were more frequently non-Caucasians (notably African Americans), and had lower age of onset and longer duration of illness. They also had more frequently short REM sleep latency (≤15 minutes) during PSG (64% vs. 23%), shorter sleep latencies (2.7 ± 0.3 vs. 4.4 ± 0.2 minutes), and more SOREMPs (3.6 ± 0.1 vs. 2.9 ± 0.1 minutes) during the MSLT. As noted, if a low level of CSF hypocretin-1 is present, the patient is still classified as NT1, even in the absence of cataplexy. If a low CSF hypocretin-1 level becomes available in a patient with NT2, the diagnosis is changed to NT1. NT2-DMC is a variant of NT2 in which a medical condition is believed to be the etiology of NT2.

Narcolepsy Due to Medical Condition (NDMC)

Narcolepsy due to a medical condition (NDMC) is a group of disorders also known as secondary or symptomatic narcolepsy (Table 32-5).[1,69-78] In the ICSD-3-TR, these disorders are listed as subtypes of NT1 (NT1-DMC) and NT2 (NT2-DMC). A diagnosis requires that the patient satisfy the diagnostic criteria for either NT1 or NT2 and have a disorder known to be associated with narcolepsy. If a patient has one of these conditions felt to cause daytime sleepiness but the criteria for narcolepsy **are not met**, the diagnosis is *Hypersomnia Due to a Medical Disorder* (HDMD). This assumes a medical condition is causing the daytime sleepiness, such as sleep apnea. The patient must report daytime sleepiness. However, in some of these disorders, the patient is quite debilitated and may not be able to participate in normal diagnostic testing. A low CSF hypocretin-1 level would be acceptable for a diagnosis of NT1-DMC. Patients with classic narcolepsy usually have a normal neurologic examination and no definite pathology on brain imaging. Patients with NDMC often have specific brain pathology or an abnormality on genetic or other testing.[71-73] The conditions associated with NT1 include those damaging the hypothalamus (hypocretin deficiency), including sarcoidosis, tumors,[73] arteriovenous malformations, or cerebrovascular accidents. Multiple sclerosis can also cause NT1. Rare genetic diseases have also been associated with NT1, including Niemann-Pick C disease, Coffin-Lowry syndrome, and perhaps Norrie disease.

Table 32-5 Medical Disorders Causing Narcolepsy Due to Medical Condition (NDMC)

NT1 NDMC

Disorders more likely NT1	Disorders that can cause NT1 but more likely NT2
• Tumors, sarcoidosis, arteriovenous malformations affecting the hypothalamus	• Head trauma
• Multiple sclerosis plaques impairing the hypothalamus	• Myotonic dystrophy
• Paraneoplastic syndrome anti-Ma2 antibodies	• Prader-Willi syndrome
• Neiman-Pick type C disease	• Parkinson disease
• Possibly Coffin-Lowry syndrome	• Multisystem atrophy

NT2 NDMC

- Head trauma
- Myotonic dystrophy
- Prader-Willi syndrome
- Parkinson disease
- Multisystem atrophy

Niemann-Pick C disease[74,75] is a lysosomal storage disease associated with accumulation of cholesterol and glycosphingolipids. The age of onset ranges from the neonatal period to adulthood, but usually the first symptoms occur at 2 to 4 years of age. Progression is relentless, and death usually occurs in the second or third decade.[5,75] Core symptoms are ataxia, dementia, and supranuclear vertical gaze palsy. Other symptoms are spasticity, dystonia, dysarthria, and, in 10% to 20% of cases cataplexy is reported. Vankova et al. found excessive daytime sleepiness in all five evaluated patients with juvenile Niemann-Pick C disease.[74] They measured CSF hypocretin-1 levels in four and found reduced levels in two; one had cataplexy and SOREMPs, and the other had levels in the lower range of normal. The authors suggested that lysosomal storage products in patients with Niemann-Pick C disease impair the function of hypocretin-secreting cells. Hypofunction of these hypocretin neurons is believed to be responsible for sleep abnormalities and cataplexy in Niemann-Pick C disease. Kanbayashi et al. found hypocretin deficiency in a patient with Niemann-Pick C disease and cataplexy.[74] The development of unexplained cataplexy (severe falls with laughter) in a patient with other neurological findings (intellectual deterioration) is a hint that Niemann-Pick disease could be present.[75] Coffin-Lowry syndrome[76] is a rare genetic disorder characterized by craniofacial (head and facial) and skeletal abnormalities, delayed intellectual development, short stature, and hypotonia. Characteristic facial features may include an underdeveloped maxilla (maxillary hypoplasia), a broad nose, protruding nostrils (nares), an abnormally prominent brow, down-slanting eyelid folds (palpebral fissures), widely spaced eyes (hypertelorism), large and low-set ears, and unusually thick eyebrows. Skeletal abnormalities may include kyphoscoliosis, dental abnormalities, and short, hyperextensible, tapered fingers. Other features may include developmental delay, hearing impairment, awkward gait, **stimulus-induced drop episodes**, and heart and kidney involvement. The disorder affects males and females in equal numbers, but symptoms are usually more severe in males. The disorder is caused by a defective gene, *RSK2*, which was found in 1996 on the X chromosome. *The episodes of cataplexy appear to overlap with stimulus-induced drop attacks.* Norrie disease[77,78] is an X-linked recessive disorder characterized by congenital blindness, progressive sensorineural hearing loss, and cognitive impairment. Cataplexy has been described, but it is controversial whether this is really a form of narcolepsy.[78]

A number of disorders can rarely be associated with NT1, although they are more likely to be associated with NT2. These include head trauma, Prader-Willi syndrome (PWS), and myotonic dystrophy (MD). These are discussed in the section on hypersomnia due to a medical disorder (hypersomnia but not meeting criteria for narcolepsy).

Narcolepsy in Children

Approximately 30% to 50% of patients diagnosed with narcolepsy have the onset of symptoms before age 15 (although diagnosis may be delayed) (Box 32-2). A meta-analysis of 235 pediatric cases derived from three studies by Challamel et al.[16] found that 34% of all patients with narcolepsy experienced onset of symptoms before the age of 15, 16% before the age of 10, and 4.5% before the age of 5. Therefore, the onset of narcolepsy before age 5 is considered rare. Detection of excessive sleepiness may be more challenging in children than in adults. It should be noted that normal prepubertal children have a mean sleep latency of around 19 minutes on an MSLT.[79] Therefore, normal prepubertal children are very alert during the day. Excessive sleepiness may manifest itself as a return to taking *daytime naps in a child that previously discontinued napping or as an increase in sleep duration*. In older children, daytime sleepiness may sometimes be manifested as symptoms similar to those of attention deficit hyperactive disorder (ADHD) with irritability, mood swings, and inattentiveness.[80] *Cataplexy is present in about two-thirds of pediatric patients with narcolepsy.*[80] *In children, not all cataplexy is associated with a clearly identifiable emotional trigger.* In one study, 9% of cataplexy appeared before daytime sleepiness in a group of children.[16] Therefore, *cataplexy can sometimes be the first symptom and often the most prominent.* Because cataplexy can be subtle, the examiner may need to ask leading questions about sudden muscle weakness in the lower extremities, neck, facial muscles, or trunk in response to laughter, fright, excitement, anger, or the anticipation of a reward. Cataplexy can be confused with syncope (except the child is awake during an attack of cataplexy) or seizure-like activity. Serra et al.[81] reported on cataplexy in 23 patients diagnosed before the age of 18 years. Forty-three percent of these patients had falls as part of their attacks. During cataplexy, knees, head, and jaw were the most frequently compromised body segments; eyelids, arms, and trunk were less commonly involved. More rarely, blurred vision, slurred speech, irregular breathing, or a sudden loss of smiling were reported. One-third of the sample presented with a previously unrecognized description of cataplexy that they termed "cataplectic facies" *consisting of a state of semipermanent eyelid and jaw weakness (droopy eye lids, mouth open), on which partial or complete cataplectic attacks were superimposed.* This last pattern was often present soon after the onset of the disorder. The usual triggering emotions, such as laughter, joking, or anger, were not always present, especially when close to often abrupt onset of narcolepsy. If cataplexy is the first symptom of narcolepsy, an evaluation of NDMC (secondary narcolepsy) is indicated (including CNS imaging and genetic testing). In one study of children with narcolepsy with cataplexy, the onset of narcolepsy was often associated with the rapid development of obesity. *Obesity is present in up to 25% of cases, and childhood narcolepsy* and nocturnal eating syndrome can be present. *The development of* ***precocious puberty*** *associated with the onset of narcolepsy has also been reported.*

Given the high sleep latency on an MSLT in prepubertal children, there is a concern that using 8 minutes as a cutoff might be too low. Some clinicians consider a mean sleep latency less than 12 minutes to be consistent with daytime sleepiness in children. However, published studies of children with narcolepsy show very short sleep latencies, well below 8 minutes.[80] In children, narcolepsy is often misdiagnosed as epilepsy (cataplexy confused as epileptic seizures), syncope, neuromuscular disorders (muscle weakness), a conversion disorder, ADHD (sleepiness manifested as inattention or irritability), depression (inattention, loss of focus, behavioral problems), or psychosis (when hypnagogic hallucinations are a prominent feature), leading to inappropriate pharmacotherapy and further complications.

Box 32-2 NARCOLEPSY IN CHILDREN

- 30% to 50% of narcolepsy diagnosed before age 15
- Cataplexy in children
  - May be the first symptom of narcolepsy – and often the most severe manifestation
  - Not always associated with emotional trigger
  - **Often associated with falls** (up to 40% of cataplexy attacks in one study)
- NT1 in children can be associated with **rapid weight gain and precocious puberty**
- Obesity in up to 25% of children with narcolepsy
- "Cataplectic facies" – state of semipermanent eyelid and jaw weakness (droopy eye lids, mouth open), on which partial or complete cataplectic attacks were superimposed.
- Prepubertal children – very high mean sleep latency (mean 19), but children with narcolepsy usually have a mean sleep latency (MSL) of ≤5 minutes
- Incorrect diagnosis (rather than cataplexy)
  - Epilepsy (cataplexy confused as epileptic seizures) or syncope
  - Neuromuscular disorders (muscle weakness)
  - Attention deficit hyperactivity disorder (sleepiness manifested an inattention or irritability)
  - Depression (inattention, loss of focus, behavioral problems)
  - Psychosis (when hypnagogic hallucinations are a prominent feature)

Treatment of Narcolepsy

Treatment of narcolepsy addresses (1) sleepiness, (2) cataplexy, (3) sleep-related hallucinations/paralysis, and (4) disturbed

Table 32-6 AASM Clinical Practice Guidelines for Treatment of Central Hypersomnolence

Recommendation	
Narcolepsy – Adults	
(Strong)	(Conditional)
• Modafinil	• Armodafinil
• Pitolisant	• Dextroamphetamine
• Sodium oxybate	• Methylphenidate
• Solriamfetol	
Idiopathic Hypersomnia – Adults	
(Strong)	(Conditional)
• Modafinil	• Clarithromycin
	• Methylphenidate
	• Pitolisant
	• Sodium oxybate
Klein-Levin Syndrome	
(Conditional)	
• Lithium	
Hypersomnia Due to Alpha-Synucleinopathies	
(Conditional)	
• Armodafinil for dementia with Lewy bodies in adults.	
• Modafinil for Parkinson disease	
• Sodium oxybate for Parkinson's disease in adults	
Posttraumatic Hypersomnia	
(Conditional)	
• Modafinil	
• Armodafinil	
Genetic Disorders	
(Conditional)	
• Modafinil for myotonic dystrophy	
Hypersomnia Caused by Brain Tumors, Infections, or Other CNS Lesions	
(Conditional)	
• Modafinil for multiple sclerosis	
Pediatric Patients With Narcolepsy	
(Conditional)	
• Modafinil	
• Sodium oxybate	

From Maski K, Trotti LM, Kotagal S, et al. Treatment of central disorders of hypersomnolence: an American Academy of Sleep Medicine clinical practice guideline. *J Clin Sleep Med.* 2021;17(9):1881-1893.

nocturnal sleep. Note that many of the medications described below can also be used to treat other causes of hypersomnia. The previous American Academy of Sleep Medicine (AASM) guideline for treatment of narcolepsy and other hypersomnias was published in 2007.[82] The 2021 AASM clinical practice guidelines for treatment of central hypersomnia[83,84] are displayed in Table 32-6. In Table 32-7, treatments approved and not approved by the U.S. Food and Drug Administration (FDA) for narcolepsy are listed.

Treatment of Daytime Sleepiness

An initial overview of medications used to treat narcolepsy will be followed by a more detailed discussion of specific medications. Medications FDA approved for treatment of sleepiness associated with narcolepsy (NT1 or NT2) include modafinil and armodafinil (R enantiomer of modafinil, Nuvigil), solriamfetol (Sunosi), certain methylphenidate and amphetamine preparations, pitolisant (Wakix), sodium oxybate (Xyrem), low sodium oxybate salts (Xywav), and extended-release sodium oxybate suspension (Lumryz).[85-90] Xyrem and Xywav are approved for children 7 years of age or older, and Lumryz is approved for adults only at the time of writing. Modafinil, armodafinil, solriamfetol are not FDA approved for use in children. Methylphenidate, amphetamine salts (Adderall), and dextroamphetamine are approved in children and adults. *Of note, only the oxybate medications and pitolisant are also FDA approved for treatment of cataplexy associated with narcolepsy.* A comparison of mediation properties is shown in Table 32-8. Additional information about these medications is shown in Tables 32-9, 32-10, and 32-11. A comprehensive discussion of treatment of sleepiness in sleep apnea provides an excellent review[91] of the medication properties of modafinil, armodafinil, solriamfetol, and pitolisant. Modafinil and armodafinil are alerting agents thought to increase dopamine signaling and are schedule IV medications (refills are allowed).[92] More information on these medications is available in Chapter 22. Armodafinil is the R enantiomer of modafinil and has a longer half-life. A generic formulation of armodafinil is available. Solriamfetol is a dopamine and norepinephrine reuptake inhibitor and is also a schedule IV medication.[93] There is no generic formulation of solriamfetol. Modafinil, armodafinil, and solriamfetol are also FDA approved to treat residual sleepiness in patients with OSA using continuous positive airway pressure (CPAP).[91] Of note, modafinil, armodafinil, solriamfetol, methylphenidate, and amphetamines are not effective treatments for cataplexy. Sodium oxybate and mixed salt oxybates (Xywav) are $GABA_B$ receptor agonists taken at night. The method of action is unknown, but by improving nocturnal sleep, they may improve daytime sleepiness. An extended-release preparation (once nightly), oxybate medication (Lumryz)[88,89,90] has been approved for treatment of daytime sleepiness and cataplexy associated with narcolepsy in adults. The oxybate medications are highly regulated (Risk Evaluation and Management System [REMS] programs) and are schedule III medications with refills. None of the medications used to treat narcolepsy are recommended for use during pregnancy.

Alerting Medications. Modafinil and armodafinil have more limited abuse potential or problems with tolerance or rebound compared with stimulants (amphetamine, methylphenidate). The clinical guideline for treatment of central hypersomnolence[84] recommends modafinil for daytime sleepiness caused by narcolepsy in both adults and children as well as for sleepiness associated with idiopathic hypersomnia, posttraumatic hypersomnia, myotonic dystrophy, and Parkinson's disease. The most common side effects are headache, nausea, dry mouth, and diarrhea. There are important potential drug interactions. Modafinil increases or decreases the hepatic metabolism of multiple medications. Modafinil may reduce the effectiveness of oral contraceptives, and an alternate method of birth control should be added. Modafinil can potentially increase the QT interval indirectly by inhibiting metabolism of certain medications. Citalopram 20 mg/day is the maximum recommended dose for patients taking CYP2C19 inhibitors because of the risk of QT prolongation. Stevens-Johnson syndrome is very rare but a potential severe side effect. Patients should stop the medication at the first sign of

Table 32-7 Treatments for Narcolepsy

Daytime Sleepiness		Cataplexy	
FDA Approved	**Not FDA Approved**	**FDA Approved**	**Not FDA Approved**
• Modafinil** • Armodafinil** • Solriamfetol** • Pitolisant** • Sodium Oxybate* • Low Sodium Oxybate* • Sodium Oxybate Extended Release Suspension** • Dextroamphetamine, Amphetamine salts (Adderall)* • Methylphenidate*	• Most long-acting forms of dextroamphetamine, Amphetamine salts, and methylphenidate	• Sodium Oxybate* • Low Sodium Oxybate*,*** • Sodium Oxybate Extended Release Suspension** • Pitolisant**	• Tricycle Antidepressants • SSRIs (Fluoxetine) • SNRIs (Venlafaxine XR) • NRIs (Atomoxetine)
Other treatments:	• Treatments for cataplexy will also treat sleep paralysis and hypnogogic hallucinations • Treat poor sleep at night with hypnotics if not on an oxybate medication • Scheduled naps • Treat anxiety or depression		

*adults and children age 7 years or older
**adults
***approved for IH in adults
NRI, norepinephrine reuptake inhibitor; *SNRI*, serotonin norepinephrine reuptake inhibitor; *SSRI*, selective serotonin reuptake inhibitor.

Table 32-8 Comparison of Properties of Medications Used to Treat Central Hypersomnia

	Schedule	Mechanism	Metabolism	Drug Interactions	Concerns	Indications
Modafinil (Provigil and Generics) Armodafinil (Nuvigil and generics)	IV	Dopamine reuptake inhibitor	Hepatic	Reduces OCP effectiveness	Headache Nausea, anxiety, Dry mouth, insomnia Skin Rash, rare Stevens-Johnson	FDA approved in adults: EDS-N, EDS-OSA, EDS-Shift work
Solriamfetol (Sunosi)	IV	Dopamine and Norepinephrine reuptake inhibitor	Renal	Use with MAOI contraindicated	Increased HR, BP	FDA approved in adults: EDS-N, EDS-OSA
Pitolisant (Wakix)	No schedule	H3 receptor antagonist inverse agonist	Hepatic	Reduces OCP effectiveness	Increase QT interval	FDA approved for adults EDS-N Cat-N
Sodium oxybate (Xyrem)	III REMS program	$GABA_B$ receptor agonist	Metabolism via Krebs cycle to CO_2 and H_2O	Combination with sedative hypnotics or alcohol contraindicated	• Administer 2 hours after eating • Reduce dose with hepatic impairment • High sodium load • Twice nightly dosing • Oxybate side effects*	FDA approved in adults and children 7 years or older EDS-N, CAT-N
Oxybate salts (Ca, Mg, K, Na) (Xywav)	III REMS program	$GABA_B$ receptor agonist	Metabolism via Krebs cycle to CO_2 and H_2O	Same as sodium oxybate	• Same as sodium oxybate except: • Lower sodium load	FDA approved in adults and children 7 years or older EDS-N, CAT-N FDA approved in adults EDS-IH
Sodium oxybate Extended release suspension (Lumryz)	III REMS program	$GABA_B$ receptor agonist	Metabolism via Krebs cycle to CO_2 and H_2O	Same as sodium oxybate	• Same as sodium oxybate (including high sodium load) except: • Once a night Dosing	FDA approved in adults: EDS-N, CAT-N

*Side effects of all oxybates: Headache, nausea, enuresis, weight loss, anxiety, hyperhidrosis, sleep terror, sleep walking, RBD. For all oxybates-contraindicated in succinic semialdehyde dehydrogenase deficiency
CAT, cataplexy; *DA*, dopamine; *EDS*, excessive daytime sleepiness; *IH*, idiopathic hypersomnia; *N*, narcolepsy; *OCP*, oral contraceptives; *RBD*, REM sleep behavior disorder.

Table 32-9 Medications for Treatment of Narcolepsy*

	Formulation	Dose	Half-Life	Side Effects
Modafinil (Provigil)	100, 200 mg	200 to 400 mg daily Can split dose morning/early afternoon	10–12 hours L- modafinil 3–4 hours R-modafinil 10–14 hours	Headache, Stevens-Johnson (rare) Interaction with OCP
Armodafinil (Nuvigil)	50, 150, 200, 250 mg	150 to 250 mg daily	15 hours	Headache, Stevens-Johnson (rare) Interaction with OCP
Solriamfetol (Sunosi)	75 mg scored, 150 mg	Start 75 mg, increase every 3 days to max 150 mg	7.1 hours	• Headache, nausea, decreased appetite, insomnia, anxiety • Contraindicated after or during MAOI
Pitolisant (Wakix)	4.45, 17.8 mg	Dose range 17.8 to 35.6 mg Wk 1, 8.9; Wk 2, 17.8; Wk 3, 35.6	20 hours	• Prolonged QT • Interaction with OCP
Sodium oxybate (Xyrem)	500 mg/ml	Start 2.25 g at bedtime and repeat in 2.5–4 hours Increase by 1.5 grams weekly Dose range 6 to 9 g per night	30–60 minutes	Nausea, confusion, anxiety, weight loss, enuresis, sleepwalking, increased sodium load concerns
Mixed salt (Ca, Mg, K, Na) oxybates (Xywav)	same	Usually same dose	same	Same, as sodium oxybagte, except much lower sodium load
Sodium oxybate Extended release suspension (Lumryz)	Granule packet 4.5 , 6.0, 7.5, 9 g	Start 4.5 g once in bed Can increase 1.5 g weekly Target dose 6–9 g	same	same as sodium oxybate including high sodium load.

*Adult dosing is indicated. For pediatric patients, see manufacturers guidelines or the section on treatment of pediatric narcolepsy. Sodium oxybate and low sodium oxybated FDA approved in adults and children 7 years or older. Modafinil, Armodafinil, Extended release sodium oxybate FDA approved for narcolepsy in adults only. g grams; OCP, oral contraceptive. Generic formulations of modafinil and armodafinil are available.

Table 32-10 Methylphenidate (MPH) Preparations

Generic (Brand Name)	Generic Available	Duration of Action (Hours)	How Supplied	Dose
MPH IR (Ritalin)*	Yes	3–4	5, 10, 20 mg	5–20 mg tid (max 60 mg)
MPH IR (Methylin)	Yes	3–4	10 mg chewable, 2.5, 5, 10 mg	same
MPH SR (Ritalin SR)*	Yes	8	20 mg generic, 10, 20 mg	10–30 mg bid
MPH ER (Metadate ER)*	Yes	8	10, 20 mg tab	10–30 mg bid
MPH ER or CD (Metadate CD)	Yes MPH ER QD	8	10, 20, 30, 40, 50, 60 mg	10–30 bid or 10 to 60 qd
MPH LA (Ritalin LA)	Yes	8–10	10, 20, 30, 40 mg Generic: 20, 30, 40 mg	10–60 qd
MPH ER OSM (Concerta)	Yes	12	18, 27, 36, 54 mg	18–54 qd

*FDA approved for narcolepsy.
ER, extended release; *LA*, long acting; *OSM*, osmotic pressure to deliver medication at a controlled rate; *SR*, sustained release.
Chavez B, Sopko MA Jr, et al. An update on central nervous system stimulant formulations in children and adolescents with attention-deficit/hyperactivity disorder. *Ann Pharmacother*. 2009;43(6):1084-1095. PMID: 19470858.

a rash. Modafinil undergoes hepatic metabolism, and the dose should be reduced in patients with significant hepatic disease. Modafinil is available in 100 and 200 mg tablets and is usually given once daily (100 to 400 mg once daily). However, some patients respond better to a split dose (200 mg qAM, 200 mg qPM). Because several studies found similar benefits on alertness as tested by the maintenance of wakefulness test from 200 mg and 400 mg daily, some insurance providers will pay for a maximum dose of 200 mg.[92] However, many patients appear to benefit from the higher dose or a split dose (morning and early afternoon).[94] Now that armodafinil is available in a generic form it may be a better choice in patients needing twice daily dosing of modafinil. Armodafinil is the R enantiomer of modafinil, has a longer half-life than L-modafinil, and is available in 50, 150, 200, and 250 mg tablets. The usual dosage is 150 or 250 mg daily. The AASM clinical guideline for treatment of narcolepsy recommends armodafinil at the conditional level (modafinil recommended at the strong level).[84]

Table 32-11 Amphetamine (AMP) Preparations

	Generic Available	Duration of Action (Hrs)	How Supplied	Dosage
D-AMP IR (Dextrostat)*	Yes	4 to 5	5, 7.5, 10, 12.5,15, 20, 30 mg tab	(5–60 mg total daily), use bid or tid dosing
D-AMP ER (Dexedrine ER)	Yes	8	5, 10, 15, 20, 25, 30 mg, ER mg capsules, Dexedrine 5 ER mg capsules not available	(5–60 mg total daily) use daily or bid dosing
MAS (Adderall)**	Yes	4 to 6	5, 7.5, 10, 12.5, 15, 30 mg	(5–60 mg total daily), use bid or tid dosing
MAS XR (Adderall XR)	Yes	10–12	5, 10, 15, 20, 25, 30 mg	5–60 qd
Lisdexamfetamine (Vyvanse)	Yes	12	20, 30, 40, 50, 60, 70 mg	20–70 qd
Methamphetamine (Desoxyn)	Yes	12	5 mg	5–25 daily, qd or bid dosing

*Brand-name IR not available.
**FDA approved for narcolepsy
ER, extended release; *IR*, immediate release; *MAS*, mixed amphetamine salts; qd daily, bid twice daily, tid three times daily.
See Chavez B, Sopko MA Jr, et al. An update on central nervous system stimulant formulations in children and adolescents with attention-deficit/hyperactivity disorder. *Ann Pharmacother.* 2009;43(6):1084-1095. PMID: 19470858.

However, this lower level of recommendation is likely because of less published evidence for armodafinil. Modafinil is the racemic form of the medication (L and R enantiomers), and after a few hours, only R-modafinil remains in the circulation. Because the R enantiomer is more potent than the L enantiomer at binding the dopamine transporter, some patients appear to respond better to armodafinil than to racemic modafinil. Side effects and precautions are similar, but insomnia is listed as a common side effect of armodafinil, perhaps due to the long duration of action.

Solriamfetol is a selective dopamine and norepinephrine reuptake inhibitor that binds to dopamine and norepinephrine transporters in vitro at concentrations inhibiting reuptake without promoting the release of monoamines.[85-87,93] The medication is FDA approved for treatment of excessive daytime sleepiness associated with narcolepsy (NT1 and NT2) or OSA. Solriamfetol improved subjective sleepiness (Epworth sleepiness scale) and improved wakefulness as measured by the objective Maintenance of Wakefulness Test (MWT) in several studies.[93,95] Although a direct comparison has not been performed, the improvements are likely greater than those from modafinil/armodafinil.[95] *Contraindications include use of a monoamine oxidase inhibitor (MAOI) – concurrent or within 14 days of the last dose of the MAOI medication.* There are two main warnings and precautions. Solriamfetol can raise both heart rate and blood pressure, and monitoring before and periodically after starting the medication is advised. The second is that there are issues with the use of solriamfetol in patients with psychosis or bipolar disorder. If mental symptoms worsen, solriamfetol should be discontinued or, at least, the dosage should be lowered. Of note, modafinil can also precipitate mania in bipolar disorder. If a patient has a mental disorder, it is always a good idea to consult with a patient's psychiatrist before starting alerting or stimulating medications, which can also increase anxiety. Solriamfetol is a schedule IV medication and has abuse potential, although less than traditional stimulants. Therefore, patients with a history of drug abuse may not be ideal candidates for the medication. The most common adverse reactions include headache, nausea, decreased appetite, insomnia, and anxiety. The drug interactions include those with drugs with dopaminergic action or those with effects on blood pressure. However, solriamfetol does not have significant interactions with hepatic enzymes metabolizing many medications. *It does not interfere with oral contraceptives.* Medication is available in 75 mg (scored) and 150 mg tablets. The initial dose is 75 mg once daily for narcolepsy and may be increased every ≥3 days. The approved dose range is 75 to 150 mg. The medication is taken once daily. The half-life of solriamfetol is 7.1 hours. The medication is excreted by the kidneys unchanged, and the dose must be adjusted for renal function. Use of solriamfetol is not recommended for end-stage renal disease (creatinine clearance (CrCl) <15 ml/min/1.73 m[1]).

Pitolisant. Pitolisant is FDA approved for treatment of excessive sleepiness and cataplexy in narcolepsy (NT1, NT2). It is *unscheduled (lack of abuse potential)*. The medication is an antagonist/inverse agonist of H3 histamine receptors (autoreceptors). This increases histaminergic neurotransmission.[44] The medication does affect hepatic enzymes metabolizing other medications and *may reduce the effectiveness of oral contraceptives*. The medication can also increase the QT interval.[91] The median half-life is 20 hours. The drug undergoes extensive hepatic metabolism. The dose should be decreased in patients with hepatic dysfunction. The dosage forms are 4.45 and 17.8 mg tablets. For narcolepsy, the recommended dosage range is 17.8 to 35.6 mg daily. The dosing is: week 1 – 8.9 mg daily, week 2 – increase to 17.8 mg daily, week 3 – may increase to 35.6 mg. The benefits for both sleepiness and cataplexy *may take several weeks*[96]. It is important to inform the patient about the delay in benefit. As pitolisant is the only alerting agent that is not a controlled substance (not scheduled), this medication is a good option for patients with a history of drug dependence or abuse.

Stimulants. Stimulants (schedule II) are effective for daytime sleepiness, but monthly prescriptions are required, and telephone prescriptions are not allowed.[97,98] The AASM clinical practice guideline for treatment of central hypersomnolence recommends dextroamphetamine and methylphenidate for treatment of narcolepsy in adults (conditional). The stimulant medications are associated with a risk for abuse, tolerance, and rebound of symptoms. Although direct head-to-head comparisons with modafinil are not available, stimulants are likely more effective in most patients.[98] Methylphenidate IR (immediate release), dextroamphetamine, and dextroamphetamine salts (Adderall and generics) are FDA approved for treatment of narcolepsy. Only two long-acting forms of methylphenidate are FDA approved for narcolepsy (metadate ER, Ritalin SR), but other long-acting formulations of dextroamphetamine and methylphenidate can be effective as off-label treatments. Lisdexamfetamine (Vyvanse and generics) is a long acting form of dextroamphetamine (the medication is a prodrug of amphetamine) administered once daily. Concerta (and generics) is a long acting formulation of methylphenidate (once daily administration) using an osmotic release mechanism. Some patients respond to one medication better than others. Methylphenidate is probably the best-tolerated stimulant but has a short duration of action requiring bid to tid dosing. As noted, long-acting (extended-release) forms of methylphenidate are available and may be better tolerated with a slower onset and offset of action. Amphetamine IR has a slightly longer half-life than methylphenidate IR. Extended-release formulations of Adderall (Adderall XR and generics) are available. Mixed amphetamine salts (Adderall and generics) contain one part D-amphetamine saccharate, one part D-amphetamine sulfate, one part racemic amphetamine aspartate, and one part racemic amphetamine sulfate (D/L isomer 3 to 1). This combination is a particularly effective form of amphetamine. Targeting the time of day with greatest sleepiness is an effective approach for the use of stimulants. A combination of immediate-release and sustained-release medication can also be useful. A small dose of immediate-acting medication in the morning in addition to a large dose of longer-acting medication may help the patient get going. A dose of immediate-release medication in the afternoon during periods of problematic sleepiness will avoid sleep disturbance from longer-acting preparations taken in the afternoon. Side effects of stimulants include anxiety, irritability, weight loss, palpitations, increased blood pressure, and disturbed sleep. Attacks of paranoia or hallucinations have been reported with amphetamines, but major psychiatric side effects are rare in the absence of underlying psychiatric disorders.

Some patients experiencing side effect with methylphenidate will tolerate amphetamine medications, and vice versa. There is an occasional patient that will actually tolerate a stimulant better than modafinil/armodafinil. Use of dextroamphetamine or methylphenidate with a monoamine oxidase (MAO) inhibitor, or within 14 days of the last MAO inhibitor dose is contraindicated.

Sodium Oxybate, Mixed Salts Oxybates. Sodium oxybate (Xyrem) (Gamma-hydroxy butyrate), lmixed salts (calcium, magnesium, potassium, and sodium) oxybates, Xywav), and extended-release sodium oxybate (Lumryz) are FDA approved for treatment of both sleepiness (both NT1 and NT2) and cataplexy (NT1) caused by narcolepsy in adults. As noted, Xyrem and Xywav are FDA approved for children 7 years of age or older. Xywav is also FDA approved for treatment of daytime sleepiness in idiopathic hypersomnia in adults.[99] Lumryz is FDA approved for treatment of narcolepsy in adults. These medications are $GABA_B$ receptor agonists. Gamma-hydroxybutyric acid (GHB) is the "date rape drug" with high abuse potential and is dispensed from only one central pharmacy under the Xyrem and Xywav REMS programs. A REMs program is also available for extended release sodium oxybate. Physicians and patients must be registered in the REMS program, but refills are permitted. Xywav has a much lower sodium content than Xyrem. Both medications are available as liquids, have a short half-life, and must be given in divided doses. Patients with the rare succinic semialdehyde dehydrogenase deficiency should not take the medication. The first dose is at bedtime, and a repeated dose is taken 2.5 to 4 hours later (alarm clock or spontaneous awakening). There are important specific dosing instructions: administer at least 2 hours after eating, prepare medicine prior to bedtime, dilute with approximately one-fourth cup of water in pharmacy-provided containers, take while in bed, and lie down after dosing. A common mistake is taking sodium oxybate after eating, which delays the onset of effects. The starting nightly dose is 4.5 grams (g) (2.25g and repeated in 2.5 to 4 hours). The dose can be slowly increased by 1.5 g nightly (increase by 0.75 g, repeated 2.5 to 4 hours later) at weekly intervals to a maximum recommended dose of 9 g per night. Slightly higher doses have been used, but most physicians are hesitant to go above 9 g. The maximum benefit from sodium oxybate on *daytime sleepiness* usually occurs at the highest recommended dose. At this dose, some patients may near normal subjective sleepiness scores. In Figure 32-9, a study of placebo versus three doses of sodium oxybate is shown. At 9 g, the change from baseline was significant, and the median value almost reached the upper limit of the normal range. In many studies of sodium oxybate, patients continued to use an alerting medication at a stable dose throughout the study. For example, some patients may benefit from a combination of modafinil and sodium oxybate, especially if they are unable to tolerate the 9-gram dose of sodium oxybate. In Figure 32-10, the results of a study of the combination of modafinil and sodium oxybate are displayed. At 6 g of sodium oxybate, the combined active treatment achieved the best result, but the difference was smaller at 9 g of sodium oxybate. Solriamfetol can also be used with sodium oxybate for patients experiencing sleepiness on the highest tolerated dose of sodium oxybate. In most patients, the nightly sodium/low sodium oxybate dose is split evenly (4.5 g twice nightly). However, some patients may benefit from uneven dosing. For example, if long midnight awakenings are an issue, one could use 5.0/4.0 g, etc.[97]

Lumryz is supplied in packets with granules that are mixed with water to create an oral suspension. The medication carton also contains a mixing cup. The dosage strengths include 4.5, 6, 7.5, and 9 g per packet of sodium oxybate. The product is taken orally as a single dose at bedtime. The usual starting dose is 4.5 g and can be increased in 1.5-g increments at weekly intervals. The recommended dosage range is 6 to 9 g nightly.

Side effects of the oxybate medications include confusion, enuresis, and sleepwalking. The REM sleep behavior disorder has also been described (but can occur with narcolepsy alone). When starting the medication, nausea can be a significant issue. Sodium oxybate can also be associated with weight loss and can significantly increase anxiety in some patients.[85-87] There is a high sodium load (sodium oxybate), and this medication may be relatively contraindicated in patients with heart

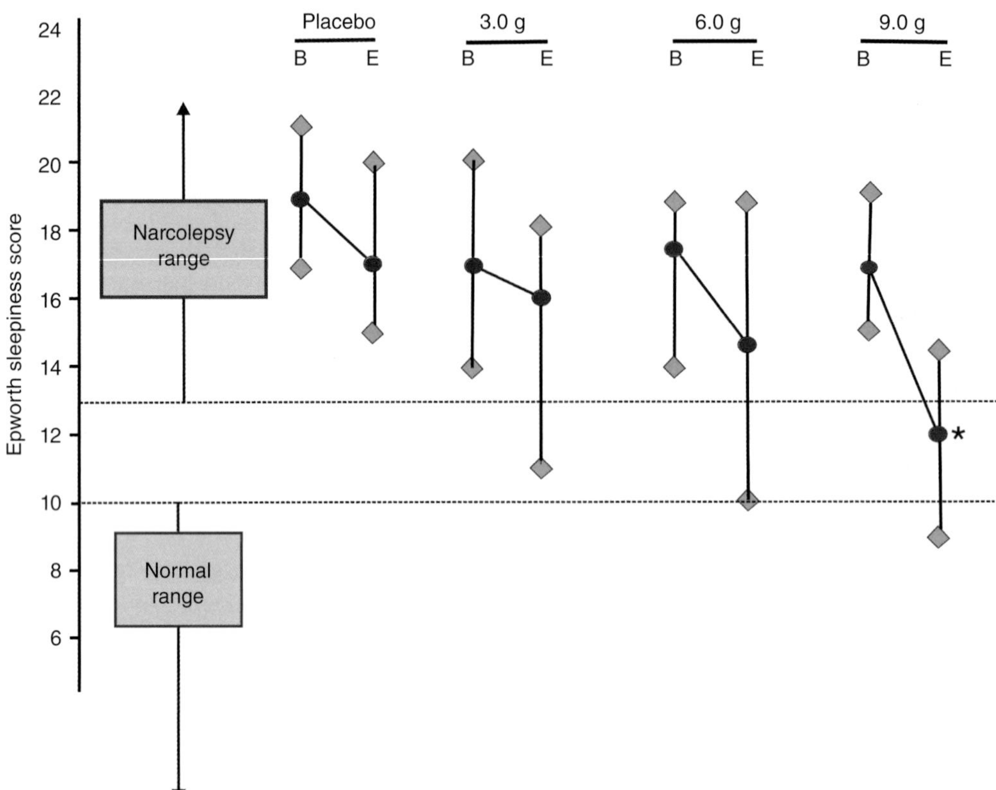

Figure 32-9 Effect of placebo and three doses of sodium oxybate on subjective sleepiness (Epworth sleepiness scale [ESS]) in narcolepsy. The solid circles are the median, and the diamonds are the 25th and 75th percentile values. For placebo and each dose of sodium oxybate, values are shown at baseline (B) and at the end of the study (E). At 9 g, the reduction in ESS from baseline was significant, and the median was just above the normal range. (From the U.S. Xyrem multicenter study group. A randomized, double blind, placebo-controlled multicenter trial comparing the effects of three doses of orally administered sodium oxybate with placebo for the treatment of narcolepsy. *Sleep*. 2002;25(1):42-49. PMID: 11833860.)

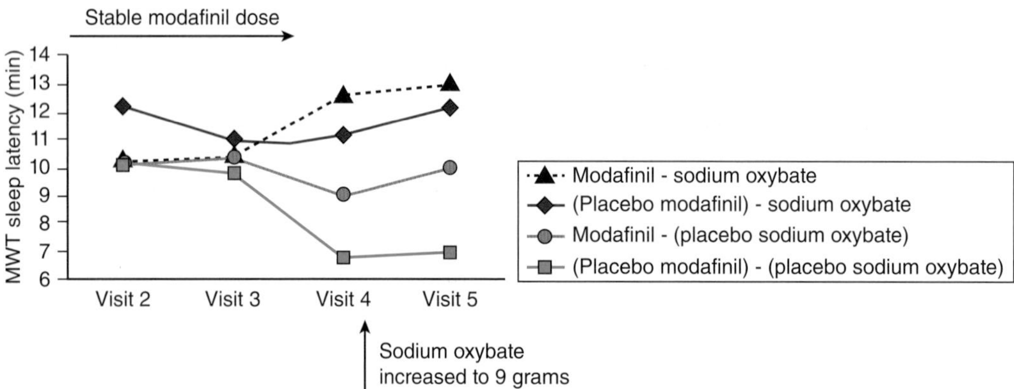

Figure 32-10 This study evaluated the combination of modafinil (MOD) and sodium oxybate (SO). Patients received unchanged doses of modafinil (with SO-placebo) during a 2-week baseline phase. Following a baseline polysomnogram and maintenance of wakefulness test (MWT), participants were randomly assigned to one of four treatment groups: (SOplacebo, MODplacebo), (SO + MODplacebo), (SOplacebo + MOD), and (SO+MOD). Sodium oxybate was administered as 6 g nightly for 4 weeks and was then increased to 9 g nightly for 4 additional weeks. At visit 4 the highest latency was in the group with both active medications. However, there was less benefit from the addition of modafinil at visit 5 after the dose of sodium oxybate was increased to 9 grams. (From Black J, Houghton WC. Sodium oxybate improves excessive daytime sleepiness in narcolepsy. *Sleep*. 2006 Jul;29(7):939-946. PMID: 16895262.)

failure. Fortunately, a lower-sodium oxybate is available. Of note, when switching from sodium oxybate to low-sodium oxybate, the dose is usually the same but may need adjustment in a minority of patients. In general, higher doses of sodium/mixed salt oxybates are needed for improvement in sleepiness than for treatment of cataplexy. Concurrent use of other sedatives, narcotics, or alcohol is potentially dangerous and should be avoided. As noted, many patients require both sodium oxybate and an alerting agent for optimal control of sleepiness. Sodium oxybate can be used in patients with both narcolepsy and OSA, but caution is advised. Ideally, patients should be on effective treatment (e.g., CPAP), and some type of monitoring should be performed to determine whether significant desaturation is present when the patient takes sodium oxybate while wearing CPAP.

Treatment of Cataplexy

Sodium oxybate, low-sodium oxybate, sodium oxybate extended-release suspension, and pitolisant are the only FDA-approved medications for the treatment of cataplexy. Other medications including tricyclic antidepressants, selective serotonin reuptake inhibitors (SSRIs), serotonin-norepinephrine reuptake inhibitors (SNRIs), and norepinephrine reuptake inhibitors (NRIs) are effective treatments in many patients but are not FDA approved for this indication. Medications with both norepinephrine and serotonin effects are the most effective. Venlafaxine XR is a useful medication for this indication (37.5 to 75 mg daily). SSRIs must be given in full dose for effectiveness. Abrupt cessation of medication used to treat cataplexy can be associated with severe withdrawal symptoms including status cataplecticus (particularly true of venlafaxine) Sodium oxybate and oxybate salts are effective for cataplexy in doses as low as 4.5 g nightly (Figure 32-11). *However, the maximum effect may take several weeks to occur.* Of interest, abrupt withdrawal of oxybate medications does not result in a suddent exacerbation of cataplexy. Medications effective for treatment of cataplexy are also effective for hypnagogic hallucinations and SP.

Treatment of Disturbed Sleep/Anxiety

Patients with narcolepsy, especially NT1, have fragmented sleep. Improvements in sleep and ensuring an adequate opportunity for sleep are important.[97] Stimulants must not be taken too close to bedtime. If taking only stimulants or alerting medications, hypnotics can be added. When taking sodium oxybate, sedative hypnotics are contraindicated. The sodium oxybate medication itself helps with sleep in many patients but can cause insomnia. One issue is waking up too early, in the middle of the night, before the second dose is scheduled. A larger first dose could be used (5 g at bedtime, with a second dose of 4 g). If a prolonged awakening between the second dose and the morning is an issue, one could use a higher dose for the second half of the night.[97] One example is a 3.5 g/5.5 g dose division. It is also important that sodium oxybate be taken on an empty stomach (avoid bedtime snacks).

Some patients with narcolepsy manifest comorbid anxiety or depression. The oxybate medications carry a risk of inducing anxiety. If needed, antidepressants or medications targeting anxiety may be used.

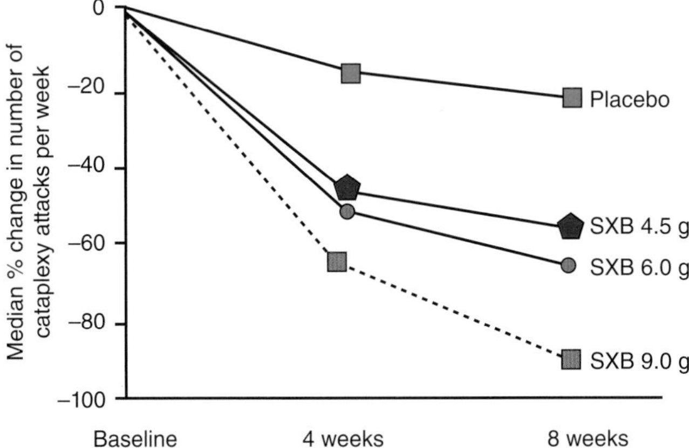

Figure 32-11 This figure shows improvement in cataplexy with various doses of sodium oxybate (SXB) at baseline, 4 weeks, and 8 weeks. A significant effect was noted at the lowest dose. Note that the full effect of each dose took 8 weeks. (From Xyrem International Study Group. Further evidence supporting the use of sodium oxybate for the treatment of cataplexy: a double-blind, placebo-controlled study in 228 patients. *Sleep Med.* 2005;6(5):415-421 PMID: 16099718.)

Pregnancy Concerns

The effects of modafinil, armodafinil, and pitolisant on the effectiveness of oral contraceptives (increased metabolism) have been mentioned, and the effects can last for a period of time after the medications have been discontinued. None of the alerting or stimulant medications used to treat narcolepsy are recommended for use during pregnancy. A publication addresses concerns about modafinil/armodafinil in pregnancy.[100]

Treatment of Narcolepsy in Children

The only FDA-approved treatment for narcolepsy in children is sodium oxybate or low-sodium oxybate (for those aged ≥7 years). These medications at appropriately reduced doses are effective for daytime sleepiness and cataplexy (see manufacturer's current dosing recommendations). For Xywav a starting nightly dose (1st dose at bedtime, 2nd dose 2.5 to 4 hours later) for 20–30 kg is (≤ 1g, ≤ 1g), for 30–45 kg is (≤ 1.5 g, ≤ 1.5g), and for ≥ 45 Kg (≤ 2.25 g, ≤ 2.25g). The maximum weekly increase for 20–30 kg is (0.5g, 0.5g), for 30 to 45 Kg is (0.5, 0.5 g) and for ≥ 45 kg (0.75,0.75g). Maximum dose for 20–30 kg is (3g, 3g), for 30–45 kg (3.75 g, 3.75 g) and for ≥ 45 Kg is (4.5g, 4.5 g). The 2021 AASM clinical practice guidelines for treatment of central hypersomnolence[84] recommend modafinil and sodium oxybate for treatment of narcolepsy in pediatric patients. Modafinil is an effective medication but is used off-label per FDA indications for the medication in children. For cataplexy, sodium/low-sodium oxybate are effective and are FDA approved for this indication for children 7 years or older. Off-label medications include SSRIs and SNRIs (venlafaxine and others).

IDIOPATHIC HYPERSOMNIA

Patients with IH complain of daytime sleepiness or the need for very long sleep duration.[101-104]

The ICSD-3-TR diagnostic criteria (A-F must be met) are as follows:

A. The patient has daily periods of irrepressible need to sleep or daytime lapses into drowsiness or sleep occurring **for at least 3 months.**

B. Cataplexy is absent.

C. PSG and MSLT findings are **not consistent** with a diagnosis of NT1 or NT2

D. The presence of at least one of the following:
   1. The MSLT performed according to current recommended protocols shows a mean sleep latency ≤8 minutes.
   2. Total 24-hour sleep time is ≥660 minutes (typically 12 to 14 hours) on 24-hour PSG recording (performed

after correction of chronic sleep deprivation) or by wrist actigraphy in association with a sleep log (averaged over at least 7 days with unrestricted sleep).

E. Insufficient sleep is ruled out *(if deemed necessary, by lack of improvement of sleepiness after an adequate trial of increased nocturnal time in bed, preferably confirmed by at least a week of wrist actigraphy).*

F. The symptoms and signs are not better explained by a circadian rhythm sleep-wake disorder or other current sleep disorder, medical disorder, mental disorder, or medication/substance use or withdrawal.

Clinical Presentation, PSG Findings, and Diagnostic Challenges

History

The typical age of onset of IH is 16 to 20 years, and constant sleepiness for many years is typical. **However spontaneous remission has been reported in up to 14%.**[3,101,102] Patients with IH do not wake up easily to alarms. The ICSD-3-TR mentions that severe and prolonged sleep inertia, known as **sleep drunkenness** (defined as prolonged difficulty waking up with repeated returns to sleep, irritability, automatic behavior, and confusion), and/or long (>1 hour) unrefreshing naps are additional supportive clinical features for a diagnosis of IH. The symptom of sleep drunkenness is reported in 36% to 66% of IH patients in several series. Important facts about IH are listed in Box 32-3.

Long (>60 minutes) naps are typical, and 46% to 78% of patients *describe the naps as unrefreshing*. This is in contrast to napping in patients with narcolepsy, which is often beneficial. *Dysfunction of the autonomic nervous system may be present*, including headaches, orthostatic disturbances, temperature dysregulation, and peripheral vascular complaints (Raynaud's-type phenomenon with cold hands and feet). In addition, hypnogogic hallucinations and SP may also be present. Self-reported total sleep time is longer than in controls and is ≥10 hours in at least 30% of patients.

Box 32-3 IMPORTANT FACTS ABOUT IH

- Long, unrefreshing naps
- Sleep drunkenness (36–66%)
- Difficulty waking up to alarms
- 24-hour sleep: >10 hours reported in 30% (often not accurate)
- Hypnogogic hallucinations and sleep paralysis are common.
- *Dysfunction of the autonomic nervous system* may be present (especially in patients with a long sleep time), including headaches, orthostatic disturbances, perception of temperature dysregulation, and peripheral vascular complaints (Raynaud's-type phenomena with cold hands and feet).
- PSG – high sleep efficiency
- PSG + MSLT ≤1 SOREMP, or 0 SOREMP on the MSLT if a PSG SOREMP present
- Mean sleep latency (MSLT) ≤8 minutes
- If MSLT not possible or mean sleep latency >8 minutes, perform 24 hour PSG (or actigraphy if 24 hour PSG not possible)
- 24-hour PSG total sleep time (or 7 days of actigraphy with unrestricted sleep) ≥660 minutes.
- Spontaneous remission can occur.

MSLT, multiple sleep latency test; *PSG*, polysomnography, *SOREMP*, sleep-onset rapid eye movement period.

PSG, MSLT, 24-Hour PSG

After a thorough history and physical, a PSG and MSLT should be ordered. It is *imperative to document adequate sleep before the testing*. A sleep diary, preferably accompanied by actigraphy for at least 7 days before testing, should eliminate the possibility of insufficient sleep syndrome. The PSG should rule out OSA.

The diagnostic criteria specify that *sleepiness must be present* ***≥3 months, and cataplexy must be absent***. The PSG and MSLT do not meet criteria for NT1 or NT2. Of note, *a high sleep efficiency (≥90%)* on the PSG preceding the MSLT is a supportive finding (as long as sleep insufficiency is ruled out). One of the following must be present: if an MSLT is performed, the mean sleep latency is ≤8 minutes (and the number of SOREMPs on the PSG/MSLT does not meet criteria for narcolepsy), or a 24-hour PSG or sleep log/actigraphy (averaged over at least 7 days of unrestricted sleep) documents a total sleep time over 24 hours of ≥660 minutes (typically 12 to 14 hours). Some patients needing a long sleep duration are unable to wake up sufficiently after the PSG to complete the usual MSLT protocol. IH is a diagnosis of exclusion, and other causes of sleepiness must be ruled out. The major exclusion before a diagnosis of IH can be made with confidence is insufficient sleep. A trial of *sleep extension* prior to the MSLT or a 24-hour PSG is needed if insufficient sleep is suspected. Documentation of adequate sleep of at least 7 days by actigraphy for 1 week prior to the MSLT or 24-hour PSG is recommended. The actigraphy results could be used to determine long sleep duration – if the patient has unrestricted sleep.

The diagnosis of IH is a challenge to many sleep centers. The ability to perform 24-hour PSG or actigraphy may not be present. Many providers will make a diagnosis of IH *only on the basis of the PSG/MSLT*. They assume that if the MSLT shows a sleep latency longer than 8 minutes, the patient does not have IH. The mean sleep latency for IH was listed as 6.2 ± 3.0 minutes in a review of the literature.[11] *Many patients with IH reporting a sleep duration >10 hours do not have a mean sleep latency ≤8 minutes on an MSLT,*[103] *and 24-hour PSG or actigraphy for 7 days to document a total sleep time ≥660 minutes is needed for a diagnosis of IH.*

Long Sleep Duration Subtype of IH

The ICSD-2[1] divided IH into those with long sleep duration (>10 hours) and without long sleep duration (<10 hours). Complicating the use of a 10-hour total sleep time to define separate groups is that patients with IH tend to overestimate their total sleep time. The ICSD-3[2] eliminated the division of IH patients on the basis of long sleep time but mentions that some clinicians may elect to retain IH with long sleep time as a subtype. The study by Vernet et al.[103] compared patients with >10 hours sleep to those with <10 hours. There were no differences in Epworth sleepiness scale scores, the percentage of individuals positive for HLA-DQB1*0602, or the percentage reporting nonrefreshing naps. The results of this study and other data informed the decision not to separate IH into two types based on total sleep duration. However, in the study by Vernet et al., there were significant differences in the MSLT sleep latency and the percentage of individuals reporting sleep drunkenness between the groups with and without reports of a long sleep time (Table 32-12).[103] Of note, prolonged PSG was used in this study to document long sleep time. A much larger percentage of the long sleep time group reported sleep drunkenness (almost two times). In addition, while 100% of the short sleep time group had a mean sleep latency less than

Table 32-12 Comparison of Controls vs IH and IH With and Without Long Sleep Time (LST)

	Controls	IH all	Without LST**	With LST	Comparison of groups with and without long sleep time (P value)
Age (years)	38.6	34	39.7	29.1	P <0.002
BMI (kg/m2)			26.1	22.8	P = 0.005
Women (%)	50	64	60	67.5	NS
ESS			15	14.9	NS
Sleep drunkenness	**0**	**36.5**	**23.1**	**50**	0.08
Hypnagogic hallucinations (%)	8.7	24	25	23.3	NS
Sleep paralysis (%)	4.3	27.6	28.6	26.7	NS
Non-refreshing naps(%)	5	46.3	45	47.6	NS
Horne-Ostberg score *	47.8	55.2	53	44	NS
BMI (Kg/m2)	24.4	24.4	26.1	22.8	NS
HLA DQB1*0602 (% +)			21.9	26.5	NS
TST	491	579	517	633	<0.0001
Sleep efficiency	88	91	89	92	0.04
TST 24-hr sleep monitoring (min)	525 ±87	695	635	747	<0.0001
MSL (min)	**15.8**	**7.8**	**5.6**	**9.6**	<0.0001
Subjects with (%)					
MSL <8 min	3.3	60.8	100%	28.6%	<0.0001
MSL 8–10 min	0.0	9.4	0%	17%	<0.0001
MSL >10 min	**97**	**29.7**	**0%**	**54%**	<0.0001

*lower score later bedtimes, difficulty getting up (Owls)
**LST long sleep time (> 600 minutes by 24 hour PSG)
MSL, mean sleep latency; *NS*, not significant; *TST*, total sleep time; *LST*, long sleep time.
From Vernet C, Arnuf I. Idiopathic hypersomnia with and without long sleep time: a controlled series of 75 patients. *Sleep*. 2009;32:753-759. PMID: 19544751.

8 minutes, *54% of the long sleep duration group had a mean sleep latency over 10 minutes*. Thus, relying only on PSG and MSLT to diagnose IH will miss the correct diagnosis in a substantial number of patients.

The differential diagnosis of IH includes NT2 with false-negative MSLT, head trauma, occult drug abuse, and sleepiness associated with a psychiatric disorder (bipolar disorder-depressive phase), neurological disorder, or structural CNS lesion. CNS imaging is suggested if there is any suspicion of a CNS lesion. Use of a urine drug screen may also be considered.

Box 32-4 TREATMENTS FOR IDIOPATHIC HYPERSOMNIA

Modafinil*, Armodafinil
Dextroamphetamine
Methylphenidate **
Clarithromycin**
Pitolisant**
Sodium oxybate**
Mixed salt oxybates (Xywav)***

2021 AASM recommendations: *strong, **conditional
***Calcium, magnesium, potassium, and sodium oxybates (Xywav) is FDA approved for treatment of IH

Treatment of IH

Many of the medications indicated for the treatment of daytime sleepiness in narcolepsy are effective at improving daytime sleepiness in IH, but many patients remain highly symptomatic. Treatments for IH are listed in Box 32-4. The 2021 AASM clinical practice parameters for treatment of central hypersomnolence[84] recommended *modafinil (strong) and clarithromycin, methylphenidate, pitolisant, and sodium oxybate (conditional)*. However, the only medication currently FDA approved for treatment of IH is mixed salts (calcium, magnesium,potassium, and sodium) oxybates (XYWAV). There is no reason to believe that armodafinil would not be effective. Amphetamines, methylphenidate, and modafinil[83] have all been used with variable success for treatment of daytime sleepiness. The 2007 AASM practice parameters for treatment of narcolepsy and other hypersomnias of central origin state that "modafinil may be effective for treatment of idiopathic hypersomnia (option)."[83] Amphetamine, methamphetamine, and methylphenidate were also listed as treatments for IH (option) in the 2007 publication. Of note, special interventions are needed for sleep drunkenness: for example, an alarm, taking bedside medication so it will start working, then another alarm to get out of bed. Some extended-release medications such as those used in ADHD might work.[105]

Clarithromycin was recommended for treatment of sleepiness in IH in the 2021 AASM clinical practice guideline for treatment of central hypersomnolence. The medication is not FDA approved for this indication, and most physicians are not familiar with the use of this medication. The usual dosage is 500 to 1000 mg taken twice daily. Use of clarithromycin is based on the hypothesis that IH may be caused by an endogenous substance that increases activity at sedating $GABA_A$ receptors in the CNS Clarithromycin is a negative allosteric modulator of $GABA_A$ receptors in the CNS and is available as an oral medication. Flumazenil is also a negative allosteric modulator of $GABA_A$ receptors, in addition to its role as a competitive antagonist at the benzodiazepine binding site but must be given intravenously. Some central hypersomnolence syndromes are associated with a positive allosteric modulator of $GABA_A$ receptors in CSF. For example, benzodiazepine receptor agonists act at the $GABA_A$ chloride ionophore complex as a positive modulator of $GABA_A$ function, increasing sedation. That is BZRA ligands increase the action of GABA binding to the complex. A negative $GABA_A$ modulator could reduce sedation. This mechanism is believed to explain the benefit of clarithromycin. The medication did improve subjective daytime sleepiness in a randomized double-blind crossover trial (10 patients had IH). Side effects include gastrointestinal symptoms, including dysgeusia, dysosmia, nausea, and diarrhea, as well as insomnia. There is an FDA warning concerning the medication increasing the risk of death in individuals with heart disease, especially in those with a history of coronary artery disease. The medication should not be used in pregnant women.

As noted above, the only medication FDA approved for treatment of IH in adults is lower-sodium oxybate (Xywav).[99]

The dosing for twice-nightly lower-sodium oxybate is similar to that used in narcolepsy. *However, there is also an option for once-nightly dosing in patients with IH (may not be able to wake for the second dose).* For once-nightly dosing, the starting dose is 3 g or less with increments of 1.5 g per week (if indicated and tolerated, up to a total dose of 6 g nightly). The option is clinically useful for patients with IH with a long sleep duration who might find it difficult to wake up for a second dose. Both dosing options were used in the studies demonstrating effectiveness in IH patients. Of interest, lower-sodium oxybate improved both subjective daytime sleepiness and the symptom of sleep inertia.

KLEINE-LEVIN SYNDROME (KLS)

The Kleine-Levin syndrome (KLS), also known as recurrent hypersomnia, is a rare disorder (one or two per million) characterized by episodes of severe hypersomnia in association with cognitive, psychiatric, and behavioral disturbances (hyperphagia, hypersexuality) that are recurrent with periods of remission (normal function) between episodes (Box 32-5).[3,106,107] A typical episode has a *median duration of 10 days* (rarely, several weeks to months). Episodes reoccur every 1 to 12 months (median interval 3 months).

ICSD-3-TR diagnostic criteria are as follows (Criteria A-E must be met):

A. The patient experiences at **least two recurrent** episodes of excessive sleepiness and sleep duration, each persisting for two days to several weeks.

B. Episodes usually recur more than once a year and at least once every 18 months.

C. The patient has normal or near normal sleep and wakefulness, cognition, behavior, and mood, between episodes, at least during the first years of the syndrome.

D. The patient must demonstrate at least one of the following during episodes:
   1. Cognitive dysfunction
   2. Derealization
   3. Major apathy
   4. Disinhibited behavior (such as hypersexuality or hyperphagia)

E. The symptoms and signs are not better explained by chronic insufficient sleep, a circadian rhythm sleep-wake disorder or other current sleep disorder, medical disorder, mental disorder, or medication/substance use or withdrawal

Box 32-5 KEY POINTS REGARDING KLEINE-LEVIN SYNDROME (KLS)

- Rare, about 1000 cases worldwide
- Men > women
- Episodes start abruptly, median duration 10 days (5 days to 5 weeks)
- Normal behavior between episodes
- Recurring episodes every 1 to 12 months (median 3 months) for years
- Can be precipitated by: infection, sleep deprivation, alcohol and other substance intake as well as medications
- Classic triad of hypersomnia, hyperphagia, and hypersexuality appears in only about 45% of patients with KLS.
- Hypersomnia – out of bed only to eat and go to bathroom
- Ravenous eating 40–60%
- Hypersexuality (usually men, 42–53%)
- Derealization (dream-like perception of environment) is the most common symptom
- Depression
- Menstrual KLS can occur
- Computed tomography, magnetic resonance imaging both normal.
- Functional imaging shows *reduced activity* (hypoperfusion, hypometabolism) in the thalamus, hypothalamus, hippocampus, and posterior association cortex, and sometimes *increased activity in the frontal lobes.* These abnormalities are found during episodes and sometimes between episodes
- Best treatment unknown. American Academy of Sleep Medicine (AASM) clinical guideline recommends lithium.
- *Spontaneous resolution common*

A flu-like illness or an infection of the upper airway (and, more rarely, gastroenteritis) is often reported immediately prior to the onset of the first episode of KLS, and, more rarely, before relapses. Other, less frequently reported triggering events include alcohol consumption, head trauma, traveling, or exposure to anesthesia. The first episode is often triggered by an infection or alcohol intake. The episodes are characterized by hypersomnia (sleep 16 to 20 hours per day) with waking or getting out of bed only to eat or go to the bathroom. It is possible to awaken these patients, but they are very irritable. When they are awake during episodes, most patients are confused, slow in speaking and answering, with anterograde amnesia. Almost all report a dream-like, altered perception of the environment (derealization). The classic description of KLS is hyperphagia, which occurs in about two-thirds of patients, though one-third of patients eat less than normal (anorexia). Other manifestations include hypersexuality (about 50%, typically men), depression (about 50%, predominantly women), and anxiety related to being left alone and seeing strangers. Patients can experience hallucinations and delusions (30%). Patients are remarkably normal between episodes with regard to sleep, cognition, mood, and eating attitude. Typically, hypersomnia is present at episode onset. The associated behavioral disturbances may not occur during each episode. The **male-to-female ratio in KLS is 2:1,** and the age of onset is typically early adolescence (second decade). Several long-term studies suggest KLS often has a benign course, with episodes lessening in duration, severity, and frequency over a median course of 14 years. The disease typically stops after a median of 14 years, except when onset is in adulthood. Of note, new studies suggest that sleep duration is longer, cognition mildly altered, and some mental disorders may be evident in 15-20% of patients during periods between episodes.

The differential diagnosis includes psychiatric disorders associated with recurrent episodes of sleepiness (depression, bipolar disorder, seasonal affective disorder, and somatoform disorder). *Birth and developmental problems, as well as Jewish heritage, are risk factors for developing the syndrome.* Computed tomography (CT) and magnetic resonance imaging (MRI) are normal. CSF hypocretin is normal. *Brain functional imaging is abnormal in most cases, with hypoperfusion/hypometabolism of the thalamus, hypothalamus, posterior association cortex, and hippocampus (temporal lobe). Some hypometabolism, frontal lobes can also be seen.*[108] These abnormalities are present both during the episode of hypersomnolence and sometimes between episodes. Hormone levels are normal, as are 24-hour secretory patterns. Key points regarding KLS are listed in Box 32-5.

Treatment of KLS

Due to the limited number of patients, no large well-controlled study exists at the time of this writing. Improvement has been reported with lithium, amantadine, lamotrigine, and valproic acid.[106,107] The AASM clinical practice guideline for treatment of disorders of central hypersomnolence recommends use of lithium (conditional level of evidence).[83]

Lithium may reduce the duration of episodes and reduce undesirable behaviors. Methylphenidate and modafinil could be used for daytime sleepiness.

HYPERSOMNIA DUE TO A MEDICAL DISORDER

In these patients, hypersomnolence is believed to be caused by a coexisting medical or neurological disorder.

Diagnostic criteria (A-C must be met) are as follows[3]:

A. The patient has daily periods of irrepressible need to sleep or daytime lapses into drowsiness or sleep occurring for at least 3 months.

B. The daytime sleepiness occurs as a consequence of a significant underlying medical or neurological condition.

C. The symptoms and signs are not better explained by chronic insufficient sleep, a circadian rhythm sleep-wake disorder or other current sleep disorder, mental disorder, or medication/substance use or withdrawal.

In patients with severe neurological or medical disorders in whom it is not possible or desirable to perform sleep studies, the diagnosis can be made by clinical criteria. If an MSLT is performed, the mean sleep latency may be ≤ 8 minutes but this is NOT required for the diagnosis of Hypersomnia Due to a Medical Disorder. In the subtype of residual hypersomnolence after treatment of OSA, the MSLT mean sleep latency is often > 8 minutes. Should criteria for narcolepsy be fulfilled, a diagnosis of NT1 or NT2 due to a medical condition should be used rather than Hypersomnia Due to Medical Disorder.

Box 32-6 DISORDERS ASSOCIATED WITH HYPERSOMNIA DUE TO A MEDICAL DISORDER

A. Posttraumatic hypersomnia
B. Hypersomnia due to Parkinson's disease
C. Genetic disorders associated with central hypersomnia
   - Niemann-Pick type C, Norrie disease, Moebius syndrome, Smith-Magenis syndrome, fragile X syndrome
D. Genetic disorders associated with central hypersomnia and SRBDs
   - Prader-Willi, Myotonic Dystrophy
E. Hypersomnia due to endocrine disorder (hypothyroidism)
F. Hypersomnia due to central nervous system lesion (infection, tumor)
G. Hypersomnia due to metabolic encephalopathy (liver or kidney failure)
I. Residual hypersomnia in patients with *adequately treated* obstructive sleep apnea

SRBD, sleep-related breathing disorder.

Daytime sleepiness is of variable severity and may resemble that of narcolepsy (i.e., refreshing effects of naps) or IH (i.e., long sleep periods or unrefreshing sleep). In these patients, hypersomnolence is believed to be the result of a medical condition. Symptoms associated with either narcolepsy or IH may be present, including sleep paralysis, hypnagogic hallucinations, or automatic behavior. If an MSLT documents sleepiness but does not meet criteria for narcolepsy, hypersomnia due to a medical disorder should be the diagnosis. In patients with both SRBD and hypersomnia due to a medical disorder, a diagnosis of hypersomnia due to a medical condition should be made *only if the hypersomnolence persists after adequate treatment* of the sleep-disordered breathing. Hypersomnia due to a medical condition is only diagnosed if the medical condition is judged to be directly causing the hypersomnolence. Hypersomnolence has been described in association with a large range of medical disorders (Box 32-6), including metabolic encephalopathy, head trauma, stroke, brain tumors, encephalitis, systemic inflammation (e.g., chronic infections, rheumatologic disorders, cancer), genetic disorders, and neurodegenerative diseases. An important point is that a diagnosis of hypersomnia due to a medical disorder assumes that there is a complaint of daytime sleepiness and that *this is not simply the result of a decreased amount of sleep.*

Posttraumatic Hypersomnia

Cases of hypersomnia secondary to head trauma are well documented and, in a **minority** of cases, result in a diagnosis of narcolepsy due to a medical condtion (NDMC, usually NT2).[109,110] However, a diagnosis of hypersomnia due to a medical disorder is more common. The cause of hypersomnia is believed to be injury to the hypocretin/orexin neurons or other wakefulness-promoting neural systems. Immediately post injury, CSF hypocretin levels may be decreased but tend to recover over 6 months. Head trauma is associated with a high prevalence of OSA, and this should be ruled out. Traumatic brain injury is discussed in Chapter 40.

Residual Hypersomnia in Patients With Adequately Treated Obstructive Sleep Apnea

This topic is discussed in Chapter 22 on medical treatment of OSA. Some patients with OSA report persistent sleepiness despite apparently adequate amounts of sleep and optimal treatment of their sleep apnea and other obvious sleep disorders. They may have moderately elevated Epworth sleepiness scores, but most have mean sleep latencies > 8 minutes on MSLT. They also report more fatigue, apathy, and depression. It is essential that sleep-disordered breathing be fully treated, confirmed by a download of CPAP machine compliance data demonstrating optimal usage, preferably at least 7 hours a night, and a PSG demonstrating elimination of essentially all sleep-disordered breathing. Other causes of sleepiness, such as insufficient sleep syndrome, psychiatric disorders, or hypersomnia related to medications or substances, must be eliminated. Modafinil, armodafinil, and solriamfetol are FDA approved for treatment of residual hypersomnia associated with adequately treated OSA.[91]

Prader Willi Syndrome (PWS)

PWS is a genetic disorder usually associated with a deletion of the long arm of chromosome 15 and is characterized by hyperphagia, obesity, hypogonadotropic hypogonadism, behavioral disorders, and sleep disorders.[111,112] Abnormal growth hormone secretion results in short stature, reduced muscle mass, and low bone density (scoliosis is common). The characteristic appearance of PWS includes a high narrow forehead, almond-shaped eyes, turned-down lips, a prominent nasal bridge, and small hands and feet. Intelligence is variable but usually ranges from low normal to mild to moderately decreased. A growth hormone deficiency is a major etiology of a number of medical problems, and growth hormone injections are commonly used to increase lean body mass and bone density. PWS typically causes low muscle tone, short stature if not treated with growth hormone, incomplete sexual development, and a chronic feeling of hunger that, coupled with a metabolism that utilizes drastically fewer calories than normal, can lead to excessive eating and life-threatening obesity, among many other medical and developmental issues.

Patients with PWS may have daytime sleepiness from a number of etiologies, including sleep apnea, narcolepsy, or the PWS itself.[112,113] SRBDs associated with PWS include sleep apnea with both obstructive and central events and hypoventilation. Unless strict dietary control is imposed, morbid obesity is common and can be associated with hypoventilation. Excessive daytime sleepiness is reported commonly in persons with PWS, may begin early in life, and has been correlated with daytime behavioral issues. In fact, excessive daytime sleepiness has been reported independent of nocturnal sleep problems (sleep apnea), suggesting it is a primary feature of PWS. Some sleepy persons with PWS meet the diagnostic criteria for narcolepsy, and PWS is considered a cause of NDMC. Abnormal sleep architecture has been reported in persons with PWS, including reduced REM latency and SOREMPs. These findings can be present in PWS patients without significant sleep-related breathing problems. Although PWS most commonly causes NDMD without cataplexy (NT2-NDMD), patients with PWS can have cataplexy[114] (accurate history is often difficult to obtain in these patients). Nevsimalova and associates[115] found reduced levels of CSF hypocretin in four patients with PWS. However, none had cataplexy. Fronczek and coworkers found no difference in the total number of hypocretin-containing neurons in seven PWS patients compared with age-matched controls.[116] If sleepiness is present in PWS but criteria for narcolepsy are not met and sleepiness is ***not*** felt to be due to sleep apnea, a diagnosis of hypersomnia due to a medical disorder is appropriate.

Hypersomnia and Neurodegenerative Disorders

Both insomnia and hypersomnia are common in Parkinson's disease, Lewy body dementia, multisystem atrophy, and Alzheimer's disease.[117,118] This is discussed in more detail in Chapter 40. The AASM clinical practice guidelines for treatment of hypersomnia recommend modafinil for sleepiness in these situations[83].

Myotonic Dystrophy (MD) Type 1

MD is an *autosomal dominant* disorder characterized by myotonia, distal muscle weakness, premature cataracts, hypogonadism, and cardiac arrhythmias. The disorder can be associated with daytime sleepiness of several causes, including OSA, NDMC, or hypersomnia due to a medical disorder.[119,120] Genetic testing is needed for definitive diagnosis. The incidence is estimated to be about 1/10,000 cases, so it is a much rarer disorder than narcolepsy. Myotonia is defined as repetitive muscle depolarization resulting in muscle stiffness and impaired relaxation. The muscles usually involved include facial, masseter, levator palpebra, forearm, hand, pretibial muscles, and the sternocleidomastoid. Pharyngeal and laryngeal and muscles of respiration including the diaphragm can be involved. Dysfunction of the hypothalamic region can result in daytime sleepiness or daytime sleepiness with SOREMPs, which may lead to the additional diagnosis of NDMC. If criteria for narcolepsy are not met, a diagnosis of hypersomnia due to a medical condition could be considered. Involvement of upper airway muscles can result in sleep apnea. In one case, a controlled study comparing age-matched groups of patients with and without MD, the patients with MD had a greater frequency of severe OSA, an elevated PLMS index, shorter mean sleep latency on the MSLT, and more frequent SOREMPs[120].

There are differences in MD presentation depending on the age of onset. Congenital MD is apparent at birth and often severe. Juvenile MD is characterized by symptoms that appear between birth and adolescence. Adult-onset MD usually appears in individuals aged 20 to 40 years and tends to be slowly progressive. Late-onset MD occurs after 40 years of age and has mild symptoms.

On physical examination, findings in MD type 1 include a narrow face, temporal wasting, premature frontal balding, distal weakness, and myotonia. MD patients have decreased strength on hand grip but then are slow to relax ("distal myopathy with myotonia"). Individuals describe muscle stiffness or difficulty releasing their grip. Patients may observe a delayed ability to open their eyes after a forceful closure or a delayed ability to extend their fingers after a firm handshake. There is wasting of hand and forearm muscles (especially hand flexors). PSG can reveal OSA, and PSG + MSLT can meet criteria for narcolepsy or simply document excessive daytime sleepiness without two SOREMPs. Decreased CSF hypocretin has been found in some patients with MD and NT1-NDMC.[121] The 2007 AASM practice parameter on the treatment of narcolepsy and other hypersomnias of central origin[82] stated, "methylphenidate and modafinil may be effective treatment for MD." The 2021 AASM clinical practice guidelines for treatment of central hypersomnolence[83] recommend treatment of daytime sleepiness in MD with modafinil. More information on MD is available in Chapter 40.

HYPERSOMNIA DUE TO A MEDICATION OR SUBSTANCE

Patients with this disorder have excessive nocturnal sleep, daytime sleepiness, or excessive napping that is believed to be caused by (1) sedating medications, (2) alcohol or drugs of abuse, or (3) withdrawal from amphetamines and other drugs.

Diagnostic criteria[3] (criteria A-C must be met) are as follows:

A. The patient has daily periods of irrepressible need to sleep or daytime lapses into sleep.

B. The daytime sleepiness occurs as a consequence of current medication or substance use or withdrawal from a wake-promoting medication or substance.

C. The symptoms are not better explained by chronic insufficient sleep, a circadian rhythm sleep-wake disorder, or other current sleep disorder, medical disorder, or mental disorder.

In chronically heavy amphetamine users, sleepiness is most severe in the first week of withdrawal and can persist for up to 3 weeks. In people who regularly consume coffee or other sources of caffeine, discontinuation can produce sleepiness, fatigue, and inattentiveness for 2 to 9 days. PSG is generally unnecessary unless a concomitant sleep disorder is suspected. PSG and MSLT results vary depending on the specific substance in question and on the timing of the most recent intake. With stimulant withdrawal, nocturnal PSG may show normal sleep, whereas the MSLT typically demonstrates a short mean sleep latency with or without multiple SOREMPs. A urine toxicology screen may be positive for the suspected substance. The diagnosis is often confirmed if symptoms resolve after the causal agent is removed.

HYPERSOMNIA ASSOCIATED WITH A MENTAL DISORDER

Patients with hypersomnia associated with psychiatric disorders may report excessive nocturnal sleep, daytime sleepiness, or excessive napping.[122,123]

Diagnostic criteria[3] (A-C must be met) are as follows:

A. The patient has daily periods of irrepressible need to sleep or daytime lapses into drowsiness or sleep occurring for at least 3 months.

B. The daytime sleepiness occurs in association with a concurrent mental disorder.

C. The symptoms are not better explained by chronic insufficient sleep, a circadian sleep-wake disorder or other current sleep disorder, medical disorder, or medication/substance use or withdrawal.

In addition, these patients often feel their sleep is of poor quality and nonrestorative. *Patients may focus on hypersomnia and ignore psychiatric symptoms and even deny depression.* Hypersomnia associated with psychiatric disorders accounts for 5% to 7% of hypersomnia cases. *Women are more susceptible than men*, and the typical age range is between 20 and 50 years.

Although insomnia rather than hypersomnia is more common in depression, hypersomnia may occur in up to one-third of cases and is often noted in atypical depression and depression associated with bipolar II disorder (at least one major depressive episode, at least one hypomanic episode, no manic episodes) and seasonal affective disorder. A short REM latency and a *long early REM period* can be seen in patients with depression. MSLT results are usually normal, but about 25% have a sleep latency less than 8 minutes but rarely less than 5 minutes. Patients with this disorder may report **long hours spent in bed.** Twenty-four-hour continuous sleep-recording studies typically show considerable time spent in bed during day and night, a behavior sometimes referred to as *clinophilia*. If associated with major depression, hypersomnia may *persist even after the depressive episode improves*, and persistent hypersomnia is associated with *increased risk of recurrent depression*.

INSUFFICIENT SLEEP SYNDROME AND LONG SLEEPER

Patients with the insufficient sleep syndrome fail to obtain sufficient nocturnal sleep to maintain daytime alertness and mental functioning.[124-127] The effects of sleep loss and recovery sleep are discussed in Chapter 9.

ICSD-3-TR diagnostic criteria are as follows (A-F must be met):

A. The patient has daily periods of irrepressible need to sleep or daytime lapses into drowsiness or sleep or, in the case of prepubertal children, there is a complaint of behavioral abnormalities attributable to sleepiness.

B. The patient's sleep time, established by personal or collateral history, sleep logs, or actigraphy is usually shorter than expected for age.

C. The curtailed sleep pattern is present on most days for at least 3 months.

D. The patient usually curtails sleep time by such measures as an alarm clock or being awakened by another person and generally sleeps longer when such measures are not used, such as on weekends or vacations.

E. Extension of total sleep time results in resolution of the symptoms of sleepiness.

F. The symptoms and signs are not better explained by a circadian rhythm sleep-wake disorder or other current sleep disorder, medical disorder, mental disorder, or medication/substance use or withdrawal.

If there is a doubt about the accuracy of personal history or sleep logs, then actigraphy should be performed, preferably for at least 2 weeks. In the case of long sleepers the sleep duration may be normal for age but insufficient for these patients. Often patients may not appreciate that their symptoms are due to insufficient sleep. Patients characteristically sleep longer on weekends and vacations. They usually report feeling more refreshed with a longer sleep period. The *evening chronotype* may predispose to insufficient sleep. The association of eveningness with insufficient sleep persists after controlling for variables like sex, age, and sleep duration.

A sleep study is not needed for diagnosis but, if performed owing to suspicion of other disorders, will often show a *short sleep latency, high sleep efficiency, and long total sleep time*. There is sometimes evidence of stage N3 or stage R rebound (high amount of those sleep stages). Note that up to 30% of normal populations have a mean sleep latency less than 8 minutes. A mean sleep latency and SOREMPs on a MSLT can be seen in some patients with insufficient sleep. Academic performance is worse among adolescents with insufficient sleep.[126] Population studies have shown SOREMPs in normal populations, and these findings are associated with shift work and short sleep duration. In one population study [127], 7% had two or more SOREMPs on the MSLT, and 22% and a mean sleep latency of less than 8 minutes.

Long sleeper is considered an isolated symptom/normal variant in the ICSD-3-TR[3]. The affected individual sleeps substantially more in 24 hours than is normal for age. In adults this is usually 10 hours or more and in children 2 hours more that age related norms. Sleep may increase to 12 hours on weekends or holidays. The prevalence of long sleepers is estimated to be 2% of men and 1.5% of women. *Long sleep (> 9 hours) has a high heritability (44%) and concordance between identical twins.* PSG is usually normal if preceded by the desired sleep duration. In contrast to patients with idiopthic hypersomnia and a long sleep time, long sleepers feel completely refreshed and alert after the long sleep period. The pattern is often established in childhood and is stable over many years. In contrast to hypersomnia due to a mental disorder, the individuals do not merely stay in bed, they actually sleep for long periods and are refreshed on awakening. *Long sleepers seek medical attention because of excessive sleepiness due societal constraints limiting their sleep.* That is, if allowed to sleep for the desired duration, long sleepers feel refreshed and deny daytime sleepiness.

SUMMARY OF KEY POINTS

1. The classification of narcolepsy as type 1 (NT1) or type 2 (NT2) is based on low or absent hypocretin-1 in the CSF (NT1) or normal levels (NT2). However, as CSF hypocretin levels are not known in most patients, clinical classification in most cases is made based on the presence (NT1) or absence of cataplexy (NT2).
2. Approximately 90% to 95% of patients with narcolepsy with cataplexy have low or absent hypocretin-1 in the CSF and severely reduced or absent hypocretin neurons in the lateral hypothalamus. Destruction of hypocretin cells is believed to be autoimmune. About 90% to 95% of patients with NT1 are positive for the HLA-DQB1*0602 antigen, but about 20% of the general population has this antigen. A patient negative for the antigen is unlikely to have NT1.
3. Only about 30% of identical twins are concordant for narcolepsy. Both genetics and acquired factors determine if narcolepsy will develop.
4. Cataplexy is characterized by temporary muscle weakness induced by emotional stimuli. The affected individual is conscious, and the duration of weakness is usually seconds to minutes. Hearing or telling a joke and laughter are the most common triggers. *Deep tendon reflexes are absent.* Strong emotion is believed to inhibit wake-on, REM-off brain areas that normally inhibit the atonia-generating neurons in the pons (sublateral dorsal nucleus). The stimulating influences of hypocretin balance the inhibition by emotion, and the wake-on, REM-off neurons still inhibit the atonia neurons. If hypocretin is absent, emotionally induced inhibition of the REM off neurons is not balanced and hypotonia/cataplexy can occur.
5. Cataplexy is the only symptom virtually specific for narcolepsy and is present in about 60% to 70% of narcolepsy cases. The onset of cataplexy typically follows the onset of daytime sleepiness. In children the onset of cataplexy can precede daytime sleepiness and may occur without a preceding emotional stimulus.
6. Other manifestations of narcolepsy include sleep paralysis, sleep-related hallucinations (hypnagogic at sleep onset, hypnopompic on awakening), automatic behavior, disturbed sleep, PLMS during REM sleep, and the RBD.
7. In the absence of the finding of low hypocretin-1 in the CSF, a diagnosis of NT1 requires daytime sleepiness the presence of cataplexy and either a SOREMP on the PSG or $2 SOREMPs on an MSLT. (This assumes another reason for these findings does not exist – e.g., prior sleep restriction, a circadian rhythm sleep-wake disorder or use or withdrawal of a medication or substance).
8. In the absence of a known CSF hypocretin-1 level, a diagnosis of NT2 requires daytime sleepiness for 3 months, the absence of cataplexy, a PSG/MSLT meeting diagnostic criteria, and absence of insufficient sleep or another current sleep disorder, circadian sleep-wake disorder, medical disorder, medication/substance use or withdrawal explaining the hypersomnolence and PSG/MSLT findings (Figure 32-12). In NT2 a SOREMP on the PSG may count as one of the two or more required SOREMPs on the MSLT.
9. FDA approved medications to treat **excessive sleepiness** in narcolepsy (NT1 or NT2) include modafinil, armodafinil, solriamfetol, pitolisant, dextroamphetamine, and methylphenidate in adults. Sodium oxybate and low-sodium (Ca^{++}, Mg^{++}, K^{+}, Na^{+}) oxybates in adults and children ≥7 years of age are FDA approved for treatment of narcolepsy. A sustained-release sodium oxybate suspension is approved in adults. The oxybate medications are approved to treat both daytime sleepiness and cataplexy.
10. FDA-approved medications for treatment of cataplexy in adults include sodium oxybate, low sodium oxybate, sustained-release sodium oxybate, and pitolisant. Non-FDA approved treatments include antidepressants (TCAs, SSRIs, or SNRIs; i.e., fluoxetine and venlafaxine XR). Medications effective for cataplexy also decrease episodes of SP of hypnogogic hallucinations. Abrupt discontinuation of the oxybates does not cause a cataplexy rebound. However, abrupt cessation of medications such as venlafaxine can cause status cataplecticus.
11. IH is diagnosed when the PSG/MLST shows 0 or 1 sleep onset REM periods and a mean sleep latency ≤8 minutes ***or*** a 24-hour PSG or actigraphy documenting a long sleep duration >660 minutes. Cataplexy must be absent and insufficient sleep ruled out. Sleep drunkenness and nonrefreshing naps are supportive.
12. Modafinil, armodafinil, or stimulants are used as treatment of IH, but the only FDA-approved medication is low-sodium oxybate.
13. When evaluating a patient for IH who reports sleeping >10 hours, the finding of a mean sleep latency on the MSLT ≥8 minutes **does not rule out IH.** A 24-hour PSG or at least 7 days of actigraphy with unrestricted sleep can make the diagnosis if the total 24-hour sleep time is ≥660 minutes.
14. The diagnosis of narcolepsy in children follows the same diagnostic criteria as in adults, but cataplexy may precede daytime sleepiness, may not always be associated with an emotional trigger, and is often associated with falls. Cataplexy may be mistaken for syncope. A return to napping is a sign of daytime sleepiness. The onset of obesity or precocius puberty may follow the onset of NT1. Cataplectic facies consisting of semipermanent eyelid and jaw weakness (droopy eye lids, mouth open) can be noted.
15. The Kleine-Levin syndrome is very rare, has a male predominance, and consists of repeated periods of hypersomnolence and mental changes (impaired cognition, derealization). Other manifestations include hyperphagia and hypersexuality. During episodes function brain imaging shows hypofunction of the thalamus and other brain ares. The episodes are separated by periods of normal behavior and function. Lithium may reduce the frequency of the episodes.

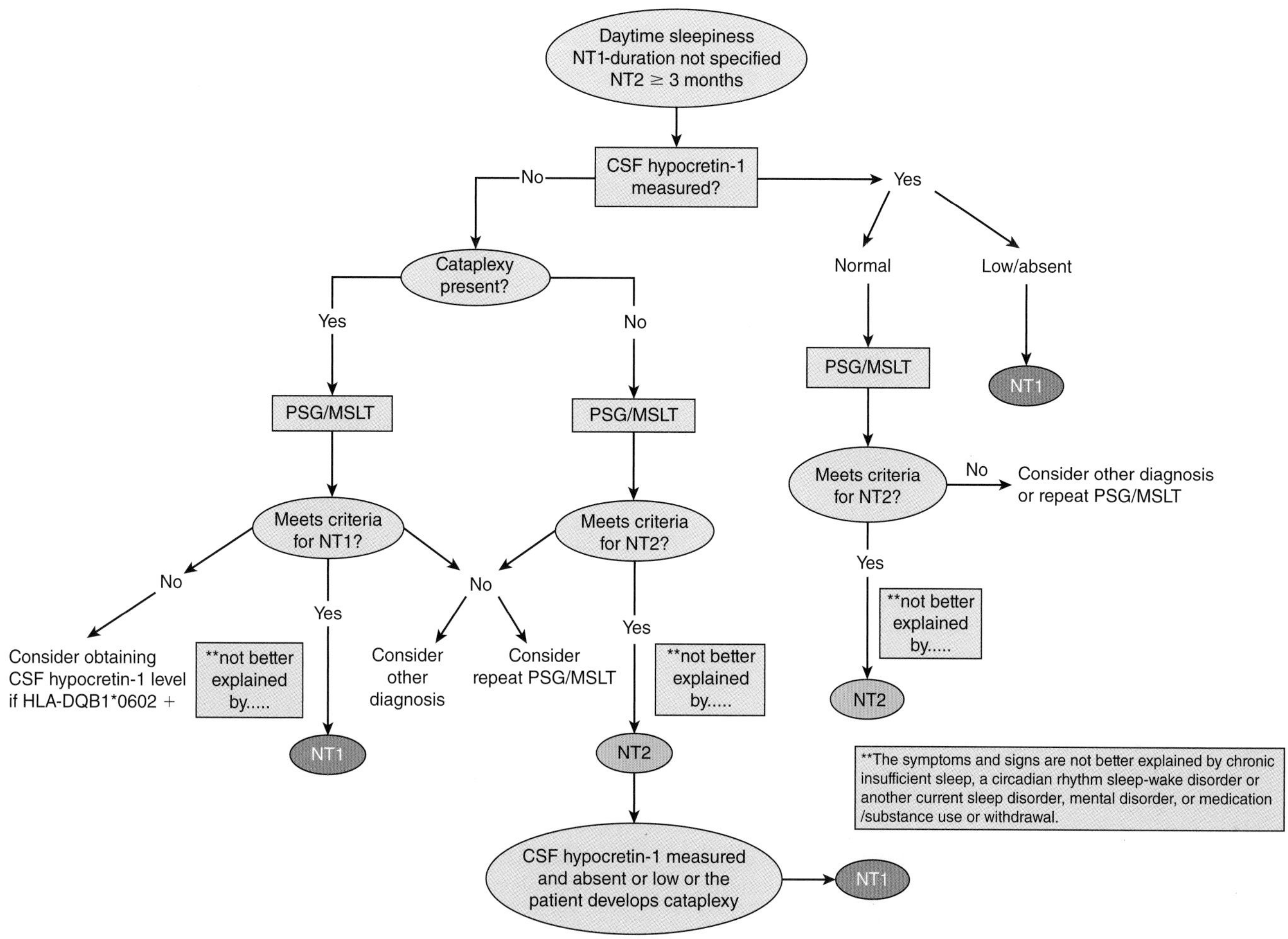

Figure 32-12 An overview of diagnostic pathways for narcolepsy type 1 (NT1) or type 2 (NT2), depending on the presence or absence of known cerebrospinal fluid (CSF) hypocretin-1 levels, the presence or absence of a history of cataplexy, polysomnography (PSG)/multiple sleep latency test (MSLT) findings, and the fact that findings are not better explained by other causes such as insufficient sleep, OSA, the circadian rhythm sleep-wake disorder, or the effect of medication or substance use or their withdrawal.

CLINICAL REVIEW QUESTIONS

1. If one member of a pair of identical twins has narcolepsy, in what percentage of twin pairs is the other twin likely to have narcolepsy?
   A. 10%
   B. 30%
   C. 50%
   D. 75%
2. Which of the following is **NOT** true about solriamfetol?
   A. It can affect the efficacy of oral contraceptives.
   B. It is a dual serotonin-norepinephrine reuptake inhibitor.
   C. It is FDA approved for treatment of excessive sleepiness in narcolepsy and OSA.
   D. Concurrent or recent use of an MAOI is contraindicated.
3. Which of the following medications (acting alone) is associated with a long QT interval?
   A. Modafinil
   B. Solriamfetol
   C. Pitolisant
   D. Sodium oxybate
4. Which of the following medications is **not scheduled** as a controlled substance?
   A. Modafinil
   B. Solriamfetol
   C. Pitolisant
   D. Methylphenidate
5. Which of the following combinations meets criteria for the **diagnosis of NT1?**

	A	B	C	D	E
Daytime sleepiness	Yes	Yes	Yes	No	Yes
Cataplexy	No	Yes	No	Yes	No
PSG/MSLT+	No	No	Yes	Yes	Yes
CSF hypocretin-1	Low	Not done	Not done	Not done	Low

PSG/MSLT+, combination of PSG and MSLT that meets criteria for narcolepsy.

   A. A, E
   B. B, D
   C. A, D
   D. B, E
6. Which of the following symptoms is most specific for narcolepsy?
   A. Daytime sleepiness
   B. Cataplexy

C. Sleep paralysis
D. Sleep-related hallucinations

7. Which of the following is **NOT** a characteristic of cataplexy?
   A. It can be asymmetrical (appearing unilateral).
   B. Deep tendon reflexes are intact
   C. Consciousness is preserved.
   D. It is associated with emotion.
   E. It can be the initial symptoms of narcolepsy.
8. Kleine-Levin syndrome is **NOT** characterized by which of the following?
   A. Recurrent episode of hypersomnia separated by periods of normal behavior
   B. Hypoperfusion of thalamus, hypothalamus, hippocampus
   C. Decreased inhibitions (increased sexuality, hyperphagia)
   D. Impaired cognition and Derealization
   E. Men > Women
   F. Never follows an infection or head trauma
   G. Spontaneous remission often occurs
9. A 25-year-old patient reports severe daytime sleepiness, frontal balding, and difficulty relaxing his grip but denies cataplexy. A PSG/MLST found an apnea-hypopnea index (AHI) of 7 events/hour with a mean sleep latency of 5 minutes, and two SOREMPs. What is the most likely cause of the daytime sleepiness?
   A. Hypersomnia due to a medical disorder
   B. Narcolepsy (NT2) due to a medical condition
   C. IH
   D. OSA
10. A patient with Prader-Willi syndrome (PWS) is being evaluated with daytime sleepiness. He denies cataplexy. PSG shows a normal REM latency and an AHI of 3 events/hour. An MSLT shows a sleep latency of 3 minutes and one SOREMP. Which of the following is the most likely diagnosis?
    A. Narcolepsy due to medical condition
    B. Narcolepsy without cataplexy
    C. Hypersomnia due to a medical disorder
    D. Idiopathic hypersomnia
11. A patient was diagnosed with NT2 on the basis of the absence of cataplexy and a compatible PSG and MSLT. A CSF hypocretin-1 level is not yet available. Which of the following would **NOT** change the diagnosis to NT1?
    A. Low CSF hypocretin-1 level
    B. Development of typical cataplexy
    C. Normal hypocretin level and development of typical cataplexy
    D. Normal CSF hypocretin-1 level

ANSWERS

1. B. About 30% of twin pairs are concordant for narcolepsy.
2. A. Solriamfetol does not affect hepatic metabolism of medications, including oral contraceptives. The other answers are correct.
3. C. Pitolisant can increase the QT interval. Modafinil can decrease the metabolism of medications which can increase the QT interval.
4. C. Pitolisant is not scheduled as a controlled substance
5. A. (Columns A and E are correct). Column A meets diagnostic criteria for NT1. Although one would expect the PSG/MSLT to meet the narcolepsy criteria in A, the test is not 100% sensitive. Daytime sleepiness and a low hypocretin level satisfy criteria for NT1. Column B does not meet diagnostic criteria for NT1 because both a history of cataplexy and a PSG/MLST meeting diagnostic criteria are needed for a diagnosis of NT1 (in the absence of a low CSF hypocretin-1 level). Column C is consistent with NT2. Column D does not meet diagnostic criteria for NT1 as the patient does not complain of daytime sleepiness. This pattern can happen if a patient with a symptom that might be cataplexy is evaluated by PSG/MSLT testing and did not have adequate sleep in the weeks preceding testing. Column E meets diagnostic criteria for NT1. Some patients with a low hypocretin-1 level do not report cataplexy.
6. B. Cataplexy is the only symptom specific for narcolepsy.
7. B. Deep tendon reflexes are absent during cataplexy because of inhibition of spinal cord motor neurons.
8. F. The onset of Kleine-Levin syndrome after infections or head trauma is often noted.
9. B. Although very mild OSA is present, the most likely cause of the picture is narcolepsy type II associated with a medical condition (associated with myotonic dystrophy). The MSLT does not meet criteria for IH. If no sleep onset REM periods were noted a diagnosis of hypersomnia due to a medical disorder would be appropriate.
10. C. The PSG/MSLT does not meet criteria for narcolepsy. It would meet criteria for IH, but in this situation there is a disorder associated with daytime sleepiness (PWS); that is, the sleepiness is not idiopathic.
11. D. A normal hypocretin level is generally thought to eliminate NT1. However, there is a small group with cataplexy and a normal hypocretin level that is considered an NT1 subtype. In the absence of cataplexy a normal hypocretin level would not change the diagnosis to NT1.

SUGGESTED READING

American Academy of Sleep Medicine. *International Classification of Sleep Disorders*. 3rd ed., text revision. Darien, IL: American Academy of Sleep Medicine; 2023.

Kushida CA, Shapiro CM, Roth T, Thorpy MJ. Once-nightly sodium oxybate (FT218) demonstrated improvement of symptoms in a phase 3 randomized clinical trial in patients with narcolepsy. *Sleep*. 2022;45(6):zsab200.

Maski K, Trotti LM, Kotagal S, Robert Auger R. Treatment of central disorders of hypersomnolence: an American Academy of Sleep Medicine clinical practice guideline. *J Clin Sleep Med*. 2021;17(9):1881-1893.

Trotti LM, Arnulf I. Idiopathic hypersomnia and other hypersomnia syndromes. *Neurotherapeutics*. 2021;18(1):20-31.

REFERENCES

1. American Academy of Sleep Medicine. *International Classification of Sleep Disorders: Diagnostic and Coding Manual*. 2nd ed. Westchester, IL: American Academy of Sleep Medicine; 2005.
2. American Academy of Sleep Medicine. *International Classification of Sleep Disorders*. 3rd ed. Darien, IL: American Academy of Sleep Medicine; 2014.
3. American Academy of Sleep Medicine. *International Classification of Sleep Disorders*. 3rd ed., text revision. Darien, IL: American Academy of Sleep Medicine; 2023.
4. Scammell TE. The neurobiology, diagnosis, and treatment of narcolepsy. *Ann Neurol*. 2003;53(2):154-166.
5. Scammell TE. Narcolepsy. *N Engl J Med*. 2015;373(27):2654-2662.
6. Burgess CR, Scammell TE. Narcolepsy: neural mechanisms of sleepiness and cataplexy. *J Neurosci*. 2012;32(36):12305-12311.
7. Mahoney CE, Cogswell A, Koralnik IJ, Scammell TE. The neurobiological basis of narcolepsy. *Nat Rev Neurosci*. 2019;20(2):83-93.

8. De Lecca L, Kilduff TS, Peyron C, et al. The hypocretins: hypothalamic specific peptides with neuroexcitatory activity. *Proc Natl Acad Sci USA.* 1998;95:322-327.
9. Sakurai T. Orexins and orexin receptors: a family of hypothalamic neuropeptides and G protein–coupled receptors that regulate feeding behavior. *Cell.* 1998;92:573-585.
10. Nishino S, Ripley B, Overeem S, et al. Hypocretin (Orexin) deficiency in human narcolepsy. *Lancet.* 2000;355:39-40.
11. Arand D, Bonnet M, Hurwitz T, et al. A review by the MSLT and MWT Task Force of the Standards of Practice Committee of the AASM. The clinical use of the MSLT and MWT. *Sleep.* 2005;28:123-144.
12. Krahn LE, Arand DL, Avidan AY, et al. Recommended protocols for the multiple sleep latency test and maintenance of wakefulness test in adults: guidance from the American Academy of Sleep Medicine. *J Clin Sleep Med.* 2021;17(12):2489-2498. Erratum in: *J Clin Sleep Med.* 2022; 18(8):2089.
13. Andlauer O, Moore H, Jouhier L, et al. Nocturnal rapid eye movement sleep latency for identifying patients with narcolepsy/hypocretin deficiency. *JAMA Neurol.* 2013;70(7):891-902. Erratum in: *JAMA Neurol.* 2013;70(10):1332.
14. Okun ML, Lin L, Pelin Z, Hong S, Mignot E. Clinical aspects of narcolepsy-cataplexy across ethnic groups. *Sleep.* 2002;25(1):27-35.
15. Longstreth WT Jr, Koepsell TD, Ton TG, Hendrickson AF, van Belle G. The epidemiology of narcolepsy. *Sleep.* 2007;30(1):13-26.
16. Challamel MJ, Mazzola ME, Nevsimalova S, Cannard C, Louis J, Revol M. Narcolepsy in children. *Sleep.* 1994;17(suppl 8):S17-S20.
17. Overeem S, van Nues SJ, van der Zande WL, Donjacour CE, van Mierlo P, Lammers GJ. The clinical features of cataplexy: a questionnaire study in narcolepsy patients with and without hypocretin-1 deficiency. *Sleep Med.* 2011;12(1):12-18.
18. Anic-Labat S, Guilleminault C, Kraemer HC, Meehan J, Arrigoni J, Mignot E. Validation of a cataplexy questionnaire in 983 sleep-disorders patients. *Sleep.* 1999;22(1):77-87.
19. Bargiotas P, Dietmann A, Haynes AG, et al. The Swiss Narcolepsy Scale (SNS) and its short form (sSNS) for the discrimination of narcolepsy in patients with hypersomnolence: a cohort study based on the Bern Sleep-Wake Database. *J Neurol.* 2019;266(9):2137-2143.
20. Pizza F, Tartarotti S, Poryazova R, Baumann CR, Bassetti CL. Sleep-disordered breathing and periodic limb movements in narcolepsy with cataplexy: a systematic analysis of 35 consecutive patients. *Eur Neurol.* 2013;70(1-2):22-26.
21. Dauvilliers Y, Rompré S, Gagnon JF, Vendette M, Petit D, Montplaisir J. REM sleep characteristics in narcolepsy and REM sleep behavior disorder. *Sleep.* 2007;30(7):844-849.
22. Schenck CH, Bassetti CL, Arnulf I, et al. English translations of the first clinical reports on narcolepsy and cataplexy by Westphal and Gelineau in the late 19th century. *J Clin Sleep Med.* 2007;3:301-311.
23. Aidie WJ. Idiopathic narcolepsy: a disease sui generis: with remarks on mechanism of sleep. *Brain.* 1926;49:257-306.
24. Compston A. Idiopathic narcolepsy. *Brain.* 2008;131(10):2532-2535. doi:10.1093/brain/awn231.
25. Yoss RE, Daly DD. Criteria for the diagnosis of the narcoleptic syndrome. *Proc Staff Meet Mayo Clin.* 1957;32:320-328.
26. Vogel G. Studies in the psychophysiology of dreams, III: the dream of narcolepsy. *Arch Gen Psychiatry.* 1960;3:421-428.
27. Juji T, Sakate M, Honda Y, Doi Y. HLA antigens in Japanese patients with narcolepsy. All patients were DR2 positive. *Tissue Antigens.* 1984; 24:316-319.
28. Mignot E, Hayduk R, Black J, et al. HLA DQB1*0602 is associated with cataplexy in 509 narcoleptic patients. *Sleep.* 1997;20:1012-1020.
29. Overeem S, Mignot E, van Dijk JG, Lammers GJ. Narcolepsy: clinical features, new pathophysiologic insights, and future perspectives. *J Clin Neurophysiol.* 2001;18:78-105.
30. Dauvilliers Y, Montplasir J, Molinari N, et al. Age of onset of narcolepsy in two large populations of patients in France and Quebec. *Neurology.* 2001;57:2029-2033.
31. Mignot E. Genetic and familial aspects of narcolepsy. *Neurology.* 1998;50(suppl 1):S16-S22.
32. Billiard M, Pasquie-Magnetto V, Heckman M, et al. Family studies in narcolepsy. *Sleep.* 1994;17(suppl 8):S54-S59.
33. Hungs M, Lin L, Okun M, Mignot E. Polymorphisms in the vicinity of the hypocretin/orexin are not associated with human narcolepsy. *Neurology.* 2001;57(10):1893-1895.
34. Ollila HM. Narcolepsy type 1: what have we learned from genetics? *Sleep.* 2020;43(11):zsaa099.
35. Mignot E, Lammers GJ, Ripley MS, et al. The role of cerebrospinal fluid hypocretin measurement in the diagnosis of narcolepsy and other hypersomnias. *Arch Neurol.* 2002;59:1553-1562.
36. Ripley BN, Overeem S, Fujiki N, et al. CSF hypocretin/orexin levels in narcolepsy and other neurological conditions. *Neurology.* 2001;57:2253-2258.
37. Mignot E, Lammers GJ, Ripley B, et al. The role of cerebrospinal fluid hypocretin measurement in the diagnosis of narcolepsy and other hypersomnias. *Arch Neurol.* 2002;59(10):1553-1562.
38. Nishino S, Kanbayashi T, Fujiki N, et al. CSF hypocretin levels in Guillain-Barré syndrome and other inflammatory neuropathies. *Neurology.* 2003;61:823-825.
39. Bourgin P, Zeitzer JM, Mignot E. CSF hypocretin-1 assessment in sleep and neurological disorders. *Lancet Neurol.* 2008;7(7):649-662. Erratum in: *Lancet Neurol.* 2008;7(9):771.
40. Krahn LE, Pankratz S, Oliver L, et al. Hypocretin (Orexin) levels in cerebrospinal fluid of patients with narcolepsy: relationship to cataplexy and HLADQB1*0602 status. *Sleep.* 2003;25:733-736.
41. Scammell TE, Winrow CJ. Orexin receptors: pharmacology and therapeutic opportunities. *Annu Rev Pharmacol Toxicol.* 2011;51:243-266.
42. Scammell TE, Arrigoni E, Lipton JO. Neural circuitry of wakefulness and sleep. *Neuron.* 2017;93(4):747-765.
43. España RA, Scammell TE. Sleep neurobiology from a clinical perspective. *Sleep.* 2011;34(7):845-858.
44. Scammell TE, Jackson AC, Franks NP, Wisden W, Dauvilliers Y. Histamine: neural circuits and new medications. *Sleep.* 2019;42(1):zsy183.
45. Thannickal T, Moore RY, Nienbus R, et al. Reduced number of hypocretin neurons in human narcolepsy. *Neuron.* 2000;27:469-474.
46. Thannickal TC, Siegel JM, Nienhuis R, Moore RY. Pattern of hypocretin (orexin) soma and axon loss, and gliosis, in human narcolepsy. *Brain Pathol.* 2003;13:340-351.
47. Crocker A, España RA, Papadopoulou M, et al. Concomitant loss of dynorphin, NARP, and orexin in narcolepsy. *Neurology.* 2005;65(8):1184-1188.
48. Overeem S, Black JL, Lammers GJ. Narcolepsy: immunological aspects. *Sleep Med Rev.* 2008;12:95-107.
49. Mahlios J, De la Herrán-Arita AK, Mignot E. The autoimmune basis of narcolepsy. *Curr Opin Neurobiol.* 2013;23(5):767-773.
50. Liblau RS, Latorre D, Kornum BR, Dauvilliers Y, Mignot EJ. The immunopathogenesis of narcolepsy type 1. *Nat Rev Immunol.* 2023. doi:10.1038/s41577-023-00902-9.
51. Lin A, Nevsimalova S, Piazzi G, et al. Elevated anti-streptococcal antibodies in patients with recent narcolepsy onset. *Sleep.* 2009;32:979-983.
52. Partinen M, Saarenpää-Heikkilä O, Ilveskoski I, et al. Increased incidence and clinical picture of childhood narcolepsy following the 2009 H1N1 pandemic vaccination campaign in Finland. *pLoS One.* 2012;7(3):e33723.
53. Sarkanen TO, Alakuijala APE, Dauvilliers YA, Partinen MM. Incidence of narcolepsy after H1N1 influenza and vaccinations: systematic review and meta-analysis. *Sleep Med Rev.* 2018;38:177-186.
54. Hallmayer J, Faraco J, Lin L, et al. Narcolepsy is strongly associated with the T-cell receptor alpha locus. *Nat Genet.* 2009;41(6):708-711. Erratum in: *Nat Genet.* 2009;41(7):859. Hong, Sheng Seung-Chul [corrected to Hong, Seung-Chul].
55. Valko PO, Gavrilov YV, Yamamoto M, et al. Increase of histaminergic tuberomammillary neurons in narcolepsy. *Ann Neurol.* 2013;74(6):794-804.
56. Nishino S, Sakurai E, Nevsimalova S, et al. Decreased CSF histamine in narcolepsy with and without low CSF hypocretin-1 in comparison to healthy controls. *Sleep.* 2009;32(2):175-180.
57. Kanbayashi T, Kodama T, Kondo H, et al. CSF histamine contents in narcolepsy, idiopathic hypersomnia and obstructive sleep apnea syndrome. *Sleep.* 2009;32(2):181-187.
58. Dauvilliers Y, Delallée N, Jaussent I, et al. Normal cerebrospinal fluid histamine and tele-methylhistamine levels in hypersomnia conditions. *Sleep.* 2012;35(10):1359-1366.
59. John J, Wu MF, Boehmer LN, Siegel JM. Cataplexy-active neurons in the hypothalamus: implications for the role of histamine in sleep and waking behavior. *Neuron.* 2004;42(4):619-634.
60. Thannickal TC, Nienhuis R, Siegel JM. Localized loss of hypocretin (orexin) cells in narcolepsy without cataplexy. *Sleep.* 2009;32(8):993-998.
61. Mahoney CE, Agostinelli LJ, Brooks JN, Lowell BB, Scammell TE. GABAergic neurons of the central amygdala promote cataplexy. *J Neurosci.* 2017;37(15):3995-4006.
62. Rogers AE, Aldrich MS, Caruso CC. Patterns of sleep and wakefulness in treated narcolepsy subjects. *Sleep.* 1994;17:590-597.
63. Broughton R, Dunham W, Newman J, et al. Ambulatory 24 hour sleep-wake monitoring in narcolepsy-cataplexy compared to matched controls. *Electroencephalogr Clin Neurophysiol.* 1988;70:473-481.

64. Aldrich MS, Chervin RD, Malow BA. Value of the multiple sleep latency test (MSLT) for the diagnosis of narcolepsy. *Sleep*. 1997;20:620-629.
65. Coelho FM, Georgsson H, Murray BJ. Benefit of repeat multiple sleep latency testing in confirming a possible narcolepsy diagnosis. *J Clin Neurophysiol*. 2011;28(4):412-414.
66. Ruoff C, Pizza F, Trotti LM, et al. The MSLT is repeatable in narcolepsy type 1 but not narcolepsy type 2: a retrospective patient study. *J Clin Sleep Med*. 2018;14(1):65-74.
67. Lopez R, Doukkali A, Barateau L, et al. Test-retest reliability of the multiple sleep latency test in central disorders of hypersomnolence. *Sleep*. 2017;40(12). doi:10.1093/sleep/zsx164.
68. Andlauer O, Moore H IV, Hong SC, et al. Predictors of hypocretin (orexin) deficiency in narcolepsy without cataplexy. *Sleep*. 2012;35(9): 1247-1255F.
69. Malik S, Boeve BF, Krahn LE, et al. Narcolepsy associated with other central nervous system disorders. *Neurology*. 2001;57:539-541.
70. Autret A, Lucas B, Henry-Lebras F, de Toffol B. Symptomatic narcolepsies. *Sleep*. 1996;17:S21-S24.
71. Nishino S, Kanbayashi T. Symptomatic narcolepsy, cataplexy, and hypersomnia, and their implications in the hypothalamic/hypocretin/orexin system. *Sleep Med Rev*. 2005;9:269-310.
72. Aldrich MS, Naylor MW. Narcolepsy associated with lesions of the diencephalon. *Neurology*. 1989;39:1505-1508.
73. Vankova J, Stepanov I, Jech R, et al. Sleep disturbances and hypocretin deficiency in Niemann-Pick disease type C. *Sleep*. 2003;26:427-430.
74. Kanbayashi T, Abe M, Fujimoto S, et al. Hypocretin deficiency in Niemann-Pick type C with cataplexy. *Neuropediatrics*. 2003;34:52-53.
75. Smit LS, Lammers GJ, Catsman-Berrevoets CE. Cataplexy leading to the diagnosis of Niemann-Pick disease type C. *Pediatr Neurol*. 2006;35(1): 82-84.
76. Pereira PM, Schneider A, Pannetier S, Heron D, Hanauer A. Coffin-Lowry syndrome. *Eur J Hum Genet*. 2010;18(6):627-633.
77. Smith SE, Mullen TE, Graham D, Sims KB, Rehm HL. Norrie disease: extraocular clinical manifestations in 56 patients. *Am J Med Genet A*. 2012; 158A(8):1909-1917.
78. Vossler DG, Wyler AR, Wilkus RJ, Gardner-Walker G, Vlcek BW. Cataplexy and monoamine oxidase deficiency in Norrie disease. *Neurology*. 1996;46(5):1258-1261.
79. Carskadon MA, Harvey K, Duke P, Anders TF, Litt IF, Dement WC. Pubertal changes in daytime sleepiness. *Sleep*. 1980;2:453-460.
80. Aran A, Einen M, Lin L, Plazzi G, Nishino S, Mignot E. Clinical and therapeutic aspects of childhood narcolepsy-cataplexy: a retrospective study of 51 children. *Sleep*. 2010;33:1457-1464.
81. Serra L, Montagna P, Mignot E, Lugaresi E, Plazzi G. Cataplexy features in childhood narcolepsy. *Mov Disord*. 2008;23(6):858-865.
82. Morgenthaler TI, Kapur VK, Brown TM, et al. Practice parameters for the treatment of narcolepsy and other hypersomnias of central origin. *Sleep*. 2007;30:1705-1711.
83. Maski K, Trotti LM, Kotagal S, et al. Treatment of central disorders of hypersomnolence: an American Academy of Sleep Medicine clinical practice guideline. *J Clin Sleep Med*. 2021;17(9):1881-1893.
84. Maski K, Trotti LM, Kotagal S, et al. Treatment of central disorders of hypersomnolence: an American Academy of Sleep Medicine systematic review, meta-analysis, and GRADE assessment. *J Clin Sleep Med*. 2021;17(9):1895-1945.
85. Thorpy MJ, Bogan RK. Update on the pharmacologic management of narcolepsy: mechanisms of action and clinical implications. *Sleep Med*. 2020;68:97-109.
86. Thorpy MJ. Recently approved and upcoming treatments for narcolepsy. *CNS Drugs*. 2020;34(1):9-27.
87. Franceschini C, Pizza F, Cavalli F, Plazzi G. A practical guide to the pharmacological and behavioral therapy of Narcolepsy. *Neurotherapeutics*. 2021;18(1):6-19.
88. Kushida CA, Shapiro CM, Roth T, et al. Once-nightly sodium oxybate (FT218) demonstrated improvement of symptoms in a phase 3 randomized clinical trial in patients with narcolepsy. *Sleep*. 2022;45(6): zsab200.
89. Roth T, Dauvilliers Y, Thorpy MJ, et al. Effect of FT218, a once-nightly sodium oxybate formulation, on disrupted nighttime sleep in patients with narcolepsy: results from the randomized phase III REST-ON trial. *CNS Drugs*. 2022;36(4):377-387.
90. Dauvilliers Y, Roth T, Bogan R, et al. Efficacy of once-nightly sodium oxybate (FT218) in narcolepsy type 1 and type 2: post hoc analysis from the phase 3 REST-ON trial. *Sleep*. 2023;46(11):zsad152. doi:10.1093/sleep/zsad152.
91. Javaheri S, Javaheri S. Update on persistent excessive daytime sleepiness in OSA. *Chest*. 2020;158(2):776-786.
92. Chapman JL, Vakulin A, Hedner J, Yee BJ, Marshall NS. Modafinil/armodafinil in obstructive sleep apnoea: a systematic review and meta-analysis. *Eur Respir J*. 2016;47(5):1420-1428.
93. Thorpy MJ, Shapiro C, Mayer G, et al. A randomized study of solriamfetol for excessive sleepiness in narcolepsy. Ann Neurol. 2019 Mar;85(3):359-370. Erratum in: *Ann Neurol*. 2020 Jan;87(1):157.
94. Schwartz JR, Nelson MT, Schwartz ER, Hughes RJ. Effects of modafinil on wakefulness and executive function in patients with narcolepsy experiencing late-day sleepiness. *Clin Neuropharmacol*. 2004;27(2):74-79. Erratum in: *Clin Neuropharmacol*. 2004;27(3):152.
95. Ronnebaum S, Bron M, Patel D, Menno D, Bujanover S. Indirect treatment comparison of solriamfetol, modafinil, and armodafinil for excessive daytime sleepiness in obstructive sleep apnea. *J Clin Sleep Med*. 2021;17(12):2543-2555.
96. Watson NF, Davis CW, Zarycranski D, et al. Time to onset of response to pitolisant for the treatment of excessive daytime sleepiness and cataplexy in patients with narcolepsy: an analysis of randomized, placebo-controlled trials. *CNS Drugs*. 2021;35(12):1303-1315.
97. Mignot EJ. A practical guide to the therapy of narcolepsy and hypersomnia syndromes. *Neurotherapeutics*. 2012;9(4):739-752.
98. Mitler MM, Hajdukovic R. Relative efficacy of drugs for the treatment of sleepiness in narcolepsy. *Sleep*. 1991;14(3):218-220.
99. Dauvilliers Y, Arnulf I, Foldvary-Schaefer N, Morse AM. Safety and efficacy of lower-sodium oxybate in adults with idiopathic hypersomnia: a phase 3, placebo-controlled, double-blind, randomised withdrawal study. *Lancet Neurol*. 2022;21(1):53-65.
100. Kaplan S, Braverman DL, Frishman I, Bartov N. Pregnancy and fetal outcomes following exposure to modafinil and armodafinil during pregnancy. *JAMA Intern Med*. 2021;181(2):275-277.
101. Trotti LM, Arnulf I. Idiopathic hypersomnia and other hypersomnia syndromes. *Neurotherapeutics*. 2021;18(1):20-31.
102. Anderson KN, Pilsworth S, Sharples RD, Smith IE, Shneerson JM. Idiopathic hypersomnia: a study of 77 cases. *Sleep*. 2007;30:1274-1281.
103. Vernet C, Arnuf I. Idiopathic hypersomnia with and without long sleep time: a controlled series of 75 patients. *Sleep*. 2009;32:753-759.
104. Ali M, Auger RR, Slocumb NL, Morgenthaler TI. Idiopathic hypersomnia: clinical features and response to treatment. *J Clin Sleep Med*. 2009;5:562-568.
105. Childress AC, Cutler AJ, Marraffino A, et al. A randomized, double-blind, placebo-controlled study of HLD200, a delayed-release and extended-release methylphenidate, in children with attention-deficit/hyperactivity disorder: an evaluation of safety and efficacy throughout the day and across settings. *J Child Adolesc Psychopharmacol*. 2020;30(1):2-14.
106. Arnulf I, Rico TJ, Mignot E. Diagnosis, disease course, and management of patients with Kleine-Levin syndrome. *Lancet Neurol*. 2012;11(10):918-928.
107. Billiard M, Jaussent I, Dauvilliers Y, Besset A. Recurrent hypersomnia: a review of 339 cases. *Sleep Med Rev*. 2011;15:247-257.
108. Ortiz JF, Argudo JM, Yépez M, Moncayo JA. Neuroimaging in the rare sleep disorder of Kleine-Levin syndrome: a systematic review. *Clocks Sleep*. 2022;4(2):287-299.
109. Castriotta RJ, Murthy JN. Sleep disorders in patients with traumatic brain injury: a review. *CNS Drugs*. 2011;25(3):175-185.
110. Castriotta RJ, Wilde MC, Lai JM, Atanasov S, Masel BE, Kuna ST. Prevalence and consequences of sleep disorders in traumatic brain injury. *J Clin Sleep Med*. 2007;3(4):349-356.
111. Butler MG, Miller JL, Forster JL. Prader-Willi syndrome - clinical genetics, diagnosis and treatment approaches: an update. *Curr Pediatr Rev*. 2019;15(4):207-244.
112. Manni R, Politini L, Nobili L, et al. Hypersomnia in the Prader-Willi syndrome: clinical, electrophysiological features, and underlying factors. *Clin Neurophysiol*. 2001;112(5):800-805. doi:10.1016/s1388-2457(01)00483-7.
113. Camfferman D, McEvoy RD, O'Donoghue F, Lushington K. Prader Willi syndrome and excessive daytime sleepiness. *Sleep Med Rev*. 2008; 12(1):65-75.
114. Tobias ES, Tolmie GJ, Stephenson JBP. Cataplexy in Prader-Willi syndrome. *Arch Dis Child*. 2002;87:170.
115. Nevsimalova S, Vankova J, Stepanova I, et al. Hypocretin deficiency in Prader-Willi syndrome. *Eur J Neurol*. 2005;12:70-72.
116. Fronczek R, Lammers GJ, Balesar R, et al. The number of hypothalamic hypocretin orexin neurons is not affected in PWS. *J Clin Endocrinol Metab*. 2005;90:5466-5470.

117. Arnulf I, Leu S, Oudiette D. Abnormal sleep and sleepiness in Parkinson's disease. *Curr Opin Neurol.* 2008;21:472-477.
118. Bruin VM, Bittencourt LR, Tufik S. Sleep-wake disturbances in Parkinson's disease: current evidence regarding diagnostic and therapeutic decisions. *Eur Neurol.* 2012;67:257-267.
119. Dauvilliers YA, Laberge L. Myotonic dystrophy type 1, daytime sleepiness and REM sleep dysregulation. *Sleep Med Rev.* 2012;16(6):539-545.
120. Yu H, Laberge L, Jaussent I, et al. Daytime sleepiness and REM sleep characteristics in myotonic dystrophy: a case-control study. *Sleep.* 2011;34(2):165-170.
121. Martinez-Rodriguez JE, Lin L, Iranzo A, et al. Decreased hypocretin-1 (orexin-A) levels in the cerebrospinal fluid of patients with myotonic dystrophy and excessive daytime sleepiness. *Sleep.* 2003;26:287-290.
122. Denton EJ, Barnes M, Churchward T, et al. Mood disorders are highly prevalent in patients investigated with a multiple sleep latency test. *Sleep Breath.* 2018;22(2):305-309.
123. Plante DT. Hypersomnia in mood disorders: a rapidly changing landscape. *Curr Sleep Med Rep.* 2015;1(2):122-130.
124. Roehrs T, Zorick F, Sicklesteel J, et al. Excessive daytime sleepiness associated with insufficient sleep. *Sleep.* 1983;6:319-325.
125. Marti I, Valko PO, Khatami R, Bassetti CL, Baumann CR. Multiple sleep latency measures in narcolepsy and behaviorally induced insufficient sleep syndrome. *Sleep Med.* 2009;10(10):1146-1150.
126. Lee YJ, Park J, Kim S, Cho SJ, Kim SJ. Academic performance among adolescents with behaviorally induced insufficient sleep syndrome. *J Clin Sleep Med.* 2015;11(1):61-68.
127. Goldbart A, Peppard P, Finn L, et al. Narcolepsy and predictors of positive MSLTs in the Wisconsin Sleep Cohort. *Sleep.* 2014;37(6):1043-1051.

Chapter 33

Insomnia Diagnosis and Treatment

CHRONIC INSOMNIA DISORDER (CID)

Insomnia is defined as **sleep difficulty** (difficulty initiating or maintaining sleep and/or early morning awakening) that is associated with **daytime consequences** with the proviso that the nighttime or daytime problems are not explained by an inadequate opportunity to sleep.[1-3] The International Classification of Sleep Disorders, 3rd edition, text revision (ICSD-3-TR) defines only three insomnia disorders (chronic insomnia disorder (CID), short-term insomnia disorder, and other insomnia disorder).[3] There are also two symptoms defined in the "isolated symptoms and normal variants" section (excessive time in bed [TIB] and short sleeper).

The diagnostic criteria for CID include (criteria A-F must be met):

A. The patient reports or the patient's parent or caregiver observes one or more of the following:
   1. Difficulty initiating sleep
   2. Difficulty maintaining sleep
   3. Final awakening earlier than desired
   4. Resistance to going to bed on appropriate schedule
   5. Difficulty sleeping without parent or caregiver presence or intervention

B. The patient reports or the patient's parent or caregiver observes one or more of the following *related to the nighttime sleep difficulty:*
   1. Fatigue/malaise
   2. Impaired attention, concentration, or memory
   3. Impaired social, family, occupational, or academic performance
   4. Mood disturbance/irritability
   5. Subjective sleepiness
   6. Behavioral problems (e.g., hyperactivity, impulsivity, aggression)
   7. Reduced motivation/energy/initiative
   8. Proneness for errors/accidents
   9. Concerns about or dissatisfaction with sleep

C. The reported sleep/wakefulness complaints cannot be explained purely by **inadequate opportunity** (i.e., time allotted for sleep) or **inadequate circumstances** (i.e., safety, darkness, quiet, and comfort) for sleep.

D. The sleep disturbance and associated daytime symptoms occur at *least three times per week.*

E. The sleep disturbance and associated daytime symptoms have been present **for at least 3 months.**

F. The sleep disturbance and associated daytime symptoms are not **solely** due to another current sleep disorder, medical disorder, mental disorder, or medication/substance use.

Other names for short-term insomnia disorder include acute insomnia (AI) and adjustment insomnia. The ICSD-2 defined eight insomnia disorders but these are now considered subtypes in ICSD-3 and ICSD-3-TR (Table 33–1).[1-3] The ICSD-3 and ICSD-3-TR include the subtypes for historical purposes and because they illustrate collections of symptoms commonly reported by insomnia patients in sleep clinic.

The DSM-V lists insomnia disorder with specifiers (nonsleep disorder comorbidity, with other medical comorbidity, with other sleep disorder) and time course specifiers (episodic, persistent, recurrent).[4] Other classifications have listed primary insomnia and secondary insomnia. However, the term *comorbid insomnia* has been used to refer to secondary insomnias, as it is often difficult to define the relationship between insomnia and the associated disorder (primary vs. secondary). For example, insomnia may precede depression, worsen during depression, and persist after remission from depression. The CID as defined in the ICSD-3-TR encompasses elements of psychophysiologic insomnia, idiopathic insomnia, paradoxical insomnia, insomnia associated with mental disorder, inadequate sleep hygiene, insomnia caused by drug or substance, insomnia caused by medical condition, and behavioral insomnias of childhood (limit setting or sleep association disorders), all of which can be considered subtypes of CID (Table 33–1). The rationale for combining subtypes into a single disorder is that the previously used subtypes could not be reliably diagnosed.[5] The same patient might be diagnosed with different subtypes by different experienced clinicians. This is not surprising, as many patients manifest overlapping symptoms. Thus, CID encompasses all subtypes of insomnia, including primary and secondary insomnia.

CID is characterized by a report of difficulty initiating or maintaining sleep or waking up too early, with associated daytime consequences occurring despite **adequate opportunity and circumstances** for sleep. The sleep difficulties must occur at least *three times per week for at least 3 months.* CID can occur in isolation but is more often comorbid with another medical disorder, mental disorder, or medication/substance use. New in the ICSD-3-TR is an additional diagnostic criterion for CID: "The sleep disturbance and associated daytime symptoms are not solely due to another current sleep disorder, medical disorder, mental disorder, or medication/substance use". This recognizes that although insomnia can be precipitated by another disorder it acquires a "life of its own" and should be considered a separate entity requiring treatment. Also new is the statement that patients who are stable on hypnotics should still be diagnosed as having CID as they often present with complaints of being unable to sleep without the medication. In the ICSD-2, only a 1-month duration was required for many insomnia disorders. However, CID requires a minimum of 3 months duration. As CID encompasses

Table 33–1 Major Characteristics of Chronic Insomnia Disorder Subtypes

Insomnia Subtype	Essential Features	Clinical Clues
Psychophysiologic	• Anxiety about sleep. • Heightened arousal when in bed. • Conditioned sleep-preventing associations (bedroom as a stimulus for wakefulness, not sleep).	• Better sleep in novel environment (away from home). • Can fall asleep outside bedroom or when not trying to sleep.
Paradoxical	• Extreme and physiologically improbable complaints: "I never sleep." • Despite report of little sleep, relatively minor daytime impairment.	• Objective sleep duration (PSG, actigraphy) much greater than reported. • No or rare naps.
Idiopathic	• Onset in infancy or childhood. • No identifiable precipitant. • No period of sustained remission.	• Lifelong insomnia without remissions. • Insidious onset.
Associated with a mental disorder	• Mental disorder has been diagnosed. • Temporally associated with mental disorder (can precede by a few days or weeks).	• Insomnia waxes and wanes with mental disorder.
Inadequate sleep hygiene	• Improper sleep scheduling. • Use of products that disturb sleep near bedtime. • Stimulating activities near bedtime. • Use of the bed for non-sleep activities.	• Variable bedtime and wake-up time. • Napping.
Behavioral insomnia of childhood sleep-association type	• Falling asleep is an extended process. • Sleep-onset associations demanded. • In absence of associated factors, sleep onset delayed.	• Nighttime awakenings require caregiver for return to sleep.
Behavioral insomnia of childhood limit-setting type	• Difficulty initiating or maintaining sleep. • Refusal to go to bed or return to bed after awakening.	• Caregiver demonstrates insufficient limit setting to establish appropriate behavior.

Adapted from Schutte-Rodin S, Broch L, Buysee D, et al. Clinical guideline for the evaluation and management of chronic insomnia in adults. *J Clin Sleep Med.* 2008;4:487-504.

insomnia in children, the diagnostic criteria wording includes "the patient's parent or caregiver observes." More details on CID are listed below. A summary of the elements of subtypes of CID is listed in Table 33–1. This terminology is widely used in the literature and illustrates the wide variability in insomnia manifestations and historical elements. Many patients have elements of more than one subtype.

Short-Term Insomnia Disorder

This disorder encompasses what was previously termed *adjustment insomnia*. The duration must be less than 3 months. There is *no requirement that manifestations be present at least 3 times per week in ICSD-3-TR*. Short-term insomnia disorder is otherwise defined by similar criteria as CID (slightly different wording) other than a duration less than 3 months and include the following[3]:

A. The patient reports or the patient's parent or caregiver observes one or more of the following: difficulty initiating or maintaining sleep, waking up earlier than desired, resistance going to bed on appropriate schedule, difficulty sleeping without parent or caregiver presence or intervention.

B. The patient reports or the patient's parent or caregiver observes one or more of the following related to nighttime sleep difficulty: fatigue, malaise; impaired attention, concentration or memory;impaired social, family, vocational, or academic performance; mood disturbance/ irritability; subjective daytime sleepiness; behavioral problems (hyperactivity, impulsivity, aggression); reduced motivation/energy/initiative; proneness for errors/accidents; concerns about or dissatisfaction with sleep.

C. The reported sleep complaints cannot be explained purely by inadequate opportunity or circumstances for sleep.

D. The sleep disturbance and associated symptoms **have been present for less than 3 months.**

E. The sleep disturbance and associated daytime symptoms are not solely due to another current sleep disorder, medical disorder, mental disorder, or medication/substance use.

Other Insomnia Disorder, Excessive Time in Bed, and Short Sleeper

Other insomnia disorder is reserved for individuals who complain of difficulty initiating and maintaining sleep yet do not meet the full criteria for either CID or short-term insomnia disorder. The ICSD-3-TR includes two diagnoses (Excessive Time in Bed and Short Sleeper) as *isolated symptoms and normal variants*. Patients with excessive time in bed do not have insomnia complaints or daytime dysfunction. Yet they spend a long time in bed. This group often includes retired individuals or individuals who feel they should get more sleep than they really need. For example an older individual who stays in bed from 9 PM until 7 AM although awakening at 4 AM. That is, the patient sleeps about 7 hours but stays in bed for 10 hours feeling that he should sleep until 7 AM. The habitual sleep duration of short sleepers sleep is ≤ 6 hours but these individuals feel refreshed when awakening. They have no daytime dysfunction after a reduced amount of sleep. A mutation in the DEC2 gene has been associated with short sleep (about 6 hours or less) without any consequences or complaints. The short sleep is not volitional (no alarm clock) and is not due to a restricted sleep schedule. The metabolic consequences of restricted sleep are not present in "normal" short sleepers. The maxima in cortisol and sleepiness exhibit a close relationship to habitual wake-up time and occur about 2.5 hours later in long sleepers (habitual sleep duration > 9 hrs) than in short sleepers.

Epidemiology of Insomnia

While intermittent complaints of insomnia occur in **30% to 50%** of the general population, the prevalence of complaints meeting criteria for CID is estimated to be *10% to 15%*.[6-9] CID is *more common among women*, those with lower socioeconomic status, and those with medical or psychiatric illness. Complaints of insomnia can occur in up to 80% to 90% of patients with depression. CID usually lasts for years to decades, with *remission rates without treatment estimated to be less than 50%*.[9] Insomnia incurs increased healthcare costs and decreased productivity.[10,11] It is estimated that more than 90% of insomnia-related costs are attributable to work absences and reduced productivity.[12]

The etiology of insomnia is complex and certainly varies among individuals.[13-15] The 3P model of Spielman[13,14] includes **predisposing, precipitating, and perpetuating** factors. Recently, Ellis et al. have added coping to these factors.[15] Patients with insomnia tend to have negative appraisals and the coping styles "Worrying" and "Punishment" are common with both acute and chronic insomnia. Worry leads to an intense focusing on the event with little constructive analysis, and "Punishment" involves reviewing the event with self-chastisement. *Punishment was the most common coping style for acute insomnia.* Predisposing factors (e.g., personality traits) run through the entire course of the disorder, making some more vulnerable to insomnia than others. Heritability is a strong predisposing factor for insomnia (an estimated 40% influence on insomnia. These predisposing factors are then compounded by a precipitating event (e.g., a stressor) that pushes the individual above an "insomnia threshold," with acute sleep disruption or acute insomnia being the result. Over time, the impact of the stressor starts to diminish but still remains the main factor fueling the insomnia (early insomnia) while perpetuating factors (e.g., learned negative associations, behaviors, and cognitions that further inhibit the sleep process) are introduced. Finally, the impact of the stressor becomes negligible, but perpetuating factors keep the individual over the insomnia threshold (chronic insomnia).

A central feature of insomnia is hyperarousal, characterized by persistent and increased somatic, cognitive, and cortical stimulation. Hyperarousal leads to a state of conditioned arousal that disrupts both sleep and daytime function. Studies have shown increases in body temperature, heart rate, electroencephalographic activity, catecholamines, and oxygen consumption as measures of metabolic rate. These findings provide evidence of increased physiologic activation in insomnia but have not been consistent.[16-18] A meta-analysis[16] found the increase in metabolic rate to be relatively minor. However, changes in regional rather than global cerebral function (persistent activation) in certain brain areas could be more important for causation of insomnia.[19] One study found reduced GABA signaling in primary insomnia,[20] and another found high-frequency activity to be elevated in older adults with insomnia.[21]

Major Components of Chronic Insomnia Disorder

1. **Sleep difficulty**: In adults, the major complaints are difficulty initiating sleep (sleep-onset insomnia [SOI]), difficulty maintaining sleep (frequent awakenings, sleep-maintenance insomnia [SMI]), and early morning awakening. In children, sleep difficulty is defined by caregiver observation of resistance to going to bed at an appropriate time and difficulty maintaining sleep without parent/caregiver presence or intervention. Isolated SOI is less common than isolated SMI, although most patients have both SOI and SMI. The Delayed Sleep-Wake Phase Disorder (a circadian rhythm sleep-wake disorder) can present with an isolated SOI complaint.[3]
2. **Daytime difficulty resulting from sleep difficulty**: Multiple complaints may be present, including fatigue, attention/concentration difficulty, impaired social or academic performance, irritability, daytime sleepiness, and reduced motivation. In children, behavioral problems such as hyperactivity, aggression, or impulsivity may be prominent. Often, the patient expresses dissatisfaction with sleep or concerns about the effects of poor sleep on their health.
3. **Frequency, duration, adequate sleep opportunity/environment**: A frequency of *at least 3 nights per week, a duration of >3 months*, and the requirement of an *adequate opportunity and environment for sleep* are requirements for the diagnosis of CID.

Insomnia Evaluation

The evaluation of a patient with insomnia complaints depends on history, the physical examination, questionnaires including sleep logs (diaries) or actigraphy, and, less commonly, polysomnography (PSG) (Table 33–2). A detailed sleep history is the cornerstone of evaluation of insomnia.[22-25] PSG is not indicated unless sleep apnea is suspected or the patient is refractory to treatment.[26] First, the nature of the **primary sleep complaint** (problems with sleep onset, sleep maintenance, or quality) should be defined and the **duration of the complaint** determined. The history and **origin** of the complaint, including age of onset, should be explored, and the life events or stressors at the start of the problem should be identified. For example, patients with the subtype idiopathic insomnia report problems since childhood or adolescence with an insidious onset. Patients with the psychophysiologic subtype of insomnia may report that chronic insomnia began after a severe illness. **Pre-sleep conditions** or activities that could affect sleep, including the bedroom environment, activities near bedtime, or mental state near bedtime, should be explored. The **bedroom environment** should be characterized by factors that might disturb sleep (noise, clock easily seen from the bed, extreme hot or cold temperature). **Activities near bedtime,** including working late on the computer, drinking caffeinated beverages or alcohol in the evening, or exercise near bedtime, may impair the ability to sleep. The **mental status at bedtime** should also be explored. Often, patients begin worrying about stressors and problems when retiring for the night. The presence or absence of **nocturnal symptoms,** including snoring, gasping during sleep, symptoms of the restless leg syndrome, and body movements, should be evaluated.

The **sleep-wake schedule** should be determined by report, including variability of bedtime and rise time and the frequency and duration of naps. Factors that worsen or improve sleep should be detailed. For example, some patients with insomnia report sleeping better in a novel environment (reverse first-night effect).[27] Patient recall can be supplemented by

Table 33–2 Evaluation of Insomnia

1. Sleep History

A. Define **primary complaint.**
- Delayed sleep onset
- Sleep maintenance problems
- Frequent awakenings/early morning awakening
- Nonrestorative sleep

B. Define **time course of complaint.**
- Age of onset
- Precipitating event or stressor.

C. Evaluate pre-sleep conditions.
- Pre-bedtime activities
- Bedroom environment
- Physical and mental status before sleep

D. **Nocturnal symptoms** (awakenings, physical or mental symptoms including snoring or body movements).

E. Sleep-wake schedule—by patient report (including variability, naps).

F. Daytime function—consequences of insomnia
- Sleepiness versus fatigue.
- Impairment of mood, cognitive dysfunction, quality of life.

G. Daytime activities relevant for sleep
- Sunlight exposure, exercise
- Napping
- Work schedule and disturbance
- Caffeine and alcohol intake

H. Medical and psychiatric conditions (e.g., chronic pain, depression) or medications that may affect sleep.

2. Physical and Mental Status Examination

A. Narrow upper airway (high Mallampati score), retrognathia

3. Supporting Information

A. Sleep/mood questionnaires
- Epworth Sleepiness Scale
- Dysfunctional Beliefs and Attitudes about Sleep
- Pittsburgh Sleep Quality Index
- Insomnia Severity Index

B. Sleep log for 2 weeks—attention to sleep and wake-up time variability, general patterns.

C. Actigraphy.

4. Polysomnography
- Not routinely indicated
- Indicated when another sleep disorder such as sleep apnea is suspected.

sleep logs and/or actigraphy. **Daytime function** should be discussed with emphasis on possible consequences of insomnia. Reports of *daytime fatigue or impaired cognition and mood* are more common than true daytime sleepiness. **True daytime sleepiness should trigger suspicion for additional sleep problems such as sleep apnea, narcolepsy, or depression.** Disturbed sleep can occur in all of these conditions. Daytime activities that may affect sleep, such as the amount of caffeine, alcohol, exercise, sunlight exposure, and napping, should be detailed. A general medical and psychiatric history is important to identify mental or medical conditions that may affect sleep. A detailed medication history including over-the-counter medications and substances of abuse is extremely important. A number of medications and substances can also disturb sleep quality (Table 33–3).[22] A more detailed discussion of medications affecting sleep can be found in Chapter 9. Although beta blocker risk for insomnia is often stated to be greater with highly lipophilic medications and those with greater 5HT receptor affinity (highest risk with propranolol and metoprolol) and lowest with atenolol), all beta blockers suppress melatonin (except for carvedilol). Melatonin administration can help with insomnia due to beta receptor blockade. Thus while some authors have stated atenolol is the beta blocker with the lowest risk (not lipophilic) others have stated that carvedilol has the lowest insomnia risk. Of interest, of the antiepileptic medications lamotrigine is the most likely to disturb sleep (can cause insomnia or sedation). The history of worsening sleep after starting a specific medication is highly suggestive of insomnia due to that medication. Patients do not associate "non-sleep" medications as possibly causing an issue. Therefore it is important to ask about all recent medication changes and the relationship with insomnia symptoms.

A physical examination and a general medical history, including appropriate laboratory tests (if not recently performed), should rule out obvious medical causes of insomnia. Examination of the upper airway showing a high Mallampati score (upper-airway narrowing)[28] might trigger suspicion of obstructive sleep apnea.

A number of other sleep disorders not included in the group of CID subtypes (Table 33–1) can also present with complaints of insomnia (Table 33–4). Sleep apnea syndromes can be associated with repetitive arousal and sleep-maintenance problems. In some patients, insomnia resolves or improves with treatment of sleep apnea. However, significant and persistent insomnia is often comorbid with sleep apnea (COMISA), and effective treatment of both components is essential for

Table 33–3 Selected Medications and Substances Known to Cause insomnia

Anticonvulsants • Lamotrigine	**Steroids** • Prednisone
Antidepressants (non-sedating) • Bupropion • Fluoxetine • Citalopram • Escitalopram • Venlafaxine	**Decongestants** • Phenylpropanolamine • Pseudoephedrine **Bronchodilators** • Theophylline • Beta agonist inhalers
Beta Blockers (risk of insomnia) • Propranolol, metoprolol. labetalol (high risk) • Pindolol, carvedilol (moderate risk) • Atenolol, bisoprolol (Low risk)	**Stimulants/Alerting Agents** • Dextroamphetamine • Methamphetamine • Modafinil
Substances • Caffeine • Alcohol: sleep-maintenance insomnia • Cannabis withdrawal	**Immunosuppressive Agents** • Interferon • Prednisone • Mycophenolate
Antibiotics/Antivirals • Efavirenz (Sustiva)	

Adapted from Schweitzer PK. Drugs that disturb sleep and wakefulness. In Kryger MH, Roth T, Dement WC (eds): *Principles and Practice of Sleep Medicine*, 4th ed. Philadelphia: Elsevier Saunders; 2005:495-518.

Table 33–4 Other Sleep Disorders Associated With Insomnia Complaints

1. Sleep apnea syndromes (COMISA)
2. Circadian rhythm sleep-wake disorders
   a. Delayed sleep-wake phase disorder—sleep-onset insomnia
   b. Advanced sleep-wake phase disorder—early-morning awakening
   c. Irregular sleep-wake rhythm disorder - at least three sleep episodes per 24 hours
   d. Non-24 hour sleep-wake rhythm disorder - alternating periods of insomnia and hypersomnia
3. Restless legs syndrome/periodic limb movement disorders

COMISA combination of OSA and comorbid insomnia

success.[29,30] In patients with sleep apnea, insomnia symptoms are more likely to be present in women than in men.[31] Circadian rhythm sleep-wake disorders (CRSWDs) can also be associated with insomnia complaints, including the Delayed Sleep-Wake Phase Disorder (SOI) and Advanced Sleep-Wake Phase Disorder (early morning awakening). In the Delayed Sleep-Wake Phase Disorder, once the affected individuals can fall asleep, they have fairly normal sleep. If undisturbed by societal demands the sleep duration is usually normal. In the Advanced Sleep-Wake Phase Disorder, individuals fall asleep early but then awaken in the early morning hours. In the Non–24-hour Circadian Sleep-Wake Rhythm Disorder, patients may report periods of insomnia alternating with hypersomnia.[3] Restless legs syndrome/periodic limb movement disorder can also be associated with symptoms of insomnia or nonrestorative sleep.

Table 33–5 Questionnaires to Evaluate Patients with Insomnia

Epworth Sleepiness Scale	Propensity to fall asleep in eight situations (0 never, 1 slight, 2 moderate, 3 high chance) with a total score 0 to 24. Normal ≥10.
Beck Depression Inventory	BDI or BDI-II is a 21-item self-report inventory used to measure depression. BDI-I scores: Minimal or no depression BDI <10, moderate to severe depression BDI ≥ 19. BDI-II scores: Minimal or no depression BDI <14, moderate to severe depression BDI ≥ 20.
Pittsburgh Sleep Quality Index	A 24-item self-report measure of sleep qualities (poor sleep associated with **global score >5**).
Insomnia Severity Index (ISI)	Seven-item self-report questionnaire assessing the nature, severity, and impact of insomnia. Each item is graded 0 to 4, with total a score of 15-21 indicating moderate insomnia and 22-28 severe insomnia
Dysfunctional Beliefs and Attitudes about Sleep Questionnaire	DBAS is a self-rating of 30 statements that is used to assess negative cognitions about sleep. A shorter version of the DBAS-16 also exists.

BDI, Beck Depression Inventory; *DBAS*, dysfunctional beliefs and attitudes about sleep; *ISI*, Insomnia Severity Index; *PSQI*, Pittsburgh Sleep Quality Index.

Questionnaires, Sleep Logs, and Actigraphy

Supporting information from questionnaires (mood, cognition about insomnia), sleep logs, and actigraphy may be helpful in evaluating patients with insomnia. These may supplement other information obtained from the sleep history. Assessing the patient's attitudes about sleep and the sleep problem is as important as documenting the degree of sleep disturbance. In addition, some patients are hesitant to admit feelings of depression. Sleep logs and actigraphy provide a more accurate estimate of the patient's sleep quantity than is possible from patient recall.

Sleep Questionnaires. Several questionnaires have been used to evaluate patients with insomnia (Table 33–5). The Epworth Sleepiness Scale is used to assess subjective estimates of the propensity to fall asleep in common situations.[32] The Pittsburgh Sleep Quality Index (PSQI)[33,34] is a 24-item self-report measure of general sleep quality that specifically addresses the preceding 1-month period. The PSQI evaluates seven domains, including the duration of sleep, sleep disturbance, sleep-onset latency (SOL), daytime dysfunction resulting from sleepiness, sleep efficiency, need for medications to sleep, and overall sleep quality. The PSQI yields a global score and seven component scores (poor sleep associated with a global score > 5). The questionnaire has been shown to discriminate healthy patients, patients with depression, and patients with sleep disorders. It was not designed specifically for insomnia but has been used in insomnia assessment and treatment studies. Detailed instructions for use and scoring of the PSQI are available at the University of Pittsburgh Sleep Medicine Institute web site, https://www.sleep.pitt.edu/instruments/.

The **insomnia severity index** (ISI) is a *seven-item self-report* questionnaire assessing the nature, severity, and impact of insomnia.[35-37] The usual recall period is the "last month" and the dimensions evaluated are: severity of sleep onset, sleep maintenance, early morning awakening problems, sleep dissatisfaction, interference of sleep difficulties with daytime functioning, noticeability of sleep problems by others, and distress caused by the sleep difficulties. A five-point Likert scale is used to rate each item (e.g., 0 = no problem; 4 = very severe problem), yielding a total score ranging from 0 to 28. The total score is interpreted as follows: absence of insomnia (0-7); sub-threshold insomnia (8-14); moderate insomnia (15-21); and severe insomnia (22-28) (Figure 33–1). An insomnia questionnaire based on two questions of the ISI has also been developed (satisfied/dissatisfied with the current sleep pattern, sleep interferes with daily function, questions 4 and 7 in the ISI).[38]

The Beck Depression Inventory (BDI-I or BDI-II)[39-41] is a 21-item self-report inventory used to measure manifestations of depression, each item being scored from 0 to 3. Higher total scores indicate more severe depressive symptoms. The BDI-II is a revision of the original BDI-I. Because primary insomnia and major depression share some daytime symptoms, the usual cutoff scores for the BDI might be less specific for depression in patients with insomnia.[41] The Dysfunctional Beliefs and Attitudes about Sleep (DBAS) Questionnaire[42,43] is a self-rating survey to assess negative cognitions about sleep. Reversal of these cognitions is a goal of the *cognitive component* of cognitive behavioral therapy (CBT). The original DBAS was a 30-item questionnaire in

Insomnia severity index (ISI)

The insomnia severity index has seven questions. The seven questions are added up to get a total score. When you have your total score look at guidelines for scoring interpretation below to see where you sleep difficulty fits.

For each question, please **circle** the number that best describes your answer.

Please rate the **current** (ie **last 2 weeks**) **severity** of your insomnia problem(s)

	None	Mild	Moderate	Severe	Very severe
1. Difficulty falling asleep	0	1	2	3	4
2. Difficulty staying asleep	0	1	2	3	4
3. Problems waking up too early	0	1	2	3	4

4. How **satisfied/dissatisfied** are you with your **current** sleep pattern?

Very satisfied	Satisfied	Moderately satisfied	Dissatisfied	Very dissatisfied
0	1	2	3	4

5. How **noticeable** to others do you think your sleep problem is in terms of impairing the quality of your life?

Not at all noticeable	A little	Somewhat	Much	Very much noticeable
0	1	2	3	4

6. How **worried/distressed** are you about your current sleep problelm?

Not at all worried	A little	Somewhat	Much	Very much worried
0	1	2	3	4

7. To what extent do you consider your sleep problem to **interfere** with you daily function (e.g. daytime fatigue, mood, ability to function at work/daily chores, concentration, memory, mood, etc) **currently?**

Not at all Interfering	A little	Somewhat	Much	Very much Interfering
0	1	2	3	4

Guidelines for scoring and interpretation:
Add scores for all seven item
Total score categories:
0–7 = No clinically significant insomnia, 8–14 subthreshold insomnia,
15–21 clinical insomnia (moderate severity), 22–28 = clinical insomnia (severe)
ISI official webpage (mapi-trust.org) used with permission Charles M. Morin, PhD, Université Laval.

Figure 33–1 The insomnia severity index.

which patients responded using an analog scale (0, strongly disagree, to 10, strongly agree). A shorter version (DBAS-16)[43] has recently been validated and is less time-consuming for patients to complete (Figure 33–2).

Sleep Logs. A sleep log (sleep diary) for at least 2 weeks is recommended when evaluating patients with insomnia. Sleep logs are often more accurate than relying on patient recall of their chronic sleep patterns. Sleep logs usually follow a question format (Figure 33–3) or time-plot graphic format (Figure 33–4). An adaptation of a basic consensus sleep log[44] is shown in Figure 33–3. The essential elements of a sleep log include the ability to assess time in bed (TIB), sleep onset latency (SOL), total sleep time (TST), and the amount of wakefulness after sleep onset (WASO). TIB is the time period from when the patient gets in bed until the final time the patient leaves the bed in the morning. WASO includes all wakefulness from sleep onset until the patient leaves the bed in the morning. The patient need report only three of these four parameters because they are related (TIB = SOL + TST + WASO). One can compute a sleep efficiency (TST × 100/TIB), with normal values exceeding 85%. Sleep logs also typically provide space to record caffeine consumption, bedtime activities, medications taken for sleep, and estimates of sleep quality. *Sleep logs are very helpful in revealing general patterns of the sleep-wake cycle, such as irregular bedtimes and wake-up times and the amount and frequency of napping.* A few characteristic patterns noted in sleep logs are listed in Table 33–6. In Figure 33–4, an example of

Name	Strongly disagree 1	2	3	4	5	6	7	8	9	Strongly agree 10
1. I need 8 hours of sleep to feel refreshed and function well during the day.										
2. When I don't get a proper amount of sleep on a given night, I need to catch up on the next day by napping or on the next night by sleeping longer										
3. I am concerned that chronic insomnia may have serious consequences on my physical health										
4. I am worried that I may lose control over my abilities to sleep										
5. After a poor nights sleep I know that it will interfere with my daily activities on the next day										
6. In order to be alert and function well during the day, I believe would be better off taking a sleeping pill rather than having a poor nights sleep										
7. When I feel irritable, depressed, or anxious during the day it is mostly because I did not sleep well the night before										
8. When I sleep poorly on one night, I know it will disturb my sleep schedule for the whole week										
9. Without an adequate night's sleep I can hardly function the next day										
10. I can't ever predict whether i'll have a good or poor night's sleep										
11. I have little ability to manage the negative consequences of disturbed sleep										
12. When I feel tired, have no energy, or just seem not to function well during the day, its generally because I did not sleep well the night before										
13. I believe insomnia is essentially the result of a chemical imbalance										
14. I feel insomnia in running my ability to enjoy life and prevents me from doing what I want										
15. Medication is probably the only solution to sleeplessness										
16. I avoid or cancel obligations (social, family) after a poor night's sleep										

Figure 33–2 The Dysfunctional Beliefs and Attitudes about Sleep (DBAS-16) questionnaire. (© Charles M. Morin. From Morin CM, Vallières A, Ivers H: Dysfunctional beliefs and attitudes about sleep (DBAS): validation of a brief version (DBAS-16). *Sleep* 2007;30:1547–1554.)

the graphical format is illustrated. The sleep log illustrates variability in go-to-bed times and out-of-bed times, sleep latency, nearly daily alcohol consumption, and napping. In Figure 33–5, the graphical sleep log shows a long sleep latency, variability in bedtime and wake-up time, and multiple wakefulness periods during the night. It also shows a prolonged TIB (in bed to out of bed) of at least 9 hours. This patient would benefit from sleep restriction therapy, to be discussed in the behavioral treatments section.

Actigraphy. Actigraphy involves use of a portable device (often resembling a watch and typically worn on the wrist) that collects movement information (activity) over an extended time period (Figure 33–6). More information on actigraphy is presented in Chapter 16. The absence of movement is assumed to be a surrogate of sleep.[45-51] The use of actigraphy is included in the ICSD-3-TR diagnostic criteria for several circadian sleep-wake rhythm disorders.[3] Practice parameters for use of actigraphy have been published by the American Academy of Sleep Medicine (AASM), with the most recent update in 2018.[46-49] While actigraphy is indicated for determining the circadian patterns of patients with insomnia, the practice parameters did not state that actigraphy was indicated as a routine evaluation of patients with insomnia.

Actigraphy does not measure sleep as defined by electroencephalography (EEG)/electro-oculography (EOG)/chin electromyography (EMG) criteria or the subjective experience of sleep (as measured by sleep logs and questionnaires). Therefore, it is not surprising that estimates of TST, wakefulness time, and the sleep latency from sleep logs and actigraphy may differ from PSG findings.[48-51] Algorithms have been developed to estimate TST and WASO from the activity data. Actigraphy estimates of sleep duration, WASO, and sleep latency are more accurate in normal individuals than in patients with insomnia. Periods of low activity in which patients lay quietly in bed but are awake may be scored as sleep by actigraphy software. When performing actigraphy, *it is essential to require patients to complete a sleep log (e.g., lights off, lights on, out of bed, actigraph off for shower; TST; sleep latency).* This information enables a correct interpretation of actigraphy tracings. *If the actigraphy estimate of TST far exceeds patient estimates, this would suggest the paradoxical insomnia subtype of CID* (Figure 33–7).

Sleep logs and actigraphy provide complementary information. Actigraphy is most valuable in determining the pattern of wakefulness and sleep. It can detect irregular bedtimes, wake-up times, and naps. Sleep logs are always filled out by patients wearing an actigraph. Sleep logs may overestimate sleep latency, while actigraphy underestimates sleep latency

Name ______

Today's date	Sample 4/5/12	1	2	3	4	5	6	7
1. What time did you get into bed last night	10:00 pm							
2. What time did you try go to sleep last night?	10:30 pm							
3. How long did it take you to fall asleep last night?	60 min							
4. How many times did you wake up, not counting your final awakening?	5 times							
5. In total, how long were you awake last night?	60 min							
6. What time was your final awakening?	6:00 am							
7. What time did you get out of bed for the day?	6:30 am							
8. In total how long did you sleep last night?	5 hours 30 min							
9. How would you rate the quality of your sleep?	☐ Very poor ☐ Poor ☐ Fair ☐ Good ☐ Very good	☐ Very poor ☐ Poor ☐ Fair ☐ Good ☐ Very good	☐ Very poor ☐ Poor ☐ Fair ☐ Good ☐ Very good	☐ Very poor ☐ Poor ☐ Fair ☐ Good ☐ Very good	☐ Very poor ☐ Poor ☐ Fair ☐ Good ☐ Very good	☐ Very poor ☐ Poor ☐ Fair ☐ Good ☐ Very good	☐ Very poor ☐ Poor ☐ Fair ☐ Good ☐ Very good	☐ Very poor ☐ Poor ☐ Fair ☐ Good ☐ Very good
10. Comments								

Figure 33–3 A typical sleep log/diary. In this format, it would be relatively easy to compute an average sleep latency, average time in bed, average total sleep time, and average sleep efficiency (total sleep time/time in bed). (Adapted from Carney CE, Buysse DJ, Ancoli-Israel S, et al. The consensus sleep diary: standardizing prospective sleep self-monitoring. *Sleep*. 2012;35(2):287-302. PMID: 22294820.)

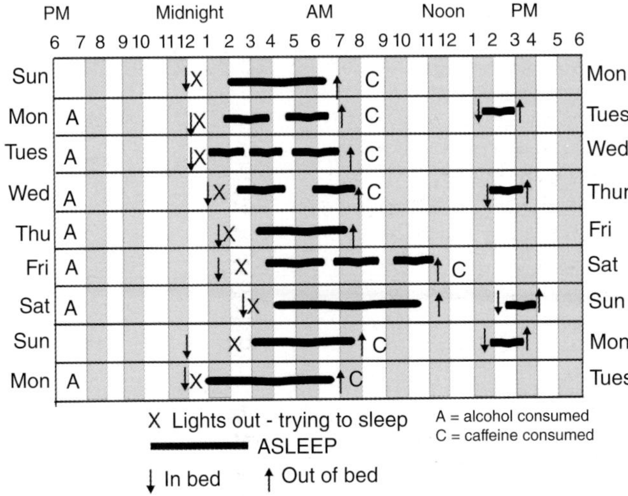

Figure 33–4 An example of a graphical sleep diary format. The periods of estimated sleep are marked by horizonal lines. The *down arrow* is time in bed, *up arrow* the time out of bed. Some formats add a symbol for trying to go to sleep. Notation is made when alcohol or caffeine (or hypnotics) are consumed/taken. The advantage of this format is that patterns of sleep and wakefulness are easily determined. However, it is more difficult to determine parameters like average sleep latency, total sleep time, and average wakefulness time during the night. In this patient, on some nights there was a long sleep latency (time from X to sleep), frequent periods of wakefulness during the night, variable wake-up and out-of-bed times, and on some nights the time in bed was much greater than the total sleep time. The patient also took several naps. Note that, on Sunday, the patient got in bed at midnight but did not try to sleep until about 2:00 AM.

Table 33–6 Some Typical Sleep-Log Patterns

Delayed sleep phase	Late bedtime or long sleep latency, few awakenings, normal sleep duration on weekends or non-work/non-school days.
Inadequate sleep hygiene	Irregular wake and rise times, naps, long time in bed.
Psychophysiologic insomnia	Long sleep latency, decreased total sleep time, frequent awakenings, long time in bed.
Paradoxical insomnia	Nights of minimal or no sleep are reported followed by no or few naps the next day.

(lying still but awake). Sleep logs may underestimate TST, and actigraphy may overestimate TST. The relationships among PSG, actigraphy, and sleep log findings also may differ depending on the characteristics of the group being studied. See Chapter 16 for additional information about actigraphy.

Polysomnography Findings in Insomnia

As noted, PSG is not indicated for the routine assessment of insomnia. The 2003 AASM practice parameters for the role of PSG in insomnia state, "*PSG is indicated when the initial diagnosis (insomnia) is uncertain, treatment fails (either behavioral or*

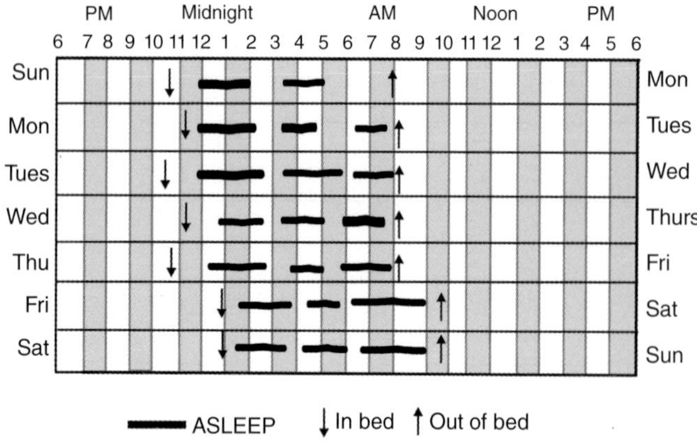

Figure 33–5 A graphical sleep log (diary) showing a pattern of variable bedtimes, variable sleep latency, frequent awakenings during the night, consistent out of bed time during the week to arrive at work by 9 AM with delayed bed time and out of bed time on the weekends.

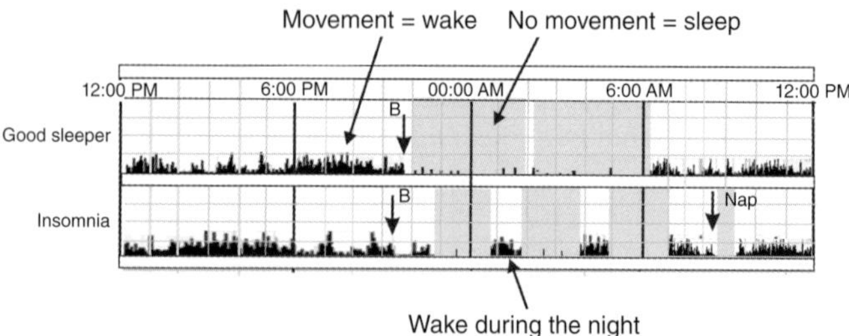

Figure 33–6 Samples of 24 hours of actigraphy in a good sleeper and a patient with insomnia showing multiple periods of wakefulness at night and a nap. B is a patient marker for lights-out time. Some actigraphy devices provide an ambient light maker allowing another estimation of lights-out time.

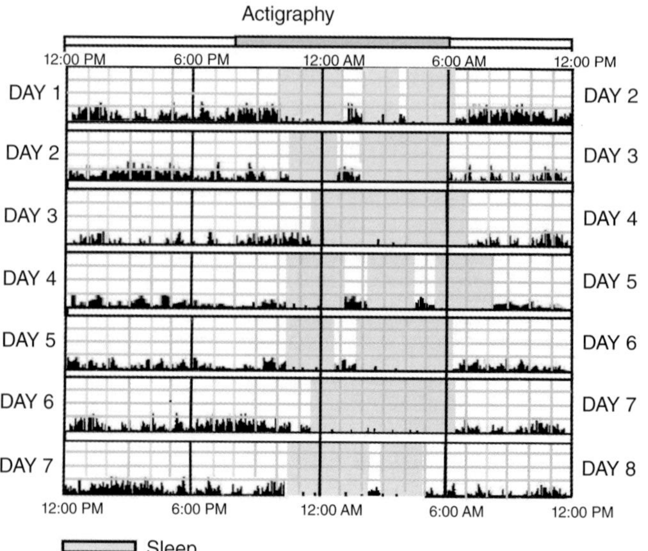

Sleep Diary

	Time in Bed	Time trying to sleep	How long to fall asleep (min)	Number of awakenings	Total sleep (hrs)	Final awakening
Day 1	9.30P	10:00P	60 min	2	3	6A
Day 2	10P	10:30P	60 min	1	3	6A
Day 3	11P	11:30P	50 min	0	2	7A
Day 4	10P	10:30P	40 min	2	2	8A
Day 5	10P	10:30P	90 min	1	3	6A
Day 6	11P	11:30P	8 hrs	0	0	6A
Day 7	10P	10:30P	60 min	1	4	5A

Figure 33–7 The sleep diary shows much shorter reported total sleep time than was apparent based on actigraphy. This pattern would be consistent with the CID subtype paradoxical insomnia.

pharmacologic), or precipitous arousals occur with violent or injurious behavior (Guideline)."[26] When PSG is performed, typical findings (Table 33–7) in patients with insomnia include a long sleep latency (>30 minutes), reduced TST, increased WASO, and reduced sleep efficiency. A long rapid eye movement (REM) latency, high arousal index, increased stage N1 sleep, and decreased stage N3 sleep may also be noted. In patients with paradoxical insomnia, the objective sleep abnormality is much less severe than reported. It is not unusual for such patients to report little or no sleep after a PSG documenting only mild to moderate decrements in TST. In some patients with psychophysiologic insomnia, the "reverse first-night effect"[27] may be noted. In these patients, the sleep quality in the sleep center is better than that reported at home. *It is essential to have patients complete a questionnaire assessing subjective sleep (estimate TST, sleep latency, sleep quality) after PSG.*

Table 33–7 Typical Polysomnography Findings in Patients With Insomnia

- Increased sleep latency (>30 minutes)
- Decreased TST
- Decreased sleep efficiency
- Increased stage N1 (%TST)
- Decreased stage N3 (%TST)
- Increased REM latency
- Decreased REM latency (depression)

REM, rapid eye movement; *TST*, total sleep time.

TREATMENT OF INSOMNIA

The two major categories of insomnia treatment include cognitive behavioral treatment for insomnia (CBT-I) and pharmacologic treatment (hypnotic medications). CBT-I is considered the treatment of choice for insomnia including insomnia comorbid with mental and medical conditions. However, CBT-I and pharmacological treatment are not mutually exclusive. In most studies, combination treatment (behavioral + medication) has not been demonstrated to be more effective than the behavioral component alone. However, a few studies have shown possible benefit of combined treatment (or combined sequential treatment) in some patients.[52-55]

Behavioral Treatment of Insomnia

Cognitive and Behavioral Treatments for Insomnia

The major categories of cognitive and behavioral treatments for insomnia and the individual types of behavioral treatments are discussed below. The precise treatments involved in CBT-I and the terminology to describe various combinations of treatments varies in the literature.[56–60] In this chapter we will use the terminology of Edinger et al[6]. Multicomponent CBT-I includes cognitive treatment (one or more techniques) plus behavioral techniques including stimulus control and sleep restriction. Other interventions such as relaxation treatment or sleep hygiene education may be included. Single component treatment includes cognitive therapy, stimulus control therapy, sleep restriction therapy, relaxation therapy, sleep hygiene (education), biofeedback, paradoxical intention, intensive sleep retraining, and mindfulness therapy. A number of other techniques exist.[6]

CBT-I is safe and effective treatment for SOI and SMI, as well as complaints of poor sleep quality (non-restorative sleep).[6,52-60] The efficacy of behavioral treatments is equal to or better than that of pharmacotherapy.[52-60] Unfortunately, many locales do not have physicians, nurses, or psychologists skilled at this form of treatment. The 2006 update of the AASM practice parameters for behavioral treatment of chronic insomnia state, "psychological and behavioral interventions are effective and recommended in the treatment of chronic primary insomnia, secondary insomnia (due or associated with other medical or psychiatric disorders), insomnia in older adults, and chronic hypnotic users (Standard)."[58] In Table 33–8, the major cognitive and behavioral treatments for insomnia are listed with the levels of recommendation according to 2021 AASM clinical practice guidelines[60]. In 2008, clinical guidelines for the evaluation and management of chronic insomnia in adults[22] recommended that CBT-I be used as initial treatment of insomnia, if possible. The 2021 AASM guidelines for management of insomnia[60] (Table 33–9) recommend "clinicians use multicomponent CBT for insomnia (Strong) for treatment of CID in adults." This

Table 33–9 2021 AASM Clinical Practice Guideline for Behavioral and Psychologic Treatments of Chronic Insomnia Disorder in Adults

1. We recommend that clinicians use *multicomponent cognitive behavioral therapy for insomnia* for the treatment of chronic insomnia disorder in adults. (Strong)
2. We suggest that clinicians use multicomponent **brief therapies** for insomnia for the treatment of chronic insomnia disorder in adults. (Conditional)
3. We suggest that clinicians use *stimulus control* as a single-component therapy for the treatment of chronic insomnia disorder in adults. (Conditional)
4. We suggest that clinicians use sleep restriction therapy as a single-component therapy for the treatment of chronic insomnia disorder in adults. (Conditional)
5. We suggest that clinicians use *relaxation therapy* as a single-component therapy for the treatment of chronic insomnia disorder in adults. (Conditional)
6. We suggest that clinicians not use sleep hygiene as a single-component therapy for the treatment of chronic insomnia disorder in adults. (Conditional)

Edinger JD, Arnedt JT, Bertisch SM, et al. Behavioral and psychological treatments for chronic insomnia disorder in adults: an American Academy of Sleep Medicine clinical practice guideline. *J Clin Sleep Med.* 2021;17(2): 255-262.

Table 33–8 Behavioral Treatments for Insomnia

Technique	Treatment Type	Level of Recommendation	Brief summary
CBT-I	Multi-component	Strong For	• Cognitive Therapy (one or more cognitive techniques) plus stimulus control and sleep restriction with or without other behavioral components including sleep education and relaxation therapy
BTI (brief behavioral treatment)	Multi-component	Conditional For	• Abbreviated versions of CBT-I (typically 1–4 sessions) emphasizing the behavior components including education about sleep sessions based on stimulus control and sleep restriction therapy
Sleep Hygiene Education	Single component	Conditional Against (when used as single component)	• Information about good sleep habits
Stimulus control therapy	Single component	Conditional For	• If not sleepy, get out of bed until sleepy • Same wake-up time every day • Bed is used only for sleep
Sleep restriction therapy	Single component	Conditional For	• Restrict time in bed so that total sleep time is ≥85% of time in bed
Relaxation therapy	Single component	Conditional For	• Progressive muscle relaxation • Guided imagery
Cognitive Treatments	Single Component	None when used alone	• Addresses dysfunctional cognitions about sleep
Biofeedback	Single component	None	• Reduce somatic tension using a device capable of providing feedback on some aspect of the patient's physiology
Paradoxical intention	Single component	None	• Passively remain awake and avoid any effort (intention) to fall asleep
Intensive sleep retraining	Single component	None	• Treatment is designed to markedly enhance homeostatic sleep drive to reduce both sleep onset difficulties and sleep misperception
Mindfulness Therapy	Single component	None	• Meditation emphasizing a nonjudgmental state of heightened or complete awareness of one's thoughts, emotions, or experiences on a moment-to-moment basis

BTI, brief behavioral treatment of insomnia; *CBT-I*, cogntive behavioral treatment for insomnia.
Adapted from Morgenthaler T, Kramer M, Alessi C, et al: Practice parameters for the psychological and behavioral treatment of insomnia: an update. *Sleep* 2006; 29:1415–1419.

recommendation was based on studies in which multicomponent treatment was administered by professionals to patients *with and without comorbid conditions*. A recommendation for use of multicomponent **brief therapies** for insomnia for the treatment of CID in adults was made at the Conditional level. Brief behavioral treatment of insomnia (BBTI), which is a type of brief behavioral treatment, will be described below. Conditional recommendations for the use of stimulus control therapy, sleep restriction therapy, or relaxation therapy as single component treatment for CID in adults were also made. A recommendation that clinicians ***not*** use sleep hygiene as a single component therapy for CID in adults was made at the Conditional level.[60]

Elements of Cognitive and Behavioral Therapy

Cognitive Therapy. Cognitive therapy is aimed toward changing the patient's belief and attitudes about insomnia.[6,22,52-60] These dysfunctional cognitions are often identified using questionnaires such as the dysfunctional beliefs about sleep questionnaire (DBAS) (Figure 33–2).[42,43] Cognitive therapy uses a psychotherapeutic method to reconstruct cognitive pathways with positive and appropriate concepts about sleep and its effects. Common cognitive distortions that are identified and addressed in the course of treatment include, "I can't sleep without medication," "I have a chemical imbalance," "If I can't sleep, I should stay in bed and rest," and "My life will be ruined if I can't sleep."[42,43]

Sleep Hygiene. Up to 30% of patients evaluated for insomnia have inadequate sleep hygiene. Although education about sleep hygiene is always used, there is no conclusive evidence that this **alone** is an effective treatment for insomnia.[6,59,60] However, education about good sleep habits is usually a part of every CBT-I program.

Relaxation Therapy (RT). Relaxation therapy (RT) is a generic term that encompasses several techniques. Progressive muscle relaxation (PMR) focuses on somatic arousal and was developed by Edmund Jacobsen. Thus, the technique is often called Jacobsen PMR. In this technique, the patient systematically goes through the parts of the body, initially tensing muscles, maintaining muscle tension, then relaxing the muscles. The patient is asked to concentrate on the sensations associated with tensing and then relaxing.[61] Guided imagery relaxation focuses on cognitive arousal and uses visualization of a relaxing setting or activity. RT is useful in patients who report or display elevated levels of arousal. The technique can be helpful with both SOI and SMI.

Stimulus Control Therapy (SCT). Stimulus control therapy (SCT) (Table 33–10) is a specific type of behavioral therapy based on the idea that arousal occurs as a conditioned response to the stimulus of the sleep (bedroom) environment.[22,58-60,62] This technique is among the most effective behavioral treatments. The standard instructions are listed in Table 33–10. The goal of SCT is to extinguish the negative association between the bed and undesirable outcomes such as wakefulness, frustration, and worry. These associations become conditioned because of prolonged efforts to fall asleep and a long time in bed while awake. SCT will replace these negative associations with positive associations of the bed with sleep.

Sleep Restriction Therapy (SRT). Sleep Restriction Therapy (SRT) limits the TIB so that (TST/TIB $\geq$ 85%, or TIB $\approx$ 1.2 $\times$ TST) as derived from sleep logs[22,57,58,63,64] (Table 33–11). A simple approach is TIB = TST + 30 to 60 in minutes).

Table 33–10 Stimulus Control Instructions

1. Lie down intending to go to sleep only when sleepy.
2. Do not use the bed for anything except sleep and sex. Do not use the bed for reading, television watching, eating, or worrying.
3. Do not watch the clock, but if you have not fallen asleep in 10 to 15 minutes, get out of bed and go into another room. Stay up as long as you wish or until you feel sleepy and then return to the bedroom.
4. If you cannot fall asleep, repeat rule 3 as often as needed.
5. Get up at the same time every morning, irrespective of how much sleep you got during the night.

Goal: Help the body acquire a consistent sleep rhythm.

6. Do not nap during the day.

From Morgenthaler T, Kramer M, Alessi C, et al. Practice parameters for the psychological and behavioral treatment of insomnia: an update. *Sleep*. 2006; 29:1415-1419; and Bootzin RR, Epstein D, Wood JM. Stimulus control instructions. In Hauri P. *Case Studies in Insomnia*. New York: Plenum Press, 1991:19-28.

Table 33–11 Sleep Restriction Instructions

1. A sleep log is kept for 1 to 2 weeks to determine the mean total sleep time (TST).
2. Set bedtime and wake-up time to achieve mean TST, with sleep efficiency >=85%.
   The minimum TIB is 5 hours.
   If TST/TIB = 0.85, then TIB = TST/0.85 = TST $\times$ 1.176.
   Example: If TST = 310 min, then goal for TIB = 364 min (bedtime 11 PM, wake time 5:04 AM.)
3. Adjustments:
   A. If TST/TIB > 0.85 for 7 days, then add 15–20 min to TIB.
   B. If TST/TIB < 0.85, decrease TIB every 7 days.

Adapted from Morgenthaler T, Kramer M, Alessi C, et al. Practice parameters for the psychological and behavioral treatment of insomnia: an update. *Sleep*. 2006;29:1415-1419; Speilman AJ, Saskin P, Thorpy MJ. Treatment of chronic insomnia by restriction of time in bed. *Sleep*. 1987;10:45-56.

The goal is to improve sleep continuity, enhancing the homeostatic sleep drive with sleep restriction. Sleep will become more consolidated when long periods in bed and napping are prohibited. As sleep continuity improves, TIB is gradually increased. When using this technique, the patient should be *cautioned about sleepiness to prevent accidents* or other mishaps. A variant of sleep restriction is termed "sleep compression."[64] Patients are asked to gradually go to bed later and/or wake up earlier so that TIB equals the reported TST. The excess TIB (TIB – TST) is gradually reduced over several weeks. For example, an excess TIB of 120 minutes would require a progressive reduction in TIB of 20 minutes per week over six sessions. The schedule is altered if TST increases. Sleep restriction could induce mania in a patient with bipolar disorder. Consultation with the patient's psychiatrist before starting this treatment is recommended.

Paradoxical Intention. Instruct the patient to passively remain awake and avoid any effort (intention) to fall asleep; the goal is to eliminate performance anxiety.

Biofeedback. Biofeedback trains the patient to control some physiologic variable through visible or auditory feedback. The goal is to reduce somatic arousal.

Intensive sleep retraining. This newly described treatment is designed to markedly enhance homeostatic sleep drive in order to reduce both sleep onset difficulties and sleep misperception. Following a night wherein the patient limits time in bed to no more than 5 hours, the treatment includes a 24-hour laboratory protocol in which the patient is given an opportunity to fall asleep every 30 minutes in sleep-conducive conditions. If sleep occurs the patient is awakened after three minutes and remains awake until the subsequent 30-minute trial. For each sleep opportunity, the patient is given feedback as to whether or not sleep occurred.[6]

Evidence for Behavioral Treatment

CBT-I for periods of 4 to 8 weeks has been proven effective by randomized, controlled trials.[6,57-59] Trials comparing CBT-I with standard care or pharmacotherapy[6,52,65,66] have found CBT-I to be at least as effective as pharmacotherapy (and in some studies better). In contrast to pharmacotherapy, the benefits persist when treatment is stopped (Figure 33–8). CBT-I

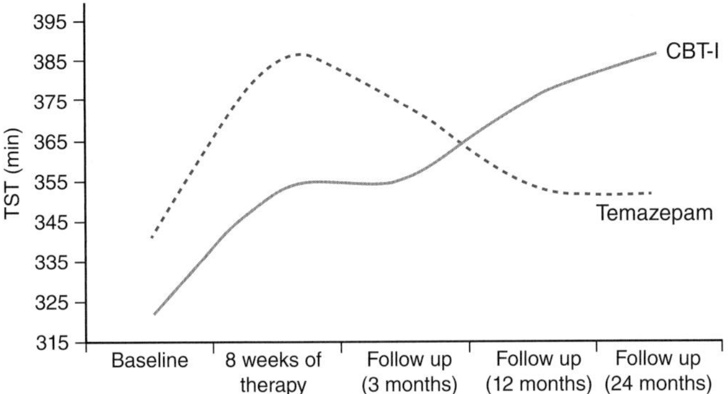

Figure 33–8 Total sleep time (TST) in groups treated with temazepam and cognitive behavioral treatment for insomnia (CBT-I). Note that after 8 weeks of treatment with temazepam, the benefits decreased (drug stopped after 8 weeks). However, the CBT-I group continued to show improvement. (From Riemann D, Perlis ML. The treatments of chronic insomnia: a review of benzodiazepine receptor agonists and psychologic and behavioral therapies. *Sleep Med Rev.* 2009;13:205-214; Data from Morin CM, Colecchi C, Stone J, et al. Behavioral and pharmacologic therapies for late life insomnia: a randomized controlled trial. *JAMA.* 1999;281:991-999.)

is effective for cases of SOI, SMI, and nonrestorative sleep. Behavioral treatment can also be effective in insomnia associated with depression or medical conditions.[67,68] Adequate treatment of the underlying condition alone can improve insomnia, but often treatment for insomnia as well as the underlying condition is the most effective approach.

Most studies have not documented an advantage for combined therapy (CBT-I + medication) versus CBT-I alone[65] (Figure 33–9). However, a few recent studies have shown a possible advantage to combination treatment or sequential treatment for those failing an initial intervention.[53-55] In some cases, addition of a hypnotic speeded the effectiveness of treatment without changing the long-term outcome. In other cases, addition of a hypnotic "rescued" a patient failing initial behavioral treatment. More studies are needed in this area with larger groups of patients. In actual clinical practice, a common scenario is a patient already on a hypnotic who undergoes CBT-I and then attempts to slowly wean the hypnotic. Use of CBT-I with respect to hypnotic weaning is discussed in the next section.

CBT-I and Hypnotic Withdrawal

CBT-I can be used in patients already on hypnotics with the possible goal of weaning the hypnotics. Using structured programs, hypnotic tapering and withdrawal is facilitated by combining the process with CBT for insomnia.[68-71] In one study by Morin and coworkers[69] comparing supervised benzodiazepine (BZ) withdrawal, CBT-I alone, and supervised withdrawal and CBT-I, all groups significantly reduced BZ use. However, more patients were BZ free in the combined group, and both groups with CBT-I had better improvements in subjective sleep quality.

Brief Behavioral Therapy for Insomnia (BBTI)

Buysse et al.[72,73] found that BBTI was effective compared to control (education about sleep only) in a group of elderly patients with insomnia. The BBTI consists of a 45- to 60-minute individual intervention session followed by a 30-minute

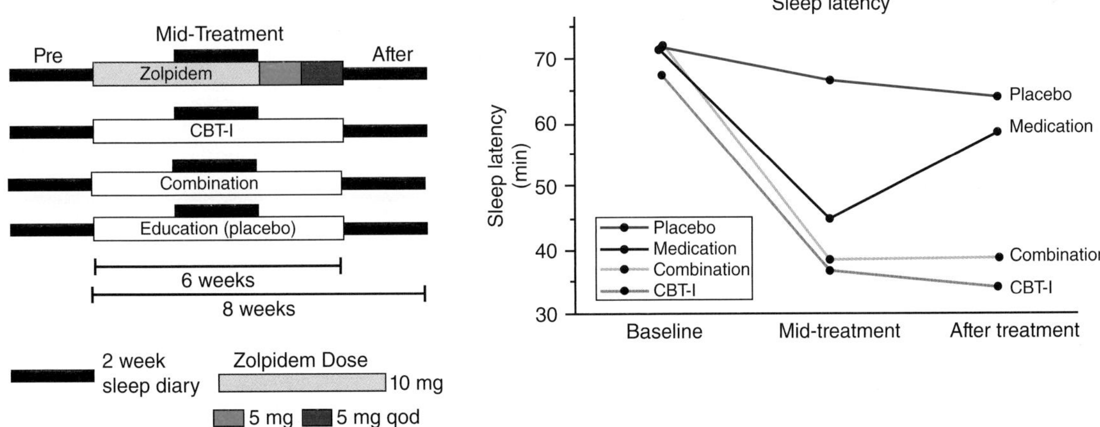

Figure 33–9 Sleep latency by sleep diary compared among four treatment arms: CBT-I, medication (zolpidem), combination treatment, and education (placebo), each for 6 weeks followed by a 2- week period without interventions during which time sleep diaries were completed (after treatment). Mid-treatment consisted of sleep diaries over weeks 3 and 4. The absolute mean values are shown. At the end of treatment the percentage decrease (not shown) in the sleep latency was significantly greater with CBT-I or combination treatment compared to medication alone or placebo. CBT-I versus medication (P=0.03) and versus placebo (P=0.02). Combination versus medication (P=0.02) and versus placebo (P= 0.001) Even at the mid-treatment time point, combined treatment was not better than CBT-I alone. (Data plotted from Jacobs GD, Pace-Schott EF, Stickgold R, Otto MW. Cognitive behavior therapy and pharmacotherapy for insomnia: a randomized controlled trial and direct comparison. *Arch Intern Med.* 2004;164:1888-1896.)

Table 33–12 Brief Behavioral Treatment of Insomnia

- Individual intervention session (45–60 minutes)
- 30-minute follow-up session (2 weeks later)
- 20-minute telephone calls after 1 and 3 weeks
- Education on rationale of interventions (homeostatic sleep drive)
- Four main interventions:
  1. Reduce time in bed (average reported sleep time plus 30 minutes, minimum 6 hours).
  2. Get up at the same time every day, regardless of sleep duration.
  3. Do not go to bed unless sleepy.
  4. Do not stay in bed unless asleep.

Other instructions: napping discouraged.

Adapted from Buysse DJ, Germain A, Moul DE, et al. Efficacy of brief behavioral treatment for chronic insomnia in older adults. *Arch Intern Med.* 2011;171(10):887-895.

follow-up session 2 weeks later and 20-minute telephone calls after 1 and 3 weeks (Table 33–12). BBTI emphasizes behavioral elements of insomnia treatment rather than the cognitive components present in CBT-I. BBTI includes sleep education and discussion of homeostatic and circadian mechanisms of human sleep regulation. This education provides the rationale for the four main interventions of BBTI: (1) reduce TIB; (2) get up at the same time every day, regardless of sleep duration; (3) do not go to bed unless sleepy; and (4) do not stay in bed unless asleep. Napping is also discouraged. These interventions derive from sleep restriction and stimulus control techniques, the efficacy of which has been well documented. TIB is limited to average self-reported sleep time plus 30 minutes, with a minimum of 6 hours. In the future, more interventions of this type may provide wider access to behavioral techniques.

New Methods of CBT-I Delivery

There are insufficient professionals trained in CBT-I to provide therapy for the large number of patients with insomnia, and they tend to be localized in urban areas. BBTI can be delivered in group settings. CBT-I delivered via the telemedicine platform has been demonstrated to be noninferior to face-to-face delivery.[74] Computer-based/web-based programs can also deliver CBT-I effectively.[75-77] For example, an Australian-based CBT-I website (https://thiswayup.org.au/programs/insomnia-program) offers both a free 4-week course and a longer paid course (free if a physician prescribes treatment).

A U.S Food and Drug Administration (FDA)-cleared web-based CBT-I program (Somryst) was available at cost to consumers with a physician's prescription.[77] The program/company has been acquired by Nox Medical and the CBI-I program will hopefully be available in the future. Smartphone-based applications such as CBT-I Coach have also been developed to complement CBT-I or allow patient-directed efforts at improvement of sleep.[78]

Behavioral Treatment of Insomnia in Children

Bedtime problems and frequent nighttime awakenings are highly prevalent in young children, occurring approximately in **20% to 30% of young children, toddlers, and preschoolers.**[79,80] One set of behaviors includes bedtime refusal/struggles (crying, getting out of bed, attention-seeking behaviors). These sleep behaviors usually fall within the clinical diagnostic category of *behavioral insomnia of childhood (BIOC), limit-setting type*, in which parents demonstrate difficulties in adequately enforcing bedtime limits. Nocturnal awakenings are problematic for caregivers if the return to sleep is difficult or prolonged or requires parental intervention. Nighttime awakenings may also fall into the *BIOC of the sleep-onset association type*. In this category of BIOC, children become dependent on *specific factors to fall asleep* (rocking, feeding, parental presence) either at bedtime or after a nocturnal awakening. AASM practice parameters for treatment of BIOC were published in 2006[79,80] (Table 33–13). An explanation of the types of behavioral treatment is presented in Table 33–14. Unmodified and graduated extinction focuses on removing reinforcement (parental attention) from unwanted behavior. Scheduled awakenings prevent reinforcement for unwanted behaviors after spontaneous awakening. The "Bed Time Pass" is another technique in which children receive a decorated note card when placed in bed. If they do not get out of bed or require parental intervention they can keep the pass and when awake the next day the pass can be redeemed for a reward (food, screen time, enjoyable activity with a parent). The pass is removed if the child gets out of bed or requires parental attention. A variant is the reward of a special sticker that can be placed on a poster or calendar documenting good bedtime behavior. More recent publications have also addressed behavioral treatment in children and adolescents,[81] including special populations (autism).[82]

Table 33–13 Recommendations for Behavioral Treatment of Insomnia of Childhood

1. Behavioral interventions are effective and recommended in the treatment of bedtime problems and night wakings in young children. (Standard)
2. **Unmodified extinction and extinction** of undesired behavior with parental presence are effective and recommended therapies in the treatment of bedtime problems and night wakings. (Standard)
3. Parent education/prevention is an effective and recommended therapy in the treatment of bedtime problems and night wakings. (Standard)
4. Graduated extinction of undesired behavior is an effective and recommended therapy in the treatment of bedtime problems and night wakings. (Guideline)
5. Delayed bedtime with removal from bed/positive bedtime routines is an effective and recommended therapy in the treatment of bedtime problems and night wakings. (Guideline) This is sometimes called "faded Bedtime with response cost" and involves taking the child out of bed for prescribed periods of time when the child does not fall asleep. Bedtime is also delayed to ensure rapid sleep initiation and that appropriate cues for sleep onset are paired with positive parent-child interactions.
6. The use of scheduled awakenings is an effective and recommened therapy in treatment of bedtime problems and night waking (Guideline)
7. Insufficient evidence was available to recommend any single therapy over another

Morgenthaler TI, Owens J, Alessi C, et al. Practice parameters for behavioral treatment of bedtime problems and night wakings in infants and young children. *Sleep.* 2006;29(10):1277-1281.

Table 33–14 Techniques Used for Behavioral Treatment of Insomnia of Childhood

Technique	Description	Rationale
Unmodified extinction	Involves parents putting the child to bed at a designated bedtime and then ignoring the child until morning (parents continue to monitor for safety issues).	Reduce undesired behaviors (e.g., crying, screaming) by eliminating parental attention (reinforcer).
Graduated extinction	Involves parents ignoring bedtime crying and tantrums for predetermined periods before briefly checking on the child. A progressive (graduated) checking schedule (e.g., 5 min, then 10 min) or fixed checking schedule (e.g., every 5 min) may be used.	Enable a child to develop "self-soothing" skills and be able to fall asleep independently without undesirable sleep associations.
Scheduled awakenings	Involves parents preemptively awakening their child, prior to a typical spontaneous awakening, and providing the "usual" responses (e.g., feeding, rocking, soothing) as if child had awakened spontaneously.	Prevents nightly reinforcement for undesirable behaviors involved with waking.
Positive routines	Parents develop set bedtime routines characterized by enjoyable and quiet activities to establish a behavioral chain leading to sleep onset.	Removes negative stimuli associated with bedtime.
Parental education and prevention	Involves parent education to prevent the development of sleep problems. Behavioral interventions are incorporated into these parent education programs.	Preventing problems before they occur.

Adapted from Mindell JA, Kuhn B, Lewin DS, et al. Behavioral treatment of bedtime problems and night wakings in infants and young children. An American Academy of Sleep Medicine review. *Sleep*. 2006;29:1263-1276.

PHARMACOLOGIC TREATMENT OF INSOMNIA

A wide variety of medications (including over-the-counter medications) are used to treat insomnia. Many of the medications are not FDA approved for this indication. The BZ receptor agonists (BZRAs), sedating antidepressants, melatonin receptor agonists, and, recently, hypocretin receptor antagonists are the major groups of FDA-approved medications. Over-the-counter medications usually contain a first-generation sedating antihistamine (diphenhydramine, doxylamine). The AASM published a clinical practice guideline for evaluation and treatment of insomnia in 2008[22] and a guideline for the pharmacologic treatment of chronic insomnia in 2017 (Table 33–15).[83] The medications listed under the "not recommended" category include some medications such as melatonin or trazodone that are widely used. However, insufficient evidence was available to recommend them. Elements of the pharmacology of BZRAs will be discussed below.

Table 33–15 Clinical Practice Guidelines for Treatment of Insomnia in Adults

Recommended			
Sleep-Onset Insomnia	Sleep-Maintenance Insomnia	Both	Not Recommended
Triazolam Temazepam Zaleplon Zolpidem Eszopiclone Ramelteon	Temazepam Zolpidem Eszopiclone Suvorexant Doxepin (3, 6 mg) (Silenor)	Temazepam Zolpidem Eszopiclone	Melatonin Tiagabine Trazodone Diphenhydramine Valerian L-Tryptophan

Data from Sateia MJ, Buysse DJ, Krystal AD, Neubauer DN, Heald JL. Clinical Practice Guideline for the Pharmacologic Treatment of Chronic Insomnia in Adults: An American Academy of Sleep Medicine Clinical Practice Guideline. *J Clin Sleep Med*. 2017 Feb 15;13(2):307-349. PMID: 27998379.

GABA–BZ–Chloride Ionophore Complex

Gamma-amino-butyric acid (GABA) is the major inhibitory neurotransmitter in the central nervous system. There are two major GABA receptor subtypes: $GABA_A$ and $GABA_B$. The $GABA_A$ receptor is associated with a chloride (Cl^-) channel ionophore located in cell membranes (Figure 33–10). Ionophores are molecular complexes located in cellular lipid membranes that allow transport/passage of compounds across the membrane. The $GABA_A$ receptor is the binding site for several drugs other than GABA, including agonists (muscimol, gaboxadol) and antagonists (bicuculline). The $GABA_A$ receptor complex also contains a receptor for benzodiazepines (BZs) and related compounds; hence, the complex is usually referred to as the $GABA_A$–BZ–chloride ionophore complex (GBC).[84,85] *When GABA binds the $GABA_A$ receptor on the complex, this allows passage of chloride ions through the membrane, resulting in hyperpolarization and reduced neuronal activity.* When medications bind to the BZ receptor on the GBC, the configuration of the GABA receptor changes to *enhance the ability of GABA binding to the $GABA_A$ receptor to open the associated chloride channel* (increased frequency). The medications are, therefore, sometimes called $GABA_A$ receptor modulators. A positive allosteric modulator (PAM) is another term for medications that modulate the ability of other compounds to bind a given receptor or **increase** the effect of binding. Medications that bind the BZ receptor and enhance the ability of GABA to open the chloride channel (a PAM) are called BZ receptor agonists (**BZRAs**). *Although BZRAs do not actually bind the GABA receptor (bind the BZ receptor on $GABA_A$ complex), they are sometimes referred to as $GABA_A$ receptor agonists.* The BZRAs include true BZ hypnotics (temazepam) and non-BZ BZRA hypnotics (zolpidem, zaleplon, eszopiclone).

The GBC is composed of five protein subunits surrounding the chloride channel (Figure 33–10). The subunits composing the GBC have different structures and are denoted as alpha, beta, gamma, epsilon, and rho.[84,85] The receptor complex is usually composed of two alpha, two beta, and one gamma

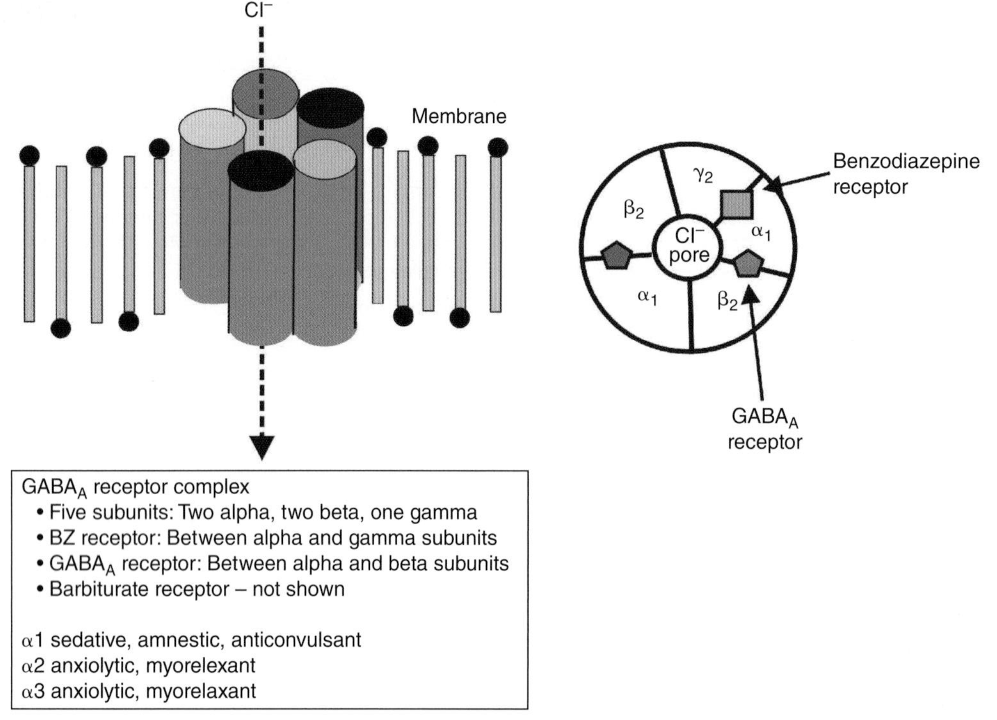

Figure 33–10 *Left,* A schematic representation of the GABA$_A$–benzodiazepine–chloride ionophore complex with five subunits arranged around the chloride pore. *Right,* A view from overhead shows the location of the GABA$_A$ receptors at the junction of the alpha1 (α1) and beta2 (β2) subunits and the benzodiazepine receptor at junction of alpha1 (α1) and gamma2 ($γ_2$) subunits.

subunit. In addition, the alpha, beta, and gamma subunits have isoforms (e.g., α1, α2, α3,...). The GABA binding site is located between alpha and beta subunits on the GBC, and the BZ receptor site is located between alpha and gamma subunits (Figure 33–10). The most common GBC receptor configuration is denoted as α1, β2, γ2 (understood to mean two α1, two β2, and one γ2 subunits) and is also known as a BZ type 1 receptor. The GBC also has receptors for barbiturates, certain anesthetics (propofol), and alcohol. The binding of GABA$_A$ BZ receptor subtypes has different actions[84] (Table 33–16). The GBCs composed of α1 subunits mediate sedation (hypnotic effect), amnesia, and anticonvulsant effects. The BZ receptor on this GBC is sometimes called an omega 1 receptor. The GBCs associated with α2 and α3 subunits mediate anxiolytic and myorelaxant effects.

Benzodiazepine Receptor Agonists

The BZRAs include BZs (triazolam, temazepam, and others) and non-BZs (zaleplon, zolpidem, eszopiclone, and others). BZs tend to have high affinity for all these BZ receptor subtypes. The non-BZ BZRAs (zolpidem, zaleplon, eszopiclone), also known as the "Z" hypnotics, have preferential binding to GBCs containing certain subunits[84-86] (Table 33–17). Zolpidem and zaleplon selectively bind GBCs containing α1 subunits and are often called *selective BZRAs.* These non-BZ BZRAs have less anxiolytic and myorelaxant activity than BZs. However, the preferential binding is only relative, and at higher doses these drugs bind to GBCs containing α1, α2, and α3 subunits. Eszopiclone is another non-BZ BZRA with receptor binding more like traditional BZs, but it has many of the same effects on sleep as the other Z hypnotics. Eszopiclone does bind

Table 33–16 GABA$_A$ Receptor Alpha Subunits and Associated Actions

	Action	Proportion of GABA$_A$ Receptors	Location
α1	Sedative, amnestic, anticonvulsant	60%	All brain regions Cortex, hippocampus
α2	Anxiolytic, myorelaxant	15–20%	Cortex, hippocampus, amygdala, forebrain, hypothalamus
α3	Anxiolytic, myorelaxant	10–15%	Cerebral cortex, thalamus (reticular nucleus)
α4, α6	Insensitive to BZ		Dentate gyrus
α5	High affinity for BZ Low affinity for zolpidem BZ tolerance		Cerebral cortex, hippocampus

BZ, benzodiazepine; *GABA,* gamma-aminobutyric acid.

Adapted from Olsen RW, Sieghart W. GABA A receptors: subtypes provide diversity of function and pharmacology. *Neuropharmacology.* 2009;56(1):141-148. PMID: 18760291.

Table 33–17 Relative Binding of Benzodiazepine Receptor Subtypes

	Alpha 1	Alpha 2	Alpha 3	Alpha 5
Zaleplon	17×	2×	2×	1×
Zolpidem	21×	1×	1×	Negligible
Eszopiclone	8×	5×	1×	8×

1× = the lowest affinity of a given drug for any receptor.
Adapted from Nutt DJ, Stahl SM. Searching for perfect sleep: the continuing evolution of GABAA receptor modulators as hypnotics. *J Psychopharmacol.* 2010;24(11):1601-1612. PMID: 19942638.

α1 subunits with higher affinity than α3 subunits but also binds α2 subunit receptors with only slightly lower affinity than α1 subunits. The clinical importance of selective receptor binding is unclear. However, in general, zolpidem and zaleplon have minimal anxiolytic or muscle relaxant activity. If a patient's insomnia has a component of anxiety, these medications may be less effective. However, eszopiclone appears to have more affinity for GBCs with α2 units than do zolpidem and zaleplon and, therefore, possibly more anxiolytic effects.[86] However, the **major property to consider in choice of a BZRA is the duration of action**. It is important to note that the *initial concentration of a medication is important*, as well as the medication's half-life, in determining whether an effective serum concentration is available at a given time. For example, both zolpidem 5 mg and 10 mg have the same half-life, but the duration of action of the 10 mg dose is longer.

BZRA Clinical Effects and Effects on Sleep. The BZRAs have a number of important clinical effects, including sedation (hypnotic), amnestic, anxiolytic, myorelaxant, and anticonvulsant (Table 33–18) side effects. The BZRAs have several notable effects on sleep[87,88] (Table 33–19). A decrease in sleep latency is common to all medications. Those with an intermediate or longer duration of action also can increase TST and decrease WASO. BZRAs can increase sleep spindle activity and the amplitude of higher EEG frequencies. The BZs reduce

Table 33–18 Benzodiazepine Receptor Agonists: Actions and Side Effects

Actions	Side Effects
• Hypnotic • Amnestic • Anxiolytic* • Myorelaxant* • Anticonvulsant	• Sedation • Anterograde amnesia (learning new material) • Tolerance* • Dependence, abuse • Rebound insomnia (especially triazolam)* • Risk of falls • Complex sleep behaviors: sleepwalking, sleep sex, sleep violence, sleep-related eating • Respiratory depression* • Daytime sedation (longer-acting agents or higher doses)

*Less prominent with zolpidem, zaleplon (eszopiclone is more like the benzodiazepines with respect to anxiolytic and muscle relaxant effects).

Table 33–19 Effects of Benzodiazepine Receptor Agonists on Sleep

- Improved sleep continuity
  - Decreased sleep latency (short-acting and intermediate-acting BZRAs)
  - Increased total sleep time (intermediate-acting BZRAs)
  - Decreased wakefulness after sleep onset (intermediate-acting BZRAs)
- Decreased stage N3 sleep
  - Reduced amplitude of slow waves (not with "Z" drugs)
  - Increased sleep spindles and faster activity
- Decrease in REM sleep: mild, less with "Z" drugs

BZRAs, benzodiazepine receptor agonists; *GABA*, gamma-aminobutyric acid; *REM*, rapid eye movement; *Z drugs*, zaleplon, zolpidem, eszopiclone.

stage N3 sleep with either no reduction or a mild reduction in REM sleep. The major effect on stage N3 sleep is via a *reduction in slow-wave amplitude*. The Z hypnotics result in no or a minimal decrease in the amount of stage N3 sleep because they do not substantially reduce the amplitude of slow waves.[89,90] The clinical importance of reduction in stage N3 sleep is still unclear.

Non-Benzodiazepine BZRAs. All three Z hypnotics (Table 33–20) are associated with less rebound insomnia or evidence of tolerance (decreased effect at the same dose) compared to BZ BZRAs. The most important differences among the three Z hypnotics are their half-lives and durations of action. The AASM practice guidelines for the pharmacologic treatment of insomnia recommend zaleplon, zolpidem, and eszopiclone for treatment of SOI and zolpidem and eszopiclone for treatment of SMI (Table 33–15). Zaleplon has a very short duration of action and may have less residual sedative effects, especially after middle-of-the-night dosing.[89,91] Generic forms of zolpidem and eszopiclone, but not zaleplon, are available in the United States. The brand-name Z hypnotics are generally quite expensive. The FDA label indication for zaleplon and zolpidem is for "short-term" treatment of insomnia, while the eszopiclone label indication omits "short-term." At the time of eszopiclone approval, a study documented effectiveness over 6 months.[90] However, all the Z hypnotics have been demonstrated to be effective for up to 12 months, and clinical experience suggests they remain effective for years. Zolpidem has a longer half-life (1.5–4 hours) than zaleplon (1 hour) but shorter than eszopiclone (6 hours).[89-91] Zolpidem may not have a sufficiently long duration of action in some patients, and for this reason zolpidem CR (zolpidem extended release) was developed.[92,93] This is a two-layered tablet with one layer for rapid release and the other for slower release. The half-life of zolpidem CR is the same as that of zolpidem, but there is a greater concentration of the medication 4 hours after drug administration (Figure 33–11). Eszopiclone has a longer half-life than zolpidem[94-96] and can be used for SMI not responding to zolpidem or zolpidem CR. However, patient responses to the different Z hypnotics are quite variable, and some patients with SMI will respond to the non-CR preparations of zolpidem. Sublingual and spray preparations of zolpidem have been developed to speed the onset of action, although the difference in sleep latency compared to zolpidem immediate release is less than half

Table 33–20 Benzodiazepine Receptor Agonist Hypnotic Medications (Non-Benzodiazepines)

Generic Name (Brand Name)* Dosage Forms	Dosage	Onset of Action (T_{max})	Duration of Action ($T_{½}$ half-life)	Indication	Selected Side Effects and Comments
Zaleplon (Sonata) 5, 10 mg capsule	10 mg qhs (max 20 mg) 5 mg qhs in women, elderly, debilitated, mild to moderate hepatic impairment, or concomitant cimetidine	10–20 min (1 hour)	Short-acting ($T_{½}$ = 1 hour)	SOI	Rescue medication if 4 hours left for sleep (not FDA approved for MOTN)
Zolpidem (Ambien)* 5, 10 mg tablets	10 mg qhs 5 mg in elderly, women, debilitated, hepatic impairment	10–20 min (1.6 hours)	Short- to intermediate-acting $T_{½}$ = 2.5 (1.5–4.5) hours	SOI > SMI	Sleep-related eating disorder and sleep-walking reported
Zolpidem CR (Ambien CR)* 6.25, 12.5 mg layered tabs	6.25–12.5 mg qhs 6.25 mg qhs in women, elderly	10–20 min (1.5 hours)	Controlled release, intermediate-acting similar half-life, higher drug level 4 hours after ingestion	SOI, SMI	Swallow whole, not crushed, cut, or chewed Higher concentrations 3 to 8 hours after ingestion than those of zolpidem IR
Zolpidem SL (Buffered) (Intermezzo) 1.75, 3.5 mg SL tablets	1.75 mg women, age >65, hepatic impairment 3.5 mg in men	10–20 min (0.6 hours)	$T_{½}$ similar to IR zolpidem	MOTNA	At least 4 hours of sleep must remain, buffering enables more rapid absorption)
Zolpidem SL (Edluar) 5, 10 mg per SL tablet	5 mg women 5 or 10 mg men	10–20 min (1.4 hours)	2.7 hrs	SOI, SMI	Slightly more rapid onset of sleep than IR zolpidem, absorbed mainly through GI tract
Eszopiclone (Lunesta)* 1, 2, 3 mg tablets	start 1 mg qhs (max 3 mg) 1 mg qhs in elderly and hepatic impairment (max 2 mg)	10–30 min (1.5 hours)	Intermediate-acting $T_{½}$ = 6 hours	SOI, SMI	Unpleasant taste a common side effect (in about 30%)

*Asterik means generic available, These medications are FDA approved as hypnotics (short-term indication, exception eszopiclone—indication not time limited). The FDA indication for zaleplon and zolpidem is sleep onset insomnia. The FDA indication for zolpidem CR and eszopiclone is for sleep onset and mainentance insomnia. The FDA indication of Intermezzo is middle of the night awakening (when at least 4 hours of bedtime remain).
The medications are all Schedule IV controlled substances
IR, immediate release; *MOTNA*, middle of the night awakening and difficulty returning to sleep; *SL*, sublingual; *SMI*, sleep-maintenance insomnia; *SOI*, sleep-onset insomnia; T_{max}, time from administration to peak drug level. $T_{½}$ half life
Data from Buysse DJ. Insomnia. *JAMA*. 2013 Feb 20;309(7):706-16.

an hour.[97] Zolpimist, an oral spray forumulation of zolpidem, has been discontinued. The only hypnotic approved by the FDA for middle-of-the-night awakening (MOTNA) is Intermezzo (a buffered sublingual zolpidem preparation).[97,98] The buffering makes absorption more rapid. As noted, zaleplon has a very short half-life and could also be used for middle-of-the-night awakening. However, zaleplon is not approved by the FDA for this indication.

Benzodiazepine BZRAs. BZ BZRAs used for insomnia are listed in Table 33–21. They are separated into those approved by the FDA for insomnia and those used off-label. The AASM clinical practice guideline recommends triazolam for SOI and temazepam for treatment of both SOI and SMI. Triazolam has a short half-life and is useful for SOI. However, triazolam is associated with rebound insomnia[22] and is no longer recommended as a first-line hypnotic. Temazepam has a longer half-life than eszopiclone and can be useful for SMI in patients not effectively treated with medications with a shorter duration of action. It has a delayed onset of action in some patients and may not be as effective as other medications for SOI. Flurazepam has a very long duration of action and is no longer available. Clonazepam, lorazepam, and alprazolam are approved by the FDA for anxiety but can be used for insomnia. There are patients with both anxiety and insomnia that may respond to these medications better than other FDA-approved hypnotics for insomnia. Note that clonazepam has a very long half-life, and lorazepam and alprazolam have half-lives longer than the Z hypnotics. Discontinuation of lorazepam and especially alprazolam can be associated with rebound insomnia.

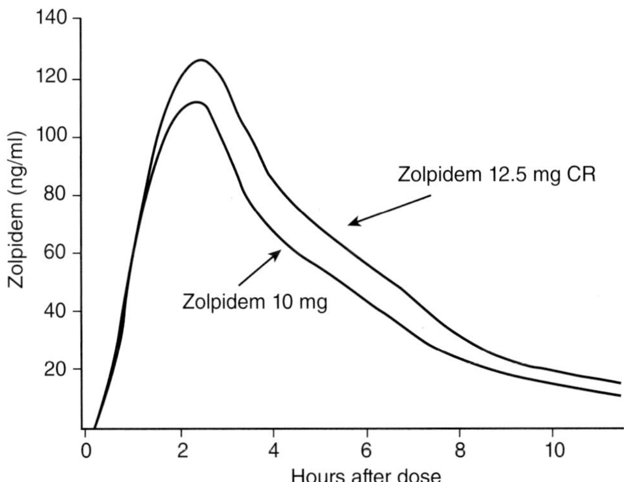

Figure 33–11 Plasma level of immediate-release zolpidem 10 mg versus zolpidem 12.5 mg controlled release. Half-life is similar but the drug level is higher 4 to 6 hours after the dose. (Modified from Greenblatt DJ, Legangneux E, Harmatz JS, et al. Dynamics and kinetics of modified release formulation of zolpidem: comparison with immediate-release standard zolpidem and placebo. *J Clin Pharmacol.* 2006:46:1469-1480.)

Side Effects of BZRAs. The BZRAs have a number of side effects (Table 33-18), including anterograde amnesia (decreased ability to learn and retain new information), ataxia (fall risk), and residual sedation during the day. Of note, eszopiclone is associated with an unpleasant (often metallic) taste in a significant number of patients (≈25-30%).[94] BZRAs can also be associated with nausea in some patients. *They are not recommended for use in nursing or pregnant women.* In 2007, the FDA required packaging information on the BZRA hypnotics to include a warning regarding several specific potential adverse effects. Current prescribing information notes that BZRAs have been associated with **complex sleep behaviors,** including sleepwalking, eating, driving, and sexual behaviors. Patients taking BZRAs should allow for adequate sleep time and ***not*** take BZRAs in combination with other sedatives, alcohol, or sleep restriction. Zolpidem is the BZRA most often associated with sleepwalking and sleep-related eating disorder, but these manifestations can happen with the other BZRAs as well. Residual sedation is another important side effect of BZRAs. In general, shorter-acting medications are less likely to cause residual sedation. In 2013, the FDA mandated revised labeling that contained a warning that

Table 33–21 Benzodiazepine Receptor Agonist Hypnotic Medications (Benzodiazepines)

Generic Name (Brand Name)* Dosage forms	Dosage	Onset of Action (T_{max})	Duration of Action	Indication	Selected Side Effects and Comments
Benzodiazepines FDA Approved as Hypnotics (Short-Term)					
Triazolam (Halcion)* 0.125, 0.25 mg	0.125–0.25 mg qhs 0.125 in elderly	10–20 min (1 to 2 hours)	Short-acting $T_{½}$ = 2–6 hours	SOI	Rebound insomnia—not a first-line hypnotic, AASM guideline approved
Estazolam (ProSom)*,** 1, 2 mg tablets	1–2 mg qhs 0.5 mg in elderly, debilitated	15–30 min (1.5 to 2 hours)	Intermediate-acting $T_{½}$ = 10–24 hours	SOI, SMI	Residual daytime sleepiness Not AASM recommended
Temazepam (Restoril)* 7.5, 15, 30 mg	15–30 mg hs 15 mg in elderly, debilitated	45–60 min (1–2 hours)	Intermediate-acting $T_{½}$ = 15–30 hours	SOI, SMI	Delayed onset of action in some patients
Flurazepam (Dalmane)**,*** 15, 30 mg	15–30 mg qhs 15 mg hours in elderly, debilitated	15–30 min (1.5 to 4.5 hours)	Long-acting $T_{½}$ = 47–100 hours	SMI	Residual daytime sleepiness Discontinued in US
Benzodiazepines NOT FDA Approved as Hypnotics					
Clonazepam (Klonopin)* 0.5, 1.0, 2.0 mg	0.25–0.5 mg qhs	(1–2.5 hours)	Long-acting $T_{½}$ = 20–40 hours	SMI	Residual daytime sleepiness Potent BZRA Not FDA approved as hypnotic
Lorazepam (Ativan)* 0.5, 1.0 mg	0.5–1.0 mg qhs Max ≤2–4 mg	(0.7–1 hours)	Long-acting $T_{½}$ = 14 hours (10 to 20)	SOI, SMI	Not FDA approved as hypnotic Wean slowly, can cause withdrawal side effects
Alprazolam (Xanax)* 0.25, 0.5, 1, 2 mg	0.25 to 0.5 mg qhs	(0.6 to 1.4 hours)	Long-acting $T_{½}$ = 11 hours (6 to 20)	SOI, SMI	Not FDA approved as hypnotic Wean slowly, can cause withdrawal side effects

*Asterik if Generic available.
**Brand discontinued in US
***Generic discontinued in US.
BZRA, benzodiazepine receptor agonists; *FDA*, U.S. Food and Drug Administration; *SMI*, sleep-maintenance insomnia; *SOI*, sleep-onset insomnia.
Data from Buysse DJ. Insomnia. *JAMA.* 2013;309(7):706-716. PMID: 23423416.

patients who take the sleep medication zolpidem extended release (either 6.25 mg or 12.5 mg) are at risk for impairment of the ability to drive or engage in other activities that require complete mental alertness the day after taking the drug. Studies have shown that zolpidem levels can remain high enough the next day to impair these activities.[99] Women metabolize zolpidem slower than men and are especially at risk for impairment. This new recommendation has been added to the warnings and precautions section of the physician label and to the patient medication guide for zolpidem extended release (Ambien CR and generic). The FDA also recommended the initial dose of immediate-release zolpidem products (zolpidem, Ambien) be 5 mg for women and either 5 mg or 10 mg for men. The recommended initial dose of zolpidem extended release (zolpidem CR, Ambien CR) is 6.25 mg for women and either 6.25 or 12.5 mg for men. If the lower doses (5 mg for immediate release, 6.25 mg for extended release) are not effective, the dose can be increased to 10 mg for immediate-release products and to 12.5 mg for zolpidem extended release. However, use of the higher dose can increase the risk of next-day impairment. A similar dose warning was issued for eszopiclone, and the recommended starting dose is 1 mg with a maximum, dose of 2 mg in older or debilitated patients. Respiratory depression caused by BZRA hypnotics alone is uncommon. However, caution is advised with the use of hypnotics in patients with hypoventilation, obstructive sleep apnea, and severe lung disease. Respiratory depression is more likely when BZRAs are combined with other central nervous system depressants such as alcohol or narcotics.

The potential for dependence and abuse resulted in BZRA hypnotics being classified as schedule 4 medications. Drugs with high receptor-binding affinity such as lorazepam, midazolam, and triazolam cause more side effects on withdrawal. As noted, triazolam has been associated with rebound insomnia. Significant rebound insomnia has ***not*** been noted in most studies of zaleplon, zolpidem, and eszopiclone. However, withdrawal side effects and rebound insomnia can potentially occur with all BZRAs, and *slow withdrawal is recommended, if possible.* There has been a concern that long-term use of BZ medications for sleep or anxiety is associated with the development of dementia. While the issue remains controversial, a study by Osler et al. did not find evidence of an association between use of these medications and development of dementia.[100]

Using BZRA Hypnotics: Choice of Medication. BZRA hypnotics (especially the Z hypnotics) are well studied, and the medications listed in Table 33–20 (non-BZ BZRAs) and Table 33–21 (BZ BZRAs) are FDA approved for treatment of insomnia unless otherwise noted. It is especially important to note the duration of action. Ideally, hypnotics should be used on a short-term or intermittent basis at the lowest effective dose. A lower dose and more caution are indicated in the elderly or in patients with impaired hepatic function because most BZRAs undergo hepatic metabolism. Studies have documented the effectiveness of some hypnotic medications (zaleplon, eszopiclone, zolpidem CR) for up to 12 months. Clinical experience also has noted continued long-term effectiveness (at least by patient report) in a number of BZRA hypnotics. However, it is recommended that BZRA hypnotics should be used in doses as low as possible for as short a time as possible. Patients should be warned about complex sleep behaviors and other complications with the use of the combination of BZRAs and alcohol or narcotics.

The major characteristic of BZRA medications to consider in choosing a hypnotic is **the duration of action.** Use of one of the Z hypnotics rather than a BZ BZRA is generally recommended given the lower incidence of rebound insomnia and shorter durations of action. However, as noted, severe side effects (sleepwalking, etc.) are not rare. The AASM clinical guidelines recommend triazolam and all the Z hypnotics for SOI and temazepam, zolpidem, and eszopiclone for SMI. Triazolam has a short duration of action but is associated with significant rebound insomnia and is not the first-line option. Zaleplon has a very short duration of action and may be useful as a "rescue medication" for middle-of-the-night dosing (as long as 4–6 hours of potential sleep remain). However, the only FDA-approved hypnotic for middle-of-the-night awakening is Intermezzo (sublingual buffered zolpidem). One study of experimental awakening during the middle of the night found morning effects with zolpidem but not with zaleplon.[89] Zolpidem has a short to intermediate action and may work for some, but not all, patients as treatment for sleep-maintenance insomnia.

Intermediate-acting medications are indicated for SOI and SMI but may cause daytime sedation in some patients. Temazepam, eszopiclone, and zolpidem CR are in this category. Of note, temazepam has a long onset of action in some patients and may not be effective for SOI in those individuals but can be tried if sleep duration is not long enough with eszopiclone. Some patients developing sleepwalking on a Z hypnotic may not experience this side effect on temazepam. Of note, *taking BZRA hypnotics with food delays the effect of these medications.* Long-acting medications have an increased risk of daytime sedation and other residual effects. It is important to note that patients who fail to respond to a given BZRA will sometimes respond to an alternate BZRA. Lorazepam (Ativan) and clonazepam are two BZ BZRAs that are not FDA approved for primary insomnia. Lorazepam is approved for treatment of anxiety and may work better than approved hypnotics if insomnia is comorbid with anxiety. Although the standard dose for anxiety is 2 to 4 mg, lower doses (0.5–1 mg) of lorazepam may work as a hypnotic. The medication has a relatively long half-life, and withdrawal symptoms may occur after long-term use. Clonazepam is a potent BZRA with a very long half-life and is commonly associated with morning grogginess. However, individual patients may respond well to this medication and not report morning sedation. Starting with the lowest possible dose (.25 mg) and having patients plan on a long sleep period is prudent. An occasional patient requires up to 2 mg of clonazepam for SMI. Alprazolam is FDA approved for treatment of anxiety and panic disorder. Although the medication's half-life is fairly long, it is often used with bid to tid dosing during the day. If used as a hypnotic, the duration of effect may not last the entire night. An extended-release preparation exists. Alprazolam can also be associated with prominent withdrawal symptoms.

Melatonin and Melatonin Agonists

Melatonin. Melatonin is a naturally occurring substance available as an over-the-counter sleeping medication. It has a short half-life, and the purity of preparations is not tightly controlled. The hypnotic dose is 3 to 5 mg. Of note, endogenous melatonin is already increased in darkness at sleep onset. The AASM clinical guidelines for treatment of insomnia[83] do not recommend use of this medication (very low quality of evidence). The use of melatonin has been analyzed with a meta-analysis[101] and had a very small effect on sleep latency and TST. Melatonin decreased sleep latency by 4 minutes and increased TST by 12 minutes. Neither of these changes is clinically significant. Another meta-analysis looked at benefits based on improvement in the PSQI. The authors concluded that there was a benefit from melatonin intervention in subjects with respiratory diseases, metabolic disorders, and primary sleep disorders, but there was no significant effect in patients with mental and neurodegenerative disorders.[102] There has been increasing interest in prolonged-release melatonin, which is more likely to benefit parameters other than sleep latency. A study of prolonged-release melatonin using a double-blind controlled design did find a decrease in sleep latency, but only in older patients.[103] Studies have documented a benefit from prolonged-release melatonin for insomnia (in TST and sleep latency) in children with autism spectrum disorder.[104] At least in the short term, prolonged-release melatonin did not affect growth.[105] There has been concern about the rapid increase in use of over-the-counter melatonin and the purity of the medication. Sometimes, the actual dose of melatonin was higher than on the label, and compounds were present that were not included on the label.[106]

Melatonin Receptor Agonists: Ramelteon (Rozerem)

Ramelteon is the first melatonin receptor agonist approved in the United States for treatment of insomnia (Table 33–22).[107,108] It is an MT1/MT2 receptor agonist. The effects at MT1 are thought to inhibit neuronal firing of the suprachiasmatic nucleus (SCN), effectively turning off the alerting signal and allowing sleep to occur. In contrast, MT2 receptor effects are thought to mediate melatonin's phase shifting effects on circadian rhythms. Ramelteon is about 17 times more potent at the MT1/MT2 receptors than melatonin. Studies have shown an absence of next-day residual effects, withdrawal, and rebound effects. The medication lacks abuse potential. Randomized, placebo-controlled studies have demonstrated efficacy of ramelteon, with most effects being on sleep latency. The medication has a short half-life. One study by Mayer and colleagues[108] demonstrated that 8 mg of ramelteon 30 minutes before bedtime reduced *subjective sleep latency* over a 6-month trial. Ramelteon also decreased latency to persistent sleep by PSG over the trial. TST was increased only during week 1 of the trial. Side effects of ramelteon include headache, nausea, dizziness, somnolence, nightmares, hallucinations, and (uncommonly) suicidal ideation. Arthralgia and myalgia can also occur. Because ramelteon has no dependence potential, it may be a good choice for patients with a history of alcohol or drug dependency. Ramelteon undergoes hepatic metabolism and should be avoided in patients with severe liver disease. Use of ramelteon is contraindicated in patients taking fluvoxamine because this antidepressant significantly increases the levels of ramelteon in the blood. Ramelteon also would be unlikely to worsen respiration, making it of potential benefit in patients with obstructive sleep apnea or lung disease. However, benefit for only sleep latency limits the enthusiasm for this use. A generic formulation of ramelteon is available.

Table 33–22 Melatonin Agonists and Dual Orexin Antagonists (DORAs): *FDA Approved for Treatment of Insomnia*

Generic Name (Brand Name)** Dosage Forms	Dosage	Onset of Action (T_{max})	Duration of Action($T_{1/2}$)	Indication	Selected Side Effects / Comments
Melatonin***	0.5 to 3 mg	(0.3–1 hrs)	$T_{1/2}$ = 0.6–1 hr	Not FDA, or AASM approved for insomnia, best use for sleep onset insomnia	MT1, MT2 agonist
Ramelteon (Rozerem) 8 mg	8 mg qhs (30 min before bedtime)	T_{max} (0.75 hours)	$T_{1/2}$ = (1 to 2.6 hours Hepatic metabolism	FDA and AASM[83] SOI	MT1, MT2 agonist Contraindicated with fluvoxamine (strong CYP1A2 inhibitor) Dizziness, fatigue
Suvorexant* (Belsomra)** 5, 10, 15, 20 mg	10–20 mg qhs Start 10 mg	T_{max} 2 hours	$T_{1/2}$ =12 hours Hepatic metabolism	FDA SOI, SMI AASM SMI	Headache, somnolence, nausea, sleep paralysis, suicidal ideation
Lemborexant* (Dayvigo)** 5 mg, 10 mg	5–10 mg qhs Start 5 mag	T_{max} 1–2 hours	$T_{1/2}$ (5 mg) = 17 hours $T_{1/2}$ (10 mg) = 19 hours Hepatic metabolism	FDA SOI, SMI	Headache, somnolence, dizziness, nausea
Daridorexant* (QuviviQ)** 25, 50 mg	25–50 mg qhs	T_{max} 1–2 hours Delayed onset if taken with food	$T_{1/2}$ = 8 hours Hepatic metabolism If moderate hepatic impairment, use 25 mg	FDA SOI, SMI	Side effects Headache, somnolence, dizziness, nausea

*Contraindicated in narcolepsy; side effects include sleep paralysis, sleep hallucinations, complex sleep behaviors.
**No generic formulations of these medications available.
***Not FDA aproved for insomnia, Data from Buysse DJ. Insomnia. *JAMA*. 2013;309(7):706-716 and references 109-116.
AASM, American Academy of Sleep Medicine; *FDA*, U.S. Food and Drug Administration; *SMI*, sleep-maintenance insomnia; *SOI*, sleep-onset insomnia.
Buysse DJ. Insomnia. *JAMA*. 2013;309(7):706-716. PMID: 23423416. Stahl SM. *Stahl's Essential Psychopharmacology*, 7th ed. Cambridge University Press.

Orexin Receptor Antagonists

Three dual orexin receptor (Hypocretin 1 and 2 receptors) antagonists (DORAs) are currently available in the United States for treatment of insomnia (Table 33–22). These include suvorexant (Belsomra),[109-113] lemborexant (Dayvigo),[114,115] and daridorexant (Quviviq).[116] These medications are FDA approved for SOI and SMI (Table 33–22). *However, the AASM clinical guidelines recommend suvorexant only for SMI.* Lemborexant and daridorexant were not released at the time the AASM guidelines were written. An interesting property of suvorexant is that the medication is less likely to inhibit arousal from sleep and might be beneficial for those needing to respond to stimuli during the night.[112] One study found that suvorexant does not appear to impair respiration in patients with obstructive sleep apnea.[113] Of note, suvorexant was effective at doses of 20/15 to 30/20 mg (non-elderly/elderly) in several studies, which is higher than the FDA-recommended starting dose of 10 mg; physicians using the medication should be aware of this fact (10 mg may not be effective). Side effects include those common with other hypnotics and can be associated with cataplexy-like episodes, sleep paralysis, and sleep-related hallucinations. These medications are contraindicated in patients with narcolepsy. *Taking with food can delay onset of action.* The lowest dose is recommended in moderate hepatic dysfunction, and use is not recommended in patients with severe hepatic dysfunction. The DORAs are schedule IV medications. Suvorexant is available in 5 and 10 mg tablets with dosages from 10 to 20 mg (starting dose 10 mg). Lemborexant is available in 5, 10, 15, and 20 mg tablets, with a starting dose of 5 mg. Dardiorexant (Quviviq™) is available in 25 and 50 mg tablets, and the recommended dosage is 25 to 50 mg taken orally within 30 minutes of going to bed (with at least 7 hours available for sleep). *The half-life of dardiorexant is considerably shorter than those of the other two DORAs*, and this could be an important property to note if morning sedation is an issue with use of suvorexant and lemborexant. However, the duration of action depends on both dose and half-life.

Sedating Antidepressants and Antipsychotics

Sedating antidepressants are widely used as hypnotics in doses lower than those used for antidepressant effects (Table 33–23). However, with the exception of low-dose doxepin, relatively little evidence has demonstrated their effectiveness as hypnotics in patients without depression. The AASM clinical guidelines do not recommend use of trazodone (insufficient evidence), while 3 or 6 mg doxepin (Silenor) nightly was recommended for SMI.[83] **Trazodone** is a sedating antidepressant with minimal anticholinergic activity that is frequently used as a hypnotic. The evidence for its efficacy as a hypnotic in patients without depression is very modest.[117,118] Trazodone was used in a study of sequential treatment

Table 33–23 Sedating Antidepressants and Antipsychotics Used "Off-Label" As Hypnotics*

Generic Name (Brand Name) Dosage Forms	Hypnotic Dose	Half-Life/Comments	Notable Side Effects
Trazodone (Desyrel)**,*** 50, 100 mg	25–100 mg qhs	Less anticholinergic side effects than TCAs $T_{1/2}$ = 9 (7–15) hours	Priapism (1/8000) Postural hypotension
Mirtazapine** (Remeron)** 15, 30 mg	7.5–15 mg qhs	$T_{1/2}$ = 30 (20–40) hours	Weight gain Higher doses may be less sedating
Sedating Tricyclic Antidepressants (TCAs)			
Amitriptyline (Elavil)** 10, 25, 50 mg	10–25 mg qhs	$T_{1/2}$ = 30 (5–45) hours metabolite active (nortriptyline)	Very anticholinergic Dry mouth, constipation QT prolongation
Doxepin (Sinequan)**,*** 10 mg, 25 mg, 50 mg, capsules, 10 mg/mL elixir	3–6 mg (elixir) 10 mg qhs	$T_{1/2}$ = 15 (10–30) hours	Dry mouth, constipation
Doxepin (Sileno)** 3, 6 mg tablet Silenor	6 mg qhs 3 mg qhs elderly	$T_{1/2}$ = 15 (10–30) hours Less anticholinergic side effects at lower doses	FDA and AASM approved for sleep-maintenance insomnia Cimetidine increases drug levels—max dose of doxepin should not exceed 3 mg if cimetidine co-administered Sertraline can also increase levels of doxepin
Sedating Antipsychotic Medications			
Quetiapine** (Seroquel)* 25, 50, 100 mg	12.5–50 mg qhs	Intermediate-acting $T_{1/2}$ = 6 hours	Headache, dizziness, constipation Neuroleptic syndrome Tardive dyskinesia Long QT Lens change

*These medications are not FDA approved as hypnotics, except for Silenor.
**Generic available.
***Brand name not available, Data from Buysse DJ. Insomnia. *JAMA*. 2013;309(7):706-716. PMID: 23423416.
FDA, U.S. Food and Drug Administration; *TCA*, tricyclic antidepressant
Data from Buysse DJ. Insomnia. *JAMA*. 2013 Feb 20;309(7):706-16.

modalities for insomnia.[55] However, a substantial number of patients seem to benefit from the medication. It is a reasonable hypnotic in comorbid depression[119] in patients with significant sleep apnea or in patients with a history of medication dependence. Its main side effects are priapism (1/8000 cases) and postural hypotension. The usual dose is 25 to 100 mg qhs. However, patients with both insomnia and anxiety may need 200 to 300 mg. The usual antidepressant dose is 150 to 600 mg. It can cause postural hypotension or increase the QT interval. Of interest, a study of prescribing in the United States found a decreasing amount of zolpidem and an increasing amount of trazodone (2011–2018).[120] **Mirtazapine** (Remeron®) is used in low doses as a hypnotic. Of interest, some clinicians feel that lower doses (7.5 and 15 mg) are sometimes more sedating than higher doses. The major side effect is weight gain. Mirtazapine is a noradrenergic and specific serotonergic antidepressant that acts by antagonizing the adrenergic alpha2-autoreceptors and alpha2-heteroreceptors and by blocking 5-HT2 and 5-HT3 receptors. It enhances the release of norepinephrine and 5-HT1A-mediated serotonergic transmission. Its sedation is believed to be a result of its antihistamine activity. *Mirtazapine is the antidepressant most likely to worsen restless leg syndrome.* **Doxepin** (Sinequan, Silenor) and amitriptyline (Elavil) are sedating tricyclic antidepressants that have been used in low doses as hypnotics. They have significant anticholinergic side effects (dry mouth, constipation, urinary retention). It is important to recall that tricyclic antidepressants are very dangerous in overdose. The brand name Sinequan is no longer available but generic doxepin formulations are available. Very low-dose doxepin (3, 6 mg) has been evaluated with randomized, controlled trials for its use as a hypnotic.[121] Lower doses avoid significant anticholinergic side effects. In these studies, the major significant effect was a decrease in WASO. The mechanism of the hypnotic action of doxepin is antagonism of histamine (H1) receptors. As noted, a preparation of doxepin (Silenor) available as 3 and 6 mg tablets is approved by the FDA for treatment of insomnia characterized by difficulties with sleep maintenance. This is the only sedating antidepressant FDA approved for treatment of insomnia. The AASM clinical practice guidelines for pharmacological treatment of insomnia recommend this medication for SMI. Silenor is expensive. Less expensive generic low dose doxepin formulations (3 mg, 6 mg) are now available but at the time of writing are still more expensive than generic BZRAs. An alternative is to use a low dose of generic doxepin (10 capsule or 5 mg using the elixir). Medications with substantial anticholinergic activity can cause urinary retention in patients with benign prostatic hypertrophy. Use of even low-dose doxepin in patients with severe urinary retention should be avoided.

Quetiapine (Seroquel) is a second-generation antipsychotic medication that antagonizes histamine, dopamine D2, and serotonin (5HT2) receptors. At low doses, the medication's main effect is as an antihistamine. Quetiapine is indicated for treatment of schizophrenia and bipolar disorder. Side effects include QT prolongation, weight gain, extrapyramidal symptoms, headache, lens changes/cataracts, and decreased white blood cell count. Even at low doses, quetiapine has been associated with significant weight gain. Due to its side effects, this medication is usually not used for insomnia in patients without significant psychiatric disorders unless other options have failed. However, it can be effective in low doses (12.5 to 25 mg) in some patients who do not respond or tolerate sedating antidepressants.

Other Mediations Used for Insomnia

Other medications with sedating effects have been used for insomnia. Gabapentin (an anticonvulsant structural analog of GABA that binds the α2-delta subunit of voltage-gated calcium channels) is used for chronic pain and restless legs syndrome. The half-life of gabapentin is approximately 5 to 9 hours, and it is excreted by the kidneys unchanged. Due to the sedative properties of gabapentin, the medication can be used as a hypnotic treatment alternative in patients who do not respond to or tolerate other medications. The usual dosage is 300 to 900 mg at bedtime. Side effects include dizziness, ataxia, and, less commonly, leukopenia. Gabapentin could potentially be useful in patients with insomnia associated with pain. Gabapentin can increase stage N3 sleep. The FDA has issued a warning about potential respiratory depression especially in patients with respiratory risk factors including chronic lung disease and co-adminstration of gabapentin with opioid medication.

Antihistamines (diphenhydramine and doxylamine) are the primary ingredients in over-the-counter sleep aids. There is some limited evidence for their efficacy. The main problem is that they have considerable anticholinergic activity (urinary retention) and can cause daytime sedation. In patients with restless legs syndrome and difficulty initiating sleep, taking an antihistamine can actually make symptoms worse and prolong sleep latency. The AASM guidelines for pharmacological treatment of insomnia did not recommend over the counter antihistamines. The half-life of diphendyramine is 4–8 hours and for doxylamine is 10 hours.[25]

Pharmacotherapy for Patients With Dependence Issues

In patients with a history of past or current alcohol or BZ dependence, the use of BZRAs is problematic. For these patients, use of melatonin, ramelteon (no abuse potential), a *low dose* of a sedating antidepressant (plus another antidepressant at an antidepressant dose if the patient is depressed), or a sedating antidepressant at an antidepressant (mirtazapine 15–45 mg qhs) dose are the best treatment options. Although DORAs are schedule IV medications (studies have shown some abuse potential, i.e., drug "liking"), clinical experience has suggested they may have less abuse potential than BZRAs.[122] This is an area of some controversy, but use of DORAs could be considered in patients with a history of drug dependence if other non-BZRA options are not successful.

Pharmacotherapy of Insomnia: Overall Strategy

An algorithm for hypnotic therapy of insomnia is illustrated in Figure 33–12. It is always important to ask patients about prior treatment failures and side effects. Drug interactions should also be considered. For patients with SOI, one could start with ramelteon or zaleplon. However, the cost of zaleplon may not be acceptable. A lower dose of a longer-acting generic medication could be tried. The duration of action depends on both the dose and the elimination half-life. If SMI is a problem, use of zolpidem, zolpidem CR, eszopiclone, or temazepam could be considered. In elderly patients, women, or patients with impaired hepatic metabolism, a lower hypnotic dose is prudent. If the duration of action is not long enough, one can switch to a longer-acting medication (e.g., from zolpidem to eszopiclone). If the duration of action is too long (morning sedation), a switch to a

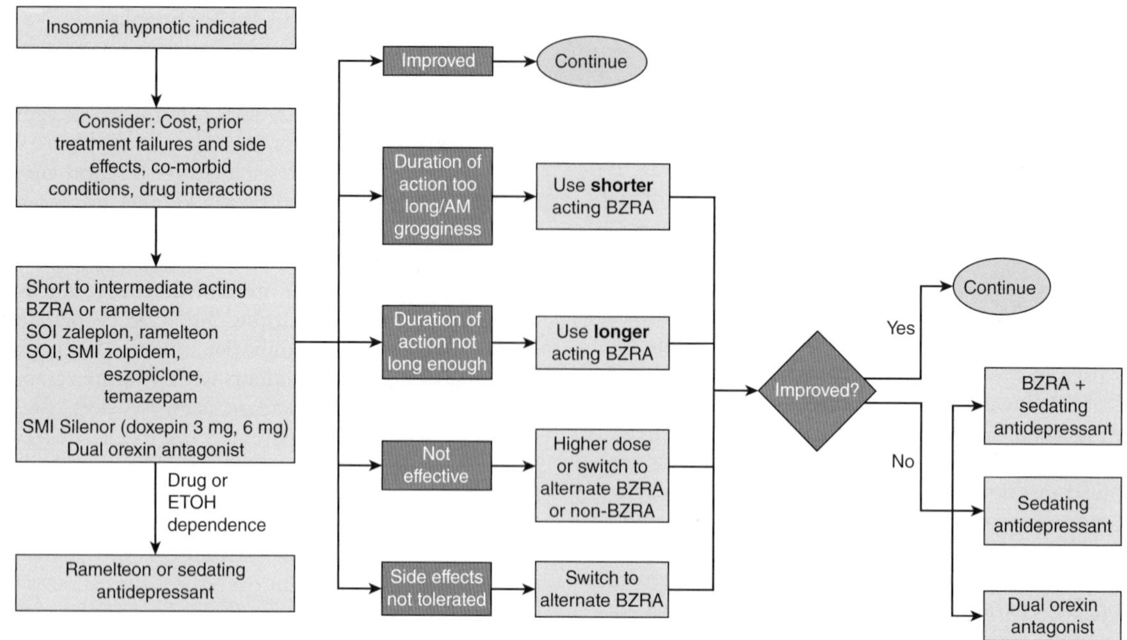

Figure 33–12 Hypnotic use pathways. Consider needed duration of action, prior drug failures, side effects, and drug interactions in choice of a hypnotic. If selection is not effective or tolerated, adjust the dose or switch to another medication. If BZRA alone is not effective, consider a sedating antidepressant alone or in combination with a BZRA or an orexin antagonist. *SMI*, sleep maintenance insomnia; *SOI*, sleep onset insomnia; *BZRA*, benzodiazepine receptor agonist. Dual orexin antagonists are FDA approved for both SOI and SMI. However, the AASM guidelines[83] recommended suvorexant only for SMI. Since the guidelines were published new dual orexin antagonists are available.

shorter-acting medication or a reduction in dosage of the current medication could be tried. If the medication is not effective, a switch to an alternate BZRA could be considered. Some patients will respond differently to alternate BZRAs. As noted, temazepam may not work well for SOI in some patients because of its longer onset of action. If anxiety is a major component of insomnia, use of a traditional BZ or eszopiclone with more anxiolytic activity might be more effective. If the current hypnotic medication is not tolerated because of side effects, a switch to an alternate BZRA could also be tried.

If treatment with standard BZRA hypnotics is not successful, one could try an orexin antagonist or sedating antidepressant. The dual orexin antagonists are relatively expensive (no generics). Given the minimal anticholinergic effects associated with trazodone, most physicians would start with this medication when using a sedating antidepressant. However, low-dose doxepin or amitriptyline may be effective in some patients. As noted, Silenor and low dose generics (3, 6 mg) are the only sedating antiderpessants FDA approved for insomnia. If sedating antidepressants are not effective (or tolerated at an effective dose), the combination of a BZRA and a sedating antidepressant could be tried (e.g., zolpidem and trazodone). If sleep onset insomnia remains an issue with the use of medication that is effective for sleep maintenance insomnia, the addition of another medication more effective for sleep onset insomnia could be tried. Another option would be to take the current medication earlier. While melatonin is not FDA or AASM approved for sleep onset insomnia, a combination of melatonin and a medication effective for SMI is an option. If there is a significant pain component to insomnia, one could try gabapentin for its sedating and analgesic effects. If anxiety is a major component of the insomnia or the traditional BZRA hypnotics are not effective, use of lorazepam, alprazolam, or clonazepam could be tried. Lastly, one could try a sedating antipsychotic (quetiapine). However, quetiapine and other atypical antipsychotic medications have major side effects and are generally avoided unless a mental disorder is present or all other options have failed. Using low dose quetiapine (12.5 or 25 mg) may reduce the risk of side effects. Adjustment of the dosage timing can also be considered if there is still difficulty with initiating sleep or morning grogginess. The timing of the dose can be important, and taking the medication 30 to 60 minutes before bedtime can help with sleep onset. Taking medications with food near bedtime can delay the onset of action of some hypnotics. If morning grogginess is an issue, decreasing the dose or taking a medication earlier than usual may be helpful.

SUMMARY OF KEY POINTS

1. Diagnosis of Chronic Insomnia Disorder (CID) requires (1) sleep difficulty, (2) daytime consequences, (3) difficulty for at least three nights per week for over 3 months, (4) adequate opportunity and environment for sleep, and (5) the sleep disturbance and associated daytime symptoms are not SOLELY due to another current sleep disorder, medical disorder, mental disorder or medication/substance abuse. The prevalence of CID is estimated to be about 10–15% of the population (30% have intermittent insomnia issues). CID is **more common in women**, those with medical, psychiatric, or substance use disorders, and those of a lower socio-economic strata. Up to 40% of OSA patients have insomnia symptoms.

2. Sleep difficulty may include problems initiating or maintaining sleep and early-morning awakening. CID is thought to be present in 10–30% of children. In children, sleep difficulties can include resistance to going to bed and difficulty sleeping or returning to sleep without caregiver presence or intervention.
3. A good sleep history is the essential tool for evaluating insomnia. PSG plays a limited role.
4. Sleep logs and actigraphy provide complementary information and can both be valuable.
5. Cognitive behavioral treatment for insomnia (CBT-I) is as effective for insomnia treatment (including comorbid insomnia) as pharmacotherapy. CBT-I is considered the treatment of choice for insomnia.
6. CBT-I is defined as cognitive therapy + stimulus control and sleep restriction therapy with or without sleep relaxation therapy.
7. The most important property of a BZRA hypnotic medication is the duration of action.
8. When the duration of the action of a hypnotic is not long enough, use either a higher dose or a longer-acting medication.
9. Longer-acting medications can cause significant morning and daytime sleepiness.
10. Hypnotics with a short duration of action are indicated to treat SOI (e.g., zaleplon, ramelteon).
11. Ensure proper timing of medication if difficulties with initiating sleep persist on medication – earlier dosing may be needed. Morning grogginess can be addressed with earlier or decreased dosing.
12. BZRAs with intermediate durations of action are indicated to treat SOI and SMI (zolpidem, zolpidem CR, eszopiclone, temazepam). The duration of action of zolpidem may be too short for SMI in some patients.
13. The non-BZ BZRAs (Z hypnotics) tend to suppress stage N3 sleep less than BZs and are less commonly associated with rebound insomnia than BZ BZRAs.
14. Rebound insomnia is less common with the "Z" BZRA hypnotics (zaleplon, zolpidem, and eszopiclone). However, it is best to wean all hypnotics to avoid rebound insomnia.
15. Triazolam is recommended for SOI by AASM guidelines but is not a first-line option, as it is associated with rebound insomnia on withdrawal. The medication is FDA approved for short term treatment of insomnia without specification of the insomnia type.
16. An unpleasant taste is a distinctive side effect of eszopiclone.
17. Sleep-related eating disorder can occur with any of the BZRAs but is most often described with zolpidem. Complex sleep behaviors (sleep walking) can occur with all the BZRAs.
18. Sublingual buffered zolpidem (Intermezzo) is FDA approved for middle-of-the-night awakening. Another option is zaleplon, a medication with an ultra-short duration of action; however, this medication is not FDA approved for middle-of-the-night awakening.
19. The dose of zolpidem should be reduced in women and the elderly (5 mg immediate release or 6.25 mg controlled release). A reduced starting dose of eszopiclone (1 mg) is also recommended by the FDA for men and women.
20. Another alternative to increase the duration of a BZRA is to add a low dose of a sedating antidepressant (e.g., trazodone 25 mg).
21. Silenor and generic doxepin (3 and 6 mg tablets) is the only sedating antidepressant FDA approved for insomnia (SMI).
22. Trazodone is a sedating antidepressant with minimal anticholinergic side effects. It is frequently used in low doses (25 to 50 mg) as a hypnotic.
23. In patients with urinary retention, treatment with sedative antidepressants or antihistamines with anticholinergic activity is relatively contraindicated. Trazodone or low-dose doxepin (3, 6 mg) can be used in this situation, as minimal anticholinergic side effects are present.
24. Patients with a history of substance or drug dependence/abuse are NOT candidates for treatment with BZRAs because of the potential for these drugs to result in dependence or abuse. Ramelteon and sedating antidepressants are an option.
25. Hypnotic medications should not be taken in the middle of the night unless at least 4 hours remain for sleep. Residual impairment of coordination or cognition in the morning may be potentiated by coadministration of other sedative medications. Women, the elderly, and patients with hepatic dysfunction are especially at risk given the slower clearance of medications such as zolpidem.
26. Zaleplon (Sonata) is used to treat sleep onset insomnia (difficulty in falling asleep). The medication has been shown to decrease the time to sleep onset for up to 30 days in clinical studies (but may be effective for a longer period of time).
27. The dual orexin receptor antagonists provide another option for hypnotics in patients who do not respond to other medications. They are contraindicated in patients with narcolepsy. Arousal from sleep may be less impaired with DORAs than with BZRAs. However, they have side effects similar to those of BZRAs (with the addition of sleep paralysis with DORAs).

CLINICAL REVIEW QUESTIONS

1. A 40-year-old man was prescribed zolpidem for insomnia complaints. His problems with sleep onset have improved, but he still is unable to sleep later than 3:00 or 4:00 AM. What medication do you prescribe?
   A. Zaleplon
   B. Eszopiclone
   C. Triazolam
   D. Ramelteon
2. Which of the following behavioral techniques has the least evidence of efficacy?
   A. Stimulus control therapy (SCT)
   B. Relaxation therapy
   C. Sleep restriction therapy (SRT)
   D. Sleep hygiene education
   E. Multimodality CBT-I
3. A 60-year-old obese man has a history of alcohol dependence, insomnia, and benign prostatic hypertrophy. What is the most appropriate medication for treatment of his insomnia?
   A. Doxepin 25 mg
   B. Amitriptyline 25 mg
   C. Zolpidem 10 mg
   D. Trazodone 50 mg
   E. Diphenhydramine 25 mg

4. A 30-year-old woman reports problems with insomnia since childhood. There have been no periods of remission. She denies sleeping better in novel environments. During the last few months, her mood and sleep complaints have worsened. What is the most likely subtype of her insomnia?
   A. Psychophysiologic insomnia
   B. Idiopathic insomnia
   C. Paradoxical insomnia
   D. Insomnia comorbid with depression
5. A 30-year-old man complains of episodes of waking up at 2:00 AM and not being able to return to sleep. These episodes occur about every 2 weeks but are not predictable. What do you prescribe? He usually does not get out of bed until 6:00 AM.
   A. Zolpidem
   B. Zaleplon
   C. Eszopiclone
   D. Temazepam
6. A 50-year-old woman is taking a hypnotic for insomnia. Recently, she has been sleepwalking and eating during sleep. Some episodes she can remember, but other times she is surprised to find evidence of food consumption when she awakens in the morning. Although the behavior could occur with almost any hypnotic, which of the following BZRAs has been most often associated with this behavior?
   A. Zaleplon
   B. Temazepam
   C. Zolpidem
   D. Eszopiclone
   E. Ramelteon
7. A 45-year-old woman complains of not sleeping at all for 2 to 3 nights each week. Other nights, it takes over an hour to fall asleep, and her estimated TST is never more than 4 hours. The patient rarely takes naps but feels terrible the next day when she does not sleep the night before. The patient describes lying in bed all night thinking about her work. She kept a sleep log and was studied with actigraphy. One night, no sleep was reported, but the actigraph estimated about 5 hours of sleep. What subtype of CID is most compatible with this history?
   A. Idiopathic insomnia
   B. Psychophysiologic insomnia
   C. Paradoxical insomnia
   D. Insomnia associated with a mood disorder
8. What of the following is **NOT** true about the $GABA_A$ receptor complex?
   A. It contains a chloride ionophore.
   B. It is composed of five protein subunits.
   C. Binding of a BZRA opens the chloride pore.
   D. The complex is usually composed of two alpha, two beta, and one gamma subunit.
9. Which of the following medications is associated with an unpleasant taste?
   A. Zolpidem
   B. Eszopiclone
   C. Ramelteon
   D. Trazodone
10. Which of the following is NOT one of the three Ps of insomnia?
    A. Precipitating
    B. Predisposing
    C. Promoting
    D. Perpetuating
11. Which of the following statements about CBT-I is **NOT** true?
    A. It consists of cognitive therapy plus two behavioral treatments (stimulus control treatment, sleep restriction treatment) with or without relaxation therapy.
    B. It continues to show benefits after the treatment period.
    C. There is no clear advantage of combination therapy (CBT-I + medication) compared to CBT-I alone. However, pharmacotherapy could be used if CBT-I is not successful.
    D. It is effective for sleep onset insomnia but not sleep maintenance insomnia or nonrestorative sleep.
12. A 5-year-old boy often awakens during the night and will not return to sleep without at least half an hour of parental presence and attention. Which diagnosis best describes the problem?
    A. Childhood behavioral insomnia—limit-setting type
    B. Childhood behavioral insomnia—sleep-association type
13. A 50-year-old man with both SOI and SMI is started on zolpidem CR. He tolerated the medication, but his sleep did not improve. Which of the following is the most appropriate next step?
    A. Eszopiclone
    B. Trazodone
    C. Quetiapine
    D. Ramelteon
    E. Zaleplon
14. Which of the following is NOT true about insomnia disorders?
    A. CID must be present for at least 3 months.
    B. Short-term insomnia disorder must be present for no more than 1 month.
    C. Short-term insomnia is often associated with an identifiable stressor.
    D. Short-term insomnia is expected to resolve spontaneously in most cases.
15. A patient complains of SOI and SMI. A sleep log reveals report of 10 hours in bed but only 6 hours of sleep. Which of the behavioral techniques would be most applicable to this patient?
    A. Relaxation therapy
    B. Stimulus control therapy
    C. Sleep hygiene education
    D. Sleep restriction therapy (SRT)

ANSWERS

1. B. A BZRA with a longer duration of action is needed. Eszopiclone has a longer duration of action than zolpidem (including zolpidem CR). Zaleplon, triazolam, and ramelteon have a short duration of action.
2. D. There is no evidence that sleep hygiene education alone is an effective treatment of insomnia.
3. D. Trazodone. Doxepin (at 25 mg), amitriptyline, and diphenhydramine all have significant anticholinergic activity and could cause urinary retention. Use of zolpidem is relatively contraindicated in a patient with current or prior substance dependence. Trazodone has minimal anticholinergic activity. Low dose doxepin (3, 6 mg, Silenor and generic Silenor) have less anticholinergic activity and are FDA approved for sleep maintenance insomnia.
4. B. Idiopathic insomnia is characteristically present since childhood without periods of remission. Psychophysiologic

and paradoxical insomnia are not present since childhood. Insomnia comorbid with depression would be a reasonable possibility, but the patient had significant insomnia many years before her mood worsened. Of note, a diagnosis of CID would be made, as idiopathic insomnia is a subtype.

5. B. Zaleplon is the only medication in the list of answers with a very short half-life. It is the most appropriate "rescue medication" for middle-of-the-night awakening. It should not be used if there are not at least 3 to 4 more hours of possible sleep, and a low dose should be used. If the patient could predict which nights were associated with middle-of-the-night awakening, use of a longer-acting medication at bedtime might also be appropriate. Of note, zaleplon is not FDA approved for treatment of middle-of-the-night insomnia. Intermezzo (sublingual zolpidem) is the only medication FDA approved to treat middle-of-the-night awakening.

6. C. Zolpidem is the BZRA most associated with sleepwalking, sleep violence, and sleep-related eating disorder. However, all BZRAs can be associated with these problems.

7. C. Paradoxical insomnia is associated with extreme reduction in reported sleep times but relatively little daytime impairment relative to the reported sleep loss. The subjective amount of sleep loss always far exceeds objective determination (PSG or actigraphy). However, a diagnosis of CID would be made, as paradoxical insomnia is considered a subtype. Since PSG was not performed, it is possible that the patient was very still and not sleeping.

8. C. BZRA binding alone is not sufficient to open the pore. Rather, BZRA binding enhances the ability of GABA binding to open the pore. BZRAs are $GABA_A$ receptor modulators (positive allosteric modulators).

9. B. Eszopiclone has a metallic taste.

10. C. Promoting. The three Ps of insomnia are predisposing, precipitating, and perpetuating.

11. D. CBT-I is effective for SOI, SMI, and nonrestorative sleep. Studies have shown that combined sequential treatment of patients not responding to CBT-I with a hypnotic may be effective. CBT-I has been shown to provide continued benefit after the therapy has been completed.

12. B. Difficulty falling asleep (or back to sleep) without parental presence is considered sleep-association type. However, in the ICSD-3-TR, behavioral insomnia of childhood is considered a subtype of CID.

13. A. Patients may respond differently to different BZRAs. Because zolpidem CR was tolerated, using another intermediate-acting BZRA is a reasonable next step. Trazodone might work, but there is less evidence for efficacy than that for another BZRA. Doxepin 3 or 6 mg (Silenor) is effective for SMI but not SOI. The patient needs treatment for SOI and SMI. Quetiapine is an antipsychotic with many side effects. Ramelteon and zaleplon are short acting and would not be appropriate for SMI. A dual orexin receptor antagonist is another option.

14. B. The duration of short-term insomnia disorder is < 3 months.

15. D. Sleep restriction treatment (SRT). Although all of these behavioral treatments could potentially be helpful, SRT is the one most indicated in accordance with the sleep pattern. The patient stays in bed almost 12 hours most days. By shortening the TIB, hopefully sleep efficiency (less WASO) will occur.

SUGGESTED READING

Buysse DJ. Insomnia. *JAMA*. 2013;309(7):706-716.

Edinger JD, Arnedt JT, Bertisch SM, et al. Behavioral and psychological treatments for chronic insomnia disorder in adults: an American Academy of Sleep Medicine clinical practice guideline. *J Clin Sleep Med*. 2021;17(2):255-262.

Sateia MJ, Buysse DJ, Krystal AD, Neubauer DN, Heald JL. Clinical practice guideline for the pharmacologic treatment of chronic insomnia in adults: an American Academy of Sleep Medicine clinical practice guideline. *J Clin Sleep Med*. 2017;13(2):307-349.

REFERENCES

1. American Academy of Sleep Medicine. *ICSD-2 International Classification of Sleep Disorders: Diagnostic and Coding Manual*. 2nd ed. Westchester, IL: American Academy of Sleep Medicine; 2005.
2. American Academy of Sleep Medicine. *ICSD-3 International Classification of Sleep Disorders: Diagnostic and Coding Manual*. 2nd ed. Darien, IL: American Academy of Sleep Medicine; 2014.
3. American Academy of Sleep Medicine. *ICSD-3 International Classification of Sleep Disorders*. 3rd ed., text revision. Darien, IL: American Academy of Sleep Medicine; 2023.
4. American Psychiatric Association. *Diagnostic and Statistical Manual of Mental Disorders*. 5th ed. Arlington, VA: American Psychiatric Association; 2013.
5. Edinger JD, Wyatt JK, Stepanski EJ, et al. Testing the reliability and validity of DSM-IV-TR and ICSD-2 insomnia diagnoses. Results of a multitrait-multimethod analysis. *Arch Gen Psychiatry*. 2011;68(10):992-1002.
6. Edinger JD, Arnedt JT, Bertisch SM, et al. Behavioral and psychological treatments for chronic insomnia disorder in adults: an American Academy of Sleep Medicine systematic review, meta-analysis, and GRADE assessment. *J Clin Sleep Med*. 2021;17(2):263-298.
7. Ohayon MM. Epidemiology of insomnia: what we know and what we still need to learn. *Sleep Med Rev*. 2002;6(2):97-111.
8. Buysse DJ, Angst J, Gamma A, Ajdacic V, Eich D, Rössler W. Prevalence, course, and comorbidity of insomnia and depression in young adults. *Sleep*. 2008;31(4):473-480.
9. Morin CM, Bélanger L, LeBlanc M, et al. The natural history of insomnia: a population-based 3-year longitudinal study. *Arch Intern Med*. 2009;169(5):447-453.
10. Wickwire EM, Tom SE, Scharf SM, Vadlamani A, Bulatao IG, Albrecht JS. Untreated insomnia increases all-cause health care utilization and costs among Medicare beneficiaries. *Sleep*. 2019;42(4):zsz007.
11. Kessler RC, Berglund PA, Coulouvrat C, et al. Insomnia and the performance of US workers: results from the America Insomnia Survey. *Sleep*. 2011;34(9):1161-1171. Erratum in: *Sleep*. 2011;34(11):1608. Erratum in: *Sleep*. 2012;35(6):725.
12. Daley M, Morin CM, LeBlancM, GrégoireJP, Savard J. The economic burden of insomnia: direct and indirect costs for individuals with insomnia syndrome, insomnia symptoms, and good sleepers. *Sleep*. 2009;32(1):55-64.
13. Spielman AJ. Assessment of insomnia. *Clin Psychol Rev*. 1986;6(1):11-25.
14. Spielman AJ, Caruso LS, Glovinski PN. A behavioral perspective on insomnia treatment. *Psychiatr Clin North Am*. 1987;10(4):541-553.
15. Ellis JG, Perlis ML, Espie CA, et al. The natural history of insomnia: predisposing, precipitating, coping, and perpetuating factors over the early developmental course of insomnia. *Sleep*. 2021;44(9):zsab095.
16. Chapman JL, Comas M, Hoyos CM, Bartlett DJ, Grunstein RR, Gordon CJ. Is metabolic rate increased in insomnia disorder? A systematic review. *Front Endocrinol (Lausanne)*. 2018;9:374.
17. Bonnet MH, Arand DL. 24-Hour metabolic rate in insomniacs and matched normal sleepers. *Sleep*. 1995;18(7):581-588.
18. Bonnet MH, Berry RB, Arand DL. Metabolism during normal, fragmented, and recovery sleep. *J Appl Physiol (1985)*. 1991;71(3):1112-1118.
19. Riedner BA, Goldstein MR, Plante DT, et al. Regional patterns of elevated alpha and high-frequency electroencephalographic activity during nonrapid eye movement sleep in chronic insomnia: a pilot study. *Sleep*. 2016;39(4):801-812.
20. Winkleman JW, Buxton OM, Jensen JE, et al. Reduced brain GABA in primary insomnia: preliminary data from 4T proton magnetic resonance spectroscopy (1H-MRS). *Sleep*. 2008;31(11):1499-1506.
21. Hogan SE, Delgado GM, Hall MH, et al. Slow-oscillation activity is reduced, and high frequency activity is elevated in older adults with insomnia. *J Clin Sleep Med*. 2020;16(9):1445-1454.

22. Schutte-Rodin S, Broch L, Buysse D, Dorsey C, Sateia M. Clinical guideline for the evaluation and management of chronic insomnia in adults. *J Clin Sleep Med.* 2008;4(5):487-504.
23. Chesson A, Hartse K, Anderson WM, et al. Practice parameters for the evaluation of chronic insomnia. *Sleep.* 2000;23:1-5.
24. Sateia MJ, Doghramji K, Hauri PJ, Morin CM. Evaluation of chronic insomnia: an American Academy of Sleep Medicine review. *Sleep.* 2000;23(2):243-308.
25. Buysse DJ. Insomnia. *JAMA.* 2013;309(7):706-716.
26. Littner M, Hirshkowitz M, Kramer M, et al. American Academy of Sleep Medicine; Standards of Practice Committee. Practice parameters for using polysomnography to evaluate insomnia: an update. *Sleep.* 2003;26(6):754-760.
27. Agnew HW, Webb WB, Williams RL. The first night effect: an EEG study. *Psychophysiology.* 1966;2:263-266.
28. Nuckton TJ, Glidden DV, Browner WS, et al. Physical examination: Mallampati as an independent predictor of obstructive sleep apnea. *Sleep.* 2006;29:903-908.
29. Ong JC, Crawford MR, Wallace DM. Sleep apnea and insomnia: emerging evidence for effective clinical management. *Chest.* 2021;159(5):2020-2028.
30. Meira E Cruz M, Kryger MH, Morin CM, Palombini L, Salles C, Gozal D. Comorbid insomnia and sleep apnea: mechanisms and implications of an underrecognized and misinterpreted sleep disorder. *Sleep Med.* 2021;84:283-288.
31. Mieno Y, Hayashi M, Sakakibara H, et al. Gender differences in the clinical features of sleep apnea syndrome. *Intern Med.* 2018;57(15):2157-2163.
32. Johns MW. Sleepiness in different situations measured by the Epworth Sleepiness Scale. *Sleep.* 1994;17:703-710.
33. Buysse DJ, Reynolds CF, Monk TH, et al. The Pittsburgh Sleep Quality Index: a new instrument for psychiatric practice and research. *Psychiatry Res.* 1989;28:193-213.
34. Buysee DJ, Reynolds CF, Monk TH, et al. Quantification of subjective sleep quality in healthy elderly men and women using the Pittsburgh Sleep Quality Index (PSQI). *Sleep.* 1991;14:331-338.
35. Morin CM, Belleville G, Bélanger L, Ivers H. The Insomnia Severity Index: psychometric indicators to detect insomnia cases and evaluate treatment response. *Sleep.* 2011;34(5):601-608.
36. Bastien CH, Vallières A, Morin CM. Validation of the Insomnia Severity Index as an outcome measure for insomnia research. *Sleep Med.* 2001;2: 297-230.
37. Morin CM. *Insomnia: Psychological Assessment and Management.* New York: Guilford Press; 1993.
38. Kraepelien M, Blom K, Forsell E, et al. A very brief self-report scale for measuring insomnia severity using two items from the Insomnia Severity Index: development and validation in a clinical population. *Sleep Med.* 2021;81:365-374.
39. Beck AT, Steer RA, Brown GK. *Manual for the Beck Depression Inventory (BDI-II).* 2nd ed. San Antonio, TX: The Psychological Association; 1996.
40. Beck AT, Ward CH, Mendelson M, et al. An inventory for measuring depression. *Arch Gen Psychiatry.* 1961;4:561-571.
41. Carney CE, Ulmer C, Edinger JD, et al. Assessing depression symptoms in those with insomnia: an examination of the Beck Depression Inventory second edition (BDI-II). *J Psychiatr Res.* 2009;43:576-582.
42. Morin CM. Dysfunctional beliefs and attitudes about sleep: Preliminary scale development and description. *The Behavior Therapist* 1994; Summer: 163-164.
43. Morin CM, Vallières A, Ivers H. Dysfunctional beliefs and attitudes about sleep (DBAS): validation of a brief version (DBAS-16). *Sleep.* 2007;30:1547-1554.
44. Carney CE, Buysse DJ, Ancoli-Israel S, et al. The consensus sleep diary: standardizing prospective sleep self-monitoring. *Sleep.* 2012;35(2):287-302.
45. Lichstenin KL, Stone KC, Donaldson J, et al. Actigraphy validation with insomnia. *Sleep.* 2006;29:232-239.
46. Littner M, Kushida CA, Anderson WM, et al. Practice parameters for the role of actigraphy in the study of sleep and circadian rhythms: an update for 2002. *Sleep.* 2003;26:337-341.
47. Morgenthaler T, Alessi C, Friedman L, et al. Practice parameters for the use of actigraphy in the assessment of sleep and sleep disorders: an update for 2007. *Sleep.* 2007;30:519-529.
48. Smith MT, McCrae CS, Cheung J, et al. Use of actigraphy for the evaluation of sleep disorders and circadian rhythm sleep-wake disorders: an American Academy of Sleep Medicine clinical practice guideline. *J Clin Sleep Med.* 2018;14(7):1231-1237.
49. Smith MT, McCrae CS, Cheung J, et al. Use of actigraphy for the evaluation of sleep disorders and circadian rhythm sleep-wake disorders: an American Academy of Sleep Medicine systematic review, meta-analysis, and GRADE assessment. *J Clin Sleep Med.* 2018;14(7):1209-1230.
50. Vallières A, Morin CM. Actigraphy in the assessment of insomnia. *Sleep.* 2003;26:902-906.
51. Sivertsen B, Omvik S, Havik OE, et al. A comparison of actigraphy and polysomnography in older adults treated for chronic primary insomnia. *Sleep.* 2006;29:1353-1358.
52. Morin CM, Colecchi C, Stone J, Sood R, Brink D. Behavioral and pharmacological therapies for late-life insomnia: a randomized controlled trial. *JAMA.* 1999;281(11):991-999.
53. Morin CM, Vallières A, Guay B, et al. Cognitive behavioral therapy, singly and combined with medication, for persistent insomnia: a randomized controlled trial. *JAMA.* 2009;301(19):2005-2015.
54. Morin CM, Beaulieu-Bonneau S, Ivers H, et al. Speed and trajectory of changes of insomnia symptoms during acute treatment with cognitive-behavioral therapy, singly and combined with medication. *Sleep Med.* 2014;15(6):701-707.
55. Morin CM, Edinger JD, Beaulieu-Bonneau S, et al. Effectiveness of sequential psychological and medication therapies for insomnia disorder: a randomized clinical trial. *JAMA Psychiatry.* 2020;77(11):1107-1115.
56. Morin CM, Hauri PK, Espie CA, et al. Nonpharmacologic treatment of chronic insomnia. *Sleep.* 1999;22:1134-1156.
57. Chesson AL, McDowell WA, Littner M, et al. Practice parameters for the non-pharmacological treatment of chronic insomnia. *Sleep.* 1999;22:28-33.
58. Morin CM, Bootzin RR, Buysse DJ, Edinger JD, Espie CA, Lichstein KL. Psychological and behavioral treatment of insomnia: update of the recent evidence (1998-2004). *Sleep.* 2006;29(11):1398-1414.
59. Morgenthaler T, Kramer M, Alessi C, et al. Practice parameters for the psychological and behavioral treatment of insomnia: an update. *Sleep.* 2006;29:1415-1419.
60. Edinger JD, Arnedt JT, Bertisch SM, et al. Behavioral and psychological treatments for chronic insomnia disorder in adults: an American Academy of Sleep Medicine clinical practice guideline. *J Clin Sleep Med.* 2021;17(2):255-262.
61. Means MK, Lichstein KL, Epperson MT, Johnson CT. Relaxation therapy for insomnia: nighttime and daytime effects. *Behav Res Ther.* 2000;38(7):665-678.
62. Bootzin RR, Epstein D, Wood JM. Stimulus control instructions. In: Hauri P, ed. *Case Studies in Insomnia.* New York: Plenum Press; 1991:19-28.
63. Spielman AJ, Saskin P, Thorpy MJ. Treatment of chronic insomnia by restriction of time in bed. *Sleep.* 1987;10(1):45-56.
64. Riedel BW, Lichstein KL, Dwyer WO. Sleep compression and sleep education for older insomniacs: self-help versus therapist guidance. *Psychol Aging.* 1995;10(1):54-63.
65. Jacobs GD, Pace-Schott EF, Stickgold R, Otto MW. Cognitive behavior therapy and pharmacotherapy for insomnia: a randomized controlled trial and direct comparison. *Arch Intern Med.* 2004;164(17):1888-1896.
66. Smith MT, Perlis ML, Park A, et al. Comparative meta-analysis of pharmacotherapy and behavior therapy for persistent insomnia. *Am J Psychiatry.* 2002;159:5-11.
67. Lancee J, van den Bout J, van Straten A, Spoormaker VI. Baseline depression levels do not affect efficacy of cognitive-behavioral self-help treatment for insomnia. *Depress Anxiety.* 2013;30(2):149-156.
68. Dopheide JA. Insomnia overview: epidemiology, pathophysiology, diagnosis and monitoring, and nonpharmacologic therapy. *Am J Manag Care.* 2020;26(suppl 4):S76-S84.
69. Morin CM, Bastein C, Guay B, et al. Randomized clinical trial of supervised tapering and cognitive behavioral therapy to facilitate benzodiazepine discontinuation in older adults with chronic insomnia. *Am J Psychiatry.* 2004;161:132-342.
70. Soeffing JP, Lichstein KL, Nau SD, et al. Psychological treatment of insomnia in hypnotic dependent older adults. *Sleep Med.* 2008;9:165-171.
71. Lichstein KL, Nau SD, Wilson NM, et al. Psychological treatment of hypnotic-dependent insomnia in a primarily older adult sample. *Behav Res Ther.* 2013;51(12):787-796.
72. Buysse DJ, Germain A, Moul DE, et al. Efficacy of brief behavioral treatment for chronic insomnia in older adults. *Arch Intern Med.* 2011;171(10): 887-895.
73. Troxel WM, Germain A, Buysse DJ. Clinical management of insomnia with brief behavioral treatment (BBTI). *Behav Sleep Med.* 2012;10(4): 266-279.
74. Arnedt JT, Conroy DA, Mooney A, Furgal A, Sen A, Eisenberg D. Telemedicine versus face-to-face delivery of cognitive behavioral therapy for insomnia: a randomized controlled noninferiority trial. *Sleep.* 2021; 44(1):zsaa136.
75. Feuerstein S, Hodges SE, Keenaghan B, Bessette A, Forselius E, Morgan PT. Computerized cognitive behavioral therapy for insomnia in a community health setting. *J Clin Sleep Med.* 2017;13(2):267-274.

76. Ritterband LM, Thorndike FP, Ingersoll KS, et al. Effect of a web-based cognitive behavior therapy for insomnia intervention with 1-year follow-up: a randomized clinical trial. *JAMA Psychiatry*. 2017;74(1):68-75.
77. Thorndike FP, Berry RB, Gerwien R, et al. Protocol for digital real-world evidence trial for adults with insomnia treated via mobile (DREAM): an open-label trial of a prescription digital therapeutic for treating patients with chronic insomnia. *J Comp Eff Res*. 2021;10(7):569-581.
78. Kuhn E, Weiss BJ, Taylor KL, et al. CBT-I coach: a description and clinician perceptions of a mobile app for cognitive behavioral therapy for insomnia. *J Clin Sleep Med*. 2016;12(4):597-606.
79. Morgenthaler TI, Owens J, Alessi C, et al. Practice parameters for behavioral treatment of bedtime problems and night wakings in infants and young children. *Sleep*. 2006;29:1277-1281.
80. Mindell JA, Kuhn B, Lewin DS, et al. Behavioral treatment of bedtime problems and night wakings in infants and young children. An American Academy of Sleep Medicine Review. *Sleep*. 2006;29:1263-1276.
81. Lunsford-Avery JR, Bidopia T, Jackson L, Sloan JS. Behavioral treatment of insomnia and sleep disturbances in school-aged children and adolescents. *Child Adolesc Psychiatr Clin N Am*. 2021;30(1):101-116.
82. Buckley AW, Hirtz D, Oskoui M, et al. Practice guideline: treatment for insomnia and disrupted sleep behavior in children and adolescents with autism spectrum disorder: Report of the Guideline Development, Dissemination, and Implementation Subcommittee of the American Academy of Neurology. *Neurology*. 2020;94(9):392-404.
83. Sateia MJ, Buysse DJ, Krystal AD, Neubauer DN, Heald JL. Clinical practice guideline for the pharmacologic treatment of chronic insomnia in adults: an American Academy of Sleep Medicine clinical practice guideline. *J Clin Sleep Med*. 2017;13(2):307-349.
84. Olsen RW, Sieghart W. GABA A receptors: subtypes provide diversity of function and pharmacology. *Neuropharmacology*. 2009;56(1):141-148.
85. Nutt DJ, Stahl SM. Searching for perfect sleep: the continuing evolution of GABAA receptor modulators as hypnotics. *J Psychopharmacol*. 2010;24(11):1601-1612.
86. Stahl SM. Selective actions on sleep or anxiety by exploiting GABA-A/benzodiazepine receptor subtypes. *J Clin Psychiatry*. 2002;63(3):179-180.
87. Krystal AD. A compendium of placebo-controlled trials of the risks/benefits of pharmacological treatments for insomnia: the empirical basis for U.S. clinical practice. *Sleep Med Rev*. 2009;13(4):265-274.
88. Mendelson W. Hypnotic medications: mechanisms of action and pharmacologic effects. In: Kryger MH, Roth T, Dement WC, eds. *Principles and Practices of Sleep Medicine*. 5th ed. St Louis, MO: Elsevier; 2011.
89. Zammit GK, Corser B, Doghramji K, et al. Sleep and residual sedation after administration of zaleplon, zolpidem, and placebo during experimental middle of the night awakening. *J Clin Sleep Med*. 2006;4:417-423.
90. Krystal A, Walsh JK, Laska E, et al. Sustained efficacy of eszopiclone over 6 months of nightly treatment: results of a randomized, double-blind, placebo-controlled study in adults with chronic insomnia. *Sleep*. 2003;26:793-799.
91. Dooley M, Plosker GL. Zaleplon: a review of its use in the treatment of insomnia. *Drugs*. 2000;60(2):413-445.
92. Roth T, Soubrane C, Titeux L, Walsh JK, Zoladult Study Group. Efficacy and safety of zolpidem-MR: a double-blind, placebo-controlled study in adults with primary insomnia. *Sleep Med*. 2006;7(5):397-406.
93. Krystal AK, Erman M, Zammit GK, et al. Long-term efficacy and safety of zolpidem extended-release 12.5mg administered 3 to 7 nights per week for 24 weeks in patients with chronic primary insomnia: a 6-month, randomized, double-blind, placebo controlled parallel-group, multi-center study. *Sleep*. 2008;31:79-90.
94. Roth T, Walsh JK, Krystal A, et al. An evaluation of the efficacy and safety of eszopiclone over 12 months in patients with chronic primary insomnia. *Sleep Med*. 2005;6:487-495.
95. Ancoli-Israel S, Krystal AD, McCall WV, et al. A 12 week, randomized, double-blind, placebo-controlled study evaluating the effects of eszopiclone 2 mg on sleep/wake function in older adults with primary and comorbid insomnia. *Sleep*. 2010;33:225-234.
96. Monti JM, Pandi-Perumal SR. Eszopiclone: its use in the treatment of insomnia. *Neuropsychiatr Dis Treat*. 2007;3:441-453.
97. Greenblatt DJ, Harmatz JS, Roth T, et al. Comparison of pharmacokinetic profiles of zolpidem buffered sublingual tablet and zolpidem oral immediate-release tablet: results from a single-center, single-dose, randomized, open-label crossover study in healthy adults. *Clin Ther*. 2013;35(5):604-611.
98. Roth T, Krystal A, Steinberg FJ, Singh NN, Moline M. Novel sublingual low-dose zolpidem tablet reduces latency to sleep onset following spontaneous middle-of-the-night awakening in insomnia in a randomized, double-blind, placebo-controlled, outpatient study. *Sleep*. 2013;36(2):189-196.
99. Kuehn BM. FDA warning: driving may be impaired the morning following sleeping pill use. *JAMA*. 2013;309(7):645-646.
100. Osler M, Jørgensen MB. Associations of benzodiazepines, z-drugs, and other anxiolytics with subsequent dementia in patients with affective disorders: a nationwide cohort and nested case-control study. *Am J Psychiatry*. 2020;177(6):497-505.
101. Brzezinski A, Vangel MG, Wurtman RJ, et al. Effects of exogenous melatonin on sleep. A meta-analysis. *Sleep Med Rev*. 2005;9:41-50.
102. Fatemeh G, Sajjad M, Niloufar R, et al. Effect of melatonin supplementation on sleep quality: a systematic review and meta-analysis of randomized controlled trials. *J Neurol*. 2022;269(1):205-216.
103. Wade AG, Ford I, Crawford G, et al. Nightly treatment of primary insomnia with prolonged release melatonin for 6 months: a randomized placebo controlled trial on age and endogenous melatonin as predictors of efficacy and safety. *BMC Med*. 2010;8:51.
104. Maras A, Schroder CM, Malow BA, et al. Long-term efficacy and safety of pediatric prolonged-release melatonin for insomnia in children with autism spectrum disorder. *J Child Adolesc Psychopharmacol*. 2018;28(10):699-710.
105. Malow BA, Findling RL, Schroder CM, et al. Sleep, growth, and puberty after 2 years of prolonged-release melatonin in children with autism spectrum disorder. *J Am Acad Child Adolesc Psychiatry*. 2021;60(2):252-261.e3.
106. Li J, Somers VK, Xu H, Lopez-Jimenez F, Covassin N. Trends in use of melatonin supplements among US adults, 1999-2018. *JAMA*. 2022;327(5):483-485. doi:10.1001/jama.2021.23652.
107. Zammit G, Erman M, Wang-Weigand S, et al. Evaluation of the efficacy and safety of ramelteon in subjects with chronic insomnia. *J Clin Sleep Med*. 2007;3:495-504.
108. Mayer G, Wang-Weigand S, Roth-Schechter B, et al. Efficacy and safety of 6 month nightly ramelteon administration in adults with chronic primary insomnia. *Sleep*. 2009;32:351-360.
109. Roehrs T, Withrow D, Koshorek G, Verkler J, Bazan L, Roth T. Sleep and pain in humans with fibromyalgia and comorbid insomnia: double-blind, crossover study of suvorexant 20 mg versus placebo. *J Clin Sleep Med*. 2020;16(3):415-421.
110. Herring WJ, Connor KM, Ivgy-May N, et al. Suvorexant in patients with insomnia: results from two 3-month randomized controlled clinical trials. *Biol Psychiatry*. 2016;79(2):136-148.
111. Herring WJ, Connor KM, Snyder E, et al. Suvorexant in patients with insomnia: pooled analyses of three-month data from phase-3 randomized controlled clinical trials. *J Clin Sleep Med*. 2016;12(9):1215-1225.
112. Drake CL, Kalmbach DA, Cheng P, et al. Can the orexin antagonist suvorexant preserve the ability to awaken to auditory stimuli while improving sleep? *J Clin Sleep Med*. 2019;15(9):1285-1291.
113. Sun H, Palcza J, Card D, et al. Effects of suvorexant, an orexin receptor antagonist, on respiration during sleep in patients with obstructive sleep apnea. *J Clin Sleep Med*. 2016;12(1):9-17.
114. Yardley J, Kärppä M, Inoue Y, et al. Long-term effectiveness and safety of lemborexant in adults with insomnia disorder: results from a phase 3 randomized clinical trial. *Sleep Med*. 2021;80:333-342.
115. Kärppä M, Yardley J, Pinner K, et al. Long-term efficacy and tolerability of lemborexant compared with placebo in adults with insomnia disorder: results from the phase 3 randomized clinical trial SUNRISE 2. *Sleep*. 2020;43(9):zsaa123.
116. Markham A. Daridorexant: first approval. *Drugs*. 2022;82(5):601-607. Erratum in: *Drugs*. 2022;82(7):841.
117. Mendelson W. A review of the evidence for the efficacy and safety of trazodone in insomnia. *J Clin Psychiatry*. 2005;66:469-476.
118. Walsh J, Erman M, Erwin CW, et al. Subjective hypnotic efficacy of trazodone and zolpidem in DSMIII-R primary insomnia. *Hum Psychopharmacol*. 1998;13:191-198.
119. Kaynak H, Kaynak D, Gözükirmizi E, et al. The effects of trazodone on sleep in patients treated with stimulant antidepressants. *Sleep Med*. 2004;5:15-20.
120. Wong J, Murray Horwitz M, Bertisch SM, Herzig SJ, Buysse DJ, Toh S. Trends in dispensing of zolpidem and low-dose trazodone among commercially insured adults in the United States, 2011-2018. *JAMA*. 2020;324(21):2211-2213.
121. Roth T, Rogowski R, Hull S, et al. Efficacy and safety of doxepin 1 mg, 3 mg, and 6 mg in adults with primary insomnia. *Sleep*. 2007;30:1555-1561.
122. Moline M, Asakura S, Beuckman C, et al. The abuse potential of lemborexant, a dual orexin receptor antagonist, according to the 8 factors of the Controlled Substances Act. *Psychopharmacology (Berl)*. 2023;240(4):699-711.

Chapter 34

Circadian Rhythm Sleep-Wake Disorders

INTRODUCTION

The word "circadian" means "about a day" and describes processes that vary over time with an approximately 24-hour period. In humans, many physiologic processes vary periodically on a nearly 24-hour schedule.[1-4] This chapter will review basics of circadian physiology, tools to assess circadian phase, and circadian rhythm sleep-wake disorders (CRSWDs). Some important facts about circadian physiology are listed in Box 34–1.

SUPRACHIASMATIC NUCLEUS

The major circadian pacemaker in mammals is the suprachiasmatic nucleus (SCN) in the anterior hypothalamus. The nucleus exists as paired structures on each side of the third ventricle above the optic chiasm.[2-6] The SCN contains cells that oscillate independently with a period *slightly longer* than 24 hours. The SCN controls the rhythms of core body temperature and sleep-wake propensity, as well as the secretion of certain hormones (melatonin, thyroid-stimulating hormone [TSH], and cortisol). The alerting signal from the SCN increases during the day to counter the increasing homeostatic sleep drive (accumulated wakefulness since the last sleep). The interaction between the homeostatic sleep drive and the SCN alerting signal is discussed below. The *period of the SCN rhythm is called tau*, and the mean value in humans is about 24.2 hours.[5] Some individuals have a slightly shorter tau, and some longer. For humans to maintain synchrony with the light-dark cycle, external stimuli must induce a slight daily advance (shift in circadian rhythms to an earlier clock time) to counteract the intrinsic tendency for phase delay resulting from a period slightly longer than 24 hours. These external stimuli, called zeitgebers ("time givers"), are said to "entrain" the SCN to the light-dark cycle. The most potent zeitgeber is non–visual light information. Other zeitgebers include exercise, food, and social activities. The light stimulus reaches the SCN via the retinohypothalamic tract (RHT) (Figure 34–1). The RHT is a monosynaptic pathway connecting the nonvisual melanopsin-containing photosensitive retinal ganglion cells (pRGCs) to the SCN. Nonvisual photoreception also mediates the pupillary light response. Some blind patients continue to be entrained by light as a result of residual function of the retinal ganglion cells. Whereas the ganglion cells are the major circadian photosensors, the rods and cones also contribute some nonvisual information via communication with the pRGCs.[4,5] *The shorter wavelengths of light (blue, about 460 nm)* have the greatest effect on circadian rhythms. The *primary neurotransmitter of the retinal ganglion cell neurons in the RHT is glutamate.* However, the neurons also release pituitary adenyl cyclase–activating peptide (PACP) as a cotransmitter that causes similar effects on the SCN neurons. The effects of glutamate are mediated by binding to N-methyl-d-aspartate (NMDA)-type glutamate receptors and the subsequent elevations of intracellular calcium and nitric oxide in the neurons of the SCN. *PACP-containing fibers* from the retinal ganglion cells also project to the *intergeniculate leaflet (IGL)*, which in turn projects to the SCN. The intergeniculate leaflet is a subdivision of the lateral geniculate area in thalamus. Neurons in the IGL use gamma-aminobutyric acid (GABA) and neuropeptide Y as cotransmitters. Neurons in the IGL may mediate some of the phase-shifting influences of exercise on the SCN. The *intensity, duration, and timing* of light exposure determine the effect of light on the circadian system. The SCN also receives input from the median raphe nucleus and ventral tegmental areas as well as the IGL and inhibitory effects of melatonin as described below.

Box 34–1 CIRCADIAN PHYSIOLOGY—IMPORTANT FACTS

- Circadian ("about a day") denotes processes with an approximately 24-hour period.
- The human period of circadian rhythms (tau) is about **24.2 hours.**
- The suprachiasmatic nucleus (SCN) is the major circadian pacemaker in humans.
- SCN function helps maintain alertness by producing an alerting signal during the day and maintaining sleep by a reduced signal at night.
- Usual human alertness:
  - Midday decrease in alertness from 2:00–4:00 PM.
  - Alertness peaks in the early evening hours.
  - Lowest levels of alertness occur from 4:00–6:00 AM (at the minimum of core body temperature, CBTmin).
- Zeitgebers (time givers) entrain the SCN to the physical environment. Some phase advance is needed daily to adjust for the intrinsic tendency to phase delay, as the tau is greater than 24 hours.
- Light (sunlight) is the major zeitgeber.
- Melanopsin-containing retinal ganglion cells are the major circadian photoreceptors and communicate the presence of light to the SCN via the retinohypothalamic tract (RHT). The neurotransmitter is glutamate.

CBTmin, minimum core body temperature.

MELATONIN

The pineal gland secretes melatonin during the dark cycle (Box 34–2).[4-11] In the *absence of light*, certain dorsal parvocellular neurons in the autonomic subdivision of the paraventricular hypothalamic nucleus (PVH) provide tonic stimulation to the pineal gland via a circuitous pathway[4-12] (Figure 34–1). These PVH glutaminergic neurons project to parasympathetic preganglionic neurons in the intermediolateral cell column (IML) of the upper thoracic spinal cord. The preganglionic sympathetic neurons provide a cholinergic projection to postganglionic neurons located in the superior cervical ganglion. The postganglionic

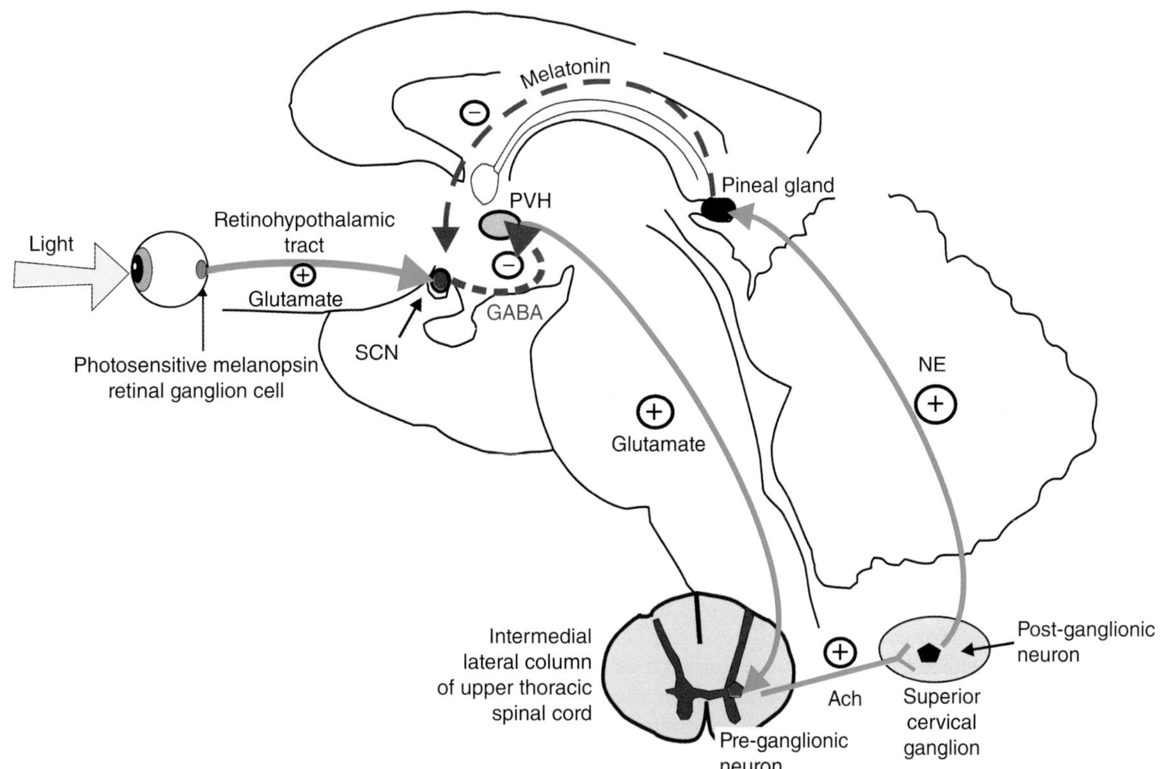

Figure 34–1 Light acting at photosensitive melanopsin containing retinal ganglion cells sends nonvisual information to the suprachiasmatic nucleus (SCN) via the retinohypothalamic tract (RHT), entraining the circadian pacemaker to the light/dark cycle. In the absence of light, dorsal parvocellular neurons in the autonomic subdivision of the paraventricular hypothalamic nucleus (PVH) send a tonic signal (glutamate), stimulating preganglionic sympathetic neurons in the thoracic spinal cord that then project to the superior cervical ganglion and stimulate postganglionic neurons using the neurotransmitter acetylcholine (Ach). These post-ganglionic noradrenergic neurons innervate the pineal gland. Norepinephrine (NE) acting at alpha and beta receptors on the pineal gland results in production and secretion of melatonin. A subset of SCN neurons project directly to the PVH neurons responsible for stimulating secretion of melatonin. When light is present, the SCN inhibits these PVH neurons using the neurotransitter gamma-aminobutyric acid (GABA). In the absence of inhibition (by light), melatonin is produced and secreted by the pineal gland. Melatonin secreted by the pineal gland inhibits SCN neurons. Thus, the SCN and pineal gland are mutually inhibitory. *Ach*, acetylcholine; *MT*, melatonin.

Box 34–2 MELATONIN SECRETION

- Melatonin is secreted by the pineal gland in darkness.
- Neurons in the paraventricular hypothalamic nucleus (PVH) provide tonic stimulation to the pineal gland (in the absence of light) via a pathway through the intermediolateral cell column of the upper thoracic spinal cord and superior cervical ganglion. Stimulation of the pineal gland increases melatonin production and secretion.
- Light acting on photosensitive retinal ganglion cells (melanopsin) sends a signal through the retinohypothalamic tract that inhibits the PVH neurons that stimulate the pineal gland to secrete melatonin. Thus, light inhibits secretion of melatonin.
- Melatonin secretion begins to increase before habitual bedtime and peaks about midway through the sleep period. **The dim light melatonin onset (DLMO)** measured in darkness defines the time at which melatonin passes a threshold (3 ug/ml for salivary melatonin) and occurs about **2 to 3 hours before habitual bedtime (or sleep time)** or 7 hours before the minimum core body temperature (CBTmin). The melatonin peak is 1 to 2 hours before the CBTmin.
- Melatonin has a short half-life 30–45 minutes
- Melatonin binding MT1 receptors on the SCN neurons decreases the SCN alerting signal.
- Melatonin binding MT2 receptors on SCN neurons shifts the circadian phase.
- The SCN and the pineal gland are mutually inhibitory.

neurons are noradrenergic and project to the pineal gland. The release of norepinephrine stimulates the pineal gland via *alpha and beta receptors* (mainly beta-1). Beta blockers can reduce the secretion of melatonin. Noradrenergic stimulation of the pineal gland results in increased cyclic adenosine monophosphate (AMP) in the pinealocytes, and this induces expression of serotonin N-acetyltransferase (also known as arylalkylamine N-acetyltransferase [AA-NAT]). This enzyme acting on serotonin catalyzes the rate-limiting step in the synthesis of melatonin. Therefore, the amount of this enzyme controls the production of melatonin. The production of melatonin begins with conversion of L tryptophan (an amino acid) to 5 hydroxytryptophan (5HTP) by the enzyme tryptophan hydroxylase (TPH). 5-HTP is the decarboxylated to serotonin (5-hydroxytryptamine or 5-HT) by the enzyme aromatic-L-amino-acid decarboxylase. Then AA-NAT converts serotonin to melatonin (the rate limiting step).

In the presence of light, some neurons of the SCN directly inhibit those neurons in the PVH that are responsible for stimulating the pineal gland to secrete melatonin. Thus, light inhibits melatonin secretion, and the absence of inhibition (absence of light) allows secretion of melatonin. Melatonin is sometimes called the "dark hormone." The melatonin secreted by the pineal gland provides *inhibitory feedback* information to SCN neurons. Therefore, the SCN and pineal gland are mutually inhibitory. Important facts about melatonin and melatonin secretion are summarized in Box 34–2.

Melatonin is not essential for circadian rhythms in humans because removal of the pineal gland has minimal effects. In other species such as birds, the pineal gland is essential. The SCN has a high density of two types of melatonin receptors (MT1 and MT2). The MT1 receptor is a G protein–coupled receptor that activates protein kinase C. When melatonin binds the MT1 receptor on SCN neurons, *this decreases the SCN alerting signal*. The MT2 receptor is a G protein–coupled receptor that inhibits the guanine cyclase pathway and results in a *shift in circadian phase*. A third type of melatonin receptor (MT3) does not affect the pineal gland. Exogenous melatonin by oral administration can also affect the SCN. The half-life of exogenous melatonin is short (30–45 min). The duration of action of oral melatonin is short unless sustained-release melatonin preparations are used. However, the duration of effect of exogenous melatonin depends on the dose of melatonin as well as the half-life. As might be expected, the effects of exogenous melatonin are largest at the time when no endogenous melatonin is being secreted.[10] Exogenous melatonin can decrease the SCN-alerting signal (hypnotic effects) and cause a phase shift of circadian rhythms. Melatonin acting on blood vessels in the skin causes vasodilatation, and increased blood flow results in heat loss and lowering of the body temperature. This may have an indirect effect favoring sleep. The circadian system has both central and peripheral pacemakers, although the SCN is the "master" pacemaker. Of note, while light and melatonin can affect the SCN, feeding, temperature cycles, and glucocorticoid signaling may affect peripheral circadian pacemaker in other part of the body such as the gastrointestinal system.

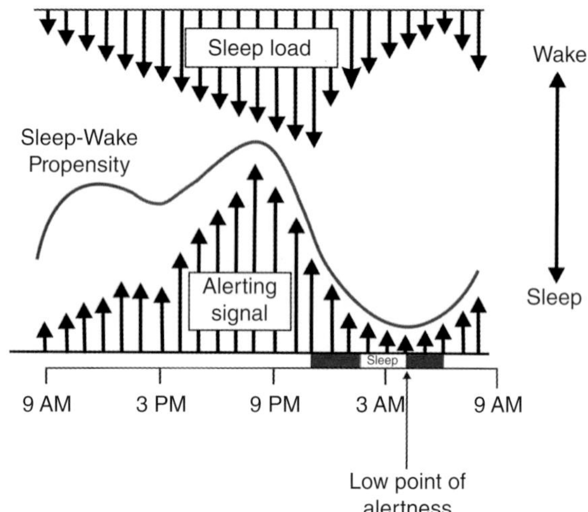

Figure 34–2 Opponent model of sleep. The sleep load (*down arrows*) increases proportional to the amount of prior wakefulness and decreases with sleep onset. It is opposed by the alerting signal from the suprachiasmatic nucleus (SCN) (*up arrows*). The alerting signal increases to a maximum just before sleep onset to help maintain wakefulness (the forbidden sleep period) but then decreases so sleep onset can occur and continues to decrease during sleep, allowing maintenance of sleep. The *solid line* is the sleep-wake propensity, with the upward direction favoring wake and downward direction favoring sleep. Note a small dip in the mid-afternoon ("siesta" time). However, the lowest point of alertness corresponds to the nadir in body temperature about 2 hours before spontaneous awakening. (Adapted from Edgar DM, Dement WC, Fuller CA. Effect of SCN lesions on sleep in the squirrel monkey: evidence for opponent processes in sleep-wake regulation. *J Neuorsci.* 1993;13:1065-1079.

CIRCADIAN RHYTHM SLEEP-WAKE DISORDERS

The SCN helps maintain alertness by producing an alerting signal during the day and helps maintain sleep by producing a reduced signal at night. The other major influence on sleep propensity is the amount of accumulated wakefulness (time since the last sleep). This homeostatic process (homeostatic sleep drive load) builds during wakefulness and then falls during sleep. As the pressure for sleep builds, the circadian signal increases to help maintain alertness despite a growing sleep debt but then decreases in the early evening so that sleep can occur (Figure 34–2). The combination of a high and rising homeostatic sleep drive and the falling alerting signal produce a "sleep gate" that allows sleep onset. The two-process model considers the interaction of process S (homeostatic sleep drive) and process C (circadian rhythms, driven in large part by the SCN). The two-process model is illustrated in Chapter 8 (Figure 8-16). The opponent model of sleep[2,11] (SCN-alerting signal vs. sleep load) is illustrated in Figure 34–2. Alertness peaks during the early evening hours and then begins falling to allow sleep to occur. There is a midday decrease in alertness from around 2:00 to 4:00 PM, and the lowest alertness is from 4:00 to 6:00 AM. The nadir in alertness coincides with the minimum in core body temperature (CBTmin). The interaction of the opponent processes (homeostatic sleep load and circadian alerting signal) allows humans to be alert during the day and to sleep at night (Table 34–1). The secretion of melatonin at night exerts an inhibitory influence on the SCN that helps maintain sleep by reducing the alerting signal. Endogenous melatonin secretion increases about 2 hours before habitual sleep onset (in darkness) and peaks about midway through the night.

The pathways by which the alerting signal of the SCN regulates sleep-wake are complex.[2,7] See Chapter 8 (Figure 8-18) for additional information. One of the major pathways is as follows: Neurons in the SCN project to neurons in the ventral subparaventricular zone (vSPZ). This area is immediately dorsal to the SCN. Neurons in the vSPZ then project to the ***dorsal medial hypothalamus* (DMH)**. Glutaminergic neurons in the DMH project to the lateral hypothalamus neurons producing hypocretin (stabilizing wakefulness-to-sleep transitions). In addition, DMH neurons using GABA as an inhibitory neurotransmitter project to the ventrolateral preoptic area (VLPO), a sleep-promoting area. These pathways mediate some of the effect of the SCN alerting signal by inhibiting sleep-promoting areas and stimulating areas stabilizing transitions from wakefulness to sleep. **The DMH is critical for circadian control of multiple processes.** Lesions of the DMH eliminate circadian variations in sleep, feeding, and locomotor activity.

The circadian phase controls both sleep/alertness propensity but also the distribution of sleep stages. Circadian influences are tied to REM sleep and the greatest REM propensity is in the early morning hours coincident with the minimum in core body temperature. Thus if sleep onset is delayed until the peak REM phase of the circadian rhythm (early morning), REM sleep can predominate and sleep onset REM periods can occur. Alterations in circadian rhythm moving the core body temperature to the morning hours (as in night shift work or the delayed sleep-wake phase disorder) can cause sleep onset REM periods in the early naps of the multiple sleep latency test.

Table 34–1 Sleep Regulation – Opponent Model

		Homeostatic Drive	Circadian Alerting Signal
Nighttime (Sleep)	First part of night	High (prior wakefulness)	Low
	Second part of night	Decreasing/Low	Low (to maintain sleep)
Daytime (Wakefulness)	First part of day	Low (prior sleep)	Increasing
	Second part of day	High and increasing (prior wakefulness)	• High (compensation) • Peak in early evening • Begins falling several hours before sleep onset

MARKERS OF CIRCADIAN PHASE

The relationship of the internal rhythms and the external environment is the circadian phase. The CBTmin and the dim light melatonin onset (DLMO) are two useful markers of the position of an individual's circadian rhythms with respect to the external environment (i.e., time of day) (Box 34–3). The CBTmin occurs about 2 hours before spontaneous awakening from nocturnal sleep (4:00–5:00 AM in most individuals) (Figure 34–3).[12-14] Of note, some publications state that CBTmin occurs about 1 to 2 hours before awakening; others state that it occurs 2 to 3 hours before spontaneous awakening. The reduction in core body temperature during the sleep period corresponds to the elevation in plasma melatonin, with *peak melatonin secretion about 2 hours before CBTmin.* The wakefulness in a sleep episode is an estimate of the wakefulness propensity; it is at a maximum in the evening before the sleep period and falls during sleep. The DLMO occurs about 2 to 3 hours before habitual bedtime or about 2 to 3 hours before habitual sleep time.[14-21] The literature varies on timing of DLMO, with some authors giving a value of 2 to 3 hours for the DLMO to bedtime interval and others DLMO to habitual sleep time. However, while many of the studies of DLMO only determined bedtime, for healthy individuals one could assume a sleep latency of less than 30 minutes; as such, DLMO to bedtime or DLMO to sleep onset are likely nearly the same. One can estimate the timing of the CBTmin as DLMO + 7 hours (Box 34–3). The DLMO is determined by interval measurement of salivary or plasma melatonin performed in dim light (5 lux; because light inhibits melatonin secretion) in the evening. A rise in melatonin level above a certain threshold defines the DLMO time (Figure 34–4). One can monitor plasma melatonin (threshold >10 pg/mL), *salivary melatonin (>3 pg/mL),* or urinary melatonin metabolite (6-sulfatoxymelatonin [aMT6s]). As noted, the *melatonin midpoint* can also be used as a circadian maker and occurs about *2 hours before* CBTmin.[12] When the circadian rhythm of the body (CBTmin or DLMO) moves to a later clock time, this is said to represent a *phase delay* in circadian rhythms. When CBTmin or DLMO move to an early clock time, this is said to represent a *phase advance.* The relationship between the timing of sleep and the circadian phase (as estimated by a circadian marker) can be quantified by the time interval (phase angle) between the two rhythms. For example, in the delayed sleep-wake phase disorder (DSWPD), there is a delay in DLMO.[22] In Figure 34–5, the progressive delay in the DLMO is evidence of a progressive delay in circadian rhythm in a patient with the non-24-hour sleep-wake rhythm disorder (N24SWRD), also called free-running disorder.[23] Use of the core body temperature as a marker of circadian rhythm is complicated by the fact that eating, activity, and sleep can affect the timing of CBTmin. In research settings, a constant routine protocol is used in which the subject is kept awake at bedrest and fed equally distributed small meals for at least 24 hours. An alternative to the constant routine protocol is to use mathematical adjustments to the temperature rhythm. Clinically, the most accurate way to determine the circadian phase is by monitoring melatonin in a dark environment to detect the DLMO. Figure 34–4 shows a DLMO onset in a normal individual and one with a delayed circadian phase. The DLMO can be affected (masked) by posture and drugs such as β-blockers and caffeine.

SHIFTING THE CIRCADIAN RHYTHMS

Phase Shifting With Light

Exposure to light before the CBTmin causes a phase delay, and light exposure after the CBTmin causes a phase advance (Figure 34–6) in circadian rhythm.[24-29] Thus, normal light exposure during the early morning induces a daily phase advance in the circadian rhythms to compensate for the intrinsic tendency to phase delay, because tau is slightly longer than 24 hours for most individuals. The amount of circadian rhythm shifting (also called phase change) depends on the timing of light as well as the intensity and duration of light (Box 34–4). In addition, the effect depends on the previous exposure to light.[27-30] For example, low light intensity may cause significant shifting of the circadian rhythm in a patient staying in a dark room for several days. Light intensity is measured in lux.

Box 34–3 MARKERS OF CIRCADIAN PHASE

- CBTmin occurs ~2 hours before spontaneous awakening from unconstrained sleep (4:00–5:00 AM)
- DLMO occurs ~2 hours before habitual bedtime (or sleep-onset time)
- CBTmin = DLMO + 7 (CBTmin occurs about 7 hours later than DLMO)
- Phase advance – circadian phase (CBTmin) moves to earlier clock time
- Phase delay – circadian phase (CBTmin) shifts to later clock time

CBTmin, minimum core body temperature; *DLMO*, dim light melatonin onset.

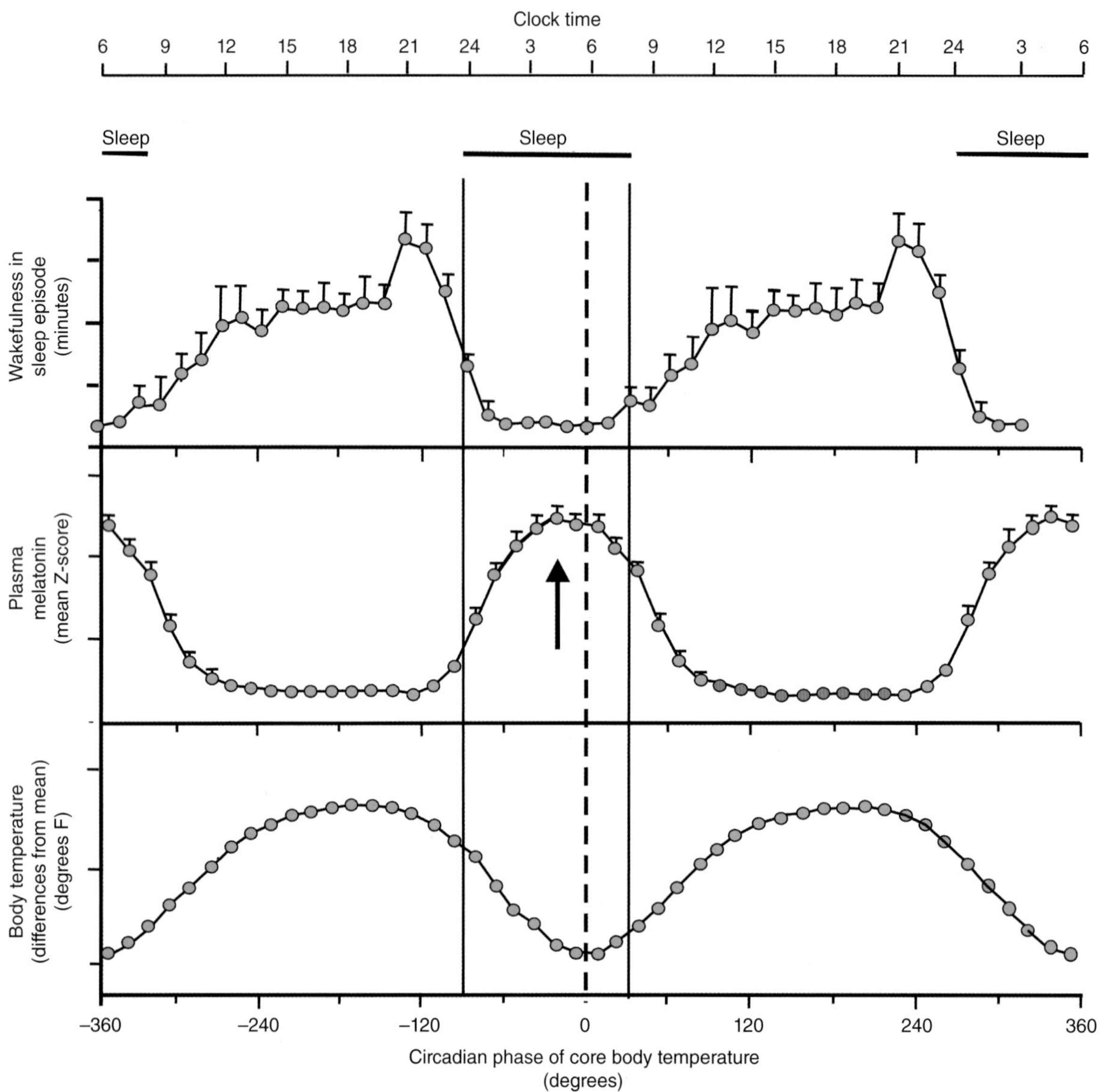

Figure 34–3 Schematic representation of the sleep period of a young adult. The minimum of core body temperature (CBTmin, depicted as the *vertical dotted line*) occurs about 2 hours before the end of the sleep period. The CBTmin also occurs about 1 to 2 hours after the midpoint of melatonin secretion (*up arrow*). The amount of wakefulness in sleep (a measure of wakefulness propensity) increases (sleep forbidden zone) just before the sleep period but falls with the onset of melatonin secretion (From Dijk DJ, Shanahan TL, Duffy JF, Ronda JM, Czeisler CA. Variation of electroencephalographic activity during non-rapid eye movement and rapid eye movement sleep with phase of circadian melatonin rhythm in humans. *J Physiol.* 1997;505(Pt 3):851-858.)

Indoor light is typically around 250 lux, and outdoor bright light has an intensity of more than 100,000 lux. For humans exposed to outside light (>10,000 lux) for a portion of each day, a relatively high light intensity is needed to shift circadian rhythms. Outside daylight is much more effective at shifting the circadian phase than indoor light. When outdoor light exposure is not practical or possible, light boxes are available (2500 lux) for therapeutic phase shifting by light. However, for patients chronically exposed to much brighter light, a higher intensity of light would be needed for maximal effect. Natural light is composed of a spectrum from 380 nm (violet) to 760 nm (red). As noted, blue light (460 nm) has greater phase-shifting properties than the rest of the visible light spectrum.[29] This may be because of properties of the melanopsin pigment that has maximum absorbance in this range. Light boxes have become available with enriched blue light to minimize the intensity or duration needed for a therapeutic response to light therapy. However, a study showed no benefit of light enriched with blue light compared with white light.[30] It is possible that light boxes with light-emitting diode (LED) emission of monochromatic blue light may be more effective. Both intermittent and continuous light are effective at resetting the circadian pacemaker.[31,32] This fact has clinical implications for delivery of light treatment when a patient cannot sit in front of a light box for long periods.

Phase Response Curve for Light

The relationship between the timing of light exposure and the amount of phase shift is best presented using a phase response curve (PRC). The curves are constructed by plotting the

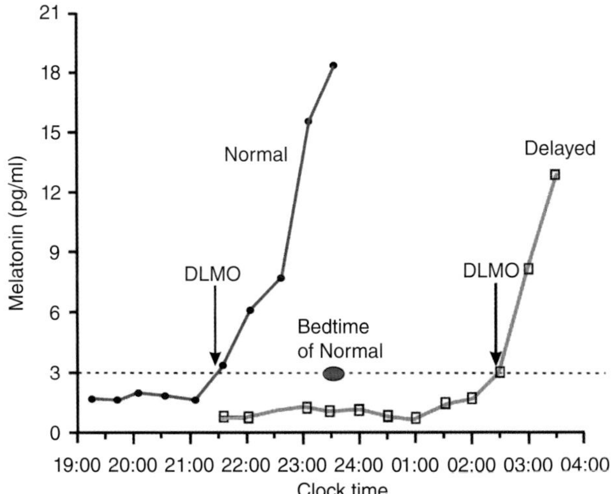

Figure 34–4 Salivary melatonin for a normal individual and one with the delayed sleep-wake phase disorder (DSWPD). The dim light melatonin onset (DLMO) is the time that melatonin reaches 3 pg/mL. This is around 9:30 PM (21:30) in the normal individual (typical sleep onset about 11:30 PM (23:30)) but is delayed to around 2:30 AM in an individual with DSWPD. The DLMO occurs about 2 hours before habitual bedtime (≈sleep onset in normal individuals). (Adapted from Wyatt JK, Stepanski EJ, Kirkby J. Circadian phase in delayed sleep phase syndrome: predictors and temporal stability across multiple assessments. *Sleep*. 2006;29:1075-1080.)

amount of phase shift versus the timing of the light stimulus (constant stimulus intensity). By convention, the *positive vertical axis represents phase advances,* and the negative axis represents phase delays. PRCs for light can look very different depending on the duration and intensity of light. For light, the magnitude of phase shifting depends on the proximity to the CBTmin (Figure 34–7). In most studies, the maximum phase shift occurs around 3 to 4 hours before (phase delay) or after (phase advance) the CBTmin (Figure 34–8). Light in the middle of the day has less phase shifting effects. However, light in the afternoon is still in the phase advance area of the PRC curve. The published PRCs for light vary somewhat depending on the methodology used to determine the PRC. For example, the PRC can be obtained by studying entrained subjects on a constant routine protocol or non-entrained subjects with a free-running routine. Typically, shifts in the DLMO are determined for different timing of light pulses. The phase shifts in circadian rhythms can also be determined by shifts in the CBTmin. However, as noted, exercise, food, and other activities can also affect CBTmin. Shifts in the DLMO or melatonin midpoint, especially if determined using a constant routine dim light protocol, assess the circadian phase more accurately than CBTmin. For example, the PRC for light shown in Figure 34–8 was determined using a constant routine, and shifts in the midpoint

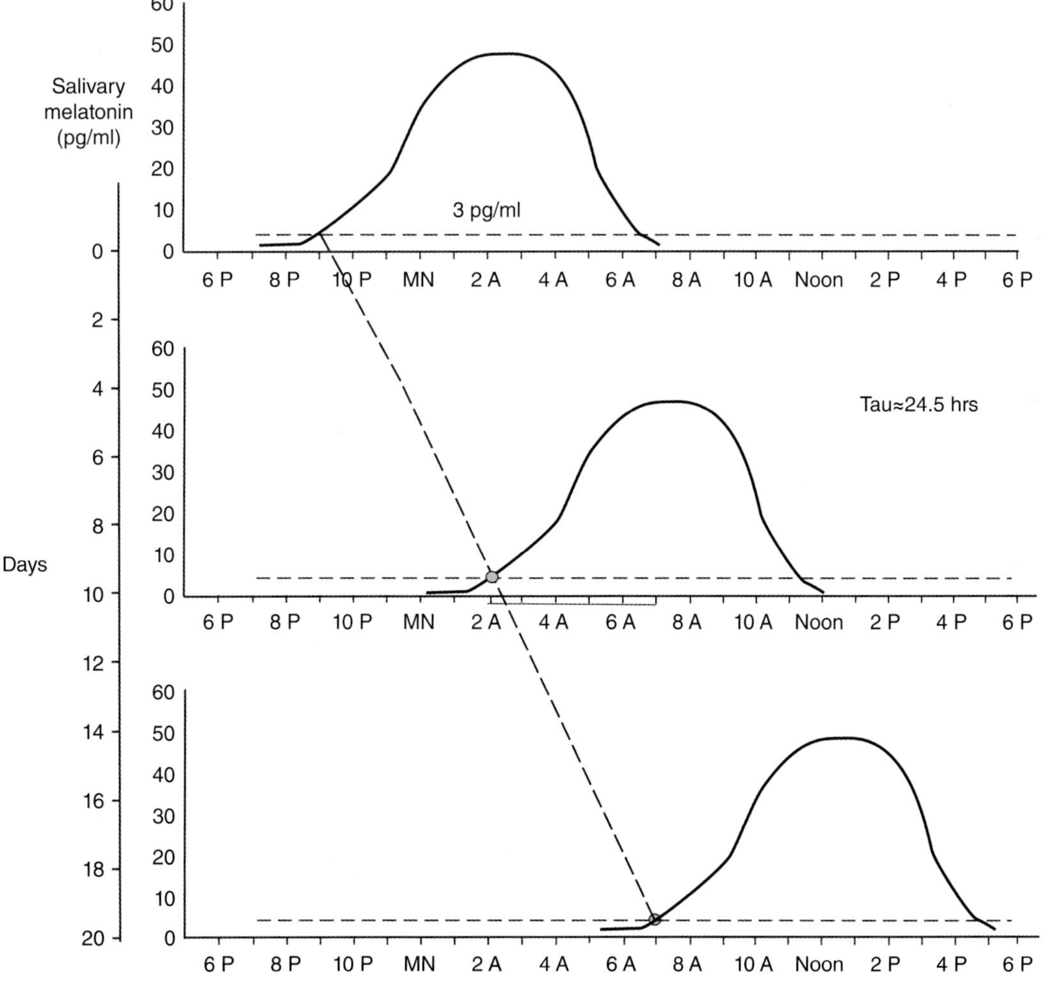

Figure 34–5 A schematic showing progressive delay in the dim light melatonin onset (DLMO) timing in a blind patient with non-24-hour sleep-wake rhythm disorder. The DLMO delays about 0.5 hours per day.

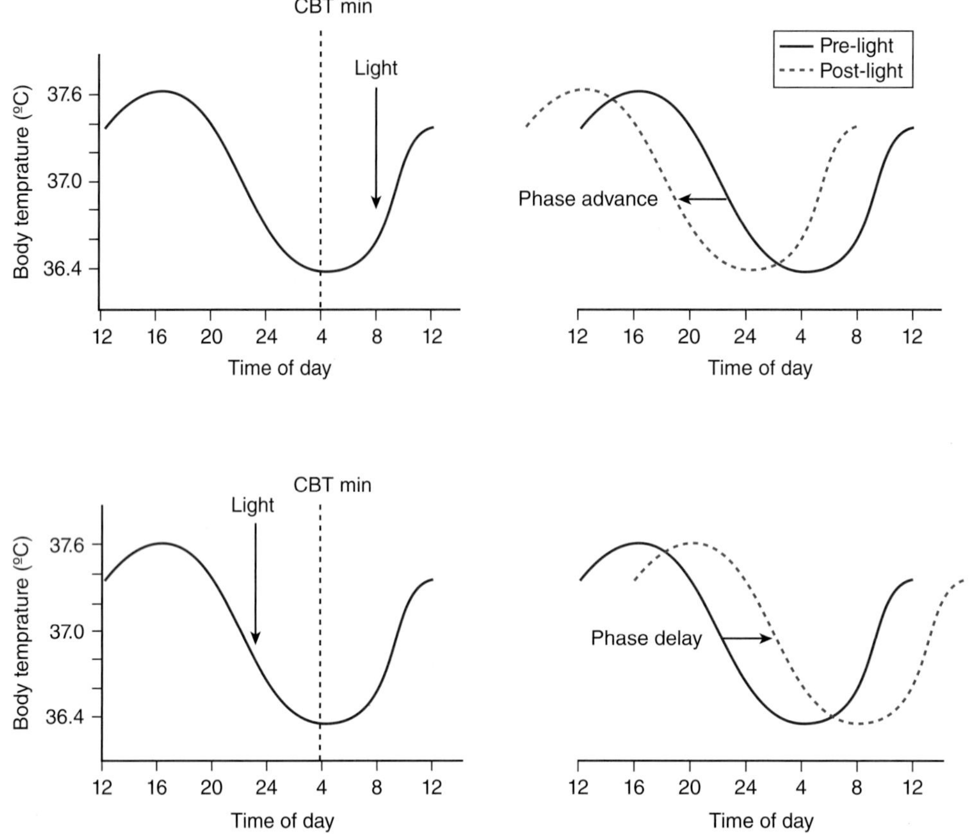

Figure 34–6 Phase shifting of the core body temperature minimum (CBTmin) with light. Light after the CBTmin phase advances and light before CBTmin phase delays. (From Berry RB. *Sleep Medicine Pearls*. 2nd ed. Philadelphia: Hanley & Belfus; 2003:344.

Box 34–4 PHASE SHIFTING WITH LIGHT

Common Light Exposures

- Bright blue midday sky >100,000 lux
- Sunrise or sunset ~10,000 lux
- Commercial light boxes up to 10,000 lux (typically 2500 lux)
- Commercial blue light boxes ~200 lux
- Normal room light ~200 to 250 lux
- Moonlight 0.1 lux

Phase Shifting With Light

- Short wavelength light (blue ~460 nm)—greatest effect on circadian phase
- Amount of phase shift depends on timing, intensity, and duration of light exposure
- Short pulses of light (intermittent) can also shift circadian rhythms
- Phase advance—light after CBTmin (peak effect about 3 hours after CBTmin)
- Phase delay—light before CBTmin (peak effect 3 hours before CBTmin)
- Light in the middle of the day—less effect

CBTmin, minimum core body temperature.

of melatonin secretion (melatonin midpoint) rather than DLMO were measured following a single pulse of 6.7 hours of light.[24] Figure 34–9 shows a PRC for light generated by a commercial light box providing monochromatic blue light using an LED.[33] The protocol used three 30-minute exposures over 2 hours. This PRC shows a broad phase advance zone following CBTmin. There is no need to allow for intrinsic phase advance during light administration, as the graph shows the difference from a baseline without light.

Phase Shifting With Exogenous Melatonin

Relatively small doses of exogenous melatonin (0.3–0.5 mg) can shift the circadian phase (Box 34–5) if taken at the correct times. As might be expected, the phase-shifting effects of exogenous melatonin are minimal during the dark period when the endogenous plasma level of melatonin is high.[34,35] Melatonin in higher doses (3–5 mg) has a direct hypnotic effect[8] as well as a chronobiotic (phase shifting) effect. However, the hypnotic effects of melatonin are limited by the drug's short half-life and the fact that, if taken at night, the endogenous plasma melatonin is already high.

Melatonin PRC Curve

The PRC curve for melatonin (Figure 34–10) is roughly 12 hours opposite (out of phase) the light PRC.[34-36] In displays of the melatonin PRC, the timing of melatonin is often expressed relative to DLMO but can also be expressed relative to the estimated CBTmin (CBTmin = DLMO + 7 hours). Melatonin, when given in the early evening before the DLMO, results in a phase advance. Melatonin given at the end of the subjective night–early subjective day causes a phase delay (Figure 34–10). As expected, the melatonin PRC has a flat region (no phase shifting) between the DLMO and the CBTmin (endogenous melatonin already high). The crossover point for melatonin (transition from phase advance to phase delay)

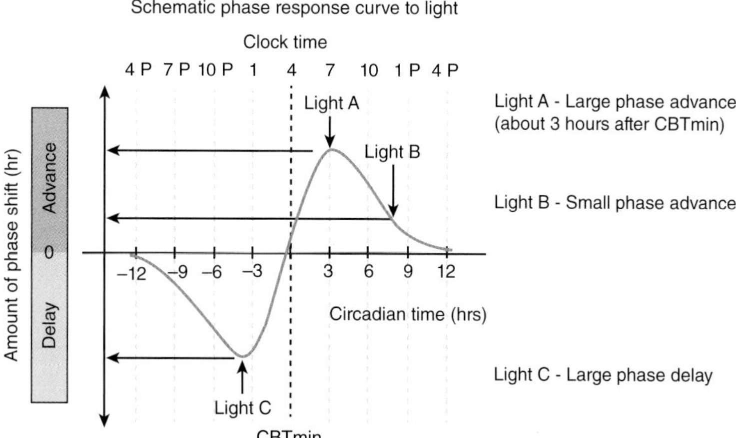

Figure 34–7 Schematic illustration of the phase response curve (PRC) to light. The normal daily phase delay (~20–30 min) is not shown. The maximum phase advance occurs about 3 hours after the core body temperature minimum (CBTmin), which is at or within 1 hour after spontaneous waking in most individuals. Light administered about 3 hours before CBTmin would cause the greatest phase delay (rarely done). The exact shape of the curve depends on the method used to make measurements. If one assumes CBTmin is at 4:00 AM, the phase advance portion of the curve extends into the early afternoon. However, from noon to early evening, there is relatively little effect of light on circadian phase based on some published PRCs to light (Figure 34–8). However, other published PRCs (Figure 34–9) have a wider phase-advance region.

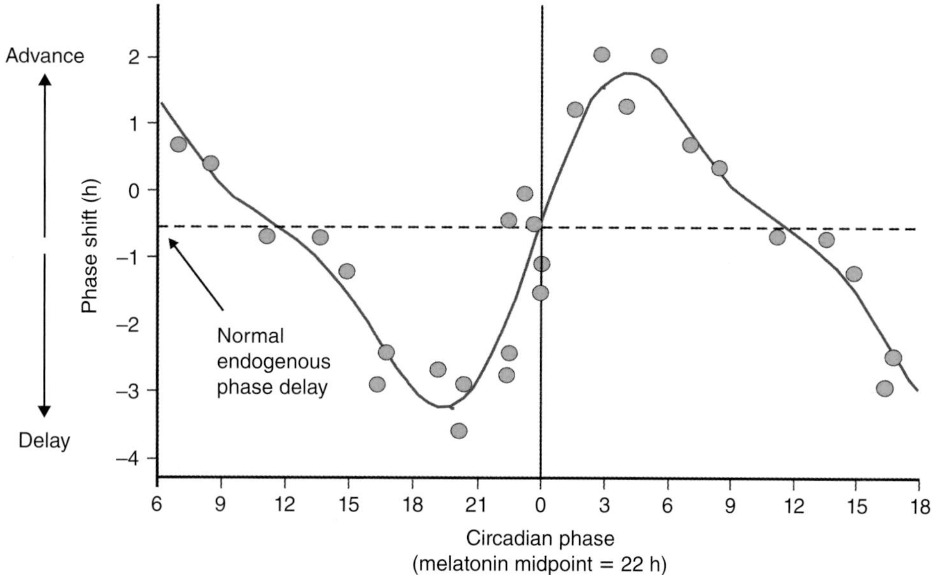

Figure 34–8 The phase response curve (PRC) to bright light using melatonin midpoints as the circadian phase marker. The determination was made using a constant routine protocol (enforced wakefulness in a semi-recumbent position). Phase advances are positive values, and phase delays are negative values. They are plotted against the time of the melatonin midpoint (dim light melatonin onset to dim light melatonin offset). The melatonin midpoint is defined as 22 hours. The core body temperature minimum (CBTmin) is assumed to be 2 hours later (0 hours). The *horizontal dashed line* represents the assumed drift in circadian phase between pre-stimulus (pre-light administration) and post-stimulus phase assessments (~3 days). (From Khalsa SBS, Jewett ME, Cajocen C, Czeisler CA. A phase response curve to single bright light pulses in human subjects. *J Physiol.* 2003;549:945-952.

is during the night but may not precisely coincide with CBTmin. In addition, the shape of the melatonin PRC appears to depend on the dose of melatonin studied and the method of PRC determination (Figure 34–11). Note that the timing of the maximum phase delay induced by melatonin is several hours after the CBTmin. Thus, taking melatonin 1 or 2 hours after spontaneous awakening causes the most phase delay. However, melatonin administration is often not used in the early morning because any hypnotic effects would not be well tolerated outside of a research setting. An exception is when morning sleep is desired by a person working a night shift.

Summary of Effects of Light and Melatonin. A summary of the effects of bright light and melatonin are summarized in Figure 34–12, with illustrations of the use of these interventions in two CRSWDs. Bright light causes a phase delay in the evening and a phase advance in the early morning. Melatonin causes a phase advance in the early evening and a

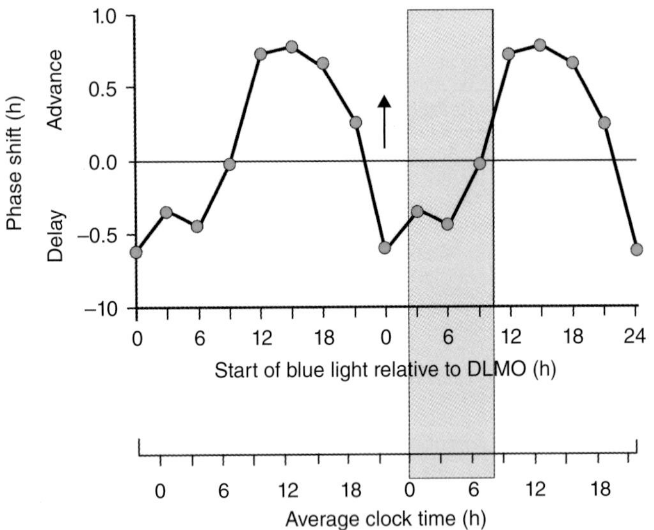

Figure 34-9 A human phase response curve to intermittent blue light using a commercially available device. The *up arrow* is dim light melatonin onset (DLMO), and the grey area is the habitual sleep period of this individual who reported sleeping from midnight to 8:00 AM. The generated curve was broader than some published curves, with the phase-advance portion extending to late afternoon. (From Revell VL, Molina TA, Eastman CI. Human phase response curve to intermittent blue light using a commercially available device. *J Physiol.* 2012;590(19):4859-4868.)

Box 34-5 PHASE SHIFTING WITH MELATONIN

- Melatonin PRC is approximately opposite to light PRC (about 12 hours out of phase).
- Reversal point (phase advance to phase delay) may be slightly before CBTmin but is always considerably after the DLMO.
- Dose-response curves may vary with dosage (0.3 mg vs. 3 mg)
- Note that, at larger doses, hypnotic effects are noted. Given closer to bedtime, melatonin may reduce SCN alerting signal (dampen wake maintenance zone)
- Exogenous melatonin half-life is about 30 to 45 min.

Maximal Phase Advance for Different Melatonin Doses (Optimal Timing)*

Dosage	0.3 to 0.5 mg	3 mg
Before DLMO	2–3 hours	5 hours
Before habitual bedtime/sleep onset	4.5–5 hours	7.5 hours
Before CBTmin	9 hours	12 hours

Maximal Phase Delay with Melatonin

- Maximal phase delay is about 10 hours after DLMO (1-2 hours after awakening)

CBTmin, minimum core body temperature; *DLMO*, dim light melatonin onset; *PRC*, phase response curve; *SCN*, suprachiasmatic nucleus.

*From Eastman CI, Burgess HJ. How to travel the world without jet lag. *Sleep Med Clin.* 2009;4:241-255.

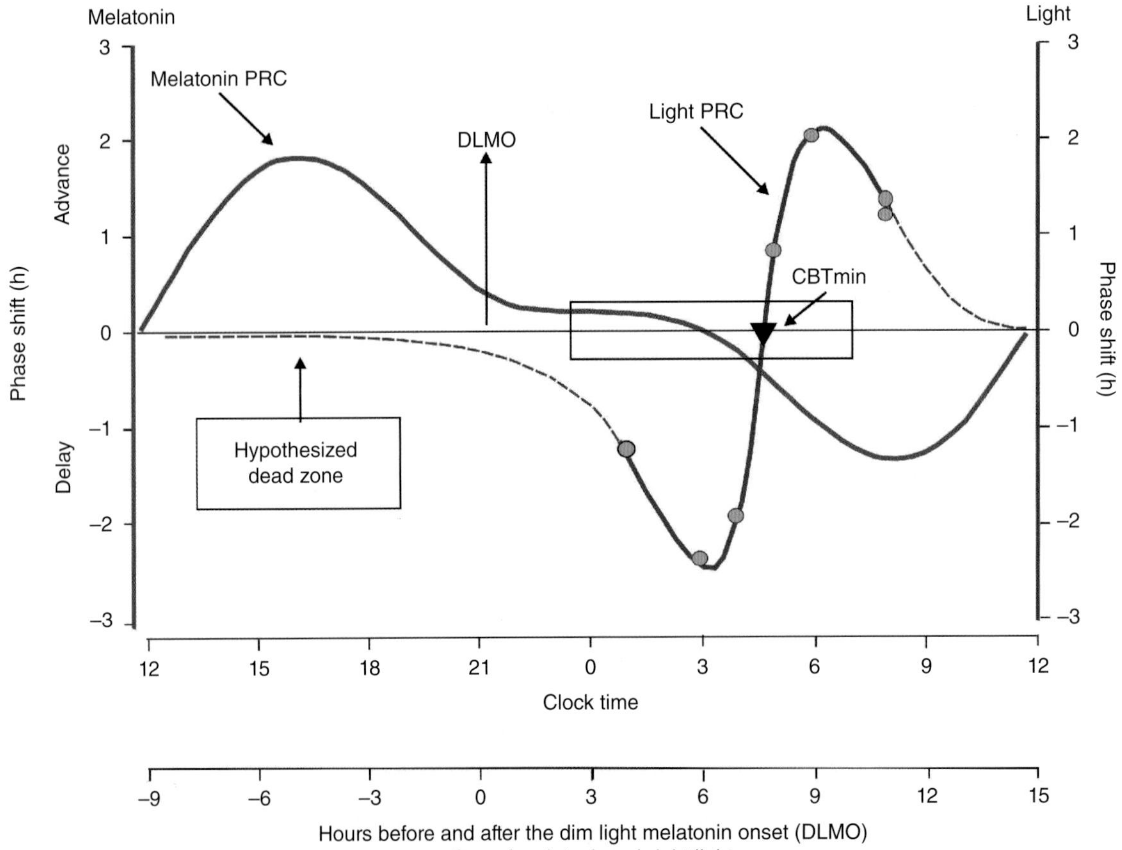

Figure 34–10 Phase response curves (PRCs) for light and melatonin (3 mg). The position of dim light melatonin onset (DLMO) and the core body temperature minimum (CBTmin, *inverted triangle*) are shown. The *rectangle* represents a period of 7.5 hours of sleep. The PRC curves of light and melatonin are approximately 12 hours out of phase. (From Eastman CI, Burgess HJ. How to travel the world without jet lag. *Sleep Med Clin.* 2009;4:241-255.)

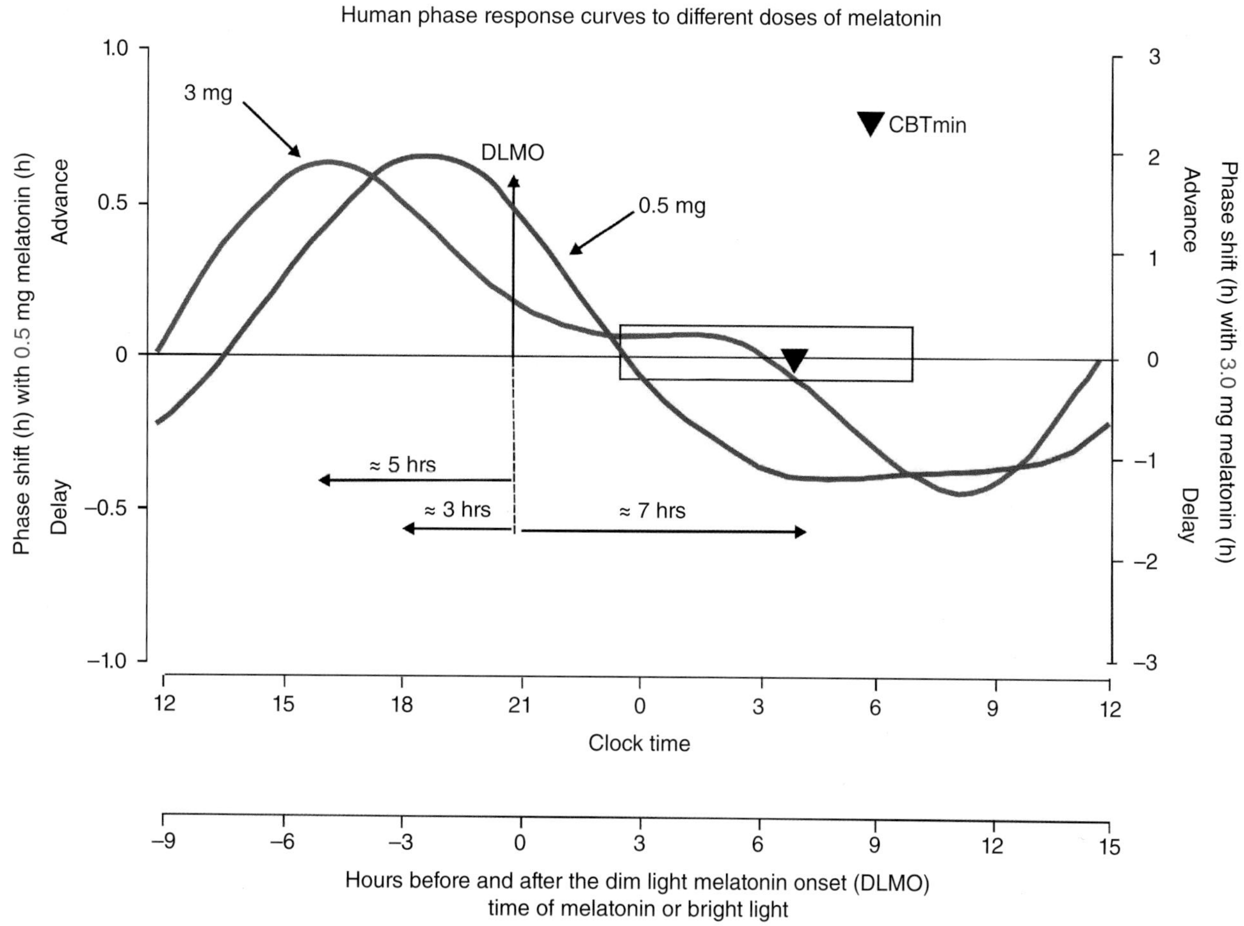

Figure 34–11 PRCs for different doses of exogenous melatonin. Note that, for the higher dose of melatonin, the maximal effect was noted at a time earlier than for the lower melatonion dose relative to the dim light melatonin onset (DLMO). The *rectangle* illustrates a typical sleep period, with the core body temperature minimum (CBTmin, *inverted triangle*) shown in the last half of the sleep period. *The maximum phase advance is about 3 to 5 hours before DLMO, depending on the dosage.* (From Eastman CI, Burgess HJ. How to travel the world without jet lag. *Sleep Med Clin.* 2009;4:241-255.)

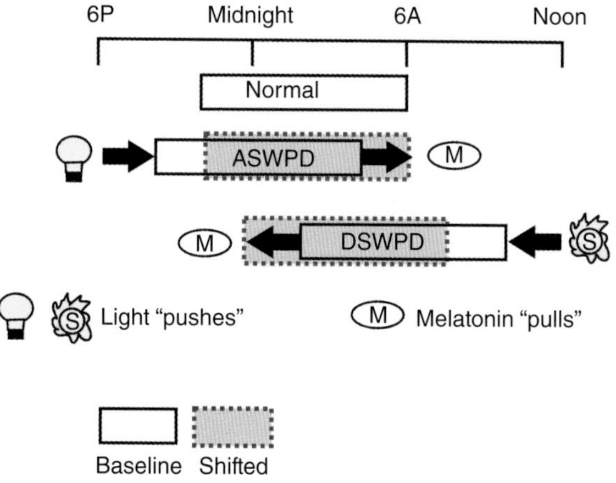

Figure 34–12 Summary of the effects of light and melatonin on the circadian phase. In patients with advanced sleep-wake phase disorder (ASWPD), melatonin in the late night/early morning phase delays, and in patients with delayed sleep-wake phase disorder (DSWPD), melatonin in the early evening phase advances. For light, the effects are opposite, with the early evening light phase delaying and the early morning light phase advancing. In summary, light "pushes" and melatonin "pulls" the circadian phase. *CBTmin*, core body temperature minimum. (Adapted from Barion A, Zee PC. A clinical approach to circadian rhythm sleep disorders. *Sleep Med.* 2007;8:566-577.)

phase delay in the early morning. A simple description of the effects of light and melatonin is that "*bright light pushes, and melatonin pulls the circadian rhythms.*" In this figure, it is assumed that the CBTmin lies within the initial sleep period of patients with advanced sleep-wake phase disorder (ASWPD) and DSWPD.

GENOMICS OF CRSWD

The intrinsic 24-hour rhythm in the SCN neurons is caused by the interactions of a number of genes.[32,33,37,38] These genes form autoregulatory feedback loops on transcription (DNA to mRNA) and translation (mRNA to proteins) that drive the cycling pattern. The feedback is provided by the protein translational products that can either stimulate or repress further gene transcription. In summary neural activity of the SCN is generated at the cellular level by a transcriptional-translational-posttranslational molecular feed back mechanism. A brief description of a few of the many molecular mechanisms responsible for the 24-hour cycle in transcription, translation, and posttranscriptional protein metabolism that drives the rhythmic cycle of the circadian clock genes is provided in Figure 34–13 and Table 34–2. By convention, small letters refer to genes and

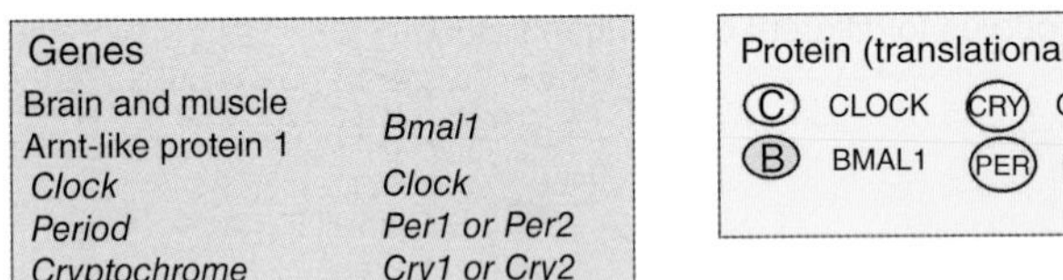

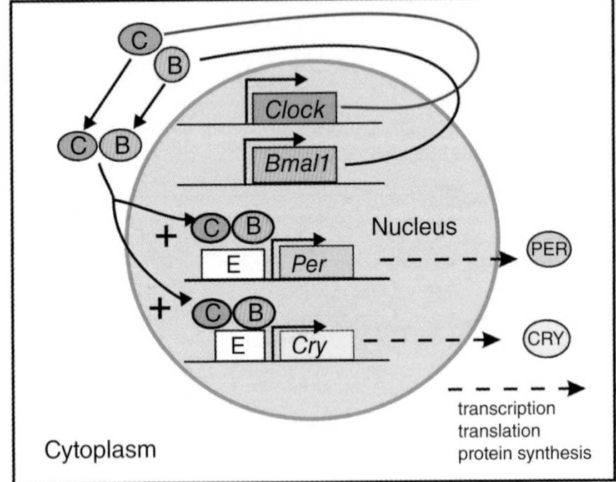

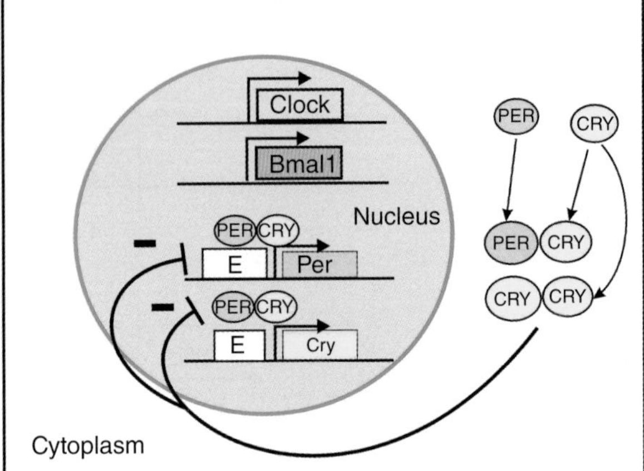

CLOCK: BMAL1 Heterodimer binds to Ebox enhancer resulting in increased transcription of Per and Cry genes

PER and CRY heterodimers and CRY homodimers suppress CLOCK and BMAL1 driven transcription of Per and Cry genes

Figure 34–13 A schematic of molecular mechanism controlling the circadian clock. Some proteins are inducers of gene transcription, and others inhibit transcription. Note that for simplicity nuclear transcription of the genes (producing messenger RNA), and translation via ribosomes in the cytoplasm producing protein are not shown. (Adapted from Vitaterna MH, Pinto LH, Turek FW. Molecular genetic basis for mammalian circadian rhythms. In: Kryger MH, Roth T, Dement WC, eds. *Principles and Practice of Sleep Medicine.* 4th ed. Philadelphia: Elsevier Saunders; 2005:363-374.)

Table 34–2 Circadian Clock Genes

	Genes	Protein
Circadian **L**ocomotor **O**utput **C**ycles **K**aput	*Clock*	CLOCK
Brain and muscle ARNT-like 1	*Bmal1*	BMAL1
Period	*Per1, Per 2, Per 3*	PER
Timeless	*Tim*	TIM
Cryptochrome	*Cry1 and 2*	CRY
Selected Genetic Polymorphisms		
DSWPD	hPer3 Arylalkylamine *N*-acetyltransferase gene (synthesis of melatonin) Cry2	
ASWPD	hPer2 mutatation in the casein kinase binding region (phosphorylation) site—reduces degradation so increased Per inhibition—shortens the circadian period. Mutations in Timeless (hTim) and Cryptochrome 2 (hCry2) in association with familial advanced sleep phase have also been identified.	

ASWPD, advanced sleep-wake phase disorder; *CRSWD*, circadian rhythm sleep-wake disorder; *DSWPD*, delayed sleep-wake phase disorder.

capital letters refer to protein translational products. For example, transcription and translation of "clock" results in production of the protein CLOCK. The human forms of genes are denoted with a preceding h (e.g., hPer2).

Proteins CLOCK and BMAL1 (synthesized from clock and Bmal1 genes) diffuse into the cytoplasm and associate as heterodimers (CLOCK:BMAL1). These heterodimers then return to the nucleus and bind the Ebox region of genes Per1, Per2, Cry1, and Cry2 and promote transcription of these genes. Ebox is a DNA sequence that usually lies upstream of a gene in a promoter region. The translational products PER and CRY proteins are negative regulators that turn off their own synthesis. The heterodimer PER:CRY and homodimer CRY:CRY diffuse back into the nucleus, inhibiting transcription of the associated genes. That is, PER:CRY and CRY:CRY repress the CLOCK:BMAL1-driven transcription of Pers and Crys. The synthesis of PER and CRY is under the influence of CLOCK:BMAL1 and can occur only when the level of intranuclear PER and CRY is low enough (after degradation of these proteins). A number of other processes alter these molecular events because PER and CRY can be phosphorylated by several enzymes, including casein kinase 1 epsilon (CK1ε), resulting in the ultimate degradation of the protein. The metabolism of PER and CRY influences the stability and rate of entry of protein dimers or heterodimers into the nucleus.

Polymorphisms of the genes are associated with certain circadian rhythm sleep-wake disorders. For example mutations in hPer2 associated with the advanced sleep-wake phase disorder and hPer3 with the delayed sleep-wake phase disorder. Differences in the in hPer3 gene can be associated with an increased ability to tolerate shift work. Specifically Per3(4/4) which means homozygous for 4 repeated sections of the gene have sleep that is less disturbed by circadian misalignment (tend to tolerate shift work better). A mutation in the gene DEC2 allows some people to be natural short sleepers.

CIRCADIAN RHYTHM SLEEP-WAKE DISORDERS

Circadian Rhythm Sleep-Wake Disorders and Terminology

The International Classification of Sleep Disorders (ICSD-3-TR)[1] lists seven CRSWDs (Box 34–6). The disorders are summarized in Figure 34–14. The word "phase" is used for DSWPD and ASWPD, as the phase of the rhythm is shifted relative to clock time but is otherwise normal. The word "rhythm" is used for irregular sleep-wake rhythm disorder (ISWRD) and N24SWRD, as the rhythm is abnormal. These four disorders are caused by alternations in the circadian timekeeping system or its entrainment—so-called intrinsic circadian disorders. Jet lag disorder and shift work disorder are caused by a misalignment of the endogenous circadian rhythm (usually normal) and the external environment. These are sometimes called *extrinsic circadian disorders.*

General criteria for the CRSWDs are:

A. A chronic or recurrent pattern of sleep-wake rhythm disruption primarily due to alteration of the *endogenous* circadian timing system or its entrainment mechanisms, or to misalignment between the endogenous circadian rhythm and the sleep-wake schedule desired or required an individual's physical environment or social/work schedules.

B. The circadian rhythm disruption leads to insomnia symptoms, excessive sleepiness, or both.

C. The sleep and wake disturbances cause clinically significant distress or impairment in mental, physical, social, occupational, educational, or other important areas of functioning.

Box 34–6 CIRCADIAN RHYTHM SLEEP-WAKE DISORDERS

1. Delayed Sleep-Wake **Phase** Disorder (DSWPD)
2. Advanced Sleep-Wake **Phase** Disorder (ASWPD)
3. Irregular Sleep-Wake **Rhythm** Disorder (ISWRD)
4. Non-24-Hour Sleep-Wake **Rhythm** Disorder (N24SWRD)
5. Shift Work Disorder (SWD)
6. Jet Lag Disorder
7. Circadian Rhythm Sleep-Wake Disorder (CRSWD)– not otherwise specified

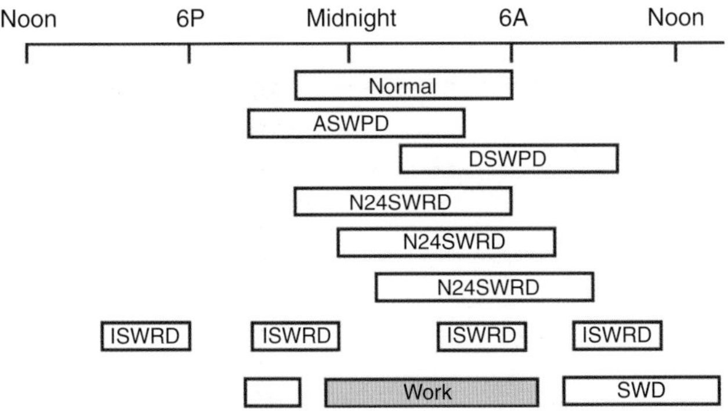

Figure 34–14 Schematic diagram of several circadian rhythm sleep disorders. *ASWPD*, Advanced Sleep-Wake Phase Disorder; *DSWPD*, Delayed Sleep-Wake Phase disorder; *N24SWRD*, Non-24-hour Sleep-Wake Rhythm Disorder; *ISWRD*, Irregular Sleep-Wake Rhythm Disorder; *SWD*, Shift-Work Disorder. (Adapted from Lu BS, Zee PC. Circadian rhythm sleep disorders. *Chest.* 2006;130:1915-1923; Barion A, Zee PC. A clinical approach to circadian rhythm sleep disorders. *Sleep Med.* 2007;8:566-577.)

Note that there must be symptoms of excessive sleepiness, insomnia symptoms, or both, as well as some type of impairment of function, to be considered a disorder. For example, if a person's normal sleep-wake phase is quite delayed but is something they desire, this would not be considered a CRSWD.[1] The ICSD-3-TR terminology emphasizes that these are disorders affect both sleep and wakefulness (hence the "sleep-wake" term). The American Academy of Sleep Medicine published an evidence review[39,40] and practice parameters[41] in 2007 for the evaluation of these disorders. A clinical practice guideline for the treatment of intrinsic CRSWD (CPGCD) was published in 2015.[42] The recommendations are summarized in Table 34–3. Because of the lack of high-quality evidence, some treatments commonly used in clinical practice were not recommended. In the discussions to follow regarding treatments for individual CRSWDs, the CPGCD recommendations will be documented in addition to common current treatment approaches. A large proportion of normal individuals experience problems with sleep or alertness secondary to shift work or jet lag at some point in their life. The boundary between what constitutes a normal response and what is an abnormal response is not well defined.

Evaluation of Patients With Suspected CRSWD

In evaluating patients for most suspected CRSWDs (jet lag is an exception), the physician uses history, a sleep log for at least 7 days (preferably 14 days), and, often, actigraphy (Box 34–7). The morningness-eveningness questionnaire (MEQ) and markers of circadian phase (DLMO) are used for research studies, but the clinical utility for routine evaluation remains to be documented. DLMO would be used more clinically if it was widely available. Polysomnography (PSG) is not indicated for evaluation of patients with CRSWD unless another sleep disorder such as sleep apnea is suspected.

Morningness-Eveningness Questionnaire

The MEQ was developed by Horne and Ostberg in 1976.[43,44] The MEQ contains 19 questions aimed to determine the natural propensity to perform certain activities during the daily temporal span ("Owls'" propensity for late evening vs. "Larks'" propensity for early morning activity). Most questions are framed in a preferential manner and require a response to specific times that an individual *would prefer* to do a certain activity (as opposed to when they actually do it). Answers to each question are labeled from 0 to 6. The sum ranges from 16 to 86. *Lower values correspond to evening types.*

Sleep Logs and Actigraphy

The 2007 AASM practice parameters state that sleep logs are indicated for evaluation of patients with suspected or known CRSWD.[41] Figure 34–14 is a schematic diagram of changes

Table 34–3 Overview of AASM Recommendations for Intrinsic CRSWD Treatment

Treatment	ASWPD	DSWPD	N24SWRD	ISWRD
Prescribed sleep-wake scheduling	No Recommendation	No Recommendation	No Recommendation	No Recommendation
Timed physical activit/exercise	No Recommendation	No Recommendation	No Recommendation	No Recommendation
Strategic avoidance of light	No Recommendation	No Recommendation	No Recommendation	No Recommendation
Light therapy	**WEAK FOR (adults)**	No recommendation	No Recommendation	**WEAK FOR** (elderly with dementia)
Sleep-promoting medications	No recommendation	No recommendation	No Recommendation	**STRONG AGAINST** (elderly with dementia)
Timed oral administration of melatonin or agonists	No recommendation	**WEAK FOR** (adults **with and without** depression) (children/adolescents **without** comorbidities) (children/adolescents **with** psychiatric comorbidity)	**WEAK FOR** (blind adults) No recommendation (sighted)	**WEAK AGAINST** (elderly with dementia) **WEAK FOR** (children/ adolescents with neurological disorders)
Wakefulness-promoting medications	No recommendation	No recommendation	No recommendation	No recommendation
Combination treeatments	No Recommendation	No Recommendation	No Recommendation	No Recommendation
Combination treatment	No recommendation	No Recommendation (adults) **WEAK FOR** (light therapy + multicomponent behavioral interventions for children/ adolescents)	No Recommendation	**WEAK AGAINST** (combination treatment of light and melatonin for demented, elderly patients

ASWPD, Advanced Sleep-Wake Phase Disorder; *DSWPD*, Delayed Sleep-Wake Phase Disorder; *ISWRD*, Irregular Sleep-Wake Rhythm Disorder; *N24SWRD*, Non-24-hour Sleep-Wake Rhythm Disorder.
Data from Auger RR, Burgess HJ, Emens JS, Deriy LV, Thomas SM, Sharkey KM. Clinical practice guideline for the treatment of intrinsic circadian rhythm sleep-wake disorders: advanced sleep-wake phase disorder (ASWPD), delayed sleep-wake phase disorder (DSWPD), non-24-hour sleep wake rhythm disorder (N24SWRD), and irregular sleep-wake rhythm disorder (ISWRD). An update for 2015. *J Clin Sleep Med.* 2015;11(10):1199-1236.

Box 34–7 EVALUATION OF PATIENTS WITH CIRCADIAN RHYTHM SLEEP-WAKE DISORDER

- History
- Polysomnography – not recommended (standard)
- Morningness-Eveningness Questionnaire (MEQ)
- Sleep log for at least 7 days (preferably 14 days)*
- Actigraphy for at least 7 days (preferably 14 days)*
- Dim light melatonin onset (DLMO), if available

* Recommended in the 2007 American Academy of Sleep Medicine practice parameters for circadian disorders (guideline): use of actigraphy to determine response to treatment (option).

in the sleep period comparing different CRSWDs with normal. In general, actigraphy or sleep logs document a habitual sleep period compared with normal that is advanced (ASWPD), delayed (DSWPD), progressively delayed (N24SWRD), irregular (ISWRD), or with a daytime major sleep episode (shift-work disorder).

Delayed Sleep-Wake Phase Disorder

In DSWPD, the timing of sleep onset is *delayed relative to clock time*. Sleep-onset time tends to be *regular but delayed* (2:00–6:00 AM). These patients represent a more extreme version of the "Owl/evening chronotype." Patients with the DSWPD complain of inability to fall asleep at a socially acceptable time—a type of sleep-onset insomnia. If allowed to maintain their own chosen schedule, they would usually sleep for a normal duration and feel rested on arising.[1,22,40,42] However, because of societal demands, they must awaken earlier than desired and are often sleepy during the day. Therefore, they complain of difficulty waking up and daytime sleepiness (short sleep duration). In contrast to behaviorally induced sleep delay, these patients cannot fall asleep earlier unless very sleep deprived. Attempts to start sleep by getting into bed at the desired time based on societal demands are unsuccessful at inducing sleep. A *delay in sleep-wake phase occurs in about 7% to 16% of normal adolescents.*

Diagnosis of DSWPD

The ICSD-3-TR diagnostic criteria are summarized here (see the ICSD-3-TR for complete criteria):

A. A significant delay in the phase of the major sleep episode in relation to the desired or required sleep time and wake-up time, as evidenced by:
- A chronic or recurrent complaint by the patient or a caregiver of inability to fall asleep
- Difficulty awakening at a desired or required conventional clock time

B. The symptoms are present for **at least 3 months**.
C. When patients are allowed to choose their ad-libitum schedule, they will exhibit improved sleep quality and duration for age and maintain a delayed phase of the 24-hour sleep-wake pattern.
D. **Sleep logs are required**, and whenever possible, actigraphy monitoring for at least 7 days (preferably 14 days) demonstrates a delay in the timing of the habitual sleep period. *Both work/school days and free days should be included within this monitoring.*
E. The sleep disturbance is not better explained by another current sleep disorder, medical disorder, mental disorder, or medication/substance use.

There must be a delay in the major sleep episode *for at least 3 m*onths. The individual complains of difficulty falling asleep or waking up at the desired or required time. In addition, if allowed to set their own schedule, patients with DSWPD usually sleep for a normal sleep duration for age and awaken feeling refreshed. Use of a sleep log or (when possible) actigraphy should document the pattern of the delayed sleep period. At least 7 days is required (preferably at least 14 days). The period should include both work/school days and free days. These document *a stable sleep-onset time that is delayed relative to clock time (usually 2:00 to 6:00 AM).* On work/school days, the sleep duration is short because of required awakening, but on free days, sleep is of a normal duration.

Differential Diagnosis DSWPD

In a study by Murray et al,[45] almost 50% of a group of patients diagnosed with the DSWPD clinically did not have a delay in their circadian rhythms (delay in DLMO) relative to their desired bedtime. Zee et al.[2] termed the group with a delayed sleep-wake phase clinically but without a delayed DLMO as "non-circadian DSWPD." The study by Murray et al.[45] illustrates the difficulty of making the diagnosis without objective circadian markers. The widespread use of electronics late into the evening and the associated phase delay is common in today's society. True DSWPD must be differentiated from sleep-onset insomnia in individuals who delay sleep for social reasons and then have trouble falling asleep when they sporadically try to go to bed earlier. These individuals have a transient sleep-wake cycle disorder caused by a self-enforced phase shift. When they maintain a regular bedtime and waketime for several days, they quickly adjust to this schedule. Patients with bipolar affective disorder in the manic or hypomanic phase also may have sleep-onset insomnia. The sleep period is short in these patients, but they have no difficulty arising at a conventional time. N24SWRD is characterized by a progressive, incremental phase delay in sleep onset and wake-up times. In the future, DLMO measurement hopefully will be more widely available and allow greater precision in the diagnosis of DSWPD.

Epidemiology

The duration of DSWPD varies from months to decades. *Adolescence is the most common age of onset*; onset after age 30 is rare. DSWPD is the most common CRSWD seen in sleep clinics. DSWPD is more common in adolescents and young adults, with an incidence of *7% to 16% in this population*. The incidence in the general population is unknown. Patients with DSWPD make up about 10% of patients seen in insomnia clinics. The mean age of onset of DSWPD is about 20 years.

As noted, there appears to be two forms of DSWPD. Individuals with circadian DSWPD have evidence of delayed DLMO. Individuals with non-circadian or motivated DSWPD do not have a delay in DLMO.

Pathophysiology

A family history is present in about 40% of patients with DSWPD.[1,3] The DSWPD has been associated with *genetic polymorphisms in circadian clock gene hPer3*,[46] AA-NAT,[47] and the Cry1 gene.[48] AA-NAT is the rate-limiting enzyme in the synthesis of melatonin resulting from modification of serotonin. Another possibility would be an intrinsically long tau. Exposure to bright light in the evening (causing phase delay) or decreased exposure to morning light can exacerbate the problem. A study by Watson and coworkers[49] found that the circadian system of patients with DSWPD has an *increased sensitivity to the delaying influence of light in the evening*. Exposure to light at the wrong time tends to perpetuate the phase delay. For example, an individual has a CBTmin at 8:00 AM but awakens at 6:00 AM to arrive at school by 8:00 AM and is exposed to light on the way to school from 7:00 to 8:00 AM. This will cause a further phase delay. Overall, a greater sensitivity to delay of evening light, decreased exposure to advancing light, and a longer intrinsic period are likely contributors to the development of DSWPD.

Sleep Logs and Actigraphy

Sleep logs (Figure 34–15) and actigraphy (Figure 34–16) typically document *a stable delay in the sleep period relative to clock time,* with a typical sleep-onset time from 1:00 to 6:00 AM and wake-up times in the late morning or early afternoon (10:00 AM–2:00 PM). During the work week or school, a forced awakening will cause a short sleep period. On the weekend or non-school or non-workdays, longer sleep until late morning/early afternoon is noted. The Horne-Ostberg questionnaire (morning-evening preference) shows a night-owl preference (eveningness). The DLMO is delayed in patients with DSWPD (at least in "circadian" DSWPD). As expected, the CBTmin is also quite delayed. Some studies found the body temperature nadir in patients with DSWPD to occur earlier during the sleep period than that of normal individuals.[50,51]

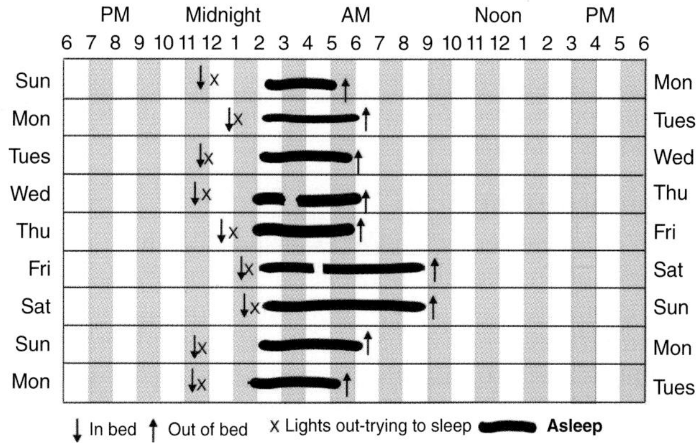

Figure 34–15 A sleep log showing the pattern typical of an individual with DSWPD. Note the stable delay in sleep-onset time (around 2 to 3 AM) despite attempts to fall asleep earlier on some nights. On the weekends, sleep continues to the late morning. Note that, once the patient is asleep, few awakenings are noted. On Friday and Saturday night the patient tried to fall asleep later and the sleep latency was shorter than on other nights.

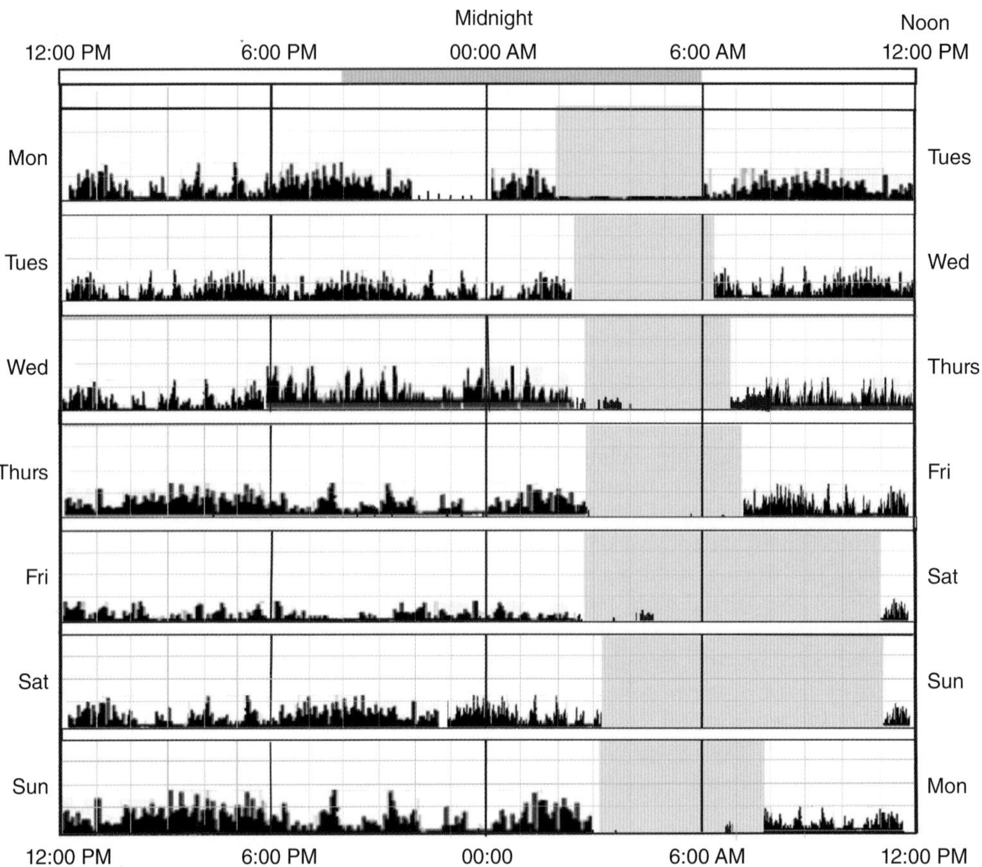

Figure 34–16 An actigraphy recording of sleep-wake activity, using wrist activity monitoring, from an individual with DSWPD. The individual consistently falls asleep around 2:00 AM and wakes up around 6:00 to 7:00 AM to get to school on time. This results in a very short total sleep time. On the weekend, the individual sleeps until about 11:00 AM. On Monday morning at the bottom of the tracing the individual was late for school.

For example, Watanabe and coworkers[51] found the CBTmin occurred near the middle of the nocturnal sleep period in patients with DSWPD, which is in contrast to normal controls in whom it occurred in the last third of the sleep period. However, Munday et al. did not find a different relationship between CBTmin and sleep period.[52] Differences in study results may result from different total sleep times and study designs. Burgess and coworkers[53] found that patients with DSWPD have greater variability in wake-up times that that of normal controls. Of note, because of the natural variability in sleep-onset and wake-up times, some researchers use the mid-point of the sleep period to estimate shifts in the circadian phase using a sleep log or actigraphy.

Treatment of DSWPD

Possible treatments for DSWPD include (1) chronotherapy (a type of sleep scheduling), (2) morning bright light, and (3) evening melatonin (Table 34–4). Chronotherapy is a prescribed progressive delay in bedtime until the desired sleep schedule is reached.[54] Basically, bedtime is delayed around the clock until it reaches an appropriate time. However, this treatment approach is not practical for most patients. The 2007 practice parameters for CRSWD state that sleep scheduling may be effective (option). The more recent 2015 clinic practice guideline for treatment of intrinsic CRSWD makes no recommendation for sleep scheduling as a treatment for DSWPD. Morning bright light and evening melatonin have both been used to advance the phase of circadian rhythms in patients with DSWPD. The 2007 AASM standards of practice parameters state that morning light exposure and properly timed evening melatonin are indicated to treat DSWPD (guideline).[41] The practice parameters state that the optimal dose and timing of light have not been determined. In contrast, the 2015 clinical practice guideline for CRSWD[42] offers no recommendation for light in DSWPD (Table 34–3) in adults. The authors did not find sufficient evidence to make a recommendation. There was a "WEAK FOR" recommendation for combination therapy (light and multicomponent behavioral interventions for children and adolescents.

In a prospective crossover study, an initial 2-week trial of light therapy at 2500 lux given for 2 hours between 6:00 and 9:00 AM in combination with evening light restriction demonstrated an advancement of CBTmin of 1.4 hours and a longer sleep latency at 9:00 AM (less sleepy).[55] A later study reported a 1.5-hour earlier sleep-onset time after 5 days of 3 hours of phototherapy given 1.5 hours after CBTmin.[56] The optimal timing, dose, and duration of bright light for treatment of DSWPD have not been defined, but common recommendations are 2500 to 10,000 lux in the morning for 1 to 2 hours. However, a pitfall of this approach is that light may be administered on the wrong side of the temperature minimum. For example, if a patient's habitual ad-libitum wake time is 10:00 AM, the CBTmin could be around 7:00 to 8:00 AM. Therefore, exposure to bright light at 6:00 to 7:00 AM

Table 34–4 Commonly Used Treatment for Delayed Sleep-Wake Phase Disorder

Chronotherapy	• Progressive phase delay
Light therapy	• 2500–10,000 lux for 30 min–2 hour. • Timing = at or slightly before habitual wake time (ad-libitum schedule). Light should be applied following the time of the CBTmin, which occurs about 2–3 hours before the habitual spontaneous (ad-libitum schedule) wake-up time. • Light administered 0.5–1 hour earlier each day (use alarm if needed). Patient also goes to bed 0.5–1 hour earlier (see example in the bottom section of this table). • Restrict light in the evening or in the morning before estimated CBTmin.
Melatonin	• 0.3–3.0 mg given 5–7 hours before habitual bedtime/sleep-onset time • 3–5 hours before DLMO. • Large melatonin dose has hypnotic effects.
Combination	• Use of light and melatonin

Sample Schedule for Phase Advancement Using Light in DSWPD

Day	Bedtime	Wake Time	Light
1	2:00 AM	10:30 AM	10:30 -11:30 AM
2	1:30 AM	10:00 AM	10:00 to 11:00 AM
3	1:00 AM	9:30 AM	9:30 to 10:30 AM
4	12:30 AM	9:00 AM	9:00 to 10:00 AM
5	12:00 AM	8:30 AM	8:30 to 9:30 AM
6	11:30 PM	8:00 AM	8:00 to 9:00 AM
7 (Target)	11:00 PM	7:30 AM	7:30 to 8:30 AM
8 (Maintenance)	11:00 PM	7:30 AM	7:30 to 8:00 AM
8 (Maintenance)	11:00 PM	7:30 AM	7:30 to 8:00 AM
8 (Maintenance)	11:00 PM	7:30 AM	7:30 to 8:00 AM

(This example assumes that, on weekends, typical bedtimes/wake-up times are 2:00 AM /11:00 AM and that the work or school schedule allows the recommended pattern of interventions.)
During maintenance, a shorter period of light exposure is sufficient.
CBTmin, core body temperature minimum; *DLMO*, dim light melatonin onset; *DSWPD*, delayed sleep-wake phase disorder.

could induce a phase delay in this individual ould induce a phase delay in this individual depending on the actual (versus estimated) CBTmin. Accurate determination of the true timing of CBTmin with DLMO testing is not widely available. A practical approach for light therapy in DSWPD is to start the light treatment at or slightly before the time of "unconstrained habitual awakening" with a light intensity of 2500 to 10,000 lux for 30 minutes to 2 hours (if possible) and advance the light treatment 30 minutes to 1 hour daily (with an alarm clock, if needed).[57] It is best to estimate the habitual awake time (and CBTmin) using ad-libitum sleep on the weekends. In fact, starting treatment on the weekends may allow appropriate light exposure at a later clock time than permitted during the school/work week. Once light treatment begins, the patient attempts to go to bed about 0.5 to 1 hour earlier each night. Once appropriate timing is reached, light treatment 1 to 2 days a week could be used for "maintenance." It is also useful to restrict light in the evening hours (to avoid phase delay). Relatively inexpensive blue light boxes are available. The advantage of blue light is that a lower intensity and shorter duration of light exposure may be effective.

Light treatment (light box) side effects include induction of hypomania, although light treatment can be used in bipolar depression with proper monitoring. Other reported side effects include nausea, eye strain, agitation, treatment-emergent headaches, and induction of migraine. Stopping light treatment resolves these issues. Patients with eye disease (especially retinal) or photosensitive skin disease should undergo artificial light treatment only in consultation with the physician treating the patient for those disorders.

Various dosages and timing of melatonin have also been used to treat DSWPD.[52,58,59] The goal is to give melatonin before DLMO to advance the phase. Mundey and colleagues[52] used both 0.3 and 3.0 mg of melatonin and found the magnitude of phase advance correlated with the time of administration (earlier was better). Of note, in this study, melatonin treatment in DSWPD had a greater effect on *wake-up time than sleep-onset time*.[52] In another study, *5 mg of melatonin* administered 5 hours before the DLMO was effective.[58] However, larger doses of melatonin are more likely to also have a hypnotic effect. A recent double-blind randomized trial examined 0.5 mg fast-release melatonin or placebo 1 hour before the desired bedtime for at least 5 consecutive nights per week. All patients received behavioral sleep-wake scheduling, consisting of a bedtime scheduled at the desired time. The primary outcome was actigraphy sleep-onset time. Sleep and symptoms improved, although the investigators believed that the major effect of melatonin was its hypnotic effect and that sleep scheduling was more effective for phase shifting than the melatonin. The 2015 AASM clinical practice guidelines did make a recommendation for scheduled melatonin (weak for) in adults *without depression*, children/adolescents *without* comorbidities, and children and adolescents *with* psychiatric comorbidity. The recommended dose was 5 mg of melatonin between 7:00 and 9:00 PM.[42] This seems like an excessive dose for phase shifting. At this dose both phase shifting and hypnotic effects would occur. Current reasonable recommendations are to administer 0.3 to 5.0 mg of melatonin 2 to 3 hours before DLMO or 5 to 7 hours before habitual bedtime (DLMO occurs 2–3 hours before habitual bedtime). One could make a case for using melatonin 0.3 to 0.5 mg to possibly minimize hypnotic effects if sleepiness at the time of administration is not desirable (Box 34–5). There is some evidence that use of the combination of light and melatonin may be more effective at inducing a phase advance than either used alone.[60] **Side effects of melatonin** *include headache, dizziness, somnolence, nausea, drowsiness, hypotension, gastrointestinal upset, nightmares, and exacerbation of alopecia areata.* At high doses, melatonin may alter growth hormone regulation or sex hormones.[8] For this reason, some clinicians are hesitant to use the medication long term in adolescents or children. Melatonin may worsen depression and alter the needed dose of warfarin.

Advanced Sleep-Wake Phase Disorder

ASWPD is thought to be quite rare if diagnostic criteria are strictly followed. Early morning awakening is a typical complaint.[1,42] Often, patients can stay awake in the evening but are unable to stay asleep until the time of desired awakening. That is they have a final awakening at 5 AM after falling asleep at 10 PM the night before. Advanced-related sleep complaints, particularly early awakening, are more common than difficulty remaining awake in the evening. Therefore, classic ASWPD (inability to stay awake in the evening and stay asleep in the early morning) is less common than complaints of early morning awakening. It may also be difficult to obtain a history of early onset of sleep, as some patients consider the time of falling asleep outside the bedroom (e.g., falling asleep for an hour in the living room) as not counting as the start of sleep. ASWPD is associated with aging, and nonaging ASWPD is rare. Early morning awakening can also be noted in depression.

Epidemiology and Pathophysiology of ASWPD

The prevalence of ASWPD is not well documented but believed to be about 1% in middle-aged populations and to increase with age. *Men and women are equally affected.* Familial ASWPD has been described, with a mutation in the circadian clock gene hPer2.[61,62] However, other familial cases do not show this pattern. Causes of ASWPD include a short endogenous circadian period or a dominant phase advance region to light. In elderly patients who take early morning walks, this behavior tends to advance the phase. The habit of taking an afternoon nap can also shorten nocturnal sleep duration by decreasing the homeostatic drive for sleep. As noted above, patients often do not complain of early bedtime but instead focus on early morning awakening.[63] A pneumonic to remember that polymorphisms of hPer2 are associated with ASWPD and hPer3 with DSWPD is that "2 is advanced compared to 3."

Diagnosis of ASWPD

The essential ICSD-3-TR criteria for diagnosis of ASWPD are (please see the ICSD-3-TR for complete criteria):

A. **A significant advance (earlier timing) in the phase of the major sleep episode** in relation to the desired or required sleep time and wake-up time, as evidenced by:
   - A chronic or recurrent complaint of profound difficulty to stay awake until the required or desired conventional clock time
   - An inability to remain asleep until the required or desired time for awakening.

B. **Symptoms are present for at least 3 months**

C. When patients are allowed to choose their ad libitum schedule, they will exhibit improved sleep quality and duration and maintain an advanced phase of the 24-hour sleep-wake pattern.

D. **Sleep logs are required,** accompanied by actigraphy monitoring whenever possible, for at least 7 days (preferably 14 days) that demonstrate a stable advance in the timing of the habitual sleep period. Both work/school days and free days should be included within this monitoring.

E. The sleep disturbance is not better explained by another current sleep disorder, medical disorder, mental disorder, or medication/substance use.

The essential requirement is that the sleep period be advanced with respect to the desired sleep and wake-up times for at least 3 months. The use of a sleep log (or actigraphy for at least 7 days if possible) is required to document a stable advance in the normal sleep period. Patients with ASWPD demonstrate a stable advance in sleep period, with sleep onset 6:00 to 9:00 PM and awakenings from 2:00 to 5:00 AM. Chronotype questionnaires (MEQ [Horne-Ostberg] questionnaire) document a "morning type," and circadian markers such as DLMO show an advance. The differential diagnosis includes poor sleep hygiene (evening or afternoon naps), caffeine abuse, alcohol, and depression (can cause early morning awakening). Napping by reducing the homeostatic sleep drive reduces total sleep time and early morning awakening.

Sleep Logs, Actigraphy, and DLMO

Patients with ASWPD demonstrate a stable advance in sleep period with sleep onset 6:00 to 9:00 PM and awakenings from 2:00 to 5:00 AM (Figure 34–17). Circadian phase makers in ASWPD patients demonstrate advanced timing.

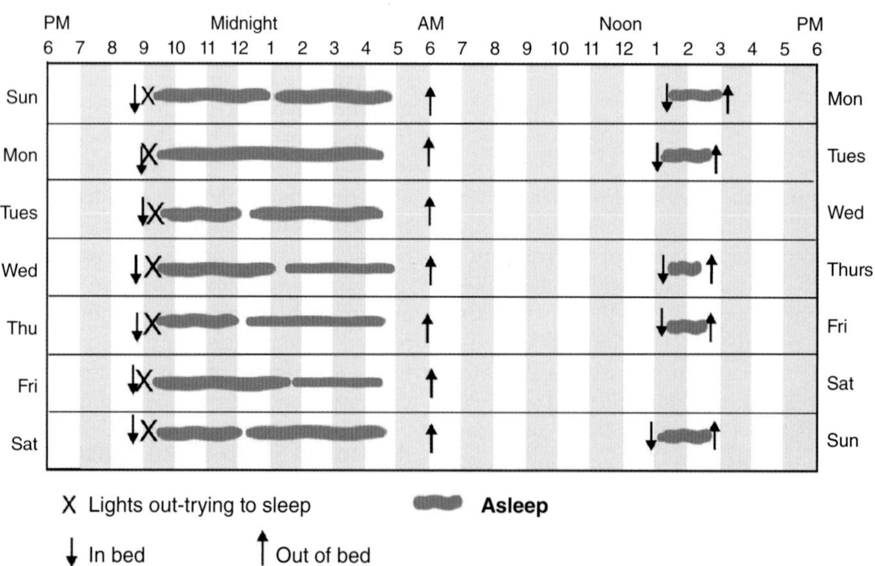

Figure 34–17 A typical sleep log pattern for a patient with advanced sleep-wake phase disorder (ASWPD). This illustrates an early bedtime and an early awakening time. The patient stayed in bed although awake for more than an hour ("to avoid getting out of bed "too early"). The patient takes naps, which may exacerbate early morning awakening by decreasing the homeostatic sleep drive.

Treatment of ASWPD

Treatment of ASWD may require only reassurance if the patient can adapt their life to their circadian rhythm. Treatment options are listed in Box 34–8. The 2015 clinical practice guidelines treatment offer no treatment recommendations for ASWPD other than a "weak for" recommendation in adults using appropriately timed (evening) light therapy. The 2007 AASM practice parameters list a planned sleep schedule, timed light exposure, and timed melatonin at the option level (lowest level of recommendation). Of note, the 2015 CRSWD clinical practice guidelines make no recommendation for either prescribed sleep-wake scheduling or avoidance of light. Chronotherapy (sleep scheduling) can be used with a progressive phase advance around the clock (going to bed earlier and earlier) until the desired bedtime is reached.[64] For most patients, this is not practical. Light exposure prior to the CBTmin and melatonin after CBTmin will cause a desired phase delay. Generally, bright light in the evening from 7:00 to 9:00 PM is recommended. As noted, the 2015 clinical guidelines for treatment of CRSWD gave a "weak for" for evening light in adults with ASWPD. Relatively few studies of ASWPD treatment exist. In one study, 4000 lux was administered for 11 consecutive days, then twice weekly for a 3-month period (maintenance).[65] Unfortunately, patients have difficulty complying with this treatment plan. Another important form of light therapy is to AVOID early morning light, which tends to cause a phase advance. Taking walks after 10:00 AM will be far enough away from the CBTmin to have less phase-advance effects. Another option would be to wear dark glasses during the walks. Although early morning melatonin would be a potential treatment (phase delay), this is not practical and may not be safe if individuals have to function in the morning. Melatonin has sedative effects, especially at higher doses and during periods when the endogenous melatonin is not elevated. The clinical practice guideline for CRSWD found no evidence for use of melatonin in ASWPD (no recommendation).

Irregular Sleep-Wake Rhythm Disorder (ISWRD)

ISWRD is characterized by lack of a clearly defined circadian rhythm of sleep and wakefulness behavior. Typically, sleep and wakefulness periods are interspersed throughout the day.[1]

Epidemiology of ISWRD

The prevalence of ISWRD is unknown. The disorder occurs most frequently in institutionalized elderly patients with dementia or institutionalized young patients with mental retardation. Precipitating factors include poor sleep hygiene and limited exposure to synchronizing zeitgebers, including outside light, exercise, and social activities. Some patients may have a decrease in the circadian amplitude of the SCN-alerting signal. *In others, absence of zeitgebers (decreased light and activity) may be important. Important risk factors for ISWRD include age, living in an institutional setting, and dementia (Alzheimer's disease) or mental retardation.*[66]

Box 34–8 TREATMENT OF ADVANCED SLEEP-WAKE PHASE DISORDER

Sleep schedule (chronotherapy)—progressive phase advance*
Avoid light after temperature minimum (early morning light)*
Bright evening light 7:00–9:00 PM**
Early morning melatonin***

* No recommendation in the 2017 American Academy of Sleep Medicine (AASM) clinical practice guidelines.
** "Weak for" recommendation in the 2017 AASM clinical practice guidelines.
***Early morning melatonin is potentially effective, but sedative effects make this impractical for most patients. Consider a low dosage to minimize sedative effects. This treatment is rarely if ever used.

Pathogenesis of ISWRD

Precipitating factors include poor sleep hygiene and limited exposure to synchronizing zeitgebers, including outside light, exercise, and social activities. Some patients may have a decrease in the circadian amplitude of the SCN-alerting signal.[66] This may be a result of damage or deterioration of the SCN. In others, absence of zeitgebers (decreased light and activity) may be more important. Important risk factors for ISWRD include age, living in an institutional setting, and dementia or mental retardation.

Factors involved in ISWRD:
1. Abnormal circadian regulation
   i. Damage or deterioration of SCN activity
   ii. Diminished response to entraining agents such as light
2. Behavioral and environmental factors
   i. Decreased exposure to bright light
   ii. Decreased physical activity and social activities
   iii. Poor sleep habits

Sleep Logs and Actigraphy in ISRWD

Actigraphy monitoring for at least 7 days demonstrates **multiple irregular sleep bouts (at least three)** during a 24-hour period (Figure 34–18). *The total sleep time over 24 hours is*

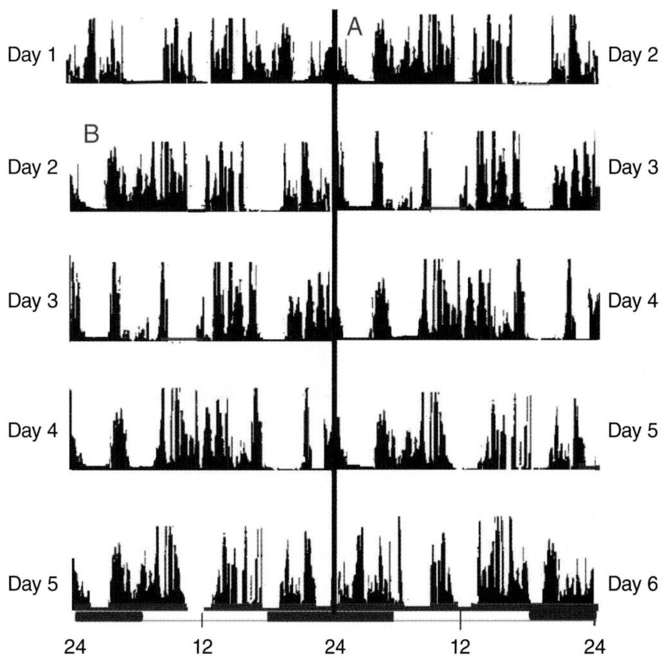

Figure 34–18 Actigraphy shows an irregular pattern of wakefulness and sleep in a nursing home patient with dementia. On the bottom, the *dark bars* represent nighttime, and the *white bars* represent daytime. Note that much of the sleep occurred during the day. At least three episodes of sleep were noted each 24 hours. This is a double plot with the second 24 hours on a given line (A), repeated as the first 24 hours on the next line of the actigraphy tracing (B). (Reproduced from Berry RB. *Fundamentals of Sleep Medicine*, 1st ed. Gainesville, FL: Elsevier Saunders; 2012:531.

typically normal for age. The 2007 AASM practice parameters for CRSWD state that actigraphy is indicated in ISWRD for diagnosis (guideline) and assessing response to treatment (option).

Diagnosis of ISWRD

The ICSD-3-TR diagnostic criteria for ISWRD[1] are:

A. The patient or caregiver reports a chronic or recurrent pattern of irregular sleep and wakefulness episodes throughout the 24-hour period, characterized by symptoms of insomnia during scheduled sleep periods (usually at night), excessive sleepiness (napping) during the day, or both.

B. Symptoms are present for at least 3 months

C. **Sleep logs are required** and actigraphy monitoring (if possible) recommended for at least 7 days, preferably 14 days, and these demonstrate *no major sleep period and multiple irregular sleep bouts (at least three)* during a 24-hour period.

Actigraphy or sleep log for at least 7 days demonstrates multiple sleep periods **(at least three)** within 24 hours with an approximately *normal amount of total sleep for age.* For most patients with ISWRD, the sleep log is problematic, and this is one setting in which actigraphy is especially helpful. Some actigraph devices also record light exposure, and decreased light exposure may be a predisposing factor for ISWRD. The diagnostic criteria also state that the sleep disturbance is not better explained by another current sleep, medical, neurological, or mental disorder, medication use, or substance use disorder.

The 2007 practice parameters for CRSWD[41] made recommendations for diagnostic procedures. As with all CRSWDs, PSG is not indicated unless another sleep disorder is suspected, and sleep logs (guideline) and actigraphy (option) are recommended by the 2007 practice parameters for ISWRD diagnosis.

Treatment of ISWRD

Treatment of patients with ISWRD aims to consolidate both sleep and wakefulness periods (Box 34–9). The 2007 practice parameters for CRSWD recommend a planned sleep schedule/mixed modality treatment and timed light exposure (bright light during the day). Mixed modality treatments include structured activities during the day to prevent napping. Timed melatonin is recommended for patients with moderate to severe mental retardation but **not** elderly patients or those with dementia (option). The 2017 AASM clinical practice guidelines give a *"weak for" recommendation for light* for elderly demented patients with the ISWRD. Of note light has alerting properties beyond effects of circadian rhythms. Timed oral melatonin or melatonin agonists were recommended for children/adolescents with neurological disorders ("weak for") but NOT recommended as *("weak against") for the elderly (especially with dementia). There was also a "weak against" recommendation against use of a combination of light and melatonin in the elderly with dementia (issues with melatonin).* There was a **strong** recommendation **against** sleep-promoting medications in elderly patients with dementia. Hypnotics have been used for ISWRD but are associated with side effects (falls or sedation) in the elderly.

Several studies have evaluated different approaches to ISRWD. Daytime light has been tried with some benefit.[67] Singer and coworkers found no benefit from use of melatonin as a hypnotic in Alzheimer's disease using a placebo-controlled trial.[68] A large randomized, controlled trial by Riemersma-ven der Lek and associates[69] compared four conditions (bright light–melatonin, dim light–melatonin, bright light–placebo, dim light–placebo) in a group of institutionalized elderly patients (87% had dementia). The light conditions included bright (1000 lux) or dim light (300 lux) between 9:00 AM and 6:00 PM. The melatonin and placebo conditions included administration of either placebo or 2.5 mg melatonin in the evening. Light had a modest benefit in improving some cognitive and non-cognitive symptoms of dementia. Melatonin (without bright light) decreased sleep latency and increased total sleep time but impaired mood. Bright light with melatonin did not impair mood but decreased sleep latency and increased total sleep time. Thus, melatonin should probably not be used alone in elderly patients in similar settings. A combination of light and melatonin might be effective. *However, use of combined light and melatonin was not recommended in the 2015 AASM practice guidelines.* Conversely, melatonin has been shown to be of benefit in some populations of younger developmentally delayed or mentally impaired individuals. A study by Pillar and coworkers[70] found that 4-week treatment with 3 mg melatonin improved sleep duration from 5.9 to 7.3 hours and sleep efficiency from 69.3% to 88% in a group of children with psychomotor retardation.

Alzheimer's disease is the most common cause of dementia (>60% of dementias). The diagnosis is one of exclusion of other causes of dementia. The hallmark is a gradual onset of short-term memory problems. Patients with Alzheimer's disease experience *sundowning,* which is defined as nocturnal exacerbation of disruptive behavior or agitation in older patients. This is likely the most common cause of institutionalization in patients with Alzheimer's disease. Donepezil (Aricept), a cholinesterase inhibitor, is used in Alzheimer's disease to improve cognition but is often associated with insomnia. Although most often prescribed at night, morning dosing is suggested to minimize sleep disturbance. The dual orexin receptor antagonist medications are now available for use as hypnotics. Studies in dementia have shown improvement in total sleep time without excessive sedation using suvorexant.[71] The use of dual orexin receptor antagonists (DORAs) for insomnia in dementia and possibly circadian rhythm disorders requires further study. Use of alerting medications during the day is a potential intervention to prevent

Box 34–9 TREATMENT OF ISWRD

Often Recommended:

- Daytime light (weak for)
- Prescribed sleep scheduling (no recommendation)
- Structured daily activity – to avoid napping (no recommendation)
- Melatonin in children and adolescents with neurological disorders (weak for)

Not Recommended:

- Sleep-promoting medications (strong against)
- Melatonin in elderly patients (weak against)
- Melatonin with multimodality in elderly patients (weak against)
- Combination of light and melatonin in elderly patients (weak against)

"Strong against," "weak against," and "weak for" from the 2017 American Academy of Sleep Medicine (AASM) clinical practice guidelines for treatment of circadian rhythm sleep-wake disorder[42]

daytime sleep lapses and improve social interaction. See Chapter 30 for information on using alerting medications in special populations. Sundowning is also discussed in Chapter 40.

Non-24-Hour Sleep-Wake Rhythm Disorder

N24SWRD was formerly called circadian rhythm sleep-wake disorder – free running type (CRSWD-FRT). The disorder is characterized by a progressive delay in sleep onset each day[1] (Figure 34–19).

The ICSD-3-TR diagnostic criteria are:

A. There is a history of insomnia, excessive daytime sleepiness, or both, which alternate with asymptomatic episodes, due to misalignment between the 24-hour light-dark cycle and the non-entrained endogenous circadian rhythm of sleep and wakefulness propensity.

B. Symptoms persist over the course of at least 3 months.

C. **Sleep logs are required**, accompanied by actigraphy monitoring whenever possible, ***for at least 14 days***, preferably longer for blind individuals. These demonstrate a pattern of sleep and wakefulness times that typically delay each day.

D. The sleep disturbance is not better explained by another current sleep, medical, neurological, or mental disorder, medication use, or substance use disorder.

Note that sleep logs are required for at least 14 days (other disorders at least 7 days and preferably 14 days) and that symptoms must be present for at least 3 months. The amount of the daily delay depends on the endogenous tau and may vary from less than 30 minutes (when tau is close to 24 hours) to more than 1 hour when the tau is longer than 25 hours. If other measures of circadian phase are obtained 2 to 4 weeks apart (DLMO), they should confirm the circadian delay.

When the endogenous circadian rhythm is out of phase with conventional sleep and wakefulness times, symptoms occur (Figure 34–20). Typically, both some degree of insomnia and daytime sleepiness are reported, alternating with periods of minimal difficulties. For example, there are periods when patients may complain of insomnia at night and daytime sleepiness (core body temperature minimum during the day, e.g., noon), early morning awakening (core body temperature early evening, e.g., 10:00 PM), sleep-onset insomnia (core body temperature at 10:00 AM), and few symptoms (core body temperature in the middle of the night). The symptoms depend on the relationship between the internal circadian rhythms and external time. When the circadian phase is aligned with a normal sleep-wake period, complaints may not be present.[1]

Epidemiology and Pathophysiology of N24SWRD

Up to 50% of totally blind patients have non-entrained circadian rhythms. About 70% have chronic sleep complaints. The cause is lack of entrainment by light. The tau of these patients is usually not abnormal. Rarely, N24SWRD occurs in sighted individuals.[72,73] The tau of these individuals may be abnormally increased. The N24SWRD has also been described after head trauma.[74] Note that there are some blind patients whose circadian systems respond to bright light, even though they have no visual perception (rods and cones in the outer retinal layer are damaged, but the layer of the retina with the photosensitive ganglion cells is intact). Some nonvisual function is still present in these patients with ganglion cells and the RHT intact. As noted, for blind individuals, the tau (internal circadian period) is usually normal[75]; they simply do not entrain to the dark-light cycle. In these patients, the daily drift may be short (30 minutes) or as long as 1 hour (if tau = 25 hours), depending on their internal circadian rhythm. In sighted individuals (often with a tau greater than 25 hours), the daily delay may be 1 to 2 hours. In one study,[72] most of the sighted patients with N24SWRD had a tau of 24.5 to 25.5 hours, though it could be as long as 26.5 hours. In another study, the delay in the midpoint of the sleep period varied from 0.8 to 1.8 hours.[73] Of interest, there was

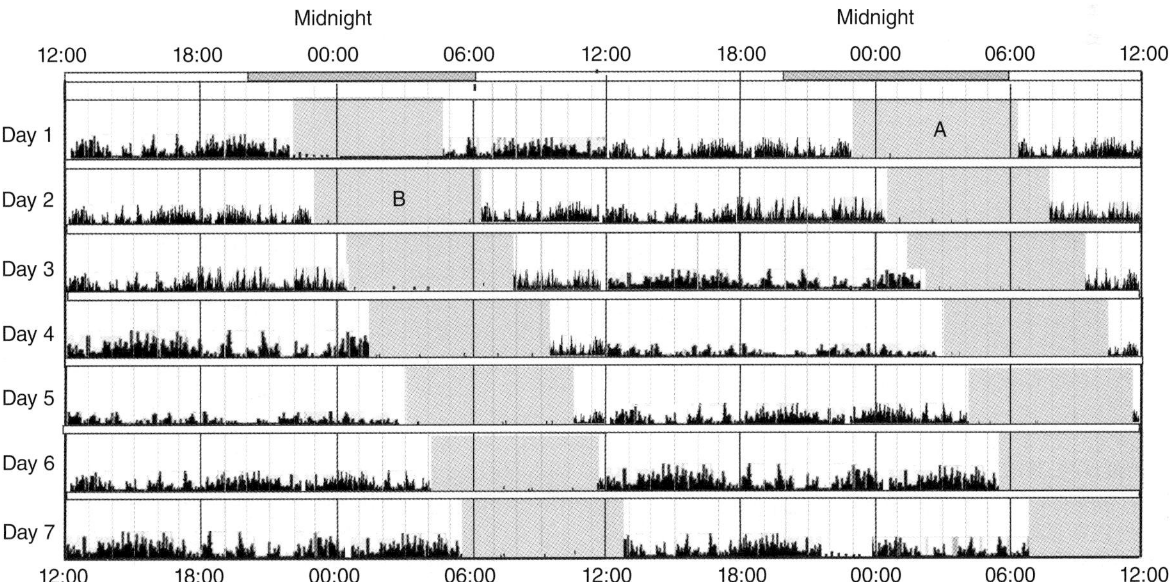

Figure 34–19 This actigraphy tracing shows a progressive delay in sleep offset with a parallel delay in sleep onset. This is characteristic of the non-24-hour sleep-wake rhythm disorder (formerly called free-running type). This is a "double plot," with each line representing 48 hours. The last 24 hours in the top line, (A) is repeated as the first 24 hours (B) on the second line. (From Berry RB, Wagner MH. *Sleep Medicine Pearls*. 3rd ed. Philadelphia: Elsevier; 2015;641)

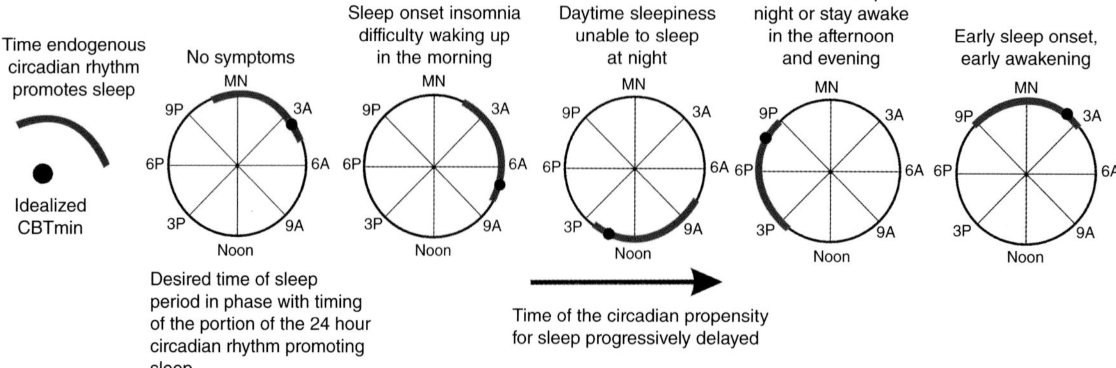

Figure 34–20 This figure illustrates the clinical manifestations in an idealized patient with the non-24-hour sleep-wake rhythm disorder associated with a progressive delay in the endogenous circadian rhythm that is out of phase with clock time. The time that the endogenous circadian rhythm has a propensity for sleep (promotes sleep) is shown in red at various positions with respect to clock time. When the circadian rhythm is in phase with clock time, there are no symptoms. With progressive delay, complaints of insomnia occur during the night (clock time), when the endogenous circadian sleep propensity does not occur at night. When the endogenous sleep period occurs during the day, a complaint of daytime sleepiness is manifested. The actual advance in circadian rhythm is much slower than illustrated and the different positions with respect to clock time are shown for illustration. Activity and the timing of food intake can also influence circadian rhythms even when the phase advancing influence of light is not present. *MN,* midnight; *CBTmin,* core body temperature minimum.

a longer time from DLMO to sleep onset (normal: 2 to 3 hours). Sighted individuals with N24SWRD have an increased incidence of psychiatric disorders and often have a long sleep duration. One cause of the N24SWRD in many sighted individuals appears to be a long tau (long internal circadian period). The delay is too large to be entrained by 0.5-hour phase advance from light. The other option is that they have poor entrainment by light. *In summary, blind individuals with N24SWRD have a fairly normal tau, but sighted individuals with N24SWRD usually have a long tau.* There appears to be an overlap between DSWPD and N24SWRD, as some patients initially diagnosed with the former condition were later noted to have a free-running pattern on actigraphy and in sleep logs.[73]

Sleep Logs, Actigraphy, CBTmin, and DLMO

Sleep logs and actigraphy (Figure 34–19) demonstrate a progressive delay in the sleep period in patients with N24SWRD. There is a progressive delay in the CBTmin and the DLMO (Figure 34–5). As noted, in blind individuals with N24SWRD, the tau is usually either normal or slightly prolonged. The major problem is lack of entrainment by light rather than a long tau. However, the longer the tau, the more difficult patients are to entrain. For sighted individuals, the tau is usually prolonged. Of note, one study[73] used the mid-point of the sleep period to estimate the daily drift in circadian rhythm and the found drift in circadian rhythm (bedtime and wake-up times) to be inconsistent as a result of societal and other influences. Therefore the melatonin mid point was the best circadian marker in these individuals.

Treatment of N24SWRD

The only recommendation in the 2017 clinical practice guidelines for N24SWRD is use of timed melatonin or melatonin agonists for blind adults. The usual treatment in blind patients includes melatonin of various dosages, usually given *about 1 hour before the desired bedtime* (Box 34–10). In one study, 10 mg of melatonin was given 1 hour before the desired bedtime.[75,76] A maintenance dose of 0.5 mg of melatonin has been used in some studies.[77] In a few patients who failed to entrain on 10 mg melatonin, there was success with a lower dose.[78] A schematic illustration of a patient entrained with a dose of melatonin about 1 hour before the desired sleep onset is shown in Figure 34–21. Tasmelteon (Hetlioz®) is approved by the U.S. Food and Drug Administration (FDA) for treatment of N24SWRD in adults.[78,79] Treatment can entrain patients with N24SWRD, but continued treatment is needed to maintain the effect.[80] The dosage is 20 mg, given 1 hour before bedtime without food. Side effects include headache, nightmares or unusual dreams, increased alanine transaminase (ALT) levels, or upper respiratory tract or urinary infections. CYP1A2 inhibitors (e.g., fluvoxamine) should not be taken with tasmelteon or melatonin, as these will increase the level of melatonin/tasmelteon. The clinical significance is unknown. Recall that the melatonin agonist binding of the melatonin receptor MT2 is believed to have more effect on shifting circadian rhythms than MT1 (hypnotic effect). Ramelteon shows an 8- to 10-fold higher affinity for MT1 than for MT2 and a 3- to 16-fold higher affinity than melatonin. Tasmelteon has a slightly higher affinity for the MT2 receptor

Box 34–10 TREATMENTS FOR NON-24-HOUR SLEEP-WAKE RHYTHM DISORDER

1. Timed oral administration of melatonin or melatonin agonists (weak for in blind adults). The timing is usually at or slightly earlier than (1 hour before) the desired bedtime. The dosage has varied from 0.5 to 5 mg melatonin. At the higher dosages, some hypnotic effects are present. It has been suggested that some patients who do not entrain with large doses of melatonin may entrain with 0.5 mg.
2. Tasmelteon (Hetlioz) is approved by the U.S. Food and Drug Administration for non-24-hour sleep-wake rhythm disorder (20 mg given 1 hour before desired bedtime).
3. For sighted individuals, the best treatment is not known.
   - Appropriately timed light to counteract the daily phase delay
   - Melatonin as for blind individuals

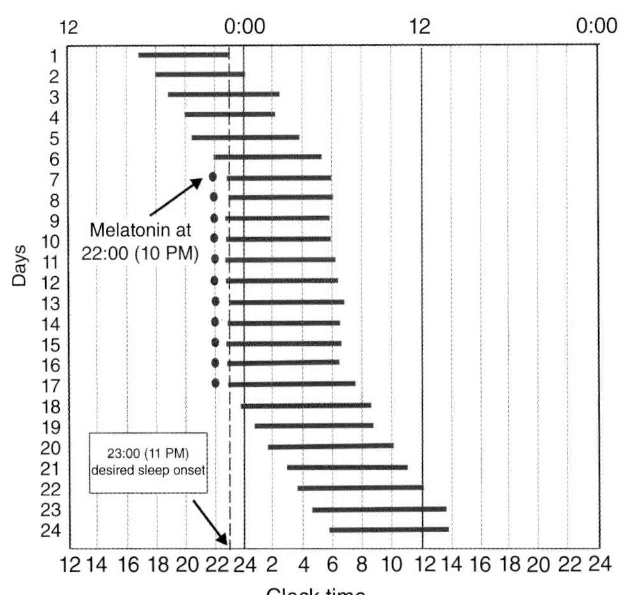

Figure 34–21 This figure illustrates a schematic of a sleep log from a blind patient with non-24-hour sleep-wake rhythm disorder and a progressive delay of the sleep period by about 1 hour. Melatonin (*red circles*) is started when the predicted sleep period coincides with the desired clock time for sleep onset. Here, the desired clock time is 11:00 PM, and melatonin is administered 1 hour earlier, at 10:00 PM. With repeated doses of melatonin, the circadian rhythm is entrained. However, once melatonin is stopped, the pattern of progressive phase delay returns. Various timing and doses of melatonin have been tried in this situation. Some patients who do not entrain with larger doses of melatonin will entrain with smaller doses (0.5 mg).

(two to four times) than MT1, although it is still considered a nonselective agonist. The medication is very expensive (over $18,000 for 30 capsules) but can be obtained at an affordable price for most patients through the HETLIOZ Solutions program if the proper paperwork if is filled out on the manufacture's website (https://hetlioz.com/hetliozsolutions). Ramelteon would be another option. A generic formulation is now available at at a much lower price than the brand name (Rozerem) but is still more expensive that some other generic hypnotics. The 2017 clinical guidelines for treatment of intrinsic CRSWD give a "weak for" recommendation for use of melatonin or melatonin agonists in blind individuals with N24SWRD.[42]

The treatment in sighted patients may include both melatonin and appropriately timed light exposure. The best treatment is unknown. A study by Malkani et al. recommended use of melatonin 0.5 to 4 mg given 2 to 4 hours before goal sleep onset and light on awakening. In their study, some patients given melatonin 1 hour before goal sleep onset developed a pattern like that of DSWPD, with a long time between melatonin dose and sleep onset. In these patients, giving the melatonin earlier was more effective. Patients were effectively entrained (circadian rhythm did not progressively advance), but only as long as a strict schedule was followed. None of the participants continued the treatment on a long-term basis because of societal and other issues. The authors concluded that this type of N24SWRD is very difficult to treat.

Light is timed to oppose the intrinsic progressive phase delay. That is, light should be timed after the CBTmin to induce a phase advance. One might begin treatment during a time when the CBTmin occurs at a normal time in the early morning (3:00 to 5:00 AM). The goal would be to maintain the CBTmin during the night. A fixed wake-up time with daily light treatment could be used for maintenance. The 2017 AASM treatment guidelines for intrinsic CRSWD made no recommendation for use of melatonin, melatonin agonists, or light for treatment of sighted individuals with the N24SWRD.[42]

Shift-Work Disorder

SWD is not considered an intrinsic CRSWD, as it is primarily caused by a work schedule overlapping with the normal sleep period. SWD[1] is characterized by excessive sleepiness or insomnia temporally associated with a recurring work schedule that overlaps the usual time for sleep.

The essential points of diagnostic criteria for SWD[1] are:

A. There is a report of insomnia, or excessive sleepiness accompanied by a reduction in total sleep time, which is associated with a recurring work schedule that overlaps the usual time of sleep.

B. The symptoms have been present and associated with the shift work schedule for **at least 3 months**.

C. **Sleep logs are required** and actigraphy monitoring recommended (whenever possible and preferably with concurrent light exposure measurement) for at least 14 days (work and free days); these demonstrate a disturbed sleep-wake pattern.

D. The sleep disturbance is not better explained by another current sleep disorder, medical disorder mental disorder, inadequate sleep hygiene, or medication/substance use.

The problem must last at least 3 months. A sleep log or actigraphy for at least 14 days (preferably with light exposure measurement) documents circadian and sleep time misalignment. The boundary between a normal and a pathologic response to circadian stress caused by an unnatural sleep schedule associated with shift work remains unclear. SWD is a common problem in industrialized countries resulting from the need for some occupations and services to function 24 hours per day.

Epidemiology of Shift-Work Disorder

Up to 20% of the populations in industrialized societies works in an occupation requiring shift work. The total number of **night-shift** workers is 2% to 5% of the population. *About 5% to 10% of shift workers experience significant insomnia or sleepiness during the shift (or day)* and qualify for this disorder.

Risk Factors for Symptoms From Shift Work

Risk factors include advancing age, *possibly female gender*, and morning light exposure (long commute home or morning social obligations, as this inhibits adaptive phase resetting). There are also limited data showing that morning types (MEQ) tend to get less daytime sleep after a night shift, but further studies are needed.

Pathophysiology

There are a number of exacerbating factors, including long shifts (fatigue) and the common practice of resuming normal daytime activities and nighttime sleep on the weekends. The sleepiness at night is often caused not only by the accumulated sleep load but, more importantly, by *loss of the circadian alerting signal*. Recall that the nadir in alertness in most individuals occurs at the time of CBTmin.

Sleep Logs, Actigraphy, and DLMO

Sleep logs tend to document the altered routine and its effect on sleep. Actigraphy is rarely needed but might document the daytime sleep pattern. *Sleep logs are required* in the diagnostic criteria in the ICSD-3-TR. While knowledge about the timing of work is known, *behavior while NOT at work (timing and amount of sleep) is not known*. Sleep-wake behavior while not at work is very important for understanding the impact of shift work in a given individual and their adaptation to an abnormal sleep period. For this reason sleep logs are more useful that might be assumed. Little data are available on the CBTmin. Note that symptoms of insomnia or sleepiness associated with reduced total sleep time (for at least 3 months) are required (but not evidence of circadian misalignment) are required for a diagnosis of SWD. Studies of DLMO suggest that night workers *are quite variable in their circadian adaptation*. Of note, *symptoms do not always correlate with whether circadian adaptation has occurred.*

Night-Shift Work

The *daytime sleep in night-shift workers is shorter than normal (5–6 hours)*. The majority of workers do not have circadian adaptation owing to societal obligations. They are typically exposed to light after their CBTmin on the drive home and, therefore, phase advance. Bright light during the start of the shift (before CBTmin) and avoiding light in the early morning (preventing phase advance) can potentially move the CBTmin to within the daytime sleep period.[81] Scheduled naps before the night shift or in the early part of the shift may improve alertness.[82,83] Two-hour naps during late afternoon before the evening shift are more effective than 2-hour naps during the shift. Figure 34–22 summarizes interventions on the return home in the morning to improve alertness during the night shift and sleep. Note that light during the shift not only causes a phase delay, but it is also *alerting*. In a simulated night-shift study over 5 consecutive nights, Crowley and colleagues[84] studied the effects of different interventions on shifts in CBTmin and performance (Figure 34–23). The groups that shifted the CBTmin to within the normal sleeping hours had improved nocturnal functioning on the psychomotor vigilance task (PVT). They used a combination of light during the simulated shift, dark glasses during the simulated drive home, and melatonin before sleep. Of interest, the groups with the **latest CBTmin** at baseline were the ones able to completely entrain to the new schedule.[84,85] Circadian phase was measured by DLMO with CBTmin = DLMO + 7 hours. Melatonin given before morning sleep after a night shift resulted in minimal change in total sleep time and added **little to circadian shifts induced by interventions with light**.[84] In another study, bright light during the start of the night shift was a very powerful phase-delaying influence. Melatonin had little effect, and dark glasses on the trip home helped *only if regular room light was used during the night shift*.[85] Smith found minimal effects of melatonin as a sleep aid for daytime sleep following a night shift.[86] One study found a significant phase advance with melatonin in the early evening for patients who desired a prolonged sleep period before the night shift.[87]

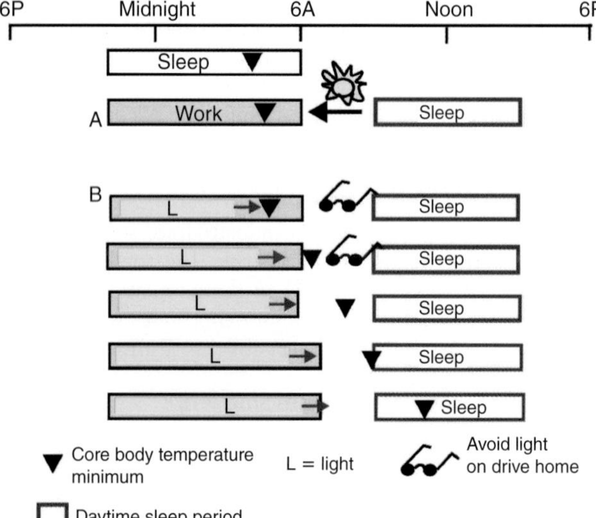

Figure 34–22 An example of interventions for night-shift work. (A) No interventions. Light exposure at work induces a slight phase delay compared to normal sleep in the dark. However this is opposed by a phase advance from light exposure on the commute home. (B) Interventions—The core body temperature minimum (CBTmin) is shifted toward daytime sleep by using **bright light in the early part of the night shift** (phase delay) and wearing dark goggles on the commute home (if in daylight). Bright light is not used at the end of the shift to avoid exposure on the advancing side of CBTmin (the position of CBT could be earlier than shown in some individuals). Note that the duration of light during the night shift can increase as the CBTmin is progressively delayed. The goal is to shift the CBTmin into the daytime sleep period. Light not only induces a phase delay, but it is also alerting. (From Berry RB. *Fundamentals of Sleep Medicine*. 1st ed. Gainsville, FL: Elsevier Saunders; 2012:539.)

A number of studies on shift work have used simulated night-shift work. However, a field study found less benefit from melatonin and light than seen in other simulated studies, possibly because, in the real world, the workers have other competing interests.[88] Sallinen and associates[82] compared four nap strategies during the night shift (nap duration/timing: 50 min/1:00 AM, 50 min/4:00 AM, 30 min/1:00 AM, 30 min/4:00 AM) to the no nap condition using an experimental night-shift protocol. Early napping improved reaction time in the later in the night but not at the end of the shift (low point circadian alertness). There was sleep inertion second half of the night. The early naps produced increased alertness (assessed by PSG sleep latency) during the second half of the night shift. Short naps (20–30 minutes) during the night shift may avoid sleep inertia but improve alterness during the shift or on the drive home. Shorter naps may avoid sleep inertia on awakening after the nap. In another study, Schweitzer and coworkers[83] showed *napping before the night shift, especially when combined with caffeine*, improved alertness as assessed by multiple sleep latency test (MSLT) and PVT.

The alerting agent modafinil (200 mg given at the start of the night shift) is FDA approved to improve alertness during shift work.[89] *However, while modafinil improved alertness, the medication still did not normalize alertness*. Armodafinil (the R enantiomer of modafinil) was also shown to be helpful in maintaining alertness during shift work.[90] Hypnotics have also been used in an attempt to improve daytime sleep. Walsh and colleagues[91] found that use of triazolam increased daytime sleep duration by about 50 minutes but did not reduce circadian sleep tendency in the early morning hours.

Rotating Shifts and Complications of Night Shifts

A number of different shift schedules exist (morning [start time 4AM to 7 AM], evening [start times 2 to 6 PM), night shift [start times 6 PM to 4 AM], or rotating shifts). Of these the least sleep loss is with evening shifts and the greatest with night shifts. There is greater sleep loss with rapidly rotating shifts than with slowly rotating shifts (slow = 3-week periods). Clockwise

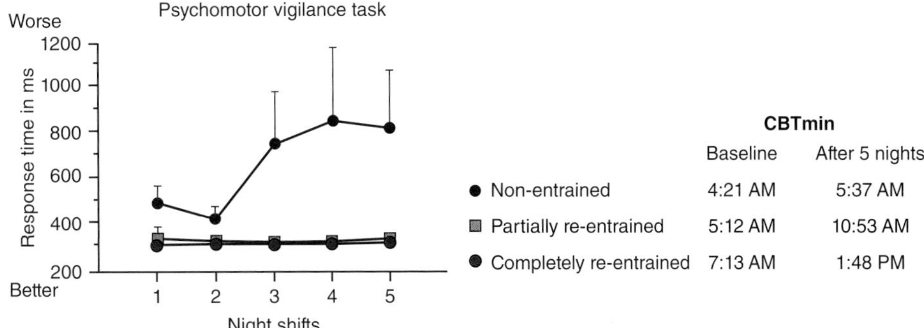

Figure 34–23 Change in psychomotor vigilance task (PVT) over 5 consecutive simulated night shifts in groups non-entrained, partially entrained, and completely re-entrained. The non-entrained group had a worsening in the PVT over 5 nights (increased response time). The other two groups did not have a deterioration over the 5 night shifts. The time of core body temperature minimum (CBTmin) is illustrated for each group at baseline and after 5 nights. The CBTmin shifted to within daytime sleep in the two groups with better function. Subjects were given different combinations of bright light/dim light during the simulated night shift, dark glasses or normal sunglasses in the morning, and melatonin or placebo before sleep time. (Adapted from Crowley SJ, Tseng CU, Fogg LF, Eastman CI. Complete or partial re-entrainment improves performance, alertness, and mood during shift-work. *Sleep*. 2004;27:1077-1087.)

rotation is better tolerated than counterclockwise rotation owing to the natural tendency to phase delay. Early morning shift workers are on the road during the low point in circadian alertness and are at risk of motor vehicle accidents. Evening shift workers may have less sleep loss but suffer from social isolation. A number of complications of shift work have been proposed, including gastrointestinal disturbances (constipation/diarrhea), obesity, miscarriage, drug dependency, and social and family life disturbances.

Treatment of Shift-Work Disorder

The recommended treatments for SWD are listed in Box 34–11. A planned sleep schedule (naps), timed bright light exposure, timed melatonin administration, stimulants (caffeine), and alerting agents (modafinil) are also listed as indicated with various levels of recommendation in the 2007 AASM circadian practice parameters.[41] The goals of treatment include interventions to (1) modify circadian rhythms to ameliorate symptoms of circadian rhythm misalignment, (2) decrease sleep load during the night (naps before the shift or hypnotics before daytime sleep), or (3) increase alertness (caffeine or modafinil). Stimulants were given the lowest level of recommendation, but evidence for their efficacy is growing. There is less convincing data for daytime melatonin than for stimulants before the shift. The rationale behind timed bright light exposure is the supposition that having the CBTmin closer to (or within) the daytime sleep period will improve sleep quality and amount (Figure 34–22). As noted, bright light also has a direct alerting effect while on the night shift. Patients should minimize light on the commute home (dark goggles, assuming it is after sunrise), if possible, because this tends to cause phase advance. If they are very sleepy on the drive home this would not be a good idea as light would be alerting at a time they need to be alert. Light very late in the shift may be after the CBTmin and cause a phase advance. Therefore, using light only during the first part of the shift would avoid administering light on the wrong side of CBTmin. Evening types may tolerate night shift work better and patients with certain polymorphisms in the hPer3 gene may have less disturbed daytime sleep while working the night shift.

Jet Lag Disorder

The jet lag type of CRSWD is due to a temporary mismatch between internal circadian rhythms (endogenous circadian clock) and external clock time required by rapid change to a new time zone. There must be a complaint of impairment of sleep and/or daytime function. Major diagnostic criteria[1] are summarized below:

- There is a complaint of insomnia or excessive daytime sleepiness, accompanied by a reduction in total sleep time, associated with transmeridian jet travel across at least two time zones.
- There is associated impairment of daytime function, general malaise, or somatic symptoms (e.g., gastrointestinal disturbance) within one to two days after travel.
- The s must last at least 3 months. A sleep log or actigraphy for at least 14 days (preferably with light exposure measurement) documents circadian and sleep time misalignment. The bound, mental disorder, or medication/substance use.

Box 34–11 TREATMENT OF NIGHT-SHIFT DISORDER

Goals

1. Treat sleep loss (short scheduled naps pre-shift or during shift, optimize daytime sleep at home).
2. Increase alertness during shift (bright light, alerting agents at start of shift).
3. Move CBTmin to the morning sleep period at home (less sleepiness associated with a low alerting signal during the shift and makes sleep easier during the day). Recall that the low point of alertness is at CBTmin.

- Bright light for 3–6 hours during the start of shift—phase delay.
- Avoid bright light on the way home in the morning (use dark goggles if after sunrise to avoiding phase advance).
- Quiet, dark sleep environment at home during sleep.
- Melatonin administered in the morning at bedtime (hypnotic and phase-delay effects).
- Go to bed as soon as possible after arriving home.
- Stimulants/alerting agents at the start of the shift
  - Caffeine (250–400 mg) during first 2 hours of the night shift.
  - Modafinil 200 mg (or armodafinil 150 mg) taken 30–60 minutes before start of the night shift. These are FDA approved for sleepiness associated with shift work.*
- Hypnotics before daytime sleep—can increase total sleep time but do not help alertness at night.

**FDA*, U.S. Food and Drug Administration approved for improving alertness during the night shift.

Epidemiology of Jet Lag Disorder

The jet lag type of CRSWD can occur in all ages, but *manifestations are worse in the elderly*. Jet lag disorder is a product of our society, with approximately 500,000 people in the air at any moment worldwide. Aircrews are more vulnerable to jet lag, with frequent phase shifting. *About one-third of travelers do not experience jet lag*.

Pathophysiology

Jet lag begins after travel across at least two time zones.[1,92,93] Desynchrony between body and local time zone is known to cause problems with sleep, alertness, and performance. The degree of dysfunction depends on (1) the number of time zones crossed, (2) the direction of travel (westward travel better tolerated, phase delay easier), (3) sleep loss during travel, (4) availability of local time cues (exposure to natural light at destination—depends on weather, business schedule, and other factors), and (5) ability to tolerate circadian misalignment (decreases with age). Some useful facts concerning jet lag are displayed in Table 34–5. Westward travel is better tolerated because the body is phase advanced compared with local time. In general, it is easier to adapt (phase delay) because of the intrinsic phase delay (tau slightly >24 hours). In *eastward travel, the body is phase delayed*. It is more difficult to undergo adaptation to the new time zone requiring a phase advance. Sleep occurs normally on the *rising phase of melatonin rhythm and the falling phase of core temperature rhythm*. It is estimated that it takes about 1 day per hour of time-zone change to adjust (maximum adaptation is a phase shift of 1 to 1.5 hour/day, depending on direction of travel). In overnight flights, some degree of sleep loss is inevitable. Flying first class (more room), wearing eye shades or ear plugs, and possibly taking a hypnotic can minimize sleep loss. If this is not possible, a short nap on arrival at the new destination may help. Drinking adequate fluids and avoiding alcohol may also help. The availability of exposure to natural light in the new destination can be influenced by time of year, weather, and schedule (indoor meetings, societal obligations). The general recommendation is to eat on the destination schedule. Individuals vary in their ability to tolerate circadian misalignment (in general, older individuals have less tolerance). *Sleep on the first night at the new destination can be better than the next night due to sleep loss from plane travel.*

Table 34–5 Jet Lag Facts

Typical internal clock resetting	• 92 min/day delay on westward flights. • 57 min/day advance on eastward flights.
Eastern travel	• Difficulty falling asleep—sleep-onset insomnia. • May not notice sleep difficulty the first night in new time zone if sleep deprived (because sleep during flight may have been poor). • Sleep fragmented, decreased REM and stage N3 sleep.
Western travel	• Less persistent symptoms. • First night: sleep quality good early in sleep period. • Increased REM in first part of the night corresponding to the last part of the night at home • Early awakenings

REM, rapid eye movement.

Antidromic Entrainment

Travel over six time zones may result in phase shifting in the opposite direction of the direction of travel (i.e., adapting "the wrong way"), so-called antidromic re-entrainment. For example, eastern flight requires a phase advance to acclimate to the new time zone. However, after an eastward flight across nine time zones, the traveler's CBTmin, normally at 5:00 AM in the old time zone, would occur at 2:00 PM in the new time zone. Thus, morning light in the new time zone would cause phase delay because light exposure occurs before CBTmin. Of note, some experts recommend that all flights that cross more than 8 to 10 time zones be treated as if they were westward travel (interventions target progressive phase delay).

Symptoms Associated With Jet Lag CRSWD

Symptoms associated with jet lag may include (1) daytime tiredness or impaired daytime alertness, (2) inability to fall asleep at night (eastward flight), and (3) early awakening (westward flight). Other symptoms may include disorientation; gastrointestinal problems (poor appetite), inappropriate timing of defecation (gut lag), excessive urination, menstrual abnormalities (flight crew), inappropriate metabolic responses (insulin and other hormones), and heart disease. Symptoms may be worsened by the stresses of airplane travel itself or use of caffeine or alcohol.

Treatment of Jet Lag

A method to determine appropriate timing of interventions is illustrated in Figure 34–24. This method allows an estimate of the timing of CBTmin in the new time zone. A number of treatments for jet lag have been recommended depending on the direction of travel (Table 34–6). Websites are available that allow the traveler to enter current and future locations. The website will supply recommendations to minimize jet lag. One difficulty with providing recommendations is in estimating the current CBTmin and also that entrainment in the new destination may depend on societal demands in the new time zone that preclude following the prescription. General sleep hygiene measures include a dark, quiet sleep environment with earplugs or eye shades, if needed. If the plane flight is long, sleeping on the flight during appropriate hours (**destination nighttime**) may be helpful. In general, daytime naps should be avoided at the destination. However, napping can improve alertness for special demands (e.g., giving a talk). Napping removes photic stimuli, so this can delay adaptation if napping occurs at a time when light exposure would shift circadian rhythms in the correct direction.

Eastward Flights. A patient flies from New York to Paris (6 time zones earlier). The patient is phase delayed (CBTmin at about 10:00–11:00 AM instead of 4:00 AM [a phase advance is required]). In Figure 34–25, the estimated CBTmin is in the early morning rather than at 4:00 AM. An example of interventions for eastward travel are shown. Light is avoided before CBTmin, but exposure to light in the early afternoon is beneficial. There is a gradual phase advance to a time within the typical sleep period in the new time zone. Here, an adaptation period of 5 days is illustrated, but it could take longer.

In Figure 34–26, an example of interventions to shorten adaptation time in a patient traveling eastward (phase delay) is displayed. The method uses an attempt to phase advance in the current time zone using morning bright light before travel begins.[93,94] At the new destination, morning light should be

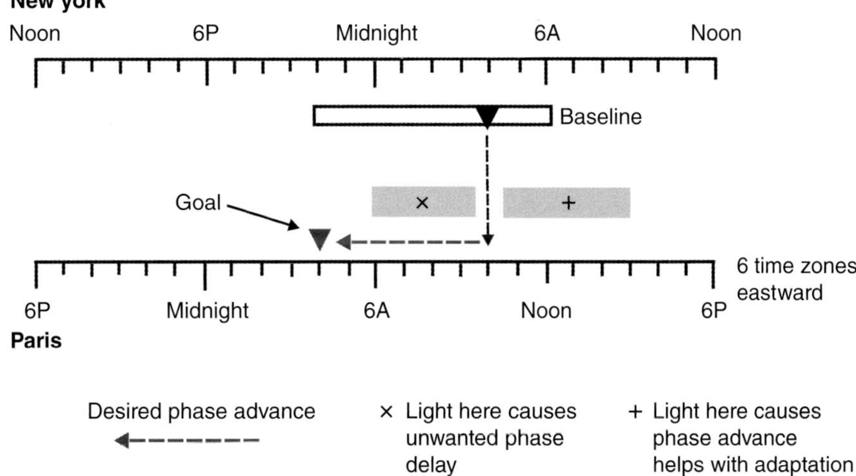

Figure 34–24 This schematic shows a method to determine the appropriate time for light exposure at a new location following eastward travel. The *top line* is the time scale for the current location (New York), and the *bottom line* is the corresponding times in the new location (Paris, 6 hours earlier). To adapt to the new location, the patient needs to phase advance. *Knowing the approximate position of CBTmin at the* ***initial*** *location, the corresponding time at the new location is noted.* Here if one assumes CBTmin is at 4 AM this corresponds to 10 AM in Paris. Then, one can determine the times light should be avoided to prevent phase delay. In this case, early morning light should be avoided. Late morning and early afternoon light would help phase advance. The goal is for CBTmin the new time zone to be at the same clock time as in the old time zone. The method can also be used for westward travel.

Table 34–6 Recommendations for Jet Lag

	Eastward Travel	Westward Travel
Phase Change/Adaptation	Internal rhythm is phase delayed. Adaptation—phase advance.	Internal rhythm is phase advanced. Adaptation—phase delay.
Before Travel Try to reset body clock to minimize necessary change.	Shift sleep 1–2 hours earlier before trip (bright light in morning).	Shift sleep 1–2 hours later before trip (bright light in evening).
During Travel During flight	Sleep, if possible—especially on long flights—to avoid sleep loss.	Sleep, if possible—especially on long flights to—avoid sleep loss.
	Sleep during time corresponding to night in the destination, if possible.	Sleep during time corresponding to night in the destination, if possible.
	Drink adequate H_2O, avoid alcohol.	Drink adequate H_2O, avoid alcohol.
On Arrival Anticipated changes in sleep.	Difficulty falling asleep. Difficulty waking up.	Difficulty staying asleep. Early awakening.
Appropriate light exposure.	Seek morning light (after CBTmin).	Seek evening light (before CBTmin).
If crossing more than eight time zones, avoid light when it may inhibit adaptation.	For the first 2 days after arrival, avoid bright light for the first 2–3 hours after dawn; starting on the 3rd day, seek exposure to bright light in the morning.	For 2–3 days, avoid bright light in the late evening (at dusk); starting on the third day, seek exposure to bright light in the evening.
Melatonin	Take 0.5–3 mg at local bedtime nightly until you adjust (phase advance).	Take 0.5 mg during the second half of the night (after CBTmin, to phase delay).
Hypnotics	Consider taking at bedtime for a few days.	Consider taking at bedtime for a few days.
Caffeine	Drink judiciously, avoid after midday.	Drink judiciously, avoid after midday.

CBTmin, minimum core body temperature.
Adapted from Sack RL. Jet lag. *N Engl J Med.* 2010;362:440-447.

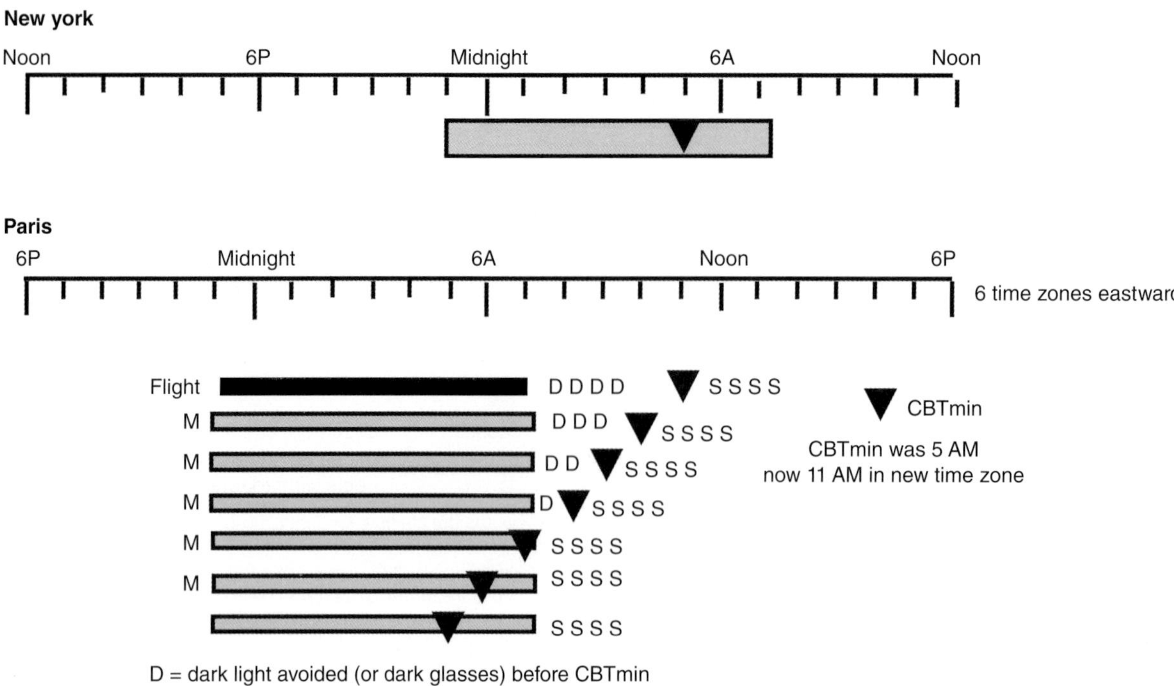

Figure 34–25 Schematic of a flight from New York to Paris (six time zones eastward). Sleep times are shown as *rectangles*, and the CBTmins as *inverted triangles*. On arrival, light is avoided (D for dark glasses) before CBTmin to prevent phase delay, and sunlight exposure is used after CBTmin (S for light exposure, ideally sunlight) to produce a phase advance. Melatonin is taken at bedtime. The circadian phase advances until the CBTmin is within the sleep period (*light blue rectangle*). However, this process takes several days. For simplicity, timing of melatonin is kept constant. A phase advance of 1 hour is shown for simplicity.

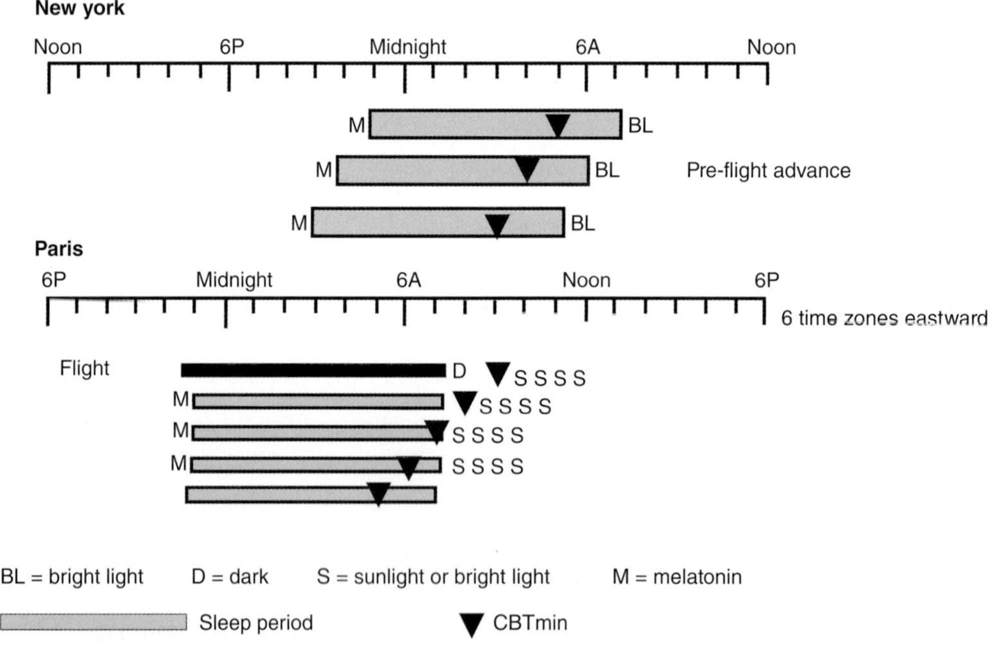

Figure 34–26 The same patient as in Figure 34–24 attempts to reduce the time required for adaptation by use of a preflight phase advance to minimize jet lag on arrival. There are fewer days until the CBTmin (*inverted triangles*) is within the desired sleep period (*light blue rectangles*). The inverted triangles are core body temperature minimum (CBTmin). At home attempts are made to go to sleep and wake up earlier. It is assumed that the phase shift is 1 hour and melatonin is given at bedtime for simplicity. In this schematic, it is also assumed that there was no change in CBTmin on the day of the flight.

sought (as long as it is after CBTmin). Evening light should be avoided on arrival at the new destination (to avoid phase delay). Melatonin before CBTmin might be useful if the hypnotic effects would not interfere with wakeful activities. Hypnotics can help with sleep but do not necessarily help with alertness the next day.[95] *Even if the individual gets adequate sleep, decreased circadian alertness will occur at the time of CBTmin.* Stimulants (caffeine) may be helpful to maintain alertness during the day in the new locale. A recent study found that 150 mg of armodafinil (R isomer of modafinil) increased wakefulness after eastward travel through six time zones.[96]

Westward Flights. The patient is phase advanced relative to local time (a phase delay is required). One could try to phase delay before travel begins (go to bed later, get up later) using evening bright light for 1 to 3 hours. Light should be avoided in the morning in the new destination (if it occurs soon after CBTmin) to prevent phase advance. Exposure to light in the evening (if before CBTmin) may be helpful (phase delay). Melatonin at bedtime in the destination, if taken before CBTmin, may have hypnotic action, but it induces phase shift in the wrong direction (phase advance). If melatonin is used, it is recommended that a small dose (to avoid prolonged hypnotic action) be taken during the last half of the night. Taking melatonin on awakening, while at the correct time for phase delay, may make the individual sleepy (counterproductive). Hypnotics at bedtime can help with sleep but do not necessarily help with alertness the next day. Even if the patients get adequate sleep, decreased circadian alertness will occur at time of CBTmin. Stimulants (caffeine) may be helpful to maintain alertness during the day in the new locale.

Crossing More Than Eight Time Zones. Exposure to light at the wrong time should be avoided because this may occur on the wrong side of CBTmin for appropriate adaptation. After **e**astward flights, avoid very **e**arly light (to avoid inappropriate phase delay); on westward flights, avoid light at dusk (to avoid inappropriate phase advance) for 2 to 3 days.[91] Thereafter, light at the usual times may help with adaptation. Conversely, as noted, some physicians recommend attempts at phase delay even if the direction of travel is eastward when more than eight time zones are crossed.

SUMMARY OF KEY POINTS

1. In humans the normal circadian period (tau) is approximately 24.2 hours (mean value). As the period is slightly longer than 24 hours, this requires a slight daily phase advance to maintain entrainment with the light-dark cycle.
2. The major circadian pacemaker in humans is the suprachiasmatic nucleus (SCN). The SCN is entrained to the light-dark cycle via light stimulation of melanopsin containing photosensitive retinal ganglion cells (pRGCs). The ganglion cells communicate via the retinohypothalamic tract (RHT) to the SCN. Blue light (short wavelength, about 460 nm) has the most potent effect. Glutamate is the major neurotransmitter of the pRGCs projecting to the SCN. Pituitary adenyl cyclase activating hormone (PACAP) is a co-neurotransmitter of pRGCs projecting to the SCN and lateral intrageniculate leaflet (IGL) in the thalamus which in turn projects to the SCN.
3. The alerting signal from the SCN increases during the day to counter the increasing homeostatic sleep drive (accumulated wakefulness since the last sleep). The alerting signal falls during the early evening to allow sleep onset and continues to fall during sleep as the homeostatic sleep drive falls. The lowest alertness occurs near the core body temperature minimum (CBTmin), about 2 hours before awakening.
4. Melatonin is secreted in darkness by the pineal gland. Light inhibits melatonin secretion by decreasing the activating influences of neurons in the paraventricular hypothalamic (PVH) nucleus. The neural pathway from the PVH neurons to the pineal gland is circuitous, passing through the spinal cord and superior cervical ganglion. Melatonin binds to receptors on the SCN and decreases the alerting signal during darkness (promoting sleep). The melatonin receptor MT1 has an effect on the alerting signal, and MT2 changes phase.
5. CBTmin occurs approximately 2 hours before the habitual wake-up time (ad-libitum schedule). The dim light melatonin onset (DLMO) occurs about 2 hours before habitual bedtime (or sleep onset) or about 7 hours before CBTmin (timing of CBTmin = DLMO + 7 hours).
6. CBTmin and DLMO can be used as markers of circadian phase. When the circadian rhythm of the body (CBTmin or DLMO) moves to a later clock time, this is said to represent a **phase delay** in circadian rhythms; to an earlier clock time, this is said to represent a **phase advance.**
7. Light after the CBTmin induces a phase advance, and light before the CBTmin induces a phase delay. Melatonin administered before the CBTmin induces a phase advance. Melatonin given after the CBTmin induces a phase delay. Bright light "pushes" and melatonin "pulls" on the circadian phase (CBTmin).
8. Sleep logs and actigraphy (for at least 7 and preferably 14 days) are used to evaluate patients with CRSWD. The sleep log and actigraphy should span at least 1 weekend or non-school/non-work period. DLMO is a very helpful marker of circadian phase, but it is not always available. The ICSD-3-TR state that sleep logs are required. A sleep log for at least 14 days is required to diagnose the Non-24-hour Sleep-Wake Rhythm Disorder.
9. DSWPD is characterized by a stable delay in sleep period relative to clock time, characterized by late sleep onset and late natural awakening. DSWPD is the most common CRSWD seen in sleep clinics. The onset is usually in adolescence or the early 20s. In DSWPD, sleep logs and actigraphy document a stable delayed sleep-onset time. Wakefulness time may vary depending on societal obligations. Up to 50% of patients with a clinical diagnosis of DSWPD do not have a delayed DLMO (non-circadian DSWPD)
10. DSWPD presents as sleep-onset insomnia or daytime sleepiness caused by short sleep period secondary to early awakening to meet obligations. If undisturbed by social obligations, patients with DSWPD have improvement in sleep quality (onset and duration) and usually awaken feeling refreshed.
11. Bright light following CBTmin or melatonin before CBTmin can induce a phase advance in patients with DSWPD, but the optimal dose and timing are unknown. The 2015 AASM clinical practice guidelines for CRSWD give a weak recommendation for appropriately scheduled melatonin for adults with or without depression or for children with or without psychiatric comorbidity. No recommendation for light treatment is provided because of the lack of controlled studies.
12. In some studies, the peak phase advance was *3 hours before DLMO for 0.5 mg melatonin and 5 hours for 3 mg melatonin.*

Only 0.3 to 0.5 mg is needed for phase shifting. Melatonin does **not** have to be given at the peak advance time for a clinical effect. In summary, melatonin should be administered *3 to 5 hours before DLMO (or about 5-7 hours before sleep onset).*

13. Typical treatments that have been used for DSPWD in small studies include bright light at or slightly before the natural (unrestricted) wake-up time (timed to follow CBTmin) or melatonin 5 to 7 hours before habitual sleep-onset time. Both melatonin and light can be used. The patient attempts to go to bed about half an hour earlier each night and awaken half an hour earlier each day. The timing of application of melatonin and light are changed to maintain the initial relationship. Once suitably shifted, appropriately timed morning light or evening melatonin can be used for maintenance. However, the most important intervention is to avoid a delay in wake-up time.
14. ASWPD is characterized by an advance in the sleep period relative to clock time characterized by early sleep onset and early awakening. It occurs most commonly in elderly individuals. Patients are more likely to complain of early morning awakening than early sleep onset. Sleep onset can be resisted for societal obligations. Sleep logs and actigraphy show a stable advance of the sleep period. Patients are "morning" types. Early morning light (e.g., early morning walks) worsen the problem by inducing further phase advance. Bright light exposure in the early morning should be avoided. Evening bright light could be tried to phase delay. Avoiding naps may also increase nocturnal sleep duration by increasing the homeostatic sleep drive. Early morning awakening can be seen in patients with depression.
15. ISWRD is characterized by at least three sleep episodes scattered throughout 24 hours. There must be a complaint of insomnia or daytime sleepiness either from the patient or caregiver. Treatments include daytime light, structured social activities, and quiet and dark at night. The 2015 clinical practice guidelines recommend light therapy (weak for) adults and melatonin in children with neurological conditions (weak for) but no melatonin in elderly patients with dementia, even if combined with light. There is a strong recommendation against use of hypnotics. If possible, administration of sedating medications should be avoided during the day and those causing insomnia avoided at night.
16. N24SWRD (free-running) is characterized by a progressive phase delay of 0.5 to 1 hour per day. It is most common in blind individuals (about 50%) but can occur in sighted individuals as well and *has been described after head trauma.* The treatment for blind patients with N24SWRD is melatonin given about 1 hour before the desired bedtime. In some studies, a lower dose (0.5 mg) was more effective than a large dose. Tasmelteon (a melatonin agonist) is an FDA-approved treatment for N24SWRD (20 mg given 1 hour before desired sleep onset). For sighted individuals, a combination of melatonin before the desired sleep onset and bright light on awakening has been successful. However, few patients appear to be able to maintain a stable schedule.
17. About 10% of patients working night shifts have complaints of difficulty staying awake at night or sleeping during the day that are severe enough to be considered a shift-work disorder (SWD). Treatment for SWD includes scheduled naps before the shift, bright light during the start of the shift, stimulants (caffeine or modafinil) at the start of the shift, dark glasses on the drive home (if after sunrise), and melatonin or hypnotics before the daytime sleep period. The major sleep period should occur soon after arriving home for work. The sleep environment should be as quiet and as dark as possible. Hypnotics may increase daytime sleep but do not seem to increase alertness at night. Decreased alertness at night is due to both decreased sleep and trying to function at the circadian time of lowest alertness.
18. Jet lag is characterized by a misalignment between endogenous circadian rhythms and local time caused by rapid travel across at least two time zones. Eastward travel requires adaptation by a phase advance, and this adaptation is more difficult than that required for westward travel. Westward travel requires adaptation by a phase delay; this adaptation is easier because of the intrinsic tendency for phase delay. Trying to avoid light at times inducing the wrong phase shift and receiving light exposure at correct times inducing the desired phase shift at the new destination is recommended. Melatonin before the desired sleep period or hypnotics may be helpful. Most individuals require about 1 day of adaptation for each time zone crossed.
19. Information from the SCN is transmitted through the ventral subparaventricular zone (vSPZ) to the dorsal medial hypothalamus (DMH). The DMH drives circadian oscillations in sleep propensity, body temperature, and hormonal secretion (cortisol).

CLINICAL REVIEW QUESTIONS

1. A 25-year-old man has difficulty falling asleep until 3:00 AM. On weekends, he sleeps until 10:30 to 11:00 AM. On workdays, he uses an alarm clock to wake up at 7:00 AM but has difficulty getting out of bed and is sleepy during the day. What time do you recommend light therapy be initially administered?
A. 6:00 AM
B. 7:00 AM
C. 8:00 AM
D. 10:00 AM

2. What is the average circadian period in humans?
A. 23.8 hours
B. 24.0 hours
C. 24.2 hours
D. 24.6 hours

3. A graph of core body temperature is shown in Figure 34–27. Bright light at which point (A, B, C, D, or E) results in the maximum phase advance?

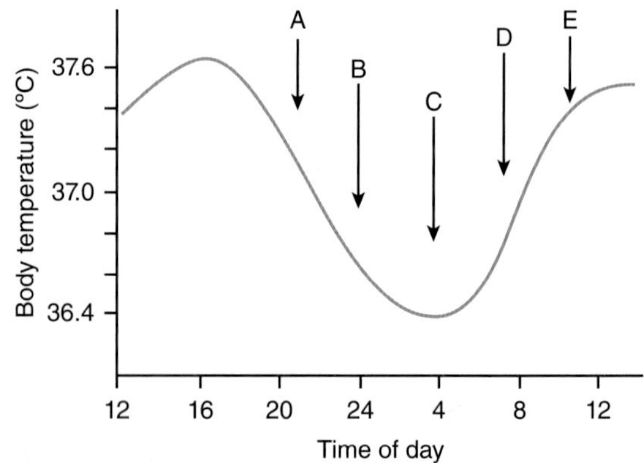

Figure 34–27 Figure for Question 3. What should the timing of light be for maximum phase advance (A, B, C, D, E)?

4. Which of the following is **NOT** true about photic input to the SCN?
   A. Nonvisual photic information travels to the SCN from the retina via the RHT.
   B. The major photosensors for entrainment of the SCN are the rods and cones.
   C. Light can entrain some blind individuals.
   D. The SCN pathway mediating inhibition of melatonin travels through the superior cervical ganglion.
   E. Blue light (wavelength 460 nm) is the most potent for phase shifting.
5. Point mutation in which gene has been associated with ASWPD?
   A. Mutation in the clock gene
   B. Mutation in the time e gene
   C. Mutation in hPer2
   D. Mutation in the alarm gene
6. What intervention would be most helpful in a patient with ASWPD?
   A. Evening light
   B. Morning light
   C. Evening melatonin
   D. Morning melatonin
7. What set of interventions in the table below would be most helpful for a **night-shift** worker? Assume that the patient gets off work and drives home after sunrise.

Possible Interventions for Night-Shift Workers

A	Bright light at the start of the shift	Dark glasses on the drive home	Nap before night shift
B	Bright light at the end of the shift	Dark glasses on the drive home	Nap before the night shift
C	Bright light at the start of the shift	Delay bedtime until 11:00 AM	Nap before drive home in the morning
D	Bright light at the end of the shift	Delay bedtime until 11:00 AM	Nap before the night shift

8. A blind patient is found to have N24SWRD. His desired bedtime is 11:00 PM. What treatment do you recommend?
   A. Melatonin 5 mg at 8 AM
   B. Melatonin 5 mg at 10 PM
   C. Melatonin 0.5 mg at 7 PM
   D. Melatonin 0.5 mg at 10 PM
9. A businessman travels 5 hours eastward. What time should light be avoided in the new time zone?
   A. 6:00 AM to 9:00 AM
   B. 11:00 AM to 2:00 PM
   C. 2:00 AM to 6:00 PM
10. A patient with DSWPD has a habitual sleep-onset time of 3:00 AM and wake-up time of 11:00 AM on the weekends. When should **melatonin** be administered?
    A. 3:00 AM
    B. 2:00 AM
    C. Midnight
    D. 9:00 PM
11. Which of the following is **NOT** true about DLMO?
    A. It occurs about 2 hours before habitual bedtime time.
    B. In DSWPD, the **DLMO** is earlier than that of a normal individual.
    C. It is measured with the subject in dim light.
    D. Typical threshold values are 3 pg/mL for salivary and 10 pg/mL for plasma melatonin.
12. A patient with DSWPD has a typical wake-up time on the weekends around 1:00 PM. He typically awakens at 8:30 AM to make a 10:00 AM class. He read that morning light is helpful for his problem and received light exposure by walking to class from approximately 9:00 AM to 10:00 AM). Unfortunately, using this regimen, he is unable to fall asleep any earlier. What do you recommend for initial treatment?
    A. Wear dark glasses on the walk to the 10:00 AM class and get bright light exposure for 1 hour starting at 3:00 PM.
    B. Wake up at 8 AM, light box for 1 hour, and light exposure on the walk to the 10:00 AM class.
    C. Wear dark glasses on the walk to the 10:00 AM class, bright light exposure after or slightly before 1:00 PM.
    D. Continue present light exposure, add melatonin 5 hours before habitual bedtime.
13. A professor is traveling from Boston to Los Angeles. What combination is true?
    A. In Los Angles he is phase advanced and to minimize jet lag should go to bed **earlier before the trip** (while in Boston).
    B. In Los Angeles he is phase delayed and should go to bed earlier **before the trip** (while in Boston) to minimize jet lag.
    C. In Los Angles he is phase advanced and should go to bed later **before the trip** (while in Boston) to minimize jet lag.
    D. In Los Angeles he is phase delayed and should go to bed later **before the trip** (while in Boston) to minimize jet lag.

ANSWERS

1. D. This patient has DSWPD. It is important to use bright light treatment after the CBTmin. The timing of the CBTmin is not known but can be estimated from the spontaneous wake-up time. In normal subjects, the CBTmin occurs about 2 hours before the spontaneous wake-up time. It may be somewhat earlier in patients with DSWPD. With a normal wake-up time (unrestricted by societal demands) of 11:00 AM, one could estimate a CBTmin around 9:00 AM or slightly earlier. Using light soon after the spontaneous wake-up time from 10:30-11:00 AM would also be appropriate. Of interest, the patient is exposed to light on his way to work (6:00–7:00 AM). This is on the phase advanced side of his temperature minimum and worsens the problem. If after sunrise, use of light-reducing glasses is an option.
2. C. 24.2 hours.

3. D. The maximum phase advance for bright light occurs about 3 to 4 hours after the CBTmin. C is at the CBTmin, the transition between the phase delay and phase advance regions. Light at A and B would phase delay. Light at E would have less of a phase-advancing effect.
4. B. The major photosensors are the retinal ganglion cells containing melanopsin.
5. C. Mutation of the hPer2 gene has been associated with familial ASWPD. A mutation in hPer3 has been associated with DSWPD. Mneumonic: hPer2 has a lower number than hPer3, and advanced comes before delay.
6. A. Evening light will cause phase delay. Morning melatonin will also cause phase delay, but the hypnotic effects are undesirable for most patients.
7. A. Bright light at the start of the shift, dark glasses on the way home, going to bed upon arrival at home, and a nap before the shift are suggested interventions. Light at the end of the shift could occur after CBTmin (exact time unknown) and is more likely to cause phase advance. Exposure to daylight on the way home or during the first hours at home could phase advance. A phase delay so that CBTmin is within the daytime sleep period is desirable.
8. D. Melatonin given 1 hour before the desired bedtime is recommended. Although 5 mg may work, some patients will fail to entrain on 5 mg but will entrain on a lower dose. However, the AASM practice parameters do not recommend a specific time or dose.
9. A. If the baseline CBTmin is assumed to be 4:00 AM, this corresponds to 9:00 AM in the new time zone. The patient must phase advance for adaptation. Light for several hours before the CBTmin induces the most significant phase delay. Light exposure should be avoided before 9:00 AM and pursued from 11:00 AM to 2:00 PM to induce the maximum phase-advancing effect. Light from 6:00 to 9:00 AM may cause phase delay. Light from 2:00 to 6:00 PM is so far away from the CBTmin that it has less effect.
10. D. Melatonin should be administered 5 to 7 hours before habitual bedtime (or sleep-onset time) or 3 to 5 hours before DLMO for phase advancement. Some studies found that, when using a higher dose of melatonin (3 mg versus 0.5 mg), administration of the higher dose at an early time compared to the lower dose (relative to DLMO) may be more effective.
11. B. DLMO occurs about 2 to 3 hours before habitual bedtime (or sleep-onset time). In DSWPD, the DLMO is later than in normal individuals. (Answer B is the incorrect statement.)
12. C. The patient's CBTmin is probably around 11:00 AM (2 hours before typical wake time on weekends). However, the exact time of the CBTmin is not known. Avoiding bright light exposure before 11:00 AM will avoid an unwanted phase delay. Seeking bright light exposure for 1 to 2 hours at or after after 1:00 PM (about 2 hours after CBTmin) should induce a phase advance. Bright light exposure at 3:00 PM will be less effective that light exposure closer to the CBTmin. Melatonin taken 5 hours before the habitual bedtime may help phase advance. However, continuing the current light exposure will induce a phase delay.
13. C. In Los Angeles he is phase advanced and needs to phase delay, he should go to bed later before the trip while in Boston and get up later if possible.

REFERENCES

1. American Academy of Sleep Medicine. *International Classification of Sleep Disorders*. 3rd ed. text revision. Darien, IL: American Academy of Sleep Medicine; 2023.
2. Zee PC, Manthena P. The brain's master circadian clock: implications and opportunities for therapy of sleep disorders. *Sleep Med Rev*. 2007;11:59-70.
3. Benarroch EE. Suprachiasmatic nucleus and melatonin: reciprocal interactions and clinical correlations. *Neurology*. 2008;71(8):594-598.
4. Zee PC, Abbott SM. Circadian rhythm sleep-wake disorders. *Continuum (Minneap Minn)*. 2020;26(4):988-1002.
5. Czeisler CA, Duffy JF, Shanahan TL, et al. Stability, precision, and nearly 24 hour period of the human circadian pacemaker. *Sleep*. 1999;284:2177-2181.
6. Gooley JJ, Saper CB. Anatomy of the mammalian circadian system. In: Kryger MH, Roth T, Dement WC, eds. *Principles and Practice of Sleep Medicine*. Philadelphia: Elsevier Saunders; 2005:335-350.
7. Dijk DJ, Archer SN. Light, sleep, and circadian rhythms: together again. *PLoS Biol*. 2009;7:1000145.
8. Brzezinski A. Melatonin in humans. *N Engl J Med*. 1997;336:186-195.
9. Reid KJ, Zee PC Circadian rhythm disorders. *Semin Neurol*. 2009;29: 393-405.
10. Emens JS, Burgess HJ. Effect of light and melatonin and other melatonin receptor agonists on human circadian physiology. *Sleep Med Clin*. 2015;10(4): 435-453.
11. Edgar DM, Dement WC, Fuller CA. Effect of SCN lesions on sleep in the squirrel monkey: evidence for opponent processes in sleep-wake regulation. *J Neuorsci*. 1993;13:1065-1079.
12. Duffy JF, Dijk DJ, Klerman EB. Czeisler CA. Later endogenous circadian temperature nadir relative to an earlier wake time in older people. *Am J Physiol*. 1998;275;R1478-R1487.
13. Czeisler CA, Buxton OM, Khalsa SBS. The human circadian timing system and sleep-wake regulation. In: Kryger MH, Roth T, Dement WC, eds. *Principles and Practice of Sleep Medicine*. 4th ed. Philadelphia: Elsevier Saunders; 2005;375-394.
14. Fahey CD, Zee PC. Circadian rhythm sleep disorder and phototherapy. *Psychiatr Clin North Am*. 2006;29:989-1007.
15. Burgess HJ, Eastman CI. The dim light melatonin onset following fixed and free sleep schedules. *J Sleep Res*. 2005;14(3):229-237.
16. Crowley SJ, Acebo C, Fallone G, Carskadon MA. Estimating dim light melatonin onset (DLMO) phase in adolescents using summer or school-year sleep/wake schedules. *Sleep*. 2006;29(12):1632-1641.
17. Burgess HJ, Savic N, Sletten T, Roach G, Gilbert SS, Dawson D. The relationship between the dim light melatonin onset and sleep on a regular schedule in young healthy adults. *Behav Sleep Med*. 2003;1(2):102-114.
18. Pandi-Perumal SR, Smits M, Spence W, et al. Dim light melatonin onset (DLMO): a tool for the analysis of circadian phase in human sleep and chronobiological disorders. *Prog Neuropsychopharmacol Biol Psychiatry*. 2007; 31(1):1-11.
19. Kennaway DJ. The dim light melatonin onset across ages, methodologies, and sex and its relationship with morningness/eveningness. *Sleep*. 2023;46(5):zsad033. doi:10.1093/sleep/zsad033.
20. Burgess HJ, Fogg LF. Individual differences in the amount and timing of salivary melatonin secretion. *PLoS One*. 2008;3(8):e3055.
21. Ruiz FS, Beijamini F, Beale AD, et al. Early chronotype with advanced activity rhythms and dim light melatonin onset in a rural population. *J Pineal Res*. 2020;69(3):e12675.
22. Wyatt JK, Stepanski EJ, Kirkby J. Circadian phase in delayed sleep phase syndrome: predictors and temporal stability across multiple assessments. *Sleep*. 2006;29:1075-1080.
23. Sack RK, Brandes RW, Kendall AR, Lewy AJ. Entrainment of free-running circadian rhythms by melatonin in blind people. *N Engl J Med*. 2000;343;1070-1077.
24. Khalsa SBS, Jewett ME, Cajocen C, Czeisler CA. A phase response curve to single bright light pulses in human subjects. *J Physiol*. 2003;549:945-952.
25. Lu BS, Zee PC. Circadian rhythm sleep disorders. *Chest*. 2006;130: 1915-1923.
26. Barion A, Zee PC. A clinical approach to circadian rhythm sleep disorders. *Sleep Med*. 2007;8:566-577.
27. Shirani A, St. Louis EK. Illuminating rationale and uses for light therapy. *J Clin Sleep Med*. 2009;5:155-163.
28. Zeitzer JM, Dijk DJ, Kronauer RE, et al. Sensitivity of human circadian pacemaker to nocturnal light: melatonin resetting and suppression. *J Physiol*. 2000;526:695-702.
29. Lockley SW, Brainard GC, Czeisler CA. High sensitivity of the human circadian melatonin rhythm to resetting by short wavelength light. *J Clin Endocrinol Metab*. 2003:88:4502-4505.

30. Smith MR, Eastman CR. Phase delaying the human circadian clock with blue-enriched polychromatic light. *Chronobiol Int*. 2009;26:709-725.
31. Rimmer DW, Boivin DB, Shanahan TL, et al. Dynamic resetting of the human circadian pacemaker by intermittent bright light. *Am J Physiol Regul Integr Comp Physiol*. 2000;279:R1574-R1579.
32. Gronifer C, Wright KP, Kronauer RE, et al. Efficacy of a single sequence of intermittent bright light pulses for delaying circadian phase in humans. *Am J Physiol Endocrinol Metab*. 2004:287:E174-E181.
33. Revell VL, Molina TA, Eastman CI. Human phase response curve to intermittent blue light using a commercially available device. *J Physiol*. 2012;590(19):4859-4868.
34. Lewy AJ, Bauer VK, Ahmed S, et al. The human phase response curve (PRC) to melatonin is about 12 hours out of phase with the PRC to light. *Chronobiol Int*. 1998;15:71-83.
35. Burgess HJ, Revell VL, Eastman CI. A three pulse phase response curve to 3 milligrams of melatonin in humans. *J Physiol*. 2008;586:639-647.
36. Eastman CI, Burgess HJ. How to travel the world without jet lag. *Sleep Med Clin*. 2009;4:241-255.
37. Vitaterna MH, Pinto LH, Turek FW. Molecular genetic basis for mammalian circadian rhythms. In: Kryger MH, Roth T, Dement WC, eds. *Principles and Practice of Sleep Medicine*. 4th ed. Philadelphia: Elsevier Saunders; 2005:335-350.
38. Piggins HD. Human clock genes. *Ann Med*. 2002;34:394-400.
39. Sack RL, Auckley D, Auger R, et al. Circadian rhythm sleep disorders: part I, basic principles, shift work and jet lag Disorders. *Sleep*. 2007;30: 1460-1483.
40. Sack RL, Auckley D, Auger R, et al. Circadian rhythm sleep disorders: part II, advanced sleep phase disorder, delayed sleep phase disorder, free-running disorder, and irregular sleep-wake rhythm. *Sleep*. 2007;30: 1484-1501.
41. Morgenthaler TI, Lee-Chiong T, Alessi C, et al. Practice parameters for the clinical evaluation and treatment of circadian rhythm sleep disorders. *Sleep*. 2007;30:1445-1459.
42. Auger RR, Burgess HJ, Emens JS, Deriy LV, Thomas SM, Sharkey KM. Clinical practice guideline for the treatment of intrinsic circadian rhythm sleep-wake disorders: advanced sleep-wake phase disorder (ASWPD), delayed sleep-wake phase disorder (DSWPD), non-24-hour sleep-wake rhythm disorder (N24SWRD), and irregular sleep-wake rhythm disorder (ISWRD). An update for 2015: an American Academy of Sleep Medicine clinical practice guideline. *J Clin Sleep Med*. 2015;11(10):1199-1236.
43. Horne JA, Ostberg O. A self-assessment questionnaire to determine morningness-eveningness in human circadian rhythms. *Int J Chronobiol*. 1976;4:97-110.
44. Wyatt JK. Delayed sleep phase syndrome: pathophysiology and treatment options. *Sleep*. 2004;27:1195-1203.
45. Murray JM, Sletten TL, Magee M, et al. Prevalence of circadian misalignment and its association with depressive symptoms in delayed sleep phase disorder. *Sleep*. 2017;40(1):zsw002.
46. Archer SN, Robillard DL, Skenen DJ, et al. A length polymorphism in the circadian clock gene Per3 is linked to delayed sleep phase syndrome and extreme diurnal preference. *Sleep*. 2003;26:413-415.
47. Hohjoh H, Takasu M, Shishikura K, et al. Significant association of the arylalkylamine N-acetyltransferase (AA-NAT) gene with delayed sleep phase syndrome. *Neurogenetics*. 2003;4:151-153.
48. Patke A, Murphy PJ, Onat OE, et al. Mutation of the human circadian clock gene CRY1 in familial delayed sleep phase disorder. *Cell*. 2017;169(2):203-215.e13.
49. Watson LA, McGlashan EM, Hosken IT, Anderson C, Phillips AJK, Cain SW. Sleep and circadian instability in delayed sleep-wake phase disorder. J Clin Sleep Med. 2020;16(9):1431-1436.
50. Uchiyama M, Okawa M, Shibui K, et al. Altered phase relation between sleep timing and core body temperature in delayed sleep phase syndrome and non-24 hour sleep-wake syndromes in humans. *Neurosci Lett*. 2000;294:101-104.
51. Watanabe T, Kajimura N, Masaaki K, et al. Sleep and circadian rhythm disturbances in patients with delayed sleep phase syndrome. *Sleep*. 2003;26:657-661.
52. Mundey K, Benloucif S, Harsanyhi K, et al. Phase-dependent treatment of delayed sleep phase syndrome with melatonin. *Sleep*. 2005;28:1271-1278.
53. Burgess HJ, Park M, Wyatt JK, Rizvydeen M, Fogg LF. Sleep and circadian variability in people with delayed sleep-wake phase disorder versus healthy controls. *Sleep Med*. 2017;34:33-39.
54. Czeisler CA, Richardson GS, Coleman RM, et al. Chronotherapy: resetting the circadian clocks of patients with delayed sleep phase insomnia. *Sleep*. 1981:4:1-21.
55. Rosenthal NE, Joseph-Vanderpool JR, Levendosky AA, et al. Phase-shifting effects of bright morning light as treatment for delayed sleep phase syndrome. *Sleep*. 1990;13:354-361.
56. Watanabe T, Kajimura N, Kato M, et al. Effects of phototherapy in patients with delayed sleep phase syndrome. *Psychiatry Clin Neurosci*. 1999;53:231-233.
57. Bjorvatn B, Pallesen S. A practical approach to circadian rhythm sleep disorders. *Sleep Med Rev*. 2009;13:47-60.
58. Nagtegall JE, Kerkhof A, Smits MG, et al. Delayed sleep phase syndrome: a placebo controlled cross-over study on the effects of melatonin administered five hour before the individual dim light melatonin onset. *J Sleep Res*. 1998;7:135-143.
59. Sletten TL, Magee M, Murray JM, et al. Efficacy of melatonin with behavioural sleep-wake scheduling for delayed sleep-wake phase disorder: a double-blind, randomised clinical trial. *PLoS Med*. 2018;15(6):e1002587.
60. Revell VL, Burgess HJ, Gazda CJ, et al. Advancing human circadian rhythms with afternoon melatonin and morning intermittent bright light. *J Clin Endocrinol Metab*. 2006;91:54-59.
61. Jones CR, Campbell SS, Zone SE, et al. Familial advanced sleep phase syndrome: a short-period circadian rhythm variant in humans. *Nat Med*. 1999;5:1062-1065.
62. Toh KL, Jones CR, Yan HE, et al. An hPer2 phosphorylation site mutation in familial advanced sleep phase syndrome. *Science*. 2001;291:1040-1043.
63. Auger RR. Advanced related sleep complaints and advanced sleep phase disorder. *Sleep Med Clin*. 2009;4:219-227.
64. Moldofsky H, Musisi S, Phillipson EA. Treatment of a case of advanced sleep phase syndrome by phase advance chronotherapy. *Sleep*. 1986;9:61-65.
65. Lack L, Wright H, Kemp K, et al. The treatment of early morning awakening insomnia with two evenings of bright light. *Sleep*. 2005;28:616-623.
66. Zee PC, Vitiello MV. Circadian rhythm disorder: irregular sleep wake rhythm. *Sleep Med Clin*. 2009;4:213-218.
67. Ancoli-Israek S, Martin JL, Kripke DF, et al. Effect of light treatment on sleep and circadian rhythms in demented nursing home patients. *J Am Geriatr Soc*. 2002;50:282-289.
68. Singer C, Trachtenberg RE, Kaye J, et al. A multicenter, placebo controlled trial of melatonin for sleep disturbance in Alzheimer's disease. *Sleep*. 2003;26:893-901.
69. Riemersma-ven der Lek RF, Swaab DF, Twisk J, et al. Effect of bright light and melatonin on cognitive and noncognitive function in elderly residents of group care facilities. *JAMA*. 2008;299:2642-2655.
70. Pillar G, Shahar E, Peled N, et al. Melatonin improves sleep wake patterns in psychomotor retarded children. *Pediatr Neurol*. 2000;23:225-228.
71. Herring WJ, Ceesay P, Snyder E, et al. Polysomnographic assessment of suvorexant in patients with probable Alzheimer's disease dementia and insomnia: a randomized trial. *Alzheimers Dement*. 2020;16(3):541-551.
72. Hayakawa T, Uchiyama M, Kamei Y, et al. Clinical analysis of sighted patients with non-24 hour sleep-wake syndrome. *Sleep*. 2005;28:945-952.
73. Malkani RG, Abbott SM, Reid KJ, Zee PC. Diagnostic and treatment challenges of sighted non–24-hour sleep-wake disorder. *J Clin Sleep Med*. 2018;14(4):603-613.
74. Boivin DB, James FO, Santo BA, et al. Non-24-hour sleep-wake syndrome following a car accident. *Neurology*. 2003;60:1841-1843.
75. Sack RL, Brandes RW, Kendall AR, Lewy AJ. Entrainment of free-running circadian rhythms by melatonin in blind people. *N Engl J Med*. 2000;343(15):1070-1077.
76. Lewy AJ, Emens JS, Lefler BJ, et al. Melatonin entrains free-running blind people according to a physiological dose response curve. *Chronobiol Int*. 2005;22:1093-1106.
77. Lewy AJ, Bauer VK, Hasler BP, et al. Capturing the circadian rhythms of free-running blind individuals with 0.5 mg of melatonin. *Brain Res*. 2001;918:96-100.
78. Lewy AJ, Emens JS, Sack RL, Hasler BP, Bernert RA. Low, but not high, doses of melatonin entrained a free-running blind person with a long circadian period. *Chronobiol Int*. 2002;19(3):649-658.
79. Lavedan C, Forsberg M, Gentile AJ. Tasimelteon: a selective and unique receptor binding profile. *Neuropharmacology*. 2015;91:142-147. doi:10.1016/j.neuropharm.2014.12.004.
80. Lockley SW, Dressman MA, Licamele L, :>et al. Tasimelteon for non-24-hour sleep-wake disorder in totally blind people (SET and RESET): two multicentre, randomised, double-masked, placebo-controlled phase 3 trials. *Lancet*. 2015;386(10005):1754-1764.
81. Boivin DB, James FO. Circadian adaptation to night-shift work by judicious light and dark exposure. *J Biol Rhythms*. 2002;17:556-567.
82. Sallinen M, Harma M, Akerstedt T, et al. Promoting alertness with a short nap during a night shift. *J Sleep Res*. 1998;7:240-247.

83. Schweitzer PK, Randazzo AC, Stone K, et al. Laboratory and field studies of naps and caffeine as practical countermeasures for sleep-wake problems associated with night work. *Sleep*. 2006;29:39-50.
84. Crowley SJ, Tseng CU, Fogg LF, Eastman CI. Complete or partial re-entrainment improves performance, alertness, and mood during shift-work. *Sleep*. 2004;27:1077-1087.
85. Crowley SJ, Tseng CY, Fogg LF, et al. Combinations of bright light, scheduled dark, sunglasses, and melatonin to facilitate circadian entrainment to night shift work. *J Biol Rhythms*. 2003;18:513-523.
86. Smith MR, Lee C, Crowley SJ, et al. Morning melatonin has limited benefit as a soporific for daytime sleep after night work. *Chronobiol Int*. 2005:22:873-888.
87. Sharkey KM, Eastman CI. Melatonin phase shift human circadian rhythms in a placebo controlled simulated night-work study. *Am J Physiol Regul Integr Comp Physiol*. 2002;282:R454-R463.
88. Bjorvatn B, Stangenes K, Oyane N, et al. Randomized placebo-controlled field study of the effects of bright light and melatonin in adaptation to shift work. *Scand J Work Environ Health*. 2007;33:204-214.
89. Czeisler CA, Walsh JK, Roth T, et al. Modafinil for excessive sleepiness associated with shift-work sleep disorder. *N Engl J Med*. 2005;353:476-486.
90. Czeisler CA, Walsh JK, Wesnew KA, et al. Armodafinil for treatment of excessive sleepiness associated with shift work disorder: a randomized controlled study. *Mayo Clin Proc*. 2009;84:958-972.
91. Walsh JK, Sugerman JL, Muehlback MJ, et al. Physiological sleep tendency on a simulated night shift: adaptation and effects of triazolam. *Sleep*. 1988;12:251-264.
92. Sack RL. Jet lag. *N Engl J Med*. 2010;362:440-447.
93. Eastman CI, Gazda CJ, Burgess HJ, et al. Advancing circadian rhythms before eastward flight: a strategy to prevent or reduce jet lag. *Sleep*. 2005;28:33-44.
94. Revell VL, Eastman CI. How to trick mother nature into letting you fly around or stay up all night. *J Biol Rhythm*. 2005;20:353-365.
95. Jamieson AO, Zammit GK, Rosenberg RS, et al. Zolpidem reduces the sleep disturbance of jet lag. *Sleep Med*. 2001;2:423-430.
96. Rosenberg RP, Bogan RK, Tiller JM, et al. A phase 3, double-blind, randomized, placebo-controlled study of armodafinil for excessive sleepiness associated with jet lag disorder. *Mayo Clin Proc*. 2010;85:630-638.

Clinical Electroencephalography and Nocturnal Epilepsy

Chapter 35

ELECTROENCEPHALOGRAPHIC (EEG) MONITORING

The location of electroencephalographic (EEG) electrodes using the international 10-20 system is illustrated in Figures 35–1 and 35–2. Each electrode is represented by a letter that refers to the underlying area or lobe of the brain (Fp = frontopolar; F = frontal; P = parietal; O = occipital; T = temporal) and numbers that specify the electrode position. The odd numbers are on the left and the even on the right, and "z" refers to electrodes in the midline. The numbers are often displayed as subscripts. The nomenclature "10-20" refers to the fact that the electrodes are positioned at 10 or 20% of the distance between landmarks such as the nasion, inion, or preauricular points (Figure 35-2).[1-6] The left and right auricular (earlobe) electrodes are A1 and A2. In sleep monitoring, these are placed on the mastoids and appropriately called M1 and M2. Figure 35–1 illustrates the new electrode nomenclature[3-5] in which T3, T4, T5, and T6 have been replaced by T7, T8, P7, and P8. In the new nomenclature, all electrodes in each sagittal plane have the same number (F7, T7, P7), and most electrodes in the same coronal plane have the same letter (P7, P3, Pz, P4, P8). However, many EEG laboratories still use the old electrode nomenclature, as does most of the published literature on epilepsy. A schematic of brain areas of interest for epilepsy and EEG monitoring[7] is shown in Figure 35–3. The central sulcus is also known as the central fissure or the Rolandic fissure and separates the frontal and parietal lobes.

BIPOLAR MONITORING AND STANDARD MONTAGES

A derivation is the voltage difference between electrodes: for example, Fp1–F3 is the voltage difference between electrodes Fp1 and F3. By EEG convention, if Fp1 is more negative than F3, the deflection is up.[5] A set of derivations is called a montage. Montages are designed with a particular purpose in mind. Standard clinical EEG montages are illustrated in Tables 35–1 and 35–2 and Figures 35–4 and 35–5.[5,8] **Bipolar longitudinal montages** sequentially compare two adjacent electrodes in chains covering the head in an anteroposterior (AP) direction ("double banana"). In the most frequently used variant (LB-18.1), the chains start at the left temporal area and then progressively move toward the right (Table 35–1 and Figure 35–4). The other commonly used montage (LB-18.3) consists of left temporal-right temporal left central-right central arrangement of derivations. Bipolar transverse montages compare two electrodes in chains in the transverse directions (Table 35–2 and Figure 35–5). **Referential montages** compare electrodes to the ipsilateral auricular electrodes A1 and A2 (actually M1 and M2, see Table 35–2 and Figure 35–5). Different laboratories may display the electrodes in a montage using different sequences. In modern digital EEG recordings, all electrodes are usually recorded against a common reference electrode (REF). Then, any two electrodes may be compared by digitally subtracting the signals (F7-REF) – (P7-REF) = F7–P7. In some systems, the reference consists of two or more linked electrodes (M1-C3-C4-M2). Using referentially recorded electrodes, one can change the display montage to show a derivation between any two referentially recorded electrodes while recording or later during study review.

Digital recording also allows one to visualize multiple time scales. The polysomnography (PSG) window to stage sleep is 30 seconds, but the clinical EEG window is 10 seconds. The 10-second time window allows detection of sharply contoured (narrow) waveforms that may signify seizure activity. In the 30-second window, a *spike* (20 to 70 milliseconds) would appear as a single vertical line. If the capacity to add a few electrodes to traditional sleep monitoring exists, one can increase the ability to detect interictal epileptiform activity (epileptiform activity between seizures). For example, one could add two electrodes (T7, T8—also known as T3, T4). The derivations F3-T7, T7-O1, F4-T8, and T8-O2 would add coverage over much of the frontal and temporal areas. These areas are the predominant foci of seizures occurring mainly during sleep. Some studies have tried to define the best minimal montage for detecting seizures with some improved detection of temporal lobe but not frontal lobe seizures.[9] Table 35–3 shows some examples of bipolar montages that can be used with typically recorded electrodes during sleep monitoring.

In sleep montages with a 30-second window, interictal activity appears sharper and often with a higher amplitude than on EEG monitoring (150 μV peak to peak during sleep monitoring vs. 200 μV peak to peak in EEG). *Interictal activity* (isolated epileptiform activity) often manifests as *repetitive occurrences of nearly identical patterns that have a sharp or spiky appearance (brief duration) that may be easier to appreciate using a 10 second compared to 30 second window.* If interictal activity is suspected, one should change to a 10-second window (the time window used in clinical EEG monitoring) and change to a bipolar montage. The 10-second window allows improved recognition of spikes and other epileptiform waveforms. Bipolar montages are useful for localization, as will be discussed.

IMPORTANCE OF VIDEO MONITORING

The addition of synchronized digital video and audio monitoring to nocturnal EEG or PSG recording greatly enhances the ability of the clinician to diagnose nocturnal events.[6,10] The EEG can be obscured by muscle artifact during a parasomnia or seizure but, the behavior during the event may help identify the type of event. If more than one event occurs during a single night, events that are manifestations of focal

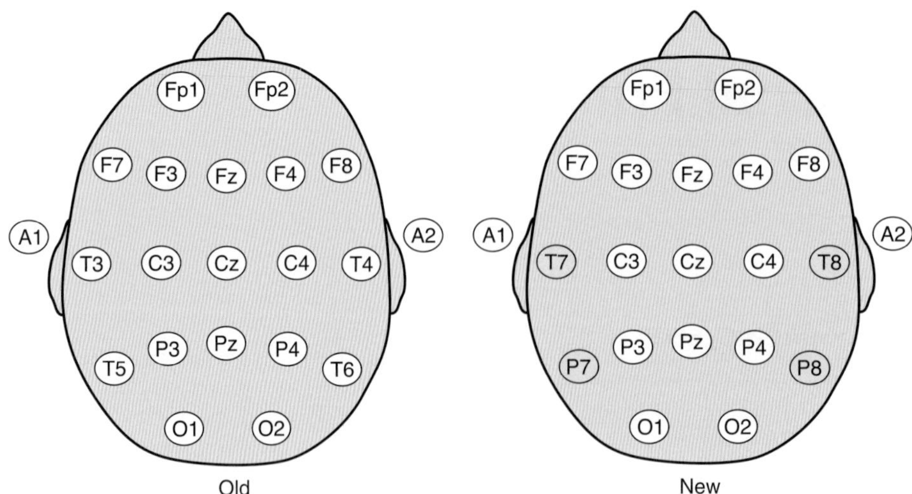

Figure 35–1 10-20 Electrode Placement. The new nomenclature renames some of the electrodes. Electrodes T3, T4, T5, and T6 are now T7, T8, P7, and P8, respectively. (From Berry RB. *Fundamentals of Sleep Medicine*. Elsevier; 2012:546.)

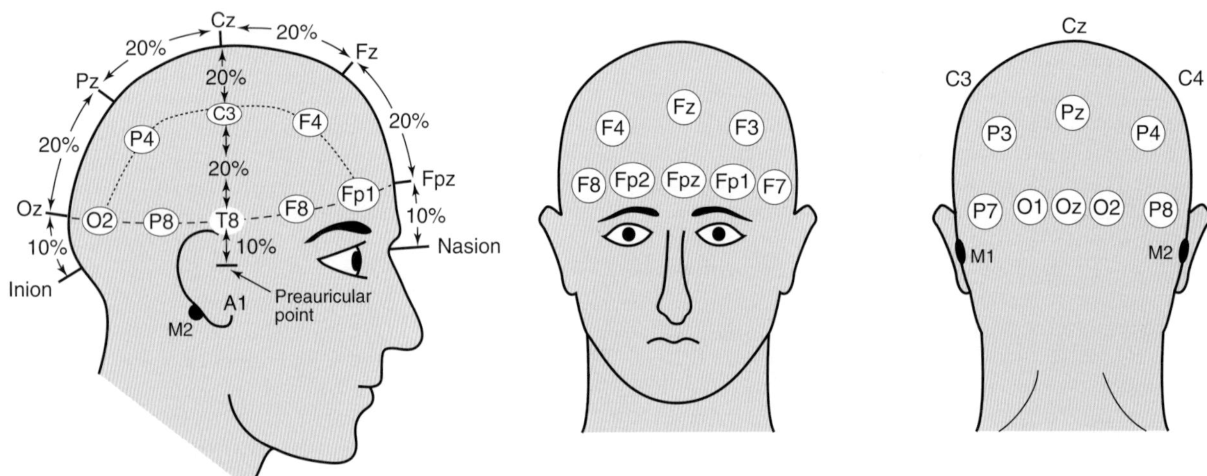

Figure 35–2 10-20 System of Electrode Placement. All electrodes are placed either 10% or 20% of the distance between two standard landmarks. (From Berry RB. *Fundamentals of Sleep Medicine*. Elsevier; 2012:546.)

seizures are nearly the same (stereotypic), while parasomnia events usually manifest variable behavior. Many nocturnal seizure disorders are not associated with scalp EEG findings, and the patient's actions during the event (semiology) may be very helpful in determining whether an episode is likely a parasomnia or nocturnal epilepsy. Some types of epilepsy manifest characteristic behaviors, and this may help provide a clue to the seizure focus.[11,12] For the physician reading a sleep study, the semiology is often more important than the EEG for differentiating typical non-rapid eye movement (NREM) parasomnias from nocturnal focal epilepsy.

WAVEFORM TERMINOLOGY

A **transient** is any isolated wave or complex that stands out compared with background activity. A **spike** is defined as a transient with a pointed peak and a duration of **20 to 70 milliseconds** (Table 35–4, Figure 35–6). On a 30-second page, spikes look like a single vertical line. A **sharp wave** is a transient with a deflection of **70 to 200 milliseconds** (measured at the base). This duration is typical of the epilepsy literature, although in the American Academy of Sleep Medicine (AASM) scoring manual, a vertex sharp wave is required to have a duration less than 0.5 seconds.[6] A **spike and wave complex** consists of a spike followed by a slow wave (usually wide and often high amplitude). Polyspike complexes often consist of multiple spikes superimposed on a slow wave. The term *epileptiform activity* literally means "EEG activity resembling that found in patients with epilepsy." This is a somewhat circular definition. Epileptiform activity includes spike, spike and wave, and polyspike complexes. Abnormal sharp waves are also considered epileptiform or interictal activity. However, sharp waves can be normal (e.g., vertex sharp waves).

Interictal and Ictal Activity

Epileptiform activity is separated into interictal and ictal discharges (Table 35–4 and Box 35–1).

As noted, **interictal activity** (interictal epileptiform discharges, or IEDs) is defined as abnormal EEG activity (epileptiform) that occurs between clinical seizures.[13-15] The activity is usually composed of spike and wave complexes or sharp waves. The activity may be transient, focal, or generalized

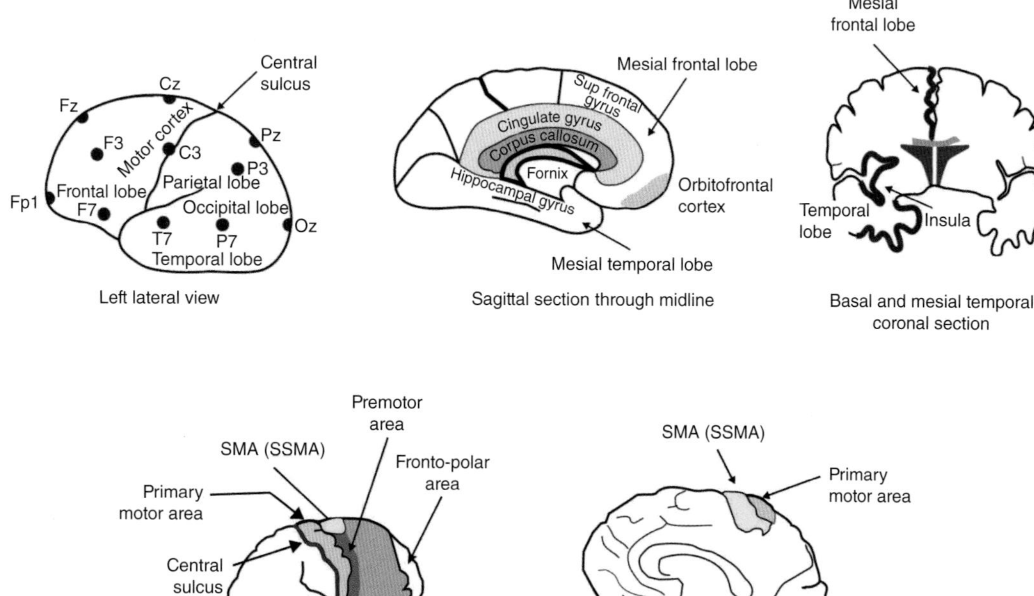

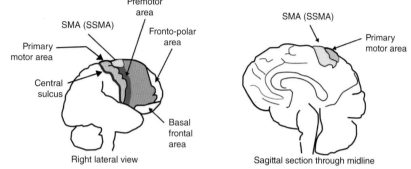

Figure 35–3 Areas of the Brain Important for Epilepsy. Note the location of the supplemental motor area (SMA), insula, and basal and mesial areas of the temporal lobe.

Table 35–1 Longitudinal Bipolar (AP Bipolar) 18 Channel "Double Banana"

LB-18.1		LB-18.2		LB-18.3	
Fp1-F7	Left temporal	Fz-Cz	Vertex	Fp1-F7	Left temporal
F7-T7		Cz-Pz		F7-T7	
T7-P7				T7-P7	
P7-O1		Fp1-F3	Left parasagittal	P7-O1	
		F3-C3			
Fp1-F3	Left parasagittal	C3-P3		Fp2-F8	Right temporal
F3-C3		P3-O1		F8-T8	
C3-P3				T8-P8	
P3-O1		Fp2-F4	Right parasagittal	P8-O2	
		F4-C4			
Fz-Cz	Vertex	C4-P4		Fp1-F3	Left parasagittal
Cz-Pz		P4-O2		F3-C3	
				C3-P3	
Fp2-F4	Right parasagittal	Fp1-F7	Left temporal	P3-O1	
F4-C4		F7-T7			
C4-P4		T7-P7		Fp2-F4	Right parasagittal
P4-O2		P7-O1		F4-C4	
				C4-P4	
Fp2-F8	Right temporal	Fp2-F8	Right temporal	P4-O2	
F8-T8		F8-T8			
T8-P8		T8-P8		Fz-Cz	Vertex
P8-O2		P8-O2		Cz-Pz	

See Figure 35–4.
American Clinical Neurophysiology Society: Guideline 6: a proposal for standard montages to be used in clinical EEG. *J Clin Neurophysiol.* 2006;23:111-117.

Table 35–2 Transverse Bipolar and Referential

Transverse – Bipolar (TB-18.1)	Transverse – Bipolar (TB-18.2)	Referential (R18-1)
F7-Fp1	Fp1-Fp2	F7-A1
Fp1-Fp2		T7-A1
Fp2-F8	F7-F3	P7-A1
	F3-Fz	
F7-F3	Fz-F4	Fp1-A1
F3-Fz	F4-F8	F3-A1
Fz-F4		C3- A1
F4-F8	A1-T7	P3-A1
	T7-C3	O1-A1
T7-C3	C3-Cz	Fz-A1
C3-Cz	Cz-C4	
Cz-C4	C4-T8	Pz-A2
C4-T8	T8-A2	Fp2-A2
		F4-A2
P7-P3	P7-P3	C4-A2
P3-Pz	P3-Pz	P4-A2
Pz-P4	Pz-P4	O2-A2
P4-P8	P4-P8	
		F8-A2
P7-O1	O1-O2	T8-A2
O1-O2		P8-A2
O2-P8		

See Figure 35-5.

discharges. In patients with known epilepsy (more than one seizure), only about 50% of EEG recordings will have abnormalities. Because seizures do not always appear during a given EEG recording (Box 35–1), the physician reading an EEG or PSG looks for spikes and/or abnormal sharp waves that may represent the interictal footprint of possible seizure activity. However, it should be noted that not all patients with spikes have seizures, and not all patients with seizures have detectable interictal activity. Sleep deprivation increases IEDs, and the frequency of IEDs is increased during NREM sleep (highest in stage N3). Spikes represent abnormal brain activity that is seen as an area of negativity at the scalp. Spikes can be localized (negativity at the scalp over one area of the brain) or appear diffusely. Focal seizures usually, though not invariably, begin at the same location as the interictal spikes. The typical spike is followed by a **slow wave**. Although most common postictally, spikes and sharp waves will occur sporadically at any time, and they may be more frequent in some patients just before or soon after a seizure. Of note, artifacts can sometimes mimic spikes or spikes and waves. In general, true spike and wave complexes have a "field" (Box 35–1).[5] That is, true spike and wave activity should be seen in derivations containing several contiguous electrodes. If a spike and wave are seen only in a single derivation, this may be an artifact. As noted, it should be appreciated that not all patients with spikes have seizures (particularly true in family members of epilepsy patients), and not all patients with seizures have interictal activity.

Ictal activity (seizure activity) is defined as EEG activity associated with a behavioral correlate of epilepsy (abnormality of movement, sensation, or mentation) and is more common in stages N1 and N2 *(NREM > wakefulness > REM)*. Ictal activity will be discussed in more detail. Observation of the video correlate of any suspicious pattern is essential.

Phase Reversal With Interictal and Ictal Activity

Localized EEG waveforms (including spikes and sharp waves) will show phase reversal if the bipolar chain crosses the area of the localized EEG activity.[5] That is, the spike or sharp wave in the adjacent derivations is out of phase (e.g., one down, the other up). *Phase reversal does not imply an abnormal waveform.* For example, K complexes and vertex sharp waves show phase reversal in montages that cross the location of origin. Phase reversal may help differentiate epileptiform activity such as a spike from artifact. As noted, epileptiform activity is usually recorded as an electronegative potential. For example, in Figure 35–7A, negative spike activity is seen under electrode T7. This results in down-going deflections in F7-T7 because T7 is more negative than F7. This pattern reverses for T7-P7, because now P7 is more positive than T7. In this figure, "s" signifies spike and "w" signifies wave. If the spike focus is located nearly equidistant between two monitoring electrodes (F8 and T8) (Figure 35–7B), the derivation containing these two electrodes may show little or no activity (F8-T8) because of cancelation, and the derivations on either side will show phase reversal ([Fp2-F8] to [T8-P8]).

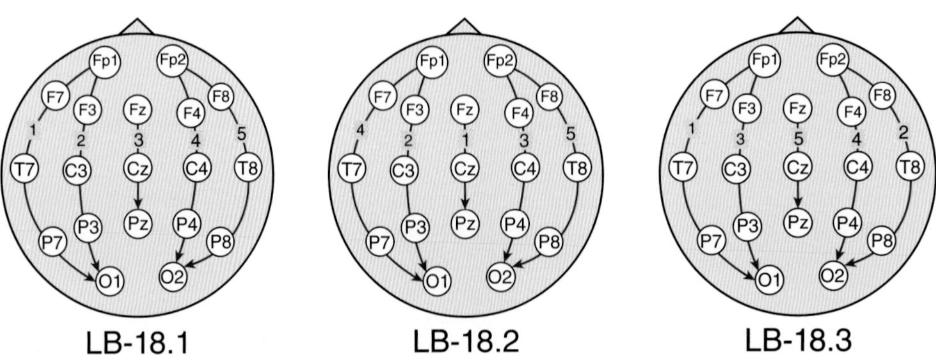

Figure 35–4 Commonly Used Longitudinal (A-P) Bipolar Montages Are Illustrated. This type of montage is often called "double banana," given the shape.

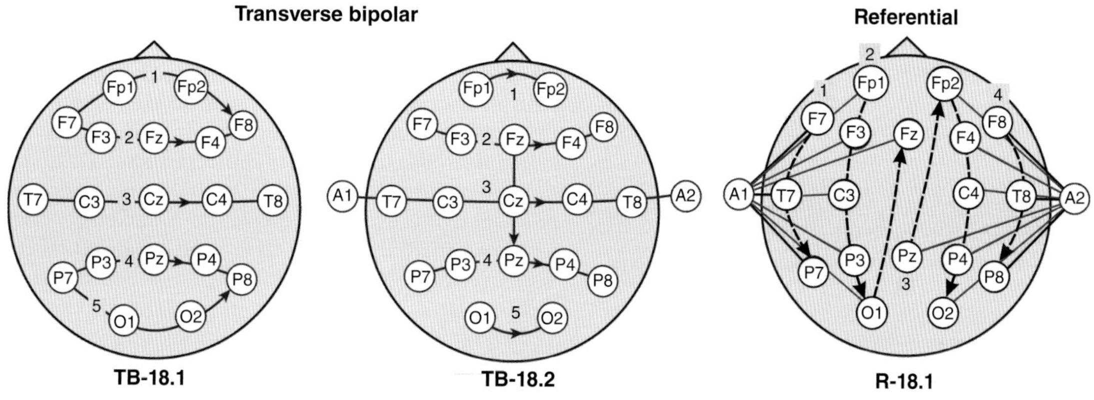

Figure 35–5 Commonly used transverse bipolar and a single referential montages are illustrated.

Table 35–3 Longitudinal Bipolar Montage With Addition of Two Temporal Electrodes

Additional electrodes T7, T8	No Additional Electrodes
F4-T4	F3-M1
T4-M2	M1-O1
M2-O2	F3-C3
F4-C4	C3-O1
C4-O2	F4-C4
F3-T3	C4-O2
T3-M1	F4-M2
M1-O1	M2-O2
F3—C3	
C3-O1	

T3, T4 are T5, T7 in new nomenclature.

Table 35–4 Waveform Terminology

Spike	Transient with a pointed peak and duration of 20–70 msec
Polyspike	Transient with multiple spikes
Sharp wave	Transient with a pointed peak and duration of 70–200 msec (measured at the base)
Spike and wave	Spike followed by a slow wave
Interictal discharge	Abnormal (epileptiform) EEG activity that occurs between seizures Can include sharp waves or, spike and wave activity
Ictal activity	EEG correlate of a seizure Rhythmic pattern of spike and wave, sharp waves, or waveforms with alpha, theta, or beta frequency

EEG, electroencephalogram.

Recall that activity that is common to the electrodes in a derivation (G1-G2) is not amplified. The difference in activity between two electrodes is amplified (common mode rejection).

Localization in Referential and PSG Montages

In referential montages, a spike has greater activity in montages containing electrodes nearer to the location of the spike.

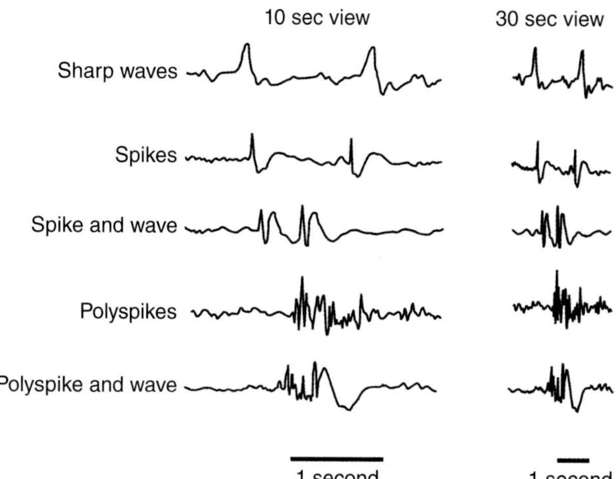

Figure 35–6 Sharp waves, spikes, spike and wave, polyspike, and polyspike and wave EEG activity. The waveforms are shown as they appear in 10 second or 30 second time windows. *EEG*, electroencephalography. (From Berry RB. *Fundamentals of Sleep Medicine*. Elsevier; 2012:550.)

In Figure 35–8, a spike focus is located between F8 and T8. On the bipolar montage, this results in the electrical activity being nearly equal in the two electrodes, resulting in minimal activity in F8-T8 but a phase reversal in adjacent bipolar pairs. However, in referential recording, the spike results in larger and nearly equal activity in F8 and T8, with less activity in adjacent electrodes. In the usual PSG montage, electrodes are referenced to the opposite mastoid.[6] Therefore, a spike located near F4 will result in greater deflection in F4-M1 than in C4-M1 or O2-M1. *It is also important to recall that the mastoid electrodes M1 and M2 are close to the left and right temporal areas, respectively*. A *right* temporal spike may be better seen in C3-M2 (spike close to M2) than in C4-M1, although C3 is on the left side. A clue to this occurrence would be visualization of the spike in derivations containing M2 but not M1.

Ictal Activity

Ictal (seizure) activity may be manifested by rhythmic activity of many types. By definition, to be considered ictal, a given burst of activity must be associated with an abnormality of movement, sensation, or mentation. However, during sleep, sensation and mentation are difficult to determine, and movement may be obscured by bed covers. Therefore, activity that

Box 35-1 INTERICTAL AND ICTAL EPILEPTIFORM DISCHARGES

Interictal EEG

- Spike and wave and sharp wave are common interictal epileptic discharges (IEDs)
- A true spike and wave complex is rarely confined to one derivation – it has a "field" of involvement (especially true if a typical bipolar clinical EEG montage is used)
- A spike and wave confined to one derivation is often an artifact
- IEDs are *most common in stage N3*, NREM > Wakefulness > REM, increased by sleep deprivation
- Present in only about 50% of cases of nocturnal epilepsy
- Repetitive similar pattern
- Visualize in 10-second window, change to bipolar montage

Ictal EEG:

- Typically, ictal EEG activity "evolves" in
  - Frequency – may increase, then exhibit postictal slowing
  - Field – amount of involved derivations increases
  - Amplitude – may increase in amplitude
- Background rhythms often suppressed
- Ictal activity most common in stage N1, N2 (NREM > Wakefulness > REM) and after awakening
- Patterns include spike and wave, rhythmic activity (delta, theta, alpha)
- Change to 10-second window, change to bipolar montage, ***observe video correlate***

EEG and Epilepsy:

- A single EEG will show epileptiform abnormalities in about 50% of adult patients with epilepsy
- Diagnostic yield increases to 70% with repeated recordings **and/or sleep EEGs**
- A normal EEG does NOT rule out epilepsy
- An abnormal EEG (epileptiform activity) does NOT rule IN epilepsy

IED, interictal epileptic discharges, *REM*, rapid eye movement; *NREM*, non-rem; EEG, electroencephalograph.

persists beyond several seconds is often considered ictal. Whereas the spike and wave activity is the most familiar waveform associated with ictal activity (Figure 35–9), the pattern of repetitive sharp waves or a pattern of rhythmic waveforms of various frequencies (rhythmic delta, theta, or alpha activity) is also common.[5,15] The postictal EEG may show slowing or interictal activity. On traditional sleep monitoring montages, ictal activity can even be mistaken for muscle artifact or normal alpha (8-13 Hz) and beta (>13 Hz) activity. Viewing the tracing in a 10-second window and observing the associated video can be helpful in this situation.

In Figure 35–10, a portion of a tracing visualized as seen in a 10-second window shows a spike and wave complex (SW) followed by rhythmic activity of 8 to 9 Hz (R). The rhythmic activity is differentiated from normal alpha rhythm by being more prominent in the eye derivations than in the occipital derivations. This is, in fact, a portion of a frontal seizure manifested by oral automatisms and loss of responsiveness. One might suspect the frontal nature because the activity is a higher amplitude in the eye leads (near the frontal lobes). A complete EEG montage documented a right frontal location (note in Figure 35–10, slightly higher amplitude in E2-M2 than in E1-M2, as E2 is nearer the right frontal area).

It is important to note that ictal activity may not be seen in scalp EEG monitoring. Seizures may begin from deeper locations (orbital frontal region, insula, or cingulate gyrus). As noted, video recording is essential because the pattern of movements (semiology) is very important for helping differentiate nonepileptic movements (parasomnias) from epileptic movements. The type of movement and the focal or generalized distribution may help define the type of seizure and/or focus in partial or partial complex seizures. Depending on the location of the onset of the seizure, the physiological correlate of the ictal activity may be manifested by motor activity (limb jerking or dystonic posturing; frontal lobe focal seizure), staring and being nonresponsive for 1 to 3 minutes (temporal lobe focal seizure), a generalized tonic-clonic seizure (GTC), myoclonic jerking, an absence seizure (brief period of

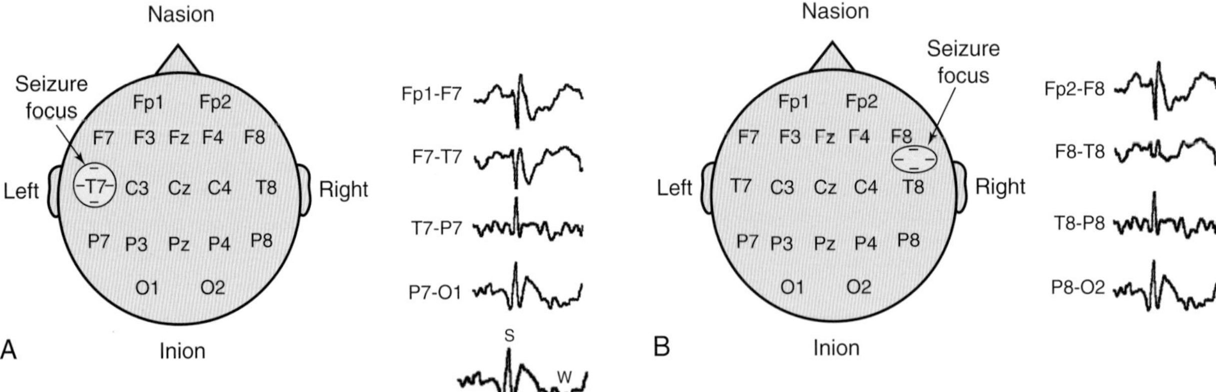

Figure 35–7 Examples of Phase Reversal. **A.** A spike (S) originates at electrode position T7, and a bipolar chain through the area shows phase reversal. *W*, wave. Note that spikes are electronegative at the scalp and, therefore, the deflection at T7-P7 is upward. **B.** Spike originated in a location between electrodes. The bipolar pair spanning the location show low amplitude due to cancellation effects (spike causes nearly equal voltage in F8 and T8), but bipolar pairs on either side show phase reversal. Recall that in the derivation G1-G2, if G1 is more negative than G2 the deflection is upward (negative up polarity). (From Berry RB. *Fundamentals of Sleep Medicine*. Elsevier; 2012:550.)

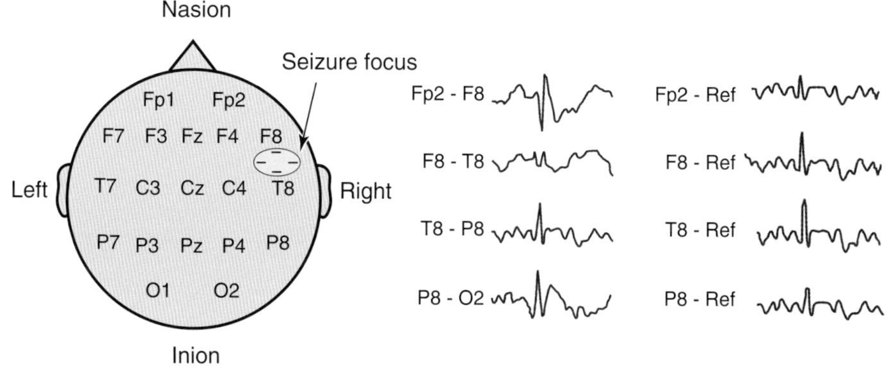

Figure 35–8 **Difference in Localization With a Bipolar or Referential Montage.** In referential montages, the electrode(s) nearest the activity in question has have the largest deflection. (From Berry RB. *Fundamentals of Sleep Medicine*. Elsevier; 2012:550.)

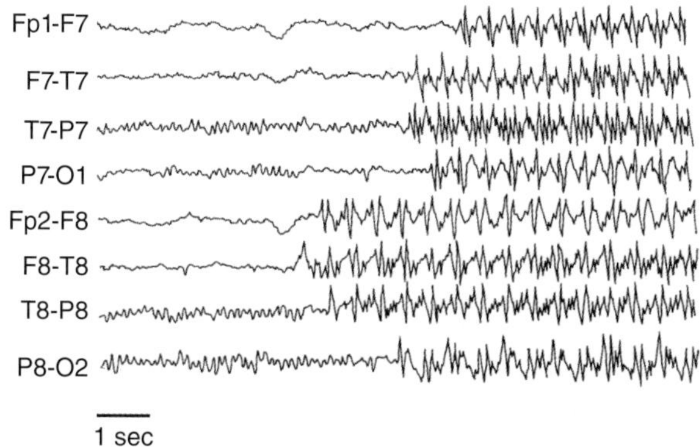

Figure 35–9 **A Seizure Beginning as Focal Activity in the Right Frontal-Temporal Areas With Secondary Generalization.** The ictal activity has a spike and wave form. (From Berry RB. *Fundamentals of Sleep Medicine*. Elsevier; 2012:555.)

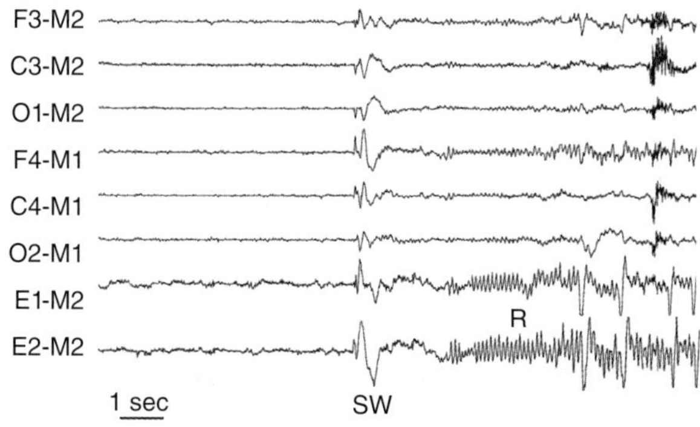

Figure 35–10 A spike and wave (SW) complex is followed by rhythmic activity (R) in the alpha frequency range that represents ictal activity in a patient with frontal lobe seizure. The origin is the right frontopolar area, and the largest amplitude is seen in the right eye derivation (E2-M2) and F4-M1. (From Berry RB. *Fundamentals of Sleep Medicine*. Elsevier; 2012:555.)

unresponsiveness), or complex motor behavior. When these symptoms occur during sleep, they may not be recognized by the patient's bedpartner. Abnormal EEG activity in scalp electrodes is not noted during a high proportion of nocturnal seizures. High-resolution magnetic resonance imaging (MRI) may identify a structural abnormality. However, if the MRI is negative intracranial electrodes placed surgically (subdural) and stereo EEG may be required for localization of the seizure focus. Ictal activity can be mistaken for a recording artifact and vice versa. Some useful characteristics of true ictal activity are noted in Box 35–1. True ictal activity evolves and changes in frequency, amplitude, and distribution during the episode.[5] The post-ictal EEG may show suppression (lower amplitude) or slowing of EEG activity. Synchronized video is very useful to determine if there are behavioral correlates (e.g., movements) temporally associated with possible ictal EEG activity. The video is also helpful in recognizing artifacts (e.g., "unusual activity" due to the patient scratching their scalp). The **postictal state** is the state after ictal activity often associated with impaired sensorium or confusion. If an episode is noted during sleep monitoring, the sleep technologist should try to communicate with the patient, as the degree of responsiveness can be helpful. However, for some seizure types, there is only a very brief or no post-ictal impairment of awareness.

Normal Sleep Waveforms in the 10-Second Window

The standard waveforms and eye movements used to stage sleep have a different appearance when viewed in a 10-second window in a standard clinical EEG montage. With digital PSG, one can change the time base (10-second to 30-second window) and montage to a typical one used for sleep recording (and vice versa) to help with waveform recognition. Figure 35–11 shows typical sleep waveforms as seen in a 10-second window using a bipolar montage.

Eye Movements in Clinical EEG Montages and Bell's Phenomenon

Bell's phenomenon describes the reflex upward movement of the front of the eyeball when the eyelids close (or blink) (Figure 35–12). Because the cornea is positive with respect to the retina, this causes a negative (downward) deflection in derivations containing electrodes placed above and near the eyes (Fp1, Fp2). Recall that, if G1 becomes positive with respect to G2, the derivation G1-G2 shows a downward deflection. Thus, eyelid closure results in downward deflections in Fp1-F7 and Fp2-F8. This is illustrated in Figure 35–13. Conjugate vertical eye movements result in characteristic deflections in bipolar derivations. The deflections depend on which electrodes are closer to the eyes. For vertical movements, the Fp1 and Fp2 electrodes are more positive (eyes up) or negative (eyes down) compared with adjacent electrodes

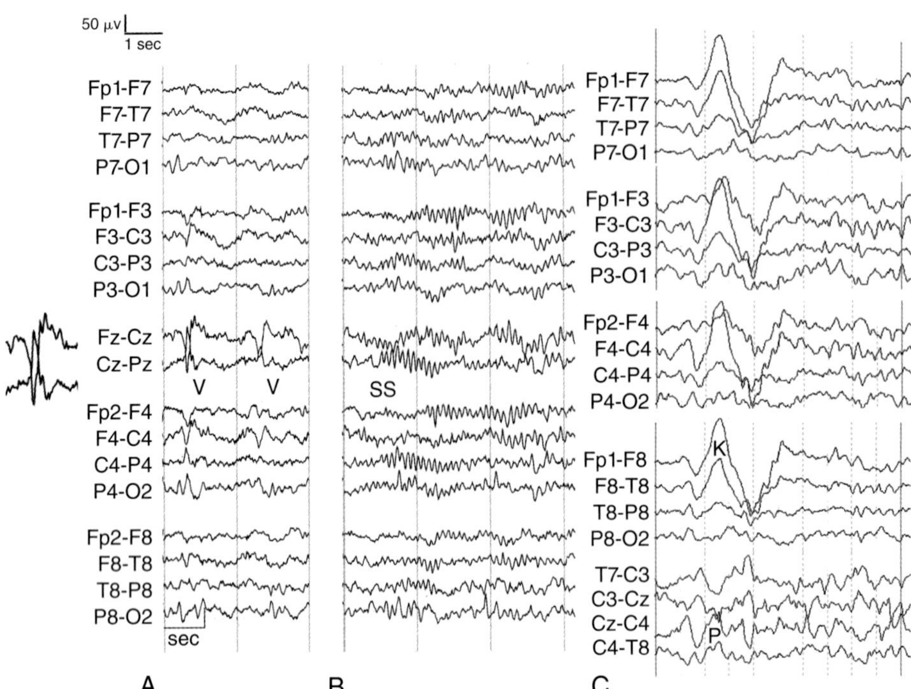

Figure 35–11 **Characteristic Waveforms During Sleep Have a Different Appearance Using a Bipolar Montage and a Time Window Duration of 10 Seconds.** Panel A: A vertex sharp wave (V) is shown as an enlargement to the left. The activity shows a phase reversal at Cz, as expected, as the location of the sharp wave is at the vertex. Panel B: Sleep spindle activity (SS) is prominent in derivations containing a frontal or central electrode (highest in central derivations). Panel C: A K complex (K) is a high amplitude waveform. The bottom four derivations are transverse chain derivations crossing at Cz. They show a phase reversal at P and relatively low amplitude due to a cancellation effect, as the K complex activity is near Cz..

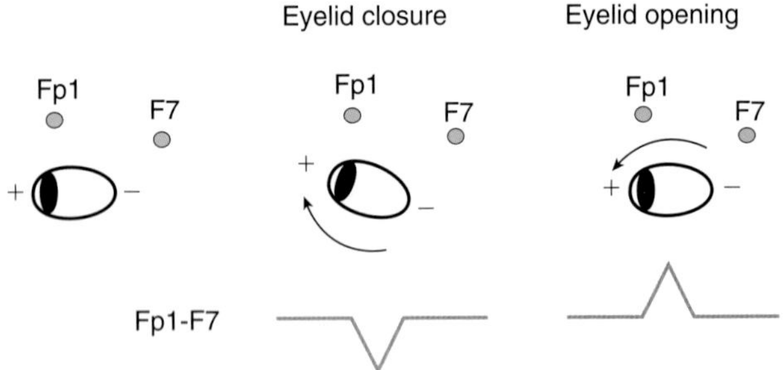

Figure 35–12 **Schematic Illustrating Bell's Phenomenon.** When eyelids close, the eyes turn upward; when eyelids open, the reverse occurs. The cornea is positive, and when moving upward, it makes Fp1, Fp2, F3, and F4 positive with respect to other electrodes so that Fp1-F7 and Fp2-F8 derivations have a downward deflection.

(Figure 35–14). For lateral eye movements, the electrodes F7 and F8 become more positive or negative than adjacent electrodes depending on the direction of lateral eye movement (Figure 35–15). Thus, in longitudinal bipolar derivations, vertical eye movements cause in-phase deflections and lateral movements result in out-of-phase deflections.

Posterior Dominant Rhythm

The term *alpha rhythm* is used to denote waveforms of 8 to 13 Hz that are prominent in occipital derivations and decrease in amplitude with eye opening.[5,6] However, the preferred term is **posterior dominant rhythm (PDR)**. The PDR of infants and children is discussed in Chapter 5. The PDR frequency is slower than 8 Hz in infants and young children. The average frequency of the PDR increases to approximately 8 Hz at 8 years of age in most individuals ("8 Hz by 8 years is OK"). With eyes closed and/or decreased visual attention, the PDR becomes prominent. With drowsiness and transition to stage N1, the occipital derivations show attenuation of the PDR and replacement with theta activity. The effect of eyes open and eyes closed on the PDR in an adult is illustrated in Figure 35–13.

Positive Occipital Sharp Transients of Sleep and Mu Rhythms

Positive occipital sharp transients of sleep (POSTS) are sharp waves that can occur normally in NREM sleep.[5] They are most prominent in occipital derivations and are positive. Therefore, in O2-M1, they would be manifested by downward deflections (O2 is positive compared with M1). In Figure 35–16, the POSTS show phase reversal across O2. The fact that the POSTS are in fact "positive" in the occipital area is documented by the fact that the deflections are up in C4-O2 and down in O2-M1.

Lambda waves have a similar morphology and location as POSTS, but *lambda waves are noted during* **wakefulness** (Table 35–5). Lambda waves are low-voltage triangular waves that appear in the occipital areas. They may be surface positive or negative (POSTS are surface positive) (Figure 35–17). **Mu rhythm** may sometimes be confused with alpha rhythm but differs in several features, listed in Table 35–6. Mu rhythm is seen in **central derivations** during wakefulness and has an

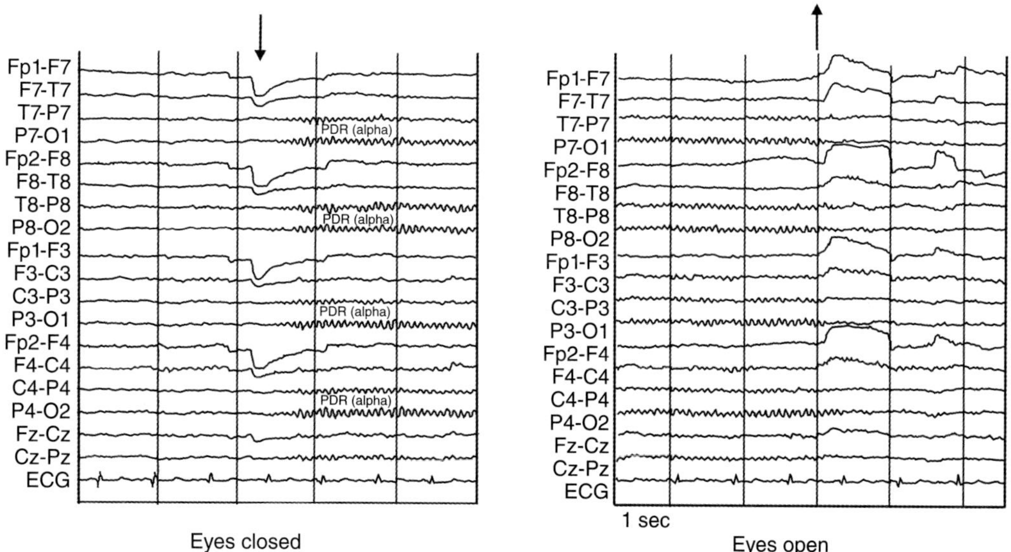

Figure 35–13 When the eyes close, the globe turns upward so the nearby electrodes are positive and there is a downward deflection in the derivations near the eyes. Also note that eye closure results in alpha activity (posterior dominant rhythm) in derivations containing occipital electrodes. In contrast, when the eyes open *(upward arrow)*, the cornea moves downward, resulting in an upward deflection in derivations close to the eyes. Alpha activity is attenuated.

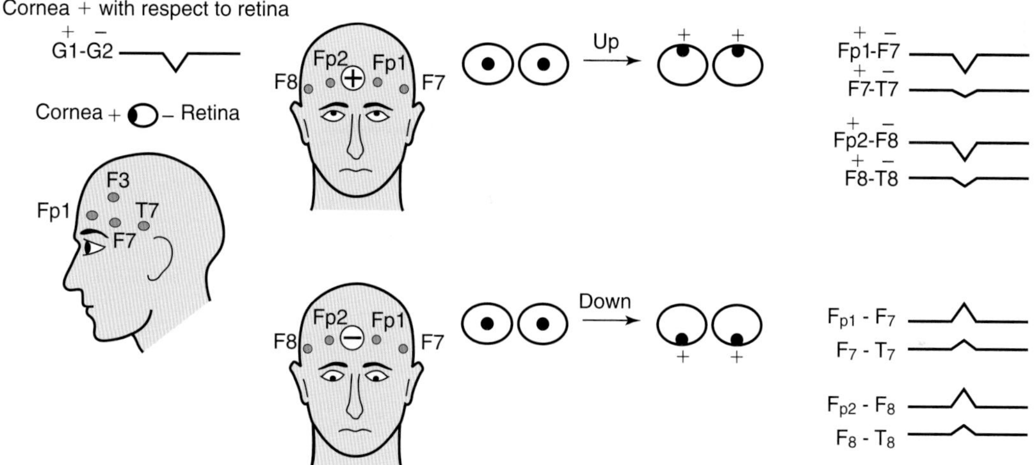

Figure 35–14 Eye Movements With the Eyes Open are Associated With Deflections in EEG Derivations Near the Eyes. The cornea is positive, so looking upward results in downward deflections in derivations Fp1-F7, F7-T7, Fp2-F8, and F8-T8, and looking downward results in positive deflections in these derivations. This assumes the EEG convention of negative polarity upward for display of EEG derivations.

"archiform" or comblike shape with rounded contour on one side and sharp contour on the other (Figure 35–18). Mu rhythm is most prominent in **central areas** (rather than occipital areas) and is reactive to movement of the contralateral hand (rather than to opening of the eyes).

CLASSIFICATION OF SEIZURES AND TERMINOLOGY

The previous classification of seizures[16] was revised in 2017 by the International League Against Epilepsy (ILAE).[17] Along with the classification, a glossary has been published to standardize terminology (Box 35–2).[18,19] Pack presents a helpful overview of the revised classification with examples.[20] Many terms, including "partial seizure," are no longer recommended. In addition, a new standardized definition of epilepsy was published in 2014.[21] Definitions of a seizure and epilepsy are as follows: "A seizure is defined as a transient occurrence of signs and/or symptoms due to abnormal excessive or synchronous neuronal activity in the brain. The manifestation may include a disturbance of mental, motor, sensory, or autonomic activity. Epilepsy is a disease of the brain defined by any of the following conditions: (1) At least two unprovoked (or reflex) seizures occurring >24 hours apart; (2) one unprovoked (or reflex) seizure and a probability of further seizures similar to the general recurrence risk (at least 60%) after two unprovoked seizures occurring over the next 10 years; (3) diagnosis of an epilepsy

Figure 35–15 As the cornea is positive, looking to the right is associated with downward deflections in EEG derivation near the eyes on the right and upward deflections in the corresponding left-sided electrodes. Looking to the left has the opposite effect.

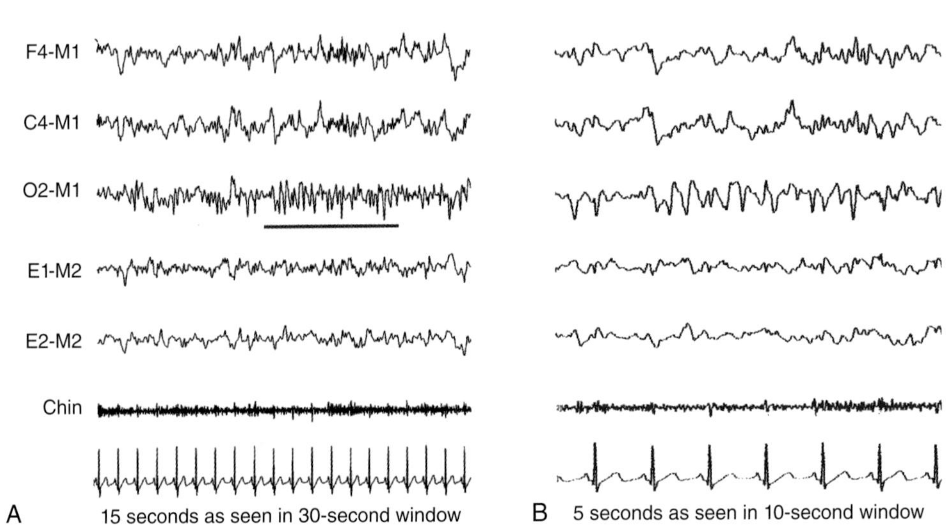

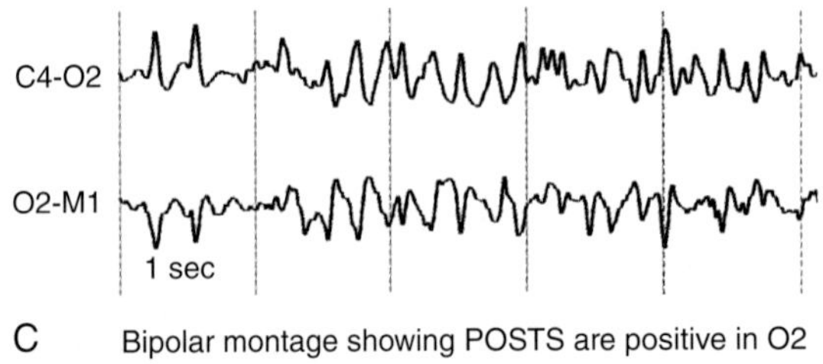

Figure 35–16 Positive occipital sharp transients of sleep (POSTS) are illustrated (*underlined area*) in the *top left panel* in a typical sleep montage as seen in a 30-second window. The same derivations are shown in the *top right panel* as seen in a 10-second window. In the bottom left panel, a 4-second bipolar arrangement illustrates that the occipital sharp waves are positive (downward deflection in O2-M1).

Table 35–5 POSTS Versus Lambda Waves

	POSTS	Lambda
Location	Posterior, occipital derivations	Same
Stage	NREM sleep	Wake
Polarity	Positive	Positive or negative
Shape	Sharp waves	Triangular
Commonly noted in sleep recording	Yes	No Seen when patient scans complex objects

POSTS, positive occipital sharp transients of sleep; *NREM*, non-rapid eye movement.

syndrome. Epilepsy is considered to be resolved for individuals who had an age-dependent epilepsy syndrome but are now past the applicable age or those *who have remained seizure free for the last 10 years with no antiseizure medicines for the last 5 years.*"

It follows that a patient with a single seizure associated with a time-limited event (medication or substance withdrawal) may not have epilepsy. It may be difficult to assess the probability of future seizures, and this decision is best left to an epileptologist. In the past, the term *symptomatic* epilepsy was used if there was an identifiable lesion or *idiopathic* epilepsy if a discrete structural abnormality is not found. The term "idiopathic" is misleading, because many seizure disorders classified as idiopathic have a genetic basis, and some have a known mechanism (autoimmune).

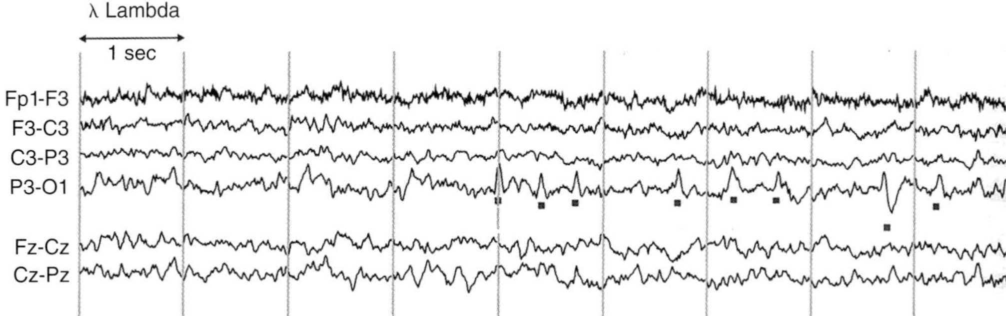

Figure 35–17 Lambda waves are noted in the P3-O1 derivation and marked by *dots under the waves*. Lambda waves are seen during stage W (wakefulness). (From Libenson MH. *Practical Approach to Electroencephalography*. Saunders Elsevier; 2010:270.)

Table 35–6 Mu Versus Alpha Rhythm

	MU	ALPHA
Stage	Wakefulness	Drowsy wakefulness
Frequency (Hz)	8–12	8–13 (adults and older children)
Location	Central (C_3, C_4)	Occipital
Reactivity, diminished with	Movement of contralateral hand	Opening eyes
Shape	Archiform comb like	Sinusoidal

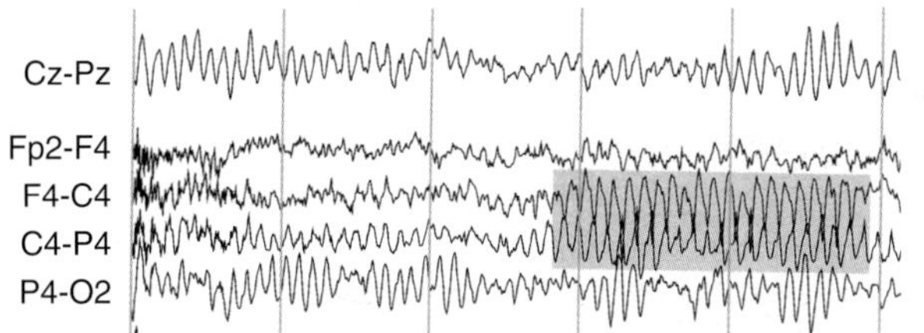

Figure 35–18 **An Example of Mu Rhythm (archiform "comb like" pattern) With a Phase Reversal at C4 During Sleep.** The vertical lines are 1 second apart. (From Libenson MH. *Practical Approach to Electroencephalography.* Saunders Elsevier; 2010:270.)

The new classification scheme for seizures is shown in Figure 35–19. The first level of classification includes **classified or unclassified seizures.** Unclassified seizures include those with inadequate information or those that cannot be placed in other categories. In the second level, seizures are grouped as **focal, generalized, or unknown onset** based on a combination of clinical features and EEG findings. **Focal onset seizures** originate within networks limited to one hemisphere. They may be discretely localized or more widely distributed. Focal seizures may originate in superficial (closer to the scalp) or deep cortical structures. Some seizures that start locally may generalize rapidly via subcortical brain networks. **Generalized seizures** originate at some point within, and rapidly engage, bilaterally distributed networks. *Generalized seizures are* ***always associated*** *with impairment of awareness.* Sometimes, it is difficult to classify a seizure as focal or generalized. Some seizures that start locally may generalize rapidly or originate in subcortical structures. Hence, the category "unknown onset" was defined. The next level of classification depends on the onset classification. For focal seizures "aware or impaired awareness" is the next level. For both focal and generalized seizures, the major divisions are **motor onset versus nonmotor onset** seizures. The classification is nonhierarchical, hence there are no lines from one level to another (e.g., a focal onset/aware/motor/hyperkinetic seizure or a focal onset/impaired awareness/motor/hyperkinetic seizure). The following terms are no longer used in the new classification: simple partial (now focal onset aware), complex partial (now focal onset impaired awareness), secondary generalized (now focal to bilateral tonic-clonic), psychic (now cognitive). The motor manifestations—atonic seizures, tonic seizures, clonic seizures, epileptic spasms, and myoclonic seizures—now appear under both focal onset and generalized onset seizure categories.

Focal Onset Seizures

These seizures are characterized by a focal onset and either motor onset or nonmotor onset. As noted, focal seizures can also generalize. If a seizure generalizes rapidly, it may be difficult to determine whether the seizure was focal and to identify the location of the focal onset.

Focal Motor Onset Seizures

The motor manifestations of focal onset seizures include automatisms; atonic, clonic, and epileptic spasms; hyperkinetic seizures; myoclonic seizures; and tonic seizures. **Automatisms** are repetitive movements that may be purposeful but serve no obvious purpose in the actual situation. Automatisms are a more or less coordinated motor activity, usually occurring when cognition is impaired and after which the subject is usually (but not always) amnesic. This often resembles a voluntary movement and may consist of an inappropriate continuation of preictal motor activity. Examples of automatisms include chewing, lip smacking, swallowing, picking at clothes with the hands, rubbing fingers together, or foot tapping. **Atonic seizures** are those with a sudden loss or diminution of muscle tone without an apparent preceding myoclonic or tonic event lasting ~1–2 seconds and involving the head, trunk, jaw, or limb musculature. **Clonic seizures** are characterized by jerking, either symmetric or asymmetric, that is regularly repetitive and involves the same muscle groups. **Tonic seizures** are associated with a sustained increase in muscle contraction lasting a few seconds to minutes. **Epileptic spasms**[19] form a new classification and are characterized as a sudden flexion, extension, or mixed extension-flexion of predominantly proximal and truncal muscles that is usually more sustained than

Box 35–2 DEFINITIONS PERTINENT TO EPILEPSY

Seizure – A transient occurrence of signs and/or symptoms due to abnormal excessive or synchronous neuronal activity in the brain

Epilepsy – Disease of the brain defined by any of the following conditions: (1) At least two unprovoked (or reflex) seizures occurring >24 h apart; (2) one unprovoked (or reflex) seizure and probability of further seizures similar to the general recurrence risk (at least 60%) after two unprovoked seizures occurring over the next 10 years; (3) diagnosis of an epilepsy syndrome

Tonic – A sustained increase in muscle contraction lasting a few seconds to minutes

Clonic – Jerking, either symmetric or asymmetric, that is regularly repetitive and involves the same muscle groups

Tonic-clonic A sequence consisting of a tonic followed by a clonic phase

Atonic – sudden loss or diminution of muscle tone without apparent preceding myoclonic or tonic event lasting about 1 to 2 seconds, involving head, trunk, jaw, or limb musculature

Aura – A subjective ictal phenomenon that, in a given patient, may precede an observable seizure

Automatism – A more or less coordinated motor activity, usually occurring when cognition is impaired and after which the subject is usually (but not always) amnesic. This often resembles a voluntary movement and may consist of an inappropriate continuation of preictal motor activity

Autonomic seizure – A distinct alteration of autonomic nervous system function involving cardiovascular, pupillary, gastrointestinal, sudomotor (autonomic nervous system control of sweat gland activity), vasomotor, and thermoregulatory functions

Dacrystic – Bursts of crying, which may or may not be associated with sadness

Dystonic – Sustained contractions of both agonist and antagonist muscles, producing athetoid or twisting movements, which may produce abnormal postures

Emotional seizure – Seizure presenting with an emotion or the appearance of an emotion as an early prominent feature, such as fear, spontaneous joy or euphoria, laughing (gelastic), or crying (dacrystic)

Eyelid myoclonia – Jerking of the eyelids at frequencies of at least 3 per second, commonly with upward eye deviation, usually lasting <10 s, often precipitated by eye closure. There may or may not be associated brief loss of awareness.

Fencer's posture seizure – A focal motor seizure type with extension of one arm and flexion at the contralateral elbow and wrist, giving an imitation of swordplay with a foil. This has also been called a supplementary motor area seizure.

Focal – Originating within networks limited to one hemisphere. They may be discretely localized or more widely distributed. Focal seizures may originate in subcortical structures.

Focal onset bilateral tonic-clonic seizure – A seizure type with focal onset, with awareness or impaired awareness, either motor or nonmotor, progressing to bilateral tonic-clonic activity. The prior term was seizure with partial onset with secondary generalization.

Gelastic – Bursts of laughter or giggling, usually without an appropriate affective tone

Generalized tonic-conic seizure – Bilateral symmetric or sometimes asymmetric tonic contraction and then bilateral clonic contraction of somatic muscles, usually associated with autonomic phenomena and loss of awareness. These seizures engage networks in both hemispheres at the start of the seizure.

Generalized – Originating at some point within, and rapidly engaging, bilaterally distributed networks

Jacksonian seizure – Traditional term indicating spread of clonic unilateral movements through contiguous body parts

Myoclonic – Sudden, brief (<100 msec), involuntary single or multiple contraction(s) of muscles(s) or muscle groups of variable topography (axial, proximal limb, distal). Myoclonus is less regularly repetitive and less sustained than clonus.

Myoclonic-tonic-clonic – One or a few jerks of limbs bilaterally, followed by a tonic–clonic seizure. The initial jerks can be considered to be either a brief period of clonus or myoclonus. Seizures with this characteristic are common in juvenile myoclonic epilepsy.

Versive – A sustained, forced conjugate ocular, cephalic, and/or truncal rotation or lateral deviation from the midline

Adapted from Fisher RS, Cross JH, D'Souza C, et al. Instruction manual for the ILAE 2017 operational classification of seizure types. *Epilepsia.* 2017;58(4):531-542.

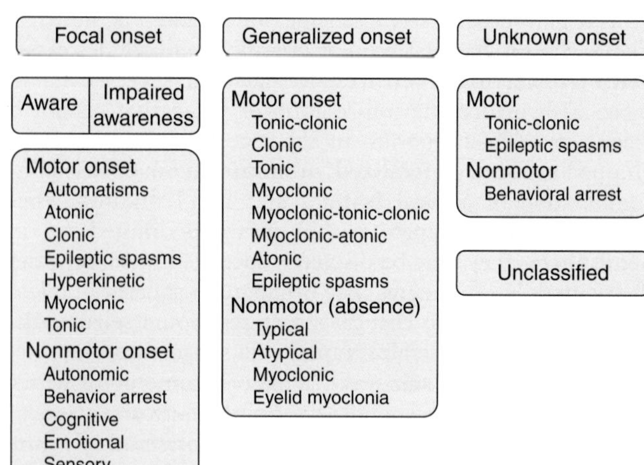

Figure 35–19 Schematic Illustrating the New Seizure Classification. The first level is the type of onset. The second level in focal onset is aware or impaired awareness, then motor or nonmotor onset. Within motor or nonmotor onset is the specific type of seizure based on its manifestation. For generalized onset, the second level is motor onset or nonmotor onset. Note that *some types of motor onset seizure types are in both the focal onset and generalized onset columns*. The designation complex partial seizure has been replaced by focal onset – impaired awareness. (From Fisher RS, Cross JH, French JA, et al. Operational classification of seizure types by the International League Against Epilepsy: position paper of the ILAE Commission for Classification and Terminology. *Epilepsia.* 2017; 58[4]:522-530. PMID: 28276060.)

a myoclonic movement but not as sustained as a tonic seizure. Limited forms may occur: grimacing, head nodding, or subtle eye movements. Epileptic spasms frequently occur in clusters. "Infantile spasms" are the best-known form, but spasms can occur at all ages. **Hyperkinetic seizures** (also known as sleep-related hypermotor epilepsy [SHE]) are characterized by motor seizures involving predominantly proximal limb or axial muscles producing *irregular sequential ballistic movements, such as pedaling, pelvic thrusting, thrashing, or rocking movements*, by an increase in ongoing movements, or by inappropriately rapid performance of a movement. While the new classification used "hyperkinetic," most authors use "hypermotor." As will be discussed, the epilepsy syndrome known as nocturnal frontal lobe epilepsy (NFLE) has been replaced by SHE.[22] **Myoclonic seizures** are characterized by sudden, brief (<100 milliseconds) involuntary *single or multiple* contraction(s) of muscles(s) or muscle groups of variable topography (axial, proximal limb, distal). Myoclonus is less regularly repetitive and **less sustained** than clonus.

Focal Nonmotor Onset Seizures

The second major category of focal onset seizures includes seizures of "nonmotor onset." The subtypes include autonomic, behavior arrest, cognitive, emotional, and sensory seizures. Autonomic seizures involve a distinct alteration of autonomic nervous system function involving cardiovascular, pupillary, gastrointestinal, sudomotor, vasomotor, and thermoregulatory functions. **Behavioral arrest** seizures involve a sudden pause in activities, freezing, and immobilization. **Cognitive seizures** (term replaced psychic seizures) involve cognitive impairment (aphasic, apraxia, neglect) as well as phenomena such as déjà vu ("already seen," previously been in this situation or place or done this before), jamais vu ("never seen," being unfamiliar with a person or situation that is actually very familiar), illusions, or hallucinations. **Emotional seizures** involve the appearance of emotions such as joy or fear without an obvious reason for the emotion. **Sensory seizures** involve a perceptual experience not caused by appropriate stimuli in the external world. **Auras** are subjective sensations such as déjà vu, epigastric sensation, or visual, olfactory, or gustatory disturbances that precede the loss of awareness in focal onset seizures with impaired awareness (formerly complex partial seizure). The *aura is a manifestation of a focal seizure* that spreads to areas that affect cognition, resulting in subsequent loss of awareness. Finally, a focal onset nonmotor seizure can either remain focal or generalize to a bilateral tonic-clonic seizure.

Focal Seizures Generalized

The **prior** term for a focal seizure that becomes generalized was "secondary generalized focal seizure." The new terminology is "focal to bilateral tonic-clonic seizure." For example, a focal onset seizure disorder might remain focal most of the time but rarely generalize (Figure 35–9).

Generalized Onset Seizures

Generalized seizures are divided into those *with and without motor manifestations*. The previous terminology was *convulsive and non-convulsive seizures*. The word **generalized** is omitted in classifications if the only type of seizure in question is generalized. For example, "absence" is used rather than "generalized absence seizure." Tonic-clonic seizures are those historically referred to as "grand-mal." Awareness is lost at the same time as the onset of tonic-clonic movements. Tonic-clonic seizures are now characterized based on the motor activity at the start of the event (e.g., myoclonic activity at the start of a tonic-clonic seizure). Thus, the myoclonic-tonic-clonic seizure type is included in the new classification.

Generalized Motor Onset Seizures

The motor subtype of generalized seizures includes tonic-clonic, clonic, tonic, myoclonic, myotonic-tonic-clonic, myoclonic-atonic, and atonic seizures and epileptic spasms. Note that atonic, clonic, tonic, and myoclonic seizures and epileptic spasms were included as motor subtypes of focal onset seizures, and the behavior has already been described in that section. *In a generalized seizure, there is impairment of awareness at the onset.* Generalized clonic seizures begin and end with sustained jerking of the limbs bilaterally and often of the head, face, and trunk. These are less common than tonic-clonic seizures. GTC seizures begin with a tonic phase, followed by a clonic phase. Generalized myoclonus differs from clonus in that it is briefer and not regularly repetitive. Generalized myoclonic seizures are characterized by brief *bilateral* muscle jerking (muscle contraction then relaxation—often involving the shoulder muscles). The postictal state (the state following ictal activity) is often associated with impaired sensorium or confusion. Myoclonic-tonic-clonic seizures begin with a few myoclonic jerks, followed by tonic-clonic activity. These seizures are commonly seen in patients with *juvenile myoclonic epilepsy* (JME). Atonic means without tone. When leg tone is lost during a generalized atonic seizure, the patient falls on the buttocks or sometimes forward onto the knees and face. Recovery is usually within seconds. While the term "drop attack" is often used to refer to atonic seizures, the term is often used to refer to any seizure type where the patient can fall and injure themselves. In contrast, *tonic or tonic-clonic seizures more typically propel the patient into a backward fall.* Epileptic spasms previously were referred to as "infantile spasms," a term that remains suitable for epileptic spasms occurring at infantile age. An epileptic spasm presents as a sudden flexion, extension, or mixed extension-flexion of predominantly proximal and truncal muscles. They commonly occur in clusters and most often during infancy.

Generalized Nonmotor Epilepsy

The nonmotor group of generalized seizures formerly called non-convulsive generalized epilepsy includes typical and atypical absence, myoclonic absence, and eyelid myoclonia. Typical absence epilepsy (AE) is associated with an abrupt impairment of consciousness (blank stare/interruption of ongoing activity, possibly a brief upward deviation of the eyes) without loss of muscle tone or posture.[5,19,20,23,24] The patient is usually unresponsive, and duration is a few to 30 seconds, with rapid recovery. *Attacks are triggered by hyperventilation and photic stimuli.* Typical AE (formerly known as "petite-mal") is characterized by spike and wave complexes of 3 per second (Figure 35–20). Typical AE starts in childhood and usually resolves by adolescence. Atypical AE is associated with slow, irregular, *generalized spike and wave activity that has a lower frequency than 3 Hz* and may be associated with combinations of impaired consciousness and motor or autonomic changes. The onset is not as abrupt as typical AE. Atypical absence

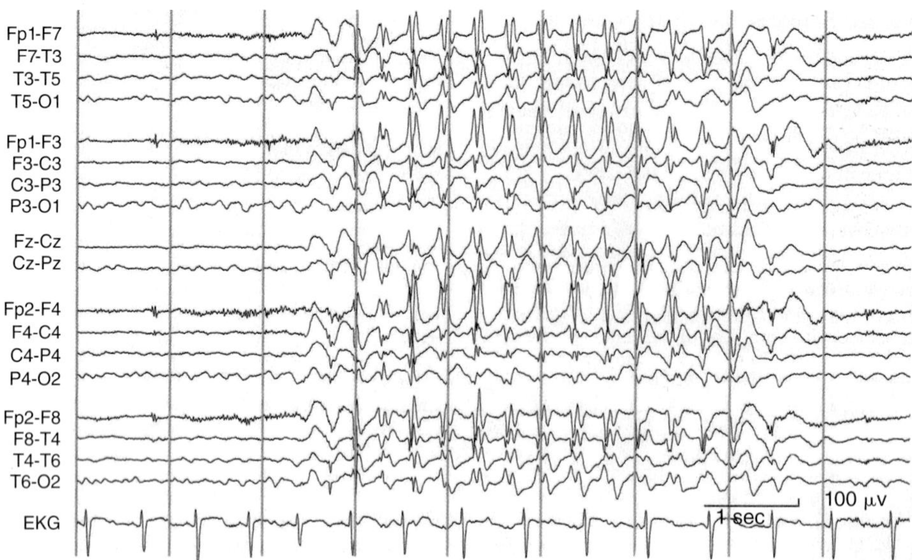

Figure 35–20 The abrupt onset and termination of a generalized absence seizure in a patient with **typical** absence epilepsy as seen in a 10-second window. The spike and wave pattern has a frequency of 3 per second. (From Libenson MH. *Practical Approach to Electroencephalography.* Saunders Elsevier; 2010:214.)

seizures are sometimes referred to a juvenile onset absence, as this type of AE occurs in older children or adolescents, in contrast to typical absence (childhood absence) that occurs in mid-childhood. Epilepsy with eyelid myoclonia is a rare form of generalized epilepsy that can have several possible seizure types, but eyelid myoclonia is the most common. Eyelid myoclonia consists of brief and repeated myoclonic jerks of the eyelids, the eyeballs may roll upward, and the head may move slightly backward. If a person has a brief loss of awareness with eyelid myoclonia, the seizure is called eyelid myoclonia with absence.

The new classification of seizure types also includes a classification of epilepsy syndromes. *An epilepsy syndrome might consist of several seizure types.* For example, temporal lobe epilepsy (TLE) may involve focal onset seizures with loss of awareness for most of the time but also less frequent GTC seizures.

SLEEP-RELATED EPILEPSY SYNDROMES

Sleep-Related Epilepsy Syndromes Overview

Seizure disorders are part of the differential diagnosis of "nocturnal spells"—episodes of abnormal motor activity during sleep. Depending on the type of patients studied, as many as *10% to 15% (10%–40% if awakening epilepsy is included) of seizures occur exclusively or mainly during sleep.* Those seizures that occur only at night are more likely to go undiagnosed or thought to be a NREM parasomnia. The lack of daytime seizure activity and the fact that automatisms or episodes of changed sensorium during sleep may not be noted by a bed partner or remembered by the patient make focal aware (simple partial) or focal impaired awareness (partial complex seizures) difficult to diagnose. Hypermotor sleep-related epilepsy (formerly called NFLE) can occur without loss of consciousness or postictal confusion (or the postictal confusion can be very brief) and be incorrectly assumed to be a parasomnia.[22]

One classification of sleep-related epilepsy includes 1) pure sleep epilepsy, 2) sleep-accentuated epilepsy, and 3) arousal epilepsy.[13] In pure sleep epilepsy, seizures occur exclusively or primarily during sleep. This category includes benign epilepsy of childhood with centrotemporal spikes and nocturnal frontal lobe/sleep-related hypermotor epilepsy. The second category is sleep-accentuated epilepsy, which can occur during wakefulness or sleep but is potentiated during sleep. This category includes epileptic encephalopathy (e.g., Lennox-Gastaut syndrome and Landau-Kleffner syndrome). The third category is arousal epilepsy (also known as **awakening epilepsy**), in which seizures are most common in the period following awakening from sleep (e.g., JME). The literature on the timing of seizures varies, likely because of variability in timing among the types of seizures. *JME and "awakening" generalized tonic-clonic seizures occur in the first hour of awakening after a night of sleep.* Frontal lobe seizures peak in the early morning hours, and temporal lobe seizures have two peaks, one in the morning and one late afternoon. In general, all manifestations of nocturnal seizure disorders are much more common in NREM than in REM sleep (NREM > wakefulness > REM). Prior sleep deprivation is believed to activate seizures; therefore, patients often undergo clinical EEG monitoring in a sleep-deprived state to increase the likelihood of recording seizure activity. As noted, *sleep deprivation does increase the frequency of IEDs.* However, recent studies suggest that prior sleep deprivation has a greater effect on generalized epilepsy (especially JME) and a lesser effect (if at all) on focal epilepsies.[13]

In Table 35–7, seizure disorders commonly associated with sleep or that typically occur soon after awakening are listed. The focal onset seizures (arising from a localized area of the brain with or without subsequent generalization) that commonly present at night are TLE and FLE. Both are usually focal seizures with impaired awareness (formerly complex partial seizures). These seizures usually arise from the mesial or lateral part of the temporal lobe but may arise from diverse parts of the frontal lobe, including the motor cortex, premotor cortex (with the supplemental motor cortex), orbital frontal areas, and prefrontal cortex (Figure 35–3). *There is an overlap in semiology between TLE and FLE.* Patients with focal seizures with impaired awareness may have no recollection of the events or only partial memory. Patients may remember an aura, a subjective sensation such as déjà vu (already experienced), epigastric sensation, or visual or olfactory disturbance that precedes the loss of awareness. The aura is initially a focal seizure without impaired awareness that spreads to areas that affect cognition, resulting in subsequent loss of awareness. In the current seizure classification, if impairment of awareness occurs during any part of a seizure, it is considered to be a seizure with impaired awareness. *TLE usually presents as impairment of consciousness with automatisms.* For example, lip smacking is a common automatism. Sleep-related hypermotor epilepsy (formerly known as NFLE) may be associated with dystonic posturing or violent movements, with consciousness often preserved. Sleep-related hypermotor epilepsy can mimic confusional arousals/sleep terrors and sleep walking. FLE most commonly presents at night, and TLE most commonly presents during the day (Figure 35–21).[25] Both FLE and TLE can generalize to tonic-clonic seizures. Daytime FLE (compared to night time FLE) is more likely to generalize. It is important to remember that *not all FLE occurs only at night;* hence, in the discussion to follow, the term FLE is used as well as SHE. One reason the term SHE is currently used rather than NFLE, is that a significant percentage of patients with SHE are found to have a seizure onset outside the frontal lobes.

Table 35–7 Epilepsy Syndromes Associated With Sleep

Epilepsy Syndrome	Time of Onset
Focal Epilepsy	
Temporal lobe epilepsy (TLE)	Late childhood to early adulthood
Sleep-related hypermotor epilepsy (SHE) Formerly nocturnal frontal lobe epilepsy (NFLE) (Including autosomal dominant frontal lobe epilepsy)	Late childhood to early adulthood
Benign centrotemporal epilepsy with centrotemporal spikes (BECTS)	3–13 yrs (peak 9–10 yrs)
Focal to generalized tonic-clonic epilepsy (Secondary generalized focal epilepsy)	Late childhood to early adulthood
Generalized Epilepsy	
Epilepsy with GTC seizures on awakening	6–25 yrs (peak 11–15 yrs)
Juvenile myoclonic epilepsy (JME)	12–18 yrs (peak 14 yrs)
Absence epilepsy	3–12 yrs (peak 6–7 yrs)
Lennox-Gastaut syndrome	1–8 yrs (peak 3–5 yrs)
Continuous spike and slow wave discharges during sleep	8 mo–11.5 yrs

Hyperkinetic versus hypermotor is used in new epilepsy classification.
GTC, generalized tonic-clonic seizures.
Malow BA. Sleep and epilepsy. *Neurol Clin.* 2005;23(4):1127-1147.

As noted, the focal seizure disorders have a higher incidence of interictal discharges or seizure activity in NREM sleep, particularly in stage N3 (ictal activity more common in stages N1 and N2) when brain activity is more synchronized.[13,14] The other focal onset epilepsy syndrome associated with sleep is benign centrotemporal epilepsy with centrotemporal spikes (BECTS). Focal seizures are uncommon during REM sleep, but if they occur, they are said to improve the ability to localize the onset.

The GTC seizures associated with sleep affect patients with generalized epilepsy and focal onset epilepsy (TLE, FLE) with generalization. Primary generalized seizures are sometimes called awakening epilepsies because they commonly occur when the patient is in a drowsy state upon awakening from sleep. Patients with both *atypical (juvenile) absence and juvenile myoclonic disorders* can have GTC seizures associated with sleep. Recall that childhood typical absence seizures start in early childhood and rarely persist into adulthood. In contrast, *juvenile atypical absence seizures start later in childhood, around 8 to 12 years old, and persist throughout adulthood.* JME typically starts in adolescence (12–18 years) and is a genetically determined condition involving myoclonic

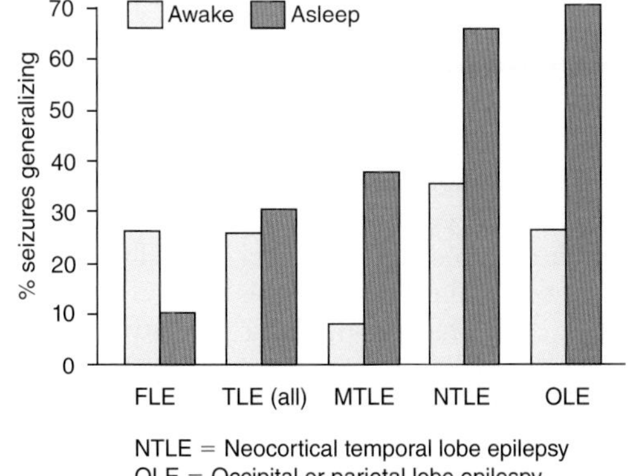

FLE = Frontal lobe epilepsy
TLE = Temporal lobe epilepsy
MTLE = Mesial temporal lobe epilepsy
NTLE = Neocortical temporal lobe epilepsy
OLE = Occipital or parietal lobe epilepsy

Figure 35–21 **Percentage of Different Seizure Types Occurring During the Night and Day.** Note frontal lobe epilepsy is more common at night. Some patients may have seizures only at night. The percentage of focal epilepsy that generalized is also shown in the *right panel*. Temporal lobe epilepsy occurring at night is more likely to generalize. Frontal lobe epilepsy occuring during the day is more likely to generalize. (From Herman ST, Walczak TS, Bazil CW. Distribution of partial seizures during the sleep-wake cycle differences by seizure onset site. *Neurology.* 2001;56[11]:1453-1459. PMID: 11402100.)

jerks in the arms shortly after awakening. It may not be appreciated until the patient has a GTC seizure.

Focal Onset Epilepsy Syndromes Associated With Sleep

Temporal and frontal lobe epilepsies are often mislabeled as other sleep-related conditions (e.g., periodic limb movements of sleep [PLMS], REM sleep behavior disorder, sleepwalking). Video PSG with synchronized video recording is very useful in making the correct diagnosis. As previously noted, some seizures are not associated with activity recorded on the scalp EEG. Therefore, capturing repetitive stereotypical events on video EEG or even home video is imperative to characterize seizure disorders, particularly those of frontal lobe origin. The type of movements that patients display during the "spell" (semiology) can be helpful. While a full clinical EEG montage is optimal, it is helpful if additional electrodes such as T7 (formerly T3) and T8 (formerly T4) are added to electrodes typically used during routine PSG. One can then have a display of the bipolar chains (F3-T7, T7-M1, F3-C3, C3-O1 and F4-T8, T8-M2, F4-C4, C4-O2) mimicking the double banana in a bipolar longitudinal montage. Optimal diagnosis of nocturnal seizures requires a full EEG montage and simultaneous synchronized video recording. As events may not happen every night, long-term EEG monitoring in a facility designed for such monitoring may be needed. The area of onset of TLE and FLE is especially difficult to document, and intracranial electrodes placed surgically (subdural) and stereo EEG may be required for localization. Some cases have no MRI abnormality. Sometimes, a diagnosis is elusive, and an empiric trial of antiepileptic medications is needed. In patients with intractable epilepsy, brain mapping is used before surgery to help identify areas of concern and important areas that should not be removed. The differential diagnosis of nocturnal seizures includes bruxism, PLMS, sleep terrors, sleepwalking, and the REM behavior disorder. Motor activity arising from focal seizures is usually simpler and more stereotypic than motor activity associated with sleepwalking, night terrors, and REM behavior disorder. However, a type of sleep-related hypermotor epilepsy termed episodic nocturnal wandering (ENW) can mimic sleepwalking.

Temporal Lobe Epilepsy

TLE accounts for about **70% to 80% of focal seizures**. It is more *common during wakefulness than sleep*. However, as TLE is more common than FLE, *TLE is the most common nocturnal seizure type*.

Temporal lobe seizures begin focally and are usually associated with impaired awareness (formerly termed complex partial seizures). Staring, orofacial or limb automatisms, and head and body movements frequently occur. TLE limb automatisms are often *ipsilateral,* while dystonic limb posturing is usually *contralateral* to the seizure focus. The ictal pattern is often characterized by a buildup of lateralized rhythmic activity in the high theta to low alpha range. Temporal lobe seizures are more common in NREM sleep but also occur at the transition from NREM to REM sleep. Interictal activity can often be seen even using traditional sleep EEG monitoring, as the *mastoid electrodes are near the temporal lobes.* Of note, no abnormal EEG activity may be observed in some patients with TLE using scalp electrodes. Temporal lobe focal onset seizures can be associated *with complex automatisms, including unusual sleepwalking episodes, vocalization, and violent behavior.* There is overlap in semiology of TLE and SHE (FLE). Brain mapping in patients with intractable epilepsy may document a temporal lobe focus that quickly involves the frontal lobe, resulting in behavior typical of NFLE/SHE. Some patients without EEG or MRI findings may respond to an empiric trial of antiepileptic medications. In others, an MRI may reveal an abnormality in the temporal lobes. Up to 30% of the cases of SHE have seizure foci that are extra-frontal (often the temporal lobes).

Mesial TLE and Neocortical TLE

In adults, hippocampal sclerosis is the most common cause of mesial TLE, whereas in children, cortical dysplasia and low-grade malignancy are most common. Typical mesial TLE consists of focal onset impaired-awareness seizures with automatisms. They start as simple partial seizures with sensory symptoms (auras). Typical auras of mesial TLE include epigastric (abdominal) and emotional auras (déjà vu, jamais vu, and fear). The motor manifestations include fine distal automatisms of finger, hands, or orobuccal movements. Interictal EEG shows temporal sharp waves maximal at anterior temporal electrodes. The ictal EEG is often a well-defined theta (5–7 Hz) rhythmic pattern from the temporal region (derivations containing T7, M1, T8, or M2 depending on the side of the body affected). High-resolution MRI enhances the diagnosis, demonstrating abnormality of the hippocampus *within the mesial temporal lobe.* Neocortical TLE epilepsy can be either focal aware or focal impaired awareness, depending on the involved area in which the seizures originate in the neocortex, part of the external surface layer of the brain.

PSG and TLE

The appearance of interictal epileptiform activity from the temporal lobe in the typical sleep montage can be misleading. The mastoid electrodes are located close to the temporal lobes. Therefore, derivations containing the mastoid electrode on the same side as the involved temporal lobe may show prominent activity, even if the other part of the derivation is on the other side of the brain. In Figure 35–22, an interictal sharp wave is noted in all derivations containing M2, as well as the derivation T4-M1. The seizure focus in this patient was located on the right near T4. The sharp wave is noted in derivations containing M2 which is near the right temporal lobe. While reviewing only the 3 recommended EEG (F4-M1, C4-M1, O2-M1) and EOG derivations is adequate for most patients, visualizing all six EEG derivations and the eye derivations is useful when evaluating a sharp wave or other suspicious activity. In Figure 35–23, prominent spike and wave complexes (inverted) are noted in derivations containing M2 derivations (M2 is near the right temporal lobe). The deflections are downward, because M2 is the second electrode in the derivation (if G2 is negative with respect to G1, the deflection in G1-G2 is downward). Spikes are surface negative, and here, M2 is negative with respect to F3, C3, and O1, resulting in downward deflections. Ictal activity is shown from the same patient (Figure 35–24) and consists of repetitive sharp waves most prominent on the right with a phase reversal at F8-T8, localizing the seizure to the right temporal area. At the normal 30-second window, the ictal activity could be mistaken for artifact.

Sleep-Related Hypermotor Epilepsy (formerly NFLE)

The classification of NFLE has been replaced in much of the current literature by the terminology sleep-related hypermotor epilepsy (also known as hyperkinetic epilepsy).[22,25-27] The reasons for the change include: 1) the attacks are *related to sleep*

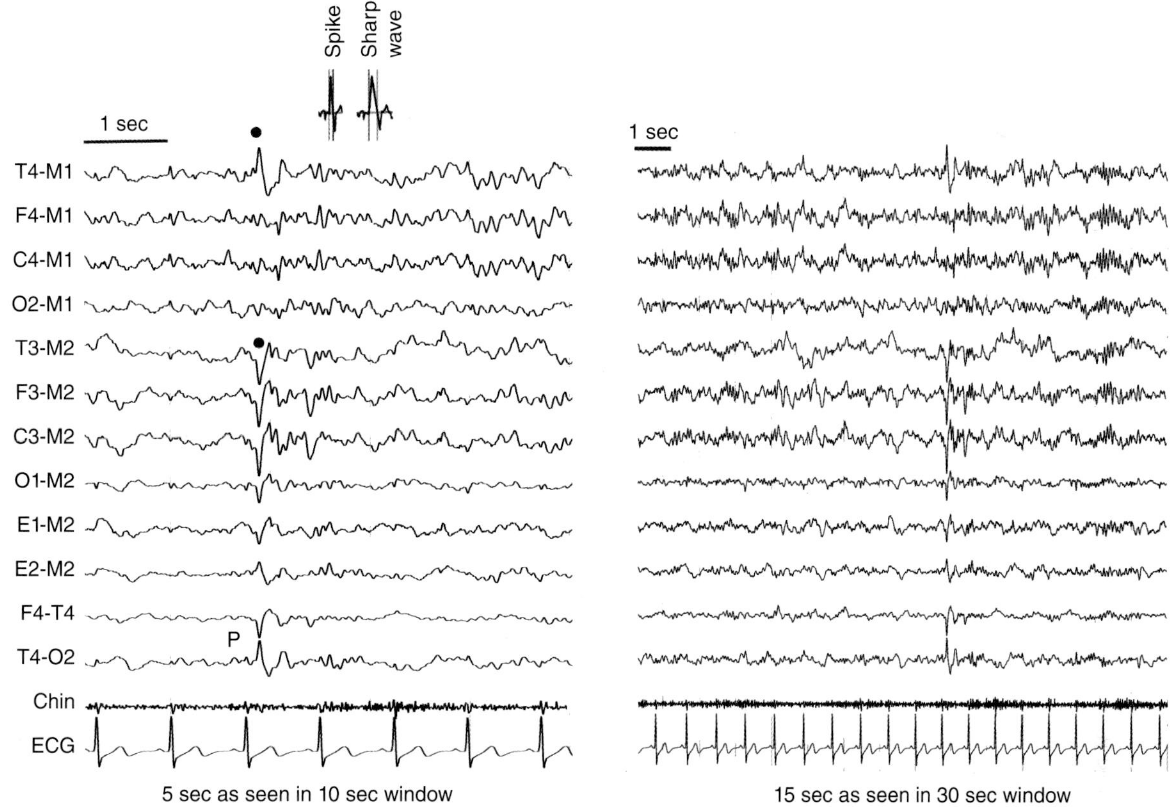

Figure 35–22 **Interictal Sharp Waves are Shown From a Patient With Temporal Lobe Epilepsy and With a Right Temporal Focus.** On the *left*, a 5-second tracing (as seen in a 10-second window) shows sharp waves *(dark circle)*. These are seen in T3-M2, F3-M2, C3-M2, and O2-M2, as the electrode M2 is near the right temporal area. As sharp waves are electronegative with respect to the scalp, electrode M2 is negative compared to the other electrodes, resulting in a downward deflection. *Note that the only right-sided derivation showing the sharp wave is T4-M1, as T4 is near the right temporal focus, making the deflection upward.* If the T4 derivation was not used, one might assume the seizure focus is on the left. Note that, using a bipolar series of electrodes (F4-T4, T4-O2) at the bottom of the tracings, a phase reversal in noted at T4. An enlargement above the tracings compares the appearance of a spike and sharp wave. In the *right panel*, the sharp wave is shown in a 15-second tracing as seen in a 30-second window. It would be easy to miss this finding.

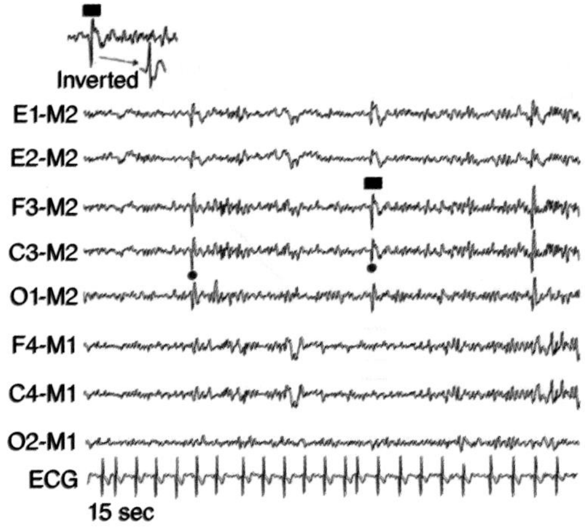

Figure 35–23 A 15-second tracing shows spikes (downward) in E1-M2, E2-M2, F3-M2, C3-M2, and O1-M2 in a patient with temporal lobe epilepsy. The small dark circles mark the location of two spikes. An inverted enlargement of a spike and wave complex marked by the short black bar is shown. When spike and wave complexes are inverted it may be more difficult to recognize the pattern. The downward spike direction in derivations containing M2 means that M2 is negative with respect to the other electrode (E1, E2, F3, C3, O1). Recall that spikes are usually electronegative with respect to the scalp. These findings suggest the seizure focus is near M2, likely in the right temporal area. However, definite localization would require a more extensive montage. A tracing from this patient is shown in Figure 35–24, confirming a right fronto-temporal seizure focus.

rather than the time of day (sleep-related vs. nocturnal), as episodes can occur during naps), 2) about *30% of seizures may arise from extra-frontal sites*, and 3) the motor aspects of the seizures are characteristic independent of the location of the focus.[22] However, not all the manifestations are truly hypermotor (hyperkinetic); they may also include dystonic posturing and episodic wandering.[26-28] FLE can occur during the day,[25] and not all FLE is sleep related. In addition, the terms FLE and NFLE have been used in the literature.[29-35] In this chapter, information about NFLE is assumed to apply to SHE with the caveat that not all SHE originates in the frontal lobe.

A consensus conference[21] defined SHE based on:

1. SHE is characterized by the occurrence of brief (<2 minutes) seizures with stereotyped motor patterns within individuals and *abrupt onset and offset.*
2. The most common clinical expression consists of hypermotor/hyperkinetic events (but can involve dystonic posturing).
3. SHE seizures occur predominantly during sleep; however, a seizure during wakefulness may occur.

In the revised epilepsy classification,[17,18] "hypermotor" has been replaced by the term hyperkinetic. However, most publications still use the former term. Hypermotor events consist of complex body movements with kicking or cycling of limbs and rocking body movements, usually with vegetative signs,

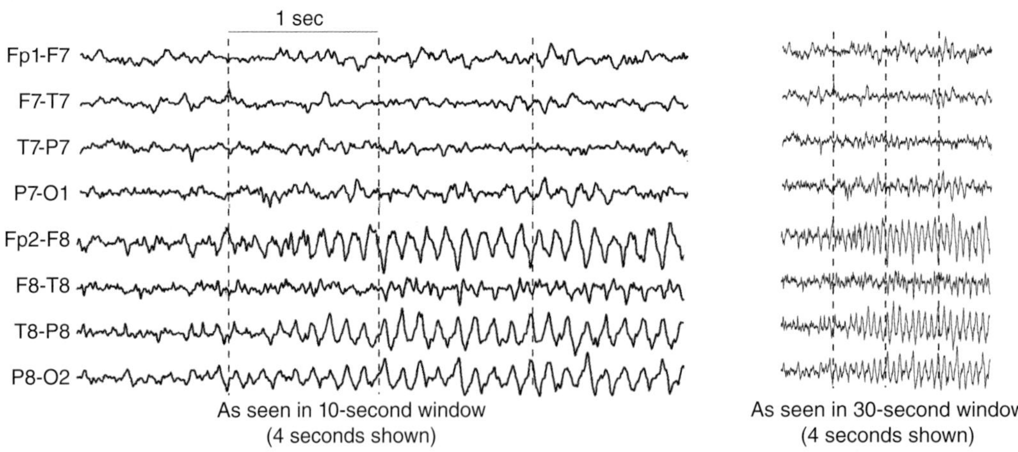

Figure 35–24 A bipolar recording shows ictal activity of approximately 8 Hz in the right frontotemporal derivations. This confirms the suspected right-sided focus noted in Figure 35–23. The low amplitude in F8-T8 suggests the focus is nearly equidistant from both electrodes (F8 and T8), so the differential signal is small (cancellation). The derivations on either side show phase reversal (Fp2-F8 and T8-P8).

vocalization, and emotional facial expressions. Asymmetric tonic/dystonic seizures with or without head/eye deviation are also observed. An example of a focal sleep-related seizure is shown in this video (video 35.1) with abrupt awakening, dystonic posturing, and only temporary impaired sensorum. Three such nearly identical episodes occurred during a single night of monitoring. No EEG correlate was visible. SHE is uncommon (1.8 per 100,000, or .0018%), but up to 10% of patients with SHE have epilepsy that does not respond to medication. The main associated pathology is cortical dysplasia. SHE events may be preceded by abrupt arousal or a distinct aura. SHE seizures typically begin in childhood and *occur nearly every night and multiple times during the night*. Of note, while SHE episodes usually occur in bed, ambulation with complex behavior mimicking sleepwalking can occur (so-called "episodic nocturnal wandering"). Gibbs et al.[12] proposed that different manifestations (semiology) could be related to the brain area of focal onset. Their publication includes informative cartoon characterization of different seizure semiology. However, linking semiology to a given brain area is beyond the scope of this chapter (and is not always reliable). The clinical manifestations of frontal lobe seizures may vary depending on localization of the epileptic focus.[12] Seizure onset in the posterior frontal lobes from the primary motor cortex may have discrete motor manifestation that have a Jacksonian march with muscle jerking that begins in the distal muscles of an extremity and moves up the extremity. Typically, seizures in patients with electrographic onset from the midline regions will involve the supplemental motor area (SMA) (Figure 35–3), which is also known as the supplemental sensorimotor area (SSMA), eliciting complex motor manifestations such as dystonic posturing, vocalizations, or speech arrest with variable loss of consciousness (sometimes awareness preserved) and minimal postictal confusion.[36-38] A classic manifestation is the "fencing posture," with the head turned toward an outstretched arm. Other behaviors associated with SSMA onset include unilateral or asymmetrical bilateral tonic posturing and may be associated with facial grimacing, vocalization, or speech arrest. SSMA seizures may be preceded by a somatosensory aura. The most dramatic movements associated with SSMA seizures include kicking, bicycling movements of the legs, laughing, or pelvic thrusting with *responsiveness often preserved*; these episodes often are misdiagnosed as non-epileptic (psychogenic) seizures. Gibbs et al. analyzed a series of patients with SHE and found that extra-frontal onset SHE (temporal and other onset) was associated with *shorter latency from EEG findings to the start of seizure behaviors, a longer duration of events, and greater postictal confusion*.

Of focal seizure disorders, approximately 20% have an onset from the frontal lobes. Sleep-related hypermotor epilepsy (about 70% with frontal focus) is associated with a wide spectrum of manifestations and is the type of epilepsy most likely mistaken as NREM or REM parasomnia.[26-35] In roughly half of SHE cases, there is no abnormality in the scalp EEG during the **episodes**, and many cases also have no interictal epileptiform activity. In some of the cases with a normal scalp EEG, abnormalities can be demonstrated by invasive EEG monitoring. The SHE episodes are confined to sleep in most cases, so they are less well observed. Patients often remain conscious, with minimal postictal confusion. Nocturnal ambulation such as walking and/or crying and autonomic activation can mimic sleepwalking and sleep terrors.[31,32,34,35] SHE/NFLE exists in familial, sporadic, symptomatic (associated with identifiable structural lesion), and idiopathic forms.

Focal seizures originating from the **orbitofrontal and insular areas as well as the cingulate gyrus** often resemble those originating from the temporal lobes with staring, nonresponsiveness, and automatisms. In addition, seizures originating from the insular area or cingulate gyrus may also have autonomic features such as tachycardia, tachypnea, pallor, and sweating. *Thus, there is considerable overlap in the manifestations of FLE and TLE.* Unfortunately, patients with frontal lobe seizures frequently do not exhibit interictal EEG activity, and ictal EEG activity is often obscured by muscle artifact (Figure 35–25).

SHE/NFLE Manifestations

Although the SHE terminology has replaced NFLE, the original description by Provini and colleagues is still useful.[29,30] They described three general manifestations of NFLE, including paroxysmal arousals (PAs), nocturnal paroxysmal dystonia (NPD), and episodic nocturnal wandering (ENW) (Table 35–8). **PAs** typically present during NREM sleep and consist of a stereotypical series of movements lasting 2 to 20 seconds in

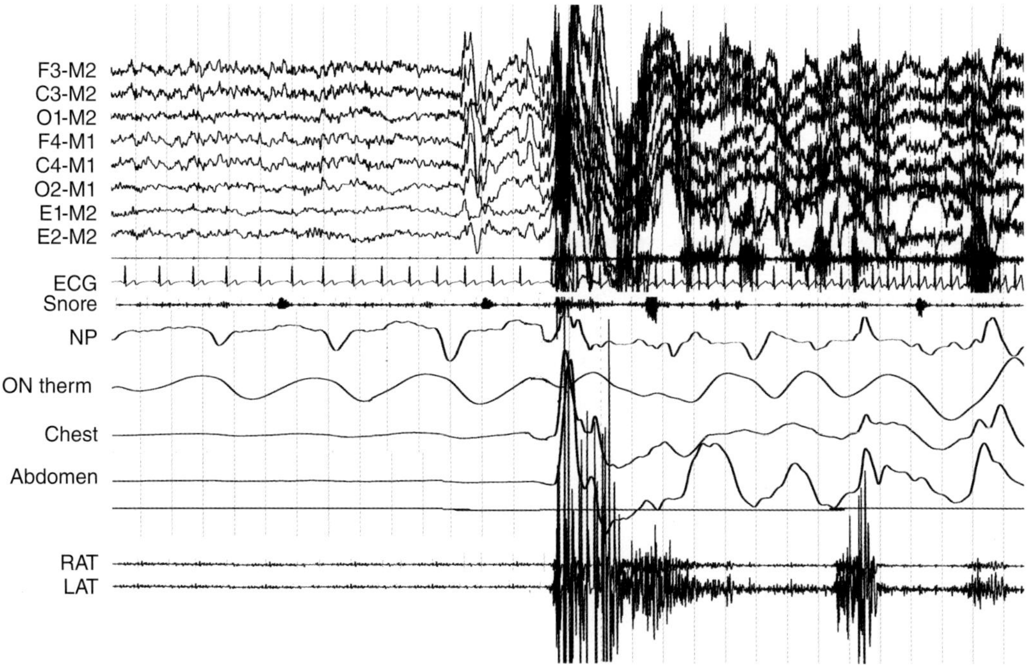

Figure 35–25 A 30-Second Tracing Showing the Start of a Frontal Lobe Focal Onset Seizure. The EEG was obscured by muscle artifact (common occurrence). No localizing EEG findings were noted before or after the event. *ON Therm*, oronasal thermal sensor; *NP*, nasal pressure.

Table 35–8 Manifestations of Different Types of Sleep-Related Hypermotor Epilepsy

	PA	Hypermotor Semiology (NPD)	ENW
Frequency	Multiple times per night (mean, 2)	Multiple times per night (mean, 3)	Multiple times (1–3 per night)
Duration of episodes	Short (20–40 sec)	More prolonged (25–98 sec)	31–180 sec
	Patients sit up and look around, confused and often scream	• Arm and leg movements • Cycling • Kicking • Dystonic posture (fencing) • Pelvic thrusting • Vocalization • Violence can occur	• Jump out of bed • Wander • Vocalize • Violent behavior
Can communicate at end of seizure	100%	44% can communicate at end of episode	100%
Can communicate during seizure	12/27	10/59 during episode	None
Stereotypical or varied	Stereotyped	Stereotyped	Stereotyped, agitated somnambulism
Daytime seizures	No	57% (49% secondarily generalized seizures)	13%
Brain structure abnormality	0%	24%	5%

NPD, nocturnal paroxysmal dystonia; *ENW*, episodic nocturnal wandering; *PA*, paroxysmal arousal.
Adapted from Provini F, Plazzi G, Tinuper P, et al. Nocturnal frontal lobe epilepsy. *Brain.* 1999;122:1017-1031.

which the individuals raise their head, sit up, look around confused with a frightened expression, then scream. Unlike typical sleep terrors, *PAs can occur many times during the night and are very stereotypical.* **NPD** (the terminology is no longer used) is characterized by nocturnal coarse movements associated with tonic spasms that often occur multiple times per night. The episodes can be violent or be associated with vocalization. Patients often move the arms and legs with cycling or kicking movements and sometimes adopt a dystonic posture of the limbs. This activity is consistent with SHE. **ENW** may present with symptoms similar to sleepwalking and sleep terrors. Patients may jump out of bed, wander, vocalize, and show violent behavior during sleep. Tuniper et al.[27] also presented a classification of SHE attacks among those mimicking sleep walking (Box 35–3): brief motor seizures, hypermotor seizures, asymmetric bilateral tonic seizures, and prolonged seizures. Gibbs and coworkers grouped SHE manifestations into four categories that correlated with an anterior to posterior gradient in the frontal lobes.[12] More anterior seizure onset was associated with more emotional manifestations (fear, anxiety, rage) and epileptic wandering.

Box 35–3 MANIFESTATIONS OF SLEEP-RELATED HYPERMOTOR EPILEPSY*

- Very brief motor seizures
  - Bilateral and axial involvement resembling a sudden arousal
  - Opening of the eyes
  - Sitting up in bed
  - Sometimes frightened expression
- Hypermotor (hyperkinetic) seizures
  - Body movements that can start in the limbs, head, or trunk
  - Complex, often violent behavior
  - Often with dystonic-dyskinetic component
  - Cycling or rocking or repetitive body movements of trunk and legs
  - Vocalization, screaming, swearing
- Asymmetric, bilateral tonic seizure
  - Sustained uncustomary forced position
- Prolonged seizures
  - Same beginning as above
  - Semi-purposeful ambulatory behavior
  - Mimics sleepwalking

*Also known as nocturnal frontal lobe epilepsy (NFLE).
Adapted from Tinuper P, Provini F, Bisulli F, Lugaresi E. Hyperkinetic manifestations in nocturnal frontal lobe epilepsy. Semeiological features and physiopathological hypothesis. *Neurol Sci.* 2005;26(Suppl 3):s210-214. PMID: 16331398.

A discussion of treatment of NFLE/SHE is beyond the scope of this chapter, though treatment with carbamazepine/oxycarbamazapine or newer anticonvulsants such as levetiracetam at bedtime is generally effective. However, roughly 10% to 30% of patients are refractory to antiepileptic medications and require surgical intervention for control. It is important to note that a significant proportion of patients with FLE do have seizures during wakefulness, generalization to tonic-clonic seizures, and a demonstrable brain abnormality. That is, not all FLE manifests as SHE.

Familial NFLE

The original description was an autosomal dominant NFLE (ADNFLE) associated with a missense mutation of the neuronal nicotinic acetylcholine receptor (nAChR) α4 subunit.[39] The associated nicotinic acetyl-choline receptor gene is also known as CHRNA4. Other mutations of the gene for the nAChR system have been found, and there is genetic heterogeneity in families with ADNFLE. Four known loci include 20q13.2, 15q24, 1q21, and 8p12.3-q12.3. Motor seizures are frequent (nearly every night), often violent, occur in clusters, and are brief (<1 minute). The age of onset is variable (2 months to 56 years), and 90% of patients present by 20 years of age.

Parasomnia Versus NFLE

Information contrasting NFLE/SHE and NREM parasomnias is listed in Table 35–9. However, *differentiation of parasomnia versus SHE can fool even expert epileptologists.* In general, SHE is associated with greater frequency (episodes per month) and is more likely to consist of multiple stereotypical episodes each night. Many patients with SHE have several episodes each night. The manifestations of NREM parasomnias also

Table 35–9 Sleep-Related Hypermotor Epilepsy Versus Non-Rapid Eye Movement Parasomnias

	Sleep-Related Hypermotor Epilepsy (SHE)*	NREM Parasomnia (Confusional Arousals, Sleep Terrors, Sleepwalking)
Age at onset (yrs ± SD)	14 ± 10 (infancy to adolescence)	<10
Gender	Male/female 7/3	M = F
Ictal EEG	NREM – sleep stage N2 Normal ictal EEG 44% (higher if only scalp electrodes used) Normal interictal EEG 51%	NREM sleep Stage N3 in children
Movement semiology	Violent, stereotypical	Complex, non-stereotypical
Family history of episodes	39%	62%–96%
Episode frequency per month	20 ± 11	<1–4
Episode frequency per night	3 ± 3 (higher with PA, NPD)*	1
Episode duration	2 sec–3 minutes	15 sec–30 min
Clinical course	Increased frequency	Tend to resolve
Triggering factors	None in 78%	Sleep deprivation, alcohol, febrile illness
Autonomic activation	Very common (tachycardia)	Yes in sleep terrors
Episode onset after sleep onset	Any time	First third of night in children
Effect of treatment	Carbamazepine abolished (20%) or improved episodes (50%)	N/A

EEG, electroencephalogram; *NREM*, non-rapid eye movement; *N/A*, not applicable; *SHE*, sleep-related hypermotor epilepsy; *SD*, standard deviation; *NPD*, nocturnal paroxysmal dystonia (this terminology is no longer used, refers to manifestation of SHE); *PA*, paroxysmal arousal.
*Previous terminology nocturnal frontal lobe epilepsy (NFLE);
Adapted from Provini F, Plazzi G, Tinuper P, et al. Nocturnal frontal lobe epilepsy. *Brain.* 1999;122:1017-1031.

vary from night to night, whereas SHE episodes have very stereotypical manifestations. They can be bizarre, but they always consist of the same activity. As noted above, EEG is not that helpful in many cases because approximately 40% to 50% of patients with SHE have no interictal or ictal EEG findings (apart from movement and muscle artifact associated with the spells). Derry and coworkers[35] analyzed a group with NREM parasomnia and NFLE/SHE episodes and found that seizures were likely to have a rapid **offset** rather than a slower emergence of full consciousness in NREM parasomnia and that *head version (involuntary forced head movement) or dystonic posturing favored seizure episodes.*

Benign Epilepsy of Childhood With Centrotemporal Spikes (BECTS)

Epileptiform discharges are found in 1% to 2% of pediatric PSGs, and the incidence may be higher in those with sleep disordered breathing.[40] Benign epilepsy with centrotemporal spikes (BECTS) is also known as benign epilepsy of childhood or benign rolandic epilepsy (BRE), accounts for 15% to 20% of childhood epilepsy and is the *most common epilepsy of childhood.*[41,42] The average age of onset is **5 to 8 years (range 3–13 years), with a male predominance.** That is, onset usually occurs by middle childhood and resolution by mid-adolescence. BECTS is considered a *genetic disorder*, as approximately 25% of patients have a family history of either febrile seizures or epilepsy. The mode of transmission is *autosomal dominant.* The cardinal features of BECTS are focal seizures consisting of unilateral facial sensory-motor symptoms (numbness tingling), oropharyngo-laryngeal symptoms (tingling or numbness of mouth, death rattle sounds, gargling, grunting, and guttural sounds), hypersalivation, tonic contractions of the ipsilateral arm and leg, and speech arrest. Hemifacial sensory-motor seizures (tingling and numbness) are mainly localized in the lower lip and may spread to the ipsilateral hand. Motor manifestations are clonic contractions sometimes concurrent with ipsilateral tonic deviation of the mouth. In speech arrest, the child is actually anarthric (unable to utter a single intelligible word and attempts to communicate with gestures). *Consciousness and recollection are fully retained in more than half (58%) of rolandic seizures.* In the remainder, consciousness becomes impaired during ictal EEG activity, and in one-third there is no recollection of ictal events. *Three-quarters of BECTS seizures occur during NREM sleep, and most commonly the onset of seizure activity is about 20 minutes to 3 hours after bedtime.* The seizures are *usually brief, lasting 1 to 3 minutes.*

By definition, centrotemporal spikes (CTS) are the hallmark of BECTS (Figure 35–26). Although called centrotemporal, these spikes are mainly localized in the C3 and C4 areas and not the temporal electrodes. In Figure 35–27, a bipolar montage using commonly recorded electrodes for sleep monitoring is shown. At the top are longitudinal chains, and at the bottom is a transverse chain across the vertex. In both approaches, there is phase reversal at C3. The CTS EEG activity is often bilateral and typically activated by drowsiness and NREM sleep, but not by hyperventilation. *Generalized seizures during sleep may occur.* Only those BECTS patients with cognitive impairment, very frequent epileptiform discharges on EEG, and a history of generalized seizures are generally treated. Such patients should undergo neurological evaluation. Given the focal nature of seizures, carbamazepine is often a first-line agent. Other medication such as oxcarbazepine, gabapentin, levetiracetam, valproate, phenytoin, lacosamide, and zonisamide have also been used.

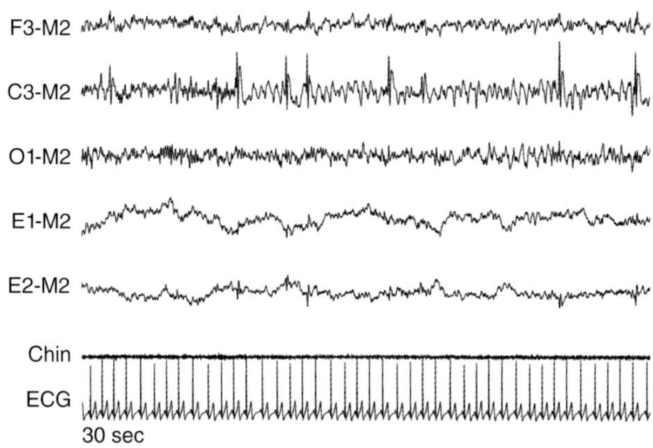

Figure 35–26 Spike and Wave Complexes Noted in C3-M2 During NREM Sleep in a Patient With BECTS. Left-sided derivations are presented, as these show the complexes most clearly. The seizure focus is near C3, as demonstrated in Figure 35–27.

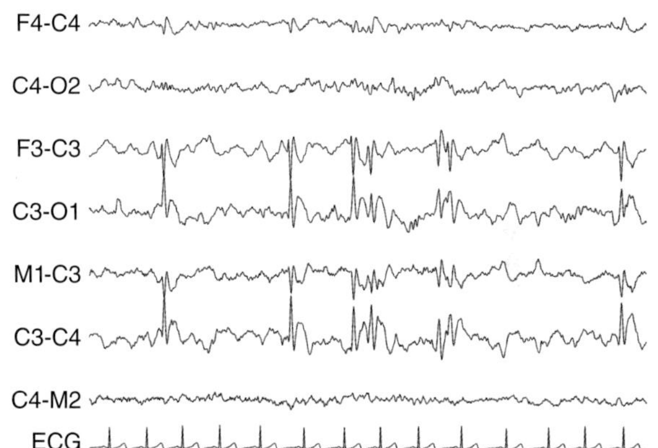

Figure 35–27 A 10-Second Tracing in the Same Patient With BECTS as Shown in Figure 35–26. The top 4 channels are a longitudinal bipolar arrangement using standard electrodes used in sleep monitoring. The bottom three derivations are a transverse bipolar arrangement across the vertex area. One can clearly see the phase reversal in spike and wave complexes at C3.

Panayiotopoulos syndrome (PS)[41,42] is another "benign," age-related focal seizure disorder occurring in early and mid-childhood. It is characterized by seizures, often prolonged, with predominantly autonomic manifestations such as nausea, retching, vomiting, pallor, incontinence of urine, hypersalivation (10%), cyanosis (12%), and mydriasis. *Unlike BECTS, the seizures are prolonged (6 minutes to many hours).* The EEG shows shifting and multiple foci, usually with **occipital predominance.**

Juvenile Myoclonic Epilepsy

JME is idiopathic (meaning no demonstrable brain lesion) and has a *genetic basis with an abnormality on the* ***short arm of chromosome 6.*** Onset is in adolescence, peaking between ages 12 and 18. This is one of the more common forms of generalized epilepsy and consists of a combination of *focal myoclonic seizures on awakening, GTC seizures, and absence seizures.*[43] The myoclonic seizures occur in clusters on awakening or shortly thereafter. Patients may not seek medical evaluation until after the first associated GTC seizure. The myoclonic seizures may subside during adulthood, but patients often have persistent GTC seizures requiring lifelong treatment. Antiepileptic medications such as valproate are quite effective, but lifelong treatment is usually needed due to persistence of GTC seizures. The interictal EEG in JME is characterized *by diffuse polyspike and slow wave complexes of 4 to 6 Hz, usually*

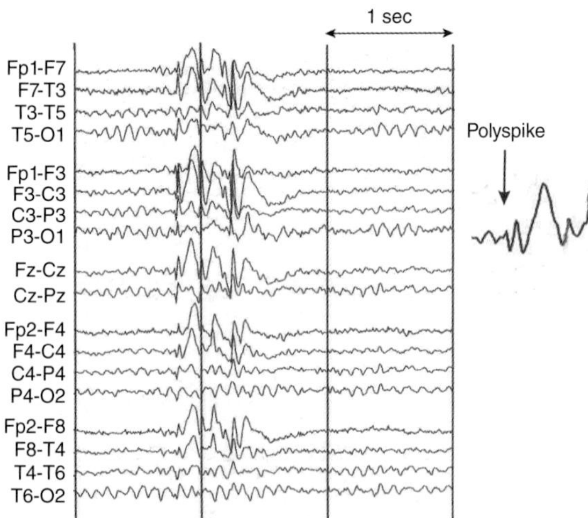

Figure 35–28 This 3-second tracing shows polyspike complexes *(enlargement to the right of the detailed tracing)* in a patient with juvenile myoclonic epilepsy. (From Berry RB, Wagner MH. *Sleep Medicine Pearls*, Elsevier; 2014:579.)

maximal at the frontal electrodes (Figure 35–28). Neurologic examination and brain MRI are usually normal.

ICTAL EFFECTS ON SLEEP

Epilepsy and sleep have a bidirectional relationship. Epilepsy has the potential to worsen sleep quality, and worse sleep quality can worsen seizure control. Several studies have found sleep-wake disorders are about 2 to 3 times more prevalent in adults with epilepsy than in the general public.[14,44] Although untreated or poorly controlled nocturnal epilepsy could impair sleep quality and prompt complaints of daytime sleepiness or insomnia, results of studies evaluating sleepiness and insomnia in patients with epilepsy have provided conflicting results. In some studies, significant fractions of patients with epilepsy complain of daytime sleepiness and insomnia. However, one large meta-analysis found no evidence of an increase in subjective daytime sleepiness but an increase in the Pittsburg Sleep Quality Index (worse sleep) in patients with epilepsy compared to normal groups.[45] Another study of excessive sleepiness in patients with epilepsy concluded that, if daytime sleepiness is present, it is more likely to be associated with untreated comorbid sleep disorders than epilepsy.[46] However, focal and primary generalized seizures can be associated with sleep fragmentation, increased sleep-stage shifts, and decreased sleep efficiency. Bazil et al.[47] found that daytime or nighttime temporal lobe seizures *decreased REM sleep on the subsequent night*. Insomnia and poor-quality sleep have been associated with poor seizure control.[48] *Although some antiepileptic drugs (AEDs) can impair sleep*,[49-51] the sleep of patients with nocturnal epilepsy is usually better on AEDs than without AEDs. *That is, seizure control improves sleep quality.*

ANTIEPILEPTIC DRUGS (AEDs) – EFFECTS ON SLEEP

The term antiseizure medication (ASM) is currently preferred to AED by some epileptologists, but the term AED commonly appears in the literature. The effects of common AEDs[49-51] on sleep are listed in Table 35–10. Published information on this topic is somewhat conflicting and often based on small studies. For most patients, the benefits of seizure control on sleep outweigh the side effects of AEDs.[51]

Table 35–10 Effects of Common Anti-Epileptic Drugs (AEDs) on Sleep

	Positive	Negative
Barbiturates (Phenobarbital)	Decreased sleep latency Increased sleep efficiency Increased stage N2	Decreased REM
Carbamazepine	None known	Decreased REM?
Phenytoin	Decreased sleep latency	Increased arousals Increased stage N1 Decreased REM
Valproic Acid	None known	Increased stage N1
Gabapentin	Increased stage N3 Decreased arousals	None
Pregabalin	Increased stage N3	None
Levetiracetam (Keppra)	Increased stage N3	None
Clobazam (Sympazan)	Decreased sleep latency and wakefulness after sleep onset	Decreased stage N3
Lacosamide (VimPAT)	None	None
Lamotrigine (Lamictal)	None	Can cause insomnia or hypersomnia, Decreased stage N3, increase number of REM periods
Medications Associated with sedation	• Higher incidence of sedation: Phenobarbital, Benzodiazepines; Moderate to mild incidence of sedation: Phenytoin, Levetiracetam, Oxcarbazepine, Carbamazapine, Topiramate, Valproic acid, Clobazam; • Least sedating: Lamotrigine, Gabapentin, Lacosamide	
Medications Most Associated with Insomnia	Lamotrigine, Felbamate	

Jain SV, Glauser TA. Effects of epilepsy treatments on sleep architecture and daytime sleepiness: an evidence-based review of objective sleep metrics. *Epilepsia*. 2014;55(1):26-37. PMID: 24299283

EPILEPSY AND OBSTRUCTIVE SLEEP APNEA

A meta-analysis of studies evaluating the presence of obstructive sleep apnea (OSA) in patients with epilepsy found that patients with epilepsy had over 2 times the risk of having OSA compared to normal controls. They also found evidence that continuous positive airway pressure (CPAP) treatment may improve seizure control.[52] A small study did find a benefit in seizure control with CPAP treatment.[53] Another retrospective analysis on a large group of patients also found a benefit[54]. However, a large, randomized controlled trial is needed to confirm benefit.

SUDDEN UNEXPECTED DEATH IN EPILEPSY (SUDEP)

Approximately 70% of sudden unexpected death in epilepsy (SUDEP) cases occur in sleep. Patients with nocturnal seizures are 6.3 times more likely to die in a prone position than those with diurnal seizures. Beside NREM activation of seizures, other physiological changes in sleep that may predispose a patient to SUDEP include reduced airway patency, lower inspiratory drive, reduced hypoxic and hypercapnic ventilatory responses, and a longer QT interval, lowering the threshold for malignant cardiac arrhythmia. Among patients with medically refractory epilepsy, the risk of SUDEP is reduced in those who undergo epilepsy surgery compared to those who continue to have seizures without surgery.[55]

SUMMARY OF KEY POINTS

1. Sleep-related epilepsy is part of the differential diagnosis of abnormal motor behavior occurring during sleep. Some patients have seizures only at night, associated with sleep, or after awakening from sleep.
2. Optimal diagnosis of nocturnal seizures requires a full EEG montage, with simultaneous synchronized video and audio recording. The ability of PSG to detect and/or localize interictal activity is enhanced by addition of temporal electrodes T7 and T8 (also known as T3 and T4) and viewing waveforms in a 10-second window. The video is often more helpful than the EEG for determining whether an event is a seizure versus an NREM parasomnia. That is, identifying semiology of different seizure types is very helpful for differentiating seizures from NREM parasomnias. The occurrence of multiple events each night with the same behavior (semiology) favors a nocturnal seizure compared to a typical NREM parasomnia. Many nocturnal seizures do not have interictal or ictal scalp EEG abnormalities.
3. Sharp EEG activity (spikes, sharp waves) noted during a routine sleep study could represent interictal epileptiform activity. It is recommended to switch to a 10-second page and/or a longitudinal bipolar montage to accurately access the activity. Remember, some sharp waves can be normal (vertex sharp waves). However, spike and wave activity is never normal unless due to artifact (video is helpful). True epileptiform activity is usually electronegative with respect to the scalp and seen in more than one derivation.
4. Identification of interictal activity on a PSG should prompt a more extensive evaluation for epilepsy, even if a clinical seizure is not recorded. Interictal activity is more frequent in NREM sleep (some references report stage N3 as having the highest frequency).
5. The incidence of epilepsy is NREM > Wakefulness > REM sleep. Most nocturnal seizures occur during stage N1 and N2 or soon after awakening.
6. SHE (formerly NFLE) consists of focal seizures primarily at night (usually out of NREM sleep), characterized by a rapid onset and offset, brief duration, a variable level of awareness, and a semiology that includes hypermotor activity (pedaling, cycling, pelvic thrusting), dystonic activity (fencing posture), brief arousals with vocalizations (mimicking sleep terrors), and rarely, prolonged events and wandering (mimicking sleepwalking). Multiple episodes each night with stereotypic behavior help differentiate SHE from NREM parasomnias. Only about 70% of SHE episodes have a frontal lobe onset. (others often temporal lobe onset) There can be preserved consciousness and partial-to-complete memory of the episodes.
7. Nocturnal epilepsy can be difficult to differentiate from parasomnias because some patients have seizures only at night, scalp EEG findings may not be visible during seizures, consciousness can be maintained with minimal postictal confusion, and behavior can be violent with some nocturnal seizures. Behavior can mimic night terrors and sleepwalking. In contrast to NREM parasomnias, SHE/NFLE episodes are more frequently out of stage N2 (vs. stage N3), multiple short episodes can occur per night (vs. one per night), and the behavior is stereotypical while behavior in NREM parasomnias is variable from episode to episode. *SHE episodes have a more rapid return to full awareness than do NREM parasomnias.*
8. TLE comprises about 70% of focal epilepsy cases. FLE accounts for about 20% of focal epilepsy cases. FLE is more likely to occur only or primarily at night than TLE. However, as TLE is more common, *TLE is the most frequent type of epilepsy occurring at night.* Daytime FLE is more likely to generalize than FLE at night. Because mastoid electrodes are near the temporal lobes, interictal activity associated with TLE can often be easily seen in standard PSG montages. For example, a left temporal spike may be visible in derivations containing M1 (M1 is near the left temporal lobe). The spike may be more prominent in C4-M1 than in C3-M2, even though the seizure focus is on the left.
9. In about 50% of cases of NFLE (SHE), scalp EEG will show neither interictal nor ictal activity. The EEG during the episode may simply show muscle and movement artifact. A significant proportion of FLE does not respond to pharmacotherapy but does respond to surgery.
10. Focal onset seizures with impaired awareness (formerly called complex partial seizures) are associated with a focal onset and impairment of consciousness. There may be associated automatisms, dystonic posturing, thrashing of arms or legs, screaming, and autonomic activation mimicking a sleep terror or complex automatisms mimicking sleepwalking.
11. TLE during sleep usually presents with focal onset seizures with impaired awareness (complex partial seizures) that may generalize. Interictal activity can often be seen even using traditional sleep EEG monitoring, as the *mastoid electrodes are near the temporal lobes*. Although, TLE is more common during the day than night, TLE is the most common seizure occuring at night. About 30% of SHE occurs from foci outside of the frontal lobes—often in the temporal lobes. Staring, orofacial or limb automatisms, and head and body movements frequently occur. There is considerable overlap in semiology between TLE and FLE.
12. BECTS should be suspected when spike and wave activity is seen prominently in the central derivations and there is a history of abnormal mouth movements, hypersalivation, and unusual vocalizations in a young child with otherwise normal neurological function. BECTS episodes are unilateral, and the patient responds but may not be able to speak. GTC seizures can occur.
13. Protracted episodes of vomiting that suddenly occur during sleep should suggest the possibility of Panayiotopoulos syndrome. Interictal discharges are commonly in the occipital areas. In contrast to BECTS, the episodes are often longer than 6 minutes.
14. Patients with JME commonly have myoclonic jerking soon after awakening. They may also have grand mal seizures. The characteristic pattern is polyspike and wave. Onset of JME is in adolescence and may not be diagnosed until the first tonic-clonic seizure.
15. Typical absence epilepsy (AE) is a generalized non-motor epilepsy characterized by 3 Hz spike and wave activity with impairment of consciousness. Typical AE has an onset in childhood and resolves by adolescence. ***Atypical*** AE has later onset, has spike and wave activity with a lower frequency than 3 Hz and does not spontaneously resolve.

CLINICAL REVIEW QUESTIONS

1. Which of the following characterizes the propensity of nocturnal seizures?
   A. NREM > REM > Wakefulness
   B. Wakefulness > REM > NREM
   C. NREM > Wakefulness > REM
   D. Wakefulness > NREM > REM
2. What is the most frequent type of nocturnal focal seizure?
   A. TLE
   B. NFLE/SHE
   C. AE
   D. JME
3. Which of the following statements about phase reversal is true?
   A. EEG events showing phase reversal are always epileptiform (abnormal).
   B. Phase reversal can help determine the location or origin of transient or focal interictal activity.
   C. A and B.
4. Which of the following statements about POSTS is **NOT** true?
   A. They are positive.
   B. They have an occipital location.
   C. They occur during wake.
   D. They consist of sharp waves.
5. Which of the following is **NOT** true about Mu rhythm?
   A. The frequency is 8 to 13 Hz.
   B. The activity is most prominent in occipital derivations.
   C. The activity is attenuated by contralateral arm movement.
   D. The rhythm has archiform morphology.
6. The terminology sleep-related hypermotor epilepsy (SHE) has replaced nocturnal frontal lobe epilepsy (NFLE) to describe focal seizure occurring primarily during sleep for all of the following reasons **EXCEPT**:
   A. The focus of the episodes can be from the non-frontal areas (often from the temporal lobes).
   B. Episodes are related to sleep rather than nighttime (ie nocturnal).
   C. All of the manifestations are hypermotor/hyperkinetic, no matter the area of focal onset.
7. An 8-year-old child has episodes of sitting up in bed with salivation, gurgling, and the inability to speak, though alert. Some facial, arm, and leg twitching is also observed. The episodes last only 2 to 3 minutes. Which of the following epilepsy types is most likely?
   A. SHE
   B. TLE with focal impaired awareness and automatisms
   C. JME
   D. BECTS
8. Which of the following characteristics of SHE is the most helpful for differentiating SHE from a NREM parasomnia?
   A. Screaming and vocalization
   B. Sudden onset
   C. Occurs during stage N2
   D. Multiple stereotypical episodes in a single night

ANSWERS

1. C. NREM > Wakefulness > REM. During NREM, seizures out of N2 are more common.
2. A. Although FLE is more likely to occur during the night than during the day, nocturnal TLE is more common than nocturnal FLE, as TLE is much more common than FLE. AE is a generalized epilepsy. JME is manifested as myoclonic jerks soon after awakening.
3. B. Phase reversal is helpful for localization but does not imply abnormality.
4. C. POSTS occur during NREM sleep (Postive Occipital Sharp Transient of **Sleep**).
5. B. Mu rhythm is more prominent in the central derivations.
6. C. Although hypermotor describes the manifestations of many of the episodes, the episodes may display other semiology such as dystonic posturing or nocturnal wandering.
7. D. BECTS
8. D. NREM parasomnias can occur in stage N2 or N3 in adults. Both can have a sudden onset, and SHE episodes can have screaming and mimic sleep (night) terrors.

SUGGESTED READING

1. Libenson MH. *Practical Approach Electroencephalography*. Philadelphia: Elsevier, 2010.
2. Tinuper P, Bisulli F, Cross JH, et al. Definition and diagnostic criteria of sleep-related hypermotor epilepsy. *Neurology*. 2016;86(19):1834-1842. PMID: 27164717.
3. Moore JL, Carvalho DZ, St Louis EK, Bazil C. Sleep and epilepsy: a focused review of pathophysiology, clinical syndromes, co-morbidities, and therapy. *Neurotherapeutics*. 2021;18(1):170-180. Erratum in: *Neurotherapeutics*. 2021;18(1):655.

REFERENCES

1. Jasper HH. The ten-twenty electrode system of the International Federation of Societies for Electroencephalography and Clinical Neurophysiology: report of the committee on methods of clinical examination in electroencephalography: ten twenty electrode system. *EEG Clin Neurophysiol*. 1958;10:371-375.
2. Klem GH, Lüders HO, Jasper HH, Elger C. The ten-twenty electrode system of the International Federation. The International Federation of Clinical Neurophysiology. *Electroencephalogr Clin Neurophysiol Suppl*. 1999;52:3-6.
3. American Clinical Neurophysiology Society. Guideline 5: Guidelines for standard electrode position nomenclature. *J Clin Neurophysiol*. 2006;23(2):107-110.
4. Acharya JN, Hani A, Cheek J, Thirumala P, Tsuchida TN. American Clinical Neurophysiology Society Guideline 2: Guidelines for standard electrode position nomenclature. *J Clin Neurophysiol*. 2016;33(4):308-311.
5. Libenson MH. *Practical Approach to Electroencephalography*. Philadelphia: Saunders Elsevier; 2010.
6. Berry RB, Quan SF, Abreu AR, et al.; for the American Academy of Sleep Medicine. *The AASM Manual for the Scoring of Sleep and Associated Events: Rules, Terminology and Technical Specifications*. Version 2.6. Darien, IL: American Academy of Sleep Medicine; 2020.
7. Kellinghaus C, Lüders HO. Frontal lobe epilepsy. *Epileptic Disord*. 2004;6(4):223-239.
8. Acharya JN, Hani AJ, Thirumala PD, Tsuchida TN. American Clinical Neurophysiology Society Guideline 3: a proposal for standard montages to be used in clinical EEG. *J Clin Neurophysiol*. 2016;33(4):312-316.
9. Foldvary N, Caruso AC, Mascha E, et al. Identifying montages that best detect electrographic seizure activity during polysomnography. *Sleep*. 2000;23(2):221-229.
10. Foldvary-Schaefer N, Alsheikhtaha Z. Complex nocturnal behaviors: nocturnal seizures and parasomnias. *Continuum (Minneap Minn)*. 2013;19(1 Sleep Disorders):104-131.
11. Jordan JW. Semiology: witness to a seizure—what to note and how to report. *Am J Electroneurodiagnostic Technol*. 2007;47(4):264-282.
12. Gibbs SA, Proserpio P, Francione S, et al. Clinical features of sleep-related hypermotor epilepsy in relation to the seizure-onset zone: a review of 135 surgically treated cases. *Epilepsia*. 2019;60(4):707-717.
13. Moore JL, Carvalho DZ, St Louis EK, Bazil C. Sleep and epilepsy: a focused review of pathophysiology, clinical syndromes, co-morbidities, and therapy. *Neurotherapeutics*. 2021;18(1):170-180. Erratum in: *Neurotherapeutics*. 2021;18(1):655.
14. Grigg-Damberger M, Foldvary-Schaefer N. Bidirectional relationships of sleep and epilepsy in adults with epilepsy. *Epilepsy Behav*. 2021; 116:107735.

15. Sammaritano M, Gigli GL, Gotman J. Interictal spiking during wakefulness and sleep and the localization of foci in temporal lobe epilepsy. *Neurology*. 1991;41(2 Pt 1):290-297.
16. Chen H, Koubeissi MZ. Electroencephalography in epilepsy evaluation. *Continuum (Minneap Minn)*. 2019;25(2):431-453.
17. Proposal for revised classification of epilepsies and epileptic syndromes. Commission on classification and terminology of the International League Against Epilepsy. *Epilepsia*. 1989;30(4):389-399.
18. Fisher RS, Cross JH, French JA, et al. Operational classification of seizure types by the International League Against Epilepsy: position paper of the ILAE Commission for Classification and Terminology. *Epilepsia*. 2017;58(4):522-530.
19. Fisher RS, Cross JH, D'Souza C, et al. Instruction manual for the ILAE 2017 operational classification of seizure types. *Epilepsia*. 2017;58(4):531-542.
20. Pack AM. Epilepsy overview and revised classification of seizures and epilepsies. *Continuum (Minneap Minn)*. 2019;25(2):306-321.
21. Fisher RS, Acevedo C, Arzimanoglou A, et al. ILAE official report: a practical clinical definition of epilepsy. *Epilepsia*. 2014;55(4):475-482.
22. Tinuper P, Bisulli F, Cross JH, et al. Definition and diagnostic criteria of sleep-related hypermotor epilepsy. *Neurology*. 2016;86(19):1834-1842.
23. Jain P. Absence seizures in children: usual and the unusual. *Indian J Pediatr*. 2020;87(12):1047-1056.
24. Guilhoto LM. Absence epilepsy: continuum of clinical presentation and epigenetics? *Seizure*. 2017;44:53-57.
25. Herman ST, Walczak TS, Bazil CW. Distribution of partial seizures during the sleep-wake cycle: differences by seizure onset site. *Neurology*. 2001;56(11):1453-1459.
26. Menghi V, Bisulli F, Tinuper P, Nobili L. Sleep-related hypermotor epilepsy: prevalence, impact and management strategies. *Nat Sci Sleep*. 2018;10:317-326.
27. Tinuper P, Provini F, Bisulli F, Lugaresi E. Hyperkinetic manifestations in nocturnal frontal lobe epilepsy. Semeiological features and physiopathological hypothesis. *Neurol Sci*. 2005;26 suppl 3:s210-s214.
28. Gibbs SA, Proserpio P, Francione S, et al. Seizure duration and latency of hypermotor manifestations distinguish frontal from extrafrontal onset in sleep-related hypermotor epilepsy. *Epilepsia*. 2018;59(9):e130-e134.
29. Provini F, Plazzi G, Tinuper P, Vandi S, Lugaresi E, Montagna P. Nocturnal frontal lobe epilepsy. A clinical and polygraphic overview of 100 consecutive cases. *Brain*. 1999;122(Pt 6):1017-1031.
30. Provini F, Plazzi G, Lugaresi E. From nocturnal paroxysmal dystonia to nocturnal frontal lobe epilepsy. *Clin Neurophysiol*. 2000;111 suppl 2:S2-S8.
31. Plazzi G, Tinuper P, Montagna P, Provini F, Lugaresi E. Epileptic nocturnal wanderings. *Sleep*. 1995;18(9):749-756.
32. Plazzi G, Vetrugno R, Provini F, Montagna P. Sleepwalking and other ambulatory behaviours during sleep. *Neurol Sci*. 2005;26 suppl 3:s193-s198.
33. McGonigal A. Frontal lobe seizures: overview and update. *J Neurol*. 2022;269(6):3363-3371.
34. Erturk Cetin O, Sirin NG, Elmali AD, Baykan B, Bebek N. Different faces of frontal lobe epilepsy: the clinical, electrophysiologic, and imaging experience of a tertiary center. *Clin Neurol Neurosurg*. 2021;203:106532.
35. Derry CP, Harvey AS, Walker MC, Duncan JS, Berkovic SF. NREM arousal parasomnias and their distinction from nocturnal frontal lobe epilepsy: a video EEG analysis. *Sleep*. 2009;32(12):1637-1644.
36. Aghakhani Y, Rosati A, Olivier A, et al. The predictive localizing value of tonic limb posturing in supplementary sensorimotor seizures. *Neurology*. 2004;62:2256-2261.
37. King DW, Smith JR. Supplementary sensorimotor area epilepsy in adults. *Adv Neurol*. 1996;70:285-291.
38. Tachibana N, Shinde A, Ikeda A, Akiguchi I, Kimura J, Shibasaki H. Supplementary motor area seizure resembling sleep disorder. *Sleep*. 1996;19(10):811-816.
39. Combi R, Dalprà L, Tenchini ML, Ferini-Strambi L. Autosomal dominant nocturnal frontal lobe epilepsy—a critical overview. *J Neurol*. 2004;251(8):923-934.
40. Capdevila OS, Dayyat E, Kheirandish-Gozal L, Gozal D. Prevalence of epileptiform activity in healthy children during sleep. *Sleep Med*. 2008;9(3):303-309.
41. Panayiotopoulos CP, Michael M, Sanders S, Valeta T, Koutroumanidis M. Benign childhood focal epilepsies: assessment of established and newly recognized syndromes. *Brain*. 2008;131(Pt 9):2264-2286.
42. Covanis A. Panayiotopoulos syndrome: a benign childhood autonomic epilepsy frequently imitating encephalitis, syncope, migraine, sleep disorder, or gastroenteritis. *Pediatrics*. 2006;118(4):e1237-e1243.
43. Baykan B, Wolf P. Juvenile myoclonic epilepsy as a spectrum disorder: A focused review. *Seizure*. 2017;49:36-41.
44. Im H-J, Park S-H, Baek S-H, et al. Associations of impaired sleep quality, insomnia, and sleepiness with epilepsy: a questionnaire-based case-control study. *Epilepsy Behav*. 2016;57(Pt A):55-59.
45. Bergmann M, Tschiderer L, Stefani A, Heidbreder A, Willeit P, Högl B. Sleep quality and daytime sleepiness in epilepsy: systematic review and meta-analysis of 25 studies including 8,196 individuals. *Sleep Med Rev*. 2021;57:101466.
46. Giorelli AS, Passos P, Carnaval T, da Mota Gomes M. Excessive daytime sleepiness and epilepsy: a systematic review. *Epilepsy Res Treat*. 2013; 2013:629469.
47. Bazil CW, Castro LH, Walczak TS. Reduction of rapid eye movement sleep by diurnal and nocturnal seizures in temporal lobe epilepsy. *Arch Neurol*. 2000;57(3):363-368.
48. Planas-Ballvé A, Grau-López L, Jiménez M, Ciurans J, Fumanal A, Becerra JL. Insomnia and poor sleep quality are associated with poor seizure control in patients with epilepsy. *Neurologia (Engl Ed)*. 2022;37(8):639-646.
49. Bazil CW. Nocturnal seizures and the effects of anticonvulsants on sleep. *Curr Neurol Neurosci Rep*. 2008;8(2):149-154.
50. Liguori C, Toledo M, Kothare S. Effects of anti-seizure medications on sleep architecture and daytime sleepiness in patients with epilepsy: a literature review. *Sleep Med Rev*. 2021;60:101559.
51. Jain SV, Glauser TA. Effects of epilepsy treatments on sleep architecture and daytime sleepiness: an evidence-based review of objective sleep metrics. *Epilepsia*. 2014;55(1):26-37.
52. Lin Z, Si Q, Xiaoyi Z. Obstructive sleep apnoea in patients with epilepsy: a meta-analysis. *Sleep Breath*. 2017;21(2):263-270.
53. Malow BA, Foldvary-Schaefer N, Vaughn BV, et al. Treating obstructive sleep apnea in adults with epilepsy: a randomized pilot trial. *Neurology*. 2008;71(8):572-577.
54. Pornsriniyom D, won Kim H, Bena J, Andrews ND, Moul D, Foldvary-Schaefer N. Effect of positive airway pressure therapy on seizure control in patients with epilepsy and obstructive sleep apnea. *Epilepsy Behav*. 2014;37:270-275.
55. Casadei CH, Carson KW, Mendiratta A, et al. All-cause mortality and SUDEP in a surgical epilepsy population. *Epilepsy Behav*. 2020; 108:107093.

Chapter 36

Parasomnias

INTRODUCTION

A parasomnia is a motor (behavioral), verbal, autonomic nervous system, or experiential phenomenon that occurs in association with sleep (at sleep onset, during sleep, or after partial or full arousal from sleep) and is often undesirable. The term *parasomnia* comes from a combination of *para* from the Greek prefix meaning "alongside of" with the Latin word *somnus*, meaning "sleep." In the usual clinical setting, the term refers to undesirable events. Some parasomnias are associated with rapid eye movement (REM) sleep, some with non-REM (NREM) sleep, and some are classified as "other parasomnias" (e.g., enuresis) because they can occur during NREM or REM sleep or during wakefulness soon after arousal from sleep.[1-6] The International Classification of Sleep Disorders, 3rd edition, text revision (ICSD-3-TR) divides parasomnias into NREM, REM, other parasomnias, and Isolated Symptoms and Normal Variants (Table 36–1).[2]

EVALUATION OF PARASOMNIAS

Evaluation of "nocturnal spells or unusual behavior" begins with a detailed history of the nature, age of onset, and timing of the episodes. Factors (sleep deprivation, stress, and medications) that may have affected the behaviors should be explored. A neurologic examination should be performed to rule out associated neurologic disorders. Not all parasomnias require evaluation by polysomnography (PSG). The indications for evaluation with PSG include: (1) potentially violent or injurious behavior, (2) behavior that is extremely disruptive to household members, (3) the parasomnia results in a complaint of excessive sleepiness, and (4) the parasomnia is associated with medical, psychiatric, or neurologic symptoms or findings.[5] Practice parameters for PSG in children[6] state that "the polysomnogram using an expanded electroencephalogram (EEG) montage is indicated in children to confirm the diagnosis of an atypical or potentially injurious parasomnia or differentiate a parasomnia from sleep-related epilepsy." Video PSG (synchronized video and audio) is the recommended method of evaluating parasomnias.[7,8] Today, virtually all digital PSG equipment manufacturers offer synchronized video and audio with their digital PSG recording systems. Additional EEG electrodes are commonly used to monitor patients with a suspected parasomnia to improve the ability to detect interictal or seizure activity. For example, the addition of T3 and T4 (new terminology T7, T8) may allow demonstration of temporal interictal or ictal EEG activity (see Chapter 35). Additional arm electromyogram (EMG) derivations (flexor digitorum superficialis, extensor digitorum communis) are often performed in addition to right and left tibialis anterior (leg) EMGs to detect transient muscle activity (TMA; phasic muscle activity) during REM sleep.[8] Some patients have more evidence of REM sleep without atonia (RWA) in arm EMG derivations (see Chapter 15 for information on limb EMG recording). One problem with monitoring a patient for a suspected parasomnia is that the events frequently do not occur every night. Multiple nights of video PSG may be needed.

NREM PARASOMNIAS

The traditional classification of NREM parasomnias includes confusional arousals, sleepwalking, and sleep terrors (Table 36–1 and Table 36–2). There is considerable overlap in these parasomnias, and individual patients may manifest behavior *consistent with all three subtypes of NREM parasomnias on different nights*.[2-4] They share a number of common features (Box 36–1). These disorders are considered disorders of arousal, with the physiological state being an admixture of wakefulness and NREM sleep.[2] Sexsomnia (sleep-related abnormal sexual behaviors)[9,10] is classified as a subtype of confusional arousal in the ICSD-3-TR,[2] as the behaviors usually occur in bed. Episodes of violent behavior during sleep are considered a subtype of sleepwalking, as the behavior usually occurs during ambulation out of bed. The ICSD-3-TR also includes sleep-related eating disorder (SRED) as an NREM parasomnia. SRED is discussed in a separate section in this chapter, as it has some unique features. This chapter will use the term "classic NREM parasomnias" to refer to a group containing confusional arousals, sleepwalking, and sleep terrors. In evaluating a patient

Table 36–1 Classification of Parasomnias[2]

NREM
• Confusional Arousals
• Sleepwalking
• Sleep Terrors
• Sleep-Related Eating Disorder
REM-Related Parasomnias
• REM Sleep Behavior Disorder
• Recurrent Isolated Sleep Paralysis
• Nightmare Disorder
Other Parasomnias
• Exploding Head Syndrome
• Sleep-Related Hallucinations
• Sleep-Related Urologic Dysfunction
• Parasomnia Due to a Medical Disorder
• Parasomnia Due to a Medication or Substance
• Parasomnia, Unspecified
Isolated Symptoms and Normal Variants
• Sleep Talking

NREM, non-REM; *REM*, rapid eye movement.

Table 36–2 Characteristics of NREM Parasomnias

	Confusional Arousal	Sleepwalking	Sleep Terrors
Sleep stage onset	Stage N3 children Stage N2, N3 adults*	Same	Same
Autonomic hyperactivity	No	No	Prominent
Loud scream	No	No	Yes
Ambulation out of bed	No	Yes	No
Confusion during episode	Yes	Yes	Yes
Amnesia (partial or complete)	Yes	Yes	Yes

A given episode can be a mixture of these three types. Some individual may have different types on different nights.
*NREM parasomnias can occur during all stages of NREM sleep but usually during stages N2 or N3.[11]
NREM. non-REM sleep, *REM*, rapid eye movement.

Box 36–1 CHARACTERISTICS OF NREM PARASOMNIAS

- Impaired cognition during event *(eyes open but glassy)*
- Amnesia for the preceding event
- In children, NREM parasomnias occur during stage N3; in adults, they occur out of stages N2 or N3 (rarely N1).
- In adults with NREM parasomnias—a high percentage (e.g., 2/3) experienced an episode in childhood
- Familial tendency
- Not usually associated with psychiatric disorders or head injury*
- Precipitating events—stress, sleep deprivation, OSA, fever in children, medications
- Can be precipitated by a loud noise, touch from another person, or other stimuli

NREM, non–rapid eye movement, *OSA*, obstructive sleep apnea.
*Psychiatric disorders are often present in adults with a NREM parasomias but the parasomnia is usually not causally linked to the mental disorder

for parasomnia, it is essential to involve the bed partner, who can provide eyewitness accounts. Patients with NREM parasomnias usually have amnesia for the nocturnal events. In REM parasomnias, the affected individual may communicate the content of dream mentation to the bed partner at the time of awakening following the event but may not remember the episode in the morning.

Common Characteristics of Classic NREM Parasomnias

To make a diagnosis of confusional arousal, sleepwalking, or sleep terror, the ICSD-3-TR[2] general diagnostic criteria for disorders of arousal from NREM sleep must be met. An adapted summary is listed here:

A. Recurrent episodes of incomplete awakening from sleep.
B. Inappropriate/absent responsiveness to efforts of others to intervene or redirect the person during the episode.
C. Limited (a single visual scene) or no associated cognition or dream imagery.
D. Partial or complete amnesia surrounding the episode.
E. The disturbance is not better explained by another current sleep disorder, medical disorder mental disorder, or medication/substance use.

The NREM parasomnias are characterized by recurrent episodes of incomplete awakening from sleep, inappropriate/absent responsiveness to effort of others to intervene or redirect the person during the episode, limited or no associated cognitive or dream imagery, and partial or complete amnesia surrounding the event. Because these episodes often occur during stage N3 sleep, they most commonly occur in the first third of the sleep period. While a lack of dream imagery is typical, complex dreaming behaviors can occur in some individuals. The disorders share similar genetic and familial patterns and similar pathophysiology (partial arousals from NREM sleep). The NREM parasomnias are generally ***not*** secondary to neuropathology or head injury. The parasomnia episodes may be triggered by sound, touch, or other stimuli. The events occur out of stage N3 sleep in children but are usually said to occur during stages N2 and N3 in adults. However, one study found that parasomnias can occur out of all stages of NREM sleep (including N1).[11] During the event, there is impaired cognition (eyes open but glassy), and communication with the individual is difficult. If patients are "awakened" (returned to a totally awake state), they are confused. There is amnesia for the episode. Stress, sleep deprivation, and treatment of sleep apnea (stage N3 rebound) may precipitate an NREM parasomnia. Untreated sleep apnea can also be associated with NREM parasomnias. *Adults* with an NREM parasomnia typically have a history of similar events as a child. However, *the onset of NREM parasomnias in adulthood can occur in up to one-third of patients* presenting for evaluation of clinically significant nocturnal behaviors.[11] The majority of NREM parasomnias are ***not*** felt to be caused by psychopathology. One study of patients with sleep terrors/sleepwalking evaluated for sleep-related injury found that 48% had evidence of current or prior psychopathology.[11,12] However, neither the onset nor the progression of sleep terrors/sleepwalking was associated with the onset or progression of any psychiatric disorder; successful treatment of the mental disorder did not usually resolve the parasomnia; and bedtime clonazepam therapy promptly controlled the sleep terrors/sleepwalking in >80% of patients. This series included patients with complicated parasomnias; therefore, a lower proportion of psychopathology might be expected if uncomplicated cases were to be included. Thus, adults with problematic sleep terrors are just as likely to not have related psychopathology as to have this problem. In addition, sleep terrors/sleepwalking and any concurrent psychopathology are usually not closely associated with respect to their onset, clinical course, or treatment response. As noted above, in contrast to REM parasomnias, dream mentation is uncommonly reported in NREM parasomnias. However, as noted previously, dream mentation can occur, and the report of dreaming does not rule out am NREM parasomnia.[13-15] For this reason, *PSG evaluation is needed in cases in which the parasomnia has significant consequences for the patient or family members to determine the type of parasomnia that is present.* Parasomnias (both NREM and REM) are often comorbid with other disorders such as obstructive sleep apnea (OSA), the restless legs syndrome (RLS)

Box 36–2 DISORDERS ASSOCIATED WITH PARASOMNIAS

- Obstructive sleep apnea (NREM and REM parasomnias)
- Restless legs syndrome (sleepwalking and sleep-related eating disorder)
- Narcolepsy Type 1 (sleepwalking and sleep-related eating disorder, REM parasomnias)
- Parkinson's disease (REM sleep behavior disorder)
- Anti-IgLON5 disease
- Hyperthyroidism (Sleep terrors)

NREM, non-REM; *REM*, rapid eye movement.

(sleepwalking and SRED), and Parkinson's disease (REM sleep behavior disorder [RBD]) (Box 36–2).[2]

Types of NREM Parasomnias

As noted, there is considerable overlap among the different types of NREM parasomnias. Here, characteristics of each will be discussed in more detail. A summary of the characteristics of the three major types is illustrated in Table 36–2.

Confusion arousals are brief episodes of partial arousal from sleep characterized by awakening with mental confusion in bed and often go unnoticed unless reported by the bed partner. Diagnostic criteria[2] include:

A. The disorder meets general diagnostic criteria for NREM disorders of arousal.
B. The episodes are characterized by mental confusion or confused behavior that occurs *while the patient is in bed.*
C. There is an absence of terror or ambulation outside of bed.

The most essential features of confusional arousals include an *absence of ambulation out of bed* and a *lack of autonomic arousal* (tachycardia, tachypnea, mydriasis, and diaphoresis). A tracing of a typical confusional arousal in shown in Figure 36–1 and in Video 36–1. During awakening, behavior may be inappropriate (especially during forced awakening) and even violent. Although behaviors are usually simple (movements in bed, thrashing about, vocalization, or inconsolable crying), they can be more complex. There is frequently an overlap between confusional arousals and sleepwalking. In contrast to sleep terrors, patients with confusional arousals do NOT exhibit autonomic hyperactivity or signs of fear or emit a blood-curdling scream. Confusional arousals are common in children, with a prevalence of 17%, and usually resolve by age 5. As noted, sexsomnia is considered a subtype of confusional arousals, as the activity typically occurs in bed.

Sleep walking (somnambulism) is defined as a series of complex behaviors that are initiated during sleep and result in ambulation (Box 36–3). Diagnostic criteria for sleepwalking include[2]:

A. The disorder meets general diagnostic criteria for NREM disorders of arousal.
B. The arousals are associated with ambulation and other complex behaviors out of bed.

Sleepwalking episodes must meet the general diagnostic criteria for NREM disorders of arousal. Abnormal behaviors during sleepwalking include routine behaviors that occur at inappropriate times, inappropriate or nonsensical behaviors, and dangerous or potentially dangerous behaviors. Of interest, the *eyes are usually open* (wide open and "glassy-eyed") during sleepwalking, but patients may be clumsy in their movements. Talking during sleep (somniloquy) can occur simultaneously. A tracing of a child having a sleepwalking episode in the sleep center is shown in Figure 36–2. A series of snap shots of his behavior as he wakes up and gets out of

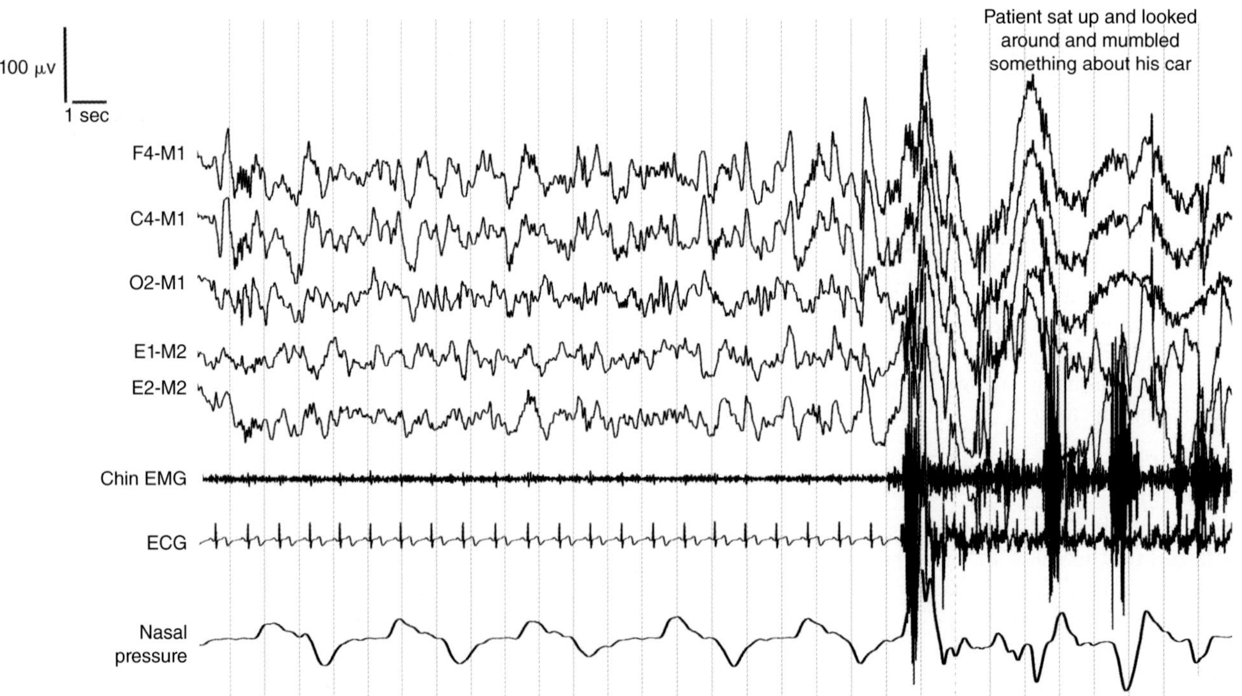

Figure 36–1 This 30-second tracing shows a patient awakening out of stage N3 sleep with a confusional arousal.

Box 36–3 SLEEPWALKING FACTS

- About 60–70% of adults with sleepwalking had episodes during childhood.
- Sleepwalking classically occurs during stage N3, in the first part of the night.
- Sleepwalking in some adults can occur in stage N2 or N3 and in the second half of the night.
- The persistence of sleepwalking into adulthood or re-emergence of sleepwalking does ***not*** usually imply sleep walking is due to an underlying psychopathology. However, a significant proportion may have current or past psychopathology.
- Prior sleep deprivation with resulting slow-wave sleep rebound (as with nasal CPAP treatment for OSA) can trigger episodes of sleepwalking.
- Violent behavior can occur during sleepwalking episodes in adults (especially in men)
- Familial influence in development of sleep walking
- Treatment of sleepwalking
  - Environmental precautions
  - Avoid sleep deprivation
  - Clonazepam and other BZRAs
  - TCAs
  - SSRIs

BZRAs, benzodiazepine receptor agonists; *CPAP*, continuous positive airway pressure; *OSA*, obstructive sleep apnea; *SSRIs*, selective serotonin reuptake inhibitors; *TCAs*, tricyclic antidepressants.

bed is shown in Figure 36–3 and the start of a sleep walking episode is shown in Video 36-2.

In addition to ambulation, the episodes have evidence of persistent sleep, altered consciousness, or impaired judgment during ambulation. Evidence of an altered state of consciousness includes difficulty arousing the person, mental confusion when awakened from an episode, amnesia (complete or partial) for the episode, and abnormal behaviors. Episodes of sleepwalking in children are rarely violent, and movements are often slow. In adults, sleepwalking episodes can be more complex, frenzied, violent, and longer in duration. Episodes of sleepwalking may be terminated by the patient returning to bed or simply lying down and continuing sleep out of bed. As noted, patients are difficult to arouse during sleepwalking episodes. When aroused during sleepwalking, patients are typically very confused. *Sleepwalking occurs in 10% to 20% of children, and the incidence peaks between the ages of 4 and 8.* The onset of sleepwalking can also occur in adulthood in up to one-third of affected individuals. However, most adult sleepwalkers had episodes during childhood (60–70%). Sleepwalking usually disappears in adolescence. However, the percentage of sleepwalking in adults that was present in childhood is variable in the literature and depends on the population being studied. One study of 100 adult patients with sleep-related injury[11] found that 33% with sleepwalking/sleep terrors had an age of onset **after** age 16 years; 70% had episodes arising from all stages of NREM sleep, while 30% had episodes arising only from stage N3. The sleepwalking behaviors varied in duration and intensity. Of interest, some of these patients reported some degree of dream mentation, and some had recall of the events. There is a *definite familial influence in the development of sleepwalking.*[16] If one or both parents have a history of sleepwalking, the risk of a child developing sleepwalking episodes is greatly increased. Fever, sleep deprivation, and certain medications (e.g., zolpidem and other benzodiazepine receptor agonists [BZRAs], phenothiazines, tricyclic antidepressants [TCAs], sodium oxybate, lithium) can precipitate the sleepwalking events. Hypermotor sleep-related epilepsy (formerly termed nocturnal frontal lobe epilepsy)[17] can be

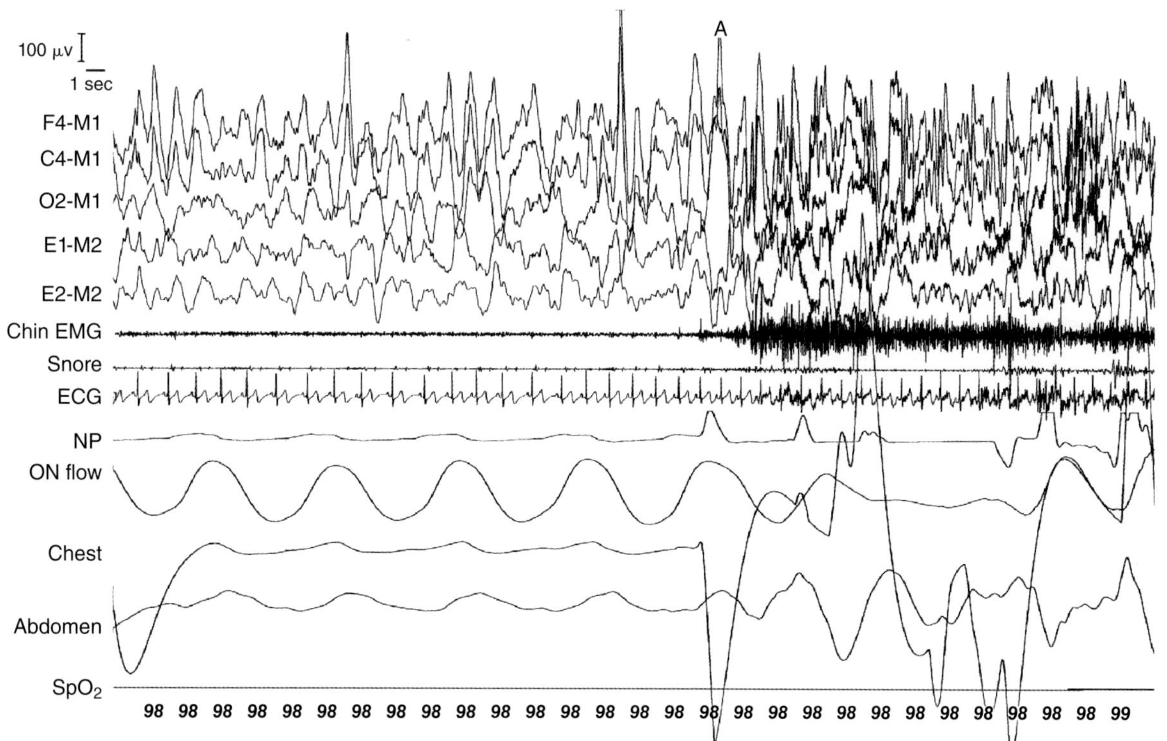

Figure 36–2 This 30-second tracing shows a child arousing from stage N3 sleep (A) and sitting up, climbing out of bed, and walking out of the room before being intercepted by a sleep technologist. Note the persistence of slow wave activity during the arousal.

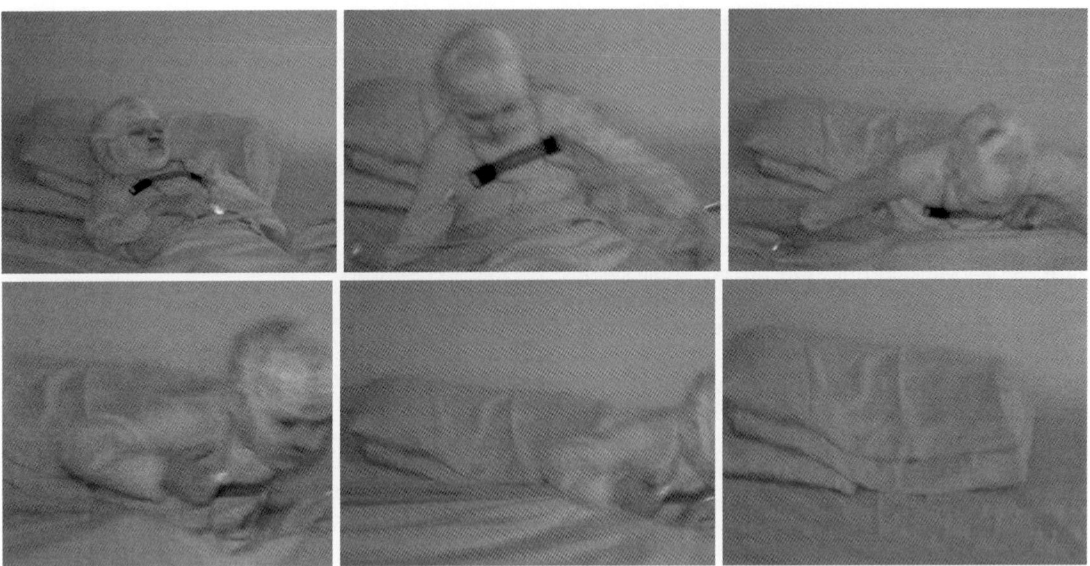

Figure 36–3 This is a series of snapshots as a child arouses from sleep, sits up in bed, and then leaves the bed, walking out of the room. The time sequence goes from left to right on the first row, then from left to right on the second row.

associated with ambulation out of bed (nocturnal wandering) with impaired consciousness. Nocturnal seizures are discussed in a later section and in Chapter 35.

Sleep terrors consist of sudden arousal from sleep accompanied by a blood-curdling scream or cry and manifestations of severe fear (behavioral and autonomic) (Box 36–4).

Diagnostic criteria for sleep terrors include:

a. The disorder meets general diagnostic criteria for NREM disorders of arousal.
b. The arousals are characterized by episodes of abrupt terror, typically beginning with an alarming vocalization such as a frightening scream.
c. There is intense fear and signs of autonomic arousal including mydriasis, tachycardia, tachypnea, and diaphoresis during an episode.

Box 36–4 SLEEP TERRORS FACTS

- In children, sleep terrors occur out of stage N3 sleep, in the first part of night.
- In adults, sleep terrors can occur from stages N2 or N3 sleep.
- Patients may manifest both sleep terrors and sleepwalking.
- In contrast to confusional arousals, patients with sleep terrors have profound autonomic hyperactivity (mydriasis [dilated pupils], diaphoresis, and tachycardia) and manifestations of fear.
- Unlike RBD or nightmares, patients with sleep terrors do not relate dream mentation associated with the event.
- The persistence of sleep terrors into adulthood, re-emergence of sleep terrors in adulthood, or onset of sleep terrors in adulthood is not necessarily evidence that psychopathology is present, or if present is causally linked to the sleep terror episodes.
- Sleep terrors have been described in adults during nasal CPAP treatment of OSA.

CPAP, continuous positive airway pressure; *OSA*, obstructive sleep apnea; *RBD*, REM sleep behavior disorder.

The affected individual is typically confused and diaphoretic, exhibits mydriasis (dilated pupils) and tachycardia, and frequently sits up in bed (children frequently stand up in bed). It is difficult or impossible to communicate with a person having a sleep terror, and total amnesia surrounding the event is usual. Patients may sleepwalk during episodes of night terrors. Sleep terrors typically occur in prepubertal children (≤3%) and subside by adolescence; they are uncommon in adults. Sleep terrors rarely begin in adulthood. The sleep clinician should be aware that paroxysmal arousal is a type of behavior that can occur with sleep-related hypermotor epilepsy (formerly nocturnal frontal lobe epilepsy) and can be characterized by sudden arousal from sleep with a scream.[17] This type of epilepsy has a focal onset, and the behavior is very stereotypical (same behavior each time). Often, individuals are almost immediately alert after the episode but can be confused. See the video clips of a sleep terror episode in an adult (Video 36–3) and in a child (Video 36–4).

PSG in NREM Parasomnias

PSG is usually not required to evaluate NREM parasomnias unless the episodes are frequent, violent, or have the potential to result in self-injury. Most clinicians feel PSG is necessary before prescribing a medication for a parasomnia. When PSG is performed, inclusion of synchronized video/audio monitoring is essential. If seizures are suspected, a complete clinical EEG montage is ideal, but at a minimum, temporal derivations should be added. A tracing of a patient with a sudden awakening from NREM sleep with confusional arousal is shown in Figure 36–1. Another tracing of the onset of a sleep walking episode in a child is shown in Figure 36–2. During NREM parasomnia episodes the chin EMG amplitude is greatly increased, and the EEG may show persistent slow-wave activity (sometimes hypersynchronous) mixed with variable amounts of alpha, theta and beta activity. At the onset of sleep terrors, the heart rate increases, but there is no pre-event increase in heart rate. Video monitoring is critical in differentiating an NREM parasomnia from frontal or temporal lobe epilepsy. Muscle artifact can obscure the EEG during events, and many nocturnal seizures are not associated with cortical EEG changes. Behavior during episodes of nocturnal focal epilepsy is usually stereotypic, and the characteristics may help identify the episodes as seizures (e.g., dystonic posturing with hypermotor/frontal lobe epilepsy).[17]

Sleep-Related Sexual Behavior and Violent Behavior During Sleep

As noted, *sleep-related sexual behavior (sexsomnia) is usually classified as a subtype of confusional arousal.* As the name implies, this disorder consists of a parasomnia in which sexual behavior occurs with limited awareness during the act, relative unresponsiveness to the external environment, and amnesia surrounding the event.[9,10] The behaviors range from sexual vocalizations to intercourse. These actions may include behaviors very atypical for the individual (e.g., anal intercourse).

Violent behavior behavior during sleep is usually classified as a subtype of sleepwalking, since behavior typically occurs out of bed. The main complications of sleepwalking are social embarrassment and danger of self-injury or injury to others. Violent behavior, including self-mutilation (parasomnia pseudo-suicide), homicide, and sexual assault (sleep sex), has been reported in association with sleepwalking episodes. Sleep-related violence occurs in a state consistent with sleepwalking/sleep terrors and is associated with an emotion of fear or anger. The violent behavior may be directed toward individuals in close proximity or toward those who confront the individual during the parasomnia episode. The patient may either awaken or go back to sleep but typically has amnesia surrounding the event. The *violence is often atypical for the individual.* Most cases of sleep-related violence occur in middle-aged men with a history of prior sleepwalking. In contrast to typical sleepwalking, these events can exceed 30 minutes in duration.

Factors Associated With NREM Parasomnias

Pressman described factors causing/associated with NREM parasomnias in categories classified as (1) predisposing (familial, genetic), (2) priming (conditions/substances that increase stage N3 sleep or make arousal from sleep more difficult (sleeping in an unfamiliar surrounding, alcohol, medications, stress, or fever), and (3) triggers (sleep-related breathing disorder, periodic limb movement disorder [PLMD], noise, or touch).[18] As noted, there is an important familial component to NREM parasomnias. This is especially true for sleepwalking and sleep terrors[16] (Table 36–3 and Box 36–4). In some studies NREM parasomnias have been associated with HLA DQB1*05:01.

As mentioned, other sleep disorders can be associated with NREM parasomnias. For example, sleepwalking has been reported to be precipitated by treatment of sleep apnea with nasal continuous positive airway pressure (CPAP),[19] and sleep terrors in adults have been reported to be precipitated by sleep apnea.[20] Sleepwalking and SRED have been associated with *each other* and with RLS.[21-23] Medications can also precipitate NREM parasomnias, especially sleepwalking.[24] Sodium oxybate has been reportedly associated with episodes of *sleep driving and sleep-related eating.*[25] Lithium,[26] amitriptyline,[27] and mirtazapine[28] have also been associated with sleepwalking. The benzodiazepines and, in particular, the non-benzodiazepine medications zolpidem, zaleplon, and eszopiclone, which are BZRAs, have been associated with sleepwalking and complex sleep behaviors with serious consequences.[29] Mechanisms of the factors favoring NREM parasomnias are summarized in Table 36–4.

Table 36–3 Factors Increasing the Incidence of Sleepwalking and Sleep Terrors

Predisposing Factors

- Genetic/familial history of sleepwalking
- Risk of sleepwalking
    - 22% if neither parent affected
    - 45% if one parent affected by sleepwalking
    - 60% if both parents have a history of sleepwalking
    - 65% if twin has sleepwalking

Priming Factors – Conditions That Increase Stage N3 or Make Arousal From Sleep More Difficult

- Sleep deprivation
- Fever
- Life stress
- Novel bedroom
- Untreated obstructive sleep apnea or with initial CPAP treatment.
- CNS disease—migraines, head injury, encephalitis
- Alcohol abuse
- Medications[24]
    - Zolpidem (all BZRAs)
    - Lithium carbonate
    - Phenothiazines
    - Second generation antipsychotics—olanzapine, quetiapine
    - Sodium oxybate
    - Bupropion
    - Paroxetine
    - Mirtazapine
    - Amitriptyline

Triggers

- Sleep-related breathing disorders
- Periodic limb movement during sleep
- Noise
- Touch by another individual

CNS, central nervous system; *CPAP*, continuous positive airway pressure, *BZRA*, benzodiazepine receptor agonist.

Table 36–4 Mechanisms of Some Factors Favoring Non-REM Parasomnias

Factors	Increased Sleep Fragmentation	Increased Sleep Inertia	Both
Examples	• Noise • Pain • RLS/PLMS	• Sleep deprivation • Circadian misalignment • Sedative-hypnotic medication	• OSA • Narcolepsy type 1

OSA, obstructive sleep apnea; *PLMS*, Periodic limb movements in sleep; *RLS*, restless legs syndrome.
Adapted From Irfan M, Schenck CH, Howell MJ. NonREM Disorders of Arousal and Related Parasomnias. Neurotherapeutics. 2021;18(1):124-139.

Differential Diagnosis of NREM Parasomnias

The differential diagnosis of NREM parasomnias includes RBD, PLMD, posttraumatic stress disorder (PTSD; which can be associated with violent movements during nightmares), nocturnal epilepsy, and nocturnal panic attacks. RBD usually occurs in the last half of the night, individuals may jump out of bed but rarely ambulate outside the bedroom, and *eyes are typically closed*. More complex dream mentation is usually associated with RBD. Nocturnal epilepsy (especially sleep-related hypermotor/frontal lobe epilepsy) can mimic NREM parasomnias, but the behavior is stereotypical, there is usually no or limited confusion after the episodes, and multiple episodes can occur each night. Differentiating nocturnal epilepsy from parasomnias will be discussed further later in this chapter. Nocturnal panic attacks occur after arousal from NREM sleep and are associated with sympathetic activation and fear but the manifestations usually peak after several minutes of wakefulness following the arousal, the affected individual is alert, amnesia for the events is usually not present, and the return to sleep is usually delayed. Most individuals with nocturnal panic attacks also have daytime episodes (see chapter 37).

Treatment of the Classic NREM Parasomnias (confusional arousals, sleepwalking, sleep terrors)

The three classic NREM parasomnias are very common in childhood, and usually reassurance and education suffice. Treatment options for confusional arousals, sleepwalking, and sleep terrors are summarized in Box 36–5. When approaching the treatment of a parasomnia, it is very important to first focus on managing triggering factors and comorbidities. Common triggering factors include untreated OSA, RLS, medications, insufficient sleep, and stress (psychological or physical). Guilleminault et al. found that CPAP treatment of OSA resolved chronic adult sleepwalking.[30] Treatment of the classic NREM parasomnias includes avoiding precipitating factors (e.g., sleep deprivation) and environmental precautions. Environmental precautions are especially important in the case of sleep walking (including locking windows and removing dangerous objects such as firearms from the bedroom/house). Medication is usually not needed, especially in children. Non-pharmacologic treatments have included sleep hygiene education, cognitive treatment of anxiety, reassurance, and scheduled awakening.[31-34] In children, *scheduled awakening* was reported to be effective for sleepwalking and sleep terrors in a small case series.[33] A similar technique has been used in adults. A sleep log over several days or weeks attempts to document the usual time of occurrence of episodes, and the affected individual is awakened 15 to 30 minutes before the timing of the typical events. *Behavioral interventions and hypnosis* have also been used to treat NREM parasomnias. Mundt described use of a case conceptualization-based, integrative approach to NREM parasomnias in three cases (two disorders of arousal and one SRED).[34] Symptoms were reduced after three to six sessions. Treatment was tailored to each individual, but common elements included education, hypnosis, and identification and reduction of priming (stress, insufficient sleep) and precipitating factors (noise, touch from bed partners). Bed or room alarms have also been used. In a retrospective review of 512 patients with NREM parasomnias, about 97% were treated successfully; about 30% of the patients were treated with nonpharmacologic measures, and 60% were treated with various medications.[35] The nonpharmacologic treatments included sleep hygiene (13%), management of sleep apnea (12%), and psychological interventions (6%). The psychological interventions included cognitive behavioral treatment and mindfulness relaxation.

Medications have frequently been used for the classic NREM parasomnias (especially in adults), but recommendations are based on case series rather than randomized controlled trials. In a study of 100 patients with injurious parasomnias, use of clonazepam was successful in about 80% of patients with sleepwalking/sleep terrors.[11] In a subsequent publication reporting on 170 patients with injurious parasomnias, both clonazepam and alprazolam were effective.[36] In the previously mentioned case series of 512 patients, 60% were managed with medication that included a benzodiazepine (about 40%), an antidepressant (about 9%), and melatonin (about 11%).[11] Typical medications that have been used for NREM parasomnias include benzodiazepines (clonazepam 0.5 to 2.0 mg qhs, alprazolam, or temazepam 30 mg qhs), TCAs, or selective serotonin reuptake inhibitors (SSRIs). If medications are used, they should be given early enough so that waking in the first cycle of NREM sleep can be prevented. Clonazepam has a long duration of action, and taking the medication earlier may reduce morning grogginess, which is a major side effect of the medication. Although benzodiazepines have been used as a treatment for parasomnias, zolpidem, a BZRA that is a non-benzodiazepine, has been associated with sleepwalking and complex behaviors during sleep. Melatonin can be used for NREM parasomnias, especially when an overlap of parasomnias is present (NREM parasomnias and RBD). A single case report found ramelteon (melatonin receptor agonist) to be effective in a child with sleepwalking and night terrors.[37]

Box 36–5 TREATMENTS FOR CONFUSIONAL AROUSALS, SLEEPWALKING, AND SLEEP TERRORS

- Interventions for inadequate sleep, anxiety, and comorbid sleep disorders (OSA, RLS)
- Environmental precautions
- Nonpharmacologic
  - Reassurance—especially in otherwise healthy children
  - Sleep hygiene
  - Cognitive behavioral treatment—treat anxiety, stress
  - Relaxation treatment
  - Scheduled awakenings
  - Hypnosis
  - CPAP for OSA
  - Bed alarms
- Medications
  - Benzodiazepines (clonazepam 0.5 to 2 mg, alprazolam)
  - Antidepressants—especially for night terrors (SSRIs, TCAs)
  - Melatonin—especially if overlap with REM sleep behavior disorder

CPAP, continuous positive airway pressure; *OSA*, obstructive sleep apnea; *RLS*, restless legs syndrome; *SSRIs*, selective serotonin reuptake inhibitors; *TCAs*, tricyclic antidepressants.
Adapted from Drakatos P, Marples L, Muza R, et al. NREM parasomnias: a treatment approach based upon a retrospective case series of 512 patients. *Sleep Med*. 2019;181-188

SLEEP-RELATED EATING DISORDER

SRED is manifested by dysfunctional eating and drinking after an arousal from sleep during the main sleep period (Boxes 36–6 and 36–7).

Box 36–6 SRED FACTS

- Strong female predominance
- Variable awareness/alertness during episodes
- Eating unusual foods (e.g., raw, frozen, toxic)
- Variable recall (partial amnesia)
- Co-morbid with other sleep disorders including OSA, eating disorders, RLS, narcolepsy, irregular sleep phase sleep-wake circadian rhythm disorder
- Medications associated with SRED: zolpidem, mirtazapine, sodium oxybate
- Treatments options: topiramate, pramipexole, and sertraline

OSA, obstructive sleep apnea; *RLS*, restless legs syndrome; *SRED*, sleep-related eating disorder.

Box 36–7 CAUSES OF SRED

1. Associated with another sleep disorder
   a. Sleepwalking—most common association
   b. Obstructive sleep apnea
   c. Narcolepsy type 1 (with cataplexy)
   d. PLMD, RLS
   e. Circadian rhythm sleep disorders (especially irregular sleep-wake type)
2. Associated with medication
   a. BZRAs: zolpidem, triazolam
   b. Psychotropic medications (lithium, olanzapine, quetiapine)
   c. Antidepressants (mirtazapine, amitriptyline)
   d. Anticholinergic medications (donepezil)
   e. Sodium oxybate
3. Idiopathic

BZRAs, benzodiazepine receptor agonists; *PLMD*, periodic limb movement disorder; *RLS*, restless legs syndrome; *SRED*, sleep-related eating disorder.

Diagnostic criteria[2] for SRED include:

A. Recurrent episodes of dysfunctional eating that occur after an arousal from sleep during the main sleep period.
B. The presence of one or more of the following in association with the recurrent episodes of involuntary eating:
   a. Consumption of peculiar forms or combinations of food or inedible or toxic substances
   b. Sleep-related injurious or potentially injurious behaviors performed while in pursuit of food or while cooking food
   c. Adverse health consequences from recurrent nocturnal eating
C. There is partial or complete loss of conscious awareness during the eating episode, with subsequent impaired recall.
D. The disturbance is not better explained by another current sleep disorder, mental disorder, medical disorder, or medication/substance use.

The eating behavior must be associated with one of the following: eating peculiar food items, sleep-related injury, potential for injury (cooking), or adverse consequences of recurrent nocturnal eating (weight gain, morning anorexia). In the past, SRED was differentiated from night eating syndrome (NES) by the level of alertness during the episodes and the degree of recall. SREDs were said to be associated with decreased awareness during the episodes, whereas NES was said to be characterized by full alertness. However, there is considerable overlap between SRED and NES.[38-41] Some clinicians consider them to be two eating disorders at the opposite ends of the spectrum of awareness (Table 36–5). The level of consciousness in SRED has typically spanned from virtual unconsciousness to various levels of partial consciousness despite a concurrent EEG pattern that is often predominantly awake, suggesting a dissociation between the EEG and the level of consciousness. A diagnosis of NES applies *when excessive eating occurs between dinner and sleep onset*, although SRED may be comorbid with NES. This pattern of NES should not apply as an exclusion criterion for patients who otherwise fulfill criteria for SRED and who consciously eat during the pre-bedtime period in a futile attempt to suppress the compulsion to eat after subsequently falling asleep.

For a diagnosis of SRED the ICSD-3-TR requires "at least partial loss of conscious awareness during the eating episode with subsequent impaired recall."[2] SRED episodes can occur during anytime of the night. The degree of alertness and recall of the eating behavior vary. Some patients cannot be brought to full consciousness during the eating events and have no recall of the event. Others are relatively alert during the episode and have considerable recall of the event the next morning. The extent of alertness can even vary between two episodes on a given night. A sensation of hunger is usually missing, and patients may eat in an "out of control" manner. As noted above, patients often eat peculiar, nonedible, or even dangerous substances. These may include frozen food, coffee grounds, and cat food. Of interest, alcoholic beverages are rarely consumed. High-calorie foods are often chosen. Often, foods not typically eaten during the day are consumed. There may be multiple episodes of eating during a single night. Some patients attempt to control weight via daytime purging.

SRED is much more common in women than in men. Women make up 66% to 83% of affected individuals in most series. The prevalence is higher among patients with other eating disorders. The typical age of onset of SRED is 20 to 30 years. The cause of SRED is unknown, but more than 50% of patients have another parasomnia, and the strong female predominance is typical of eating disorders. An idiopathic form does exist in which no obvious cause or association is identified. SRED is commonly associated with sleepwalking but can occur with PLMD, RLS,[21,22,40-42] OSA,[19] narcolepsy,[43] and circadian rhythm disorders. *Sleepwalking is the most common sleep disorder associated with sleep-related eating*, although once eating becomes part of the behavioral repertoire, it quickly becomes the predominant, if not the exclusive, nocturnal "sleepwalking" behavior. In a recent case-controlled study of 65 patients with narcolepsy-cataplexy, 32% of the patients had SRED (SRED-NC) vs. 2% of the controls. Nocturnal smoking was present in 33% of patients with SRED and narcolepsy with cataplexy and in 16% of patients with narcolepsy-cataplexy but without SRED.[43]

Medication-induced SRED has been reported with BZRAs, including zolpidem[44] and triazolam, and psychotropic medications, including quetiapine,[45] olanzapine,[46] and risperidone.[47] SRED episodes have also been reported in patients taking sodium oxybate.[25] Zolpidem-associated SRED is especially common if patients escalate the dose in an attempt to sleep. Patients also report triggering of SRED episodes by stress, cigarette smoking cessation, and cessation of the use of alcohol or other drugs of abuse.

The diagnosis of SRED is usually based on observations by a significant other finding evidence of nocturnal eating behavior (e.g., open food packages, dirty plates), videotaping, and self-report (in patients with some recall). If SRED is medication

Table 36–5 Characteristics Sleep-Related Eating Disorder and Nocturnal Eating Syndrome

	Sleep-Related Eating Disorder	Nocturnal Eating Syndrome
State of consciousness	Partial to full arousal state	Fully awake during compulsive eating
Timing of onset	Onset out of sleep period	Eating between evening meal and onset of nocturnal sleep or Eating during complete awakenings from sleep
Food	Unusual foods or toxic substances Preference for high-caloric foods Foods NOT typically preferred during daytime (e.g., raw food, cat food, frozen food)	Absence of bizarre or atypical foods
Recall	Partial or complete amnesia	Compete recall
State in the morning	Morning anorexia and abdominal distention	Morning anorexia and bulimia can occur
Associated disorders	Sleepwalking, OSA, PLMD	Eating and psychiatric disorders
Gender	Women 60–80%	Women ≈ 60% (less female predominance compared to SRED)

Note: The ICSD-3 requires at least a partial loss of consciousness during the eating episodes with subsequent impaired recall for diagnosis of sleep-related eating disorder.
OSA, obstructive sleep apnea; *PLMD*, periodic limb movement disorder.

associated (zolpidem), the medication should be withdrawn. Patients may not have the behavior with another medication in the same class (e.g., switch from zolpidem to temazepam). Sometimes, medication-induced SRED will continue, at least temporarily, even with discontinuation of the offending medication. There have been reports of success with a few medications.[48] Topiramate appears to be the best-documented treatment, although sertraline, carbidopa/levodopa, and pramipexole have been used successfully. In contrast to the classic NREM parasomnias, randomized controlled trials of medications have been performed for SRED. Winkelman et al. evaluated topiramate for SRED using a placebo-controlled randomized trial.[49] The study medication was titrated over a 9-week period starting at 25 mg and increasing by 25 mg every week up to 150 mg and then by 50 mg every week up to a maximum of 300 mg/day or the participant's minimum effective dose. The topiramate group had reduction in SRED and lost significantly more weight than the placebo group (about 8.5 pounds). The most common side effects were paresthesias and cognitive dysfunction. A typical dosage of topiramate is 25 to 200 mg at bedtime. Many patients may note an improvement at a 100-mg dosage. The side effects of topiramate include weight loss, paresthesia, *renal calculi*, cognitive dysfunction, and orthostasis. In one series, up to 41% of patients discontinued the medication because of side effects. If SRED is associated with sleepwalking, clonazepam has sometimes been effective for both disorders. Other medications used for SRED include pramipexole[50] and sertraline.[51,52] A placebo-controlled randomized trial (flexible dose study) found sertraline 50 to 200 mg to be more effective than placebo at improving SRED. Of interest, improvement in SRED was reported using low-dose sertraline (25 mg) in two patients.[52] This treatment could prove useful in patients unable to tolerate topiramate or clonazepam. Sertraline has also been used for the nocturnal eating syndrome.

NREM PARASOMNIA IN ANTI-IGLON-5 DISEASE

This novel neurological disorder was identified in 2014 and consists of a distinct sleep pattern including RBD, NREM parasomnia (diffuse intentional behavior – but not a disorder of arousal), and sleep apnea.[53,54] The nocturnal episodes (described by bed partners) may consist of vocalizations, limb movements, and purposeful-looking gestures during sleep, as well as snoring and apneas. Dysarthria, stridor, and sialorrhea can be present. There are serum/cerebrospinal fluid (CSF) autoantibodies against the neuronal protein IgLON5. There is a strong human leukocyte antigen (HLA) association but no comorbid autoimmune disorders. Important features of the disorder are listed in Box 36–8.

Box 36–8 ANTI-IGLON5 DISEASE

- Antibodies against IgLON5 (a neuronal cell adhesion protein)
- Haplotypes DQB1*0501, DRB1*1001
- Tauopathy involving brainstem and hypothalamus
- Men = women, age >50
- Daytime findings:
  - Gait instability
  - Dystonia
  - Upward gaze palsy
  - Dysphagia
  - Dementia
  - Hoarseness
- Sleep findings
  - Obstructive sleep apnea
  - Hypersialorrhea during sleep
  - Inspiratory stridor (vocal cord palsy)
  - Abnormal sleep architecture—poorly defined N1, N2
  - Diffuse intentional behaviors in NREM sleep but only mild RBD (body jerks, but minimal complex behaviors)
- Treatment—no effective treatment

NREM, non–rapid-eye movement; *RBD*, REM sleep behavior disorder.

NOCTURNAL EPILEPSY VERSUS NREM PARASOMNIA

Definitive differentiation of NREM parasomnias from focal-onset epilepsy occurring out of sleep with variable loss of

Table 36–6 Comparison of Sleep-Related Hypermotor Epilepsy and NREM Parasomnias

	Sleep-Related Hypermotor Epilepsy	NREM Parasomnias
Daytime episodes	Can occur	No
Movement semiology	Often violent, stereotypical	Complex, non-stereotypical
Episodes per night	3 or more common	One or two
Autonomic activation	Very common (tachycardia)	Only in sleep terrors
EEG	Episodes out of NREM sleep Ictal: normal 50% with scalp electrodes Interictal EEG: normal in about 50%	Stage N3 children Stages N2, N3 adults NREM sleep with arousal
Clinical Course	Increasing or stable frequency	Tends to resolve

EEG, electroencephalography; *NREM*, non–rapid eye movement. The terminology Sleep-related hypermotor epilepsy was previously Nocturnal Frontal Lobe Epilepsy. Adapted from Provini F, Plazzi G, Tinuper P, et al. Nocturnal frontal lobe epilepsy. *Brain.* 1999;122:1017-1031.

awareness is difficult without complete video and EEG monitoring.[17,55,56] Sleep-related epilepsy is discussed in detail in Chapter 35. Sleep-related hypermotor epilepsy[17] is a focal epilepsy confined primarily to sleep and this terminology replaces nocturnal frontal lobe epilepsy, since the temporal lobe can be the actual focus and the episodes are closely associated with sleep rather than the time of day (can occur in naps during the day). Seizures tend to be more stereotypic than NREM parasomnias and may also occur during the day (Table 36–6). Provini and colleagues[55,56] described three general manifestations of nocturnal frontal lobe epilepsy that also applies to sleep-related hypermotor epilepsy, including paroxysmal arousals, nocturnal paroxysmal motor behaviors (formerly called nocturnal paroxysmal dystonia), and episodic nocturnal wandering (ENW). Paroxysmal arousals typically present during NREM sleep consisting of a stereotypical series of movements lasting 2 to 20 seconds in which the individuals raise their head, sit up, and look around confused with a frightened expression and then screams. Unlike typical sleep terrors, paroxysmal arousals can occur many times during the night and are very stereotypic. The motor behaviors associated with sleep-related hypermotor epilepsy include periods of coarse movements, dystonic posturing, and violent movements, sometimes with vocalization that can occur multiple times per night, often with only transient or no impairment of awareness. Patients often move their arms and legs in cycling or kicking movements.

Episodic nocturnal wanderings (ENWs) may present with symptoms like sleepwalking and sleep terrors. Patients may jump out of bed, wander, vocalize, and show violent behavior during sleep. In summary, sleep-related hypermotor epilepsy can mimic confusional arousals, sleep terrors, sleepwalking, and RBD. The fact that multiple episodes occur in one night and that all the episodes are very similar differentiates these events from NREM or REM parasomnias. Episodes of nocturnal epilepsy usually occur out of NREM sleep (more common in stage N2), and frequently no EEG abnormality other than muscle artifact is noted (in over 50%, no ictal activity can be detected). The nature of the behavior as recorded with video is extremely important, as semiology rather than the EEG may be most helpful in sleep-related hypermotor epilepsy. Synchronized video is recommended for evaluation of parasomnia in the American Academy of Sleep Medicine (AASM) scoring manual.[8]

SLEEP-RELATED DISSOCIATIVE DISORDERS

Sleep-related dissociative disorders (SRDD) comprise a sleep-related variant of dissociative disorders defined as "a disruption in the usually integrated functions of consciousness, memory, identity, or perception of the environment." Often, there is a history of abuse or PTSD. Diagnostic criteria for these disorders are not included in ICSD-3-TR but were included in the ICSD-2.[1] Adapted diagnostic criteria include:

A. A dissociative disorder characterized by a disruption of the usually integrated functions of consciousness, memory, identity, or perception of the environment that emerges in close association with the main sleep period.
B. One of the following is present:
   a. PSG demonstrates a dissociative episode or episodes that *emerge during sustained EEG wakefulness*, either in the transition from wakefulness to sleep or after an awakening from NREM or REM sleep.
   b. In the absence of a PSG-recorded episode of dissociation, the history provided by observers is compelling for SRDD, particularly if the sleep-related behaviors are similar to observed daytime dissociative behaviors.

The behavior may resemble a confusional arousal or sleepwalking (moving, falling out of bed, ambulation) ***except*** that the *episode occurs out of wakefulness.*[57] That is, it does ***not*** occur at the transition from NREM to wakefulness but during a period of definite wakefulness. There is a *female predominance*, and most patients have daytime dissociative disorder episodes. Many patients with dissociative disorders have a history of physical or sexual trauma. This entity is included here, as most physicians will encounter a patient with unusual behavior during a sleep study that happens out of sustained wakefulness. Patients with dissociative disorders need psychiatric treatment, but environmental precautions for the behaviors are indicated.

PARASOMNIAS USUALLY ASSOCIATED WITH REM SLEEP

Parasomnias usually associated with REM sleep (stage R) include RBD, recurrent isolated sleep paralysis, and nightmare disorders. RBD has two variants: overlap parasomnia and status dissociatus.

REM Sleep Behavior Disorder (including variants)

RBD is characterized by a loss of the normal muscle atonia associated with REM sleep (REM without atonia, RWA), with body movements that are often associated with dream mentation.[58-62] This is referred to as dream-enactment behavior (oneirism). Limb and body movements are often violent (e.g., hitting a wall, kicking) and may be associated with emotionally charged utterances. The movements can be related to dream content ("kicking an attacker"), but the patient may or may not remember associated dream material when awakened during an episode. Serious injury to the patient or the bed partner can result from these episodes, which typically occur one to four times a week. Because the episodes occur during REM sleep, they are most common during the early morning hours (the second half of the night). There is a strong male predominance in most studies, and the median age of onset is about 50 years. However, some studies show that the *male predominance may result from a milder form of RBD in women that is less likely to result in a complaint to a physician.*[63] A milder prodrome of sleep talking, simple limb-jerking, or vividly violent dreams may precede the full-blown syndrome. The pathophysiology of RBD includes dysfunction of areas of the brain responsible for atonia during REM sleep as well as other areas of the brain (limbic system and others) involved with generation of the violent dreams. The neurobiology of RWA is discussed in Chapter 8.

Screening Questionnaires for RBD

Several screening questionnaires have been devised for detection of possible RBD. The simplest is the RBD1Q,[64] which consists of a single question, answered "yes" or "no," as follows:

> *"Have you ever been told, or suspected yourself, that you seem to 'act out your dreams' while asleep (for example, punching, flailing your arms in the air, making running movements, etc.)?"*

One study found the positive and negative predictive values of 88% and 93%, respectively, in 484 participants consisting of 242 patients with known RBD and 242 controls (48 normal, 194 other sleep disorders). However, this is certainly an enriched study population. The Mayo Questionnaire uses one question (yes or no), and then five additional questions if the answer is yes. This questionnaire is given to the bed partner.[65] Other questionnaires have also been developed.[66] It is important to question the bed partner, and today, prolonged episodes can be captured by the bed partner using the camera in a smartphone.

Box 36–9 CLASSIFICATION AND CAUSES OF RAPID EYE MOVEMENT BEHAVIOR DISORDER

Acute RBD

- Alcohol withdrawal
- Substance abuse or withdrawal (benzodiazepines, barbiturates)
- Medication toxicity (caffeine, MAOIs, TCAs)

Chronic RBD

- **Isolated (≈ 60% when first evaluated)**
- **Associated with other sleep disorders (≈ 30%)**
- **Narcolepsy with cataplexy (up to 30% of these patients)**
- **Neurodegenerative Disorders**
  - Alpha synucleinopathy disorders – preceding or following diagnosis
    - Idiopathic Parkinson disease (25 to 54% of cases)
    - Dementia with Lewy Bodies (50–70% of cases)
    - Multiple system atrophy (90–100% of cases)
  - Progressive Supranuclear Palsy
- **Other Neurological** Disorders – CVA, traumatic encephalopathy
- **Autoimmune Disorders**
  - Anti-Ma1 and Ma2 encephalitis
  - Anti-IgLON5 disease (100%)
  - Multiple Sclerosis
- **Medications***
  - Common:
    - SSRIs (fluoxetine, paroxetine)
    - SNRIs (venlafaxine, duloxetine)
    - Mirtazapine
    - TCAs (imipramine)
    - Monoamine oxidase inhibitors
  - Rare:
    - Beta blockers
    - Cholinesterase inhibitors
    - Orexin receptor antagonists

MAOIs = monoamine oxidase inhibitors; *RBD* = rapid eye movement sleep behavior disorder; *SSRIs* = selective serotonin reuptake inhibitors; *TCAs* = tricyclic antidepressants.
SNRIs selective serotonin and norepinephrine reuptake inhibitors
*RBD Associated or worsened with medications

RBD: Causes and Associations

Common causes of RBD are listed in Box 36–9. An acute form of RBD can occur after withdrawal from REM suppressants, such as ethanol. Even after extensive evaluation, about 60% of cases of chronic RBD are classified as isolated (iRBD) when first evaluated. In the literature the terminology idiopathic RBD has been used but in the ICSD-3-TR the terminology is "isolated" RBD. *That is, a neurological disorder known to be associated with RBD is not present.* Chronic RBD can be associated with a number of neurologic disorders[61,62] including narcolepsy,[67] multiple sclerosis, subarachnoid hemorrhage, dementia, ischemic cerebrovascular disease, and brainstem neoplasms and α-synucleinopathies including Parkinson's disease, diffuse Lewy body dementia (DLBD), and multiple system atrophy. RBD has also been associated with the post-traumatic stress disorder. Drug-induced or exacerbated cases of RBD[68] have been reported with the use of monoamine-oxidase inhibitors, TCAs (e.g., imipramine), SSRIs (e.g., fluoxetine), selective serotonin norepinephrine reuptake inhibitors (SNRIs; venlafaxine, duloxetine), and other antidepressants (mirtazapine). Serotonergic antidepressants can also cause isolated RWA (RWA without clinical manifestations of RBD).[69] Bupropion has not been associated with RBD. However, a study found evidence of RWA associated with that medication.[70] Medications rarely causing RBD, include β-blockers (bisoprolol, atenolol),[71] anticholinesterase inhibitors (rivastigmine in Alzheimer's disease),[72] orexin antagonists (suvorexant in Parkinson's disease),[73] and selegiline. While rivastigmine, a cholinesterase inhibitor used for treatment of dementia, has been reportedly associated with RBD,[72] the medication has been used to treat refractory RBD in patients with Parkinson's disease[74] and in those with isolated RBD and mild cognitive impairment.[75] It is important to note that there can also be a sudden exacerbation of RBD when the dosages of medications associated with RBD are increased. The ICSD-3-TR[2] states that drug-induced RBD should be classified as isolated RBD unless a neurological disorder is present in which case the classification would be secondary RBD.

RBD is often a precursor of a number of neurodegenerative diseases. Delayed onset (often a decade or more) of a neurodegenerative disease is common after the emergence of isolated RBD in men over 50 years of age. An updated analysis[76] of a cohort of elderly men found that 81% of

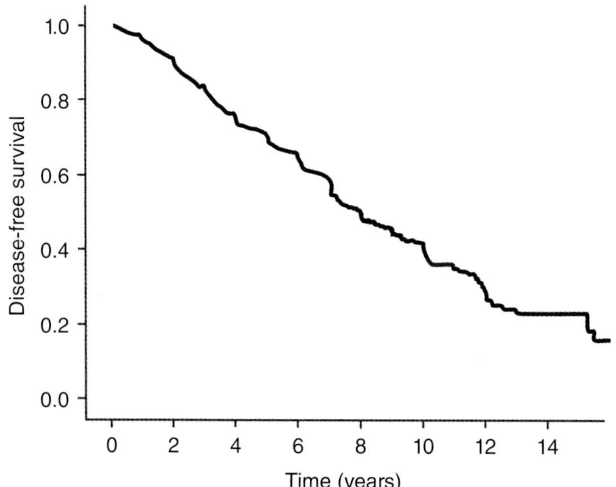

Figure 36–4 A Kaplan-Meier plot of neurological disease-free survival (no development of Parkinsonian disorder or dementia) in patients with idiopathic (isolated) REM sleep behavior disorder. Approximately 70% of patients developed a neurological disorder within 12 years of the diagnosis of idiopathic RBD. The cohort consisted of 1280 individuals (mean age 63.3 years [92% age 55 years or older] and 82% male) at diagnosis of RBD. (From Postuma RB, Iranzo A, Hu M, et al. Risk and predictors of dementia and parkinsonism in idiopathic REM sleep behaviour disorder: a multicentre study. *Brain*. 2019;142(3):744-759.)

patients originally diagnosed with idiopathic (isolated) RBD later developed Parkinson's disease or atypical Parkinson's syndromes, with a mean time interval of 13 years. A large multicenter study followed 1280 patients with RBD and determined the conversion rate to Parkinson's disease or dementia.[77] The overall conversion rate from iRBD to an overt neurodegenerative syndrome was 6.3% per year, with 73.5% converting after 12-year follow-up. In Figure 36–4, a Kaplan-Meier survival plot is shown of the conversion of the group of patients with RBD to a parkinsonian disorder or dementia. The rate of conversion was significantly increased, with abnormal quantitative motor testing, an abnormal objective motor examination, an olfactory deficit, mild cognitive impairment, erectile dysfunction, motor symptoms, an abnormal DAT scan (dopamine-transporter single photon emission tomography), color vision abnormalities, constipation, and older age. In atypical Parkinson's syndromes (DLBD, multisystem atrophy), RBD is more likely to be present either just before or soon after the diagnosis. RBD is much more common in these disorders compared to Parkinson's disease and presents earlier in the course of the disease[78-80] (Table 36–7). In these disorders, the rate of overall disease progression is more rapid than that in Parkinson's disease. However, if RBD is present in a patient with PD, it is associated with more rapid cognitive decline. The acute onset of RBD in a middle-aged woman with other neurological complaints should raise the possibility of multiple sclerosis. RBD emerging before age 50 has less male predominance and the associated nocturnal behaviors are typically less violent. As discussed below, the occurrence of RBD in childhood suggests the presence of narcolepsy (usually type 1).

Polysomnography in RBD

PSG reveals a normal number of REM periods, normal REM cycling, a normal amount of REM sleep as a percentage of total sleep time, and normal REM latency (except with narcolepsy comorbid with RBD). A few studies have found an increase in stage N3 sleep, but this is not a universal finding. A single study found that the duration of each period of REM sleep and the number of rapid eye movements per duration of REM sleep increased over the night in normal controls but not in RBD patients. Autonomic system activation (tachycardia) is uncommon during REM sleep motor activity (in contrast to NREM parasomnias). There is evidence of RWA in the chin and leg EMG channels.[81-83] Synchronized video PSG and recording both leg and arm EMG is recommended.[8] Some patients with RBD display evidence of transient EMG activity during REM sleep, mainly in the arms. The combination of chin EMG and flexor digitorum EMG has been recommended as a simple and sensitive combination.[82] A 30-second tracing from a 70-year-old man with RBD is shown in Figure 36–5. Transient muscle activity is noted in the chin EMG and both anterior tibial EMG channels. A given PSG study may or may not reveal an episode of abnormal behavior/body movements, because most patients do not have nightly attacks. For this reason, some sleep centers perform multiple sleep studies if the diagnosis remains unclear. However, even if abnormal behavior is not documented by a given PSG, evidence of RWA (tonic or phasic EMG abnormality during REM sleep) is usually present. Guidelines

Table 36–7 RBD and Neurogenerative Disorders (α-synucleinopathy)

Parkinson's Disease (PD)
• RBD in 15–50% of PD
• RBD precedes PD (45–65%)
• Latency (1 to 30 years)
• PD patients with RBD usually non-tremor type (rigidity, gait dysfunction)
Multisystem Atrophy (MSA)
• RBD present 90–100% MSA (RBD diagnosed by PSG)
• Only 69% complain of dream enactment, no male predominance
• RBD may precede MSA (44%)
• Latency RBD to MSA (mean 1–19 years)
Diffuse Lewy Body Dementia (DLBD)
• RBD present in ≈ 80% of patients with DLBD
• RBD may precede DLBD (77%)
• Latency RBD to DLBD (mean 9 years)
Predictors of Development of a Neurodegenrative Disorder in RBD patients
• Impaired olfaction (decreased smell)
• Impaired color vision
• Autonomic Dysfunction (orthostatic hypotension, constipation)
• Absent/decreased Dopamine Tracer (DAT) uptake – reduced striatal uptake using DAT-SPECT scanning
• Increased Echogenicity (hyper-echogenicity) in substantia nigra
• Abnormalities in MRI and PET scanning

DAT, dopamine tracer; *DLBD*, Diffuse Lewy Body Dementia; *MRI*, magnetic resonance imaging; *MSA*, multisystem atrophy; *PD*, Parkinson's disease; *PET*, positron emission tomography; *PSG*, polysomnography; *RBD*, REM sleep behavior disorder; *SPECT*, single-proton emission tomography.
Adapted from Howell MJ, Schenck CH. Rapid Eye Movement Sleep Behavior Disorder and Neurodegenerative Disease. *JAMA Neurol.* 2015 Jun;72(6):707-12.

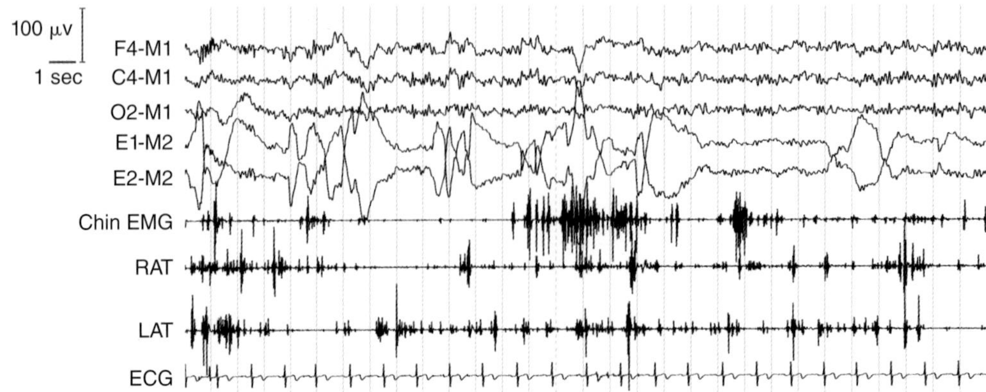

Figure 36–5 This 30-second epoch displays REM sleep without atonia. Transient muscle activity is seen in both the chin and leg electromyography (EMG). Using any chin EMG criteria (tonic or phasic), more than 50% of sequential 3-second min-epochs have either chin or leg activity present (in this case, 10/10 3-second mini-epochs contain activity). See Chapter 15 for rules and examples of scoring REM sleep without atonia. *LAT* and *RAT*, left and right anterior tibial EMG channels.

concerning a decision to withhold treatment before PSG for patients already on treatment for presumed RBD are not available. Continuing RBD medications on the night of the PSG has the potential to decrease the diagnostic accuracy. However, sudden withdrawal of clonazepam (especially at high doses) has the potential to cause significant withdrawal effects. Weaning the medication before the study is one option. Another option might be using a lower dose on the night of the study. Many clinicians would stop melatonin especially as this medication decreases REM sleep without atonia. However, some benefit from melatonin may persist for a variable time period after stopping the medication[96].

The AASM scoring manual provides criteria for scoring the EMG activity associated with RBD[8] (see Chapter 15 for examples). Sustained EMG activity may be noted in the chin EMG during stage R. Excessive phasic activity (TMA) may be noted in the chin EMG or limb EMGs (anterior tibial, flexor digitorum superficialis, extensor digitorum), or both. Monitoring of at least one set (left and right) of arm EMG activity is recommended. Some studies suggest that increased EMG activity in the arm muscles is more specific than leg EMG activity for discriminating patients with RBD from normal individuals. When the chin EMG muscle activity is not reduced (e.g., in RBD), identification of REM sleep (versus stage W) may be challenging. Epochs could potentially be scored as stage W (REMs + increased chin EMG). Clues that abnormal REM sleep is present include the presence of sawtooth waves in the EEG, excessive TMA in the chin and/or limb EMGs, and alterations in airflow associated with bursts of eye movements. The heart rate also may remain constant, despite the sudden appearance of increased EMG tone (as opposed to an awakening). TMA can also be mistaken for PLMS activity. However, TMA usually contains many more brief spikes of activity. *Of interest, during RBD body movements, video monitoring of the face will often show closed eyes but obvious movements of the eyes under the eyelids consistent with REMs*. In contrast, during confusional arousals or sleepwalking, the eyes are typically open with a blank stare and dilated pupils (affected individuals are minimally responsive). See the video clips 36-5 to 36-11 for examples of behavior and body movements associated with RBD.

The AASM scoring manual provides criteria to determine whether a given epoch has sufficient activity in the chin and limb EMGs during REM sleep to be classified as abnormal or excessive.[8] However, the number of such epochs (as a percentage of the total amount of REM sleep) that is considered abnormal (sufficient to support a diagnosis of RBD) is not specified. To date, *no widely accepted* method of defining the amount of RWA to diagnose RBD exists. A study by Montplaisir et al.[81] suggested that RBD is supported by the PSG findings of either (a) tonic chin EMG activity in >30% of REM sleep or (b) phasic chin EMG activity in >15% REM sleep, scored in 20-second epochs. Some studies found that inclusion of arm/hand muscle EMG improved the ability to detect RWA. An analysis by Frauscher et al.[82] suggested that the combination of "any (tonic/phasic)" chin EMG activity combined with bilateral phasic activity of the flexor digitorum superficialis muscles for greater than 50% of the epoch of stage R (scored in 3-second mini epochs) was an effective method to determine the percentage of REM epochs having RWA. Using this combination, RWA in 27% of 30-second REM epochs (or 32% of 3-second mini-epochs without regard to the epoch in which they occurred) was 100% specific as a cutoff for the diagnosis of RBD. The equivalent cutoff using any chin EMG and bilateral anterior tibial EMG was 46%. This illustrates the fact that EMG activity in the arms may be more specific for detecting RWA than EMG of the legs. However, in these studies, some normal individuals showed abnormal activity, and some with RBD did not exhibit sufficient RWA to be classified as abnormal. McCarter and coworkers[83] compared patients with RBD associated with Parkinson's disease with normal individuals and patients with OSA (including split studies). Using slightly different criteria for tonic and phasic (transient) activity, they found that, using a combined "any chin" and leg EMG activity, a cutoff value of 43% of REM RWA epochs had a 95% sensitivity and 97% specificity. Using "any" chin activity, a cutoff of 21.6% of 3-second mini-epochs was 85% sensitive and 97% specific. In summary, the best criteria for determining sufficient RWA to make a diagnosis of RBD remains to be determined. The muscles included in the analysis of RWA will likely change cutoff values, as will the method used to define RWA epochs.

Of note, increased chin EMG and leg EMG activity can occur in normal individuals on SSRIs.[69] *Antidepressants increase RWA in individuals with or without RBD.*[70] A study of 118 normal individuals without parasomnias using the chin and anterior tibial EMG to detect RWA found that older men were more likely to exhibit isolated RWA.[84]

Diagnosis of RBD

The ICSD-3-TR criteria for RBD are:

A. Repeated episodes of sleep-related vocalization and/or complex motor behaviors

B. The behaviors are documented by PSG to occur during REM sleep or, based on clinical history of dream enactment, are presumed to occur during REM sleep.

C. PSG indicates REM sleep without atonia.

D. The disturbance is not better explained by another current sleep disorder or mental disorder.

The major points are demonstration of vocalization or complex motor behaviors (usually violent) during REM sleep (as recorded on video PSG or based on clinical history), and demonstration of RWA. The ICSD-3-TR includes some important notes concerning the diagnostic criteria. First criterion A can be fulfilled by documenting multiple episodes of a single night of video-PSG. There should be an absence of EEG epileptiform activity during REM sleep. Nocturnal seizures are much less likely to occur during REM sleep. Seizure disorders can present with manifestations virtually identical to those of RBD. Therefore, *making a diagnosis of RBD without PSG monitoring is not recommended.* Absence of RWA and/or body movements occuring only during NREM sleep would be inconsistent with RBD. Nocturnal epilepsy occurs most commonly out of NREM sleep but can rarely occur out of REM sleep (NREM > wakefulness > REM). A detailed neurological evaluation of patients suspected of having RBD is indicated with attention to symptoms and signs of associated neurological disorders such as Parkinson's disease. Magnetic resonance imaging (MRI) of the brain (to rule out structural causes) and a full clinical EEG (preferably during sleep) are usually performed *if manifestations are atypical or patients do not respond to therapy.* Note that while a history of *dream enactment* is common (behaviors associated with dream mentation), it is not required for a diagnosis of RBD. If patients awaken, they may report to a bed partner the dream mentation. However, if they quickly return to sleep, they may not remember the dream in the morning. About 8% to 35% of patients with RBD (especially those with neurodegenerative disorders) are not aware of dream-enacting behaviors. *Documenting behaviors during REM sleep on video PSG establishes the behaviors are occuring during REM sleep even if a history of dream enactment is not present.* An important clue that one is dealing with RBD versus an NREM parasomnia is that when awakened, individuals with *RBD are nearly instantly alert*, but individuals with NREM parasomnias are confused. In NREM parasomnias, the *eyes are open* during the behaviors, but during RBD behavior the *eyes are closed.* A summary of important facts about RBD is presented in Box 36–10.

There are a few special situations that merit discussion. A diagnosis of RBD can be made even if the patient is taking medication known to have neurological effects. Certain medications are associated with RWA and may also predispose a patient to RBD manifestations. For example, a patient may develop RBD manifestations when started on an antidepressant. That is, certain medications could unmask underlying isolated RBD. Some clinicians would classify the disorder as medication-induced RBD. However, such patients may develop RBD in the future even if the causative medication is withdrawn. The ICSD-3-TR suggests that a diagnosis of isolated RBD is justified (rather than medication induced RBD), pending future longitudinal studies. The second situation is when a patient manifests movements during REM sleep consistent with RBD but has minimal evidence of RWA (or the amount is insufficient to confidently diagnose RWA). The ICSD-3-TR suggests one could provisionally diagnose RBD based on clinical judgment.

Box 36–10 REM SLEEP BEHAVIOR DISORDER FACTS

- Male predominance (80–90%)*
- Older age (mean age ~50 years)
- Sleep-related injury common
- Dream enactment (common but not required)
- Altered dream process and content—violent and combative
- Tonic and phasic (transient muscle activity) EMG activity during REM sleep
- Preserved sleep architecture (normal amount of REM sleep, stage N3 can be increased)**
- Periodic limb movements during NREM sleep
- Efficacy of clonazepam treatment (>80%)
- Delayed development of neurodegenerative disorder in a large percentage of patients with isolated RBD onset after age 50.

EMG, electromyogram; *NREM*, non-REM; *RBD*, REM sleep behavior disorder; *REM*, rapid eye movement.
* less male predominance in RBD emerging before age 50.
** the duration of REM periods did not increase over the night in one study.[96]
Adapted from Schenck CH, Mahowald MW. REM sleep behavior disorder: clinical, developmental, and neuroscience perspective 16 years after its formal identification in sleep. *Sleep*. 2002;25:120-138.

Differential Diagnosis of RBD

When there is a history of violent motor activity in bed, the differential diagnosis includes night terrors in an adult, periodic leg movements during REM sleep (usually associated with narcolepsy or RBD), nocturnal epilepsy, and PTSD. One article reported on a group of patients with PLMD mimicking RBD.[85] Another publication discussed dream-enactment behavior associated with traumatic dreams in PTSD.[86] A study identified a group of patients with severe OSA who manifested violent movements during sleep but did not have evidence of RWA (pseudo-RBD).[87]

Variants of RBD

In the ICSD-3-TR, two variants of RBD are listed: parasomnia overlap disorder (POD) and status dissociatus. However, a few additional subtypes are listed here, as they have some unique features.

Parasomnia Overlap Disorder (POD). POD (Box 36–11) consists of a combination of RBD and NREM parasomnias (confusional arousals, sleepwalking, sleep terrors).[88,89] Diagnostic criteria for both RBD and one or more of the NREM parasomnias must be met. Most patients with POD had some manifestation of an NREM parasomnia in childhood. POD

Box 36–11 PARASOMNIA OVERLAP SYNDROME

- A subtype of REM sleep behavior disorder in the ICSD-3-TR
- Presentation at a younger age than RBD
- NREM parasomnias are present and may account for the predominant episodes
- PSG findings of RBD, RWA (can be less prominent)
- Causes: narcolepsy, multiple sclerosis, brain tumors, alcohol withdrawal, traumatic brain injury

ICSD-3-TR, International Classification of Sleep Disorders, 3rd edition, text revision; *NREM*, non-REM; *PSG*, polysomnography; *REM*, rapid eye movement; *RBD*, REM sleep behavior disorder; *RWA*, REM sleep without atonia.
Dumitrascu O, Schenck CH, Applebee G, Attarian H. Parasomnia overlap disorder: a distinct pathophysiologic entity or a variant of rapid eye movement sleep behavior disorder? A case series. *Sleep Med.* 2013;14:1217-1220.

can be idiopathic or associated with narcolepsy, multiple sclerosis, brain tumor, or psychiatric disorders. The disorder may respond to treatments used for RBD, such as clonazepam.

Status Dissociatus. This is an extreme form of state dissociation without identifiable sleep stages but with sleep and dream behaviors resembling those in RBD.[2,90] The disorder is a major breakdown of the PSG markers of wakefulness, NREM sleep, and REM sleep. The involved individual thinks they are awake but appears to observers to be acting out a dream. Dream enactment (oneirism) associated with a dissociated wakefulness–REM sleep like state is a manifestation of agrypnia excitata, which includes low stage N3 sleep and marked motor and sympathetic activation. This can be seen with delirium tremens or fatal familial insomnia. This condition is both a severe parasomnia and a severe insomnia disorder. Status dissociatus should not be confused with SRDD (not included as a separate parasomnia in the ICSD-3-TR), which is discussed in a previous section in this chapter and is a condition with *recognizable sleep stages but confused behavior occurring during a period of wakefulness in the major sleep period.*[1]

Isolated REM Sleep Without Atonia. This variant includes findings of RWA without a clinical history or video findings consistent with RBD.[83,84] There can be limb twitching without overt body movements. This is common in patients taking SSRIs. There is some evidence that these patients can go on to develop RBD.

RBD in Children. Narcolepsy with cataplexy is the most common cause of RBD in children (RBD onset may precede narcolepsy with cataplexy by months).[91,92] RBD may also manifest during treatment of cataplexy or depression with a medication (e.g., an SSRI such as venlafaxine). RBD in children has also been seen in association with *neurodevelopmental disorders* (autism, attention deficit hyperactive disorder [ADHD]) and brain-stem tumors with manifestation of both NREM and REM parasomnias (similar to POD). The etiology is distinct from that of common childhood arousal parasomnias and RBD in adults. Some investigations suggest that RWA in children is a biomarker for narcolepsy type 1 (NT1).[93] Of interest, there is a report of RBD in children with NT1 responding to sodium oxybate.[94] Sodium oxybate and low-sodium (calcium, magnesium, potassium, and sodium) oxybates are now approved for treatment of narcolepsy in children ages 7 years and older. RBD in children is modestly responsive to to benzodiazepines or melatonin.

RBD in Narcolepsy With Cataplexy

RBD occurs in patients with narcolepsy and cataplexy (NT1) in about 30% to 60% of cases. *Those experiencing frequent cataplexy attacks are more likely to have RBD.* RBD can also occur in patients with narcolepsy without cataplexy. RBD in narcolepsy with cataplexy is characterized by *greater gender parity* and an early age of onset (including children).[67] In general, there is a lower frequency of RBD episodes and less complex/aggressive behaviors. In contrast to isolated RBD, patients with *RBD associated with narcolepsy with cataplexy are NOT at increased risk of developing neurodegenerative disorders.*

RBD in Neurodegenerative Disorders. As noted, adult patients with RBD emerging after age 50 years (majority men) are at risk of developing a neurodegenerative disorder. On the other hand, a significant proportion of patients with α-synucleinopathy develop RBD. The latency to development of Parkinson's disease following a diagnosis of isolated RBD can be long (median over 13 years). Some patients with Parkinson's disease also manifest RBD after a diagnosis of Parkinson's disease is made and, in general, have more severe Parkinson's disease. A much higher percentage of patients with DLBD and multisystem atrophy (MSA) develop RBD (compared to PD).[78-79] (Table 36–7). The time from the onset of RBD to the onset of DLBD or MSA is variable but is often shorter than for Parkinson's disease. As noted, RBD often develops closer to the onset of these disorders (onset can be either slightly before or after the disorder manifests). The risk of developing a neurodegenerative disorder for patients with emergence of isolated RBD at an age less than 50 years (especially those taking antidepressant medication) remains to be determined.

Pseudo-RBD. As mentioned in the section on the differential diagnosis of RBD, a group of patients with a history of dream-enactment behavior and daytime sleepiness were found to have OSA on PSG but no evidence of RWA.[87] Treatment with CPAP eliminated the behaviors. It is possible that increased pressure for REM sleep (prior REM sleep fragmentation) overwhelmed normal REM atonia processes in these cases. Of note, patients with both true RBD and OSA may also exhibit fewer RBD episodes when adequately treated with CPAP. As RWA can be absent on a given night, the diagnosis of pseudo-RBD is presumptive.

Treatment of RBD

There have been no randomized, controlled clinical trials for treatment of RBD. A best clinical practice guide to treatment of RBD developed by the Standards of Practice Committee of the AASM was published in 2010 following a systematic review of the published literature.[95] A more recent AASM clinical practice guideline for RBD treatment was published in 2022.[96] A summary of the recommendations is provided in Box 36–12. Environmental precautions are an essential first step in RBD treatment because, even with effective treatment with medications, breakthrough episodes do occur. Environmental precautions include having the bedmate sleep in a separate room or bed, closed and locked windows and doors, removal of furniture with sharp edges, and use of a mattress or pads on the floor near the bed (avoiding a high bed).

The most evidence for effective RBD treatment is for the use of clonazepam. Successful treatment of RBD has been achieved with 0.25 to 2 mg clonazepam (≤4 mg) given

Box 36–12 TREATMENTS FOR THE RAPID EYE MOVEMENT SLEEP BEHAVIOR DISORDER

General Measures

- Environmental Precautions
  - Removal of objects that could be thrown or firearms
  - Sharp furniture like nightstands should be moved away or their edges and headboard should be padded.
  - To reduce the risk of injurious falls, a soft carpet, rug, or mat should be placed next to the bed.
  - Patients with severe, uncontrolled RBD should be recommended to sleep separately from their partners, or at the minimum, to place a pillow between themselves and their partners
- Patient education
- Evaluation for Disorders associated with RBD if indicated

AASM Clinical Practice Guideline Recommendations*:

- Adults with Isolated RBD
- Clonazepam
- Melatonin (immediate release) 3–15 mg
- Pramipexole
- Transdermal rivastigmine in adults with mild cognitive impairment
- Adults with secondary RBD due to medical condition
  - Clonazepam
  - Melatonin (immediate release) 3–15 mg
  - Transdermal rivastigmine in adults with RBD and Parkinson Disease
  - Against use of deep brain stimulation
- Adults with drug induced RBD
  - Drug discontinuation

Other Treatments:**

- Sustained release melatonin
- Combination of melatonin and clonazepam
- Non-clonazepam BZRAs (temazepam, triazolam, alprazolam)
- SSRIs
- Bed alarms

BZRAs, benzodiazepine receptor agonists.
*level of recommendation conditional.
**no recommendation concerning these in the AASM clinical practice guidelines (insufficient evidence).
Adapted from Antelmi E, Filardi M, Pizza F, Vandi S, et al. REM Sleep Behavior Disorder in Children With Type 1 Narcolepsy Treated With Sodium Oxybate. Neurology. 2021 Jan 12;96(2):e250-e254.

30 minutes before bedtime in approximately 80% to 90% of patients. Clonazepam dramatically reduced episode frequency or severity, but in most studies, *did not eliminate the finding of REM sleep without atonia*[96]. The medication also does not work by decreasing the amount of REM sleep. A lower dose range was mentioned in the AASM practice guidelines for treatment of RBD (0.25 to 1.0 mg).[96] Clonazepam may modify dream content or inhibit the brainstem locomotor pattern generators. Clonazepam has a half-life of 30 to 40 hours and can cause early morning sedation, confusion, motor incoordination, or memory dysfunction. It may also increase the risk of falls or worsen OSA. A response hierarchy with increasing doses has been described: vigorous violent behavior > complex non-vigorous behavior > simple limb jerking > excessive EMG twitching in stage R. Unfortunately, a significant proportion of patients with RBD treated with clonazepam have one or more significant side effects. The 2022 AASM clinical practice guideline for RBD treatment recommends use of clonazepam and immediate-release melatonin in isolated RBD and RBD associated with a medical condition.[96] Melatonin in doses of 3 to 15 mg has also been found to be effective treatment of RBD either as a sole agent or as an add-on to clonazepam.[96-98] Side effects of melatonin include hallucinations, morning headaches, nightmares, and morning sleepiness. The AASM guideline specifies immediate-release melatonin rather than sustained release. Melatonin has a short half-life, and this may explain the need for high doses. Some patients may respond to a sustained-release form of the medication. Sustained release melatonin was not recommended in the AASM treatment guidelines due to insufficient evidence. Unfortunately, the quality of melatonin is variable and is not under the same scrutiny by regulatory agencies as prescription medications. *In contrast to clonazepam, some studies suggest that melatonin decreases the number of stage R epochs without atonia.* The benefits of melatonin may persist for awhile even if the medication is stopped. Patients with RBD do not exhibit the usual increase in duration of REM episodes over the night and melatonin restores more of this REM feature[96]. A combination of melatonin and clonazepam is another RBD treatment option. This is especially useful when treatment of melatonin alone, is not adequate. Combination treatment may avoid the need for a high dose of clonazepam. The AASM clinical practice guideline recommends *pramipexole in isolated* RBD but not in RBD associated with another medical disorder.[96] Many clinicians would still use melatonin versus pramipexole in isolated RBD, especially if it is well tolerated. In patients with dementia, any sedation should be avoided, if possible. If melatonin is used, the dosage should be as low as possible. Transdermal rivastigmine is recommended for adults with isolated RBD and mild cognitive impairment and in RBD caused by a medical condition (Parkinson's disease).[96] As noted above, this medication is an acetylcholinesterse inhibitor used for treatment of dementia. Side effects of rivastigmine include nausea, vomiting, diarrhea, stomach pain, loss of appetite, or weight loss. The transdermal patch appears to be better tolerated than oral preparations. Successful treatment of RBD has also been reported (case reports with small patient numbers) with paroxetine, BZRAs other than clonazepam (temazepam, triazolam, alprazolam), clozapine (an atypical antipsychotic that can be associated with severe neutropenia), Yi-Gan San (an herbal medication), and carbamazepine.[95] Of interest, the use of a bed alarm with a recorded calming voice was found to be helpful in a patient with RBD.[99]

Because adult patients with RBD are at risk of developing a neurodegenerative disorder, many clinicians feel they should be informed of this fact. Even if not discussed, the patients may find this information on the internet or via other sources. In contrast, other clinicians feel that disclosure may cause undue anxiety and stress. At the time of this writing, there is no treatment to prevent the onset of neurodegenerative disorders. There are efforts to define RBD patients at increased risk for conversion to a neurodegenerative disorder[77]. More information on this topic is presented in Chapter 40. Clinical judgment is needed, and the decision to disclose the risk of conversion to a neurodegenerative disorder should be individualized on a case-by-case basis[96].

Recurrent Isolated Sleep Paralysis

Recurrent isolated sleep paralysis[2,100] (Box 36–13) is characterized by the inability to move at sleep onset (hypnogogic) or upon awakening (hypnopompic).

Box 36–13 RECURRENT ISOLATED SLEEP PARALYSIS FACTS

- Sleep paralysis can be associated with hallucinations
- Timing
  - Sleep onset hypnogogic
  - Upon awakening—hypnopompic (most common)
- Associations/precipitating factors
  - Prior sleep deprivation or fragmentation
  - Withdrawal from REM-suppressing medications
- Treatment
  - Avoid sleep deprivation
  - Medications that treat cataplexy are effective:
    TCAs (imipramine)
    SSRIs
    SNRIs

REM, rapid eye movement; *SNRIs*, selective serotonin and norepinephrine reuptake inhibitors; *SSRIs*, selective serotonin reuptake inhibitors; *TCAs*, tricyclic antidepressants.

Diagnostic criteria[2] are:

A. A recurrent inability to move the trunk and all the limbs at sleep onset or upon awakening from sleep.
B. Each episode lasts from seconds to a few minutes.
C. The episodes cause clinically significant distress, including bedtime anxiety or fear of sleep.
D. The disturbance is not better explained by another current sleep disorder (especially narcolepsy), medical disorder, mental disorder, or medication/substance use.

Patients are awake and have full recall of the event. Although diaphragmatic function is not affected, a sensation of dyspnea is common. Episodes can be aborted by the affected individual being touched or spoken to or by making intense efforts to move. Sleep paralysis is also common in patients with narcolepsy and idiopathic hypersomnia. The term "isolated" refers to the fact that other sleep disorders such as narcolepsy or idiopathic hypersomnia are **not** present. The frequency of sleep paralysis episodes is quite variable—from once per lifetime to several per month. Hallucinatory experiences accompany sleep paralysis in 25% to 75% of affected individuals. Studies of students suggest 15% to 40% experience at least one episode of sleep paralysis. Sleep disruption, irregular sleep periods, sleep deprivation, and stress are known triggers. In most cases, treatment with medications is not needed. Avoiding sleep deprivation and following a regular sleep pattern may help prevent isolated sleep paralysis: SSRI medications (in antidepressant doses) and TCAs (low doses) are usually effective treatment for isolated sleep paralysis. None of these medications are approved by the U.S. Food and Drug Administration (FDA) for this indication. There is a report of use of escitalopram, which is a well-tolerated SSRI, in two patients with isolated sleep paralysis.[101]

Nightmare Disorder

Nightmare disorder (dream anxiety attacks)[2,100] is characterized by recurrent nightmares, which are disturbing mental experiences that usually occur during REM sleep and often result in an awakening. Nightmares can follow acute trauma (acute stress disorder [ASD]) or occur 1 month or more after trauma (PTSD). The dreams of PTSD can occur out of NREM stages N2 or N3, during REM sleep, and at sleep onset. A number of medications can also be associated with nightmares[102,103] (Box 36–14), including

Box 36–14 MEDICATIONS COMMONLY ASSOCIATED WITH NIGHTMARES

- β-blockers—propranolol, metoprolol
- Cholinergic agonists—donepezil
- Antibiotics—levofloxacin (Levaquin)
- Antiviral agents—amantadine, gancyclovir
- Dopamine agonists—ropinirole, pramipexole
- Antidepressants—fluoxetine, paroxetine
- Antiretroviral—efavirenz (Sustiva)
- Benzodiazepine receptor agonists—zolpidem
- Melatonin agonist—ramelteon
- Ethanol withdrawal—REM rebound

REM, rapid eye movement.

efavirenz, pramipexole, donepezil, and varenicline. Fifty percent to 80% of adults report occasional nightmares. Ten percent to 50% of children 3 to 5 years of age experience nightmares severe enough to for them to disturb their parents. Nightmares within 3 months of trauma are present in up to 80% of patients with PTSD. Few PSG studies of nightmares exist, but typically, accelerated heart rate and respiratory rate precede awakening from REM sleep with report of a nightmare.

Diagnosis of Nightmare Disorder

The ICSD-3-TR diagnostic criteria[2] for nightmare disorder are:

A. Repeated occurrences of extended, extremely dysphoric, and well-remembered dreams that usually involve threats to survival, security, or physical integrity.

B. On awakening from the dysphoric dreams, the person rapidly becomes oriented and alert.

C. The dream experience, or the sleep disturbance produced by awakening from it, causes clinically significant distress or impairment in social, occupational, or other important areas of functioning as indicated by the report of at least one of the following:
   1. Mood disturbance (e.g., persistence of nightmares affect anxiety, dysphoria).
   2. Sleep resistance (e.g., bedtime anxiety, fear of sleep/subsequent nightmares).
   3. Negative impact on caregiver or family functioning (e.g., nighttime disruption).
   4. Behavioral problems (e.g., bedtime avoidance, fear of the dark).
   5. Daytime sleepiness.
   6. Fatigue or low energy.
   7. Impaired occupational or educational function.
   8. Impaired interpersonal/social function.

Note that repeated episodes and adverse consequences are both required. One would probably not classify the rare occurrence of a nightmare as a disorder given the high percentage of normal individuals experiencing an occasional nightmare. A diagnosis of nightmare disorder requires that the dreams/awakenings cause significant distress or impairment of social function, including mood disturbance and resistance going to sleep.

Treatment of Nightmare Disorder

The AASM published a best practice guideline for treatment of nightmare disorder in adults in 2010,[104] with an update in

2018.[105] The 2018 publication discusses several behavioral techniques (exposure, relaxation, and rescripting; eye movement desensitization, and reprocessing) that are beyond the scope of this chapter. The reader is referred to the AASM publication for a detailed discussion of these treatments. If a medication is temporally associated with nightmares, a trial of medication discontinuation or change is prudent. Cognitive behavioral treatments have been used to treat nightmares with some success.[106-108] One behavioral technique called imagery rehearsal therapy[107-108] has proved successful in several studies of nightmares associated with PTSD. Patients are asked to rewrite their previous dreams with a positive outcome. In the past, use of medications for nightmares had limited success. Several studies have reported success with the alpha-1 blocker prazosin in nightmares associated with PTSD.[109] However, a large randomized trial[110] failed to show a benefit. One explanation for this unexpected finding is that the trial excluded unstable individuals (who may benefit the most). Doses of 2 to 12 mg have been used (usually 3 to 6 mg). Note that, when prazosin is started, the drug should be initiated with a dose of 1 mg at bedtime to avoid severe first-dose hypotension (often orthostatic hypotension). The drug can then be titrated upward slowly over several nights.

OTHER PARASOMNIAS

The ICSD-3-TR category of other parasomnias is composed of exploding head syndrome, sleep-related hallucinations, sleep-related urological disorder, parasomnia due to a medical disorder, parasomnia due to a medication or substance, and parasomnia unspecified. This section will also discuss *catathrenia* (included in the sleep breathing disorders section of the ICSD-3-TR), as this disorder is usually considered in the differential diagnosis of other parasomnias.

Exploding Head Syndrome

Patients with exploding head syndrome report a sudden loud noise or sense of explosion in the head that is not painful.[2,111]

Diagnostic criteria include:

A. There is a complaint of a *sudden loud noise or sense of explosion* in the head either at the wakefulness-sleep transition or upon waking during the night.

B. The individual experiences *abrupt arousal following the event, often with a* ***sense of fright.***

C. The experience is ***not*** associated with significant complaints of pain.

The exploding head episodes occur as the individual falls asleep or upon awakening from sleep. The sensation may be a loud bang or a clash of a cymbal associated with a flash of light. The individual may awaken with a sense of fright. *More than one episode can occur during a single night.* In some patients, the episodes occur in clusters over several nights. Exploding head syndrome is *more common in women than in men.* The differential diagnosis of exploding head syndrome is presented in Box 36–15. In contrast to sleep-related migraines, cluster headaches, nocturnal paroxysmal hemicrania, and hypnic headaches, exploding head syndrome is painless.

Hypnic headache is an uncommon headache characterized by awakening with a generalized or lateralized headache that lasts at least 15 minutes (usually 30-60 minutes). Nausea is often

Box 36–15 DIFFERENTIAL DIAGNOSIS OF EXPLODING HEAD SYNDROME

- Conditions to consider include sleep-related headaches (see below). In contrast to other headache syndromes, exploding head syndrome is usually painless.
- Simple partial seizures can present with sensory phenomena but do not usually occur predominantly at sleep onset.
- Nocturnal panic attacks can awaken a person from sleep but are not usually associated with a sense of noise or explosion.
- Recurrent nightmares are characterized by recall of more complex and longer-lasting visual imagery.
- Hypnic jerks (sleep starts) occur at the wakefulness-sleep transition but are predominantly a motor phenomenon with sudden myoclonic jerks rather than an emphasis on sensory symptoms.
- Sudden-onset headache syndromes (see text):
  - Idiopathic stabbing headache
  - Thunderclap headache
  - Hypnic headache syndrome
  - Cluster headaches
  - Nocturnal paroxysmal hemicrania
  - Migraines

present. Onset is after age 50, with a frequency of at least 15 per month. Hypnic headaches tend to occur out of REM sleep. They often occur in a regular pattern and awaken patients 4 to 6 hours after sleep onset ("alarm clock headache"). Treatment is with lithium, indomethacin, or caffeine.[112] *Idiopathic stabbing headache* (icepick headache) is a benign syndrome involving the sensation of brief stabs of pain on the side of the head. Although the headaches can occur at sleep onset, they are more common during wakefulness. *Thunderclap headache* is a very severe sudden-onset headache characteristic of subarachnoid hemorrhage but also results from other causes and, occasionally, as a benign symptom. *It does not usually occur at sleep onset. Cluster headaches* occur at the same hour every day usually between 9 PM and 10 AM. The attacks are strongly related to REM sleep. They are severe unilateral periorbital or temporal headaches of a relatively short duration (average about one hour). Cluster headaches occur in clusters with the cluster period lasting from one week to a year. Then there is a pain-free period, known as remission, for three months or longer before the next headache cluster begins. Nocturnal paroxysmal hemicrania is characterized by severe unilateral headaches of short duration that occur at least five times per day (often associated with REM sleep), and are very responsive to indomethacin. Migraines are severe unilateral throbbing headaches associated with nausea, vomiting, or photophobia. *Migraines occur during wakefulness or sleep, but about 50% start between 4 AM and 9 AM.* The reader is referred to a more complete discussion of sleep-related headache and its management.[113]

Sleep-Related Hallucinations

Sleep-related hallucinations (SRH) can occur when falling asleep (hypnogogic) or upon awakening (hypnopompic) (Box 36–16).[2] SRH can be associated with sleep paralysis, and both are common in patients with narcolepsy. However, SRH can occur in normal individuals and can be associated with isolated sleep paralysis.

The ICSD-3-TR diagnostic criteria are:

A. There is a complaint of recurrent hallucinations experienced just prior to sleep onset or upon awakening during the night or in the morning.

Box 36–16 SLEEP-RELATED HALLUCINATION FACTS

- Sleep-related hallucinations are predominantly visual but may include auditory, tactile, or kinetic phenomena.
- Hallucinations at sleep onset (hypnagogic hallucinations) may be difficult to differentiate from sleep-onset dreaming.
- Hallucinations upon awakening in the morning (hypnopompic hallucinations) may arise out of a period of REM sleep, and patients also may be uncertain whether they represent waking or dream-related experiences.

B. The hallucinations are predominantly visual.
C. The disturbance is not better explained by another sleep disorder (especially narcolepsy), mental disorder, medical disorder, or medication/substance use.

Obtaining adequate sleep is often an effective treatment. If necessary, medications used for isolated sleep paralysis[100] (TCAs, SSRIs) can be effective. SRH in patients with neurodegenerative disorders are a manifestation of the underlying disease. Patients with Parkinson's disease often have daytime or sleep-related hallucinations.[114] *Complex nocturnal hallucinations*[2,115] characterize a state of dream mentation that occurs either at sleep onset or offset. The hallucinations are usually visual, vivid, multicolored, and distorted. They occur in wakefulness after sudden arousal from sleep and occur in the setting of idiopathic hypersomnia, diffuse lewy body dementia, anxiety, and macular degeneration. Medication-induced SRH can occur with alcohol (withdrawal) or β-blockers. Charles Bonnet hallucinations consist of visual hallucination resulting from damage of the brain visual pathways (often in blind individuals). These hallucinations tend to be bizarre but seldom disturbing. The images include inanimate objects, animals, and people.[115]

Sleep-Related Urologic Dysfunction (Including Sleep-Related Enuresis)

Sleep-related urologic dysfunction is divided into three categories in ICSD-3-TR[2]: sleep enuresis (SE), nocturia, and nocturnal urinary urge incontinence. A summary of the diagnostic criteria include:

Sleep Enuresis

A. The patient exhibits recurrent involuntary voiding during sleep, occurring at least once per month.
B. The condition has been present for at least 3 months.
C. **The patient is older than 5 years.**

Nocturia

A. The patient exhibits three or more nightly episodes of urination arising from sleep.
B. Each episode of urination is followed by sleep or the intention to sleep.
C. The condition has been present for at least 3 months.
D. **The patient is older than 5 years.**

Nocturnal Urinary Urge Incontinence

A. The patient or care provider reports or observes urinary urgency and leakage (wetting bedding, bedclothes, or undergarments) after arising from sleep.
B. Sleep-related wetness episodes must occur at least once per week.
C. The condition has been present for at least 3 months.

SE (voiding during sleep) has traditionally been divided into *primary and secondary SE based on whether the patient had been previously consistently dry.* The ICSD-3[116] included separate criteria for primary and secondary SE (no longer specified in the ICSD-3-TR). Criteria for primary SE included age >5 years, involuntary voiding during sleep at least twice weekly for at least 3 months, and the patient has never been consistently dry during sleep. Criteria for secondary SE included: age >5 years, involuntary voiding during sleep at least twice weekly for at least 3 months, and the patient must have been previously consistently dry for at least 6 months. New criteria for SE are noted above. At least one episode per month for at least 3 months is now required with an age >5 years. The International Children's Continence Society[117] recommend use of the term monosymptomatic enuresis when no lower urinary tract symptoms are present and non-monosymptomatic when manifestations such as daytime incontinence, urinary tract infection, bowel dysfunction, or difficulty urinating are present. SE is called frequent if >4 episodes per week are noted.

Important SE facts are displayed in Box 36–17. A limit of 5 years of age for primary SE is somewhat arbitrary. The spon-

Box 36–17 SLEEP-RELATED ENURESIS (SRE) FACTS

Diagnostic Considerations:

- Monosymptomatic SE
  - SE occurs in 15 to 20% of five year old children (spontaneous cure rate about 15% per year)
  - 3/2 ratio boys/girls (more common in boys)
  - SRE is hereditary: prevalence 77% if both parents had SE and 44% if one parent had SRE
- Non-monosymptomatic SE
  - Lower urinary tract symptoms, urinary tract infection, bowel dysfunction, daytime incontinence, underactive bladder (straining to urinate), anatomic abnormality of urinary tract
- PSG in SE.
  - SE can occur in all stages of sleep, during wake episodes during the night or associated with arousal from sleep

Causes of Sleep Enuresis

- Late maturation - SE in 15–20% of normal five year old children
- OSA has been reported in 4 to 6% of children with SRE
- Psychological stress (parental divorce, physical or sexual abuse
- Urinary tract infection or structural abnormalities
- Inability to concentrate urine (DI, nephrogenic DI, sickle cell anemia)
- Increased urine production (caffeine, medications)
- Chronic constipation and encopresis (bulging colon constricts bladder capacity)
- Neurologic disorders: seizures, neurogenic bladder
- Diabetes
- Nocturnal epilepsy

Treatments for Sleep Enuresis

- Reassurance (especially if mono-symptomatic)
- Behavioral treatments (frequent daytime voiding, fluid restriction at night).
- Alarm treatments (wet bed triggers alarm).
- Evaluation for sleep apnea and genitourinary pathology if indicated.
- Drug therapy: vasopressin, anticholinergics (oxybutynin), tricyclic antidepressants.

DI, diabetes insipidus; *OSA*, obstructive sleep apnea; *UTI*, urinary tract infection.

taneous *"cure" rate for SE after age 5 is approximately 15% per year*. The prevalence of SE is approximately 15 to 20% of five year olds, up to 15% at age 7 year, 10% at age 10 years, and about 2% for adolescents. There is a *strong familial component to primary SE* and a high prevalence of SE in parents or siblings of a child with primary SE. The risk of SE is 77% if both parents had SE and 44% when one parent had SE. There is a *male-to-female ratio of 3:2 in* primary SE. For secondary SE, in addition to having been previously dry for 6 months and older than 5 years, the condition must occur at least twice a week for at least 3 months. *Episodes of SE can occur in all stages of sleep, during wakefulness, and following arousal from sleep*. Common causes of secondary SE are listed in Box 36–17. Urinary tract infection and structural abnormalities should be ruled out. Parental questioning should assess the situation for causes of psychological stress. Inability to concentrate the urine should raise the question of diabetes insipidus (DI) or nephrogenic DI. *Another possibility is that SE is a manifestation of untreated OSA*. The possibility of OSA-induced SE should be suspected in children with obesity or a history of snoring and disturbed sleep.[118] Nocturnal enuresis can occur in adults and is often associated with identifiable conditions.

Treatment options[119] (Box 36–17) include reassurance (especially if the child is less than 5 years of age). *However, some children may not become dry until a later age*. If OSA is present, effective treatment may improve SE. Behavioral treatment, alarm treatments, and medications are other options. Medications include vasopressin, anticholinergics such as oxybutynin, or TCAs.

The upper limit of normal for urination episodes during the night is controversial but here nocturia is defined as 3 or more urination episodes during the night. *Urinary urge incontinence* is when an individual awakens at night with urinary urgency but cannot reach the bathroom before an episode of urinary incontinence occurs. The is typically in elderly debilitated individuals.

Parasomnia Caused by a Medical Disorder

The essential feature of this diagnosis is the presence of a parasomnia that is attributable to an underlying neurological or medical condition.[2] RBD is the parasomnia most commonly associated with an underlying neurological condition ("symptomatic RBD"). However, when diagnostic criteria for RBD are met, the more specific diagnosis of RBD should be made. An example of a parasomnia caused by a medical disorder is complex nocturnal sleep-related visual hallucinations.[2,115] This disorder can occur with neurological disorders such as narcolepsy, Parkinson's disease, DLBD, vision loss (Charles Bonnet hallucinations), and midbrain and diencephalic pathology (peduncular hallucinations).

Parasomnia Caused by a Medication or Substance

The essential feature of this diagnosis is the close temporal relationship between exposure to a drug, medication, or biological substance and the onset of the signs and symptoms of that disorder.[2] A likely causal relationship can be inferred if signs and symptoms of the parasomnia disappear when the drug or substance is withdrawn.

ISOLATED SYMPTOMS AND NORMAL VARIANTS

Sleep Talking (somniloquy)

Sleep talking can occur as an isolated symptom but can also be part of NREM and REM parasomnias. For example, during episodes of RBD, some talking is common and can be conversational in nature.

Catathrenia

In the ICSD-3-TR,[2] catathrenia (sleep-related groaning) is classified in the isolated symptoms and normal variants section under *sleep-related breathing disorders*. Others have classified the disorder as a parasomnia, as the complaint usually does ***not*** come to clinical attention as a breathing disturbance. Diagnostic criteria for catathrenia are not specified in the ICSD-3-TR although common manifestations are discussed. Some important facts about catathrenia are displayed in Box 36–18. Catathrenia is a chronic (often nightly) disorder characterized by expiratory groaning during NREM or REM sleep.[120-126] The initial descriptions of catathrenia reported groaning out of REM sleep (especially during REM episodes in the second part of the night). Others found catathrenia to occur out of both NREM and REM sleep or predominantly out of NREM sleep. *The ICSD-3-TR states the disorder occurs predominantly out of REM sleep*.[2] The sleep stage predominance may vary among patients. Episodes may be associated with bradypneic episodes (slow respiratory rate) with long exhalations. Typically, a large inspiration is followed by protracted expiration during which a monotonous vocalization ("mournful moaning or groaning") is produced. See Video 36-12 for an example of an episode of catathrenia. Catathrenia events tend to occur in clusters and are often associated with bradycardia. Patients are usually unaware of the groaning. The disorder is thought to be benign, and its main complication is disturbance of the bed partner. Catathrenia is very rare, with onset usually in adolescence or early adulthood (mean age 19 years, with a range of 5 to 36 years). *The prevalence of catathrenia is greater in men than in women*. Catathrenia has been reportedly associated with sodium oxybate treatment of narcolepsy.[123]

Catathrenia events may occur in clusters *resembling a run of central apneas*.[124] An EEG arousal with or without body movement often marks the end of the event. Clusters of catathrenia events can be confused with central apneas. However, in central apneas, an exhalation precedes the long inspiratory pause. In contrast, in catathrenia, a deep inspiration precedes the long expiratory pause (Figure 36–6). Mild bradycardia during the exhalation is common. Of note, atypical catathrenia has been described, consisting of expiratory groaning without prolonged inspiration or exhalation.

The differential diagnosis of catathrenia includes stridor, sleep-related laryngospasm, and sleep talking. Stridor can be inspiratory or expiratory, typically occurs with every breath, and does not have a prolonged expiratory phase. Sleep-related

Box 36–18 CATATHRENIA FACTS

- Expiratory groaning
- Men > women
- Can occur during NREM and REM sleep (some studies found REM > NREM, others NREM > REM). The ICSD-3-TR states that more episodes occur from REM sleep
- Typical pattern: large inspiration, prolonged expiration while groaning
- *Can be confused with central apnea*
- CPAP beneficial to some patients

CPAP, continuous positive airway pressure; *NREM*, non-REM; *REM*, rapid-eye movement.

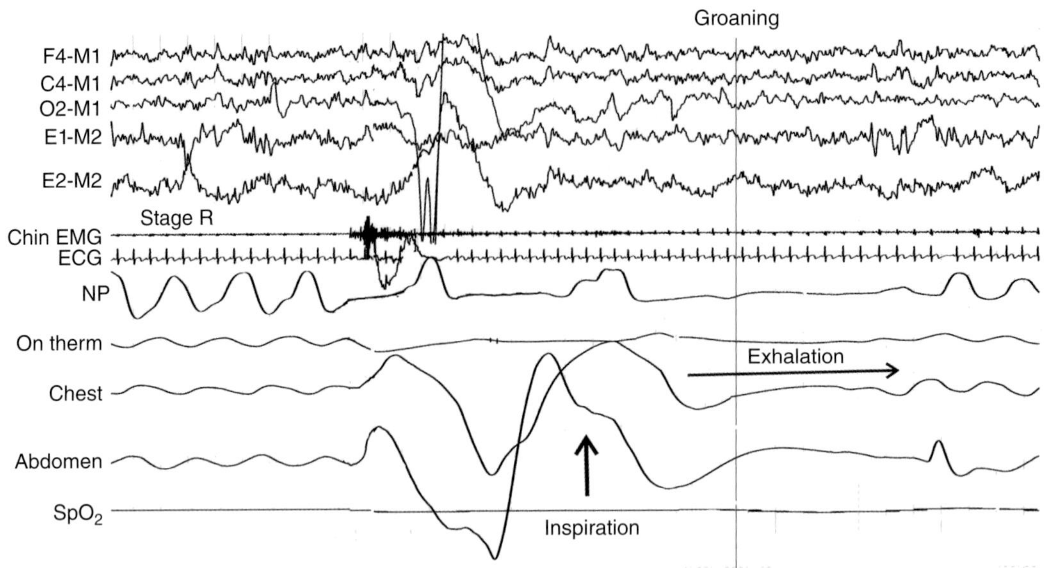

Figure 36–6 This 30-second tracing shows an episode of expiratory groaning following a large inspiration occuring during stage R (REM sleep). At first glance, this appears to be a central apnea, but the event started with the exhalation immediately following the big inspiration. ON Therm is the oronasal thermal airflow sensor channel. Inspiration is upward.

laryngospasm is associated with a sense of suffocation. Sleep talking consists of words rather than groans. Not all cases of catathrenia require treatment. Multiple medications have been tried without success. CPAP treatment has been effective in some patients but ineffective in others.[125,126] Some of the reported patients improving with CPAP had both OSA and catathrenia.

SUMMARY OF KEY POINTS

1. If PSG is indicated for evaluation of a patient with suspected parasomnia, use of video PSG (synchronized video and audio) is essential. The use of additional arm EMG electrodes may help more accurately determine whether RWA is present, and additional EEG electrodes may help detect interictal seizure activity (e.g., adding temporal electrodes).
2. The classic NREM parasomnias include confusional arousals (awakening with confusion), sleepwalking (ambulation during sleep), and sleep terrors (awakening with a loud scream and intense fear). The sleep-related eating disorder is also classified as an NREM parasomnia in the ICSD-3 and ICSD-3-TR.
3. In children, NREM parasomnias occur out of stage N3 sleep (first part of the night) but in adults can occur out of stages N2 or N3 (during any part of the night). Approximately 60% to 70% of adults with an NREM parasomnia experienced one or more NREM parasomnias in childhood.
4. The classic NREM parasomnias have characteristics in common, including amnesia following the event, limited dream recall, eyes open during the episode (glassy eyes), and impaired cognition during the event It is difficult to communicate with the affected individual during the event. Precipitating events include stress, sleep deprivation, OSA, fever in children, and medication use.
5. REM parasomnias include RBD, nightmare disorder, and recurrent sleep paralysis.
6. Diagnostic criteria for RBD include:
   A. Repeated episodes of sleep-related vocalization or complex motor behaviors.
   B. The behaviors are documented by video-polysomnography to occur during REM sleep or, based on clinical history of dream enactment are presumed to occur during REM sleep.
   C. PSG demonstrates REM sleep without atonia (RWA),
   D. The disturbance is not better explained by another current sleep disorder or mental disorder.
7. Treatments for isolated RBD include environmental precautions, clonazepam, and/or immediate release melatonin (often in high doses). Clonazepam is effective but can cause daytime sedation. Pramipexole has also been recommended. The cholinesterase inhibitor rivastigmine has been recommended as a treatment for RBD in patients with isolated RBD and mild cognitive impairment and in RBD associated with Parkinson's disease. Clonazepam and melatonin are also recommended in RBD associated with a medical disorder.
8. The Parasomnia Overlap Disorder consists of manifestations of both an NREM parasomnia and RBD.
9. Isolated RBD (formerly idiopathic RBD) refers to the disorder without an association with another neurological disorder. Secondary RBD has been associated with several neurological disorders including narcolepsy with cataplexy, Parkinson's disease, diffuse lewy body dementia, multiple system atrophy, and multiple sclerosis.
10. A significant proportion (over 80%) of patients with isolated RBD emerging after age 50 years later develop Parkinson's disease or another neurodegenerative disorder. In one study, the mean latency was about 13 years. In another study, about 70% converted in about 12 years. Risk factors for development of a neurodegenerative disorder include impaired olfaction, color vision deficits, and constipation.
11. Nocturnal seizures may mimic parasomnias, especially sleep-related hypermotor epilepsy (SHE). Features favoring epilepsy over a parasomnia include stereotypical behavior (same manifestations each time) and more than one episode per night.

12. The sleep-related eating disorder (SRED) is manifested by eating and drinking during the main sleep period and is associated with a variable degree of alertness and recall of the eating behavior. The behavior must be associated with one or more of several manifestations including eating peculiar food items, associated with insomnia caused by sleep disturbance from the eating episodes, sleep-related injury, dangerous behaviors in pursuit of food, morning anorexia, or adverse consequences of binge eating. Treatments include topiramate or SSRI medications.

13. SRED can be associated with sleepwalking, RLS, narcolepsy, or medications. Medication-induced SRED has been reported with BZRAs, including zolpidem and triazolam, psychotropic medications (lithium, quetiapine, mirtazapine, risperidone), and sodium oxybate. Any BZRA can cause SRED, but zolpidem is the medication most commonly reported. *SRED is more common in women than in men.*

14. Catathrenia is characterized by a deep inspiration and long expiratory groan, most commonly during REM sleep. The episodes can occur out of either NREM or REM sleep. *Catathrenia is seen more commonly in men.* Treatment is not always needed, but CPAP has been effective in some studies.

15. The ICSD-3-TR diagnostic category Sleep-Related Urologic Dysfunction includes sleep-related enuresis (SE), Nocturia, and Nocturnal Urinary Urge Incontinence. The previous terminology of primary and secondary enuresis (no longer separate diagnostic categories in the ICSD-3-TR) is still widely used. Primary SE is defined as SE in a child over 5 years of age that has never been dry. Secondary SE is defined as the onset of SE in a patient who has previously been dry for at least 6 months. *The diagnosis of OSA should be considered in all children who snore and have secondary SE.* Heritable factors are present in primary SE.

16. Exploding head syndrome is characterized by a sudden loud imagined noise or sense of violent explosion in the head occurring as the patient is falling asleep (drowsy but awake) or upon waking during the night. The event is **painless**, but patients usually awaken with **fright**.

CLINICAL REVIEW QUESTIONS

1. Which of the following is **NOT** true about sleepwalking in adults?
   A. About 60% to 70% had a history of sleepwalking in childhood.
   B. Can be precipitated by sleep deprivation
   C. Adult sleep walking can be more violent and the episodes longer than in children.
   D. Always occurs out of stage N3 sleep

2. Which of the following disorders is NOT commonly associated with RBD?
   A. Narcolepsy
   B. Parkinson's disease
   C. Diffuse Lewy Body Dementia
   D. Alzheimer's disease
   E. Multiple system atrophy
   F. Multiple sclerosis

3. Which of the following medications are associated with RBD?
   A. Fluoxetine
   B. Venlafaxine
   C. Mirtazapine
   D. Tricyclic antidepressants
   E. All of the above

4. Which of the following is true about RBD?
   A. Typically occurs in the first half of the night
   B. Women > men
   C. Responds to clonazepam in about 80% of patients
   D. Responds to 0.3 to 0.5 mg of melatonin
   E. Dream recall is always present.

5. What characteristic(s) are true about nocturnal panic attacks?
   A. Associated with autonomic hyperactivity, tachycardia
   B. The patient is awake and alert during the panic attack.
   C. Amnesia surrounding the event
   D. B and C
   E. A and B

6. Which of the following factors favor nocturnal epilepsy over a parasomnia?
   A. Confusion following the event
   B. Stereotypic behavior (all events similar)
   C. One episode per night
   D. Amnesia surrounding the event

7. Which of the following is true concerning SRED?
   A. Patients are never alert during events.
   B. Amnesia surrounding SRED events is always present.
   C. Prevalence of SRED: Men > women
   D. Zolpidem is the medication most often associated with SRED.
   E. Normal foods are usually eaten.

8. Which of the following does **NOT** characterize events associated with exploding head syndrome?
   A. Painless
   B. Men > women
   C. Occurs during transitions from wakefulness to sleep or upon awakening
   D. Associated with fright
   E. Often associated with the sensation of a loud noise

9. In which of the following situations would a diagnosis of RBD be indicated?
   A. REM sleep without atonia (RWA), history of dream enactment with complex movements or vocalizations
   B. RWA, complex body movements or vocalizations on video PSG during REM sleep
   C. RWA, no complex body movements during PSG, no history of dream enacting behavior
   D. A and B
   E. A and C

10. Which of the following patterns is **NOT** considered compatible with RBD?
   A. Chin EMG: sustained tonic activity during REM sleep
   B. Chin EMG: transient muscle activity (phasic) during REM sleep
   C. Leg EMG: sustained tonic activity
   D. Leg EMG: transient muscle activity (phasic)
   E. Chin EMG: sustained tonic activity and transient muscle activity during REM sleep

11. Which of the following describes catathrenia?
   A. Deep inspiration, prolonged expiratory groan, slow breathing rate
   B. NREM > REM sleep
   C. Women > Men
   D. Patient complains of disturbed sleep

12. A child was age 8, has nocturnal enuretic episodes. He also was noted to snore loudly and to have difficulty concentrating in classes. Which of the following are true?
   A. Enuretic episodes can occur in all stages of sleep and following arousal from sleep.
   B. One of his parents likely had sleep enuresis.
   C. OSA should be considered.
   D. The episodes must occur at least three times per month for at least 3 months
   E. A, B. and C

ANSWERS

1. D. Sleepwalking in adults can occur out of stages N2 and N3. One study found it can also occur out of stage N1 (that is all stages of NREM sleep). Adult sleep walking in adults can be more violent and episodes longer than in children.
2. D. Although RBD can occur in patients with Alzheimer's disease, it is not typical.
3. E. All of the above.
4. C. RBD responds to clonazepam in about 80% of cases, although many patients experience side effects. Melatonin, often in doses of 5 to 15 mg, may be effective. RBD is typically a disorder of men over 50 years of age. As this parasomnia occurs out of REM sleep, the usual timing is in the second part of the night. Dream recall is not aways present in the morning. If asked immediately after the episode ends, the patient may tell the bed partner about dream mentation. A history of dream enactment is not required to make a diagnosis of RBD if video PSG shows behaviors during REM sleep and REM sleep without atonia.
5. E. Unlike in NREM parasomnias, during panic attacks, patients are alert and do not have amnesia surrounding the event. Panic attacks may occur out of NREM sleep and be associated with autonomic hyperactivity and intense fear. The patient may awaken abruptly from NREM sleep with the panic attack in progress, but ongoing symptoms are experienced when the patient is alert.
6. B. Stereotypical behaviors (same manifestations with every episode) and several episodes per night are more common with nocturnal epilepsy. Confusion following the event and amnesia can occur both with NREM parasomnias and many types of nocturnal seizures.
7. D. Zolpidem is the medication most often associated with SRED. Alertness during the event and recall of the event are highly variable. SRED is much more common in women than in men. Although normal foods (especially those high in carbohydrates) may be eaten, frozen foods and non-foods are also sometimes consumed.
8. B. Exploding head syndrome is more *common in women than in men* in clinical series but approximately equal prevalence in survey studies according to the ICSD-3-TR. In any case, the prevalence is not higher in men (**B** is not correct). Exploding head episodes are **painless,** may be associated with the sensation of a loud noise, occur during drowsiness or upon awakening, and are associated with **fright**.
9. D. (A and B). A diagnosis of RBD requires PSG evidence of RWA and either body movements during REM sleep noted on a PSG or a history of dream enactment. A PSG showing evidence of RWA without other findings does not meet diagnostic criteria. Isolated RWA can simply mean that the patient is taking an SSRI or similar medication. In pseudo-RBD (severe untreated OSA), body movements can be noted during REM sleep with ***no*** evidence of RWA.
10. C. Sustained leg EMG activity is not considered evidence of RWA.
11. A. Catathrenia is more common in REM than in NREM sleep (in most but not all of the literature) and is characterized by a deep inspiration followed by a prolonged expiratory groan/moan, often with a slow breathing rate. **Catathrenia is more common in men than in women.** This parasomnia is believed to have no direct consequences for the patient but can significantly disturb the sleep of the bed partner.
12. E. (A. B, and C are correct). Sleep enuresis (SE) can occur during any stage of sleep or following arousal from sleep. A diagnosis of sleep enuresis requires at least one episode per month for at least 3 months (Answer D is not correct). Heritable factors are associated SE and SE can be a manifestation of OSA. A diagnosis of sleep enuresis requires at least one episode per month (not 3 episodes per month) for at least 3 months. Therefore D is not correct.

SUGGESTED READING

Postuma RB, Iranzo A, Hu M, et al. Risk and predictors of dementia and parkinsonism in idiopathic REM sleep behaviour disorder: a multicentre study. *Brain*. 2019;142(3):744-759.

Winkelman JW, Wipper B, Purks J, Mei L, Schoerning L. Topiramate reduces nocturnal eating in sleep-related eating disorder. *Sleep*. 2020;43(9): zsaa060.

Drakatos P, Marples L, Muza R, et al. NREM parasomnias: a treatment approach based upon a retrospective case series of 512 patients. *Sleep Med*. 2019;53:181-188.

Frauscher B, Iranzo A, Gaig C, et al. Normative EMG values during REM sleep for the diagnosis of REM sleep behavior disorder. *Sleep*. 2012;35(6): 835-847.

Troester MM, Quan SF, Berry RB, et al. *The AASM Manual for the Scoring of Sleep and Associated Events: Rules, Terminology and Technical Specifications. Version* 3. Darien, IL: American Academy of Sleep Medicine; 2023.

Howell M, Avidan AY, Foldvary-Schaefer N, et al. Management of REM sleep behavior disorder: an American Academy of Sleep Medicine clinical practice guideline. *J Clin Sleep Med*. 2023;19(4):759-768.

REFERENCES

1. American Academy of Sleep Medicine. *International Classification of Sleep Disorder, 2nd ed: Diagnostic and Coding Manual*. Westchester, Illinois: American Academy of Sleep Medicine; 2005.
2. American Academy of Sleep Medicine. *International Classification of Sleep Disorders, 3rd ed, text revision*. Darien, IL: American Academy of Sleep Medicine; 2023.
3. Irfan M, Schenck CH, Howell MJ. NonREM disorders of arousal and related parasomnias: an updated review. *Neurotherapeutics*. 2021;18(1): 124-139.
4. Leung AKC, Leung AAM, Wong AHC, Hon KL. Sleep terrors: an updated review. *Curr Pediatr Rev*. 2020;16(3):176-182.
5. Kushida CA, Littner MR, Morgenthaler T, et al. Practice parameters for the indications for polysomnography and related procedures: an update for 2005. *Sleep*. 2005;28(4):499-521.
6. Aurora RN, Lamm CI, Zak RS, et al. Practice parameters for the non-respiratory indications for polysomnography and multiple sleep latency testing for children. *Sleep*. 2012;35(11):1467-1473.
7. Berry RB, Quan SF, Abreu AR, et al. *The AASM manual for the scoring of sleep and associated events: rules, terminology and technical specifications*. Version 2.6. Darien, IL: American Academy of Sleep Medicine; 2020.
8. Troester MM, Quan SF, Berry RB, et al. *The AASM manual for the scoring of sleep and associated events: rules, terminology and technical specifications*. Version 3. Darien, IL: American Academy of Sleep Medicine; 2023.

9. Muza R, Lawrence M, Drakatos P. The reality of sexsomnia. *Curr Opin Pulm Med.* 2016;22(6):576-582.
10. Schenck CH, Arnulf I, Mahowald MW. Sleep and sex: what can go wrong? A review of the literature on sleep related disorders and abnormal sexual behaviors and experiences. *Sleep.* 2007;30(6):683-702.
11. Schenck CH, Milner DM, Hurwitz TD, Bundlie SR, Mahowald MW. A polysomnographic and clinical report on sleep-related injury in 100 adult patients. *Am J Psychiatry.* 1989;146(9):1166-1173.
12. Schenck CH, Mahowald MW. On the reported association of psychopathology with sleep terrors in adults. *Sleep.* 2000;23(4):448-449.
13. Rocha AL, Arnulf I. NREM parasomnia as a dream enacting behavior. *Sleep Med.* 2020;75:103-105.
14. Uguccioni G, Golmard JL, de Fontréaux AN, et al. Fight of flight? Dream content during sleep walking/sleep terrors vs rapid eye movement sleep behavior disorder. *Sleep Med.* 2013;14(5):391-398.
15. Oudiette D, Leu S, Pottier M, Buzare MA, Brion A, Arnulf I. Dreamlike mentations during sleepwalking and sleep terrors in adults. *Sleep.* 2009; 32(12):1621-1627.
16. Petit D, Pennestri MH, Paquet J, et al. Childhood sleep walking and sleep terrors: a longitudinal study of prevalence and familial aggregation. *JAMA Pediatr.* 2015;169(7):653-658.
17. Wan H, Wang X, Chen Y, Jiang B, et al. Sleep-related hypermotor epilepsy: etiology, electro-clinical features, and therapeutic strategies. *Nat Sci Sleep.* 2021;3:2065-2084.
18. Pressman MR. Factors that predispose, prime and precipitate NREM parasomnias in adults: clinical and forensic implications. *Sleep Med Rev.* 2007;11(1):5-33.
19. Millman RP, Kipp GJ, Carskadon MA. Sleepwalking precipitated by treatment of sleep apnea with nasal CPAP. *Chest.* 1991;99;750-751.
20. Pressman MR, Meyer TJ, Kendrick-Mohamed J, et al. Night terrors in adults precipitated by sleep apnea. *Sleep.* 1995;18:773-775.
21. Howell MJ. Restless eating, restless legs, and sleep related eating disorder. *Curr Obes Rep.* 2014;3(1):108-113. doi: 10.1007/s13679-013-0083-6.
22. Howell MJ, Schenck CH. Restless nocturnal eating: a common feature of Willis-Ekbom syndrome (RLS). *J Clin Sleep Med.* 2012;8:413-419.
23. Brion A, Flamand M, Oudiette D, Voillery D, Golmard JL, Arnulf I. Sleep-related eating disorder versus sleepwalking: a controlled study. *Sleep Med.* 2012;13:1094-1101.
24. Stallman HM, Kohler M, White J. Medication induced sleepwalking: a systematic review. *Sleep Med Rev.* 2018;37:105-113.
25. Wallace DM, Maze T, Shafazand S. Sodium oxybate-induced sleep driving and sleep-related eating disorder. *J Clin Sleep Med.* 2011;7(3):310-311.
26. Landry P, Montplaisir J. Lithium-induced somnambulism. *Can J Psychiatry.* 1998;43(9):957-958.
27. Ferrándiz-Santos JA, Mataix-Sanjuan AL. Amitriptyline and somnambulism. *Ann Pharmacother.* 2000;34(10):1208.
28. Yeh YW, Chen CH, Feng HM, Wang SC, Kuo SC, Chen CK. New onset somnambulism associated with different dosage of mirtazapine: a case report. *Clin Neuropharmacol.* 2009;32(4):232-233.
29. Harbourt K, Nevo ON, Zhang R, Chan V, Croteau D. Association of eszopiclone, zaleplon, or zolpidem with complex sleep behaviors resulting in serious injuries, including death. *Pharmacoepidemiol Drug Saf.* 2020;29(6):684-691.
30. Guilleminault C, Kirisoglu C, Bao G, Arias V, Chan A, Li KK. Adult chronic sleepwalking and its treatment based on polysomnography. *Brain.* 2005;128(Pt 5):1062-1069.
31. Galbiati A, Rinaldi F, Giora E, Ferini-Strambi L, Marelli S. Behavioural and cognitive-behavioural treatments of parasomnias. *Behav Neurol.* 2015; 2015:786928.
32. Ntafouli M, Galbiati A, Gazea M, Bassetti CLA, Bargiotas P. Update on nonpharmacological interventions in parasomnias. *Postgrad Med.* 2020;132(1):72-79.
33. Frank NC, Spirito A, Stark L, Owens-Stively J. The use of scheduled awakenings to eliminate childhood sleepwalking. *J Pediatr Psychol.* 1997; 22(3):345-353.
34. Mundt JM, Baron KG. Integrative behavioral treatment for NREM parasomnias: a case series. *J Clin Sleep Med.* 2021;17(6):1313-1316.
35. Drakatos P, Marples L, Muza R, et al. NREM parasomnias: a treatment approach based upon a retrospective case series of 512 patients. *Sleep Med.* 2019;53:181-188.
36. Schenck CH, Mahowald MW. Long-term, nightly benzodiazepine treatment of injurious parasomnias and other disorders of disrupted nocturnal sleep in 170 adults. *Am J Med.* 1996;100(3):333-337.
37. Sasayama D, Washizuka S, Honda H. Effective treatment of night terrors and sleepwalking with ramelteon. *J Child Adolesc Psychopharmacol.* 2016; 26(10):948.
38. Vetrugno R, Manconi M, Ferini-Strambi L, Provini F, Plazzi G, Montagna P. Nocturnal eating: sleep-related eating disorder or night eating syndrome? A video-polysomnographic study. *Sleep.* 2006;29:949-954.
39. Vinai P, Ferri R, Ferini-Strambi L, et al. Defining the borders between sleep-related eating disorder and night eating syndrome. *Sleep Med.* 2012;13:686-690.
40. Schenck CH, Hurwitz TD, Bundlie SR, Mahowald MW. Sleep-related eating disorders: polysomnographic correlates of a heterogeneous syndrome distinct from daytime eating disorders. *Sleep.* 1991;14:419-431.
41. Howell MJ, Schenck CH, Crow SJ. A review of nighttime eating disorders. *Sleep Med Rev.* 2009;13:23-34.
42. Provini F, Antelmi E, Vignatelli L, et al. Association of restless legs syndrome with nocturnal eating: a case-control study. *Mov Disord.* 2009; 24(6):871-877.
43. Palaia V, Poli F, Pizza F, et al. Narcolepsy with cataplexy associated with nocturnal compulsive behaviors: a case-control study. *Sleep.* 2011;34(10): 1365-1371.
44. Morgenthaler TI, Silber MH. Amnestic sleep-related eating disorder associated with zolpidem. *Sleep Med.* 2002;3(4):323-327.
45. Tamanna S, Ullah MI, Pope CR, Holloman G, Koch CA. Quetiapine-induced sleep-related eating disorder-like behavior: a case series. *J Med Case Rep.* 2012;6(1):380.
46. Paquet V, Strul J, Servais L, Pelc I, Fossion P. Sleep-related eating disorder induced by olanzapine. *J Clin Psychiatry.* 2002;63(7):597.
47. Lu ML, Shen WW. Sleep-related eating disorder induced by risperidone. *J Clin Psychiatry.* 2004;65(2):273-274.
48. Howell MJ, Schenck CH. Treatment of nocturnal eating disorders. *Curr Treatment Options Neurol.* 2009;11:333-339.
49. Winkelman JW, Wipper B, Purks J, Mei L, Schoerning L. Topiramate reduces nocturnal eating in sleep-related eating disorder. *Sleep.* 2020;43(9): zsaa060.
50. Provini F, Albani R, Vetrugno R, et al. A pilot double-blind placebo-controlled trial of low-dose pramipexole in sleep-related eating disorder. *Eur J Neurol.* 2005;12:432-436.
51. O'Reardon JP, Allison KC, Martino NS, Lundgren JD, Heo M, Stunkard AJ. A randomized, placebo-controlled trial of sertraline in the treatment of night eating syndrome. *Am J Psychiatry.* 2006;163(5):893-898.
52. Varghese R, Rey de Castro J, Liendo C, Schenck CH. Two cases of sleep-related eating disorder responding promptly to low-dose sertraline therapy. *J Clin Sleep Med.* 2018;14(10):1805-1808.
53. Sabater L, Gaig C, Gelpi E, et al. A novel non-rapid-eye movement and rapid-eye-movement parasomnia with sleep breathing disorder associated with antibodies to IgLON5: a case series, characterization of the antigen, and post-mortem study. *Lancet Neurol.* 2014;13(6):575-586. Erratum in: *Lancet Neurol.* 2015;14(1):28.
54. Gaig C, Graus F, Compta Y, et al. Clinical manifestations of the anti-IgLON5 disease. *Neurology.* 2017;88(18):1736-1743.
55. Provini F, Plazzi G, Tinuper P, Vandi S, Lugaresi E, Montagna P. Nocturnal frontal lobe epilepsy. A clinical and polygraphic overview of 100 consecutive cases. *Brain.* 1999;122(Pt 6):1017-1031.
56. Provini F, Plazzi G, Lugaresi E. From nocturnal paroxysmal dystonia to nocturnal frontal lobe epilepsy. *Clin Neurophysiol.* 2000;111(suppl 2):S2-S8.
57. Schenck CH, Cramer Bornemann M, Kaplish N, Eiser AS. Sleep-related (psychogenic) dissociative disorders as parasomnias associated with a psychiatric disorder: update on reported cases. *J Clin Sleep Med.* 2021;17(4): 803-810.
58. Schenck CH, Bundlie SR, Patterson AL, et al. Rapid eye movement sleep behavior disorder: a treatable parasomnia affecting older males. *JAMA.* 1987;257:1786-1789.
59. Schenck CH, Mahowald MW. REM sleep behavior disorder: clinical, developmental, and neuroscience perspective 16 years after its formal identification in sleep. *Sleep.* 2002;25:120-138.
60. Högl B, Stefani A, Videnovic A. Idiopathic REM sleep behaviour disorder and neurodegeneration - an update. *Nat Rev Neurol.* 2018;14(1):40-55.
61. Boeve BF, Silber MH, Saper CB, et al. Pathophysiology of REM sleep behavior disorder and relevance to neurodegenerative disease. *Brain.* 2007;130:2770-2788.
62. Zhang F, Niu L, Liu X, et al. Rapid eye movement sleep behavior disorder and neurodegenerative diseases: an update. *Aging Dis.* 2020;11(2): 315-326.
63. Bodkin CL, Schenck CH. Rapid eye movement sleep behavior disorder in women: relevance to general and specialty medical practice. *J Womens Health (Larchmt).* 2009;18(12):1955-1963.
64. Postuma RB, Arnulf I, Hogl B, et al. A single-question screen for rapid eye movement sleep behavior disorder: a multicenter validation study. *Mov Disord.* 2012;27(7):913-916.

65. Boeve BF, Molano JR, Ferman TJ, et al. Validation of the Mayo Sleep Questionnaire to screen for REM sleep behavior disorder in a community-based sample. *J Clin Sleep Med.* 2013;9(5):475-480.
66. Stiasny-Kolster K, Mayer G, Schäfer S, Möller JC, Heinzel-Gutenbrunner M, Oertel WH. The REM sleep behavior disorder screening questionnaire—a new diagnostic instrument. *Mov Disord.* 2007;22(16):2386-2393.
67. Antelmi E, Pizza F, Franceschini C, Ferri R, Plazzi G. REM sleep behavior disorder in narcolepsy: a secondary form or an intrinsic feature? Sleep Med Rev. 2020;50:101254.
68. Hoque R, Chesson Jr AL. Pharmacologically induced/exacerbated restless legs syndrome, periodic limb movements of sleep, and REM behavior disorder/REM sleep without atonia: literature review, qualitative scoring, and comparative analysis. *J Clin Sleep Med.* 2010;6(1):79-83.
69. Winkleman JW, James L. Serotonergic antidepressants are associated with REM sleep without atonia. *Sleep.* 2004;27:317-321.
70. McCarter SJ, St Louis EK, Sandness DJ, et al. Antidepressants increase REM sleep muscle tone in patients with and without REM sleep behavior disorder. *Sleep.* 2015;38(6):907-917.
71. Morrison I, Frangulyan R, Riha RL. Beta-blockers as a cause of violent rapid eye movement sleep behavior disorder: a poorly recognized but common cause of violent parasomnias. *Am J Med.* 2011;124(1):e11.
72. Yeh SB, Yeh PY, Schenck CH. Rivastigmine-induced REM sleep behavior disorder (RBD) in a 88-year-old man with Alzheimer's disease. *J Clin Sleep Med.* 2010;6(2):192-195.
73. Tabata H, Kuriyama A, Yamao F, Kitaguchi H, Shindo K. Suvorexant-induced dream enactment behavior in Parkinson disease: a case report. *J Clin Sleep Med.* 2017;13(5):759-760.
74. Di Giacopo R, Fasano A, Quaranta D, Della Marca G, Bove F, Bentivoglio AR. Rivastigmine as alternative treatment for refractory REM behavior disorder in Parkinson's disease. *Mov Disord.* 2012;27(4):559-561.
75. Brunetti V, Losurdo A, Testani E, et al. Rivastigmine for refractory REM behavior disorder in mild cognitive impairment. *Curr Alzheimer Res.* 2014;11(3):267-273. doi:10.2174/1567205011666140302195648.
76. Schenck CH, Boeve BF, Mahowald MW. Delayed emergence of a Parkinsonian disorder or dementia in 81% of older males initially diagnosed with idiopathic REM sleep behavior disorder (RBD): 16 year update on a previously reported series. *Sleep Med.* 2013;14:744-748.
77. Postuma RB, Iranzo A, Hu M, et al. Risk and predictors of dementia and parkinsonism in idiopathic REM sleep behaviour disorder: a multicentre study. *Brain.* 2019;142(3):744-759.
78. Chan PC, Lee HH, Hong CT, Hu CJ, Wu D. REM sleep behavior disorder (RBD) in dementia with lewy bodies (DLB). *Behav Neurol.* 2018; 2018:9421098.
79. Stang CD, Mullan AF, Hajeb M, et al. Timeline of rapid eye movement sleep behavior disorder in overt alpha-synucleinopathies. *Ann Neurol.* 2021;89(2):293-303.
80. Howell MJ, Schenck CH. Rapid eye movement sleep behavior disorder and neurodegenerative disease. *JAMA Neurol.* 2015;72(6):707-712.
81. Montplaisir J, Gagnon JF, Fantini ML, et al. Polysomnographic diagnosis of idiopathic REM sleep behavior disorder. *Mov Disord.* 2010;25(13): 2044-2051.
82. Frauscher B, Iranzo A, Gaig C, et al. Normative EMG values during REM sleep for the diagnosis of REM sleep behavior disorder. *Sleep.* 2012;35(6):835-847.
83. McCarter SJ, St Louis EK, Duwell EJ, et al. Diagnostic thresholds for quantitative REM sleep phasic burst duration, phasic and tonic muscle activity, and REM atonia index in REM sleep behavior disorder with and without comorbid obstructive sleep apnea. *Sleep.* 2014;37(10):1649-1662.
84. Feemster JC, Jung Y, Timm PC, et al. Normative and isolated rapid eye movement sleep without atonia in adults without REM sleep behavior disorder. *Sleep.* 2019;42(10):zsz124.
85. Gaig C, Iranzo A, Pujol M, Perez H, Santamaria J. Periodic limb movements during sleep mimicking REM sleep behavior disorder: a new form of periodic limb movement disorder. *Sleep.* 2017;40(3). doi:10.1093/sleep/zsw063.
86. Barone DA. Dream enactment behavior-a real nightmare: a review of post-traumatic stress disorder, REM sleep behavior disorder, and trauma-associated sleep disorder. *J Clin Sleep Med.* 2020;16(11):1943-1948.
87. Iranzo A, Santamaria J. Severe obstructive sleep apnea/hypopnea mimicking REM sleep behavior disorder. *Sleep.* 2005;28:203-206.
88. Schenck CH, Boyd JL, Mahowald MW. A parasomnia overlap disorder involving sleepwalking, sleep terrors, and REM sleep behavior disorder in 33 polysomnographically confirmed cases. *Sleep.* 1997;20(11):972-981.
89. Dumitrascu O, Schenck CH, Applebee G, Attarian H. Parasomnia overlap disorder: a distinct pathophysiologic entity or a variant of rapid eye movement sleep behavior disorder? A case series. *Sleep Med.* 2013;14(11): 1217-1220.
90. Schenck CH. REM sleep behavior disorder as a complex condition with heterogeneous underlying disorders: clinical management and prognostic implications [Commentary]. *Sleep Breath.* 2022;26(3):1289-1298. doi:10.1007/s11325-022-02574-6.
91. Lloyd R, Tippmann-Peikert M, Slocumb N, Kotagal S. Characteristics of REM sleep behavior disorder in childhood. *J Clin Sleep Med.* 2012;8(2):127-131.
92. Nevsimalova S, Prihodova I, Kemlink D, Lin L, Mignot E. REM behavior disorder (RBD) can be one of the first symptoms of childhood narcolepsy. *Sleep Med.* 2007;8(7-8):784-786.
93. Bin-Hasan S, Videnovic A, Maski K. Nocturnal REM sleep without atonia is a diagnostic biomarker of pediatric narcolepsy. *J Clin Sleep Med.* 2018;14(2):245-252.
94. Antelmi E, Filardi M, Pizza F, et al. REM sleep behavior disorder in children with type 1 narcolepsy treated with sodium oxybate. *Neurology.* 2021;96(2):e250-e254.
95. Aurora RN, Zak RS, Maganti RK, et al. Standards of Practice Committee; American Academy of Sleep Medicine. Best practice guide for the treatment of REM sleep behavior disorder (RBD). *J Clin Sleep Med.* 2010;6(1):85-95. Erratum in: J Clin Sleep Med. 2010;6(2): table of contents.
96. Howell M, Avidan AY, Foldvary-Schaefer N, et al. Management of REM sleep behavior disorder: an American Academy of Sleep Medicine clinical practice guideline. *J Clin Sleep Med.* 2023;19(4): 759-768.
97. Arnaldi D, Latimier A, Leu-Semenescu S, et al. Loss of REM sleep features across nighttime in REM sleep behavior disorder. *Sleep Med.* 2016;17:134–137.
98. McGrane IR, Leung JG, St Louis EK, Boeve BF. Melatonin therapy for REM sleep behavior disorder: a critical review of evidence. *Sleep Med.* 2015;16(1):19-26.
99. Howell MJ, Arneson PA, Schenck CH. A novel therapy for REM sleep behavior disorder (RBD). *J Clin Sleep Med.* 2011;7(6):639-644A.
100. Stefani A, Högl B. Nightmare disorder and isolated sleep paralysis. *Neurotherapeutics.* 2021;18(1):100-106.
101. Hintze JP, Gault D. Escitalopram for recurrent isolated sleep paralysis. *J Sleep Res.* 2020;29(6):e13027.
102. Pagel JF, Helfter P. Drug induced nightmares—an etiology based review. *Hum Psychopharmacol.* 2003;18(1):59-67.
103. Natter J, Yokoyama T, Michel B. Relative frequency of drug-induced sleep disorders for 32 antidepressants in a large set of Internet user reviews. *Sleep.* 2021;44(12):zsab174.
104. Aurora RN, Zak RS, Auerbach SH, et al. Best practice guide for the treatment of nightmare disorder in adults. *J Clin Sleep Med.* 2010;6(4): 389-401.
105. Morgenthaler TI, Auerbach S, Casey KR, et al. Position paper for the treatment of nightmare disorder in adults: an American Academy of Sleep Medicine Position Paper. *J Clin Sleep Med.* 2018;14(6):1041-1055.
106. Gieselmann A, Ait Aoudia M, Carr M, et al. Aetiology and treatment of nightmare disorder: state of the art and future perspectives. *J Sleep Res.* 2019;28(4):e12820.
107. Krakow B, Hollifield M, Johnston L, et al. Imagery rehearsal therapy for chronic nightmares in sexual assault survivors with post-traumatic stress disorder. *JAMA.* 2001;286:537-545.
108. Harb GC, Cook JM, Phelps AJ, et al. Randomized controlled trial of imagery rehearsal for posttraumatic nightmares in combat veterans. *J Clin Sleep Med.* 2019;15(5):757-767.
109. Raskind MA, Peskind ER, Hoff DJ, et al. A parallel group placebo-controlled study of prazosin for trauma nightmares and sleep disturbance in combat veterans with post-traumatic stress disorder. *Biol Psychiatry.* 2007;61:928-934.
110. Raskind MA, Peskind ER, Chow B, et al. Trial of prazosin for post-traumatic stress disorder in military veterans. *N Engl J Med.* 2018;378(6): 507-517.
111. Sharpless BA, Denis D, Perach R, French CC, Gregory AM. Exploding head syndrome: clinical features, theories about etiology, and prevention strategies in a large international sample. *Sleep Med.* 2020;75: 251-255.
112. Liang JF, Wang SJ. Hypnic headache: a review of clinical features, therapeutic options and outcomes. *Cephalalgia.* 2014;34(10):795-805. doi:10.1177/0333102414537914.
113. Singh NN, Sahota P. Sleep-related headache and its management. *Curr Treat Options Neurol.* 2013;15(6):704-722.
114. Komagamine T, Suzuki K, Kokubun N, et al. Sleep-related hallucinations in patients with Parkinson's disease. *PLoS One.* 2022;17(10): e0276736.

115. Silber MH, Hansen MR, Girish M. Complex nocturnal visual hallucinations. *Sleep Med.* 2005;6(4):363-366.
116. American Academy of Sleep Medicine. *International Classification of Sleep Disorders, 3rd ed.* Darien, IL: American Academy of Sleep Medicine; 2014.
117. Nevéus T, von Gontard A, Hoebeke P, et al. The standardization of terminology of lower urinary tract function in children and adolescents: report from the Standardisation Committee of the International Children's Continence Society. *J Urol.* 2006;176(1):314–324.
118. Shafiek H, Evangelisti M, Abd-Elwahab NH, Barreto M, Villa MP, Mahmoud MI. Obstructive sleep apnea in school-aged children presented with nocturnal enuresis. *Lung.* 2020;198(1):187-194.
119. Robson WL. Clinical practice. Evaluation and management of enuresis. *N Engl J Med.* 2009;360(14):1429-1436.
120. Vetrugno R, Provini F, Plazzi G, Vignatelli L, Lugaresi E, Montagna P. Catathrenia (nocturnal groaning): a new type of parasomnia. *Neurology.* 2001;56:681-683.
121. Ramar K, Olson EJ, Morgenthaler TI. Catathrenia. *Sleep Med.* 2008;9: 457-459.
122. Abbasi AA, Morgenthaler TI, Slocumb NL, et al. Nocturnal moaning and groaning-catathrenia or nocturnal vocalizations. *Sleep Breath.* 2012;16: 367-373.
123. Poli F, Ricotta L, Vandi S, et al. Catathrenia under sodium oxybate in narcolepsy with cataplexy. *Sleep Breath.* 2012;16(2):427-434.
124. Siddiqui F, Walters AS, Chokroverty S. Catathrenia: a rare parasomnia which may mimic central sleep apnea on polysomnogram. *Sleep Med.* 2008;9:460-461.
125. Iriarte J, Alegre M, Urrestarazu E, et al. Continuous positive airway pressure as treatment for catathrenia (nocturnal groaning). *Neurology.* 2006;66:609-610.
126. Songu M, Yilmaz H, Uucetruk AV, et al. Effect of CPAP therapy on catathrenia and OSA: a case report and review of the literature. *Sleep Breath.* 2008;12:401-405.

Chapter 37

Psychiatry and Sleep

INTRODUCTION

Psychiatric disorders are among the most common health problems, with 15% to 20% of Americans being treated for a significant psychiatric illness in any given year.[1-5] Anxiety disorders, followed by mood disorders, are the most common. Almost one-third of individuals with significant complaints of insomnia or hypersomnia show evidence of psychiatric disorders.[2-5] Major depression is a very common disorder, with a lifetime prevalence of 29.9% and a prevalence of 8.6% in the last 12 months in American adults[4] and an increased risk (odds ratio 1.7) in women.[3] Psychiatric disorders account for the largest diagnostic category for patients with sleep complaints.[1-6] Conversely, sleep complaints are a part of the diagnostic criteria for many psychiatric disorders[5] and are a source of considerable morbidity. The psychiatric disorders commonly affecting sleep (or vice versa) are listed in Box 37–1.

MOOD DISORDERS AND MOOD EPISODES

Anxiety disorders and mood disorders (including depressive disorders and bipolar disorders, Box 37–2) are the first and second most common categories of psychiatric disorders, respectively, according to national surveys. The Diagnostic and Statistical Manual of Mental Disorders, 5th edition (DSM-V) has separate chapters for depressive disorders and bipolar disorders (Box 37–2).[5] The major mood disorders include major depressive disorder (MDD) and bipolar I (BP-I) and bipolar II (BP-II) disorders. These disorders are diagnosed based on **mood episodes**. The DSM-V has diagnostic criteria for major depressive episodes (MDEs), manic episodes (MEs), and hypomanic episodes (HMEs). The mixed episode defined in the DSM-IV is not present in the DSM-V. The time duration criteria for the episodes includes 2 weeks for MDEs, 1 week for MEs (or any duration requiring hospitalization), and 4 consecutive days for HMEs. Each of the mood episodes, including their diagnostic criteria, will be discussed below.

Box 37–1 PSYCHIATRIC DISORDERS COMMONLY AFFECTING SLEEP

Mood Disorders

- Major depressive disorder
- Bipolar Disorder I (BP-I)
- Bipolar Disorder II (BP-II)

Anxiety Disorders

- Panic disorder
- General anxiety disorder
- Posttraumatic stress disorder

Box 37–2 MOOD DISORDERS

Depressive Disorders

- Disruptive mood dysregulation disorder (DMDD)
- Major depressive disorder (MDD) – Unipolar depression
- Persistent depressive disorder (Dysthymia) (PDD)
- Premenstrual dysphoric disorder
- Substance/medication induced depressive disorder
- Depressive disorder due to another medical condition
- Other specified depressive disorder

Bipolar Disorders

- Bipolar Disorder I (BP-I)
- Bipolar Disorder II (BP-II)
- Cyclothymic disorder

DEPRESSIVE DISORDERS

The depressive disorders to be discussed in this chapter include major depresssive disorder (MDD), also known as unipolar depression, disruptive mood dysregulation disorder (DMDD) diagnosed in children, and persistent depressive disorder (PDD). DMDD was added in the DSM-V to describe a mood disturbance in childhood (temper outbursts and irritability) to avoid overdiagnosis of bipolar disorder in this age group. Most children with the symptoms characterized by DMDD either have resolution of symptoms or develop MDD or an anxiety disorder rather than bipolar disorder as they mature. PDD (also known as dysthymia) combines dysthymia with elements of a major depressive episode (MDE) to describe patients with long-lasting depressive symptoms (somewhat milder than those of MDEs) without remission.[5] PDD may evolve into MDD, prompting patients to seek medical attention. The DSM-V includes two new specifiers for depressive disorders and bipolar disorders. Now, the specifier "with mixed symptoms" allows for the presence of hypomanic and manic symptoms as part of depressive episodes in patients who do not meet the criteria for HMEs/MEs. "With anxious distress" has also been added as a specifier because the presence of anxiety may impact treatment choices and the patient's response.

Diagnosing a Mood Disorder and Useful Questionnaires

Patients do not come to sleep clinics for help with mental health issues but rather with complaints about sleep. The challenge for sleep physicians is to determine whether there is a mental health disorder that needs diagnosis and treatment before sleep can improve. Some patients are already on treatment for depression or anxiety, but sometimes the *treatment is not completely effective* (persistent depression). Collaboration with the primary physician and/or psychiatrist is important. In addition, sometimes the type of depression is not specified, and the medications may be a clue that bipolar disorder is being treated. In some circumstances, a sleep physician may start an antidepressant if there is no active

Box 37–3 IMPORTANT HISTORICAL ELEMENTS FOR DIAGNOSIS OF MOOD DISORDERS

A. Historical elements common to all mood disorders
- Family history of depression, bipolar disorders (mental breakdowns), hospitalization for mental issues, suicide
- Current or past medications for mood disorders
- Sleep disturbance – hypersomnia, insomnia, decreased need for sleep

B. Historical elements for diagnosis of depression
- SIGECAPS for symptoms of depression
  - Sleep (**insomnia or hypersomnia**)
  - Interest
  - Guilt
  - Energy (decreased)
  - Concentration (difficulty concentrating)
  - Appetite
  - Psychomotor retardation
  - Suicidality

C. Symptoms Common to Both Manic and Hypomanic Episodes
- Grandiosity, inflated self esteem
- **Decreased need for sleep** (well-rested on 3 hours of sleep)
- Pressure to keep talking, more talkative than usual
- Flight of ideas, thoughts racing
- Easily distracted (especially to irrelevant stimuli)
- Increased goal directed activity (school, work, school, sexuality) or psychomotor agitation
- Involvement in high risk activities (buying sprees, sexual affairs, foolish business investments)

D. Important Differences Manic Episodes (ME) versus Hypomanic Episodes (HME)
- HME do NOT cause severe impairment , hospitalization, and have no psychotic feasture
- ME cause severe impairment (including hospitalization) and can include psychotic features

primary care physician involvement or suggest psychiatric referral. A general knowledge of the medications used to treat depression is very useful.

Important historical elements useful for recognizing the presence of a mood disorder are listed in Box 37–3. Because of the stigma of having a mental health disorder, patients may not accept the fact that a disorder is present. Simply asking if they are depressed often results in a false negative response. Patients, particularly men, will say they just feel tired or "blah" rather than sad or down. Exploring the *absence of positive feelings is helpful.* A key diagnostic sign of depression is difficulty feeling pleasure. "Are you able to enjoy things that should make you feel good?" Patients may manifest signs of excess negative emotion – easily upset, frustrated, anxious, worried, guilty, worthless. The pneumonic SIGECAPS (Sleep, Interest, Guilt, Energy, Concentration, Appetite, Psychomotor retardation/agitation, Suicidality) is useful for eliciting symptoms consistent with depression. *Psychomotor retardation* is the slowing down or hampering of mental or physical activities. Manifestations include slow thinking, slow speech, or slow body movements. Obtaining a family history is very important. *Genetic factors account for 33% of the risk of major depression and more than 85% of the risk of bipolar disorder.*[7,8]

The major characteristics of a MDE are listed here (see the DSM-V for complete diagnostic criteria). It is important to remember that *MDEs can occur with MDD, BP-I, and BP-II disorders.*

Essential diagnostic criteria for Major Depressive Episode (MDE) [5]:

- ≥5 of the 9 symptoms listed below during the same 2-week period Symptoms must include either depressed mood or loss of interest of pleasure.
- Symptoms:
  - Depressed mood
  - Markedly diminished interest or pleasure
  - Weight loss (not dieting), weight gain, or loss or increase in appetite nearly every day
  - **Insomnia or hypersomnia (nearly every day)**
  - Psychomotor agitation or retardation (observable)
  - Fatigue or loss of energy
  - Feelings of worthlessness or guilt (excessive, inappropriate)
  - Diminished ability to think or concentrate
  - Recurrent thoughts of death
- Symptoms cause impairment

Because MDEs can occur with BP-I or BP-II (MDEs can be the first manifestation of a bipolar disorder), it is important to screen for a history of past HMEs or MEs and a family history of bipolar disorder. Bipolar disorders are highly heritable. Because there is an increased risk of suicide in patients with bipolar disorder, it is important to ask about a family history of attempted or completed suicide.

The major characteristics of a ME are listed here (see the DSM-V for complete diagnostic criteria).

Essential diagnostic criteria for a Manic Episode (ME)[5]:

- A distinct period of **abnormally and persistently elevated, expansive, or irritable mood** and abnormal/persistent goal-directed behavior or energy
- **Duration of at least 1 week** (or any duration if hospitalization is necessary).
- ≥3 of the following symptoms (≥4 if mood is only irritable):
  - Grandiosity, inflated self esteem
  - Decreased need for sleep (well-rested on 3 hours of sleep)
  - Pressure to keep talking, more talkative than usual
  - Flight of ideas/thoughts racing
  - Easily distracted (especially to unimportant or irrelevant stimuli)
  - Increased goal-directed activity (social, work, school, sexual) or psychomotor agitation
  - Involvement in high-risk activities (buying sprees, sexual affairs, foolish business investments)
- Mood disturbance causes marked impairment or hospitalization (harm to self or others), psychotic features

Typical questions to screen for prior MEs include: "Have you needed hospitalization for an emotional problem ('mental breakdown')?" "Have you ever been on medicines such as Lithium, Depakote, Lamictal, Seroquel?" These medicines are commonly used for the treatment of bipolar disorders. "Did you have a period when you felt rested on only 3 hours of sleep?" MEs cause severe impairment and can result in a divorce, a patient being fired, or catastrophic financial loss. Typical questions to ask are, "Have you had a period of great energy, extended partying, uncharacteristic sexual episodes with undesirable consequences, buying sprees, or a decreased need for sleep? If you had one of these periods, how long did it last?" MEs must last for at least a week or any duration requiring hospitalization.

Some major aspects of diagnostic criteria for a hypomanic episode (HME). See DSM-V for full diagnostic criteria[5]:

- A distinct period of abnormally and persistently elevated, expansive, or irritable mood and abnormally and persistently increased activity or energy lasting **at least 4 consecutive days** and present most of the day, nearly every day.
- During the period of mood disturbance and increased energy and activity, three (or more) of the following symptoms (four if the mood is only irritable) have persisted, represent a noticeable change from usual behavior, and have been present to a significant degree. These symptoms include grandiosity, decreased need for sleep, pressure to keep talking (more talkative than usual), flight of ideas, easily distracted, increased goal directed activity, and involvement in high-risk activities. The symptoms are the same seven manifestations included in the diagnostic criteria for a ME.
- The episode is associated with an unequivocal change in functioning that is uncharacteristic of the individual when not symptomatic.
- The disturbance in mood and the change in functioning are observable by others.
- The episode is **NOT** severe enough to cause marked impairment in social or occupational functioning or to necessitate hospitalization. If there are psychotic features, the episode is, by definition, manic.

A HME must only be present for 4 consecutive days to meet criteria. Asking about HMEs is more difficult than asking about mania, as patients may actually be more productive. The change in mood must be observable by others, and the episode must represent a noticeable change from prior behavior. HMEs do not cause marked impairment, have psychotic features, or result in hospitalization. Because a diagnosis of BP-II *requires at least one HME and one MDE*, it is important to inquire about both periods of great energy and periods of depression. A summary of the mood episodes required for a diagnosis of MDD, BP-I, and BP-II is presented in Table 37–1.

Screening for a history of MEs or HMEs in a patient with depression is important. It is not uncommon for a patient to be diagnosed with MDD (unipolar depression) when in fact they are exhibiting a MDE and have BP-I or BP-II (that is, they have bipolar depression). The medications used to treat bipolar depression are often different than those used to treat unipolar depression. In addition, treatment of a patient with bipolar depression with an antidepressant can precipitate a ME.

A number of depression scales are available for use by the sleep clinician to help evaluate patients for possible depression or measure improvements with treatment. The Beck Depression Inventory was mentioned in Chapter 33 on insomnia.[9] The Hamilton Depression Scale (HAMD) is a 17-, 21-, or 24-question instrument that is widely used for research.[10] The Montgomery-Åsberg Depression Rating Scale (MADRS) is a 10-item diagnostic questionnaire used to measure the severity of depressive episodes in patients.[11] It was developed to be sensitive to the changes brought on by antidepressants and other forms of treatment. The Patient Health Questionnaire (PHQ-9) is a short 9-question instrument[12] that the patient can quickly fill out and is easy to use. The PHQ-9 has been validated and may be used to screen patients with sleep disorders for depression. A shorter screening version, the PHQ-2, has also been validated (Table 37–2).[13]

Major Depressive Disorder

The diagnostic criteria for MDD require at least one MDE meeting criteria with a duration of at least 2 weeks (current or prior). The symptoms are associated with the presence of significant distress or impairment, the disorder is not attributable to schizophrenia or other psychotic disorder, and *there has never been a ME or HME* (not attributable to a substance or

Table 37–1 Mood Disorders and Associated Episodes

Major Depressive Disorder	• **At least one major depressive episode** (current or prior) • **No history of manic or hypomanic episodes** • Symptoms cause significant distress or impairment • Disorder not attributable to schizophrenia or psychotic disorder
Bipolar I Disorder	• **At least one manic episode** (current or prior) • Major depressive episodes, hypomanic episodes **may occur** (usually present) • In manic episodes, the disturbance is sufficiently *severe to cause marked impairment* in occupational function or usual social activities or relationships with others or to *necessitate hospitalization to prevent harm to self or others* or there are *psychotic features*
Bipolar II Disorder	• At least **one hypomanic and one major depressive episode** (current or prior) • **No manic episodes** • The symptoms of depression or unpredictability caused by frequent alternation between periods of depression and hypomania cause clinically *significant distress or impairment in social, occupational, or other import areas of functioning.*
Minimum Duration of Mood Episodes	
Major Depressive Episode	2 weeks
Manic Episode	1 week or any duration requiring hospitalization
Hypomanic Episode	4 consecutive days

Table 37–2 Patient Health Questionnaires (PHQ2, PHQ9)

PHQ-2

1. During the past 2 weeks, have you often been bothered by little interest or pleasure in doing things? (☐ Yes ☐ No)
2. During the past 2 weeks, have you often been bothered by feeling down, depressed, or hopeless? (☐ Yes ☐ No)

If the answer to both questions is no, the screen is negative for depression (rescreen if indicated). If yes was selected for one or both questions, please consult appropriate discipline to complete the PHQ-9.

PHQ-9

Question: Over the last 2 weeks, how often have you been bothered by any of the following problems? (Use "✓" to indicate your answer)	Not at all	Several days	More than half the days	Every day
1. Little interest or pleasure in doing things	0	1	2	3
2. Feeling down, depressed, or hopeless	0	1	2	3
3. Trouble falling or staying asleep, or sleeping too much	0	1	2	3
4. Feeling tired or having little energy	0	1	2	3
5. Poor appetite or overeating	0	1	2	3
6. Feeling bad about yourself — or that you are a failure	0	1	2	3
7. Trouble concentrating on things, such as reading	0	1	2	3
8. Moving or speaking so slowly that other people could have noticed; or the opposite — being so fidgety or restless that you have been moving around a lot more than usual	0	1	2	3
9. Thoughts that you would be better off dead or of hurting yourself in some way	0	1	2	3

Total Score 0-27
0-4 minimal depression
5-9 mild
10-14 moderate
15-19 moderately severe
20-27 severe

If you checked any box, how difficult did these problems make it for you to do your work, take care of things at home, or get along with other people?
( ) not difficult at all ( ) somewhat difficult ( ) very difficult ( ) extremely difficult

Developed by Drs. Robert L. Spitzer, Janet B.W. Williams, Kurt Kroenke, and colleagues, with an educational grant from Pfizer Inc. No permission was required to reproduce, translate, display, or distribute this information.

medical condition). As mentioned, MDD is also known as unipolar depression. The MDE requires five or more of the nine symptoms listed in the diagnostic criteria for a MDE during the **same 2-week period** and representing a **change from previous functioning**; at least one of the symptoms is (1) depressed mood or (2) loss of interest or pleasure (DSM-V).[5] A MDE can occur with bipolar disorders. *Note that insomnia or hypersomnia nearly every day is one of the symptoms of depression.*

Specifiers for Depressive Disorders

The reader is referred to the DSM-V for a complete list of specifiers and a detailed discussion of each specifier. Here, specifiers most relevant to sleep physicians will be discussed. There are severity/time course specifiers for MDD, including (not a complete list) severity (mild, moderate, severe), presence of psychotic features, in partial remission (symptoms of depression still present but does not meet depressive episode criteria), or in full remission (at least 2 months after previous episode without significant signs or symptoms of depression). There are symptom type specifiers: "with anxious distress," "with mixed features," "with melancholic features," "with atypical features," "with mood-congruent psychotic features (delusions and hallucinations consistent with depression)," "with mood incongruent psychotic features (delusions and hallucination not consistent with depression)," and "with catatonic features". The specifiers have clinical importance, as they may affect the choice of treatment. A few of the specifiers most relevant for sleep physicians will be discussed in more detail here.

"With melancholic features" requires one the following: loss of pleasure in most all activities or lack of reactivity to pleasurable stimuli. In addition, ≥3 of the following should be present: profound despondency, worse depression in the morning, *early morning awakening* (at least 2 hours before regular awakening), psychomotor agitation or retardation, anorexia or weight loss, and excessive/inappropriate guilt (Table 37–3). The "with atypical features" specifier requires that the patient exhibit mood reactivity (mood brightens in response to positive events) and two or more of the following: weight gain or increase in appetite, hypersomnia, leaden paralysis (feeling arms and legs are weighted down), and interpersonal rejection sensitivity (fear of negative social evaluation resulting in social or occupational impairment).

Unipolar depressive episodes more commonly have melancholic features (insomnia features, especially early morning

Table 37–3 Melancholic or Atypical Features of Major Depressive Episodes

Melancholic Features	Atypical Features
A. One or more of the following are present during the most severe period: 1. Loss of pleasure 2. Lack of mood reactivity B. Three or more of the following: 1. Depressed mood with despondency, despair, moroseness, or empty mood 2. Worsened in the morning 3. Early morning awakening 4. Marked psychomotor agitation or retardation 5. Significant anorexia or weight loss 6. Excessive or inappropriate feelings of guilt	A. Mood reactivity must be present (Can be better or even normal in social situations) B. Two or more of the following: 1. Significant weight gain or increase in appetite 2. Hypersomnia 3. Leaden fatigue 4. Rejection sensitivity – fear of negative social evaluation resulting in social or occupational impairment

awakening), while bipolar depressive episodes are more likely to have atypical features.

"With mixed features" is specified when at least three of the following hypomanic/manic symptoms are present: elevated expansive mood, inflated self-esteem, pressure to speak, flight of ideas, and increased energy or goal-directed activity (social, work, sexual).

"With seasonal pattern" applies to patients with recurrent MDD in which there is a regular relationship between season and onset of the depressive episode (often fall or winter).

Box 37–4 SLEEP AND MAJOR DEPRESSIVE EPISODES

Symptoms

- 80% to 90% have sleep complaints
- 60% to 80% of those with sleep complaints report insomnia
  - Difficulty falling asleep or staying asleep
  - Early-morning awakening
  - Frequent awakening
- 15% to 20% of those with sleep complaints report hypersomnia (More likely with bipolar, seasonal, and atypical depression)
- Sleep abnormalities may precede a major depressive episode or persist after remission of the episode
- Persistent sleep abnormalities may be associated with a risk of recurrence (some but not all studies)

Polysomnography Findings

A. Major depressive episode with insomnia
- Prolonged sleep latency
- Decreased total sleep time
- Increased wake, early-morning awakening, frequent awakenings
- Decreased stage N3, decreased N3 in the early part of the night
- REM abnormalities
  - Short REM latency
  - Increased REM density
  - Increased REM early in the night
  - Increased REM (% total sleep time)

B. Major depressive episode with hypersomnia
- Increased total sleep time or time in bed
- Short REM latency
- Multiple sleep latency test, if performed, does ***not*** usually demonstrate severe objective sleepiness, even if hypersomnia is the complaint

Depression and Sleep

Depression and sleep have a bidirectional relationship, with depression affecting sleep quality and the presence of insomnia associated with an increased risk of developing depression; when insomnia is present in a patient with depression, it tends to perpetuate the depression. The effects of a MDE (or MDD) on sleep are summarized in Box 37–4. A sleep complaint (insomnia or hypersomnia) is one of the primary diagnostic criteria for a MDE. About 80% to 90% of patients with depression have some type of sleep complaint.[13-18] Insomnia is the most common sleep complaint and is estimated to occur in about 75% of adult patients with depression. It is believed that about 15% to 20% complain of hypersomnia. The complaint may depend on age and gender. Nutt et al. found that about three-quarters of patients with depression have insomnia symptoms, and hypersomnia is present in about 40% of young adults with depression and 10% of older patients with depression, with a preponderance in women.[16] The insomnia complaints include early-morning awakening and frequent awakenings. It is important to rule out obstructive sleep apnea in a patient with depression and hypersomnia, as up to 20% of patients with depression have some type of sleep apnea (although only roughly half report hypersomnia).

Polysomnography (PSG) findings in those with MDEs (Box 37–4)[17-21] include a prolonged sleep latency, increased wakefulness after sleep onset, decreased stage N3 sleep, and rapid eye movement (REM; stage R) abnormalities. The stage R abnormalities include a short REM latency, an increased length of the first REM episode, and increased REM density in the early part of the night. Recall that REM density (number of REMs per time) is typically low during the first REM episodes. However, the findings are neither sensitive nor specific enough for PSG to be used to diagnose depression.[21] PSG abnormalities or symptoms of insomnia may persist after remission of depression.[19-21] Rush and coworkers[19] found a short REM latency (< 65 minutes) in 11 of 13 patients during active depression; of those 11 patients, a short REM latency persisted in 8 after clinical remission. Some studies have suggested that the persistence of sleep disturbance during remission from depression is predictive of relapse.[21,22] Dombrovski and colleagues[23] found that anxiety and possibly residual sleep disturbance (as determined by PSQI) predicted early recurrence while assessment of depression (Hamilton Depression Rating scale, HAM-D) did not. In addition, insomnia is the most common residual complaint in patients who have recovered from depression.[22,24] However, Yang and associates[25] did not find that persistent sleep disturbance predicted recurrence. Patients having a response to fluoxetine during an open-label study received placebo or fluoxetine during withdrawal. Sleep components of the HAM-D group were used to determine whether residual sleep complaints correlated with an increased chance of relapse. No sleep complaint was associated with a higher rate of relapse of depression. However, a more specific sleep questionnaire such as that used by Dombrovski and coworkers[23] may have demonstrated an association between a sleep complaint and relapse of depression.

Even if patients with MDD complain of hypersomnia, the multiple sleep latency test (MSLT) does not usually reveal severe sleepiness or sleep-onset REM periods.[26] The differential diagnosis of sleep disturbance in MDD includes chronic insomnia disorder (psychophysiologic insomnia) or inadequate sleep hygiene. If hypersomnia complaints are prominent, one should consider obstructive sleep apnea, narcolepsy, or insufficient sleep.

Depression and insomnia appear to have a reciprocal relationship, as insomnia frequently precedes the onset of depression and has been found to be predictive of future depressive episodes in some studies. Individuals with persistent insomnia have been found to be 4 to 10 times more likely to subsequently develop depression than those with short-term insomnia or no insomnia.[27] Pigeon et al.[28] found that patients with depression and persistent insomnia on treatment are 1.8 to 3.5 times more likely to remain depressed than patients with no insomnia. That is, insomnia is a perpetuating factor in depression. Of interest, sleep deprivation or restriction has been found to have an *acute antidepressant effect* on patients with unipolar depression.[29-31] With recovery sleep, 50% to 80% of patients have a relapse. As noted, sleep loss can also precipitate mania in some patients.[32]

Persistent Depressive Disorder

PDD represents a consolidation of DSM-IV–defined chronic MDD and dysthymic disorder. The disorder describes the course of individuals with persistent symptoms of a depressed mood for most of the day, for more days than not, for at least 2 years. Depressed mood and two or more of the following symptoms should be present: poor appetite or overeating, insomnia or hypersomnia, low energy or fatigue, low self-esteem, poor concentration or difficulty making decisions, and feelings of hopelessness.

Note that, in MDEs, at least four symptoms must present. In PDD, symptoms may be milder (loss of appetite rather than weight loss). Depressive symptoms can be present continuously, or there may be brief periods of absent symptoms; however, these periods must be less than 2 months in duration. There is no history of HMEs or MEs, criteria have never been met for cyclothymic disorder, the symptoms are not better explained by a psychotic disorder, there must be significant impairment, and the symptoms are not caused by a substance/medication or medical disorder.

Disruptive Mood Dysregulation Disorder (DMDD)

As noted, this is a new diagnosis in the DSM-V.[5] The diagnosis should not be made before 6 years of age or after 18 years of age. Symptoms should have been present before age 10. Manifestations include severe temper outbursts, physical aggression, and irritable mood between outbursts. The new diagnosis was added to avoid diagnosing bipolar disorder in children. As they mature, most individuals will develop either unipolar depression or an anxiety disorder.

BIPOLAR DISORDERS

The bipolar disorders include BP-I, BP-II, cyclothymia, substance/medication induced bipolar and related disorders, and bipolar and related disorders caused by another medical condition. Bipolar disorders affect 1% to 3% of the population, have a chronic course with periods of relapse and remission, and are associated with premature mortality.[33] The typical age of onset of bipolar disorders is between 15 and 30 years, although the bipolar nature of the disorder may not be recognized for several years. *It is estimated that about 40% of individuals with a bipolar disorder are initially diagnosed with unipolar depression.* In the United States the lifetime prevalence of BP-I and BP-II is each estimated to be about 1% (2% combined) with men and women equally affected. However, the degree of impairment is estimated to be **severe** in about 80% of the affected individuals.

BP-I and BP-II Diagnostic Criteria

The diagnostic criteria for BP-I are summarized in Table 37–1 (see the DSM-V for complete diagnostic criteria[5]). Criteria must be met for at least one ME (current or previous), and the ME cannot be better explained by a psychotic disorder or ingestion of a substance or medication. *MDEs or HMEs may be present before or after the defining ME.* While most patients with BP-I have repeated manic and depressive episodes, *the presence or history of a MDE is not required to diagnose BP-I* (Figure 37–1).

The essential diagnostic criteria for BP-II are summarized in Table 37–1. At least one HME and one MDE must be present. There is no history of a ME (or the diagnosis would be BP-I). The diagnosis of the HMEs and MDEs is not better explained by a psychotic disorder or a substance/medication. For BP-II, an additional requirement is *one of impairment.* "The symptoms of depression or unpredictability caused by frequent alternation between periods of depression and hypomania causes clinically *significant distress or impairment in social, occupational, or other important areas of functioning.*" This additional criterion is not needed for BP-I, as *impairment* is present in the definition of a ME.

	Major depressive disorder	Bipolar I	Bipolar II
Manic episode	None	At least one	None
Hypomanic episode	None	Often occurs	At least one
Major depressive episode	At least one	Often occurs	At least one

Figure 37–1 A summary of requirements for diagnosis of major depressive disorder, bipolar I disorder, and bipolar II disorder with respect to occurrence of mood episodes. For major depressive disorder, there must be at least one major depressive episode and no manic or hypomanic episodes. For bipolar I, there must be at least one manic episode. However, hypomanic and depressive episodes often occur. In bipolar II, there must be at least one hypomanic episode and one major depressive episode. There can be no manic episodes.

Characteristics of Mood Episodes in Bipolar Disorders

This section will describe details and characteristics of the three episodes describing bipolar disorders. Some of the information on ME and HME is repeated for emphasis. Note that MDE, ME, and HME can all occur in BP-I, but only MDE and HME in BP-II. While the same diagnostic criteria for MDEs apply for bipolar disorders, some characteristics of depression unique to bipolar disorders are present.

Manic Episodes

MEs are distinct periods of abnormally and persistently elevated, expansive, or irritable mood, **lasting at least 1 week** (or any duration if hospitalization is necessary). Three of the core symptoms must be present. If the mood is only irritable, four of the core symptoms must be present. The core symptoms include: 1. Grandiosity, inflated self esteem, 2. Decreased need for sleep (well-rested on 3 hours of sleep), 3. Pressure to keep talking, more talkative than usual, 4. Flight of ideas, thoughts racing, 5. Easily distracted (especially to irrelevant stimuli), 6. Increased goal directed activity (school, work, sexuality) or psychomotor agitation, and 7. Involvement in high risk activities (buying sprees, sexual affairs, foolish business investments).

In MEs, the disturbance is sufficiently *severe to cause marked impairment* in occupational function or usual social activities or relationships with others or to *necessitate hospitalization to prevent harm to self or others*, or there are *psychotic features*. Note that symptoms in MEs are essentially the same for HMEs, but the manifestations are more severe in MEs.

Hypomanic Episodes

A HME is a distinct period of persistently elevated, expansive, or irritable mood, lasting at **least 4 consecutive days**, that is clearly different from the usual nondepressed mood.[5] During the period of mood disturbance, three (or more) of the symptoms listed in the previous information on hypomanic episodes (four if the mood is only irritable) are present to a significant degree. HMEs are associated with an *unequivocal change in functioning that is uncharacteristic of the person when not symptomatic.* Of note, the disturbance in mood and change in functioning are observable by others. Although the HME criteria are similar to those of MEs, an important feature that differentiates hypomania from mania is that hypomania is *not severe enough to cause marked impairment, does not require hospitalization,* and there are ***no** psychotic features* (such as delusions or hallucinations). Diagnosis of *a HME requires a consecutive 4-day duration, whereas a ME requires symptoms for a week (or any duration with hospitalization).* Patients with BP-I commonly have hypomanic episodes as well as manic episodes, and a diagnosis may be changed from BP-II to BP-I if a patient previously diagnosed with BP-II (no prior manic episode) develops a manic episode.

Bipolar Depression (MDE in patients with Bipolar Disorders)

Non-psychiatrists are well aware of manic or hypomanic episodes in patients with bipolar disorder. However, the time spent in major depressive episodes is usually much greater than that spent in manic or hypomanic episodes over the lifetime course of the disease, and major depressive episodes are the greatest cause of morbidity and mortality (associated with a high rate of suicide).[33,34] Patients with bipolar disorder have a *20% to 30% higher lifetime risk of suicide* than the normal population, and most suicides occur during depressive phases of the disease. About 4% to 19% of patients with bipolar disorder will complete suicide, while 20% to 60% will make at least one attempt in their lifetime. The bipolar disorders are also associated with high rates of alcoholism or other substance abuse disorders. A diagnosis of major depressive disorder (unipolar depression) is sometimes made in a patient who actually has a bipolar disorder if the first episode is a major depressive episode rather than a manic or hypomanic episode. Treatment with typical antidepressants used for unipolar depression can precipitate mania or hypomania.[35-38] It is important to question patients carefully about prior symptoms consistent with mania or hypomania before antidepressant treatment is started. There are no pathognomonic characteristics of bipolar depression compared to those of unipolar depression. Table 37–4 presents characteristics that are more probable in each category.[39]

Effects of Bipolar Depression, Mania, and Hypomania on Sleep

Hypersomnia complaints are typical of *bipolar depression* and are associated with increased total sleep time, increased time in bed, and a short REM latency. MEs are associated with marked insomnia, but the patient awakens refreshed after a few hours of sleep (Box 37–5). PSG findings include reduced stage N3, a short REM latency, and increased REM density.[40,41] The fact that sleep loss can precipitate mania[32] is an important reason to treat insomnia associated with bipolar depression or hypomania. In hypomania, a complaint of insomnia (mainly short sleep duration) or decreased need for sleep is common. In general, patients with hypomania report similar sleep symptoms as those with mania but with less severity and less distress. In fact, patients may enjoy having more energy and the lower sleep requirement.

Specifiers in Bipolar Disorders

Specifiers for bipolar disorders include (incomplete list): "with anxious distress," "manic or hypomanic episodes with mixed features," "depressive episode (MDE in a bipolar patient) with mixed features," "with rapid cycling," "with melancholic features (MDE in a bipolar patient)," and "with atypical features (MDE in a bipolar patient)." The "with melancholic features" and "with atypical features" are similar to those discussed in the section on MDD. "With *atypical features*" applies to MDEs in patients with bipolar disorder associated with mood reactivity (mood improves with positive events), hypersomnia, significant weight gain, and rejection sensitivity. The "with melancholic features" in a patient with bipolar depression

Table 37–4 Manifestations of Patients With Bipolar and Unipolar Depression

Bipolar I Depression More Likely	Unipolar Depression More Likely
Hypersomnia	Prominent insomnia
Hyperphagia	Reduced appetite, weight loss
Psychomotor retardation	Normal activity levels
Earlier age of onset of first episode	Later age of onset of first episode
Psychotic features (pathologic guilt)	Somatic complaints
Lability of mood	No family history of bipolar disorder
Family history of bipolar disorder	

Mitchell PB, Goodwin GM, Johnson GF, Hirschfeld RMA. Diagnostic guidelines for bipolar depression: a probabilistic approach. *Bipolar Disord.* 2008;10:144-152.

Box 37–5 MANIC/HYPOMANIC EPISODES AND SLEEP*

Manic Episodes

- Marked insomnia
- Refreshed with only a few hours of sleep
- Polysomnography findings:
  - Reduced stage N3
  - Short REM latency
  - Increased REM density
- Sleep loss can trigger mania.

Hypomanic Episodes

- Report of decreased need for sleep
- Polysomnography findings similar to those in mania may occur.

* Depressive episodes in BP disorders are often associated with complaints of hypersomnia

characterizes a MDE with loss of pleasure in almost all activities, marked psychomotor retardation, depression worse in the morning, early-morning awakening, anorexia or weight loss, and feelings of guilt. "With anxious distress" describes patients who are tense, restless, have difficulty concentrating, and fear they may lose control. Patients who experience at least four episodes (MDE, ME, or HME) during a 12-month period are classified as **rapid cycling**.[5] "With mixed features" can apply to a ME or HME associated with depressive symptoms or a MDE with hypomanic/manic features. The seasonal specifier describes MDEs that can occur with MDD, BP-I, or BP-II. The MDEs have a seasonal pattern; these patients may have depression that begins and ends during a specific season every year (with full remittance during other seasons) for at least 2 years and may have more seasons of depression than seasons without depression over a lifetime. Seasonal pattern disorders occur most frequently in winter, although they can also occur in summer. This circumstance is also known as *seasonal affective disorder*. The "with catatonia" specifier can apply to MEs or MDEs with symptoms that can include not responding to anything, not being able and/or willing to talk, rigid muscles, repeating what someone just said, grimacing, moving around with no purpose, and resisting movement. The psychotic features include delusions or hallucinations characteristic (congruent) or not characteristic (incongruent) of the current episode.

The reader is referred to the DSM-V for a complete discussion.

Episodes in Bipolar I and II and Bipolar Disorder Prognosis

The major difference between BP-I and BP-II is that at least one lifetime ME (current or previous) is required for BP-I (duration 1 week or shorter with hospitalization). No MDE is required. In contrast, BP-II must include at least one HME (minimum duration 4 consecutive days) and one MDE. No MEs (prior or current) is also required for a diagnosis of BP-II. It should be emphasized that patients with BP-I can have HMEs as well as MEs and usually have frequent MDEs, which can occur before or after the defining ME. In BP-II, a MDE episode may also precede the qualifying HME. As noted, if a ME occurs in a patient with a previous diagnosis of BP-II, the diagnosis is changed to BP-I.

It is important to appreciate that it is the MDEs in the bipolar disorders rather than the HMEs and MEs that cause the most morbidity. Examples of time courses of MDD, BP-I, and BP-II are shown in schematic form in Figure 37–2. Approximately 60% to 70% of the HMEs that occur in patients with BP-II occur immediately before or after a MDE, with characteristic patterns that are unique to each individual. Depressive episodes last about 3 months, while episodes of mania typically last 1.5 months. In Figure 37–3, the duration of episodes (until recovery) is shown. It is obvious that depressive episodes are longer than MEs and HMEs are shorter than MEs. In BP-I, episodes of depression are very disabling. Most patients with BP-I have repeated MDEs as well as MEs. The increased risk of suicide during MDEs in patients with BP is worth a second mention. Treatment of depression in patients with bipolar disorder with typical antidepressants can send the patient into mania unless they are on a mood stabilizer (anti-manic medication). Treatment of depression in bipolar disorder requires an entirely different approach. Of interest, pregnancy is an important risk factor for relapse in bipolar disorders. *The presence of postpartum depression should alert the clinician to the possibility of the presence of a bipolar disorder*. In summary, in most patients with BP-I and all patients with BP-II, the depression is by far the most disabling part of the disorder.

Even with good care, the long-term prognosis of patients with bipolar disorders is uncertain. The suboptimal effectiveness of

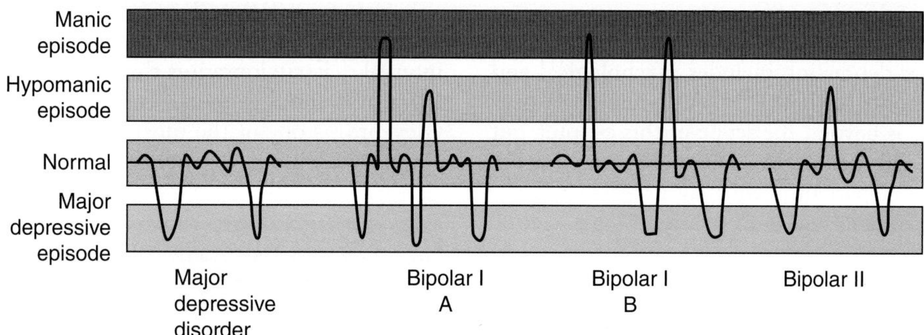

Figure 37–2 Schematic graphs show the time course of major depressive disorder with two examples of bipolar I and one example of bipolar II. For bipolar I, there must be at least one manic episode. However, hypomanic episodes and major depressive episodes commonly occur. Note that, in example A of bipolar I, the first episode of mania followed a major depressive episode. In example B of bipolar I, the time spent in depression was greater than that in mania. In bipolar II, there is one episode of hypomania following an initial major depressive episode. The time in depressive episodes is greater than the time in hypomania.

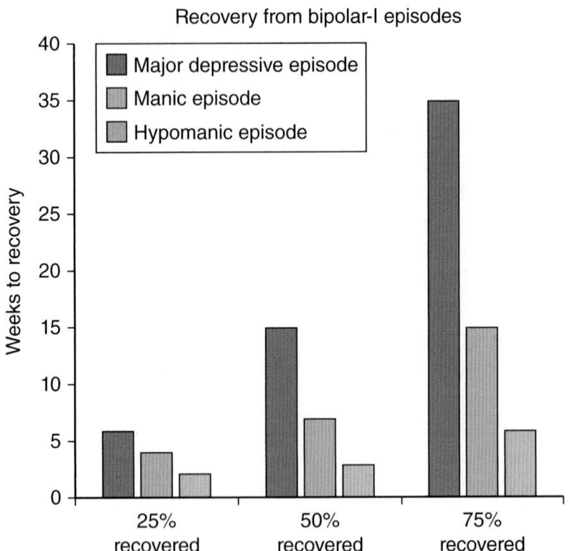

Figure 37–3 Time to recovery of various types of episodes in bipolar-I disorder. The time for 25%, 50%, and 75% of episodes to recover is shown. (Data plotted from Solomon DA, Leon AC, Coryell WH, et al. Longitudinal course of bipolar I disorder: duration of mood episodes. *Arch Gen Psychiatry.* 2010;67(4):339-347.PMID: 20368510.)

treatments for bipolar disorders is underscored by evidence indicating the relapse rate for individuals who recover from first-episode mania is approximately 40% to 60% within 1 to 2 years.[42-44] *As previously noted recurrent MDSs often follow episodes of mania or hypomania.* While some patients achieve long-term remission, many others have repeated episodes. *A clinical course composed of frequent MDEs is associated with a greater time being ill, while one characterized by mainly MEs is associated with frequent hospitalizations.*

Cyclothymic Disorder

This disorder describes periods of both hypomanic and depressive symptoms over a 2-year period that do not meet criteria for HMEs or MDEs. The symptoms have been present for most of the 2-year period, with no more than 2 months without symptoms. There is also **no history** of a period meeting criteria for a HME or MDE.[5]

TREATMENT OF UNIPOLAR DEPRESSION

Treatment of unipolar depression includes psychological and pharmacologic treatments (or both).[45,46] A discussion of psychological treatments is beyond the scope of this chapter, but these interventions may be preferred in mild to moderate depression and in older patients who may experience more side effects and drug interactions with pharmacologic agents.

Antidepressants

Many antidepressants are available.[45-65] Often, the choice is based on side effects, drug interactions, cost, and which symptoms are most prominent (anxiety, fatigue).[45-49] Individual patients may respond to different medications if treatment with an initial antidepressant is not successful. It is important to obtain a thorough drug history. *If a patient previously responded to a medication, he or she is likely to have a good response again* (Box 37–6).

Monoamine oxidase inhibitors (MAOIs) are very effective as antidepressants (increase both serotonin and norepinephrine signaling) but are rarely used because of their side effects and the need for dietary restrictions to avoid a hypertensive crisis. Use of selective serotonin reuptake inhibitors (SSRIs) is contraindicated in combination with MAOIs. The MAOIs approved by the U.S. Food and Drug Administration (FDA) for depression are selegiline (patch), phenelzine, tranylcypromine, and isocarboxazid. They are very effective for treatment refractory depression and atypical depression. If changing from an SSRI to a MAOI, the SSRI should be tapered over 2 to 4 weeks and then stopped for at least 2 weeks (longer with fluoxetine) before starting the MAOI. If stopping an MAOI and switching to an SSRI, a similar process is needed, with 2 weeks off the MAOI before starting the SSRI.[50-52]

The tricyclic antidepressants (TCAs) block the reuptake of serotonin (5HT) and norepinephrine (NE) and are effective treatments for depression.[53,54] However, the TCAs are not selective in the blockade of 5HT and NE receptors and are associated with prominent anticholinergic side effects (constipation, dry mouth). They are also lethal in overdose (Table 37–5). They may be more effective for melancholic depression and severe or refractory depression. In some meta-analysis, amitriptyline, and imipramine were among the most effective antidepressants. Amitriptyline, imipramine, and doxepin are more sedating and likely to cause weight gain compared to desipramine and nortriptyline, which are often better tolerated.

The SSRIs are safer in overdose than the TCAs and in general have fewer side effects than the TCAs (Table 37–6). Note that some SSRIs are FDA approved for disorders other than MDD, although others can be used off-label for many of these disorders. The efficacy of all SSRIs for depression is fairly similar, but they vary considerably in half-life, side effects, and drug interactions. One study evaluated 12 newer antidepressants for efficacy and tolerability.[48] Escitalopram and sertraline had the best combination of efficacy and tolerability, but some other antidepressants were more effective. A similar study of 21 antidepressants found that amitriptyline, escitalopram, mirtazapine, venlafaxine, and vortioxetine were among the most effective antidepressants. Citalopram, escitalopram, fluoxetine, sertraline, and vortioxetine were among those better tolerated.[49] The SSRIs can cause either daytime sedation or insomnia. If they cause insomnia, they should be given in the morning. If they cause sedation, they should be given at bedtime. SSRIs may also have prominent sexual side effects or result in weight gain in some patients. *They can promote hyponatremia, especially in the elderly.*[55] Some antidepressants can increase the QT interval.[56] Escitalopram is the S stereoisomer of racemic citalopram (R and S isomers). There is evidence that escitalopram (Lexapro) is one of the most effective and well tolerated and is now available as a generic medication.[49,57] Escitalopram is

Box 37–6 CHOOSING AN ANTIDEPRESSANT

- Which symptoms are most troubling? (anxiety, fatigue, depressed mood, lack of energy)
- History of a previous response or non-response to antidepressants
- Side effects (sexual, weight gain)
- History of previous side effects
- Type of depression (melancholic, atypical)
- Family history of response to medication

Table 37–5 Tricyclic Antidepressants

Advantages

- More effective for melancholic depression than SSRIs
- More effective than SSRIs for severe, refractory depression
- Equally effective for atypical depression
- Both serotonin and norepinephrine reuptake inhibitor actions
- Some sedating TCAs can be used in low doses for sleep (amitriptyline, doxepin, imipramine)
- Some TCAs useful for pain, neuropathy, migraine prophylaxis (nortriptyline)

Disadvantages

- Lethal in overdose
- Can increased QT interval
- Block multiple receptors
- Histamine (weight gain, sedation)
- Muscarinic (anticholinergic side effects like dry mouth and constipation)
- Alpha-1 adrenergic receptors (postural hypotension)
- Not first-line treatments for depression

Receptor Affinity for Selected Tricyclic Antidepressants (FDA approved for treatment of depression)

Drug	Amine type	NET	SERT	Ach	Histamine	Alpha 1
Amitriptyline (Elavil)	Tertiary	+	++	+++	+++	+++
Doxepin (Sinequan)	Tertiary	+	+	+++	++++	++
Imipramine (Tofranil)	Tertiary	+	++	+++	+++	+++
Desipramine (Norpramin)	Secondary	+++	+	+	+	++
Nortriptyline (Pamelor)	Secondary	++	+	+	+	+

Drug	Comments
Amitriptyline	Sedating, very effective for depression, used in fibromyalgia (often at low doses)
Doxepin	Sedating (used in low doses for insomnia)
Imipramine	Sedating, very effective for depression, used for enuresis
Desipramine	More NE activity, used for ADHD, fewer side effects
Nortriptyline	More NE activity, *used for pain and fibromyalgia, fewer side effects*

Ach, acetylcholine (muscarinic); *ADHD*, attention deficit hyperactive disorder; *Alpha-1*, alpha-1 adrenergic; *FDA*, U.S. Food and Drug Administration; *NE*, norepinephrine; *NET*, norepinephrine transporter; *SERT*, serotonin transporter; *SSRI*, selective serotonin reuptake inhibitor.

From Plattner A, Dantz B. The tricyclics: more than just antidepressants. *Psychiatric Annals.* 2011:41(3);159-165; Schneider J, Patterson M, Jimenez XF. Beyond depression: other uses for tricyclic antidepressants. *Cleve Clin J Med.* 2019;86(12):807-814. doi: 10.3949/ccjm.86a.19005. PMID: 31821138.

among the most selective of the SSRIs, without significant affinity for muscarinic, dopamine, or norepinephrine receptors. Escitalopram has fewer drug interactions than many other antidepressants (low potential to affect hepatic cytochrome 450 enzymes) *but can be associated with withdrawal symptoms (gradually discontinue)*. Concerns about QT prolongation limit the maximum dose to 20 mg. As generic escitalopram is now available, use of the racemic form (citalopram) has decreased. Citalopram may be less effective than escitalopram and has more side effects. Citalopram (at high doses, especially in combination with medications such as modafinil) can cause QT prolongation. Sertraline is an effective medication available as a generic that also has relatively few drug interactions and is generally well tolerated (some weight gain). As it has some dopaminergic effect it is activating and has advantages in treatment of depression with melacholic features. Sertraline is FDA approved for treatment of posttraumatic stress disorder (PTSD) as well as depression and is often used for PTSD treatment. It is also approved for *premenstrual dysphoric disorder*. Fluoxetine has a long half-life and is good for patients who skip doses or experience SSRI withdrawal symptoms on other medications. Fluoxetine is FDA approved for MDD and a wide range of other disorders (Table 37–6). It can be associated with significant sexual side effects. Paroxetine is the most potent SSRI but has a high rate of side effects including withdrawal, weight gain, and sedation. It has anti-anxiety benefits and is FDA approved for MDD as well as several other conditions.

Of note, the sexual side effects of SSRIs include erectile dysfunction, delayed ejaculation, or difficulty reaching orgasm. These side effects may respond to the phosphodiesterase-5 inhibitors (PDE5-I) including sildenafil (Viagra) or tadalafil (Cialis).[60] Although most studies have been performed in men, the medications can also be useful in women who have difficulty becoming sexually aroused or having an orgasm. Both men and women with sexual side effects on an SSRI may benefit from adding bupropion to their treatment. This medication has been found to counter SSRI-induced sexual dysfunction, boost sexual drive and arousal, and increase the intensity or duration of an orgasm.[61] In some people, the anti-anxiety drug buspirone (BuSpar) may help increase libido and restore the ability to have an orgasm.[62]

The serotonin/norepinephrine reuptake inhibitors (SNRIs) approved for MDD are listed in Table 37–7. The drugs have

Table 37–6 Selective Serotonin Reuptake Inhibitors

Advantages
- Safe in overdose
- Effective for both anxiety and depression
- Effective in comorbid panic disorder, GAD, OCD, SAD

Disadvantages
- Sexual side effects
- Some weight gain
- Withdrawal symptoms in some
- Hyponatremia in the elderly

Commonly Used SSRIs

Escitalopram (Lexapro)
- Good first choice, some withdrawal symptoms
- Highest response rate in some meta-analysis
- Favorable side effect profile/low drug interactions
- FDA approved for MDD, GAD (acute Rx)

Sertraline (Zoloft)
- High response rate, activating, some dopaminergic effect
- Well tolerated (some weight gain), few drug interactions
- Effective in premenstrual dysphoric disorder (PMDD)
- FDA approved for MDD, OCD, PD, PTSD, PMDD

Fluoxetine (Prozac)
- In addition to SSRI effects, weak norepinephrine reuptake inhibition, antagonist at $5HT_{2C}$ receptors which may explain increases in NE and dopamine in prefrontal cortex
- Long half-life, can be used for SNRI withdrawal, good for patients who miss doses
- Less potent, significant sexual side effects
- FDA approved for MDD, acute and maintenance treatment of OCD, acute treatment of Panic Disorder with or without agoraphobia. The medication combined with olanzapine is approved for acute depressive episodes associated with bipolar I disorder and treatment-resistant depression.

Paroxetine (Paxil)
- Most potent
- High rate of side effects including withdrawal, weight gain, sedation
- Anti-anxiety benefits
- FDA approved for MDD, OCD, PD, Social anxiety disorder (SAD), GAD, PTSD

Citalopram (Celexa)
- Racemic of escitalopram; escitalopram generally preferred
- Can increase QT interval in high doses
- FDA approved for MDD

GAD, generalized anxiety disorder; *MDD*, major depressive disorder; *OCD*, obsessive compulsive disorder; *PD*, panic disorder; *PMDD*, premenstrual dysphoric disorder; *PTSD*, posttraumatic stress disorder; *SAD*, social anxiety disorder; *SNRI*, selective norepinephrine reuptake inhibitors; *SSRI*, selective serotonin reuptake inhibitors.

mainly serotonin reuptake activity at lower doses and more norepinephrine reuptake activity at higher doses.[58] When a patient does not respond to an SSRI, an SNRI is often effective. Milnacipran (Savella) is a SNRI but is only approved for treatment of fibromyalgia. All of the SNRI medications can increase heart rate and blood pressure. Venlafaxine can have significant withdrawal side effects, and the XR preparation is almost always used. The medication is useful when there is comorbid anxiety and also in patients with hot flashes. Desvenlafaxine is a metabolite of venlafaxine *available as an extended-release preparation.* It has *less withdrawal, sexual, and weight-gain side effects than venlafaxine.*

Table 37–7 Serotonin/Norepinephrine Reuptake Inhibitors

Venlafaxine (Effexor)
- XR formulation preferred
- Significant withdrawal side effects
- Good for comorbid anxiety, hot flashes
- Can increase blood pressure and heart rate
- FDA approved for MDD, GAD, SAD, and Panic Disorder (PD)

Desvenlafaxine (Pristiq)
- A metabolite of venlafaxine, available in extended release capsules
- Minimal withdrawal, less weight gain and sexual side effects than venlafaxine
- Can increase blood pressure and heart rate
- FDA approved for MDD

Duloxetine (Cymbalta)
- Possibly best all-around SNRI
- Good side effect profile
- Good for pain
- FDA approved for MDD, GAD, fibromyalgia, chronic pain, diabetic neuropathy

GAD, generalized anxiety disorder; *MDD*, major depressive disorder; *PD*, panic disorder; *SAD*, social anxiety disorder; *SNRI*, selective norepinephrine reuptake inhibitors.

Duloxetine may have the best combination of potency and fewer side effects of the SNRIs, has a good side effect profile, and is *effective for pain.*

Several other antidepressants are often characterized as atypical (Table 37–8). Bupropion is a unique medication with norepinephrine and dopamine uptake blocking effects. It has fewer sexual side effects than SSRIs, and weight gain is not a problem. It must be taken two or three times a day unless used in the extended-release form (Wellbutrin XL). *It should not be used in patients with a seizure disorder.* Although some reviews suggest the medication should be avoided in patients with comorbid anxiety, other studies have found bupropion to be effective in patients with depression and anxiety.[58,59] Another option would be to use a *combination of an SSRI and bupropion* in a patient with both anxiety and the need for an activating antidepressant. Patients with emotional blunting ("feeling blah") on an SSRI may improve with addition of bupropion. Mirtazapine is a unique medication that blocks histamine 1 receptors, central alpha 2 receptors, and some serotonin receptors ($5HT_2$, $5HT_3$). In low doses (7.5–15 mg), mirtazapine is sedating and can be used for insomnia. The typical effective antidepressant dose is 30 to 45 mg. Mirtazapine, like bupropion, is less likely to cause sexual side effects *but can cause significant weight gain.* Mirtazapine may help patients with anxiety. Blockade of the $5HT_2$ receptors may improve sleep quality.[58] Mirtazapine is one of the most *effective antidepressants and has a rapid onset of action.* It is the *most likely of all antidepressants to worsen the restless legs syndrome.* Trazodone is included here, but it is rarely used as an antidepressant because of significant sedation. The medication is classified as an SARI ($5HT_2$ antagonist/serotonin reuptake inhibitor). Trazodone potently blocks serotonin 2A receptors ($5HT_{2A}$) and is a less-potent inhibitor of serotonin reuptake. Its antihistamine activity is responsible for its sedative effects, although $5HT_{2A}$ blockade may be beneficial for sleep and trazodone can increase stage N3 sleep. Priapism, a long-lasting painful erection, occurs in about 1/8000 males. The medication can prolong the QT interval and can cause postural hypotension (some blockage of alpha-1

Table 37–8 Other Antidepressants

Bupropion (Wellbutrin) • Need to use XL to avoid multiple doses • Possibly less effective in depression (especially if anxiety) • Best side effect profile (no weight gain, lower sexual side effects), *good second choice for initial treatment* • Increases NE and dopamine (noradrenergic reuptake inhibitor, mild dopaminergic effect)
Mirtazapine (Remeron) • Central alpha-2 receptor antagonist, blocks $5HT_2$, $5HT_3$, histamine receptors • Possibly antidepressant with quickest action, increases 5HT1 stimulation, NE • Good for anxiety, one of the most effective (more than SSRIs) • Minimal anticholinergic side effects • Good for patients with insomnia • *Significant sedation (antihistamine activity) and weight gain*
Trazodone (Desyrel – brand name no longer available in United States; generic available) • SARI (serotonin antagonist and reuptake inhibitor), $5HT_{2A}$ antagonist, weak SSRI, sedation due to antihistamine activity • Very sedating, used as hypnotic 25 to 100 mg • Can increase QT interval, postural hypotension (alpha-1 blockade) • Priapism in 1/8000 cases (painful persistent erection)
Vilazodone (Viiybryd) • Serotonin reuptake inhibitor and $5HT_{1A}$ partial agonist • Has SSRI and antianxiety activity • Low rate of sexual dysfunction • Can cause nausea and diarrhea • Now available as generic
Vortioxetine (Trintellix, formerly Brintellix) • Novel mechanism of action, SSRI, $5HT_{1A}$ agonist, $5HT_{1B}$ partial agonist, antagonist of $5HT_{1D}$, $5HT_3$, $5HT_7$ receptors • **Nausea can be severe** • Long half-life (no withdrawal syndrome) • May work when other antidepressants have not been effective • No generic formulation, more expensive

NE, norepinephrine; *SNRI*, selective norepinephrine reuptake inhibitors; *SSRI*, selective serotonin reuptake inhibitors. Generic formulations of bupropion, mirtazapine, trazodone, vilazodone are available. Vortioxetine available as brand name only.

adrenergic receptors). Its lack of anticholinergic properties make it more attractive as a hypnotic in low doses compared to sedating tricyclic antidepressants. Trazodone is one of the most frequently used medications for insomnia (usually in doses of 25 to 100 mg). Antidepressant doses are typically 150 to 300 mg.

Two newer medications include vilazodone (Viiybryd) and vortioxetine (Trintellix). Of the two medications, only vilazodone is currently available as a generic medication. Patients not responding to older antidepressants may respond to one of these. Vilazodone[63] is both an SSRI and partial $5HT_{1A}$ agonist. The medication has a *low rate of sexual dysfunction* but can cause nausea and diarrhea. Vortioxetine[64,65] has a novel mechanism of action at multiple receptors in addition to SSRI activity (Table 37–8). The medication has a long half-life and *may work when no other medication has been effective*. However, it is associated with very severe nausea in many individuals.

An approach for choosing an antidepressant for treatment of unipolar depression is listed in Table 37–9. If the patient has prominent melancholic versus atypical features, different

Table 37–9 Approach for Unipolar Depression Treatment: *General Approach*

Step 1 Escitalopram (Lexapro) • Highest response rate in some meta-analyses • Favorable side effect profile and few drug interactions • Some withdrawal can occur OR Bupropion XL • Possibly less effective than SSRIs, activating • Best side effects profile – no weight gain and minimal sexual side effects OR Sertraline (Zoloft) • Fluoxetine (Prozac) - less likely to cause weight gain, prominent sexual side effects, long half life - no withdrawal • Effective, activating, well tolerated, relatively few drug interactions OR Other SSRIs: citalopram, paroxetine (sedating may be helpful in anxiety)
Step 2 Venlafaxine, desvenlafaxine (fewer issues than venlafaxine), or duloxetine (good for pain)
Step 3 Combination of SNRI and SSRI – OR – Bupropion and SSRI – OR – SNRI and mirtazapine Mirtazapine – very effective, use if insomnia prominent, weight gain an issue Consider psychiatric referral
Step 4 Consider psychiatric referral Vortioxetine Vilazodone Augmentation* of previous medication with SGA (Abilify) Consider other augmentation*
Melancholic Features TCA classic treatment: many side effects, lethal in overdose Try Bupropion XL, SNRIs, mirtazapine (may help appetite and sleep) Augmentation* based on symptoms; consider modafinil, armodafinil
Atypical Features Monoamine oxidase inhibitors classic treatment – many issues, cannot use with SSRIs SSRI + augmentation* usually needed (bupropion XL, aripiprazole, modafinil, armodafinil, or traditional stimulants). Some references state sertraline may be the best SSRI for depression with atypical features.

SGA, second generation antipsychotic; *SNRI*, serotonin norepinephrine reuptake inhibitor; *SSRI*, selective serotonin reuptake inhibitor; *TCA*, tricyclic antidepressant. *Augmentation refers to the addition of a second agent to an existing antidepressant regimen with the aim of achieving improved clinical response. Bupropion and mitrazapine are sometimes used for augmentation with SSRIs. The SGAs aripiprazole, brexpiprazole, cariprazine, and quetiapine XR are FDA approved for augmentation and have demonstrated consistent efficacy when used as augmentation to SSRIs/SNRIs for major depressive disorder. Risperidone, olanzapine may also be effective. The combination of fluoxetine and olanzapine (Symbax) is FDA approved for resistance major depression and depression associated with BP-I
See also reference for CANMAT algorithms[47].

medications may be considered for initial treatment. If the patient does not respond to the recommended target dose of the initial medication or the medication is not tolerated, a trial of another medication in the same class or starting a medication in another class are options. The addition of another agent (augmentation) could be considered. Note that *serotonin syndrome* (agitation, tachycardia, hyperthermia) can rarely occur when two medications blocking serotonin reuptake are used together. The goal of treatment is remission not just improvement. It is estimated that 30-40% of patients on an antidepressant still have significant depression after treatment with an adequate dose and duration of treatment. Changing to another medication, adding a medication for augmentation, or psychiatric referral are indicated.

Patients with severe or refractory depression may benefit from the addition of augmenting medications.[66-71] A detailed discussion of the use of second-generation antipsychotics (SGAs)[68,69] (e.g., quetiapine, aripiprazole) or alerting agents (modafinil)[71] for augmentation of treatment of depression is beyond the scope of this chapter. However, the reader should be aware that such medications are being used for this purpose. Aripiprazole (Abilify) is FDA approved for adjunctive therapy of major depression. This medication tends to cause less metabolic side effects (weight gain) than other SGAs. Quetiapine XR (Seroquel XR) is approved as both an adjunctive medication[69,70] and a single-agent treatment for depression.[72] Brexpiprazole (Rexulti) is an SGA approved for depression augmentation[73] (as well as treatment of schizophrenia). The medication is a dopamine D_2 receptor partial agonist and has been described as a "serotonin–dopamine activity modulator." Like aripiprazole, it causes less weight gain than quetiapine and others and possibly less akathisia and extrapyramidal symptoms than aripiprazole, but no head-to-head comparisons have been performed. Both are FDA approved for treatment of schizophrenia and as adjunctive treatments of major depression.

Effects of Antidepressants on Sleep

A discussion of the effects of antidepressants on sleep (Table 37–10) is complicated by the fact that the results can vary depending on whether normal or depressed individuals are studied. The acute and chronic effects may also vary.[74-76] The literature is somewhat conflicting on the effects of some medications. In general, antidepressants increase the REM latency and

Table 37–10 Effects of Antidepressants on Sleep

	Continuity	Stage N3	REM	REM Latency	Sedation
TCAs					
Amitriptyline	↑↑↑	↑	↓↓↓	↑	++++
Doxepin	↑↑↑	↑↑↑	↓↓	↑	+++
Imipramine	↑↔	↑	↓↓	↑	++
Nortriptyline	↑	↑	↓↓	↑	++
Desipramine	↔	↑	↓↓	↑	+
Clomipramine	↑↔	↑	↓↓↓↓	↑	↔
MAOIs					
Phenelzine	↓	↔	↓↓↓↓	↑↑↑↑	↔
SSRIs					
Fluoxetine	↓	↓	↓	↑	±
Paroxetine	↓↓	↓	↓↓	↑	++
Sertraline	↔	↔↓	↓	↑	+
Citalopram	↔	↓	↓	↑	+
Escitalopram	↔	↓	↓	↑	+
SNRIs					
Venlafaxine	↓	↔↓ or ↑	↓↓	↑↑	+
Desvenlafaxine	Same	↔↓ or ↑	Same	Same	↔
Duloxetine	Same	↔↓ or ↑	Same	Same	↔
Atypical					
Bupropion	↓↔	↔	↔↑	↔ or ↓ or ↑**	↔
Trazodone	↑	↔↑	↔↓	↑	4+
Mirtazapine	↑	↔↑	↔↓	↔	3+

**Bupropion data limited and conflicting.
Up arrows, increased; *down arrows*, decreased; *double longitudinal arrows*, no or minimal change, *1 to 4+*, increasing amount of sedation.
MAOIs, monoamine oxidase inhibitors; *REM*, rapid eye movement; *SNRIs*, selective norepinephrine reuptake inhibitors; *SSRIs*, selective serotonin reuptake inhibitors; *TCAs*, tricyclic antidepressants.
Stahl SM. *Stahl's Essential Psychopharmacology*. 7th ed. New York: Cambridge Press; 2021 and Gursky JT, Krahn LE. The effects of antidepressants on sleep: a review. *Harvard Rev Psychiatry*. 2000;8:298-306.

decrease the amount of REM sleep. Bupropion is one of the few medications that can actually increase the amount of REM sleep, although it slightly increased the REM latency (at least in one study in depressed patients).[77-79] Nefazodone is a sedating antidepressant that also tends to increase REM sleep but can cause severe hepatotoxicity and is no longer available.[80] The medication is mentioned here because a study comparing nefazodone and fluoxetine found that both improved depression and subjective sleep quality, but only nefazodone improved sleep architecture determined using PSG. *Satisfaction with sleep* may improve in some patients on an antidepressant, even if sleep architecture determined by PSG does not improve. An improvement in mood may improve subjective sleep quality.

Mirtazapine and trazodone have been reported to be associated with no or only mild reduction in the amount of REM sleep. MAOIs are less commonly used but are the most powerful suppressors of REM sleep. In general, sedating antidepressants have a beneficial effect on sleep efficiency, whereas nonsedating antidepressants tend to decrease sleep efficiency. As noted, if patients respond to an antidepressant, their subjective estimate of their sleep quality may improve, even if objective sleep quality by PSG does not.

Pharmacotherapy for Comorbid Insomnia of Psychiatric Disorders

Patients with MDD frequently have prominent comorbid insomnia. In such patents, one might choose to use (1) a sedating antidepressant at antidepressant doses (e.g., mirtazapine 30–45 mg nightly), (2) the combination of an effective nonsedating antidepressant (at antidepressant doses) and a sedating antidepressant at low doses, (3) the combination of an effective nonsedating antidepressant and a benzodiazepine receptor agonist ([BZRA] hypnotic), or (4) the combination of an antidepressant and a sedating atypical antipsychotic (quetiapine). Sedating antidepressants and antipsychotics commonly used for their hypnotic effects are listed in Table 37–11. For information on BZRA hypnotics, see Chapter 33.

Several sedating antidepressants are used in lower than antidepressant doses for their sedating properties. Doxepin is a sedating antidepressant but has anticholinergic side effects. It has been used in low doses (25 mg) as a hypnotic. It is approved by the FDA for sleep maintenance in very low doses (3, 6 mg as Silenor). At these low doses significant anticholinergic side effects are not present. Low dose doxepin (3 mg, 6 mg) is available as a generic but is more expensive than generic higher dose doxepin formulations (10 mg, 25 mg, 50 mg, 10 mg/mL). One approach is to use doxepin 10 mg or to use 0.6 mL of the elixir (6 mg). As mentioned, trazodone is used in low doses (25–50 mg) as a hypnotic but rarely in higher doses as an antidepressant. Trazodone can be used in combination with an SSRI to reduce antidepressant-associated insomnia.[81] Trazodone has *minimal anticholinergic* side effects compared with sedating TCAs. Because of the lack of anticholinergic side effects, trazodone is widely used as a hypnotic. As discussed in Chapter 33, the evidence for its hypnotic efficacy in patients who are not depressed is limited.

The combination of an antidepressant and a BZRA has been studied using placebo-controlled trials. Fava and coworkers[82] studied a group of patients with both MDD and insomnia. The combination of fluoxetine and placebo was compared with

Table 37–11 Antidepressants and Atypical Antipsychotics Used for Sleep*

Generic Name (Brand Name)	Dose Forms	Hypnotic Dose	Comments	Notable Side Effects
Trazodone (Desyrel)**	50, 100 mg	25–100 mg qhs	Less anticholinergic side effects than TCAs $T_{1/2}$ 9 (3–14) hours	Priapism Postural hypotension
Mirtazapine (Remeron)	15, 30 mg	7.5–15 mg qhs	$T_{1/2}$ 20–40 hours	Weight gain Higher doses less sedating
Tricyclic Antidepressants (TCAs)				
Amitriptyline (Elavil)	10, 25, 50 mg	10–25 mg qhs	$T_{1/2}$ 10-26 hours metabolite active (nortriptyline)	Dry mouth, constipation QT prolongation
Doxepin (Sinequan)**	10, 25, 50 10 mg/ml	1–10 mg (elixir) 25mg qhs	$T_{1/2}$ 6–8 hours	Dry mouth, constipation
Doxepin (Silenor)***	3, 6 mg	6 mg qhs 3 mg qhs elderly	$T_{1/2}$ 6–8 hours	FDA approved for sleep maintenance insomnia Cimetidine increases drug levels – max dose of doxepin should not exceed 3 mg Sertraline can also increase levels of doxepin
Sedating Antipsychotic Medications				
Quetiapine (Seroquel)	25, 50, 100 mg	12.5–50 mg qhs	$T_{1/2}$ 6 hours Intermediate acting	Headache, dizziness Neuroleptic syndrome Tardive dyskinesia Long QT Lens change

* generic trazodone, mirtazapine, and quetiapine are available
** brand names Desyrel and Sinequan no long available
*** generic 3, 6 mg doxepin now available
Stahl SM. *Stahl's Essential Psychopharmacology.* 7th ed. New York: Cambridge Press; 2021.

fluoxetine + 3 mg of eszopiclone. Coadministration of eszopiclone resulted in improved subjective sleep latency, wakefulness after sleep onset (WASO), and total sleep time compared with fluoxetine alone. Although this result was not unexpected, a surprising finding was that treatment with the combination of fluoxetine and eszopiclone resulted in greater improvement in depression (Hamilton depression scale) at 4 weeks with progressive improvement at 8 weeks and more responders and remitters than treatment with placebo + fluoxetine (Figure 37–4). A similar trial with zolpidem found improvement in sleep but no evidence of greater improvement in depression.[83]

In patents with a history of past or current alcohol or benzodiazepine dependence, the use of BZRAs is problematic. For these patients, use of ramelteon (a melatonin receptor agonist with no abuse potential) or a sedating antidepressant may be the best treatment option. Ramelteon is approved only for sleep-onset insomnia and is not useful to improve sleep maintenance. It should ***not*** be used with the SSRI fluvoxamine, which causes increased melatonin levels.

Quetiapine (Seroquel) is a second generation antipsychotic (SGA) medication that antagonizes histamine, dopamine D2, and serotonin 5HT2 receptors. At low doses, the medications' main effect is as an antihistamine. Therefore, it can be used in low doses as a hypnotic. Quetiapine is indicated for treatment of schizophrenia and mania in bipolar disorders. As noted, quetiapine XR has been used as a second medication (augmentation) in treatment-resistant depression or as a single antidepressant medication for bipolar disorders. Side effects of quetiapine include QT prolongation, weight gain, extrapyramidal symptoms, headache, and a decreased white blood cell count. Even at low doses, quetiapine has been associated with significant weight gain.

Behavioral treatment (cognitive behavioral treatment of insomnia, CBT-I) can also be used to treat insomnia comorbid with depression.[84,85] While it effectively treats insomnia, it is not clear whether separate treatment of insomnia improves the overall success of antidepressant treatment. As noted, successful treatment of depression can also improve symptoms of insomnia, although objective findings (PSG) may not confirm an objective improvement in sleep quality.

TREATMENT OF BIPOLAR DISORDERS

The treatment of bipolar disorders is complex.[86-89] Most sleep physicians who are not psychiatrists will probably not be the primary physician treating a patient for bipolar disorder. However, an understanding of the approach is important. The treatment of bipolar disorders is usually grouped into three treatment phases: acute bipolar mania, bipolar depression, and bipolar maintenance (Table 37–12). The medications FDA approved for the different treatment phases are shown along with other medications commonly used for treatment of bipolar disorder. The major medication groups used include mood stabilizers (lithium, valproate), anticonvulsants (carbamazepine, lamotrigine), and SGAs. Antidepressants can be used for BP-I depression but usually only after several other medications have failed and always in combination with one or more anti-mania medications (mood stabilizers of an SGA). Studies have not shown benefit from the addition of an antidepressant to a mood stabilizer in unselected patients.[90] However, some patients may benefit. In patients with BP-II who have not displayed a HME over many years of depressive episodes, some clinicians will use an antidepressant without a mood stabilizer. It is worth mentioning that psychological treatments and psychoeducation are important parts of the treatment of bipolar disorders and are discussed in several guidelines.[86,87]

Acute Mania

The newer SGA drugs such as risperidone (Risperdal), quetiapine (Seroquel), aripiprazole (Abilify), ziprasidone (Geodon), cariprazine (Vraylar), and olanzapine (Zyprexa) are often used in acute mania because these medications have a rapid onset of psychomotor inhibition, which may be lifesaving in the case of a violent or psychotic patient. These medications are approved for use in acute mania alone or in combination with lithium or

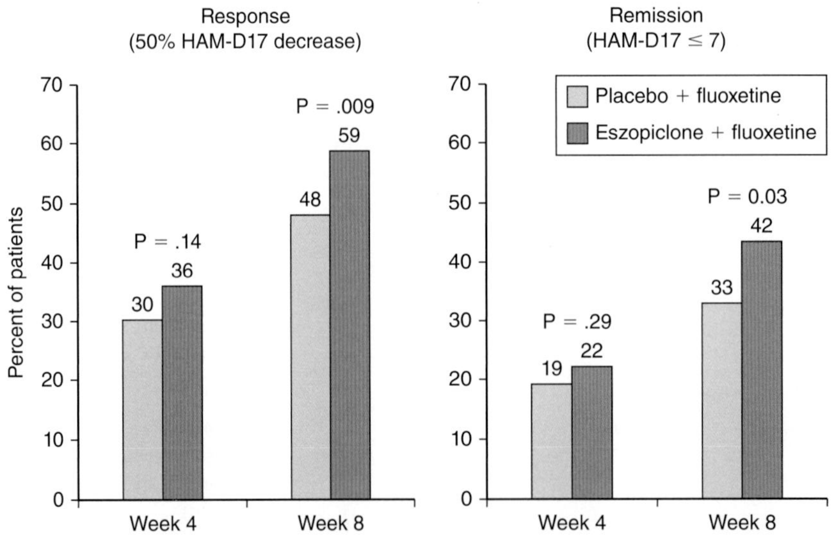

Figure 37–4 Eszopiclone + fluoxetine resulted in a significantly greater improvement in the Hamilton depression scale (HAM) at 8 weeks, as determined by both relapse and remission compared with placebo + fluoxetine. (Reprinted by permission of Elsevier from Fava M, McCall V, Krystal A, et al: Eszopiclone co-administered with fluoxetine in patients with insomnia coexisting with major depressive disorder. Biol Psychiatry 2006;59:1052–1060. © 2006 by the Society of Biological Psychiatry.)

Table 37–12 Treatments for Bipolar Disorder

Bipolar Phase	Mania	Maintenance	Depression
Goal	• Rapid onset of action • Relief of symptoms • No depression induction	• Prevent depression or mania/hypomania	• Relief of symptoms • No mania induction
Medication Options	*Valproic acid/valproate Or *Lithium Or SGAs • Quetiapine (Seroquel)* • Aripiprazole* (Abilify) • Risperidone* (Risperdal) • Ziprasidone* (Geodon) • Olanzapine* (Zyprexa) • Azepine (Saphris)* • Cariprazine (Vraylar)* Other Medications • Haloperidol • Carbamazepine*	*Lamotrigine *Lithium – only medication reducing suicide risk Valproic acid/valproate *Aripiprazole (Abilify Maintena) *Ziprasidone (Geodon) as monotherapy or in combination with lithium or valproate *Olanzapine in BP-I (Zyprexa)	BP-I • Olanzapine + Fluoxetine (Symbyax)* • Lurasidone (Latuda)* alone or in combination with lithium or valproate • Quetiapine XR (Seroquel XR)** • Cariprazine (Vraylar)* • Lumateperone (Caplyta)* alone or in combination with lithium or valproate BPI, BPII depression • Lithium (takes time to reach effective level) • Lamotrigine (better for preventing depression) • Valproic acid/valproate BP-II • Lithium, Valproic acid/Valproate • Lamotrigine (better for preventing depression) • Quetiapine XR (Seroquel XR)** • Lumateperone (Caplyta)* alone or in combination with lithium or valproate BP-II > BP-I • If monotherapy with mood stabilizer or SGA not satisfactory add bupropion, fluoxetine
Comments	SGAs can be used as monotherapy for rapid action or used as combined therapy with lithium or valproate	Lamotrigine better for preventing depression, not anti-mania	In BP-I use antimanic medication if using antidepressant, BP-II antidepressants alone may work in some patients

* FDA approved for this indication, SGA Second generation antipsychotic, **Quetiapine XR FDA approved for depressive episodes in bipolar disorders (BP-I or BP-II not specified)

divalproex. The approved mood stabilizers for mania also include lithium, divalproex (Depakote), and carbamazepine (Tegretol). Divalproex is an enteric-coated formulation of sodium valproate and valproic acid in a 1:1 molar ratio. Valproic acid and injectable sodium valproate are other available formulations. Divalproex is available in a long-acting preparation (Depakote ER), allowing once-daily dosing. The combination of an atypical antipsychotic and a mood stabilizer is also often used for severe mania. Lithium must be titrated up slowly and is not the drug of choice for acute severe mania. Anti-mania effects occur after 1 to 3 weeks of lithium at therapeutic doses. If lithium is used for acute mania, it usually requires the addition of another medication. Lithium side effects are experienced by up to 30% of patients taking this medication and include tremor, nausea, weight gain, fatigue, and mild cognitive impairment. A number of medications have important drug interactions with lithium. For example, diuretics and nonsteroidal antiinflammatory drugs (NSAIDs) can reduce renal clearance (increase lithium levels). Lithium levels must be followed closely. Divalproex is probably the mood stabilizer of choice for acute mania in this situation because it can be titrated up fairly rapidly (20–30 mg/kg/day on a TID schedule). In less urgent cases, the medication is started at 250 mg with a meal on day 1, then increased to 250 mg TID for 3 to 6 days. Mania typically begins improving 1 to 4 days after drug levels exceed 50 μg/ml. Side effects of divalproex include nausea, vomiting, dyspepsia, and diarrhea. When titrated up rapidly, divalproex can also cause sedation. Rare but very severe side effects include hepatotoxicity, leukopenia, thrombocytopenia, and pancreatitis. Drug levels can be obtained before the morning dose with a therapeutic range of 50 to 125 μg/ml (commonly felt that >75 μg/ml is needed for mania). *Both lithium and divalproex have been associated with an increased risk of birth defects.* Of note, *lithium increases stage N3 sleep and decreases REM sleep.*

More recently, many clinicians favor use of SGAs as monotherapy. Although some analyses have favored one medication over another in general, they all are effective, and the choice may depend on potential side effects. In picking a drug, avoid lithium in renal disease, avoid valproate in liver disease, avoid olanzapine, quetiapine, and risperidone in obesity, and avoid aripiprazole and risperidone in those with sensitivity to extrapyramidal side effects.

Maintenance Treatment

The goal of maintenance treatment is to prevent relapse of mania and depressive episodes. *The cumulative rate of relapse after an episode of mania in the absence of maintenance treatment is 50% at 12 months and nearly 90% at 60 months.* Lithium and lamotrigine (Lamictal) are the two mood stabilizers that are FDA approved for maintenance treatment. Divalproex is ***not*** FDA approved for maintenance treatment but is also widely used for this application. Lithium also has the advantage of preventing bipolar depression and reducing suicide risk (the only medication documented to do this). It appears to have an advantage over divalproex in these respects. Lamotrigine may be used as a mood stabilizer for maintenance but is not an antimanic medication. Lamotrigine has equivocal antidepressant effects but is useful in maintenance to prevent bipolar depression. This medication requires a slow upward titration (over 6 weeks) to avoid a significant skin rash. It can be associated with Stevens-Johnson syndrome. Lamotrigine is ***not*** approved for acute mania. *Aripiprazole (Abilify Maintena), Olanzapine (Zyprexa) and ziprasidone (Geodon) as an adjunct to lithium or valproate are the only antipsychotic medications currently FDA approved for maintenance.* Aripiprazole is a partial dopamine D2 agonist and serotonin 5HT1A agonist, as well as an antagonist at the 5HT2A receptors. Ziprasidone antagonizes dopamine D2 receptors and serotonin 5HT2 receptors. Olanzapine blocks dopamine D2 receptors and 5HT2A receptors. Of note, even with maintenance treatment, relapse of mania or depression may occur in up to 40% of patients with BP-I in the first year and up to 75% over 5 years.

Bipolar Depression

Treatment of bipolar depression is often challenging (Table 37–13).[86-89] An increasing number of SGAs are approved for treatment of depression in bipolar disorders. Quetiapine XR, a combination of olanzapine and fluoxetine with the brand name Symbyax, lurasidone (Latuda) (alone or in combination with lithium or valproate), cariprazine (Vraylar), and lumateperone (Caplyta) alone or in combination with lithium or valproate are FDA approved for treatment of depression in BP-I. Lumateperone and Quetiapine XR are approved for treatment of depression in BP-II. One problem with the olanzapine/fluoxetine combination is that fluoxetine has a very long half-life. If mania occurs, the residual effects can be problematic. *Olanzapine is the SGA with the greatest tendency for weight gain.* Divalproex/valproate and lithium are not FDA approved for bipolar depression but commonly used. In fact, traditionally many treatment algorithms used a mood stabilizer (lithium or divalproex) as the initial step. Lithium is generally more effective for bipolar depression than divalproex. Many clinicians would next add lamotrigine, which has equivocal antidepressant activity but *is effective for preventing relapse of depression.* If a patient is not on a mood stabilizer and develops depression, starting with quetiapine XR or lurasidone is an option, as lithium and valproate must be titrated up slowly. In general, the SGAs are used in lower doses for depression than typically used for schizophrenia. In BP-II an antidepressant less likely to precipitate mania can be used (bupropion, fluoxetine).

Most studies have not documented an advantage of the addition of a standard antidepressant to a mood stabilizer in the treatment of bipolar depression.[90] The use of an antidepressant in a patient with a bipolar disorder *can worsen anxiety, increase mood instability, or trigger a switch to mania.* In most algorithms, an antidepressant is added only after other combinations have been tried. However, individual patients may benefit from the long-term combination of a mood stabilizer and an antidepressant. If an antidepressant is used, the activating ones such as venlafaxine or duloxetine are more likely to cause switches (mania). Bupropion or an SSRI (usually fluoxetine) are typically used. As noted, some very stable patients with BP-II who have not had a HME for years might be treated with an antidepressant alone.

Table 37–13 Treatment of Bipolar Depression – One Approach

Assumes no antimanic drug (lithium, valproate, SGA , but not lamotrigine) is currently being used

Step 1
- Quetiapine or lurasidone monotherapy

Step 2
- Olanzapine plus fluoxetine
- Valproate monotherapy
- Combination: quetiapine or lurasidone + lithium or valproate
- Lithium + valproate or lamotrigine

Step 3
- Monotherapy lamotrigine, lithium, olanzapine
- Monotherapy carbamazepine or cariprazine (Vraylar)
- Combination of lithium or valproate and an antidepressant (SSRI; [eg. fluoxetine] or buproprion)
- Combination of a SGA (usually quetiapine, lurasidone, or olanzapine) and an antidepressant

This list is not inclusive of all medications used for bipolar depression. Adapted from Shelton RC, Bobo WV. Bipolar depression in adults: choosing treatment. https://www.uptodate.com/contents/bipolar-major-depression-in-adults-choosing-treatment?search=BIPOLAR%20DEPRESSION&source=search_result&selectedTitle=1~150&usage_type=default&display_rank=1. Accessed 10/28/2022.

ANXIETY DISORDERS AFFECTING SLEEP

Anxiety disorders are listed in a separate chapter in the DSM-V. Disorders relevant to sleep medicine will be discussed herein, including panic disorder (PD), general anxiety disorder (GAD), and PTSD. A detailed discussion of the disorders is beyond the scope of this chapter, but relevant topics will be discussed.

Panic Disorder

Panic disorder is characterized by recurrent **unexpected panic attacks**, and at least one of the attacks has been followed by 1 month or more of one or both of the following: a persistent concern about additional panic attacks and/or a significant maladaptive change in behavior related to the attacks. The disturbance is not attributable to the effects of a substance or medication and not better explained by another mental disorder. Note that the DSM-V lists panic disorder and agoraphobia as separate disorders[5]. *A panic attack is not a diagnosis but is a component of the criteria for the diagnosis of panic disorder.*

A panic attack and the panic disorder have the following characteristics (see the DSM-V for complete diagnostic criteria for panic disorder).[16]

- Recurrent unexpected panic attacks. A panic attack is an abrupt surge of intense fear or intense discomfort that reaches a peak within minutes and during which time **four (or more) of the following symptoms occur****:
  1. Palpitations, pounding heart, or accelerated heart rate
  2. Sweating
  3. Trembling or shaking
  4. Sensations of shortness of breath or smothering
  5. Feelings of choking
  6. Chest pain or discomfort
  7. Nausea or abdominal distress
  8. Feeling dizzy, unsteady, light-headed, or faint
  9. Chills or heat sensations

10. Paresthesias (numbness or tingling sensations)
11. Derealization (feelings of unreality) or depersonalization (being detached from oneself)
12. Fear of losing control or "going crazy"
13. Fear of dying

** **Note:** The abrupt surge can occur from a calm state or an anxious state.

- At least **one of the attack**s has been followed **by 1 month (or more)** of one or both of the following:
  1. Persistent concern or worry about additional panic attacks or their consequences (e.g., losing control, having a heart attack, "going crazy").
  2. A significant maladaptive change in behavior related to the attacks (e.g., behaviors designed to avoid having panic attacks, such as avoidance of exercise or unfamiliar situations).
- The disturbance is not attributable to the physiological effects of a substance (e.g., a drug of abuse, a medication) or another medical condition (e.g., hyperthyroidism, cardiopulmonary disorders).

Four or more of the 13 manifestations listed must be present to meet criteria for a panic attack. The *unexpected characteristic* refers to the fact that the panic attack comes "from out of the blue" without any cue (e.g., the patient is relaxing or has awoken from sleep – nocturnal panic attack). The presence of *expected* panic attacks does not rule out the panic disorder, and *about 50% of patients with panic disorder have expected panic attacks.* **Nocturnal panic attacks** are characterized by awakening from sleep in a panic, but the symptoms are experienced while fully awake. Nocturnal panic attacks occur at least one time in about one-fourth to one-third of patients with panic disorder. *The majority of patients with nighttime panic attacks also have daytime panic attacks.* However, *some patients have only nocturnal panic attacks.* Note that panic attacks can occur in any other anxiety disorder as well as depressive disorders. The DSM-V adds the following diagnostic criteria for panic disorder: "The disturbance is not better explained by another mental disorder (e.g., the panic attacks do not occur only in response to feared social situations, as in social anxiety disorder; in response to circumscribed phobic objects or situations, as in specific phobia; in response to obsessions, as in obsessive-compulsive disorder; in response to reminders of traumatic events, as in PTSD; or in response to separation from attachment figures, as in separation anxiety disorder)."[5]

Sleep and Panic Disorder

Some key points concerning sleep and panic disorder are listed in Box 37–7. A nocturnal panic attack is in the differential diagnosis of parasomnias including night terrors. The majority of patients with panic disorder have a history of at least one nocturnal panic attack. *About one-third of patients with panic disorder have recurrent nocturnal panic attacks.* Of those patients with panic disorder who experience nocturnal panic attacks, up to two-thirds report insomnia often associated with fear of returning to sleep.[91,92] The symptom of *dyspnea appears to be more common in nocturnal panic attacks.* The attacks occur from non-REM (NREM) sleep, commonly at the transition from stage N2 to stage N3 sleep. In most patients, sleep architecture is normal (normal REM latency and sleep efficiency). However, some patients may develop sleep phobia—and this can be associated with findings consistent with insomnia.

Box 37–7 SLEEP AND PANIC DISORDER

- Most patients with nocturnal panic attacks also have daytime panic attacks.
- The majority of patients with panic disorder have at least one nocturnal panic attack.
- One-third or more of patients with panic disorder have recurrent nocturnal panic attacks.
- Nocturnal panic attacks occur during NREM, commonly at transition from N2 to N3.
- Up to two-thirds of patients with panic disorder report sleep-onset and sleep-maintenance insomnia (fear of returning to sleep).
- In contrast to an NREM parasomnia, the patient is fully awake when experiencing the symptoms.
- **In contrast to nightmares, there is no dream recall.**
- If an SSRI is started, the initial dose should be low to avoid an exacerbation.
- Some patients will need an anti-anxiety medication until an effective dose of the SSRI is reached.

NREM, non-rapid eye movement, *SSRI*, selective serotonin reuptake inhibitor.

The differential diagnosis of nocturnal panic attacks includes sleep terrors, nightmares, PTSD, and the REM behavior disorder (Box 37–8). Sleep terrors usually begin in childhood, and during the episodes, the individual is not aware of their surroundings (not alert) and does not remember the episodes in the morning. In **panic attacks, the patient is awake and aware of their surroundings**. In night terrors, the patient usually quickly returns to sleep, but in panic disorder, the return to sleep can be quite delayed. In nightmares, the patient usually is aware of a frightening dream. In contrast, patients with panic attacks remember the episode but typically do not report a terrifying dream. In nocturnal laryngospasm, the patient wakes up choking with near-total cessation of airflow with stridor.[93] However, the episodes usually last less than 60 seconds.

Treatment of Panic Disorder

Treatments of panic attacks include cognitive behavioral therapy (CBT) with or without relaxation techniques and pharmacotherapy.[91,92,94-98] Although benzodiazepines (e.g., alprazolam, clonazepam) are the classic treatments for panic disorder, *the long-term treatment of choice for panic disorder is an antidepressant.* The SSRIs FDA approved for treatment of panic disorder included fluoxetine, paroxetine, and sertraline. A network analysis found escitalopram and sertraline to be the most effective for panic disorder.[95] Paroxetine is the SSRI

Box 37–8 DIFFERENTIAL DIAGNOSIS OF NOCTURNAL PANIC ATTACKS

1. Medical disorder (hyperthyroidism, pheochromocytoma)
2. Paroxysmal nocturnal dyspnea (CHF)
3. Arousal from OSA
4. Arousal from GERD
5. Nocturnal laryngospasm
6. NREM parasomnia—sleep terrors
7. PTSD
8. REM sleep behavior disorder

CHF, congestive heart failure; *GERD*, gastroesophageal reflux disease; *NREM*, non-REM; *OSA*, obstructive sleep apnea; *PTSD*, posttraumatic stress disorder; *REM*, rapid eye movement.

most frequently used for panic disorder in the past and may be suited for nocturnal panic attacks, as it is sedating and usually taken at night.[97] It does have prominent anticholinergic side effects. The benzodiazepines approved for treatment of panic disorder are alprazolam or clonazepam. SSRIs must be started at a very low dose, or the panic disorder initially may be exacerbated. For example, paroxetine is started at 10 mg daily or escitalopram at 5 mg daily. The doses are slowly increased as tolerated. Because improvements may take 4 to 6 weeks or longer, many physicians add benzodiazepines during the early course of therapy. Alprazolam (Xanax) has a short half-life, and many psychiatrists prefer to use clonazepam, which has a long duration of action. This is especially true for patients requiring anti-anxiety treatment during the day. Unfortunately, clonazepam can be quite sedating in some patients. Alprazolam is available in an extended-action preparation (Xanax XR), which prevents the need for repeated dosing. Once SSRI treatment reaches a target dose, the benzodiazepines can be weaned. Alprazolam is associated with particularly severe withdrawal symptoms in some patients as a result of its high potency and short half-life.[98] In summary, approximately one-half of patients with panic disorder report experiencing nocturnal panic attacks at some point during the course of their illness. Some studies estimate that up to one-third of patients with the panic disorder experience recurrent nocturnal panic attacks. However, a lack of daytime panic attacks does not rule out nocturnal panic attacks.

GENERALIZED ANXIETY DISORDER

GAD is characterized by excessive anxiety and worry occurring more days than not for a period of at least 6 months about a number of events or activities.[5] The individual finds it difficult to control their worry. The anxiety and worry are associated with at least three of the following six symptoms, with at least one symptom present for more days than not over the previous 6 months: (1) restlessness or feeling on edge, (2) easily fatigued, (3) difficulty concentrating or mind going blank, (4) irritability, (5) muscle tension, and (6) sleep disturbance, including difficulty falling/staying asleep or restless nonrestorative sleep. The worry, anxiety, or physical symptoms cause significant distress or impairment. The symptoms are not better explained by another mental disorder, medical condition, or medication.

Sleep in GAD

Chronic subjective sleep disturbance is common among people with GAD. Few PSG results are available but usually describe *prolonged sleep latency, reduced sleep efficiency and total sleep time*, as well as disturbance of sleep continuity and reduced slow-wave sleep. Fava and coworkers[99] compared the combination of extended-release zolpidem and escitalopram with placebo and escitalopram in a group of patients with insomnia and comorbid GAD. The group with the addition of zolpidem had improvement in insomnia (subjective total sleep time) and next-day symptoms (but not anxiety symptoms). Note that zolpidem is a BZRA hypnotic without anti-anxiety activity. Medications such as clonazepam and lorazepam could be used for sleep in patients with GAD for both their hypnotic and anti-anxiety effects. Alprazolam is another alternative, although it may have less hypnotic activity because it tends to be less sedating. Clonazepam, lorazepam, and alprazolam are not FDA approved for use as hypnotics. The differential diagnosis of patients with anxiety and sleep disturbance includes those with chronic insomnia disorder and patients anxious about a medical condition, or both anxiety and sleep disturbance due to a substance. Many patients with the chronic insomnia disorder report anxiety and worry, but their anxiety is usually less intense than in GAD and their worries are less generalized (*anxiety is focused on sleep*).

Treatment of GAD

Treatments include psychotherapy, benzodiazepines (alprazolam, lorazepam, diazepam, clonazepam), and SSRI/SNRIs. The antidepressant medications with demonstrated effectiveness include citalopram, escitalopram, paroxetine, and sertraline.[100-102] Some patients may feel more anxious when starting an SSRI, and benzodiazepines can be used during the first 4 to 6 weeks of treatment. A discontinuation syndrome has been described with alprazolam after only 6 to 8 weeks of treatment. In general, all benzodiazepines should be weaned rather than abruptly discontinued.

POSTTRAUMATIC STRESS DISORDER

An in-depth discussion of PTSD is beyond the scope of this chapter. However, a brief discussion with an emphasis on sleep is included given the impact of PTSD on the sleep of many patients seen in sleep clinics. The DSM-V diagnostic criteria for PTSD are very extensive; only the most important points are summarized below.

In PTSD, symptoms occur after exposure to an extremely traumatic stressor involving (1) direct personal experience of an event that involves actual or threatened death, serious injury, or other threat to ones' physical integrity; (2) witnessing an event that involves death, injury, or a threat to the physical integrity of another person; (3) learning about unexpected or violent death, serious harm, or threat of death or injury experienced by a family member or close friend; or (4) exposure to aversive details of traumatic events (e.g., first responders collecting human remains or police officers with repeated exposure to details of child abuse). The characteristic symptoms resulting from exposure to the extreme trauma include persistent re-experience of the traumatic event, persistent avoidance of stimuli associated with the trauma, numbing of general responsiveness, and *persistent symptoms of increased arousal.*

Marked arousal and reactivity associated with the traumatic events is typically present. For example, angry outbursts, hypervigilance, reckless or self-destructive behavior, and irritability are common symptoms of PTSD. *Sleep disturbance includes sleep-onset and maintenance insomnia. The post-event manifestations must be present for at least 1 month.*

Sleep and PTSD

Recurrent distressing dreams (i.e., nightmares) of the traumatic event are one of the diagnostic features of PTSD. For many patients with PTSD, the associated nightmares represent one of the most frequently occurring and problematic aspects of the disorder. Persistent nightmares may also be one of the most enduring symptoms in PTSD. A high percentages of patients (70–90%) describe subjective sleep disturbance with or without nightmares. However, PSG studies of patients with PTSD have yielded variable and inconclusive findings. In regard to abnormalities in REM sleep, controlled studies have not found consistent abnormalities in sleep architecture. However, increased rates of sleep-related breathing disturbance have been reported in trauma victims.

Symptoms of PTSD can begin immediately after the event or have a delayed onset (up to years later). Patients with PTSD also report a heightened startle response. Given a common exposure to a traumatic event, PTSD appears to *occur more frequently in women than in men*. Patients with PTSD also may have depression and may abuse ethanol or other substances.

Differential Diagnosis of Nocturnal Event Caused by PTSD

Patients with PTSD often report waking up associated with anxiety and autonomic activation. The differential of awakening with anxiety includes nocturnal panic disorder, REM sleep behavior disorder, and sleep terrors. Unlike patients with nocturnal panic attacks, patients with PTSD can recount a dream of a specific traumatic event. In contrast to sleep terrors, patients become alert quickly after awakening. As noted, sleep studies in patients with PTSD have produced conflicting results. The duration of REM latency and the amount of REM sleep have varied among studies. These variations in findings may be caused by the fact that some patients with PTSD also have depression. Several studies have found an increase in REM density in patients with PTSD (as in depression),[103] an increase in body movements during sleep, and the presence of periodic limb movements in sleep (PLMs).[104,105] Some patients may have REM sleep without atonia, but some are already on SSRIs that can cause this finding. *As noted, studies have found high rates of sleep apnea in patients with PTSD (50–90%).*

Treatment of PTSD: General Considerations

Based on a large meta-analysis,[106] the first-line therapy for PTSD is trauma-focused psychotherapy (TFP), and medications are second line. Some of the TFPs include prolonged exposure therapy (PET), cognitive reprocessing therapy, eye movement desensitization and reprocessing (EMDR), and written exposure therapy. Detailed discussion is beyond the scope of this chapter. However, PET will be discussed briefly. PET is a specific type of cognitive behavioral therapy that teaches individuals to gradually approach trauma-related memories, feelings, and situations. Prolonged exposure is typically provided over a period of about 3 months with weekly individual sessions, resulting in 8 to 15 sessions overall. Sixty- to 120-minute sessions are usually needed for the individual to engage in exposure (oral and written details of experience slowly discussed). The idea is exposure and habituation will help the individual sufficiently process the experience. Therapists begin with an overview of treatment and understanding the patient's past experiences. Therapists continue with psychoeducation and then will generally teach a breathing technique to manage anxiety. Generally, after the assessment and initial session, exposure begins. As this is very anxiety-provoking for most patients, the therapist works hard to ensure that the therapy relationship is perceived to be a safe space for encountering very scary stimuli.

As for medications, the meta-analysis found the most evidence for sertraline, paroxetine, fluoxetine, and venlafaxine. Of these, sertraline has consistently performed well in a number of analyses. Sertraline and venlafaxine were most effective, but benefits of venlafaxine decreased over time. Of note, *only sertraline and paroxetine are FDA approved for the treatment of PTSD*. Escitalopram has also been used for PTSD.[107] Benzodiazepines and atypical antipsychotics were not recommended for treatment of PTSD. A randomized trial of prolonged exposure versus sertraline treatment was performed. Patients were shown the rationales behind treatments. After randomization to choice or no-choice groups, they underwent treatment. Those in the no-choice group were randomized to prolonged exposure or sertraline. Prolonged exposure and sertraline conferred significant benefits for PTSD, with some evidence of an advantage for prolonged exposure. Giving patients with PTSD their preferred treatment also conferred important benefits, including enhancing adherence.[108] A study suggested that continuous positive airway pressure (CPAP) treatment of obstructive sleep apnea (if present) is beneficial to PTSD symptoms.[109]

With respect to PTSD associated nightmares, image rehearsal therapy (IRT) and a number of other behavioral treatments have been used effectively. The position paper by the AASM on treatment of the nightmare disorder recommends both medication and a wide variety of behavioral treatments.[110] One of the best-known and most-studied techniques is IRT. It is a modified cognitive behavioral therapy technique that involves altering the content of a nightmare by creating a new set of positive images and rehearsing the rewritten dream scenario for 10 to 20 minutes per day while awake.[111]

Several observational studies and small randomized controlled trials showed a benefit of prazosin, a centrally acting alpha-1 blocker.[112] However, a very large, randomized trial (PACT) did not show a benefit of prazosin for nightmares or sleep compared to placebo.[113] Quite high doses of prazosin were used in the PACT study (about 14 mg). The study had some limitations. First, only screening questions were used to identify untreated obstructive sleep apnea, which can have a large effect (if not diagnosed and treated). The groups studied were very stable. The previous studies did not exclude patients still in distress. For these reasons, most clinicians still feel prazosin is effective in many patients. A meta-analysis published since the PACT trial used the PACT data and data from previous studies and concluded that prazosin was beneficial for nightmares but did not improve sleep or overall PTSD symptoms.[114] The AASM position paper on treatment of nightmares continued to recommend prazosin but at a lower level of certainty. When using prazosin, it is important to start with a very low dose (1 mg) and increase slowly.

The FDA approved a device called NightWare for the treatment of nightmares to be used in conjunction with other therapies.[115] After establishing a sleep profile for the patient using a proprietary algorithm, the watch will detect nightmares based on heart rate and body movement, providing vibration to awaken the patient. Based on its review of all data submitted by the company, in November 2020, the FDA cleared NightWare for the reduction of sleep disturbance related to nightmares in adults 22 years of age or older who have nightmare disorder or nightmares from PTSD. It is not intended to be used alone and should not be used by patients who have acted out their nightmares (i.e., sleepwalking, violence). At the time of this writing, the device is available only through the U.S. Department of Veterans Affairs and the Department of Defense (https://nightware.com/product/).

SUMMARY OF KEY POINTS

1. A significant proportion of patients with a sleep complaint have a psychiatric illness, and a significant number of patients with a psychiatric illness have a sleep complaint.
2. MDD, BP-I, and BP-II are defined by mood episodes. A summary of duration criteria for the mood episodes:
   - Major depressive episode (MDE): 2 weeks
   - Manic episode (ME): 1 week or any duration resulting in hospitalization
   - Hypomanic episode (HME): 4 days
3. Insomnia or hypersomnia nearly every day is one of the nine major criteria for diagnosis of a Major Depressive Episode (MDE).
4. During a MDE, approximately 80% of patients complain of symptoms of insomnia (frequent awakenings, early-morning awakening), and 20% complain of hypersomnia.
5. PSG during a MDE shows a long sleep latency, reduced sleep efficiency, reduced stage N3, a short REM latency, a longer first REM period, and a higher REM density early in the night. Early-morning awakening may also be present.
6. Insomnia can precede a MDE and is often the last symptom of depression to resolve. Some but not all studies suggest that the persistence of sleep complaints is a risk factor for relapse of depression.
7. The major depressive disorder (MDD) is defined by at least one depressive episode and no current or past MEs or HMEs.
8. During Manic Episodes (MEs), the patient reports a decreased need for sleep (feeling rested on a few hours of sleep). Sleep loss can precipitate a ME.
9. Hypomanic Episodes (HMEs) have characteristics similar to those of Manic Episodes (MEs) except for the following three conditions: severe impairment is not present, hospitalization is not necessary, and there are no psychotic features. If any of the three are present, the episode is considered a ME.
10. BP-I diagnosis requires at least one current (or prior) ME. The ME may have been preceded by and may be followed by HMEs or MDEs. The ME is not better explained by a schizophrenic/psychotic disorder. Recurrent MDEs are typical and are the most disabling part of the disorder (but not required for a diagnosis of BP-I). HMEs can also occur in BP-I.
11. BP-II diagnosis requires at least **one Hypomanic episode (HME)** and **one Major Depressive Episode (MDE)**. There has never been a ME. The HME and MDE are not better explained by a schizophrenic/psychotic disorder, and there is clinically significant distress or impairment in social, occupational, or other important areas of functioning.
12. The lifetime risk of suicide in bipolar disorders is as high as 25% to 30%.
13. Relapse rates for bipolar disorder patients are very high, even on maintenance therapy.
14. If the first mood episode of a patient with bipolar disorder is a MDE, an incorrect diagnosis of unipolar depression is likely. Treatment with the usual antidepressants can precipitate a ME and are often not effective. *A family history of bipolar disorder is an important clue that bipolar depression may be present.*
15. Selection of an antidepressant for treatment of unipolar depression depends on which symptoms are most troublesome, prior history of what was or was not effective, side effect profile, and cost.
16. With exception of sedating antidepressants, most antidepressants disturb sleep. Sedating tricyclic antidepressants (amitriptyline, imipramine, doxepin [low dose]), mirtazapine, and trazodone (low dose) may improve sleep quality. Most antidepressants, with the exception of mirtazapine and trazodone, significantly increase the REM latency. There is conflicting and limited data on bupropion but this medication also has relatively minor effects on REM sleep.
17. Most patients with nocturnal panic attacks have similar episodes during the day. However, panic attacks can occur mainly at night and must be differentiated from NREM parasomnias such as sleep terrors. The patient awakens with a panic attack but *experiences the attack in an awake state.* Unlike in sleep terrors, the patient experiencing a nocturnal panic attack is not confused, and unlike a sleep terror, the return to sleep is delayed. *A panic attack is not a disorder but an episode frequently occurring in patients with panic disorder.*
18. The treatment of panic disorder includes cognitive-behavioral psychotherapy/relaxation techniques, an SSRI (e.g., paroxetine or sertraline), and an anti-anxiety medication such as alprazolam or clonazepam. The SSRI is typically started in a low dose in combination with an anti-anxiety medication to prevent initial worsening of symptoms. The anti-anxiety medication can later be tapered in many cases.
19. The first-line treatment of PTSD is behavioral techniques *including prolonged exposure therapy.* Medications are second line. Recommended medications are sertraline, venlafaxine, fluoxetine, and paroxetine. Sertraline has the most consistent evidence of effectiveness. Only sertraline and paroxetine are FDA-approved medications for PTSD.
20. Disturbing nightmares are a significant problem impairing sleep in PTSD. Behavioral treatments such as image rehearsal therapy are effective therapy for nightmares. Treatment with prazosin may be effective in some patients.

CLINICAL REVIEW QUESTIONS

1. Which of following is true about a MDE?
   A. Insomnia complaints in about 80% of patients
   B. Hypersomnia complaints in about 50% of patients
   C. Hypersomnia complaints in 60% of patients
   D. Insomnia complaints in 40% of patients

2. Which of the following is a common PSG finding during a MDE?
   A. Short sleep latency
   B. Short REM latency
   C. Increased total sleep time
   D. Short initial REM period, with few REMs

3. The most common misdiagnosis in the first episode of bipolar depression is:
   A. Anxiety disorder
   B. Substance abuse
   C. Personality disorder
   D. Unipolar depression

4. Treatment of BP-I with antidepressants may lead to:
   A. Anxiety
   B. Greater mood instability
   C. Mania induction
   D. B and C
   E. A, B, and C

5. The family of a 50-year-old man reports a recent change in his behavior for 2 weeks. He has been sleeping 5 hours per

night but seems well rested. The patient "never stops talking" and switches from one topic to another. He starts many new projects that he never completes. The patient has continued to work and manage his home responsibilities. However, the behavior is causing difficulty getting along with his wife and coworkers. He had an episode of depression about 1 year ago. What is the most likely disorder?
   A. BP-I
   B. BP-II
   C. MDD
   D. Cyclothymic disorder
6. Which of the following would be more typical for bipolar depression than for unipolar depression?
   A. Loss of appetite
   B. Hypersomnia
   C. Normal activity
   D. No family history of bipolar disorder
7. During PSG, a patient suddenly has an arousal from stage N2 sleep, sits up in bed, and appears awake. He does not return to sleep and develops tachycardia. He signals for the technologist, who comes to evaluate him. The patient is trembling and sweaty but completely alert and responsive. He reports feeling like he is about to die. What is the most likely diagnosis?
   A. Confusional arousal
   B. Nocturnal frontal lobe epilepsy
   C. Panic attack
   D. A sleep terror
8. Which of these antidepressants is associated with both a low incidence of side effects and no weight gain?
   A. Mirtazapine
   B. Bupropion
   C. Fluoxetine
   D. Escitalopram
9. What is the first-line treatment of choice for PTSD?
   A. Venlafaxine
   B. Clonazepam
   C. Prazosin
   D. Trauma-focused psychotherapies

ANSWERS

1. A. A MDE is characterized by complaints of insomnia in a majority of patients. About 20% complain of hypersomnia.
2. B. PSG in MDE shows short REM latency, long sleep latency, decreased total sleep time, and more REM sleep in the first part of the night. The first REM period may be relatively long in duration (normally short) with many eye movements (a high REM density). The first episode of REM sleep normally has few eye movements.
3. D. Unipolar depression is often diagnosed because the first mood episode in bipolar disorders may be a major depressive episode. In addition the history of a prior episode of mania or hypomania may not be elicited by the treating clinician.
4. E. Treatment with a typical antidepressant (especially without a mood stabilizer) can cause mania, mood instability, and anxiety.
5. B. The patient is able to work and is not disabled, but there has been a significant acute change in his behavior that is causing significant impairment (difficulty with relationships). He had a prior episode of depression. The best diagnosis based on information supplied in the question is BP-II given the current HME and history compatible with a previous MDE. Cyclothymic disorder is characterized by less severe symptoms for 2 years.
6. B. Hypersomnia can occur with unipolar MDD with atypical features but is more typical of bipolar depression. Hyperphagia or absence of loss of appetite is more common with bipolar then unipolar depression.
7. C. Panic attack. Panic attacks may occur abruptly out of sleep (including after arousals from sleep), but the patient experiences the symptoms while fully awake with manifestations of pounding heart, diaphoresis, and often chest pain or choking. Unlike in NREM parasomnia, the patient is not confused, and the return to sleep is usually delayed.
8. B. Bupropion is not associated with weight gain or prominent sexual side effects. Mirtazapine causes significant weight gain, and the SSRIs (fluoxetine, escitalopram) are associated with sexual side effects. Escitalopram, sertraline, and bupropion are among the best-tolerated antidepressants. However, escitalopram and sertraline can be associated with weight gain.
9. D. Trauma-focused psychotherapies such as prolonged exposure therapy are considered the first-line treatment for PTSD.[97]

SUGGESTED READING

American Psychiatric Association. *Diagnostic and Statistical Manual of Mental Disorders*. 5th ed. Arlington, VA: American Psychiatric Publishing; 2013.

Bobo WV. The diagnosis and management of bipolar i and ii disorders: clinical practice update. *Mayo Clin Proc*. 2017;92(10):1532-1551.

Boyce P, Ma C. Choosing an antidepressant. *Aust Prescr*. 2021;44(1):12-15.

Cipriani A, Furukawa TA, Salanti G, et al. Comparative efficacy and acceptability of 12 new-generation antidepressants: a multiple-treatments meta-analysis. *Lancet*. 2009;373(9665):746-758.

Kessler RC, Petukhova M, Sampson NA, et al. Twelve-month and lifetime prevalence and lifetime morbid risk of anxiety and mood disorders in the United States. *Int J Methods Psychiatr Res*. 2012;21(3):169-184.

Lee DJ, Schnitzlein CW, Wolf JP, Vythilingam M, Rasmusson AM, Hoge CW. Psychotherapy versus pharmacotherapy for posttraumatic stress disorder: systematic review and meta-analyses to determine first-line treatments. *Depress Anxiety*. 2016;33(9):792-806.

REFERENCES

1. Kessler RC, Demler O, Frank RG, et al. Prevalence and treatment of mental disorders, 1990 to 2003. *N Engl J Med*. 2005;352(24):2515-2523.
2. Kessler RC, Berglund P, Demler O, et al. National Comorbidity Survey Replication. The epidemiology of major depressive disorder: results from the National Comorbidity Survey Replication (NCS-R). *JAMA*. 2003;289(23):3095-3105.
3. Kessler RC, Berglund P, Demler O, Jin R, Merikangas KR, Walters EE. Lifetime prevalence and age-of-onset distributions of DSM-IV disorders in the National Comorbidity Survey Replication. *Arch Gen Psychiatry*. 2005;62(6):593-602. Erratum in: *Arch Gen Psychiatry*. 2005;62(7):768. Merikangas, Kathleen R [added].
4. Kessler RC, Petukhova M, Sampson NA, Zaslavsky AM, Wittchen HU. Twelve-month and lifetime prevalence and lifetime morbid risk of anxiety and mood disorders in the United States. *Int J Methods Psychiatr Res*. 2012;21(3):169-184.
5. American Psychiatric Association. *Diagnostic and Statistical Manual of Mental Disorders*. 5th ed. Arlington, VA: American Psychiatric Association; 2013.
6. Benca RM, Obermeyer WH, Thisted RA, et al. Sleep and psychiatric disorders: a meta-analysis. *Arch Gen Psychiatry*. 1992;49:651-668.
7. McGuffin P, Rijsdijk F, Andrew M, et al. The heritability of bipolar affective disorder and the genetic relationship to unipolar depression. *Arch Gen Psychiatry*. 2003;60:497-502.
8. McIntyre RS, Berk M, Brietzke E, et al. Bipolar disorders. *Lancet*. 2020;396(10265):1841-1856.
9. Beck AT, Steer RA, Brown GK. *Manual for the Beck Depression Inventory*. 2nd ed (BDI-II). San Antonio, TX: The Psychological Association; 1996.

10. Hamilton M. A rating scale for depression. *J Neurol Neurosurg Psychiatry.* 1960;23:56-62.
11. Montgomery SA, Åsberg M. A new depression scale designed to be sensitive to change. *Br J Psychiatry.* 1979;134:382-389.
12. Kroenke K, Spitzer RL, Williams JBW. The PHQ-9. Validity of a brief depression severity measure. *J Gen Intern Med.* 2001;16:606-613.
13. Kroenke K, Spitzer RL, Williams JB. The Patient Health Questionnaire-2: validity of a two-item depression screener. *Med Care.* 2003;41(11): 1284-1292.
14. Murphy MJ, Peterson MJ. Sleep disturbances in depression. *Sleep Med Clin.* 2015;10(1):17-23.
15. Franzen PL, Buysse DJ. Sleep disturbances and depression: risk relationships for subsequent depression and therapeutic implications. *Dialogues Clin Neurosci.* 2008;10(4):473-481.
16. Nutt D, Wilson S, Paterson L. Sleep disorders as core symptoms of depression. *Dialogues Clin Neurosci.* 2008;10(3):329-336.
17. Plante DT. Hypersomnia in mood disorders: a rapidly changing landscape. *Curr Sleep Med Rep.* 2015;1(2):122-130.
18. Dauvilliers Y, Lopez R, Ohayon M, Bayard S. Hypersomnia and depressive symptoms: methodological and clinical aspects. *BMC Med.* 2013; 11:78.
19. Rush AJ, Erman MK, Giles DE, et al. Polysomnographic findings in recently drug-free and clinically remitted depressed patients. *Arch Gen Psychiatry.* 1986;43:878-884.
20. Medina AB, Lechuga DA, Escandón OS, Moctezuma JV. Update of sleep alterations in depression. *Sleep Sci.* 2014;7(3):165-169.
21. Arfken CL, Joseph A, Sandhu GR, Roehrs T, Douglass AB, Boutros NN. The status of sleep abnormalities as a diagnostic test for major depressive disorder. *J Affect Disord.* 2014;156:36-45.
22. Reynolds CF III, Frank E, Houck PR, et al. Which elderly patients with remitted depression remain well with continued interpersonal psychotherapy after discontinuation of antidepressant medication? *Am J Psychiatry.* 1997;154:958-962.
23. Dombrovski AY, Mulsant BH, Houck PR, et al. Residual symptoms and recurrence during maintenance treatment of late life depression. *J Affect Disord.* 2007;103:77-82.
24. Reynolds CF III, Kupfer DJ. Sleep research in affective illness: state of the art circa 1987. *Sleep.* 1987;10(3):199-215.
25. Yang H, Sinicropi-Yao L, Chuzi S, et al. Residual sleep disturbance and risk of relapse during the continuation/maintenance phase treatment of major depressive disorder with the selective serotonin reuptake inhibitor fluoxetine. *Ann Gen Psychiatry.* 2010;9:10.
26. Nofzinger EA, Thase ME, Reynolds CF III, et al. Hypersomnia in bipolar depression: a comparison with narcolepsy using the multiple sleep latency test. *Am J Psychiatry.* 1991;148(9):1177-1781.
27. Taylor DJ, Lichstein KL, Durrence HH, Reidel BW, Bush AJ. Epidemiology of insomnia, depression, and anxiety. *Sleep.* 2005;28(11): 1457-1464.
28. Pigeon WR, Hegel M, Unützer J, et al. Is insomnia a perpetuating factor for late-life depression in the IMPACT cohort? *Sleep.* 2008;31(4):481-488.
29. Vogel GW, Vogel F, McAbee RS, Thurmond AJ. Improvement of depression by REM sleep deprivation. New findings and a theory. *Arch Gen Psychiatry.* 1980;37(3):247-253.
30. Giedke H, Schwärzler F. Therapeutic use of sleep deprivation in depression. *Sleep Med Rev.* 2002;6(5):361-377.
31. Riemann D, Krone LB, Wulff K, Nissen C. Sleep, insomnia, and depression. *Neuropsychopharmacology.* 2020;45(1):74-89.
32. Wehr TA. Sleep loss as a possible mediator of diverse causes of mania. *Br J Psychiatry.* 1991;159:576-578.
33. Dome P, Rihmer Z, Gonda X. Suicide risk in bipolar disorder: a brief review. *Medicina.* 2019;55:403. Available at: https://doi.org/10.3390/medicina55080403.
34. Miller JN, Black DW. Bipolar disorder and suicide: a review. *Curr Psychiatry Rep.* 2020;22(2):6.
35. Goldberg JF, Truman CJ. Antidepressant-induced mania: an overview of current controversies. *Bipolar Disord.* 2003;5(6):407-420.
36. Bond DJ, Noronha MM, Kauer-Sant'Anna M, Lam RW, Yatham LN. Antidepressant-associated mood elevations in bipolar II disorder compared with bipolar I disorder and major depressive disorder: a systematic review and meta-analysis. *J Clin Psychiatry.* 2008;69(10):1589-1601.
37. McInerney SJ, Kennedy SH. Review of evidence for use of antidepressants in bipolar depression. *Prim Care Companion CNS Disord.* 2014;16(5):10.4088/PCC.14r01653.
38. Baldessarini RJ, Faedda GL, Offidani E, et al. Antidepressant-associated mood-switching and transition from unipolar major depression to bipolar disorder: a review. *J Affect Disord.* 2013;148(1):129-135.
39. Mitchell PB, Goodwin GM, Johnson GF, Hirschfeld RMA. Diagnostic guidelines for bipolar depression: a probabilistic approach. *Bipolar Disord.* 2008;10:144-152.
40. Hudson JI, Lipinski JF, Keck Jr PE, et al. Polysomnographic characteristics of young manic patients: comparison with unipolar depressed patients and normal control subjects. *Arch Gen Psychiatry.* 1992;49:378-383.
41. Hudson JI, Lipinski JF, Frankenburg FR, et al. Electroencephalographic sleep in mania. *Arch Gen Psychiatry.* 1988;45:267-273.
42. Uher R, Pallaskorpi S, Suominen K, Mantere O, Pavlova B, Isometsä E. Clinical course predicts long-term outcomes in bipolar disorder. *Psychol Med.* 2019;49(7):1109-1117.
43. Altamura AC, Mundo E, Dell'Osso B, Tacchini G, Buoli M, Calabrese JR. Quetiapine and classical mood stabilizers in the long-term treatment of Bipolar Disorder: a 4-year follow-up naturalistic study. *J Affect Disord.* 2008;110(1-2):135-141.
44. Kessing LV, Andersen PK, Vinberg M. Risk of recurrence after a single manic or mixed episode: a systematic review and meta-analysis. *Bipolar Disord.* 2018;20(1):9-17.
45. Boyce P, Ma C. Choosing an antidepressant. *Aust Prescr.* 2021;44(1):12-15.
46. Kok RM, Reynolds CF III. Management of depression in older adults: a review. *JAMA.* 2017;317(20):2114-2122.
47. Kennedy SH, Lam RW, McIntyre RS, et al. CANMAT Depression Work Group. Canadian Network for Mood and Anxiety Treatments (CANMAT) 2016 clinical guidelines for the management of adults with major depressive disorder: section 3. Pharmacological treatments. *Can J Psychiatry.* 2016;61(9):540-560. Erratum in: *Can J Psychiatry.* 2017;62(5):356.
48. Cipriani A, Furukawa TA, Salanti G, et al. Comparative efficacy and acceptability of 12 new-generation antidepressants: a multiple-treatments meta-analysis. *Lancet.* 2009;373(9665):746-758.
49. Cipriani A, Furukawa TA, Salanti G, et al. Comparative efficacy and acceptability of 21 antidepressant drugs for the acute treatment of adults with major depressive disorder: a systematic review and network meta-analysis. *Lancet.* 2018;391(10128):1357-1366.
50. Sabri MA, Saber-Ayad. *MAO Inhbitors.* StatPealrs. Available at: https://www.ncbi.nlm.nih.gov/books/NBK557395/.
51. Suchting R, Tirumalajaru V, Gareeb R, et al. Revisiting monoamine oxidase inhibitors for the treatment of depressive disorders: a systematic review and network meta-analysis. *J Affect Disord.* 2021;282:1153-1160.
52. Shulman KI, Herrmann N, Walker SE. Current place of monoamine oxidase inhibitors in the treatment of depression. *CNS Drugs.* 2013;27(10):789-797. doi:10.1007/s40263-013-0097-3.
53. Gillman PK. Tricyclic antidepressant pharmacology and therapeutic drug interactions updated. *Br J Pharmacol.* 2007;151(6):737-748.
54. Schneider J, Patterson M, Jimenez XF. Beyond depression: other uses for tricyclic antidepressants. *Cleve Clin J Med.* 2019;86(12):807-814.
55. Gandhi S, Shariff SZ, Al-Jaishi A, et al. Second-generation antidepressants and hyponatremia risk: a population-based cohort study of older adults. *Am J Kidney Dis.* 2017;69(1):87-96.
56. Behlke LM, Lenze EJ, Carney RM. The cardiovascular effects of newer antidepressants in older adults and those with or at high risk for cardiovascular diseases. *CNS Drugs.* 2020;34(11):1133-1147.
57. Ali MK, Lam RW. Comparative efficacy of escitalopram in the treatment of major depressive disorder. *Neuropsychiatr Dis Treat.* 2011;7:39-49.
58. Kent JM. SNaRIs, NaSSAs, and NaRIs: new agents for the treatment of depression. *Lancet.* 2000;355:911-918.
59. Berigan TR. The many uses of bupropion and bupropion sustained release (SR) in adults. *Prim Care Companion J Clin Psychiatry.* 2002;4(1): 30-32. doi:10.4088/pcc.v04n0110a.
60. Luft MJ, Dobson ET, Levine A, Croarkin PE, Strawn JR. Pharmacologic interventions for antidepressant-induced sexual dysfunction: a systematic review and network meta-analysis of trials using the Arizona sexual experience scale. *CNS Spectr.* 2021:1-10.
61. Coleman CC, King BR, Bolden-Watson C, et al. A placebo-controlled comparison of the effects on sexual functioning of bupropion sustained release and fluoxetine. *Clin Ther.* 2001;23:1040-1058.
62. Landén M, Eriksson E, Agren H, Fahlén T. Effect of buspirone on sexual dysfunction in depressed patients treated with selective serotonin reuptake inhibitors. *J Clin Psychopharmacol.* 1999;19(3):268-271.
63. Reed CR, Kajdasz DK, Whalen H, Athanasiou MC, Gallipoli S, Thase ME. The efficacy profile of vilazodone, a novel antidepressant for the treatment of major depressive disorder. *Curr Med Res Opin.* 2012;28(1):27-39.
64. Connolly KR, Thase ME. Vortioxetine: a new treatment for major depressive disorder. *Expert Opin Pharmacother.* 2016;17(3):421-431.
65. D'Agostino A, English CD, Rey JA. Vortioxetine (brintellix): a new serotonergic antidepressant. *P T.* 2015;40(1):36-40.

66. Ionescu DF, Rosenbaum JF, Alpert JE. Pharmacological approaches to the challenge of treatment-resistant depression. *Dialogues Clin Neurosci.* 2015;17(2):111-126.
67. Nuñez NA, Joseph B, Pahwa M, et al. Augmentation strategies for treatment resistant major depression: a systematic review and network meta-analysis. *J Affect Disord.* 2022;302:385-400.
68. McIntyre RS, Filteau MJ, Martin L, et al. Treatment-resistant depression: definitions, review of the evidence, and algorithmic approach. *J Affect Disord.* 2014;156:1-7.
69. Chen J, Gao K, Kemp DE. Second-generation antipsychotics in major depressive disorder: update and clinical perspective. *Curr Opin Psychiatry.* 2011;24:10-17.
70. Anderson IM, Sarsfield A, Haddad PM. Efficacy, safety and tolerability of quetiapine augmentation in treatment resistant depression: an open-label, pilot study. *J Affect Disord.* 2009;117:116-119.
71. Abolfazli R, Hosseini M, Ghanizadeh A, et al. Double-blind randomized parallel-group clinical trial of efficacy of the combination fluoxetine plus modafinil versus fluoxetine plus placebo in the treatment of major depression. *Depress Anxiety.* 2011;28:297-302.
72. Bortnick B, El-Khalili N, Banov M, et al. Efficacy and tolerability of extended release quetiapine fumarate (quetiapine XR) monotherapy in major depressive disorder: a placebo- controlled, randomized study. *J Affect Disord.* 2011;128:83-94.
73. Cha DS, Luo X, Ahmed J, Becirovic L, Cha RH, McIntyre RS. Brexpiprazole as an augmentation agent to antidepressants in treatment resistant major depressive disorder. *Expert Rev Neurother.* 2019;19(9):777-783.
74. Mayers AG, Baldwin DS. Antidepressants and their effect on sleep. *Hum Psychopharmacol.* 2005;20:533-559.
75. Winokur A, Gary KA, Rodner S, et al. Depression, sleep physiology, and antidepressant drugs. *Depress Anxiety.* 2001;14:19-28.
76. Gursky JT, Krahn LE. The effects of antidepressants on sleep: a review. *Harvard Rev Psychiatry.* 2000;8:298-306.
77. Nofzinger EA, Reynolds CF III, Thase ME, et al. REM sleep enhancement by bupropion in depressed men. *Am J Psychiatry.* 1995;152(2):274-276. doi:10.1176/ajp.152.2.274.
78. Rye DB, Dihenia B, Bliwise DL. Reversal of atypical depression, sleepiness, and REM-sleep propensity in narcolepsy with bupropion. *Depress Anxiety.* 1998;7(2):92-95.
79. Ott GE, Rao U, Lin KM, Gertsik L, Poland RE. Effect of treatment with bupropion on EEG sleep: relationship to antidepressant response. *Int J Neuropsychopharmacol.* 2004;7(3):275-281.
80. Gillin JC, Rapaport M, Erman MK, et al. A comparison of nefazodone and fluoxetine on mood and on objective, subjective, and clinician-rated measures of sleep in depressed patients. *J Clin Psychiatry.* 1997;58:186-192.
81. Nierenberg AA, Adler LA, Peselow E, et al. Trazodone for antidepressant-associated insomnia. *Am J Psychiatry.* 1994;151:1069.
82. Fava M, McCall WV, Krystal A, et al. Eszopiclone co-administered with fluoxetine in patients with insomnia coexisting with major depressive disorder. *Biol Psychiatry.* 2006;59(11):1052-1060.
83. Fava M, Asnis GM, Shrivastava RK, et al. Improved insomnia symptoms and sleep-related next-day functioning in patients with comorbid major depressive disorder and insomnia following concomitant zolpidem extended-release 12.5 mg and escitalopram treatment: a randomized controlled trial. *J Clin Psychiatry.* 2011;72(7):914-928.
84. Carney CE, Edinger JD, Kuchibhatla M, et al. Cognitive behavioral insomnia therapy for those with insomnia and depression: a randomized controlled clinical trial. *Sleep.* 2017;40(4):zsx019.
85. Manber R, Buysse DJ, Edinger J, et al. Efficacy of cognitive-behavioral therapy for insomnia combined with antidepressant pharmacotherapy in patients with comorbid depression and insomnia: a randomized controlled trial. *J Clin Psychiatry.* 2016;77(10):e1316-e1323.
86. Goodwin GM, Haddad PM, Ferrier IN, et al. Evidence-based guidelines for treating bipolar disorder: revised third edition recommendations from the British Association for Psychopharmacology. *J Psychopharmacol.* 2016; 30(6):495-553.
87. Yatham LN, Kennedy SH, Parikh SV, et al. Canadian Network for Mood and Anxiety Treatments (CANMAT) and International Society for Bipolar Disorders (ISBD) 2018 guidelines for the management of patients with bipolar disorder. *Bipolar Disord.* 2018;20(2):97-170.
88. Geddes JR, Miklowitz DJ. Treatment of bipolar disorder. *Lancet.* 2013;381(9878):1672-1682.
89. Malhi GS, Bell E, Boyce P, et al. The 2020 Royal Australian and New Zealand College of psychiatrists clinical practice guidelines for mood disorders: bipolar disorder summary. *Bipolar Disord.* 2020;22(8): 805-821. doi:10.1111/bdi.13036.
90. Sachs GS, Nierenberg AA, Calabrese JR, et al. Effectiveness of adjunctive antidepressant treatment for bipolar depression. *N Engl J Med.* 2007;356:1711-1722.
91. Mellman TA, Uhde TW. Patients with frequent sleep panic: clinical findings and response to medication treatment. *J Clin Psychiatry.* 1990;51(12):513-516.
92. Craske MG, Tsao JC. Assessment and treatment of nocturnal panic attacks. *Sleep Med Rev.* 2005;9(3):173-184.
93. Thurnheer R, Henz S, Knoblauch A. Sleep-related laryngospasm. *Eur Respir J.* 1997;10(9):2084-2086.
94. Nutt DJ. Overview of diagnosis and drug treatments of anxiety disorders. *CNS Spectr.* 2005;10(1):49-56.
95. Chawla N, Anothaisintawee T, Charoenrungrueangchai K, et al. Drug treatment for panic disorder with or without agoraphobia: systematic review and network meta-analysis of randomised controlled trials. *BMJ.* 2022;376:e066084.
96. Ziffra M. Panic disorder: a review of treatment options. *Ann Clin Psychiatry.* 2021;33(2):124-133.
97. Zhang B, Wang C, Cui L, et al. Short-term efficacy and tolerability of paroxetine versus placebo for panic disorder: a meta-analysis of randomized controlled trials. *Front Pharmacol.* 2020;11:275.
98. Ait-Daoud N, Hamby AS, Sharma S, Blevins D. A review of alprazolam use, misuse, and withdrawal. *J Addict Med.* 2018;12(1):4-10.
99. Fava M, Asnis GM, Shrivastava R, et al. Zolpidem extended-release improves sleep and next-day symptoms in comorbid insomnia and generalized anxiety disorder. *J Clin Psychopharmacol.* 2009;29(3):222-230.
100. Goodwin GM, Stein DJ. Generalised anxiety disorder and depression: contemporary treatment approaches. *Adv Ther.* 2021;38(suppl 2):45-51.
101. Davidson JR, Zhang W, Connor KM, et al. A psychopharmacological treatment algorithm for generalised anxiety disorder (GAD). *J Psychopharmacol.* 2010;24(1):3-26.
102. Schrader C, Ross A. A review of PTSD and current treatment strategies. *Mo Med.* 2021;118(6):546-551.
103. Ross RJ, Ball WA, Dinges DR, et al. Rapid eye movement sleep disturbance in posttraumatic stress disorder. *Biol Psychiatry.* 1994;35:195-202.
104. Mellman TA, Nolan B, Hedding J, et al. A polysomnographic comparison of veterans with combat-related PTSD, depressed men, and non-ill controls. *Sleep.* 1997;20:46-51.
105. Brown TM, Boudewyns PA. Periodic limb movements of sleep in combat veterans with posttraumatic stress disorder. *J Trauma Stress.* 1996;9:129-136.
106. Lee DJ, Schnitzlein CW, Wolf JP, Vythilingam M, Rasmusson AM, Hoge CW. Psychotherapy versus pharmacotherapy for posttraumatic stress disorder: systematic review and meta-analyses to determine first-line treatments. *Depress Anxiety.* 2016;33(9):792-806.
107. Robert S, Hamner MB, Ulmer HG, et al. Open-label trial of escitalopram in the treatment of posttraumatic stress disorder. *J Clin Psychiatry.* 2006;67:1522-1526.
108. Zoellner LA, Roy-Byrne PP, Mavissakalian M, Feeny NC. Doubly randomized preference trial of prolonged exposure versus sertraline for treatment of PTSD. *Am J Psychiatry.* 2019;176(4):287-296.
109. Orr JE, Smales C, Alexander TH, et al. Treatment of OSA with CPAP is associated with improvement in PTSD symptoms among veterans. *J Clin Sleep Med.* 2017;13(1):57-63.
110. Morgenthaler TI, Aurebach S, Casey KR, et al. Position paper for the treatment of nightmare disorder in adults: an American Academy of Sleep Medicine position paper. *J Clin Sleep Med.* 2018;14(6): 1041-1055.
111. Krakow B, Hollifield M, Johnston L, et al. Imagery rehearsal therapy for chronic nightmares in sexual assault survivors with post traumatic stress disorder. *JAMA.* 2001;286:537-545.
112. Raskind MA, Peskind ER, Hoff DJ, et al. A parallel group placebo-controlled study of prazosin for trauma nightmares and sleep disturbance in combat veterans with post-traumatic stress disorder. *Biol Psychiatry.* 2007;61:928-934.
113. Raskind MA, Peskind ER, Chow B, et al. Trial of prazosin for post-traumatic stress disorder in military veterans. *N Engl J Med.* 2018;378(6): 507-517.
114. Zhang Y, Ren R, Sanford LD, et al. The effects of prazosin on sleep disturbances in post-traumatic stress disorder: a systematic review and meta-analysis. *Sleep Med.* 2020;67:225-231.
115. *FDA Permits Marketing of New Device Designed to Reduce Sleep Disturbance Related to Nightmares in Certain Adults.* Available at: https://www.fda.gov/news-events/press-announcements/fda-permits-marketing-new-device-designed-reduce-sleep-disturbance-related-nightmares-certain-adults.

Chapter

38 Sleep and Nonrespiratory Physiology

INTRODUCTION

This chapter reviews aspects of endocrine, gastrointestinal, and renal physiology of interest to the sleep clinician. It is not a comprehensive review of any area. The emphasis is on the interaction between sleep and physiology.

ENDOCRINE PHYSIOLOGY AND SLEEP

The timing of the secretion of important hormones with respect to sleep and circadian control is briefly reviewed. The secretion of some hormones is tied to sleep, whereas others are under circadian control[1,2] (Table 38–1). A common strategy to determine whether sleep or circadian influence predominates is to move the timing of sleep and determine what happens to the pattern of hormone secretion.

Growth Hormone

Growth hormone (GH) is secreted by somatotroph cells of the anterior pituitary under hypothalamic control. GH secretion is increased by GHRH (growth hormone releasing hormone) and decreased by somatostatin, both secreted by the hypothalamus. GH secretion is also increased by acylated ghrelin (ghrelin is secreted by the stomach) (Figure 38–1). The most reliable burst of GH secretion is associated with the first slow wave sleep (SWS) cycle (any time of the day).[1-7] This is associated with increased GHRH and *decreased* somatostatin. Somatostatin is also known as growth hormone–inhibiting hormone (GHIH). Estrogens also play an important role in modulating GH secretion. Integrated 24-hour GH concentration is significantly higher in women than in men and greater in young versus older adults.

Table 38–1 Summary of Control of Major Hormones		
Hormone	**Primary**	**Secondary**
GH	Sleep (stimulatory, onset stage N3)	Weak positive circadian effect (increased GH secretion at night)—low somatostatin?
Prolactin	Sleep (stimulatory)	Circadian effect—sleep is more stimulatory when it occurs at night
ACTH, cortisol	Circadian (peaks around 7 am)	Sleep inhibitory
TSH	Circadian (peaks around 2 am)	Sleep inhibitory

The mnemonic GPSATC represents **G**rowth Hormone/**P**rolactin—**S**leep, **A**drenal/**T**hyroid—**C**ircadian. *ACTH,* Adrenocorticotropic hormone; *GH,* growth hormone; *TSH,* thyroid-stimulating hormone.

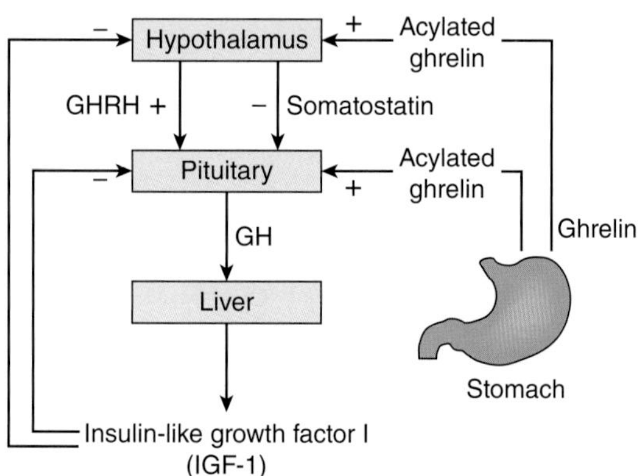

Figure 38–1 Schematic of the control of growth hormone (GH) secretion. Acylated ghrelin is the active form of ghrelin that increases GH secretion. *GHRH,* Growth hormone releasing hormone.

Box 38–1 GROWTH HORMONE AND SLEEP

Men: Sleep-onset GH pulse is generally the largest, and often the only, secretory pulse observed over the 24-hour span.

Women: Daytime GH pulses are more frequent, and the sleep-associated pulse, although still present in the vast majority of individual profiles, does not account for the majority of the 24-hour secretory output.

- GH secretion is tied to **sleep onset** (start of stage N3 sleep) rather than time of day.
- Amount of GH secretion correlates with length of stage N3 episodes.
- Weak circadian effect (increased GH secretion at night).

GH, Growth hormone.

In healthy adults, the 24-hour profile of plasma GH consists of stable low levels abruptly interrupted by bursts of secretion (Box 38–1; Figures 38–2 and 38–3). The most reproducible GH pulse occurs shortly after sleep onset with maximum levels within a few minutes of the onset of stage N3 sleep. In men, the sleep-onset GH pulse is the largest and often the only secretory pulse over the 24-hour day. In women, daytime GH pulses are more frequent, and the sleep-onset pulse does not account for the majority of the 24-hour secretory output (Figure 38–2). The amount of GH released is proportional to slow wave activity. Figure 38–3 shows a large burst of GH secretion after sleep onset in a male individual. During the next nighttime period, the subject is awake and there is only a small increase in GH secretion (during the same nighttime period). The subject is allowed to sleep at 10 AM, and sleep onset is followed by a large burst in GH secretion. This pattern is consistent with a sleep-related GH secretion (rather than

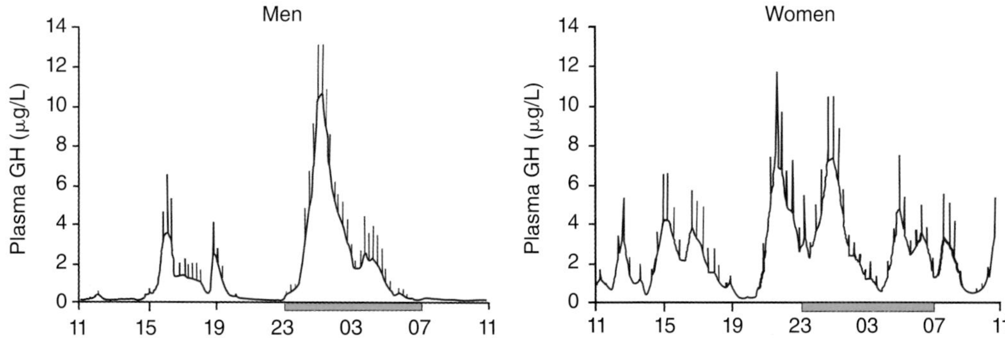

Figure 38–2 Growth hormone (GH) secretion in a group of young men *(left)* and women *(right)*. The plots are mean values. The *light blue bar* is the sleep period. Men have most of their GH secretion during sleep, but in women, bursts during the day are more common. (From Van Cauter E, Plat L, Copinschi G. Interrelations between sleep and the somatotropic axis. *Sleep*. 1998;21:553-566.)

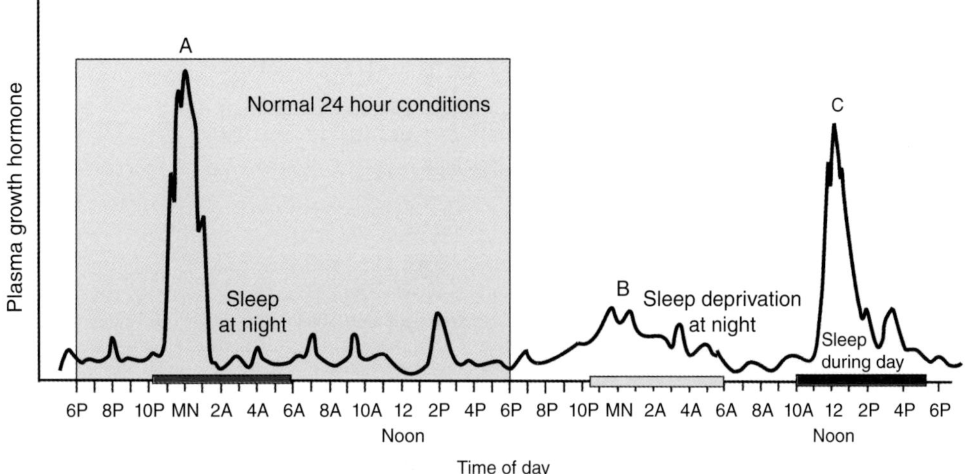

Figure 38–3 A schematic illustrating the pattern of growth hormone (GH) secretion in a male individual. **(A)** A large burst of GH secretion is seen soon after sleep onset. The following night **(B)** the individual is kept awake and there is only a small increase in GH secretion. However, when the individual is allowed to sleep during the following day **(C)**, there is a large burst of secretion of GH shortly after sleep onset. This pattern shows GH secretion is mainly associated with sleep rather than the time of day. There is a smaller circadian component increasing GH secretion at night. The red bar is sleep at night, the grey bar sleep deprivation at night, and the blue bar sleep during the day.

circadian or time of day). Even in individuals without daytime napping, after sleep deprivation, the blunting of the normal sleep-related GH pulse is compensated during the day. Consequently, the amount of GH secreted during a 24-hour period is similar whether or not a person has slept during the night.

Etiology of Sleep-Related GH Burst

The sleep-related burst of GH secretion is due to increased GHRH activity during stage N3 sleep and decreased somatostatin. There is a *secondary circadian peak in GH* at the time of normal sleep (slight increase in GH secretion occurs at night even when individuals are awake) likely due to a decrease in somatostatin. Of interest, ghrelin is also highest at night (peaks during first part of the night) and could contribute to the weak circadian component to control of GH release. An acetyl chain (octanoate residue) is added to ghrelin by the enzyme ghrelin-O-acyltransferase before it can bind GH secretagogue receptors. Acylated ghrelin does increase slightly with sleep at night but much less than total ghrelin, and one study felt this represents inhibition of acylated ghrelin production by sleep[5] (Figure 38–4).

GHRH and GH—Effects on Sleep

Injections of **GHRH** increased the amount of stage N3 sleep and slow wave activity (electroencephalogram [EEG] spectral power in the delta range) in animal studies.[8] In humans the findings are discrepant. The effects of GHRH may depend on the timing of administration, the dose, and the duration of administration. A major issue is that GHRH also increases GH, which has effects on sleep. A review published in 2004 concluded that GHRH likely increases NREM sleep and that the increase in REM sleep in some studies depends on the increase of GH by GHRH[9].

Medications that increase stage N3 sleep increase GH secretion. Conversely, injections of **GH** appear to consistently enhance rapid eye movement (REM) sleep in animal models. However, in normal human studies results have been inconsistent.[4,9] Mendelson et al.[8] found an increase in REM sleep after GH injection 15 minutes before bedtime. Another study in human participants administered intravenous GH three hours before bedtime found no change in sleep architecture.[4]

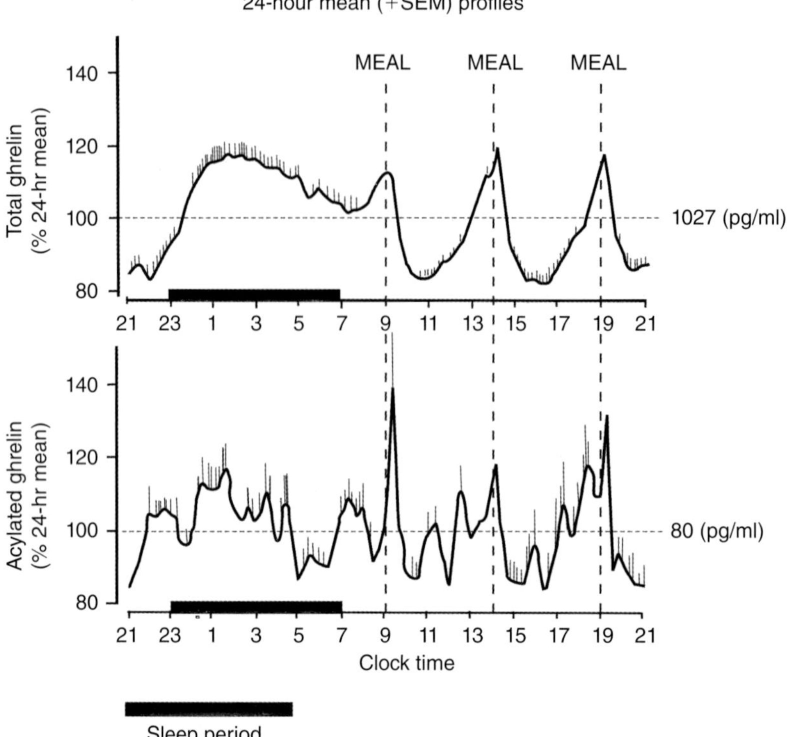

Figure 38–4 The 24-hour profile (time course) of ghrelin and acylated ghrelin during a controlled experiment with evenly spaced meals. Values are expressed as a proportion of the 24 hour mean. Total *ghrelin increases at night during sleep (dark bar).* Note the large drop after meals. However, acylated ghrelin (the active form) increases only slightly at night suggesting an inhibitory effect of sleep. (From Spiegel K, Tasali E, Leproult R, Scherberg N, Van Cauter E. Twenty-four-hour profiles of acylated and total ghrelin: relationship with glucose levels and impact of time of day and sleep. *J Clin Endocrinol Metab.* 2011;96(2):486-493.)

Changes in GH Secretion With Age

The nocturnal increase in GH decreases with age in parallel with the decrease in the amount of stage N3 sleep (Figure 38–5).[4]

Sleep and the Corticotropic Axis

The adrenal glands secrete cortisol under the control of **pituitary** adrenocorticotropic hormone (ACTH).[1,2] Secretion of ACTH is stimulated by hypothalamic corticotropin-releasing hormone (CRH) (Figure 38–6). There is strong circadian control of ACTH secretion (and cortisol secretion). The plasma levels of cortisol and ACTH *peak in the early morning* and decline during the day (Box 38–2; Figure 38–7). *The nadir of cortisol and ACTH levels is during the first part (one-third) of sleep.* The levels start to climb a few hours before waking. During shifted sleep, the cortisol rhythm remains tied to clock time. There is a weak sleep-related component. The *presence of sleep causes slight inhibition* and maintains low levels early in the sleep period (Figure 38–8). Sleep onset is reliably associated with a short-term inhibition of cortisol secretion. Under normal conditions, because cortisol secretion is already quiescent in the late evening, this inhibitory effect of sleep, which is temporally associated with stage N3 sleep,[10] prolongs the

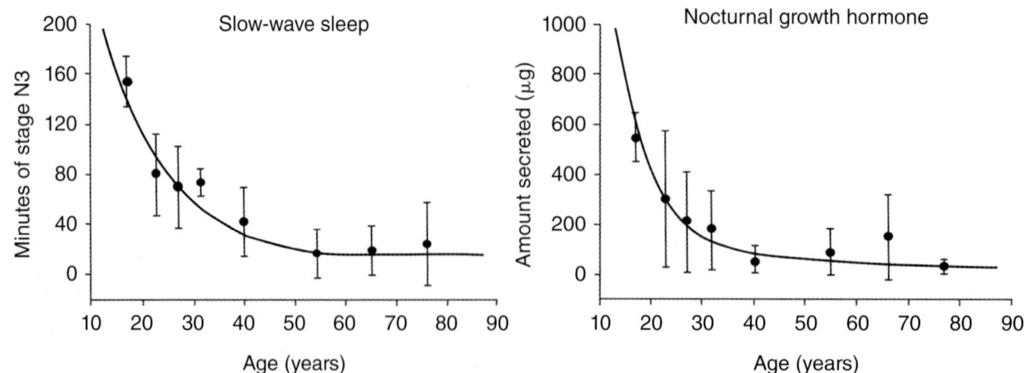

Figure 38–5 Patterns of the amount of slow wave sleep (SWS, stage N3) and nocturnal growth hormone (GH) secretion throughout aging, obtained in 102 healthy nonobese men, ages 18 to 83 years, who were grouped according to age bracket (mean ± SEM for each age bracket). GH decreases with age in parallel to the amount of SWS. (Data from Van Cauter E, Plat L, Copinschi G. Interrelations between sleep and the somatotropic axis. *Sleep.* 1998;21:553-566.)

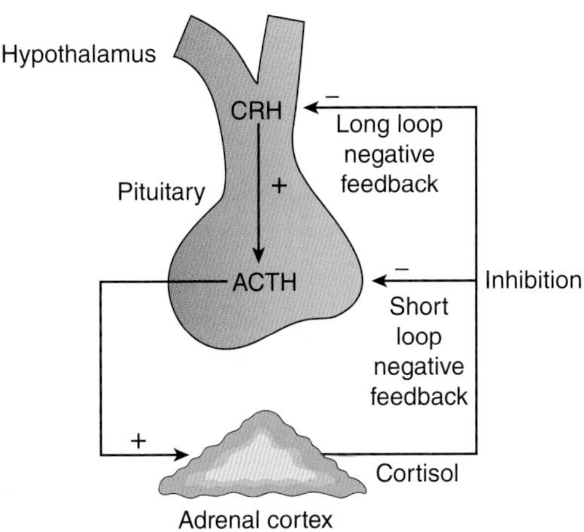

Figure 38–6 Schematic of control of adrenocorticotropic hormone (ACTH) and cortisol secretion. *CRH*, Corticotropin-releasing hormone.

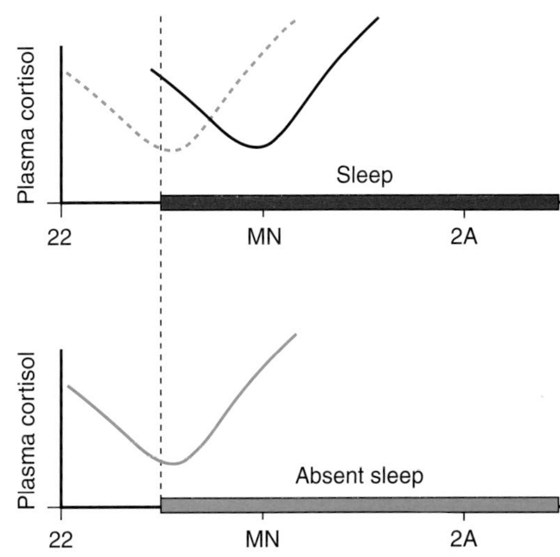

Figure 38–8 A schematic illustrating that sleep is inhibitory for cortisol secretion. Two examples of the same time of night. When sleep is present, it is inhibitory on cortisol secretion. When sleep is absent, the rise in cortisol starts earlier.

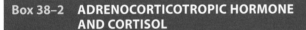

Box 38–2 ADRENOCORTICOTROPIC HORMONE AND CORTISOL

- Under circadian control
- Nadir shortly after the typical time of sleep onset (does not depend on sleep)
- Peak levels in the early morning then decline over the day
- The overall shape of the corticotropic profile is not markedly affected by the absence of sleep or by sleep at an unusual time of day
- During sleep deprivation, the nocturnal cortisol is higher (amplitude of oscillation is reduced, i.e., early night not as low, early morning not as high)

quiescent period. Conversely, awakening at the end of the sleep period is consistently followed by a pulse of cortisol secretion, often referred to as the "cortisol awakening response."[11]

Sleep Deprivation and Sleep Loss on Cortisol

Sleep deprivation induces a 15% decrease in amplitude of the 24-hour cortisol rhythm (i.e., the peak to trough of excursion is smaller). The rapid effects of sleep onset and sleep offset on corticotropic activity are absent. The nadir of cortisol level is slightly higher than during nocturnal sleep deprivation (because of the absence of the inhibitory effects of the first hours of sleep), and the morning maximal peak is slightly lower (because of the absence of the stimulating effects of morning awakening). A night of sleep deprivation induces less recovery (less impact on morning stimulation by ACTH) but is associated with higher evening cortisol levels (Figure 38–9; see also Box 38–2).[12,13] Older adults tend to have higher evening cortisol levels.[14]

Sleep and the Thyroid Axis

TSH stimulates the thyroid gland to secrete the hormones thyroxine (T4) and triiodothyronine (T3). TSH production is controlled by thyrotropin-releasing hormone (TRH), which is manufactured in the hypothalamus and transported to the anterior pituitary gland where it stimulates TSH production and release[2] (Figure 38–10). Somatostatin is also produced by the hypothalamus and has an opposite effect on the pituitary production of TSH, decreasing or inhibiting its release.

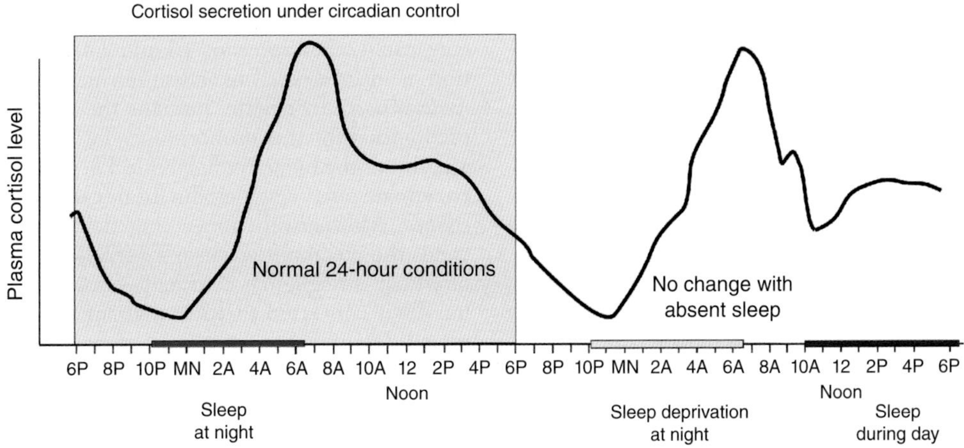

Figure 38–7 A schematic showing cortisol secretion versus time of day and sleep. The plasma cortisol remains largely synchronized to clock time even when sleep is shifted, indicating a predominant role of circadian rhythmicity in the control of hypothalamus-pituitary-adrenal axis activity.

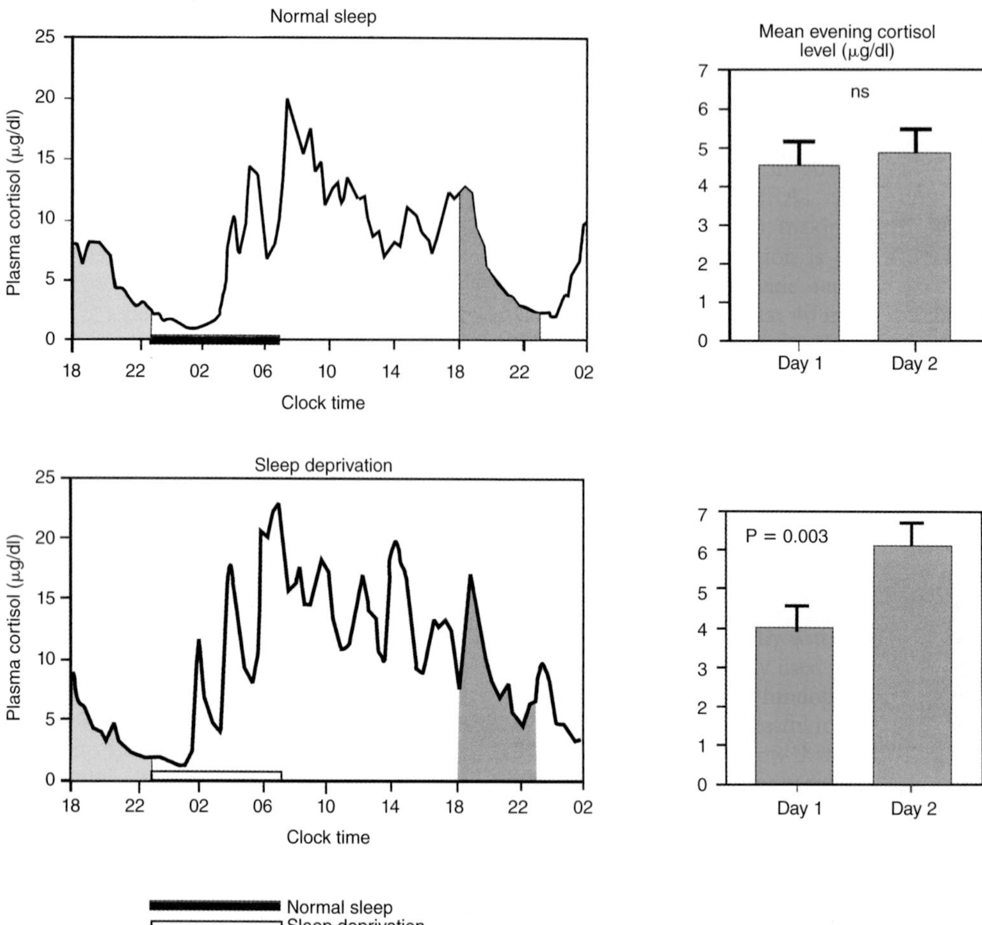

Figure 38–9 During sleep deprivation, the nocturnal cortisol is greater. Mean profiles of plasma cortisol for two groups of healthy young subjects during a 32-hour period with normal sleep *(upper panel)* and sleep deprivation *(lower panel)*. The *dark blue bar* represents the sleep period. The *shaded areas* represent cortisol secretion between 18:00 and 23:00 on Day 1 *(light blue)* and Day 2 *(gray)* before and after the night of normal sleep or the night of sleep deprivation. The mean of these areas determines the mean evening cortisol level *(bar graphs)*. In the *top panel*, the mean of the two *shaded areas* is virtually identical (bar graph to the right of the upper panel). In the *bottom panel*, sleep deprivation results in an increase in the mean evening cortisol level (bar graph to the right of the bottom panel). Thus sleep deprivation results in a higher late evening cortisol level. (From Van Cauter E. Endocrine physiology. In: Kryger MH, Roth T, Dement WC, eds. *Principles and Practice of Sleep Medicine.* Elsevier; 2005.)

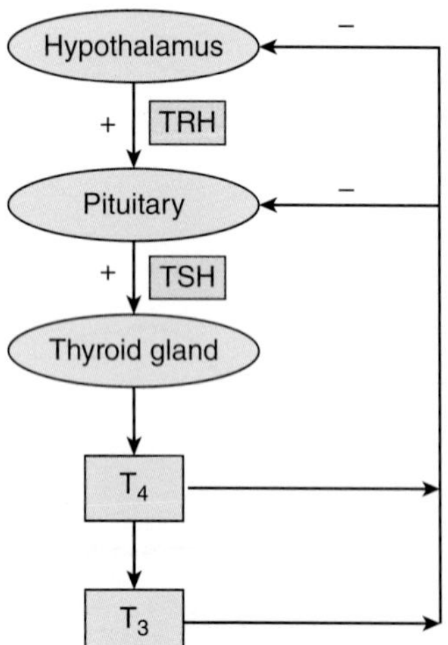

Figure 38–10 Schematic of the control of thyroid-stimulating hormone (TSH) secretion. There is negative feedback from the produced thyroid hormone at the pituitary and hypothalamic levels. *TRH,* Thyrotropin-releasing hormone; *T3,* triiodothyronine; *T4,* thyroxine.

The level of thyroid hormones (T3 and T4) in the blood has an effect on the pituitary release of TSH. When the levels of T3 and T4 are low, the production of TSH is increased, and conversely, when levels of T3 and T4 are high, TSH production is decreased. This effect creates a *regulatory negative feedback loop*. In healthy humans the thyroid gland produces predominantly the prohormone T4 together with a small amount of the bioactive hormone T3. Most T3 is produced by enzymatic outer ring deiodination (ORD) of T4 in peripheral tissues. Alternatively, inner ring deiodination (IRD) of T4 yields the metabolite reverse T3 (rT3), the thyroidal secretion of which is negligible. Normally, about one-third of circulating T4 is converted to T3 and about one-third to rT3.[15] The remainder of T4 is metabolized by different pathways, in particular glucuronidation and sulfation.

TSH Secretion

Daytime levels of plasma TSH are low and relatively stable. There is a rapid elevation of TSH starting in the early evening and culminating in a nocturnal maximum occurring around the end of the first third (beginning) of the sleep period (Box 38–3; Figure 38–11).[2] The latter part of the sleep period is associated with a progressive decline in TSH. *Because the nocturnal rise in TSH occurs well before the time of sleep onset, it likely reflects a circadian effect. Sleep exerts an inhibitory influence on TSH secretion*, and sleep deprivation relieves this inhibition resulting in higher TSH during the normal time of sleep. The inhibition of TSH by sleep is greatest during stage N3 sleep, and the inhibition is greater on recovery sleep from prior sleep deprivation (more stage N3, higher delta power).

The suppression of TSH by sleep depends on the time of day. When sleep occurs during daytime hours, TSH secretion is not suppressed significantly below normal daytime levels. Thus the inhibitory effect of sleep on TSH secretion appears to be operative when the nighttime elevation has taken place, indicating an interaction of the effects of circadian time and the effects of sleep. Awakenings interrupting nocturnal sleep appear to relieve the inhibition of TSH and are consistently associated with a short-term TSH elevation.

Thyroid Hormone Levels

Circadian and sleep-related variations in thyroid hormones have been difficult to demonstrate. Thyroid hormones are bound to serum proteins, and thus peripheral concentrations are affected by diurnal variations in hemodilution caused by postural changes. However, under conditions of sleep deprivation, the increased amplitude of the TSH rhythm may result in a detectable increase in plasma T3 levels, paralleling the nocturnal TSH rise.

Box 38–3 THYROID-STIMULATING HORMONE AND THE THYROID AXIS

- Circadian control
- Peak in the first third of the typical sleep period (around midnight to 1 AM)
- Stable level during the day
- Sleep inhibitory at night (higher at night if no sleep)

Prolactin Secretion and Sleep

Prolactin Secretion

Prolactin is a polypeptide hormone responsible for lactation and breast development. Pituitary prolactin (PRL) secretion is regulated by neuroendocrine neurons in the hypothalamus, the most important ones being the neurosecretory tuberoinfundibular (TIDA) neurons of the arcuate nucleus, which secrete dopamine to act on the dopamine-2 receptors on lactotrophs, *causing inhibition of PRL secretion* (Figure 38–12).[2] Neurons in the hypothalamus also produce thyrotropin-releasing factor (TRH), which has a stimulatory effect on PRL release. In the absence of pregnancy (ie, high estrogen) or lactation in sexually mature females, prolactin is constitutively inhibited by dopamine, and the effect of dopamine trumps the effect of minimal stimulatory effects of TRH. Dopamine antagonists can increase PRL secretion. Dopamine agonists can reduce PRL secretion. PRL levels

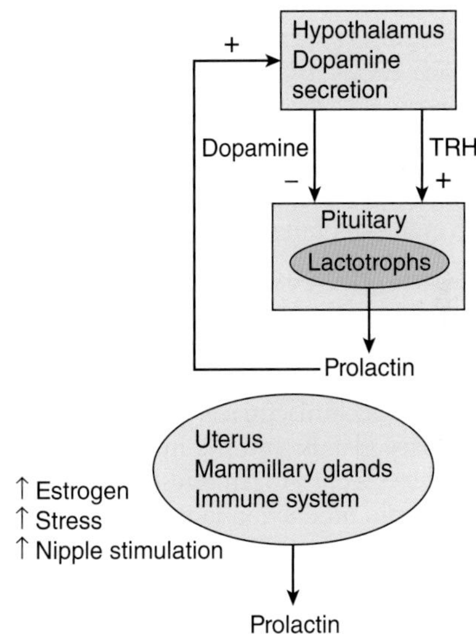

Figure 38–12 Schematic of control of prolactin secretion. Prolactin secretion is chronically inhibited by dopamine signaling from the hypothalamus. Thyrotropin-releasing hormone (TRH) stimulates release. Some prolactin is secreted by the uterus, mammillary glands and immune system (lymphocytes).

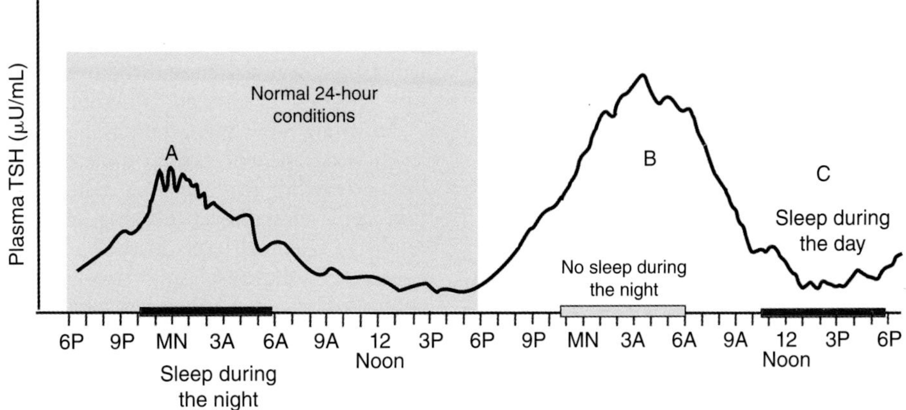

Figure 38–11 Schematic illustrating secretion of thyroid-stimulating hormone (TSH) in a male individual. **(A)** TSH levels start to rise before sleep and peak during the first third of the sleep period, falling until the next upswing in the late afternoon/early evening. **(B)** The absence of sleep at night increases levels, consistent with an inhibitory effect on TSH from sleep. **(C)** The inhibitory effects of sleep on TSH secretion depend on the time of day. Daytime sleep does not significantly alter (inhibit) TSH levels, which are already low at that time of day because of circadian influences. In summary TSH is under circadian control but is inhibited by sleep at night.

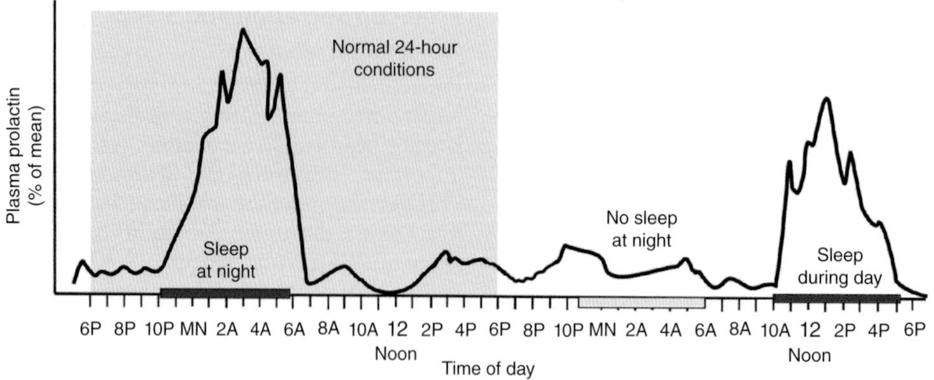

Figure 38–13 A schematic illustrating the secretion of prolactin (PRL). During nocturnal sleep, levels are increased. During nocturnal sleep deprivation, there is no increase in the PRL level. However, during daytime sleep, PRL levels increase. That is, daytime sleep is associated with PRL secretion. Sleep has a stimulatory effect on PRL secretion.

Box 38–4 SLEEP AND PROLACTIN

- PRL—timing of secretion is primarily sleep related (sleep stimulatory)
- Sleep more stimulatory at night (circadian effect)
- PRL secretion has a possible role in circadian control of REM sleep and in the amount of stage N3 sleep

PRL, Prolactin; *REM,* rapid eye movement.

are low in males and non-lactating females. Vasoactive intestinal peptide and the peptide histidine isoleucine also stimulate PRL secretion in humans. Prolactin can also be produced in the uterus, mammillary glands, and the immune system (lymphocytes). Increased levels of estrogen, stress, and nipple stimulation can increase prolactin production in the uterus (increased estrogen) and mammillary glands (nipple stimulation).

PRL levels show a bimodal pattern. They are minimal around noon, increase somewhat during the afternoon, and then increase shortly before sleep onset (Figure 38–13). During sleep the PRL levels remain elevated. Decreased dopaminergic inhibition of PRL during sleep is likely to be the primary mechanism underlying nocturnal PRL elevation. In adults of both sexes, the nocturnal maximum corresponds to an average increase of more than 200% above the minimum level. Morning awakenings and awakenings interrupting sleep are consistently associated with a rapid inhibition of PRL secretion. *Studies of the PRL profiles during daytime naps or after shifts of the sleep period have consistently demonstrated that sleep onset, irrespective of the time of day, has* ***a stimulatory effect*** *on PRL release* (Box 38–4). Sleep is more stimulatory at night (circadian effect).

Evidence for the Role of PRL in Regulation of Sleep

Several studies have examined the possible relationship between pulsatile PRL release during sleep and the alternation of REM and non–rapid eye movement (NREM) stages. Using power spectral analysis of the EEG, a close temporal association between increased PRL secretion and delta wave activity is apparent.[2] Awakenings inhibit nocturnal PRL release. Thus fragmented sleep generally is associated with lower nocturnal PRL levels. Studies in rodents have demonstrated a stimulation of REM sleep by PRL. The effect may be observed 1 to 2 hours after treatment. The stimulatory effect of PRL on REM sleep depends on time of day (observed only during light—the inactive period in rodents).

There is evidence for involvement of PRL in stage N3 regulation. Stage N3 is enhanced in patients with hyperprolactinemia and in women who breastfeed and have high PRL levels compared with women who bottle-feed their infants.[16,17]

A summary of the control of secretion of GH, cortisol, TSH, and PRL is listed in Table 38–1. The table highlights that the secretion of some hormones is tied to sleep and others to circadian factors (time of day). There are also secondary control mechanisms.

Sleep and the Gonadal Axis

The 24-hour patterns of gonadotropin release and gonadal steroid levels vary according to the stage of life and are sex dependent.[16,17] In prepubertal children, luteinizing hormone (LH) and follicle-stimulating hormone (FSH) are secreted in pulses of low amplitude, and *a sleep onset–augmentation effect* is present in the majority of both girls and boys. As the child approaches puberty, the amplitude of the nocturnal pulses increases, and the diurnal rhythm becomes more evident. Studies have shown that both sleep and circadian rhythmicity contribute to this nocturnal elevation.[18] In pubertal boys, the nocturnal rise of testosterone parallels the elevation of gonadotropins, whereas in pubertal girls, higher concentrations of estradiol occur during the daytime instead of the nighttime.[19] It has been proposed that the lack of parallelism between the diurnal variation of gonadotropins and estradiol reflects a 6- to 10-hour delay between gonadotropin stimulation and the ovarian response related to the time required for aromatization of estradiol.

In young adult men, the day-night variation of plasma LH levels is dampened or even undetectable,[20] whereas a marked diurnal rhythm in circulating testosterone levels persists with minimal levels in the late evening, and a clear nocturnal elevation results in maximal levels in the early morning.[21,22] This robust circadian rhythm of plasma testosterone appears to be partially controlled by factors other than LH. One possible explanation is a circadian variation in the sensitivity of the gonads to circulating levels of gonadotropins.[20] Alternatively, intrinsic effects of *sleep on testosterone release may be involved because the nocturnal testosterone increase is temporally linked to the REM latency.*[22]

In elderly men, the *morning level of testosterone* depends on the amount of sleep. Higher levels correlate with more sleep. A study indicated that the amount of nighttime sleep is a strong predictor of morning testosterone levels in healthy older men[23] (Figure 38–14).

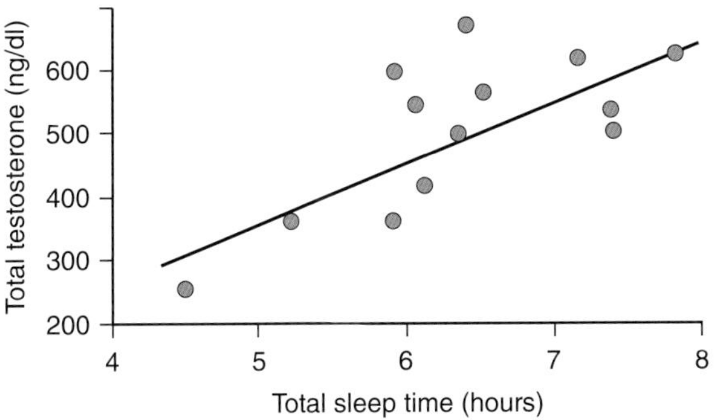

Figure 38–14 Morning levels of plasma total testosterone in healthy older men in relation to the amount of their nocturnal total sleep measured by polysomnography. A superimposed *best-fit* line illustrates the unadjusted bivariate correlation of these variables. Total sleep time is highly correlated with the total testosterone the following morning. (From Penev PD. Association between sleep and morning testosterone levels in older men. *Sleep.* 2007;30:428, with permission.)

Leptin and Ghrelin

Appetite is regulated by the interaction between metabolic and hormonal signals and neural mechanisms.[24,25] The arcuate nucleus of the hypothalamus has two opposing sets of neuronal circuitry, appetite-simulating and appetite-inhibiting, and several peripheral hormonal signals have been identified that affect these neuronal regions.[26] The peripheral signals include leptin and ghrelin[27,28] (Box 38–5). Leptin is primarily secreted by adipose tissue and appears to promote satiety.[28] Ghrelin is a peptide released primarily from the stomach.[27] Studies in humans also indicate that ghrelin increases appetite and food intake. *Plasma ghrelin levels are rapidly suppressed by food intake and then rebound after 1.5 to 2 hours*, paralleling the resurgence in hunger. Thus leptin and ghrelin exert opposing effects on appetite. Animal studies suggest that leptin and ghrelin also have opposing effects on energy expenditure (leptin increasing energy expenditure), but the picture is less clear in humans. Under normal conditions, the 24-hour profile of human plasma leptin levels shows a marked nocturnal rise. When leptin levels were studied with continuous enteral nutrition, leptin levels still rose at night.[28] Ghrelin levels typically rise during the first half of the night, then decrease in the second half even in the fasting condition (Figure 38–4).[29]

Box 38–5 SLEEP LOSS, LEPTIN, AND GHRELIN

Sleep Loss Is Associated With:

- Impaired glucose metabolism.
- Lower leptin levels (leptin reduces appetite).
- Higher ghrelin levels (increases appetite).
- Increased risk of obesity (chronic short sleep duration).

Leptin (Peptide):

- Is secreted by adipose tissue.
- Promotes satiety.
- Levels rise at night.

Ghrelin (Peptide):

- Is secreted by the stomach.
- Increases appetite.
- Secretion is suppressed by food intake.
- Levels increase in the first part of the night then fall in the second part.

There have been several studies of the effect of sleep loss on ghrelin and leptin levels. Some of the studies varied in their findings. However, in general, sleep loss leads to increased ghrelin and decreased leptin.[24] This would tend to increase food intake and perhaps decrease energy usage. Some of the variable findings from studies may have been due to the fact that nocturnal sleep times were not very reduced or that variable degrees of obesity were present in the populations studied.

Sleep Duration and Obesity

Sleep curtailment along with the emergence of the obesity epidemic over the last few decades has spurred many to question whether there may be a direct connection between the two. Numerous cross-sectional population studies have tried to determine whether obesity is associated with sleep loss.[30-35] Although different studies have yielded inconsistent findings, one consistent finding is the strong relationship between short sleep duration and obesity in children and younger adults.[32,33] Patel and Hu[32] looked at 36 publications in their systematic review on short sleep duration and weight gain. They found an independent association between short sleep duration and weight gain, particularly in younger age groups. Moreover, Hasler et al.[34] looked at 496 young adults and analyzed the association between sleep and body mass index (BMI) over a 13-year period. Participants were interviewed at ages 27, 29, 34, and 40 years. In this study they found that the odds ratio for sleep duration predicting obesity was 0.50; this means that every hour of increase of sleep duration was associated with a 50% reduction in the risk of obesity. Analysis of data from the first National Health and Nutritional Examination Survey (NHANES I) indicated that subjects between the ages of 32 and 49 with self-reported sleep durations at baseline of less than 7 hours had higher average BMIs and were more likely to be obese than subjects with sleep duration of 7 hours.[35] Other studies are not consistent with this finding. For example, in the CARDIA (Coronary Artery Risk Development in Young Adults)[36] and SWAN (Study of Women's Health Across the Nation)[37] cohorts, there was no association between sleep duration and weight gain.

In recent years the mechanism behind shorter sleep duration and weight gain has started to take shape. Historically, weight gain via increased hormone levels of ghrelin and decreased leptin in shorter sleep duration have been used to explain the relationship. Recent studies, however, seem to support short sleep duration yielding more opportunity to eat and greater sensitivity to food reward as the explanation (see Figure 38–15).[38] It is therefore thought that part of the tendency for weight gain after sleep loss is that there is increased time for calorie consumption. Chaput et al. concluded that **excess energy intake** associated with not getting adequate sleep suggests that hedonic rather than hormonal factors are to blame.[38] Hedonic eating is for pleasure rather than energy balance. Sleep restriction increases 2-AG (2-arachidonylglycerol), a ligand of the endocannabinoid (eCG) system that increases hedonic eating.[2] Sleep restriction at night increases 2-AG levels in the afternoon and early evening. In summary, insufficient sleep may be a risk factor for weight gain, as the sleep-deprived individual has more access to food and is less able to control eating behavior, often tends to have less physical activity, and the net increase in calorie intake exceeds the caloric demands of extended wakefulness.

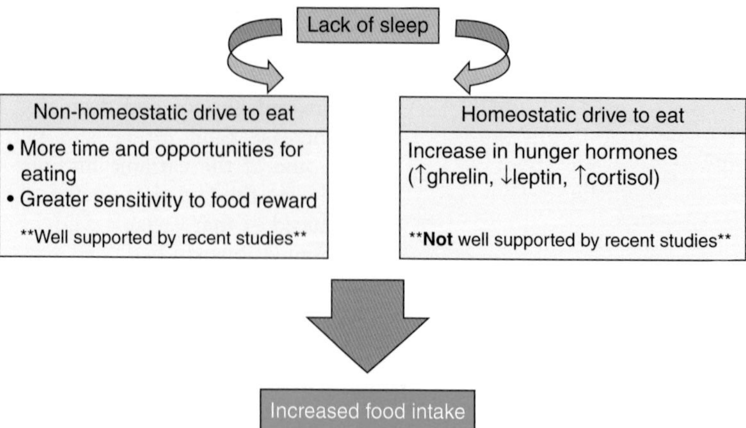

Figure 38–15 Proposed pathways by which insufficient sleep increases caloric consumption. (Reproduced under Creative Commons license from Chaput JP, St-Onge MP. Increased food intake by insufficient sleep in humans: are we jumping the gun on the hormonal explanation? *Front Endocrinol (Lausanne)*. 2014;5:116.)

Sleep and Glucose Tolerance

Sleep has important effects on glucose metabolism, suggesting that sleep disturbances may adversely affect glucose tolerance. Normally constant plasma glucose levels are maintained during sleep despite a 7 to 8 hour fast. In a study by Scheen and coworkers,[39] *subjects received a constant glucose infusion* during (1) nocturnal sleep, (2) nocturnal sleep deprivation, and (3) daytime recovery sleep. The investigators analyzed plasma glucose levels, insulin secretion rates (ISRs), and plasma GH and cortisol levels. The constant glucose infusion (decreases endogenous glucose production) means that change in plasma glucose represents change in glucose utilization. Plasma glucose and ISR markedly increased during early nocturnal sleep and returned to presleep levels during late sleep. These changes in glucose and ISR appeared to reflect the predominance of slow wave activity (stage N3) in early sleep and of REM and wake stages in late sleep. Major differences in glucose and ISR profiles were observed during sleep deprivation as glucose and ISR remained essentially stable during the first part of the night and then decreased significantly, despite the persistence of bedrest and constant glucose infusion.

During daytime recovery sleep, slow wave activity (stage N3) was increased, glucose levels peaked earlier than during nocturnal sleep, and the decreases of glucose and ISR in late sleep were reduced by one-half. Thus sleep has important effects on brain and tissue glucose utilization, suggesting that sleep disturbances may adversely affect glucose tolerance. The findings suggest both sleep and circadian influences on glucose metabolism. Spiegel and colleagues[40] studied 11 healthy volunteers using a protocol of experimental sleep restriction (4 hr/night × 6 nights) followed by a recovery period (12 hr/night × 6 nights). The findings included decreased glucose tolerance in the sleep-debt condition compared with the fully rested condition. Evening cortisol concentrations were elevated, and activity of the sympathetic nervous system was increased in the sleep-debt condition. Gottlieb and associates[41] analyzed a subsample of the population from the Sleep Heart Health Study (1486 subjects: 722 men and 764 women). The usual sleep time was obtained by self-report. Statistical adjustments were made for numerous covariates including age, gender, race, apnea-hypopnea index (AHI), and waist girth. Lower sleep time was associated with impaired glucose tolerance and diabetes mellitus based on serum glucose measurements (fasting and 2 hour).

Chapter 20 discusses the evidence that obstructive sleep apnea (OSA) is associated with impaired glucose tolerance and an increased risk of developing diabetes. The major confounder is the presence of obesity. Possible reasons that OSA impairs glucose tolerance include increased sympathetic nervous activity (may promote hyperglycemia), intermittent hypoxia may damage beta cells (reducing insulin release), and excessive daytime sleepiness promotes sedentary behavior (reducing brain glucose utilization). A cross-sectional analysis of the Sleep Heart Health data[42] was performed (2588 participants aged 52 to 96 years; 46% men) on individuals without known diabetes. Sleep-disordered breathing (SDB) was defined as a respiratory disturbance index of 10 events/hr or greater. Impaired fasting glucose (IFG), impaired glucose tolerance (IGT), occult diabetes, and body weight were classified according to accepted guidelines. Participants with and without SDB were compared on prevalence and odds ratios for measures of impaired glucose metabolism (IGM) after adjusting for age, sex, race, BMI, and waist circumference. SDB was observed in 209 non-overweight and 1036 overweight/obese participants. SDB groups had significantly higher adjusted prevalence and adjusted odds of IFG, IGT, IFG plus IGT, and occult diabetes. The adjusted odds ratio for all subjects was 1.3 for IFG, 1.2 for IGT, 1.4 for IFG plus IGT, and 1.7 for occult diabetes. SDB was associated with occult diabetes, IFG, and IFG plus IGT after adjusting for age, sex, race, BMI, and waist circumference. The magnitude of these associations was similar in nonoverweight and overweight participants. The consistency of associations across all measures of IGM and body habitus groups and the significant association between SDB and IFG plus IGT, a risk factor for rapid progression to diabetes, cardiovascular disease, and mortality suggests the importance of SDB as a risk factor for clinically important levels of metabolic dysfunction. *This and other studies suggest that the prevalence of OSA in patients with type 2 diabetes exceeds 50%.*[43]

Chapter 20 discusses studies showing that continuous positive airway pressure (CPAP) may improve glucose control in some patients with both OSA and diabetes. The results are somewhat conflicting. At least in some studies, CPAP treatment has more significant effects in patients who are not obese.[43]

SLEEP AND GASTROINTESTINAL PHYSIOLOGY AND DISORDERS

The two biggest factors controlling GI tract function are circadian rhythms and food intake. Daily variation of gut motility, endocrine and exocrine gut function, and microbial barrier integrity is among the many functions affected by the circadian clock and are primarily modified by timing of food intake.[44-47] Dyssynchrony between circadian rhythms and food intake or sleep can cause multiple changes including alterations in the gut flora (microbiome).[46]

Gastric and Intestinal Function

Moore found that there is a *peak in acid secretion that occurs between 10 PM and 2 AM.*[48] Acid secretion then decreases during the night to basal awake levels, and then begins increasing again in the evening. Acid secretion does increase after arousals from sleep. Stacher studied only four heathy subjects and found basal acid secretion levels were lower during sleep than wake with a trend for a decrease in the deeper stages of NREM and lowest in REM sleep.[49] However, there is no conclusive evidence of change in acid secretion with sleep stage. Basal waking acid secretion is minimal during wake unless stimulated by food. The general consensus is that *peak in acid secretion is under circadian control and* is *not altered by sleep or sleep stage.*[44,45] There is delayed gastric emptying during sleep. *Intestinal and colonic activity is generally decreased during sleep.* Rectal activity and motor activity increase during sleep, but propulsion is retrograde. This and the fact than anal sphincter tone (though reduced) remains higher than rectal tone prevent anal leakage during sleep.

Gastroesophageal Reflux and Sleep

Gastroesophageal reflux (GER) and sleep have a bidirectional relationship. GER can impair sleep quality due to awakenings with GER symptoms as well as sleep fragmentation from arousals that are not remembered (amnestic arousals).[45] Conversely, any process that causes awakenings or arousal can increase GER episodes (see below), and sleep impairs the ability to neutralize acid after reflux episodes. Sleep disturbance can affect GI tract function, and GI disease can negative impact sleep quality.

Normal Gastroesophageal Physiology

The lower esophageal sphincter (LES) prevents reflux of stomach contents into the esophagus. In the upright position, postprandial gastric distention causes brief relaxation of the LES with transient reflux that is quickly cleared. A number of factors assist in clearance or neutralization of stomach contents: (1) volume clearance, in which two or three swallows induce clearance of reflux material; and (2) acid neutralization, in which saliva itself buffers the acidity of refluxed material. These mechanisms quickly return the distal esophagus to pH 5.5 to 6.5 (normal esophageal pH) (Boxes 38–6 and 38–7).

Nocturnal Gastroesophageal Reflux

GER during sleep is common, with up to 10% of the population reporting symptoms of nocturnal reflux in survey studies.[50,51] In a Gallup poll of heartburn patients, 79% reported *nighttime heartburn*, of which 75% noted that heartburn negatively affected their sleep. Despite medical therapy for GER, only 49% had adequate control of their nocturnal symptoms.[50,51] *Nocturnal GER is potentially more injurious than diurnal GER because acid clearance mechanisms are impaired during sleep.*

Box 38–6 IMPORTANT FACTS ABOUT GASTROESOPHAGEAL REFLUX

GER and Sleep

- 45–50% of patients with GER have nocturnal symptoms
  - Prolonged sleep latency
  - Frequent awakenings
- GER is common in OSA patients (50–75%)
- Fewer but longer GER episodes at night

GER and Pulmonary Complications

- Exacerbation of nocturnal asthma
- Nocturnal pulmonary aspiration
- Increased incidence of GERD in pulmonary fibrosis
- Sleep-related laryngospasm (possible role for GER)

GER and Gastrointestinal Complications

- Erosive esophagitis
- Increased risk for Barrett esophagus (?)
- Increased risk esophageal carcinoma (?? Unproven.)
- Nocturnal GER
  - May increase risk of GER complications
  - Can cause significant sleep disturbance

Nocturnal Mechanisms Worsening Damage From GER

- Swallowing decreased during sleep
- Decreased primary and secondary esophageal peristalsis
- Swallowing occurs only after arousal from sleep
- Saliva production virtually stops during sleep
- Decreased perception of intraesophageal stimuli
- Decreased *upper* esophageal sphincter pressure
- Transient LES relaxation after arousal from sleep or during wake (most sleep-related reflux occurs during arousal from stage N2 sleep)
- Increased gastric secretion in early portion of sleep period
- Decreased gastric emptying
- Combined effects of the above factors = Prolonged acid contact time (ACT)

ACT, Acid contact time; *GER,* gastroesophageal reflux; *GERD,* gastroesophageal reflux disease; *LES,* lower esophageal sphincter; *OSA,* obstructive sleep apnea.

Box 38–7 pH MONITORING DEFINITIONS

pH Probe Position

1. pH probe placed 5 cm H_2O above LES (GE junction about 42 cm from nares).
2. LES pressure determined by pressure transducers.
3. LES position determined by pH measurement. Probe is inserted until pH drops to 1.5–2.5, is slowly withdrawn until pH = 4, and then slowly withdrawn to 5–7 cm above this point.

pH Monitoring Definitions

1. Reflux episodes—pH drops below 4.
2. Clearance defined as the point when pH returns to 4.
3. Clearance interval—time from initial pH drop below 4 until return to above 4.
4. Acid contact time—time below pH of 4
   Expressed as % of time in 24 hours, normally 4–6%.

Eastwood and associates found that the **upper** esophageal sphincter (UES) pressure progressively declines with deeper stages of sleep, resulting in an increased risk of reflux reaching the larynx, pharynx, and pulmonary system.[52] Thus sleep decreases the effectiveness of the UES to act as a barrier to pharyngoesophageal reflux, particularly during stage N3. UES pressure varies with respiration, with minimal values observed during expiration. Hence barrier function of the UES appears most impaired during stage N3 and during the expiratory phase of the respiratory cycle. The LES pressure and its barrier pressure also vary with respiration, being least during expiration. **However, unlike the UES, the function of the LES was unaffected by sleep.**[52]

Freidin and coworkers[53] compared normal subjects and patients with reflux esophagitis with nocturnal monitoring of pH, esophageal manometry, and sleep stage. The LES pressures were similar in normal subjects and patients. Both groups had similar LES pressure during both wakefulness and sleep. The patients had many more reflux episodes. *However, most nocturnal reflux episodes occurred during wake periods, and some occurred after brief arousals from sleep.* Transient lower esophageal sphincter relaxations (TLESRs) accounted for most of these episodes. Transient lower esophageal sphincter (LES) relaxation and gastroesophageal reflux occur primarily during transient arousals from sleep or when patients are fully awake.[54] In a study of recumbent asymptomatic individuals Dent and coworkers[54] found that GER is related to transient inappropriate LES relaxations rather than to low steady-state basal LES pressure, and that primary peristalsis is the major mechanism that clears the esophagus of refluxed material. Furthermore, acid reflux events may occur during either prolonged periods of wakefulness or brief arousals from sleep.[53] Of interest, they found that the LES basal pressure is not affected during sleep.

Frazzoni et al.[55] found that complicated reflux disease (erosive esophagitis, Barrett esophagus [BE]) is characterized by high levels of supine nocturnal percentage acid reflux time. BE is characterized by a change in the mucosal lining of the distal esophagus whereby the squamous epithelium of the esophagus is replaced by the metaplastic columnar epithelium. It is a premalignant lesion associated with esophageal adenocarcinoma. However, a very low percentage of patients with BE develop esophageal cancer. Even so, patients with gastroesophageal reflux disease who have additional risk factors (White, male sex, age > 50 years, tobacco use, alcohol, and central obesity) might benefit from surveillance endoscopy. Because symptomatic reflux is a risk factor for the development of BE,[56] nocturnal GER may play a significant role in the development of BE. One study of GER patients found that a history of nocturnal reflux increased the risk of having BE.[57] Other studies, however, did not replicate this finding.[58] Symptoms of nocturnal GER include multiple awakenings, substernal burning or chest discomfort, indigestion, and heartburn. Other symptoms include a sour or bitter taste in the mouth, regurgitation, water brash, coughing, and choking.

pH Monitoring

Esophageal pH testing is used to diagnose GER and has a sensitivity and specificity of approximately 90% (Box 38–7).[59] It can be performed as an ambulatory study or integrated with polysomnography (sleep monitoring) for temporal correlation of sleep-related events such as arousals. Esophageal pH testing is performed by placing a pH probe in the distal esophagus (5 cm above the LES). Many laboratories include dual pH probes, in which a proximal pH probe is also placed at the UES or in the pharynx. A GER episode is defined by the presence of material that has a pH less than 4. Figure 38–16 shows a GER event after an arousal from sleep. GER episodes should be suspected on routine polysomnography if there is an arousal followed by a prolonged period of increased chin electromyogram (manifestation of swallowing).

Sleep Deficiency and GER

GER disrupts sleep and may lead to sleep deficiency. It has been proposed that sleep deficiency may also worsen GER symptoms through increased sensitivity to reflux (hyperalgesic effect). In addition, one study found that poor sleep quality on the night prior to pH testing was associated with more acid exposure the following day. Thus there may be a bidirectional

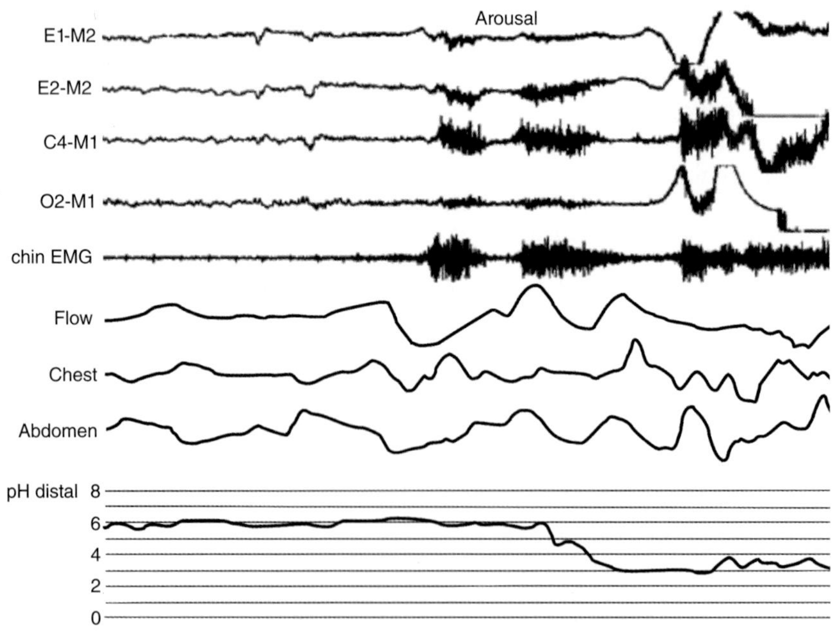

Figure 38–16 An episode of gastroesophageal reflux follows an arousal from sleep. Note that the pH drops below 4. *EMG*, Electromyogram. (From Berry RB, Harding SM. Sleep and medical disorders. *Med Clin North Am.* 2004;88:679-703.)

impact of sleep and GER.[60] It is also possible that improving sleep may improve GER. However, one study found that although zolpidem[61] did reduce the arousal response to GER, duration of the reflux events increased. Prolonged acid exposure increases the risk of GER complications. Another study in patients with GER found that ramelteon[62] improved sleep and a GER symptoms score. In summary, interventions that improve sleep may be useful if they do not worsen acid exposure.

Nocturnal Asthma and GER

There has been considerable interest in the relationship between nocturnal GER and asthma. Some experimental evidence suggests that GER can worsen airway function with or without aspiration into the lungs. Jack and colleagues[63] monitored both tracheal and esophageal pH in four nocturnal asthmatics with GER. There were 37 episodes of esophageal reflux of which 5 episodes were associated with a fall in tracheal pH. Tracheal acid episodes were associated with prolonged reflux episodes, nocturnal awakenings, and bronchospasm during the night. Aspiration, however, may not be required to trigger changes in bronchial tone. Afferent vagal fibers are present in the lower esophagus and could trigger changes in bronchial tone when stimulated by gastric contents. Cuttitta and associates[64] evaluated spontaneous reflux episodes and airway patency during the night in seven asthmatics with GER. Multiple stepwise linear regression analysis revealed that the most important predictor of change in lower respiratory resistance was the duration of esophageal acid exposure. Both long and short GER episodes (those <5 min and those >5 min) were associated with higher respiratory resistance compared with baseline. These data collectively suggest that esophageal acid is able to elicit nocturnal bronchoconstriction. Given these findings, an important question is whether or not treatment of nocturnal GER can improve asthma. One uncontrolled study found a benefit in asthma with aggressive treatment of GER.[65] A large parallel-group, randomized, double-blind study of esomeprazole for treatment of poorly controlled asthma (patient did **not** complain of GER) found no difference in episodes of asthma exacerbations.[66] GER was found in 40% of patients using pH monitoring (asymptomatic). No subgroup of patients could be identified in which treatment of GER improved asthma. The investigators concluded that GER is unlikely to be a major factor in uncontrolled asthma. However, this group of patients *did not have GER symptoms*. Treatment of patients with asthma and symptomatic GER could be considered with the goal to improve GER symptoms, but may also help asthma in individual patients (or when a patient does not respond to asthma treatment).

GER and Obstructive Sleep Apnea

Given the negative intrathoracic pressure during obstructive apnea and the frequent arousals from sleep, one would suspect that nocturnal GER is common in patients with OSA. Green and coworkers[67] prospectively examined 331 OSA patients. Significant nighttime GER was found in 62% of subjects before OSA treatment. Patients compliant with CPAP had a 48% improvement in their nocturnal GER symptoms. There was no change in nighttime reflux symptoms if patients did not use CPAP. Furthermore, there was a strong correlation between higher CPAP pressure and the amount of improvement in nocturnal GER symptom scores (with patients with higher CPAP pressures demonstrating a greater improvement in nocturnal GER score). This study shows that nocturnal reflux is common in OSA patients and that CPAP decreases the frequency of nocturnal GER symptoms.

Of note, the fact that nocturnal GER is common in OSA patients and that CPAP reduces GER does not necessarily prove that OSA causes GER. In some studies, episodes of GER were not correlated with apneic events.[68] By increasing the pressure gradient between the thorax and the stomach, *CPAP may also reduce GER independent of the effects of CPAP on OSA*. A few studies have documented a benefit with CPAP in patients with OSA and GER. Kerr et al.[69] found CPAP reduced nighttime esophageal pH events in five subjects. Tawk and colleagues[70] performed 24-hour pH monitoring and analyzed data from 4 PM to 4 AM before and after 1 week of CPAP. The final monitoring was performed with the subjects wearing CPAP at night. The acid contact time (ACT) fell, as did the number of reflux episodes. Eighty-one percent of subjects had ACT reduced to normal range (<4%) (Figure 38–17).

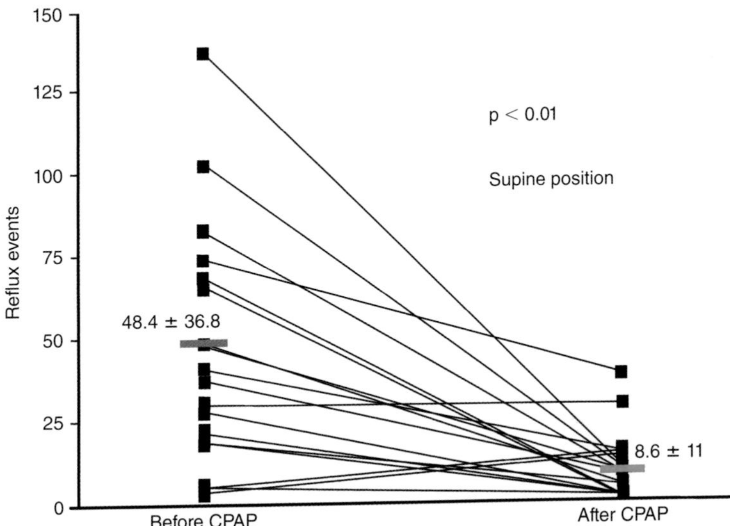

Figure 38–17 Continuous positive airway pressure (CPAP) reduced the reflux events in the supine position in patients with obstructive sleep apnea and gastroesophageal reflux. (From Tawk M, Goodrich S, Kinasewitz G, Orr W. The effect of 1 week of continuous positive airway pressure treatment in obstructive sleep apnea patients with concomitant gastroesophageal reflux. *Chest.* 2006;130:1003-1008.)

Ing et al.[71] found that CPAP reduces GER parameters nonspecifically (in patients with GER both with and without OSA). A meta-analysis of the effects of CPAP on GER in OSA patients concluded that CPAP does decrease reflux events in OSA patients with GER.[72] Another study evaluated the effect of CPAP on OSA patients with GER who complained of chronic cough and found a benefit on both GER and cough.[73]

GER and Sleeping Position

Sleeping in the left lateral position or with the head elevated decreases GER.[74] A trial of a positional treatment device (using both head inclination and the **left lateral** sleeping position) improved GER symptoms (questionnaire) in a group of proton pump inhibitor (PPI)-refractory patients.[75]

GER and Sleep-Related Laryngospasm

GER also has a role in sleep-related laryngospasm. Patients abruptly awaken with an intense feeling of suffocation often accompanied with stridor and choking sensations.[76] Other features include intense anxiety, rapid heart rate, sensation of impending death, and residual hoarseness. The differential diagnosis for sleep-related laryngospasm includes OSA, epilepsy, sleep choking syndrome, sleep terrors, vocal cord dysfunction, and other upper airway pathologies. Thurnheer and associates[77] noted that 9 of 10 patients with sleep-related laryngospasm had GER documented by esophageal pH testing. Six patients responded to antireflux therapy, showing that GER may be associated with sleep-related laryngospasm.

Treatment of Nocturnal GER

A combination of lifestyle changes and medications is used to treat nocturnal GER (Box 38–8).[45,78] Patients should not eat for at least 2 to 3 hours before bedtime and avoid foods that promote GER, including high-fat foods, caffeine, chocolate, mint, alcohol, tomato products, citrus, and sodas. Medications that promote reflux should be avoided, including calcium channel blockers, theophylline, prostaglandins, and bisphosphonates. Smoking significantly decreases LES pressure, so all patients should be encouraged to stop smoking. Patients should lose weight if they are obese and should sleep in loose-fitting clothing. Positional therapy can also be used. Sleeping with the head of the bed elevated 6 inches with a full-length wedge or placing blocks under the head of the bed may be useful. The right lateral decubitus position worsens GER, whereas the *left lateral decubitus posture seems to be the best sleep position for sleep-related GER.*[74] Medications to treat sleep-related GER include antacids for acute symptom control, H2 receptor antagonists (H2RAs), proton pump inhibitors (PPIs), and prokinetic agents.[78,79] H2RAs provide heartburn relief in 60% of patients and can be given before sleep onset. H2RAs competitively block histamine-stimulated acid secretion, making them fundamentally less potent because acid secretion is also stimulated by gastrin and acetylcholine. PPIs provide superior gastric acid suppression. One study found that that 40 mg of omeprazole before dinner, or 20 mg omeprazole before breakfast and before dinner, resulted in better gastric acid suppression than giving 40 mg before breakfast only.[80] PPIs should be taken *before the evening meal* rather than before bedtime to treat nocturnal GER. Some data suggest there may be nocturnal acid breakthrough despite PPI therapy.[81] Whether nocturnal gastric acid breakthrough is clinically important in GER is not known. Metoclopramide (Reglan and generic formulations) is the only prokinetic agent available in the United States and has a high prevalence (20–50%) of central nervous system side effects. Prokinetic agents can be used concomitantly with gastric acid–suppressive agents. Metoclopramide is rarely used because of its side effects. Antireflux surgery, primarily fundoplication (both open and laparoscopic methods), is successful in 80% to 90% of patients. Long-term results, however, show that many surgically treated patients use antireflux medications regularly.[82]

Box 38–8 TREATMENT OF GER

Lifestyle Modifications

- Elevate head of the bed (or full length wedge)
- Avoid right decubitus position
- Avoid late-night snacks (3 hours between last food and bedtime)
- Improve sleep hygiene (minimize sleep disturbance)
- Smoking cessation and avoid alcohol

Pharmacological and Surgical Treatment

- PPI before breakfast
- PPI before supper (if PPI reflux mainly at night, NOT before bedtime)
- PPI before breakfast and supper
- Add histamine 2 antagonist (H2RA), Carafate or Gaviscon, before bedtime
- Surgical options—after failure of medical management

Adapted from references 44 and 75.
PPI, Proton pump inhibitor.

Sleep and Inflammatory Bowel Disease

Circadian disruption and sleep are directly linked to inflammatory bowel disease (IBD) manifestations. Patients with IBD are more likely to have acute flares and are at higher risk for hospitalization when sleep is disrupted.[83] Conversely, patients with IBD report poor sleep[84] often as a consequence of their disease. Active IBD may contribute to dysregulation of circadian CLOCK genes.[85] A study by Weintraub and coworkers found that young, newly diagnosed, untreated patients with IBD have reduced expression of CLOCK genes in inflamed and noninflamed intestinal mucosal samples, and also in blood cells, compared with healthy individuals. This suggests a possible route for potentiation of disease through a circadian pathway. Sleep disruption or sleep loss is associated with upregulation of inflammatory genes with increased release of inflammatory cytokines such as TNF-α (tumor necrosis factor alpha) and interleukins. Both vedolizumab (a monoclonal antibody that binds to α4β7 integrin on blood monocytes, thereby inhibiting their ability to enter the intestinal epithelium) and anti-TNF-alpha biological therapies were associated with improvement in sleep and mood quality in IBD.[86] The reader is referred to a discussion by D'Souza et al [45] for more details about the interface between IBD and sleep.

SLEEP AND RENAL PHYSIOLOGY

Renin and Aldosterone and Sleep

Water and sodium homeostasis depends on coordination of a number of factors, including several hormones. Arginine vasopressin (AVP) is secreted by the posterior pituitary and is also known as antidiuretic hormone (ADH). AVP is secreted in bursts but is independent of sleep stage. AVP results in reabsorption of water from the collecting duct of the kidney. Renin is secreted by the juxtaglomerular cells of the kidney, and aldosterone secreted by the adrenal cortex (Figure 38–18). Renin hydrolyzes angiotensinogen (produced by the liver) to produce angiotensin I. Angiotensin I is metabolized by lung endothelial cells containing angiotensin-converting enzyme (ACE) to angiotensin II. Angiotensin II is a potent vasoconstrictor and also stimulates the adrenals to produce aldosterone. Aldosterone causes absorption of sodium and water and excretion of potassium. Atrial natriuretic peptide (ANP) is secreted by the atrial myocytes in response to stretch and other influences. ANP causes an increase in the renal excretion of sodium and is a mechanism to respond to fluid overload. ANP is elevated in untreated sleep apnea (negative intrathoracic pressure swings stretch the atria), resulting in nocturia. Patients with untreated OSA have nocturnal naturesis.[87,88] However, factors other than increased ANP, such as nondipping blood pressure in untreated OSA, may play a role. CPAP reduces nocturia in some OSA patients.[88] Of note, urine volume and electrolyte secretion is normally lower at night. In particular, REM sleep is associated with decreased urine flow and increased osmolality.

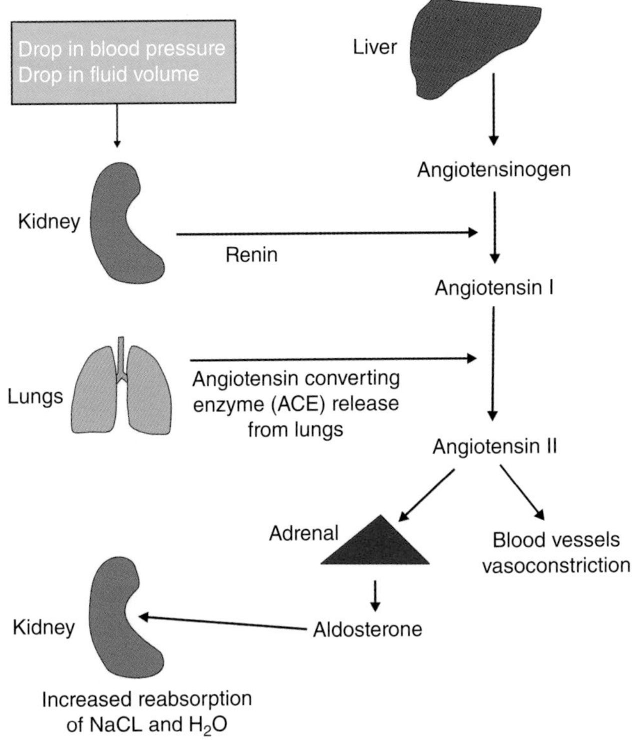

Figure 38–18 A schematic of the renin-angiotensin-aldosterone system.

Plasma renin activity (PRA) and aldosterone levels are elevated during sleep.[89-92] This effect is mainly related to sleep rather than circadian factors. The usual nocturnal rise in PRA and aldosterone is blunted by sleep deprivation[93] (Figure 38–19). *PRA increases during NREM sleep and decreases during REM sleep.* REM sleep is associated with increased sympathetic tone, which increases renin. This seems inconsistent with lower renin during REM sleep. However, the dip in renin during REM sleep may occur from lower blood pressure and sympathetic tone during NREM sleep. *Renin activity is already sharply decreasing before REM sleep occurs.* At the transition from REM sleep to NREM sleep, renin levels are already rising. A study of experimental recurrent circadian disruption found that total sodium excretion increased and total potassium excretion decreased during circadian disruption without a change in total aldosterone secretion.[94] This suggests that factors other than aldosterone may affect total body sodium balance.

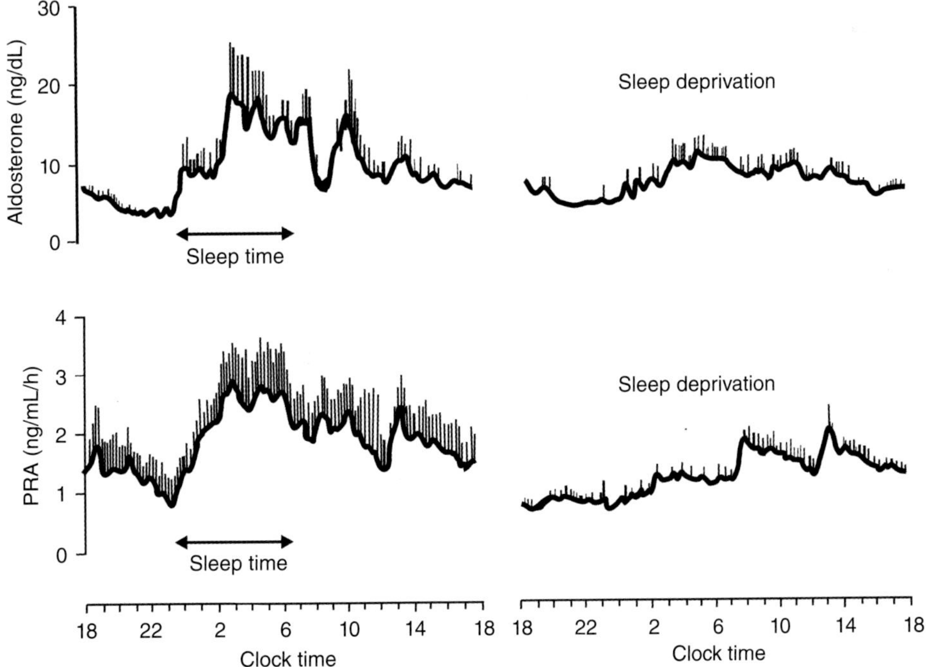

Figure 38–19 Mean 24-hour profiles of plasma renin activity (PRA) and aldosterone in eight normal young men during normal nocturnal sleep and acute sleep deprivation. The vertical bar at each time point represents the standard error of the mean (SEM). Sleep deprivation blunts the nocturnal increase in PRA and aldosterone. (Charloux A, Gronfier C, Chapotot F, et al. Sleep deprivation blunts the nighttime increase in aldosterone release in humans. *J Sleep Res.* 2001;10(1):27-33.)

SUMMARY OF KEY POINTS

1. The secretion of GH and PRL by the pituitary is controlled mainly by the timing of sleep. GH secretion in men is tightly tied to the first cycle of stage N3 sleep. PRL secretion is increased during sleep and inhibited by wakefulness. (see Table 38-1)
2. The secretion of ACTH, cortisol, and TSH is mainly controlled by circadian timing (time of day) influences with weaker sleep-related effects. The secretion of ACTH and cortisol peaks soon after awakening. TSH secretion is under circadian control (peaks during the night). Sleep inhibits TSH secretion.
3. Ghrelin is a hormone secreted by the stomach that stimulates the appetite and is *increased by sleep loss*. Leptin is a hormone secreted by adipose tissue that increases satiety. Leptin is *decreased by sleep loss*. Some studies suggest that individuals with decreased total sleep time have an increased risk of developing obesity.
4. Studies consistently show a strong relationship between short sleep duration and obesity in children and younger adults.
5. Tendency for weight gain after sleep loss is thought to be due to increased time for calorie consumption as well as greater sensitivity to food reward.
6. The normal defense mechanisms to minimize the detrimental effects of GER are not present during sleep. Saliva secretion virtually stops and reflex swallowing to clear refluxed material is not present. This results in prolonged acid contact time. The absence of symptoms does not eliminate the presence of GER. Esophageal pH monitoring often shows significant GER episodes in asymptomatic patients.
7. Sleep decreases the *upper* esophageal sphincter tone and impairs the ability to protect the upper airway. Sleep does **not** reduce the baseline LES tone. However, reflux episodes occur due to transient LES reduction associated with arousal and wakefulness during sleep. Sleep disturbance worsens GER, and GER worsens sleep quality.
8. Nocturnal GER is common in parents with OSA and is improved with CPAP treatment.
9. Lifestyle modifications to reduce GER include elevating the head of the bed, avoiding the right lateral decubitus position, no eating near bedtime, ceasing smoking, avoiding alcohol or foods that worsen GER, and practicing good sleep hygiene (avoiding arousals from sleep). Medical treatments include PPI before breakfast, before supper, or before both breakfast and supper.
10. Untreated obstructive sleep apnea is associated with natriuresis and nocturia. CPAP treatment may reduce the frequency of episodes.
11. PRA and aldosterone levels are elevated during sleep. This effect is mainly related to sleep rather than circadian factors. The usual nocturnal rise in PRA and aldosterone is blunted by sleep deprivation.

CLINICAL REVIEW QUESTIONS

1. Secretion of GH is most closely tied to which of the following?
   A. First period of stage N3.
   B. First REM period.
   C. Time of day (circadian).
   D. Time of awakening.
2. Which of the following about PRL secretion is true?
   A. There is a major circadian influence on the timing of secretion.
   B. It is inhibited by sleep.
   C. It is stimulated by sleep.
   D. It is increased by dopaminergic signaling from the hypothalamus.
   E. It is inhibited by TRH.
3. Which of the following is true about cortisol secretion?
   A. It is closely tied to timing of sleep versus time of day.
   B. Nocturnal levels are increased by sleep deprivation.
   C. Lowest levels are in the morning.
   D. Highest levels are in the early evening.
4. Which of the following is true about TSH secretion?
   A. TSH secretion is stimulated by sleep.
   B. TSH secretion is inhibited by sleep.
   C. TSH stimulation is under circadian control.
   D. A and B.
   E. B and C.
5. Which of the following are **NOT** true about leptin and ghrelin?
   A. Sleep loss increases ghrelin and decreases leptin.
   B. Leptin stimulates the appetite.
   C. Eating reduces ghrelin secretion.
   D. Acylated ghrelin increases growth hormone secretion.
   E. Ghrelin levels are higher at night.
6. A GER episode during esophageal pH monitoring is defined by a pH less than which number?
   A. 3.
   B. 4.
   C. 5.
   D. 6.
7. Which of the following statements are true concerning nocturnal GER episodes?
   A. They occur during sleep.
   B. They occur at night during wake or after arousals.
   C. Acid clearance at night is normal.
   D. Acid clearance at night is abnormal.
   E. B and D.
8. In which of the following groups do studies show a clear link between short sleep duration and obesity?
   A. All humans, irrespective of age.
   B. Adults aged >40 years.
   C. Children and young adults.
   D. Adults aged >65 years.
9. Which of the following is true about acid secretion?
   A. Highest during REM sleep.
   B. Constant during the night.
   C. Equal to awake daytime levels.
   D. Maximum 10 PM to 2 AM.
10. Which of the following is a treatment for nocturnal GER?
    A. Avoid right decubitus position.
    B. PPI before bedtime.
    C. No eating within 1 hour of bedtime.

ANSWERS

1. A. GH secretion is linked to the first period of stage N3.
2. C. Sleep stimulates PRL secretion. Therefore answer B is not correct. Answer A is not correct as the occurrence of sleep rather than time of day is the major influence on the timing of secretion. D and E are not correct as dopamine inhibits PRL secretion, and TRH increases PRL secretion.

3. B. Cortisol secretion is under circadian control. The lowest levels are in the early evening and the first part of sleep. The highest cortisol levels are around 7 AM. Sleep deprivation increases nocturnal cortisol levels (on the night following sleep deprivation).
4. E. TSH secretion is under circadian control but is inhibited by sleep.
5. B. Leptin induces satiety. The other answers are correct: sleep loss increases ghrelin and decreases leptin, ghrelin stimulates appetite, ghrelin falls after meals, and ghrelin levels are higher at night.
6. B. pH = 4.
7. E. GER occurs after arousals during transient LES relaxation. Acid clearance is reduced as saliva secretion stops during sleep and swallowing does not occur.
8. C.
9. D. Maximum acid secretion is 10 PM to 2 AM and then decreases over the night. Acid secretion can increase after arousals (possibly vagally mediated). Acid secretion is not sleep stage dependent.
10. A. Avoiding the right lateral decubitus position reduces GER. PPI should be given before meals either before breakfast, before breakfast and supper, or before supper—not before bedtime. Eating should be avoided for 3 hours before bedtime.

SUGGESTED READING

D'Souza SM, Fass R, Shibli F, Johnson DA. Sleep and gastrointestinal health. In: Kryger M, Roth T, Goldstein CA, Dement WC, eds. *Principles and Practice of Sleep Medicine*. 7th ed. Elsevier; 2022:1557-1564.

Hanlon EC, Van Cauter E, Tasalt E, Broussard JL. Endocrine physiology in relation to sleep and sleep disturbances. In: Kryger M, Roth T, Goldstein CA, Dement WC, eds. *Principles and Practice of Sleep Medicine*. 7th ed. Elsevier; 2022:284-300.

Khoury RM, Camacho-Lobato L, Katz PO, et al. Influence of spontaneous sleep positions on nighttime recumbent reflux in patients with gastroesophageal reflux disease. *Am J Gastroenterol*. 1999;94:2069-2073.

Knutson KL, Spiegel K, Penev P, Van Cauter E. The metabolic consequences of sleep deprivation. *Sleep Med Rev*. 2007;11:163-178.

Reutrakul S, Mokhlesi B. Obstructive sleep apnea and diabetes: a state of the art review. *Chest*. 2017;152(5):1070-1086.

Tawk M, Goodrich S, Kinasewitz G, Orr W. The effect of 1 week of continuous positive airway pressure treatment in obstructive sleep apnea patients with concomitant gastroesophageal reflux. *Chest*. 2006;130:1003-1008.

REFERENCES

1. Van Cauter E, Spiegel K. Circadian and sleep control of hormones. In: Turek FW, Zee PC, eds. *Regulation of Sleep and Circadian Rhythms*. Marcel Dekker; 1999:399.
2. Hanlon EC, Van Cauter E, Tasalt E, Broussard JL. Endocrine physiology in relation to sleep and sleep disturbances. In: Kryger M, Roth T, Goldstein CA, Dement WC, eds. *Principles and Practice of Sleep Medicine*. 7th ed. Elsevier; 2022:284-300.
3. Pannain S, Van Cauter E. Modulation of endocrine function by sleep-wake homeostasis and circadian rhythmicity. *Sleep Med Clin*. 2007;2:147-159.
4. Van Cauter E, Plat L, Copinschi G. Interrelations between sleep and the somatotropic axis. *Sleep*. 1998;21:553-566.
5. Spiegel K, Tasali E, Leproult R, Scherberg N, Van Cauter E. Twenty-four-hour profiles of acylated and total ghrelin: relationship with glucose levels and impact of time of day and sleep. *J Clin Endocrinol Metab*. 2011;96(2):486-493.
6. Latta F, Leproult R, Tasali E, et al. Sex differences in nocturnal growth hormone and prolactin secretion in healthy older adults: relationships with sleep EEG variables. *Sleep*. 2005;28(12):1519-1524.
7. Brandenberger G, Gronfier C, Chapotot F, Simon C, Piquard F. Effect of sleep deprivation on overall 24 h growth-hormone secretion. *Lancet*. 2000;356(9239):1408.
8. Mendelson WB, Slater S, Gold P, Gillin JC. The effect of growth hormone administration on human sleep: a dose-response study. *Biol Psychiatry*. 1980;15:613-618.
9. Obal Jr F, Krueger JM. GHRH and sleep. *Sleep Med Rev*. 2004;8(5):367-377.
10. Bierwolf C, Struve K, Marshall L, Born J, Fehm HL. Slow wave sleep drives inhibition of pituitary-adrenal secretion in humans. *J Neuroendocrinol*. 1997;9(6):479-484.
11. Stalder T, Kirschbaum C, Kudielka BM, et al. Assessment of the cortisol awakening response: expert consensus guidelines. *Psychoneuroendocrinology*. 2016;63:414-432.
12. Leproult R, Copinschi G, Buxton O, Van Cauter E. Sleep loss results in an elevation of cortisol levels the next evening. *Sleep*. 1997;20(10):865-870.
13. Leproult R, Van Cauter E. Impact of sleep debt on metabolic and endocrine function. *Lancet*. 1999;354(9188):1435-1439.
14. Van Cauter E, Leproult R, Plat L. Age-related changes in slow wave sleep and REM sleep and relationship with growth hormone and cortisol levels in healthy men. *JAMA*. 2000;284(7):861-868.
15. Peeters RP, Visser TJ. Metabolism of thyroid hormone. [Updated 2017 Jan 1]. In: Feingold KR, Anawalt B, Blackman MR, et al., eds. *Endotext* [Internet]. MDText.com, Inc.; 2000. Available at: https://www.ncbi.nlm.nih.gov/books/NBK285545.
16. Frieboes RM, Murck H, Stalla GK, et al. Enhanced slow-wave sleep in patients with hyperprolactinemia. *J Clin Endocrinol Metab*. 1998;83:2706-2710.
17. Blyton DM, Sullivan CE, Edwards N. Lactation is associated with an increase in slow-wave sleep in women. *J Sleep Res*. 2002;11:297-303.
18. Van Cauter E, Copinschi G. Endocrine and other biological rhythms. In: DeGroot LJ, Jameson JL, eds. *Endocrinology*. Vol. 1. Elsevier Saunders; 2006:341-372.
19. Goji K. Twenty-four-hour concentration profiles of gonadotropin and estradiol (E2) in prepubertal and early pubertal girls: the diurnal rise of E2 is opposite the nocturnal rise of gonadotropin. *J Clin Endocrinol Metab*. 1993;77:1629-1635.
20. Fehm HL, Clausing J, Kern W, et al. Sleep-associated augmentation and synchronization of luteinizing hormone pulses in adult men. *Neuroendocrinology*. 1991;54:192-195.
21. Luboshitzky R, Zabari Z, Shen-Orr Z, et al. Disruption of the nocturnal testosterone rhythm by sleep fragmentation in normal men. *J Clin Endocrinol Metab*. 2001;86:1134-1139.
22. Luboshitzky R, Herer P, Levi M, et al. Relationship between rapid eye movement sleep and testosterone secretion in normal men. *J Androl*. 1999;20:731-737.
23. Penev P. Association between sleep and morning testosterone levels in older men. *Sleep*. 2007;30:427-432.
24. Knutson KL, Spiegel K, Penev P, Van Cauter E. The metabolic consequences of sleep deprivation. *Sleep Med Rev*. 2007;11:163-178.
25. Mullington JM, Haack M, Toth M, Serrador JM, Meier-Ewert HK. Cardiovascular, inflammatory, and metabolic consequences of sleep deprivation. *Prog Cardiovasc Dis*. 2009;51(4):294-302.
26. Gale SM, Castracane VD, Mantzoros CS. Energy homeostasis, obesity and eating disorders: recent advances in endocrinology. *J Nutr*. 2004;134:295-298.
27. van der Lely A, Tschop M, Heiman M, Ghigo E. Biological, physiological, pathophysiological, and pharmacological aspects of ghrelin. *Endocr Rev*. 2004;25:426-457.
28. Simon C, Gronfier C, Schlienger JL, Brandenberger G. Circadian and ultradian variations of leptin in normal man under continuous enteral nutrition: relationship to sleep and body temperature. *J Clin Endocrinol Metab*. 1998;83:1893-1899.
29. Dzaja A, Dalal MA, Himmerich H, et al. Sleep enhances nocturnal plasma ghrelin levels in healthy subjects. *Am J Physiol Endocrinol Metab*. 2004;286:E963-E967.
30. Ogilvie RP, Patel SR. The epidemiology of sleep and obesity. *Sleep Health*. 2017;3(5):383-388.
31. Theorell-Haglow J, Lindberg E. Sleep duration and obesity in adults: what are the connections? *Curr Obes Rep*. 2016;5(3):333-343.
32. Patel SR, Hu FB. Short sleep duration and weight gain: a systematic review. *Obesity (Silver Spring)*. 2008;16(3):643-653.
33. Li L, Zhang S, Huang Y, Chen K. Sleep duration and obesity in children: a systematic review and meta-analysis of prospective cohort studies. *J Paediatr Child Health*. 2017;53(4):378-385.
34. Hasler G, Buysse DJ, Klaghofer R, et al. The association between short sleep duration and obesity in young adults: a 13-year prospective study. *Sleep*. 2004;27(4):661-666.

35. Gangwisch JE, Malaspina D, Boden-Albala B, Hemsfield SB. Inadequate sleep as a risk factor for obesity: analyses of the NHANES I. *Sleep.* 2005;28(10):1289-1296.
36. Lauderdale DS, Knutson KL, Rathouz PJ, et al. Cross-sectional and longitudinal associations between objectively measured sleep duration and body mass index: the CARDIA Sleep Study. *Am J Epidemiol.* 2009;170(7):805-813.
37. Appelhans BM, Janssen I, Cursio JF, et al. Sleep duration and weight change in midlife women: the SWAN sleep study. *Obesity (Silver Spring).* 2013;21(1):77-84.
38. Chaput JP, St-Onge MP. Increased food intake by insufficient sleep in humans: are we jumping the gun on the hormonal explanation? *Front Endocrinol (Lausanne).* 2014;5:116.
39. Scheen AJ, Byrne MM, Plat L, et al. Relationships between sleep quality and glucose regulation in normal humans. *Am J Physiol.* 1996;271:E261-E270.
40. Spiegel K, Leproult R, Van Cauter E. Impact of sleep debt on metabolic and endocrine function. *Lancet.* 1999;354:1435-1439.
41. Gottlieb DJ, Punjabi NM, Newman AB, et al. Association of sleep time with diabetes mellitus and impaired glucose tolerance. *Arch Intern Med.* 2005;165:863-867.
42. Seicean S, Kirchner HL, Gottlieb DJ, et al. Sleep-disordered breathing and impaired glucose metabolism in normal-weight and overweight/obese individuals: the Sleep Heart Health Study. *Diabetes Care.* 2008;31:1001-1006.
43. Reutrakul S, Mokhlesi B. Obstructive sleep apnea and diabetes: a state of the art review. *Chest.* 2017;152(5):1070-1086.
44. Orr WC. Gastrointestinal physiology. In: Kryger M, Roth T, Dement WC, eds. *Principles and Practice of Sleep Medicine.* Elsevier; 2005: 283-291.
45. D'Souza SM, Fass R, Shibli F, Johnson DA. Sleep and gastrointestinal health. In: Kryger M, Roth T, Goldstein CA, Dement WC, eds. *Principles and Practice of Sleep Medicine.* 7th ed. Elsevier; 2022:1557-1564.
46. Bron R, Furness JB. Rhythm of digestion: keeping time in the gastrointestinal tract. *Clin Exp Pharmacol Physiol.* 2009;36(10):1041-1048.
47. Vaughn B, Rotolo S, Roth H. Circadian rhythm and sleep influences on digestive physiology and disorders. *ChronoPhysiology Ther.* 2014;4: 67-77.
48. Moore JG. Circadian dynamics of gastric acid secretion and pharmacodynamics of H2 receptor blockade. *Ann N Y Acad Sci.* 1991;618: 150-158.
49. Stacher G, Presslich B, Stärker H. Gastric acid secretion and sleep stages during natural night sleep. *Gastroenterology.* 1975;68(6):1449-1455.
50. Farup C, Kleinman L, Sloan S, et al. The impact of nocturnal symptoms associated with gastroesophageal reflux disease on health-related quality of life. *Arch Intern Med.* 2001;161:45-70.
51. Shaker R, Castell DO, Schoenfeld PS, Spechler SJ. Nighttime heartburn is an underappreciated clinical problem that impacts sleep and daytime function: the results of a Gallup survey conducted on behalf of the American Gastroenterological Association. *Am J Gastroenterol.* 2003;98: 1487-1493.
52. Eastwood PR, Katagiri S, Shepherd KL, Hillman DR. Modulation of upper and lower esophageal sphincter tone during sleep. *Sleep Med.* 2007;8(2): 135-143.
53. Freidin N, Fisher MJ, Taylor W, et al. Sleep and nocturnal acid reflux in normal subjects and patients with reflux oesophagitis. *Gut.* 1991;32: 1275-1279.
54. Dent J, Dodds WJ, Friedman RH, et al. Mechanism of gastroesophageal reflux in recumbent asymptomatic human subjects. *J Clin Invest.* 1980;65(2): 256-267.
55. Frazzoni M, De Micheli E, Savarino V. Different patterns of oesophageal acid exposure distinguish complicated reflux disease from either erosive reflux oesophagitis or non-erosive reflux disease. *Aliment Pharmacol Ther.* 2003;18(11-12):1091-1098.
56. Lagergren J, Bergstrom R, Lindgren A, Nuyren O. Symptomatic gastroesophageal reflux as a risk factor or esophageal adenocarcinoma. *N Engl J Med.* 1999;340:825-831.
57. Gerson LB, Edson R, Lavori PW, Triadafilopoulos G. Use of a simple symptom questionnaire to predict Barrett's esophagus in patients with symptoms of gastroesophageal reflux. *Am J Gastroenterol.* 2001;96: 2005-2012.
58. Eloubeidi MA, Provenzale D. Clinical and demographic predictors of Barrett's esophagus among patients with gastroesophageal reflux disease: a multivariable analysis in veterans. *J Clin Gastroenterol.* 2001;33:306-309.
59. Kahrilas PJ, Quigley EMM. Clinical esophageal pH recording: a technical review for practice guideline development. *Gastroenterology.* 1996;110: 1982-1996.
60. Shibli F, Skeans J, Yamasaki T, et al. Nocturnal gastroesophageal reflux disease (GERD) and sleep, and important relationship that is commonly overlooked. *J Clin Gastroenterol.* 2020;54:663-674.
61. Gagliardi GS, Shah AP, Goldstein M, et al. Effect of zolpidem on the sleep arousal response to nocturnal esophageal acid exposure. *Clin Gastroenterol Hepatol.* 2009;7(9):948-952.
62. Jha LK, Fass R, Gadam R, et al. The effect of ramelteon on heartburn symptoms of patients with gastroesophageal reflux disease and chronic insomnia: a pilot study. *J Clin Gastroenterol.* 2016;50(2):e19-e24.
63. Jack CIA, Calverley PMA, Donnelly RJ, et al. Simultaneous tracheal and oesophageal pH measurement in asthmatic patients with gastro-oesophageal reflux. *Thorax.* 1995;50:201-204.
64. Cuttitta G, Cibella F, Visconti A, et al. Spontaneous gastroesophageal reflux and airway patency during the night in adult asthmatics. *Am J Respir Crit Care Med.* 2000;161:177-181.
65. Harding SM, Richter JE, Guzzo MR, et al. Asthma and gastroesophageal reflux: acid suppressive therapy improves asthma outcomes. *Am J Med.* 1996;100:395-405.
66. ALA Asthma Clinical Research Centers. Efficacy of esomeprazole for treatment of poorly controlled asthma. *N Engl J Med.* 2009;360: 1487-1499.
67. Green BT, Broughton WA, O'Connor JB. Marked improvement in nocturnal gastroesophageal reflux in a large cohort of patients with obstructive sleep apnea. *Arch Intern Med.* 2003;163:41-45.
68. Graf KI, Karaus M, Heinemann S, et al. Gastroesophageal reflux in patients with sleep apnea syndrome. *Z Gastroenterol.* 1995;33:689-693.
69. Kerr P, Shoenut JP, Millar T, Buckle P, Kryger MH. Nasal CPAP reduces gastroesophageal reflux in obstructive sleep apnea syndrome. *Chest.* 1992;101(6):1539-1544.
70. Tawk M, Goodrich S, Kinasewitz G, Orr W. The effect of 1 week of continuous positive airway pressure treatment in obstructive sleep apnea patients with concomitant gastroesophageal reflux. *Chest.* 2006;130:1003-1008.
71. Ing AJ, Ngu MC, Breslin AB. Obstructive sleep apnea and gastroesophageal reflux. *Am J Med.* 2000;108(suppl 4a):120S-125S.
72. Li C, Wu ZH, Pan XL, Yuan K. Effect of continuous positive airway pressure on gastroesophageal reflux in patients with obstructive sleep apnea: a meta-analysis. *Sleep Breath.* 2021;25(3):1203-1210.
73. Su J, Fang Y, Meng Y, et al. Effect of continuous positive airway pressure on chronic cough in patients with obstructive sleep apnea and concomitant gastroesophageal reflux. *Nat Sci Sleep.* 2022;14:13-23.
74. Khoury RM, Camacho-Lobato L, Katz PO, et al. Influence of spontaneous sleep positions on nighttime recumbent reflux in patients with gastroesophageal reflux disease. *Am J Gastroenterol.* 1999;94:2069-2073.
75. Allampati S, Lopez R, Thota PN, Ray M, Birgisson S, Gabbard SL. Use of a positional therapy device significantly improves nocturnal gastroesophageal reflux symptoms. *Dis Esophagus.* 2017;30(3):1-7.
76. American Academy of Sleep Medicine. *International Classification of Sleep Disorders.* 3rd ed. American Academy of Sleep Medicine; 2014.
77. Thurnheer R, Henz S, Knoblauch A. Sleep-related laryngospasm. *Eur Respir J.* 1997;10:2084-2086.
78. Sandhu DS, Fass R. Current trends in the management of gastroesophageal reflux disease. *Gut Liver.* 2018;12(1):7-16.
79. Katzka DA, Kahrilas PJ. Advances in the diagnosis and management of gastroesophageal reflux disease. *BMJ.* 2020;371:m3786.
80. Kuo B, Castell DO. Optimal dosing of omeprazole 40 mg daily: effects on gastric and esophageal pH and serum gastrin in healthy controls. *Am J Gastroenterol.* 1996;91:1532-1538.
81. Peghini PL, Katz PO, Bracy NA, et al. Nocturnal recovery of gastric acid secretion with twice-daily dosing of proton pump inhibitors. *Am J Gastroenterol.* 1998;93:763-767.
82. Spechler SJ, Lee E, Ahnen D, et al. Long-term outcome of medical and surgical therapies for gastroesophageal reflux disease: follow-up of a randomized controlled trial. *JAMA.* 2001;285:2331-2338.
83. Sofia MA, Lipowska AM, Zmeter N, et al. Poor sleep quality in Crohn's disease is associated with disease activity and risk for hospitalization or surgery. *Inflamm Bowel Dis.* 2020;26(8):1251-1259.
84. Zargar A, Gooraji SA, Keshavarzi B, Haji Aghamohammadi AA. Effect of irritable bowel syndrome on sleep quality and quality of life of inflammatory bowel disease in clinical remission. *Int J Prev Med.* 2019;10:10.
85. Weintraub Y, Cohen S, Chapnik N, et al. Clock gene disruption is an initial manifestation of inflammatory bowel diseases. *Clin Gastroenterol Hepatol.* 2020;18(1):115-122.e1.
86. Stevens BW, Borren NZ, Velonias G, et al. Vedolizumab therapy is associated with an improvement in sleep quality and mood in inflammatory bowel diseases. *Dig Dis Sci.* 2017;62(1):197-206. Erratum in: *Dig Dis Sci.* 2017;62(2):552.

87. Umlauf MG, Chasens ER, Greevy RA, Arnold J, Burgio KL, Pillion DJ. Obstructive sleep apnea, nocturia and polyuria in older adults. *Sleep*. 2004;27(1):139-144.
88. Wang T, Huang W, Zong H, Zhang Y. The efficacy of continuous positive airway pressure therapy on nocturia in patients with obstructive sleep apnea: a systematic review and meta-analysis. *Int Neurourol J*. 2015;19(3): 178-184.
89. Brandenberger G, Krauth MO, Ehrhart J, et al. Modulation of episodic renin release during sleep in humans. *Hypertension*. 1990;15:370-375.
90. Schüssler P, Yassouridis A, Uhr M, et al. Sleep and active renin levels: interaction with age, gender, growth hormone and cortisol. *Neuropsychobiology*. 2010;61(3):113-121.
91. Luthringer R, Brandenberger G, Schaltenbrand N, et al. Slow wave electroencephalographic activity parallels renin oscillations during sleep in humans. *Electroencephalogr Clin Neurophysiol*. 1995;95:318-322.
92. Charloux A, Gronfier C, Lonsdorfer-Wolf E, et al. Aldosterone release during the sleep wake cycle in humans. *Am J Physiol*. 1999;276: E43-E49.
93. Charloux A, Gronfier C, Chapotot F, et al. Sleep deprivation blunts the nighttime increase in aldosterone release in humans. *J Sleep Res*. 2001;10(1): 27-33.
94. McMullan CJ, McHill AW, Hull JT, et al. Sleep restriction and recurrent circadian disruption differentially affects blood pressure, sodium retention, and aldosterone secretion. *Front Physiol*. 2022;13:914497.

Chapter 39

Sleep in Medical Disorders and Pregnancy

INTRODUCTION

This chapter covers sleep in a variety of medical disorders as well as in pregnancy. For some topics, a brief background may be given, as they may apply to sleep, but it is beyond the scope of this chapter to provide detailed information on the diagnosis, management, and treatment of these conditions.

ACROMEGALY

Basics and Clinical Manifestations of Acromegaly

Acromegaly is a disorder caused by excess growth hormone secretion from somatotrophic cells in the pituitary. Secretion is under regulation of the hypothalamus, which secretes growth hormone–releasing hormone (GHRH) and somatostatin (growth hormone–inhibiting hormone). Growth hormone induces the synthesis of insulin-like growth factor 1 (IFG-1) in the liver, which mediates the anabolic action of growth hormone. Growth hormone also binds growth hormone receptors on numerous target organs, including the liver, kidneys, bone, cartilage, skeletal muscle, and adipose cells.[1] More than 90% of patients with acromegaly have a benign growth hormone–secreting pituitary adenoma.[2] The clinical manifestations of acromegaly range from subtle to obvious and depend on the age of presentation. Adenomas occurring in younger patients are usually fast growing, presenting before the closure of epiphyseal bone and resulting in quick growth and gigantism. Adenomas presenting later in life are slower growing and have more subtle physical changes. Manifestations of acromegaly include local tumor effects from pituitary enlargement, soft tissue thickening in the hands and feet (acral enlargement), gigantism, prognathism, frontal bone hypertrophy, visceromegaly (including tongue enlargement), and many effects on other organ systems.[1]

Sleep and Acromegaly

Grunstein and colleagues[3] studied 53 patients with acromegaly and found 81% had sleep apnea. Snoring was present in nearly all study subjects. Hypertension in acromegaly was strongly associated with sleep apnea. Of those with sleep apnea, *67% had obstructive sleep apnea, and 33% had central sleep apnea (CSA).* Upper airway growth and soft tissue swelling are thought to contribute to the obstructive component. Patients with CSA had higher IGF-1 levels and higher mean random glucose levels, indicating hypersecretion was associated with CSA.[3] Increased ventilatory responsiveness in these patients and elevated hormonal parameters of disease activity were both found to contribute to CSA in these patients.[4] Davi et al. looked at 36 patients with acromegaly, including 18 with active disease and 18 with controlled disease. Their analysis showed that the prevalence of sleep apnea was higher in the group with active disease than that in the control group (55% vs. 39%), with an overall incidence of 47% in their study group. The severity of sleep apnea was also decreased in the control group. They showed that a higher IGF-1 level, male gender, older age, higher body mass index (BMI), and disease duration were associated with sleep apnea. In a longitudinal portion of their study on six subjects, the severity of sleep apnea improved but did not resolve with treatment in five of the six.[5] Octreotide, a somatostatin analog, is used to treat acromegaly by suppressing growth hormone secretion. Six months of treatment with octreotide was shown to improve sleep apnea in patients with acromegaly. Indices including respiratory disturbance index (RDI), % total apnea time, and oxygen desaturation all improved on octreotide. It is thought that octreotide decreases obstructive sleep apnea (OSA) in these patients by decreasing soft tissue swelling in the upper airway. In addition, octreotide likely improves CSA by decreasing ventilatory responsiveness. Improvement in indices was seen even in partial biochemical remission, but sleep apnea was seen to persist even with normalization of growth hormone levels.[6] Rosenow and colleagues studied patients with treated acromegaly to understand the prevalence of sleep apnea. They found an incidence of sleep apnea of at least 21% in this group. In this study, Rosenow et al. studied patients with an ambulatory device that recorded oxygen saturation, heart rate, snoring, and body position. Oxygen desaturations of >4% were counted towards a desaturation index and sleep apnea was defined as >10 desaturations per hour in the presence of snoring and a sawtooth pattern.[7] The incidence of sleep apnea was likely underestimated in this study for multiple reasons (e.g., airflow was not obtained to define respiratory events, actual sleep time was not known, events with 4% desaturations were not included, and the desaturation cutoff to define apnea does not match up with currently defined indices for measuring SDB).

CANCER

Sleep and Cancer

Büttner-Teleagă et al. performed a systematic review yielding 8073 studies and ultimately analyzed 89 on the topic of sleep and sleep disorders in cancer. They found that sleep disturbances and/or sleep disorders were noted in up to 95% of patients with cancer. Sleep disturbances can be noted during diagnosis, treatment, and even years after treatment. *The most common sleep disorder in those with cancer is insomnia,* followed by sleep-related breathing disorders (SRBDs). Restless leg syndrome, narcolepsy, and rapid eye movement (REM) sleep behavior disorder (RBD) were much less common.[8]

Historically, studies looking at insomnia in cancer have included only small sample sizes or were limited to a specific kind or site of cancer. In recent years, however, longitudinal studies have looked at large sample sizes and various cancer types. Savard et al. looked at the prevalence and natural course of insomnia comorbid with cancer over an 18-month period.[9] They studied 962 patients with cancer (mixed sites) who were scheduled to receive curative surgery for a first diagnosis of nonmetastatic cancer. These patients were approached at their preoperative visit to participate in the study, and data were collected at that visit, then at 2, 6, 10, 14, and 18 months after surgery. Participants were categorized into three groups: *good sleepers* (no subjective sleep difficulties or use of hypnotics <1 night per week), *patients with insomnia symptoms* (reported sleep difficulties not meeting criteria for insomnia syndrome or use of hypnotics 1 to 2 nights per week), and patients with clinical *insomnia* disorder (subjective report of sleep difficulties, sleep latency, or wakefulness after sleep onset 30 or more minutes, 3 or more nights per week for 1 month or more, associated with impaired daytime function or use of hypnotics 3 or more nights per week for 1 month or more). Patients in this study had high rates of insomnia symptoms at baseline (59%), including 28% with insomnia. Over the course of 18 months, those with insomnia symptoms not meeting criteria for clinical insomnia were more likely to become good sleepers from interval to interval than those with clinical insomnia. Those individuals meeting criteria for clinical insomnia at the beginning of the study were likely to still have it at the end of the study.[9] Insomnia was therefore considered a lasting problem in these patients, and early evaluation of these patients for insomnia symptoms and treatment directed at the underlying cause may be beneficial.

Screening of patients with cancer for sleep disturbances with a validated method, such as the Insomnia Severity Index (ISI), is considered best practice for routine oncology care. Positive screens merit further evaluation of the patient's symptoms, and an individualized treatment plan should be directed at the patient's individual scenario. For example, sleep disturbances from comorbid depression, oncologic pain, or treatment side effects may call for different, specific treatments.[10] Given the superiority of cognitive-based therapy for insomnia (CBTI) compared to medications, CBTI is recommended as a first-line treatment for insomnia.[11] See Chapter 33 for a discussion of the ISI as well as the diagnosis and treatment of insomnia.

Cancer-Related Fatigue

Cancer-related fatigue is one of the most common and bothersome symptoms in cancer, and there is significant variability in how and when (before, during, or after treatment) it manifests in individual patients. There is increasing evidence that inflammatory pathways play a role in this fatigue, and specific genes related to inflammation suggest a genetic contribution. Risk factors for cancer-related fatigue include depression, sleep disturbance, physical inactivity, and dysfunctional expectations or beliefs about fatigue. It is important to note that symptoms experienced from cancer-related fatigue are not necessarily proportional/specific to the specific cancer treatment, so two patients undergoing the same treatment can experience very different levels of fatigue.[12]

While there are varying approaches to treatment, increasing physical activity via exercise is the most common initial approach, and studies have documented its benefits. Other interventions aimed at strengthening the mind-body connection, such as yoga, mindfulness, and acupuncture, as well as psychosocial treatment via cognitive behavioral therapy, have also been shown to be beneficial.[12] Pharmacological treatment via stimulants (e.g., dextroamphetamine/amphetamine, methylphenidate) or wakefulness-promoting medications (e.g., modafinil, armodafinil) is recommended in active or advanced disease, per recent guidelines.[12,13] Regarding those who have been treated and are now disease free, guidelines suggest there is no firm evidence in the literature that supports treatment with stimulants or wakefulness-promoting medications in these patients.[12,13] That being said, some clinicians will try these medications as an off-label use in cases of severe fatigue when the benefits are felt to outweigh the risks of medication.

MYALGIC ENCEPHALOMYELITIS (ME)/CHRONIC FATIGUE SYNDROME (CFS)

Background and Diagnostic Criteria of ME/CFS

Over the last few decades, the diagnostic criteria for chronic fatigue syndrome (CFS) have gone through multiple revisions, most recently in 2015 with an effort to make diagnosis more straightforward. This revision also included the addition of post-exertional malaise (PEM), the hallmark symptom of this syndrome.[14,15] The 2015 criteria were published by the U.S. National Academy of Medicine[14] and afterward were adopted by the U.S. Centers for Disease Control and Prevention. These criteria are described below. The current nomenclature for CFS is myalgic encephalitis (ME). ME/CFS affects between 0.23% and 2.6% of the adult population.[16] *Women are affected three times more than men,* with patients developing symptoms as early as their teens and as late as their 70s, but most often in their 30s. Symptoms of ME/CFS significantly impair occupational, educational, social, and personal activities. There is a spectrum of severity that can vary from mild (mobile, able to perform self-care and continue working) to very severe (unable to carry out most activities of daily living, mostly bedridden).[15] The exact etiology of ME/CFS is unclear but is felt to be multifactorial.[15,16] Most recently evidence has suggested that central sensitization, autonomic dysregulation, and/or dysregulation of the hypothalamic pituitary adrenal axis are involved.[16] A precipitating event such as viral infection or major life event may have occurred.[15,16] In cases in which viral illness occurred, the exact virus is often not known because of an initial self-limited event. Occasionally, the inciting virus may be known if symptoms occur after a documented infection with Epstein-Barr virus or mononucleosis.[16] Predisposing factors can include a history of abuse, mood disorder, and emotional distress.[15,16]

Diagnostic criteria for ME/CFS at the time of this writing are:

Patients ***must*** have the following three symptoms:

1. Substantial reduction or impairment in the ability to engage in pre-illness levels of occupational, educational, social, or personal activities, persisting for >6 months, accompanied by fatigue that is new or of definite onset (not lifelong), is not due to ongoing excessive exertion, and is not substantially alleviated by rest, and
2. Post-exertional malaise (hallmark symptom), and
3. Unrefreshing sleep.

At least one of the following two manifestations is also required:

1. Cognitive impairment or
2. Orthostatic intolerance.[14]

Sleep in ME/CFS

Unrefreshing sleep is part of the required diagnostic criteria for ME/CFS. Patients will often describe nonrestorative sleep or reduced sleep quality. These symptoms remain despite what should be an adequate or even extended total sleep time (TST) for their age. Some patients may report difficulty with initiating or maintaining sleep, but once these problems are addressed, sleep remains unrefreshing.[15,17] Recent studies looking at heart rate variability (HRV) in sleep have linked autonomic nervous system activity in sleep with unrefreshing sleep in these patients.[15,17,18] Decreased HRV *because of decreased parasympathetic activity* is thought to suggest hypervigilant sleep. Fatt et al. showed that diminished HRV indicating autonomic hypervigilance during slow-wave sleep (stage N3) was associated with poorer-quality sleep. Patients with CFS in that study had delayed sleep onset, more awakenings, and reduced parasympathetic signaling during deeper sleep compared to healthy controls.[18] Previous studies of sleep architecture in patients with ME/CFS have shown some slight deviations in sleep indices (sleep efficiency and REM latency) from healthy controls; however, no consistent patterns have emerged. Further complicating the picture in these studies is difficulty in controlling for subjective symptom severity in these patients. Despite no clear pattern in sleep architecture differences in these patients, Gotts et al.[16] examined 343 patients with CFS with a single night of polysomnography (PSG) in an effort to identify whether sleep-specific phenotypes exist in this population. Of the 343, 103 (30.3%) were found to have a primary sleep disorder (sleep-disordered breathing or periodic limb movement disorder). Of the remaining 239, 89.1% were found to have at least one objective sleep problem. Upon analysis, four different phenotypes emerged and are shown in Table 39–1. This may indicate that a single night of PSG in patients with ME/CFS is enough to identify a potential phenotype to tailor specific sleep-based treatments.[16]

Treatment of ME/CFS

Bateman et al. noted that, while there is no treatment approved by the U.S. Food and Drug Administration (FDA) for ME/CFS, there is still much that can be done to treat it. Treatment of ME/CFS begins with validating the patient's experience through patient and family education, as well as assessing their needs and providing support (e.g., handicap placards, work or educational accommodations, disability benefits). Treatment is then directed at the individual symptoms experienced, which can include postexertional malaise, orthostatic intolerance, sleep issues, cognitive difficulties, immune dysfunction, pain, and gastrointestinal issues. A full discussion of all of the treatments for ME/CFS is beyond the scope of this chapter; however, the treatments directed at sleep issues will be discussed in brief. Any known primary sleep disorders, such as sleep apnea, should be fully treated. Measures to address external disruptions such as light, sound, or stressors can be addressed with eye masks or blue light filters, ear plugs, and meditation and relaxation exercises, respectively. Hypnotics can also be used to address issues with difficulty initiating or maintaining sleep, as appropriate.[15]

FIBROMYALGIA

Manifestations of Fibromyalgia

Fibromyalgia (FM) is a syndrome comprising complex symptomatology including chronic widespread pain (CWP), fatigue, and sleep disturbances. While CWP, fatigue, and sleep disturbances are the cardinal features, other common features include autonomic disturbances, cognitive dysfunction, psychiatric symptoms, regional pain syndromes, hypersensitivity to external stimuli, and stiffness.[19] Criteria to define and diagnose FM have been revised in recent years. In 2016, the American College of Rheumatology provided their revisions[20] to the 2010/2011 diagnostic criteria.[21] These revisions

Table 39–1 Sleep-Specific Phenotypes in CFS

Sleep Phenotype	Central Differential Features	Associated Diagnostic Features	How This May Present Subjectively
1	Long sleep onset latency, long REM latency, high amounts of slow wave (stage N3) sleep and low amounts of REM	Low amounts of stage N2 sleep	Problems in sleep initiation, but when asleep, few awakenings. The sleep that is obtained is of normal quality.
2	Same as phenotype 1, columns 2 and 3 are different than phenotype 1	High number of arousals per hour and high amounts of stage N2 sleep	No difficulty in sleep initiation and few awakenings but feelings or evidence of a 'restless' night sleep.
3	High total sleep time, low amounts of time awake during the night and low number of wake periods during the night	High amounts of REM sleep, short sleep onset latency, few awakenings, short REM latency, and decreased amounts of stage N1 sleep	No difficulties in sleep initiation and few awakenings but feelings of being unrefreshed on waking despite a significant amount of time in bed asleep.
4	Highest number of wake periods during the night and highest amounts of time awake during the night	Low total sleep time, low number of arousals per hour during the night, and low amounts of slow wave sleep	Short sleep duration and although no difficulties in sleep inititation, many awakenings for significant periods of time. Also increased feelings of daytime sleepiness.

Table adapted and reproduced under Creative Commons.

Source: Gotts ZM, Deary V, Newton J, et al. Are there sleep-specific phenotypes in patients with chronic fatigue syndrome? A cross-sectional polysomnography analysis. *BMJ Open*. 2013. 3:3002000. Doi: 10.1136/bmjopen-2013-002999.

were made to emphasize generalized (multi-site) pain.[19] These criteria define FM when the following conditions are met:

1. Generalized pain, defined as pain in at least four of five regions, is present;
2. Symptoms have been present at a similar level for at least 3 months;
3. Widespread pain index (WPI) ≥7 and symptom severity scale (SSS) score ≥5 OR WPI of 4 to 6 and SSS score ≥9; and
4. A diagnosis of FM is valid irrespective of other diagnoses. A diagnosis of FM does not exclude the presence of other clinically important illnesses.[20]

In previous versions, noting tenderness at ≥11 of 18 specific sites (tender points) had been used as criteria,[22] but the 2010 criteria replaced this with pain in specific body regions. The prevalence of FM was shown to be between 2% and 8%, depending on the diagnostic criteria used.[19,23,24] *FM is more common in women*, with a female:male ratio of 2:1[23] to 3:1.[19] The pathophysiology of FM is very complex; it is thought to be caused by mechanisms resulting in neuromorphologic modifications and pain dysperception.[19]

Sleep in FM

Sleep complaints in FM are common and include nonrestorative sleep, fragmented sleep, and insomnia.[19,25] Poor sleep seems to worsen pain symptoms in these patients and pain often worsens sleep (bidirectional).[19] Poor sleep, in fact, is thought to play a role in the pathophysiology of FM, as demonstrated by Lentz et al.[26] and Smith et al.[27] Lentz et al.[26] deprived 12 healthy female subjects (middle aged, sedentary, and without muscle discomfort) of stage N3 for 3 consecutive nights. They showed that the disruption of stage N3, in the absence of reduction TST or sleep efficiency, was associated with a decreased pain threshold and increased fatigue, discomfort, and inflammatory response in the skin.[26] Smith et al.[27] found similar findings. They studied 32 healthy women for 7 nights with PSG. On nights 1 and 2, they slept without disruption for 8 hours. After night 2, they were randomized to a forced awakening (FA) group (one forced awakening per hour) and reduced sleep opportunity (RSO) group on nights 3 through 5. On night 6, both groups began 36 hours of sleep deprivation, followed by 11 hours of recovery sleep. Sleep deprivation had no effect on pain thresholds, but during partial sleep deprivation, the FA group demonstrated a significant loss of pain inhibition and increased spontaneous pain. This suggests that **interruptions in sleep continuity**, rather than simple sleep deprivation, may play a pathophysiological role in the development of chronic pain.[27]

Analysis of PSG in patients with FM have shown variable results. Older studies showed decreased TST, decreased stage N3, and increased arousals. A more recent study found decreased sleep efficiency and increased stage N1.[25] An interesting electroencephalography (EEG) pattern (alpha sleep or alpha-NREM anomaly) was first described in patients with FM by Roizenblatt and coworkers[28] and Branco and colleagues.[29] This is characterized by prominent alpha activity (8-13 Hz) persisting into NREM sleep (alpha intrusion). Alpha activity is normally present during relaxed wakefulness and after brief awakenings (arousals) but is normally virtually absent during stages N2 and N3, except as associated with arousals. Alpha intrusion into stage N3 (slow wave or delta sleep) is called alpha-delta sleep. Since that time, it has been recognized that the alpha-NREM anomaly is not specific for FM and is not present in all patients with FM. Other groups in which the alpha-NREM sleep anomaly can be found include patients with chronic pain syndromes, depression, and diverse causes of nonrestorative sleep. Indeed, alpha sleep has been seen in up to 15% of normal subjects.[30] In a variant of alpha sleep (phasic alpha activity), alpha intrusion is seen mainly during stage N3 rather than being present diffusely in NREM sleep. In one study, phasic alpha activity seemed to be present in patients with FM with prominent sleep disturbance, subjective feelings of superficial sleep, and more pain and stiffness.[28] Chapter 4 contains sleep tracings illustrating the alpha anomaly. Of note, *patients with FM have a higher prevalence of restless leg syndrome than that of controls.*[31]

Treatment of FM

As interrupted sleep plays a significant role in the pathophysiology of FM, screening for (and treating) primary sleep disorders should be considered. Sleep hygiene and sleep extension to ensure adequate sleep are also indicated. Treatment of FM is best accomplished with a comprehensive, often multidisciplinary approach. Sarzi-Puttini et al. propose a treatment regimen for FM that is divided into four pillars: *patient education, fitness, pharmacologic treatment,* and *psychotherapy*. Fitness includes physical activity, weight loss, and a nutritional program. Psychotherapy includes cognitive behavioral therapy, hypnosis, and/or relaxation techniques. Pharmacologic treatment is recommended beginning at diagnosis, as most patients with FM have had symptoms for years prior to diagnosis[19] (Table 39–2).

Some FM patients have clinical improvement with low doses of antidepressants, whereas others require the usual doses needed for an antidepressant effect. Traditionally, low doses of tricyclic antidepressants (both serotonin and norepinephrine

Table 39–2 Treatments for Fibromyalgia*

- Patient education
- Fitness
  - Physical activity
  - Weight loss
  - Nutritional program
- Psychotherapy
  - Cognitive behavioral treatment
  - Hypnosis
  - Relaxation techniques
- Pharmacological Treatments
  - Anticonvulsants
    - Pregabalin** (Lyrica)
    - Gabapentin (Neurontin)
  - Muscle relaxants
    - Baclofen
    - Cyclobenzaprine
  - Antidepressants
    - TCAs
      - Amitriptyline (25–50mg)
    - SSRIs (if associated depression)
    - SNRIs
      - Venlafaxine (Effexor)
      - Duloxetine** (Cymbalta)
      - Milnacipran** (Savella)

*Based on the four pillars of treatment Suggested by Sarzi-Puttini[19])
**FDA approved for treatment of fibromyalgia
FDA, U.S. Food and Drug Administration; *SNRI*, selective norepinephrine reuptake inhibitor; *SSRIs*, selective serotonin reuptake inhibitors; *TCAs*, tricyclic antidepressants

reuptake inhibitors) such as amitriptyline 25 to 50 mg qhs have been used for FM.[32] The selective serotonin reuptake inhibitors (SSRIs) have not been very effective as treatment for FM unless depression is present. Two medications selectively blocking reuptake of both serotonin and norepinephrine (SNRI) are FDA approved for treatment of FM. These medications are duloxetine (Cymbalta) and milnacipran (Savella) (Table 39–2). Venlafaxine (Effexor, also an SNRI) has also been used but is not FDA approved for FM. The SNRIs appear to work in both depressed and nondepressed patients with FM.[33–36] Pregabalin (Lyrica) is an anticonvulsant that has also been FDA approved for FM. Gabapentin is another anticonvulsant that has been used for chronic pain syndromes, including FM (not FDA approved for FM). Both pregabalin and gabapentin have been shown to benefit patients with FM.[37,38] Muscle relaxants such as cyclobenzaprine have also been used.[39] Studies have shown benefit from treatment of FM with sodium oxybate.[40,41]

Sodium oxybate is believed to work in FM by improving sleep quality. Sodium oxybate is currently FDA approved for treatment of narcolepsy (cataplexy and daytime sleepiness). An application was made to the FDA for an indication for the use of sodium oxybate as a treatment for FM. However, this application was rejected, in part because of the large FM population and the potential for abuse of medication ("date rape drug"). No studies have been done to date on Xywav (calcium/magnesium/potassium/sodium oxybate, currently FDA approved for cataplexy and daytime sleepiness in narcolepsy and idiopathic hypersomnia) as a treatment for FM.

CHRONIC KIDNEY DISEASE (CKD)

Sleep in CKD

Chronic kidney disease (CKD) is present in nearly one in seven (~15%) adults in the United States, with hypertension (HTN) and diabetes mellitus (DM) being the biggest risk factors.[42] CKD results from kidney damage or decreased function resulting in a glomerular filtration rate (GFR) <60 mL/min/1.73 m^2 for ≥3 months. Stage 1 represents normal or high GFR, Stage 2 GFR <60, and the stages of CKD increase as GFR (renal function) decreases, culminating in Stage 5 or end-stage renal disease (ESRD) with a GFR <15 or requiring dialysis.[43] Nearly 2 in every 1000 adults in the United States live with ESRD, 71% of those being on dialysis via hemodialysis (HD) or peritoneal dialysis (PD) and the other 29% living with a kidney transplant.[44] Sleep disturbances are common in those on HD and are noted in up to 80%.[44] Holley et al. studied sleep disorders in 48 patients on chronic HD. *Restless legs were reported in 84%, sleep-onset insomnia in 76%, nighttime awakenings in 76%, and early morning awakenings in 72%.*[45] In addition to these sleep disturbances, changes in sleep architecture have been noted in these patients. Elias et al. studied 57 patients with ESRD using PSG and matched them to 57 controls without ESRD who had already undergone PSG according to age, BMI, periodic limb movement (PLM) index, and apnea-hypopnea index (AHI). They showed that ESRD was independently associated with a reduced TST and REM sleep time after controlling for sleep apnea and other variables. They hypothesized that reduced sleep times in patients with ESRD could be in part from uremia or fluid overload (or both).[46] Indeed, fluid status plays a role in sleep disordered breathing (SDB).

Sleep Disorders in CKD

Insomnia, RLS, PLM in sleep (PLMS), and *SDB* are all common in patients with ESRD.[47,48] Holley et al. showed that insomnia is present in 52% of patients on HD and 50% patients on PD, compared to 12% in matched healthy controls.[49] This manifests objectively on PSG as decreased TST, fragmented sleep, and decreased sleep efficiency.[46,49] Treatment of insomnia in these patients is geared toward what is thought to be the underlying cause—treatment of RLS if thought to be causing prolonged sleep latency (sleep-onset insomnia), treatment of PLMS if thought to be contributing to fragmented sleep as in PLM disorder (PLMD), and treatment of SDB if present, as it can manifest as decreased TST and fragmented sleep. Loewen et al. note it is important to keep in mind that patients with ESRD and SDB may have causes of sleep fragmentation that are beyond apnea (e.g., PLMS); if left untreated, this may compromise the goal of treating SDB (by preventing consolidated sleep).[50] The type of dialysis can also play a role, as patients undergoing PD were noted to have more fragmented sleep, and lower oxygen levels from SDB on nights fluid was present in their abdomen.[48]

The prevalence of RLS is increased in those with CKD compared to controls (3.5% vs. 1.5%, respectively).[51] *In ESRD, the prevalence is even higher, with up to 80% reporting symptoms.* PLMS symptoms are reported in up to 50% of patients with ESRD. RLS symptoms will typically be present in the evening, but also occur *during the daytime more than in patients without ESRD.* RLS in patients on hemodialysis (HD) is not more common in women than men. PLMS can fragment sleep but can be difficult to isolate as the definite cause—treatment is geared toward reduction of PLMS and symptomatic improvement (more consolidated sleep).[47] Iron deficiency and uremia are often causes of RLS in those with CKD. Treatment directed toward the underlying etiology is the proper approach. Treatment of anemia with erythropoietin, if appropriate, has shown to help in this population via reduction in RLS symptoms, PLMS, arousals from sleep, and sleep fragmentation; this facilitates more restorative sleep and improved daytime symptoms.[52] Pharmacologic therapy for RLS in these patients should be approached with attention to proper renal dosing according to renal function. It may be necessary to completely avoid renally cleared medications for an alternate mode of metabolism. For example, ropinirole may be preferred over pramipexole, as the former is metabolized in the liver whereas the latter depends on renal clearance. Though HD and PD do not treat RLS or PLMS, kidney transplantation has been shown to improve both[53,54] in these patients. A reduced dose of gabapentin can also be used to treat RLS in patients with ESRD. Please see Chapter 31 for a detailed discussion of treatment of RLS, including that for patients on dialysis.

The prevalence of SDB is increased in those with CKD compared to the general population for both OSA and CSA. Prevalence depends on the AHI cutoff used to define sleep apnea in individual studies, but while OSA is present in 10% and CSA in <1% of the general population, they are present in 27% to 57% and 10% of those with CKD, respectively.[43] Although the prevalence of SDB is increased in ESRD, the clinical presentation is different from that in the general population—*snoring is often less robust, witnessed apneas are less common, and the patients are often not overweight.*[47,55] It is increasingly clear that there is a bidirectional interaction between SDB and CKD—each contributing to the other. Nicholl et al. showed that as renal function declines, the prevalences of SDB and nocturnal hypoxia both increase.[56]

The mechanisms by which CKD contributes to the progression of SDB is tied to the increases in uremia, hypervolemia, and altered chemosensitivity as renal function declines. Uremia contributes to increased upper airway collapsibility and decreased upper airway dilator function. *Hypervolemia contributes to SDB through nocturnal rostral fluid shift, which results in upper airway edema and subsequently increased OSA.*[57,58] Fluid from the legs also results in pulmonary fluid accumulation and is thought to stimulate stretch receptors, leading to hyperventilation and CO_2 levels below the apneic threshold and resulting in central apnea and cycles of hyperventilation followed by apnea.[57] Altered chemosensitivity from renal disease leads to ventilatory instability, resulting in SDB. The SDB contribution to CKD is multifactorial. SDB resulting in hypoxia and oxidative damage, activation of the sympathetic nervous system and hypertension, and activation of the renin-angiotensin system and resulting arterial stiffness and endothelial dysfunction all contribute to CKD.[43] *It should be appreciated that patients with ESRD using continuous positive airway pressure (CPAP) may have variability in the treatment response (changes in the machine estimate of the AHI).* Increased volume pre-dialysis can predispose patients to development of a component of central apnea or periodic breathing. Others may need higher pressure because of upper airway edema.

HUMAN IMMUNODEFICIENCY VIRUS (HIV)

Sleep in Human Immunodeficiency Virus (HIV)

Poor-quality sleep and sleep disturbances are present in approximately 73% of people living with human immunodeficiency virus (PLWH).[59,60] Faraut et al. noted sleep disturbances in the form of greater sleep latency and high sleep fragmentation in PLWH compared to gender- and age-matched controls[61] (although it should be emphasized that sleep was estimated by actigraphy rather than by EEG, electrooculography [EOG], and electromyography [EMG] in PSG). Norman et al. used PSG to study PLWH, demonstrating variations in sleep architecture in this population. Their study of 24 men (14 with HIV and 10 aged-matched controls without HIV) showed that wakefulness, SWS, and REM sleep were more evenly dispersed throughout the night than in controls. **Stage N3 in particular was more prevalent in the second half of the night.** PLWH had more subjective sleep complaints, including difficulty with initiating sleep, difficulty maintaining sleep, and daytime sleepiness; however, no correlation was found with the PSG-derived data.[62] Though the presence of HIV infection goes hand in hand with sleep disturbances, it has also been shown that increasing severity of HIV (decreasing CD4 counts) is correlated with increasing sleep disturbance. Darko et al. showed that those with mild HIV infection (CD4 >400 cells/mm^3) had more mild symptoms of insomnia and fatigue, and PSG showed *increased* stage N3 and alpha intrusion. In those with moderate infection (CD4 200-400 cells/mm^3), insomnia and fatigue were more significant, and PSG yielded *decreased* stage N3. Finally, those with severe HIV infection (CD4 <200 cells/mm^3) were more fatigued, slept more during the day, and commonly experienced severe insomnia. PSG in these patients yielded absent stage N3 and fragmented sleep.[62,63] Patients on pharmacologic therapy for HIV, including the non-nucleoside reverse transcriptase inhibitors (NNRTIs) *efavirenz and nevirapine, often report vivid dreams.*[64]

PREGNANCY

Sleep in Pregnancy

Pregnancy involves significant anatomical, hormonal, and physiological changes in the mother that must take place for a healthy pregnancy and delivery. A full detail of these changes is outside the scope of this chapter, but owing to these changes, sleep disturbances are common and increase as the pregnancy moves from the first through third trimesters and following delivery.[65] Many expectant mothers report sleep disturbances. The exact proportion that report disturbances varies widely in the literature.[66] This variation is in part because studies seeking to quantify the exact changes in sleep in pregnancy have been challenged by different (subjective vs. objective) methods of data collection (self-report vs. actigraphy vs. home sleep testing vs. PSG), different points in gestation of those being studied, and different points in menstrual cycles for those being studied as controls for comparison.[65] Sedov et al. conducted a meta-analysis to quantify the prevalence of poor sleep quality in pregnancy. Data analyzed in their study included the Pittsburg Sleep Quality Index (PSQI) values of 11,002 pregnant women. The average PSQI in these women was 6.07 (scores ≥5 differentiated poor from good sleepers). *Sleep quality had a significant decrease from the second to the third trimester.*[66] Though parsing between normal and abnormal sleep in pregnancy may be difficult, it is an important distinction to make, as *poor sleep has been tied to adverse outcomes including postpartum depression, longer labor duration, and increased frequency of cesarean deliveries.*[67] Additionally, sleep deficiency is tied to gestational diabetes and hypertensive disorders in pregnancy.[68] Balserak et al. wrote extensively on sleep in pregnancy. A summary of sleep patterns, nocturnal changes, and daytime symptoms in each trimester and during labor and delivery is provided in Table 39–3.[65]

Sleep Disorders in Pregnancy

SDB, insomnia, RLS, and narcolepsy in pregnancy will be covered in this section.

SDB is more likely in expectant mothers than in the non-pregnant population. This is because of multiple physiologic changes that begin in the first semester and continue throughout the pregnancy, resulting in narrowing in the upper airway.[67] Increased estrogen and progesterone effects on capillaries yield mucosal swelling in the upper airway.[69] The resultant narrowing leads to airflow resistance and a higher Mallampati score.[70] SDB is more common as gestation progresses and has been linked to adverse pregnancy outcomes. These include gestational hypertensive disorders, gestational diabetes, and cesarean deliveries. Patients with a diagnosis of SDB who are already on treatment prior to pregnancy should continue it for the duration of the pregnancy.[67,71] Since weight gain is expected during pregnancy, the patient's pressure requirement on positive airway pressure (PAP) will increase. Generally, an increase of 1 to 3 cm H_2O will be required, and a switch to auto-titrating mode on the patient's device is a straight-forward and quick way to address this issue.[72] There are limited data regarding the effect of CPAP therapy on pregnancy outcomes for those diagnosed with SDB during pregnancy. Small studies suggest that CPAP treatment of SDB is associated with lower

Table 39–3 Sleep Pattern, Nocturnal Features, and Daytime Symptoms in Each Trimester, Labor, and Delivery

	First Trimester	Second Trimester	Third Trimester	Labor, Delivery
Pattern	↑TST ↑Number of naps ↑WASO ↓SE ↓SWS	↓TST ↓SWS ↓WASO ↑SE REM (no change)	↑TST ↑Number of naps ↑WASO ↑N1 ↓SE ↓SWS ↓REM	↓TST ↓SE ↓NREM ↓REM
Nocturnal Features	• Urinary frequency • Physical discomfort (tender breasts/back pain)	Toward end of the trimester: • Snoring • RLS • Irregular uterine contractions • Heartburn • Vivid dreams • Back, neck, and joint pain	• Urinary frequency • Physical discomforts • Heartburn • Irregular uterine contractions • Fetal movements • Muscle/leg cramps • Shortness of breath • Vivid dreams/nightmares • Snoring • RLS	• Anxiety • Forceful uterine contractions
Daytime Symptoms	• Fatigue • Drowsiness • Nausea • Mood changes	• Nasal congestion	• Fatigue • Drowsiness • Impaired vigilance • Nasal congestion	• Fatigue • Anxiety • Pain

NREM, Non-rapid eye movement; *REM*, rapid eye movement; *SWS*, slow wave sleep; *TST*, 24-hour total sleep time; *WASO*, wake after sleep onset.

Adapted from Balserak BI, O'Brien LM, and Bei B. (2022). Sleep and sleep disorders associated with pregnancy. In M Kryger, T Roth, C Goldstein, et al (Eds.), *Principles and Practice of Sleep Medicine, 7th Edition*. Vol 2, p1754. Elsevier.

rates of preterm deliveries, unplanned cesarean sections, and neonatal intensive care unit admissions.[73] Use of an auto-titrating device with a modem is ideal and can speed up treatment and adjustments, if needed. Initiating treatment with an oral appliance during pregnancy is not recommended given the time it takes for construction of the device, adjustment, and testing for efficacy.[71,72]

Insomnia symptoms are prevalent throughout pregnancy and can persist into the postpartum period.[72] *By the third trimester, insomnia is present in 60% of expectant mothers*, while 55% experience it in the postpartum period.[73] Thus pregnancy related insomnia is more likely to persist following delivery than pregancy related RLS. It cannot be stressed enough that distinguishing between normal and abnormal sleep disturbances is vital. This is because of adverse pregnancy outcomes, detailed in the above section on "Sleep in Pregnancy." It should be noted that, in addition, *poor sleep quality in pregnancy is associated with more depression and anxiety in the postpartum period.*[74] Diagnosis of insomnia during pregnancy is associated with a twofold higher risk of early preterm (<34 weeks) birth.[75] The clinical presentation often depends on the trimester. Table 39–3 details the common nocturnal features found in each trimester. Treatment should be directed toward the underlying etiology (e.g., acid reflux, RLS, positional discomfort, etc.), if possible. Some nocturnal features cannot be helped (e.g., fetal movements, uterine contractions, etc). Of course, the nocturnal features mentioned herein may be present but may not be the underlying cause of the insomnia, and a thorough history is necessary. Given the lack of risk to both the mother and developing baby, cognitive behavioral therapy for insomnia (CBTI) is the preferred treatment for insomnia in these patients. Pharmacologic treatment can be considered for those who fail or are not willing to go through CBTI. The severity of symptoms, risks, benefits, and evidence for efficacy must all be considered for any medication considered. Doxylamine is safe in pregnancy and as a first-generation antihistamine; its sedative properties can help with sleep onset. However, this medication can worsen RLS. If insomnia symptoms are severe and a prescription hypnotic is indicated, first-line treatment would be doxepin or zolpidem, given their efficacy, but their side effect profiles should be kept in mind.[72]

RLS is present in 2% to 3% of the general population[76] and *is two to three times more likely during pregnancy.*[77] Prevalence increases with gestational age, and after delivery, symptoms resolve in 50% of patients within 1 month.[78] In the other 50% of patient, symptoms persist and improve over the following year. Patients most likely to have persistent symptoms are those with RLS prior to pregnancy or with a strong family history.[72] The evaluation and treatment of RLS, including specific information on RLS in pregnancy, are discussed in detail in Chapter 31. It is appropriate, however, to note that antihistamines that block H1 receptors such as doxylamine, diphenhydramine, and hydroxyzine all classically exacerbate RLS symptoms, and all may be used as sleep aids, especially in the pregnant population, in which sleep disturbances are common. In many cases, it is not until the patient takes one of these medications that RLS symptoms are significant. It should also be noted that RLS symptoms can be exacerbated by low iron stores, even in the absence of anemia. In the pregnancy population, in which iron shifts occur and patients are more prone to iron deficiency anemia, the appropriate evaluation for low iron stores and supplementation if low (traditional ferritin goal >75 μg/L) can be very effective. A ferritin goal of >50 μg/L is more appropriate during pregnancy. There are limited data on the relationship between RLS and pregnancy outcomes; however, some analyses noted an association between gestational RLS and increased risk of peripartum depression, gestational hypertension, and preeclamsia.[72]

There is very little published data on narcolepsy in pregnant patients. It should be noted that since narcolepsy is often diagnosed in the early 20s, it is often discovered before the reproductive peak; as such, many are diagnosed before becoming pregnant. For patients with narcolepsy Type 1 (narcolepsy with cataplexy), a thorough history of cataplexy and usual triggers can be important, as pain, sudden contractions, or the labor process can potentially cause cataplexy. Avoiding any scenarios in which falling asleep could be potentially injurious to the patient or others is of course necessary. Scheduled napping during pregnancy and educating/preparing the partner about facilitating more sleep for the mother in the postpartum period is important as well. When considering stimulants or wakefulness-promoting medications, most clinicians do not prescribe these medications because of the pregnancy class and possible risks of the medication. It is important that the history include whether the mother intends to breastfeed, as some medications will be present in the breast milk.[67] Some patients may decide not to breastfeed if it means being able to resume medication for their symptoms. Weighing severity of symptoms, risks, and benefits is recommended.

EFFECT OF COVID-19 ON SLEEP AND ALERTNESS

Sleep and COVID-19

The emergence of the global pandemic in December 2019 triggered by the novel severe acute respiratory syndrome coronavirus 2 (SARS-CoV-2), the virus that causes coronavirus disease 2019 (COVID-19), has served as a major stressor and precipitating factor for sleep disturbances.[79] In response to the pandemic, many countries implemented lockdowns to contain the virus, thereby significantly altering the daily routines of many millions, perhaps billions, of people. Mendelkorn et al. sought to identify which populations experienced changes in sleeping patterns during the pandemic and to what extent. They analyzed online surveys completed by 2562 adults in 49 countries. Average sleep duration prior to the pandemic was 6.9 hours ± 1.1 hours, with 42% reporting <7 hours of sleep. At the time of the pandemic, average sleep duration was 7.2 hours ± 1.5 hours, with 35% reporting <7 hrs of sleep. *New complaints of insomnia, altered circadian rhythm, and daytime dysfunction were reported in one-third of responders.*[80] Genta et al. studied 94 *high school students in Brazil* who went through school closure and home confinement as a result of the pandemic. In this group, *bedtimes and wake-up times were delayed, and these individuals' chronotypes shifted to "eveningness" with school closure and home confinement.*[81] Conoy et al. looked at the effects of the COVID-19 stay-at-home order on sleep, health, and working patterns in U.S. healthcare workers. They found that *71% reported a change in sleep habits.* These changes included reduced TST in those working in person (essential employee status), whereas those who worked from home reported no change in sleep duration. Regardless of work location, worsened mood and increased bedtime screen time were reported in most participants.[82] Post-COVID-19 syndrome, also known as long COVID or long-haul COVID, is increasingly being studied. Overall, this illness is poorly understood and can affect any COVID-19 survivor. Fatigue and dyspnea can last for months after infection, and other symptoms can include cognitive symptoms, joint pain, palpitations, headache, smell and taste dysfunction, and gastrointestinal or cardiac issues.[83,84] No other etiology is found to explain the symptoms in these patients. These patients are increasingly referred to sleep clinicians for evaluation of a potential sleep disorder that may play a role in the fatigue they experience.

Sleep Disorders and COVID-19

SDB and COVID-19

The literature has begun to shed some light on sleep disorders and COVID-19. Strausz et al. studied 445 individuals with COVID-19 and performed a meta-analysis of previous studies.[85] Severe COVID-19 in this study was defined as illness requiring hospitalization. *OSA was associated with COVID-19 hospitalization independent of age, sex, and comorbidities.* The risk of contracting COVID-19 was the same for patients with OSA as for those without. *Among COVID-19-positive patients, OSA was associated with a higher risk of hospitalization and development of respiratory failure.* It should be noted that severe COVID-19 and OSA share similar risk factors-high BMI, diabetes, older age, and male gender. Thus far, no studies have shown a clear risk for increased mortality between OSA and COVID-19. There has been conflicting information about mortality, as both OSA and increased mortality are associated with risk factors such as obesity and metabolic syndrome. That is, many,[86] but not all,[87] studies have documented that OSA increases the risk of mortality as a result of COVID-19. One study of patients with OSA on auto-adjusting PAP (APAP) treatment[88] found that, after COVID-19, pressure requirements increased. This suggests long-term upper-airway changes are present after COVID-19 infection. The pandemic was associated with increased use of telehealth in sleep medicine with remote CPAP setup and mask fitting by computer programs. An increase in telehealth in sleep medicine will likely persist (or even increase) in the future.

Hypersomnias and COVID-19

Rodrigues Aguilar et al. sought to understand the effects of the COVID-19 pandemic on patients with narcolepsy[89]. They studied 76 patients (52 with narcolepsy Type 1 [NT1], 24 with narcolepsy Type 2 [NT2]) at a sleep clinic in Brazil using a questionnaire of 36 questions, including the Epworth Sleepiness Scale (ESS) during a 3-month quarantine period. *Bedtime and wake-up time both shifted later in this population.* During the pandemic, 60.5% of patients reported increased scheduled naps, and 52.6% reported worsened sleepiness, while 51.3% reported worsened quality of life during the pandemic. Nigam et al.[90] performed a similar study on patients with NT1, NT2, and idiopathic hypersomnia (IH) in France and noted decreased symptoms of the central hypersomnias. In surveys completed by 851 patients, 25.7% reported a *mean increase in night sleep time and a mean decrease of ESS during lockdown.* Bedtime was delayed in 46.1% of participants, and wake-up time was delayed in 59.6%, mainly in participants with IH. Cataplexy improved in 54.1% of participants. *The authors concluded that patients with NT1, NT2, and IH may benefit from a decrease in social and professional constraints on their sleep-wake habits.*

SUMMARY OF KEY POINTS

1. Sleep apnea is very common in patients with acromegaly (47–81%, depending on the study). The prevalence of sleep apnea is higher with active disease. Of those with acromegaly and sleep apnea, two-thirds have OSA and one-third have CSA. Hypertension in acromegaly is strongly associated with sleep apnea.
2. Increased ventilatory responsiveness and insulin-like growth factor-1 (IGF-1) are higher in patients with acromegaly and CSA than in those with OSA.
3. The severity of sleep apnea has been shown to improve, but not resolve, in most cases with treatment of acromegaly.
4. Patients with cancer commonly experience insomnia symptoms, and screening for insomnia with a validated method, such as the ISI, is considered best practice for routine oncologic care.
5. CBTI is recommended as the first-line treatment of insomnia. Sleep disturbances secondary to comorbid depression, oncologic pain, or treatment side effects may call for different, specific treatments directed toward the etiology.
6. **Cancer-related fatigue** is one of the most common and bothersome symptoms in cancer, and the degree of symptoms will vary among patients and clinical scenarios.
7. Criteria for the diagnosis of ME/CFS have been revised in recent years. *Post-exertional malaise is considered the hallmark symptom. Unrefreshing sleep is also one of the required criteria.*
8. Symptoms of ME/CFS significantly impair occupational, educational, social, and personal activities, and the degree of impairment may be anywhere from very mild to severe.
9. Decreased HRV as a result of decreased parasympathetic activity is thought to suggest hypervigilant sleep in those with ME/CFS.
10. From a sleep perspective, treatment of ME/CFS includes fully treating any primary sleep disorders, if present, and addressing external disruptions, if present. Hypnotics can be considered.
11. Criteria for the diagnosis of FM were revised in 2016. Sleep complaints in FM are common and include nonrestorative sleep, fragmented sleep, and insomnia.
12. Studies of PSG in FM have shown decreased sleep efficiency, increased stage N1, and increased awakenings.
13. Alpha-delta sleep is characterized by alpha intrusion into stage N3 (slow-wave or delta) sleep. Though this finding can be seen in FM, it is not specific to FM, nor is it found in all patients with FM.
14. Patients with CKD commonly report sleep disturbances, including RLS symptoms, sleep-onset insomnia, nighttime awakenings, and early morning awakenings. PSG in these patients has objectively shown decreased TST, fragmented sleep, and decreased sleep efficiency.
15. ESRD is associated with reduced TST and REM sleep after controlling for sleep apnea. Reduced sleep times in patients with ESRD is thought to be in part from uremia or fluid overload (or both).
16. OSA is common in patients with CKD but patients with OSA and CKD may be thinner and report less snoring than patients with OSA who do not have CKD.
17. RLS is increased in patients with CKD compared to controls. The incidence of RLS is highest in ESRD.
18. While HD and PD do not treat RLS or PLMS, kidney transplantation has been shown to improve both in these patients.
19. CKD and SDB have a bidirectional relationship – each contributes to the other in multiple ways. In patients on hemodialysis, the effective level of CPAP can increase during periods of fluid overload which can upper airway edema and also cause instability in ventilatory control.
20. Poor sleep quality and sleep disturbances are common in PLWH. In studies of PSG in these patients, SWS was more prevalent in the second half of the night.
21. Increasing sleep disturbances go hand in hand with increasing severity of HIV infection (decreasing CD4 counts).
22. Patients with severe HIV infection (CD4 <200 cells/mm^3) were found to be more fatigued and slept more during the day. PSG in these patients shows **absent SWS and fragmented sleep.**
23. Sleep disturbances are common in pregnancy and tend to increase while sleep quality decreases with gestational age.
24. Poor sleep, poor sleep quality, and short sleep duration are all associated with adverse pregnancy outcomes. It is therefore important for the clinician to be able to distinguish between normal and abnormal sleep in the expectant mother. Many individuals with pregnancy related insomnia will have persistent insomnia in the post-partum period.
25. Physiological changes on the upper airway in pregnancy contribute to increased risk of developing SDB, and there is increasing risk of SDB up until delivery.
26. RLS is common in pregnancy and increases with gestational age. It will resolve within 1 month after delivery in 50% of patients and improves over the next 6 to12 months in the other 50%. Of note, some studies show a quicker resolution of RLS after delivery. The presence of RLS during pregnancy (even if not present before pregnancy) is a risk factor for development of RLS in future pregnancy. There are special considerations for treatment of RLS in pregnancy (see Chapter 31).
27. The emergence of the global pandemic and subsequent lockdowns and quarantines imposed to restrict virus spread had significant impacts on daily routines, including sleep and wake-up times. Later bedtimes and wake-up times, increased mood disturbances, and increased screen time are a few of the changes in habits that have been noted.
28. The COVID-19 pandemic resulted in an increase in sleep disorders and complaints such as insomnia, nightmares, and posttraumatic stress disorder (PTSD)–like syndrome among *uninfected* caregivers and the public.
29. OSA is a risk factor for severe COVID-19 (SARS-CoV-2 infection requiring hospitalization or development of respiratory failure). *CPAP pressure requirements may increase* after SARS-CoV-2 infection.
30. The decrease in social and professional constraints on sleep-wake habits associated NT1, NT2, and IH likely results from the ability to take more naps or increase sleep duration.
31. Phenotypes of patients with long COVID include those with cognitive symptoms often manifested as brain fog, respiratory symptoms such as shortness of breath, neurological symptoms manifested by fatigue, and mixed phenotypes of all three.

CLINICAL REVIEW QUESTIONS

1. HTN in acromegaly is strongly associated with which of the following sleep disorders?
   A. Insomnia
   B. RLS
   C. SDB
   D. RBD
   E. NT1
2. Which of the following is the most common initial approach to treating cancer-related fatigue, as studies have documented its benefits in this population?
   A. Sleep extension
   B. Increasing physical activity via exercise
   C. Initiating wakefulness-promoting medications or stimulants
   D. Transfusion of red blood cells
3. Which of the following is the "hallmark symptom" of ME/CFS?
   A. Substantial reduction or impairment in the ability to engage in pre-illness levels of occupational, educational, social, or personal activities persisting for >6 months and accompanied by fatigue that is new or of definite onset (not lifelong), is not caused by ongoing excessive exertion, and is not substantially alleviated by rest.
   B. Post-exertional malaise
   C. Unrefreshing sleep
   D. Cognitive impairment
   E. Orthostatic intolerance
4. A common finding on PSG in patients with FM is which of the following?
   A. Increased sleep spindles
   B. REM-rebound
   C. Increased sleep efficiency
   D. Alpha-delta sleep
   E. Decreased amount of stage N1 sleep.
5. Which of the following is **NOT** true regarding patients with CKD compared to the general population when presenting with SDB?
   A. Snoring is often less robust compared to OSA patients without CKD.
   B. Witnessed apneas are less common.
   C. They are often not overweight.
   D. Neck circumference is often higher.
6. Which of the these populations would you expect to have the most sleep disturbances?
   A. Patients with mild HIV infection (CD4 count >400 cells/mm^3)
   B. Patients with moderate HIV infection (CD4 200–400 cells/mm^3)
   C. Patients with severe HIV infection (CD4 <200 cells/mm^3)
7. What percent of pregnant women experience a resolution in RLS symptoms by 1 month after delivery?
   A. 10%
   B. 25%
   C. 50%
   D. 95%
8. SDB in pregnancy has been linked to which of the following adverse pregnancy outcomes?
   A. Gestational hypertension
   B. Gestational diabetes
   C. Cesarean deliveries
   D. A and B
   E. A, B, and C
9. Which of the following was NOT a common finding during the COVID-19 pandemic?
   A. An earlier bedtime
   B. Benefit from a longer sleep duration in some patients with hypersomnia disorders
   C. Insomnia
   D. Obesity as a risk factor for severe COVID-19
   E. Nightmares, dreams with negative emotion
10. Which statement describes the relationship between OSA and COVID-19?
   A. The presence of OSA is not related to COVID-19 manifestations.
   B. PAP settings remain stable during SARS-CoV-2 infection.
   C. Patients with OSA appear to have worse COVID-19-related outcomes, including hospitalization and respiratory failure

ANSWERS

1. C. SDB.
2. B. Increasing physical activity via exercise.
3. B. Post-exertional malaise.
4. D. Alpha-delta sleep. However, this finding is not specific to patients with FM and is not found in all patients with FM. Sleep efficiency is decreased and the amount of stage N1 is increased. in patients with fibromyalgia.
5. D. Neck circumference if often higher (this is false).
6. C. Patients with severe HIV infection (CD4 <200 cells/mm^3).
7. C. 50%. (Although some studies show a much higher percentage.)
8. E. A, B, and C.
9. A. A later bedtime was common during the pandemic.
10. C. There may be higher CPAP requirements after COVID-19. The presence of OSA increases the risk of being hospitalized or developing respiratory failure with COVID-19. There is conflicting information regarding the presence of OSA increasing mortality risk in patients with COVID-19.

SUGGESTED READING

Facco FL, Chan M, Patel SR. Common sleep disorders in pregnancy. *Obstet Gyencol.* 2022;140(2):321-339. doi:10.1097/AOG.0000000000004866.

Lin CH, Lurie RC, Lyons OD. Sleep apnea and chronic kidney disease: a state-of-the-art review. *Chest.* 2020;157(3):673-685.

Melmed S. Acromegaly. *N Engl J Med.* 2006;355:2558-2573.

Sarzi-Puttini P, Giorgi V, Marotto D, Atzeni F. Fibromyalgia: an update on clinical characteristics, aetiopathogenesis and treatment. *Nat Rev Rheumatol.* 2020;16:645-660. doi:10.1038/s41584-020-00506-w.

REFERENCES

1. Melmed S. Acromegaly. *N Engl J Med.* 2006;355:2558-2573.
2. Sanno N, Teramoto O, Osamura RY, et al. Pathology of pituitary tumors. *Neurosurg Clin N Am.* 2003;14:25-39.
3. Grunstein RR, Ho KY, Sullivan CE. Sleep apnea in acromegaly. *Ann Intern Med.* 1991;115:527-532.
4. Grunstein RR, Ho KY, Berthon-Jones M, et al. Central sleep apnea is associated with increased ventilatory response to carbon dioxide and hypersecretion of growth hormone in patients with acromegaly. *Am J Respir Crit Care Med.* 1994;150:496-502.

5. Davi MV, Carbonare LD, Giustina A, et al. Sleep apnoea syndrome is highly prevalent in acromegaly and only partially reversible after biochemical control of the disease. *Eur J Endocrinol.* 2008;159:533-540.
6. Grunstein RR, Ho KY, Sullivan CE. Effect of octreotide, a somatostatin analog, on sleep apnea in patients with acromegaly. *Ann Intern Med.* 1994;121:478-483.
7. Rosenow F, Reuter S, Deub U, et al. Sleep apnoea in treated acromegaly: relative frequency and predisposing factors. *Clin Endocrinol.* 1996;45: 563-569.
8. Büttner-Teleagă A, Kim YT, Osel T, Richter K. Sleep disorders in cancer – a systematic review. *Int J Environ Res Public Health.* 2021;18:11696. Available at: https://doi.org/10.3390/ijerph182111696.
9. Savard J, Ivers H, Villa J, Caplette-Gingras A, Morin CA. Natural course of insomnia comorbid with cancer: an 18-month longitudinal study. *J Clin Oncol.* 2011;29:3580-3586. doi:10.1200/JCO.2010.33.2247.
10. Howell D, Oliver TK, Keller-Olaman S, et al. Sleep disturbance in adults with cancer: a systematic review of evidence for best practices in assessment and management for clinical practice. *Ann Oncol.* 2014;25:791-800. doi:10.101093/annonc/mdt506.
11. Mitchell MD, Gehrman P, Perlis M, Umscheid CA. Comparative effectiveness of cognitive behavioral therapy for insomnia: a systematic review. *BMC Fam Pract.* 2012;13(40):1-11. Available at: http://www.biomedcentral.com/1471-2296/13/40.
12. Bower JE. Cancer-related fatigue: mechanisms, risk factors, and treatments. *Nat Rev Clin Oncol.* 2014;11(10):597-609. doi:10.1038/nrclinonc.2014.127.
13. Bower JE, Bak K, Berger A, et al. Screening, assessment, and management of fatigue in adult survivors of cancer: an American Society of Clinical Oncology clinical practice guideline adaptation. *J Clin Oncol.* 2014;32:1840-1850. doi:10.1200/JCO.2013.53.4495.
14. U.S. Institute of Medicine. *Beyond Myalgic Encephalomyelitis/Chronic Fatigue Syndrome: Redefining an Illness.* Washington, DC: National Academies Press; 2015. doi:10.17226/19012.
15. Bateman L, Bested AC, Bonilla HF, et al. Myalgic encephalomyelitis/chronic fatigue syndrome: essentials of diagnosis and management. *Mayo Clin Proc.* 2021:96(11):2861-2878. doi:10/1016/j.mayocp.2021.07.004.
16. Gotts ZM, Deary V, Newton J, et al. Are there sleep-specific phenotypes in patients with chronic fatigue syndrome? A cross-sectional polysomnography analysis. *BMJ Open.* 2013;3:3002000. doi:10.1136/bmjopen-2013-002999.
17. Jackson ML, Bruck D. Sleep abnormalities in chronic fatigue syndrome/myalgic encephalomyelitis: a review. *J Clin Sleep Med.* 2012;8(6):719-728.
18. Fatt SJ, Beilharz JE, Joubert M, et al. Parasympathetic activity is reduced during slow-wave sleep, but not resting wakefulness, in patients with chronic fatigue syndrome. *J Clin Sleep Med.* 2020;16(1):19-28.
19. Sarzi-Puttini P, Giorgi V, Marotto D, Atzeni F. Fibromyalgia: an update on clinical characteristics, aetiopathogenesis and treatment. *Nat Rev Rheumatol.* 2020;16(11):645-660. doi:10.1038/s41584-020-00506-w.
20. Wolfe F, Clauw DJ, Fitzcharles MA, et al. 2016 revisions to the 2010/2011 fibromyalgia diagnostic criteria. *Semin Arthritis Rheum.* 2016; 45(3):319-329.
21. Wolfe F, Clauw DJ, Fitzcharles MA, et al. The American College of Rheumatology preliminary diagnostic criteria for fibromyalgia and measurement of symptom severity. *Arthritis Care Res.* 2010;62(5): 600-610.
22. Wolfe F, Smythe HA, Yunus MB, et al. The American College of Rheumatology 1990 criteria for the classification of fibromyalgia. Report of the multicenter criteria committee. *Arthritis Rheum.* 1990;33(2):160-172. doi:10.1002/art.1780330203.
23. Clauw DJ. Fibromyalgia: a clinical review. *JAMA.* 2014;311(15):1547-5155. doi:10.1001/jama.2014.3266.
24. Arnold LM, Bennett RM, Crofford LJ, et al. AAPT diagnostic criteria for fibromyalgia. *J Pain.* 2019;20(6):611-628. doi:10.1016/j.jpain.2018.10.008.
25. Diaz-Piedra C, Catena A, Sánchez AI, et al. Sleep disturbances in fibromyalgia syndrome: the role of clinical and polysomnographic variables explaining poor sleep quality in patients. *Sleep Med.* 2015 Aug;16(8):917-25.
26. Lentz MJ, Landis CA, Rothermel J, Shaver JL. Effects of slow wave sleep disruption on musculoskeletal pain and fatigue in middle aged women. *J Rheumatol.* 1999;26(7):1586-1592.
27. Smith MT, Edwards RR, McCann UD, Haythornthwaite JA. The effects of sleep deprivation on pain inhibition and spontaneous pain in women. *Sleep.* 2007;30(4):494-505.
28. Roizenblatt S, Moldofsky H, Benedito-Silva AA, Tufik S. Alpha sleep characteristics in fibromyalgia. *Arthritis Rheum.* 2001;44:222-230.
29. Branco J, Atalaia A, Paiva T. Sleep cycles and alpha-delta sleep in fibromyalgia syndrome. *J Rheumatol.* 1994;21:1114-1117.
30. Mahowald ML, Mahowald MW. Nighttime sleep and daytime functioning (sleepiness and fatigue) in less well-defined chronic rheumatic diseases with particular reference to the "alpha-delta NREM sleep anomaly". *Sleep Med.* 2000;1:195-207.
31. Yunus MB, Aldag J. Restless legs syndrome and leg cramps in fibromyalgia syndrome: a controlled study. *BMJ.* 1996;312:1339.
32. Goldenberg D, Mayskiy M, Mossey C, et al. A randomized, double-blind crossover trial of fluoxetine and amitriptyline in the treatment of fibromyalgia. *Arthritis Rheum.* 1996;39:1852-1859.
33. Mease PJ, Clauw DJ, Gendreau RM, et al. The efficacy and safety of milnacipran for treatment of fibromyalgia: a randomized, double-blind, placebo-controlled trial. *J Rheumatol.* 2009;36:398-409.
34. Choy EHS, Mease PJ, Kajdasz DK, et al: Safety and tolerability of duloxetine in the treatment of patients with fibromyalgia: pooled analysis of data from five clinical trials. *Clin Rheumatol* 2009;28:1035-1044.
35. Iyengar S, Webster AA, Hemrick-Luecke SK, et al: Efficacy of duloxetine, a potent and balanced serotonin-norepinephrine reuptake inhibitor in persistent pain models in rats. *J Pharmacol Exp Ther* 2004;311:576-584.
36. Arnold LM, Rosen A, Pritchett YL, et al. A randomized, double-blind, placebo-controlled trial of duloxetine in the treatment of women with fibromyalgia with or without major depressive disorder. *Pain.* 2005;119:5-15.
37. Hauser W, Bernardy K, Uceyler N, et al. Treatment of fibromyalgia syndrome with gabapentin and pregabalin: a meta-analysis of randomized controlled trials. *Pain.* 2009;145:69-81.
38. Arnold LM, Goldenberg DL, Stanford SB, et al. Gabapentin in the treatment of fibromyalgia: a randomized, double-blind, placebo-controlled, multicenter trial. *Arthritis Rheum.* 2007;56:1336-1344.
39. Tofferi JK, Jackson JL, O'Malley PG. Treatment of fibromyalgia with cyclobenzaprine: a meta-analysis. *Arthritis Rheum.* 2004;51:9-13.
40. Scharf MB, Baumann M, Berkowitz DV. The effects of sodium oxybate on clinical symptoms and sleep patterns in patients with fibromyalgia. *J Rheumatol.* 2003;30:1070-1074.
41. Moldofsky H, Inhaber NH, Guinta DR, Alvarez-Horine SB. Effects of sodium oxybate on sleep physiology and sleep/wake-related symptoms in patients with fibromyalgia syndrome: a double-blind, randomized, placebo-controlled study. *J Rheumatol.* 2010;37:2156-2166.
42. Centers for Disease Control and Prevention. *Chronic Kidney Disease in the United States, 2021.* Atlanta, GA: U.S. Department of Health and Human Services, Centers for Disease Control and Prevention; 2021.
43. Lin CH, Lurie RC, Lyons OD. Sleep apnea and chronic kidney disease: a state-of-the-art review. *Chest.* 2020;157(3):673-685.
44. Parker KP. Sleep disturbances in dialysis patients. *Sleep Med Rev.* 2003;7(2): 131-143. doi:10.1053/smrv.2001.0240.
45. Holley JL, Nespor S, Rault R. Characterizing sleep disorders in chronic hemodialysis patients. *ASAIO Trans.* 1991;37(3):M456-M457.
46. Elias RM, Chan CT, Bradley TD. Altered sleep structure in patients with end-stage renal disease. *Sleep Med.* 2016;20:67-71. Available at: http://dx.doi.org/10.1016/j.sleep.2015.10.022.
47. Hanly P. Sleep disorders and end-stage renal disease. *Curr Opin Pulm Med.* 2008;14:543-550. doi:10.1097/MCP.0b013e3283130f96.
48. Berry RB, Harding SM. Sleep and medical disorders. *Med Clin N Am.* 2004;88:679-703.
49. Holley JL, Nespor S, Rault R. A comparison of reported sleep disorders in patients on chronic hemodialysis and continuous peritoneal dialysis. *Am J Kidney Dis.* 1992;19(2):156-161. doi:10.1016/s0272-6386(12) 70125-7.
50. Loewen A, Siemens A, Hanly P. Sleep disruption in patients with sleep apnea and end-stage renal disease. *J Clin Sleep Med.* 2009;5(4): 324-329.
51. Aritake-Okada S, Nakao T, Komada Y, et al. Prevalence and clinical characteristics of restless legs syndrome in chronic kidney disease patients. *Sleep Med.* 2011;12:1031-1033.
52. Benz RL, Pressman MR, Hovick ET, et al. A preliminary study of the effects of correction of anemia with recombinant human erythropoietin therapy on sleep, sleep disorders, and daytime sleepiness in hemodialysis patients (The SLEEPO study). *Am J Kidney Dis.* 1999;34(6):1089-1095. doi:10.1016/S0272-6386(99)70015-6.
53. Molnar MZ, Novak M, Ambrus C, et al. Restless legs syndrome in patients after renal transplantation. *Am J Kidney Dis.* 2005;45(2):388-396. doi:10.1053/j.ajkd.2004.10.007.
54. Beecroft JM, Zaltzman J, Prasad R, et al. Improvement of periodic limb movements following kidney transplantation. *Nephron Clin Pract.* 2008; 109(3):c133-c139. doi:10.1159/000145456.

55. Beecroft J, Pierratos A, Hanly P. Clinical presentation of obstructive sleep apnea in patients with end-stage renal disease. *J Clin Sleep Med.* 2009;5(2):115-121.
56. Nicholl DDM, Ahmed SB, Loewen AHS, et al. Declining kidney function increases the prevalence of sleep apnea and nocturnal hypoxia. *Chest.* 2012;141(6):1422-1430. doi:10.1378/chest.11-1809.
57. Yumino D, Redolfi S, Ruttanaumpawan P, et al. Nocturnal rostral fluid shift: a unifying concept for the pathogenesis of obstructive sleep apnea and central sleep apnea in men with heart failure. *Circulation.* 2010; 121(14):1598-1605. doi:10.1161/circulationaha.109.902452.
58. Elias RM, Chan CT, Paul N, et al. Relationship of pharyngeal water content and jugular volume with severity of obstructive sleep apnea in renal failure. *Nephrol Dial Transplant.* 2013;28(4):937-944.
59. Rubinstein ML, Selwyn PA. High prevalence of insomnia in an outpatient population with HIV infection. *J Acquir Defic Syndr Hum Retrovirol.* 1998;19(3):260-265.
60. Gutierrez J, Tedaldi EM, Armon C, et al. Sleep disturbances in HIV-infected patients associated with depression and high right of obstructive sleep apnea. *SAGE Open Med.* 2019;7:2050312119842268. doi:10.1177/2050312119842268.
61. Faraut B, Tonetti L, Malmartel A, et al. Sleep, prospective memory, and immune status among people living with HIV. *Int J Environ Res Public Health.* 2021;18:438. doi:10.3390/ijerph18020438.
62. Norman SE, Chediak AD, Freeman C, et al. Sleep disturbances in men with asymptomatic human immunodeficiency (HIV) infection. *Sleep.* 1992;15(2):150-155. doi:10.1093/sleep/15.2.150.
63. Darko DF, McCutchan JA, Kripke DF, et al. Fatigue, sleep disturbance, disability, and indices of progression of HIV infection. *Am J Psychiatry.* 1992;149(4):514-520. doi:10.1176/ajp.149.4.514.
64. Morlese JF, Qazi NA, Gazzard BG, et al. Nevirapine-induced neuropsychiatric complications, a class effect of non-nucleoside reverse transcriptase inhibitors? *AIDS.* 2002;16(13):1840-1841.
65. Balserak BI, O'Brien LM, Bei B. Sleep and sleep disorders associated with pregnancy. In: Kryger M, Roth T, Goldstein C, et al., eds. *Principles and Practice of Sleep Medicine.* 7th ed., Vol. 2. Elsevier; 2022:1751-1763.
66. Sedov ID, Cameron EE, Madigan S, et al. Sleep quality during pregnancy: a meta-analysis. *Sleep Med Rev.* 2018;38:168-176. doi:10.1016/j.smrv.2017.06.005.
67. Oyiengo, D, Louis M, Hott B, et al. Sleep disorders in pregnancy. *Clin Chest Med.* 2014;35(3):571-587. doi:10.1016/j.ccm.2014.06.012.
68. Delgado A, Louis JM. Sleep deficiency in pregnancy. *Clin Chest Med.* 2022;43(2):261-272. doi:10.1016/j.ccm.2022.02.004.
69. Izci B, Riha RL, Martin SE, et al. The upper airway in pregnancy and pre-eclampsia. *Am J Resp Crit Care Med.* 2003;167(2):137-140. doi:10.1164/rccm.200206-590OC.
70. Pilkington S, Carli F, Dakin MJ, et al. Increase in Mallampati score during pregnancy. *Br J Anaesth.* 1995;74(6):638-642. doi:10.1093/bja/74.6.638.
71. Facco F, Louis J, Knauert MP, et al. Sleep-disordered breathing in pregnancy. In: Kryger M, Roth T, Goldstein C, et al., eds. *Principles and Practice of Sleep Medicine.* 7th ed., Vol. 2. Elsevier; 2022:1764-1772.
72. Facco FL, Chan M, Patel SR. Common sleep disorders in pregnancy. *Obstet Gyencol.* 2022;140(2):321-339. doi:10.1097/AOG.0000000000004866.
73. Siversten B, Hysing M, Dorheim SK, et al. Trajectories of maternal sleep problems before and after childbirth: a longitudinal population-based study. *BMC Pregnancy Childbirth.* 2015;15:129. doi:10.1186/s12884-015-0577-1.
74. Okun ML, Mancuso RA, Hobel CJ, et al. Poor sleep quality increases symptoms of depression and anxiety in postpartum women. *J Behav Med.* 2018;41(5):703-710. doi:10.1007/s10865-018-9950-7.
75. Felder JN, Baer RJ, Rand L, et al. Sleep disorder diagnosis during pregnancy and risk of preterm birth. *Obstet Gynecol.* 2017;130(3):573-581.
76. Allen RP, Walters AS, Montplaisir J, et al. Restless legs syndrome prevalence and impact: REST general population study. *Arch Intern Med.* 2005;165(11):1286-1292. doi:10.1001/archinte.165.11.1286.
77. Manconi M, Govoni V, De Vito A, et al. Restless legs syndrome and pregnancy. *Neurology.* 2004;63(6):1065-1069. doi:10.1212/01.wnl.0000138427.83574.a6.
78. Chen SJ, Shi L, Bao YP, et al. Prevalence of restless legs syndrome during pregnancy: a systematic review and meta-analysis. *Sleep Med Rev.* 2018;40:43-54. doi:10.1016/j.smrv.2017.10.003.
79. Kryger M, Goldstein CA. Covid-19 and sleep. In: Kryger M, Goldstein A, Roth T, Dement WC, eds. *Principles and Practice of Sleep Medicine.* Philadelphia: Elsevier; 2023:1999-2009.
80. Mandelkorn U, Genzer S, Choshen-Hillel S, et al. Escalation of sleep disturbances amid the COVID-19 pandemic: a cross-sectional international study. *J Clin Sleep Med.* 2021;17(1):45-53. doi:10.5664/jcsm.8800.
81. Genta FD, Rodrigues NGB, Sunfeld JPV, et al. COVID-19 pandemic impact on sleep habits, chronotype, and health-related quality of life among high school students: a longitudinal study. *J Clin Sleep Med.* 2021;17(7):1371-1377. doi:10.5664/jcsm.9196.
82. Conroy DA, Hadler NL, Cho E, et al. The effects of COVID-19 stay-at-home order on sleep, health, and working patterns: a survey study of US health workers. *J Clin Sleep Med.* 2021;17(2):185-191. doi:10.5664/jcsm.8808.
83. Yong SJ. Long-haul COVID-19: putative pathophysiology, risk factors, and treatments. *Infect Dis (Lond).* 2021;53(10):737-754. doi:10.1080/23744235.2021.1924397.
84. Writing Committee for the COMEBAC Study Group, Morin L, Savale L, et al. Four-month clinical status of a cohort of patients after hospitalization for COVID-19. *JAMA.* 2021;325(15):1525-1534. doi:10.1001/jama.2021.3331. Erratum in: *JAMA.* 2021;326(18):1874.
85. Strausz S, Kiiskinen T, Broberg M, et al. Sleep apnoea is a risk factor for severe COVID-19. *BMJ Open Respir Res.* 2021;8(1):3000845. doi:10.1136/bmjresp-2020-000845.
86. Hariyanto TI, Kurniawan A. Obstructive sleep apnea (OSA) and outcomes from coronavirus disease 2019 (COVID-19) pneumonia: a systematic review and meta-analysis. *Sleep Med.* 2021;82:47-53.
87. Wang H, Shao G, Rong L, et al. Association between comorbid sleep apnoea-hypopnoea syndrome and prognosis of intensive care patients: a retrospective cohort study. *BMJ Open.* 2021;11(6):e048886.
88. Fidan V, Koyuncu H, Akin O. Alteration of auto-CPAP requirements in obstructive sleep apnea patients with COVID-19 history. *Am J Otolaryngol.* 2021;42(3):102919.
89. Rodrigues Aguilar AC, Frange C, Huebra L, et al. The effects of the COVID-19 pandemic on patients with narcolepsy. J Clin Sleep Med. 2021 Apr 1;17(4):621-627. Doi: 10.5664/jcsm.8952.
90. Nigam M, Hippolyte A, Dodet P, et al. Sleeping through a pandemic: impact of COVID-19 – related restrictions on narcolepsy and idiopathic hypersomnia. J Clin Sleep Med. 2022 Jan 1;18(1):255-263. Doi: 10.5664/jcsm.9556.

Chapter 40

Sleep and Neurological Disorders

INTRODUCTION

This chapter is not meant to be a comprehensive discussion of sleep and sleep disorders in all neurological disorders; it concentrates on neurodegenerative disorders, stroke, and traumatic brain injury (TBI). Some discussion of sleep and neuromuscular disorders appears in Chapter 30, sleep and epilepsy in Chapter 35, and sleep and neurological disorders associated with hypersomnia in Chapter 32. Myotonic dystrophy is a muscle disorder but is included here, as it considered to be a cause of central hypersomnia and may present with daytime sleepiness and distal muscle weakness (or wasting).

NEURODEGENERATIVE DISORDERS AND SLEEP

Sleep complaints are very common in patients with neurodegenerative disorders (Box 40–1). Some basic knowledge about these disorders is essential for the sleep clinician. The major neurodegenerative disorders are discussed briefly with an emphasis on their effects on sleep.

Synucleinopathies

The synucleinopathies are chronic and progressive disorders associated with a decline in cognitive, behavioral, and autonomic functions.[1,2] The two major categories are tauopathies and alpha synucleinopathies (Table 40–1). The tauopathies are disorders associated with intracellular disposition of abnormally phosphorylated tau (a microtubule-associated protein) usually expressed as neurofibrillary tangles, neutrophil threads, and abnormal tau filaments (Pick bodies). Tau proteins are involved in maintaining the cell shape and serve as tracks for axonal transport. The tauopathy disorders include Alzheimer's disease (AD), progressive supranuclear palsy (PSP), corticobasal degeneration (CBD), frontotemporal dementia (FTD), and Pick's disease. Alpha synuclein is a protein that helps in the transportation of dopamine-laden vesicles from the cell body to the synapses. The alpha synucleinopathies include Parkinson's disease (PD), diffuse Lewy body dementia (DLBD), and multiple system atrophy (MSA).

DEMENTIAS

Dementia is defined as a clinical syndrome characterized by acquired loss of cognitive and emotional abilities severe enough to interfere with daily functioning.[1-3] Sometimes the terms mild cognitive impairment (MCI) and three or more stages of dementia are used (early/mild, middle/moderate, late/severe) to classify the severity of dementia. A dementia classification scale based on the global deterioration scale has also been used.[4] Both MCI and mild dementia are characterized by objective evidence of cognitive impairment. The main distinctions between MCI and mild dementia are that in the latter, more than one cognitive domain is involved and *substantial interference with daily life is evident*. In the *Diagnostic and Statistical Manual of Mental Disorders* (DSM-5) the term *major neurocognitive disorder* is used rather than *dementia*.[3] In this disorder there is evidence of significant cognitive decline from a previous level of performance in one or more cognitive domains: learning and memory, language, executive function, complex attention, perceptual-motor, and social cognition. The cognitive deficits interfere with the ability to independently carry out the tasks of everyday life.

In evaluating any patient with dementia, it is important to rule out treatable causes including medication side effects, hypothyroidism, vitamin B_{12} deficiency, depression, and occult obstructive sleep apnea (OSA). Pseudodementia of the elderly is due to depression and can be associated with a short rapid eye movement (REM) latency and high REM density. In contrast, patients with Alzheimer's Disease (AD) tend to have a low REM density, a long REM latency, and a reduction in amount of REM sleep. AD is by far the most common cause of dementia with DLBD the next most common cause (Box 40–2).

Alzheimer's Disease

AD is the most common cause of dementia (>60% of dementias). The diagnosis is one of exclusion. The hallmark is a *gradual onset of short-term memory problems*. AD affects 5% to 10% of people older than 65 years, and 50% of those older than 85 years. Nonmodifiable risk factors for AD include female sex, Black race, Hispanic ethnicity, and genetic factors such as the specific allele (ϵ4) of the apolipoprotein E gene. In the early stages of Alzheimer's disease, an MRI scan of the brain may be normal. In later stages, MRI may show a decrease in the size of different areas of the brain (mainly affecting the temporal and parietal lobes. The brains of people with AD bear two cellular hallmarks: clumps of amyloid-β, known as plaques, that form outside cells; and strings of a protein called tau, associated with neurofibrillary tangles, that form inside cells. Some clinicians consider AD an amyloidopathy rather than a tauopathy as amyloid deposition typically appears before tau. *Sleep disturbance worsens in parallel with cognitive dysfunction.* Patients with AD suffer from sundowning (Box 40–3), which is defined as nocturnal exacerbation of disruptive behavior or agitation in older patients. This is likely the most common cause of institutionalization in patients with AD. Some of the key points concerning AD are listed in Box 40–4.

Sleep Disturbances in AD

A number of sleep-related manifestations disturbances are present in AD[1,2,5] and vary with the course of the illness (Table 40–2). These include insomnia, circadian rhythm sleep-wake disorders, and OSA. *Insomnia is the most common issue in AD*. Early in the illness, there is disruption of sleep-wake

Box 40–1 SLEEP DISORDERS IN NEURODEGENERATIVE DISORDERS

- Insomnia—sleep onset, sleep maintenance, fragmented sleep
- Hypersomnia
  - Sleep apnea syndromes
  - Hypersomnia due to the neurological disorder
  - Narcolepsy due to a medical condition
- Excessive nocturnal motor activity
- Circadian rhythm sleep disorders (irregular sleep-wake rhythm)
- Sundowning
- REM sleep behavior disorder

RBD, Rapid eye movement sleep behavior disorder.

Table 40–1 Neurodegenerative Disorders

Tauopathies

- Alzheimer's disease (AD)
- Progressive supranuclear palsy (PSP)
- Corticobasal degeneration (CBD)
- Frontotemporal dementia (FTD)
- Pick's disease*

Alpha Synucleinopathies

- Parkinson's disease (PD)
- Diffuse Lewy body dementia (DLBD)
- Multiple system atrophy (MSA)

*(specific type of FTD usually persons under 65)

Box 40–2 MAJOR DEMENTIAS

- Alzheimer's disease (60–80%)
- Diffuse Lewy body dementia (20%)
- Others (vascular, metabolic)

Box 40–3 SUNDOWNING

- *Definition:* Nocturnal exacerbation of disruptive behavior or agitation in older patients
- Factors
  - Early bedtime
  - Use of sedatives
  - Advanced cognitive impairment
  - Associated medical conditions

Box 40–4 ALZHEIMER'S DISEASE FACTS

- Most common cause of dementia (60% of cases of dementia)
- Progressive intellectual deterioration in middle to late adult life
- RBD much **less** common than in other causes of dementia
- Insomnia a major issue
- Daytime sleepiness
- Sundowning common
- OSA common, CPAP may improve mood and function
- Circadian rhythm and orexin dysregulation
- Treatment is with central anticholinesterase inhibitor medications and Memantine (Namenda)

CPAP, Continuous positive airway pressure; *OSA,* obstructive sleep apnea; *RBD,* rapid eye movement sleep behavior disorder.

Table 40–2 Sleep Disturbance in AD

- Insomnia
- Circadian rhythm sleep-wake disorders
- Daytime sleepiness
- OSA
- Medication side effects

Early AD	Late AD
• Disruption of sleep-wake rhythms • Increased nocturnal awakenings • Decreased stage N3	• Reduction in REM • Increased REM latency • EDS and daytime napping—not associated with OSA or medications

AD, Alzheimer's disease; *EDS,* excessive daytime sleepiness; *OSA,* obstructive sleep apnea; *REM,* rapid eye movement.

rhythms, nocturnal awakenings, and a decrease in stage N3 sleep. Late in the disease course, there is a reduction in REM sleep and an increased REM latency as well as excessive daytime sleepiness (EDS). The pattern is one of excessive nocturnal awakenings and increased daytime napping. Whereas both OSA, sleep loss, and medications (e.g., donepezil) can contribute to daytime sleepiness in AD patients, sleepiness can occur simply as a manifestation of AD.

AD is associated with circadian rhythm dysfunction. Degeneration of neurons in several areas important for normal circadian rhythms has been documented, including the optic nerve, retinal ganglion cells, the suprachiasmatic nucleus (SCN), and the pineal gland. The dysfunction of these brain areas may contribute to circadian rhythm disturbances in AD.[5-7] There is a decreased amplitude in circadian rhythmicity and a delayed phase in temperature and some hormonal rhythms. These patients may manifest the *irregular sleep-wake rhythm disorder (ISWRD)* characterized by multiple bouts of sleep spread over the day and night.[7] Institutional factors can worsen circadian rhythm disorders by decreasing normal zeitgebers (decreased light and activity) and disturbing nocturnal sleep (noise). Poor sleep hygiene including daytime sleeping and decreased physical activity may also impair sleep-wake rhythms. The disruption of the sleep-wake rhythms manifests itself with large amounts of daytime sleep and often an irregular sleep-wake pattern. A decrease in melatonin MT1 receptors in the SCN has been demonstrated.[7] This could be one reason for the poor response to melatonin in AD. A large multicenter trial of melatonin *did not* show an improvement in elderly patients in group facilities.[8] However, another study in elderly residents of group facilities found that combined bright light and melatonin decreased aggressive behavior and modestly improved sleep efficiency and decreased nocturnal restlessness.[9] The 2015 American Academy of Sleep Medicine (AASM) clinical practice guideline for treatment of circadian rhythm sleep wake disorders[10] recommended that ISRWD in elderly patients with dementia be treated with light therapy but **that sleep promoting medications and melatonin be avoided**. Deterioration in brain centers responsible for the control of wake and sleep also contributes to abnormal wake and sleep. *Early autopsy studies showed reduced hypocretin producing cells in the hypothalamus in patients with AD.* Other studies found an increased level of hypocretin in cerebrospinal fluid (CSF). The nature of hypocretin secretion could vary over the course of the disease. Whereas the story of hypocretin in AD is still unfolding, there appears to be *dysregulation* *of orexin secretion in AD, which is normally high during the day and low at night.*[11]

Obstructive Sleep Apnea in AD

OSA is common among patients with AD, and several studies have suggested that continuous positive airway pressure (CPAP) treatment of AD patients with OSA can slow the deterioration of cognition and improve sleep and mood.[12,13]

Treatment of AD

Patients with AD have reduced cerebral production of choline acetyl transferase, which leads to a decrease in acetylcholine synthesis and impaired cortical cholinergic function. Cholinergic medications (cholinesterase inhibitors) are used to treat AD and are mildly beneficial.[1,2] However, cholinergic medications can cause sleep disturbance (insomnia). The cholinergic medications used to treat AD include *donepezil (Aricept), rivastigmine (Exelon), and galantamine (Razadyne)*. The cholinesterase inhibitors tend to *increase REM sleep*. Donepezil is indicated for all stages of AD, and rivastigmine (Exelon) and galantamine (Razadyne) for mild to moderate AD. Rivastigmine is available as capsules, a solution, and a transdermal patch. Side effects of the cholinesterse inhibitors include nausea, vomiting, loss of appetite, and weight loss.

Memantine (Namenda), an *N*-methyl-D-aspartate (NMDA) receptor antagonist, is approved for treatment of moderate to severe AD. It is thought to prevent excitotoxicity from excessive glutamate actions at NMDA receptors that can cause neuronal dysfunction. Memantine's side effects include hallucinations and dizziness (most common side effect). Treatment with memantine can be combined with a cholinesterase inhibitor. Some studies have shown a benefit from combined treatment.

It has been increasingly recognized that amyloid deposition in the brain may be an important factor in development of AD. Aducanumab (Aduhelm)[14] and lecanemab (Leqembi)[15] are two amyloid-targeting monoclonal antibodies delivered by monthly intravenous infusions that remove beta-amyloid. The new treatments are approved by the U.S. Food and Drug Administration (FDA) for treatment of patients with AD and MCI or mild dementia. Use of these treatments is associated with a risk of infusion-related reactions known as amyloid-related imaging abnormalities (ARIA) on MRI that are characterized by brain edema (ARIA-E) and microhemorrhages (ARIA-H).

Medication-Induced Insomnia in AD

Donepezil (Aricept) (usual maximum dose of 10 mg) has been associated with incident insomnia up to 18% of patients taking this medication. Morning dosing of donepezil is recommended to minimize insomnia, nightmares, and vivid dreams.[16,17] Whereas donepezil is a once-a-day medication, rivastigmine is administered two or three times daily and must be titrated up slowly. Rivastigmine and galantamine have more gastrointestinal side effects than donepezil. The sleep of some AD patients may improve with evening doses of galantamine or rivastigmine. Stahl and coworkers[18] reviewed the results of double-blind studies of galantamine and found no higher incidence of sleep side effects than with placebo. Rivastigmine improved sleep complaints in some studies.[19,20] Whereas transdermal rivastigmine has been used to treat the REM sleep behavior disorder (RBD) in patients with mild cognitive dysfunction and Parkinson's disease,[21] rivastigmine has also been reported to cause RBD in a patient with AD.[22]

Treatment of Insomnia in AD

Interventions for insomnia in AD include good sleep hygiene and habits. This includes light and structured activities during the day (to prevent napping) and a quiet environment at night. Hypnotics must be used with great caution. A small, randomized, placebo-controlled study found benefit with low–dose (50-mg) trazodone.[23] Another placebo-controlled randomized study found benefit with prolonged-release melatonin.[24] As mentioned previously, the AASM guidelines for treatment of the ISWRD discouraged use of any type of sleeping medication in patients with dementia.

Progressive Supranuclear Palsy (PSP)

PSP is characterized by a *supranuclear extraocular gaze palsy*. Manifestations include a pseudobulbar palsy (upper neuron lesion to corticobulbar tract with dysarthria and choking), akinetic rigidity, ataxic gait and falling, limb and axial rigidity, and frontal lobe–type dementia. Dysarthria refers to difficult with speech due to weakness of the muscles involved with speech. PSP patient display both Parkinsonism (rigidity, akinesia, postural instability) and frontal lobe dementia. While AD presents with memory loss, frontal lobe dementia presents with behavior or language abnormalities. PSP patients have issues with speech and swallowing. In PSP patients there is a lack of response to dopaminergic medications.[1,2] Sleep disturbance will be present in most patients (Box 40–5). *Severe insomnia is the most common complaint* **(worse than in AD or PD).** Patients have an absence or a drastic reduction in REM sleep. *Nocturia is a common problem.* One study comparing patients with AD and PSP found occult OSA in around 50% of both groups.[25] A high and nearly equal percentage of both groups had REM sleep without atonia. However, *clinical* RBD was less common in PSP than PD (7/20 versus 13/20).[26] If RBD is present in PSP, it presents concomitantly with other findings. In contrast, RBD can occur many years before the onset of PD. Patients with PSP have a mean age of 63, and the *mean survival from symptom onset is 9 years*. Tau-positive neurofibrillary tangles are present in multiple subcortical nuclei including the locus coeruleus. There is relative preservation of the hippocampus and cortex. The physical examination in PSP shows *impaired voluntary vertical gaze, especially in the downward direction*. This early finding is useful to differentiate PSP from other Parkinson's disorders.

Sleep in PSP

PSP patients have severe sleep-maintenance insomnia (worse than PD). Sleep complaints in PSP include an increased

Box 40–5 SLEEP DISTURBANCE IN PROGRESSIVE SUPRANUCLEAR PALSY

- Sleep disturbance present in most patients (>50%)
- Insomnia is the most common sleep disorder (more severe than in AD or PD)
- RBD occurs (13–30%)—tends to **start concomitantly or soon after onset of** PSP (unlike RBD in PD, which starts BEFORE manifestations of motor and cognitive dysfunction)
- Factors leading to insomnia
  - Immobility in bed
  - Difficulty with transfer
  - Frequent nocturia

AD, Alzheimer's disease; *PD*, Parkinson's disease; *PSP*, progressive supranuclear palsy; *RBD*, rapid eye movement sleep behavior disorder.

sleep latency, increased arousals, increased awakening frequency, decreased REM sleep, and increased REM latency.[27] *Polysomnography (PSG) reveals absence of vertical eye movements during REM sleep.* Horizontal movements are present but are slower.

Corticobasal Degeneration

CBD is a neurodegenerative disorder characterized by progressive asymmetrical rigidity, apraxia, and other findings reflecting cortical and basal ganglia dysfunction.[1-2] *Apraxia* is characterized by loss of the ability to execute or carry out learned purposeful movements, despite having the desire and the physical ability to perform the movements. It is a disorder of motor planning, which may be acquired or developmental but may not be caused by incoordination. Another diagnostic feature of CBD is the **alien limb phenomenon,** which refers to *involuntary motor activity of a limb in conjunction with the feeling of estrangement from that limb.* Tau-positive astrocytic threads and oligodendroglial coiled bodies are noted. Oligodendrocytes are a type of glial cells that are responsible for myelination of axons in the central nervous system (CNS).

Frontotemporal Dementia

FTD is a type of cortical dementia with a slow onset like AD.[1,2] However, early FTD is associated with personality change versus short term memory loss in AD. FTD is characterized by insidious onset, early loss of insight, social decline, emotional blunting, *relative preservation of perception and memory*, perseverance, and echolalia. *Disinhibition and personality change are also characteristic.* Computed tomography (CT) and magnetic resonance imaging (MRI) show *frontal or anterior temporal atrophy.*

Pick's Disease

Pick's disease is a type of frontal lobe dementia *usually not associated with memory loss in early stages* (unlike AD).[1,2] The age of onset of Pick' Disease is earlier than AD. Pick's disease is especially *known for the aphasia or the speech difficulty* it causes (hesitant speech, difficulty articulating, stuttering, ungrammatical speech, difficulty recalling words or names). That is, there is progressive aphasia in this disorder. Definitive diagnosis is demonstration of Pick bodies in the brain (tangles of tau proteins inside cells).

PARKINSONISM SYNDROMES (PD, PD+)

The term *parkinsonism* is used to refer to a group of manifestations including tremor, rigidity, bradykinesia, and postural instability. Parkinsonism is found in both PD and Parkinson's Plus (PD+) disorders (Box 40–6).[28-32] The PD+ disorders (sometimes called atypical PD) include those characterized by parkinsonism and other manifestations. *The PD+ disorders include progressive supranuclear palsy (PSP), diffuse lewy body disease (DLBD), corticobasal degeneration (CBD), and multisystem atrophy (MSA).* Of note, the *brains of PD patients do have Lewy bodies* (Figure 40–1), but in DLBD, the distribution of Lewy bodies is more dense and more diverse. DLBD patients have *more prominent dementia, which occurs earlier in the disease course.* However, there is overlap between PD and DLBD. The PD+ disorders tend to progress more quickly than PD. Typically, anti-Parkinson's medications are either less effective or completely ineffective in PD+ disorders. Some PD+ patients

Box 40–6 DISORDERS ASSOCIATED WITH PARKINSONISM

Parkinsonism = tremor, rigidity, bradykinesia, and postural instability
Disorders with parkinsonism
- PD: idiopathic Parkinson's disease
- PD+: disorders **with parkinsonism** + other manifestations
  - Progressive Supranuclear Palsy (PSP)
  - Corticobasal Degeneration (CBD)
  - Diffuse Lewy Body Dementia (DLBD)
  - Multiple System Atrophy (MSA)
- Medication-induced parkinsonism (medication side effects, dopamine blockers)
- Wilson's disease (hereditary copper accumulation)—presents in younger patients with parkinsonism features, diagnosis by slit lamp examination showing Kayser-Fleischer rings

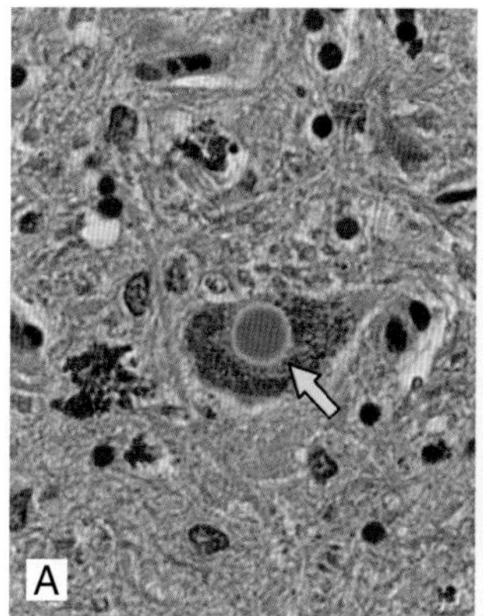

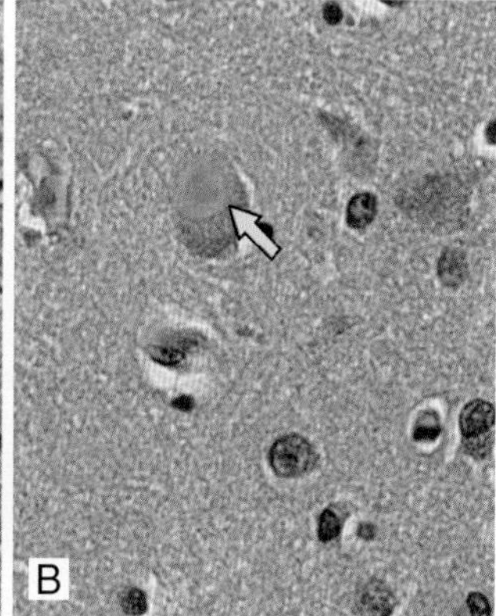

Figure 40–1 Examples of Lewy bodies *(arrows)* using hematoxylin and eosin staining. A classical Lewy body is an eosinophilic cytoplasmic inclusion consisting of a dense core surrounded by a halo of 10-nm–wide radiating fibrils, the primary structural component of which is alpha-synuclein. (A) Lewy body in substantia nigra. (B) Cortical type Lewy body in the superior temporal cortex. (From Koga S, Sekiya H, Kondru N, Ross OA, Dickson DW. Neuropathology and molecular diagnosis of synucleinopathies. *Mol Neurodegener.* 2021;16(1):83.)

(DLBD) are also very sensitive to dopamine blockers (can develop severe rigidity).

Parkinson's Disease

PD is also called primary parkinsonism or idiopathic PD. The term idiopathic means "no secondary systemic cause." The etiology of PD is partially understood and, in this sense, is not truly idiopathic. PD is a chronic neurodegenerative disorder associated with a *loss of dopaminergic neurons* (substantia nigra and other sites). PD moves through stages (Braak stages)[33] from the brainstem to midbrain (substantia nigra), to cortex. It is characterized by bradykinesia (slowing of physical movement), akinesia (loss of physical movement), rigidity, resting tremor, postural instability, and a good response to levodopa (LD) (Box 40–7).[28-32] The mnemonic TRAP can be used (<u>T</u>remor, <u>R</u>igidity, <u>A</u>kinesia, <u>P</u>ostural instability). The Movement Disorders Society[34] published diagnostic criteria using only three main elements including bradykinesia and either or both of rest tremor or rigidity. The criteria did not include postural instability, as this is not nonspecific for PD. The disorder *often starts unilaterally.* Movements are slow and reduced

Box 40–7 PARKINSON'S DISEASE MANIFESTATIONS

- Bradykinesia/akinesia—slowing/absence of physical movement
- Rigidity
- Rest tremor (pill rolling)
- Postural instability
- Glabellar reflex (sensitive but not specific)—breakdown of frontal lobe inhibition characterized by continued blinking after tapping the forehead
- Masklike facies
- Small handwriting (micrographia)
- Walking without arm swinging
- Flexed forward posture when walking with small shuffling steps
- Good response to levodopa
- Sleep disorders
  - RBD in 20–30%—often precedes PD manifestations, sometimes by 10–20 years
  - Insomnia in 50%
  - OSA very common
  - Excessive daytime sleepiness (PD, medications, OSA, nocturia, PD motor manifestations disturbing sleep)
  - Nightmares

OSA, Obstructive sleep apnea; *PD*, Parkinson's disease; *RBD*, rapid eye movement sleep behavior disorder.

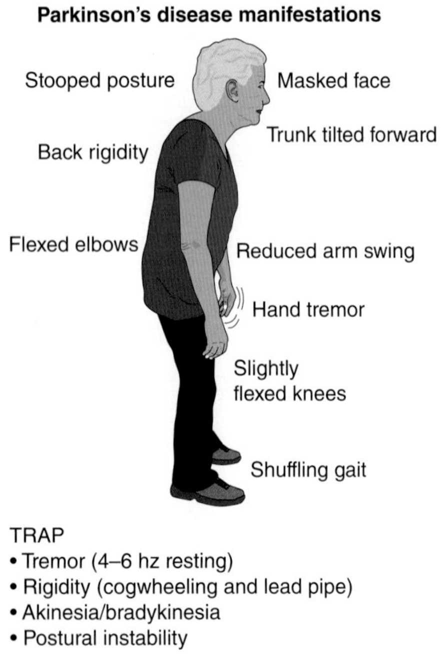

Parkinson's disease manifestations

Stooped posture
Masked face
Trunk tilted forward
Back rigidity
Flexed elbows
Reduced arm swing
Hand tremor
Slightly flexed knees
Shuffling gait

TRAP
- Tremor (4–6 hz resting)
- Rigidity (cogwheeling and lead pipe)
- Akinesia/bradykinesia
- Postural instability

Figure 40–2 A representation of some of the manifestations of Parkinson's disease. The TRAP mnemonic (Tremor, Rigidity, Akinesia, Postural instability) may also be helpful in remembering some key findings. The nonmotor manifestations (see Figure 40–3) are also problematic for the patients.

facial expressiveness is noted (masklike facies) with infrequent blinking and a monotonous voice. Gait is slow and shuffling with small steps (Figure 40–2). The tremor in PD is a *resting tremor*, maximal when limb is at rest and disappearing with voluntary movement and sleep. Secondary symptoms may include cognitive dysfunction and subtle language problems.

Nonmotor manifestations of PD include sleep disorders, constipation, dementia, orthostatic hypotension, oily skin, and seborrheic dermatitis (Figure 40–3). The sleep disorders in PD

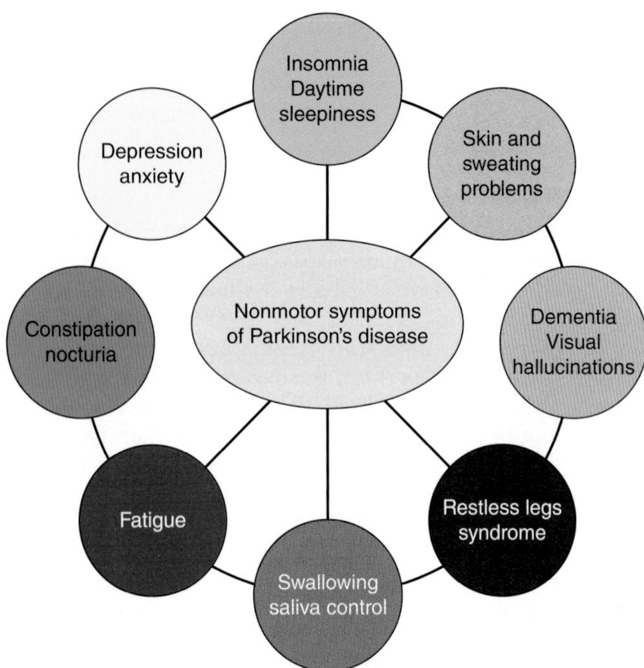

Figure 40–3 Nonmotor manifestations of Parkinson's disease. In some patients these are prominent and cause a reduced quality of life.

can occur due to medications but are also a primary manifestation of the disorder. PD patients have a sixfold increased risk of dementia. Physical findings in PD include resting pill rolling tremor, glabellar tap (tap of forehead elicits continued blinking [a frontal lobe sign]), and cogwheel rigidity (joint stiffness and increased muscle tone). Imaging of the CNS (MRI, CT scan) is typically normal. The neuropathology of PD includes the presence of Lewy bodies. A major component of the Lewy body is alpha synuclein. Secondary parkinsonism can occur secondary to drugs such as dopamine blockers (phenothiazines and butyrophenones) or head trauma.

Differential Diagnosis of PD

1. Essential tremor—Responds to beta blocker, worse on intention, improved with alcohol.
2. PD+ disorders—If cognitive dysfunction occurs early in the course (within the first year) of the suspected PD disorder, then DLBD should be suspected. If postural instability + vertical gaze palsy are prominent early, then PSP should be suspected. If autonomic dysfunction is prominent early (erectile dysfunction or syncope), MSA should be suspected.
3. CBD—If CT or MRI shows prominent asymmetry with patchy changes and cortical deficits (apraxia) are prominent, CBD should be suspected.
4. Wilson's disease—a disorder of hereditary copper accumulation. The typical presentation is a young person who has parkinsonian features. Diagnosis is made by performing a slit lamp examination for Kayser-Fleischer rings.

Treatment of PD

A detailed discussion of the treatment of PD is beyond the scope of this chapter. A number of guidelines have been published.[28,34,35] There is no proven neuroprotective treatment, so for patients with very mild disease, a wait-and-see approach (no treatment) may be useful. However, if symptoms are impacting the quality of life, treatment is indicated. Before treatment is started, the potential sleep disturbance should be discussed, as well as medication side effects. Side effects of medications play a major role in manifestation of PD related to sleep and daytime alertness. A number of different medications have been used to treat PD (Table 40–3). The reader is referred to the references for dosage.[28,34,35] The usual treatment of PD is with carbidopa/levodopa (CD/LD). Levodopa is a precursor to dopamine (DA). CD (does not pass the blood-brain barrier) prevents peripheral metabolism of LD to dopamine, thus reducing side effects and allowing for more LD to reach the CNS. The medication is effective early in disease, but efficacy slowly wanes over time. The immediate-release formulation is generally preferred. A sustained-release preparation CD/LD CR is available currently only as a generic. The brand Sinemet-CR is no longer available in the United States. The CD/LD CR formulation is poorly and slowly absorbed, with a delayed effect. The main use is for mildly affected patients in whom a slow onset is acceptable or for use during the night. CD/LD ER is a new formulation (Rytary) that has IR and CR beads and can replace the IR and CR forms. However, it is expensive. Eventually, patients treated with CD/LD will have "on times," referring to periods of time when symptoms go away or improve markedly, and "off times," referring to periods of time when symptoms return. "Wearing-off time" refers to times when symptoms are under less control, usually at the end of the expected medication duration.[28] As the number of DA neurons decreases, there is less dopamine produced for the same amount of precursor. *Dyskinesias, manifested by sudden jerky or uncontrolled movements of the limbs and neck, are a major side effect of* CD/LD treatment. Dystonia consisting of abnormal posture or cramps of the extremities or trunk can occur.

Dopamine agonists are less likely to cause dyskinesia but have some dose-dependent side effects of their own. In low doses, dopamine agonists tend to cause sleepiness or promote sleep in PD patients. Ropinirole or pramipexole have dopamine D2/D3 receptor activity and can stimulate auto receptors to decrease dopamine release. In high doses, dopamine agonists can cause insomnia, an impulse control disorder, frequent awakenings, nightmares, and a reduction in the amount of stage N3. Another serious side effect of dopamine agonist treatment of PD patients is the *often unpredictable sudden onset of severe daytime sleepiness.* Most clinicians prefer CD/LD to dopamine agonists, but the longer duration of action of dopamine

Table 40–3 Medications Used to Treat Parkinson's Disease

CD/LD Carbidopa/Levodopa 10/100, 25/100, 25/250 mg	• Very effective for akinetic symptoms or tremor • Levodopa (LD), a dopamine precursor • Carbidopa (CD) prevents peripheral conversion of LD to dopamine (decarboxylase inhibitor)
CD/LD ER (25/100, 50/200 ER) mg Sinemet CR no longer available, but generics are	• Poorly and slowly absorbed, 30% higher dose needed for same effect, time to onset unpredictable • Very low dose of LD/CD ER can cause nausea owing to inadequate CD • Possibly useful overnight • Used for mild disease when a delayed onset is acceptable.
CD/LD ER (Rytary)	• Expensive • Contains IR and ER CD/LD beads • Can replace IR and CR
Dopamine Agonists • Ropinirole (Requip) • Pramipexole (Mirapex)	• Less likely to cause dyskinesias than LD • Can cause sudden episodes of severe sleepiness • Dopamine dysregulation syndrome/impulse control disorder may occur
COMT Inhibitors • Entacapone (Comtan) • Opicapone (Ongentys) • Tolcapone (Tasmar)	• These medications prolong the effect of LD and can allow a reduction in dose • COMT inhibition reduces the peripheral methylation of LD or dopamine, which increases the plasma half-life of LD, thus prolongs action of LD • Entacapone: peripheral inhibition of COMT • Tolcapone: peripheral and central inhibition of COMT • Tolcapone: deaths from hepatotoxicity have been noted
MAOIs (type B) • Selegiline (Eldepryl): adjunct • Safinamide (Xadago): adjunct • Rasagiline (Azilect): monotherapy, adjunct	• Reduce metabolism of dopamine • Reduce "wearing-off time" • Monotherapy: mild effect, safinamide not effective as monotherapy according to FDA label • Adjunct with L-dopa useful in patients with fluctuations and wearing off
Amantadine	• Antiviral • May improve rigidity, akinesia, and tremor • Monotherapy or combined in lower doses with LD
Trihexyphenidyl (Artane) Benztropine (Cogentin)	• For younger patients with predominant tremor • Side effects: cognitive impairment and typical anticholinergic side effects (dry mouth, urinary retention, constipation)

CD, Carbidopa; *COMT,* catechol-*O*-methyl transferase; *DAs,* dopamine agonists; *ER,* extended release; *LD,* levodopa; *MAOI,* monoamine oxidase inhibitor. MAO-A inhibition reduces the breakdown of serotonin, norepinephrine, dopamine, and tyramine (dietary). MAO-A is found in the liver and intestine and important for breakdown of dietary tyramine. Dietary intake of foods rich in tyramine must be restricted. MAO-B inhibition reduces the breakdown mainly of dopamine and phenethylamine and to a lesser extent tyramine. Most MAO in the brain is type B.

agonists might make them useful for sleep (assuming insomnia or nightmares do not occur).

Catechol-*O*-methyl transferase (COMT) inhibitors have also been used as adjunctive medications in PD.[34,35] This enzyme is involved in degrading neurotransmitters including dopamine. The COMT inhibitors available include entacapone, opicapone, and tolcapone. Entacapone is only peripherally active, whereas tolcapone is active in both the peripheral and the CNS. Tolcapone can be hepatotoxic, whereas entacapone is not. These medications can permit LD effects to last longer or maintain higher levels of effectiveness. It may be possible to reduce the LD dose. Monoamine oxidase inhibitors (MAO) type B are another class of medications used in PD.[36] The enzyme MAO-A metabolizes serotonin and norepinephrine as well as dopamine. MAO-B metabolizes phenylethylamine and dopamine. MAO-B inhibitors prolong the effect of CD/LD. Selegiline is an irreversible selective MAO-B inhibitor. Amphetamine is a metabolite of selegiline, but this does not seem to be an issue. It is FDA approved as an adjunct to CD/LD and mildly prolongs the effects of CD/LD. Safinamide is a reversible highly selective MAO-B inhibitor but approved only to be used in combination with CD/LD. Rasagiline is an irreversible MAO-B selective inhibitor approved for monotherapy or to be used with CD/LD. The MAOI-B selectivity of selegiline and rasagline is dose dependent (selective at lower doses). The COMT inhibitors and MAO inhibitors are useful in advanced patients with fluctuating motor symptoms on CD/LD. Anticholinergic agents are typically used in younger patients without cognitive impairment *in whom tremor is the major feature*. The concept behind the use of these agents is that PD has upset the cholinergic-dopaminergic balance in the basal ganglia due to loss of dopaminergic neurons. Anticholinergic drugs restore the balance. The anticholinergic drugs do not work for other PD manifestations. Note that CD/LD is usually very effective for tremor. The two anticholinergic drugs most commonly used include trihexyphenidyl (Artane) and benztropine (Cogentin). Side effects of these medications including memory impairment and hallucinations limit their use. The anticholinergic side effects include dry mouth, constipation, and urinary retention.

Amantadine is an antiviral agent that can improve rigidity, akinesia, or tremor in about two-thirds of PD patients. *However, most commonly the medication is used to target dyskinesias.* The mechanism of action is unknown. Side effects include confusion, hallucinations, insomnia, and *nightmares.*

Sleep-Related Manifestations and Daytime Sleepiness in PD

Patients with PD have several sleep-related manifestations and disturbances (Box 40–8).[37-41] A meta-analysis of polysomnographic findings in PD[37] found evidence of significant reductions in total sleep time, sleep efficiency, N2 percentage, slow wave (stage N3) sleep, REM sleep percentage, and **increases** in wake time after sleep onset, the N1 percentage of total sleep time, the REM latency, the apnea-hypopnea index (AHI), and periodic limb movement in sleep index in PD patients compared with controls. There were no remarkable differences in sleep continuity or sleep architecture between PD patients with and without RBD. Treating the nocturnal manifestations of PD can be challenging. Sleep disturbance can occur due to motor manifestations, and sleep can affect some of the motor manifestations. Some factors disturbing sleep in PD and possible interventions[38,42] are listed in Table 40–4. Tremor is worse during wakefulness (Figure 40–4) and usually decreases or is abolished during sleep. Tremor often stops with the onset of alpha activity during drowsiness even before the onset of stages N1 or N2. Tremor is rare during stage N3. However, in some patients, motor manifestations persist during sleep. Examples of motor findings associated with sleep include repeated eye blinking at onset of sleep, blepharospasm at the onset of REM sleep, and prolonged tonic contractions of limb extensor or flexor muscles during non–REM (NREM) sleep. Because of rigidity, patients with PD have difficulty changing body position during the night. Early-morning akinesia and painful dystonia as medication is wearing off can be problematic. Although CD/LD can improve symptoms during sleep in some patients, it has a short duration of action. Repeat dosing during the night or use of a continuous release preparation are possible interventions. However, there is conflicting data about the benefits of LD during sleep, and it likely varies from patient to patient. In a study by Gros et al. CD/LD CR reduced the AHI.[43] In another study higher doses of LD were associated with worse sleep[44] without any change in perceived body movements. In patients with significant dyskinesias on CD/LD, a higher dose of nocturnal medication could worsen sleep if dyskinesias during the night are more frequent. The dopamine agonists have a longer duration of action and potentially could be useful in patients with motor manifestations during sleep. Another approach would be to use LD with a COMT or MAO-B inhibitor to prolong medication effect.[45] In patients with severe dyskinesias deep brain stimulation (DBS) is often used. A review of the effect of DBS on sleep determined that significant benefits were present including longer sleep and less sleep fragmentation.[46]

Box 40–8 INSOMNIA AND HYPERSOMNIA IN PARKINSON'S DISEASE

Insomnia

- Sleep maintenance insomnia - in about 50% of patients
- Causes of insomnia
  - Motor symptoms (cramps, stiffness, impaired turning in bed)
  - Nocturia
  - Depression/anxiety
  - Inadequate sleep hygiene
  - Restless legs syndrome
  - Medications
  - Circadian rhythm sleep-wake disorders
  - Nightmares

Hypersomnia

- Excessive Daytime Sleepiness- persistent throughout the day
- Sleep attacks (up to 14%, either due to PD, or dopamine agonists)
- Causes of Hypersomnia
  - PD- the disorder itself
  - Sleep Apnea
  - Medication side effects (dopamine)
  - Loss of hypocretin neurons (low hypocretin)
  - Insufficient sleep
  - Circadian rhythm sleep-wake disorders
  - RLS
  - REM sleep behavior disorder

PD, Parkinson's disease; *RLS*, restless legs syndrome.

Table 40–4 Factors Causing Sleep Disturbance in Parkinson's Disease

Pathophysiology	Manifestation	Treatment
Changes in cholinergic and monoaminergic systems	Impaired wake-sleep control Decreased REM sleep	Cautious use of sedating antidepressants and hypnotics
Bradykinesia and rigidity	Decreased body shifts during sleep → discomfort and increased awakenings Impaired ability to use the bathroom	Sustained-release CD/LD or DAs, some still prefer multiple doses of IR CD/LD
Tremor	Arousals Insomnia	Sustained release CD/LD, repeated doses of IR CD/LD or a dopamine agonist
Drug-induced dyskinesia	Jerks, arousals	Decrease evening CD/LD or use dopamine agonist
Abnormal motor control of respiratory and upper airway muscles	OSA (BMI often normal)	CPAP
RBD	Disturbed REM sleep Injury to self or bed partner May precede other findings by years Prevalence 15–30%	Clonazepam Melatonin Transdermal Rivastigmine
PLMS, RLS	Arousals, difficulty sleep onset	Gabapentin, dopamine agonists
Depression and anxiety	Insomnia Difficulty with sleep onset Early morning awakening	Cautious use of hypnotics and antidepressants
Dementia	Nocturnal confusional episodes	Aricept
Nocturnal Hallucinations and Psychosis	Nocturnal hallucinations and delusions associated with PD Psychosis	Quetiapine or Pimavanserin (Nuplazid)

BMI, Body mass index; *CD,* carbidopa; *DAs,* dopamine agonists; *IR,* immediate release, *LD,* levodopa; *OSA,* obstructive sleep apnea; *PLMS,* periodic limb movements during sleep; *RBD,* rapid eye movement sleep behavior disorder; *REM,* rapid eye movement; *RLS,* restless legs syndrome.
Adapted from Comella CL. Sleep disorders in Parkinson's disease. *Curr Treat Options Neurol.* 2008;10:215-221.

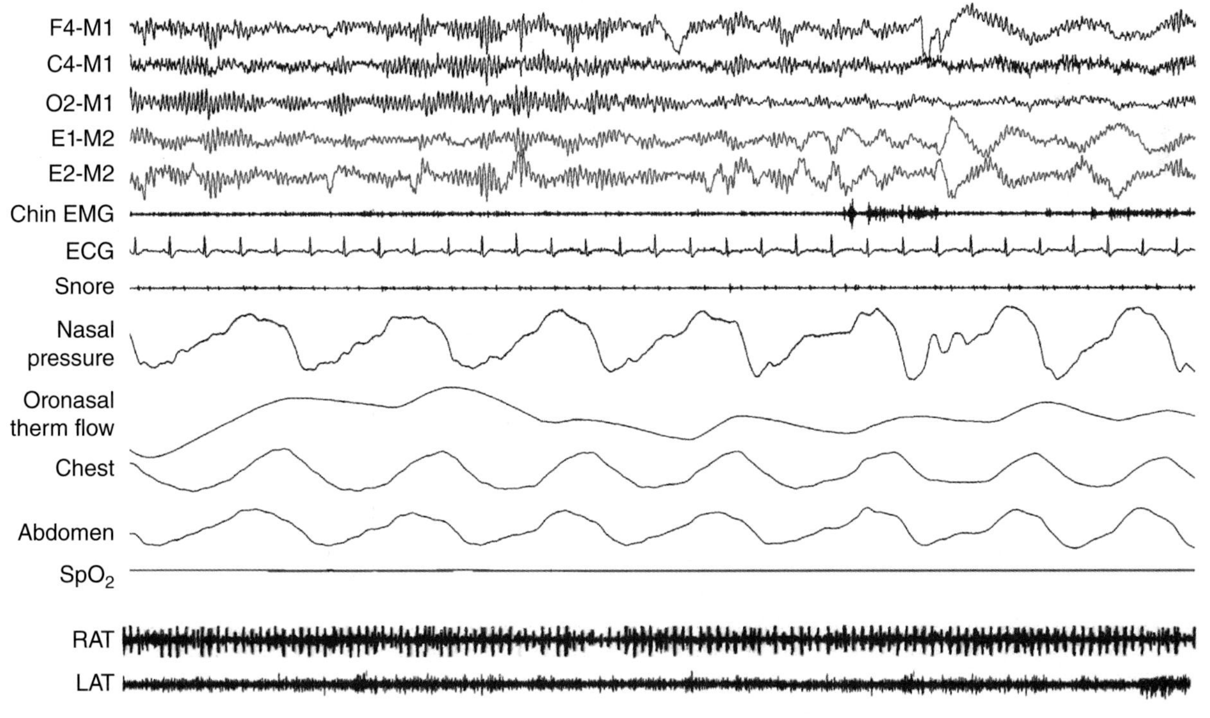

Figure 40–4 A 4-Hz resting tremor seen in the right anterior tibial (RAT) electromyogram (EMG) in this patient with Parkinson's disease. In this patient the tremor was present during wake (even during the presence of alpha rhythm). The tremor did decrease in stage N1 and was absent in stage N2. Oronasal therm flow is the signal from a thermal flow sensor.

Daytime Sleepiness in PD

Excessive daytime sleepiness (EDS) not due to OSA or medications is a well-known phenomenon in PD. The possibility of OSA should be eliminated. Sleep attacks were once thought due to side effects from dopamine agonists. Most recent studies suggest medications used to treat PD may worsen EDS but that the underlying disease process is the most common cause of EDS in PD. *Studies have reported 50% loss of hypocretin neurons in patients with PD.*[47] Treatment of EDS (in addition to treatment of OSA) in PD patients includes modafinil, bupropion, and traditional stimulants. The 2021 AASM clinical practice guideline for treatment of central hypersomnia[48] recommended the use of modafinil for sleepiness associated with PD (conditional level of recommendation). Rodriguez et al. performed a meta-analysis of studies of modafinil in PD and found evidence of a benefit.[49] However, the evidence from studies of the effects of modafinil in PD is somewhat conflicting.[49-52] Fatigue can also be a major complaint in PD. Using a double-blind, placebo-controlled design, Lou and coworkers[53] noted no improvement in fatigue symptoms or improvement in the Epworth sleepiness scale with modafinil. As noted previously, treatment with DAs can be associated with sudden attacks of severe daytime sleepiness. One case report found that the addition of modafinil to pramipexole therapy reduced the severity of the pramipexole sleepiness side effect.[54] A randomized double-blind study found that sodium oxybate was beneficial for daytime sleepiness and sleep disturbance in patients with Parkinson's disease.[55] The 2021 AASM guidelines for treatment of central hypersomnia[48] also recommended sodium oxybate in Parkinson's patients with EDS. However, the medication is not FDA approved for this indication.

Nocturnal Behavior: RBD, Nocturnal Hallucinations, and Nocturnal Psychosis

The RBD occurs in 30% to 50% of patients with PD (Box 40–9). It can be the earliest manifestation, occurring many years before other PD symptoms and signs (see Chapter 36). In general, treatment options for RBD in PD are similar to those for isolated (idiopathic) RBD. Dopamine agonists have been reported to be effective treatment of RBD in some patients. Pramipexole was recommended for treatment of isolated RBD (RBD not due to a medical disorder) by the 2023 AASM practice guidelines.[21] Clonazepam, immediate-release melatonin, and transdermal rivastigmine were recommended for treatment of RBD in patients with Parkinson's disease.[21]

Nocturnal hallucinations can occur in PD and disturb sleep.[56,57] A recent study compared sleep between groups of PD patients with and without visual hallucinations. Although both groups slept poorly, *the group with visual hallucinations had much poorer sleep.*[57] *Drug-induced psychosis* is a major problem in PD. It can occur in up to 22% and is a major cause of placing patients in a chronic care facility. Treatments have included reducing the dose of anti-Parkinson's medication, adding a neuroleptic drug, or discontinuing PD treatment for a period of time. Low-dose clozapine (an atypical antipsychotic) was found effective even if anti-Parkinson's medications were still taken and did not worsen tremor. In this study, doses of 6.25 to 50 mg were used (far lower than the 300–900 mg used for schizophrenia). The drug can cause leukopenia, and careful monitoring is needed.[58] Quetiapine is commonly used for psychosis in PD, although convincing evidence for a benefit is lacking and the medication can cause problems with glucose control and sedation.[59] However, most clinicians would try quetiapine before clozapine. Pimavanserin (Nuplazid) has recently been approved to treat hallucinations and delusions related to PD psychosis.[60] This medication is an atypical antipsychotic and is a 5HT2A serotonin receptor inverse agonist/antagonist with no known *dopamine receptor–blocking activity* (unlike other atypical antipsychotic medications), and is indicated for the treatment of hallucinations and delusions associated with PD psychosis.[60] All antipsychotics have a black box warning of increased risk of death in the use of antipsychotics to treat dementia-related symptoms in the elderly.

Box 40–9 PREVALENCE OF RBD IN NEURODEGENERATIVE DISORDERS

- Parkinson's disease—30–50% (other references 20–40%)
- Dementia with Lewy bodies—50–80%
- Multiple system atrophy—80–95%
- In patients with RBD emerging after 50 years of age, 81–90% will eventually develop a neurodegenerative disorder

RBD, Rapid eye movement sleep behavior disorder.
Data from Howell MJ, Schenck CH. Rapid Eye Movement Sleep Behavior Disorder and Neurodegenerative Disease. *JAMA Neurol.* 2015 Jun;72(6):707-12.

Dementia in PD

The Movement Disorders Society published an update on recommended treatment of nonmotor symptoms of PD. Rivastigmine was the only medication recommended for PD dementia and is the only medication FDA approved for treatment of dementia in PD.[61] A study by Trieschmann et al. found modest benefit from donepezil, and the drug did not cause worsening of PD.[62] A study by Thomas and coworkers found donepezil to be equally effective for dementia in PD and DLBD.[63] Another study has reported some benefit from memantine in patients with PD with dementia or DLBD.[64]

Diffuse Lewy Body Dementia

DLBD is also known as dementia with Lewy bodies (DLB), Lewy body dementia, or diffuse Lewy body disease. DLBD is a type of dementia characterized on histologic exam by the presence of Lewy bodies, clumps of alpha synuclein and ubiquitin proteins in neurons. In this disorder, loss of cholinergic neurons results in cognitive dysfunction and loss of dopamine neurons results in parkinsonism (Box 40–10). If dementia occurs more than 1 year after other symptoms in PD, the disorder is called PD with dementia. If dementia occurs within the first year of parkinsonism, the diagnosis is DLBD. DLBD tends to progress much more rapidly than PD.

Manifestations of DLBD

The major manifestations of DLBD[65-68] include (1) *fluctuating cognition* with great variation in attention and alertness from day to day and hour to hour, (2) recurrent visual hallucination (75% of patients with DLBD), (3) motor features of parkinsonism (tremor less common in DLBD than in PD), (4) RBD (50–80%), and (5) problems with orthostasis, including repeated falls, syncope, and transient loss of consciousness. The *RBD can have an onset years before the other*

Box 40–10 DIFFUSE LEWY BODY DEMENTIA

- Fluctuating cognition and alertness
- Visual hallucinations in 70%
- Orthostasis and frequent falls
- Motor manifestations of parkinsonism (rigidity, tremor less common than in PD)
- Onset of dementia within 1 year of symptoms of parkinsonism
- Insomnia and daytime sleepiness common
- RBD is very common (50–80%)
- Life-threatening rigidity with dopamine blockers

PD, Parkinson's disease; *RBD,* rapid eye movement sleep behavior disorder.

manifestations of DLBD (similar to PD) but often is first noted at a time near the onset of the other manifestations of DLBD. Patients with DLBD have a *transient or no response to LD treatment.* Sleep complaints include moderate to severe EDS and disturbed sleep at night due to confusion, nightmares/RBD, and hallucinations. A variant of dementia with Lewy bodies and RBD but without parkinsonism or hallucinations has been reported.[68]

Visual Hallucinations in DLBD

The most common reported *hallucination is of people or animals.* The patient may misinterpret what they see: for example, the patient may open a drawer full of socks but see snakes.

Sensitivity to DA Blockers

An important characteristic of DLBD is exquisite sensitivity to dopamine blockers. When given dopamine blockers, patients with DLBD can develop life-threatening rigidity or malignant neuroleptic syndrome. Anticholinergic drugs such as diphenhydramine (Benadryl) or terazosin (Hytrin) can worsen dementia.

Treatment of DLBD

Treatment of DLBD is generally supportive. Parkinsonian symptoms have a limited response to LD. All the cholinesterase inhibitors used for AD and memantine can be used for PD dementia[62,63] and are as effective for dementia in DLBD as in PD. *Some clinicians feel that in general the cholinesterase inhibitors are more efficacious in DLBD than in AD.* While improvement may be limited, use of the medications may be associated with slower worsening of cognition. As stated above, rivastigmine is the only anticholinesterase inhibitor approved for dementia in PD. The patch formulation appears to have fewer gastrointestinal side effects compared to the oral preparation. The AASM clinical practice guidelines for treatment of central hypersomnia recommended armodafinil for treatment of daytime sleepiness in patients with DLBD.[48] Modafinil (the racemic form of armodafinil) would likely be as effective.

Multiple System Atrophy (MSA)

MSA is a neurodegenerative disorder characterized by a combination of parkinsonism, dysautonomia, cerebellar dysfunction, and features of pyramidal tract dysfunction (Box 40–11).[69,70] Some patients have more prominent dysfunction in one category. *Hallucinations and dementia do not occur.* MSA is sometimes divided into three separate conditions (Table 40–5). These include (1) striatonigral degeneration, (2) olivopontocerebellar degeneration, and (3) progressive autonomic failure (Shy-Drager syndrome). The second MSA consensus conference[69] recommended new MSA terminology (MSA-P, primarily parkinsonism; MSA-C, primarily cerebellar ataxia), and the term *Shy-Drager* was not used in the recent classification, although it is widely used in the literature. The typical age of onset of MSA is 50 to 60 years. The pathology of MSA involves alpha synuclein oligodendroglial inclusions in the brainstem, cerebellum, and spinal cord. Glial cytoplasmic inclusions (Papp-Lantos bodies) appear in the brain centers involved with control of movement, balance, and autonomic control centers. The disease course is fairly rapid with onset to death in about 9 years. The disorder progresses more rapidly than PD. It is helpful to think of MSA symptoms/manifestations in three groups.

Box 40–11 MANIFESTATIONS MSA

- Age of onset 50–60 years
- Onset to death in 9 years
- **Not seen—hallucinations and dementia**
- Orthostatic hypotension a major problem
- Variants
    - Striatonigral degeneration—rigidity, bradykinesia
    - Olivopontocerebellar atrophy—prominent ataxia, postural instability
    - Shy-Drager—autonomic dysfunction
- Stridor—poor prognostic sign, normal awake laryngeal examination does not exclude, can be presenting feature
- Sleep disorders very common (>70%)
- RBD very common (80–95% of patients)
- OSA
- CSA including Cheyne-Stokes breathing, rare nocturnal hypoventilation

CSA, Central sleep apnea; *MSA,* Multiple System Atrophy; *OSA,* obstructive sleep apnea; *RBD,* rapid eye movement sleep behavior disorder.

Symptom Groups in MSA

1. Autonomic dysfunction (erectile dysfunction, bladder control/urgency, incomplete emptying, constipation, abnormal breathing during sleep, orthostatic hypotension).
2. Parkinsonism: rigidity (with or without tremor), bradykinesia, and postural instability. The tremor of MSA is irregular and *usually not a pill rolling tremor* as seen in PD.
3. Ataxia (poor coordination/unsteady walking) may be a presenting symptom.

Diagnosis Classification

As noted above, the second consensus conference on MSA defined two categories of MSA based on the predominant symptoms at the time of evaluation (Table 40–5)[69,70]:

1. MSA-P: MSA with predominant parkinsonism (also called striatonigral degeneration, parkinsonian variant).
2. MSA-C: MSA with predominant cerebellar features. MSA in which cerebellar features predominate is also called sporadic olivopontocerebellar atrophy.

Table 40–5 Classifications of Multiple System Atrophy

	Characteristics	1996 Consensus Conference	2007 Consensus Conference
Striatonigral degeneration	Predominantly Parkinson's type symptoms	MSA-P	MSA-P
Sporadic OPCA	Progressive ataxia (an inability to coordinate voluntary movements) of the gain and arms and dysarthria (difficulty in articulating words)	MSA-C	MSA-C
Shy-Drager syndrome	Characterized by parkinsonism + pronounced failure of the autonomic nervous system	MSA-A	No longer used

MSA, Multiple system atrophy; *OPCA*, sporadic olivopontocerebellar atrophy.
Adapted from Gillman S, Wenning P, Low PA, et al. Second consensus statement of the diagnosis of multiple system atrophy. *Neurology.* 2008;71:670-676.

Vocal Cord Palsy and Stridor in MSA

Stridor may occur in up to 30% of patients with MSA. It can be much worse during sleep. A normal laryngeal examination during wakefulness does not rule out the problem.[71,72] The presence of stridor is associated with a poor prognosis (compared with MSA patients without stridor) and has traditionally been managed by tracheostomy. CPAP has been used to assist with stridor at night.[72,73] Of note, patients with MSA often have OSA as well as worsening stridor during sleep. The etiology of stridor is controversial but is likely due to overactivity of the vocal cord adductors (close vocal cords) and underactivity of vocal cord abductors (posterior cricoarytenoid muscles [PCA]). A neuropathy of the recurrent laryngeal nerves that innervate the PCA muscles may be involved. The syndrome of stridor in many patients is a dystonia rather than vocal cord paralysis. In others, there is complete vocal cord immobility. Sudden death has been reported in patients with stridor even though treated with tracheostomy or CPAP.[74,75] A consensus conference on stridor in MSA concluded that the ability to improve survival with CPAP treatment is uncertain.[76]

Central Sleep Apnea and Cheyne-Stokes Breathing

Central sleep apnea, nocturnal hypoventilation, Cheyne-Stokes breathing (CSB), and complex sleep apnea have been reported in MSA, especially in patients with prominent autonomic features.[77-79] The use of adaptive servoventilation in MSA patients with CSB has been reported.[80]

Treatment of MSA

The treatment of MSA is mostly supportive. There is usually no or only a short initial response to CD/LD. Patients with stridor can be treated with CPAP or tracheostomy (although sudden death can still occur at night).

OTHER NEURODEGENERATIVE DISORDERS

Fatal Familial Insomnia

Fatal familial insomnia (FFI) is a *familial autosomal dominant prion disorder* associated with the D178N mutation and *methionine-methionine* genotype at codon 129 in the prion protein gene on chromosome 20.[81,82] Of note, the D178N mutation and valine-valine genotype at codon 129 are associated with familial Creutzfeldt-Jakob disease (CJD). The methionine-methionine genotype at codon 129 produces dorsomedial and anteroventral thalamic dysfunction, whereas the valine-valine genotype of CJD is associated with more general cortical involvement.

FFI manifestations include *insomnia, dementia, ataxia, dysarthria, dysautonomia, hallucinations, and hypersomnolence.* The duration from onset to death varies from a few months to 4 years. Features of FFI are discussed in the *International Classification of Sleep Disorders,* 3rd edition, text revision (ICSD-3-TR)[83] in Appendix A: Sleep Related Medical and Neurological Disorders. However, no diagnostic criteria are specified.

Essential features of FFI include difficulties falling/staying asleep and spontaneous lapses from quiet wakefulness into sleep with enacted dreams, leading to cognitive dysfunction with progression to coma and death. Patients with FFI often have loss of endocrine circadian rhythms and autonomic hyperactivity (pyrexia, salivation, dyspnea, tachypnea, tachycardia). Dysarthrias, dysphagia, tremor, myoclonus, ataxia, dystonic posturing, and hallucinations may be seen. The dream enactment is often mimicking daily activities such as combining hair.

The age of onset of FFI is 36 to 62 years, and the disorder is rare. *Males and females are equally affected.* The PSG in FFI reveals severe disruption of the sleep-wake cycle, reduction in stage N3 and stage R, as well as reduced sleep efficiency. As the disease progresses, there may be loss of the defining features of the different sleep stage such as loss of sleep spindles. REM sleep without atonia can occur. *Positron emission tomography (PET) reveals* ***nearly absent or very low activity of the thalamus.***

Both sporadic (rarer) and familial patterns of FFI can occur. The familial form is characterized by autosomal dominant genetics associated with a mutation at codon 178 of prion protein gene (PRNP). A missense GAC to AAC mutation at codon 17 of the PRNP gene (d178N) co-segregating with the methionine polymorphism at codon 129 of the PRNP on the mutated allele is found (this mutation is absent in sporadic FFI). Patients who are methionine homozygous at the 129 codon (versus methionine-valine) present at an early age and have a rapid course.

FFI should be considered in any patient with prominent sleep-wake disturbance and dementia. A family history of dementia occurring at an early age with a rapid course to death is suggestive of FFI.[84] The differential diagnosis of FFI includes RBD, dementia, CJD, Morvan fibrillary chorea, delirium tremens, and schizophrenia.

Treatment is supportive. The course of FFI shows a relentless worsening of symptoms from confusion, to stupor, to coma and death in 8 to 72 months.

Myotonic Dystrophy

Myotonic dystrophy (MD) comprises myotonic dystrophy type 1 (MD-1) and myotonic dystrophy type 2 (MD-2). The two forms of the disease are genetically distinct. MD-1 is caused by an expanded CTG triplet in the MD-1 protein kinase (DMPK) gene on chromosome 19, while MD-2 is caused by the expansion of a CCTG tetramer on the cellular nucleic acid-binding protein (CNBP) gene on chromosome 3. Patients with MD-1 have weakness and atrophy in *distal* muscles while MD-2 patient have *proximal* muscular weakness and muscular atrophy. MD-2 often is manifested after age 45. Myotonic dystrophy type 1 (MD-1) patients may present with excessive daytime sleepiness as well as muscle weakness.[85-87] MD-1 (also known as Steinert's disease) is an *autosomal dominant disorder characterized by myotonia, distal muscle weakness, premature cataracts, hypogonadism, and cardiac arrythmias*. Muscles involved include the masseter, levator palpebra, forearm, hand, pretibial muscles, and sternocleidomastoid. Sleep-related issues include daytime sleepiness and a risk for nocturnal hypoventilation.

As noted above, the genetic defect in MD-1 results from an amplified trinucleotide CTG repeat in the 3′ untranslated region of a protein kinase gene (DMPK) on chromosome 19. The pathogenesis of myotonic dystrophy is related to trinucleotide repeat expansions that produce toxic mutant mRNA with subsequent interference of RNA-splicing mechanisms. Definitive diagnosis depends on genetic testing of the DNA of leukocytes. The incidence is estimated to be about 1/10,000, so it is a much rarer disorder than narcolepsy. Myotonia is defined as repetitive muscle depolarization resulting in muscle stiffness and impaired relaxation. Pharyngeal and laryngeal muscles of respiration including the diaphragm can be involved. Dysfunction of the hypothalamic region can result in daytime sleepiness or daytime sleepiness with SOREMPs consistent with a diagnosis of **narcolepsy due to a medical condition**. If criteria for narcolepsy are **not** met, a diagnosis of hypersomnia due to a medical disorder is appropriate. Involvement of upper airway muscles can result in sleep apnea. Some patients have abnormal ventilatory control and hypoventilation. Involvement of the cardiac condition system can occur (heart block, prolonged QRS or PR intervals). In one case-controlled study comparing age-matched groups of patients with and without MD-1, the patients with MD-1 had a greater frequency of severe OSA, an elevated PLMS index, shorter mean sleep latency on the multiple sleep latency test (MSLT), and more frequent SOREMPs, with one and two SOREMPs being present in 47.5% and 32.5%, respectively. More stage N3 and stage R and a higher REM density were noted in MD-1.[86] Another study found poor correlation between reports of daytime sleepiness and findings on the MSLT.[87]

There are differences in MD-1 presentation depending on the age of onset. Congenital MD-1 is apparent at birth and often severe. Juvenile MD-1 is a characterized by symptoms the appear between birth and adolescence. Adult-onset MD-1 usually appears in individuals aged 20 to 40 and tends to be slowly progressive. Late-onset MD-1 occurs after 40 and has mild symptoms. On physical examination, findings in MD-1 include a narrow face, temporal wasting, premature frontal balding, distal weakness, and myotonia. MD-1 patients have decreased strength on hand grip but then are slow to relax ("distal myopathy with myotonia"). *Symptomatic myotonia* typically *precedes* muscle weakness in MD-1. Individuals describe muscle stiffness or difficulty releasing their grip. Patients may observe a delayed ability to open their eyes after a forceful closure or a delayed ability to extend their fingers after a firm handshake. There is wasting of hand and forearm muscles (especially hand flexors). PSG can reveal OSA, and PSG + MSLT can meet criteria for narcolepsy or simply document excessive daytime without two SOREMPs. As noted above, there is poor correlation between subjective symptoms and objective findings.[87] The 2021 AASM clinical practice guideline for treatment of central hypersomnia recommended use of *modafinil for EDS* in patients with myotonic dystrophy.[48]

SLEEP DISTURBANCES IN STROKE

Important points concerning stroke and sleep are listed in Box 40–12. Sleep-disordered breathing (SDB) occurs in 50% to 70% of stroke patients (defined as AHI > 10/hour).[88-93] A recent review reports prevalence of sleep apnea poststroke as 71% for AHI > 5/hour and 30% for AHI > 30/hour.[93] Central sleep apnea (CSA) including CSA with Cheyne-Stokes Breathing (CSB) can be noted, especially soon after stroke, but tends to decrease with time. CSB in some chronic stroke patients is associated with heart failure.[88-93] Other patients with stroke and CSA have occult heart failure.[94] However, *OSA is the most common sleep apnea disorder after cerebrovascular accident (CVA)*. OSA also tends to improve with time, but a substantial number of patients still have OSA at 2 to 3 months after stroke. The presence of sleep apnea after a CVA raises questions about the temporal relationship with stroke. Does brain damage from CVA cause sleep apnea, or did sleep apnea precede the stroke? If the latter is true, is the presence of sleep apnea an independent risk factor for the development of a CVA? *The Sleep Heart Health Study did show an increased risk of having a CVA (prevalence) if OSA is present.*[95] *In another study, Redline and colleagues*[96] *evaluated the Sleep Heart Health data and found an increased risk for incident ischemic stroke in* ***men with mild to moderate OSA***. In this study, data were adjusted for a number of confounders that complicate the analysis including obesity. *McDermott and Brown report that OSA was associated with a twofold risk of incident stroke.*[93] If there is a causal role for OSA in stroke, what are the mechanisms? OSA could predispose a patient to atherosclerosis, hypertension, and early-morning hemoconcentration. These factors would increase the risk of stroke. During sleep apnea, there are increases in intracranial pressure (ICP) and decreases in cerebral blood flow.[97,98] Because cerebral perfusion is proportional to the mean arterial pressure (MAP) less the ICP, increases in ICP

Box 40–12 SLEEP DISTURBANCE IN STROKE

- Sleep-disordered breathing found in 50–70% poststroke
- OSA most common; CSA can occur, including CSA with Cheyne-Stokes breathing
- OSA is a risk factor for incident CVA (up to 2×)
- Observational studies report reduced mortality in patients with stroke who are treated with CPAP
- Insomnia and daytime sleepiness can occur depending on area of stroke
- New-onset RLS can occur after stroke

CPAP, Continuous positive airway pressure; *CSA,* central sleep apnea; *CVA,* cerebrovascular accident; *OSA,* obstructive sleep apnea; *RBD,* rapid eye movement sleep behavior disorder; RLS, restless legs syndrome.

may reduce perfusion pressure even if MAP also rises. Studies of cerebral blood flow velocity using Doppler monitoring have shown that flow velocity increases in early apnea, then has approximately a 25% fall below baseline at end apnea.[98]

There is evidence that the presence of OSA in patients who have had a CVA is a poor prognostic sign regardless of whether OSA precedes or follows the CVA. Good and associates[99] found that the Barthel index (a multifaceted scale measuring mobility and activities of daily living that is used to assess patients after stroke) was significantly lower in patients with OSA and CVA compared with those with no evidence of OSA after CVA. The presence of OSA was determined at discharge, and the Barthel index was lower at 3 and 12 months in the OSA-CVA group. Martinez-Garcia and coworkers[100] found that CPAP treatment reduced mortality in patients found to have OSA after an ischemic stroke. This study suggests that physicians need to be more aggressive about ruling out OSA in patients with a recent CVA. McDermott and Brown suggest that detection of OSA should be done by physiologic testing rather than questionnaire.[93] Unfortunately, CPAP adherence with treatment after CVA is often suboptimal.

After stroke, other sleep-wake disorders may impair recovery. Insomnia can occur, but treatment should be cautious unless sleep apnea is excluded. Daytime sleepiness can occur even if sleep apnea is not present. *Poststroke hypersomnia* can be found after subcortical (caudate-putamen), thalamic/mesencephalic, medial pontomedullary, and cortical strokes. **In one study, *up to 12% of patients developed new-onset restless legs syndrome after stroke*.**[101] Pontine-tegmental strokes can lead to RBD.

TRAUMATIC BRAIN INJURY (TBI)

TBI is defined as a complex pathophysiological process affecting the brain induced by traumatic biomechanical forces.[102] Causes of TBI include the head being struck by an object, the head striking an object, acceleration/deceleration of the brain without direct external impact, a foreign body penetrating the brain, force from a blast/explosion, and other forces yet to be defined. Concussion is another term for mild TBI. TBI is a major problem and cause of long-term disability in millions of individuals in both military and civilian populations. Sleep disturbances after TBI are estimated to occur in 30% to 70% of head-injured patients, often impairing the resumption of normal activities (Table 40–6). *Patients suffering from TBI of any severity, in both the acute and chronic phases, commonly report EDS, increased sleep need, insomnia, and sleep fragmentation.* The prevalence of sleep disorders in individuals with TBI is very high yet often unrecognized. There has been a change in the epidemiology of TBI. TBI after falls has surpassed motor vehicle accidents as the leading cause of head injury.[103] Currently, most emergency department visits and hospitalizations from TBI are from falls in patients over 75 years of age. In adolescents, TBI from motor vehicle accidents is predominant. TBI is common in combat veterans exposed to blasts from explosive devices. Theodorou and Rice noted that 59% of blast-exposed veterans of the Afghanistan/Iraq conflict had TBI.[104] TBI severity is most commonly classified according to the Glasgow Coma Scale (GCS),[105] where a GCS score of 13 to 15 is considered mild injury, 9 to 12 is moderate injury, and 8 points or fewer is severe TBI.

Common sleep disorders associated with head trauma are listed in Box 40–13. Up to 50% of all chronic TBI patients have

Table 40–6 Sleep and Traumatic Brain Injury

Overview: Sleep and TBI

- Sleep disturbance in 30–70% of TBI
- PSG and MSLT evaluation needed in about 50%
- Chronic TBI—50% have a sleep disorder

Sleep Disorders in TBI

- **Hypersomnia** ≈ 50%
    - Transient in many, resolves over 6 months
    - *Tends to occur with more severe brain injury*
    - 25% symptoms at 1 year
    - Sleep apnea (23% of all TBI patients), obstructive, central, complex SA
    - Posttraumatic hypersomnia (11%)—hypersomnia due to a medical disorder
    - Narcolepsy (6%) due to medical condition
    - Periodic limb movement disorder (7%)
- **Insomnia** ≈ 30–50%
    - More common in milder TBI
    - Some due to circadian rhythm sleep-wake disorder
    - Anxiety, depression comorbid
- **Parasomnias** ≈ 25%, RBD most common
- **Circadian rhythm sleep-wake disorders**—delayed sleep phase, non–24-hour sleep-wake rhythm disorder (esp. injury to eyes)
- **Increased sleep need** (pleiosomnia)
- **RLS/PLMD**

Acute Phase

Mild TBI: Sleep-wake complaints in about one-third within the first 10 days after mild TBI and up to 50 percent at 6 weeks postinjury

Severe TBI: ≈ 80% had sleep-wake disturbances upon admission; 66% continued to have disturbances at one month postinjury

Chronic Phase

- In observational studies of survivors of TBI, the most common sleep disturbances reported in the chronic phase (>3 months after injury) are:
    - Insomnia (50%)
    - Difficulty maintaining sleep (50%)
    - Poor sleep efficiency on PSG (49%)
    - Early morning awakenings (38%)
    - Nightmares (27%)

Hypocretin in TBI

- Low hypocretin for first 6 months in moderate to severe TBI
- Hypocretin tends to normalize, levels normal in posttraumatic hypersomnia
- Hypocretin levels low—narcolepsy with cataplexy due to medical condition (if tested)

MSLT, Multiple sleep latency test; *PLMD,* periodic limb movement disorder; *PSG,* polysomnography; *RBD,* rapid eye movement sleep behavior disorder; *RLS,* restless legs syndrome; *SA,* sleep apnea; *TBI,* traumatic brain injury.

Box 40–13 CAUSES OF HYPERSOMNIA AFTER TBI

- OSA (the most common cause of hypersomnia after TBI)
- Narcolepsy type 1 (with cataplexy) due to a medical condition
- Narcolepsy type 2 (without cataplexy) due to a medical condition
- Hypersomnia due to a medical disorder
    - Posttraumatic hypersomnia
- Inadequate sleep
- Medications

OSA, Obstructive sleep apnea; *TBI,* traumatic brain injury.

sleep disorders, which may require nocturnal PSG and the MSLT for diagnosis. Castriotta and colleagues prospectively studied 87 adults at least 3 months after TBI *without* specific sleep complaints. PSG and MSLT were administered to all subjects; 46% had abnormal sleep studies. The authors diagnosed 23% with OSA, 11% with posttraumatic hypersomnia, 7% with periodic limb movements in sleep, and 6% with narcolepsy.[106]

The type of sleep disorder after head trauma may depend on the area of brain that is injured. Posttraumatic hypersomnia is seen when areas involved in the maintenance of wakefulness are damaged. These regions include the brainstem reticular formation, posterior hypothalamus, and the area surrounding the third ventricle. Hypothalamic injury with decreased levels of wake-promoting neurotransmitters such as hypocretin (orexin) may be involved in the pathophysiology of daytime sleepiness. *Low CSF hypocretin-1 levels are found in most cases of narcolepsy with cataplexy after head trauma, but normal levels are typically seen in hypersomnia due to trauma (posttraumatic hypersomnia).* Most patients with moderate to severe TBI have low or intermediate hypocretin-1 levels in the acute injury phase. Hypocretin levels tend to normalize (become >200 pg/mL) 6 months after the injury, which may explain why *post-TBI sleepiness resolves in many over time*,[107] However, hypocretin-1 levels were lower at 6 months after TBI in patients with EDS. *High cervical cord lesions have also been known to cause sleepiness and OSA.* In addition, whiplash may cause hypersomnia by precipitating SDB.[108] Coup-contrecoup brain injury after head trauma occurs most frequently at the base of the skull in areas of bony irregularities (especially the sphenoid ridges), with consequent damage to the inferior frontal and anterior temporal regions, including the basal forebrain (an area involved in sleep initiation). As a result, insomnia is a common symptom after injuries from this mechanism. Closed head injury can involve the SCN or its output tracts, leading to disturbance of circadian rhythmicity with concomitant hypersomnia and insomnia.

HYPERSOMNIA AND TBI

Hypersomnia is most common with moderate to severe TBI. Whereas *hypersomnia after TBI is most commonly associated with OSA*,[106] less common causes are hypersomnia due to medical disorder (posttraumatic hypersomnia) and narcolepsy due to medical condition.[84,106] A study of 87 patients at least 3 months after TBI with PSG and MSLT found 46% had an abnormal sleep study, 23% with OSA, 11% with posttraumatic hypersomnia, 6% with narcolepsy, and 7% with periodic limb movements in sleep. Of all subjects, 25% had evidence of objective hypersomnia (mean sleep latency ≤ 8 min). The mean sleep latency was not correlated with subjective sleepiness complaints. In this study posttraumatic hypersomnia was defined as a mean sleep latency < 10 minutes and fewer than 2 SOREMPs (and no history of hypersomnia before TBI).

The essential diagnosis criteria for hypersomnia due to medical disorder include the following (see ICSD-3-TR for complete criteria):

- The patient has daily periods of irrepressible need to sleep or daytime lapses into drowsiness or sleep occur for at least 3 months.
- The daytime sleepiness occurs as a consequence of an underlying medical or neurological condition.
- Symptoms and signs not explained by chronic insufficient sleep, circadian disorder, another sleep disorder, mental disorder, or medication/substance use or withdrawal.

In posttraumatic hypersomnia, the symptoms are not believed due to OSA, and if an MSLT is performed the findings may document a short mean sleep latency (≤8 min) but 0 or 1 SOREMP. Note that whereas a short mean sleep latency would document objective daytime sleepiness, a diagnosis of posttraumatic hypersomnia does not require a short mean sleep latency. Narcolepsy due to TBI (narcolepsy due to medical condition) requires that patients meet the usual diagnostic criteria for narcolepsy. Narcolepsy after TBI is usually associated with hypocretin deficiency. *In both conditions hypersomnia must be present for at least 3 months.* The role of wake-promoting agents and CNS stimulants for the sleepiness involved with TBI is still evolving. The 2021 AASM clinical practice guideline for treatment of central disorders of hypersomnolence recommended both modafinil and armodafinil for posttraumatic hypersomnia (conditional).[48] For patients with narcolepsy there was a strong recommendation for use of modafinil, pitolisant, sodium oxybate, solriamfetol, and a conditional recommendation of methylphenidate, dextroamphetamine, and armodafinil.

Increased sleep need (pleiosomnia)[109] and fatigue are also common after TBI. It is often difficult to differentiate between sleepiness and fatigue. Objective testing with PSG and MSLT can be useful in objectively documenting sleepiness. Fatigue after TBI is more common in women than men.

Head trauma has been reported to precipitate a few cases of Kleine-Levin syndrome, a rare disorder consisting of recurrent hypersomnia and cognitive or behavioral disturbances,[83] hypersexuality, and compulsive eating. The Klüver-Bucy syndrome[110] (a rare behavioral impairment that causes people to put objects in their mouths and engage in inappropriate sexual behavior) is more common after head trauma than Kleine-Levin.

INSOMNIA AND TBI

Insomnia is the most common complaint in chronic TBI and is more commonly associated with mild TBI. Insomnia often persists long-term in TBI survivors. In one study, insomnia was present in approximately one-quarter of patients 5 years after injury. Sleep onset and sleep maintenance issues are reported as well as early awakening. Those TBI patients with prominent insomnia often have associated depression and anxiety, which can contribute to insomnia. Head trauma occasionally triggers parasomnias, including *sleepwalking, sleep terrors, and RBD.* These can all disturb sleep. *PTSD is also common, but whether this is due to TBI or the incident causing the TBI is difficult to determine.* The usual treatments for PTSD are often effective. Nightmares associated with PTSD are a significant cause of sleep disturbance in patients.

Standard treatment regimens of sleep disorders appear to be effective in TBI patients, including CPAP for sleep apnea, the usual treatments for RLS, and cognitive behavioral therapy for insomnia (CBT-I). CBT-I is the preferred treatment of insomnia. Benzodiazepines should be avoided in the early recovery phase. There is some evidence that they could impair brain recovery.[111] The Z drugs (zolpidem, eszopiclone) are recommended only for temporary use. Sedating antidepressants can also be used. Diphenhydramine is also not recommended (has anticholinergic activity). A summary of treatments for sleep disorders in TBI is shown in Table 40–7.[112]

Table 40–7 Treatment of Sleep Disorders in Traumatic Brain Injury

OSA	CPAP
Insomnia	CBT-I Avoid BZ, especially in early period (may impair healing) Z drugs for short-term use only Trazodone, mirtazapine, amitriptyline Prazosin if PTSD nightmares
Hypersomnia	Posttraumatic hypersomnia—modafinil, armodafinil Narcolepsy—modafinil, armodafinil, sodium oxybate, pitolisant, solriamfetol, amphetamine, methylphenidate
RLS	Usual treatments
PTSD	Cognitive therapy, SSRIs, image rehearsal therapy, prazosin for nightmares

BZ, Benzodiazepines; *CBT-I,* cognitive behavioral disorder for insomnia; *CPAP,* chronic obstructive pulmonary disorder; *OSA,* obstructive sleep apnea; *PTSD,* post-traumatic stress disorder; *RLS,* restless legs syndrome; *SSRI,* selective serotonin uptake inhibitor.

SUMMARY OF KEY POINTS

1. A summary of neurodegenerative disorder properties is included in Table 40–8.
2. AD is the most common cause of dementia and can be associated with the ISWRD and sundowning. In early AD there is a decrease in stage N3. In late AD there is a decrease in REM sleep and increase in REM latency.
3. OSA is common in AD patients and, if successfully treated with CPAP, can improve sleep quality and mood as well as slow the rate of cognitive decline.
4. Donepezil (Aricept), a cholinesterase inhibitor, is used in AD to improve cognition but is often associated with insomnia. Morning dosing is suggested to minimize sleep disturbance. Some studies have suggested that evening doses of rivastigmine and galantamine can improve sleep quality. Cholinesterase inhibitors and cholinergic medications in general tend to increase REM sleep. Rivastigmine has been reported to cause RBD in AD patients. However, transdermal Rivastigmine is also recommended for RBD in Parkinson's Disease or patients with mild cognitive impairment (MCI).
5. PSP is characterized by *vertical gaze palsy and prominent sleep maintenance insomnia* (worse than in AD) and nocturia. PSP patients have a large reduction in the amount of REM sleep. *PSG will often show absence of vertical eye movements during REM sleep.* RBD occurs in about 13% to 30% of PSP patients.
6. Diagnostic criteria for PD include bradykinesia and one or more of either tremor or rigidity. Postural instability was often included as a major criteria but is not used in the most

Table 40–8 Summary of Properties of Neurodegenerative Disorders

	AD	PSP	PD	DLBD	MSA
Dementia	60% of dementia	Frontal lobe dementia (recent memory intact)	Yes, but starts over 1 year after PD onset	• 30% of all dementia • Starts early—within 1 year of PD symptoms	No dementia
Tau/alpha	Tauopathy	Tauopathy	• Alpha synucleinopathy • Some Lewy bodies	• Alpha synucleinopathy • Many Lewy bodies	Alpha synucleinopathy
Useful symptoms/findings	• Loss of recent memory • Sundowning	• Vertical gaze palsy (worse looking down) • Early postural instability • Nocturia • No vertical EM on PSG	• Nocturnal Hallucinations • Drug psychosis • Slower course • TRAP	• Fluctuating cognition • Visual hallucinations in 75% • Repeated falls	• Erectile dysfunction • Bladder symptoms • Syncope • Ataxia • Stridor • Rapid course
Parkinsonism symptoms	No	• Yes • Ataxic gait, falling	Yes	Yes, less tremor	Yes
Sleep complaints	Insomnia, ISWRD EDS	Severe insomnia (worse than AD or PD)	Insomnia and EDS	• Insomnia and EDS • Hallucinations	• Stridor • OSA, CSA • Hypoventilation can occur
Response to Levodopa	n/a	No	Yes	• Minimal/none • Rigidity with dopamine blockers	No
RBD	Uncommon	Yes, starts near disease onset	• Yes (30–35%) • Can precede PD by many years	Yes (50–75%)	Yes (80–95%)

AD, Alzheimer's disease; *DLBD,* diffuse Lewy body dementia; *EDS,* excessive daytime sleepiness; *EM,* eye movements; *ISWRD,* irregular sleep-wake rhythm disorder; *MSA,* Multiple system atrophy; *PD,* Parkinson's disease; *PSG,* polysomnography; *PSP,* progressive supranuclear palsy; *RBD,* rapid eye movement sleep behavior disorder; *TRAP,* Tremor, Rigidity, Akinesia, Postural instability.

recent guidelines. The mnemonic TRAP (tremor, rigidity, akinesia, postural instability) is useful.

7. The sleep of patients with PD is impaired by rigidity, tremor (tends to resolve with sleep onset), dyskinesias, OSA, RBD, nocturia, nightmares, and nocturnal hallucinations. Patients with PD can manifest EDS even if OSA is not present. Modafinil and sodium oxybate are recommended as treatment for daytime sleepiness in PD patients by the 2021 AASM practice guidelines for treatment of central hypersomnia.[48]

8. PD+ disorders are manifested by parkinsonism (bradykinesia and rigidity), no or decreased response to LD, sensitivity to dopamine blockers, and a more rapid downhill course than PD. PD+ disorders include **PSP**, DLBD, and MSA.

9. Patients with DLBD have prominent dementia much earlier in the disease course compared with PD (within 1 year). These patients frequently have *visual hallucinations and are exquisitely sensitivity to dopamine blockers (can develop severe rigidity).* Fluctuation of cognition, visual hallucinations, and postural instability are core symptoms. The RBD is very common in patients with DLBD. *Armodafinil was recommended for daytime sleepiness in patients with DLBD by* the 2021 AASM clinical practice guidelines for treatment of central hypersomnia.

10. Multiple system atrophy (MSA) patients have various amounts of striatonigral degeneration (rigidity and bradykinesia), olivopontocerebellar degeneration (cerebellar dysfunction, ataxia, falls), and autonomic dysfunction (erectile dysfunction, orthostatic hypotension, bladder dysfunction). The RBD is very common in MSA patients and often starts concurrently with other manifestations.

11. Stridor (especially during sleep) is a well-known manifestation of MSA and denotes a poor prognosis. CPAP is often used but has not been proven to prevent sudden death during sleep.

12. Fatal familial insomnia (FFI) is a familial autosomal dominant prion disease with progressive insomnia, dementia, and death within a few years. PET scan shows characteristic *absent or very low activity of the thalamus.*

13. There is a high prevalence of sleep apnea in patients who have had a recent stroke. OSA is the most common form of sleep apnea but CSA (including CSA with Cheyne-Stokes Breathing) can occur. If OSA is present, this is associated with a worse prognosis, but observational studies suggest that CPAP treatment may improve symptoms and outcomes. Adequate CPAP adherence is an issue.

14. Consider a diagnosis of myotonic dystrophy if a patient presents with complaints of muscle weakness in the hands/arms and daytime sleepiness. Good physical examination tests for myotonia include a delay in the ability to open eyes after a forceful closure or a delayed ability to extend their fingers after a firm handshake—that is, delayed relaxation after a firm handshake.

15. The sleepiness associated with myotonic dystrophy can be due to sleep apnea, narcolepsy due to a medical condition, or hypersomnia due to a medical disorder. Treatment of sleepiness in patients with myotonic dystrophy may respond to modafinil or traditional stimulants. The 2021 AASM clinical practice guidelines for treatment of central hypersomnia recommended modafinil for hypersomnia associated with myotonic dystrophy.

16. A high percentage of TBI patients suffer from sleep disorders. Hypersomnia is more common in moderate to severe TBI. Up to 50% of patients may need a PSG and MSLT to evaluate hypersomnia. The most common cause is obstructive sleep apnea, but posttraumatic hypersomnia (hypersomnia due to a medical disorder) or narcolepsy (narcolepsy due to medical condition) do occur. Hypocretin levels are low after moderate to severe TBI but recover over 6 months in most individuals. *Those with narcolepsy after TBI are usually hypocretin deficient.*

17. Insomnia is very common in TBI and tends *to be most prominent in those with mild TBI.* Insomnia in these patients could be due to damage of the sleep promoting areas of the brain or those involved with circadian control. Circadian rhythm sleep-wake disorders including the delayed sleep-wake phase disorder and the non-24-hour sleep-wake rhythm disorder have been described.

18. The AASM practice guidelines for treatment of central hypersomnia recommended modafinil and armodafinil for treatment of posttraumatic hypersomnia and the usual medications for treatment of narcolepsy secondary to TBI (modafinil, armodafinil, sodium oxybate, pitolisant, solriamfetol, amphetamines, and methylphenidate).

19. The treatment of choice for insomnia in TBI is CBT-I and in the early recovery stage after TBI the use of sleeping medications is not recommended. The Z drugs can be used later on a limited basis and other medication such as trazodone or amitriptyline could be tried. Sedating atypical antipsychotics and diphenhydramine are not recommended.

CLINICAL REVIEW QUESTIONS

1. In which of the following dementias is the REM sleep behavior disorder (RBD) relatively **uncommon?**
A. Progressive supranuclear palsy (PSP)
B. Alzheimer's disease (AD)
C. Parkinson's disease (PD)
D. Multiple system atrophy (MSA)
E. Diffuse Lewy body dementia (DLBD)

2. What neurodegenerative disorder is not an alpha synucleinopathy?
A. PSP
B. MSA
C. PD
D. DLBD

3. Which of these neurodegenerative disorders is frequently associated with stridor?
A. PD
B. AD
C. PSP
D. DLBD
E. MSA

4. In which of the following disorders is sundowning a prominent feature?
A. AD
B. PD
C. PSP
D. MSA

5. Which of the following is NOT a PD+ disorder?
A. PSP
B. AD
C. MSA
D. DLB
E. CBD

6. Which of the following is true about PD+ disorders compared with PD?
   A. There is a good response to LD.
   B. They have a slower downhill course than PD.
   C. Some PD+ disorders are very sensitive to dopamine blockers.
   D. Dementia early in the course is less common than in PD.
7. Which of the following is true about patients with DLBD?
   A. Dopamine blockers can cause life-threatening rigidity.
   B. Dementia starts about 2 years after rigidity and loss of balance.
   C. Visual hallucinations occur in 5%.
   D. They respond well to CD/LD.
8. What medication is recommended for treatment of daytime sleepiness (not due to narcolepsy) in PD, myotonic dystrophy, and posttraumatic hypersomnia in the 2021 AASM guidelines for treating central hypersomnia?
   A. Amphetamine
   B. Methylphenidate
   C. Modafinil
   D. Sodium oxybate
9. Which of the following is common in patients with PSP?
   A. Vertical gaze palsy, especially downward
   B. Severe insomnia
   C. Nocturia
   D. Dysarthria or choking
   E. All of the above
10. What is the more common type of sleep apnea found in patients after a stroke?
   A. Obstructive sleep apnea
   B. Central sleep apnea

ANSWERS

1. B. RBD is uncommon in AD. RBD is very common in PD, DLB, and MSA and tends to precede other neurologic manifestations. In PD the manifestations of RBD can occur many years before PD manifestations. In DLBD and MSA onset of RBD usually occurs shortly before or after other manifestations appear. RBD occurs in about 13% of PSP patients and tends to start concomitantly with other manifestations.
2. A. Progressive supranuclear palsy is a tau disorder.
3. E. MSA is associated with stridor.
4. A. Sundowning is common in AD.
5. B. AD is not a PD+ disorder.
6. C. DLBD patients are very sensitive to dopamine blockers. PD+ disorders have a more rapid course than PD, they have minimal response to LD, and dementia can be prominent early (DLBD).
7. A. Dopamine blockers can cause life-threatening rigidity. Visual hallucinations are very common—up to 70%. Dementia starts with or within 1 year of manifestations of Parkinsonism (tremor, bradykinesia, postural instability)
8. C. Modafinil (see Table 40–9). Sodium oxybate was recommended for hypersomnia due to PD but not myotonic dystrophy or posttraumatic hypersomnia.
9. E. All of the above.
10. A.

Table 40–9 Recommendations for Treatment of Central Hypersomnia Not Due to Narcolepsy

Parkinson's disease	Modafinil, Sodium oxybate
Diffuse Lewy body dementia	Armodafinil
Posttraumatic hypersomnia	Modafinil, Armodafinil
Myotonic dystrophy	Modafinil

Data from Maski K, Trotti LM, Kotagal S, Auger R et al. Treatment of central disorders of hypersomnolence: an American Academy of Sleep Medicine clinical practice guideline. *J Clin Sleep Med.* 2021 Sep 1;17(9):1881-1893.

SELECTED READINGS

Armstrong MJ. Lewy body dementias. *Continuum (Minneap Minn).* 2019;25(1):128-146.

Armstrong MJ, Okun MS. Diagnosis and treatment of Parkinson disease: a review. *JAMA.* 2020;323(6):548-560.

Arvanitakis Z, Shah RC, Bennett DA. Diagnosis and management of dementia: review. *JAMA.* 2019;322(16):1589-1599.

Malhotra RK. Neurodegenerative disorders and sleep. *Sleep Med Clin.* 2018; 13(1):63-70.

Pringsheim T, Day GS, Smith DB, et al; Guideline Subcommittee of the AAN. Dopaminergic therapy for motor symptoms in early Parkinson disease practice guideline summary: a report of the AAN Guideline Subcommittee. *Neurology.* 2021;97(20):942-957.

REFERENCES

1. Malhotra RK. Neurodegenerative disorders and sleep. *Sleep Med Clin.* 2018;13(1):63-70.
2. Arvanitakis Z, Shah RC, Bennett DA. Diagnosis and management of dementia: review. *JAMA.* 2019;322(16):1589-1599.
3. American Psychiatric Association. *Diagnostic and Statistical Manual of Mental Disorders, Fifth Edition* (DSM-5). American Psychiatric Association; 2013.
4. Reisberg B, Ferris SH, de Leon MJ, Crook T. The global deterioration scale for assessment of primary degenerative dementia. *Am J Psychiatry.* 1982;139:1136-1139.
5. Kent BA, Feldman HH, Nygaard HB. Sleep and its regulation: an emerging pathogenic and treatment frontier in Alzheimer's disease. *Prog Neurobiol.* 2021;197:101902.
6. Wu YH, Swaab DF. Disturbance and strategies for reactivation of the circadian rhythm system in aging and Alzheimer's disease. *Sleep Med.* 2007;8(6):623-633.
7. Zee PC, Vitiello MV. Circadian rhythm sleep disorder: irregular sleep-wake rhythm type. *Sleep Med Clin.* 2009;4:213-218.
8. Singer C, Tractenberg RE, Kaye J, et al. A multicenter, placebo-controlled trial of melatonin of sleep disturbance in Alzheimer's disease. *Sleep.* 2003;26:893-901.
9. Riemersma–van der Lek RF, Swaab DF, Twisk J. Effect of bright light and melatonin on cognitive and noncognitive function in elderly residents of group care facilities. *JAMA.* 2008;299:2647-2655.
10. Auger RR, Burgess HJ, Emens JS, et al. Clinical practice guideline for the treatment of intrinsic circadian rhythm sleep-wake disorders: advanced sleep-wake phase disorder (ASWPD), delayed sleep-wake phase disorder (DSWPD), non-24-hour sleep-wake rhythm disorder (N24SWD), and irregular sleep-wake rhythm disorder (ISWRD). An update for 2015: An American Academy of Sleep Medicine clinical practice guideline. *J Clin Sleep Med.* 2015;11(10):1199-1236.
11. Gao F, Liu T, Tuo M, Chi S. The role of orexin in Alzheimer disease: from sleep-wake disturbance to therapeutic target. *Neurosci Lett.* 2021;765:136247.
12. Cooke JR, Ayalon L, Palmer BW, et al. Sustained use of CPAP slows deterioration of cognition, sleep, and mood in patients with Alzheimer's disease and obstructive sleep apnea: a preliminary study. *J Clin Sleep Med.* 2009;5:305-309.
13. Chong MS, Ayalon L, Marler M, et al. Continuous positive airway pressure reduces subjective daytime sleepiness in patients with mild to moderate Alzheimer's disease with sleep disordered breathing. *J Am Geriatr Soc.* 2006;54(5):777-781.
14. Cummings J, Aisen P, Apostolova LG, Atri A, Salloway S, Weiner M. Aducanumab: appropriate use recommendations. *J Prev Alzheimers Dis.* 2021;8(4):398-410.

15. Van Dyck CH, Swanson CJ, Aisen P, et al. Lecanemab in early Alzheimer's disease. *N Engl J Med.* 2023;388(1):9-21.
16. Agboton C, Mahdavian S, Singh A, et al. Impact of nighttime donepezil administration on sleep in the older adult population: a retrospective study. *Mental Health Clinician.* 2014;4(5):257-259.
17. Song HR, Woo YS, Wang HR, Jun TY, Bahk WM. Effect of the timing of acetylcholinesterase inhibitor ingestion on sleep. *Int Clin Psychopharmacol.* 2013;28(6):346-348.
18. Stahl SM, Markowitz JS, Papadopoulos G, Sadik K. Examination of nighttime sleep-related problems during double-blind, placebo-controlled trials of galantamine in patients with Alzheimer's disease. *Curr Med Res Opin.* 2004;20:517-524.
19. Gauthier S, Juby A, Dalziel W, et al; EXPLORE Investigators. Effects of rivastigmine on common symptomatology of Alzheimer's disease (EXPLORE). *Curr Med Res Opin.* 2010;26:1149-1160.
20. Grossberg G, Irwin P, Satlin A, Mesenbrink P, Spiegel R. Rivastigmine in Alzheimer disease: efficacy over two years. *Am J Geriatr Psychiatry.* 2004;12(4):420-431. Erratum in: *Am J Geriatr Psychiatry.* 2004;12(6):679.
21. Howell M, Avidan AY, Foldvary-Schaefer N, et al. Management of REM sleep behavior disorder: an American Academy of Sleep Medicine clinical practice guideline. *J Clin Sleep Med.* 2023;19(4):759-768.
22. Yeh SB, Yeh PY, Schenck CH. Rivastigmine-induced REM sleep behavior disorder (RBD) in a 88-year-old man with Alzheimer's disease. *J Clin Sleep Med.* 2010;15:192-195.
23. Camargos EF, Louzada LL, Quintas JL, Naves JO, Louzada FM, Nóbrega OT. Trazodone improves sleep parameters in Alzheimer disease patients: a randomized, double-blind, and placebo-controlled study. *Am J Geriatr Psychiatry.* 2014;22(12):1565-1574.
24. Wade AG, Farmer M, Harari G, et al. Add-on prolonged-release melatonin for cognitive function and sleep in mild to moderate Alzheimer's disease: a 6-month, randomized, placebo-controlled, multicenter trial. *Clin Interv Aging.* 2014;9:947-961.
25. Sixel-Döring F, Schweitzer M, Mollenhauer B, Trenkwalder C. Polysomnographic findings, video-based sleep analysis and sleep perception in progressive supranuclear palsy. *Sleep Med.* 2009;10:407-415.
26. Arnulf I, Merino-Andreu M, Bloch F, et al. REM sleep behavior disorder and REM sleep without atonia in patients with progressive supranuclear palsy. *Sleep.* 2005;28:349-354.
27. Boini SY, Mahale R, Doniparthi Venkata S, et al. Oculomotor abnormalities and its association with sleep stages in progressive supranuclear palsy. *Sleep Med.* 2022;98:34-38.
28. Armstrong MJ, Okun MS. Diagnosis and treatment of Parkinson disease: a review. *JAMA.* 2020;323(6):548-560.
29. Halli-Tierney AD, Luker J, Carroll DG. Parkinson disease. *Am Fam Physician.* 2020;102(11):679-691.
30. Jankovic J. "Parkinson's disease": clinical features and diagnosis. *J Neurol Neurosurg Psychiatry.* 2008;79:368-376.
31. Reichmann H. Clinical criteria for the diagnosis of Parkinson's disease. *Neurodegener Dis.* 2010;7:284-290.
32. Postuma RB, Berg D, Stern M, et al. MDS clinical diagnostic criteria for Parkinson's disease. *Mov Disord.* 2015;30(12):1591-1601.
33. Braak H, Del Tredici K, Rüb U, de Vos RA, Jansen Steur EN, Braak E. Staging of brain pathology related to sporadic Parkinson's disease. *Neurobiol Aging.* 2003;24(2):197-211.
34. Pringsheim T, Day GS, Smith DB, et al; Guideline Subcommittee of the AAN. Dopaminergic therapy for motor symptoms in early Parkinson disease practice guideline summary: a report of the AAN Guideline Subcommittee. *Neurology.* 2021;97(20):942-957.
35. Grimes D, Fitzpatrick M, Gordon J, et al. Canadian guideline for Parkinson disease. *CMAJ.* 2019;191(36):e989-e1004.
36. Jost WH. A critical appraisal of MAO-B inhibitors in the treatment of Parkinson's disease. *J Neural Transm (Vienna).* 2022;129(5-6):723-736.
37. Zhang Y, Ren R, Sanford LD, et al. Sleep in Parkinson's disease: a systematic review and meta-analysis of polysomnographic findings. *Sleep Med Rev.* 2020;51:101281.
38. Comella CL. Sleep disorders in Parkinson's disease. *Curr Treat Options Neurol.* 2008;10:215-221.
39. Stefani A, Högl B. Sleep in Parkinson's disease. *Neuropsychopharmacology.* 2020;45(1):121-128.
40. Lajoie AC, Lafontaine AL, Kaminska M. The spectrum of sleep disorders in Parkinson disease: a review. *Chest.* 2021;159(2):818-827.
41. Zahed H, Zuzuarregui JRP, Gilron R, Denison T, Starr PA, Little S. The neurophysiology of sleep in Parkinson's disease. *Mov Disord.* 2021;36(7):1526-1542.
42. Wallace DM, Wohlgemuth WK, Trotti LM, et al. Practical evaluation and management of insomnia in Parkinson's disease: a review. *Mov Disord Clin Pract.* 2020;7(3):250-266.
43. Gros P, Mery VP, Lafontaine AL, et al. Obstructive sleep apnea in Parkinson's disease patients: effect of Sinemet CR taken at bedtime. *Sleep Breath.* 2016;20(1):205-212.
44. Schaeffer E, Vaterrodt T, Zaunbrecher L, et al. Effects of levodopa on quality of sleep and nocturnal movements in Parkinson's disease. *J Neurol.* 2021;268(7):2506-2514.
45. Park KW, Jo S, Lee SH, et al. Therapeutic effect of levodopa/carbidopa/entacapone on sleep disturbance in patients with Parkinson's disease. *J Mov Disord.* 2020;13(3):205-212.
46. Zuzuárregui JRP, Ostrem JL. The impact of deep brain stimulation on sleep in Parkinson's disease: an update. *J Parkinsons Dis.* 2020;10(2):393-404.
47. Thannickal TC, Lai YY, Siegel JM. Hypocretin (orexin) cell loss in Parkinson's disease. *Brain.* 2007;130:1586-1595.
48. Maski K, Trotti LM, Kotagal S, et al. Treatment of central disorders of hypersomnolence: an American Academy of Sleep Medicine clinical practice guideline. *J Clin Sleep Med.* 2021;17(9):1881-1893.
49. Rodrigues TM, Castro Caldas A, Ferreira JJ. Pharmacological interventions for daytime sleepiness and sleep disorders in Parkinson's disease: systematic review and meta-analysis. *Parkinsonism Relat Disord.* 2016;27:25-34.
50. Ondo WG, Fayle R, Atassi F, Jankovic J. Modafinil for daytime somnolence in Parkinson's disease: double blind, placebo controlled parallel trial. *J Neurol Neurosurg Psychiatry.* 2005;76(12):1636-1639.
51. Högl B, Saletu M, Brandauer E, et al. Modafinil for the treatment of daytime sleepiness in Parkinson's disease: a double-blind, randomized, crossover, placebo-controlled polygraphic trial. *Sleep.* 2002;25(8):905-909.
52. Nieves AV, Lang AE. Treatment of excessive daytime sleepiness in patients with Parkinson's disease with modafinil. *Clin Neuropharmacol.* 2002;25:111-114.
53. Lou JS, Dimitrov DM, Park BS, et al. Using modafinil to treat fatigue in Parkinson disease: a double-blind, placebo-controlled pilot study. *Clin Neuropharamacol.* 2009;32:305-310.
54. Hauser RA, Walha MN, Anderson WM. Modafinil treatment of pramipexole associated somnolence. *Mov Disord.* 2000;15:1269-1271.
55. Büchele F, Hackius M, Schreglmann SR, et al. Sodium oxybate for excessive daytime sleepiness and sleep disturbance in Parkinson disease: a randomized clinical trial. *JAMA Neurol.* 2018;75(1):114-118.
56. Manni R, Terzaghi M, Repetto A, et al. Complex paroxysmal nocturnal behaviors in Parkinson's disease. *Mov Disord.* 2010;25:985-990.
57. Barnes J, Connelly V, Wiggs L, et al. Sleep patterns in Parkinson's disease patients with visual hallucinations. *Int J Neurosci.* 2010;120:564-569.
58. Parkinson Study Group. Low-dose clozapine for the treatment of drug-induced psychosis in Parkinson's disease. *N Engl J Med.* 1999;340(10):757-763.
59. Cummings J, Ritter A, Rothenberg K. Advances in management of neuropsychiatric syndromes in neurodegenerative diseases. *Curr Psychiatry Rep.* 2019;21(8):79.
60. Cummings J, Isaacson S, Mills R, et al. Pimavanserin for patients with Parkinson's disease psychosis: a randomised, placebo-controlled phase 3 trial. *Lancet.* 2014;383(9916):533-540. Erratum in: *Lancet.* 2014;384(9937):28.
61. Seppi K, Ray Chaudhuri K, Coelho M, et al; The collaborators of the Parkinson's Disease Update on Non-Motor Symptoms Study Group on behalf of the Movement Disorders Society Evidence-Based Medicine Committee. Update on treatments for nonmotor symptoms of Parkinson's disease—an evidence-based medicine review. *Mov Disord.* 2019;34(2):180-198. Erratum in: *Mov Disord.* 2019;34(5):765.
62. Trieschmann MM, Reichwein S, Simuni T. Donepezil for dementia in Parkinson's disease: a randomised, double-blind, placebo-controlled, crossover study. *J Neurol Neurosurg Psychiatry.* 2005;76:934-939.
63. Thomas AJ, Burn DJ, Rowan EN, et al. A comparison of the efficacy of donepezil in Parkinson's disease with dementia and dementia with Lewy bodies. *Int J Geriatr Psychiatry.* 2005;20(10):938-944.
64. Emre M, Tsolaki M, Bonuccelli U, et al; 11018 Study Investigators. Memantine for patients with Parkinson's disease dementia or dementia with Lewy bodies: a randomised, double-blind, placebo-controlled trial. *Lancet Neurol.* 2010;9(10):969-977.
65. McKeith IG, Boeve BF, Dickson DW, et al. Diagnosis and management of dementia with Lewy bodies: fourth consensus report of the DLB Consortium. *Neurology.* 2017;89(1):88-100.
66. Gomperts SN. Lewy body dementias: dementia with Lewy bodies and Parkinson disease dementia. *Continuum (Minneap Minn).* 2016;22(2 Dementia):435-463.

67. Armstrong MJ. Lewy body dementias. *Continuum (Minneap Minn).* 2019;25(1):128-146.
68. Ferman T, Boeve B, Smith G, et al. Dementia with Lewy bodies may present as dementia with REM sleep behavior disorder without parkinsonism or hallucinations. *J Int Neuropsychol Soc.* 2002;8:907-914.
69. Gillman S, Wenning P, Low PA, et al. Second consensus statement of the diagnosis of multiple system atrophy. *Neurology.* 2008;71:670-676.
70. Wenning GK, Stankovic I, Vignatelli L, et al. The Movement Disorder Society criteria for the diagnosis of multiple system atrophy. *Mov Disord.* 2022;37(6):1131-1148.
71. Iranzo A. Management of sleep-disordered breathing in multiple system atrophy. *Sleep Med.* 2005;6:297-300.
72. Videnovic A. Management of sleep disorders in Parkinson's disease and multiple system atrophy. *Mov Disord.* 2017;32(5):659-668.
73. Kuźniar TJ, Morgenthaler TI, Prakash UBS, et al. Effects of continuous positive airway pressure on stridor in multiple system atrophy—sleep laryngoscopy. *J Clin Sleep Med.* 2009;5:65-67.
74. Silber MH, Levine S. Stridor and death in multiple system atrophy. *Mov Disord.* 2000;15(4):699-704.
75. Sadaoka T, Kakitsub N, Fujiwara Y, et al. Sleep-related breathing disorders in patients with multiple system atrophy and vocal fold palsy. *Sleep.* 1996;19:479-484.
76. Cortelli P, Calandra-Buonaura G, Benarroch EE, et al. WG. Stridor in multiple system atrophy: consensus statement on diagnosis, prognosis, and treatment. *Neurology.* 2019;93(14):630-639.
77. Cormican LJ, Higgins S, Davidson AC, Howard R, Williams AJ. Multiple system atrophy presenting as central sleep apnoea. *Eur Respir J.* 2004;24(2):323-325.
78. Garcia-Sanchez A, Fernandez-Navarro I, Garcia-Rio F. Central apneas and REM sleep behavior disorder as an initial presentation of multiple system atrophy. *J Clin Sleep Med.* 2016;12(2):267-270.
79. Ralls F, Cutchen L. Respiratory and sleep-related complications of multiple system atrophy. *Curr Opin Pulm Med.* 2020;26(6):615-622.
80. Hamada S, Takahashi R, Mishima M, Chin K. Use of a new generation of adaptive servo ventilation for sleep-disordered breathing in patients with multiple system atrophy. *BMJ Case Rep.* 2015;2015:bcr2014206372.
81. Lugaresi E, Tobler I, Montagna P, et al. Fatal familial insomnia and dysautonomia with selective degeneration of thalamic nuclei. *N Engl J Med.* 1986;315:997-1003.
82. Montagna P, Gambetti P, Cortelli P, Lugaresi E. Familial and sporadic fatal insomnia. *Lancet Neurol.* 2003;2:167-176.
83. American Academy of Sleep Medicine. *International Classification of Sleep Disorders.* 3rd ed., text revision. American Academy of Sleep Medicine; 2023.
84. Turpen K, Thornbury A, Wagner M, et al. A patient with rapidly progressing early-onset dementia and insomnia. *J Clin Sleep Med.* 2017; 13(11):1363-1364.
85. Berry RB, Wagner MH. A patient with possible narcolepsy and weakness in his hands. In: *Sleep Medicine Pearls.* 3rd ed. Saunders; 2015: 530-532.
86. Yu H, Laberge L, Jaussent I, et al. Daytime sleepiness and REM sleep characteristics in myotonic dystrophy: a case-control study. *Sleep.* 2011; 34(2):165-170.
87. Sansone VA, Proserpio P, Mauro L, et al. Assessment of self-reported and objective daytime sleepiness in adult-onset myotonic dystrophy type 1. *J Clin Sleep Med.* 2021;17(12):2383-2391.
88. Hermann DM, Bassetti CL. Sleep-related breathing and sleep wake disturbances in ischemic stroke. *Neurology.* 2009;73:1313-1322.
89. Turkington P, Bamfor J, Wanklyn P, et al. Prevalence and predictors of upper airway obstruction in the first 24 hours after acute stroke. *Stroke.* 2002;33:2037-2041.
90. Para O, Arboix A, Bechichi S, et al. Time course of sleep-related breathing disorders in first-ever stroke or transient ischemic attack. *Am J Respir Crit Care Med.* 2000;161:375-380.
91. Siccoli MM, Valko PO, Hermann DM. Central periodic breathing during sleep in 74 patients with acute ischemic stroke—neurogenic and cardiogenic factors. *J Neurol.* 2008;255:1687-1692.
92. Hermann DM, Siccoli M, Kirov P, et al. Central periodic breathing during sleep in ischemic stroke. *Stroke.* 2007;38:1082-1084.
93. McDermott M, Brown DL. Sleep apnea and stroke. *Curr Opin Neurol.* 2020;33:4-9.
94. Nopmaneejumruslers C, Kaneko Y, Hajek V, et al. Cheyne-Stokes respiration in stroke: relationship to hypocapnia and occult cardiac dysfunction. *Am J Respir Crit Care Med.* 2005;171:1048-1052.
95. Shahar E, Whitney CW, Redline S, et al. Sleep-disordered breathing and cardiovascular disease: cross-sectional results of the Sleep Heart Health Study. *Am J Respir Crit Care Med.* 2001;163:19-25.
96. Redline S, Yenokyan G, Gottlieb DJ, et al. Obstructive sleep apnea-hypopnea and incident stroke: the Sleep Heart Health study. *Am J Respir Crit Care Med.* 2010;182:269-277.
97. Sugita Y, Susami I, Yoshio T, et al. Marked episodic elevation of cerebral spinal fluid pressure during nocturnal sleep in patients with sleep apnea hypersomnia syndrome. *Electroencephalogr Clin Neurophysiol.* 1985;60: 214-219.
98. Balfors EM. Impairment of cerebral perfusion during obstructive sleep apneas. *Am J Respir Crit Care Med.* 1994;150:1587-1591.
99. Good DC, Henkle JQ, Gelber D, et al. Sleep disordered breathing and poor functional outcome after stroke. *Stroke.* 1996;27:252-259.
100. Martinez-Garcia MA, Soler-Cataluna JJ, Ejarque-Martinez L, et al. Continuous positive airway pressure treatment reduces mortality in patients with ischemic stroke and obstructive sleep apnea: a five-year follow-up. *Am J Respir Crit Care Med.* 2008;180:36-41.
101. Lee SJ, Kim JS, Song IU, et al. Post-stroke restless legs syndrome and lesion location. Anatomical considerations. *Mov Disord.* 2008;24:77-84.
102. Menon DK, Schwab K, Wright DW, et al; Demographics and Clinical Assessment Working Group of the International and Interagency Initiative toward Common Data Elements for Research on Traumatic Brain Injury and Psychological Health. Position statement: definition of traumatic brain injury. *Arch Phys Med Rehabil.* 2010;91(11): 1637-1640.
103. Roozenbeek B, Maas AI, Menon DK. Changing patterns in the epidemiology of traumatic brain injury. *Nat Rev Neurol.* 2013;9(4):231-236.
104. Theodorou AA, Rice SA. Is the silent epidemic keeping patients awake? *J Clin Sleep Med.* 2007;3(4):347-348.
105. Teasdale G, Jennett B. Assessment of coma and impaired consciousness. A practical scale. *Lancet.* 1974;2(7872):81-84.
106. Castriotta RJ, Wilde MC, Lai JM, et al. Prevalence and consequences of sleep disorders in traumatic brain injury. *J Clin Sleep Med.* 2007; 3(4):349-356.
107. Baumann CR, Werth E, Stocker R, Ludwig S, Bassetti CL. Sleep-wake disturbances 6 months after traumatic brain injury: a prospective study. *Brain.* 2007;130(Pt 7):1873-1883.
108. Guilleminault C, Yuen KM, Gulevich MG, Karadeniz D, Leger D, Philip P. Hypersomnia after head-neck trauma: a medicolegal dilemma. *Neurology.* 2000;54(3):653-659.
109. Sommerauer M, Valko PO, Werth E, Baumann CR. Excessive sleep need following traumatic brain injury: a case-control study of 36 patients. *J Sleep Res.* 2013;22(6):634-639.
110. Clay FJ, Kuriakose A, Lesche D, et al. Klüver-Bucy syndrome following traumatic brain injury: a systematic synthesis and review of pharmacological treatment from cases in adolescents and adults. *J Neuropsychiatry Clin Neurosci.* 2019;31(1):6-16.
111. Larson EB, Zollman FS. The effect of sleep medications on cognitive recovery from traumatic brain injury. *J Head Trauma Rehabil.* 2010; 25(1):61-67.
112. Capizzi A, Woo J, Verduzco-Gutierrez M. Traumatic brain injury: an overview of epidemiology, pathophysiology, and medical management. *Med Clin North Am.* 2020;104(2):213-238.

Index

Note: Page numbers followed by f refer to figures; page numbers followed by t refer to tables; page numbers followed by b refer to boxes.

B

C

D

E

F

G

N